HANDBOOK OF NONPRESCRIPTION DRUGS

An Interactive Approach to Self-Care

18th Edition

Editor-in-Chief

Daniel L. Krinsky, MS, RPh
Associate Professor, Department of Pharmacy Practice, Northeast Ohio Medical University, Rootstown, Ohio; Manager, Medication Therapy Management (MTM) Services, Department of Pharmacy, Giant Eagle, Ravenna, Ohio

Associate Editors

Stefanie P. Ferreri, PharmD, CDE, FAPhA
Clinical Associate Professor and Director, PGY-1 Community Pharmacy Residency Program, UNC Eshelman School of Pharmacy, The University of North Carolina at Chapel Hill

Brian Hemstreet, PharmD, FCCP, BCPS
Assistant Dean for Student Affairs and Associate Professor, Regis University School of Pharmacy, Denver, Colorado

Anne L. Hume, PharmD, FCCP, BCPS
Professor of Pharmacy, Department of Pharmacy Practice, University of Rhode Island College of Pharmacy, Kingston; Adjunct Professor of Family Medicine, Brown University/Memorial Hospital of Rhode Island, Providence

Gail D. Newton, PhD, RPh
Associate Professor, Department of Pharmacy Practice, Purdue University College of Pharmacy, West Lafayette, Indiana

Carol J. Rollins, MS, RD, PharmD, BCNSP
Coordinator, Nutrition Support Pharmacy and Director, PGY2 Nutrition Support Pharmacy Residency, The University of Arizona Medical Center, Tucson; Clinical Professor, Department of Pharmacy Practice and Science, The University of Arizona College of Pharmacy, Tucson

Karen J. Tietze, PharmD
Professor of Clinical Pharmacy, Department of Pharmacy Practice and Pharmacy Administration, Philadelphia College of Pharmacy, University of the Sciences, Philadelphia, Pennsylvania

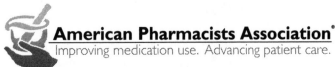

American Pharmacists Association®
Improving medication use. Advancing patient care.

APhA

Washington, DC

MANAGING EDITOR
Linda L. Young

EDITORIAL SERVICES
Linda L. Young, Mary Coe, Publications Professionals, LLC

COMPOSITION SERVICES
Circle Graphics

COVER DESIGNER
Richard Muringer, APhA Creative Services

ANATOMIC DRAWINGS
Aaron Hilmers, Gray Matter Studio, Walter Hilmers, Jr.

© 2015 by the American Pharmacists Association
APhA was founded in 1852 as the American Pharmaceutical Association.

Published by the American Pharmacists Association
2215 Constitution Avenue, NW,
Washington, DC 20037-2985
www.pharmacist.com   www.pharmacylibrary.com
All rights reserved.

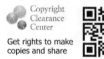

To comment on this book via e-mail, send your message to the publisher at aphabooks@aphanet.org.

Library of Congress Cataloging-in-Publication Data
Main entry under the title: Handbook of Nonprescription Drugs
ISSN 0889-7816
ISBN-978-1-58212-225-0

How to Order This Book

Online: www.pharmacist.com/shop
By phone: 800-878-0729 (770-280-0085 from outside the United States and Canada)
VISA®, MasterCard®, and American Express® cards accepted.

CONTENTS

vi

section
VIII DERMATOLOGIC DISORDERS
Editors: Stefanie P. Ferreri (32–35, 41–44) and Gail D. Newton (36–40)

section
IX OTHER MEDICAL DISORDERS
Editors: Karen J. Tietze (45), Anne L. Hume (46), and Daniel L. Krinsky (47)

FOREWORD

Publication of the eighteenth edition of the American Pharmacists Association's (APhA) *Handbook of Nonprescription Drugs: An Interactive Approach to Self-Care* continues a tradition of providing comprehensive content to pharmacists and other health care providers so they can assist patients with the self-care process.

The United States is the world's largest market for non-prescription products, with retail sales of $33.1 billion, (http://www.chpa.org/PR_OTCRetailSales.aspx). These sales figures include all outlets (food, drug, mass, convenience, and military stores, as well as select club and dollar store retailers). Other similar surveys confirm the increased use of nonprescription medications. The anticipated increase in the number of prescription medications that will be reclassified as nonprescription will provide new treatment options but will also further confound the patient's dilemma in selecting appropriate self-treatment.

A provision of the Patient Protection and Affordable Care Act of 2010 unintentionally created a problem for self-treating patients by removing nonprescription medications, except insulin, from the list of medical items covered by health flexible spending plans if the medications were purchased without a prescription (www.irs.gov/newsroom/article/0,,id=227308,00.html). The intent of the provision was to save $5 billion over 10 years by reducing unnecessary drug purchases; however, it actually resulted in increased medical costs as patients made appointments with health care providers solely to obtain prescriptions for nonprescription medications. A bipartisan bill titled Restoring Access to Medication Act of 2013 was introduced in the U.S. House of Representatives on July 25; in November 2013, similar legislation was introduced in the U.S. Senate (http://blog.euromonitor.com/2014/06/correcting-contradictions-restoring-otc-coverage-to-health-spending-accounts-in-the-us.html). APhA supports the pending bipartisan legislation to repeal this provision.

The use of complementary and alternative medicine (CAM) therapies, dietary supplements, nondrug measures, diagnostic tests, and medical devices is also integral to self-care. However, there is a paucity of clinical evidence as to their safety and effectiveness, and the potential for serious adverse events when these products are combined with prescription or non-prescription medications demands that health care providers be knowledgeable about alternatives to traditional medications and be able to provide therapeutic information and guidance to the consumer. Unlike nonprescription medications, no federal regulatory agency evaluates the safety and effectiveness of CAM therapies.

Numerous other factors have contributed to the growing self-care movement in the United States, including an increase in direct-to-consumer advertising of prescription and nonprescription medications. Information obtained from television commercials, newspaper and magazine advertisements, the Internet, and health-related articles serves to empower consumers to make decisions about their health care. However, individuals who wish to self-treat minor health disorders are faced with a staggering number of single-entity and combination nonprescription products, and they may not have adequate information to determine whether their medical disorder is amenable to self-treatment and whether the self-selected treatment is appropriate for the disorder.

All health care providers should be able to assist individuals in managing their self-care. However, because of their accessibility and expertise with respect to nonprescription and prescription medications, pharmacists are in a unique position to fulfill the self-care needs of most individuals with minor health ailments. Thus, providing a self-care curriculum for pharmacy students with learning outcomes that ensure appropriate knowledge and skills is now more important than ever. The importance of this objective is reflected in the most recent Accreditation Council for Pharmacy Education's (ACPE) Accreditation Guidelines (www.acpe-accredit.org/deans/standards.asp) and the Competency Statements of the North American Pharmacist Licensure Examination (NAPLEX) taken by all United States pharmacy graduates prior to licensure (www.nabp.net/programs/examination/-naplex/naplex-blueprint/).

The information in this edition is also available online through the subscription-based PharmacyLibrary portal (www.pharmacylibrary.com). Here you will find the complete *Handbook* content along with many other complementary resources. Through PharmacyLibrary we are also introducing additional case studies to reinforce key concepts discussed in the chapters.

The eighteenth edition of the APhA *Handbook of Nonprescription Drugs: An Interactive Approach to Self-Care* is an excellent and up-to-date resource for all health care educators, students, and providers engaged in self-care.

THOMAS E. MENIGHAN, BSPHARM, MBA
Executive Vice President & CEO
American Pharmacists Association

PREFACE

The newly revised and updated eighteenth edition of the *Handbook of Nonprescription Drugs: An Interactive Approach to Self-Care* is a comprehensive and authoritative textbook on self-care and nonprescription medications. The goals for this edition were to:

- Enhance the content from the previous edition with up-to-date information beneficial to all health care providers and students.
- Update the universal objectives to complement the content in the chapters focused on medical disorders.
- Rewrite Chapter 2, "Patient Assessment and Consultation," so that the content is more applicable and practical to the self-care/nonprescription product environment, and add case studies that illustrate the use of a more abbreviated problem-solving model.

This edition remains true to the spirit of previous editions, namely to assist health care providers and students in developing knowledge and problem-solving skills needed to:

- Assess a patient's health status, medical problems, and current practice of self-treatment, including nonprescription and prescription medications, dietary supplements, and other self-care measures.
- Determine whether self-care and/or self-testing and monitoring are necessary and/or appropriate.
- If appropriate, recommend safe and effective self-care measures, taking into account the patient's treatment preferences.

Written and reviewed by experts in practice and academia, this edition of the *Handbook* continues to serve as an authoritative source for students and health care providers who guide and care for individuals undertaking self-treatment. The major changes for this edition include:

- Redesigned and rewritten Chapter 2, which discusses patient assessment processes and focuses more on applicability in the self-care/nonprescription environment.
- Revised reference format.
- Inclusion of current pregnancy risk categories for drugs and some natural products, where appropriate.
- Inclusion of references for exclusions for self-treatment, in both the running text and the algorithm box.
- An online version of the book that resides on APhA's digital platform PharmacyLibrary (www.pharmacylibrary.com), allowing updating and/or revision of chapters as needed.

- Incorporation of vaccine information into certain chapters where the content is synergistic.
- Two new comprehensive patient cases per chapter for the print version that are based on the revised seventeenth edition case format.
- Additional cases based on the abbreviated case format, introduced in the seventeenth edition, again will be included only in the online version of the book.

Self-care opportunities exist for many individuals with myriad health disorders. The content presented in this text that is focused on these disorders lends itself to the following objectives. The editors encourage you to review and utilize these objectives to help you gain the greatest benefit from the information presented in the disorder-related chapters. For each patient complaint:

- Identify its most likely underlying cause(s).
- Identify common signs and symptoms.
- Determine whether the complaint is amenable to self-care, the patient requires referral, or nothing needs to be done.
- Identify the Food and Drug Administration (FDA) monograph active ingredients in a given nonprescription drug category.
- Determine common side effects for a given category of nonprescription drugs.
- Determine contraindications to the use of a given category of nonprescription drugs or devices.
- Distinguish indications and limitations for use of nonprescription drugs or devices in a given category.
- Explain nondrug measures commonly used in treatment or prevention.
- Develop an appropriate plan for a given patient who seeks self-care advice.
- Formulate a list of key counseling points to educate a patient on the appropriate use of nonprescription drugs, nondrug measures, or a device.

Highlights of New Features and Revisions

Considerable time and effort have been invested in improving this edition. We are hopeful that the following changes improve the quality and usability of the book, as well as provide increased clarity and convenience. Key enhancements in this edition include:

- Vaccine information: where appropriate, vaccine information is included in a primary chapter. Examples include: human papillomavirus virus (HPV) and hepatitis B virus in Chapter 10, "Prevention of Pregnancy and Sexually Transmitted Infections"; rotavirus vaccines in Chapter 16, "Diarrhea"; tetanus vaccine in Chapter 40, "Minor Burns, Sunburn, and Wounds"; and influenza, varicella zoster, MMR (measles, mumps, and rubella), and pneumococcal polysaccharide vaccine, polyvalent (Pneumovax-23) vaccines in Chapter 45, "Self-Care Components of Selected Chronic Disorders."

- A rewrite of Chapter 2 to make the content more applicable to and practical for the self-care/nonprescription product environment. The new authors include information about both comprehensive and abbreviated problem-solving models, each providing advantages based on the experience of the provider. Part of our responsibility as educators is to expose our students to multiple options for assessing patients for self-care. Although the traditional approach in the *Handbook* was to focus solely on the very complex process, we realized other approaches, such as those that better fit situations when health care providers have more experience and/or limited time to interact with a patient, are important to discuss. One of these abbreviated processes, QuEST/SCHOLAR-MAC, is used as the basis for the electronic cases written to enhance the application of content in the disorder-related chapters. These supplemental cases are available on APhA's digital subscription product PharmacyLibrary at www.pharmacylibrary.com. In addition, two new comprehensive patient cases are included in each chapter.

- Chapter 5, "Headache," and Chapter 6, "Fever," added information about the FDA recommendation that health care professionals no longer prescribe or dispense prescription products containing more than 325 mg acetaminophen per dosage unit (capsule, tablet, etc).

- Chapter 5 contains new information about:
  - Availability of new Advil film-coated tablets, a potentially faster-acting version than standard ibuprofen propionic acid tablets.
  - A warning for prescription and nonprescription products containing acetaminophen regarding its association with rare but serious cutaneous adverse reactions (SCAR).

- Chapter 7, "Musculoskeletal Injuries and Disorders," has information about the potential for serious burns associated with nonprescription topical analgesics.

- Chapter 10 discusses the nonprescription availability of Plan B One-Step

- Chapter 11, "Colds and Allergy," and Chapter 27, "Ophthalmic Disorders," have information about potentially severe adverse events in children if they accidentally ingest decongestants found in ocular and nasal preparations.

- Chapter 11 includes information about:
  - Tamper-resistant pseudoephedrine products.
  - Potential infection risk from improper use of neti pots and other nasal irrigation devices.
  - Approval of Nasacort Allergy 24 HR (triamcinolone acetonide), an intranasal glucocorticoid used to treat nasal symptoms caused by allergic rhinitis, for nonprescription use.

- Chapter 11 and Chapter 45 discuss options for recording sales of nonprescription ephedrine, pseudoephedrine, and phenylpropanolamine products.

- Chapter 13, "Heartburn and Dyspepsia," has added information about:
  - Availability of Nexium 24HR (esomeprazole magnesium 22.3 mg), the most recent proton pump inhibitor (PPI) to be granted nonprescription product status by FDA.
  - Safety labeling changes to PPIs regarding concomitant use with methotrexate sodium for injection.
  - The potential for increased risk of Clostridium difficile–associated diarrhea (CDAD) in individuals using nonprescription PPIs.
  - New labeling requirements for nonprescription PPI products.

- Chapter 15, "Constipation," now includes information regarding a warning for the potential side effects of nonprescription sodium phosphate drugs commonly used to treat constipation.

- Chapter 30, "Prevention of Hygiene-Related Oral Disorders," includes information about a safety warning concerning potential serious injury associated with use of *all* models of the Spinbrush Powered Toothbrush.

- Chapter 37, "Acne," includes updated information about the potential for serious allergic reactions associated with nonprescription topical acne products.

- Chapter 44, "Hair Loss," has information about the approval of Women's Rogaine (5% minoxidil) Topical Aerosol for the nonprescription treatment of female pattern hair loss/androgenetic alopecia on the top of the scalp.

- Chapter 45 also has updated information about:
  - The possibility of the GenStrip Blood Glucose Test reporting false results during routine use due to a manufacturing issue.
  - The availability of new versions of influenza vaccines.
  - Asthmanefrin, a new nonprescription racemic epinephrine solution for inhalation.

- Chapter 47, "Tobacco Cessation," discusses the changes in labeling regarding warnings and limitations for nonprescription nicotine replacement therapy products.

- Chapter 48, "Home Testing and Monitoring Devices," includes information about a new test, available to consumers, for the detection of human immunodeficiency virus (HIV) antibodies to determine HIV status at home.

- Chapter 49, "Adult Urinary Incontinence and Supplies," includes information about Oxytrol for Women, a new nonprescription oxybutynin transdermal system.

- Complementary and alternative medicine (CAM) chapters: The CAM section consists of three chapters that have been significantly enhanced. These changes provide the reader with a broad overview of the different health systems/healing practices that a consumer may be using.

- Appendixes: This edition includes an updated version of the two appendixes that discuss the safe use of nonprescription medications, nutritional supplements, and natural products (herbal and amino acid dietary supplements) during pregnancy:
  - Appendix I, "FDA Pregnancy Risk Categories for Selected Nonprescription Medications and Nutritional Supplements"
  - Appendix II, "Safety Issues with the Use of Selected Natural Products in Pregnancy"

- Case studies: New cases were developed for each disorder-related chapter.

Chapter Content

All disorder-related chapters in this edition include the following features and information:

- Up-to-date information on nonprescription medications, including indications, dosages, interactions, supportive evidence for efficacy and safety, medical disorders or symptoms amenable to self-treatment, prescription-to-nonprescription reclassifications, and nonprescription drug withdrawals from the market.
- Treatment algorithms that outline triage and treatment.
- Controversies in self-care therapeutics.
- Self-care treatment or prevention guidelines.
- Product tables with examples of specific nonprescription products.
- New nonprescription medications and dietary supplements, including nutrition-related dietary supplements, such as vitamins and minerals, which are discussed in the nutrition section of the book.

Chapter Features

Most chapter features remain unchanged and are intended to promote an interactive approach to self-care. Students and health care providers can use these features to develop or improve problem-solving and critical thinking skills.

- Disorder-related chapters are grouped primarily according to body systems. These chapters begin with a discussion of the epidemiologic, etiologic, and pathophysiologic characteristics and the clinical manifestations of the disorder. These discussions are followed by a comprehensive discussion of self-care options. The inclusion of dietary supplements, as well as nonpharmacologic and preventive measures, completes the discussion of self-care options.
- Case studies, treatment algorithms, comparisons of self-treatments, patient education boxes, and product selection guidelines foster an interactive therapeutic approach to learning.
- Sections on the evaluation of patient outcomes reinforce follow-up of patients who are self-treating. This section defines the parameters for confirming successful self-treatment and those that indicate the need for medical referral.
- Chapters include tables that list interactions (drug–drug, drug–supplement, drug–nutrient), as well as dosage and administration guidelines.
- At the end of each chapter, authors provide a list of key points. These are intended to serve as a summary of critical information in the chapter and can be an excellent resource for educators.
- Authors provide comparisons of agents based on clinical studies of safety and efficacy, as well as product selection guidelines based on patient factors and preferences.
- Authors discuss the role of nonprescription therapies among the available treatment options for a specific disorder and describe other options in the event that nonprescription therapy fails or is not appropriate.

- The book's organization and content allow students and health care providers to quickly identify the information needed to make a treatment recommendation and to counsel patients.

Acknowledgments

This edition marked another significant turning point in the history of the Handbook. This is the first edition in over 20 years that Rosemary Berardi has not been an active contributor as an author, reviewer, or editor. However, her influence is still evidenced in this edition, with some of her previous contributions continuing to offer value in the self-care/nonprescription product arena. Again, the editorial team and APhA staff want to recognize Rosemary for her sustained contributions to this very important publication. Her vision for the Handbook had a great impact in terms of consistency and high-quality standards, and her insight and dedication will remain an inspiration long after her tenure as EIC and Editor Emerita has passed. We welcome a new Associate Editor, Brian Hemstreet, to the eighteenth edition. Brian brings with him over 15 years of experience in practice and academia, with a primary focus on gastrointestinal pharmacotherapy. Brian has myriad experience in research, publication, and practice, and he brings a valuable perspective to the content of the Handbook.

We would like to acknowledge the many individuals who contributed to the new edition of this textbook. We are grateful to the 72 authors and coauthors and more than 140 reviewers who contributed to this comprehensive and authoritative textbook. These individuals were selected from many practice settings and health professions throughout the country. Their scholarship and clinical experience reflect a broad perspective and interdisciplinary approach to patient care. The dedication of the authors and reviewers in ensuring that chapters were accurate, comprehensive, balanced, and relevant to practice and of the highest quality is deeply appreciated.

The editors of this edition also want to acknowledge the contributions of previous editors, authors, reviewers, and the many health care providers, students, residents, and others who have helped make the Handbook the premier resource for self-care content.

We would like to convey a special thanks to Linda Young, our managing editor. Ms. Young provided invaluable guidance and support to the editors and authors in all aspects related to the publication of this edition of the textbook. She contributed to the copyediting of chapters, and managed the design, editorial, and composition stages of the book. Without her experience and attention to detail, the improvements in this edition would not have been possible.

We are confident that the combined efforts of these individuals will ensure that the *Handbook of Nonprescription Drugs: An Interactive Approach to Self-Care* continues to serve as the worldwide practice and teaching resource on self-care and nonprescription products.

STEFANIE P. FERRERI
BRIAN HEMSTREET
ANNE L. HUME
DANIEL L. KRINSKY
GAIL D. NEWTON
CAROL J. ROLLINS
KAREN J. TIETZE

CONTRIBUTORS

Authors

Note: Numbers in parentheses denote the chapter(s) authored or coauthored.

Donna M. Adkins, BS Pharm, PharmD, CGP, FASCP (42)
Chair, Department of Pharmacy Practice and Associate Professor of Pharmacy Practice, Appalachian College of Pharmacy, Oakwood, Virginia

Nicole Paolini Albanese, PharmD, CDE, BCACP (31)
Clinical Assistant Professor, Department of Pharmacy Practice, The State University of New York at Buffalo School of Pharmacy and Pharmaceutical Sciences; PGY1 Pharmacy Residency Director, Buffalo Medical Group, PC, Buffalo, New York

Cedric B. Baker, PharmD, RPh (23)
Adjunct Clinical Assistant Professor of Pharmacy Practice, Department of Pharmacy Practice/Center for Clinical Research CCR-15, Mercer University College of Pharmacy and Health Sciences, Atlanta, Georgia; Walmart Health and Wellness: Pharmacy Division Clinical Natural Product Pharmacist-Georgia/North Florida, Atlanta, Georgia

Cathy L. Bartels, PharmD (26)
Clinical Pharmacist, Pharmacy Educator, Children's Hospital & Medical Center, Omaha, Nebraska

Kimberley W. Benner, PharmD, BCPS, FASHP, FPPAG (32)
Professor of Pharmacy Practice, McWhorter School of Pharmacy, Samford University, Birmingham, Alabama; Clinical Pharmacy Specialist, Children's of Alabama, Birmingham

Daphne B. Bernard, PharmD, CACP (40)
Associate Dean of Academic Affairs and Assessment, Howard University College of Pharmacy, Washington, DC

Tricia M. Berry, PharmD, BCPS (44)
Professor, Department of Pharmacy Practice, St. Louis College of Pharmacy, St. Louis, Missouri

Mary M. Bridgeman, PharmD, BCPS, CGP (22)
Clinical Associate Professor, Ernest Mario School of Pharmacy, Rutgers, The State University of New Jersey, Piscataway

Geneva Clark Briggs, PharmD, BCPS (48)
President, Briggs and Associates, Richmond Virginia

Wayne Buff, PharmD (36)
Associate Dean and Clinical Associate Professor, Department of Pharmacy and Outcomes Sciences, South Carolina College of Pharmacy, University of South Carolina Campus, Columbia, South Carolina

Juliana Chan, PharmD, FCCP, BCACP (17)
Clinical Pharmacist, University of Illinois Medical Center at Chicago; Clinical Associate Professor, Department of Pharmacy Practice, College of Pharmacy, and Department of Medicine, Sections of Digestive Diseases and Nutrition and Section of Hepatology, University of Illinois at Chicago

Aleda M. H. Chen, PharmD, MS, PhD (28)
Vice Chair and Assistant Professor of Pharmacy Practice, Cedarville University School of Pharmacy, Cedarville, Ohio

M. Petrea Cober, PharmD, BCNSP (25)
Pharmacy Clinical Coordinator, Neonatal Intensive Care Unit, Akron Children's Hospital One, Akron, Ohio; Associate Professor of Pharmacy Practice, Northeast Ohio Medical University College of Pharmacy, Rootstown, Ohio

Cynthia W. Coffey, PharmD (37, 43)
Pharmacy Manager, Publix Pharmacy, Lawrenceville, Georgia

Kimberly M. Crosby, PharmD, BCPS, CGP, CDE, BC-ADM (38, 39)
Associate Professor, Department of Clinical and Administrative Sciences, The University of Oklahoma College of Pharmacy–Tulsa Campus; Adjunct Associate Professor, Department of Family Medicine–Tulsa Campus, The University of Oklahoma School of Community Medicine

Barbara Insley Crouch, PharmD, MSPH (20)
Executive Director, Utah Poison Control Center; Professor (Clinical), Department of Pharmacotherapy, University of Utah College of Pharmacy, Salt Lake City

Patricia L. Darbishire, PharmD (34)
Clinical Associate Professor, Department of Pharmacy Practice, Purdue University College of Pharmacy, West Lafayette, Indiana; Director of Introductory Pharmacy Practice Experiences

Cathi Dennehy, PharmD (50)
Professor in the Department of Clinical Pharmacy, University of California, San Francisco, School of Pharmacy

Holly Divine, PharmD, BCACP, CGP, CDE, FAPhA (2)
Clinical Associate Professor, Pharmacy Practice and Science, University of Kentucky College of Pharmacy, Lexington

Holly Duhon, PharmD (48)
Assistant Dean of Experiential Education, The Ben and Maytee Fisch College of Pharmacy, The University of Texas at Tyler

Shareen Y. El-Ibiary, PharmD, FCCP, BCPS (10)
Professor of Pharmacy Practice, Midwestern University, College of Pharmacy–Glendale, Glendale, Arizona

Patricia H. Fabel, PharmD, BCPS (36)
Assistant Professor, Department of Clinical Pharmacy and Outcomes Sciences, South Carolina College of Pharmacy, University of South Carolina Campus, Columbia

Brett M. Feret, PharmD (6)
Clinical Associate Professor, University of Rhode Island College of Pharmacy, Kingston

Stefanie P. Ferreri, PharmD, BCACP, CDE, FAPhA (19)
Clinical Associate Professor and Director, PGY-1 Community Pharmacy Residency Program, UNC Eshelman School of Pharmacy, The University of North Carolina at Chapel Hill

Richard G. Fiscella, PharmD, MPH (27)
Clinical Professor Emeritus, Department of Pharmacy Practice, University of Illinois at Chicago College of Pharmacy; Former Adjunctive Assistant Professor, Department of Ophthalmology, University of Illinois at Chicago

Daniel Forrister, PharmD (30)
Clinical Assistant Professor and Pharmaceutical Care Lab Coordinator, UNC Eshelman School of Pharmacy–Asheville Campus, The University of North Carolina

Karla T. Foster, PharmD, BCPS (37, 43)
Pharmacist, Walgreens Company, Ridgeland, Mississipi

Tracy R. Frame, PharmD, BCACP (28)
Assistant Professor of Pharmacy Practice, Belmont University College of Pharmacy, Nashville, Tennessee

Jeffery A. Goad, PharmD, MPH, FAPhA (18)
Professor and Chair, Department of Pharmacy Practice, Chapman University School of Pharmacy, Harry and Diane Rinker Health Science Campus, Irvine, California

Jean-Venable "Kelly" R. Goode, PharmD, BCPS (15)
Professor, Department of Pharmacotherapy and Outcome Science, Virginia Commonwealth University School of Pharmacy, Medical College of Virginia Campus, Richmond

Nicholas E. Hagemeier, PharmD, PhD (35)
Assistant Professor of Pharmacy Practice, East Tennessee State University Gatton College of Pharmacy, Johnson City

Metta Lou Henderson, RPh, PhD (1)
Professor Emerita of Pharmacy, Raabe College of Pharmacy, Ohio Northern University, Ada; Research Professor, Department of Pharmacy Practice and Science, The University of Arizona College of Pharmacy, Tucson

Richard N. Herrier, PharmD (33)
Professor of Pharmacy Practice and Science, The University of Arizona College of Pharmacy, Tucson

Michael K. Jensen, RPh, MS (27)
Clinical Pharmacist, Team Lead, OR Pharmacy, Utah Valley Regional Medical Center-Intermountain Healthcare, Provo, Utah

Cynthia K. Kirkwood, PharmD, BCPP (46)
Professor of Pharmacy and Vice Chair for Education, Virginia Commonwealth University, Richmond

Wendy Klein-Schwartz, PharmD, MPH (20)
Coordinator of Research and Education, Maryland Poison Center, Baltimore; Associate Professor, Department of Pharmacy Practice and Science, University of Maryland School of Pharmacy, Baltimore

Daniel L. Krinsky, MS, RPh (45)
Associate Professor, Department of Pharmacy Practice, Northeast Ohio Medical University College of Pharmacy, Rootstown, Ohio; Manager, Medication Therapy Management (MTM) Services, Department of Pharmacy, Giant Eagle, Ravenna, Ohio

Nicole M. Lodise, PharmD (8)
Associate Professor of Pharmacy Practice-Women's Health/Tobacco Cessation, Albany College of Pharmacy and Health Sciences, Albany, New York; Clinical Pharmacy Specialist, Albany Medical Center, Albany, New York

Beth A. Martin, RPh, BSPharm, MS, PhD (47)
Associate Professor (CHS), University of Wisconsin School of Pharmacy, Madison

Cydney E. McQueen, PharmD, MSHP (51)
Clinical Associate Professor, Pharmacy Practice and Administration, University of Missouri-Kansas City School of Pharmacy

Sarah T. Melton, PharmD, BCPP, BCACP, CGP, FASCP (46)
Associate Professor of Pharmacy Practice, East Tennessee State University Bill Gatton College of Pharmacy, Johnson City

Sarah J. Miller, PharmD, BCNSP (26)
Professor of Clinical Pharmacy, Department of Pharmacy Practice, University of Montana Skaggs School of Pharmacy, Missoula

Edith Mirzaian, PharmD (18)
Assistant Professor of Clinical Pharmacy, Titus Family Department of Clinical Pharmacy, Pharmaceutical Economics and Policy, University of Southern California School of Pharmacy, Los Angeles

Mark Newnham, PharmD, BCPS, BCNSP (24)
Clinical Pharmacist, Lawnwood Regional Medical Center and Heart Institute, Fort Pierce, Florida

Gail D. Newton, PhD, RPh (2, 41)
Associate Professor, Department of Pharmacy Practice, Purdue University College of Pharmacy, West Lafayette, Indiana

Julie L. Olenak, PharmD (7)
Associate Professor of Pharmacy Practice, Wilkes University Nesbitt School of Pharmacy, Wilkes-Barre, Pennsylvania

Katherine S. O'Neal, PharmD, MBA, BCACP, CDE, BC-ADM, AE-C (38, 39)
Assistant Professor, Department of Clinical and Administrative Sciences, The University of Oklahoma College of Pharmacy–Tulsa Campus

Christine K. O'Neil, PharmD, BCPS, FCCP, CGP (49)
Professor of Pharmacy Practice and Director, Curriculum Development, Duquesne University Mylan School of Pharmacy, Pittsburgh, Pennsylvania

Katherine Kelly Orr, PharmD (51)
Clinical Associate Professor, University of Rhode Island College of Pharmacy, Kingston

Kimberly S. Plake, PhD (34)
Associate Professor, Department of Pharmacy Practice, Purdue University College of Pharmacy, West Lafayette, Indiana

Erin C. Raney, PharmD, BCPS (10)
Professor, Department of Pharmacy Practice, Midwestern University College of Pharmacy, Glendale Campus, Glendale, Arizona

Edward D. Rickert, BS Pharm, JD (4)
Partner, Quarles & Brady LLP, Chicago, Illinois; Adjunct Professor, Pharmacy Law, University of Illinois at Chicago College of Pharmacy

Jennifer Robinson, PharmD (14)
Director of Student Services and Clinical Assistant Professor, Washington State University College of Pharmacy, Pullman

Magaly Rodriguez de Bittner, PharmD, BCPS, CDE (3)
Chair and Professor, Department of Pharmacy Practice and Science, University of Maryland School of Pharmacy, Baltimore

Carol J. Rollins, MS, RD, PharmD, BCNSP (22, 23)
Coordinator, Nutrition Support Pharmacy and Director, PGY2 Nutrition Support Pharmacy Residency, The University of Arizona Medical Center, Tucson; Clinical Professor, Department of Pharmacy Practice and Science, The University of Arizona College of Pharmacy, Tucson

Kelly L. Scolaro, PharmD (11)
Clinical Assistant Professor and Director of Pharmaceutical Care Laboratory, Division of Practice Advancement and Clinical Education, UNC Eshelman School of Pharmacy, The University of North Carolina at Chapel Hill

Joan Lerner Selekof, BSN, RN, CWOCN (21)
Manager, WOCN Team and Certified Wound Ostomy Continence Nurse, University of Maryland Medical Center, Baltimore, Maryland

Leslie A. Shimp, PharmD, MS (9)
Professor of Pharmacy, Department of Clinical, Social and Administrative Sciences, The University of Michigan College of Pharmacy, Ann Arbor, Michigan

Jeri J. Sias, PharmD, MPH (3)
Clinical Associate Professor, The University of Texas at El Paso/ UT Austin Cooperative Pharmacy Program

Judith B. Sommers Hanson, PharmD, FAPhA (29)
Manager, Clinical Program Development, Walgreen Company, Deerfield, Illinois

Karen J. Tietze, PharmD (12)
Professor of Clinical Pharmacy, Department of Pharmacy Practice and Pharmacy Administration, Philadelphia College of Pharmacy, University of the Sciences, Philadelphia, Pennsylvania

Candy Tsourounis, PharmD (50)
Professor of Clinical Pharmacy, Department of of Clinical Pharmacy, University of California, San Francisco School of Pharmacy

Timothy R. Ulbrich, PharmD, RPh (45)
Associate Professor, Department of Pharmacy Practice and Associate Dean, Workforce Development and Practice Advancement, Northeast Ohio Medical University College of Pharmacy, Rootstown, Ohio

Catherine Ulbricht, PharmD, MBA [c] (52)
Founder, Natural Standard Research Collaboration and Journal of Dietary Supplements, Somerville, Massachusetts; Senior Attending Pharmacist, Massachusetts General Hospital, Boston

Paul C. Walker, PharmD, FASHP (16)
Clinical Professor and Director, Experiential Education and Community Engagement College of Pharmacy, Department of Clinical Sciences, The University of Michigan College of Pharmacy, Ann Arbor; Manager, Pharmacy Patient Outcomes, Department of Pharmacy, The University of Michigan Health System, Ann Arbor

Kristin W. Weitzel, PharmD, CDE, FAPhA (15)
Associate Director, UF Health Personalized Medicine Program and Clinical Associate Professor, Department of Pharmacotherapy and Translational Research, University of Florida College of Pharmacy, Gainesville

Adam C. Welch, PharmD, MBA, BCACP, FAPhA (19)
Associate Professor, Department of Pharmacy Practice, Wilkes University Nesbitt School of Pharmacy, Wilkes-Barre, Pennsylvania

Tara Whetsel, PharmD, BCACP, BC-ADM (13)
Clinical Associate Professor, Department of Clinical Pharmacy, West Virginia University School of Pharmacy, Morgantown

Julie J. Wilkinson, PharmD, M.S., BCPS (5)
Associate Dean and Professor of Pharmacy Practice, Lake Erie College of Osteopathic Medicine School of Pharmacy, Bradenton, Florida

Sharon Wilson, PharmD, BCPS (21)
Clinical Specialist-Surgery Critical Care, University of Maryland Medical Center, Baltimore; Clinical Assistant Professor, Department of Pharmacy Services, University of Maryland School of Pharmacy, Baltimore

Maria C. Wopat, PharmD, BCACP, TTS (47)
Clinical Pharmacist and Tobacco Cessation Coordinator, William S. Middleton Memorial Veterans Hospital, Madison, Wisconsin

Ann Zweber, BS Pharm (13)
Senior Instructor, Department of Pharmacy Practice, Oregon State University College of Pharmacy, Corvallis

Reviewers

Note: Numbers in parentheses denote the chapter(s) reviewed.

W. Renee Acosta, RPh, MS (12)
Clinical Associate Professor of Health Outcomes & Pharmacy Practice, The University of Texas at Austin College of Pharmacy

Rebecca K. Baer, BS, PharmD (39)
Pharmacist, Sanford Health, Sioux Falls, South Dakota; Formerly Associate Professor, South Dakota State University College of Pharmacy, Brookings

Danial E. Baker, PharmD, FASHP, FASCP (2)
Associate Dean for Clincial Programs, Professor of Pharmacotherapy, Department of Pharmacotherapy, Washington State University Spokane College of Pharmacy

Veronica T. Bandy, PharmD, MS (29)
Director of IPPE Programs and Clinical Associate Professor, Pharmacy Practice Department, University of the Pacific Thomas J. Long School of Pharmacy and Health Sciences, Stockton, California

Forrest Batz, PharmD (51)
Associate Professor of Pharmacy Practice, The Daniel K. Inouye College of Pharmacy, University of Hawai'i at Hilo

Renee Anne Bellanger, PharmD, BCNSP (50)
Associate Professor, Department of Pharmacy Practice, University of the Incarnate Word Feik School of Pharmacy, San Antonio, Texas; Pharmacy Faculty, Children's Hospital of San Antonio, San Antonio, Texas

Elizabeth Weeks Blake, PharmD, BCPS (35, 38)
Clinical Assistant Professor, Director of Interprofessional Education, South Carolina College of Pharmacy, University of South Carolina Campus, Columbia; Clinical Pharmacy Specialist, Primary Care, Palmetto Health Richland, Columbia, South Carolina

Sara Elizabeth Bliss, PharmD, BCPS, BCNSP (22, 25)
Surgery/Nutrition Support Pharmacist, Wake Forest University Baptist Medical Center, Winston-Salem, North Carolina

KarenBeth H. Bohan, PharmD, BCPS (43)
Associate Professor, Wilkes University Nesbitt College of Pharmacy and Nursing, Wilkes-Barre, Pennsylvania

Heather S. Boon, BScPhm, PhD (51)
Professor and Dean, Leslie Dan Faculty of Pharmacy, University of Toronto, Toronto, Ontario, Canada

Alaina Borries, PharmD, BCACP (25)
Assistant Professor, Wingate University School of Pharmacy, Wingate, North Carolina

Ashley Branham, PharmD, BCAP (34)
Adjunct Assistant Professor and Preceptor, Community Pharmacy Residency Program, UNC Eshelman School of Pharmacy, The University of North Carolina at Chapel Hill; Director of Clinical Services, Moose Professional Pharmacy, Concord, North Carolina; Clinical Pharmacist, Cabarrus Family Medicine, Kannapolis, North Carolina

Mary M. Bridgeman, PharmD, BCPS, CGP (24)
Clinical Associate Professor, Rutgers, The State University of New Jersey, Ernest Mario School of Pharmacy, Piscataway

Kristy L. Brittain, PharmD, BCPS (4)
Assistant Professor, Department of Clinical Pharmacy and Outcome Sciences, South Carolina College of Pharmacy, Charleston

Kimberly Broedel-Zaugg, RPh, MBA, PhD (1)
Professor and Chair, Pharmacy Practice, Administration, and Research, Marshall University, Huntington, West Virginia

Wayne Buff, PharmD (1)
Associate Dean and Clinical Associate Professor, Department of Pharmacy and Outcomes Sciences, South Carolina College of Pharmacy, University of South Carolina Campus, Columbia, South Carolina

Stephen M. Caiola, MS, FRSH (14, 48)
Adjunct Associate Professor, Division of Practice Advancement and Clinical Education, UNC Eshelman School of Pharmacy, The University of North Carolina at Chapel Hill

Jay S. Campbell, BS Pharm, JD (4)
Executive Director, North Carolina Board of Pharmacy and Adjunct Assistant Professor, UNC Eshelman School of Pharmacy, The University of North Carolina at Chapel Hill

Ann Canales, PharmD, BCPS (6)
Part Time Clinical Staff Pharmacist, Healix Infusion Therapy, Inc., Sugar Land, Texas

Mary Chavez, PharmD (52)
Professor and Chair of Pharmacy Practice, Texas A&M Health Science Center Rangel College of Pharmacy, Kingsville

Peter A. Chyka, PharmD (20)
Professor and Executive Associate Dean, Professor and Executive Associate Dean, Department of Clinical Pharmacy, University of Tennessee Health Science Center College of Pharmacy–Knoxville Campus

Lisa Clayville-Martin, PharmD, CDE (33, 34)
Clinical Assistant Professor, Department of Pharmacotherapy and Translational Research, University of Florida College of Pharmacy–Orlando Campus, Apopka

Valerie B. Clinard, PharmD (32, 42)
Vice Chairman for Experiential Education and Associate Professor of Pharmacy Practice, Campbell University College of Pharmacy and Health Sciences, Buies Creek, North Carolina

Martha D. Cobb, MS, MEd, CWOCN, ACNS-BC (21)
Clinical Associate Professor (Emeritus), The University of Arizona College of Nursing, Tucson; Wound, Ostomy Nurse Educator, Private Practitioner, Tucson, Arizona

M. Petrea Cober, PharmD, BCNSP (6)
Clinical Pharmacy Coordinator, Neonatal Intensive Care Unit, Akron Children's Hospital, Akron, Ohio; Associate Professor of Pharmacy Practice, Northeast Ohio Medical University College of Pharmacy, Rootstown

Andrea Lynn Coffee, PharmD, MBA, BCPS (9)
Pharmacy Clinical Specialist, Inpatient Pharmacy, Scott & White Healthcare, Temple, Texas

Janice C. Colwell, MS, RN, CWOCN, FAAN (21)
Department of General Surgery, University of Chicago Medical Center, Chicago, Illinois

Steven J. Crosby, BSP, RPh, MA, FASCP (44)
Assistant Professor of Pharmacy Practice and Assistant Coordinator of Advanced Practice Management Laboratories, Massachusetts College of Pharmacy and Health Sciences School of Pharmacy–Boston

Altaf S. Darvesh, M Pharm, PhD (16)
Assistant Professor, Pharmaceutical Sciences, Psychiatry, Northeast Ohio Medical University College of Pharmacy, Rootstown, Ohio

Heather Brooke F. DeBellis, PharmD, CDE (44)
Associate Professor, Department of Pharmacy Practice, South University School of Pharmacy, Savannah, Georgia

Mark Anthony Della Paolera, BS, RPh, PharmD, BCPS, BCACP (42)
Assistant Professor, Pacific University School of Pharmacy, Hillsboro, Oregon

Gladys Garcia Duenas, PharmD (45)
Assistant Professor of Clinical Pharmacy, Department of Pharmacy Practice and Pharmacy Administration, Philadelphia College of Pharmacy, University of the Sciences in Philadelphia, Philadelphia, Pennsylvania

Kaelen C. Dunican, PharmD, RPh (42, 44)
Associate Professor of Pharmacy Practice, Massachusetts College of Pharmacy and Health Sciences School of Pharmacy–Worcester/Manchester

Herbert L. DuPont, MD (16)
Chief, Internal Medicine Service, St. Luke's Episcopal Hospital, Houston, Texas; Director, Center for Infectious Diseases, The University of Texas School of Public Health–Houston Campus; Clinical Professor and Vice-Chairman, Department of Medicine, Baylor College of Medicine, Houston

Melissa Jean Durham, PharmD (16)
Assistant Professor, Clinical Pharmacy and Pharmaceutical Economics and Policy, University of Southern California School of Pharmacy, Los Angeles

Lana Dvorkin Camiel, PharmD (51)
Professor of Pharmacy Practice, Natural Products Division Coordinator of Center for Drug Information and Natural Products, and Director of Applied Natural Products Programs, Massachusetts College of Pharmacy and Health Sciences School of Pharmacy–Boston

Christine Eisenhower, PharmD, BCPS (46)
Clinical Assistant Professor, Department of Pharmacy Practice, University of Rhode Island College of Pharmacy, Kingston

Patricia M. Elsner, PharmD (40)
Pharmacist, Walgreens Company, West Lafayette, Indiana

Danielle C. Ezzo, PharmD, BCPS, CGP (32)
Clinical Associate Professor, Department of Clinical Pharmacy Practice, St. John's University College of Pharmacy and Health Sciences, Queens, New York; Clinical Coordinator of Ambulatory Care and Resident Preceptor of Ambulatory Care Rotation, Long Island Jewish Medical Center, New Hyde Park, New York; Pharmacist, Per-diem, Target Pharmacy, Long Island Region, New York

Patricia H. Fabel, PharmD, BCPS (19)
Clinical Assistant Professor, Department of Clinical Pharmacy and Outcomes Sciences, South Carolina College of Pharmacy, University of South Carolina Campus, Columbia

Stefanie P. Ferreri, PharmD, CDE, FAPhA, BCACP (15)
Clinical Associate Professor and Director, PGY-1 Community Pharmacy Residency Program, UNC Eshelman School of Pharmacy, The University of North Carolina at Chapel Hill

Karla T. Foster, PharmD, BCPS (19)
Pharmacist, Walgreens Company, Ridgeland, Mississippi

Andrea S. Franks, PharmD, BCPS (17)
Associate Professor, Department of Clinical Pharmacy and Assistant Dean, Assessment and Education, University of Tennessee Health Science Center College of Pharmacy–Knoxville Campus; Associate Professor, Department of Family Medicine, University of Tennessee Graduate School of Medicine, Knoxville

Randolph V. Fugit, PharmD, BCPS (13)
Internal Medicine Clinical Specialist, Denver Veterans Affairs Medical Center, Denver, Colorado; Clinical Associate Professor, University of Colorado Health Sciences Center, Denver

April Gardner, MSBS, PA-C (5, 41)
Assistant Professor, Associate Program Director, and Academic Coordinator, Department of Physician Assistant Studies, University of Toledo College of Medicine Graduate Programs, Toledo, Ohio

Lauren Garton, Pharm D, BCACP (13)
Assistant Professor of Pharmacy Practice, South University School of Pharmacy, Savannah, Georgia

Jennifer Goldman-Levine, PharmD, CDE, BC-ADM, FCCP (45)
Professor of Pharmacy Practice, Massachusetts College of Pharmacy and Health Sciences School of Pharmacy–Boston; Clinical Pharmacy Faculty, Tufts University Family Medicine Residency, Malden, Massachusetts

Justin Gollon, RN, PharmD, BCPS, BCNSP (24)
Clinical Staff Pharmacist, The University of Arizona Medical Center, Tucson

William C. Gong, PharmD, FASHP, FCSHP (2)
Associate Professor of Clinical Pharmacy and Director of Residency and Fellowship Training, University of Southern California School of Pharmacy, Los Angeles

Maqual Graham, PharmD (36)
Professor, Division of Pharmacy Practice and Director, Applied Therapeutics and Professional Skills, University of Missouri–Kansas City School of Pharmacy

Nicholas E. Hagemeier, PharmD, PhD (38, 40)
Assistant Professor, Department of Pharmacy Practice, East Tennessee State University Gatton College of Pharmacy, Johnson City, Tennessee

Yolanda Hardy, PharmD (3)
Associate Professor of Pharmacy Practice, Chicago State University College of Pharmacy, Chicago, Illinois

Karl M. Hess, PharmD, FCPhA (4, 18)
Associate Professor of Pharmacy Practice and Administration, Western University of Health Sciences College of Pharmacy, Pomona, California

Michelle L. Hilaire, PharmD, CDE, BCPS (27)
Clinical Associate Professor, Department of Pharmacy Practice, University of Wyoming School of Pharmacy, Laramie; Clinical Pharmacist, Fort Collins Family Medicine Residency Program, Fort Collins, Colorado

Thomas J. Holmes, PhD (42)
Director and Professor, Pharmaceutical Science Programs, Campbell University College of Pharmacy and Health Sciences, Buies Creek, North Carolina

Marcella Honkonen, PharmD, BCPS (26)
Assistant Professor, Department of Pharmacy Practice and Science, The University of Arizona College of Pharmacy, Tucson

Amanda Marie Howard-Thompson, PharmD, BCPS (7, 18)
Associate Professor, Department of Clinical Pharmacy, College of Pharmacy and Associate Professor, Department of Family Medicine, College of Medicine, University of Tennessee Health Science Center–Memphis Campus

Yvonne Huckleberry, RD, PharmD, BCPS (22)
Clinical Staff Pharmacist, The University of Arizona Medical Center, Tucson

Timothy R. Hudd, BS, PharmD, RPh, AE-C (29)
Associate Professor of Pharmacy Practice, Massachusetts College of Pharmacy and Health Sciences School of Pharmacy–Boston; Clinical Pharmacist, Greater Lawrence Family Health Center, Lawrence, Massachusetts; Pharmacist (part-time), Walgreens Company, Danvers, Massachusetts

Anita N. Jackson, PharmD (3)
Clinical Assistant Professor of Pharmacy Practice, University of Rhode Island College of Pharmacy, Kingston; Clinical Pharmacist, Eleanor Slater Hospital, Rhode Island Department of Behavioral Healthcare, Developmental Disabilities and Hospitals, Cranston

Courtney Izzo Jarvis, PharmD (9)
Associate Professor of Pharmacy Practice, Massachusetts College of Pharmacy and Health Sciences School of Pharmacy–Worcester/Manchester

Pramodini B. Kale-Pradhan, PharmD (12)
Professor (Clinical), Department of Pharmacy Practice, Wayne State University Eugene Applebaum College of Pharmacy and Health Sciences, Detroit, Michigan; Clinical Specialist - Infectious Diseases, Department of Pharmacy Services, St. John Hospital and Medical Center, Detroit, Michigan

William D. King, RPh, MPH, DrPH (19)
Division Director and Professor of Pediatrics, Department of Pediatrics, The University of Alabama at Birmingham

Erika L. Kleppinger, PharmD, BCPS, CDE (28)
Associate Clinical Professor, Department of Pharmacy Practice, Auburn University Harrison School of Pharmacy, Auburn, Alabama

Jeffrey Kreitman, PharmD (6)
Regional Pharmacy Director, AmeriHealth Caritas Family of Companies, Harrisburg, Pennsylvania

Thomas E. Lackner, PharmD (49)
Director of Pharmacy Services, Univita Health, Eden Prairie, Minnesota

Karen W. Lee, PharmD, BCPS (11)
Director of Clinical Operations and Quality Assurance, Regional Clinical Director, and Residency Program Director, Comprehensive Pharmacy Services, Tewksbury, Massachusetts

Ginger Lemay, PharmD, CDOE, CVDOE (8)
Clinical Assistant Professor, Community Pharmacy Practice, University of Rhode Island College of Pharmacy, Kingston; Community Pharmacist, MTM Specialist, and Diabetes Educator, Rite Aid 10257, Providence, Rhode Island

Thomas L. Lenz, PharmD, MA, PAPHS (24)
Associate Professor, Director of Pharmacy Distance Pathway, and Clinical Director of Creighton CVD/Diabetes Risk Reduction Program, Creighton University School of Phamacy and Health Professions, Omaha, Nebraska

Roberto W. Linares, Bpharm (29)
Senior Instructor, Department of Pharmacy Practice, Oregon State University College of Pharmacy, Corvallis

Janene Marie Madras, BS Pharm, PharmD, BCPS, BCACP (31)
Director of Student Services and Professor of Pharmacy Practice, Lake Erie College of Osteopathic Medicine School of Pharmacy, Erie, Pennsylvania

Michele L. Matthews, PharmD, CPE, BCACP (7)
Associate Professor of Pharmacy Practice, Massachusetts College of Pharmacy and Health Sciences School of Pharmacy–Boston; Advanced Pharmacist Practitioner – Pain Management, Brigham and Women's Hospital, Boston, Massachusetts

Jamie Lynn McConaha, PharmD, CGP, TTS, BCACP, CDE (39)
Assistant Professor of Pharmacy Practice, Duquesne University Mylan School of Pharmacy, Pittsburgh, Pennsylvania

Marsha McFalls, PharmD, MSEd, RPh (40)
Assistant Professor of Pharmacy Practice and Director, Academic Research Center for Pharmacy Practice, Department of Clinical, Social, and Administrative Sciences, Duquesne University Mylan School of Pharmacy, Pittsburgh, Pennsylvania

Rebekah Jackowski McKinley, PharmD (2)
Assistant Professor, Midwestern University College of Pharmacy–Glendale, Glendale, Arizona

Bella H. Mehta, PharmD, FAPhA (52)
Associate Professor of Pharmacy and Family Medicine, Department of Pharmacy Practice and Administration and Director, Clinical Partners Program, The Ohio State University College of Pharmacy, Columbus

Jill E. Michels, PharmD, DABAT (20)
Managing Director, Palmetto Poison Center and Clinical Assistant Professor, South Carolina College of Pharmacy, University of South Carolina, Columbia

Brad A. Miller, PharmD (5)
Clinical Specialist–Emergency Medicine, Pharmacy Department, Spectrum Health, Grand Rapids, Michigan

Amee D. Mistry, PharmD (33)
Associate Professor of Pharmacy Practice, Massachusetts College of Pharmacy and Health Sciences School of Pharmacy–Boston; Community Practice Pharmacist, Walgreens Company, Waltham, Massachusetts

Anna K. Morin, PharmD, RPh (46)
Associate Dean and Associate Professor, Department of Pharmacy Practice, Massachusetts College of Pharmacy and Health Sciences School of Pharmacy–Worcester/Manchester

Leigh Anne Nelson, PharmD, BCPP (46)
Associate Professor, Division of Pharmacy Practice and Administration, University of Missouri-Kansas City School of Pharmacy

Monika Majer Nuffer, PharmD (50)
Academic and Experiential Program Coordinator, Distance Degrees and Programs and Senior Instructor, Department of Clinical Pharmacy, University of Colorado Skaggs School of Pharmacy and Pharmaceutical Sciences, Aurora; Clinical Pharmacist/Herbal Specialist, The Center for Integrative Medicine at the University of Colorado Hospital, Aurora

Wesley A. Nuffer, PharmD, BCPS, CDE (26)
Assistant Director of Experiential Programs and Assistant Professor, University of Colorado Skaggs School of Pharmacy and Pharmaceutical Sciences, Aurora

Shanna O'Connor, PharmD (33)
Faculty Fellow, Kelley-Ross Pharmacy, Seattle, Washington; Acting Assistant Professor, University of Washington School of Pharmacy, Seattle

Rachel R. Ogden, BS Pharm, Pharm.D., MS, CGP (12)
Associate Professor of Pharmacy Practice and Associate Dean of Accelerated Pathway, Lake Erie College of Osteopathic Medicine School of Pharmacy, Erie, Pennsylvania; Clinical Pharmacist, Lake Erie College of Osteopathic Medicine Institute for Successful Aging, Erie, Pennsylvania

Anne C. Pace, PharmD (3)
Community Experiential Director and Assistant Professor, Department of Pharmacy Practice, University of Arkansas for Medical Sciences College of Pharmacy, Little Rock

Sarah Parnapy Jawaid, PharmD (11)
Associate Professor of Pharmacy Practice and Vice Chair, Department of Pharmacy Practice, Shenandoah University Bernard J. Dunn School of Pharmacy–Winchester Campus, Winchester, Virginia

Dhiren K. Patel, PharmD, CDE, BC-ADM, BCACP (7)
Associate Professor of Pharmacy Practice, Massachusetts College of Pharmacy and Health Sciences School of Pharmacy–Boston; Clinical Pharmacy Specialist, VA Boston Healthcare System

Rupal Patel Mansukhani, PharmD (41, 43)
Clinical Assistant Professor, Rutgers, The State University of New Jersey Ernest Mario School of Pharmacy–Busch Campus, Piscataway; Clinical Pharmacist, Morristown Medical Center, Morristown, New Jersey

Karen Steinmetz Pater, PharmD, BCPS, CDE (5)
Assistant Professor, Department of Pharmacy and Therapeutics, University of Pittsburgh School of Pharmacy, Pittsburgh, Pennsylvania

Denise L. Walbrandt Pigarelli, PharmD, BC-ADM (42)
Associate Professor of Pharmacy (CHS), University of Wisconsin–Madison School of Pharmacy; Clinical Pharmacist, William S. Middleton Memorial VA Hospital, Madison, Wisconsin

Matthew K. Pitlick, PharmD, BCPS (28)
Assistant Professor of Pharmacy Practice, St. Louis College of Pharmacy, St. Louis, Missouri

Kimberly S. Plake, PhD (49)
Associate Professor, Department of Pharmacy Practice, Purdue University College of Pharmacy, West Lafayette, Indiana

Barbara Poetzsch, PhD, RPA-C (34)
Associate Professor and Pre-Clinical Coordinator, Center for Physician Assistant Studies, Albany Medical College, Albany, New York

Charles D. Ponte, BS, PharmD, DPNAP, FAADE, FAPhA, FASHP, FCCP (37)
Professor of Clinical Pharmacy and Family Medicine, Departments of Clinical Pharmacy and Family Medicine, Schools of Pharmacy and Medicine, West Virginia University Robert C. Byrd Health Sciences Center, Morgantown, West Virginia

Traci M. Poole, PharmD, BCACP, CGP (15)
Assistant Professor of Pharmacy Practice, Belmont University College of Pharmacy, Nashville, Tennessee

Cathy Ramey, PharmD, CGP (32, 34)
Assistant Professor of Pharmacy Practice, Butler University College of Pharmacy and Health Sciences, Indianapolis, Indiana

Celtina K. Reinert, PharmD (52)
Staff Pharmacist, HealthScripts of America–Kansas City, Kansas City, Missouri; Staff Pharmacist, CVS/Pharmacy, North Kansas City, Missouri

Lorraine M. Reiser, PhD, CRNP, FAANP (25, 26)
Region 3 Director, American Academy of Nurse Practitioners, Pittsburgh, Pennsylvania

Pamela Ringor, MBA, RPh (36, 38)
Pharmacy Manager, PayLess Pharmacy, Lafayette, Indiana

Ronald J. Ruggiero, PharmD (9, 10)
Clinical Professor, Departments of Clinical Pharmacy and Obstetrics, Gynecology, and Reproductive Sciences, Schools of Pharmacy and Medicine, The Medical Center at University of California, San Francisco

Jill S. Sailors, PharmD (17)
Assistant Professor of Pharmacy Practice, St. Louis College of Pharmacy, St. Louis, Missouri

Marissa C. Salvo, PharmD, BCACP (8)
Assistant Clinical Professor, Department of Pharmacy Practice, University of Connecticut School of Pharmacy, Storrs

G. Blair Sarbacker, PharmD (27)
Associate Professor, Department of Pharmacy Practice, University of the Incarnate Word Feik School of Pharmacy, San Antonio, Texas

Morgan Sayler, PharmD (41, 43)
Assistant Professor (Clinical), University of Utah College of Pharmacy, Salt Lake City; Clinical Pharmacist, University of Utah Greenwood Health Center Pharmacy, Midvale

Tara Schmitz, PharmD (43)
Assistant Professor of Practice, Department of Pharmacy Practice, North Dakota State University College of Pharmacy, Nursing, and Allied Sciences, Fargo; Owner, Tara's Thrifty White Pharmacy, Oakes, North Dakota; Director of Pharmacy, Oakes Community Hospital, Oakes, North Dakota

Stacey Schneider, PharmD (31)
Associate Professor of Pharmacy Practice, Northeast Ohio Medical University College of Pharmacy, Rootstown

Emmanuelle Schwartzman, PharmD, CDE, BCACP (37)
Director, Residency and Fellowship Training and Associate Professor of Pharmacy Practice and Administration, Western University of Health Sciences College of Pharmacy, Pomona, California

Kelly L. Scolaro, PharmD (48)
Clinical Assistant Professor and Director of Pharmaceutical Care Laboratory, Division of Practice Advancement and Clinical Education, UNC Eshelman School of Pharmacy, The University of North Carolina at Chapel Hill

Kayce M. Shealy, PharmD, BCPS, BCACP, CDE (15)
Assistant Professor of Pharmacy Practice, Presbyterian College School of Pharmacy, Clinton, South Carolina

Justin J. Sherman, PharmD, MCS (47)
Associate Professor of Pharmacy Practice and Family Medicine, University of Mississippi Schools of Pharmacy and Medicine, University of Mississippi Medical Center Campus, Jackson

Kelly M. Shields, PharmD (50)
Associate Professor of Pharmacy Practice, Ohio Northern University Raabe College of Pharmacy, Ada

Debra Sibbald, BSc Phm, RPh, ACPR, MA (Adult Education), PhD (Curriculum, Teaching and Learning) (35)
Director of Assessment Services, Centre for the Evaluation of Health Professionals Educated Abroad, Toronto, Ontario, Canada; Senior Lecturer and Coordinator, Pharmacotherapy II: Dermatology and EENT, University of Toronto, Leslie Dan Faculty of Pharmacy, Toronto, Ontario, Canada

Dorothy L. Smith, PharmD (2)
President and CEO, Consumer Health Information Corporation, McLean, Virginia; Academic Cross-appointments with 40 Schools of Pharmacy, P4 Patient Adherence/Patient Education Rotation Site

Jeanie Smith, PharmD (34)
Associate Professor of Pharmacy Practice, Harding University College of Pharmacy, Searcy, Arkansas

Jennifer D. Smith, PharmD, CPP, BC-ADM, CDE (45)
Associate Professor, Campbell University College of Pharmacy and Health Sciences, Buies Creek, North Carolina; Clinical Pharmacist Practitioner, Wilson Community Health Center, Wilson, North Carolina

Susan Claire Smolinske, PharmD, BCPS, DABAT (20)
Professor of Medicine, Pediatrics, Wayne State University, Detroit, Michigan; Director, Children's Hospital of Michigan Regional Poison Center, Detroit

Jenelle L. Sobotka, PharmD (1)
Staff, Professor, and Endowed Chair, Department of Pharmacy Practice, Ohio Northern University Raabe College of Pharmacy, Ada, Ohio

Phillip S. Springer, DMD (30, 31)
Clinical Assistant Professor, Department of Oral Medicine, University of Pennsylvania School of Medicine, Philadelphia; Private Practitioner (General Dentistry), Philadelphia, Pennsylvania

Sneha Baxi Srivastava, PharmD, BCACP (32)
Clinical Associate Professor, Chicago State University College of Pharmacy, Chicago, Illinois

Erin L. St. Onge, PharmD (46)
Assistant Dean/Campus Director and Clinical Associate Professor, Department of Pharmacotherapy and Translational Research , University of Florida College of Pharmacy–Orlando Campus, Apopka

Donald L. Sullivan, PhD (48)
Professor of Pharmacy Practice, Ohio Northern University College of Pharmacy, Ada

Jeff G. Taylor, PhD (11)
Professor of Pharmacy, University of Saskatchewan College of Pharmacy and Nutrition, Saskatoon, Saskatchewan, Canada

Renee Ahrens Thomas, PharmD, MBA (17)
Adjunct Associate Professor of Pharmacy Practice, Shenandoah University Bernard J. Dunn School of Pharmacy–Winchester Campus, Winchester, Virginia

Dominick P. Trombetta, PharmD, BCPS, CGP, FASCP (41)
Associate Professor of Pharmacy Practice, Wilkes University Nesbitt School of Pharmacy, Wilkes-Barre, Pennsylvania; Allied Services Rehabilitation Hosptial & Outpatient Centers, Scranton, Pennsylvania

Timothy R. Ulbrich, PharmD, RPh (47)
Associate Dean, Workforce Development and Practice Advancement and Associate Professor of Pharmacy Practice, Northeast Ohio Medical University College of Pharmacy, Rootstown

Tanya Vadala, PharmD (33)
Assistant Professor, Ambulatory Care, Albany College of Pharmacy and Health Sciences, Albany, New York[1]

Jesse C. Vivian, BS Pharm, JD (4)
Professor of Pharmacy Practice, Wayne State University School of Pharmacy and Health Sciences, Detroit, Michigan

Ty Vo, PharmD, BCPS, CDE (49)
Associate Professor, Department of Pharmacy Practice, Pacific University Oregon School of Pharmacy, Hillsboro

Lucio Volino, PharmD (41, 43)
Clinical Assistant Professor, Rutgers, The State University of New Jersey Ernest Mario School of Pharmacy, Piscataway; Clinical Pharmacist, The Great Atlantic and Pacific Tea Company, Kenilworth, New Jersey

Paul C. Walker, PharmD, FASHP (35)
Clinical Professor and Director, Experiential Education and Community Engagement, College of Pharmacy, Department of Clinical Sciences, The University of Michigan College of Pharmacy, Ann Arbor; Manager, Pharmacy Patient Outcomes, Department of Pharmacy, The University of Michigan Health System, Ann Arbor

Kristina E. Ward, BS, PharmD, BCPS (10)
Clinical Associate Professor and Director of Drug Information Services, University of Rhode Island College of Pharmacy, Kingston

C. Wayne Weart, PharmD, BCPS, FASHP, FAPhA (13)
Professor Emeritus, Department of Clinical Pharmacy and Outcome Sciences, South Carolina College of Pharmacy, Medical University of South Carolina Campus, Charleston; Professor of Family Medicine, Medical University of South Carolina, Charleston

Miranda Wilhelm, PharmD (35)
Clinical Associate Professor of Pharmacy Practice, Southern Illinois University-Edwardsville School of Pharmacy

Jennifer A. Wilson, PharmD, BCACP (44)
Assistant Professor of Pharmacy, Wingate University School of Pharmacy, Wingate, North Carolina

Supakit Wongwiwatthananukit, PharmD, PhD (47)
Associate Professor of Pharmacy Practice, The Daniel K. Inouye College of Pharmacy, University of Hawai'i at Hilo

Tonja M. Woods, PharmD (8)
Associate Dean of Academic Affairs and Student Affairs and Clinical Associate Professor, University of Wyoming School of Pharmacy, Laramie; Clinical Pharmacist, Adult & Geriatric Medical Specialties, Laramie, Wyoming

Mark J. Wrobel, PharmD (30)
Clinical Assistant Professor, University at Buffalo School of Pharmacy and Pharmaceutical Sciences, Buffalo, New York

John R. Yuen, PharmD, BCNP (28)
Board Certified Nuclear Pharmacist, Los Angeles County and USC Medical Center, Los Angeles, California; Adjunct Assistant Professor of Pharmacy Practice, University of Southern California School of Pharmacy, Los Angeles

Kathy Zaiken, PharmD (37)
Associate Professor of Pharmacy Practice, Massachusetts College of Pharmacy and Health Sciences School of Pharmacy–Boston

Deborah Zeitlin, PharmD (30, 31)
Assistant Professor of Pharmacy Practice, Butler University College of Pharmacy and Health Sciences, Indianapolis, Indiana

Ann Zweber, BS Pharm (14)
Senior Instructor, Department of Pharmacy Practice, Oregon State University College of Pharmacy, Corvallis

[1] Position held at the time the contributor reviewed the chapter.

THE PRACTITIONER'S ROLE IN SELF-CARE

SELF-CARE AND NONPRESCRIPTION PHARMACOTHERAPY

Metta Lou Henderson

Self-Care

Self-care is the independent act of preventing, diagnosing, and treating one's illnesses without seeking professional advice. Preventive self-care involves maintaining well-being and appearance through exercise and a healthy lifestyle. For many individuals, a healthy lifestyle includes controlling their diet; taking vitamins, minerals, and herbal supplements; participating in regular exercise and keeping fit; and maintaining their appearance by using dental, skin, and hair care products. However, sickness self-care for individuals involves diagnosing their conditions and obtaining products for the goal of mitigating illness and relieving symptoms. Examples of sickness self-care include use of dietary options (e.g., warm soup for a cold); use of devices for both disease assessment (e.g., home blood glucose meters and pregnancy tests) and treatment (e.g., ice packs, first-aid bandages, vaporizers, and nasal strips); and use of nonprescription medications. The use of sickness self-care products is limited to mild illness or short-term management of illness, and most products warn users to contact a health care provider if conditions do not improve within a short period of time.

For the provision of sickness self-care, one individual from each household usually plays a leading role in adopting a course of action. This individual must determine whether a health care provider should be consulted or whether the use of home remedies and self-care will suffice. Furthermore, the number of individuals involved in choosing the most appropriate self-care option is increasing because of the growth of the U.S. geriatric population, whose members are known as high users of nonprescription medications.[1]

Individuals responsible for providing self-care for themselves or family members rely on knowledge and experience to guide their decisions. For better or worse, there is no shortage of information, given the wealth of health-related self-help books, newspaper feature articles, magazine and television advertisements, magazine articles, radio programs, instructional tapes and CDs, DVDs, and Internet sites—all of which provide self-care advice. The availability of coupons indirectly provides information and encourages cost savings for trying a product. The abundance of available health-related information, especially from the Internet, helps individuals become more "self-empowered" to address their health care issues and leads to aggressive marketing and use of self-care alternatives. The quality of the information ranges from excellent to very poor. Although it is more accepted today for individuals to attempt to manage their health-related issues rather than to consult a health care provider, the concern

is whether they are making appropriate and informed decisions. Furthermore, all this health information can become overwhelming, driving some individuals to seek advice from family and friends. This well-intentioned advice can be problematic because it is often biased, and most individuals are not sufficiently informed or qualified to consider another's health conditions or medications before making a recommendation. They simply state what has worked best for them and fail to consider how their approach might apply to someone else.

Commercial products used for preventive or sickness self-care are often classified together as health and beauty care (HBC) products. Staggering numbers of HBC products are available. Although access to quality HBC products is crucial to the goal of self-care, the vast number of similar, competing products makes appropriate selection difficult. Yet, in one consumer poll in which 66% of adults believed that the wide range of competing products made selection difficult, less than half (43%) said they consulted a pharmacist before making a purchase.[2] The pharmacist plays a crucial role in assisting patients who are seeking both preventive and sickness self-care products. The practicing pharmacist has the expertise to screen patient health information and apply his or her knowledge and training to select products according to individual health care needs. Therefore, for pharmacies to provide pharmacist-assisted self-care, only quality HBC products should be stocked, and a pharmacist should be readily available for patients seeking assistance. More and more pharmacies are changing their floor layout and design and staffing to ensure that a pharmacist is available and easily accessible to patients seeking advice in the nonprescription drug aisles. At times, this change coincides with the implementation of a retail clinic staffed by a nurse practitioner or a physician assistant as a primary care provider.

Self-Medication

Self-medication is often the most sought-after first level of self-care. As self-care has increased, so has the practice of self-medication with vitamins (i.e., nutritional dietary supplements), natural products (i.e., herbal/botanical and nonherbal dietary supplements [e.g., glucosamine]), and nonprescription medications. Factors that help drive reliance on self-medication include (1) growth of the aging population, (2) decreased availability of primary care providers, (3) increased costs of health care, and (4) high proportion of underinsured or uninsured people in the United States. Easy accessibility, convenience, and cost-effectiveness of self-medication products ensure their essential role in the U.S. health care system.

Results of a 2002 survey conducted for the National Council on Patient Information and Education (NCPIE)[3] illustrate how ubiquitous the use of nonprescription medications has become. According to the survey, 59% of Americans had taken at least one nonprescription medication in the preceding 6 months. Table 1–1 illustrates some of the conditions that are self-treatable with nonprescription medications. Conditions and symptoms commonly treated with nonprescription medications include the following:

- Pain (78%)
- Cough/cold/flu/sore throat (52%)
- Allergy/sinus problems (45%)
- Heartburn/indigestion (37%)
- Constipation/diarrhea/gas (21%)
- Minor infections (12%)
- Skin problems (10%)

Approximately 20% of Americans believe that they are consuming more nonprescription medications and taking them more frequently than they did 5 years earlier.[3] This increase in nonprescription drug use may reflect a consumer belief that self-medication is safe.

Additional data collected in the survey "Your Health at Hand: Perceptions of Over-the-Counter Medicine in the U.S." supports the view that consumers and physicians are confident in their use of nonprescription medications.[4] These survey results show the following:

- 93% of physicians believe it is important that medications for minor ailments be available over the counter.
- 96% of consumers believe nonprescription medications make it easy to care for minor medical ailments.
- 87% of physicians and 89% of consumers believe nonprescription medications are an important part of overall and family health care.
- 93% of adults prefer to treat minor ailments with nonprescription medications before seeking professional care.
- 88% of physicians recommend patients address minor ailments with self-care, including nonprescription medications before seeking professional care.

A major 2012 survey of more than 3200 individuals provides information regarding the value of nonprescription medications

---

table 1–1   Selected Medical Disorders Amenable to Nonprescription Drug Therapy[a]

Abrasions	Cold sores	Gastritis	Ostomy care
Aches and pains (general, mild-moderate)	Colds (viral upper respiratory infection)	Gingivitis	Ovulation prediction
Acidity, stomach	Congestion (chest, nasal)	Hair loss	Periodontal disease
Acne	Constipation	Halitosis	Pharyngitis
Allergic reactions (mild)	Contact lens care	Hangover relief, morning	Pinworm infestation
Allergic rhinitis	Contraception	Head lice	Premenstrual syndrome
Anemia (after diagnosis by a health care provider)	Corns	Headache	Prickly heat
Arthralgia	Cough	Heartburn	Psoriasis
Asthma (after diagnosis by a health care provider)	Cuts (superficial)	Hemorrhoids	Ringworm
Athlete's foot	Dandruff	Herpes	Seborrhea
Bacterial infection (dermatologic, mild)	Decongestant, nasal	Impetigo	Sinusitis
Blisters	Dental care	Indigestion	Smoking cessation
Blood pressure monitoring	Dermatitis (contact)	Ingrown toenails	Sprains
Boils	Diabetes mellitus (insulin, monitoring equipment, supplies)	Insect bites and stings	Strains
Bowel preparation (diagnostic)	Diaper rash	Insomnia	Stye (hordeolum)
Burns (minor, thermal)	Diarrhea	Jet lag	Sunburn
Calluses	Dry skin	Jock itch	Teething
Candidal vaginitis	Dyslipidemia	Migraine	Thrush
Canker sores	Dysmenorrhea	Motion sickness	Toothache
Carbuncles	Dyspepsia	Myalgia	Vomiting
Chapped skin	Fever	Nausea	Warts (common and plantar)
	Flatulence	Nutrition (infant)	Xerostomia
		Obesity	Wound care
		Occult blood, fecal (detection)	

[a] The pertinent nonprescription medication(s) for a particular disorder may serve as primary or major adjunctive therapy.

Source: U.S. Food and Drug Administration. Status of OTC rulemaking. February 17, 2011. Accessed at http://www.fda.gov/Drugs/DevelopmentApprovalProcess/DevelopmentResources/Over-the-CounterOTCDrugs/StatusofOTCRulemakings/default.htm, June 2014.

and their contribution to cost savings and quality care in our health care system.[5] These data showed the following:

- Availability of nonprescription products provides $102 billion in annual savings relative to alternatives and increased access to medications.
- Each dollar spent on nonprescription medications saves $6–$7 for the health care system.
- In the previous 12 months, 79% of consumers (or approximately 240 million people) took a nonprescription drug in the categories of allergy, analgesics, antifungals, cough/cold/flu, lower gastrointestinal, upper gastrointestinal, and medicated skin.
- 180 million individuals would seek treatment from a primary care provider if nonprescription medications were not available.

Self-medication plays an increasing role as adjunctive therapy for chronic diseases that are managed with prescription medications. Examples include low-dose aspirin for reducing heart attack risk, fish oil (omega-3 fatty acids) to help manage certain dyslipidemias, and glucosamine with chondroitin to help relieve symptoms of osteoarthritis. However, the use of nonprescription products as adjunctive therapy comes with potential risks associated with incorrect product selection. For example, many patients who require daily low-dose aspirin do not fully understand the differences between the many aspirin products. There are various strengths (low dose, regular, and extra strength) and products (chewable, buffered, and enteric coated). Selection of the wrong product could result in adverse reactions (e.g., gastritis or ulcer) or drug–drug interactions (e.g., warfarin and blood pressure medications). The pharmacist plays an important role in helping patients select the correct products for their condition.

Options for Self-Medication

Three general categories of products are available for self-medication: (1) nonprescription medications, (2) nutritional dietary supplements, and (3) natural products and homeopathic remedies.

Nonprescription Medications

Nonprescription medications are regulated by the Center for Drug Evaluation and Research, a division of the U.S. Food and Drug Administration (FDA)—the same agency that regulates prescription drug products. As such, nonprescription medications are held to the same drug product formulation (e.g., purity and stability), labeling, and safety (benefits outweigh risks) standards as those for prescription medications. A complete discussion of the monograph system can be found in Chapter 4. It is worth noting that, although nonprescription medications are regulated in a manner equivalent to that of prescription medications, the sales of nonprescription medications are not limited to pharmacies. They are also available in retail establishments such as discount stores, supermarkets, and gas station quick stops and on a plethora of Internet sites.

The provisions of the 1951 Durham–Humphrey Amendment to the Food, Drug, and Cosmetic Act of 1938 gives FDA the final authority to categorize a medication as prescription or nonprescription. FDA deems nonprescription medications safe and effective when they are used without a prescriber's directive and oversight. In addition, these products have the following characteristics: they have a low potential for misuse and abuse; patients can use them for self-diagnosed conditions; they are adequately labeled; and they do not require access to a health care provider for safe and effective use.[6] The estimated number of available FDA-approved nonprescription drug products is 100,000, including more than 1000 active ingredients that cover more than 80 therapeutic categories. *Your Health at Hand Book: Guide to OTC Active Ingredients in the United States* provides an extensive list of active ingredients, therapeutic categories, and examples of brand name products.[7] Sales of nonprescription medications in 2011 were estimated at $17.4 billion dollars.[8] Sales of the top 15 therapeutic categories of nonprescription medications for 2011 are shown in Figure 1–1.[9] Not surprisingly, the dollars spent, as shown in this figure, correspond to what consumer surveys have reported as the most common conditions managed with self-care. For example, in a survey in which consumers were asked what health problems they had experienced in the preceding 6 months, the most frequent responses were muscle/back/joint pain and cough/cold/flu/sore throat (both categories at 48%), with headache and heartburn/indigestion trailing at 43% and 32%, respectively.[10] The correlation between common types of illnesses and dollars spent implies that many Americans provide self-care for those conditions using nonprescription medications.

Nutritional Dietary Supplements

The Dietary Supplement Health and Education Act of 1994 amended the 1983 Food, Drug, and Cosmetic Act to establish standards with respect to dietary supplements. The amendment defined dietary supplements as products that are intended to supplement the diet and that bear or contain one or more of the following dietary ingredients: (1) a vitamin, (2) a mineral, (3) an herb, or (4) an amino acid. Results from a recent National Health and Nutrition Survey indicate that more than 50% of adults used one or more dietary supplements between 2003 and 2006.[11] A survey of college students found that almost three-quarters (71%) had used an herbal or nutritional supplement and that 61% had used both a nonprescription product and a nutritional or herbal supplement within the past year.[12] (See Chapters 50–52 for further information on dietary supplements.)

Natural Products and Homeopathic Remedies

Because of factors such as high health care costs and restricted access to conventional health care providers, many patients seek care from providers of complementary and alternative medicine (CAM). The National Center for Complementary and Alternative Medicine and the National Center for Health Statistics reported survey results on Americans' use of CAM.[13] Approximately 38% of adults and 12% of children reported receiving some form of CAM therapy in 2007. Some of the most common forms of CAM therapy were natural products (18%), deep breathing (13%), meditation (9%), chiropractic and osteopathic care (9%), massage (8%), and yoga (6%). Adults spent approximately $34 billion out of pocket to visit CAM providers and purchase products.[14]

Self-care is a component of many CAM therapies. By definition, the term *dietary supplement* includes both herbal and natural products. In 2011, the total estimated sales of herbal products were $5.03 billion, with the top-selling supplements

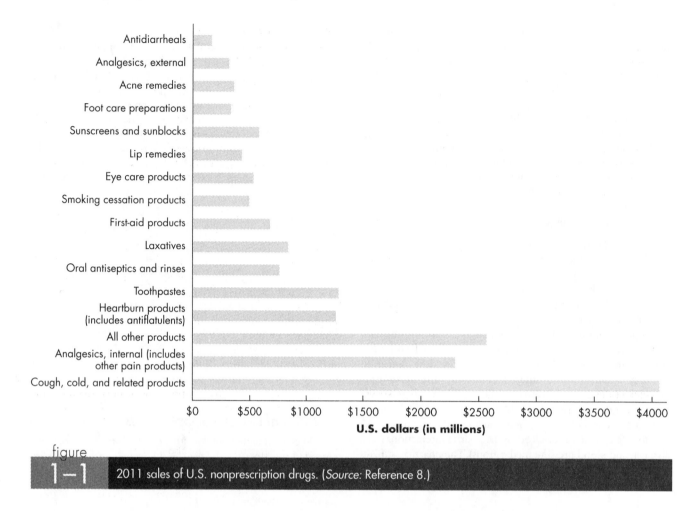

1–1   2011 sales of U.S. nonprescription drugs. (*Source:* Reference 8.)

being cranberry, soy, saw palmetto, garlic, and echinacea.[15] A 2002 National Health Survey indicated that about 13% of elderly patients had used an herbal supplement during the preceding year.[16] The use of combined herbal and conventional therapy raises safety concerns because 51% of patients failed to inform their health care provider about their herbal therapy.[11] These safety concerns include the potential for herbal supplement–drug interactions. Lexi-Comp's Lexi-Interact database (Hudson, Ohio, Lexi-Comp, Inc., 2013) lists several hundred herb–drug interactions, with garlic, St. John's wort, the various ginseng products, and *Ginkgo biloba* leading the way. Therefore, individuals who take prescription or nonprescription medications should consult with a pharmacist or other health care provider before self-medicating with herbal supplements.

Influences on Self-Medication
Costs

Patients often seek self-care and nonprescription medications to avoid the costs associated with a primary care provider visit. Pharmacists can help these individuals by triaging to determine the appropriateness of self-care (see Chapter 2). Although nonprescription products can reduce overall costs, federal legislation eliminated one of the benefits. Nonprescription medications purchased over the counter can no longer be paid for by flexible

spending accounts and health savings accounts. However, the Affordable Care Act of 2010 included a provision allowing reimbursement for nonprescription medications if they are prescribed. Various private health insurance plans and Medicare and state Medicaid programs are continually making decisions regarding payment/reimbursement for nonprescription products. For accurate and up-to-date answers regarding the tax status of nonprescription medication purchases, individuals should consult with their tax advisor for additional information. Many people have medical and prescription insurances with higher copays and deductibles; therefore, the patient's copay for a physician office visit may be comparable to or even higher than the cost of nonprescription treatment. This lower cost may result in even more self-care and nonprescription medication use in the future.

Aging Population

The results of the 2010 census found the number of people 65 years old or older has increased 15.1% since 2000, compared with a total population increase of 9.7%.[17] The average life expectancy for Americans has increased, with individuals reaching age 65 years expected to live an additional 18.6 years. The percentage of older Americans is increasing sharply as the baby boom generation approaches the age of 65. By 2030, 72.1 million people in the United States will be 65 years or older, up from 39.6 million in 2009. The fastest-growing segment of the elderly is individuals older than 85 years. These patients will have a bigger impact on the future of the U.S. health care system because they tend to be in poorer health and require more services than patients between the ages of 65 and 85 years require.[18]

In a major 2005–2006 study of older adults, researchers found that 81% used at least one prescription drug, 42% used at least one nonprescription drug, and 49% used a dietary supplement. Almost half (46%) of older adults using prescription drugs also used nonprescription medications, with 4% at risk for major drug–drug interactions.[19] One study in elderly nursing home patients showed that use of nonprescription medications (93.9%) was only slightly less than that of prescription medications (98.2%). This study noted that, on average, nursing home residents used 8.8 unique medications per month, one-third (2.8) of which were nonprescription medications.[20] The elderly population's increased use of nonprescription medications can be attributed to the following:

- Conditions for which nonprescription medications are used, such as arthritis pain, insomnia, and constipation, become more prevalent with advancing age.
- Nonprescription medications provide low-cost alternatives to more expensive primary care provider visits and prescription medications.
- Accessibility to pharmacists in the community setting makes nonprescription medications an acceptable alternative to scheduling visits with primary care providers.

Elderly patients who use nonprescription medications have heightened safety concerns because of the greater likelihood for multiple disease states and concurrent use of prescription medications. For example, one study documented the use of nonprescription medications and dietary supplements in 45 elderly patients (average age of 85 years) residing in assisted-living facilities.[21] The results showed that elderly residents used an average of 3.4 nonprescription products, with the most common being nutritional dietary supplements (32%), gastrointestinal products (17%), pain relievers (16.3%), and herbal products (14.4%). Potential safety concerns of drug duplication (70%)

and drug–disease–food interactions (20.8%) were identified in more than one-half of these patients.

Gender Differences

As is true worldwide, there are more women than men in the United States. The gender gap widens dramatically with age. For example, in 2009 the overall percentage of males (49%) and females (51%) was almost equal.[17] For ages 65–69, the female-to-male ratio is 114 women to 100 men; for ages 85 and older, the ratio is 216 women to 100 men.[18] The preponderance of elderly women has a considerable influence on self-medication. In the Self-Care in the New Millennium survey, women consistently reported that they had a variety of health problems in the past 6 months more frequently than did men.[10] Figure 1–2 shows that, across the board, more women than men report having each of the six ailments. Women were also more likely (82%) than men (71%) to report using nonprescription medications. This gender difference was also observed in dietary supplement use, which was reported by 30% of women but only 23% of men.[10] Therefore, the increasing population of older women should increase demand for nonprescription products in the future.

There are also gender-specific self-medication concerns, such as the use of nonprescription medications during pregnancy. The ability of pregnant women to self-medicate safely is limited because most products state, "if pregnant or breast-feeding, ask a health care professional before use." Pharmacists are trained to assess whether a nonprescription medication is safe for use during pregnancy, yet women often make these decisions independently.

Breast-feeding mothers are also faced with difficult choices when selecting nonprescription medications. As an example, all four primary nonprescription pain relievers (i.e., aspirin, acetaminophen, naproxen, and ibuprofen) have the potential to enter breast milk. Pharmacists can make the following recommendations to help avoid problems in women who are breast-feeding[22]:

- Advise using nonpharmacologic therapy, if possible.
- Advise taking medications immediately after nursing or before the infant's longest sleep period.

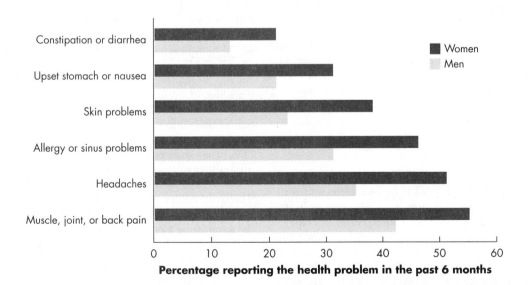

1–2   Selected ailments self-treated by men and women. (*Source:* Reference 10.)

- Avoid recommending any medications that are extra strength, maximum strength, or long acting.
- Avoid recommending combination products.
- Counsel about potential side effects that could occur in the child.

Determining the nonprescription status of an emergency contraception product (e.g., Plan B One-Step) is another example of an issue for which female patients will need direct access to the pharmacist. The pharmacist plays an important role in terms of ensuring timely access to the medication. A 2013 federal decision changed the status of Plan B One-Step, and it must now be readily available to all.

Access to Nonprescription Drug Products for Self-Medication

The major benefits of nonprescription medications are accessibility and convenience. As mentioned earlier, these products are readily available at numerous locations, including pharmacies, supermarkets, and discount stores, thereby saving time for the consumer. The Consumer Healthcare Products Association released a white paper that provides a long list of benefits for the use of nonprescription products, including the following[23]:

- Numerous conditions can be treated effectively with these products, and products can be kept in the home to provide quick access. A number of national medical associations now provide guidelines for use. Households are being encouraged to have a stock of preparations for earwax removal; products for relieving sore throats, coughs, heartburn, diarrhea, skin rashes, allergies, and cold sores; and first-aid supplies. Pharmacists have an important role in advising individuals on which products to purchase and explaining the products' correct use.
- A variety of products and dosage forms allows patients to select the best choice to meet their needs.
- These products can be used to manage a condition or disease while waiting to see a health care provider. Cost is also a factor in determining whether to see a provider or attempt to treat at home.

The benefits of these products will occur only if they are used safely and effectively (the right product for the condition). Nonprescription drug labels include a significant amount of information that can assist the patient in product selection and use.

Web-Based Drug Information and Internet Pharmacies

As people live longer, work longer, and take on a more active role in their health care, they need to become better informed about self-care options and how to safely self-medicate. Web-based health care–related information is easily and rapidly accessed in the privacy and comfort of one's home. According to a 2011 Pew Internet and American Life Project report, 80% of American Internet users, or 59% of U.S. adults, have searched for online health information.[24] Individuals who were most likely to search for health information online were women, non-Hispanic whites, adults younger than 65 years, and those with higher levels of education as well as higher income.

Popular search topics were a specific disease/medical problem (66%), certain medical treatments/procedures (56%), exercise and fitness (27%), and various questions regarding drugs (24%) often combined with specific medical problems.

Dependence on the Internet for self-care information can be problematic. No single organization is accountable for the quality or accuracy of health-related information available on Web sites. The sheer number and diversity of Internet sources increases the likelihood that patients may unknowingly view biased or outdated information. Relatively new sources of information include social media sites such as Facebook, Twitter, YouTube, and My Space. Sixty-two percent of the responders to the Pew report accessed those sites.[24] Because many sites contain inadequate, outdated, or incomplete information, it is not safe to simply "surf" and self-medicate. For example, one study that evaluated the suitability of written supplemental materials available on the Internet for nonprescription medications determined that most manufacturer-sponsored Web sites intended for consumers had information that scored poorly in the areas of reading level and use of uncommon words.[25] A number of valid Internet sources are available to provide information on nonprescription drugs, including the National Institutes of Health (www.nlm.nih.gov/medlineplus) and sites such as the Cleveland Clinic (www.clevelandclinicmeded.com), WebMD (www.webmd.com), and Mayo Clinic (www.mayoclinic.com).

Purchasing drugs online has become an issue in terms of safety, legality, quality, and effectiveness. In response to public safety concerns, the National Association of Boards of Pharmacy (NABP) evaluates the credentials of online pharmacies (also known as e-pharmacies) through the Verified Internet Pharmacy Practice Sites (VIPPS) program.[26] The VIPPS program is voluntary, and an e-pharmacy must agree to strict conditions, including NABP inspections, to be certified under its auspices. Use of the VIPPS logo on Web pages confers credibility to each e-pharmacy that meets the NABP standards. As of April 2013, 32 VIPPS-approved online pharmacies are in the United States.[27] Although prescription medications are available at all of the sites, some sites also sell nonprescription medications, nutritional dietary supplements, herbal products, and medical devices, in addition to providing "on-site" medical/pharmaceutical information.

Rx-to-OTC Switch

An *Rx-to-OTC* switch is defined as over-the-counter (OTC) marketing of a drug product that was once a prescription (Rx) drug for the same indication with the same strength, dose, duration of use, dosage form, and route of administration.[28] Pharmaceutical companies can benefit financially by requesting that FDA switch from prescription to nonprescription status a medication that is about to potentially lose market share because of patent expiration and subsequent generic drug competition. The much-longer period of sales generated as a nonprescription medication can offset the decreased revenue associated with the agent being a prescription medication in competition with generic entities. However, FDA has the final word in reclassifying a drug from prescription to nonprescription status. FDA considers a medication for Rx-to-OTC switch if the following types of questions can be answered affirmatively:

- Can the patient adequately self-diagnose the clinical abnormality?
- Can the clinically abnormal condition be successfully self-treated?

Is the self-treatment product safe and effective for consumer use under conditions of actual use?

Since 1976, more than 106 ingredients, indications, or dosage strengths have been switched from prescription to nonprescription status, resulting in more than 700 nonprescription products on the market.[29] These products include single-ingredient and combination agents. Table 1–2 shows examples of pharmaceuticals switched from prescription to nonprescription status between 2007 and 2013.[30] Consumers benefit from Rx-to-OTC switches because they broaden access to important medications. In addition, the nonprescription versions are usually cost-effective for consumers and third-party insurers. Examples of the cost benefits of Rx-to-OTC switches include the following:

In one scenario, a female patient saves money by using a nonprescription vaginal antifungal product for a yeast infection. A nonprescription drug can be obtained for less than $20; however, a physician's visit and prescription-only vaginal antifungal drug can cost almost $100. Savings can be even greater when indirect costs (e.g., travel and lost time from work) are considered.

A survey found that consumers save up to $750 million a year as a result of using nonprescription cough/cold medications that once were available only by prescription. The same study demonstrated that physician visits for the common cold dropped by 110,000 a year between 1976 and 1989.[29]

The pharmacist is ideally situated to advise patients on appropriate choices of switched medications. In 1996, an entirely new nonprescription drug category called "smoking cessation aids" was created when Nicorette chewing gum, NicoDerm CQ transdermal patch, and Nicotrol transdermal patch were switched from prescription to nonprescription status. A 10-year review of the effect of nonprescription nicotine replacement therapy (NRT) concluded that "Studies over the decade of OTC nicotine replacement therapy (NRT) availability demonstrate that OTC availability increased access and utilization of treatment, while also demonstrating that the projected adverse effects of OTC switch have not materialized: OTC NRT is being used safely and effectively, without substantial misuse or abuse."[31] NRT is an example of a nonprescription product category that is perfectly positioned for pharmacist interaction with potential purchasers.

Behind-the-Counter Medications

FDA continues to explore whether to expand the use of a third drug class, which would not require a prescription but would be kept behind the pharmacy counter and require a pharmacist to dispense it. Behind-the-counter (BTC) medications are also sometimes referred to as "pharmacist only" or "Schedule 3" medications. This class of medications could provide patients greater access to medications that require safeguards for their use. Pharmacists could ensure appropriate drug selection while screening for potential overlap and drug–disease or drug–drug interactions. Other countries such as Canada and the United Kingdom already have a BTC category of drugs (the statins, specifically simvastatin, used to lower cholesterol).

Recently, FDA has begun to explore expanding the definition of a new group of drugs that may otherwise require a prescription but might be available as nonprescription items. New criteria for use would include special conditions such as talking with a pharmacist, undergoing additional diagnostic testing, and, possibly, requiring the original prescription but not requiring the physician's agreement regarding renewals.

One current example of a BTC medication in the United States is pseudoephedrine (PSE). Nonprescription PSE has some therapeutic value, but it also has the potential for abuse. Because it is used to manufacture methamphetamine illicitly, PSE has become a major public health concern. PSE-containing products were moved behind the counter on the recommendation of the Drug Enforcement Administration to combat shoplifting and the sale of bulk quantities, which are needed to manufacture methamphetamine. Federal and state regulations require record keeping by the pharmacist. Purchasers must provide the pharmacy staff with photographic identification and a signature (in a logbook or via electronic documentation) when purchasing PSE-containing products. Quantities of PSE-containing

table 1–2	Examples of Prescription-to-Nonprescription Switches, 2007–2013		
Year of Approval	**Ingredient**	**Brand Name**	**Use**
2007	Cetirizine	Zyrtec	Allergy symptoms
2007	Cetirizine, pseudoephedrine	Zyrtec-D	Allergy symptoms
2007	Orlistat	Alli	Weight-loss aid
2009	Lansoprazole	Prevacid 24 HR	Acid reducer, heartburn
2009	Levonorgestrel	Plan B One-Step	Contraception
2009	Omeprazole, sodium bicarbonate	Zegerid OTC	Acid reducer, heartburn
2010	Ibuprofen, phenylephrine	Advil Congestion Relief	Pain relief, nasal congestion
2011	Fexofenadine	Allegra	Allergy symptoms
2011	Fexofenadine, pseudoephedrine	Allegra D 12-Hour, Allegra D 24-Hour	Allergy symptoms
2013	Oxybutynin	Oxytrol for women	Overactive bladder

Source: Reference 30.

products available for single purchase are limited as are quantities available for purchase over a certain period of time.

Another example of making a nonprescription medication BTC is Plan B One-Step, an emergency contraceptive. In this instance, FDA wanted to ensure that Plan B One-Step was available without a prescription to all ages of females, so the agency classified it as BTC.

Despite the potential advantages, several strong lobbying groups oppose the expansion of BTC medications. Manufacturers of nonprescription medications oppose the creation of BTC medications because the restriction would reduce the number of retail outlets for their products and thereby reduce sales. Some grocery stores and other mass retailers without pharmacies that have traditionally sold nonprescription medications would be unable to sell BTC medications. A 2009 Government Accounting Office report, "Nonprescription Drug Considerations Regarding a Behind-the-Counter Drug Class," states that three factors need to be considered: (1) the ability of the pharmacist to provide the necessary counseling, (2) an appropriate infrastructure in place in pharmacies to protect consumer privacy, and (3) cost issues.[32] The BTC discussion will continue and changes may or may not occur.

Self-Medication and the Safe Use of Nonprescription Drug Products

Informed, appropriate, and responsible use of nonprescription medications is crucial for effective self-medication. Casual or inappropriate use of nonprescription medications can lead to serious adverse effects (e.g., liver toxicity with prolonged intake of high doses of acetaminophen), drug–drug interactions (e.g., warfarin and naproxen), and indirect effects (e.g., from delay in seeking appropriate medical attention).

In 2007, FDA issued an initial warning for consumers to avoid treating children younger than 2 years with nonprescription cough and cold products because of an increased risk of overdose that requires emergency medical treatment. FDA cited studies estimating that during a 2-year period, 1519 children younger than 2 years were admitted to emergency departments for evaluation after known or possible exposure to cough/cold products. A large percentage of these incidents were related to dosing and use of the drug that differed from labeling instructions. In response to the warning, the manufacturers changed labels to state not to use the products in children under the age of 4 years and to ask a physician for dosing in children ages 4–6 years. Pharmacists can take a prominent role in ensuring the safe use of cough/cold medications in children by counseling parents to (1) carefully determine their child's dose according to weight, not age; (2) avoid mistakenly duplicating ingredients if giving multi-ingredient products (e.g., adding a dose of Tylenol after administering a cough/cold medication that contains acetaminophen); and (3) use the provided dosing device correctly to measure the amount needed.

A major challenge exists because of the numerous combination products that are available. Consumers may not be aware that they are using a single-entity product (i.e., acetaminophen) and also a combination product containing the same ingredient. The use of multiple combination products may contribute to duplicate therapies. The reality of drug–food interactions or drug–drug interactions (between different nonprescription products or between a nonprescription product and a prescription product) can lead to serious problems.

Pharmacists can combat misuse of nonprescription medications through the following measures:

- Be actively involved in helping patients with their self-care opportunities (see Chapter 2 for a discussion of patient assessment processes).
- Ensure that patients are able to read and understand product labeling, and provide supplemental educational materials where appropriate.
- Help patients avoid drug interactions.
- Warn patients about potential allergic reactions and side effects.
- Discuss appropriate drug storage and handling.

Nonprescription Drug Labeling

The Omnibus Budget Reconciliation Act of 1990 mandates that pharmacists "offer to counsel" on the prescription medications they dispense. However, nonprescription medications are exempt from this provision, so it is typically the consumer's responsibility to seek information from the pharmacist when he or she has a question. In the absence of this consultation, the consumer is on his or her own to understand what is written on the product label and to ensure proper use.

To assist consumers in understanding product labels, FDA mandated the use of a standard label format for nonprescription medications. The standard product label for nonprescription medications, titled "Drug Facts," has specific sections detailing active ingredients, uses, warnings, when to use the product, directions, and inactive ingredients (see Chapter 4). The label is designed to be easy to read, with all relevant information about taking the drug appearing in the same sequence on all package labels. This consistency enables patients to find information in a familiar spot on the label regardless of the use for the product (e.g., pain, cough/cold, or diarrhea). Initiated in 2002, the Drug Facts label has been on all nonprescription medications since May 15, 2005. Other products such as herbs and dietary supplements do not use the Drug Facts label format.

NCPIE commissioned a survey to determine whether the Drug Facts label has helped to promote the message that nonprescription medications must be taken with care.[33] Results of this survey of a little more than 1000 adult Americans included the following:

- As for reading the label: 44% looked for the active ingredient; 20% read about possible side effects; and 8% read nothing on the label.
- As for following the dosing recommendations: 48% of respondents confided that, if they needed to increase product effectiveness, they would take more than the recommended dose by either taking the next dose sooner than directed (35%), taking more than the recommended amount at a single time (32%), or taking the medication more times during the day than recommended (18%).
- Providers cited nonprescription medications being used incorrectly in the following ways: combining of nonprescription and prescription medications (51%), chronic use of a nonprescription medication (44%), use of a nonprescription drug for a prescription indication (32%), and use of more than one nonprescription product with the same active ingredient (27%).

The likelihood of inappropriate nonprescription drug use resulting from misreading of product labels increases when patients have limited reading skills or language barriers. The National Assessment of Adult Literacy found that a majority (53%) of adults were at an intermediate level of health literacy, 12% were proficient, and the remaining 35% were either at a basic or below basic level.[34] In another survey, 40%–70% of parents made errors when giving nonprescription medications to their children.[35] Effects of health illiteracy are particularly profound for adults ages 65 or older. Such a low level of literacy could be expected to adversely affect health care in patients using nonprescription medications. Other factors that can impair the ability to read nonprescription drug labeling include the size of type and critical information being covered by price or antitheft tags.[36,37] The U.S. Department of Health and Human Services is now undertaking a national action plan to improve literacy. This plan is designed to restructure the methods of creating and disseminating health information.[34] Despite literacy concerns, studies have concluded that nonprescription medications are being used safely. For example, appropriate use of nonprescription medications to treat upper gastrointestinal symptoms has been documented.[38]

Nonprescription Drug Product Reformulation

FDA sometimes initiates reformulation of nonprescription drug products because of safety or efficacy concerns. At times, this reformulation is also known as brand name extension. For example, Kaopectate is a brand-name antidiarrheal product that has been on the market for many years and has strong name recognition. The name *Kaopectate* was originally derived from its active ingredients, kaolin and pectin. However, in 1992 it was reformulated with attapulgite because FDA banned the use of pectin in nonprescription products because of insufficient data regarding its safety and efficacy. The product was reformulated again in 2003 to contain bismuth subsalicylate because all attapulgite-containing medications were discontinued. Despite all these reformulations, the product maintained its original brand name, Kaopectate.

Confusion and misuse can occur when a nonprescription drug product is reformulated to contain different active ingredient(s) but does not change its brand name. Although reformulated products may be labeled as being "new and improved," the packaging may not indicate that the active ingredient is entirely different. Again using Kaopectate as an example, before its reformulation in 2003, the product could be used in children and had pediatric dosing instructions on the label. However, in 2004, FDA ruled that antidiarrheals containing bismuth subsalicylate could be labeled for use by only adults and children ages 12 years and older. Therefore, the most recent version of the Kaopectate label does not include pediatric dosing information. As a result of all these formulation changes, there was a time in 2004 when patients had the option of purchasing up to three different types of Kaopectate: one containing attapulgite, one with bismuth subsalicylate and pediatric dosing information, and one with bismuth subsalicylate and no pediatric dosing information. In addition, patients with aspirin or salicylate allergies who may have previously taken the old formulation of Kaopectate could not take the new version because it contained bismuth subsalicylate. The Kaopectate example shows that a potentially serious adverse reaction can occur in patients who do not carefully recheck the label of a "new and improved" product that they have used safely in the past.

Another example of a brand-name extension is the Pepto-Bismol products. Pepto-Bismol is a very recognizable name, yet it is used for myriad products that contain different active ingredients such as bismuth subsalicylate (adult liquid and chewable tablets) and calcium carbonate (kid's chewable tablets). Each of these products is an example of a product line extension in which the manufacturer uses a well-known brand name for many nonprescription medications that have different ingredients and indications. This example is additional evidence and support for encouraging patients to read labels carefully and often.

It is also important to note that drug manufacturers can reformulate products for their own reasons. Changes to PSE-containing products are an example of a drug manufacturer–driven product reformulation. When the government restricted the sale of PSE-containing products to BTC status, many large pharmaceutical companies rushed to reformulate their brand-name products to contain a different decongestant, phenylephrine, which is not restricted. In most cases, the brand names of these products did not change. This therapeutic switch was not related to safety or efficacy concerns; rather, manufacturers feared that BTC restrictions would decrease sales. In fact, before the reformulation, phenylephrine was not widely used because of its limited effectiveness. Health care providers need to remain current with product reformulations and help patients understand how these changes affect self-care.

Drug Interactions

The risk for drug interactions increases as patients use more nonprescription medications. Diet and lifestyle can also have considerable effects on a medication's ability to work in the body. Certain foods, beverages (e.g., grapefruit juice), alcohol, caffeine, herbal supplements, and even cigarette smoking can interact with medications. These interactions may increase or decrease the effectiveness of certain medications, or they may cause dangerous side effects or other therapeutic problems. For example, one study concluded that older adults were unaware of the adverse risks associated with concurrent use of nonprescription pain medications, alcohol, high blood pressure medications, and regular caffeine use; the study also concluded that health care providers need to increase their educational efforts.[39] The increasing use of herbal supplements creates the potential for interactions between nonprescription and prescription medications. A survey conducted in a rural community found that 91% of the individuals using one or more herbs/natural products were also using at least one prescription or nonprescription medication and that 21% of those individuals were using a combination of products with a possibility of an interaction.[40] The public is being made aware of potential problems through articles in magazines, newspapers, and online information. However, to avoid drug interactions, patients should consult pharmacists before selecting herbal products, nutritional dietary supplements, or nonprescription medications. Table 1–3 lists some commonly used nonprescription medications and their interactions with food, alcohol, certain medical conditions, and other nonprescription medications.

Allergies to Active or Inactive Ingredients

Although the likelihood is low, any medication can cause an allergic reaction. For example, allergic reactions have occurred in patients taking common nonprescription pain relievers, such

table

1–3   Potential Interactions with Selected Nonprescription Drugs

Drug–Drug Interactions

OTC Drug	Drug	Potential Adverse Effect
Aluminum-containing antacids	Ascorbic acid	Increases aluminum absorption and excretion, primarily in patients with renal dysfunction
Aluminum-containing antacids	Bisacodyl	Decreases effect of bisacodyl
Aspirin	Products containing aluminum, calcium, or magnesium	Decreases blood aspirin concentration by increasing aspirin elimination
Iron (ferrous sulfate)	Products containing aluminum, calcium, or magnesium	Decreases iron absorption
Mineral oil	Docusate	Increases mineral oil absorption
Psyllium	Digoxin	Decreases digoxin absorption
Psyllium	Lithium	Decreases lithium absorption

Drug–Food/Beverage Interaction

OTC Drug	Food/Beverage	Potential Adverse Effect
Aspirin	Garlic	Increases risk of bleeding

Drug–Disease Interactions

OTC Drug	Condition	Mechanism
Aspirin	Hyperuricemia/gout	Decreases renal excretion of uric acid (with smaller aspirin doses)
Aspirin, naproxen, ibuprofen	Gastrointestinal disease	Alters gastric mucosal barrier
Doxylamine succinate, phenylephrine HCl	Glaucoma, increased intraocular pressure	Obstructs aqueous outflow
Pheniramine maleate/naphazoline HCl, pseudoephedrine, nicotine	Hypertension	Increases vascular resistance

Drug–Alcohol Interactions

OTC Drug	Potential Adverse Effect	Mechanism
Aspirin	Increased gastrointestinal blood loss	Increases gastrointestinal mucosal damage
Diphenhydramine HCl	Increased sedation	Depresses central nervous system
Insulin	Increased hypoglycemia	Decreases hepatic gluconeogenesis
Ketoconazole (topical)	Vomiting, tachycardia	Causes disulfiram-like reaction
Yohimbine	Increased blood pressure	Increases norepinephrine level

Key: HCl = Hydrochloric acid; OTC = over-the-counter.
Source: Lexi-Drugs Online™ [subscription database]. Hudson, OH: Lexi-Comp, Inc.; 2013. Accessed at http://online.lexicomp, August 1, 2013; Facts and Comparisons E Answers [subscription database]. St. Louis, MO: Wolters Kluwer Health, Inc.; 2013. Accessed at http://www.factsandcomparisons.com, August 1, 2013; and Caspi D, Lubart E, Graff E, et al. The effect of mini-dose aspirin on renal function and uric acid handling in elderly patients. *Arthritis Rheum.* 2000;43(1):103–8.

as aspirin, ibuprofen, and naproxen. Patients should always be counseled about the signs and symptoms of an allergic reaction (e.g., itching, hives, and trouble breathing) and instructed to seek medical care immediately. Both active and inactive ingredients can cause allergic reactions and side effects. Inactive ingredients in nonprescription medications (e.g., binders, disintegrants, fillers, and preservatives) can cause reactions in a few individuals. Therefore, for safety reasons, FDA requires that inactive ingredients also be listed on the label. Table 1–4 lists some of the

common inactive ingredients used in drug formulations and their known adverse effects.

Handling and Storage of Nonprescription Medications

Appropriate product handling, from the time it leaves the manufacturing facility to when it gets into a patient's home, is critical to ensure consistent potency. Patients reasonably assume that

table

1—4 Adverse Effects of Some Inactive Ingredients Used in Drug Preparations

Inactive Ingredient	Use	Where Found	Adverse Reactions
Aspartame	Sweetener	Liquid sucrose-free preparations	Headaches, caution in patients with PKU
Benzalkonium chloride	Preservative	Antiasthmatic drugs, nasal decongestants	Airway constriction, contact dermatitis, contact lens discoloration, allergic reactions
Benzyl alcohol	Preservative	Liquid preparations	Neonatal deaths, severe respiratory and metabolic complications, erythema, pruritus, eye irritation
Lactose	Filler	Capsules and tablets	Diarrhea, dehydration, cramping
Propylene glycol	Solubilizer	Liquid preparations	Respiratory problems, irregular heartbeat, low blood pressure, seizures, skin rashes, metabolic acidosis, hyperglycemia
Saccharin	Sweetener	Liquid preparations	Possible cross-sensitivity with sulfonamides, dermatologic reactions, pruritus, nausea, vomiting, diarrhea, alterations in taste, gastrointestinal irritation
Sulfites	Antioxidant	Antiasthmatic drugs; anti-inflammatory drugs	Wheezing, breathing difficulties, nausea, vomiting, diarrhea, abdominal pain, hypotension, seizures, tachycardia, dermatologic reactions
Yellow tartrazine	Coloring agent	Solid/liquid preparations	Allergic reaction similar to that of aspirin; minimal dermatologic and gastrointestinal effects

Key: PKU = Phenylketonuria.
Source: Micromedex 2.0. Englewood, CO: Thomson Reuters; 2010.

because nonprescription drug products are under the aegis of FDA, they are pure and have their stated potency. Although this is almost always the case, recalls of nonprescription medications because of impurity, contamination, or other issues can occur. Patients should be aware of some clues that should arouse suspicion about a nonprescription product, including abnormal odors, color changes, texture differences, and abnormal shape of a solid dosage form. Patients should avoid taking any drug product they suspect is bad and call their pharmacist for guidance. Pharmacists should also remove any recalled drug product from their shelves and post notices that inform patients of the recall and tell them what action they should take.

Before any product is used, especially one that was purchased quite some time ago, patients should check the expiration date that appears on the product label. Health care providers should be aware of conflicting information about the real meaning of a drug product expiration date. Pharmacists should help patients understand that after the expiration date, the product is no longer under the manufacturer's warranty and may no longer work.

Drugs must be stored properly to maintain their potency. Prescription and nonprescription medications are often mistakenly stored in bathroom cabinets, usually above the sink. Humidity and heat from the shower and sink are easily trapped in the cabinet, accelerating the degradation of the medications, even if they are in a prescription vial or bottle. Patients need to be aware that all medications should be stored away from high humidity in a cool, dark place. Furthermore, all medications should be stored in places to ensure they are kept out of a child's reach. This precaution is especially important for the many nonprescription medications that are not packaged in child-resistant containers. Examples of this type of packaging include blister packs, lozenges, topical creams or ointments, spray canisters, and bulk powder containers (e.g., laxatives).

Table 1–5 lists some nonprescription medications and health care products that are generally kept on hand to treat minor ailments or injuries; storage recommendations are also listed. Patients should be encouraged to check product expiration dates and purge medication cabinets at least once every 6 months.

table

1—5 Recommended Storage Places of Selected Nonprescription Health Care Products

Closet/Kitchen Cabinet or Shelf	Bathroom Medicine Cabinet
Analgesics (relieve pain)	Adhesive bandages
Antacids (relieve upset stomach)	Adhesive tape
Antibiotic ointments (reduce risk of infection)	Alcohol wipes
Antihistamines (relieve allergy symptoms)	Calibrated measuring spoon
Antipyretics (reduce fever; adult and child formulations)	Dental floss
Antiseptics (help prevent infection)	Disinfectant
Decongestants (relieve stuffy nose and cold)	Gauze pads
Hydrocortisone (relieves itching and inflammation)	Thermometer

Source: Adapted from Lewis C. Your medicine cabinet needs an annual checkup, too. *FDA Consum.* 2000;34(2):25–8.

Pharmacists' Role in Nonprescription Drug Therapy

The public's ability to discern critical information about the condition being treated and the clinical risk–benefit of a nonprescription drug is highly variable. Many individuals are confused by the array of product choices; line extensions; and overstated, vague, or misleading marketing messages. Generally, package labeling is limited in the breadth and depth of the message it communicates; it can never address the informational needs of all patients. Therefore, the pharmacist–patient interaction is vital for ensuring the best possible outcome from nonprescription drug therapy. In 2007, *U.S. Pharmacist* published survey results concerning chain and independent pharmacists and their roles in counseling on nonprescription medications.[41] More than 90% of the pharmacists stated that they had an active role in counseling patients on nonprescription medications, with more than 40% recommending 6–10 products per day. Table 1–6 shows how pharmacists ranked the importance of various counseling topics. Pharmacists clearly feel they should help each patient select the most appropriate drug for his or her condition and counsel on how to avoid drug interactions.

A study in two community pharmacies found that consumers widely accepted a pharmacist intervention in their nonprescription therapy.[42] Of the consumers who completed a follow-up phone call from a pharmacist and claimed adherence to the previous advice, 83% experienced "great relief" and 75% stated the follow-up was very helpful. However, only 45% would be willing to pay for a pharmacist's advice.

The underlying goal of pharmacists' counseling is to ensure that the patient receives accurate, practical information written at the consumer level and that the patient understands it in the context of the ailment being treated. Validation of the patient's understanding is also critically important. The pharmacist should always encourage the patient to ask questions and learn more. During the initial encounter with a patient who is seeking assistance with nonprescription medications, the pharmacist should do the following:

- Assess, by interview and observation, the patient's physical complaint/symptoms and medical condition (Chapter 2).

table

1–6   Pharmacist Ranking of Nonprescription Drug Counseling Topics

Survey Question: "Which of the following counseling topics are most important when discussing OTC-related products with patients?"	Average Rank (1 = highest importance; 5 = lowest importance)
Selection of right product	1.5
Rx-to-OTC drug interactions	2.5
Side effects/adverse reactions	3.0
Directions/instructions	3.0
Cost	4.4

Key: OTC = Over-the-counter; Rx = prescription.
Source: Reference 41.

- Differentiate self-treatable conditions from those requiring referral to a primary care provider or emergency department.
- Advise and counsel the patient on the proper course of action (i.e., no drug treatment, self-treatment with nonprescription medications, or referral to another health care provider or emergency department).
- Advise the patient on the outcome of the selected course of action.
- Assure the patient that the desired therapeutic outcome can be achieved if the selected/recommended nonprescription medications are taken as directed on the label and/or as directed by the primary care provider or pharmacist.
- Reinforce the concept that the pharmacist and primary care provider are qualified to perform a follow-up assessment of the treatment.
- If self-care with a nonprescription medication is in the best interest of the patient, pharmacists can help in the following ways:
  - Assess patient risk factors (e.g., contraindications, warnings, precautions, comorbidities, age, and organ function).
  - Assist in product selection.
  - Counsel the patient about proper drug use (e.g., dosage, administration technique, monitoring parameters, and duration of self-therapy).
  - Maintain an accurate patient drug profile that includes prescription, nonprescription, nutritional and dietary supplement, and herbal products.
  - Assess the potential of nonprescription medications to mask symptoms of a more serious condition.
  - Educate the patient on when to seek medical attention if the recommended nonprescription medication is ineffective or if symptoms worsen.

Key Points for Self-Care and Nonprescription Pharmacotherapy

➤ Self-care will play an increasingly important role in health care, and self-medication represents a significant element in the self-care process.

➤ Nonprescription medications are used by millions of Americans each year because they offer safe and effective relief for a variety of common health care ailments.

➤ Health care providers and FDA agree that nonprescription medications, although safe and effective, have some risks that are associated with patients not reading and closely following the label instructions when taking the medications.

➤ Patients, manufacturers, governmental agencies, and particularly pharmacists should become even more intent on recognizing that each group fulfills essential functions in ensuring the safe, appropriate, effective, and economical use of nonprescription medications.

REFERENCES

1. U.S. Census Bureau and U.S. Department of Commerce, Economics and Statistics Administration. Population distribution and change: 2000 to 2010. March 2011. Accessed at http://www.census.gov/prod/cen2010/briefs/c2010br-01.pdf, April 22, 2013.

2. National Council on Patient Information and Education. Uses and attitudes about taking over-the-counter medicines: findings of a 2003 national opinion survey conducted for the National Council on Patient Information and Education. Accessed at http://www.bemedwise.org/survey/summary_survey_findings.pdf, April 1, 2013.

3. National Council on Patient Information and Education. Attitudes and beliefs about the use of over-the-counter medicines: a dose of reality. January 2002. Accessed at http://www.bemedwise.org/survey/final_survey.pdf, April 1, 2013.

4. Consumer Healthcare Products Association. Your health at hand: perceptions of over-the-counter medicine in the U.S. November 24, 2010. Accessed at http://www.yourhealthathand.org/images/CHPA_YNH_Survey_062011.pdf, April 16, 2013.

5. Consumer Healthcare Products Association. The value of OTC medicine to the United States. January 2012. Accessed at http://www.yourhealthathand.org/images/uploads/The_Value_of_OTC_Medicine_to_the_United_States_BoozCo.pdf, March 30, 2013.

6. U.S. Food and Drug Administration. Regulation of nonprescription products. Accessed at http://www.fda.gov/AboutFDA/CentersOffices/OfficeofMedicalProductsandTobacco/CDER/ucm093452.htm, February 4, 2014.

7. Consumer Healthcare Products Association and American Pharmacists Association. Your health at hand book: guide to OTC active ingredients in the United States. *Pharm Today.* 2010;15(10 suppl):1–18.

8. Consumer HealthCare Products Association. OTC retail sales: 1964–2012. Accessed at http://www.chpa.org/OTCRetailSales.aspx, March 30, 2013.

9. Consumer HealthCare Products Association. OTC sales by category: 2009–2011. Accessed at http://www.chpa.org/OTCsCategory.aspx, March 30, 2013.

10. Consumer Healthcare Products Association. *Self-Care in the New Millennium: American Attitudes toward Maintaining Personal Health and Treatment.* Harrison, NY: Roper Starch Worldwide; 2001. Accessed at http://www.chpa.org/WorkArea/DownloadAsset.aspx?id=1483, February 4, 2014.

11. Centers for Disease Control and Prevention. Dietary supplement use among U.S. adults has increased since NHANES III (1988–1994). Accessed at http://www.cdc.gov/nchs/data/databriefs/db61.htm, February 4, 2014.

12. Stasio MJ, Curry K, Sutton-Skinner KM, et al. Over-the-counter medication and herbal or dietary supplement use in college: dose frequency and relationship to self-reported distress. *J Am Coll Health.* 2008;56(5):535–47.

13. National Center for Complementary and Alternative Medicine. The use of complementary and alternative medicine in the United States. Accessed at http://nccam.nih.gov/news/camstats/2007/camsurvey_fs1.htm, April 23, 2013.

14. National Center for Complementary and Alternative Medicine. The use of complementary and alternative medicine in the United States: cost data. Accessed at http://nccam.nih.gov/news/camstats/costs/costdatafs.htm, February 4, 2014.

15. Blumenthal M, Lindstrom A, et al. Herbal supplement sales increase 4.5% in 2011. *HerbalGram* 2012;95:60–4.

16. Bruno JJ, Ellis JJ. Herbal use among US elderly: 2002 national health interview survey. *Ann Pharmacother.* 2005;39(4):643–8.

17. U.S. Census Bureau and U.S. Department of Commerce, Economics and Statistics Administration. The older population: 2010. November 2011. Accessed at http://www.census.gov/prod/cen2010/briefs/c2010br-09.pdf, March 31, 2013

18. U.S. Department of Health and Human Services, Administration on Aging. A profile of older Americans: 2010. Accessed at http://www.aoa.gov/aoaroot/aging_statistics/profile/2010/docs/2010profile.pdf, February 4, 2014.

19. Qato DM, Alexander GC, Conti RM, et al. Use of prescription and over-the-counter medications and dietary supplements among older adults in the United States. *JAMA.* 2008;300(4):2867–78.

20. Simoni-Wastila L, Stuart BC, Shaffer T. Over-the-counter drug use by Medicare beneficiaries in nursing homes: implications for practice and policy. *J Am Geriatr Soc.* 2006;54(10):1543–9.

21. Lam A, Bradley G. Use of self-prescribed nonprescription medications and dietary supplements among assisted living facility residents. *J Am Pharm Assoc.* 2006;46(5):574–81.

22. Nice FJ, Synder JL, Kotansky BC. Review: breastfeeding and over-the-counter medications. *J Hum Lact.* 2000;16(4):319–31.

23. Consumer Healthcare Products Association's Clinical/Medical Committee. White paper on the benefits of OTC medicines in the United States. *Pharm Today.* 2010;16(10):68–79.

24. Fox S. The social life of health information, 2011. May 12, 2011. Pew Internet and American Life Project Web site. Accessed at http://www.pewinternet.org/Reports/2011/Social-Life-of-Health-Info.aspx, February 4, 2014.

25. Wallace LS, Rogers ED, Turner LW, et al. Suitability of written supplemental materials available on the Internet for nonprescription medications. *Am J Health Syst Pharm.* 2006;63(1):71–8.

26. National Association of Boards of Pharmacy. VIPPS criteria. Accessed at http://www.napb.net/programs/accreditation/vipps/vipps-criteria, April 1, 2013.

27. National Association of Board of Pharmacy. Find a VIPPS online pharmacy. Accessed at http://www.nabp.net/programs/accreditation/vipps/find-a-vipps-online-pharmacy, April 1, 2013.

28. Mahecha LA. Rx-to-OTC switches: trends and factors underlying success. *Nature Rev Drug Discov.* 2006;5(5):380–5.

29. Consumer Healthcare Products Association. Briefing information on the Rx-to-OTC switch process. October 22, 2012. Accessed at http://www.chpa.org/SwitchProcess.aspx, February 4, 2014.

30. Consumer Healthcare Products Association. Ingredients and dosages transferred from Rx-to-OTC status (or new OTC approvals) by the Food and Drug Administration since 1975. October 16, 2013. Accessed at http://www.chpa.org/SwitchList.aspx, February 4, 2014.

31. Shiffman S, Sweeney CT. Ten years after the Rx-to-OTC switch of nicotine replacement therapy: what have we learned about the benefits and risks of non-prescription availability? *Health Policy* 2008;86(1):17–26.

32. U.S. Government Accountability Office. Nonprescription drugs: considerations regarding a behind-the-counter drug class. GAO-09-245. Accessed at http://www.gao.gov/assets/290/286263.html, February 4, 2014.

33. National Council on Patient Information and Education. The new drug facts label. Accessed at http://www.bemedwise.org/label/drug_label_print.pdf, April 1, 2013.

34. U.S. Department of Education National Center for Education Statistics. The health literacy of America's adults: results from the 2003 National Assessment of Adult Literacy. September 2006. Accessed at http://nces.ed.gov/pubs2006/2006483.pdf, April 1, 2013.

35. Yin HS, Parker RM, Wolf MS, et al. Health literacy assessment of labeling of pediatric nonprescription medications: examination of characteristics that may impair parent understanding. *Acad Pediatr.* 2012;12(4):288–96.

36. Sansgiry SS, Pawaskar MD. Obstruction of critical information on over-the-counter medication packages by external tags. *Ann Pharmacother.* 2005;39(2):249–54.

37. Wogalter MS, Vigilante WJ. Effects of label format on knowledge acquisition and perceived readability by younger and older adults. *Ergonomics* 2004;46(4):327–44.

38. Mehuys E, Van Bortel L, De Bolle, L, et al. Self-medication of upper gastrointestinal symptoms: a community pharmacy study. *Ann Pharmacother* 2009;43(5):890–8.

39. Amoaka EP, Richardson-Campbell L, Kennedy-Malone L. Self-medication with over-the-counter drugs among elderly adults. *J Gerontol Nurs.* 2003;29(8):10–5.

40. Blalock SJ, Gregory PJ, Patel RA, et al. Factors associated with potential medication-herb/natural product interactions in a rural community. *Altern Ther Health Med.* 2009;15(5):26–34.

41. Pharmacists take center stage in OTC counseling. *US Pharm.* 2007;32(7):4–6.

42. Bosse N, Machado M, Mistry A. Efficacy of an over-the-counter intervention follow-up program in community pharmacies. *J Am Pharm Assoc.* 2012;52(4):535–40.

chapter 2

PATIENT ASSESSMENT AND CONSULTATION

Gail D. Newton and Holly Divine

Self-care, self-diagnosis, and self-medication are important components of the health care system in the United States. Instead of seeking the advice of a health care provider, many people self-diagnose and treat their symptoms using a vast array of self-care options, ranging from nonprescription medications, herbal products, and home remedies to yoga, meditation, and spiritual healing. Survey data show that about 80% of Americans who have conditions that can be treated with nonprescription medications would purchase a specific nonprescription drug if advised by their pharmacist.[1] Nonprescription medications allow individuals to manage their medical problems rapidly, economically, and conveniently. In addition, they may prevent unnecessary visits to a primary care provider or specialist. Patients often believe medications that move from prescription to nonprescription status are more effective than older nonprescription medications, and one study showed that 9 of 10 Americans believe that nonprescription medications are a key part of their family health care.[2] The demand for and shift toward self-medication are further described and documented in Chapter 1.

The appropriate use of a nonprescription product, as with any medication, requires attention to the intended use, effectiveness, safety, and convenience of administration. Although warnings are required on the labels of these products, labeling alone may be insufficient. The patient may need assistance in selecting and properly using a nonprescription medication. Inappropriate use and misuse of nonprescription medications can increase the risk of drug misadventures,[3] resulting in increased health care costs and more serious illness. Further, because 23% of all drug therapy problems in the general population involve one or more nonprescription drug products,[4] health care providers must assume a crucial role in helping patients to use self-treatment options safely and effectively.

Self-Care Problem Solving Processes

Interacting with a patient regarding self-treatment is a primary care activity that carries a great professional responsibility. Patients with self-care needs present differently from those who have already received a treatment decision from a health care provider.

To determine which recommendation is most appropriate for a patient, the health care provider must complete the following problem-solving steps (Figure 2-1 provides more detail):

- Collect and assess patient-specific information relative to each health problem.
- Create and implement a care plan to resolve each health problem.
- Evaluate the results of the care plan and make adjustments when the outcome is less than optimal.[4]

Health care providers must use systematic, comprehensive, and efficient cognitive processes to ensure that their patients realize optimal therapeutic outcomes. A variety of approaches to ensure optimal results is documented in the literature, and selected examples are outlined in Table 2-1. Although the approaches differ in terms of level of specificity and terminology, they are all designed to address the previous problem-solving steps. In addition, a technique described as LEARN can be used in conjunction with any self-care problem-solving model to ensure that patient-specific cultural characteristics are taken into account during therapeutic decision making. Details are described in Chapter 3.

This chapter describes two self-care problem-solving approaches. The comprehensive method is useful for students who are novice problem solvers, whereas the abbreviated approach is more suited to health care providers who are experienced problem solvers. The primary difference between these approaches relates to their levels of structure and specificity.

Educational research asserts that novice problem solvers, such as students, require explicit instruction with ample opportunities for practice and feedback. As students become more proficient problem solvers, they require less structure and can eventually adapt to problem-solving methods that are little more than brief prompts to the initiation of complex problem-solving steps.[5] In contrast, experienced problem solvers have created cognitive structures that enable them to complete the steps in solving problems with few prompts and in a much more timely fashion. They view explicit approaches as cumbersome and unworkable for use in their busy practices.[5]

Comprehensive Problem-Solving Model

The comprehensive problem-solving model is based on the guided-design instructional format that models the steps of decision making. The detailed processes facilitate student development of a framework for organizing and applying acquired

---

Editor's Note: This chapter is based on the 17th edition chapter of the same title, written by Lawrence M. Brown and Brian J. Isetts.

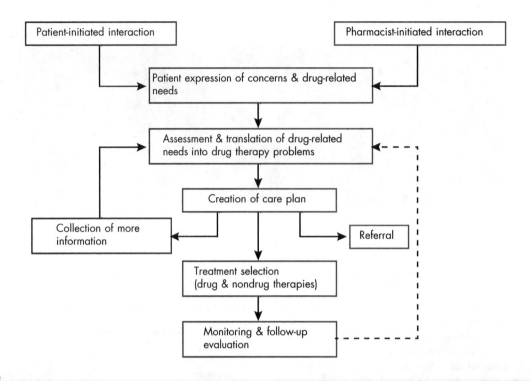

figure
2–1   Patient–pharmacist consultation process.

table
2–1   **Selected Self-Care Problem-Solving Formats**

QuEST/SCHOLAR-MAC
QuEST: **Qu**ickly assess, **E**stablish self-care appropriateness (using SCHOLAR-MAC), **S**uggest care, **T**alk to patient
SCHOLAR: **S**ymptoms, **C**haracteristics, **H**istory, **O**nset, **L**ocation, **A**ggravating factors, Remitting factors
MAC: **M**edications, **A**llergies, **C**onditions

WWHAM method
Who, **W**hat, **H**ow long, **A**ctions taken, **M**edications taken

AS METTHOD
Age, **S**elf or someone else, **M**edicines taken, **E**xact symptoms, **T**ime of symptoms, **T**aken anything, **H**istory of disease, **O**ther symptoms, **D**oing anything to alleviate or worsen the situation

PQRST
Palliation, **Q**uality, **R**egion, **S**igns and symptoms, **T**emporal relationship

CHAPS-FRAPS
Chief complaint, **H**istory of illness, **A**llergies, **P**ast medical history, **S**ocial history – **F**amily history, **R**eview of symptoms, **A**ssessments, **P**lan and **S**OAP note summary

Source: Buring SM, Kirby J, *Educ.* 2007;71(1):8. Accessed at http://www.ncbi.nlm.nih.gov/pmc/articles/PMC1847542/, May 17, 2013; Conrad WF. A structured approach for teaching students to counsel self-care patients. *Am J Pharm Educ.* 2007; 71(1):8. Accessed at http://www.ncbi.nlm.nih.gov/pmc/articles/PMC1847542/, May 17, 2013.

information to the solving of novel problems.[6] The basic steps used in the comprehensive problem-solving model are as follows:

1. Gather information.
2. Perform assessment and triage.
3. Prepare and implement a plan.
4. Educate the patient.
5. Evaluate patient outcomes.

Step 1: Gather Information

When a patient presents to a health care provider and is in need of self-care advice, the provider must collect information about the patient that is pertinent to solving the patient's problem. This information falls into two general categories: (1) information about the symptoms that prompted the patient to seek assistance and (2) information about the patient's background characteristics.

It may be argued that it is unnecessary to collect all the patient's background characteristics to solve every patient problem. However, it should be remembered that novice problem solvers do not yet have the expertise to selectively elicit the information most pertinent to a specific situation. Therefore, this model provides prompts to ask about all of the listed characteristics to avoid overlooking information that is critical to the solution of the problem.

Step 2: Assessment and Triage

The second step involves the assessment of information gathered in step 1 to identify the patient's problem, its severity, and its most probable cause. Clear articulation of the problem is critical (1) to assist with differentiation among conditions with similar symptoms and (2) to determine the goals of self-treatment. Comparing the patient's symptoms to those of a particular condition will help to differentiate and determine the most likely primary problem. For example, it is inadequate to conclude simply that a patient's problem is a common cold. In this instance, the therapeutic goal—to relieve the cold—is too vague to be useful because there are many symptoms that may or may not be associated with a common cold. Further, this goal offers little in the way of guidance relative to the type of nonprescription product that may be indicated. On the other hand, if the patient's problem is nasal congestion secondary to a common cold, the goal would be to relieve the congestion. This goal is much more focused and allows evaluation of a more limited set of potential therapeutic options.

Step 1 also involves assessment of patient data to identify exclusions for self-treatment. It may not be appropriate for an individual to self-treat for several reasons, including:

1. The symptoms require medical referral (e.g., eye pain).
2. The patient is not an appropriate candidate for self-care (e.g., a woman with diabetes who develops a vaginal candidal infection).
3. The symptoms are too severe or long lasting for self-treatment.
4. Effective nonprescription therapy is not available.
5. Nonprescription dosages or duration of treatment is inadequate to treat the condition.

Finally, the first step involves formulating a list of all possible solutions to the patient's problem. At this point, nothing should be ruled in or out. Four general options are available to health care providers who are advising patients about self-care: (1) recommend self-care with drug, nondrug, and/or alternative/complementary therapies; (2) refer the patient to another health care provider for treatment; (3) recommend self-care until another health care provider can be consulted; or (4) take no action. In the context of self-treatment, all potential product categories, dosage forms, and nondrug products and measures should be included in the list. Similarly, all potential sources of primary care (e.g., urgent care clinic, physician, physician assistant, nurse practitioner, dentist, or emergency department) should be considered.

Critics of this approach have sometimes indicated that including no action as an option is unconscionable or not in the best interest of patients. In fact, taking no action may be preferred in some situations. For example, consider a situation involving a patient with a limited income who suffers from an asymptomatic, common wart that is in a location where it is neither noticeable nor likely to be spread easily to others. Because most common warts resolve spontaneously without treatment and the patient has limited income to pay for a nonprescription product, taking no action may indeed be the best solution in this instance. Furthermore, it is important to remember that, at this point in the decision-making process, all ideas are listed and none are prejudged. This approach is taken because the comprehensive problem-solving model is targeted at novice problem solvers who have little experience in identifying alternative therapeutic options. Therefore, the model prompts those with less experience in patient assessment to formulate a list of all alternatives to prevent them from prematurely ruling out appropriate options.

Step 3: Prepare and Implement a Plan

In step 3, each of the plausible solutions is evaluated to determine whether and to what extent each achieves the intended goal(s) and also is concordant with the patient's preferences in terms of therapeutic goals, cost, and overall approach, including personal philosophy and health beliefs for self-care. Next, the optimal therapeutic alternative is identified on the basis of patient-specific and therapy-specific variables. Patient-specific variables include age, gender, medication history, medical conditions, allergies, social habits (alcohol, tobacco use), patient preferences, family/home dynamics, and economic status. Therapy-specific variables include dosage forms, ingredients, side effects, adverse effects, potential interactions, relative effectiveness, flavor, and price. Step 3 also involves communication of the therapeutic plan to the patient. The plan should include an explanation of the condition, the treatment recommendation(s), and the rationale for the treatment recommendation(s).

Step 4: Educate the Patient

Patient education is designed to provide a clear and concise description of the treatment and its administration, any side effects and precautions, expected outcome and time to achieve it, and guidelines for appropriate use, as well as the appropriate health care provider to contact if a problem occurs or if the expected outcome is not achieved. Where applicable, the plan should also include nondrug measures, lifestyle changes, and additional information resources. Including family members in this process may be appropriate to ensure the best chance for a positive outcome.

The health care provider should ensure that the patient understands the plan by having the patient repeat it and by correcting any misunderstandings. Finally, after answering any remaining questions, the provider should document the interaction in the patient's profile and encourage the patient to call or return if the symptoms fail to resolve.

Step 5: Evaluate Patient Outcomes

In some instances, patients do not realize the full intended benefit from their health care provider's recommendations. If further treatment is needed, the patient and health care provider can come together to begin the problem-solving cycle anew. For example, a patient who does not achieve the desired outcome with the proper use of a particular nonprescription product may realize the goal with another product or referral. It may be prudent to obtain the patient's telephone number so the health care provider can contact the patient to evaluate outcomes. Cases 2-1 and 2-2 illustrate the application of this model to self-care problem solving.

Abbreviated Problem-Solving Model

The abbreviated problem-solving model is better known as the QuEST/SCHOLAR method. It was first presented by Leibowitz and Ginsburg at the inaugural 2002 Self-Care Institute of the American Pharmacists Association. This method employs simple acronyms to prompt health care providers to complete key steps in the self-care problem-solving process. Although no published studies have compared QuEST/SCHOLAR with other problem-solving models, the easy-to-remember acronyms may expedite completion of the problem-solving process relative to more structured models that contain no such prompts.

case
2–1

Relevant Evaluation Criteria	Scenario/Model Outcome

Information Gathering

1. Gather essential information about the patient's symptoms and medical history, including:

   a. description of symptom(s) (i.e., nature, onset, duration, severity, associated symptoms)

   Patient complains of difficulty sleeping. He describes difficulty falling asleep about 2–3 nights a week and has early awakening with inability to fall back to sleep 5–7 days a week. "I just don't sleep very well anymore, and I wonder if there's something I can take that will help." Symptoms started approximately 1 month ago.

   b. description of any factors that seem to precipitate, exacerbate, and/or relieve the patient's symptom(s)

   He sometimes, but not always, has "better sleep" if he sleeps upright in a recliner chair instead of the bed.

   c. description of the patient's efforts to relieve the symptoms

   He tried melatonin 3 mg each evening last week for 3–4 nights with no relief.

   d. patient's identity

   James Markum

   e. age, sex, height, and weight

   81 years old, male, 5 ft 9 in. tall, 170 lb

   f. patient's occupation

   Retired railroad worker

   g. patient's dietary habits

   Normal balanced diet; three cups of caffeinated coffee daily; no alcohol

   h. patient's sleep habits

   Averages 5–6 hours per night. Naps one to two times per day in morning and/or afternoon.

   i. concurrent medical conditions, prescription and nonprescription medications, and dietary supplements

   Gastroesophageal reflux disease: omeprazole 20 mg daily; hypertension: hydrochlorothiazide 25 mg daily, lisinopril 20 mg daily; depression: sertraline 100 mg daily; Alzheimer's dementia: donepezil 5 mg daily

   j. allergies

   NKA

   k. history of other adverse reactions to medications

   None

   l. other (describe) _____

   None

Assessment and Triage

2. Differentiate patient's signs/symptoms and correctly identify the patient's primary problem(s).

   Insomnia, possibly secondary to current medical conditions

3. Identify exclusions for self-treatment.

   ≥65 years old, chronic insomnia (>3 weeks), sleep disturbances possibly secondary to medical disorders

4. Formulate a comprehensive list of therapeutic alternatives for the primary problem to determine if triage to a health care provider is required, and share this information with the patient or caregiver.

   Options include:

   (1) Refer patient to his primary care provider.

   (2) Recommend self-care with lifestyle modifications for good sleep hygiene and diphenhydramine.

   (3) Recommend self-care until patient can see his primary care provider.

   (4) Take no action.

Plan

5. Select an optimal therapeutic alternative to address the patient's problem, taking into account patient preferences.

   Patient should consult his primary care provider.

6. Describe the recommended therapeutic approach to the patient or caregiver.

   "I recommend you see your primary care provider for treatment of your sleep problems."

7. Explain to the patient or caregiver the rationale for selecting the recommended therapeutic approach from the considered therapeutic alternatives.

   "This is the best option for you since you have had the sleep problems for several weeks and your situation may be related to your current medical conditions. Also, the over-the-counter medications we typically use to treat sleep problems are not the best option for you. You may require prescription medications or adjustments of your current medications by your primary care provider."

case
2–1   *continued*

Relevant Evaluation Criteria	Scenario/Model Outcome
Patient Education	
8. When recommending self-care with nonprescription medications and/or nondrug therapy, convey accurate information to the patient or caregiver.	Criterion does not apply in this case.
Solicit follow-up questions from the patient or caregiver.	"Are there any drugs I can take to help until I get an appointment with my physician?"
Answer the patient's or caregiver's questions.	"No. You tried the melatonin and it didn't work. There are no other over-the-counter medications that are safe and effective for your sleep problems. I recommend seeing your physician as soon as possible. If you are unable to see your physician immediately, you can try to improve sleep by avoiding or reducing caffeine, avoiding daytime naps, and participating in something relaxing prior to bedtime, such as reading."
Evaluation of Patient Outcome	
9. Assess patient outcome.	Contact the patient in 1–2 days to ensure that he sought medical care for insomnia.

Key: NKA = No known allergies.

case
2–2

Relevant Evaluation Criteria	Scenario/Model Outcome
Information Gathering	
1. Gather essential information about the patient's symptoms and medical history, including:	
a. description of symptom(s) (i.e., nature, onset, duration, severity, associated symptoms)	Patient complains of a burning sensation in her stomach and throat that is often accompanied by feeling of fullness and "acid in my throat." The burning occurs after a heavy meal no more than once weekly. Symptoms last 2–4 hours after a meal and began about 1 month ago.
b. description of any factors that seem to precipitate, exacerbate, and/or relieve the patient's symptom(s)	Symptoms occur after eating lunch out with coworkers or after potlucks at work and last 2–4 hours after the meal.
c. description of the patient's efforts to relieve the symptoms	Peppermint candy did not help symptoms. She tried Tums (calcium carbonate 500 mg) once without full symptomatic relief.
d. patient's identity	Jill Golden
e. age, sex, height, and weight	43 years old, female, 5 ft 4 in., 175 lb
f. patient's occupation	Office assistant
g. patient's dietary habits	Normal balanced diet; 4 or 5 cups of caffeinated coffee daily; 3 or 4 alcoholic beverages once per week
h. patient's sleep habits	Averages 7–9 hours per night
i. concurrent medical conditions, prescription and nonprescription medications, and dietary supplements	No concurrent medical conditions; multivitamin daily
j. allergies	NKA
k. history of other adverse reactions to medications	None
l. other (describe) _____	Weight gain of 10 pounds in the past 3 months
Assessment and Triage	
2. Differentiate patient's signs/symptoms and correctly identify the patient's primary problem(s).	Infrequent postprandial burning sensation is consistent with uncomplicated heartburn. Patient denies pregnancy.

case

2–2   *continued*

Relevant Evaluation Criteria	Scenario/Model Outcome
3. Identify exclusions for self-treatment.	None
4. Formulate a comprehensive list of therapeutic alternatives for the primary problem to determine if triage to a health care provider is required, and share this information with the patient or caregiver.	Options include: (1) Refer patient to her primary care provider. (2) Recommend self-care with lifestyle modifications and nonprescription acid-reducing medication. (3) Recommend self-care until patient can see her primary care provider. (4) Take no action.

Plan

5. Select an optimal therapeutic alternative to address the patient's problem, taking into account patient preferences.	A nonprescription acid-reducing medication along with lifestyle modifications should be effective.
6. Describe the recommended therapeutic approach to the patient or caregiver.	"There are a number of things you can do on your own to decrease your symptoms. In addition, I recommend that you use the acid-reducer famotidine 20 mg for additional relief."
7. Explain to the patient or caregiver the rationale for selecting the recommended therapeutic approach from the considered therapeutic alternatives.	"Referral to a primary care provider may not be necessary if adequate relief is achieved from the recommended medication. Because the heartburn is predictable with large meals, primarily after lunch, using the famotidine on an as-needed basis should be sufficient."

Patient Education

8. When recommending self-care with nonprescription medications and/or nondrug therapy, convey accurate information to the patient or caregiver.	
a. appropriate dose and frequency of administration	"Swallow one tablet at any time from 10–60 minutes before eating food or drinking beverages that cause heartburn."
b. maximum number of days the therapy should be employed	"You can use this for up to 14 days in a row, if needed. If you think you need it for a longer period of time, call your primary care provider for further evaluation. From what you said, I can't imagine you'll need this more than once a week, if that."
c. product administration procedures	"Be sure to take this with a full glass of water."
d. expected time to onset of relief	"You should feel better a few hours after you take this. Often the relief happens sooner."
e. degree of relief that can be reasonably expected	"You should expect at least some relief; often patients get complete relief with a dose."
f. most common side effects	"Some of the more common side effects are headache, diarrhea, dizziness and constipation, but these don't happen too often and are rarely serious."
g. side effects that warrant medical intervention should they occur	"If you experience any unusual bleeding or bruising, be sure to call your primary care provider and stop using this medicine."
h. patient options in the event that condition worsens or persists	"If this situation worsens please consult a primary care provider."
i. product storage requirements	"Store this medicine in a cool dry place out of the reach of children."
j. specific nondrug measures	"Other things that can help you include eating smaller, more frequent meals and avoiding or reducing consumption of foods and drinks that trigger symptoms."
Solicit follow-up questions from the patient or caregiver.	"May I take the medication after I start the meal if I have forgotten to take it prior?"
Answer the patient's or caregiver's questions.	"Yes, but the medication may not be as effective in prevention of heartburn symptoms because of the delayed onset of action."

Evaluation of Patient Outcome

9. Assess patient outcome.	To evaluate efficacy of the treatment, advise the patient to call the pharmacy after using the as-needed medication for heartburn prevention.

Key: NKA = No known allergies.

Each letter in the acronym QuEST represents an ordered step in the problem-solving process as follows[7]:

- *Qu*ickly and accurately assess the patient.
- *E*stablish that a patient is an appropriate self-care candidate (using the SCHOLAR–MAC questioning process described here).
- *S*uggest appropriate self-care strategies.
- *T*alk with the patient.

Similarly, each letter in SCHOLAR represents information that the health care provider should elicit from each patient or caregiver, and includes:

- *S*ymptoms: What are the patient's symptoms?
- *C*haracteristics: What are the symptoms like?
- *H*istory: What has been done so far?

- *O*nset: When did the symptoms begin?
- *L*ocation: Where are the symptoms occurring?
- *A*ggravating factors: What makes the symptoms worse?
- *R*emitting factors: What makes the symptoms better?

Because nothing in the SCHOLAR line of questioning is specific to an individual's medical history, the MAC acronym was added to QuEST/SCHOLAR and is intended to prompt users to collect the following additional key patient information:

- *M*edications: prescription and nonprescription as well as alternative and complimentary therapies
- *A*llergies: to medications and other substances
- *C*onditions: coexisting health conditions

Cases 2–3 and 2–4 illustrate the application of this model to self-care problem solving.

case

2-3

A mother of a 3-month-old boy calls the pharmacy requesting advice for her son who has had several watery stools since yesterday.

Information to Obtain from the Patient	What the Parent Told You
Quickly and accurately assess the patient: Ask about the current problem (SCHOLAR).	
Symptoms What are the main and associated symptoms?	"My son has had watery diarrhea since yesterday."
Characteristics What is the situation like? Is it changing?	"The stool is very thin and has no consistency at all. He's breast-fed, and he has stopped eating the last few hours. He seems more tired and has not had a wet diaper for several hours."
History What has been done so far?	"I haven't given him anything to stop the diarrhea."
Onset When did it start?	"About 24 hours ago."
Location Where is the problem?	"Just diarrhea. No vomiting."
Aggravating factors What makes it worse?	"Nothing."
Remitting factors What makes it better?	"Nothing."
Ask about other **Medications, Allergies, and Conditions (MAC):** Within reason, get as much detail as possible to assist in the decision-making process.	- "My son takes D-Vi-Sol Vitamin D drops daily." - "He's not allergic to anything that I know of." - "He is otherwise very healthy. This is the first time he has been sick."

The "E.S.T." pieces of QuEST: Establish, Select, and Talk	Your assessment, recommendation, and counseling
Establish that the patient is an appropriate self-care candidate: - Any severe symptoms? - Any symptoms that persist or return repeatedly? - Is the patient self-treating to avoid medical care?	The child's symptoms are severe given that he is under 6 months old with diarrhea and signs of moderate-severe dehydration. He is not a candidate for self-care.
Suggest appropriate self-care strategies.	"Ma'am, there are no appropriate self-care strategies for your son because he is so young. I strongly suggest you call your son's pediatrician as soon as possible to decide what to do. Your son may need rehydration that could be done only in an emergency department.
Talk with the patient about: - Medication action, administration, and adverse effects - What to expect from the treatment - Appropriate follow-up	Key Counseling Points: "Because your child is so young and has diarrhea, you should seek medical attention immediately to ensure that he gets adequately hydrated to prevent complications."

case
2–4

A 35-year-old female is a regular patient of yours. She was walking into your pharmacy from her car to pick up a prescription and was stung by a bee. She wants to know what she should do to stop the burning.

Information to Obtain from the Patient	What the Patient Told You
Quickly and accurately assess the patient: Ask about the current problem (SCHOLAR).	
Symptoms What are the main and associated symptoms?	"Pain from a bee sting on my right hand."
Characteristics What is the situation like? Is it changing?	"Burning, itching, and redness."
History What has been done so far?	"Nothing."
Onset When did it start?	"Five minutes ago as I was walking from my car to the pharmacy."
Location Where is the problem?	"Palm of my right hand."
Aggravating factors What makes it worse?	"When I touch the bee sting area."
Remitting factors What makes it better?	"Nothing has been tried yet."
Ask about other Medications, Allergies, and Conditions (MAC): Within reason, get as much detail as possible to assist in the decision-making process.	▪ "I take levothyroxine 50 mcg every day." ▪ "I'm not allergic to any medications." ▪ "This is the first time I've ever had a bee sting."

The "E.S.T." pieces of QuEST: Establish, Select, and Talk	Your assessment, recommendation, and counseling
Establish that the patient is an appropriate self-care candidate: ▪ Any severe symptoms? ▪ Any symptoms that persist or return repeatedly? ▪ Is the patient self-treating to avoid medical care?	▪ Symptoms are mild and localized to the right hand. Because she is experiencing her first bee sting, the risk of hypersensitivity is low. ▪ She is not exhibiting any signs of an anaphylactic reaction, such as hives, swelling, dizziness, weakness, or difficulty breathing.
Suggest appropriate self-care strategies.	▪ Nondrug: Remove the stinger by scraping with a credit card immediately; then apply an ice pack or cold compress. ▪ Medication: Apply local anesthetic such as benzocaine 20% aerosol spray to affected area 3–4 times daily for up to 7 days to reduce itching and burning.
Talk with the patient about: ▪ Medication action, administration, and adverse effects ▪ What to expect from the treatment ▪ Appropriate follow-up	Key Counseling Points: ▪ "I think you can do a few things to help this situation. Benzocaine is a topical anesthetic that will help relieve itching and irritation associated with the bee sting. Spray the affected area 3–4 times daily for up to 7 days. If the site becomes more irritated or redness increases, stop using the spray." ▪ "The benzocaine should provide immediate relief. The symptoms should resolve over time and should not last longer than 1 week." ▪ "If you experience any hives, excessive swelling, dizziness, vomiting, or difficulty breathing, seek medical attention immediately. If the condition worsens or is not resolved by 1 week, seek medical attention." ▪ "Keep the area clean by washing regularly with soap and water; do this before each application of benzocaine."

High-Risk and Special Patient Groups

Providing appropriate self-care recommendations is especially important for vulnerable populations. Certain groups of patients—infants and children, older persons (≥65 years of age), and pregnant and breast-feeding women—may experience a higher incidence of drug therapy problems. Because these problems can have dire consequences, high–risk patients require special attention. Awareness of the physiologic state, possible pathologic conditions, and social context of high–risk patients is necessary to properly assess their medical conditions and recommend appropriate treatment.

In many respects, infants, children, and persons of advanced age require surprisingly similar considerations. They all have a need for drug dosages that differ from those for other age groups because of the following features:

- They have altered pharmacokinetic parameters.
- Their ability to cope with illness or adverse drug events is decreased because of physiologic changes associated with either child development or normal aging.
- Their patterns of judgment are impaired because of either immaturity or altered sensory function.
- They experience drug effects and potential adverse reactions that are unique to their age groups.
- They have a need for special consideration with medication administration.

Yet, because each of these patient groups is heterogeneous, it is important to consider these features individually for each patient.

Special Considerations in Infants and Children

A study of the prevalence of nonprescription medication use in 3-year-old children found that 53.7% had been given a nonprescription medication within the preceding 3 months. The most commonly used medications were acetaminophen and cough or cold products. Analysis of vitamin supplement use found that 54.4% of 3-year-olds in the United States were given vitamin and mineral supplements within the preceding 3 months.[8] Providing self-care recommendations for pediatric patients is challenging because of differences in physiology and pharmacokinetics, lack of clinical data, insufficient drug labeling, and problems associated with drug dosing and administration.[9]

For most products, the Food and Drug Administration (FDA) recommends against self-medication in children younger than 2 years and against the use of cough and cold products in children younger than 4 years.[10] Some package labeling provides dosage guidelines by weight rather than by age group. Pharmacists can provide recommendations regarding medications that are FDA approved for children (e.g., acetaminophen products), but they should recommend referral to a primary care provider for medical conditions or medications that extend beyond the FDA-approved labeling for nonprescription products.

Physiologic and Pharmacokinetic Differences

Pediatric patients are at risk for drug therapy problems because their body and organ functions are in a continuous state of development. Not only do the pharmacokinetic properties of medications differ between children and adults, these properties also can undergo rapid change as children grow and mature.[11] Furthermore, illness in children is potentially more serious than in adults, given that the physiologic state of children is less tolerant of changes. For example, fever, vomiting, and diarrhea represent greater potential risks because children are more susceptible to the effects of fluid loss. Therefore, the pharmacist should consider referral to another health care provider sooner for children with certain conditions than for an adult with the same condition.

Potential Drug Therapy Problems

The health care provider should be sensitive to the potential for drug therapy problems among children. In some illnesses such as diarrhea (see Chapter 16), nondrug therapy is often more appropriate than therapy with nonprescription antidiarrheals.

In some situations, specific medications are contraindicated; for example, aspirin should not be administered to young children with certain viral illnesses (especially influenza and varicella) because of its association with Reye's syndrome (see Chapter 5). For younger children, solid dosage forms are inappropriate and the health care provider will need to guide parents to liquid or chewable formulations.

Inaccurate Dosing

Labeling for nonprescription medications generally uses age-based guidelines to determine dosages; however, many products do not provide dosage information for children younger than 6 years. Applying label instructions designed for dosing children older than 6 years to a younger child can result in excessive dosing and potential toxicity for the younger child. Inaccurate dosing by parents can result from determining an incorrect dose from the label instructions, by measuring an incorrect amount, or both. A study of 200 children, 10 years of age and younger, who had been given a dose of acetaminophen or ibuprofen in the preceding 24 hours, found that 51% of them had been given an incorrect dose by their caregiver.[12] Pharmacists must help parents interpret labels and better educate them about accurate dosing.

Improper Administration/Dosage Forms

Selecting the proper medication and dosage is not beneficial unless the medication is actually administered correctly. Proper administration of medications to pediatric patients requires that health care providers and caregivers have an appreciation of available dosage forms, delivery methodologies, routes of administration, palatability, and how to use measuring devices.

A young child can swallow liquid formulations more easily than other dosage forms, and the dose can be titrated to the patient's weight/age; therefore, liquids are often used in pediatric populations. Because elixirs and syrups can have high alcohol and sugar content, respectively, these liquid formulations may be less desirable than suspensions and solutions. A suspension also may mask the disagreeable taste of a medication. Refrigeration also may improve the flavor of liquid formulations.

Problems with drug administration can result in the child receiving the wrong dose. In a mock dosing scenario in which caregivers had the choice of using teaspoons, tablespoons, syringes, droppers, measuring cups, and measuring tubes, only 67% of the caregivers accurately measured the dose they intended to administer.[12] The volume delivered by household teaspoons ranges from 2.5 to 7.8 mL and may also vary greatly when the same spoon is used by different individuals. The American Academy of Pediatrics Committee on Drugs highly recommends the use of appropriate devices for liquid administration, such as a medication cup, cylindrical dosing spoon, oral dropper, or oral syringe. Ease of administration and accuracy should be considered when choosing a dosing device. Plastic medication cups are fairly accurate for volumes of exact multiples of 5 mL (5 mL, 10 mL, 15 mL, etc.). An oral syringe is preferable to the other oral dosing devices for higher viscosity liquids because the syringe completely expels the total measured dose. Potent liquid medications should be administered with an oral syringe to ensure that the correct dose is given. The health care provider should demonstrate to caregivers how to read and use all these devices.

In response to the problem of inaccurate measurement of doses, FDA released in May 2011 guidelines for liquid nonprescription drug products that include any type of dispensing device, such as a dropper, cup, syringe, or spoon.[13,14] These products include liquid analgesics, liquid cough and cold products, and lactase replacement drops. The following recommendations are the key points of the guidance:

- A dosing device should be included with all oral liquid nonprescription products.
- The device should be calibrated to the dose recommended in the product directions.
- The device should be used only with the product in which it is packaged.
- The markings should remain visible even when the liquid is in the device.

In May 2011, the Consumer Healthcare Products Association also announced that its member companies would voluntarily convert nonprescription single-ingredient liquid pediatric acetaminophen medications to just one concentration (160 mg/5 mL) for use in all children younger than 12 years. Most concentrated infant drops (80 mg/0.8 mL; 80 mg/1 mL) were being phased out starting mid-2011. Infant products will include flow restrictors and will be packaged with oral syringes for more accurate dosing. Products for children ages 2 to younger than 12 years will still be packaged with dosing cups. Because both concentrations will be available during the transition period, parents and caregivers should carefully read and follow product labeling, and health care providers should pay special attention to this issue during the education step.[15]

A child older than 4 years can usually swallow tablets or capsules. Tablets that are neither sustained-release nor enteric-coated formulations may be crushed. Most capsules may be opened and the contents sprinkled on small amounts of food (e.g., applesauce, jelly, or pudding) to improve palatability. If the child does not eat the full portion, underdosing can occur. If multiple medications are necessary, the child may be more cooperative if allowed to choose what flavored drink to use and which medication to take first. Table 2–2 presents selected guidelines for administering oral medications to pediatric patients.

Adverse Drug Effects

Adverse reactions are another potential drug therapy problem in children. Adverse drug events in children may differ from those in adults. Antihistamines and central nervous system (CNS) depressants may cause excitation in children. In contrast, sympathomimetics such as pseudoephedrine may cause drowsiness in children. In the United States, drug-induced acute liver failure is most commonly caused by acetaminophen, and about 18% of these cases were a result of accidental overdose. In addition, administration of acetaminophen at doses above the recommended daily dose over a period of 2–4 days can result in hepatotoxicity in children.[16]

Nonadherence

Nonadherence may occur when children refuse to take medication, when caregivers give up before the child receives the entire dose, or when caregivers just forget to give a dose. Adherence

---

table
2–2   Selected Administration Guidelines for Oral Medications

Infants

- Use a calibrated dropper or oral syringe.
- If a medicine dropper is used, the medication should be squirted into the side of the cheek and not straight back into the throat so that the infant does not choke.
- Do not place the child's medication in the formula because the baby might not like the taste of the formula and might refuse to take this formula in the future.
- Support the infant's head while holding the infant in the lap.
- Give small amounts of medication at a time to prevent choking.
- If desired, crush non–enteric-coated or non–sustained-release tablets into a powder and sprinkle them on small amounts of food.
- Provide physical comfort while administering medications to help calm the infant.

Toddlers

- Allow the toddler to choose a position in which to take the medication.
- If necessary, disguise the taste of the medication with a small volume of flavored drink or small amounts of food. A rinse with a flavored drink or water will help remove an unpleasant aftertaste.
- If the medication is not palatable, ask the pharmacist whether the pharmacy offers a flavoring service and can add flavoring to the child's medication. Refrigeration also may help.
- Make sure that the medication is not referred to as candy.
- Use simple commands in the toddler's jargon to obtain cooperation.
- Allow the toddler to choose which medication (if multiple) to take first.
- Provide verbal and tactile responses to promote cooperative taking of medication.
- Allow the toddler to become familiar with the oral dosing device.

Preschool Children

- If possible, place a tablet or capsule near the back of the tongue; then provide water or a flavored liquid to aid the swallowing of the medication.
- If the child's teeth are loose, do not use chewable tablets.
- Use a follow-up rinse with a flavored drink to help minimize any unpleasant medication aftertaste.
- Allow the child to help make decisions about dosage formulation, place of administration, which medication to take first, and type of flavored drink to use.

may be improved by recommending a sweetly flavored product because children may be more willing to take a medication if they like the flavor, consistency, or texture.[17] However, it is important to stress to caregivers to keep all medications out of the reach of children, especially those that taste good and could be mistaken as "candy" by the child. Nonadherence also can occur when caregivers do not understand instructions or do not pass them on to day care providers, teachers, or school nurses. A 2003 study that surveyed 82 child day care centers found that 52% of centers reported forgetting to give a dose of medication to a child in their care during the preceding year, and 49% reported that the child's medication was not available.[18]

Assessment and Consultation

Assessment and consultation for pediatric patients usually involve the parents or caregivers but may involve the child directly. A 2003 article by Sleath and coworkers[19] lists six overall steps for communicating with children and improving their medication use process (Table 2–3). One should remember that it is important to include the child and parent or caregiver during the patient counseling process, and that the child's and parents' or caregivers' concerns or fears about the medication should be considered and addressed.

Special Considerations in Persons of Advanced Age

Social, economic, physiologic, and age-related health factors place persons of advanced age at high risk for medical problems and predispose them to consume large numbers of nonprescription medications. This population as a group consumes more medications than any other age segment of our society. Individuals ages 65 years or older take on average 1.8 nonprescription medications daily, and factors that affect this number include geographic area, race/ethnicity, and gender.[20] Nonprescription drug use in this population is highest in residents of the Midwestern United States, Caucasians, and women. Analgesics, laxatives, and nutritional supplements are the most common nonprescription medications used by persons of advanced age. A study in 86 women who were 65 years of age or older reported an average use of 3.8 nonprescription medications per person and, in the 45% of women who used herbal products, an average number of 2.5 herbal products.[21]

table 2-3 Six Steps for Improving Medication Use in Children

Pharmacists should use a patient-centered style that focuses on the following steps:

1. Educating both the child and parents about the medication.
2. Investigating any concerns or fears that the child or parents may have about the medication.
3. Asking the child and parents about priorities for improved quality of life.
4. Following up with the child and parents to learn whether they consider the child's treatment effective.
5. Offering to follow up with the pediatrician to improve the child's therapy (if needed).
6. Encouraging the child or parents to ask questions about the medication.

Source: Reference 19.

The response to drug therapy by older patients is more scattered and unpredictable than that of other populations. Pharmacokinetic, pharmacodynamic, and various nonpharmacologic factors predispose older patients to potential problems with nonprescription medications. Preexisting medical conditions in older persons may affect the use of some nonprescription medications. For example, antihistamines should be avoided in patients with emphysema, bronchitis, glaucoma, and urinary retention from prostatic hypertrophy. Although nasal and oral decongestants can be used without adverse effect in many older persons, caution may be necessary in some patients with heart disease, hypertension, thyroid disease, and diabetes because of potential adverse effects of sympathomimetics on heart rate, blood pressure, and blood glucose.

The American Geriatrics Association's 2012 Beers criteria is a valuable source of information about safe prescription and nonprescription medication use by older patients. The evidence-based criteria identify drugs that pose risks in the elderly population, and this update included more nonprescription medications than in previous versions.[22]

Physiologic and Pharmacokinetic Differences

Persons of advanced age often have impaired vision (e.g., difficulty reading small print and differentiating colors of similar contrast) and hearing loss. Health care providers should be aware of patient behaviors that indicate visual or hearing loss and should consider these impairments when communicating with older patients. Additional instructions for nonprescription medications may need to be provided in larger, high-contrast, dark print. Asking the patient to repeat counseling instructions can ensure that the directions were heard correctly and understood.

Subtle changes in mental status, such as confusion, may be anticipated in older patients, especially those who are anxious about their state of health. Older patients with cognitive impairments may have difficulty comprehending directions. Patients may not remember the names of all their medications or may not be able to remember instructions. Because of memory lapses, some older patients may require special drug delivery systems (e.g., transdermal patches or sustained-release preparations) to help them adhere to their dosage regimen. Older patients with cognitive impairments are less likely to read and interpret labels correctly,[23] which further emphasizes their need for special dosage form considerations.

Misbeliefs about the health problems can cause elderly patients to underreport their symptoms.[23] For example, they may attribute treatable symptoms to simply growing older. In addition, older patients are often reluctant to share health information with others. Accurate perception and reporting of symptoms are vital to the successful selection and use of any medication. Therefore, health care providers must take special care to establish rapport and carefully question older patients to recommend appropriate care.

The aging process and many chronic diseases can alter a patient's nutritional status. Older patients who are most at risk for undernourishment or malnutrition are homebound patients and nursing home residents. Limited income, poverty, multiple chronic diseases, mental status changes, multiple drug therapy, or a combination of these factors may cause malnutrition in older patients. The patient's nutritional status and weight are important because these factors can alter pharmacokinetics and pharmacodynamics. For example, a recent study demonstrated that malnourishment in elderly patients with diabetes is associated with a higher incidence of hypoglycemia independent of the use of insulin and sulphonylureas.[24]

Aging alters the absorption, distribution, metabolism, and elimination of certain medications, increasing the susceptibility of older patients to drug therapy problems. Pharmacokinetic changes, which are well described in the literature, are caused not only by advancing age but also by the effects of disease states and often by multiple drug use. For example, there has been concern that prolonged use of proton pump inhibitors will lead to vitamin B_{12} deficiency. This is because vitamin B_{12} requires stomach acid for absorption. There is no evidence that long-term omeprazole use by young, healthy adults leads to vitamin B_{12} deficiency. In contrast, older patients are at risk because stomach acid and vitamin B_{12} absorption normally decrease with age.[25]

Older persons appear to have a greater sensitivity to some medications, particularly anticholinergic medications, which may relate in part to alterations in cholinergic transmission. Nonprescription medications with anticholinergic effects (e.g., certain antihistamines) may worsen preexisting medical conditions and symptoms such as congestive heart failure, diabetes mellitus, glaucoma, constipation, angina, urinary dysfunction, sleep disturbance, and dementia.[26] The risk of accidents, such as falls, also may increase as a result of sedation or pupillary dilation induced by anticholinergic medications and the inability to accommodate the effect.

Both subjective and objective evidence indicates that older patients have an enhanced CNS sensitivity to medications, especially CNS depressants such as sedatives.[22] Increased brain sensitivity and other changes (e.g., decreased coordination, prolongation of reaction time, and impairment of short-term memory) manifest as increased frequency of confusion, urinary incontinence, and number of falls, especially among older women. Co-administered medications may exaggerate all these changes, particularly if they are taken in the usual adult dose or if multiple medications are used.

Control of bowel and bladder function lessens with advancing age. A further decrease in bowel efficiency is likely with laxative use. Anticholinergic and CNS medications may reduce neurologic control. Antihistamines have sedative properties that may reduce bladder control in older persons.[27] Adverse effects of nonprescription medications often increase when these medications are added to an existing medication regimen through interactions with other therapies and health conditions.

NSAIDs are widely used, especially by patients with chronic pain, osteoarthritis, and rheumatoid arthritis. The incidence of NSAID-related toxicity is greater for older patients because of their frequent use of NSAIDS and the increased prevalence of comorbid conditions and concomitant drug therapies. These patients may be especially susceptible to NSAID-associated peptic ulcer disease as well as congestive heart failure.

Other Potential Drug Therapy Problems

Duplicate Therapy

Older patients may receive unnecessary drug therapy when medications are added to their regimen without an assessment to determine whether an existing medication can be stopped. For example, patients may be taking a prescription proton pump inhibitor such as Nexium and be unaware that their newly purchased nonprescription stomach medicine, Prilosec OTC, is in the same drug class. Duplicate therapy also may occur if

patients are seeing multiple health care providers for various medical problems or using multiple pharmacies. Use of a single pharmacy can significantly lower the risk of inappropriate drug combinations. Nonprescription medications commonly involved in drug interactions in older persons include aspirin, other NSAIDs, antacids, cimetidine, and antihistamines.[28] Certain illnesses or medications may contraindicate the use of other medications. Many older patients have conditions such as coronary artery disease, renal dysfunction, and congestive heart failure, which can be aggravated by concurrent therapy for other acute problems. In addition it is important to consider whether an older patient is requesting a nonprescription medication to treat an adverse reaction from another medication. This assessment is best performed by a pharmacist.

Inaccurate Dosing/Dosage Forms

Normal doses of certain medications such as analgesics and sedating antihistamines may be too high for older patients because they have diminished hepatic and renal function. These situations may necessitate either lowering the dose or increasing the dosing interval. Furthermore, because of physical limitations, older patients may experience difficulty with some dosage forms (e.g., swallowing large calcium or vitamin tablets). Arthritis or tremors may make it difficult for older patients to open and close containers. Child-resistant containers may be especially difficult for older patients to open if they have deficits in manual dexterity. A pharmacist should direct older patients to products without child-resistant containers but also warn them of the potential poisoning hazard for unintended users, such as visiting grandchildren or other young individuals in the household.

Nonadherence

The prevalence of nonadherence with medications is high in the older population and is often the result of their inadequate understanding of their medication regimen. Poor adherence may result from difficulty swallowing or other administration procedures. It also may result from an inability to afford the medication because of a limited or fixed income. Older patients may lack an adequate social support network to provide assistance in managing a complex group of illnesses. Health care providers may need to involve caregivers in administering certain types of medications (e.g., suppositories and eye drops) to patients to help ensure adherence.

Special Considerations in Pregnant Patients

Drug therapy during pregnancy may be necessary to treat medical conditions or to manage common complaints of pregnancy, such as vomiting or constipation. Because most medications cross the placenta to some extent, a mother who ingests a medication is likely to expose her fetus. Therefore, the desire to ease the mother's discomfort must be balanced with concern for the developing fetus.

A 2001 study[29] found that 13% of pregnant women from an academic setting birthing center used dietary supplements. Of these women, 25% reported using supplements to relieve nausea and vomiting, and 25% reported stopping the use of these products because of concern for their fetus. The authors concluded that, although the use of dietary supplements was low among these women, the lack of safety data for the products is of concern. In another study,[30] women attending an antenatal clinic reported using an average of 2.3–2.6 nonprescription medications in the three pregnancy trimesters, which was slightly higher than nonprescription drug use in the 3 months before pregnancy. The most frequently consumed medications were analgesics, vitamin and mineral supplements, and gastrointestinal preparations. In addition, approximately 10% of pregnant women used herbal products.

Potential Drug Therapy Problems

Pregnant women should never presume that a nonprescription medication is safe to use during pregnancy. They should first consult with a health care provider to determine whether a medication is teratogenic (i.e., causes abnormal embryonic development). Nausea and vomiting during pregnancy can cause another medication-related problem: difficulty in taking oral dosage forms of medications. There are ways to address this problem as well, but it requires the involvement of a health care provider to work with the patient to explore options and solutions.

Teratogenic Effects

Several factors are important in determining whether a medication taken by a pregnant woman will adversely affect the fetus. Two such factors are the stage of pregnancy and the ability of the medication to pass from maternal to fetal circulation through the placenta. The first trimester, when organogenesis occurs, is the period of greatest risk for inducing major anatomic malformations. However, exposure at other periods of gestation may be no less important because the exact critical period depends on the specific medication in question. Patients should work closely with their health care provider to evaluate the risks and benefits of each situation.

Drug therapy problems are also important considerations for pregnant patients. Although dosage guidelines for some prescription medications (e.g., phenytoin) differ for pregnant patients, no information on dosage adjustments exists for nonprescription medications. Unnecessary drug therapy should be avoided. Nondrug therapy (e.g., use of a humidifier or vaporizer for relief of nasal congestion secondary to a common cold) is often more appropriate than drug therapy for pregnant women. Use of cigarettes and ingestion of alcohol should be avoided because they have been associated with increased risk to the fetus.[31] Consumption of moderate doses of caffeine appears to be safe.[32]

In pregnant patients, the primary concern is drug safety. All nonprescription medications have a Drug Facts label, which is arranged the same way on all nonprescription medications. One section of the Drug Facts label is for pregnant women. With nonprescription medications, the label usually tells a pregnant woman to speak with a health care provider before using the medicine. Some nonprescription medications are known to cause certain problems in pregnancy. The labels for these medications give pregnant women facts about why and when they should not use the medications. For example, aspirin can cause fetal and maternal hemorrhage if taken during the third trimester. Thus, the labeling on aspirin products warns against this practice.[33]

Nonadherence

Nausea and vomiting associated with pregnancy are probably the leading causes of nonadherence in pregnant women because they prevent consumption of most oral medications on a consistent basis. Health care providers can recommend eating small meals, frequent snacks, and crackers to alleviate or minimize

nausea and vomiting. The patient should avoid foods, smells, or situations that cause vomiting. If necessary, the use of an effervescent glucose or buffered carbohydrate solution or ginger may be effective.[34] If ginger ale is used, it should be verified that the product actually includes ginger. Only if these measures are ineffective should an antihistamine or antiemetic be considered. Consultation with a primary care provider may be indicated at this point. It is very important for providers to be cognizant of potential adherence issues during pregnancy and to take a proactive role in helping to prevent them.

Management of the Pregnant Patient

The health care provider can assist the self-treating pregnant woman in deciding which drug or nondrug treatments she should consider and when self-treatment may be harmful to her or her unborn child. When the health care provider has more than one medication option, the preferred medication will be the one that has the best efficacy and safety profiles. Ascertaining the trimester of pregnancy is important because it is a factor in determining whether some nonprescription medications can be used safely. Health care providers should discourage pregnant women from self-medicating with nonprescription medications without receiving counseling from a primary care provider or pharmacist. The assessment and management of the pregnant patient requires observation of the following principles:

1. The health care provider must be alert to the possibility of pregnancy in any woman of childbearing age who has certain key symptoms of early pregnancy, such as nausea, vomiting, and frequent urination. Any woman who fits this profile should be warned not to take a medication that might be of questionable safety until her pregnancy status is confirmed.
2. The health care provider should generally advise the pregnant patient to avoid using medications at any stage of pregnancy unless the patient's primary care provider deems the use essential. In addition, because the safety and effectiveness of homeopathic and herbal remedies in pregnancy have not been established, their use should be discouraged.
3. The health care provider should advise the pregnant patient to increase her reliance on nondrug modalities as treatment alternatives (see the section Nonadherence).
4. The health care provider should refer the patient to a primary care provider for certain problems that carry increased risk of poor outcomes in pregnancy (e.g., high blood pressure, vaginal bleeding, urinary tract infections, severe nausea and vomiting, rapid weight gain, and edema).

Special Considerations in the Nursing Mother

A mother's drug use while breast-feeding can have an adverse effect on the infant. The concentration of a medication in the mother's milk depends on a number of factors, including the medication's concentration in the mother's blood; the medication's molecular weight, lipid solubility, degree of ionization, and degree of binding to plasma and milk protein; and the extent of the medication's active secretion into the milk. Other important considerations include the relationship between the time of taking a medication and the time of breast-feeding, as well as the medication's potential for causing toxicity in infants. In addition, some medications such as decongestants may decrease milk supply.[32]

When advising a nursing mother on self-care, the health care provider should first decide whether a medication is really necessary. Then, if a medication is indicated, the safest one (e.g., acetaminophen instead of aspirin) is recommended, and the mother is advised to take the medication just after breast-feeding or just before the infant's lengthy sleep periods to minimize infant exposure during subsequent nursing periods.[35,36] It is preferable to select a medication that has been in use for a long time and that has shown no apparent harm to nursing infants. If appropriate, topical or local therapy may be preferred to oral, systemic therapy. In general, advise against medications that are extra strength, maximum strength, or long acting, or products that contain a variety of active ingredients.[36]

When taken in therapeutic doses, most medications are not present in breast milk in sufficient concentrations to cause significant harm to the infant.[32] However, several medications are contraindicated for use while breast-feeding, and others should be used with caution by nursing mothers. The amount of caffeine in caffeine-containing beverages is not harmful, but higher doses (i.e., >1 gram daily) have been reported to cause irritability and poor sleep patterns in infants.[34] Many nonprescription medications have no data on their transfer into breast milk and their possible clinical effects.

Nonprescription medications that are usually considered compatible with breast-feeding include the following[32,37]:

- *Analgesics:* acetaminophen, ibuprofen, and naproxen
- *Antacids*
- *Antidiarrheals:* loperamide
- *Antihistamines:* brompheniramine, chlorpheniramine, diphenhydramine, and triprolidine
- *Antisecretory agents:* famotidine and ranitidine
- *Cough preparations:* dextromethorphan
- *Cromolyn sodium*
- *Decongestants:* pseudoephedrine
- *Fluoride*
- *Laxatives:* bran type, bulk-forming type, docusate, glycerin suppositories, magnesium hydroxide, and senna
- *Vitamins*

CAM Use in Special Populations

Special consideration should be given to the risk–benefit assessment of complementary and alternative medicine (CAM) use in children, older persons, and pregnant and nursing women because the level of use is high in these populations. Herbal use in a study population of children ages 3 weeks to 18 years was 45% during the year before they were surveyed.[38] In the adult population, use of herbal products is estimated to be about 57%; only 33% of the patients told their health care provider about their use of herbal products.[39]

During a typical patient medication interview, the emphasis is usually on prescription and nonprescription medications. Although patients may not even consider herbal and home remedies to be therapeutic agents, their use also may cause drug therapy problems. Therefore, specific questions need to be asked to assess the current use of such remedies. Patients have a tendency to view herbal products as safe for use because they are natural products and not drugs. In the previously mentioned study of herbal use, "77% of patients or caregivers did not believe or were uncertain if herbal products had any side effects and only 27% could name a potential side effect. Sixty-six percent were unsure or thought that herbal products did not interact with other medications."[38]

It is imperative that a specific assessment of herbal use be completed. In this context, the health care provider should ask about herbal use but also include examples. One might say, "Okay, now I am going to ask you about any herbal or natural products you may be taking. This would be things like St. John's wort, echinacea, ginseng, ginkgo, cod liver oil, or even home remedies that you might use." Phrased this way, the question leaves little doubt as to the type of products to which the health care provider is referring. Furthermore, it takes patients off the defensive, while still expressing the health care provider's need to know about the use of such products.

Key Points for Patient Assessment and Consultation

The use of nonprescription medications represents an important component of the health care system. Under ideal conditions, consumers can diagnose their own symptoms, select a nonprescription product, and monitor their own therapeutic response. If properly used, nonprescription medications can relieve patients' minor physical complaints and permit primary care providers to concentrate on more serious illnesses. If used improperly, however, nonprescription products can create a multitude of drug therapy problems. The key points discussed in this chapter include the following:

➤ Twenty-three percent of all drug therapy problems experienced by patients are either caused or resolved by nonprescription medications.

➤ Health care providers should use systematic cognitive processes to effectively address patients' self-care needs.

➤ The consistent and systematic patient care process helps providers be complete and concise when assuming responsibility for a patient's self-care needs.

➤ There are special drug-related needs associated with high-risk groups, such as infants and children, older persons, and pregnant and breast-feeding women.

To be of greatest service to patients, health care providers must continually expand their therapeutic knowledge and work to improve their interpersonal communication skills. As providers strive to fulfill their responsibilities and continue to expand their patient care services, people will learn of the services and seek their assistance whenever they are in doubt about self-treatment. The result will be better informed patients who will use the expertise of their health care providers to experience better outcomes with their self-care interventions.

REFERENCES

1. National Council on Patient Information and Education (NCPIE). Uses and attitudes about taking over-the-counter medicines: 2003 national opinion survey conducted for the National Council on Patient Information and Education. Accessed at http://www.bemedwise.org/survey/summary_survey_findings.pdf, May 21, 2013.
2. Consumer Healthcare Products Association. Understanding trust in OTC medicines: Consumer and healthcare provider perspectives. Accessed at http://www.yourhealthathand.org/images/uploads/CHPA_OTC_Trust_Survey_White_Paper.pdf, June 3, 2014.
3. Manasse HR Jr., Speedie MK. Summary: pharmacists, pharmaceuticals, and policy issues shaping the work force in pharmacy. *Am J Health Syst Pharm.* 2007;64(12):1292–3.
4. Cipolle RJ, Strand LM, Morley PC. *Pharmaceutical Care Practice: The Patient-Centered Approach to Medication Management.* 3rd ed. New York, NY: McGraw-Hill Companies; 2012:1–33.

5. Halpern DF. *Thought and Knowledge: An Introduction to Critical Thinking.* Hillsdale, NJ: Lawrence Earlbaum Associates, Inc.; 1984:109–202.

6. McKeachie WJ, Hofer BK. *McKeachie's Teaching Tips: Strategies, Research, and Theory for College and University Teachers.* 11th ed. Boston, MA: Houghton Mifflin Company; 2002:196–203.

7. Leibowitz K, Ginsburg D. Counseling self-treating patients quickly and effectively. Proceedings of the APhA Inaugural Self-Care Institute, May 17–19, 2002, Chantilly, VA.

8. Kogan MD, Pappas G, Yu SM, et al. Over-the-counter medication use among U.S. preschool-age children. *JAMA.* 1994;272(13):1025–30.

9. Food and Drug Administration. Drug research in children. Accessed at http://www.fda.gov/drugs/resourcesforyou/consumers/ucm143565.htm, September 20, 2013.

10. Food and Drug Administration. Using over-the-counter cough and cold products in children. Accessed at http://www.fda.gov/ForConsumers/ConsumerUpdates/ucm048515.htm, May 17, 2013.

11. Skaer TL. Dosing considerations in the pediatric patient. *Clin Ther.* 1991; 13(5):526–44.

12. Weinkle DA. Over-the-counter medications. Do parents give what they intend to give? *Arch Pediatr Adolesc Med.* 1997;151(7):654–6.

13. Food and Drug Administration. FDA issues final guidance for liquid OTC drug products with dispensing devices [news release]. May 4, 2011. Accessed at http://www.fda.gov/NewsEvents/Newsroom/PressAnnouncements/ucm254029.htm, May 17, 2013.

14. Food and Drug Administration. *Guidance for Industry: Dosage Delivery Devices for Orally Ingested OTC Liquid Drug Products.* Rockville, MD: U.S. Department of Health and Human Services, Food and Drug Administration, Center for Drug Evaluation and Research; May 2011. Accessed at http://www.fda.gov/downloads/Drugs/GuidanceComplianceRegulatoryInformation/Guidances/UCM188992.pdf, May 17, 2013.

15. Consumer Healthcare Products Association. OTC industry announces voluntary transition to one concentration of single-ingredient pediatric liquid acetaminophen medicines. CHPA Executive Newsletter. 2011; Issue No. 05-11. Accessed at http://www.chpa.org/WorkArea/DownloadAsset.aspx?id=962, June 1, 2014.

16. Larsen OM, Ostapowicz G, Fontana RJ, et al. Outcome of acetaminophen-induced liver failure in the USA in suicidal vs accidental overdose: preliminary results of a prospective multicenter trial. *Hepatology.* 2000;32(suppl):396A.

17. Compounding for the pediatric patient. *Pharm Compound.* 1997;1:84–6.

18. Sinkovits HS, Kelly MW, Ernst ME. Medication administration in day care centers for children. *J Am Pharm Assoc.* 2003;43(3):379–82.

19. Sleath B, Bush PJ, Pradel FG. Communicating with children about medicines: a pharmacist's perspective. *Am J Health-Syst Pharm.* 2003;60(6):604–7.

20. Hanlon JT, Fillenbaum GG, Ruby CM, et al. Epidemiology of over-the-counter drug use in community dwelling elderly: United States perspective. *Drugs Aging.* 2001;18(2):123–31.

21. Yoon SJ, Horne CH. Herbal products and conventional medicine used by community-residing older women. *J Adv Nurs.* 2001;33(1):51–9.

22. The American Geriatrics Society. American geriatrics society updated Beers criteria for potentially inappropriate medication use in older adults. Accessed at http://www.americangeriatrics.org/files/documents/beers/2012BeersCriteria_JAGS.pdf, September 20, 2013.

23. Sirey JA, Greenfield A, Weinherger MI. Medication beliefs and self-reported adherence among community-dwelling older adults. *Clin Ther.* 2013;35(2):153–60

24. Maggi S, Noale M, Pilotto A, et al. The METABOLIC Study: multi-dimensional assessment of health and functional status in older patients with type 2 diabetes taking oral antidiabetic treatment. *Diabetes Metabol.* 2013;39(3):236–43.

25. Heidelbaugh JJ. Proton pump inhibitors and risk of vitamin and mineral deficiency: evidence and clinical implications. *Therapeut Advances Drug Saf.* 2013;4(3):125–33.

26. Mintzer J, Burns A. Anticholinergic side-effects of drugs in elderly patients. *J R Soc Med.* 2000;93(9):457–62.

27. Hall SA, Chiu GR, Kaufman DW, et al. Associations of commonly used medications with urinary incontinence in a community based sample. *J Urol.* 2012;188(1):183–9.

28. Seymour RM, Routledge PA. Important drug-drug interactions in the elderly. *Drugs Aging.* 1998;12(6):485–94.

29. Tsui B, Dennehy CE, Tsourounis C. A survey of dietary supplement use during pregnancy at an academic medical center. *Am J Obstet Gynecol.* 2001;185(2):433–7.

30. Henry A, Crowther C. Patterns of medication use during and prior to pregnancy: the M A P study. *Aust N Z J Obstet Gynaecol.* 2000;40(2):165–72.

31. Wagner CL, Katikaneni LD, Cox TH, et al. The impact of prenatal drug exposure on the neonate. *Obstet Gynecol Clin North Am.* 1998;25(1):169–94.

32. Briggs GG, Freeman RK, Yaffe SJ. *Drugs in Pregnancy and Lactation: A Reference Guide to Fetal and Neonatal Risk.* 5th ed. Baltimore, MD: Williams & Wilkins; 1998:73a–81a, 125c–31c, 254c–5c, 524i–6i, 757n–8n.

33. Food and Drug Administration. OTC drug facts label. Accessed at http://www.fda.gov/drugs/resourcesforyou/consumers/ucm143551.htm, September 20, 2013.

34. Ehrlich SD. Ginger. Complementary and Alternative Medicine Guide, University of Maryland Medical Center. Reviewed November 17, 2008. Accessed at http://www.umm.edu/altmed/articles/ginger-000246.htm, May 17, 2013.

35. American Academy of Pediatrics Committee on Drugs. Transfer of drugs and other chemicals into human milk. *Pediatrics.* 2001;108(3):776–89.

36. Dillon AE, Wagner CL, Wiest D, et al. Drug therapy in the nursing mother. *Obstet Gynecol Clin North Am.* 1997;24(3):675–96.

37. Nice FJ, Snyder JL, Kotansky BC. Breastfeeding and over-the-counter medications. *J Hum Lact.* 2000;16(4):319–31.

38. Lanski SL, Greenwald M, Perkins A, et al. Herbal use in a pediatric emergency department population: expect the unexpected. *Pediatrics.* 2003;111(5 pt 1):981–5.

39. Kennedy J. Herb and supplement use in the U.S. adult population. *Clin Ther.* 2005;27(11):1847–58.

DEVELOPING CULTURAL COMPETENCY FOR SELF-CARE

Magaly Rodriguez de Bittner and Jeri J. Sias

Culture influences beliefs about the health care system and may impact patients' decisions regarding self-care. This chapter explores cultural competency in health care to help guide health care providers in promoting self-care and in counseling patients from diverse backgrounds and cultures. If cultural issues are not considered during the patient interview, the health care provider may be less able to assess and/or counsel a patient effectively.

Providers may be able to formulate a more appropriate self-care plan for a given health issue if they understand the patient's cultural point-of-view and incorporate the patient's health care beliefs into the plan. In this chapter, major demographic shifts in the composition of the U.S. population are outlined to illustrate the relevance of diversity in health and the overall delivery of health care. Emphasis is placed on defining and listing important cultural terms and theoretical frameworks for cross-cultural care so that providers are able to better understand the cultural context in which patients may make self-care decisions related to overall health. General characteristics found in major racial and ethnic groups in the United States are discussed, as well as differences in cultural approaches to seeking care, particularly self-care. Attention is given to cultural assessment techniques and communication strategies to assist health care providers in communicating effectively with patients of diverse cultures and in developing a more culturally competent treatment plan.

The terms *Western, American,* and *conventional medicine* often are used synonymously to mean therapies regulated by the Food and Drug Administration (FDA), including prescription and nonprescription products. The terms *complementary, alternative,* and *traditional* are referred to as complementary and alternative medicine (CAM). In general, CAM encompasses a broad array of health practices from all over the world. Examples include magnet therapy, acupuncture, herbs, mind and body techniques, homeopathy, and massage therapy. The concept of CAM is introduced in this chapter to encourage health care providers to consider the use of these modalities among diverse patient populations. (See Chapters 50 through 52 for an in-depth discussion of CAM.)

Rationale for Cultural Competency in Self-Care

Demographic Changes in the U.S. Population

For statistical purposes, the U.S. Census Bureau classifies five races: (1) Black or African American, (2) Asian, (3) Native Hawaiian and other Pacific Islander, (4) American Indian and Alaska Native, and (5) White.[1] Individuals who identify as Hispanic (considered to be an ethnicity by the U.S. Census Bureau) may be of any race(s); race and Hispanic origin are considered separate categories. For example, individuals may classify themselves as non-Hispanic White, Hispanic White, non-Hispanic Black, or Hispanic Black.

The heterogeneity of the classification options should be recognized. For example, the groups included under Asian (e.g., Vietnamese, Filipino, and Indian) and Pacific Islander (e.g., Fijian and Samoan) exhibit great variability. This is also true for the Hispanic classification, which includes four diverse groups: Mexican Americans, Puerto Ricans, Cubans, and others (e.g., Central Americans, South Americans, and Spaniards). People in the United States increasingly identify themselves as belonging to two or more racial groups, making the issue of race and ethnic background complex.[1,2]

The reported number of racial and ethnic minorities has resulted in a shift in the composition of the U.S. population (Table 3–1).[1-4] In 2010, there were nearly 39.8 million foreign-born inhabitants, with Latin America as the leading region of origin.[1] In perspective, one of every three U.S. residents identifies with a race or ethnicity that is not White. The largest racial and ethnic minority group is Hispanic followed by Black or African American and Asian.

Other changes in health care delivery include aging of the baby boomer generation and people 65 years and older, comprising 13% of the population.[1,2] Although people in all U.S. geographical areas are aging, those in certain regions are becoming younger, which may partially be attributed to the lower median childbearing age in some minority and foreign immigrant groups. Current trends in migration patterns have created unevenly distributed racial and ethnic diversity across the United States. Therefore, transformation and diversity in ethnic consumer markets will be more pronounced in certain regions. The U.S. population is also diverse according to sex, physical disabilities, religious preference, and sexual orientation. The religious landscape of the United States indicates that about 78% of the population is Christian, 16% is not affiliated with any religion, and about 5% is aligned with non-Christian faiths.[5] These demographic changes have penetrated most areas in the United States that previously were considered homogeneous in culture, making the importance of cultural competence a national issue. Providers in every practice setting are likely to interact with patients from diverse cultures and backgrounds.

table
3-1 Changes in Racial, Ethnic, Social, and Economic Characteristics in the United States (2000, 2010)

Characteristic	Percentage of Total Population[a]	
	2000	**2010 & Estimates**
Total population[b]	100.0 (281.4 million)	100.0 (308.7 million)
White	75.1	72.4
Hispanic	12.5	16.3
Black or African American	12.3	12.6
Asian	3.6	4.8
American Indian and Alaska Native	0.9	0.9
Native Hawaiian and Pacific Islander	0.1	0.2
Other Demographic Markers[c]		
Population 65 years and older	12.4	13.0
Education below 12th grade	19.6	14.6
Born outside of the United States	11.1	12.8
Language other than English spoken at home	17.9	20.3
Families (poverty level)	9.2	10.5

[a] Total adds up to greater than 100% because of some cross-classification in Census data.

[b] Total is based on race "alone or in combination with one or more other races."

[c] The median age of the population is 35.3 years for 2000 and 37.2 years for 2010 and estimates.

Source: References 1–4.

table
3-2 Health Disparities among Racial and Ethnic Groups in the United States

Disparity Focus	Examples
Infant mortality	Higher death rates exist in African American (2.5 times), American Indian, and Puerto Rican infants compared with white infants.
Heart disease and stroke	Heart disease and stroke rates of death are 29% and 40% higher, respectively, among African American adults than whites.
Diabetes	American Indians and Alaskan Natives are 2.6 times as likely to have diabetes as non-Hispanic whites.
HIV/AIDS	African Americans and Hispanic Americans represent 66% of adults with AIDS.
Immunizations	Hispanic and African American adults ages 65 years and older are less likely than whites of the same age to receive influenza and pneumococcal vaccination.
Hepatitis	In 2000, about 50% of people with Hepatitis B in the United States identify as Asian Americans and Pacific Islanders.

Key: AIDS = Acquired immunodeficiency syndrome; HIV = human immunodeficiency syndrome.
Source: Reference 7.

Health Disparities

Although the health of some racial and ethnic groups has improved, health disparities persist.[6] In many cases, health disparities cannot be explained solely on the basis of information about the biologic and genetic characteristics of racial and ethnic groups. Health disparities often result from "complex interactions among genetic variations, environmental factors, socioeconomic factors, and specific health beliefs and behaviors."[6]

Individuals from some minority groups do not equally experience long life spans, good health, and access to health services. Low rates of cancer screening and treatment among racial and ethnic minority groups are attributed to cultural and linguistic barriers, as well as limited access to health services. Heart disease and stroke are the leading causes of death for all U.S. racial and ethnic groups (Table 3–2).[7]

Factors linked to health disparities include race, socioeconomic status, health practices, psychosocial stressors, lack of resources, environmental exposures, discrimination, and access to health care.[6] These factors will continue to influence future patterns of disease, disability, and health care utilization unless they are addressed. For instance, Hispanics and American Indians under 65 years of age are more likely to be uninsured than those in other racial and ethnic groups. Persons living in poverty are more likely to be in fair or poor health and to have disabling conditions.[8]

In an effort to create a healthier society and develop strategies to decrease the gap in health care, the U.S. government has guided public health policy over three decades through the Healthy People initiative.[9] By setting health care priorities and measurable health objectives, Healthy People 2020 provides a foundation for the health care agenda for the next decade. The overarching goals address how the United States can strive for health equity and improved health across the population, promote behaviors and environments that are healthy, and help achieve a higher quality of life.[9]

Several specific objectives within Healthy People 2020 are linked to self-care such as self-monitoring blood glucose in diabetes, taking measures to prevent sunburn, and quitting smoking. This initiative is a road map to better health and can be used by different people, states, communities, professional organizations, and groups to improve overall health.

Health Care Provider Competencies and Workforce Issues

One of the factors identified by government agencies and health care groups as a cause of health disparities is the lack of awareness of cultural issues and health disparities among health care providers. This problem may be attributed to limited formal education on cultural issues among health profession schools. To ensure effective delivery of culturally and linguistically appropriate care in cross-cultural settings, providers should understand basic cultural issues related to health and illness, health disparities among different groups, and communication strategies for culturally diverse patients.[10] Although cultural competency and diversity education are required as part of accreditation in health professional training, lack of workforce diversity still exists in health care.

The current racial and ethnic composition of health care professionals in the United States does not reflect the general population. For example, only 4.4% and 6.6% of Doctor of Pharmacy graduates in 2011 were Hispanic and African American, respectively.[11] Health care providers who share the same racial and/or ethnic minority and socioeconomic backgrounds with their patients are more likely than providers from different backgrounds to

- Provide cultural and/or linguistic concordance (e.g., when patients can consult providers from their primary racial, ethnic, and/or language background)
- Improve trust and comfort for follow-up and partnership
- Provide advocacy and leadership for policies and programs aimed at improvements for vulnerable populations

This shared identity may improve access to care, quality of provider-patient communication, and outcomes.[12]

These issues highlight the need for providers of all races to understand the influences of culture in health care and for health sciences curricula to incorporate content on cultural competency.[13] The Health Resources and Services Administration (HRSA) also provides information on the rationale and resources for cultural competence in diverse health professional programs such as dentistry, medicine, and nursing.[12,14]

In 2000, the Office of Minority Health developed the National Standards for Culturally and Linguistically Appropriate Services (CLAS) in Health Care.[15] These standards, which were updated in 2013, are based on an in-depth review of the literature, regulations, laws, and standards currently used by federal and state agencies. The new 15 standards are divided into four main sections that address: (1) the principal standard; (2) governance, leadership, and workforce; (3) communication and language assistance; and (4) engagement, continuous improvement, and accountability.

One intended purpose of the national standards is to provide criteria that credentialing and accreditation agencies can use to ensure the level and quality of culturally appropriate care that providers and institutions deliver and to accredit many health organizations. Some of these agencies include the Joint Commission,[16] the National Committee for Quality Assurance, professional organizations such as the American Medical Association and American Nurses Association, and quality review organizations such as peer review organizations.

Research in Minorities, Pharmacogenomics, and Drug Response

Historically, culturally diverse populations have been underrepresented in clinical research trials. This problem has been addressed in part by the National Institutes of Health (NIH) Revitalization Act of 1993, amended in October 2001. This act requires ethnic minorities and women to be included in clinical studies funded by the NIH.[17] In addition, the NIH has a National Institute on Minority Health and Health Disparities to help address research among racial and ethnic groups.

Although research exists on the potential pharmacokinetic and pharmacodynamic differences among varied racial and ethnic groups, more information is needed. In addition, little data exist on differences in response to nonprescription drugs among individuals from diverse racial and cultural groups.

The field of pharmacogenomics uses genome-wide approaches to study the inherited basis of differences between persons in the response to drugs.[18] Although unique opportunities exist to target drug choices and dosages based on a person's genes, there are challenges in understanding the relationship of the social environment, behaviors, diet, and access to genomic testing among various races and ethnicities. Prospects exist to enhance therapies, but more data are needed to clarify the clinical implications of pharmacogenomics for diverse patient populations.

Definitions
Culture

What is culture? Cultural identity is developed on the basis of characteristics such as ethnicity, sex, age, race, country of origin, language, sexual orientation, and religious and spiritual beliefs. One definition of *culture* is an "integrated pattern of human behavior that includes thoughts, communications, languages, practices, beliefs, values, customs, courtesies, rituals, manners of interacting and roles, relationships and expected behaviors of a racial, ethnic, religious or social group."[19] Culture can influence all aspects of human behavior. Of particular importance is the role of culture in help seeking and health maintenance behaviors, and the way these health beliefs and practices are passed from generation to generation.

Another definition of *culture* is the sum of socially inherited characteristics of a human group. This definition includes assumptions learned from family and society about the nature of the physical, social, and supernatural world, as well as the goals of life and the permissible means that one can take to achieve them.[20] Culture, as a learned set of values, beliefs, and meanings, guides patient decisions, attitudes, and actions.

Unique individuals with slightly different characteristics or beliefs may belong to the same cultural group. Individual differences must be considered when working with patients from specific ethnic or cultural groups. There is a great risk in stereotyping and assuming that a person within a group will always behave in the same manner. Stereotyping may be viewed as an assumption about behaviors or characteristics exhibited by a group of people.[21] Generalizations may be based on documented or self-described behaviors or characteristics found in groups of people or cultures and may be used as a starting point for understanding cultures. For example, a stereotype would be that all racial and ethnic minorities use CAM. A generalization would be that high CAM use is documented in many racial and ethnic minorities. During each consultation, the patient should be treated as an individual with unique beliefs and values. However, having a general idea of behaviors and characteristics of groups of people can help providers be aware of potential health beliefs and behaviors. Providers should still avoid stereotyping and be cautious if making generalizations about groups of people.

Acculturation

Variations in behaviors among members of a group become more important when people belonging to a specific cultural group migrate to and live in places that have a different, but dominant, culture. In this case, the effect of acculturation or assimilation can be observed. *Acculturation* is a process by which members of a specific cultural group adopt the beliefs and behaviors of a dominant group, but they may still value and practice their own traditional beliefs and behaviors when in the presence of their own group members.[20]

One model of acculturation creates four identities based on the degree that individuals retain a home culture and adapt to a (new) host culture.[22] Individuals who are able to function well in both their home and host culture and/or language have been able to *integrate* both cultures. These persons are often able to navigate back and forth between cultures. Persons who adopt the new host culture but let go of their original home culture *assimilate*. They function well in the host culture but may have little knowledge or understanding of the cultural heritage or language of their forebearers. Some individuals may live between cultures and feel *separated* because they do not fit into either the new host culture or the home culture. Older individuals who have moved to a new country but hold onto their home culture and/or language and never fully adopt the new host culture or language may feel *marginalized*. In the acculturation process, people who are influenced by the host culture may behave differently from the norms found in their home culture.

Although acculturation is often directed at a minority group adopting habits and language patterns of the dominant group, the outcomes of acculturation can be reciprocal. The dominant group may also adopt patterns typical of the minority group. Adopting ethnic slang words, enjoying ethnic foods and dances, and dressing in a manner that represents different cultures are examples of reciprocal acculturation practices. When individuals lose or modify their cultural identity to acquire a new identity that differs from their original cultural group (*assimilation*), these behaviors and adaptations may cause internal conflicts among members of the cultural group. For example, conflicts can arise when younger members of a cultural group (e.g., second- or third-generation immigrants) do not follow traditions of the older generation and start to exhibit behaviors and beliefs more consistent with the host culture. In some instances, the children of immigrants may not speak their parents' native language.

Culture and acculturation can influence an individual's beliefs and attitudes toward health, illness, and treatment, which will influence the person's decisions regarding health and self-care issues. When providers do not understand a patient's culture, the effective delivery of patient-centered care and, consequently, the achievement of optimal health outcomes may be impeded. Incongruent beliefs and expectations between the provider and the patient may lead to misunderstandings, confusion, and, ultimately, undesirable therapeutic outcomes.

Cultural Competence

Cultural competence has been defined as a set of congruent behaviors and attitudes among professionals that enables them to work effectively in cross-cultural situations.[23] Cultural competence is a continuous process undertaken to ensure that care is delivered in an effective manner among diverse populations of patients and providers while avoiding cultural assumptions.

Several cultural competency models have been used by providers and educators to better understand stages and processes of cultural competency. Common models (Table 3–3) describe cultural competency as a process versus an achievement and were developed by Terry Cross,[24] Larry Purnell,[25] and Josepha Campinha-Bacote.[26] The Cultural Competence Continuum (Cross) explores six stages of cultural competency from cultural destructiveness to cultural proficiency. As providers and educators gain more experience and develop their skills and knowledge they may move toward cultural proficiency.[24]

The Purnell model, which is based in several disciplinary theories (e.g., organizational, family development, religion, and political science), describes the inter-relationship of several cultural domains such as heritage, family roles, workforce issues, and high-risk behaviors (Figure 3–1).[25] In this model, the providers go through a zigzag process from "unconscious incompetence," where they may not realize that they lack knowledge and skills to work in diverse cultures, toward "unconscious competence," where they have a positive attitude and a more developed foundation of knowledge and skills to adapt care in an efficient manner.

Cultural awareness, cultural knowledge, cultural skills, and cultural encounters are the primary constructs in the cultural competence process developed by Campinha-Bacote.[26] These constructs are interdependent, and at the core, where they intersect, is "The Process of Cultural Competence." Overlapping these constructs is cultural desire—a concept that providers are caring and *want* to gain knowledge and skills to navigate across cultures. In this model, providers would also accept an attitude of *cultural humility,* recognizing that they will be in a state of learning about cultures throughout their lives. Health care providers can use these models as a framework for working with diverse cultures and developing cultural competency.

Barriers to Self-Care Management

Differences in language, health literacy, and culture pose barriers that health care providers may encounter every day in their practice. In some cases, small differences in the interpretation of language, gesture, or eye contact may lead to misunderstandings between people of different cultures and their health care providers. The provider's lack of cultural competency may impede the delivery of appropriate care.

Fear and Mistrust of Health Care Providers

Mistrust of providers may create barriers to self-care management, including reduced preventive and follow-up care. Patients may feel that providers did not consider their concerns; therefore, their expectations were not met. The disparities for racial and ethnic minorities, as historically found in African Americans, American Indians, and other groups, have been associated with discriminatory treatment and systemic racism. Many negative institutionalized health care policies and social aspects of provider–patient relationships remain as barriers to effective care. Racism is insidious, cumulative, and chronic; its effects can be felt

table
3–3 Cultural Competency Models and Applied Examples for Self-Care

Model	Attributes	Applied Examples in Self-Care
Cultural Competence Continuum (Terry Cross)	*Cultural Destructiveness* (Beginning of the continuum and the most negative stage.) ▪ Attitudes and policies support bigotry, racism, discrimination, and exploitation harmful to cultures and patients. ▪ Behavior is intentional or unintentional. In the Tuskegee study, the U.S. Public Health Service withheld syphilis treatment from African American men.	A health care provider judges a patient who is using CAM and assumes patient is not well educated or informed.
	Cultural Incapacity ▪ Organizations or providers do not have any programs or services to respond to needs of patients from other cultures. ▪ Ethnocentrism (dominant culture makes assumptions about other cultures) often exists.	A pharmacy may not carry candles requested by several patients. This common, inexpensive noninvasive adjunct self-care therapy (prayer and candles) is perceived to not be important.
	Cultural Blindness ▪ Organizations or individuals try to remain unbiased. ▪ Assumption exists that culture or race makes no difference; treat everyone "equally." ▪ Organizations have programs, but do not tailor them to address cultural needs of different groups.	Bandage is "flesh" colored and would be camouflaged on anyone, regardless of skin tone.
	Cultural Precompetence (Toward positive end of continuum) ▪ Health care organizations or individuals recognize that cultural differences exist. ▪ Organizations may reach out to cultures by hiring diverse workforce, interpreters, or translators for written materials. ▪ Organizations limit their efforts to several initiatives and may become frustrated with lack of progress.	Providers might be quick to point to an herbal product line available in their pharmacy targeted for a specific cultural group and assume that this action suffices to care for different cultures.
	Cultural Competence ▪ Ongoing acceptance and respect exist for differences among cultural groups. ▪ Providers and organizations continually increase their cultural competence knowledge and skills. ▪ Implement models to deliver culturally appropriate care—true commitment to improve outcomes of patients from diverse cultures. ▪ Providers strive to assess personal cultural biases and beliefs. ▪ Concerted efforts are made to meet and work with people of diverse backgrounds in the community. ▪ Ongoing assessments occur to improve care for different cultures.	Organizations may be committed to training their personnel to better understand the self-care needs of patients from different cultural groups.
	Cultural Proficiency (Highest level in the continuum) ▪ Organizations and providers have a true commitment to culturally competent practices. They engage in research, evaluate new approaches to care, publish and disseminate findings, advocate for improvements, and conduct trainings. ▪ Organizations and providers continually work to achieve cultural proficiency. They value the positive effect and transformation of understanding and engaging different cultures.	Organizations and providers may work with community members to identify commonly used self-care and herbal products. They provide ongoing training for staff and students on community health beliefs and values.
Purnell model	*Unconsciously Incompetent* Providers do not realize what they do not know about other cultures or the influence of culture across person, family, and community.	A provider encourages influenza vaccine for an individual without recognizing that the family home is multigenerational and everyone could be vaccinated.
	Consciously Incompetent Providers recognize that they have challenges working with persons from diverse backgrounds.	A provider realizes that different values about contraception may exist in a Nigerian culture and takes time to research information about the beliefs.

(continued)

table

3–3 Cultural Competency Models and Applied Examples for Self-Care *(continued)*

Model	Attributes	Applied Examples in Self-Care
	Consciously Competent Providers are aware of their effort to work effectively within or across different cultures.	A provider trains the entire staff on a new refugee population resettled in the community and invites key cultural leaders to help role-play and address potential cultural beliefs and practices.
	Unconsciously Competent Providers are more easily able to navigate within a different culture or across new cultures; their approach may seem effortless.	A provider has worked with Mexican American patients with diabetes over time and understands different cultural barriers to self-management.
Campinha-Bacote model	*Cultural Awareness* Providers explore their own culture and profession through a process of understanding personal biases and assumptions about different cultures.	Providers acknowledge cultural differences in home remedies and self-care treatments such as chicken soup and hot tea with lemon to alleviate cold symptoms.
	Cultural Knowledge Process involves gaining more information about diverse cultures, values, beliefs, and practices.	Providers learn about common herbs and alternative therapies used in the Vietnamese-American Buddhist population living in the neighborhood surrounding the pharmacy or clinic.
	Cultural Skill Providers can collect, assess, evaluate, and adapt cultural information from diverse patients to improve care.	Providers recognize that when supplying information about religion and culture in the social history, a woman who identifies as Islamic may prefer to have a female provider to discuss medication for a yeast infection.
	Cultural Encounters Providers actually have the opportunity to interact with one or more patients and families of diverse cultures to enrich their awareness, knowledge, and skills.	Providers are able to see multiple patients who are Hispanic each day and over time understand the importance of family in making decisions about diet and diabetes management.
	Cultural Desire Providers are sincerely motivated to grow in their capacity and skill to navigate across cultures.	In addition to working with patients from the large Catholic parish nearby, the Hindu provider volunteers at the parish community and outreach events.

Key: CAM = Complementary and alternative medicine.
Source: References 24–26.

in health care organizations, providers, and patients. Ongoing mistrust and perceptions by patients can adversely affect patient satisfaction and health outcomes.[27]

The NIH mandates for inclusion of racial and ethnic minorities have succeeded in encouraging accountability in research design, institutional review board approval, and federal research funding.[27] However, recruitment and retention of minority groups in research studies remains inadequate. This lack of participation has also been linked to barriers in the optimal use of health care facilities, willingness to seek care, and follow-up on treatment recommendations.

Persons from racial and ethnic minority groups may also differ in their perceptions about research and research participation. For example, in many African American and other communities, mistrust of research exists as a result of the Tuskegee study conducted by the U.S. Public Health Service (USPHS) for 40 years between 1932 and 1972.[28] In the study, African

American men, with ($n = 399$) and without ($n = 201$) syphilis, were enrolled, without informed consent, for "free" medical examinations and meals while researchers monitored the effects of the disease. Even when penicillin was discovered as a treatment for syphilis, subjects were not informed of the treatment option nor were they offered the antibiotic. Because of the unethical decisions of that study, many African Americans who are not recent immigrants are unwilling to participate in clinical trials and other aspects of the medical system. Fear persists that unfair treatment and further abuses will occur.[27–28]

American Indians have also survived a past that includes government policies and wars that resulted in damaging a people and culture. Some American Indians have sustained cultural traditions through family and clan relationships, kinships with homelands, religious ceremonies, and ancient rituals.[27]

The long history of American Indians and African Americans with public health services has led these populations to often

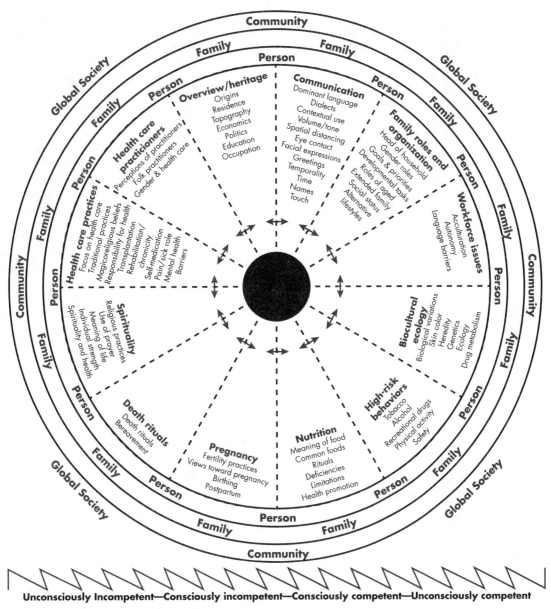

Unconsciously Incompetent—Consciously incompetent—Consciously competent—Unconsciously competent

Variant cultural characteristics: age, generation, nationality, race, color, gender, religion, educational status, socioeconomic status, occupation, military status, political beliefs, urban versus rural residence, enclave identity, marital status, parental status, physical characteristics, sexual orientation, gender issues, and reason for migration (sojourner, immigrant, undocumented status)

Unconsciously incompetent: not being aware that one is lacking knowledge about another culture
Consciously incompetent: being aware that one is lacking knowledge about another culture
Consciously competent: learning about the client's culture, verifying generalizations about the client's culture, and providing culturally specific interventions
Unconsciously competent: automatically providing culturally congruent care to clients of diverse cultures

figure
3-1 Purnell Model for Cultural Competence. (*Source:* Reprinted with permission from reference 25.)

mistrust providers and health systems. This patient perception may exist on the basis of multiple aspects:

- Feelings of prejudice against them
- Fear that their best interests are not considered and that they are treated differently from other patients
- Apprehension that their concerns and problems are not heard

- Concern that their traditional medical practices and beliefs will not be affirmed and will be called primitive
- Lack of confidence in the health care providers' skills because of the quality of the historical resources provided by the USPHS or through the Indian Health Services.[29]

Other minorities such as Hispanics or Asian Americans may also have perceptions of mistrust, but the mistrust is often derived from sources in their history outside the United States. Many immigrants have experienced political oppression or government policies that fostered suspicion or unfair practices. Fears may be centered on deportation if they entered the country undocumented, or skepticism may be present because of experiences and language barriers.

Reducing mistrust of the health care system requires repeated positive encounters over time. Some key practices that health care providers can adopt to foster trusting relationships include one-on-one outreach and frequent involvement of the provider with the targeted community. Volunteering and partnering with community leaders such as clergy or other spiritual leaders can help form networks and establish program approval at the earliest stage of the health care–planning process.[29]

Training of community health workers can be an effective strategy for garnering trust in the community, especially when time and resources are limited. Community liaisons can help diffuse health messages, integrate culturally and linguistically diverse prevention programs, provide information about new health technologies, and conduct screenings in the language and the context that the group understands. Health care providers should embrace cultural competency training to gain knowledge and skills to better tailor patients' self-care plans and deliver culturally appropriate health messages.

Language Barriers

Many patients who cannot speak or read English have difficulty in communicating with their health care providers or reading instructions on prescription and nonprescription labels. Limited English proficiency creates a significant barrier to seeking self-care or the advice of a health care provider such as the pharmacist. Because of language barriers, patients may rely on television advertisements on channels in their language of origin or on the recommendations of family members or relatives.

In many cultures, patients may express their symptoms in a different manner than what is typically encountered in a Western medical system. For example, patients from different cultural groups may express pain differently from patients raised in a Western culture. In some Asian heritage cultures, patients may not request analgesics even when they are in extreme pain, which may lead to undertreatment.

Literacy and Health Literacy

Studies have documented a relationship between poor reading skills and poor health.[30] People who cannot read often hide their illiteracy because of shame, embarrassment, low self-esteem, and fear. As a result, many health care providers often overlook this potential source of misinformation concerning nonprescription products and nonadherence to prescription drugs.

To detect literacy problems, the provider should be sensitive to cues that indicate the patient has difficulty reading. For example, patients may say they "forgot their glasses" when asked to read. People who read poorly may never join a group education class. Instead, such patients may prefer one-on-one consultations with their health care providers.

Health literacy, or "the degree to which individuals have the capacity to obtain, process, and understand basic health information and services needed to make appropriate health decisions," is also an important skill to self-management and decision making about nonprescription products.[30] A person may have high reading literacy but not functional health literacy (i.e., be able to make good decisions about their health).

In different cultures, styles of communication and belief systems can affect health literacy.[30] Health illiteracy is more common in minority groups and may be linked to general literacy levels and/or language. For example, some immigrants may have completed only a third or fourth grade education because of prolonged military conflicts and poverty in their home country. Overall low health literacy makes it difficult for providers to rely on nonprescription labels, drug information pamphlets, or prescription labels produced by the pharmacy computer systems. Through verbal communication with the patient, an interpreter, or an adult family member, providers must ensure that the patient understands the instructions and/or prescription label directions.

The prerequisite requirements of the FDA Durham–Humphrey (1951) and Kefauver–Harris (1962) amendments, used in evaluating New Drug Applications for proposed nonprescription drugs, demonstrate the need for improved health literacy. The criteria for nonprescription drug approval include evidence that (1) patients can recognize and diagnose themselves for the condition specified in the proposed indication, (2) patients can read the product label and extract the key information necessary to use the drug properly, (3) the drug is effective when used as recommended, and (4) the drug is safe when used as instructed. The consumer must be able to read and understand the information on the label to know the proper dosage, recognize warnings and contraindications, and determine whether contraindications apply.

FDA labeling requirements implemented in 2002 were intended to allow patients to read and understand nonprescription drug labels more easily. The standard product label for nonprescription drugs, titled "Drug Facts," has specific sections for active ingredients, uses, warnings, when to use the product, directions, and inactive ingredients (see Chapters 1 and 4). Manufacturers are required to use large print, simple language, and an easy-to-read format on the labels to help patients with product selection and dosage instruction. In addition to these requirements, providers should be alert to the educational needs of all patients, particularly those with poor reading skills.

To ensure that patients understand aspects of their condition and their responsibility for self-care, providers may improve clinical outcomes by integrating the following tips. First, the provider should never take for granted that the patient can comprehend fully all instructions whether written or spoken. Providers should be aware of the potential for shame and treat the patient with respect. Patient education specialists suggest using the teach-back method to ensure the clarity of the message. This method involves using phrases such as "Tell me in your own word how you are going to take this medicine." Gaps in the patient's interpretation will provide additional opportunities to explain the process again or to correct gaps using different methods to deliver the message. Counseling should be followed with materials such as pictures or demonstration products.[31]

Sociocultural Framework for Self-Care Practices

Self-care behaviors have been defined as "the range of health and illness behaviors undertaken by individuals on behalf of their own health."[32] However, these behaviors have not been well described among various racial and ethnic minorities. Factors that influence self-care behaviors can include understanding the cultural context of health and attitudes toward taking responsibility for one's own health and illness.[33,34] Further, religious beliefs, family and social contacts, cultural expectations, educational training, and personal experiences affect self-care behaviors. These interpretations are within the foundations of an ethnomedical model of care.[35]

According to Kleinman,[35] the patient's understanding of a disease is based on a consensus of beliefs, information, and expectations pertaining to the illness that are shared with a social network. This understanding helps a patient interpret healing and sickness. Normative beliefs are generated by social interaction and personal experiences, which may differ completely from evidence-based medicine and the use of technology to diagnose and treat patients (biomedical model).[35] For example, some cultures may view hypertension as caused by "bad nerves" or "high excitement" and may not understand that the disease is the chronic elevation of arterial blood pressure.

Providers who do not consider a patient's beliefs and expectations may encounter resistance to their professional advice. Expecting a patient to respond to the provider's advice solely on the basis of biomedical principles may evoke considerable frustration for the patient and the provider. Each patient may have different social support needs and concerns related to making decisions about self-care behaviors and medication use. Providers should remember the significance of "groupness" in minority populations' self-care behaviors. One classic example involves patients who are neither able nor willing to modify their dietary intake of certain foods (e.g., high fat, salty, and/or low fiber) so as not to impose these restrictions on the whole family. These patients are willing to sacrifice their own health to avoid inconveniencing their family.

Normative beliefs based on the group's experiences may also assist the individual in making the decision whether to seek care from the health system or to use CAM.[36] Self-care practices of many cultural groups involve use of home remedies, herbs, or other treatments that are passed from generation to generation. Communicating within the framework of the patient's culture helps break down barriers, while also facilitating trust and understanding between the patient and health care provider. Through this knowledge, the provider can lead a patient successfully away from harmful practices and provide safe, culturally appropriate alternatives. Subsequently, the provider can develop interventions, even biomedical ones, within the context of the patient's belief system. If the folk practices are not harmful or are even beneficial to the patient, the provider may be able to accept them as part of a monitored treatment plan.

For example, a patient who is being monitored and treated through Western medicine might also use a folk or traditional healer. Some common healing methods include prayers, massage, and aromatherapy. Because these practices may be harmless and potentially additive to Western medicine, the provider may accept and even encourage their use. Providers should maintain open and consistent communication with the patient, traditional healer, and other health care providers regarding new information on CAM.

Patients and/or their family members are responsible for the day-to-day management of their illness. Consequently, better methods are needed to determine the patient's health-seeking behaviors, informational needs, preferences, and expectations about treatment management approaches.

Providers are encouraged to develop a framework for understanding how patients interpret their illness experiences. This framework, according to Kleinman,[35] goes beyond discrete medical episodes of "controlling the biological malfunctioning of disease" to include the psychosocial dynamics of family-based care, healer–client transactions, spiritualism, shamanic cures, and other important holistic approaches based on the patient's world view as mentioned earlier. Using this approach reduces the adverse effect of miscommunication, misinformed decisions, and harmful health behaviors.

General Description of Beliefs by Different Population Groups

Some common themes have emerged in the literature related to chronic illness and self-care behaviors in the social context of older adults from African American, American Indian, Asian American, and Hispanic backgrounds.[33] These self-care behaviors may be found more often among racial and ethnic groups whose identities are rooted in their home culture and who may have less identity with Western culture and values. The following concepts highlight how self-care practices may be connected to various cultural ideals or beliefs:

1. *Concepts of independence and interdependence.* In Western medicine, independence, self-determination, and autonomy may be linked to increased self-care. Among African Americans, particularly women, values of self-reliance and independence are consistent with self-care. Among older American Indians and Hispanics, family needs may supersede the importance of individual health. Messages of self-care in these populations may need to focus on helping the overall family structure. Among older Asian Americans, a mixed phenomenon may occur because of a higher emphasis on self-discipline consistent with self-care, but family needs may be valued over those of an individual.

2. *Acceptance of intergenerational households.* European American households are less likely than those of other racial and ethnic groups to have older family members living in a household. When households have several generations living together, different dynamics of social and family support for self-care may exist. The literature is unclear whether this influence is positive or negative.

3. *Gender roles within the family structure.* Across cultures, the woman is often given the role of the "health manager" in the family, even if the household is patriarchal. When family units are intact, wives may have a greater role in influencing self-care practices of the family. When an older married man is widowed, for example, he may have a decreased ability for self-care practices, which may be noted especially among African American and Hispanic men.

4. *Family traditions related to CAM use.* In general, older adults and immigrants from African, American Indian, Asian, and Hispanic cultures more often use CAM as part of self-care compared with whites. Older Asian Americans may use more CAM because of the tendency for friends to provide health-related help.

5. *Role of friends.* Friends, godparents, and "fictive kin" (very close friendships that are family-like) can be relied on for support as much as family. For example, in some African American communities, women will rely strongly on each other to help provide child care. Hispanics, American Indians, and Asian Americans also have strong extended friendships that are closely connected to the family.

6. *Religious and spiritual beliefs of cultures.* The role of God and spiritual healing may influence how persons from a cultural group use and/or accept self-care practices. In some American Indian cultures, physical health is not as important as spiritual or emotional health. In some African American communities, churches have a central role that is sometimes of a familial nature.

Differences in health beliefs and behaviors, as well as the interplay of biological and societal influences, are documented in the literature.[20,36,37] Table 3–4 lists some of the characteristics found to be shared among people in major racial and ethnic minority groups in the United States. Not every member of an ethnic or cultural group will conform to these attitudes and beliefs. This chapter uses these examples to help sensitize providers to aspects of health behavior they may encounter; however, each patient should be evaluated individually. Awareness of this diversity may help providers deliver more effective care with increased cultural competence.

Religious beliefs are also important in patients' acceptance of the diagnosis and treatment. A set of beliefs, attitudes, and expectations of illness and treatment based on religion may cause friction with the health care system and the health care team. For example, a person whose religious background is Jewish or Islamic may have restrictions on the use of certain nonprescription products. Omega-3 fatty acids and other animal-based or gelatin-containing products may or may not ascribe to strict religious guidelines (kosher or halal) regarding consumption of animal-based products.[38,39]

Individuals from different cultures may choose to treat illnesses by using different rituals and religious items that are outside the realm of Western medicine. For example, patients who identify as Hispanic may use home remedies or other artifacts recommended by spiritual healers, sometimes called *curanderos*. These healers may use a combination of herbal remedies and religious rituals. When providers are nonjudgmental, they can better understand how and when the patient plans to use drug therapy or another alternative treatment. Knowing this information can help providers determine what treatments the patient used previously or is going to use or whether major interactions exist between the nonprescription product and the patient's alternative treatment.

Use of Nonprescription Medications by Culturally Diverse Patients

Limited data are available on the use of nonprescription products among patients of diverse cultural groups or among patients with diverse sexual or religious preferences. For many cultural groups, especially those without prescription drug coverage, nonprescription products represent the most frequently used treatments prior to consulting a provider.[40] Because of financial constraints, fear of the health care system, lack of health care access, and cultural beliefs, some immigrants may use the pharmacist as the first source of care. In many countries, the pharmacist plays a significant role in assessing symptoms and triaging the patient to appropriate medical care.

Because of the limited access to health care in many countries, pharmacists have served as primary care providers. Many patients from other countries might seek this same level of pharmacist involvement in their care while in the United

table 3–4	Examples of Cultural Behaviors That May Be Observed among Selected Racial and Ethnic Groups[a]
Group	**General Characteristics**
African American (not recent immigrant)	▪ Recognize importance of family ▪ May use home remedies and folk medicine ▪ May distrust the health care system because of previous experiences with system ▪ Recognize importance of religion in achieving cure
American Indian	▪ May use sweat lodges as a method of cure ▪ May use herbal medicine and natural roots ▪ May use prayer for cure of illnesses ▪ May believe that health is a harmony with "Mother Earth" ▪ May use healer (medicine man)
Asian heritage	▪ Recognize importance of family ▪ May believe that balance between forces may define health (*yin and yang*) ▪ May believe that illnesses may be caused by an imbalance of cold and hot forces ▪ May use alternative medicine ▪ May use Chinese herbal products ▪ May distrust Western medicine
Hispanic heritage	▪ Recognize importance of family (family members may be deeply involved in the care of the patient) ▪ May use *curanderos/curanderas* (traditional healers) ▪ May use home remedies—mostly teas or herbal remedies ▪ May use religious medals for good luck ▪ May believe that health is a matter of luck ▪ May have an attitude toward recovery that is pessimistic (fatalism) ▪ May believe that illnesses are classified as hot and cold with treatment chosen depending on the classification of the disease

[a] The described behaviors have been observed in these racial and ethnic groups and are meant solely as a guide and not as stereotypes.

Source: Seidl HM, Ball JW, Dains JE, et al. Cultural awareness. In: *Mosby's Guide to Physical Examination.* 6th ed. St. Louis, MO: Mosby; 2006.

States. For example, evidence is consistent about a link between health-seeking behaviors and antibiotic use among patients accustomed to over-the-counter access found in some pharmacies in Mexico.[20] Patients' expectations may include that the pharmacist will provide them with antibiotics as nonprescription products. Failure to do so may negatively influence the patients' expectations of the pharmacist. Understanding these beliefs can help providers communicate to the patient the rationale for the therapeutic recommendations.

Suboptimal Responses to Nonprescription Drug Therapy

The improper use of nonprescription products places vulnerable populations at an increased risk for adverse drug reactions, drug–drug interactions, and toxicities from long-term exposure. Therefore, the misuse and abuse of drugs that are available for self-treatment may outweigh the benefit–risk ratio in some patients. Increased use of nonprescription products by minority groups may create another self-care challenge.

Self-care is important for patients with chronic illnesses. The need for quick relief may prompt more frequent use of nonprescription medicines, thus raising the risk of overmedication and a tendency for people to self-medicate for conditions. Lowered tolerance for discomfort can also lead people to rely on drug therapy, especially nonprescription pain relievers, instead of seeking long-term behaviorally oriented prevention strategies. Another example is the use of vitamins, laxatives, and antacids to counteract poor eating habits. Poor self-management practices can mask more serious symptoms and complicate the diagnosis of serious diseases.

Low-income patients are often vulnerable to the harmful effects of overuse of nonprescription products for several reasons. First, patients who are chronically ill and have inadequate health insurance may restrict use of prescription drugs when their costs increase.[41] Many uninsured patients use nonprescription products as alternatives to prescription drugs simply because of cost.[42] These same patients may seek medical care only for the most urgent symptoms, delaying routine visits to their primary care provider's office. Health care providers who counsel patients on the use of nonprescription products can help prevent delays in seeking medical care. Conditions such as hypertension and hyperlipidemia are often not recognized because of lack of symptoms.[43] Nonprescription products may be used by patients to treat minor symptoms associated with these conditions such as headache or chest discomfort. The key problem with a suboptimal response to a nonprescription medication is that a more serious condition may not be diagnosed until the patient experiences a complication.

Communication with Culturally Diverse Groups
Data Gathering

When interacting with patients from different cultures, providers should use specific communication skills aimed at identifying the patient's cultural beliefs. These communication skills include (1) an openness to alternative viewpoints and approaches; (2) a clear understanding of one's own prejudices and biases (self-awareness); (3) engagement to identify the patient's beliefs, expectations, and barriers to treatment; (4) an understanding of how the patient's beliefs and attitudes may influence the treatment plan; and (5) an ability to negotiate treatment that is acceptable to the patient and the provider. Trust is essential to gaining awareness of the issues involved in the interaction, and appropriate language is crucial to effective communication.[15]

Diverse techniques have been suggested to improve communication and care in cross-cultural settings. One classic model

has been described for individual and institutional cross-cultural development.[44] This technique, described by the acronym "LEARN," may be used in clinical encounters. The primary steps (Table 3–5) in LEARN are as follows:

- **L**isten with sympathy and understanding to the patient's perception of the problem.
- **E**xplain your perceptions of the problem.
- **A**cknowledge and discuss the differences and similarities.
- **R**ecommend treatment.
- **N**egotiate a treatment plan that is mutually agreed upon.

Within "L" of LEARN, providers can apply the 4C's of the patient understanding of illness that have been adapted from Kleinman's Patient Explanatory Model.[21] With the 4C's, providers elicit the following from the patient (and/or family):

1. What do you *call* the problem? (perception)
2. What do you think *caused* the problem? (beliefs regarding source of illness)
3. How do you *cope* with the problem? (use of CAM or other treatments)
4. What *concerns* do you have about the problem or treatment? (understanding of fears; may also address adherence)

table 3–5	Examples of Ways to Use LEARN

Listen with sympathy to patient's perception. A woman from Somalia is reluctant to give her mother medication for pain. When asked, she explains that she would prefer to help her mother's pain through massage.[a]

Explain your perceptions of the problem. A pharmacist encounters a patient from Iraq who has received U.S. refugee assistance. The patient has upper respiratory sneezing and coughing and requests an antibiotic because of antibiotics' wider availability in pharmacies in Iraq without a prescription. The pharmacist tries to explain (1) the differences in pharmacy practice in the two countries, and (2) health care providers' concern that overprescribed antibiotics are not working because of resistance. The pharmacist recommends appropriate nonprescription symptomatic therapy. Further, she suggests that the patient see a primary care provider and helps the patient find a provider.[b]

Acknowledge, **R**ecommend, and **N**egotiate: A patient from Cambodia complains that her 7-year-old child has had a "fever" for several days. In the pharmacy, the pharmacist has read that the word for "fever" in Cambodian may not necessary mean an elevated temperature. Rather, the term may refer only to not feeling well. The pharmacist clarifies with the mother that the child actually has had a common cold and no elevated temperature.[c] Together they find an appropriate over-the-counter therapy to treat the symptoms. The mother agrees with the plan.

[a] Lewis T, Mooney J, Shepodd G. Somali cultural profile. Ethnomed. 2009. Accessed at http://ethnomed.org/culture/somali/somali-cultural-profile, July 30, 2014.

[b] Regester K, Parcells A, Levine Y. Iraqi refugee health cultural profile. Ethnomed. 2012. Accessed at http://ethnomed.org/culture/iraqi, July 30, 2014.

[c] Graham EA. Clinical pearl: "fever" in SE Asians. Does it really mean an elevated body temperature? Ethnomed. 1997. Accessed at http://ethnomed.org/clinical/culture-bound-syndromes/pearl_fever, July 30, 2014.

table

3–6 Recommended Actions to Develop Effective Cross-Cultural Communication

- Acknowledge that diversity exists.
- Understand that culture is part of what makes individuals unique.
- Respect people or cultures that may be unfamiliar or different from one's own.
- Conduct a self-assessment to identify one's own cultural beliefs and biases.
- Recognize differences in the way people define and value health and illness.
- Be patient, flexible, and willing to modify health care delivery to meet patients' cultural needs.
- Allow for differences among members of the same cultural group. (Do not expect all individuals from a cultural group to behave identically at all times.)
- Appreciate the richness of culture.
- Embrace diversity.
- Understand that cultural beliefs and values are difficult to change and, in many instances, are learned from birth.

Source: Adapted with permission from Schrefer S. *Quick Reference to Cultural Assessment.* St. Louis, MO: Mosby; 1994:IV.

Table 3–6 provides guidelines to help the provider communicate better with culturally diverse patients. In many instances, the communication barrier may include the patient's inability to speak the provider's language. Several Web sites provide tips for providers to work with health care interpreters and with patients who have limited English proficiency (Table 3–7).

An interpreter provides a means of addressing a language barrier, but this approach has limitations. Problems may arise when family members are used as interpreters because the patient and family members may be put in an uncomfortable position. This situation becomes more critical when a younger family member, sometimes a child, is asked to interpret for older family members, such as parents or grandparents, in a clinical encounter. Putting a child in a position of responsibility is not acceptable and can lead to family conflicts by altering the hierarchy within the family. It also places an undue burden on the child, so this situation should be avoided.

Using family members or untrained personnel to interpret may lead to receiving or transmitting inaccurate information. The health care provider may fail to detect relevant and critical information, or the interpreter and/or patient may misinterpret the information. These problems can be avoided when the health care provider uses personnel who are trained in medical language interpretation and are familiar with the providers.

To assist with communication, the Agency for Healthcare Research and Quality has a Web site exploring health literacy issues in a pharmacy setting.[45,46] Educational materials should be at a sixth grade reading level or below and a variety of media used to convey a health message.[46]

Assessment of Cultural Issues on Patient Adherence

Providers can better assess the role that culture may play in a patient's acceptance of the diagnosis and treatment of an

table

3–7 Resources for Developing a More Culturally Competent Health Care Environment

Resource	Web Site
Limited English Proficiency (LEP) Resources for Effective Communication	www.hhs.gov/ocr/civilrights/resources/specialtopics/hospital communication/eclep.html
Self-Assessments	nccc.georgetown.edu/resources/assessments.html
Curricula Enhancement Module Series	ncccurricula.info
Office of Minority Health, U.S. Department of Health and Human Services	minorityhealth.hhs.gov
National Standards for Culturally and Linguistically Appropriate Services (CLAS) in Health and Health Care	www.thinkculturalhealth.hhs.gov/pdfs/EnhancedNational CLASStandards.pdf
Provider Guide to Quality & Culture	www.innovations.ahrq.gov/content.aspx?id=942
Cultural and Linguistic Competence Policy Assessment	www.clcpa.info/documents/CLCPA.pdf
Ethnomed: Integrating Cultural Information into Clinical Practice	www.ethnomed.org

illness if they learn about cultural health beliefs and values, gain insight into the patient's understanding of the disease state (e.g., Patient Explanatory Model), and improve cross-cultural communication skills. For example, patients from some Latin American cultures may have the perception that injectable dosage forms are more effective than oral tablets. This belief is probably based on the practice of primary care providers in some Latin American countries using injectable drugs with repository drug delivery formulations to provide more sustained drug delivery. These injectable drugs may be available for purchase and administration without a prescription from a pharmacy in those countries and can be a form of self-care. This technique is sometimes used because of the geographic distances many patients must travel to receive care and helps achieve a more predictable duration of treatment. Furthermore, this form of drug delivery ensures adherence with treatment. Because a cure is often achieved with this repository of products such as antibiotics, the patient may associate the effectiveness of care with this method of drug administration. Because injectable dosage forms are not routinely used in outpatient settings in the United States, Hispanic patients may leave a health care facility with a prescription for an oral product believing that the treatment is not going to be effective. This lack of confidence in the therapy may affect adherence and the achievement of a cure. If providers are aware of this cultural belief and assess the patient's preferences or beliefs for a variety of treatments, they can modify the treatment or educate the patient about the benefits of oral dosage forms. Although this approach seems simplistic, time and individual assessment of the patient's beliefs and preferences are required.

Decision Making and Nonprescription Products

Patient autonomy concerning health care extends to taking part in the decision making for the need for treatment; monitoring of treatment progress; and use of nonprescription medications, home monitoring devices, and diagnostic kits at intervals during the treatment process. Because rates of chronic conditions[9] are higher among minority populations, drugs, including nonprescription products, may be more widely used.

Development of a Self-Care Plan

Self-care activities include a range of individual health behaviors such as health maintenance, use of preventive services, symptom evaluation, self-treatment, interaction with health care providers, and seeking of advice through lay and alternative care networks.[47] In general, providers should encourage their patients' and their families' participation in self-care behaviors to promote patient empowerment. Unfortunately, some health care providers do not encourage self-care behaviors because they are not aware of appropriately targeted techniques, strategies, and support systems that patients can use.

When assisting patients in their self-care behaviors and self-medication, providers can help initiate dialogue with the patient for informed decision making. Providers can also participate in health screening programs to identify health risks in the community and lead health awareness campaigns.[48]

The self-care plan should include the cultural differences and beliefs identified by the patient. These beliefs, as well as the role of the family in the patient's care, will help dictate the most appropriate recommendation. The provider must then use this information to develop self-care recommendations and patient education strategies. Communication with other health care providers about the patient's cultural beliefs and preferences is essential. A collaborative approach helps ensure that all providers are aware of the patient's preferences. For example, when developing a plan of care for the treatment of a self-limiting illness that requires nonprescription drug therapy, the provider can synthesize other providers' knowledge and skills by expanding on "Negotiating a Treatment Plan" from the LEARN model. When negotiating a plan, providers can evaluate the following:

- Communication styles and needs (e.g., interpreter, family support)
- Patient beliefs, perceptions (4C's and Patient Explanatory Model), and relevant restrictions related to religion or culture
- Prior treatments (prescription, nonprescription, and CAM) and acceptance of these therapies
- Use of tools to help patients understand and apply a recommendation (e.g., medication calendar, pictograms, and dosing reminders)
- Appropriate follow-up support (e.g., adverse event, worsening of condition, or need to see provider)

Ensuring Cultural Competence in Health Care
Organizational Commitment

Even the most culturally competent providers will find it difficult to optimize care for patients without having organizational commitment and support. Both providers and health system leaders should have a commitment to change, hold a real conviction of the significance of the task, and conduct in-depth self-assessments of the beliefs and attitudes of the personnel and the institution.

Organizations can conduct self-assessments of the level of cultural competence in the institution and the care being provided. The Georgetown University National Center for Cultural Competence (NCCC) developed a survey aimed at assessing the level of cultural competence in institutions and of the health care provider.

Ongoing organizational support for cultural competency training within the workforce provides a path for continuous improvement. In 2013, five states had legislative requirements to provide cultural competency training to part or all of their health care workforce.[49]

To develop targeted health service programs that are culturally competent, the provider may follow the recommendations and guidelines from NCCC, which include planning guides, policy briefs, monographs, and multimedia products. The resource materials are designed to assist meeting and conference planners in infusing principles, content, and themes related to cultural and linguistic competence into their service delivery systems (Table 3–7).

Cases 3–1 and 3–2 illustrate aspects of culturally competent care in the area of self-care. These cases are examples of issues that may be observed in community practice.

Key Points for Multicultural Aspects of Self-Care

➤ Cultural issues affect patients' attitudes and behaviors toward health and illness, as well as their acceptance and adherence to treatment plans.

➤ Major shifts in the demographics of the U.S. population are affecting the delivery of care to patients.

➤ Racial and ethnic minority populations have experienced a range of health disparities compared with their white counterparts. A disproportionately high number of minority patients continue to experience increased rates of complications with chronic diseases compared with other populations.

➤ The inability of health care providers to deliver culturally competent care can affect the health outcomes of diverse populations.

➤ Health care providers should evaluate their biases and prejudices and acquire knowledge and skills to effectively care for patients from diverse cultures. Delivering culturally competent care should be a goal of every health care provider, particularly in the area of self-care.

➤ Self-care lends itself very well to the practice of culturally competent care. Many racial and ethnic minority groups seek nonprescription products, as well as CAM therapies, as their main source of care.

case

3-1

Cultural Competence in Self-Care (Referral)

Patient Complaint and History

Mr. Jackson is a 54-year-old African American man. He and his wife request information about over-the-counter products for constipation. Mr. Jackson looks uncomfortable and indicates that he has experienced constipation over the past month or two. For the past 2 weeks, he has increased water and fiber intake in his diet through fresh fruit, oatmeal, and whole grains. Mr. Jackson's last bowel movement was 2 days ago, but he states that he didn't think he really emptied his bowels. Mr. Jackson's wife says that he has seems to be weaker in the past couple days. When you offer different laxatives and probiotics, both Mr. Jackson and his wife don't really seem interested.

Upon further discussion, the couple acknowledges that they have heard information in the news about the importance of detoxifying the bowels periodically because toxins can build up and lead to constipation (cause). Mr. Jackson has tried to increase his water and fiber intake by eating more fresh fruits and whole grains (cope). Further, they reveal that 2 days ago he had a colon cleansing using oral herbs and laxative preparations. Since that day, he has felt a little week and nauseated. He has also noted some blood in the rectal area.

Clinical and Cultural Considerations

Although not endorsed by the Food and Drug Administration or the medical community, colon cleansings have been promoted to detoxify the body, with some marketing specifically targeted African American populations. Cleansings may be available via oral, enema, or more invasive colonic irrigation routes. Because Mr. Jackson was experiencing constipation, he and his wife may have decided to explore this perceived "natural" remedy. They may also be confused between a colon preparation for medical colonoscopy versus a detoxification in the lay and natural health communities. These cleansings can cause nausea and weakness, may deplete natural flora from the colon, cause electrolyte imbalances, and increase risks for infection and dehydration, leading to more serious complications. Because Mr. Jackson has experienced weakness and noted blood in the stool, he should be referred to a primary care provider for evaluation.

According to the National Cancer Institute, colorectal cancer incidence (62.1% in African Americans versus 51.6% across all racial and ethnic groups) and mortality rates (26.7% in African Americans versus 19.4% across all racial and ethnic groups) are higher among African Americans compared with all racial and ethnic groups combined. Mr. Jackson, as a 54-year-old, has been eligible for colorectal screenings since the age of 50, and some expert panels within the American Society of Gastroenterologists recommend screening starting at age 45 for African Americans. By receiving a referral to a provider, Mr. Jackson can be evaluated for any potential negative effects of the natural colon cleansing, for constipation, and for colonoscopy screening. His wife may be eligible for screening as well.

case

3-2

Cultural Competence in Self-Care

Patient Complaint and History

Mrs. Morales comes into the pharmacy today complaining of increased urination and thirst. She has a history of type 2 diabetes and hypertension and was started on insulin yesterday.

Clinical and Cultural Considerations

Mrs. Morales has been started on insulin, but after your interview you discovered that the patient is not planning to fill the prescription. She has come to the pharmacy to get your advice on which over-the-counter medications can help control her diabetes. In your approach to the patient you should reflect a level of acknowledgment of her desire to seek treatment for her diabetes and her symptoms and demonstrate a level of *respeto* (respect) and *confianza* (trust). It is important to rule out acute symptoms of infection or other causes of hyperglycemia. It is also important to acknowledge and identify the reasons that the patient is unwilling to fill her insulin prescription and to try to help the patient understand the need to treat her symptoms and diabetes. In this case, the patient states that in her culture, insulin use is associated with "end stage" diabetes and foot amputations. She explains that everyone in her family who started using insulin ultimately had an amputation and that she is unwilling to use insulin and end up with an amputation. It is important to explain to the patient that diabetes is a progressive disease and, in many cases the patient may require insulin to prevent further deterioration and complications. This approach may require that you dispel the "myth" or "belief" that may have deep-rooted cultural implications. In this case, the identification of peers (ideally of the same cultural group) who are using insulin will prove to be an important clinical tool. It will also be important to seek the support of the patient's family to reinforce the need to dispel the myth. In addition, the patient could benefit from receiving educational material about diabetes, as well as insulin and its benefits. Developing a culturally sensitive approach to manage the patient's diabetes is critical. Collaboration with the patient's primary care provider and sharing of information are essential.

REFERENCES

1. U.S. Census Bureau. Community facts: United States foreign-born population, popular tables for this geography. Accessed at http://factfinder2.census.gov/faces/nav/jsf/pages/community_facts.xhtml, February 17, 2014.

2. U.S. Census Bureau. 2008–2012. American community survey 5-year estimates: demographic and housing estimates. Accessed at http://factfinder2.census.gov/faces/tableservices/jsf/pages/productview.xhtml?pid=ACS_12_5YR_DP05, February 17, 2014.

3. U.S. Census Bureau. Selected social characteristics in the United States: 2007–2011. American community survey 5-year estimates. Accessed at http://factfinder2.census.gov/faces/tableservices/jsf/pages/productview.xhtml?src=bkmk, February 17, 2014.

4. U.S. Census Bureau. Census 2000. Table DP-1. Profile of general demographic characteristics: 2000. Geographic area: United States. Accessed at http://censtats.census.gov/data/US/01000.pdf, February 17, 2014.

5. Pew Forum on Religion and Public Life. *U.S. Religious Landscape Survey—Religious Affiliation: Diverse and Dynamic*. Washington, DC: Pew Research Center; 2008. Accessed at http://religions.pewforum.org/pdf/report-religious-landscape-study-full.pdf, February 17, 2014.

6. Office of Minority Health and Health Disparities. Disease burden & risk factors. Last modified 2007. Accessed at http://www.cdc.gov/omhd/AMH/dbrf.htm, February 17, 2014.

7. Office of Minority Health and Health Disparities. Eliminating racial and ethnic health disparities. Last modified March 17, 2009. Accessed at http://www.cdc.gov/omhd/About/disparities.htm, February 17, 2014.

8. National Council on Disability. *The Current State of Health Care for People with Disabilities.* Washington, DC: National Council on Disability; 2009. Accessed at http://www.ncd.gov/publications/2009/Sept302009, February 17, 2014.

9. U.S. Department of Health and Human Services. Healthy People 2020. Accessed at http://www.healthypeople.gov/2020, February 17, 2014.

10. Betancourt JR, Green AR, Carrillo JE, et al. Cultural competence and health care disparities: key perspectives and trends. *Health Aff.* 2005; 24(2):499–505.

11. Taylor D, Taylor J. The pharmacy student population: applications received 2010–11, degrees conferred 2010–11, fall 2011 enrollments. *Am J Pharm Educ.* 2012;76(6 (S2)):1–16.

12. Health Resources and Services Administration. Executive summary. In: *The Rationale for Diversity in the Health Professions: A Review of the Evidence.* Washington, DC: Health Resources and Services Administration; 2006. Accessed at http://bhpr.hrsa.gov/healthworkforce/reports/diversityreviewevidence.pdf, February 17, 2014.

13. Shaya F, Gbarayor C. The case for cultural competence in health professions education. *Am J Pharm Educ.* 2006;70(6):124.

14. Health Resources and Services Administration. Culture, language, and health literacy. Accessed at http://www.hrsa.gov/culturalcompetence/index.html, February 17, 2014.

15. U.S. Department of Health and Human Services, Office of Minority Health. National standards for culturally and linguistically appropriate services in health and health care. 2013. Accessed at https://www.thinkculturalhealth.hhs.gov/pdfs/EnhancedNationalCLASStandards.pdf, February 17, 2014.

16. The Joint Commission's Division of Quality Measurement and Research. *Culture and Linguistic Care in Area Hospitals.* Oakbrook Terrace, IL: The Joint Commission; 2010. Accessed at http://www.jointcommission.org/assets/1/18/FINAL_REPORT_MARCH_2010.pdf, February 17, 2014.

17. National Institutes of Health. NIH policy and guidelines on the inclusion of women and minorities as subjects in clinical research—amended October 2001. Accessed at http://grants.nih.gov/grants/funding/women_min/guidelines_amended_10_2001.htm, February 17, 2014.

18. Kahn J. The troubling persistence of race in pharmacogenomics. *J Law Med Ethics.* 2012;40(4):873–85.

19. Goode TD, Dunne C. *Definitions of Cultural Competence.* Curricula Enhancement Module Series. Washington, DC: National Center for Cultural Competence, Georgetown University Center for Child and Human Development; 2004. Accessed at http://www.nccccurricula.info/culturalcompetence.html, February 17, 2014.

20. Spector RE. *Cultural Diversity in Health and Illness.* 8th ed. Upper Saddle River, NJ: Prentice Hall; 2012.

21. Galanti G. *Caring for Patients from Different Cultures.* 4th ed. Philadelphia, PA: University of Pennsylvania Press; 2008.

22. Berry J. Acculturation as varieties of adaptation. In: Padilla AM, ed. *Acculturation: Theory, Models, and Some New Findings.* Boulder, CO: Westview Press; 1980.

23. Cohen E, Goode TD. *Policy Brief 1: Rationale for Cultural Competence in Primary Health Care.* Washington, DC: National Center for Cultural Competence; 1999.

24. Cross T, Bazron B, Dennis K, et al. *Towards a Culturally Competent System of Care: Volume I.* Washington, DC: CASSP Technical Assistance Center, Georgetown University Child Development Center; 1989.

25. Purnell L. The Purnell Model for Cultural Competence. *J Transcult Nurs.* 2002;13(3):193–6.

26. Campinha-Bacote J. The process of cultural competence in the delivery of healthcare services: a model of care. *J Transcult Nurs.* 2002;13(3):181–4.

27. Benkert R, Peters R, Clark R, et al. Effects of perceived racism, cultural mistrust and trust in providers on satisfaction with care. *J Natl Med Assoc.* 2006;98:1532–40.

28. Centers for Disease Control and Prevention. U.S. public health service syphilis study at Tuskegee. The Tuskegee timeline. June 2011. Accessed at http://www.cdc.gov/tuskegee/timeline.htm, February 17, 2014.

29. Calderon L, Baker RS, Fabrega H. An ethno-medical perspective on research participation: a qualitative pilot study. *Medscape Gen Med.* 2006;8(2):23.

30. National Library of Medicine. Health literacy. July 2013. Accessed at http://nnlm.gov/outreach/consumer/hlthlit.html, February 17, 2014.

31. Villaire M, Mayer G. Low health literacy. *Prof Case Manag.* 2007;12:213–6.

32. Dean K. Health-related behavior: concepts and methods. In: Ory MG, Abeles RP, Lipman DP, eds. *Aging, Health and Behavior.* Newbury Park, CA: Sage; 1992:27–56.

33. Gallant MP, Spitze G, Grove JG. Chronic illness self-care and the family lives of older adults: a synthetic review across four ethnic groups. *J Cross Cult Gerontol.* 2010;25:21–43.

34. Ory MG. The resurgence of self-care research: addressing the role of context and culture. *J Cross Cult Gerontol.* 2008;23:313–7.

35. Kleinman A. *Patients and Healers in the Context of Culture.* Berkeley, CA: University of California Press; 1980.

36. Brashers DE, Goldsmith DJ, Hsieh E. Information seeking and avoiding in health contexts. *Hum Commun Res.* 2002;28:258–71.

37. Institute of Medicine. *Health and Behavior: The Interplay of Biological, Behavioral, and Societal Influence.* Washington, DC: National Academies Press; 2001.

38. Tanenbaum Center for Interreligious Understanding. *The Medical Manual for Religio-cultural Competence: Caring for Religiously Diverse Populations.* New York, NY: Tanenbaum Center for Interreligious Understanding; 2009.

39. Queensland Health and Islamic Council of Queensland. *Healthcare Providers' Handbook on Muslim Patients.* 2nd ed. Brisbane, Queensland, Australia: Division of the Chief Health Officer, Queensland Health; 2010. Accessed at http://www.health.qld.gov.au/multicultural/health_workers/hbook-muslim.asp, February 17, 2014.

40. The Commonwealth Fund. *2001 Health Quality Survey.* New York, NY: The Commonwealth Fund; 2002. Pub No. 523.

41. Heisler M, Wagner TH, Piette JD. Patient strategies to cope with high prescription medication costs: who is cutting back on necessities, increasing debt, or underusing medications? *J Behav Med.* 2005;28(1):43–51.

42. Covington TR. Nonprescription drug therapy: issues and opportunities. *Am J Pharm Educ.* 2006;70(6):137.

43. Oborne CA, Luzac ML. Over-the-counter medicine use prior to and during hospitalization. *Ann Pharmacother.* 2005;39:268–73.

44. Berlin EA, Fowkes WC. A teaching framework for cross-cultural health care. *West J Med.* 1983;139:934–8. Accessed at http://www.ncbi.nlm.nih.gov/pmc/articles/PMC1011028/pdf/westjmed00196-0164.pdf, February 17, 2014.

45. Agency for Healthcare Research and Quality. AHRQ Pharmacy Health Literacy Center. Accessed at http://www.ahrq.gov/legacy/pharmhealthlit/index.html, February 17, 2014.

46. DeWalt Da, Callahan LF, Hawk VH, et al. *Health Literacy Universal Precautions Toolkit.* AHRQ Publication 10-0046-EF. Rockville, MD; Agency for Healthcare Research and Quality; April 2010. Accessed at http://www.ahrq.gov/professionals/quality-patient-safety/quality-resources/tools/literacy-toolkit/healthliteracytoolkit.pdf, February 17, 2014.

47. Answers.com. Gale encyclopedia of public health: self-care behavior. Accessed at http://www.answers.com/topic/self-care, February 17, 2014.

48. Nichols-English G, Poirier S. Optimizing adherence to pharmaceutical care plans. *J Am Pharm Assoc.* 2000;40:475–85.

49. U.S. Department of Health and Human Services, Office of Minority Health. CLAS legislation map. Accesssed at https://www.thinkcultural health.hhs.gov/Content/LegislatingCLAS.asp, February 17, 2014.

LEGAL AND REGULATORY ISSUES IN SELF-CARE PHARMACY PRACTICE

Edward D. Rickert

This chapter analyzes the federal laws and regulations that govern the manufacturing, distribution, labeling, and marketing of the products that patients commonly use for self-care. Theories of civil liability, negligence, and breach of warranty are also discussed. Nonprescription drugs are regulated differently than prescription drugs and other consumer health care products, such as dietary supplements and homeopathic medicines. It is important that health care providers have a basic understanding of these regulations so they can respond to their patients' questions and concerns about the self-care products they use.

Regulation of Nonprescription Drugs

The first major federal legislation enacted in the United States to regulate drugs was the Pure Food and Drugs Act of 1906.[1] Under this act, drugs were required to meet only the standards of strength, quality, and purity claimed by the manufacturers. "Unsafe" and "nonefficacious" drug products were not actually prohibited by the statute. Federal law did not mandate drug safety until passage of the 1938 Federal Food, Drug, and Cosmetic Act (FDC Act).[2]

In 1951, the Durham–Humphrey amendment to the FDC Act established two classes of drugs: prescription-only and non-prescription (also referred to as over-the-counter, or OTC).[3] Before that time, manufacturers were free to determine whether to market their drug products as prescription or nonprescription items. Under the Durham–Humphrey amendment, only drugs that could be used safely without medical supervision and had labeling that included adequate directions for use could be marketed without a prescription.

The next major change in federal law occurred in 1962, when the FDC Act was again amended through passage of the Kefauver–Harris Act.[4] This amendment required that all new drugs be shown to be effective as well as safe for their intended uses. As a result of this amendment, the Food and Drug Administration (FDA) undertook a review of the effectiveness of 4500 new drug products, including 512 nonprescription drugs that had been approved only for safety since 1938.

In 1972, FDA initiated a massive scientific review of the 700 active ingredients in 300,000 nonprescription drug formulations to ensure that they were safe and effective and also bore fully informative labeling. This review process, which is still under way, is often referred to as the "OTC Drug Review."[5]

FDA is also responsible for the labeling of nonprescription drugs and reclassifying (i.e., switching) drugs from prescription to nonprescription status. Consequently, nonprescription drugs that are on the market today fall into one of the three following categories:

- Approved through the drug approval process and either (1) reclassified from prescription to nonprescription status or (2) approved directly as a nonprescription drug.
- Marketed in accordance with the OTC monograph for that ingredient (see the online section titled OTC Monograph Process).[6]
- On the market pending a determination under the OTC Drug Review monograph process of the drug's disposition.

Drug Approval Process

The FDC Act of 1938, as amended in 1962, requires that all new drugs introduced for marketing be cleared in advance through a New Drug Application (NDA) that proves the drug safe and effective for human use. Products marketed before 1938 were exempted from the NDA requirement under a grandfather clause. However, FDA's Office of Nonprescription Products has evaluated, or is in the process of evaluating, all nonprescription drugs for safety, effectiveness, and labeling, regardless of the date of marketing entry.[6]

A new chemical entity never before marketed in the United States is classified as a new drug and, in most cases, would be approved initially for prescription use only. An NDA for a nonprescription drug product can also be approved directly (without reclassification), as occurred with ibuprofen 200 mg (a dose that was never available by prescription). When a new drug is used for many years by many patients (referred to in the FDC Act as "used for a material time and material extent"), it may be considered generally recognized as safe and effective and qualify for marketing as a nonprescription drug. In addition, certain data regarding the safety, efficacy, and use of the product in a foreign country can be used to determine whether a drug can be marketed as a nonprescription product in the United States.[7]

Some drugs are available in the same strength as prescription-only and nonprescription products, but they are marketed for different uses. For example, nonprescription meclizine is available for motion sickness, which is easy to self-diagnosis. It is also available as a prescription drug for the management of vertigo, which should be diagnosed and treated by a primary care provider.

New Drug Application

An NDA is the vehicle through which persons or entities, referred to in the regulations as "sponsors," apply to FDA to seek approval of a new pharmaceutical for sale and marketing in the United States. The data gathered during the animal studies and human clinical trials of an Investigational New Drug (IND) become part of the NDA. The goals of the NDA are to provide FDA with enough information to determine, among other things, whether (1) the drug is safe and effective for its proposed use(s); (2) the benefits of the drug outweigh the risks; and (3) the methods and controls used in manufacturing the drug are adequate to preserve the drug's identity, strength, quality, and purity.[8] During this process a determination is also made as to whether the drug product is a candidate for nonprescription status.

The approved NDA is manufacturer specific and allows only the sponsor to market the product. Any other manufacturer interested in marketing a similar product would first need to seek FDA approval through its own NDA. If a second manufacturer seeks to manufacture a prescription drug product that is essentially a copy of a previously-FDA-approved product, a full NDA is not necessary; an Abbreviated NDA (ANDA) may be submitted instead, eliminating the need for duplicative testing. The second manufacturer, and any subsequent manufacturer, must demonstrate that its product is bioequivalent to the original product.

All NDAs must contain, among other things, complete labeling information; the final printed labeling is usually the last step before approval (see the section "Drug Facts" Labeling for Nonprescription Drugs in this chapter).

OTC Monograph Process

An OTC monograph is developed for therapeutic classes of ingredients that are generally recognized as safe and effective (also referred to as "GRASE"). A manufacturer desiring to market a product that contains an ingredient covered under an OTC monograph need not seek FDA's prior approval. In this case, marketing is not exclusive; any manufacturer may market a similar product without specific approval.

Under the monograph approach, all data and information supporting safety and efficacy of the ingredient and its nonprescription status are publicly available. The FDA Office of Nonprescription Products has established the monographs through a complex administrative process called "rulemaking," which allows the general public, manufacturers, and other interested parties to comment on proposed rules. Each individual rulemaking has resulted in an extensive administrative record. Figure 4–1 illustrates the process by which the OTC drug monographs are reviewed.

Under a final OTC monograph, the manufacturer has considerable flexibility in labeling. All the required monograph labeling (requirements vary for each therapeutic class) must be included; for example, antacids must include terms such as *heartburn, acid indigestion,* and *sour stomach.* In addition, certain language not included in the monograph may be used in specific places on the label without prior approval. For example, *hospital-tested* or *pleasant-tasting antacid* are terms considered outside the scope of the monograph but are permissible in antacid labeling. However, even though these permissible terms are not preapproved, they are subject to the general labeling provision of the FDC Act and may not be false or misleading.

Monographs primarily address active ingredient(s) in the product, and in most cases final formulations are not subject to monograph specifications. Manufacturers are free to include any inactive ingredients that serve a pharmaceutical purpose, provided those ingredients are safe and do not interfere with either product effectiveness or any required final product testing. With regard to final product testing, although FDA prior approval of a product covered under an OTC monograph is not required, the monograph itself may require additional testing of the product prior to marketing. This is true even though the product contains GRASE ingredients; for example, antacids must pass an acid-neutralizing test.

Laws and regulations require the manufacturer, packer, or distributor whose name appears on the label of a nonprescription medication to report certain adverse events associated with the drug.[9,10] FDA's MedWatch program, a safety information and adverse event reporting system for medical products, including nonprescription drugs, is addressed later in this chapter, under Adverse Event Reporting.[11]

Labeling and Packaging Issues
"Drug Facts" Labeling for Nonprescription Drugs

It is essential that the labeling of nonprescription drug products clearly communicates to the consumer the important information on how to use the product safely and effectively. For many years, FDA and consumers have been concerned about the adequacy of labeling for nonprescription drugs.[12] This concern is heightened because an increasing number of prescription drugs are being reclassified from prescription to nonprescription status. Many of these reclassified drugs require the patient to perform more sophisticated self-diagnostic and self-monitoring evaluations. Therefore, a greater number of sophisticated messages must be communicated through the nonprescription label to provide adequate directions and safety information.

Recognizing these concerns, FDA has changed nonprescription drug labeling requirements. FDA regulations now require a standardized content and format for the labels on all nonprescription drugs on the market.[13] Nonprescription drug labels have an area on the package designated as the "Drug Facts" box (Figure 4–2), which contains the information required by FDA to be on the label.[14] A nonprescription product that lacks this labeling feature may be considered misbranded and subject to the same enforcement approach that FDA can take with other misbranded drugs, including issuance of a warning letter, product seizures, and injunctions.

The nonprescription labeling regulations are intended to improve the consumer's ability to read and understand information about the product's benefits and risks and its directions for use. The Drug Facts labeling also helps consumers select the right product to meet their needs. The format enables them to determine readily and easily whether a product contains ingredients they need, do not need, or should not take. It also allows consumers to compare similar products to determine the appropriate ingredients for their symptoms or personal health situation.

The Drug Facts labeling format, with standardized headings and subheadings, also uses terms that are familiar to consumers (e.g., *uses* instead of *indications*). Lay terms are also used instead of medical terminology (e.g., *lung* instead of *pulmonary*).

The population of persons 65 years of age or older is increasing. Older people are significant users of nonprescription products, and they may have greater difficulty reading product labels

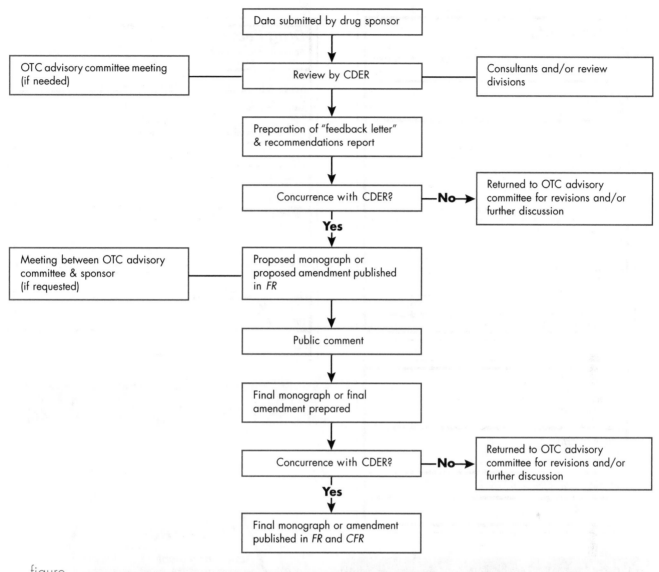

figure

4–1 OTC drug monograph review process, showing how CDER determines the safety and effectiveness of OTC drug products. Key: CDER, Center for Drug Evaluation and Research; *CFR, Code of Federal Regulations; FR, Federal Register;* OTC, over-the-counter. (*Source:* Adapted from U.S. Food and Drug Administration, Center for Drug Evaluation and Research. *The CDER Handbook.* Rockville, MD: Department of Health and Human Services, U.S. Food and Drug Administration, Center for Drug Evaluation and Research; 1998. Accessed at http://www.fda.gov/downloads/AboutFDA/CentersOffices/CDER/UCM198415.pdf, August 15, 2011.)

because of decreasing visual functioning. The labeling requirements set a minimal type size for labels, ranging from 6 point Helvetica type for text to 14 point for certain headings. An easy-to-read font style is also required, as are other graphic features such as bold type and bullet points that enhance the ability to read the information on the label clearly.

Health care providers, particularly pharmacists, should be familiar with the Drug Facts format. It is an essential counseling tool for nonprescription drugs. This format allows pharmacists to readily find information on the label and point it out to the patient. Figures 4–3 and 4–4 show examples of product labels in the Drug Facts format.

Dietary supplements are not regulated as "drugs" under the FDC Act. Consequently, they do not follow the Drug Facts format. Dietary supplements must be labeled in accordance with the regulations discussed in Chapter 50 and illustrated in Figure 50–1.

Expiration Date Labeling

Most nonprescription drug products are required to include an expiration date on the labeling.[15] This is the date beyond which the product should not be used because the stability, potency, strength, or quality may change over time. FDA regulations govern how this date is determined and tested. Most nonprescription drug product labels must also include any special storage conditions or requirements for the product. Nonprescription drug products that do not have a dosage limit and are stable for at least 3 years are exempt from the requirement to include the expiration date on the label. These products include some topical drugs, skin protectants, lotions, and astringents.

Health care providers should remind patients to check their nonprescription drug product labels periodically to ensure that the expiration date has not passed. Patients often ask whether

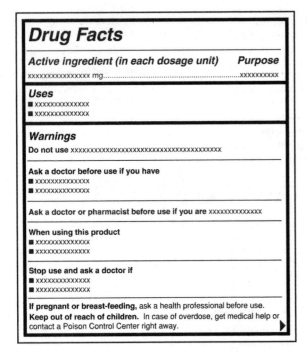

Drug Facts

Active ingredient (in each dosage unit)   **Purpose**

xxxxxxxxxxxxxxx mg...xxxxxxxxx

Uses
- xxxxxxxxxxxxxx
- xxxxxxxxxxxxxx

Warnings

Do not use xxxxxxxxxxxxxxxxxxxxxxxxxxxxxxxxxxxxxx

Ask a doctor before use if you have
- xxxxxxxxxxxxxx
- xxxxxxxxxxxxxx

Ask a doctor or pharmacist before use if you are xxxxxxxxxxxxxx

When using this product
- xxxxxxxxxxxxxx
- xxxxxxxxxxxxxx

Stop use and ask a doctor if
- xxxxxxxxxxxxxx
- xxxxxxxxxxxxxx

If pregnant or breast-feeding, ask a health professional before use.
Keep out of reach of children. In case of overdose, get medical help or contact a Poison Control Center right away. ▶

Drug Facts (continued)

Directions
- xxxxxxxxxxxxxx
- xxxxxxxxxxxxxx

Other information
- xxxxxxxxxxxxxx
- xxxxxxxxxxxxxx

Inactive ingredients xxxxxxxxxxxxxx

Questions? 123-555-1234

figure 4–2   Drug facts labeling outline. (*Source:* Reference 14.)

Drug Facts

Active ingredient (in each tablet)   **Purpose**

Chlorpheniramine maleate 2 mg.................................Antihistamine

Uses temporarily relieves these symptoms due to hay fever or other upper respiratory allergies: ■ sneezing ■ runny nose ■ itchy, watery eyes ■ itchy throat

Warnings
Ask a doctor before use if you have
- glaucoma ■ a breathing problem such as emphysema or chronic bronchitis
- trouble urinating due to an enlarged prostate gland

Ask a doctor or pharmacist before use if you are taking tranquilizers or sedatives

When using this product
- you may get drowsy ■ avoid alcoholic drinks
- alcohol, sedatives, and tranquilizers may increase drowsiness
- be careful when driving a motor vehicle or operating machinery
- excitability may occur, especially in children

If pregnant or breast-feeding, ask a health professional before use.
Keep out of reach of children. In case of overdose, get medical help or contact a Poison Control Center right away.

Directions

adults and children 12 years and over	take 2 tablets every 4 to 6 hours; not more than 12 tablets in 24 hours
children 6 years to under 12 years	take 1 tablet every 4 to 6 hours; not more than 6 tablets in 24 hours
children under 6 years	ask a doctor ▼

Drug Facts (continued)

Other information ■ store at 20-25°C (68-77°F)   ■ protect from excessive moisture

Inactive ingredients D&C yellow no. 10, lactose, magnesium stearate, microcrystalline cellulose, pregelatinized starch

figure 4–3   Drug facts labeling sample 1. (*Source:* Reference 14.)

a nonprescription drug product they have at home is still good if the expiration date has passed. Safety issues rarely arise from using a drug that is modestly past its expiration date; however, the patient should be advised that the product may have reduced efficacy and that the product should be discarded.

Tamper-Evident Packaging

In the wake of several high-profile tampering incidents involving nonprescription drug products, such as Tylenol in the 1980s, FDA instituted several packaging, labeling, and manufacturing requirements to protect consumers. Historically, the term "tamper-resistant" described methods used to prevent tampering. The focus has shifted to "tamper-evident" to heighten consumer awareness of any evidence of tampering, rather than attempt to make products difficult to breach or tamper-proof.

With few exceptions (dermatologic, dentifrice, insulin, and lozenge products), nonprescription drug products must have one or more barriers to entry that, if breached or missing from the package, provide consumers with evidence that tampering may have occurred.[16] Packages must contain unique designs or other

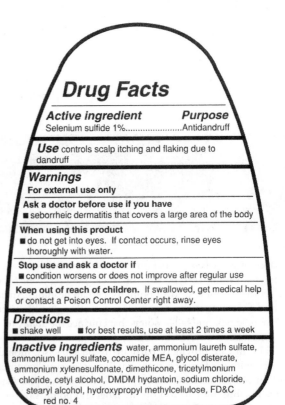

Drug Facts

Active ingredient   **Purpose**

Selenium sulfide 1%.....................Antidandruff

Use controls scalp itching and flaking due to dandruff

Warnings
For external use only

Ask a doctor before use if you have
- seborrheic dermatitis that covers a large area of the body

When using this product
- do not get into eyes. If contact occurs, rinse eyes thoroughly with water.

Stop use and ask a doctor if
- condition worsens or does not improve after regular use

Keep out of reach of children. If swallowed, get medical help or contact a Poison Control Center right away.

Directions
- shake well ■ for best results, use at least 2 times a week

Inactive ingredients water, ammonium laureth sulfate, ammonium lauryl sulfate, cocamide MEA, glycol disterate, ammonium xylenesulfonate, dimethicone, tricetylmonium chloride, cetyl alcohol, DMDM hydantoin, sodium chloride, stearyl alcohol, hydroxypropyl methylcellulose, FD&C red no. 4

figure 4–4   Drug facts labeling sample 2. (*Source:* Reference 14.)

characteristics that typically cannot be duplicated. In addition, to alert the consumer to the specific tamper-evident features, the retail package must contain a statement that identifies the feature. The statement must be prominently placed on the package in a way that it will be unaffected if the tamper-evident feature is missing or breached. For example, the statement on a bottle with a shrink band might say "For your protection, this bottle has an imprinted seal around the neck."

Patients should be educated to check for the tamper-evident features on every nonprescription drug product they purchase and, if the features are missing or look suspicious, to return the product as soon as possible to the pharmacy or store where it was purchased.

Drug Reclassification: Prescription-to-Nonprescription (OTC) Switch

Traditionally, a prescription-to-nonprescription (OTC) switch occurs in one of three ways:

- The drug is switched through the nonprescription drug review process.

- The manufacturer requests the switch by submitting a supplemental application to its approved NDA.
- The manufacturer or other party petitions FDA.

Through the nonprescription drug review process, panels of nongovernment experts are reviewing the prescription drug products that were on the market before 1962 to determine whether some are appropriate for nonprescription marketing. This ongoing process has produced more than 40 reclassifications from prescription–only to nonprescription status since the 1970s. See Table 4–1.[17]

Another common way that a prescription drug is switched to nonprescription status is for the manufacturer to submit data to FDA, in the form of a supplemental NDA, demonstrating that the drug is appropriate for self-administration. Typically, these applications include studies showing that the product's labeling can be read, understood, and followed by a consumer without the guidance of a health care provider.[18] FDA reviews this information, along with any information known about the drug from its prescription use history. All of this information is usually presented to FDA's Nonprescription Drugs Advisory Committee, which comprises nongovernment experts. This committee serves as a forum for the exchange of ideas and recommends to FDA whether the

table
4–1   Selected List of Reclassified Drugs

Ingredient	Indication(s)	Ingredient	Indication(s)
Acidulated phosphate fluoride	Dental rinse	Loperamide HCl	Antidiarrheal
Brompheniramine maleate	Antihistamine	Miconazole nitrate	Antifungal
Butoconazole nitrate	Antifungal	Minoxidil	Baldness
Cetirizine	Antihistamine	Naproxen	Analgesic
Chlorpheniramine maleate	Antihistamine	Nicotine	Smoking cessation
Cimetidine	Heartburn	Nicotine polacrilex	Smoking cessation
Clemastine fumarate	Antihistamine	Omeprazole	Heartburn (proton pump inhibitor)
Clotrimazole	Antifungal	Omeprazole and sodium bicarbonate	Heartburn
Cromolyn sodium	Allergy prevention/treatment	Orlistat	Weight-loss aid
Dexbrompheniramine maleate	Antihistamine	Oxybutynin	Overactive bladder
Diphenhydramine HCl	Antihistamine	Oxymetazoline HCl	Decongestant
Docosanol	Cold sore/fever blister	Phenylephrine HCl	Decongestant
Doxylamine succinate	Sleep aid	Polyethylene glycol 3350	Laxative
Dyclonine HCl	Oral anesthetic	Pseudoephedrine HCl	Decongestant
Famotidine	Heartburn	Pyrantel pamoate	Pinworm treatment
Fexofenadine hydrochloride (NDA)	Antihistamine	Ranitidine	Heartburn
Guaifenesin	Expectorant	Sodium fluoride	Dental rinse
Hydrocortisone	Antipruritic, anti-inflammatory	Stannous fluoride	Dental rinse or gel
Ibuprofen	Analgesic	Terbinafine HCl	Antifungal
Ketoconazole	Antifungal (shampoo only)	Tolnaftate	Antifungal
Ketotifen	Antihistamine	Triclosan	Antigingivitis
Lansoprazole	Heartburn, reflux	Triprolidine HCl	Antihistamine
Levonorgestrel	Contraception	Xylometazoline HCl	Decongestant
Loratadine	Nonsedating antihistamine		

drug in question should be switched to nonprescription status. The FDA is not bound by the committee's recommendation, but the agency usually follows the committee's advice.

Overall, more than 700 nonprescription drug products on the market today use ingredients or dosages once available only by prescription.[19] The categories of drug products that have seen the most activity in this area are analgesics, H_1 and H_2 histamine-receptor antagonists, antifungal medications, smoking cessation agents, and topical medications used to treat minor skin conditions. Drug products in these categories are good candidates for prescription-to-nonprescription reclassification because they are used to treat self-limiting conditions that are easily identified by laypersons, with or without the assistance of a health care provider.

A company, usually the manufacturer, can also petition FDA to switch a drug or class of drugs to nonprescription status. In recent years, however, FDA has received petitions that originated not from the drug's manufacturer, but from third party payers.[20] These third party payers, citing FDA's statutory authority under Section 503(b) of the FDC Act to remove the prescription requirement for a drug when doing so will not create a threat to public health, have petitioned FDA to switch certain drugs from prescription to nonprescription status.

It is easy to understand why third party payers, employers, and state and federal health care programs have taken a strong interest in increasing the number of prescription-to-OTC switches. The availability of nonprescription drug products for self-treatment may save consumers millions of dollars in health care costs by reducing the number of physician visits, preventing unnecessary sick days from work, and decreasing costs associated with the advancement of disease states that could have been limited by treatment with a nonprescription product. Medicare Part D is another area in which patients may benefit by purchasing a nonprescription rather than a prescription medication to slow progression to the coverage gap. That said, out-of-pocket expenditures may increase for many consumers if employers, insurers, and other third party payers no longer cover the cost of the medications as the result of a prescription-to-OTC switch. Nevertheless, it will be important for health care providers to stress to their patients the importance of continuing needed drug therapy, even if the cost of the medication is no longer covered by insurance.

Exact standards or switch criteria are very difficult to set because many factors must be carefully considered. The information that must be gathered from the expert opinions of advisors and consultants regarding a drug's classification as nonprescription includes, but is not limited to, the following:

- Is the condition self-diagnosable?
- Is the condition self-treatable?
- Does the product possess misuse and/or abuse potential?
- Is the product habit forming?
- Do methods of use preclude nonprescription availability?
- Do the benefits of availability outweigh the risks?
- Can adequate directions for use be written?

Further scientific scrutiny typically addresses the following questions:

- Does the reclassification candidate have an adequate margin of safety?
- Has the reclassification candidate been used for a sufficiently long time (e.g., 3–5 years) on the prescription market to yield a full characterization of its safety profile?
- Has a vigorous risk analysis been performed? If so, what are the results?

- Has the efficacy literature been reviewed in a way that supports the expected use and labeling of the reclassification candidate?
- Have potential drug interactions for the reclassification candidate been characterized?

FDA has explored the benefits and regulatory and legislative issues related to behind-the-counter availability of drugs in the United States.[21] Products in this class would be available without a prescription, but they would be stored behind the pharmacy counter and sold only by a pharmacist. Such a class of drugs may address concerns surrounding the desire for increased availability of certain drug products, while also ensuring oversight of a health care provider, particularly a pharmacist, to ensure that these medications are used appropriately.

A de facto third class of drugs has been created and currently exists, however. For example, under federal law and the laws of most states, the sale of certain Schedule V controlled substances, such as codeine-based cough and cold products, is permitted without a prescription, but only from a pharmacist. Pseudoephedrine is also an example of a behind-the-counter product that is sold without a prescription but with pharmacist oversight. In addition, many states have passed laws permitting pharmacists to furnish prescription medications to patients without a prescription in certain circumstances, often through a standing order, protocol, or collaborative practice arrangement with a physician. Products furnished under this model retain prescription-only status, but their availability directly from the pharmacist without a visit to the physician improves patient access to needed medications. Evidence that consumers have benefited and pharmacists have successfully managed risks in these areas could be used as support for a broader, federally sanctioned third class of drugs.

In 2012, FDA took a step toward the creation of this third class of drugs when it proposed a new paradigm under which the agency would approve certain prescription drugs for OTC use under conditions of safe use. Because the undertreatment of many common diseases or conditions is recognized as a public health problem, making certain medications more accessible as nonprescription drugs in health care settings such as pharmacies may improve patient outcomes. The required conditions of safe use would be drug-product specific and, according to FDA, might include using innovative technologies in addition to requiring pharmacist intervention. Medications discussed as potential candidates for OTC approval include those used for treatment of hyperlipidemia, hypertension, migraine headaches, asthma, and allergic reactions.[22]

Activity in the area of prescription-to-OTC switches seems certain to increase in the coming years. Health care providers can reasonably expect that more prescription drugs will be subjected to review, as payers, the pharmaceutical industry, and FDA continue to grapple with the difficult task of balancing economic pressures with safety concerns. As more drugs are switched to nonprescription status, health care providers will be called on to play a greater role in assessing the need for treatment and monitoring the use of these drugs.

Case Study—Levonorgestrel Rx-to-OTC Switch

In July 2013, a prescription (Rx)-to-OTC switch occurred, not as the result of pressure from a third party payer, but as the result of litigation in federal court over the issue of whether levonorgestrel-based emergency contraceptives should be sold without a prescription and without point-of-sale or age restrictions. The product's manufacturer originally petitioned FDA in 2003 to market its levonorgestrel-based emergency contraceptives for use without a prescription for women 15 years of age and older.[23] A Citizen's Petition seeking to remove all age restrictions followed. FDA finally granted this petition when, after several amendments, further research, and much litigation, the United States District Court for the Eastern District of New York issued a landmark opinion that granted the OTC sale of levonorgestrel-based emergency contraceptives to all women and girls, regardless of age.[24] As a result of the decision, FDA agreed to allow certain levonorgestrel-based products to be distributed over the counter to women and girls of all ages.[25] This represents one of the most substantial changes from prescription to nonprescription status over the past decade.

Regulation of Methamphetamine Precursors

Over the past several years, state and federal regulators have increased the regulation of nonprescription products that contain pseudoephedrine and other methamphetamine precursors. These laws were enacted to combat the growing problem of illicit methamphetamine laboratories, operated by "garage chemists" who use pseudoephedrine as the precursor in the manufacturing process. Although the federal government has passed laws that directly regulate retail sales of products containing pseudoephedrine, many states have passed more stringent laws, and it is important that retail sellers be familiar with both state and federal regulations.

Under federal law, the Comprehensive Methamphetamine Control Act of 1996 and the Combat Methamphetamine Epidemic Act of 2005 regulate the sale of products containing pseudoephedrine by limiting the quantities that can be purchased at retail and by imposing certain record-keeping and reporting requirements on sellers, including pharmacies.[26] Key requirements concerning the sale of pseudoephedrine-containing products under the federal laws include the following requirements:

- These products must be kept behind the counter or in a locked cabinet.
- Individuals may not purchase more than 3.6 grams of pseudoephedrine in 1 day and not more than 9 grams in any 30-day period or, if purchased from a mail-order pharmacy or a "mobile vendor," no more than 7.5 grams in any 30-day period.
- Purchasers must present a state or federal government–issued photo identification card at the time of purchase.
- Sellers must maintain either a written or an electronic logbook as follows:
  — All pseudoephedrine transactions for a period of not less than 2 years from the date of purchase are recorded.
  — Specific information, including the name and address of the purchaser, the name of the product, the quantity purchased, and the date and time of the transaction, must be included.
  — Products packaged for individual sale that contain less than 60 mg of pseudoephedrine are exempt from the logbook requirements but still must be kept behind the counter.
- The person selling the pseudoephedrine must confirm that the information provided by the purchaser matches that provided on the identification card.

- The purchaser must provide a signature verifying that the information provided is correct.

The Combat Methamphetamine Enhancement Act of 2010[27] requires retail sellers of methamphetamine precursors, except pharmacies that are DEA registrants, to submit to the U.S. Attorney General a self-certification, stating that the seller understands each of the requirements under the federal methamphetamine precursor laws. The Attorney General will develop and make available on the Drug Enforcement Administration (DEA) Web site a list of all self-certified retailers or persons and will require that all distributors of methamphetamine precursors sell those products only to retailers or persons registered with the DEA or included on the self-certification list.

In addition to federal law, nearly every state has enacted its own laws to regulate the sale of methamphetamine precursors.[28] The regulatory approach varies from state to state, and many state laws are more stringent than federal law. Retailers and other persons are required to comply with the most stringent law; therefore, it is essential that they be familiar with the methamphetamine precursor laws in their states.

Marketing Issues
Product Line Extensions

Product line extensions are becoming more commonplace in the nonprescription drug market. Product line extensions include new strengths, formulations, combinations of ingredients, and even a totally different therapeutic entity of a brand-name product that was originally marketed as a single-ingredient product at a specific dose to treat a specific symptom. In developing product line extensions, manufacturers hope to capitalize on the loyalty created by consumer recognition and trust of a brand name.

Product line extensions can create consumer confusion and inappropriate drug selection and use.[29] Health care providers must be familiar with the range of products within a brand name to recommend them safely and correctly and to counsel patients on these products. Particular care must be taken with respect to the active ingredients because these often differ within a product line. Some product line extensions carry the original brand name on the label and retain the active ingredient of the original product, but strengths may vary. Some manufacturers with many product line extensions continue to use the original brand name on the label, but the product line extensions contain none of the active ingredients of the original products and have a suffix attached to the brand name for differentiation (e.g., PM, EX, DM, AF, Cold and Flu, Non-Drowsy, Extra, Allergy-Sinus-Headache, Advanced Formula, PH, Day/Night, and Plus).

Nonprescription Drug Advertising

FDA handles most matters involving the labeling, as opposed to the advertisement, of nonprescription drugs, whereas the Federal Trade Commission (FTC) is responsible for matters involving claims made in advertisements for nonprescription drug products.[30] In the 1970s, the Federal Trade Commission Act (FTC Act) was amended to prohibit advertisers from using language to describe the therapeutic benefits of a nonprescription drug product that differs from language approved by FDA for use in the product labeling.

The FTC Act requires that advertising be truthful and forthright. Depending on the claim, advertisers may be required to back up their representations with competent and reliable scientific evidence, including tests, studies, or other objective data.

In 1973, the National Association of Broadcasters and the Consumer Healthcare Products Association developed a code of guidelines for manufacturers to follow in creating television advertisements for nonprescription drugs.[31] The guidelines, which are updated periodically, set standards for truthfulness and honesty and suggest that an advertisement should, among other things, do the following:

- Comply with all relevant applicable laws and regulations.
- Urge the consumer to read and follow label directions.
- Contain no claims of product effectiveness that are unsupported by clinical or other scientific evidence, responsible medical opinion, or experience through use.
- Present no information in a manner that suggests the product prevents or cures a serious condition that must be treated by a licensed health care provider.
- Emphasize the uses, results, and advantages of the particular product.
- Reference no physicians, hospitals, or nurses, unless such representations can be supported by independent evidence.
- Present no negative or unfair reflections about competing nonprescription drug products, unless those reflections can be supported scientifically and presented in a manner that consumers can perceive differences in the uses.

Consumers should be analytical when listening to or reading marketing messages, particularly because some can be subjective, superficial, vague, or potentially misleading. Health care providers, particularly the pharmacist and the primary care provider, are well positioned to assist patients in separating fact from ambiguity with regard to nonprescription drug use and to serve the public interest as an objective, informed source of nonprescription drug information.

Vitamins, Minerals, Botanical Medicines, and Other Dietary Supplements

Dietary supplements are regulated under the federal Dietary Supplement Health and Education Act of 1994 (DSHEA). This act became law in recognition that many consumers believe dietary supplements have health benefits. The law represents a balance between consumer access to dietary supplements and the authority of FDA to withdraw dangerous products and address false and misleading claims. FDA's authority to regulate dietary supplements is significantly less than that for prescription and nonprescription products. A thorough discussion of dietary supplements, including regulatory issues, clinical issues, and patient assessment issues, can be found in Chapter 50.

Homeopathy

Homeopathic drugs are recognized as drugs under the FDC Act, which defines the term *drug* as "articles recognized in the official United States Pharmacopoeia, official Homeopathic Pharmacopoeia of the United States ('HPUS'), or official National Formulary, (i) or any supplement to any of them."[32] Furthermore,

the act provides that whenever a drug is recognized in both the *United States Pharmacopoeia* and the *HPUS,* it is subject to the requirements of the *United States Pharmacopoeia,* unless it is labeled and offered for sale as a homeopathic drug, in which case it is subject to the provisions of the *HPUS.* A discussion of homeopathic products can be found in Chapter 52.

Drug–Cosmetic Products

Some nonprescription drug products are also considered cosmetic products.[33] The claim(s) made for the product determine whether it is a drug, a cosmetic, or a drug–cosmetic. Labeling and marketing requirements differ depending on how a product is classified. Often this distinction is not apparent to consumers, so they may wonder why a product they consider to be a cosmetic contains Drug Facts labeling. If a product has a drug-intended use and a cosmetic-intended use, it is considered a drug–cosmetic. For example, a nonmedicated shampoo is a cosmetic because its intended use is to clean the hair, which is a cosmetic claim. An antidandruff shampoo is a drug because its intended use is to treat dandruff, which is considered a drug claim. Therefore, an antidandruff shampoo that claims to clean the hair and treat dandruff would be a drug–cosmetic and bear OTC Drug Facts labeling. Other drug–cosmetic products include toothpastes that contain fluoride, deodorants that are also antiperspirants, moisturizers, and some cosmetics that are marketed with sun-protection claims.

Identifying and Removing Potentially Dangerous Products from the Market
Adverse Event Reporting

Pharmacists play a critical role in helping FDA, consumers, and the pharmaceutical industry manage the risks associated with regulated products. To fulfill this responsibility, pharmacists and other health care providers must understand FDA's adverse event reporting system.

The FDA MedWatch program is a voluntary adverse event reporting system that allows health care providers and consumers to report serious adverse drug reactions directly to the agency.[34] FDA analyzes trends and correlations between drug use and adverse reports from information submitted to MedWatch. There is no cost to either the provider or the consumer for filing a report. Although the program is voluntary, it is ineffective unless properly used. Providers should take their role in patient safety seriously and, as part of that responsibility, make sure that serious adverse drug reactions suspected to be associated with drugs are reported to FDA. Official reporting forms are available from FDA by calling 1-800-FDA-1088. Reports can also be submitted online by accessing the MedWatch Web site (www.fda.gov/medwatch/index.html). FDA safety alerts and product recall information are also accessible at this site.

It is important to understand that submitting a report to FDA does not constitute a legal claim, nor does it in any way constitute an acknowledgment that there has even been an adverse drug reaction associated with use of the product. The identities of the providers and the patients are confidential. Providers are encouraged to report all suspected adverse reactions and to ensure effective review of the reports. FDA asks that providers describe the reaction, the exposure to the regulated product, the time between exposure and reaction, and the underlying disease.

Product Recalls

When a product regulated by FDA is identified as a potential risk to the public, removal of the product from the market may be necessary. Products may pose a risk for a variety of reasons, including adulteration, misbranding, or discovery of an unacceptable risk of adverse effects through postmarket surveillance.

FDA has two methods available to force the removal of a product from the market. First, if the drug is misbranded or adulterated or is an unapproved new drug, the FDC Act allows FDA to seize the product and order that it be held pending a review by the court.[35] Second, FDA can also seek a court injunction, preventing further distribution or sale of the product. Both of these remedies are potentially expensive and time consuming and, more important, do not address the issue of retrieving drugs that have already been purchased.

A third avenue that FDA may pursue is to request that the manufacturer recall the product from the market. FDA has no statutory authority to order a recall, but when potentially serious health risks are associated with the use of a drug product, manufacturers typically are willing to institute a recall. If a recall is instituted, FDA does have the authority to prescribe the procedures to which the recall must conform. This cooperation between FDA and its regulated industries has proven over the years to be the quickest and most reliable method for removing potentially dangerous products from the market. This method has been successful because it is in the interest of both FDA and the industry to remove unsafe and defective products from consumer hands as soon as possible. FDA guidelines governing product recalls make clear that FDA expects manufacturers to take full responsibility for product recalls, including follow-up checks to ensure that recalls are successful. Under the guidelines, manufacturers are expected to notify FDA when recalls are started, make reports to FDA on their progress, and undertake recalls when asked to do so.[36]

The guidelines categorize all recalls into one of three classes according to the level of hazard associated with the product at issue:

■ *Class I* recalls are for dangerous or defective products that predictably could cause serious health problems or death.
■ *Class II* recalls are for products that might cause a temporary health problem or pose only a slight threat of a serious nature.
■ *Class III* recalls are for products that are unlikely to cause any adverse health reaction but violate FDA labeling or manufacturing regulations.

The manufacturer is responsible for notifying sellers of the recall. The sellers, including pharmacists, are responsible for contacting customers, if necessary. A pharmacist is also responsible for knowing what drugs or other regulated products have been recalled. Failing to remove a recalled product from the shelf and subsequently providing the product to a consumer may violate the FDC Act and also expose the pharmacist to civil liability if someone is injured by use of the product.

FDA issues general information about new recalls that it is monitoring through FDA Enforcement Reports, a weekly publication available on FDA's Web site (www.fda.gov/Safety/Recalls/EnforcementReports/default.htm).

Patient Protection and Affordable Care Act

The most recent federal legislation to affect the health care industry, including nonprescription drug products, is the Affordable Care Act (ACA).[37] The ACA was signed into law on March 23, 2010, with most provisions effective January 2014. Section 9003, however, became effective January 1, 2011. This section affects the regulation and purchase of nonprescription drug products by further revising the definition of medical expenses. According to Section 9003, any nonprescription drug products purchased without a prescription may no longer be paid for or reimbursed under health flexible spending arrangements (FSAs), health reimbursement arrangements (HRAs), health savings accounts (HSAs), or Archer Medical Savings Accounts (Archer MSAs). The exception to this is insulin, which will remain reimbursable through FSAs, HRAs, HSAs, and Archer MSAs. Therefore, the only way an individual may pay or be reimbursed for nonprescription drug products through such account is by obtaining a prescription for such drug products. This restriction does not apply to items that are not drug products, such as devices, supplies, and other similar medical-related items.

Nonprescription Drug Products and Civil Liability

Nonprescription drug products are, by nature, deemed to be safe and effective for use by the general public for self-care, without the oversight of a health care provider. However, no drug, whether prescription or nonprescription, is completely safe. As with any product, injuries can result from the use of a nonprescription product. For example, a patient can have an allergic reaction to an ingredient in a nonprescription product, can become injured as a result of an interaction between a nonprescription product and another drug, or suffer injury resulting from a side effect associated with the use of the drug. The fact that these types of injuries can and do occur, however, does not mean that the drugs causing the problem are inherently dangerous or unsafe, or that they should not be available without a prescription.

Whether a health care provider can be held liable for money damages for recommending or selling a nonprescription drug product that causes an injury is an issue that is decided under state law, and the legislation varies from state to state. A complete analysis of the nuances of the various theories of liability is beyond the scope of this chapter. There are, however, some general principles that health care providers may find useful to understand and guard against potential civil liability.

It is important to note that regardless of what a court may decide in any given case, the primary obligation of a health care provider is to provide health care. This obligation may include recommending or selling appropriate nonprescription drug products for patient self-care. A health care provider who refuses to recommend or sell a product for fear of incurring civil liability is not providing health care and is doing a disservice to himself or herself, the profession, and the patient.

Theories of Civil Liability

The body of law concerning civil liability is guided by the general principle that, in a civilized society, people are responsible for their actions. If one's actions cause an injury to another person, the law may require that the injured person be compensated.

In the U.S. justice system, an injured person who seeks compensation for the injuries that he or she has sustained as a result of another's actions has the right to bring a civil lawsuit against the person who caused the injury. Typically, the injured party (the plaintiff) will ask the court to award money damages to be paid by the party causing the injury (the defendant). For example, a plaintiff who sustains an injury after taking a nonprescription medication recommended by a pharmacist can file a lawsuit against the pharmacist, seeking monetary compensation for the injuries. The plaintiff may seek compensation for the past, present, and future medical bills that he or she has incurred or will incur as a result of the injury; any income lost from missing work; the pain and suffering endured; and any permanent injury or damage.

The mere fact that an injury occurred does not, however, entitle the plaintiff to damages. The plaintiff has the burden of proving that he or she has satisfied each of the elements required to be proved under the theory of liability alleged in the complaint. The theories of liability that can be alleged against a health care provider in connection with an injury caused by a nonprescription drug product include negligence, breach of warranty, and strict product liability.

Negligence

The sole fact that an injury has occurred does not mean that a party can be found liable for negligence. Similarly, even if a health care provider makes a mistake, that action alone does not necessarily entitle the injured party to compensation. To prevail in a case alleging negligence of a health care provider, the plaintiff must prove four elements: (1) the defendant owed the plaintiff a duty of care; (2) the defendant by his or her conduct breached that duty; (3) the breach caused the plaintiff's injury; and (4) in fact, the plaintiff sustained some cognizable injury or damage. If the plaintiff cannot prove all of these elements, there can be no liability.

The first element, duty, is decided by the court. The relevant inquiry is whether the health care provider failed to exercise the degree of care that a reasonable and prudent person would have used under similar circumstances. Courts will examine the relationship between the parties; the foreseeability that the defendant's actions, or failure to act, could cause an injury; and the gravity of harm that resulted from the act or failure to act. After the court defines the duty, the jury will decide whether the duty has been breached by the health care provider.

In a historical case that addressed liability for injuries resulting from a pharmacist's recommendation of a nonprescription drug product, the court defined the duty as requiring the pharmacist to exercise a high degree of care in advising the purchaser of the injurious effects of the recommended nonprescription product.[38] In that case, the patient presented the pharmacist with a prescription for a product to treat poison ivy. The pharmacist advised the patient to use a nonprescription product instead of the product prescribed by the physician. A reaction between the nonprescription ointment and a residue present on the patient's skin caused the skin to turn black. The court stated:

> In the discharge of their functions, druggists, apothecaries, and other persons dealing in drugs, poisons, and medicines, are required, not only to be skillful, but also exceedingly cautious and prudent, in view of the terrific consequences which may attend the least inattention on their part. The highest degree of care known among practical men must be used

by them to prevent injury from the use of their compounds, and they are held to a special degree of responsibility corresponding with their superior knowledge and are generally held liable for the slightest negligence.

The court sustained a jury verdict awarding money damages to the plaintiff, finding that the recommendation of the nonprescription drug product and the recommendation that the plaintiff continue to use the product even after she began to notice that her skin was turning black constituted a breach of the standard of care owed to the patient.

Although each state's law differs and the ruling in any case is dependent on the facts presented, courts likely will hold pharmacists and other health care providers to a high standard of care in connection with the recommendation of nonprescription drug products. For example, a reasonable pharmacist likely would not recommend that a patient discontinue all antidepressant medications and take St. John's wort to treat clinical depression. Nor would a reasonable health care provider recommend that a patient take aspirin if it is known that the patient is also on warfarin therapy. The health care provider must act reasonably and make recommendations that are in the patient's best interest. If, despite the exercise of due care, an injury results, a provider likely would not be held liable for negligence.

Even if a duty and a breach were found, the provider would not be liable for injuries that were not caused by the negligent conduct. If, for example, the evidence in the poison ivy case described above showed that the patient's skin turned black not because of any reaction between the product recommended by the pharmacist but because of some inherent condition the patient suffered from, which coincidentally manifested itself at the same time that the patient began using the nonprescription ointment, the pharmacist would not be held liable. Again, the plaintiff must prove all four elements—duty, breach, causation, and injury—to prevail.

Breach of Warranty

Liability for breach of warranty is based on the theory that the defendant violated either an express or implied agreement concerning the quality of the product in connection with its sale. Express warranties arise out of specific statements made by the seller, whereas implied warranties are created by and imposed by law. Keep in mind that warranty liability can arise only if the health care provider sold the product that fails to perform. Therefore, a recommendation by a provider that the patient buy a certain cough and cold preparation that causes injury will not result in warranty liability if the provider merely recommended but did not sell the product.

The Uniform Commercial Code (UCC), which has been adopted by nearly every state, defines an express warranty as "an affirmation of fact or promise made to the buyer that relates to the goods and becomes a basis of the bargain."[39,40] In one of the few published cases addressing the breach of an express warranty made by a pharmacist in connection with the sale of a drug product, the court found the representation that the product sold "was the same as what the plaintiff's prescription called for" created an express warranty, and when the product sold was in fact different—and caused an injury—the pharmacist was held liable.[40] As an example, the pharmacist in the poison ivy case advised the plaintiff that the blackened skin that resulted after the first use of the nonprescription product would clear up with continued use of the ointment. Instead, it worsened. On those facts, the plaintiff likely could have stated a claim for breach of express warranty.

Express warranties should not be confused with "sales talk," or puffery, which are statements made to induce a sale that do not specifically relate to the ability of the product. For example, a statement such as "this is the best ointment you will ever buy" would likely be viewed as sales talk, not an express warranty.

Implied warranties are created by law. Two implied warranties included in the UCC should most concern health care providers who sell goods: (1) the implied warranty of fitness for a particular purpose and (2) the implied warranty of merchantability. When a seller recommends a particular product to meet the buyer's specific needs, it is implied that the product recommended is fit for that purpose. Therefore, for example, if a health care provider recommends and sells a product to treat a specific condition, and it turns out that the product should not have been used for that purpose, the plaintiff could claim the provider breached the warranty of fitness for a particular purpose.

The implied warranty of merchantability states that the product sold is fit for all general purposes for which the product typically is sold. Included within this warranty is the understanding that the products sold and their containers meet certain minimum quality standards. If a pharmacist sells a product that is outdated, contaminated, or subpotent, he or she has breached the implied warranty of merchantability.

Warranty claims often are brought against not only the immediate seller of the product but also the product's manufacturer. However, if the condition that has rendered the product unfit for ordinary purposes was caused by the manufacturer, and not the seller, the seller is not necessarily relieved of responsibility. State laws vary in this area, with some states having laws that limit the liability of the seller in those circumstances. In general, to avoid warranty liability, the provider must be mindful of the source and origin of the products it sells.

Strict Product Liability

Unlike a negligence or warranty theory, strict liability is imposed when a product causes an injury to the user, even if the seller was not negligent and made no express or implied representations regarding the product. Although this type of case is typically brought against the manufacturer, it remains a viable theory of recovery against retail sellers of products in many states. The theory is based on the idea that a seller of a product that has profited from the sale should also be required to compensate victims who are injured by the product, even if the seller was not in any way negligent in causing the injury. The mere sale of a product that is found to be defective, even if the defect is unknown or even unknowable to the seller, can form the basis for imposing strict liability.

When the product involved is a prescription drug product, courts have almost universally held that pharmacists cannot be held strictly liable for injuries caused by products they dispense. However, when a pharmacist acts as a retailer and sells goods that cause injuries, the theory may remain viable. Again, many states have laws that will automatically pass liability up the chain, past the retailer to the manufacturer.

Again, the most important rule that a pharmacist or any health care provider can follow to avoid civil liability is simply to practice health care as it should be practiced. Caring for the patient and acting in the patient's best interest to improve the patient's health and well-being should be the primary concern of all health care providers. More often than not, adherence to that general principle will provide a defense if a patient claims that the provider's conduct in connection with the recommendation or sale of a product caused an injury.

Key Points for Legal and Regulatory Issues in Self-Care Pharmacy Practice

➤ Although nonprescription drug products are readily available, they are subject to regulatory and legal requirements to ensure their safety and efficacy.

➤ The Drug Facts labeling panel is a useful consumer counseling tool for health care providers.

➤ Dietary supplements and homeopathic products are not subject to all the regulations that govern prescription and nonprescription drugs.

➤ Health care providers play a critical role in helping FDA, consumers, and industry manage risks associated with nonprescription drug products and should voluntarily report adverse events to FDA's MedWatch program or the manufacturer.

➤ With increasing frequency, FDA is approving product switches from prescription to nonprescription status. Health care providers play a crucial role in educating their patients as to the safe and proper use of recently switched products.

➤ Although liability risks may be associated with the sale of a nonprescription drug product, health care providers must remember that their primary role is to provide health care and that the best way to protect themselves is to act reasonably and in the best interest of their patient when recommending a nonprescription product.

REFERENCES

1. The Pure Food and Drug Act of 1906. Pub L No. 59-386, 34 Stat 768 (1906) (repealed in 1938 by 21 USC §329(a)).
2. Federal Food, Drug, and Cosmetic Act, 21 USC §301 et seq.
3. Durham–Humphrey Drug Prescriptions Act. Pub L No. 82-215, 65 Stat 648–9 (1951) (amending 21 USC §353(b)).
4. Kefauver–Harris Amendments to the Federal Food, Drug, and Cosmetic Act of 1938. Pub L No. 87-781, 76 Stat 780 (1962) (codified in 21 USC §502(n)).
5. Food and Drug Administration. Over-the-counter (OTC) drug product review process. Accessed at http://www.fda.gov/Drugs/Development ApprovalProcess/SmallBusinessAssistance/ucm052786.htm, June 24, 2013.
6. Food and Drug Administration, Center for Drug Evaluation and Research. Status of OTC rulemakings. Accessed at http://www.fda.gov/Drugs/ DevelopmentApprovalProcess/DevelopmentResources/Over-the-CounterOTCDrugs/StatusofOTCRulemakings/default.htm, June 24, 2013.
7. Additional Criteria and Procedures for Classifying Over-the-Counter Drugs as Generally Recognized as Safe and Effective and Not Misbranded. Final rule. *Federal Regist.* January 23, 2002;67(15):3060–76 (codified at 21 CFR §330.14).
8. Food and Drug Administration, Center for Drug Evaluation and Research. New Drug Application (NDA). Accessed at http://www.fda.gov/Drugs/ DevelopmentApprovalProcess/HowDrugsareDevelopedandApproved/ ApprovalApplications/NewDrugApplicationNDA/default.htm, June 24, 2013.
9. Serious Adverse Event Reporting for Nonprescription Drugs, 21 USC §379aa.

10. Postmarketing reporting of adverse drug experiences. CFR: Code of Federal Regulations. Title 21, Part 314, Section 314.80; Postmarketing reports. CFR: Code of Federal Regulations. Title 21, Part 314, Section 314.98.

11. Food and Drug Administration. Reporting serious problems to FDA. U.S. Accessed at http://www.fda.gov/Safety/MedWatch/HowToReport/default.htm, June 24, 2013.

12. U.S. Food and Drug Administration. Over-the-counter human drugs; proposed labeling requirements. *Federal Regist.* February 27, 1997; 62(39):9024–61. Accessed at http://www.fda.gov/downloads/Drugs/DevelopmentApprovalProcess/DevelopmentResources/Over-the-CounterOTCDrugs/StatusofOTCRulemakings/UCM106775.pdf, February 4, 2014.

13. U.S. Food and Drug Administration. Over-the-counter human drugs; labeling requirements. *Federal Regist.* March 17, 1999;64(51):13254–303. Accessed at http://frwebgate.access.gpo.gov/cgi-bin/getdoc.cgi?dbname=1999_register&docid=99-6296-filed.pdf, June 24, 2013.

14. Format and content requirements for over-the-counter (OTC) drug product labeling. CFR: Code of Federal Regulations. Title 21, Part 201, Section 201.66.

15. Expiration dating. CFR: Code of Federal Regulations. Title 21, Part 211, Section 211.137.

16. Tamper-evident packaging requirements for over-the-counter (OTC) human drug products. Title 21, Part 211, Section 211.132.

17. Consumer Healthcare Products Association. Ingredients & dosages transferred from Rx-to-OTC status by the Food and Drug Administration since 1975. October 16, 2013. Accessed at http://www.chpa.org/SwitchList.aspx, December 24, 2013.

18. Nordenberg T. Now available without a prescription. *FDA Consum.* 1996;30(9):6.

19. U.S. Food and Drug Administration. *Over-the-Counter Medicines: What's Right for You?* Washington, DC: U.S. Food and Drug Administration; 2003. Accessed at http://www.fda.gov/Drugs/ResourcesForYou/Consumers/BuyingUsingMedicineSafely/UnderstandingOver-the-Counter Medicines/Choosingtherightover-the-countermedicineOTCs/ucm150299.htm, June 24, 2013.

20. Newton GD, Benninghoff AJ, Popovich NG. New OTC drugs and devices: a selective review. *J Am Pharm Assoc.* 2002;42:267–77.

21. U.S. Food and Drug Administration. Transcript of FDA press conference on behind the counter availability of certain drugs. November 14, 2007. Accessed at http://www.fda.gov/downloads/NewsEvents/Newsroom/MediaTranscripts/ucm122281.pdf, June 24, 2013.

22. U.S. Food and Drug Administration. Using innovative technologies and other conditions of safe use to expand which drug products can be considered nonprescription; public hearing. *Federal Regist.* February 28, 2012; 77(39):12059–62. Accessed at http://www.gpo.gov/fdsys/pkg/FR-2012-02-28/pdf/2012-4597.pdf, July 25, 2013.

23. Princeton University, Office of Population Research. History of Plan B OTC. Accessed at http://ec.princeton.edu/pills/planbhistory.html, July 15, 2013.

24. U.S. Food and Drug Administration. FDA approves Plan B One-Step emergency contraceptive for use without a prescription for all women of child-bearing potential [press release]. June 20, 2013. Accessed at http://www.fda.gov/NewsEvents/Newsroom/PressAnnouncements/ucm358082.htm, July 15, 2013.

25. *Tummino v Hamburg,* 2013 WL 1348656 (ED NY April 5, 2013).

26. U.S. Department of Justice. Combat Methamphetamine Epidemic Act 2005. Title VII of USA Patriot Improvement Reauthorization Act of 2005. Pub L No. 109-177, 120 Stat 192 (2006). Accessed at http://www.deadiversion.usdoj.gov/meth/index.html, June 24, 2013.

27. U.S. Department of Justice. Combat Methamphetamine Enhancement Act of 2010. Pub L No. 111–268, 124 Stat 2847. (2010). Accessed at http://frwebgate.access.gpo.gov/cgi-bin/getdoc.cgi?dbname=111_cong_public_laws&docid=f:publ268.111.pdf, June 24, 2013.

28. National Association of State Controlled Substances Authorities. Impact of state laws regulating pseudoephedrine on methamphetamine tracking and abuse: a white paper of the National Association of State Controlled Substances Authorities. April 2012. Accessed at http://www.nascsa.org/pdf/NASCSApseudoephedrineWhitePaper4.12.pdf, May 31, 2014.

29. Institute for Safe Medical Practices. Maalox brand extension may cause confusion. *Medicat Safe Alert.* 2005;4(12):1. Accessed at http://www.ismp.org/Newsletters/ambulatory/Issues/community200512.pdf, June 24, 2013.

30. Food and Drug Administration. Memorandum of Understanding between the Federal Trade Commission and the Food and Drug Administration. MOU 225-71-8003. U.S. Accessed at http://www.fda.gov/AboutFDA/PartnershipsCollaborations/MemorandaofUnderstandingMOUs/DomesticMOUs/ucm115791.htm, June 24, 2013.

31. Consumer Healthcare Products Association. CHPA voluntary codes and guidelines: advertising practices for nonprescription medicines. Accessed at http://www.chpa.org/VolCodesGuidelines.aspx, May 31, 2014.

32. Definitions; Generally, 21 USC §321(g)(1).

33. U.S. Food and Drug Administration. Is it a cosmetic, a drug, or both? (Or is it soap?). July 8, 2002. Accessed at http://www.fda.gov/cosmetics/guidanceregulation/lawsregulations/ucm074201.htm, June 24, 2013.

34. USCA §379aa-1, et seq. [The Dietary Supplement and Nonprescription Drug Consumer Protection Act was enacted on December 22, 2006. Public Law No. 109-462 amends the Federal Food, Drug, and Cosmetic Act (the Act) to add safety reporting requirements for OTC drug products that are marketed without an approved application under Section 505 of the Act (21 USC §355).]

35. Seizure, 21 USC §334.

36. Recall policy. CFR: Code of Federal Regulations. Title 21, Part 7, Section 7.40.

37. Internal Revenue Service. Notice 2010-59. [Guidance is provided on §9003 of the Patient Protection and Affordable Care Act revising the definition of medical expenses as it relates to over-the-counter drugs.] Accessed at http://www.irs.gov/pub/irs-drop/n-10-59.pdf, June 24, 2013.

38. *Fuhs v Barber,* 36 P2d 962 (Kan 1934).

39. Uniform Commercial Code. Article 2, §2313.

40. *Jacobs Pharmacy Co v Gibson,* 159 SE2d 171 (Ga 1967).

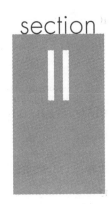

PAIN AND FEVER DISORDERS

HEADACHE

Julie J. Wilkinson

Worldwide, 47% of the population suffers from headache at any given time, and 66% will suffer from headache at some point in their lives. Migraine headache is more severe and debilitating compared with tension-type headache. However, the overall disease burden to society is similar between the two headache types because 38% of the population suffers from tension-type headache and 10% from migraine.[1]

Many headache sufferers self-treat with nonprescription remedies rather than seek medical attention. As much as two-thirds of nonprescription analgesic use may be for headache.[2] One study[2] found that 24% of patients chronically overused medication and only 14.5% had ever been advised to limit their intake of acute headache treatments. Clearly, an opportunity to improve medication use exists among patients self-treating for various pain syndromes.

Headaches are generally classified as primary or secondary. Primary headaches (approximately 90% of headaches) are not associated with an underlying illness. Examples include episodic and chronic tension-type headaches, migraine headache with and without aura, cluster headaches, and medication-overuse headaches. Secondary headaches are symptoms of an underlying condition, such as head trauma, stroke, substance abuse or withdrawal, bacterial and viral diseases, and disorders of craniofacial structures.

This chapter focuses on the most common headaches that are amenable to self-treatment: tension-type, diagnosed migraine, and sinus headaches. Nonprescription analgesics are useful in treating headache, either as monotherapy or as adjuncts to non-pharmacologic or prescription therapy.

Tension-type headaches, also called stress headaches, can be episodic or chronic. Chronic headaches occur 15 or more days per month for at least 3 months.[1] The prevalence of tension-type headache is greatest in the age range 40–49 years, occurs in a ratio of 5:4 of women to men, and increases with higher levels of education.[3]

The prevalence of migraine headache in the United States is about 18% for women and 6% for men. Onset usually begins in the first three decades of life, with greatest prevalence at around age 40. Among children, boys and girls are affected equally, but attacks usually greatly decrease in boys after puberty.[4] Migraine without aura (i.e., neurologic symptoms that precede the head pain) occurs almost twice as frequently as migraine with aura, and many individuals may have both types of headaches. Up to 70% of patients with migraine have family histories of migraine, suggesting that this disease is influenced by heredity.

The economic impact of migraine headache is substantial. Direct costs for medical services have been estimated at $1 billion in the United States. A greater burden comes from lost productivity and wages, with migraine costing $13 billion for American employers. Migraine headaches affect health-related quality of life in a manner similar to that of depression.[4]

Headache is a frequently reported symptom in patients with acute sinusitis. These patients also experience other sinus symptoms such as toothache in the upper teeth, facial pain, nasal stuffiness, and nasal discharge. The prevalence of sinus headache is low, and up to 90% of patients who believe they have sinus headache may actually be experiencing migraine headache.[5]

Pathophysiology of Headache

Tension-type headaches often manifest in response to stress, anxiety, depression, emotional conflicts, and other stimuli. The episodic tension-type headache subtype is thought to have a peripheral pain source, whereas the chronic tension-type headache has a central mechanism. A genetic component appears to influence the presence or absence of tension type headache. Furthermore, it is likely that tension-type and migraine headache share pathophysiologic features, making them more similar than distinct.[6] *Migraine headaches* probably arise from a complex interaction of neuronal and vascular factors. Stress, fatigue, irregular sleep patterns, fasting or a missed meal, vasoactive substances in food, caffeine, alcohol, changes in female hormones, changes in barometric pressure and altitude, lights, odor, neck pain, exercise, and sexual activity may trigger migraine.[7] Medications (e.g., reserpine, nitrates, oral contraceptives, and postmenopausal hormones) can also trigger migraine. Although their role in migraine headache is still debated, personality features of migraine sufferers include perfectionism, rigidity, and compulsiveness. Menstrual migraines appear at the menstrual stage of the ovarian cycle and occur in less than 10% of women. For some women, these migraine headaches occur at specific times before, after, or during the menstrual cycle.

Most investigation into the pathophysiology of headache has centered on migraine headache. The best evidence suggests that migraine occurs through dysfunction of the trigeminovascular system. Neuronal depolarization that spreads slowly across the cerebral cortex is observed during the aura phase. Magnesium deficiency may contribute to this state. During the headache phase, stimulation (by an axon reflex) of trigeminal sensory fibers in the large cerebral and dural vessels causes neuropeptide release with concomitant neurogenic inflammation, vasodilation, and activation of platelets and mast cells. Menstrual migraine pathophysiology occurs through estrogen withdrawal followed by serotonin withdrawal. Decreased serotonin is associated with increased calcitonin gene–related peptide and substance P from trigeminal nerves, which lead to vasodilation of vessels and sensitivity of the trigeminal nerves. Estrogen may also influence nitric oxide, magnesium, or prostaglandins, which may contribute to the menstrual migraine.[8,9] *Sinus headache* occurs when infection or blockage of the paranasal sinuses causes inflammation or distension of the sensitive sinus walls (see Chapter 11). Pathophysiologic mechanisms at work during migraine headache can produce prominent sinus congestion.

Medication-overuse headache results from a rebound effect after the withdrawal of an analgesic. This type of headache differs from a headache related to a medication side effect. Some patients who suffer from migraine or tension headaches receive some relief from nonprescription medication, and over time may increase their use of the nonprescription treatment, which can lead to medication-overuse headaches. These headaches are usually associated with frequent use (more than twice weekly) for 3 months or longer and occur within hours of stopping the agent; re-administration of the agent provides relief.[10] Agents associated with medication-overuse headaches are acetaminophen, some nonsteroidal anti-inflammatory drugs (NSAIDs), aspirin, caffeine, triptans, opioids, butalbital, and ergotamine formulations.[10] Symptomatology shifts from the baseline headache type to a nearly continuous headache, particularly noticeable on awakening.

Clinical Presentation of Headache

Headaches can be differentiated by their signs and symptoms; the major defining characteristics are listed in Table 5–1. The severity of pain associated with tension-type headaches is highly variable. Some headaches are so mild they do not require treatment, whereas others are sufficiently severe to be disabling. Shivering or cold temperatures may increase pain from tension-type headaches. Chronic tension-type headaches occurring at least 15 days per month for at least 6 months may be a manifestation of psychological conflict, depression, or anxiety. These headaches may be associated with sleep disturbances, shortness of breath, constipation, weight loss, fatigue, decreased sexual drive, palpitations, and menstrual changes.

Migraine headaches are classified as migraine with or without aura. Aura manifests as a series of neurologic symptoms:

shimmering or flashing areas, blind spots, visual and auditory hallucinations, muscle weakness that is usually one sided, and difficulty speaking (rarely). These symptoms may last up to 30 minutes, and the throbbing headache pain that follows may last from several hours to 2 days. Migraines without aura begin immediately with throbbing headache pain. Both forms of migraine often are associated with nausea, vomiting, photophobia, phonophobia, sinus symptoms, tinnitus, light-headedness, vertigo, and irritability, and are aggravated by routine physical activity. Premonitary (prodrome) symptoms in migraine can be neuropsychiatric (e.g., anxiety, irritability, yawning, unhappiness, and insomnia), sensory (e.g., phonophobia, photophobia, focusing difficulties, and speech difficulties), digestive (e.g., food craving, nausea, vomiting, diarrhea, and constipation), and general (e.g., asthenia, tiredness, fluid retention, and urinary frequency).[11]

Sinus headache is usually localized to facial areas over the sinuses and is difficult to differentiate from migraine without aura. The pain quality of a sinus headache is typically a dull and pressure-like sensation. Stooping or blowing the nose often intensifies the pain of sinus headache, but the headache is not accompanied by nausea, vomiting, or visual disturbances. Persistent sinus pain and/or discharge suggests possible infection and requires referral for medical evaluation.

Treatment of Headache
Treatment Goals

The goals of treating headache are (1) to alleviate acute pain, (2) to restore normal functioning, (3) to prevent relapse, and (4) to minimize side effects. For chronic headache, an additional goal is to reduce the frequency of headaches.

General Treatment Approach

Most patients with episodic headaches respond adequately to self-treatment with nonpharmacologic interventions, nonprescription medications, or both. However, some patients with episodic headaches and most with chronic headaches are candidates for prescription treatments. Throughout this chapter, the abbreviation *NSAID* will be used to denote the class of nonsalicylate nonsteroidal anti-inflammatory drugs (e.g., ibuprofen and naproxen).

table 5–1	Characteristics of Tension-Type, Migraine, and Sinus Headaches		
	Tension-Type Headache	**Migraine Headache**	**Sinus Headache**
Location	Bilateral Over the top of the head, extending to base of skull	Usually unilateral	Face, forehead, or periorbital area
Nature	Varies from diffuse ache to tight, pressing, constricting pain	Throbbing; may be preceded by an aura	Pressure behind eyes or face; dull, bilateral pain; worse in the morning
Onset	Gradual	Sudden	Simultaneous with sinus symptoms, including purulent nasal discharge
Duration	Minutes to days	Hours to 2 days	Days (resolves with sinus symptoms)
Non-headache symptoms	Scalp tenderness	Nausea	Nasal congestion

Episodic tension-type headaches often respond well to nonprescription analgesics, including acetaminophen, NSAIDs, and salicylates, especially when taken at onset of the headache. If nonprescription analgesics are used to treat chronic headache, frequency of use should be limited to less than 3 days per week to prevent medication-overuse headache. When medication-overuse headache is suspected, the use of offending agent(s) should be tapered and subsequently eliminated. Most often, tapering of an agent should be done with medical supervision because use of prescription therapies may be needed to combat the increased headaches that temporarily ensue during the days to weeks of the withdrawal period.[10] In addition to nonprescription or prescription medication, chronic tension-type headaches may benefit from physical therapy and relaxation exercises. Figure 5–1 outlines the self-treatment of headaches and lists exclusions for self-treatment.

A medical diagnosis of migraine headache is required before self-treatment can be recommended. Taking an NSAID or salicylate at the onset of symptoms can abort mild or moderate migraine headache. Once a migraine has evolved, analgesics are less effective. Patients with migraines who can predict the occurrence of the headache (e.g., during menstruation) should take an analgesic (usually an NSAID) before occurrence of the event known to trigger the headache, as well as throughout the duration of the event. For patients with coexisting tension and migraine headaches, treatment of the initiating headache type can abort the mixed headache.

Sinus headaches respond well to decongestants (e.g., pseudo-ephedrine or phenylephrine), which are useful for sinus drainage (see Chapter 11). Concomitant use of decongestants and nonprescription analgesics can relieve sinus headache pain.

Nonpharmacologic Therapy

Chronic tension-type headaches may respond to relaxation exercises and physical therapy that emphasizes stretching and strengthening of head and neck muscles. General treatment measures for migraine include maintaining regular sleeping, eating, and exercise schedules, stress management, biofeedback, and cognitive therapy.[7] Some patients benefit from applying ice or cold packs combined with pressure to the forehead or temple areas to reduce pain associated with acute migraine attacks.

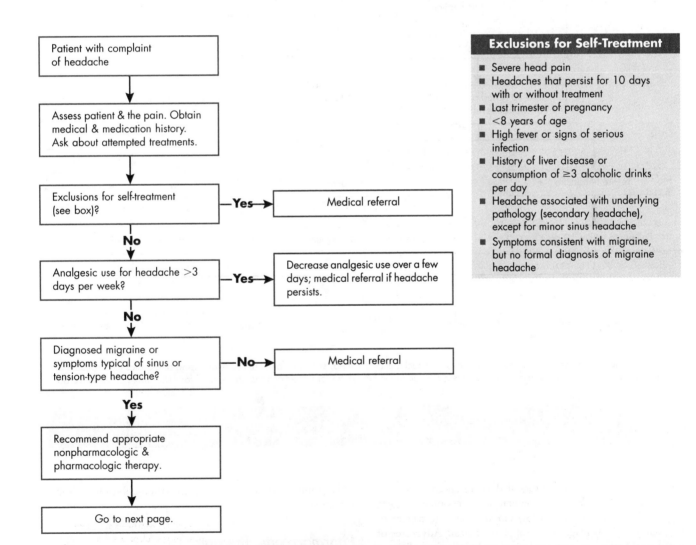

Exclusions for Self-Treatment

- Severe head pain
- Headaches that persist for 10 days with or without treatment
- Last trimester of pregnancy
- <8 years of age
- High fever or signs of serious infection
- History of liver disease or consumption of ≥3 alcoholic drinks per day
- Headache associated with underlying pathology (secondary headache), except for minor sinus headache
- Symptoms consistent with migraine, but no formal diagnosis of migraine headache

[Flowchart:]

Patient with complaint of headache → Assess patient & the pain. Obtain medical & medication history. Ask about attempted treatments. → Exclusions for self-treatment (see box)? —**Yes**→ Medical referral

No → Analgesic use for headache >3 days per week? —**Yes**→ Decrease analgesic use over a few days; medical referral if headache persists.

No → Diagnosed migraine or symptoms typical of sinus or tension-type headache? —**No**→ Medical referral

Yes → Recommend appropriate nonpharmacologic & pharmacologic therapy. → Go to next page.

figure
5–1 Self-care of headache. Key: CHF = Congestive heart failure; GI = gastrointestinal; HBP = high blood pressure; NSAID = nonsteroidal anti-inflammatory drug; OTC = over-the-counter. *(continued on next page)*

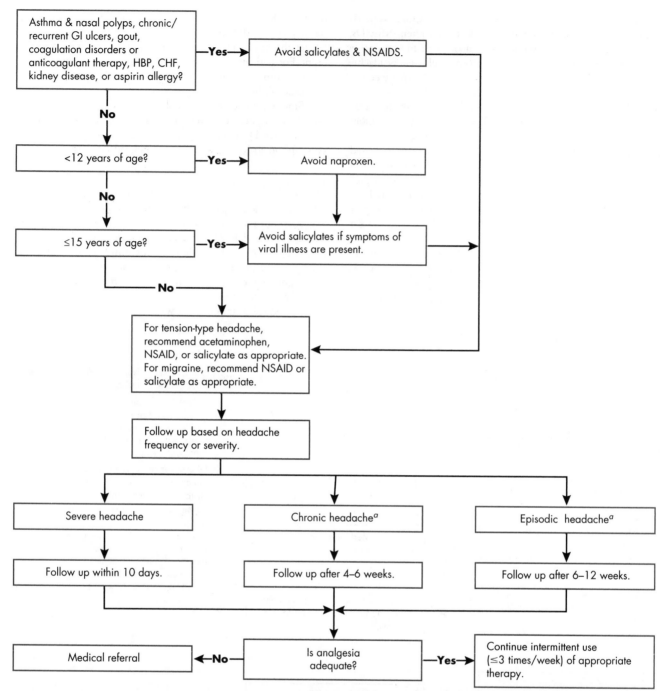

^a Once a diagnosis of chronic tension-type or episodic headache is established, self-care can resume. Avoid using analgesics more often than 3 days per week. Seek medical attention if there is a change in the headache, or if medications are needed for 10 or more consecutive days.

figure
5–1   Self-care of headache. Key: CHF = Congestive heart failure; GI = gastrointestinal; HBP = high blood pressure; NSAID = nonsteroidal anti-inflammatory drug; OTC = over-the-counter. *(continued)*

Nutritional strategies are intended to prevent migraine and are based on (1) dietary restriction of foods that contain triggers, (2) avoidance of hunger and low blood glucose (a trigger of migraine), and (3) magnesium supplementation. Advocates of nutritional therapy recommend avoiding known food allergies and foods with vasoactive substances, such as nitrites; tyramine (found in red wine and aged cheese); phenylalanine (found in the artificial sweetener aspartame); monosodium glutamate (often found in Asian food); caffeine; and theobromines (found in chocolate).

Pharmacologic Therapy

Available nonprescription analgesics for management of headache include acetaminophen, NSAIDs (ibuprofen and naproxen), and salicylates (aspirin and magnesium salicylate).

Acetaminophen

Acetaminophen is an effective analgesic and antipyretic. Acetaminophen produces analgesia through central inhibition of prostaglandin synthesis.

Acetaminophen is rapidly absorbed from the gastrointestinal (GI) tract and extensively metabolized in the liver to inactive glucuronic and sulfuric acid conjugates. Acetaminophen is also metabolized by the cytochrome P450 enzyme system to a hepatotoxic intermediate metabolite that is detoxified by glutathione. When given by suppository, rectal bioavailability of acetaminophen is approximately 50%–60% of that achieved with oral administration. Onset of analgesic activity of acetaminophen is about 30 minutes after oral administration. Duration of activity is about 4 hours and is increased to 6–8 hours with an extended-release formulation.

FDA-approved uses for nonprescription acetaminophen include reducing fever and relieving mild-moderate pain. It is effective in relieving mild-moderate pain of nonvisceral origin (i.e., pain that is not organ related). Randomized, double-blind studies have documented the effectiveness of acetaminophen 1000 mg compared to placebo in patients with migraine and tension-type headache.[12]

Recommended children and adult dosages of acetaminophen are provided in Tables 5–2 and 5–3. Table 5–2 provides more stringent nonprescription acetaminophen dosing for children younger than 12 years old. Table 5–4 lists selected trade-name products. Acetaminophen is available for administration in various oral and rectal dosage forms.

Recent changes implemented to decrease pediatric dosing errors with liquid acetaminophen formulations include having only one concentration (160 mL/5 mL) available for all children younger than 12 years.[13] Acetaminophen oral capsules contain tasteless granules that can be emptied onto a spoon containing a small amount of cold beverage (hot beverages result in a bitter taste) or soft food. Capsule contents should not be added to a cup of liquid because large numbers of granules may adhere to the cup.

Acetaminophen is potentially hepatotoxic in doses exceeding 4 g/day, especially with chronic use. Patients should be cautioned against exceeding the dose limit. More conservative dosing (i.e., ≤2 g/day) or avoidance may be warranted in patients at increased risk for acetaminophen-induced hepatotoxicity, including those with diagnosed liver disease, concurrent use of other potentially hepatotoxic drugs, poor nutritional intake, or ingestion of three or more alcoholic drinks per day.[14] One alcoholic drink is defined as 12 ounces of beer, 5 ounces of wine, or 1.5 ounces 80-proof liquor.

In 2011, FDA mandated placement of a boxed warning on acetaminophen products indicating that more than 4 g/day may cause severe liver damage. At that time, FDA *recommended* reduction of acetaminophen maximum daily dosage of 3900–4000 mg to 3000–3250 mg in efforts to reduce the risk of accidental overdose. The manufacturer of Tylenol responded to the agency's suggestion and volunteered to reduce their maximum daily dosage for Regular Strength Tylenol to 3250 mg (10 tablets) and Extra Strength Tylenol to 3000 mg (6 tablets). However, most generic manufacturers continued to follow the mandated maximum daily dosage of 4 g/day. Several acetaminophen 650 mg products (tablets and suppositories) are available with labeling that includes a maximum daily dosage of 3900 mg (6 doses).[15] In January 2014, FDA urged health care professionals to no longer prescribe or dispense prescription products containing more than 325 mg acetaminophen per dosage unit. The agency also stated that it intended, in the near future, "to institute proceedings to withdraw approval of prescription combination drug products containing >325 mg of acetaminophen per dosage unit that remain on the market."[16]

Acetaminophen poisoning is a major reason for contacting poison control centers and the leading cause of acute liver failure in the United States.[17] Hepatotoxicity from acetaminophen is probably dose related and is uncommon at recommended doses.[18] Unintended chronic overdose comprises about half of the cases

table

5–2 FDA-Approved Dosages for Nonprescription Analgesics in Children Younger than 12 Years[a]

Age (years)	Weight (lb)	Ibuprofen (mg) Dose by Body Weight (mg/kg) 5–10 mg/kg	Acetaminophen (mg) 10–15 mg/kg	Aspirin (mg) 10–15 mg/kg
<22	<24	Ask a doctor[a]	Ask a doctor[a]	Ask a doctor[a]
2–3	24–35	100	160	160
4–5	36–47	150	240	240
6–8	48–59	200	320	320
9–10	60–71	250	400	400
11	72–95	300	480	480

[a] OTC labeling limits use to children over age 3. For patients seeking dosing advice for younger children, weight-based dosing is recommended.

table

5–3 Recommended Dosages of Nonprescription Analgesics for Adults and Children 12 Years and Older

Agent	Dosage Forms	Usual Adult Dosage (maximum daily dosage)
Acetaminophen[a,b]	Immediate-release, extended-release, effervescent, disintegrating, rapid-release, and chewable tablets; capsules; liquid drops; elixir; suspension; suppositories	325–1000 mg every 4–6 hours (suggested 3250 mg[a])
Ibuprofen	Immediate-release and chewable tablets; capsules; suspension; liquid drops	200–400 mg every 4–6 hours (1200 mg)
Naproxen sodium	Tablets	220 mg every 8–12 hours (660 mg) Over age 65 years: 220 mg every 12 hours (440 mg)
Aspirin	Immediate-release, buffered, enteric-coated, film-coated, effervescent, and chewable tablets; suppositories	650–1000 mg every 4–6 hours (4000 mg)
Magnesium salicylate	Tablets	650 mg every 4 hours or 1000 mg every 6 hours (4000 mg)

[a] The manufacturer's voluntary dosing reductions in 2011 resulted in the following dosage Extra Strength Tylenol: 2 tablets (500 mg each) every 6 hours with a maximum daily dosage of 3000 mg (6 tablets). The maximum daily dosage for Regular Strength Tylenol was reduced to 3250 mg. However, a maximum daily dosage of 4000 mg is allowed for acetaminophen labeling.[15]

[b] In January 2014, FDA urged health care professionals to no longer prescribe or dispense prescription products containing >325 mg acetaminophen per dosage unit. The agency also stated that it intended, in the near future, "to institute proceedings to withdraw approval of prescription combination drug products containing >325 mg of acetaminophen per dosage unit that remain on the market.[16]

table

5–4 Selected Single-Entity Nonprescription Acetaminophen Products

Trade Name	Acetaminophen Content
Pediatric Formulations	
Children's Tylenol Meltaway Tablets	80 mg
FeverAll Infants' Suppositories	80 mg
FeverAll Children's Suppositories	120 mg
FeverAll Junior Strength Suppositories	325 mg
Jr Tylenol Meltaway Tablets	160 mg
Children's Tylenol Oral Suspension	160 mg/5 mL
Infants' Tylenol Oral Suspension	160 mg/5 mL
Adult Formulations	
Tylenol Arthritis Pain Extended Release Caplets	650 mg
Tylenol 8 hour Extended Release Caplets	650 mg
Tylenol Extra Strength Caplets	500 mg
Tylenol Rapid Blast Liquid	500 mg/15 mL
Tylenol Regular Strength Tablets	325 mg

of acetaminophen-induced acute liver failure. Contributing factors include repeated dosing in excess of package labeling, use of more than one product containing acetaminophen, and alcohol ingestion.[19]

Early symptoms of acetaminophen intoxication can include nausea, vomiting, drowsiness, confusion, and abdominal pain, but these symptoms may be absent, belying the potential severity of the exposure. Serious clinical manifestations of hepatotoxicity begin 2–4 days after acute ingestion of acetaminophen and include increased plasma aspartate aminotransferase (AST) and alanine aminotransferase (ALT); increased plasma bilirubin with jaundice; prolonged prothrombin time; and obtundation. In the majority of cases, hepatic damage is reversible over a period of weeks or months, but more severe cases may require liver transplant or result in fatal hepatic necrosis.

Because of the potential seriousness of acetaminophen overdose, all cases should be referred to a poison control center or emergency department. Supportive care is provided along with activated charcoal to reduce acetaminophen absorption in patients who present within 1 hour after ingestion. When acetaminophen serum levels, related to time since ingestion, exceed those known to cause hepatic injury, prompt administration of acetylcysteine is warranted to supplement glutathione, which is essential for deactivation of a toxic intermediate metabolite of acetaminophen. Acetylcysteine's effectiveness decreases if it is administered more than 8 hours after acute ingestion. For patients with chronic ingestions of greater than 4 g/day, administration of acetylcysteine is indicated until liver toxicity is ruled out by assessment of liver function tests.

Asymptomatic elevations in serum ALT have been reported in otherwise healthy individuals taking acetaminophen 4 g/day.

In a prospective study, 39% of patients experienced ALT elevations greater than three times the upper limit of normal. These elevations generally appeared in the first week of use, with some resolution despite continued dosing. The clinical significance of this observation is uncertain.[20]

Patients with glucose-6-phosphate dehydrogenase deficiency, a hereditary disease that causes premature breakdown of red blood cells, should use caution when taking acetaminophen. Patients with hypersensitivity to acetaminophen are contraindicated for future use.

Rare but serious cutaneous adverse reactions (SCAR) have been found to be associated with use of acetaminophen as well as other analgesics including NSAIDs. Skin reactions may occur in either new or ongoing users of the drug and have the potential to progress into life-threatening rash such as Stevens-Johnson syndrome and toxic epidermal necrolysis. Although these events are very rare, it is important to be aware of the possibility and refer patients for further evaluation.[21]

Clinically important drug interactions of acetaminophen are listed in Table 5–5. For patients taking warfarin, acetaminophen is considered the analgesic of choice; however, it has been associated with increases in international normalized ratio (INR). Regular acetaminophen use should be discouraged in patients on warfarin. Patients who require higher scheduled doses (e.g., those with osteoarthritis) should have their INR monitored and warfarin adjusted as acetaminophen doses are titrated.

table
5–5   Clinically Important Drug–Drug Interactions with Nonprescription Analgesic Agents

Analgesic/ Antipyretic	Drug	Potential Interaction	Management/Preventive Measures
Acetaminophen	Alcohol	Increased risk of hepatotoxicity	Avoid concurrent use if possible; minimize alcohol intake when using acetaminophen.
Acetaminophen	Warfarin	Increased risk of bleeding (elevations in INR)	Limit acetaminophen to occasional use; monitor INR for several weeks when acetaminophen 2–4 grams daily is added or discontinued in patients on warfarin.
Aspirin	Valproic acid	Displacement from protein-binding sites and inhibition of valproic acid metabolism	Avoid concurrent use; use naproxen instead of aspirin (no interaction).
Aspirin	NSAIDs, including COX-2 inhibitors	Increased risk of gastroduodenal ulcers and bleeding	Avoid concurrent use if possible; consider use of gastroprotective agents (e.g., PPIs).
Ibuprofen	Aspirin	Decreased antiplatelet effect of aspirin	Aspirin should be taken at least 30 minutes before or 8 hours after ibuprofen. Use acetaminophen (or other analgesic) instead of ibuprofen.
Ibuprofen	Phenytoin	Displacement from protein-binding sites	Monitor free phenytoin levels; adjust dose as indicated.
NSAIDs (several)	Bisphosphonates	Increased risk of GI or esophageal ulceration	Use caution with concomitant use.
NSAIDs (several)	Digoxin	Renal clearance of digoxin inhibited	Monitor digoxin levels; adjust dose as indicated.
Salicylates and NSAIDs (several)	Antihypertensive agents, beta-blockers, ACE inhibitors, vasodilators, diuretics	Antihypertensive effect inhibited; possible hyperkalemia with potassium-sparing diuretics and ACE inhibitors	Monitor blood pressure, cardiac function, and potassium levels.
Salicylates and NSAIDs	Anticoagulants	Increased risk of bleeding, especially GI	Avoid concurrent use, if possible; risk is lowest with salsalate and choline magnesium trisalicylate.
Salicylates and NSAIDs	Alcohol	Increased risk of GI bleeding	Avoid concurrent use, if possible; minimize alcohol intake when using salicylates and NSAIDs.
Salicylates and NSAIDs (several)	Methotrexate	Decreased methotrexate clearance	Avoid salicylates and NSAIDs with high-dose methotrexate therapy; monitor levels with concurrent treatment.
Salicylates (moderate–high doses)	Sulfonylureas	Increased risk of hypoglycemia	Avoid concurrent use, if possible; monitor blood glucose levels when changing salicylate dose.

Key: ACE = Angiotensin-converting enzyme; COX = cyclooxygenase; GI = gastrointestinal; INR = international normalized ratio; NSAID = nonsteroidal anti-inflammatory drug; PPI = protein pump inhibitor.

Nonsteroidal Anti-Inflammatory Drugs

NSAIDs relieve pain through central and peripheral inhibition of cyclooxygenase (COX) and subsequent inhibition of prostaglandin synthesis.

All nonprescription NSAIDs are rapidly absorbed from the GI tract with consistently high bioavailability. They are extensively metabolized, mainly by glucuronidation, to inactive compounds in the liver. Elimination occurs primarily through the kidneys. Onset of activity for naproxen sodium and standard ibuprofen is about 30 minutes. Ibuprofen sodium dehydrate is absorbed more rapidly and has a slightly shorter onset of action than that of standard ibuprofen. Duration of activity for naproxen sodium is up to 12 hours and 6–8 hours for ibuprofen. FDA-approved uses for nonprescription NSAIDs include reducing fever and relieving minor pain associated with headache, the common cold, toothache, muscle ache, backache, arthritis, and menstrual cramps. NSAIDs have analgesic, antipyretic, and anti-inflammatory activity, and they are useful in managing mild-moderate pain of nonvisceral origin. Naproxen sodium and ibuprofen became available for nonprescription use in 1994 and 1984, respectively, and both are propionic acid derivatives. Although FDA approved ketoprofen for nonprescription use, no commercially available nonprescription analgesics currently contain this agent.

Recommended children and adult dosages of nonprescription NSAIDs are provided in Tables 5–2 and 5–3. Table 5–6 lists selected trade-name products. Unfortunately, liquid formulations of ibuprofen have the same pediatric dosing errors mentioned earlier for acetaminophen, but no changes have been implemented to mitigate the dosing errors for ibuprofen. A dose–effect relationship has been demonstrated for ibuprofen analgesia in the range of 100–400 mg.

NSAID overdoses usually produce minimal symptoms of toxicity and are rarely fatal. In a prospective study of 329 cases of ibuprofen overdose, 43% of ibuprofen-overdose patients were asymptomatic. Among patients with symptoms, GI and central nervous system (CNS) symptoms were most common (in 42% and 30% of patients, respectively) and included nausea, vomiting, abdominal pain, lethargy, stupor, coma, nystagmus, dizziness, and light-headedness. Hypotension, bradycardia, tachycardia, dyspnea, and painful breathing were also reported.[22]

The most frequent adverse effects of NSAIDs involve the GI tract and include dyspepsia, heartburn, nausea, anorexia, and

table 5–6	Selected Single-Entity Nonprescription Nonsteroidal Anti-Inflammatory Drugs
Trade Name	**Primary Ingredients**
Pediatric Formulations of Ibuprofen Products	
Children's Advil Suspension	Ibuprofen 100 mg/5 mL
Children's Motrin Suspension	Ibuprofen 100 mg/5 mL
Infants' Motrin Concentrated Drops	Ibuprofen 50 mg/1.25 mL
Junior Strength Motrin Chewable Tablets	Ibuprofen 100 mg
Adult Formulations of Ibuprofen Products	
Advil Migraine Solubilized Capsules	Ibuprofen 200 mg
Advil Tablets/Caplets/Gel Caplets/ Film-Coated Tablets[a]	Ibuprofen 200 mg
Motrin IB Tablets/Caplets	Ibuprofen 200 mg
Naproxen Products	
Aleve Tablets/Caplets/Liquid Gels/ Gel Caps	Naproxen sodium 220 mg
Midol Extended Relief Caplets	Naproxen sodium 220 mg

[a] Provided as 256 mg of ibuprofen sodium.

epigastric pain, even among children using pediatric formulations. NSAIDs may be taken with food, milk, or antacids if upset stomach occurs. Tablets should be taken with a full glass of water, suspensions should be shaken thoroughly, and enteric-coated or sustained-release preparations should be neither crushed nor chewed. Other adverse effects include dizziness, fatigue, headache, and nervousness. Rashes or itching, photosensitivity, and fluid retention or edema may occur in some patients; however, at normal doses, these effects are usually rare.

GI ulceration, perforation, and bleeding are uncommon but serious complications of NSAID use. Risk factors include

a word about
NSAIDs and Stomach Bleeding

In 2010, FDA approved a label warning concerning stomach bleeding for nonprescription products that contain NSAIDs in adult doses:

Stomach bleeding warning: This product contains an NSAID, which may cause severe stomach bleeding. The chance is higher if you:

- Are age 60 or older.
- Have had stomach ulcers or bleeding problems.
- Take a blood thinning (anticoagulant) or steroid drug.
- Take other drugs containing prescription or nonprescription NSAIDs (aspirin, ibuprofen, naproxen, or others).
- Have 3 or more alcoholic drinks every day while using this product.
- Take more or for a longer time than directed.

Ask a doctor before use if the stomach bleeding warning applies to you:

- You have a history of stomach problems, such as heartburn.
- You have high blood pressure, heart disease, liver cirrhosis, or kidney disease.
- You are taking a diuretic.

Stop use and ask a doctor if:

- You experience any of the following signs of stomach bleeding:
  - Feel faint.
  - Vomit blood.
  - Have bloody or black stools.[34]
  - Have stomach pain that does not get better.

age older than 60 years, prior ulcer disease for GI bleeding, concurrent use of anticoagulants (including aspirin), higher dose or longer duration of treatment, and moderate use of alcohol. Package labeling for NSAIDs includes warnings about stomach bleeding with adult doses (see the box A Word about NSAIDs and Stomach Bleeding).[23]

NSAIDs are associated with increased risk for myocardial infarction, heart failure, hypertension, and stroke. The mechanism by which the risk is conferred is not clear, but it may be related to increased thromboxane A2 activity and suppressed vascular prostacyclin synthesis, resulting in vasoconstriction and platelet aggregation. According to results from a meta-analysis of randomized trials, the cardiovascular risk of nonselective NSAIDs appears to depend on dose and duration. In addition, the risk differs between individual nonselective NSAIDs. For instance, ibuprofen has been associated with a significant increase in cardiovascular risk, whereas naproxen has not; thus, naproxen is considered the preferred, safer option.[24]

The American Heart Association recommends that patients with or at high risk for cardiovascular disease (e.g., hyperlipidemia, hypertension, diabetes, or other macrovascular disease) avoid NSAIDs. Low-risk patients should exercise caution in using NSAIDs by taking the minimum dose for the shortest duration needed to control symptoms. Clinical evidence has shown that the use of NSAIDs in patients who have a past history of myocardial infarction will increase their risk of future cardiovascular events indefinitely.[25]

Clinically important drug–drug interactions of NSAIDs are listed in Table 5–5. Ibuprofen increases bleeding time by reversibly inhibiting platelet aggregation. Patients taking aspirin for cardiovascular prophylaxis should take it at least 1 hour before or 8 hours after ibuprofen to avoid a pharmacodynamic interaction that inhibits the antiplatelet effect of aspirin. In doses of 1200–2400 mg/day, ibuprofen does not appear to affect the INR in patients taking warfarin. However, ibuprofen should not be recommended for self-treatment in patients who are concurrently taking anticoagulants because its antiplatelet activity could increase GI bleeding.

Patients who ingest three or more alcoholic drinks per day should be cautioned about the increased risk of adverse GI events, including stomach bleeding. They also should be referred to their primary care provider for monitoring of their NSAID use.

NSAIDs may decrease renal blood flow and glomerular filtration rate as a result of inhibition of renal prostaglandin synthesis. Consequently, increased blood urea nitrogen and serum creatinine values can occur, often with concomitant sodium and water retention. Advanced age, hypertension, diabetes, atherosclerotic cardiovascular disease, and use of diuretics appear to increase the risk of renal toxicity with ibuprofen use. Therefore, patients with a history of impaired renal function, congestive heart failure, or diseases that compromise renal hemodynamics should not self-medicate with NSAIDs.

Salicylates

Salicylates inhibit prostaglandin synthesis from arachidonic acid by inhibiting both isoforms of the COX enzyme (COX-1 and COX-2). The resulting decrease in prostaglandins reduces the sensitivity of pain receptors to the initiation of pain impulses at sites of inflammation and trauma. Although some evidence suggests that aspirin also produces analgesia through a central mechanism, its site of action is primarily peripheral.

Salicylates are absorbed by passive diffusion of the non-ionized drug in the stomach and small intestine. Factors affecting absorption include dosage form, gastric pH, gastric-emptying time, dissolution rate, and the presence of antacids or food. Absorption from immediate-release aspirin products is complete. Rectal absorption of a salicylate suppository is slow and unreliable, as well as proportional to rectal retention time.

Once absorbed, aspirin is hydrolyzed in the plasma to salicylic acid in 1–2 hours. Salicylic acid is widely distributed to all tissues and fluids in the body, including the CNS, breast milk, and fetal tissue. Protein binding is concentration dependent. At concentrations lower than 100 mg/mL, approximately 90% of salicylic acid is bound to albumin, whereas at concentrations greater than 400 mg/mL, approximately 75% is bound. Salicylic acid is largely eliminated through the kidney. Urine pH determines the amount of unchanged drug that is eliminated, with urinary concentrations increasing substantially in more alkaline urine (pH ~8).

Dosage form alterations include enteric coating, buffering, and sustained release. These formulations were developed to change the rate of absorption and/or reduce the potential for GI toxicity. Enteric-coated aspirin is absorbed only from the small intestine; its absorption is markedly slowed by food, which is attributed to prolonged gastric-emptying time. Hypochlorhydria from acid-suppressing agents (especially proton pump inhibitors) may result in dissolution of enteric-coated products in the stomach, negating any potential benefit on local gastric toxicity. For patients requiring rapid pain relief, enteric-coated aspirin is inappropriate because of the delay in absorption and the time to analgesic effect.

Buffered aspirin products are available in both tablet and effervescent forms. Although buffered products are absorbed more rapidly than are nonbuffered products, time to onset of effect is not improved appreciably. Common buffers include aluminum hydroxide; magnesium carbonate, hydroxide, or oxide; calcium carbonate; and sodium bicarbonate (in effervescent formulations). Some effervescent aspirin solutions contain large amounts of sodium and must be avoided by patients who require restricted sodium intake (e.g., patients with hypertension, heart failure, or renal failure). Sustained-release aspirin is formulated to prolong duration of action by slowing dissolution and absorption. Magnesium salicylate is available as a tablet or capsule. Sodium salicylate is approved for nonprescription use, but it is not currently available in a commercial product.

FDA-approved uses for salicylates include treatment of symptoms for osteoarthritis, rheumatoid arthritis, and other rheumatologic diseases, as well as temporary relief of minor aches and pains associated with backache or muscle aches. Salicylates also are effective in treating mild-moderate pain from musculoskeletal conditions and fever. Because of its inhibitory effects on platelet function, aspirin is also indicated for prevention of thromboembolic events (e.g., myocardial infarction and stroke) in high-risk patients.

Recommended children and adult dosages of nonprescription salicylates are provided in Tables 5–2 and 5–3. Table 5–7 provides selected salicylate products. Aspirin dosages ranging from 4–6 g/day are usually needed to produce anti-inflammatory effects. The maximum analgesic dosage for self-medication with aspirin is 4 g/day; therefore, anti-inflammatory activity often will not occur unless the drug is used at the high end of the acceptable dosage range.

table 5-7	Selected Adult Formulations of Nonprescription Single-Entity Salicylate Products

Trade Name	Primary Ingredients
Bayer Low-Dose Aspirin Tablets	Aspirin 81 mg
St. Joseph 81 mg Chewable Aspirin	Aspirin 81 mg
Ecotrin Regular Strength Safety Enteric-Coated Tablets	Aspirin 325 mg
Genuine Bayer Aspirin Tablets	Aspirin 325 mg
Bayer Plus Extra Strength	Aspirin 500 mg
Extra Strength Doan's Caplets	Magnesium salicylate 580 mg
Percogesic Maximum Strength Backache Relief Coated Caplets	Magnesium salicylate tetrahydrate 580 mg

Mild salicylate intoxication (salicylism) occurs with chronic toxic blood levels, generally achieved in adults who take 90–100 mg/kg/day of a salicylate for at least 2 days. Conditions that predispose patients to salicylate toxicity include (1) marked renal or hepatic impairment (e.g., uremia, cirrhosis, or hepatitis); (2) metabolic disorders (e.g., hypoxia or hypothyroidism); (3) unstable disease (e.g., cardiac arrhythmias, intractable epilepsy, or poorly controlled diabetes); (4) status asthmaticus; and (5) multiple comorbidities. Symptoms include headache, dizziness, tinnitus, difficulty hearing, dimness of vision, mental confusion, lassitude, drowsiness, sweating, thirst, hyperventilation, nausea, vomiting, and occasional diarrhea. These symptoms can all be reversed by lowering the plasma concentration to a therapeutic range. Tinnitus, typically one of the early signs of toxicity, should not be used as a sole indicator of salicylate toxicity.

Acute salicylate intoxication is categorized as mild (ingestion of <150 mg/kg), moderate (ingestion of 150–300 mg/kg), or severe (ingestion of >300 mg/kg). Symptoms depend on the concentration and include lethargy, nausea, vomiting, dehydration, tinnitus, hemorrhage, tachypnea and pulmonary edema, convulsions, and coma. Acid–base disturbances are prominent and range from respiratory alkalosis to metabolic acidosis. Initially, salicylate affects the respiratory center in the medulla, producing hyperventilation and respiratory alkalosis. In severely intoxicated adults and in most salicylate-poisoned children younger than 5 years, respiratory alkalosis progresses rapidly to metabolic acidosis. Children are more prone than are adults to develop high fever in salicylate poisoning. Hypoglycemia resulting from increased glucose utilization may be especially serious in children. Bleeding may occur from the GI tract or mucosal surfaces, and petechiae are a prominent feature at autopsy.

Emergency management of acute salicylate intoxication is directed toward preventing absorption of salicylate from the GI tract and providing supportive care. Activated charcoal should be used at home only if recommended by poison control center or emergency department personnel. In an emergency department setting, gastrointestinal decontamination with gastric lavage or activated charcoal may be undertaken. Enhancing renal elimination can be accomplished through alkalinization of the urine. Dosing recommendations for the use of activated charcoal are included in Chapter 20.

Aspirin is known to commonly cause dyspepsia, which may be minimized by taking it with food. In addition, aspirin is associated with gastritis and ulceration of the upper GI tract. It produces GI mucosal damage by penetrating the protective mucous and bicarbonate layers of the gastric mucosa and permitting back diffusion of acid, thereby causing cellular and vascular erosion. Two distinct mechanisms cause this problem: (1) a local irritant effect resulting from the medication contacting the gastric mucosa and (2) a systemic effect from prostaglandin inhibition. Lack of upper abdominal pain or discomfort is not a reliable indicator for the absence of gastrointestinal damage associated with use of aspirin or other NSAIDs.[26]

The use of aspirin has been shown to increase the risk for serious upper GI events two- to fourfold.[26] It is recommended that the lowest effective dose be used for cardioprotection (usually 81 mg) and that the use of proton pump inhibitors may be indicated for gastric protection.[26] Patients with risk factors for upper GI bleeding should avoid self-treatment with aspirin. These risk factors include (1) history of uncomplicated or bleeding peptic ulcer; (2) age older than 60 years; (3) concomitant use of aspirin or other NSAIDs, anticoagulants, antiplatelet agents, bisphosphonates, selective serotonin reuptake inhibitors, or systemic corticosteroids; (4) infection with *Helicobacter pylori;* (5) rheumatoid arthritis; (6) NSAID-related dyspepsia; and (7) concomitant use of alcohol.[27]

Various aspirin formulations may have different rates of GI side effects. Enteric coating may decrease local gastric irritation. However, with regard to the risk of major GI ulceration and bleeding, no difference has been identified among plain, enteric-coated, and buffered products.

Serious aspirin intolerance is uncommon and consists of two types: cutaneous (urticaria and angioedema) or respiratory (bronchospasm, laryngospasm, and rhinorrhea). The mechanism is not immunologically mediated. Risk factors for serious aspirin intolerance include chronic urticaria (for the cutaneous type) and asthma with nasal polyps (for the respiratory type). Ten percent of people diagnosed with asthma have aspirin sensitivity.[28] Severity of the intolerance is variable, ranging from minor to severe. Patients with aspirin intolerance generally are advised to avoid aspirin and other NSAIDs. However, the nonacetylated salicylates (magnesium salicylate) are considered safe, and acetaminophen will not cause cross-sensitivity.[28]

Nonprescription salicylates interact with several other important drugs and drug classes. Clinically important drug interactions of salicylates are listed in Table 5–5. When monitoring therapy in patients who are taking high-dose salicylates, health care providers should review current drug interaction references for newly identified interactions.

Aspirin ingestion may produce positive results on fecal occult blood testing; therefore, its use should be discontinued for at least 3 days before testing. Similarly, aspirin should be discontinued 2–7 days before surgery and should not be used to relieve pain after tonsillectomy, dental extraction, or other surgical procedures, except under the close supervision of a health care provider. Aspirin can potentiate bleeding from capillary sites such as those found in the GI tract, tonsillar beds, and tooth sockets.

Because of the effect on hemostasis, aspirin is contraindicated in patients with hypoprothrombinemia, vitamin K deficiency, hemophilia, history of any bleeding disorder, or history of peptic ulcer disease. Patients with compromised renal function have the potential for decreased renal excretion of magnesium, allowing accumulation of toxic levels when taking magnesium salicylate. The maximum 24-hour dose of magnesium salicylate contains 264 mg (11 mEq) of magnesium.

All salicylates should be avoided in patients with a history of gout or hyperuricemia because of dose-related effects on renal uric acid handling. Dosages of 1–2 g/day inhibit tubular uric acid secretion without affecting reabsorption and may increase plasma uric acid levels, which can precipitate or worsen a gout attack. Moderate dosages of 2–3 g/day have little effect on uric acid secretion. More than 5 g/day may decrease plasma uric acid by increasing its renal excretion, but because these salicylate doses are toxic, they should not be used in the clinical management of gout or hyperuricemia.

Reye's syndrome is an acute illness occurring almost exclusively in children 15 years of age or younger. The cause is unknown, but viral and toxic agents, especially salicylates, have been associated with the syndrome. Onset usually follows a viral infection with influenza (type A or B) or varicella zoster (chickenpox). Reye's syndrome is characterized by progressive neurologic damage, fatty liver with encephalopathy, and hypoglycemia. The mortality rate may be as high as 50%.

The American Academy of Pediatrics, FDA, the Centers for Disease Control and Prevention, and the Surgeon General have issued warnings that aspirin and other salicylates (including bismuth subsalicylate and nonaspirin salicylates) should be avoided in children and teenagers who have influenza or chickenpox. The following contraindication is listed on labels of nonprescription aspirin and aspirin-containing products:

> Aspirin should not be used in children and teenagers for viral infections, with or without fever, because of the risk of Reye's syndrome with concomitant use of aspirin in certain viral illnesses.

Although a simple viral upper respiratory infection (e.g., a common cold) is not a contraindication to aspirin use, it can be difficult to differentiate symptoms of this type of infection from those of influenza and chickenpox. Many health care providers, therefore, recommend a conservative approach of avoiding aspirin whenever symptoms resembling those of influenza are present. The use of aspirin as a pediatric antipyretic has all but ceased in the United States, as have reports of Reye's syndrome.

FDA requires a warning label regarding alcohol use on all nonprescription analgesic/antipyretic products for adult use. Concurrent use of aspirin with alcohol increases the risk of adverse GI events, including stomach bleeding. Patients who consume three or more alcoholic drinks daily should be counseled about the risks and referred to their primary care provider before using aspirin.

Combination Products

Many nonprescription analgesics are available in combination products (Table 5–8).

Caffeine is used as an adjunct to analgesics for tension-type and migraine headaches. It also may have its own analgesic properties and is known to cause withdrawal headache when taken regularly. Combination dosage forms containing a decongestant and either acetaminophen or an NSAID are also available. These combinations appear logical for use in sinus headaches or other indications for which both analgesia and decongestion are needed.

table 5–8 **Selected Nonprescription Combination Analgesic Products**

Trade Name	Primary Ingredients
Acetaminophen-Containing Products	
Excedrin Tension Headache	Acetaminophen 500 mg; caffeine 65 mg
Excedrin PM	Acetaminophen 500 mg; 38 mg
Excedrin Sinus	Acetaminophen 325 mg; phenylephrine 5 mg
Goody's PM Powder	Acetaminophen 500 mg; diphenhydramine 38 mg
Percogesic Original Strength	Acetaminophen 325 mg; diphenhydramine 12.5 mg
Percogesic Extra Strength	Acetaminophen 500 mg; diphenhydramine 12.5 mg
Sudafed PE Pressure + Pain	Acetaminophen 325 mg; phenylephrine 5 mg
Tylenol PM	Acetaminophen 500 mg; diphenhydramine 25 mg
Tylenol Sinus Congestion and Pain	Acetaminophen 325 mg; phenylephrine 5 mg
NSAID-Containing Products	
Advil Cold & Sinus	Ibuprofen 200 mg; pseudoephedrine 30 mg
Advil Congestion Relief	Ibuprofen 200 mg; phenylephrine 10 mg
Aleve-D Sinus & Headache	Naproxen sodium 220 mg; pseudoephedrine 120 mg
Motrin PM	Naproxen sodium 200 mg; diphenhydramine 38 mg
Sudafed 12h Pressure + Pain	Naproxen sodium 220 mg; pseudoephedrine 120 mg
Aspirin-Containing Products	
Anacin Maximum Strength	Aspirin 500 mg; caffeine 32 mg
Anacin Regular Strength	Aspirin 400 mg; caffeine 32 mg
Bayer Cafiaspirina	Aspirin 500 mg; caffeine 40 mg
Excedrin Extra Strength or Excedrin Migraine	Aspirin 250 mg; acetaminophen 250 mg; caffeine 65 mg
Goody's Cool Orange Powder	Aspirin 500 mg; acetaminophen 325 mg; caffeine 65 mg
Goody's Extra Strength Headache Powder	Aspirin 500 mg; acetaminophen 260 mg; caffeine 32.5 mg
Goody's Extra Strength or Goody's Migraine Relief caps	Aspirin 250 mg; acetaminophen 250 mg; caffeine 65 mg

Key: NSAID = Nonsteroidal anti-inflammatory.

Enhanced analgesia has been reported for various antihistamine/analgesic combinations, including orphenadrine/acetaminophen and phenyltoloxamine/acetaminophen. Although these combinations have demonstrated superior efficacy in acute pain, compared with acetaminophen alone, their use is limited by the sedating effects of the antihistamines.

Pharmacotherapeutic Comparison
Aspirin versus Nonacetylated Salicylates

Although definitive clinical data are lacking, aspirin and nonacetylated salicylates are believed to be equal in anti-inflammatory potency; however, aspirin is thought to be a superior analgesic and antipyretic.

Aspirin versus Acetaminophen

Numerous controlled studies have demonstrated the equivalent analgesic efficacy of aspirin and acetaminophen on a milligram-for-milligram basis; however, statistical methods used to compare effectiveness between different studies show that acetaminophen may not be quite as effective in some types of pain.[29]

Aspirin versus NSAID

Ibuprofen has been shown to be at least as effective as aspirin in treating various types of pain, including dental extraction pain, dysmenorrhea, and episiotomy pain. Because aspirin must be dosed near the self-care maximum to achieve anti-inflammatory effects, NSAIDs may be preferred for self-treatment of inflammatory disorders such as rheumatoid arthritis or acute muscle injury.[29]

NSAID versus Acetaminophen

For episodic tension-type headache, acetaminophen 1000 mg appears to provide relief that is equivalent to naproxen 375 mg.[30] For moderate-severe dental or sore throat pain in children, single doses of acetaminophen 7–15 mg/kg produced pain relief similar to that of ibuprofen 4–10 mg/kg. Ibuprofen was a more effective antipyretic, and both drugs were well tolerated.[31] A review of evidence comparing ibuprofen with acetaminophen for headache treatment in children and adults found that only two trials had shown a modest advantage for ibuprofen, and the researchers concluded that the two agents should be considered equally effective.[32] Acetaminophen does not have anti-inflammatory properties, which may limit its effectiveness in some conditions, including dysmenorrhea.[29]

Naproxen versus Ibuprofen

Naproxen sodium 220 mg and ibuprofen 200 mg appear to have similar efficacy. The onset of activity also is similar between the two NSAIDs. Duration of action of naproxen is somewhat longer than that of ibuprofen, but the clinical significance of this difference is not clear. Nonetheless, some patients report better response to one NSAID than to another for reasons that are unclear.

Product Selection Guidelines
Special Population Considerations

Age is an important consideration in the selection of an appropriate nonprescription medication for self-treatment of headache. Parents of children younger than 8 years should consult a pediatrician prior to giving their children nonprescription medications. Children 2 years and older may use acetaminophen or ibuprofen. Children 12 years and older may use naproxen. To decrease the risk of Reye's syndrome, parents should not use aspirin or aspirin-containing products in children ages 15 years or younger, unless directed to do so by a primary care provider.

Older adults are at increased risk for many adverse effects of salicylates and NSAIDs. Comorbidities, impaired renal function, and use of other medications contribute to the increased risk. Older adults are more vulnerable to serious GI toxicity, hypertensive, and renal effects of salicylates and NSAIDs.[33] For this reason, acetaminophen is generally recognized as the treatment of choice for management of mild-moderate pain in older adults.

When aspirin's effect on hemostasis is a concern and peripheral anti-inflammatory activity is not needed, acetaminophen is an appropriate analgesic for self-medication. Alternatively, if a peripheral anti-inflammatory agent is indicated, prescription salicylate compounds (e.g., salsalate and choline magnesium trisalicylate) are reasonable alternatives.

Acetaminophen crosses the placenta but it is considered safe for use during pregnancy (FDA pregnancy category B). Acetaminophen appears in breast milk, producing a milk-to-maternal plasma ratio of 0.5:1.0. A 1-gram maternal dose has an estimated maximum infant dose that is 1.85% of the maternal dose. The only adverse effect reported in infants exposed to acetaminophen through breast milk is a rarely occurring maculopapular rash, which subsides upon drug discontinuation. Acetaminophen use is considered compatible with breast-feeding.

No evidence exists that NSAIDs are teratogenic in either humans or animals. However, use of these agents is contraindicated during the third trimester of pregnancy because all potent prostaglandin synthesis inhibitors can cause delayed parturition, prolonged labor, and increased postpartum bleeding. Ibuprofen and naproxen are pregnancy categories B and C, respectively, in the first trimester and pregnancy category D in the third trimester. These agents also can have adverse fetal cardiovascular effects (e.g., premature closure of the ductus arteriosus). Lactating women taking up to 2.4 grams of ibuprofen per day showed no measurable excretion of ibuprofen into breast milk; therefore, ibuprofen is considered compatible with breast-feeding. Naproxen also is considered compatible with breast-feeding.

Aspirin should be avoided during pregnancy, especially during the last trimester, and during breast-feeding. Aspirin is pregnancy category D during the last trimester; its ingestion during pregnancy may produce maternal adverse effects, such as anemia, antepartum or postpartum hemorrhage, and prolonged gestation and labor. Regular aspirin ingestion during pregnancy may increase the risk for complicated deliveries, including unplanned cesarean section, breech delivery, or forceps delivery. However, definitive data supporting this concern are lacking.

Aspirin readily crosses the placenta and can be found in higher concentrations in the neonate than in the mother. Salicylate elimination is slow in neonates because of the liver's immaturity and underdeveloped capacity to form glycine and glucuronic acid conjugates and because of reduced urinary excretion resulting from low glomerular filtration rates.

Fetal effects from in utero aspirin exposure include intrauterine growth retardation, congenital salicylate intoxication, decreased albumin-binding capacity, and increased perinatal mortality. In utero mortality results, in part, from antepartum hemorrhage or premature closure of the ductus arteriosus. In utero aspirin exposure within 1 week of delivery can produce neonatal hemorrhagic episodes and/or pruritic rash. Reported neonatal bleeding complications include petechiae, hematuria, cephalhematoma, subconjunctival hemorrhage, and bleeding after circumcision. An increased incidence of intracranial hemorrhage in premature or low-birth-weight infants associated with maternal aspirin use near the time of birth also has been reported.[34] An association between maternal aspirin ingestion, oral clefts, and congenital heart disease has been reported. However, the relationship between maternal aspirin ingestion and congenital malformation remains unresolved, and studies have failed to confirm a relationship between maternal ingestion of aspirin and increased risk for fetal malformation.

Aspirin and other salicylates are excreted into breast milk in low concentrations. After single-dose oral salicylate ingestion, peak milk levels occur at about 3 hours, producing a milk-to-maternal plasma ratio of 3:8. Although no adverse effects on platelet function in nursing infants exposed to aspirin via breast milk have been reported, these agents still must be considered a potential risk.[34]

Patients with renal impairment should exercise caution when using salicylates. Clinically important alterations in renal blood flow resulting in acute reduction in renal function can result from use of even short courses of salicylates. Renally impaired patients should be referred for medical evaluation for assistance in selecting an analgesic.

Patient Factors

Nonprescription analgesics are available in a number of dosage forms. During patient assessment, health care providers should determine which dosage form will provide an optimum outcome for the patient. If rapid response is desired, then immediate-release oral dosage forms would be preferred over coated or extended-release forms. For patients experiencing migraine headache with severe nausea, rectal dosage forms may be preferred. Liquid dosage forms often are used in children or adult patients who have difficulty swallowing solid dosage forms.

Use of acetaminophen in the pediatric population is complicated by the various available strengths and formulations. Unintended over- or underdosing can occur when parents switch between infant drops (80 mg/0.8 mL) and elixir (160 mg/5 mL), incorrectly assuming that they are the same concentration.

Other issues with pediatric doses of acetaminophen were discussed at a joint meeting of the Nonprescription Drugs Advisory Committee and the Pediatric Advisory Committee; the committees recommended (1) a single concentration for solid-dose, single-ingredient acetaminophen products for children, (2) the addition of weight-based dosing for children ages 2–12, and (3) the addition of new label directions for children ages 6 months to 2 years that would include the indication for fever reduction.

In addition, rapidly growing infants quickly outgrow previous dose requirements. Therefore, recalculation of the pediatric dose according to present age and body weight is recommended at the time of each treatment course.

Patients with significant alcohol ingestion (three or more drinks per day) should avoid self-treatment with nonprescription analgesics.

Patients who are intolerant to aspirin also may cross-react with other chemicals or drugs. Up to 15% of patients who are intolerant to aspirin may cross-react when exposed to tartrazine (Food Drug and Cosmetic Yellow Dye No. 5), which can be found in many drugs and foods. Among those with the respiratory type of aspirin sensitivity, the rate of cross-reaction between aspirin and acetaminophen, ibuprofen, and naproxen in documented aspirin-intolerant patients is 7%, 98%, and 100%, respectively.[34] High cross-reaction rates also are reported with some prescription NSAIDs. The proposed mechanism of cross-sensitivity between aspirin and NSAIDs involves shunting arachidonic metabolism down the lipoxygenase pathway (because of inhibition of the COX-1 enzyme pathway), resulting in accumulation of leukotrienes that can cause bronchospasm and anaphylaxis. Acetaminophen and nonacetylated salicylates are weak inhibitors of COX-1 at moderate doses. Therefore, patients with a history of aspirin intolerance should be advised to avoid all aspirin- and NSAID-containing products, and to use acetaminophen or a nonacetylated salicylate, with the caveat that acetaminophen does not offer anti-inflammatory properties.

Patient Preferences

Consideration of dosing frequency in product selection may improve outcomes for individual patients. Naproxen can be taken 2–3 times daily and may improve patient adherence. Conversely, acetaminophen, ibuprofen, and salicylates may require dosing as frequently as every 4 hours. Because of the delayed absorption of sustained-release aspirin, this dosage form is not useful for rapid pain relief but may be useful as a bedtime medication.

Complementary Therapies

Butterbur, feverfew, riboflavin, and coenzyme Q10 commonly are used for the prevention of migraine headaches and are discussed in depth in Chapter 51. These natural products are generally ineffective for the treatment of headaches. Other unproven remedies include peppermint oil applied to the forehead and temples for treatment of tension headache, magnesium for treatment and prevention of migraine, and riboflavin for prevention of migraine headache.

Acupuncture has been used to prevent migraine and tension-type headache. Evaluation of acupuncture is complicated by difficulties in blinding and differences in identifying acupuncture points. Overall, results have been variable, but several randomized, placebo-controlled trials found acupuncture effective in reducing frequency and severity of headache.[35]

Assessment of Headache: A Case-Based Approach

Before self-treatment of headache can be recommended, the health care provider must assess the patient's headache as to type, severity, location, frequency, intensity over time, and age at onset. The next step is to obtain a medical and psychosocial history. All current medications should be inventoried, and all past and present headache treatments should be reviewed, with emphasis on determining which treatments, if any, were successful or preferred.

Secondary headaches, other than minor sinus headache, are excluded from self-treatment. Headache associated with seizures, confusion, drowsiness, or cognitive impairment may be a sign of brain tumor, ischemic stroke, subdural hematoma, or subarachnoid hemorrhage. Headache accompanied by nausea, vomiting, fever, and stiff neck may indicate brain abscess or meningitis. Headache with night sweats, aching joints, fever, weight loss, and visual symptoms (e.g., blurring) in patients with rheumatoid arthritis may indicate cranial arteritis. Headache associated with localized facial pain, muscle tenderness, and limited motion of the jaw may indicate temporomandibular joint disorder.

Cases 5–1 and 5–2 illustrate assessment of a patient with headache.

Patient Counseling for Headache

To optimize outcomes from therapy, the provider should instruct patients to take an appropriate dose of analgesic early in the course of the headache. The use of nonprescription analgesics to preempt or abort migraine headaches also should be explained to patients with migraines whose headaches are predictable. Patients who have headaches with some frequency should be encouraged to keep a log of their headaches to document triggers, frequency, intensity, duration of episodes, and response to treatment. This record also may be helpful in identifying factors that can improve headache prevention and treatment. Patients should be advised that continuing or escalating pain can be a sign of a more serious problem and that prompt medical attention is warranted. Appropriate drug and nondrug measures for

case

5–1

Relevant Evaluation Criteria	Scenario/Model Outcome
Information Gathering	
1. Gather essential information about the patient's symptoms and medical history, including:	
a. description of symptom(s) (i.e., nature, onset, duration, severity, associated symptoms)	Patient states that a severe headache took place yesterday and incapacitated him for almost 8 hours. The pain eventually subsided, but nothing he could do would make it stop. This type of headache has happened several times in the past 2 months.
b. description of any factors that seem to precipitate, exacerbate, and/or relieve the patient's symptom(s)	Bright light and loud sounds made the pain worse. Even slight movements of his head resulted in discomfort.
c. description of the patient's efforts to relieve the symptoms	He states that the only thing he could do was to lie down on his bed with the curtains drawn and the door shut. Acetaminophen has not been helping.
d. patient's identity	Dom Rugolo
e. age, sex, height, and weight	26 years old, male, 6 ft 1 in., 245 lb
f. patient's occupation	Produce manager at a grocery store
g. patient's dietary habits	He eats healthy some of the time but does like fruits and vegetables. He sometimes has difficulty eating regularly. He skips breakfast a lot because of his busy schedule and often eats frozen dinners because they are quick and easy.
h. patient's sleep habits	He has no problems sleeping. Because of the nature of his work, he has to be up at 5 am most days, but he tries to compensate for the early rising by going to bed at a decent hour.
i. concurrent medical conditions, prescription and nonprescription medications, and dietary supplements	He has mild acne on his face that is currently being treated with tretinoin cream 0.025% applied topically daily.
j. allergies	Bactrim caused a bad rash a few years ago.
k. history of other adverse reactions to medications	None
l. other (describe) _____	He does not smoke but does drink infrequently with friends (1 or 2 beers every few weeks).
Assessment and Triage	
2. Differentiate patient's signs/symptoms and correctly identify the patient's primary problem(s) (Table 5–1).	Mr. Rugolo might be having migraine headaches as indicated by intense pain that is exacerbated by bright lights, sounds, and head movement.
3. Identify exclusions for self-treatment (Figure 5–1).	Undiagnosed migraine is an exclusion for self-treatment.
4. Formulate a comprehensive list of therapeutic alternatives for the primary problem to determine if triage to a medical practitioner is required, and share this information with the patient or caregiver.	Options include: (1) Refer Mr. Rugolo to an appropriate health care provider. (2) Recommend self-care with a nonprescription analgesic. (3) Recommend self-care until Mr. Rugolo can see an appropriate health care provider. (4) Take no action.

Relevant Evaluation Criteria	Scenario/Model Outcome

Plan

5. Select an optimal therapeutic alternative to address the patient's problem, taking into account patient preferences.

Referral to a health care provider is appropriate for Mr. Rugolo. He may need a prescription-only therapy that is specific for migraines. Until a health care provider can be seen, the patient should take ibuprofen 200 mg every 4–6 hours. The dosage can be increased to 400 mg if necessary but is limited to 6 tablets per day. The patient should take the medication as soon as he feels the headache begin.

6. Describe the recommended therapeutic approach to the patient or caregiver.

"What you have been experiencing may be migraine headaches. It is recommended that you seek evaluation by your primary care provider to determine appropriate treatment. Take ibuprofen at the onset of headache until you can see your health care provider."

7. Explain to the patient or caregiver the rationale for selecting the recommended therapeutic approach from the considered therapeutic alternatives.

"Ibuprofen may be a good alternative to the acetaminophen you were taking because it is in a different class of medication and exerts its therapeutic action in a different manner. The most benefit will be seen if the ibuprofen is taken at the earliest sign of headache, rather than waiting for the pain to become severe."

Patient Education

8. When recommending self-care with nonprescription medications and/or nondrug therapy, convey accurate information to the patient or caregiver:

   a. appropriate dose and frequency of administration

"Take ibuprofen 200 mg, 1 tablet every 4–6 hours. This dosage may be increased to 400 mg (2 tablets) every 4–6 hours if needed. Do not exceed 6 tablets in a 24-hour period."

   b. maximum number of days the therapy should be employed

"Use this medication only until you are able to see your health care provider. Self-care for a headache should not exceed 10 days. Also, limit treatment to 3 days per week."

   c. product administration procedures

"Start ibuprofen at the first sign of headache."

   d. expected time to onset of relief

"Relief should begin in 30–60 minutes."

   e. degree of relief that can be reasonably expected

"Complete resolution of your symptoms is unlikely. For this reason, you will need to see your health care provider."

   f. most common side effects

"Stomach upset. Taking ibuprofen with food may help prevent that."

   g. side effects that warrant medical intervention should they occur

"Ibuprofen should be stopped if there is severe stomach pain, bloody vomit, black stool, abnormal bruising or bleeding, or allergic reaction (swelling of the face or throat, difficulty breathing)."

   h. patient options in the event that condition worsens or persists

"Follow up with the health care provider."

   i. product storage requirements

"Store ibuprofen in a closed container at room temperature away from moisture and children."

   j. Specific nondrug measures

"Keep track of events prior to the headaches to try and determine possible triggers."

Solicit follow-up questions from the patient or caregiver.

"Are there effective treatments for these headaches that my doctor can give me? I don't want to keep having my life disrupted by them."

Answer the patient's or caregiver's questions.

"Multiple prescription medications for migraine headaches that have established safety and efficacy are available. Your health care provider will determine the appropriate course of treatment to help you minimize the effects that the headaches have on your life."

Evaluation of Patient Outcome

9. Assess patient outcome.

Call the patient in a few days to determine whether he is receiving further medical care.

case
5-2

Relevant Evaluation Criteria	Scenario/Model Outcome

Information Gathering

1. Gather essential information about the patient's symptoms and medical history, including:

   a. description of symptom(s) (i.e., nature, onset, duration, severity, associated symptoms)

   Patient states that she has had two mild headaches in the past few weeks. Both times the pain went from the top to the base of her head. The pain lasted only a few hours and went away by itself, but it was significant enough to prevent her from getting her work done for class. She wants to plan ahead for the next headache so she does not have to sacrifice study time.

   b. description of any factors that seem to precipitate, exacerbate, and/or relieve the patient's symptom(s)

   The headaches have been happening before exams when her stress is at its peak.

   c. description of the patient's efforts to relieve the symptoms

   She states that she stopped focusing on her work and relaxed until she fell asleep.

   d. patient's identity

   Marta Schuler

   e. age, sex, height, and weight

   22 years old, female, 5 ft 8 in., 130 lb

   f. patient's occupation

   Full-time student

   g. patient's dietary habits

   She tries to eat healthy but is often on the run and skips breakfast frequently. For lunch she usually grabs a bagel and tea from the cafeteria. Dinner is usually a wrap or a salad, and she snacks on cashews throughout the day.

   h. patient's sleep habits

   She tries to go to bed by midnight because she has class at 8 am. She sometimes stays up late studying, but that happens infrequently and usually does not disrupt her normal sleep pattern.

   i. concurrent medical conditions, prescription and nonprescription medications, and dietary supplements

   She has mild asthma for which she has an emergency inhaler that she has not needed in months.

   j. allergies

   None

   k. history of other adverse reactions to medications

   None

   l. other (describe) _____

   Ms. Schuler drinks socially on the weekend and says that she has a couple of drinks to unwind. She does not smoke.

Assessment and Triage

2. Differentiate patient's signs/symptoms and correctly identify the patient's primary problem(s) (Table 5–1).

   Ms. Schuler is having a tension headache that is most likely due to the stress of school.

3. Identify exclusions for self-treatment (Figure 5–1).

   Ms. Schuler has no exclusions for self-treatment.

4. Formulate a comprehensive list of therapeutic alternatives for the primary problem to determine if triage to a medical practitioner is required, and share this information with the patient or caregiver.

   Options include:

   (1) Refer Ms. Schuler to an appropriate health care provider.

   (2) Recommend self-care with a nonprescription analgesic.

   (3) Recommend self-care until Ms. Schuler can see an appropriate health care provider.

   (4) Take no action.

Plan

5. Select an optimal therapeutic alternative to address the patient's problem, taking into account patient preferences.

   Ms. Schuler should use a nonprescription analgesic to help relieve her headache pain. Acetaminophen is an appropriate medication for short-term treatment for her symptoms.

6. Describe the recommended therapeutic approach to the patient or caregiver.

   "What you have been experiencing may be tension headaches. It is likely a result of the stress you are experiencing from school. Taking acetaminophen will help to relieve the symptoms."

7. Explain to the patient or caregiver the rationale for selecting the recommended therapeutic approach from the considered therapeutic alternatives.

   "When taken as directed, acetaminophen can provide quick relief of headache symptoms and has a lower chance of gastrointestinal side effects compared with NSAIDs."

case

5–2 *continued*

Relevant Evaluation Criteria	Scenario/Model Outcome

Patient Education

8. When recommending self-care with nonprescription medications and/or nondrug therapy, convey accurate information to the patient or caregiver:

a. appropriate dose and frequency of administration

"Take acetaminophen 500 mg, 1 tablet every 6 hours. This dosage may be increased to 2 tablets every 6 hours, if needed. Do not take more than 6 tablets (3000 mg) in a 24-hour period. Note that many nonprescription and prescription products include acetaminophen, so avoid taking more than one product containing acetaminophen."

b. maximum number of days the therapy should be employed

"Take the acetaminophen for no more than 10 days. Also, limit future treatment to 3 days per week."

c. product administration procedures

"Start acetaminophen when you feel a headache starting. Take the medication with a full glass of water."

d. expected time to onset of relief

"Relief should begin in 30–60 minutes."

e. degree of relief that can be reasonably expected

"Complete resolution of your symptoms is possible."

f. most common side effects

"Nausea and vomiting are the most common side effects."

g. side effects that warrant medical intervention should they occur

"Acetaminophen should be stopped if you experience yellowing of the skin or eyes, bloody vomit, black stool, abnormal bruising or bleeding, or allergic reaction (hives, swelling of the face, difficulty breathing)."

h. patient options in the event that condition worsens or persists

"If acetaminophen does not relieve your headache, you also may try a nonsteroidal anti-inflammatory drug such as ibuprofen or naproxen. Otherwise, seek advice from your health care provider."

i. product storage requirements

"Store acetaminophen in a closed container at room temperature away from moisture and children."

j. Specific nondrug measures

"Managing your stress may help you avoid tension headaches. Relaxation exercises can help with stress management."

Solicit follow-up questions from the patient or caregiver.

"Can I consume alcohol with this medication?"

Answer the patient's or caregiver's questions.

"Consuming alcohol while taking acetaminophen should be avoided. The combination can increase the risk of liver damage."

Evaluation of Patient Outcome

9. Assess patient outcome.

To evaluate efficacy of the treatment, advise patient to call the pharmacy after using the recommended medication.

---

treating headaches should be explained to the patient. Frequent use of nonprescription analgesics is not appropriate because of the risk for medication-overuse headache. Providers should convey the message that nonprescription analgesics are potent medications with accompanying potential adverse effects, interactions, and precautions/warnings. The box Patient Education for Headache lists specific information to provide patients.

patients should seek medical attention if headaches persist longer than 10 days or worsen despite self-treatment.

One-quarter of migraine patients will benefit from preventive therapy but many do not receive it.[36] Patients with migraine headaches who are not adequately self-treated should be referred for a medical evaluation because effective prescription therapies are available to substantially limit pain and disability.

Evaluation of Patient Outcomes for Headache

Appropriate follow-up will depend on headache frequency and severity, as well as patient factors. For patients with episodic headaches, a trial of 6–12 weeks may be needed to assess efficacy of treatment. For chronic headache, follow-up after 4–6 weeks should be adequate to assess treatment efficacy. For severe headaches, patients should be contacted within 10 days of initiation of self-treatment to assess efficacy and tolerability. In all cases,

Key Points for Headache

➤ Most tension-type, migraine, and sinus headaches are amenable to treatment with nonprescription medications.

➤ Patients with symptoms suggestive of secondary headaches (except for minor sinus headache) or undiagnosed migraine headaches should be referred for medical attention.

➤ Many patients with frequent headaches may experience improvement by identifying and modifying environmental, behavioral, nutritional, or other triggers for their headaches.

➤ The choice of nonprescription analgesic for an individual patient depends on patient preferences, presence of precautionary or contraindicating conditions, concomitant medications, cost, and other factors.

➤ Pharmacists have been identified as key sources of information on nonprescription analgesics to reduce risk for acetaminophen-induced hepatotoxicity and NSAID-induced GI bleeding, cardiovascular events, and nephrotoxicity.

➤ Use of nonprescription analgesics for headache should be limited to 3 days per week to prevent medication-overuse headache.

patient education for
Headache

The objectives of self-treatment are to (1) relieve headache pain, (2) prevent headaches when possible, and (3) prevent medication-overuse headaches by avoiding chronic use of nonprescription analgesics. Carefully following product instructions and the self-care measures listed here will help ensure the best results.

Tension-Type Headaches

▪ Nonprescription pain relievers (analgesics) are usually effective in relieving tension-type headaches. However, consult your primary provider before using them for chronic tension-type headaches that occur more than 15 days per month for 6 months.

▪ If nonprescription pain relievers are used for chronic headaches, keep records of how often they are used, and share this information with your provider.

Migraine Headache

▪ Avoid substances (food, caffeine, alcohol, and medications) or situations (stress, fatigue, oversleeping, fasting, and missing meals) that you know can trigger a migraine.

▪ Use the following nutritional strategies to prevent migraine:
  - Avoid foods or food additives known to trigger migraines, including red wine, aged cheese, aspartame, monosodium glutamate, coffee, tea, cola beverages, and chocolate.
  - Avoid foods to which you are allergic.
  - Eat regularly to avoid hunger and low blood sugar.
  - Consider taking magnesium supplements.

▪ If onset of migraines is predictable (e.g., headache occurs during menstruation), take aspirin, ibuprofen, or naproxen to prevent the headache. Start taking the analgesic 2 days before you expect the headache and continue regular use during the time the headache might start.

▪ Try to stop a migraine by taking aspirin, acetaminophen, or a nonsteroidal anti-inflammatory agent (NSAID) at the onset of headache pain.

▪ If desired, use an ice bag or cold pack applied with pressure to the forehead or temples to reduce the pain associated with acute migraine attacks.

Sinus Headache

▪ Consider using a combination of a decongestant and a nonprescription analgesic to relieve the pain of sinus headache.

Precautions for Nonprescription Analgesics

▪ If you are pregnant or breast-feeding, consult your primary care provider before taking any nonprescription medications.

▪ If you have a medical condition or are taking prescription medications, obtain medical advice before taking any of these medications. Nonprescription analgesics are known to interact with several medications.

▪ Do not take nonprescription analgesics longer than 10 days unless a medical provider has recommended prolonged use.

▪ Do not take these medications if you consume three or more alcoholic beverages daily.

▪ Do not exceed recommended dosages.

▪ Products containing aspartame and/or phenylalanine (usually chewable tablets) should not be given to individuals with phenylketonuria.

Salicylates (Aspirin and Magnesium Salicylate) and NSAIDs (Ibuprofen and Naproxen)

▪ Do not take aspirin during the last 3 months of pregnancy unless a primary care provider is supervising such use. Unsupervised use of this medication could harm the unborn child or cause complications during delivery.

▪ Do not give aspirin or other salicylates to children 15 years of age or younger who are recovering from chickenpox or influenza. To avoid the risk of Reye's syndrome, a rare but potentially fatal condition, use acetaminophen for pain relief.

▪ Do not take aspirin or NSAIDs if you are allergic to aspirin or have asthma and nasal polyps. Take acetaminophen instead.

▪ Do not take aspirin or NSAIDs if you have stomach problems or ulcers, liver disease, kidney disease, or heart failure.

▪ Do not take NSAIDs if you have or are at high risk for heart disease or stroke unless the use is supervised by a health care provider.

▪ Do not take aspirin if you have gout, diabetes mellitus, or arthritis unless the use is supervised by a health care provider.

▪ Do not take salicylates or NSAIDs if you are taking anticoagulants.

▪ Do not take magnesium salicylate if you have kidney disease.

▪ Do not give naproxen to a child younger than 12 years.

When to Seek Medical Attention

▪ Stop taking salicylates or NSAIDs and seek medical attention if any of the following symptoms occur:
  - Headache, dizziness, ringing in the ears, difficulty in hearing, dimness of vision, mental confusion, lassitude, drowsiness, sweating, thirst, hyperventilation, nausea, vomiting, or occasional diarrhea. These symptoms indicate mild salicylate toxicity.
  - Dizziness, nausea and mild stomach pain, constipation, ringing in the ears, or swelling in the feet or legs. These symptoms are common side effects of salicylates and NSAIDs.
  - Rash or hives, or red, peeling skin; swelling in the face or around the eyes; wheezing or trouble breathing; bloody or cloudy urine; unexplained bruising and bleeding; or signs of stomach bleeding such as bloody or black tarry stools, severe stomach pain, or bloody vomit (see the box A Word about NSAIDs and Stomach Bleeding). These symptoms require immediate medical attention.

Acetaminophen

▪ To avoid possible damage to the liver, do not take more than 4 grams of acetaminophen a day from all nonprescription and prescription single-ingredient or combination products containing acetaminophen.

▪ Do not drink alcohol while taking this medication.

▪ Follow dosage instructions for acetaminophen carefully if you have glucose-6-phosphate dehydrogenase deficiency.

When to Seek Medical Attention

▪ Stop taking acetaminophen and seek medical attention if you develop nausea, vomiting, drowsiness, confusion, or abdominal pain.

REFERENCES

1. Stovner LJ, Hagen K, Jensen R, et. al. The global burden of headache: a documentation of headache prevalence and disability worldwide. *Cephalgia.* 2007; 27(3):193–210.

2. Mehuys E, Paemeleire K, Van Hees T, et. al. Self-medication of regular headache: a community pharmacy-based survey. *Eur J Neurol.* 2012, 19(8):1093–99.

3. Loder E, Rizzoli P. Tension-type headache. *BMJ.* 2008;336(7635):88–92.

4. Lipton RB. Migraine: epidemiology, impact, and risk factors for progression. *Headache.* 2005;45(suppl 1):S3–13.

5. Cady RK, Dodick DW, Levine HL, et al. Sinus headache: a neurology, otolaryngology, allergy, and primary care consensus on diagnosis and treatment. *Mayo Clin Proc.* 2005;80(7):908–16.

6. Vargas BB. Tension-type headache and migraine: two points on a continuum? *Curr Pain Headache Rep.* 2008;12(6):433–6.

7. Kelman L. The triggers or precipitant of the acute migraine attack. *Cephalagia.* 2007; 27(5):394–404.

8. Martin VT, Behbehani M. Ovarian hormones and migraine headache: understanding mechanisms and pathogenesis–part 1. *Headache.* 2006;45(1):3–3.

9. Martin VT, Behbehani M. Ovarian hormones and migraine headache: understanding mechanisms and pathogenesis–part 2. *Headache.* 2006;46(3):365–86.

10. Dodick D, Freitag F. Evidence-based understanding of medication-overuse headache: clinical implications. *Headache.* 2006; 46(suppl 4): S202–211.

11. Quintela E, Castillo J, Muñoz P, et al. Premonitory and resolution symptoms in migraine: a prospective study in 100 unselected patients. *Cephalalgia.* 2006; 26(9):1051–60.

12. Derry S, Moore RA. Paracetamol (acetaminophen) with or without an antiemetic for acute migraine headache in adults. *Cochrane Database Syst Rev.* 2013;4:CD008040. DOI:10.1002/14651858. CD008040.pub2. Accessed at http://www.thecochranelibrary.com/view/0/index.html.

13. Consumer HealthCare Products Association. OTC industry announces voluntary transition to one concentration of single-ingredient pediatric liquid acetaminophen medicines. CHPA Executive Newsletter. May 2011; Issue No. 5-11. Accessed at http://www.chpa.org/WorkArea/Download Asset.aspx?id=962, June 1, 2014.

14. Krahenbuhl S, Brauchli Y, Kummer O, et al. Acute liver failure in two patients with regular alcohol consumption ingesting paracetamol at therapeutic dosage. *Digestion.* 2007;75(4):232–77.

15. Krenzelok EP, Royal MA. Confusion: acetaminophen dosing changes based on NO evidence in adults. *Drugs R D.* 2012;12(2):45–8.

16. U.S. Food and Drug Administration. FDA recommends health care professionals discontinue prescribing and dispensing prescription combination drug products with more than 325 mg of acetaminophen to protect consumers. Accessed at http://www.fda.gov/Drugs/DrugSafety/ucm381644.htm, June 1, 2014.

17. Bronstein AC, Spyker DA, Cantilena LR Jr, et al. 2006 Annual Report of the American Association of Poison Control Centers' National Poison Data System (NPDS). *Clin Toxicol* (Phila). 2007;45(8):815–917.

18. Dart RC, Bailey E. Does therapeutic use of acetaminophen cause acute liver failure? *Pharmacotherapy* 2007;27(9):1219–30.

19. Larson AM, Polson J, Fontana RJ, et al. Acetaminophen-induced acute liver failure: results of a United States multicenter, prospective study. *Hepatology.* 2005;42(6):1364–72.

20. Watkins PB, Kaplowitz N, Slattery JT, et al. Aminotransferase elevations in healthy adults receiving 4 grams of acetaminophen daily. *JAMA.* 2006;296(1):87–93.

21. U.S. Food and Drug Administration. FDA Drug Safety Communication: FDA warns of rare but serious skin reactions with the pain reliever/fever reducer acetaminophen [news release]. August 8, 2013. Accessed at http://www.fda.gov/downloads/ Drugs/DrugSafety/UCM363052.pdf, August 8, 2013.

22. McElwee N, Veltri JC, Bradford DC, et al. A prospective, population-based study of acute ibuprofen overdose: complications are rare and routine serum levels not warranted. *Ann Emerg Med.* 1990;19(6):657–62.

23. Food and Drug Administration. Labeling requirements regarding stomach bleeding; labeling requirements for NSAIDs. CFR: Code of Federal Regulations. Title 21, Part 201, Section 201.326. Updated April 1, 2010. Accessed at http://www.fda.gov, August 15, 2011.

24. Antman EM, Bennett JS, Daugherty A, et al. Use of nonsteroidal anti-inflammatory drugs: an update for clinicians. *Circulation.* 2007;115:1634–42.

25. Olsen AM, Fosbøl EL, Lindhardsen J, et.al. Long-term cardiovascular risk of nonsteroidal anti-inflammatory drug use according to time passed after first-time myocardial infarction: a nationwide cohort study. *Circulation.* 2012;126(16):1955–63.

26. Bhatt DL, Scheiman J, Abraham NS, et.al. ACCF/ACG/AHA 2008 expert consensus document on reducing the gastrointestinal risks of antiplatelet therapy and NSAID use: a report of the American College of Cardiology Foundation Task Force on Clinical Expert Consensus Documents. *Circulation.* 2008;118:1894–909.

27. Lanas A, Hunt R. Prevention of anti-inflammatory drug-induced gastrointestinal damage: benefits and risks of therapeutic strategies. *Ann Med.* 2006;38(6):415–28.

28. Can individuals with aspirin sensitivity take NSAIDs? *Pharmacist's Letter/Prescriber's Letter* 2010;26(10).

29. Blondell RD, Azadfard M, Wisniewski AM. Pharmacologic therapy for acute pain. *Am Fam Physician.* 2013;87(11):766–72.

30. Prior MJ, Cooper KM, May LG, et al. Efficacy and safety of acetaminophen and naproxen in the treatment of tension-type headache: a randomized, double-blind, placebo-controlled trial. *Cephalgia.* 2002;22(9):740–8.

31. Perrott DA, Piira T, Goodenough B, et al. Efficacy and safety of acetaminophen vs ibuprofen for treating children's pain or fever. *Arch Pediatr Adolesc Med.* 2004;158(6):521–6.

32. Manzano S, Doyon-Trottier E, Bailey B. Myth: ibuprofen is superior to acetaminophen for the treatment of benign headaches in children and adults. *CJEM.* 2010;12(3):220–2.

33. Tielemans MM, Eikendal T, Jansen JBMJ, et al. Identification of NSAID users at risk for gastrointestinal complications: a systematic review of current guidelines and consensus agreements. *Drug Saf.* 2010;33(6):443–53.

34. Briggs G, Freeman R, Yaffe S, eds. *Drugs in Pregnancy and Lactation.* 8th ed. Baltimore, MD: Lippincott Williams & Wilkins; 2008.

35. Linde K, Allais G, Brinkhaus B, et al. Acupuncture for migraine prophylaxis. *Cochrane Database Syst Rev.* 2009;1:CD001218. doi:10.1002/14651858. CD001218.pub2. Accessed at http://www.thecochranelibrary.com/view/0/index.html, August 8, 2014.

36. Jenkins C, Costello J, Hodge L. Systematic review of prevalence of aspirin induced asthma and its implications for clinical practice. *BMJ.* 2004; 328(7437):434–40.

FEVER

6

Brett M. Feret

Fever is a common reason for visits to pediatrician offices, with the National Ambulatory Medical Care Survey estimating that 6% of all ambulatory visits to pediatricians are related to fever.[1] Fever is also the leading cause of visits to the emergency room for children younger than 15 years.[2] In 2009, patients complaining primarily of fever made approximately 12.5 million medical office visits, with men making a slightly greater number of visits.[3] Children have more reported fevers compared with adults: the rate of reported fevers in children younger than 5 years is 10 in 100 persons versus the rate of 0.5 in 100 adults. Nonetheless, the rate of fever does not seem to differ significantly when distinguishing among gender, race, or geographic area of residence in the United States.[4]

Most fevers are self-limited and nonthreatening; however, fever can cause a great deal of discomfort and, in some cases, may indicate serious underlying pathology (e.g., acute infectious process) for which prompt medical evaluation is indicated. The principal reason for treating fever is to alleviate discomfort, but the underlying cause should be identified and treated appropriately. Fever must be distinguished from hyperthermia and hyperpyrexia. Fever is defined as a body temperature higher than the normal core temperature of 100°F (37.8°C). Fever is a regulated rise in body temperature maintained by the hypothalamus in response to a pyrogen. It is a sign of an increase in the body's thermoregulatory set point.

Hyperthermia, in contrast, represents a malfunctioning of the normal thermoregulatory process at the hypothalamic level caused by excessive heat exposure or production.[5] Because of their different mechanisms, treatment of fever versus hyperthermia also varies.

Hyperpyrexia is a body temperature greater than 106°F (41.1°C) that typically results in mental and physical consequences. Hyperpyrexia may result from either a fever or hyperthermia.

Pathophysiology of Fever

Core body temperature is controlled by the hypothalamus and is regulated by a feedback system that involves information transmitted between the thermoregulatory center in the anterior hypothalamus and the thermosensitive neurons in the skin and central nervous system (CNS). Physiologic (e.g., sweating and vasodilation) and behavioral mechanisms regulate body temperature within the normal range. Although skin temperature may fluctuate greatly in response to environmental conditions, the core temperature is regulated within a narrow range.[6]

Normal thermoregulation prevents wide fluctuations in body temperature; the average temperature is usually maintained between 97.5°F and 98.9°F (36.4°C and 37.2°C), although the commonly accepted core body temperature is usually 98.6°F (37°C). Temperature maintained in this range is considered to be the "set point," or the point at which the physiologic or behavioral mechanisms are not activated.

Pyrogens are fever-producing substances that activate the body's host defenses, resulting in an increase in the set point. Pyrogens can be exogenous (e.g., microbes or toxins) or endogenous (e.g., immune cytokines). Exogenous pyrogens do not independently increase the hypothalamic temperature set point. They stimulate the release of endogenous pyrogens and thereby increase the core temperature. Endogenous pyrogens are products released in response to or from damaged tissue such as interleukins, interferons, and tumor necrosis factor.[6-8]

Prostaglandins of the E_2 series (PGE_2) are produced in response to circulating pyrogens and elevate the thermoregulatory set point in the hypothalamus. Within hours, body temperature reaches the new set point, and fever occurs. During the period of upward temperature readjustment, the patient experiences chills caused by peripheral vasoconstriction and muscle rigidity to maintain homeostasis.[6]

An increase in body temperature may be idiopathic or can be caused by a variety of mechanisms, including an infectious process, pathologic processes, a response to certain drugs, or vigorous activity.

Most febrile episodes are caused by microbial infections (e.g., viruses, bacteria, fungi, yeasts, or protozoa). There is no basis for differentiating viral from bacterial infections according to the magnitude of the fever or the temperature reduction from antipyretic drug therapy. Fever is often less pronounced in elderly patients and neonates. Consequently, infection may not be recognized easily in older patients if fever is the primary assessment criterion.[9]

Noninfectious pathologic causes of increases in temperature include malignancies, tissue damage (e.g., myocardial infarction or surgery), antigen–antibody reactions, dehydration, heat stroke, CNS inflammation, and metabolic disorders such as hyperthyroidism or gout. Many of these processes actually may cause hyperthermia rather than fever because they interfere with the hypothalamic regulation of temperature.

Drug fever is simply defined as a febrile response to the administration of a medication. Its incidence is unknown in an ambulatory setting, but the incidence among hospitalized patients is approximately 10% (Table 6–1). Drug-induced fevers usually

table
6-1   **Selected Medications That Induce Hyperthermia**

Anti-Infectives	Antineoplastics	Cardiovascular	CNS Agents	Other Agents
Aminoglycosides	Bleomycin	Epinephrine	Amphetamines	Allopurinol
Amphotericin B	Chlorambucil	Hydralazine	Barbiturates	Atropine
Cephalosporins	Cytarabine	Methyldopa	Benztropine	Azathioprine
Clindamycin	Daunorubicin	Nifedipine	Carbamazepine	Cimetidine
Chloramphenicol	Hydroxyurea	Procainamide	Haloperidol	Corticosteroids
Imipenem	l-Asparaginase	Quinidine	Lithium	Folate
Isoniazid	6-Mercaptopurine	Streptokinase	MAOIs	Inhaled anesthetics
Linezolid	Procarbazine		Nomifensine	Interferon
Macrolides	Streptozocin		Phenytoin	Iodides
Mebendazole			Phenothiazines	Metoclopramide
Nitrofurantoin			SNRIs	Propylthiouracil
Para-aminosalicylic acid			SSRIs	Prostaglandin E_2
Penicillins			Sumatriptan	Salicylates
Rifampin			Trifluoperazine	Tolmetin
Streptomycin			Thioridazine	
Sulfonamides			TCAs	
Tetracyclines				
Vancomycin				

Key: CNS = Central nervous system; MAOIs = monoamine oxidase inhibitors; SNRIs = serotonin-norepinephrine reuptake inhibitors; SSRIs = selective serotonin reuptake inhibitors; TCAs = tricyclic antidepressants.

Source: References 5, 11, and Musselman ME, Saely S. Diagnosis and treatment of drug-induced hyperthermia. *Am J Health-Syst-Pharm.* 2013;70(1):34–42.

range from 98.9°F (37.2°C) to as high as 109°F (42.8°C). Drug fever should be suspected in patients without an obvious source of fever. Drug fever often goes unrecognized because of inconsistent signs and symptoms, yet failure to discontinue the offending drug can result in substantial morbidity and mortality.[10,11]

Drug fever may be differentiated from other causes by establishing a temporal relationship between the fever and the administration of a medication, as well as by observing a temperature elevation despite improvement of the underlying disorder.

The management of drug fever involves discontinuing the suspected medication whenever possible. If feasible, all medications should be temporarily discontinued. If the hyperthermia is drug-induced, the patient's temperature will generally decrease within 24 to 72 hours after the offending agent is withdrawn. After the patient's safety has been considered and the offending medication has been identified and discontinued, each medication may be restarted, one at a time, while monitoring for fever recurrence.[11]

Clinical Presentation of Fever

Because the symptoms of fever are nonspecific and do not occur in all patients, the etiology of a fever is difficult to determine from the symptomatology. The most important sign of fever is an elevated temperature; therefore, accurate temperature measurement

is paramount. Fever is a symptom of a larger underlying process, whether the process is an infection or abnormal metabolism or is drug induced. Once the symptom of fever is established, investigation into the underlying cause is important. Signs and symptoms that typically accompany fever and cause a great deal of discomfort include headache, diaphoresis, generalized malaise, chills, tachycardia, arthralgia, myalgia, irritability, and anorexia. Most children will tolerate a fever well, so if they continue to be alert, play normally, and stay hydrated, the fever is not of great concern. However, high body temperature dulls intellectual function and causes disorientation and delirium, especially in individuals with preexisting dementia, cerebral arteriosclerosis, or alcoholism.

Detection of Fever

Subjective assessment of fever typically involves feeling a part of the body, such as the forehead, for warmth. Although this method may identify an increase in skin temperature, it does not accurately detect a rise in core temperature. The most accurate method of detecting fever is to use a thermometer properly to measure body temperature. The patient's age and level of physical and emotional stress, the environmental temperature, the time of day, and the anatomical site at which the temperature is measured are important considerations, given that each factor can affect the results of temperature measurement.

Core temperature is estimated with various types of thermometers used at the rectal, axillary, oral, temporal, or tympanic sites. Rectal temperature has long been considered the gold standard measurement; however, its utility has been challenged.[12] Many patients prefer other methods of temperature measurement because of comfort and ease of use. Body temperature should be measured with the same thermometer at the same site over the course of an illness because the readings from different thermometers or sites may vary (Table 6–2). The discrepancy among the various sites of temperature measurement is normal and should not be ascribed to improper measurement technique. On average, a rectal temperature greater than 100.4°F (38.0°C), an oral temperature greater than 99.7°F (37.6°C), an axillary temperature greater than 99.3°F (37.4°C), a tympanic temperature greater than 100.0°F (37.8°C), or a temporal measurement greater than 100.1°F (37.8°C) is considered elevated.[13] The variation in temperatures at the different sites verifies a simple conception about temperature measurement among the public: add 1 degree to an oral temperature to get a rectal or tympanic measurement, and subtract 1 degree from an oral temperature for an axillary measurement. Normal body temperature may range 1.8°F–2.5°F (1°C–1.4°C) from these norms. Diurnal rhythms cause variances in body temperature during the day, with higher temperatures typically in the late afternoon to early evening. Because the Food and Drug Administration (FDA) regulates thermometers as medical devices, all approved types of thermometers are accurate and reliable, if used appropriately. Providers should not recommend mercury-in-glass thermometers for use at this point because of environmental concerns with mercury.[14]

Electronic probe thermometers are available for oral, rectal, and axillary temperature measurements. The probes have an electronic transducer that provides a temperature reading in about 10–60 seconds. The oral electronic probes are mostly available in either pen or pacifier shapes, although infant probes can be a different shape. The pacifier-shaped electronic thermometer is for oral use only and is useful in infants who are unable to hold probes under their tongues. The amount of time the pacifier needs to stay in the child's mouth varies depending on the manufacturer, but the time can range from 3 to 8 minutes.[15,16] The pen-shaped probe may be used in the oral, rectal, or axillary area. Because of their electronic digital temperature displays, electronic thermometers provide quick readings, eliminate the possibility of glass breakage, and are easier to read compared with traditional glass thermometers. The use of disposable probe covers with electronic thermometers also reduces the need for disinfection after their use. Disinfection should still occur if the thermometer is being used for multiple patients. A thermometer that is used rectally should not be used subsequently for oral measurement.

Infrared thermometers are available for tympanic artery and temporal artery temperature measurements. These thermometers use infrared technology to detect heat from the arterial blood supply. They must be placed directly in the line of a blood supply, whether near the temporal artery or the tympanic membrane. Infrared thermometers measure body temperature in less than 5 seconds and are considered very accurate, if used appropriately. The major problem with infrared thermometers is that they are not always placed appropriately and consequently may give inaccurate readings. Infrared thermometers are relatively expensive and require batteries, but many families with young children prefer them because of their convenience and noninvasive nature. New technology also includes no-touch infrared thermometers, which offer the advantage of not having to wake a sleeping child to take a temperature.[16,17]

Color-change thermometers are easy to use, but they are not sufficiently accurate or reliable. The thermometer is an adhesive strip containing heat-sensitive material that changes color in response to different temperature gradients. The strip may be placed anywhere on the skin, but the forehead is used most often because the forehead shows less variation in temperature than other parts of the body. Although this method may detect changes in skin temperature, it does not reliably detect changes in core temperature.

Patient-related factors may preclude the use of a particular type of thermometer through a given route. Although there are a variety of routes of temperature measurement, rectal temperature measurement historically has been the standard because the site is not influenced by ambient temperatures, and it can be used in patients of varying ages.[13] Oral, tympanic, axillary, and temporal routes are all appropriate for temperature measurements if the proper procedure is followed.

Table 6–3 describes the proper methods of taking rectal temperatures in children and adults. Rectal temperature measurement has a predictable rise in temperature and a high sensitivity and specificity compared with the body's core temperature. Although the rectal route is the closest estimate of the core temperature, its intrusive nature can be very frightening and possibly psychologically harmful to older children. In children younger than 3 months, however, rectal temperature is the preferred method of estimating fever and should be recommended if caregivers are confident they can safely use this route.[16] Risks associated with taking a rectal temperature include retention of the thermometer, rectal or intestinal perforation, and peritonitis. Rectal temperature measurement is also very time consuming, and the patient should never be left unattended while the rectal thermometer remains in place; a positional change may cause the thermometer to be expelled or broken. Rectal temperature measurement is relatively contraindicated in patients who are

table **6–2**	**Body Temperature Range Based on Site of Measurement**	
Site of Measurement	**Normal Range**[a]	**Fever**[a]
Rectal	97.9°F–100.4°F (36.6°C–38°C)	>100.4°F (38.0°C)
Oral	95.9°F–99.5°F (35.5°C–37.5°C)	>99.5°F (37.5°C)
Axillary	94.5°F–99.3°F (34.7°C–37.4°C)	>99.3°F (37.4°C)
Tympanic	96.3°F–100°F (35.7°C–37.8°C)	>100°F (37.8°C)
Temporal	97.9°F–100.1°F (36.6°C–37.8°C)	>100.7°F (38.1°C) for 0–2 months old >100.3°F (37.9°C) for 3–47 months old >100.1°F (37.8°C) for >4 years old

[a] Conversion formulas: Celsius = 5/9(°F – 32); Fahrenheit = (9/5 × °C) + 32.

Source: References 13 and 16.

table 6-3   Guidelines for Rectal Temperature Measurements Using Electronic Thermometers

1. Cover the tip of thermometer with a probe cover.
2. Turn on the thermometer and wait until it is ready for use.
3. Apply a water-soluble lubricant to tip of thermometer to allow for easy passage through the anal sphincter and to reduce risk of trauma.
4. For infants or young children, place child face down over your lap, separate the buttocks with the thumb and forefinger of one hand, and insert the thermometer gently in the direction of the child's umbilicus with the other hand. For infants, insert the thermometer to the length of the tip. For young children, insert it about 1 inch into the rectum.
5. For adults, have the patient lie on one side with the legs flexed to about a 45° angle from the abdomen. Insert the tip 0.5–2 inches into the rectum by holding the thermometer 0.5–2 inches away from the tip and inserting it until the finger touches the anus. Have the patient take a deep breath during this process to facilitate proper positioning of the thermometer.
6. Hold the thermometer in place until it beeps and a temperature is displayed.
7. Remove the thermometer.
8. Dispose of probe cover and clean thermometer with an antiseptic such as alcohol or a povidone/iodine solution by wiping away from the stem toward tip. Rinse with cool water.
9. Wipe away any remaining lubricant from the anus.

neutropenic, have had recent rectal surgery or injury, or have rectal pathology (e.g., obstructive hemorrhoids or diarrhea). In addition, rectal temperature measurement is slow to measure rapid changes in body temperature because of the large muscle mass and poor blood flow to the area.[13,16,18]

Table 6–4 describes the proper methods of taking oral measurements with electronic thermometers.[16] Oral temperature

table 6-4   Guidelines for Oral Temperature Measurements Using Electronic Thermometers

Digital Probe

1. Wait 20–30 minutes after drinking or eating.
2. Place a clean disposable probe cover over tip.
3. Turn on the thermometer and wait until it is ready for use.
4. Place tip of thermometer under tongue.
5. Close mouth and breathe through nose.
6. Hold thermometer in place until it beeps and temperature has been recorded (usually after 5–30 seconds).
7. Record the displayed temperature.
8. Remove and dispose of probe cover.

Digital Pacifier Thermometer

1. Wait 30 minutes after drinking or eating.
2. Inspect the pacifier for any tears or cracks. Do not use if worn.
3. Press the button to turn on thermometer.
4. Place the pacifier in child's mouth.
5. Have the child hold pacifier in mouth without moving, if possible, for time specified on packaging of thermometer (2–6 minutes).
6. Record temperature when thermometer beeps.

Source: References 15 and 16.

should not be obtained when an individual is mouth breathing or hyperventilating; has recently had oral surgery; is not fully alert; or is uncooperative, lethargic, or confused. Oral digital probe thermometers may not be appropriate for use in most children younger than 3 years. Children this young may find it difficult to maintain a tight seal around the thermometer and keep the thermometer under the tongue, in which case pacifier thermometers may be recommended. Pacifier thermometers provide reliable temperature readings compared with rectal measurements; however, in children younger than 3 months, pacifier thermometers are less accurate.[19,20] To ensure reliable measurement, the patient should neither smoke, engage in vigorous physical activity, nor drink hot or cold beverages for a minimum of 20 minutes before the temperature is measured.

Table 6–5 describes the proper method of using tympanic thermometers, which varies slightly depending on the age of the patient.[16] Tympanic thermometers have digital readouts, and many can be set to provide either a rectal or an oral temperature equivalent. The tympanic membrane is close to the hypothalamus, and the blood supply to both anatomical areas is at the same temperature, providing an accurate reading of the core body temperature. The thermometer must be positioned in the ear canal properly to ensure that the measured infrared radiation is from the tympanic membrane and not from the ear canal or adjacent areas. In clinical trials, accuracy of tympanic thermometers has varied compared with rectal and oral routes.[21,22] Variations in temperature assessment have been attributed to cerumen impaction, inflammation in the ear canal (e.g., otitis media), age of patient (size of ear canal), and inappropriate technique.[16] Tympanic thermometers are not recommended in infants younger than 6 months; their ear canals are not developed fully, leading to inappropriate technique and inaccurate readings. Although not as reliable as the rectal method in children, if used correctly, tympanic thermometry has been found to be more accurate than axillary or oral thermometry in estimating core temperature.[18]

Temporal touch thermometers are placed on the side of the forehead directly over the temporal artery and moved across the forehead (Table 6–6). The temporal artery is directly supplied by the hypothalamus and is near the surface of the skin at the side of the head, thereby allowing surface measurement with infrared technology to be possible. The thermometer is capable of providing a temperature reading in a few seconds. Its rapid, noninvasive nature makes it a preferable route of temperature

table 6-5   Guidelines for Tympanic Temperature Measurements

1. Place a clean disposable lens cover over ear probe.
2. Turn on thermometer and wait until it is ready for use.
3. For children younger than 1 year, pull ear backward to straighten ear canal. Place ear probe into canal, and aim the tip of the probe toward patient's eye.
4. For patients older than 1 year, pull ear backward and up to straighten ear canal. Place the ear probe into canal, and aim the tip of probe toward patient's eye.
5. Press the button for temperature measurement (usually for only 1–5 seconds).
6. Read and record temperature.
7. Discard lens cover.

Source: Reference 16.

<table>
<tr><td>

table 6-6

Guidelines for Temporal Artery Temperature Measurements

1. Allow thermometer to acclimatize to the environment for about 30 minutes, if you moved the thermometer from a hot room to a cold room or vice versa.
2. Place probe on one side of forehead (near temporal area).
3. Depress button and hold while scanning for the temporal artery temperature.
4. Sweep thermometer across forehead to the hairline on the opposite side of the head. Ensure that probe remains in contact with skin at all times, and hold button down until finished scanning.
5. If there is sweat on the forehead, sweep the thermometer as normal, but nestle the thermometer on the neck directly behind the ear lobe before releasing the button.
6. Lift thermometer, release the button, and document the recorded temperature.

</td></tr>
</table>

Source: References 16 and 17.

measurement for individuals, and the temporal thermometer is significantly more sensitive than the tympanic thermometer for detecting fever.[23] However, in a recent study, the temporal temperature measurement still did not show superiority or greater reliability compared with the rectal method.[21] Temporal temperature measurement may differ from rectal temperature measurement by ±2.3°F (1.3°C).[20,21] The presence of hair near the temporal area may confound the temperature reading, so hair must be pushed away before a reading is obtained.

No-touch infrared thermometers do not require contact with the patient for measurement. Temperature is measured by aiming the thermometer at the center of the forehead. Certain models may also allow for alternative sites such as the navel and neck, although these sites are less accurate.[16] Although no-touch infrared thermometers are convenient and less invasive, a study of children ages 1 month to 4 years treated in the emergency room found infrared thermometers to be less accurate and reliable than rectal measurement.[24]

Axillary temperature measurement is frequently used by caregivers and in ambulatory settings because it is relatively noninvasive. However, axillary measurement performed with digital thermometers (Table 6–7) is not as reliable for detecting fever compared with oral and rectal routes.[25,26] Reported large variations in temperatures taken by the axillary method are attributable to inappropriate placement of the thermometer, movement of arms during measurement leading to a poor seal

<table>
<tr><td>

table 6-7

Guidelines for Axillary Temperature Measurements Using Electronic Thermometer

1. Place a clean disposable probe cover over tip.
2. Turn on thermometer and wait until it is ready for use.
3. Place tip of thermometer in armpit. Ensure that armpit is clean and dry. Thermometer must be touching skin, not clothes.
4. If taking a child's temperature, hold child close to secure the thermometer under armpit, if necessary.
5. Read and record temperature when thermometer beeps.

</td></tr>
</table>

Source: Reference 16.

around the thermometer, and measurements being taken for too short a period of time. Axillary temperature should not be taken directly after vigorous activity or bathing because both can affect body temperature temporarily without altering the thermoregulatory set point at the hypothalamus. If a fever is detected with the axillary method, a confirmation reading using another method is recommended.

Complications of Fever

The presence of fever is a cause of great concern, although in most cases fever may be self-limiting, and serious complications are rare. In one study, 73% of caregivers were "very concerned" about the potential complications of fever, and 88% were "very concerned" when a child's fever was not reduced by antipyretics. There is less concern about complications of fever now than 20 years ago; however, interviewed caregivers still list seizures (32%), brain damage (15%), and death (16%) as the main complications of fever.[27] Overall, the major risks of fever are rare but may include acute complications such as seizures, dehydration, and change in mental status.

Febrile seizure is defined as a seizure accompanied by fever in infants or children who do not have an intracranial infection, a metabolic disturbance, or a defined cause.[28] Febrile seizures occur in 2%–5% of all children from the ages of 6 months to 5 years, with the peak occurrence in children ages 18–24 months. Risk factors for a first febrile seizure include day care attendance, developmental delay, a family history of febrile seizure, and a neonatal hospital stay of more than 30 days. The height of the fever and rate of increase also appear to be critical determinants in the precipitation of a first febrile seizure.[29] The most common seizures associated with fever are simple febrile seizures, which are characterized by nonfocal movements, generally of less than 15 minutes in duration, with only one occurrence in a 24-hour period. Significant neurologic sequelae (e.g., impaired intellectual development or epilepsy) are unlikely after a single pediatric febrile seizure. The risk of recurrence is increased in children who have had multiple febrile seizures, are younger than 1 year at the time of their first seizure, and have a family history of epilepsy. Antipyretics are generally recommended to make the child more comfortable, although they do not reduce the risk of recurrent febrile seizures.[28,30,31] Prophylaxis against simple febrile seizures with antiepileptic or antipyretic drugs is not recommended by the American Academy of Pediatrics.[28]

Serious detrimental effects (e.g., dehydration, delirium, seizures, coma, or irreversible neurologic or muscle damage) occur more often in patients with hyperpyrexia (temperatures > 106°F [41.1°C]), which is usually associated with hyperthermia and not fever. Because of the homeostatic mechanisms of the hypothalamus, a febrile person with a core temperature exceeding 106°F (41.1°C) is rare. However, even lower body temperature elevations may be life threatening in patients with heart disease and pulmonary dysfunction. Increased risk of complications exists in infants and patients with brain tumors or hemorrhage, CNS infections, preexisting neurologic damage, and a decreased ability to dissipate heat attributed to lower tolerance of elevated body temperature. Elderly patients are at a higher risk for fever-related complications because of their decreased thirst perception and perspiration ability.[6,32]

Treatment of Fever

Fever is a sign of an underlying process. Treatment should focus on the primary cause rather than on the temperature reading. No correlation exists between the magnitude and pattern of temperature elevation (i.e., persistent, intermittent, recurrent, or prolonged) and the principal etiology or severity of the disease. Therefore, trying to determine the cause of the fever on the sole basis of the temperature reading is difficult. The decision to treat fever is based on a patient-specific risk–benefit ratio and the desire to improve comfort.[33] Fever is not associated with many harmful effects unless the temperature exceeds 106°F (41.1°C); most fevers are of short duration and may actually have beneficial effects on host-defense mechanisms (e.g., antigen recognition, T-helper lymphocyte function, and leukocyte motility). Certain microbes are thermolabile, and their growth may be impaired by higher-than-normal temperatures. Therefore, overtreatment of fever for viral and bacterial infections may actually be detrimental.[33] Other arguments against treatment include the generally benign and self-limited course of fever, the delayed identification of the diagnosis, and the untoward effects of antipyretic medications.[34]

Treatment Goals

The major goal of self-treatment is to alleviate the discomfort of fever rather than treating to a specific temperature.[33,35]

General Treatment Approach

Treatment of fever using antipyretics (see Chapter 5, Tables 5–2 and 5–3) is most often indicated for patients with elevated temperatures who also have discomfort. Fever associated with discomfort may be treated with antipyretic agents as well as nonpharmacologic measures.

Self-care measures, including antipyretics, are appropriate initial therapy, unless a patient has exclusions for self-treatment (Figure 6–1). In addition, parents should be urged to call their child's pediatrician immediately or seek urgent medical care if their child has a history of seizure; refuses to stay hydrated; develops a rash; has a rectal temperature of 104°F (40.0°C) or higher or its equivalent; or is very sleepy, irritable, or difficult to wake. Children younger than 3 months should be referred for medical evaluation at rectal temperatures of 100.4°F (38.0°C) or higher. Children younger than 3 months have immature immune systems and are prone to more serious bacterial infections. In all cases, self-care measures should be started while medical evaluation is being sought.[33,35,36]

Nonpharmacologic Therapy

Nonpharmacologic therapy consists mainly of adequate fluid intake to prevent dehydration. Sponging or baths have limited utility in the management of fever. Body sponging with tepid water may facilitate heat dissipation, given that only a small temperature gradient between the body and the sponging medium is necessary to achieve an effective antipyretic response. However, sponging is not routinely recommended for those with a temperature less than 104°F (40°C); sponging is usually uncomfortable and often induces shivering, which could further raise the temperature. Bathing with ice water or sponging with hydroalcoholic solutions

(e.g., isopropyl or ethyl alcohol) is uncomfortable, dangerous, and not recommended. Alcohol poisoning can result from cutaneous absorption or inhalation of topically applied alcohol solutions. Infants and children are at a higher risk of alcohol poisoning because of their smaller body mass. Unlike acetaminophen and nonsteroidal anti-inflammatory drugs (NSAIDs), sponging does not reduce the hypothalamic set point; therefore, sponging should follow oral antipyretic therapy by 1 hour to permit the appropriate reduction of the hypothalamic set point and a more sustained temperature-lowering response.[37]

Other nonpharmacologic interventions, regardless of the temperature, include wearing lightweight clothing, removing blankets, maintaining a comfortable room temperature of approximately 68°F (20°C), and drinking sufficient fluid to replenish insensible losses. Because a fever will cause a child to lose fluids more rapidly, sufficient fluid intake is recommended. Fluid intake in febrile children should be increased by at least 30–60 mL (1–2 ounces) of fluids per hour (e.g., sports drinks, fruit juice, water, balanced electrolyte replacement products, or ice pops) and by at least 60–120 mL (3–4 ounces) of fluids per hour in adults, unless fluids are contraindicated. Caution should be exercised in recommending fruit juice and sport drinks to patients with diarrhea; drinks with high sugar loads may worsen concurrent diarrhea.

Pharmacologic Therapy

Antipyretics inhibit PGE_2 synthesis, which decreases the feedback between the thermoregulatory neurons and the hypothalamus, thereby reducing the hypothalamic set point during fever. All antipyretics decrease the production of PGE_2 by inhibiting the cyclooxygenase (COX) enzyme. NSAIDs and aspirin inhibit the COX enzyme in the periphery and CNS, whereas acetaminophen mainly inhibits the COX enzyme in the CNS.[38] Chapter 5 provides an in-depth discussion of the pharmacokinetics, dosing, adverse effect profile, interactions, contraindications, and precautions of nonprescription antipyretic agents.

Acetaminophen typically reaches a maximum temperature reduction at 2 hours at the usual recommended dosing of 10–15 mg/kg every 4–6 hours, with a maximum of 5 doses per day (see Chapter 5, Tables 5–2 and 5–3). Approximately 80% of children will experience a reduction in their fever with that dose.[33] Adult dosing ranges from 325–1000 mg every 4–6 hours up to a maximum of 4000 mg per day. Some providers have recommended loading doses of acetaminophen for the reduction of fever at 30 mg/kg per dose, after a small study found a faster (one-half hour) and more significant (0.9°F [0.5°C]) decrease compared with a traditional dose.[39] This practice is not recommended, however, because of the size and limitations of the study and the lack of any follow-up evidence for the practice.

Acetaminophen is also available as a rectal suppository. Although a suppository may be an advantage for caregivers who have problems giving their children oral medications, or for children who are vomiting or are having a febrile seizure, the suppository's absorption is erratic, and studies on its antipyretic activity are conflicting.[40]

Ibuprofen is the most common NSAID used as an antipyretic; it typically reaches a maximum temperature reduction at 2 hours at the recommended dosing of 5–10 mg/kg per dose every 6–8 hours, with a maximum of 4 doses per day (see

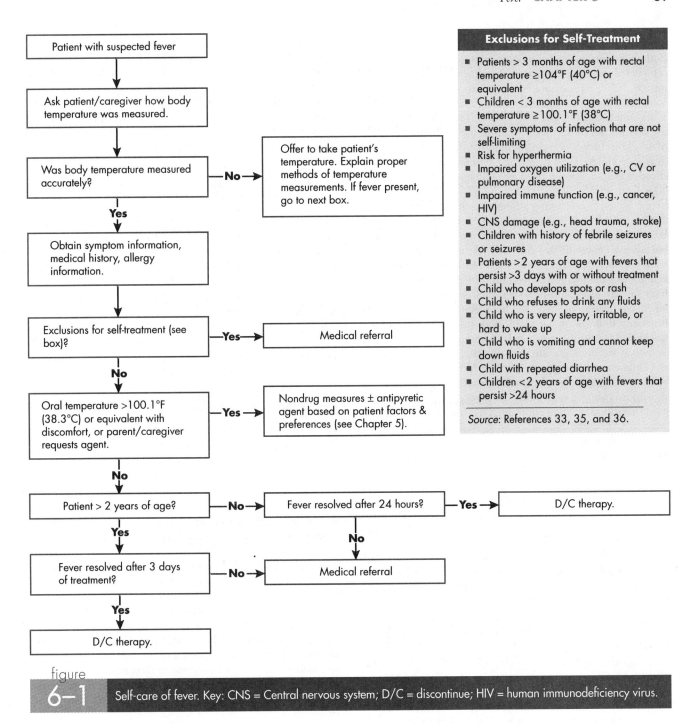

figure

6–1 Self-care of fever. Key: CNS = Central nervous system; D/C = discontinue; HIV = human immunodeficiency virus.

Chapter 5, Tables 5–2 and 5–3). Note that ibuprofen is approved for the reduction of fever only in patients older than 6 months. Adult dosing ranges from 200 to 400 mg every 4–6 hours up to a maximum of 1200 mg per day.

Although NSAIDs and acetaminophen are safe and effective when used at low doses for a short duration, they should not be used more than 3 days to treat fever without referral for further evaluation to determine the underlying cause. Common medication errors associated with over-the-counter antipyretics include overdosing or duplicating therapy attributed to using multiple products with similar ingredients, and inappropriate dosing for pediatric patients attributed to mathematical errors in calculating a weight-based dose. One study has shown that only 30% of parents were able to measure an accurate dose of acetaminophen, and another study demonstrated that 51% of the study's pediatric patients received an inaccurate dose of medication (62% for acetaminophen and 26% for ibuprofen).[41] Because of these alarming statistics, health care providers should provide an appropriate measuring device and/or demonstrate to patients and caregivers proper dosing and measurement of the medications. In addition, patients should be educated on the appropriate dosing interval and the avoidance of combining cold and cough products containing either acetaminophen or ibuprofen.

Pharmacotherapeutic Comparison

Both ibuprofen and acetaminophen are more effective than placebo in reducing fever, with both showing reductions of approximately 1–2 degrees within 30 minutes to 1 hour. Clinical trials comparing the antipyretic effects of ibuprofen to acetaminophen in recommended dosages have produced variable results, making conclusions on superiority of one agent difficult. A review of 14 clinical trials comparing ibuprofen and acetaminophen in febrile children did find that ibuprofen was slightly more effective than acetaminophen in reducing fever after a single dose; furthermore, ibuprofen was found to be more effective after 6 hours, thus showing a longer duration of action.[42] The same review found that multiple-dose studies failed to show any statistically significant clinical difference. The risk of serious adverse effects did not differ between the medications. The authors concluded that the efficacy and safety between acetaminophen and ibuprofen are similar in recommended dosages, with slightly more benefit shown with ibuprofen in terms of onset and duration of action and fever reduction; however, more conclusive findings are needed. A meta-analysis looking at both children and adults also concluded that ibuprofen was more efficacious than acetaminophen in the reduction of fever in both adults and children and was equally as safe.[43] Although ibuprofen has been studied most frequently, other NSAIDs (e.g., naproxen and aspirin) may also be appropriate as antipyretics in adults.

Alternating different antipyretics has become a widespread practice. A survey of 256 caregivers showed that 67% alternated acetaminophen and ibuprofen, and 81% of them stated that their health care provider or pediatrician advised them to do so. Although alternating the antipyretics was recommended, only 61% of caregivers received any type of written instructions on how to dose the medications, and the dosing intervals varied from 2 to 6 hours.[41] Despite those practices and clinical trials showing lower temperatures at 4 or more hours with combination therapy, the American Academy of Pediatrics at this time does not recommend alternation of antipyretics because of the risk of overdose, medication errors resulting from the complexity of the regimens, and increased side effects.[33,41] In addition, only one study actually showed less stress and time missed from daycare with alternating therapy.[44] Health care providers should continue to counsel patients and caregivers on the practical application of this practice if patients are instructed to alternate doses by their providers. For example, caregivers should be encouraged to write down the generic name, dose of the medication, and time of administration to minimize the likelihood of duplicate dosing and adverse effects.

The use of antipyretics immediately after vaccine administration is a widespread practice meant to reduce anticipated discomfort and fever. Recently, two open-label, randomized trials found that administration of acetaminophen was effective in reducing febrile episodes, but it also significantly reduced the antibody response to several vaccines, although all levels were still considered protective. Even though the clinical significance of these antibody reductions is still unknown, prophylactic antipyretics either before or immediately after vaccine administration should be discouraged; however, symptomatic post-vaccination reactions may still be treated with antipyretics until additional data says otherwise.[45]

Product Selection Guidelines

Age is an important consideration in the selection of an antipyretic, particularly among neonates. Parents and caregivers of children younger than 3 months of age should seek medical evaluation at rectal temperatures or equivalent of 100.4°F (38.0°C) or higher. Children older than 3 months with a rectal temperature or equivalent of 104°F (40.0°C) or higher should also be referred. Ibuprofen should be used only in children older than 6 months; because of the risk of Reye's syndrome, children younger than 15 years of age should avoid using aspirin or aspirin-containing products as an antipyretic. A detailed description of additional criteria for the appropriate use of antipyretic agents is available in Chapter 5.

The choice of an antipyretic depends on the patient. Both acetaminophen and ibuprofen are available in a variety of dosage forms for both children and adults, including tablets, chewable tablets, suspensions, and even suppositories. Selection of a dosage form can be left to patient preference. Consideration of palatability and the taste of the different ibuprofen and acetaminophen suspensions may improve outcomes and adherence of antipyretic regimens in children. A variety of flavors are available for both ibuprofen and acetaminophen liquids. The dosing frequency of ibuprofen at once every 6–8 hours versus acetaminophen at once every 4–6 hours may also improve adherence and be considered in product selection, especially in children who have difficulty taking medicine.

Complementary Therapies

Currently, insufficient evidence exists to recommend any dietary supplement or other complementary therapy for the treatment of fever.

Assessment of Fever: A Case-Based Approach

The first step in assessing a patient with a complaint of fever is to obtain an objective temperature measurement to determine whether fever is actually present. Subjective or inaccurate temperature measurement must be ruled out. If fever is present, assessment of its severity, the seriousness of the underlying cause, and other associated symptoms is indicated. Children who are capable of providing and understanding information should be included in any dialogue concerning their care.

Cases 6–1 and 6–2 are examples of the assessment of patients presenting with fever.

Patient Counseling for Fever

Although fever is a common symptom, it often is misunderstood and poorly treated. Studies suggest that fever is incorrectly considered a disease associated with detrimental consequences rather than a symptom, is frequently treated inappropriately, and is evaluated improperly.[46] Many parents and caregivers have "fever phobia" that results in heightened anxiety and inappropriate treatment of fever.[27] Health care providers can improve patient outcomes by educating patients and caregivers about fever and by teaching patients self-assessment skills (e.g., the proper methods for measuring body temperature using the variety of thermometers available, as well as proper interpretation of the results). If patients

case

6–1

Relevant Evaluation Criteria	Scenario/Model Outcome

Information Gathering

1. Gather essential information about the patient's symptoms and medical history, including:

   a. description of symptom(s) (i.e., nature, onset, duration, severity, associated symptoms)

   Nate Connor's mother noticed his forehead felt warm when he woke up this morning for the start of the weekend. Normally a high-energy child, Nate wasn't acting himself, which worried her. He also complained of having a slight headache and feeling uncomfortable.

   b. description of any factors that seem to precipitate, exacerbate, and/or relieve the patient's symptom(s)

   Nate's mom took his temperature with an oral thermometer, which was 102.4°F. She did not notice any other symptoms other than a slight stuffy nose.

   c. description of the patient's efforts to relieve the symptoms

   She hadn't tried anything to treat his fever up to this point.

   d. patient's identity

   Nate Connor

   e. patient's age, sex, height, and weight

   7 years old, male, 4 ft 2 in., 58 lb

   f. patient's occupation

   Nate attends first grade

   g. patient's dietary habits

   Normal diet

   h. patient's sleep habits

   Normal sleep patterns

   i. concurrent medical conditions, prescription and nonprescription medications, and dietary supplements

   No medical conditions; Flintstones Multivitamin

   j. allergies

   NKDA

   j. history of other adverse reactions to medications

   None

   k. other (describe) _____

   Nate is not his usual high-energy self. His mother reported he is still playing and eating some, but not at his usual levels. You retake his temperature in the pharmacy using a temporal thermometer, and it reads 102.0°F.

Assessment and Triage

2. Differentiate the patient's signs/symptoms and correctly identify the patient's primary problem(s).

   Nate has a fever and his decreased activity level and headache indicate that he is in some discomfort. He most likely has a virus transmitted through contact with classmates at school. He has no other signs or symptoms of a bacterial infection.

3. Identify exclusions for self-treatment (Figure 6–1).

   None

4. Formulate a comprehensive list of therapeutic alternatives for the primary problem to determine if triage to a health care provider is required, and share this information with the caregivers.

   Options include:

   (1) Refer Nate for immediate medical attention.

   (2) Monitor his symptoms and fever and recommend nondrug measures only.

   (3) Recommend a medication alone or in combination with nondrug measures.

   (4) Take no action.

Plan

5. Select an optimal therapeutic alternative to address the patient's problem, taking into account patient preferences.

   Nate has a fever and is in discomfort, most likely from a viral infection. He has no exclusions for self-care at this time (Figure 6–1); therefore, treatment with either acetaminophen or ibuprofen is warranted. Drug therapy should be used in conjunction with nondrug measures. Nate prefers liquid medications, specifically cherry-flavored acetaminophen. He should not receive any aspirin-containing medications.

6. Describe the recommended therapeutic approach to the caregivers.

   See Table 5–2 in Chapter 5 for recommended doses. If fever persists >72 hours with or without treatment, Nate should be seen by a health care provider.

7. Explain to the caregivers the rationale for selecting the recommended therapeutic approach from the considered therapeutic alternatives.

   Nate has a fever that is causing some discomfort, so minimizing the fever with an antipyretic medication, either acetaminophen or ibuprofen, should help. He currently does not need to see a health care provider, but you should contact one if his fever persists for >72 hours or if he complains of other symptoms, such as a stiff neck, severe headache or sore throat, severe ear pain, an unexplained rash, or he has repeated vomiting or diarrhea.

case
6–1   *continued*

Relevant Evaluation Criteria	Scenario/Model Outcome
Patient Education	
8. When recommending self-care with nonprescription medications and/or nondrug therapy, convey accurate information to the caregivers:	
a. appropriate dose and frequency of administration	"You can give Nate acetaminophen liquid (160 mg/5 mL). Give 2 teaspoonfuls or 10 mL (320 mg) every 4–6 hours. Do not exceed 5 doses per 24 hours."
b. maximum number of days the therapy should be employed	"Do not give Nate the medication for more than 3 days."
c. product administration procedures	"Measure liquid using appropriate dosing syringe or cup and have Nate swallow liquid."
d. expected time to onset of relief	"A reduction in fever is usually seen within ½–1 hour. Maximum reduction is usually seen within 2 hours."
e. degree of relief that can be reasonably expected	"A 1–2 degree reduction in temperature is expected, but complete resolution of symptoms may vary, depending on the underlying cause of the fever."
f. most common side effects	"Side effects are rare but gastrointestinal effects or rash is possible. Nate can take medication with food if gastrointestinal effects occur."
g. side effects that warrant medical intervention, should they occur	"Contact a health care provider if signs of an allergic reaction, such as a rash or trouble breathing, occur after a dose is given."
h. patient's options in the event that condition worsens or persists	"Contact a health care provider in 72 hours if the fever persists or if symptoms worsen."
i. product storage requirements	"Keep medication in a tightly secured container away from any extreme temperatures and out of reach of children."
j. specific nondrug measures	"Maintain room temperature at 68°F. Maintain adequate fluid intake and dress him in lightweight clothing."
Solicit follow-up questions from caregivers.	"Can I alternate ibuprofen with the acetaminophen for Nate?"
Answer caregivers' questions.	"You should not. The American Academy of Pediatrics does not recommend alternating ibuprofen and acetaminophen because of the increased risk of medication errors and side effects."
Evaluation of Patient Outcome	
9. Assess patient outcome.	Contact Nate's mother in 1–2 days to see if his fever is improving.

Key: NKDA = No known drug allergies.

are still using mercury-in-glass thermometers, they should be urged to dispose of them according to their local environmental standards. Health care providers should also explain the appropriate nonpharmacologic and pharmacologic treatments for fever and when to seek further medical care. Discussions of pharmacologic treatments should highlight methods for safe use of antipyretics and the avoidance of complementary therapies. The box Patient Education for Fever provides specific information to give the patient.

Evaluation of Patient Outcomes for Fever

The primary monitoring parameters for febrile patients include temperature and discomfort. In one study, 32% of caregivers said they would check a febrile patient's temperature at least every hour.[27] Overaggressive monitoring may result from fever phobia. Because fever may actually be of benefit, the ultimate goal of antipyretic therapy is not to normalize temperature as much, but to improve overall comfort and well-being.[33] Associated symptoms (e.g., headache, diaphoresis, generalized malaise, chills, tachycardia, arthralgia, myalgia, irritability, and anorexia) should also be monitored daily. Although most patients demonstrate a reduction in temperature after each individual dose of an antipyretic, pharmacologic therapy for fever may take up to 1 day to result in a decrease in temperature. If symptoms are not improving or are worsening over the course of 3 days with self-treatment, regardless of a drop in temperature, a health care provider should be consulted either by phone or appointment for further evaluation.[36] Timeliness of patient follow-up with medical care is important in determining the presence of a non–self-limiting underlying cause.

case
6-2

Relevant Evaluation Criteria	Scenario/Model Outcome

Information Gathering

1. Gather essential information about the patient's symptoms and medical history, including:

   a. description of symptom(s) (i.e., nature, onset, duration, severity, associated symptoms)

   A mother calls the pharmacy claiming her newborn, Alison, is spiking a fever. Alison has not been eating as usual today. Alison's mother decided to take the baby's temperature rectally, and Alison had a temperature of 102.1°F.

   b. description of any factors that seem to precipitate, exacerbate, and/or relieve the patient's symptom(s)

   The mother just noticed that Alison had a fever; the baby was fine the previous night when she went to bed.

   c. description of the patient's efforts to relieve the symptoms

   The mother has not tried anything at all at this point. She has not noticed any other symptoms, and she denies that the baby has any rash or coughing.

   d. patient's identity

   Alison Woods

   e. patient's age, sex, height, and weight

   10 weeks old, female, 13 lb

   f. patient's occupation

   None

   g. patient's dietary habits

   Breast milk every 3–4 hours

   h. patient's sleep habits

   Sleeps most of the day and night; awakes to eat every few hours.

   i. concurrent medical conditions, prescription and non-prescription medications, and dietary supplements

   No significant medical conditions

   j. allergies

   NKDA

   k. history of other adverse reactions to medications

   No medications

   l. other (describe) _____

   NA

Assessment and Triage

2. Differentiate the patient's signs and symptoms and correctly identify the patient's primary problem(s).

   Alison has a fever that is concerning because of her age.

3. Identify exclusions for self-treatment (Figure 6–1).

   Age < 3 months with a fever > 100.1°F

4. Formulate a comprehensive list of therapeutic alternatives for the primary problem to determine if triage to a health care provider is required, and share this information with the caregivers.

   Options include:

   (1) Refer Alison to her pediatrician

   (2) Refer Alison to the emergency room for immediate medical attention.

   (3) Monitor her symptoms and fever and recommend nondrug measures only.

   (4) Recommend a medication alone or in combination with nondrug measures.

   (5) Take no action.

Plan

5. Select an optimal therapeutic alternative to address the patient's problem, taking into account patient preferences.

   Alison has an exclusion for self-care based on her age of 10 weeks and the temperature that was reported. Alison's mother should contact her pediatrician immediately to rule out any infectious etiology.

6. Describe the recommended therapeutic approach to the caregivers.

   "No medication recommended at this time. Immediate medical referral."

7. Explain to the caregivers the rationale for selecting the recommended therapeutic approach from the considered therapeutic alternatives

   "Alison has a fever and is at high risk for an infection because of her immature immune system. Infants < 3 months also have yet to develop many of the signs that can be used to judge clinical appearance."

case

6-2 *continued*

Relevant Evaluation Criteria	Scenario/Model Outcome

Patient Education

8. When recommending self-care with nonprescription medications and/or nondrug therapy, convey accurate information to the caregivers:

   a. appropriate dose and frequency of administration

      None recommended

   b. patient's options in the event that condition worsens or persists

      "If fever worsens or does not improve, you should take Alison to a hospital emergency department after speaking with the pediatrician."

   c. specific nondrug measures

      "Maintain room temperature at 68°F, and dress her in lightweight clothing"

Solicit follow-up questions from caregivers.

      "I have ibuprofen (Advil) liquid at home. Is that OK to give her for now until I get to the pediatrician?"

Answer caregivers' questions.

      "Ibuprofen is not recommended in children < 6 months of age. Please call your pediatrician immediately."

Evaluation of Patient Outcome

9. Assess patient outcome.

      Contact Alison's mother in 1–2 days to ensure that she sought medical care for Alison.

Key: NA = Not applicable; NKDA = no known drug allergies.

patient education for

Fever

The primary objectives of treating fever are to (1) relieve the discomfort of fever and (2) prevent complications associated with fever. For most patients, carefully following product instructions and the self-care measures listed here will help to ensure optimal therapeutic outcomes.

Temperature Measurement

- Do not rely on feeling the body to detect fever. Take a temperature reading with an appropriate thermometer.
- For children up to 3 months of age, the rectal method of temperature measurement is preferred (Table 6–3). Use of a tympanic thermometer is not recommended in children younger than 6 months because of the size and shape of the infant's ear canal.
- For children ages 6 months to 3 years, the rectal, oral, tympanic, or temporal method may be used if proper technique is followed (Tables 6–3 through 6–6).
- For individuals older than 3 years, the oral, tympanic, or temporal method is appropriate (Tables 6–4 through 6–6).

Nondrug Measures

- Do not use isopropyl or ethyl alcohol for body sponging. Alcohol poisoning can result from skin absorption or inhalation of topically applied alcohol solutions.
- For all levels of fever, wear lightweight clothing, remove blankets, and maintain room temperature at 68°F.
- Unless advised otherwise, drink or provide sufficient fluids to replenish body fluid losses. For children, increase fluids by at least 1–2 ounces per hour; for adults, increase fluids by at least 2–4 ounces per hour. Sports drinks, fruit juice, a balanced electrolyte formulation, or water is acceptable.

Nonprescription Medications

- Nonprescription analgesics/antipyretics (see Chapter 5, Tables 5–2 and 5–3) help in alleviating discomfort associated with fever and reducing the temperature.

- Nonprescription analgesics/antipyretics typically take 30 minutes to 1 hour to begin to decrease temperature and discomfort.
- Monitor level of discomfort and body temperature using the same thermometer at the same body site two to three times per day during a febrile illness.
- Use single-entity nonprescription analgesics/antipyretics at low doses for up to 3 days for treatment of fever (see Chapter 5, Tables 5–2 and 5–3 for dosages), unless you have exclusions for self-care (Figure 6–1).
- Avoid alternating antipyretics because of the complexity of the dosing regimens, increased risk of medication errors, and adverse effects.
- Dosing of either ibuprofen or acetaminophen in children should be based on body weight, not age.
- To avoid incorrect dosing, use a measuring device such as a syringe, dosing spoon, or medicine cup when administering liquid medication.
- If you are pregnant or have uncontrolled high blood pressure, congestive heart failure, renal failure, or an allergy to aspirin, avoid use of NSAIDs (ibuprofen and naproxen sodium) or aspirin-containing products.
- Avoid using aspirin and aspirin-containing products for fever in children younger than 15 years because of the possible risk of Reye's syndrome.

When to Seek Medical Attention

- Seek medical attention if fever or discomfort persists or worsens after 3 days of drug treatment.

Key Points for Fever

➤ Fever is self-limiting and rarely poses severe consequences unless the core temperature is greater than 106°F (41.1°C).

➤ The main treatment goal for fever is to eliminate the underlying cause as well as to alleviate the associated discomfort.

➤ Fever should be confirmed only by using a thermometer, which is an FDA-regulated medical device.

➤ Patients should be educated on the proper measurement techniques for the thermometry they utilize.

➤ Patients should be referred for further evaluation if their rectal temperature or its equivalent is greater than 104°F (40°C), they have a history of febrile seizures, they have comorbid conditions compromising their health, or they are younger than 3 months with a temperature exceeding 100.4°F (38.0°C).

➤ Sponge baths using topical isopropyl or ethyl alcohol to reduce fever should be discouraged.

➤ Referral for further medical evaluation is appropriate to detect an underlying cause if 3 days of self-treatment are not successful in a patient older than 2 years of age and for more than 24 hours in a child younger than 2 years of age.

➤ Health care providers should counsel patients on the proper use of nonprescription antipyretic agents (including appropriate use of measuring devices) to limit medication errors and side effects. If a patient has been instructed to alternate antipyretic therapies by their health care provider, they should be counseled on the importance of recording the generic name of the drug given, the dose, and the time of administration to avoid any adverse effects.

REFERENCES

1. Cohee L, Crocetti MT, Serwint JR, et al. Ethnic differences in parental perceptions and management of childhood fever. *Clin Pediatr.* 2010; 49(3):221–7.

2. Niska R, Bhuiya F, and Xu J. *National Hospital Ambulatory Medical Care Survey: 2007 Emergency Department Summary.* National Health Statistics Reports; No. 26. Hyattsville, MD: National Center for Health Statistics; 2010. DHHS Publication No. (PHS) 2010–1250. Accessed at http://www.cdc.gov/nchs/data/nhsr/nhsr026.pdf, April 19, 2013.

3. Centers for Disease Control and Prevention. *National Ambulatory Medical Care Survey: 2008 Summary Tables.* Accessed at http://www.cdc.gov/nchs/data/ahcd/namcs_summary/2008_namcs_web_tables.pdf, April 20, 2013.

4. Rehm KP. Fever in infants and children. *Curr Opin Pediatr.* 2001;13(1):83–8.

5. Halloran LL, Bernard DW. Management of drug-induced hyperthermia. *Curr Opin Pediatr.* 2004;16(2):211–5.

6. Dinarello CA, Porat R. Fever and hyperthermia. In: Fauci AS, Kasper DL, Jameson JL, Longo DL, Hauser SL, eds. *Harrison's Principles of Internal Medicine.* 18th ed. New York: McGraw-Hill; 2012. Accessed at http://www.accesspharmacy.com/content.aspx?aID=9095580, April 19, 2013.

7. Bartfai T, Conti B. Fever [serial online]. *Sci World J.* 2010;10:490–503. Accessed at http://www.hindawi.com/journals/tswj/2010/636738/abs, July 25, 2013.

8. Barrett KE, Barman SM, Boitano S, Brooks HL. Hypothalamic regulation of hormonal functions. In: Barrett KE, Barman SM, Boitano S, Brooks HL, eds. *Ganong's Review of Medical Physiology.* 24th ed. New York: McGraw-Hill; 2012. Accessed at http://www.accesspharmacy.com/content.aspx?aID= 56262421, April 19, 2013.

9. Norman DC. Fever in the elderly. *Clin Infect Dis.* 2000;31(1):148–51.

10. DiPiro JT. Allergic and pseudoallergic drug reactions. In: Talbert RL, DiPiro JT, Matzke GR, Posey LM, et al., eds. *Pharmacotherapy: A Pathophysiologic Approach.* 8th ed. New York: McGraw-Hill; 2011. Accessed at http://www.accesspharmacy.com/content.aspx?aID=7995862, April 19, 2013.

11. Cuddy, ML. The effects of drugs on thermoregulation. *ACCN Clin Issues.* 2004;15(2):238–53.

12. Schuh S, Komar L, Stephens D, et al. Comparison of the temporal artery and rectal thermometry in children in the emergency department. *Pediatr Emerg Care.* 2004;20(11):736–41.

13. El-Radhi AS, Barry W. Thermometry in paediatric practice. *Arch Dis Child.* 2006;91(4):351–6.

14. U.S. Environmental Protection Agency. Mercury thermometers. Accessed at http://www.epa.gov/mercury/thermometer-main.html, April 19, 2013.

15. Kaz Inc. Vicks digital pacifier thermometer Model V925P product manual. Accessed at http://www.kaz.com/kaz/thermometers/products/vicks-digital-pacifier-thermometer-v925p-a, April 19, 2013.

16. Thermometer comparison. *Pharm Lett Prescrib Lett.* 2010;26.

17. Exergen Corporation. Exergen Temporal Artery Thermometer instructions for use. Accessed at http://www.exergen.com//medical/PDFs/tat2000instrev7.pdf, July 24, 2013.

18. Robinson JL, Seal RF, Spady DW, et al. Comparison of esophageal, rectal, axillary, bladder, tympanic, and pulmonary artery temperatures in children. *J Pediatr.* 1998;133(4):553–6.

19. Braun CA. Accuracy of a pacifier thermometer in young children. *Pediatr Nurs.* 2006;32(5):413–8.

20. Callanan D. Detecting fever in young infants: reliability of perceived, pacifier, and temporal artery temperatures in infants younger than 3 months of age. *Pediatr Emerg Care.* 2003;19(4):240–3.

21. Paes BF, Vermeulen K, Brohet RM, et al. Accuracy of tympanic and infrared skin thermometers in children [serial online]. *Arch Dis Child.* 2010;95(12):974–8.

22. Craig JV, Lancaster GA, Taylor S, et al. Infrared ear thermometry compared with rectal thermometry in children: a systematic review. *Lancet.* 2002;360(9333):603–9.

23. Greenes DS, Fleisher GR. Accuracy of a noninvasive temporal artery thermometer for use in infants. *Arch Pediatr Adolesc Med.* 2001;155(3):376–81.

24. Fortuna EL, Carney MM, Macy M, et al. Accuracy of non-contact infrared thermometry versus rectal thermometry in young children evaluated in the emergency department for fever. *J Emerg Nurs.* 2010;36(2):101–4.

25. Stine CA, Flook DM, Vincze DL. Rectal versus axillary temperatures: Is there a significant difference in infants less than 1 year of age? *J Pediatr Nurs.* 2012;27(3):265–70.

26. Klein M, DeWitt TG. Reliability of parent-measured axillary temperatures. *Clin Pediatr.* 2010;49(3):271–3.

27. Poirier MP, Collins EP, McGuire E. Fever phobia: a survey of caregivers of children seen in a pediatric emergency department. *Clin Pediatr.* 2010; 49(6):530–4.

28. Steering committee on quality improvement and management, subcommittee on febrile seizures. Febrile seizures: clinical practice guidelines for the long-term management of the child with simple febrile seizures. *Pediatrics.* 2008;121(6):1281–6.

29. Millar JS. Evaluation and treatment of the child with febrile seizure. *Am Fam Physician.* 2006;73(10):1761–4.

30. Strengell T, Uhari M, Tarkka R, et al. Antipyretic agents for preventing recurrences of febrile seizures. *Arch Pediatr Adolesc Med.* 2009;163(9): 799–804.

31. Lux AL. Treatment of febrile seizures: historical perspective, current opinions, and potential future directions. *Brain Develop.* 2010;32(1):42–50.

32. High KP, Bradley SF, Gravenstein S, et al. Clinical practice guideline for the evaluation of fever and infection in older adult residents of long-term care facilities: 2008 update by the Infectious Diseases Society of America. *J Am Geriatr Soc.* 2009;57(3):375–94.

33. Section on Clinical Pharmacology and Therapeutics, Committee on Drugs, Sullivan JE, Farra HC. Fever and antipyretic use in children. *Pediatrics.* 2011;127(3):580–7.

34. Mackowiak PA. Concepts of fever. *Arch Intern Med.* 1998;158(17):1870–81.

35. Aver JR. Acute fever. *Pediatr Rev.* 2009;30(1):5–13.

36. American Academy of Pediatrics. Fever and your child. Accessed at http://www.healthychildren.org/English/health-issues/conditions/fever/pages/When-to-Call-the-Pediatrician.aspx, April 23, 2013.

37. Axelrod P. External cooling in the management of fever. *Clin Infect Dis.* 2000;31(suppl 5);S224–9.

38. Aronoff DM, Neilson EG. Antipyretics: mechanisms of action and clinical use in fever suppression. *Am J Med.* 2001;111(4):304–15.

39. Treluyer JM, Tonnelier S, d'Athis P, et al. Antipyretic efficacy of an initial 30-mg/kg loading dose of acetaminophen versus a 15-mg/kg maintenance dose. *Pediatrics.* 2001;108(4);E73.

40. Goldstein LE, Berlin M, Berkovitch M, et al. Effectiveness of oral vs. rectal acetaminophen. *Arch Pediatr Adolesc Med.* 2008;162(11):1042–6.

41. Wright AD, Liebelt EL. Alternating antipyretics for fever reduction in children: an unfounded practice passed down to parents from pediatricians. *Clin Pediatr.* 2007;46(2):146–50.

42. Goldman RD, Ko K, Linett LJ, et al. Antipyretic efficacy and safety of ibuprofen and acetaminophen in children. *Ann Pharmacother.* 2004;38(1):146–50.

43. Pierce CA, Voss B. Efficacy and safety of ibuprofen and acetaminophen in children and adults: A meta-analysis and qualitative review. *Ann Pharmacother.* 2010;44(3):489–506.

44. Sarrell EM, Wielunsky E, Cohen HA. Antipyretic treatment in young children with fever. *Arch Pediatr Adolesc Med.* 2006;160(2):197–202.

45. Prymula R, Siegrist CA, Chlibek R, et al. Effect of prophylactic paracetamol administration at time of vaccination on febrile reactions and antibody response in children: two open-label, randomized controlled trials. *Lancet.* 2009;374(9698):1339–50.

46. Lagerlov P, Helseth S, Holager T. Childhood illnesses and the use of paracetamol: a qualitative study of parents' management of common childhood illnesses. *Fam Pract.* 2003;20(6):717–23.

chapter 7

MUSCULOSKELETAL INJURIES AND DISORDERS

Julie L. Olenak

Pain is one of the most common symptoms to prompt a visit to a health care provider. Because pain is a common symptom of disease or injury, patients often seek medical attention, although many seek to relieve the pain by self-treating with nonprescription analgesics. Much of the pain for which people attempt self-treatment arises from the musculoskeletal system. Musculoskeletal pain may be felt in the affected tissue itself or referred from another anatomic source (e.g., hip pain referred from its primary source in the low back).[1]

Musculoskeletal pain arises from the muscles, bones, joints, and connective tissue. The development of musculoskeletal pain can be acute, such as sport injuries (e.g., tendonitis, sprains, and strains), or it can stem from the exacerbation of a condition (e.g., osteoarthritis). Acute pain is typically defined as pain lasting less than 4 weeks. Pain lasting at least 3 months is considered chronic pain and may arise from degenerative joint disease, osteoarthritis, or chronic tendonitis (e.g., carpal tunnel).[2]

Use of nonprescription systemic and topical analgesics remains high, with more than $3,893 million and $516 million spent, respectively, per year in the United States on such remedies.[3] Ideally, a patient experiencing pain will ask a provider to assist in selecting a nonprescription product. Providers need to communicate effectively to understand the types of pain for which patients are seeking treatment to better understand the nature of their pain complaints. Providers must also be ready to offer reasonable recommendations for either treatment or further evaluation.

Musculoskeletal complaints result in a significant amount of lost work days, work limitations, loss of employment, and increased utilization of the health care system. These complaints are believed to be the greatest contributors to the economic burden of chronic pain, costing state and federal agencies $100 billion annually. The total annual cost of persistent pain for adults in the United States, both noninstitutionalized and nonmilitary personnel, is estimated to be between $560 and $635 billion dollars.[4,5] More than 100 million adults in the United States battle chronic pain.[5]

Pathophysiology of Musculoskeletal Injuries and Disorders

The musculoskeletal system includes the muscles, tendons, ligaments, cartilage, and bones. Muscles are attached to bones by tendons, and ligaments connect bone to bone. Tendons and ligaments normally have limited ability to stretch and twist. Because of their tensile strength, tendons and ligaments rarely rupture unless subjected to intense forces, but they may become damaged when hyperextended or overused. Synovial bursae are fluid-filled sacs located between joint spaces to provide lubrication and cushioning. Cartilage functions as protective pads between bones in joints and in the vertebral column.[6]

Skeletal, or striated, muscle is composed of cells (myocytes) in which two constituents (actin and myosin) are primarily responsible for contraction. Muscle contraction also involves several electrolytes within the muscle tissue, including calcium and potassium. Pain receptors are located in skeletal muscle and the overlying fascia, and those receptors can be stimulated as a result of overuse or injury to the muscle or surrounding structures.[1,6]

Somatic pain occurs when pain impulses are transmitted from peripheral nociceptors to the central nervous system (CNS) by nerve fibers. Common sites of origin are muscles, fascia, and bones. Somatic pain is most commonly myofascial (e.g., muscle strain) or musculoskeletal (e.g., arthritis).[1] (See Chapter 5 for discussion of transduction, transmission, perception, and modulation of pain.)

Mechanoreceptors and chemoreceptors mediate muscle pain. These nerve endings are heterogeneous: only a single chemical can stimulate some endings, whereas a variety of chemical, mechanical, and thermal triggers can stimulate others.[1,6]

Erythema (redness), edema, and hyperalgesia (an exaggerated pain response to minor amounts of noxious stimuli[5]) at the affected site characterize the inflammatory response, which develops through participation of multiple mediators, including histamine, bradykinin, serotonin, leukotrienes, and prostaglandin E.[1] Muscle injuries can be categorized as delayed-onset muscle soreness (e.g., overexertion), myalgia, strains, tendonitis, bursitis, and sprains. Low back pain and osteoarthritis are common conditions associated with musculoskeletal complaints. *Overexertion* or *repeated unaccustomed eccentric muscle contraction* is associated with delayed-onset (8 hours or more) muscle soreness, which can last for days, usually peaking at 24–48 hours. This pain reflects muscle damage that was presumably initiated by force generated in the muscle fibers; the pain is thought to be induced by inflammation, acidosis, muscle spasms, and/or microlesions. Prolonged tonic contraction produced by exercise, tension, or poor posture and by body mechanics can also produce muscle pain. Overexertion is common in individuals who do not exercise regularly but then begin an exercise regimen at a level of high intensity.

Myalgia, or *muscle pain,* can result from systemic infections (e.g., influenza, coxsackievirus, measles, and other illnesses), chronic disorders (e.g., fibromyalgia and polymyalgia rheumatica), and medications (e.g., some cholesterol-lowering agents such as HMG-CoA reductase inhibitors). Abuse of alcohol may precipitate acute alcoholic myopathy. Bone and muscle pain related to a vitamin D deficiency (osteomalacia) may also occur.[1]

Strains are a result of an injury to a muscle or a tendon. A strain can be caused by an acute injury, or with prolonged overuse, a strain can become a chronic condition. The movements that cause a strain involve twisting or pulling. Tendons can become strained when their stretch capacity is exceeded (e.g., hyperextension injury of an arm or leg). The strain injury is caused by eccentric contraction of the muscle while the muscle is lengthening. A tear of the muscle or tendon can also occur.[7]

Tendonitis is the inflammation of a tendon, which results from acute injury or from chronic repetitive movements of a body part. An example of an overuse injury is carpal tunnel syndrome, a condition characterized by tingling or numbness of the first digits of the hand caused by repetitive use of the hands and wrists. Tendon sheaths become inflamed and constrict the median nerve as it passes through a narrow channel between the wrist bones.[6] Tendonitis can also commonly occur in the Achilles tendon, which connects the calf muscle to the heel.

Common terms that describe sports-related tendonitis from overuse include tennis or golfer's elbow, swimmer's shoulder, and jumper's knee. In sports-related overuse injuries, contributing factors for tendonitis can include increased age, poor technique, improper conditioning, exercise of prolonged intensity or duration, and poorly designed equipment for specific activities (e.g., poor cushioning of athletic shoes).

Finally, certain medications (e.g., fluoroquinolone antimicrobials) are associated with the development of tendonitis or tendon rupture and carry a boxed warning.[8]

Bursitis is a common cause of localized pain, tenderness, and swelling, which is worsened by any movement of the structure adjacent to the bursa, in the joint. Bursitis generally results from an acute injury to the joint or over-repetitive joint action. When pain is accompanied by the presence of a puncture site (possibly from intra-articular injection), an adjacent source of infection, or severe inflammation, an infectious cause should be suspected and ruled out before recommending self-treatment.

Sprains are the most common problem with ligaments. Sprains are graded by their characteristics, with grade I sprains resulting from excessive stretching, grade II sprains resulting from a partial tear, and grade III sprains involving a complete tear of the tissue. Grade II and III sprains typically result in moderate-severe pain, loss of function of the affected limb, and an inability to bear weight. Tears and ruptures are more common in ligaments than in tendons. Sprains commonly occur during physical activity. Approximately 628,000 sprains occur annually in the United States.[7]

Low back pain is the fifth most likely reason for a physician visit; the lifetime prevalence of developing low back pain approaches 80%.[6,9] The National Institute of Arthritis and Musculoskeletal and Skin Disease reports that 25% of people report at least 1 day of back pain in a 3-month period.[10]

Main risk factors for the development of low back pain include sedentary lifestyle (particularly one disrupted by bursts of activity), poor posture, improper shoes, excessive body weight, poor mattress and sleeping posture, and improper technique when lifting heavy objects. Most patients recover within a few days to a few weeks, even without treatment; if pain persists for more than

3 months, it is classified as chronic low back pain.[2,11] Other causes of low back pain include congenital anomalies, osteoarthritis, vertebral fractures and compressions, spinal tuberculosis, and referred pain from diseased kidneys, pancreas, liver, or prostate.[1]

Osteoarthritis is characterized by a gradual softening and destruction of the cartilage between bones. Cartilage and bone are destroyed in the joint spaces and regenerated, causing a rearrangement of the synovial architecture. Often referred to as "degenerative joint disease," osteoarthritis is caused by genetic, metabolic, and environmental factors. Heavy physical activity, repetitive movement, and lifting of heavy weights may aggravate this condition, whereas light-moderate activity does not and is generally helpful.[12,13] Approximately 27 million people in the United States have a diagnosis of osteoarthritis; by 2030, that number is expected to increase to 67 million.[14]

Clinical Presentation of Musculoskeletal Injuries and Disorders

Table 7–1 lists many of the presenting signs and symptoms of musculoskeletal disorders and also differentiates other factors. Pain is a common symptom among all these disorders.

In addition to the pain induced by a sprain, patients have variable degrees of joint function. If a sprain patient has limited joint function, the injury is most likely a grade II or grade III sprain that requires proper workup to rule out a fracture or tear. If a joint is visibly deformed, it requires emergency assistance.

Patients with carpal tunnel syndrome often experience a diminished ability to feel heat or cold; a sense that their hands are swollen, even when they are not; a weakness in the hands; and a tendency to drop things. Symptoms persist during sleep and even when the hand is not being used, a characteristic that can be used to distinguish this disorder from others.

The pain of osteoarthritis does not correlate directly with the degree of joint damage. Pain is often referred, and proximal muscles can be involved if a person with osteoarthritis guards the affected joint by changing his or her gait to reduce discomfort. The pain caused by chronic osteoarthritis often limits the patient's activities of daily living (ADLs) (e.g., inability to grip containers or walk more than a short distance).

Low back pain can also be neuropathic in nature, involving the sciatic nerve, causing sharp referred pain into one or both of the patient's legs. Low back pain can often limit a patient's ability to bend, move, sit, or walk.

Complications of untreated pain-inducing injuries include further tissue damage and (in advanced arthritis) bone and cartilage remodeling. Pain is associated with significant limitations, including a reduction in ADLs, disability, loss of work time, and physical impairments (e.g., insomnia). Be sure to look for warning signs and symptoms that preclude self-treatment of such disorders. (See exclusions for self-treatment in Figure 7–1.)

Treatment of Musculoskeletal Injuries and Disorders

Acute pain is the body's alarm system; it signals injury by trauma, disease, muscle spasms, or inflammation. Chronic pain, conversely, may or may not be indicative of injury and requires a primary care provider's assessment before treatment is initiated.

table

7–1   Comparison of Musculoskeletal Disorders

	Myalgia	Tendonitis	Bursitis	Sprain	Strain	Osteoarthritis
Location	Muscles of the body	Tendon locations around joint areas	Inflammation of the bursae within joints; common locations include knee, shoulder, big toe	Stretching or tearing of a ligament within a joint	Hyperextension of a muscle or tendon	Weight-bearing joints, knees, hips, low back, hands
Signs	Possible swelling (rare)	Warmth, swelling, erythema	Warmth, edema, erythema, and possible crepitus	Swelling, bruising	Swelling, bruising	Noninflammatory joints, narrowing of joint space, restructuring of bone and cartilage (resulting in joint deformities), possible joint swelling
Symptoms	Dull, constant ache (sharp pain relatively rare); weakness and fatigue of muscles also common	Mild-severe pain generally occurring after use; loss of range of motion	Constant pain that worsens with movement or application of external pressure over the joint	Initial severe pain followed by pain, particularly with joint use; tenderness; reduction in joint stability and function	Initial severe pain with continued pain upon movement and at rest; muscle weakness; loss of some function	Dull joint pain relieved by rest; joint stiffness <20–30 minutes; localized symptoms to joint; crepitus
Onset	Varies depending on cause (i.e., trauma = acute, but drug-induced = insidious)	Often gradual, but can develop suddenly	Acute with injury; recurs with precipitant use of joint	Acute with injury	Acute with injury	Insidious development over years
Modifying Factors	Elimination of cause; use of stretching, rest, heat, topical analgesics, systemic analgesics	Elimination of cause; use of stretching, rest, ice, heat, topical analgesics, systemic analgesics	Joint rest; immobilization; topical analgesics; systemic analgesics	RICE; stretching; use of protective wraps (e.g., ankle tape, knee brace, cane); topical counterirritants; systemic analgesics	RICE; stretching; use of protective wraps; topical counterirritants; systemic analgesics	Continuous exercise (light-moderate activity); weight loss, analgesic medication; topical pain relievers

Key: RICE = rest, ice, compression, elevation (Table 7–2).

Treatment Goals

Treatment of the patient with musculoskeletal complaints encompasses many different goals, including (1) decreasing the subjective intensity (severity) of pain; (2) decreasing the duration of pain, when possible; (3) restoring function of the affected area; (4) preventing re-injury and disability (i.e., improve ADLs); and (5) preventing acute pain from becoming chronic persistent pain.

General Treatment Approach

Patients with musculoskeletal injuries present with common symptoms (especially pain and swelling of the affected area) and have similar self-treatment approaches. Nonpharmacologic therapy consisting of rest, ice, compression, and elevation (RICE) along with nonprescription oral analgesics and/or topical analgesics during the first 1–3 days following injury is helpful.[7] Before treatment can be recommended, however, the patient should be carefully screened to ensure appropriateness of self-treatment. The algorithm in Figure 7–1 presents a stepwise approach to self-management of pain for patients who are not excluded for self-care.

Patients with acute low back pain are candidates for self-treatment. Management of acute back pain includes rest for 1–2 days and nonprescription oral or topical analgesics. Chronic low back pain requires medical evaluation before initiating therapy.[15]

Pain associated with osteoarthritis is approved for self-treatment after an initial medical diagnosis. The general treatment

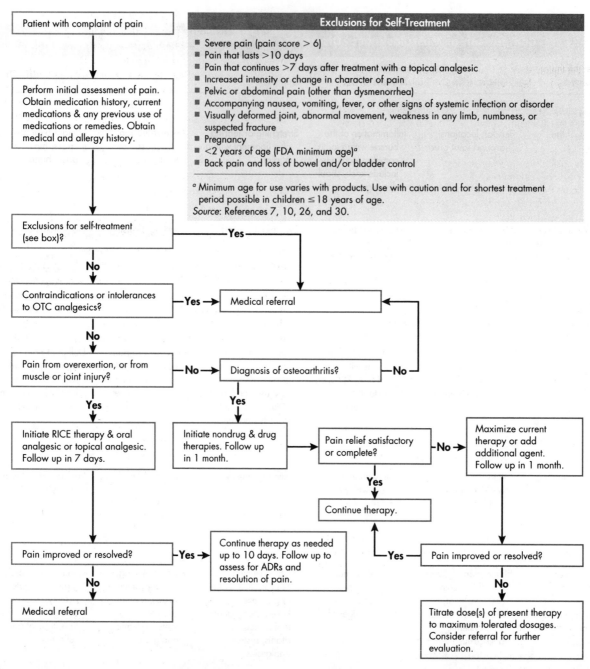

Exclusions for Self-Treatment

- Severe pain (pain score > 6)
- Pain that lasts >10 days
- Pain that continues >7 days after treatment with a topical analgesic
- Increased intensity or change in character of pain
- Pelvic or abdominal pain (other than dysmenorrhea)
- Accompanying nausea, vomiting, fever, or other signs of systemic infection or disorder
- Visually deformed joint, abnormal movement, weakness in any limb, numbness, or suspected fracture
- Pregnancy
- <2 years of age (FDA minimum age)[a]
- Back pain and loss of bowel and/or bladder control

[a] Minimum age for use varies with products. Use with caution and for shortest treatment period possible in children ≤18 years of age.
Source: References 7, 10, 26, and 30.

figure 7-1 Self-care of musculoskeletal injuries and disorders. Key: ADR = Adverse drug reaction; FDA = Food and Drug Administration; OTC = over-the-counter; RICE = rest, ice, compression, elevation. (*Source:* Adapted from Self-care of self-limited pain. In: Albrant DH, ed. *The American Pharmaceutical Association Drug Treatment Protocols.* 2nd ed. Washington, DC: American Pharmaceutical Association; 2001:424–5.)

approach includes appropriate lifestyle changes (including physical activity and weight loss) and use of an analgesic, which may be a nonprescription medication.[13]

Nonpharmacologic Therapy

Injury from playing sports or exercising can be prevented by warming up and stretching muscles before physical activity, ensuring proper hydration, and wearing appropriate footwear. Stretching must be done cautiously—without bouncing—to avoid muscle strain. For muscle cramps, stretching and massaging

the affected area followed by immediate rest will loosen the muscle. For electrolyte depletion, oral supplementation of wasted electrolytes is appropriate, including fluids containing potassium, sodium, and magnesium (e.g., sports drinks or enhanced waters).

RICE therapy promotes healing and helps reduce swelling and inflammation associated with muscle and joint injuries (Table 7–2). Ice should not be applied for more than 15–20 minutes because excessive icing causes considerable vasoconstriction and reduces vascular clearance of inflammatory mediators from the damaged area. Ice therapy can also be recommended for patients with osteoarthritis experiencing

table
7–2
Guidelines for RICE Therapy

- Rest the injured area and continue until pain is reduced (generally 1–2 days). Slings, splints, or crutches can be used, if necessary.
- As soon as possible, apply ice to the injured area in 15- to 20-minute increments, at least 3–4 times a day. Continue the ice-pack therapy until swelling subsides (usually 1–3 days, depending on the severity of injury).
- Apply compression to the injured area with an elastic support or an elasticized bandage as follows:
  - Choose the appropriate size bandage for the injured body part. If preferred, purchase a product specifically designed for the injured body part.
  - If ice is also being applied to the injured area, soak the bandage in water to aid the transfer of cold.
  - Wrap the injured area by overlapping the previous layer of bandage by about one-third to one-half its width.
  - Wrap the point most distal from the injury (e.g., if the ankle is injured, begin wrapping just above the toes).
  - Decrease the tightness of the bandage as you continue to wrap. If the bandage feels tight or uncomfortable, or if circulation is impaired, remove the compression bandage and rewrap it. Cold toes or swollen fingers indicate that the bandage is too tight.
  - After using the bandage, wash it in lukewarm, soapy water; do not scrub it. Rinse the bandage thoroughly and allow to air dry on a flat surface.
  - Roll up the bandage to prevent wrinkles, and store it in a cool, dry place. Do not iron the bandage to remove wrinkles.
- Elevate the injured area at or above the level of the heart 2–3 hours a day to decrease swelling and relieve pain.

Key: RICE = Rest, ice, compression, elevation.

pain and/or swelling.[13,16] Both ice and heat, at temperatures outside the skin's threshold for tolerance, can be damaging and can result in blistering or burning; therefore, neither therapy should be applied directly to the skin.

Heat therapy is an alternative for patients who develop pain of a noninflammatory nature. It has been studied in the treatment of acute low back pain with favorable effects.[9,15] In addition, osteoarthritis guidelines recommend heat as adjunct nonpharmacological treatment for pain and stiffness.[13,16] Although its mechanism of action is not fully understood, heat may alleviate pain by increasing blood flow, reducing muscle spasm, and improving stiffness. Heat should be applied for 15–20 minutes, 3–4 times a day. Heat should not be applied to inflamed areas because it can intensify vasodilation and exacerbate vascular leakage.[17] Furthermore, heat should not be used with topical analgesics or over broken skin.

Heat should be applied to the affected area in the form of a warm wet compress, heating pad, or hot-water bottle. Ease of use favors newer, heat-generating adhesive and wrap products (e.g., ThermaCare, Precise, and various generic brands), which can be worn on the affected area up to 8 hours (some products can be used for 12 hours). The products come in various shapes, including back, hip, neck, knee, wrist and hand, shoulder, elbow, and lower abdomen. For nonadhesive products, the darker side of the heat cells should be placed toward the skin.

The adhesive products should be applied on dry skin that is free of lotion. There are product exceptions to this that have unique directions (e.g., ThermaCare menstrual product, BodiHeat), such as placing the adhesive side on the undergarment or clothing.

Heating devices should not be used on areas of skin with decreased sensation, a practice that can lead to a skin burn. Specifically, ThermaCare heat-generating products should not be placed on the back of the knee or inside the bend of the arm.[18]

Although not generally associated with many side effects, at least two brands of heat-generating patches have been recalled for causing burns along with skin irritation.[19,20] Patients should be advised to remove the patch immediately if they have any pain or discomfort, itching, or burning. Heat wraps should be worn over a towel or layer of clothing in patients older than 55 years; heat wraps should not be used during sleep.

Limited scientific information is available regarding contrast therapy (alternating heat and ice) to aid in sports injury recovery. Anecdotally, some individuals report relief, but insufficient scientific evidence exists to recommend this therapy.[21,22]

Transcutaneous electrical nerve stimulation (TENS) therapy is used widely by various practitioners (e.g., physical therapists, physicians, and chiropractors) in the treatment of pain. FDA has approved TENS therapy for nonprescription use as a class II medical device for the relief of pain associated with sore, aching muscles; joint pain; or chronic intractable pain.[23–25] Pain relief is thought to come from two mechanisms: alteration of pain transmission and an increase in the production of natural endorphins. A TENS device is typically used for an interval of 15–30 minutes up to 3 times daily. The electrode pads can be placed on various areas of the body for pain relief (e.g., back, legs, ankles, arms, and shoulders), but placement is product dependent. Because of safety concerns patients should avoid placing the electrodes on the throat, chest, or head or over the carotid arteries. The electrodes also should not be placed on open wounds, rashes, inflamed skin, cancerous lesions, or areas of skin with altered sensation, or over topical analgesics. Patients with internal or attached medical devices (e.g., pacemakers, defibrillators, electrocardiograms, and respirators); pregnant patients; and the pediatric population should not use nonprescription TENS devices.[24,25] The directions for proper and safe use of these devices are product specific, so the health care provider should review the directions with the patient.

Proper posture and the use of ergonomic controls (e.g., a chair with back support or an ergonomic keyboard) improve function and reduce pain. Heel lifts and better-fitting shoes are recommended for patients with Achilles tendonitis or low back pain. Approaches to chronic low back pain also include therapeutic interventions such as heat therapy, massage with traction, and, most important, mobilization with exercise or physical therapy. Chiropractic manipulation and acupuncture are also commonly used for the treatment of back pain.[15]

Pharmacologic Therapy
Systemic Analgesics

NSAIDs and acetaminophen are commonly used nonprescription analgesics; they are often employed in the initial treatment of musculoskeletal injuries. Systemic analgesic therapy should be limited to 10 days of self-care use,[26] and patients should seek appropriate medical care if the condition continues beyond this period or worsens during the course of treatment. (See Chapter 5 for dosages, safety, and properties of nonprescription systemic analgesics.)

For the treatment of osteoarthritis of the hip and knee, acetaminophen (rather than NSAIDs) has been recommended historically by some organizations as first-line therapy, despite data suggesting that NSAIDs provide slightly improved pain relief.[12,27] This initial treatment recommendation is made on the basis of drug safety rather than efficacy. Chronic use of NSAIDs leads to more severe and prevalent side effects (e.g., nephropathy, gastrointestinal ulcerations and bleeding, and the potential for cardiac events). Recent recommendations published by the American College of Rheumatology (ACR), however, include both acetaminophen and NSAIDs among their initial therapy options. They recommend that if NSAIDs are used chronically for the management of osteoarthritis, a proton-pump inhibitor should be considered for gastrointestinal protection. See Chapter 13 for further information on risks of long-term use of proton-pump inhibitors. The ACR guidelines do express a strong recommendation to consider using topical NSAIDS rather than systemic NSAIDs in patients 75 years of age and older.[13]

Topical Products

Topical analgesics may have local analgesic, anesthetic, antipruritic, and/or counterirritant effects. Nonprescription topical analgesics are approved specifically for the topical treatment of minor-moderate aches and pains of muscles and joints (e.g., simple backache, arthritis pain, strains, bruises, and sprains).[28] They are recommended as adjuncts to pharmacologic and nonpharmacologic therapy of musculoskeletal injuries and disorders.

Counterirritants

Topical counterirritants are applied to the skin to relieve pain.[28,29] Counterirritation is the paradoxical pain-relieving effect achieved by producing a less severe pain to counter a more intense one. The pain relief results more from nerve stimulation than depression.[28,29] When applied to the skin at pain sites, counterirritants produce a mild, local inflammatory reaction, which provides relief to the site underlying the skin surface being treated. These induced sensations distract from the deep-seated pain in muscles, joints, and tendons. Pain is only as intense as it is perceived to be, and the perception of other sensations caused by the counterirritant or its application (e.g., massage, warmth, or redness) causes the sufferer to disregard the sensation of pain.[29] On the basis of

their topical effects, counterirritants are classified into four types (Table 7–3). Table 7–4 lists examples of commercially available products.

All regulations and labeling for topical counterirritants are based on the detailed previous proposed rulemaking documents published in the *Federal Register* in 1979 and 1983.[28,30] FDA has recognized the ingredients in Table 7–3 as safe and effective (Category I) counterirritants for use in adults and in children ages 2 years and older.[30] Note that many topical nonprescription analgesic products have age limits older than 2 years.

Labels for most counterirritants indicate that the product is to be used for "the temporary relief of minor-moderate aches and sprains of muscles and joints." In addition, the labeling recommended by most of FDA's review panels includes claims for "simple backache, arthritis pain, strains, bruises, and sprains."[30] In September 2012, FDA issued a Drug Safety Communication about serious burns associated with nonprescription topical counterirritants. Forty-three case reports of chemical burns were identified in FDA's Adverse Event Reporting System (AERS) database and medical literature. Most of the second- and third-degree burn cases were associated with topical counterirritant products with higher concentrations of menthol as the single ingredient or with a combination product containing greater than 3% menthol and 10% methyl salicylate. In many of the case reports, the reactions occurred with only one application, and the resulting injury occurred within 24 hours.[31,32] FDA recommendations for users of nonprescription topical analgesic products are presented in Table 7–5. In the consumer version of the communication, FDA states that, although a feeling of warmth or coolness is normal with topical counterirritant use, patients should seek medical attention if burning pain or blistering occurs.[32]

Table 7–3 provides dosing information for the various counterirritants.

The following sections describe the commonly used counterirritants currently available in the United States.

Methyl Salicylate. Methyl salicylate occurs naturally as wintergreen oil or sweet birch oil; gaultheria oil, teaberry oil, and mountain tea are other names for the compound. Methyl

table

7–3   Classification and Dosage Guidelines[a] for Nonprescription Counterirritant External Analgesics

Group	Ingredients	Concentration (%)	Mechanism of Action	Frequency and Duration of Use
A	Allyl isothiocyanate Ammonia water Methyl salicylate Turpentine oil	0.5–5.0 1.0–2.5 10–60 6–50	Rubefacients (increase blood flow)	For all counterirritants: Apply no more than 3–4 times/day for up to 7 days
B	Camphor Menthol	3–11 1.25–16.0	Produce cooling sensation	As above in group A
C	Histamine dihydrochloride Methyl nicotinate	0.025–0.1 0.25–1.0	Cause vasodilation	As above in group A
D	Capsicum Capsicum oleoresin Capsaicin	0.025–0.25 0.025–0.25 0.025–0.25	Incite irritation without rubefaction; are as potent as group A ingredients	For acute pain: As above in group A; For chronic pain: Apply 3–4 times/day for duration of pain (often long-term use with medical supervision)

[a] Dosages approved for adults and for children 2 years and older.
Source: Reference 28.

table

7–4 Selected External Analgesic Products

Trade Name	Primary Ingredients
Menthol-Containing Products	
Aspercreme Heat Pain Relieving Gel	Menthol 10%
Bengay Ultra Strength Pain Relieving Patch	Menthol 5%
Icy Hot No Mess Applicator	Menthol 16%
Mineral Ice	Menthol 2%
Camphor-Containing Products	
JointFlex Pain Relieving Cream	Camphor 3.1%
Capsaicin-Containing Products	
Capzasin Arthritis Pain Relief No-Mess Applicator	Capsaicin 0.15%
Capzasin-HP Arthritis Pain Relief Cream	Capsaicin 0.1%
Zostrix Hot and Cold Therapy	Capsaicin 0.025%
Zostrix-HP Arthritis Pain Relief Cream	Capsaicin 0.075%
Histamine Dihydrochloride–Containing Products	
Australian Dream Pain Relieving Arthritis Cream	Histamine dihydrochloride 0.025%
Trolamine Salicylate–Containing Products	
Aspercreme Cream/Lotion	Trolamine salicylate 10%
Sportscreme Deep Penetrating Pain Relieving Rub Cream	Trolamine salicylate 10%
Combination Products	
ActivOn Topical Analgesic Ultra Strength Arthritis	Histamine dihydrochloride 0.025%; menthol 4.127%
Arthritis Hot Cream	Methyl salicylate 15%; menthol 10%
Bengay Ultra Strength Pain Relieving Cream	Methyl salicylate 30%; menthol 10%; camphor 4%
Flexall Ultra Plus Relieving Gel	Menthol 16%; methyl salicylate 10%; camphor 3.1%
Icy Hot Cream Extra Strength/Precise Pain Relieving Cream	Methyl salicylate 30%; menthol 10%
Mentholatum Ointment	Camphor 9%; natural menthol 1.3%
Mentholatum Deep Heating Extra-Strength Pain Relieving Rub Cream	Methyl salicylate 30%; menthol 8%
Salonpas Pain Relief Patch	Methyl salicylate 10%; menthol 3%
Sloan's Liniment	Turpentine oil 47%; capsaicin 0.025% (from capsicum oleoresin)
Tiger Balm Arthritis Rub Cream	Camphor 11%; menthol 11%

table

7–5 FDA Recommendations for Application of Nonprescription Topical Analgesic Products

- If pain, swelling, or blistering of the skin occurs after application of a topical analgesic, patients should immediately discontinue use of the product and seek medical attention.
- Do not bandage the area tightly where the product has been applied.
- Do not use any heat where the product has been applied.
- Do not apply to wounded, damaged, broken, or irritated skin.
- Do not allow these medications to come in contact with the eyes, or inside the nose, mouth, or genitals.

Source: References 31 and 32.

salicylate is usually combined with other ingredients (e.g., menthol and/or camphor).

As a rubefacient, methyl salicylate causes vasodilation of cutaneous vasculature, thereby producing reactive hyperemia. This increase in blood pooling and/or flow is hypothesized to be accompanied by an increase in localized skin temperature, which in turn may exert a counterirritant effect. Because of its rubefacient action, methyl salicylate is responsible for the "hot" action in many topical counterirritant products.[29]

In addition to the mechanisms described previously, topically applied methyl salicylate products inhibit both central and peripheral prostaglandin synthesis. Studies on the rate and extent of percutaneous absorption of various commercially available methyl salicylate preparations show direct tissue penetration rather than redistribution by the systemic blood supply, indicating a localized effect of the topical product.[29]

Localized reactions (e.g., skin irritation or rash) and systemic reactions (e.g., salicylate toxicity) may occur with the use of methyl salicylate. Strong irritation may cause local reactions such as erythema, blistering, neurotoxicity, or thermal hyperalgesia. In addition, heat exposure and exercise after applying methyl salicylate have been shown to cause a threefold increase in systemic absorption of salicylate, which can lead to increases in adverse systemic reactions.[33] Table 7–5 reviews appropriate precautions to take when using topical analgesics. Because percutaneous absorption of salicylate can occur, methyl salicylate should be avoided in children and used with caution in individuals who are sensitive to aspirin. Concomitant use of salicylate-containing topical analgesics and maintenance warfarin therapy has been implicated in prolonging prothrombin time.[29] Chapter 5 describes other potential drug interactions related to systemically absorbed salicylates.

The report of the American Association of Poison Control Centers documents 10,000 encounters of methyl salicylate exposure in children ages 6 years and younger.[34] In children of that age, just a teaspoon of wintergreen oil can cause death.[34] Although an FDA survey found that oral ingestion of methyl salicylate in ointment form caused no deaths and that few cases manifested severe symptoms,[28] regulations require the use of child-resistant containers for liquid preparations containing concentrations greater than 5%.

Camphor.

Although camphor occurs naturally and is obtained from the camphor tree, approximately three-fourths of the camphor used is prepared synthetically.

In concentrations of 0.1%–3.0%, camphor depresses cutaneous receptors and is used as a topical analgesic, anesthetic, and antipruritic. In concentrations exceeding 3%, particularly when combined with other counterirritant ingredients, camphor stimulates the nerve endings in the skin and induces relief of pain and discomfort by masking moderate-severe deeper visceral pain, with a milder pain arising from the skin at the level of innervation. When applied vigorously, it produces a rubefacient reaction.

Concentrations higher than those recommended are not more effective and can cause more serious adverse reactions if accidentally ingested.[30] The risk of toxicity relates to both the concentration of camphor in the ingested product and the extent of absorption of camphor into the body. CNS toxicity, expressed primarily as tonic–clonic seizures, is the major toxicity and begins to occur as early as 10 minutes following ingestion. High doses of camphor can cause nausea, vomiting, colic, headache, dizziness, delirium, convulsion, coma, and death.

Case reports of camphor toxicities in children continue.[35,36] In 2009, the American Academy of Pediatrics Committee on Drugs reaffirmed their statement on camphor, noting that although nonprescription camphor-containing preparations cannot exceed concentrations of 11%, camphor toxicity continues. The academy advised parents to be aware of this potential danger and recommended use of modalities that do not contain camphor.[37]

Menthol.

Menthol is either prepared synthetically or extracted from peppermint oil (which contains a 30%–50% concentration of menthol). Menthol may be used safely in small quantities as a flavoring agent and has found wide acceptance in candy, chewing gum, cigarettes, cough drops, toothpaste, nasal sprays, and liqueurs. It is also used as a permeability enhancer to increase absorption of other topically administered medications.[38]

At concentrations less than 1%, menthol depresses cutaneous receptor response (i.e., acts as an anesthetic); at concentrations greater than 1.25%, menthol stimulates cutaneous receptor response (i.e., acts as a counterirritant).

Recent studies have led to the identification of heat- and cold-sensitive receptors within sensory neurons called transient receptor potential (TRP) cation channels. Topically applied menthol activates the TRPM8 menthol receptor, triggering the sensation of cold.[38] The resultant cold sensation travels along pathways similar to the somatic pain sensations from the affected muscle or joint, which distracts from the sensation of pain. The initial feeling of coolness is soon followed by a sensation of warmth.

Menthol is contraindicated in patients with hypersensitivity or sensitization to the agent (e.g., urticaria, erythema, and other cutaneous lesions).[38] Treatment should be discontinued if the patient develops irritation, rash, burning, stinging, swelling, or infection.

Methyl Nicotinate.

Although nicotinic acid is inactive topically, methyl nicotinate readily penetrates the cutaneous barrier. Vasodilation and elevation of skin temperature result from very low concentrations, with higher penetration rates seen with hydrophilic mediums (i.e., gels). One study showed that indomethacin, ibuprofen, and aspirin significantly depress the skin's vascular response to methyl nicotinate. Because these three drugs suppress prostaglandin biosynthesis, the vasodilator response to methyl nicotinate is mediated, at least in part, by prostaglandin biosynthesis.[39]

Generalized vascular dilation can occur when methyl nicotinate passes through the skin into the circulatory system. Therefore, persons who apply methyl nicotinate over large areas may experience a drop in blood pressure, a decrease in pulse rate, and syncope caused by generalized vascular dilation.[27]

Capsicum Preparations.

Capsicum preparations (capsaicin, capsicum, and capsicum oleoresin) are derived from the fruit of various species of plants of the nightshade family. Capsicum contains about 1.5% of an irritating oleoresin, the major component of which is capsaicin (0.02%). Capsaicin is the major pungent ingredient of hot (chili) peppers.

When applied to normal skin, capsaicin elicits a transient feeling of warmth through stimulation of the TRPV1 receptor. The mechanism of action is thought to be directly related to capsaicin's effects on the depletion of substance P. This substance is found in slow-conducting, unmyelinated type C neurons that innervate the dermis and epidermis. It is released in the skin in response to endogenous (e.g., stress) and exogenous (e.g., trauma or injury) factors. It appears that pruritic stimuli along with pain impulses are conveyed to central processing centers by type C fibers in the skin, for which capsaicin has selective activity. Local application of capsaicin to the peripheral axon appears to deplete substance P from sensory neurons. The depletion occurs both peripherally and centrally, presumably as the result of impulse initiation. When substance P is released, burning pain occurs but abates with repeated applications. The diminishing sensation experienced with repeated applications can lead to adherence-related failures; health care providers should inform their patients about such effects and the importance of continuing therapy.[40]

Capsaicin has additional indications in comparison to other counterirritants. Capsaicin is used to reduce the pain—but not the inflammation—of rheumatoid arthritis and osteoarthritis; it is also used in a wide variety of other pain disorders (e.g., postherpetic neuralgia, psoriasis, and diabetic neuropathy).

The optimal dose of capsaicin varies among patients. The efficacy of capsaicin decreases (and local discomfort increases) when capsaicin is applied less often than directed because the drug's duration of action is 4–6 hours. Pain relief is usually noted within 14 days after therapy has begun, but relief will occasionally be delayed by as much as 4–6 weeks.

Once topical nonprescription capsaicin has begun to relieve pain, its use must continue regularly 3 or 4 times a day. If capsaicin treatment is stopped and the pain returns, treatment can be resumed. Capsaicin may produce a sensation of burning or stinging pain. However, as a result of tachyphylaxis, this local effect diminishes in intensity with repeated applications, typically within a few days but as long as 1–2 weeks.[40–42] To reduce the likelihood of capsaicin reaching topically sensitive areas (e.g., mucous membranes), patients should be instructed to use a glove for application and to wash their hands following use.[40] If the hands are the site of application, the patient should wait 30 minutes after application and then wash his or her hands. During use, capsaicin should not come in contact with the eyes or other sensitive areas of the body, as it will cause a burning sensation.[40] Capsaicin is available in a roll-on applicator or patch formulation, which may be preferred by some patients because of their ease of application. Patients using such formulations should still be instructed to wash their hands after handling the product.

Use in patients with hypersensitivity to capsaicin is contraindicated. The agent should be discontinued temporarily if skin breaks down (i.e., skin is weeping and red; small ulcers are present), and the agent should not be applied to wounds or damaged skin.

In addition to skin reactions, capsaicin has also been associated with a cough, runny nose, or sneezing if particles are inhaled.[40] Overdose with use of capsaicin has not been reported, but more serious and intense side effects are reported with higher concentrations.[43]

Capsaicin is also available in a prescription patch formulation (Qutenza 8%) approved for the treatment of postherpetic neuralgia.[43]

Additional Counterirritants

Allyl isothiocyanate, ammonia water, turpentine oil, and histamine dihydrochloride are also classified as Category I counterirritants by FDA, but few counterirritant preparations contain those ingredients. Most products that contain them also contain other topical analgesics, making any beneficial action or side effects of the products indistinguishable from other ingredients. In addition, very little evidence supports the efficacy of such compounds. Allyl isothiocyanate, ammonia water, and turpentine oil are rubefacients, so they should be expected to have effects similar to those of methyl salicylate. However, histamine dihydrochloride causes vasodilation, similar to the action of methyl nicotinate.

Pharmacotherapeutic Efficacy and Recommendations for Counterirritants

Literature regarding the efficacy of counterirritants is conflicting; given their age, in some instances, current studies are lacking. However, Cochrane reviews evaluating the use of counterirritants in specific conditions and current guidelines for osteoarthritis provide some guidance on their use.

A 2009 Cochrane review reports that topical rubefacients (those specifically containing salicylates) are not supported by enough evidence to be recommended for use in acute or chronic pain. The authors noted that studies in assessing acute pain were limited; however, the studies included showed a 50% pain reduction in 1 in 3 patients treated after 1 week and a 50% pain reduction for 1 in 6 patients treated after 2 weeks. For chronic pain, however, the study concluded that topical rubefacients compare poorly with topical NSAIDs.[44]

After the Cochrane review, one study evaluated the use of a nonprescription combination methyl salicylate and menthol patch for the treatment of mild-moderate muscle strain; the results showed that pain relief was approximately 40% better in those using the 8-hour patch versus placebo.[45] These patches (Salonpas Pain Relief Patch and Salonpas Arthritis Pain Patch) are the only nonprescription analgesic patches to undergo FDA approval of a New Drug Application, which was granted in 2009.

Conflicting recommendations exist with capsaicin. An updated Cochrane Review in 2012 focused on reevaluating low concentration (<1%) capsaicin products for the treatment of chronic neuropathic pain. This review was conducted because the authors believed the 2009 conclusion might have been biased and ultimately may have overestimated capsaicin's efficacy. They utilized a stricter approach to the evaluation of evidence for inclusion in the updated review. The 2012 review states that there is insufficient evidence to make a conclusion about low-dose capsaicin in treating neuropathic pain but that it unlikely has any "meaningful effect."[42]

The National Institute for Health and Clinical Excellence guidelines for osteoarthritis do not support the use of rubefacients, with the exception of capsaicin.[16,46] The 2012 ACR guidelines for the management of osteoarthritis conditionally recommend topical capsaicin as an initial option for the hand. The guidelines also conditionally recommend that capsaicin should not be used in the management of osteoarthritis of the knee. They do not make any recommendations regarding nonprescription topical analgesics in the management of osteoarthritis of the hip.[13]

Other Topical Analgesics

Trolamine Salicylate

Trolamine salicylate is a category III ingredient (insufficient data are available to establish safety and efficacy). Despite this designation, several nonprescription products contain trolamine salicylate as the primary ingredient (Table 7–4).

Trolamine salicylate, or triethanolamine salicylate, is not a counterirritant analgesic. It has been suggested that trolamine salicylate is absorbed through the skin and results in synovial fluid salicylate concentrations below those of oral aspirin. The recommended topical dosage of trolamine salicylate for adults and for children 2 years and older is a 10%–15% concentration applied to the affected area not more than 3 or 4 times a day. There are no recent studies published regarding the efficacy of topical trolamine salicylate.

Trolamine salicylate is still available over the counter and may be most useful to those patients who do not favor the localized irritation or the scent of Category I counterirritants. ACR guidelines conditionally recommend trolamine salicylate as an option for osteoarthritis of the hand.[13]

Trolamine salicylate has the same drug interactions and contraindications as other salicylates (see Chapter 5). During use, the agent should not contact the eyes or mucous membranes.

Topical NSAIDs

Traditional topical NSAIDs are not currently available for nonprescription use in the United States, but they are available for prescription use (e.g., diclofenac). Their application on acute soft tissue strains and sprains, where the target tissue is situated closer to the skin surface, is reported to provide the benefits of oral NSAIDs with minimal systemic side effects. A 2010 Cochrane review recognizes the effectiveness of topical NSAIDs to treat acute musculoskeletal pain,[47] and a 2012 Cochrane review supports their use in the management of chronic pain from osteoarthritis.[48] Several guidelines recommend topical NSAIDs to be considered early in treatment for osteoarthritis.[13,16,27]

Combination Products

General guidelines for nonprescription drug combination products state that Category I active ingredients from the same therapeutic category should not ordinarily be combined, unless the combination is deemed safer or more effective and has enhanced patient acceptance or quality of formulation.[30] Four separate chemical and/or pharmacologic groups of counterirritants provide four qualitatively different types of irritation. Many marketed preparations aim for at least two such effects when greater potency is desired, provided that each active ingredient is from a different group.

Combining counterirritants with skin protectants is irrational; the protectants oppose and may nullify counterirritant effects.

Preparation labels must list the active ingredients, including their concentrations, and must identify them by their officially recognized, established names. In addition, manufacturers voluntarily list ingredients on the label. Many manufacturers of combination products list only some of the active ingredients under the "active" heading, and they list many of the other pharmacologically viable products in the inactive ingredients section (e.g., BenGay Vanishing Scent Gel lists camphor and Aspercreme Heat Pain Relieving Gel lists capsaicin under inactive ingredients). Although the concentrations of inactive ingredients are not listed, they are generally below therapeutically determined amounts and are added for reasons other than pain-relieving effects. The manner of use and the frequency of applications should also be indicated.[28]

Product Selection Guidelines

Special Populations

No significant variability in response has been noted among patients of different ages or racial backgrounds.

Variability related to the minimum age of patients does exist in product labeling. According to the tentative final monograph published in the *Federal Register* in 1983, use of external analgesics, as labeled within the confines of the statement, is to be avoided in children younger than 2 years.[30] However, most available products elect to label the minimum age as older than 12 years, and some products (particularly capsaicin products) list 18 years and older. Providers should follow labeling instructions for the products used. These products should be used cautiously, or avoided, in populations who cannot effectively communicate side effects they are experiencing after application of a topical analgesic. Of particular concern is use of such products in young children.

Musculoskeletal complaints are common in pregnancy, but complications may occur; therefore, patients should be evaluated by their primary care provider.[49] Limited information is available regarding use of nonprescription topical analgesics in pregnancy. Capsaicin, in the prescription patch formulation, is pregnancy category B. One source lists the nonprescription formulation as category C, but limited data are available to determine a pregnancy classification.[50] Camphor, menthol, methyl salicylate, trolamine salicylate, and methyl nicotinate are not categorized. Topical camphor is suggested to be compatible during pregnancy based on a determination of limited data that it is low risk.[51] Definitive recommendations are not available because of the limited—or in some cases, complete lack of—data that are

available on topical use in pregnancy. Consideration should be given to the systemic absorption of topical salicylates, particularly in the third trimester. Information regarding salicylates in pregnancy can be found in Chapter 5.

Patient Factors

The choice of treatment for acute pain syndromes and chronic conditions such as osteoarthritis is patient dependent. In addition to nonpharmacologic treatment, oral drug therapy is often employed. One should consider a patient's history (taking note of exclusions for self-treatment), other medications the patient is taking, and any known allergies to medications. Topical analgesics are used as an adjunct or substitute to oral drug therapy. If a counterirritant is selected, one with Category I ingredients should be recommended. Product concentrations are variable; in general, the lowest effective dose should be recommended for the shortest duration needed.

Patient Preferences

Factors that impact product selection include dosage form, ease of use, cost, and even odor of the preparation. Dosage forms available include solutions, liniments, gels, lotions, ointments, creams, and patches. Oleaginous preparations (ointments and oil-based liniments) have increased absorption compared with solutions, gels, lotions, and creams, but they are greasy and generally less acceptable to patients. The use of patches is becoming more popular because of their simple application and long duration of action. With the exception of patches and solutions, topical products should be rubbed into the skin.

Complementary Therapies

The most common dietary supplement used for osteoarthritis contains glucosamine and chondroitin. Published data regarding these supplements are conflicting because of population size, trial duration, preparations used, and outcomes measured (i.e., quality of life, pain indices, and radiologic changes). The National Institutes of Health and National Center for Complementary and Alternative Medicine has provided the largest study, the Glucosamine/Chondroitin Arthritis Intervention Trial (GAIT).[52] Initial results from this 6-month study showed no benefit in mild pain but showed a statistically significant reduction with moderate-severe pain. However, only 22% of patients enrolled in the study were categorized as having moderate-severe pain; therefore, the GAIT trial concluded that further studies are needed because of the small population size. A 2-year follow-up using patients from the GAIT trial showed no clinical difference in reduction of pain and function and joint space width compared with placebo.[53,54] The new ACR guidelines conditionally recommend that patients with osteoarthritis of the hip and knee should not use glucosamine or chondroitin sulfate.[13] These products and other complementary therapies are discussed in greater detail in Chapter 51.

Assessment of Musculoskeletal Injuries and Disorders: A Case-Based Approach

Routinely, the health care provider should inventory all patient medications, including pain medications, and should note the patient's satisfaction with or preference for past treatments. In addition, the health care provider should ask about aspects of the patient's medical history that relate directly to the origin or treatment of pain.

Before an attempt is made to treat a pain complaint, the health care provider should qualify and quantify the pain. Inquiry about the cause, duration, location, and severity of pain, as well as factors that relieve and exacerbate the pain, will help assess the pain. Chapter 2 outlines effective strategies for obtaining information from patients about specific complaints. Using a pain scale helps to quantify the intensity of a patient's pain. With the numerical pain scale, the health care provider asks the patient to rank the present pain on a scale of 0–10, with 0 being no pain and 10 being the worst pain the patient can imagine. Typically, mild pain is defined as 1–3, moderate pain 4–6, and severe pain 7–10 on the numerical pain scale.[1] Initially, pain scores establish a baseline for pain before treatment. In addition, a high pain score can be used to screen for patients who would be better served by seeking an appropriate medical evaluation. Pain scores also serve as a measuring device for therapeutic outcomes. Other scales are available for pain rating in children (Wong-Baker FACES Pain Scale), adolescents, people who do not speak English, and other special populations.

A chronic painful condition presents a different set of challenges. An observant health care provider should intervene with a patient who regularly purchases nonprescription analgesics. If additional interviewing indicates an inadequately treated pain problem, additional workup by an appropriate provider should be made. Education should be offered regarding the risks of inadequate treatment as well as the overuse of medications.

Cases 7–1 and 7–2 are examples of the assessment of patients with musculoskeletal injuries and disorders.

case 7–1

Relevant Evaluation Criteria	Scenario/Model Outcome
Information Gathering	
1. Gather essential information about the patient's symptoms and medical history, including:	
a. description of symptom(s) (e.g., nature, onset, duration, severity, associated symptoms)	Patient presents with a complaint that his back is really hurting him and that he is having difficulty moving around without pain. He reports that his pain right now is a 4 out of 10.
b. description of any factors that seem to precipitate, exacerbate, and/or relieve the patient's symptom(s)	Yesterday he was working outside in the yard all day for the first time this spring.
c. description of the patient's efforts to relieve the symptom(s)	He has tried a heat patch, which he wore for 8 hours; he has not experienced any significant relief.
d. patient's identity	Alexander Smith
e. age, sex, height, and weight	70 years old, male, 5 ft 11 in., 205 lb
f. patient's occupation	Retired
g. patient's dietary habits	He eats a diet high in carbohydrates and red meat. He does not eat a balanced diet, avoiding vegetables, poultry, and fish.
h. patient's sleep habits	He finds that it is getting more difficult to sleep through the whole night; on average, he sleeps about 7 hours a night.
i. concurrent medical conditions, prescription and nonprescription medications, and dietary supplements	He has a history of osteoarthritis, diabetes, coronary artery disease, uncontrolled hypertension, dyslipidemia, and anemia. He occasionally has problems with his back. His current medications include acetaminophen arthritis formulation, 1300 mg every 8 hours, 2–3 doses a day; metformin 1000 mg twice a day; metoprolol succinate 25 mg once daily; enalapril 10 mg once daily; aspirin 81 mg once daily; pravastatin 40 mg once daily; and B12 injections monthly.
j. allergies	Penicillin
k. history of other adverse reactions to medications	None
l. other patient preferences	He prefers patch formulations for convenience.
Assessment and Triage	
2. Differentiate patient's signs/symptoms and correctly identify the patient's primary problem(s).	Patient is experiencing acute back pain as a result of his burst of activity yesterday with his yard work.
3. Identify exclusions for self-treatment (Figure 7–1).	Patient does not have any exclusions for self-care. If his pain were more severe (>6 on pain scale), a referral would be recommended.

Relevant Evaluation Criteria	Scenario/Model Outcome
4. Formulate a comprehensive list of therapeutic alternatives for the primary problem to determine if triage to a medical provider is required, and share this information with the patient or caregiver.	Options include: (1) Refer patient to PCP for further assessment and treatment. (2) Continue nondrug measures (heat). (3) Continue APAP alone. (4) Recommend an NSAID. (5) Recommend adjunct topical analgesic, single or combination product (methyl salicylate, trolamine salicylate, camphor, menthol, or capsaicin). (6) Take no action.

Plan

5. Select an optimal therapeutic alternative to address the patient's problem, taking into account patient preferences.	Recommend nondrug measures, including 1–2 days of rest. Recommended therapy would include a topical counterirritant in a patch formulation because the patient prefers that. Continue APAP, which is a regular scheduled medication for his osteoarthritis that is a systemic analgesic. Patient has uncontrolled hypertension, so avoid systemic NSAIDs.
6. Describe the recommended therapeutic approach to the patient or caregiver.	"A topical analgesic medication to treat the pain is appropriate, and we can select a patch formulation."
7. Explain to the patient or caregiver the rationale for selecting the recommended therapeutic approach from the considered therapeutic alternatives.	"An oral nonsteroidal anti-inflammatory should not be used because you regularly have elevated blood pressure readings. A topical analgesic will help treat your muscle pain."

Patient Education

8. When recommending self-care with nonprescription medications and/or nondrug therapy, convey accurate information to the patient or caregiver:	
a. appropriate dose and frequency of administration	"Apply Salonpas original patch (methyl salicylate 6.3%, menthol 5.7%, and camphor 1.2%) 3–4 times a day."
b. maximum number of days the therapy should be employed	"This medication can be used for up to 7 days."
c. product administration procedures	"Apply the patch to your back on clean, dry skin where the pain is occurring. A new patch can be applied 3–4 times per day. Do not wear a patch for more than 8 hours. Wash hands before and after you apply the patch. It is not recommended to use heat when you are using this medication."
d. expected time to onset of relief	"You should experience some improvement shortly after application."
e. degree of relief that can be reasonably expected	"This medication will help reduce the pain but not eliminate it."
f. most common side effects	"It is normal to feel warmth in the area where the medication is applied. Some minor skin irritation may occur."
g. side effects that warrant medical intervention should they occur	"Immediately remove the product and contact your primary care provider if you experience any symptoms that would indicate a severe reaction (e.g., excessive redness, blistering, rash, burning, or stinging)."
h. patient options in the event that condition worsens or persists	"If this topical medication does not adequately relieve pain, please contact me to recommend a different topical medication."
i. product storage requirements	"Keep out of children's reach."
j. specific nondrug measures	"Rest for a day or two so as not to further aggravate your condition. Do not use heat over this medicated patch."
Solicit follow-up questions from the patient or caregiver.	"Does the Tylenol that I take for my arthritis help my back?"
Answer the patient's or caregiver's questions.	"Yes, Tylenol is a medication that can help with pain from any cause, but it does not reduce inflammation."

Evaluation of Patient Outcome

9. Assess patient outcome.	Monitor for a reduction in the patient's reported pain level using a pain scale. In addition, monitor for improved mobility.

Key: APAP = Acetaminophen; NA = not applicable; NKA = no known allergies; NSAID = nonsteroidal anti-inflammatory drug; PCP = primary care provider.

case
7–2

Relevant Evaluation Criteria	Scenario/Model Outcome

Information Gathering

1. Gather essential information about the patient's symptoms and medical history, including:

   a. description of symptom(s) (e.g., nature, onset, duration, severity, associated symptoms)

   Patient presents with a complaint that she hurt her ankle during her basketball game last night. She reports that her pain is an 8 out of 10. She is struggling to walk in the pharmacy and is favoring her right ankle. Upon examination, you observe that her ankle is very swollen and discolored.

   b. description of any factors that seem to precipitate, exacerbate, and/or relieve the patient's symptom(s)

   During the game last night, she collided with another player, and her ankle rolled when she fell.

   c. description of the patient's efforts to relieve the symptom(s)

   She has been icing while awake for 15 minutes on and then 15 minutes off. She also slept with her ankle elevated.

   d. patient's identity

   Madison Jones

   e. age, sex, height, and weight

   17 years old, female, 5 ft 5 in., 140 lb

   f. patient's occupation

   High school student

   g. patient's dietary habits

   She does not eat a regular diet outside of dinner with her family.

   h. patient's sleep habits

   Sleeping habits are erratic because of her schedule and social activities. She sleeps 8 hours on school nights but likes to sleep in on the weekends.

   i. concurrent medical conditions, prescription and nonprescription medications, and dietary supplements

   She is currently experiencing acne. Her current medications include a multivitamin daily and adapalene gel applied at bedtime.

   j. allergies

   NKA

   k. history of other adverse reactions to medications.

   None

   l. other (describe) _____

   NA

Assessment and Triage

2. Differentiate patient's signs/symptoms and correctly identify the patient's primary problem(s) (Table 7–1).

   Patient appears to have at least sprained her ankle but may have a more serious injury such as a fracture or torn tendons around her ankle.

3. Identify exclusions for self-treatment (Figure 7–1).

   Patient is experiencing pain that is severe (8 out of 10 on pain scale) and is having significant difficulty putting weight on it.

4. Formulate a comprehensive list of therapeutic alternatives for the primary problem to determine if triage to a medical provider is required, and share this information with the patient or caregiver.

   Options include:

   (1) Refer patient to PCP for further assessment and treatment.

   (2) Recommend nondrug measures (ice initially).

   (3) Recommend systemic analgesic.

   (4) Recommend topical analgesic, single or combination product (methyl salicylate, trolamine salicylate, camphor, menthol, or capsaicin).

   (5) Take no action.

Plan

5. Select an optimal therapeutic alternative to address the patient's problem, taking into account patient preferences.

   Refer patient to PCP for further evaluation because of the severity of pain. Recommend to continue nondrug measures including rest, elevation, compression, and ice (Table 7–2).

6. Describe the recommended therapeutic approach to the patient or caregiver.

   "Self-treatment is not appropriate for your condition. You should contact your primary care provider."

7. Explain to the patient or caregiver the rationale for selecting the recommended therapeutic approach from the considered therapeutic alternatives.

   The severity of your pain requires further evaluation by your primary care provider.

case
7–2   *continued*

Relevant Evaluation Criteria	Scenario/Model Outcome
Patient Education	
8. When recommending self-care with nonprescription medications and/or nondrug therapy, convey accurate information to the patient or caregiver:	Criterion does not apply in this case.
Solicit follow-up questions from the patient or caregiver.	"Do you think they will want me to get an x-ray?"
Answer the patient's or caregiver's questions.	"Your primary care provider may recommend an x-ray to rule out the possibility that you fractured a bone. Your primary care provider will be able to make that determination once he or she examines your ankle."
Evaluation of Patient Outcome	
9. Assess patient outcome.	Follow up with patient to determine the outcome of her visit with her primary care provider.

Key: NA = Not applicable; NKA = no known allergies; PCP = primary care provider.

Patient Counseling for Musculoskeletal Injuries and Disorders

Consultation with the patient should include explanation of the expected benefit of any recommended medication, the appropriate dose and drug administration schedule, application directions, potential adverse reactions, potential drug–drug or drug–disease interactions, and self-monitoring techniques for assessing response to therapy. Printed materials reinforce verbal information. Many such pamphlets or single-page handouts are available from national professional societies (e.g., www.arthritis. org). These materials offer advice on exercise, diet, and sleep habits, as well as the advantages and disadvantages of pharmacologic therapy.

In acute pain management, early administration of nonprescription analgesics should be employed to prevent escalating pain, with downward tapering of the analgesic doses as pain severity allows. Patients should be assessed for the appropriateness of nonprescription oral analgesics (Chapter 5).

Patients should be instructed to notify their primary care provider if the pain worsens in quality or severity, or if new acute pain develops. Other sudden uncharacteristic pains may be harbingers of new tissue damage.

The box Patient Education for Musculoskeletal Injuries and Disorders lists specific information about topical analgesics, as well as preventive and nondrug measures to provide patients.

Evaluation of Patient Outcomes for Musculoskeletal Injuries and Disorders

The primary indicator of treatment effectiveness is the patient's perception of pain relief. If a patient reports the pain is still present or has worsened after 7 days of using topical nonprescription analgesics,[30] the health care provider should refer the patient for further evaluation. In many instances, the lack of a return visit indicates a successful treatment regimen (the provider may call the patient in a few days to determine whether the complaint has resolved). However, a patient who returns with signs of continued swelling, pain, or inflammation should be referred for medical evaluation. The continued pain may indicate an ongoing process that could lead to long-term disability or decreased mobility.

Key Points for Musculoskeletal Injuries and Disorders

➤ Self-treatment of patients presenting with pain secondary to an injury or a disorder of the musculoskeletal system should be limited to those with mild–moderate pain who have no exclusions for self-treatment (Figure 7–1).

➤ Self-treatment of acute musculoskeletal injuries should include nondrug therapy, such as rest, ice, compression, and elevation (RICE). Heat therapy may also provide benefit after symptoms of inflammation have abated.

➤ Systemic analgesics are valid first-line agents to treat the majority of musculoskeletal injuries and disorders. Acetaminophen is preferred in noninflammatory diseases, whereas NSAIDs are preferred if inflammation is present. Side effects and drug interactions should be considered before therapy is chosen (see Chapter 5).

➤ Health care providers should counsel patients on the discussion points listed in Table 7–5 to avoid chemical burns with topical nonprescription analgesics.

➤ Health care providers should monitor the outcome of self-treatments and advise patients who self-treat their acute musculoskeletal injury with nonprescription topical analgesics to seek medical attention if their symptoms do not improve after 7 days. Patients who experience pain for greater than 10 days, regardless of treatment, should also be referred.

Musculoskeletal Injuries and Disorders

The objectives of self-treatment are to (1) reduce the severity of pain; (2) reduce the duration of pain, when possible; (3) restore function to the affected area; (4) prevent re-injury and disability; and (5) prevent acute pain from becoming chronic persistent pain. Certain nondrug measures and nonprescription counterirritants can relieve pain symptoms from a sudden and recent muscle, tendon, or ligament injury; an overuse injury (e.g., tendonitis, bursitis, or repetitive stress injury); low back pain; or arthritis. For most patients, carefully following product instructions and the self-care measures listed here will help ensure optimal therapeutic outcomes.

Preventive Measures

- To prevent muscle or joint strains and sprains, do warm-up and stretching exercises before playing sports or exercising, and wrap injured muscle or joint with protective bandage or tape.
- To prevent repetitive strain, exercise the muscles that are vulnerable to the injury, and use ergonomic controls to adjust posture, stresses, motions, and other damaging physical factors.
- To prevent tendonitis and cramps, warm up and stretch muscles before physical activity, drink sufficient fluids, and do not exercise to the point of exhaustion. To help prevent nocturnal leg cramps, raise the foot of the bed. For Achilles tendonitis, wearing better-fitting shoes with heel lifts may help reduce the symptoms.
- To prevent or reduce the occurrence of low back pain, do exercises to strengthen the muscles of the low back and abdomen, and use assistive devices (i.e., cane or walker), if needed.
- To prevent or reduce the occurrence of osteoarthritis, avoid a sedentary lifestyle; keep joints active; lose weight, if overweight; and use assistive devices, if needed.

Nondrug Measures

- For pain related to muscle or joint injuries, begin treatment with RICE therapy (Table 7–2).
- For periodic muscle cramps, stretch and massage the affected area immediately; then rest or reduce activity of the muscle to allow it to loosen.
- For stiffness, apply heat to the affected area in the form of a warm wet compress, a heating pad, or a hot-water bottle.
- For osteoarthritis, try a combination of nondrug measures, including applying heat or cold to the affected area, supporting the area with splints, and doing range-of-motion and strength-maintenance exercises.

Nonprescription Medications

- For mild-moderate muscle pain, take a nonprescription systemic analgesic for no longer than 10 days[23] (see Chapter 5 for a listing of nonprescription analgesics), and/or use a topical counterirritant

for no longer than 7 days[27] (Table 7–3 provides recommended dosages of counterirritants).
- Do not use counterirritants if your skin is abraded, sunburned, or otherwise damaged.
- When using counterirritants, especially capsaicin, wash your hands after application and before touching your eyes and mucous membranes, or before handling contact lenses.
- Gently rub a thin layer of counterirritant product into affected muscles or joints until you cannot see the product. Thick application of the product does not make the product work better.
- Do not put a tight bandage or dressing over an area treated with a counterirritant. Do not use heat/warming devices with counterirritants.
- Do not treat a child 2 years of age or younger with counterirritants unless a primary care provider supervises the use. Follow age limits on product labeling.
- If you have asthma, and symptoms of wheezing and shortness of breath worsen while you are using a mentholated formulation, stop using it.
- If you are receiving anticoagulation therapy (especially warfarin), do not use products containing salicylates (including aspirin, methyl salicylate, and trolamine salicylate).
- If a counterirritant causes excessive redness and blistering or hives and vomiting, stop using it.

When to Seek Medical Attention

- A feeling of warmth or coolness is normal; however, if burning pain or blistering occurs, seek medical attention.
- If you experience nausea, vomiting, colic, and other unusual symptoms while using a product containing camphor, seek medical care immediately.
- If the pain has been present for more than 10 days or has worsened, consult a primary care provider.
- If the symptoms persist after more than 7 days of treatment with a topical product, or if the pain is constant and felt in any position, consult a primary care provider.

REFERENCES

1. Mense S, Gerwin R. *Muscle Pain: Diagnosis and Treatment*. New York, NY: Springer; 2010:1–84.
2. Chou R, Qaseem A, Snow V, et al. Diagnosis and treatment of low back pain: a joint clinical practice guideline from the American College of Physicians and the American Pain Society. *Ann Intern Med*. 2007;147(7): 478–91.
3. Consumer Healthcare Products Association. OTC sales by category 2009–2012. August 2013. Accessed at http:chpa-info.org, August 26, 2013.
4. Gaskin DJ, Richard P. The economic costs of pain in the United States. *J Pain*. 2012;13(8):715–24.
5. Institute of Medicine. Relieving pain in America: a blueprint for transforming prevention, care, education, and research. June 2011. Accessed at http://iom.edu/Reports/2011/Relieving-Pain-in-America-A-Blueprint-for-Transforming-Prevention-Care-Education-Research. aspx, April 13, 2013.
6. Buckwalter J. Musculoskeletal tissues and musculoskeletal system. In: Weinstein S, Buckwalter J, eds. *Tureks Orthopaedics: Principles and Their*

Application. 6th ed. Philadelphia, PA: Lippincott Williams and Wilkins; 2005:3–72.
7. National Institute of Arthritis and Musculoskeletal and Skin Disease. Questions and answers about sprains and strains. July 2012. Accessed at http://www.niams.nih.gov/Health_Info/Sprains_Strains/default.asp, August 6, 2013.
8. U.S. Food and Drug Administration Web site. Information for healthcare professionals: fluroquinolone antimicrobial drugs. May 29, 2010. Accessed at http://www.fda.gov/Drugs/DrugSafety/PostmarketDrugSafety InformationforPatientsandProviders/ucm126085.htm, April 6, 2013.
9. French SD, Cameron M, Walker BF, et al. Superficial heat or cold for low back pain. *Cochrane Database Syst Rev* 2006;1:CD004750. doi: 10. 1002/14651858.CD004750.pub2. Accessed at http://www.thecochrane library.com/view/0/index.html.
10. National Institute of Arthritis and Musculoskeletal and Skin Disease. Handout on health: back pain. April 2012. Accessed at http://www. niams.nih.gov/Health_Info/Back_Pain/default.asp, July 28, 2013.
11. Sprouse R. Treatment: current treatment recommendations for acute and chronic undifferentiated low back pain. *Prim Care*. 2012;39(3):481–6.

12. Zhang W, Doherty M, Arden N, et al. EULAR evidence based recommendations for the management of hip osteoarthritis: report of a task force of the EULAR Standing Committee for International Clinical Studies Including Therapeutics (ESCISIT). *Ann Rheum Dis.* 2005;64(5):669–81.

13. Hochberg MC, Altman RD, April KT, et al. American College of Rheumatology 2012 recommendations for the use of nonpharmacologic and pharmacologic therapies in osteoarthritis of the hand, hip, and knee. *Arthritis Care Res.* 2012;64(4):465–74.

14. National Institute of Arthritis and Musculoskeletal and Skin Disease. Handout on health: osteoarthritis. July 2010. Accessed at http://www.niams.nih.gov/Health_Info/Osteoarthritis/default.asp, April 10, 2013.

15. Chou R, Huffman LH. Nonpharmacologic therapies for acute and chronic low back pain: a review of the evidence for an American Pain Society/American College of Physicians clinical practice guideline. *Ann of Intern Med.* 2007;147(7):492–504.

16. Conaghan PG, Dickson J, Grant RL. Care and management of osteoarthritis in adults: summary of NICE guidance. *BMJ.* 2008;336(7642):502–3.

17. Brosseau L, Yonge KA, Robinson V, et al. Thermotherapy for treatment of osteoarthritis. *Cochrane Database Syst Rev.* 2011;4:CD004522. doi: 10.1002/14651858.CD004522. Accessed at http://www.thecochranelibrary.com/view/0/index.html.

18. ThermaCare.com. ThermaCare frequently asked questions. Accessed at http://www.thermacare.com/faqs, April 7, 2013.

19. U.S. Food and Drug Administration Web site. Pfizer Consumer Healthcare issues voluntary recall of one lot of ThermaCare HeatWraps Menstrual product. September 29, 2010. Accessed at http://www.fda.gov/Safety/Recalls/ucm227658.htm, April 7, 2013.

20. U.S. Food and Drug Administration. Chattem issues URGENT voluntary nationwide recall of Icy Hot® Heat Therapy™ products. February 8, 2008. Accessed at http://www.fda.gov/Safety/Recalls/ArchiveRecalls/2008/ucm112369.htm, April 7, 2013.

21. Hing WA, White SG, Bouaaphone A, et al. Contrast therapy–a systematic review. *Phys Ther Sport.* 2008;9(3):148–61.

22. Bahnert A, Norton K, Lock P. Association between post-game recovery protocols, physical and perceived recovery, and performance in elite Australian football league players. *J Sci Med Sport.* 2013;16(2):151–6.

23. U.S. Food and Drug Administration. Product classification. August 11, 2014. Accessed at http://www.accessdata.fda.gov/scripts/cdrh/cfdocs/cfPCD/classification.cfm?ID=3434, August 17, 2014.

24. IcyHotSmartRelief [product information]. Chattam, Inc., Chattanooga, TN. Accessed at http://www.smartrelief.com/wp-content/uploads/2014/02/IH_SmartRelief_Inst_Manual.pdf, August 16, 2014.

25. TENS pain relief systems. AccuRelief Web site. Accessed at http://www.accurelief.com/products.php, August 17, 2014.

26. U.S. Food and Drug Administration. Internal analgesic, antipyretic, antirheumatic drug products for over-the-counter human use; tentative final monograph. *Federal Register.* 1988;53:46204–60. Accessed at http://www.fda.gov/downloads/Drugs/DevelopmentApprovalProcess/DevelopmentResources/Over-the-CounterOTCDrugs/StatusofOTCRulemakings/UCM078460.pdf, August 26, 2013.

27. American Geriatrics Society panel on the pharmacological management of persistent pain in older persons. *J Am Geriatr Soc.* 2009;57(8):1331–46.

28. U.S. Food and Drug Administration. External analgesic products for over-the-counter human use; establishment of a monograph and notice of proposed rulemaking. *Federal Register.* 1979;44(234):69768–874. Accessed at http://www.fda.gov/downloads/Drugs/DevelopmentApprovalProcess/DevelopmentResources/Over-the-CounterOTCDrugs/StatusofOTCRulemakings/UCM077916.pdf, August 26, 2013.

29. Methyl Salicylate. In: Sweetman S, ed. *Martindale—The Complete Drug Reference.* 37th ed. Gurnee, IL: Pharmaceutical Press; 2011:89–90.

30. U.S. Food and Drug Administration. External analgesic drug products for over-the-counter human use: tentative final monograph. *Federal Register.* 1983;48(27):5852–69. Accessed at http://www.fda.gov/downloads/Drugs/DevelopmentApprovalProcess/DevelopmentResources/Over-the-CounterOTCDrugs/StatusofOTCRulemakings/UCM077928.pdf, August 26, 2013.

31. U.S. Food and Drug Administration. FDA drug safety communication: rare cases of serious burns with the use of over-the-counter topical muscle and joint pain relievers. September 13, 2012. Accessed at http://www.fda.gov/Drugs/DrugSafety/ucm318858.htm, April 15, 2013.

32. U.S. Food and Drug Administration. For consumers: topical pain relievers may cause burns. September 12, 2012. Accessed at http://www.fda.gov/ForConsumers/ConsumerUpdates/ucm318674.htm, April 15, 2013.

33. Danon A, Ben-Shimon S, Ben-Zvi Z. Effect of exercise and heat exposure on percutaneous absorption of methyl salicylate. *Eur J Clin Pharmacol.* 1986;31(1):49–52.

34. Davis JE. Are one or two dangerous? Methyl salicylate exposure in toddlers. *J Emerg Med.* 2007;32(1):63–9.

35. Khine H, Weiss D, Graber N, et al. A cluster of children with seizures caused by camphor poisoning. *Pediatrics.* 2009;123(5):1269–72.

36. Michiels EA, Mazor SS. Toddler with seizures due to ingesting camphor at an Indian celebration. *Pediatr Emerg Care.* 2010;26(8):574–5.

37. American Academy of Pediatrics. Policy Statement—AAP Publications Retired and Reaffirmed. *Pediatrics* 2009;124:845.

38. Patel T, Ishiuji Y, Yosipovitch G. Menthol: a refreshing look at this ancient compound. *J Am Acad of Dermatol.* 2007;57(5):873–8.

39. Wilkin JK, Fortner G, Reinhardt LA, et al. Prostaglandins and nicotinate-provoked increase in cutaneous blood flow. *Clin Pharmacol Ther.* 1985;38(3):273–7.

40. Capsaicin. In: Sweetman S, ed. *Martindale—The Complete Drug Reference.* 37th ed. Gurnee, IL: Pharmaceutical Press; 2011:33–4.

41. Stanos SP. Topical agents for the management of musculoskeletal pain. *J Pain Symptom Manage.* 2007;33(3):342–55.

42. Derry S, Moore RA. Topical capsaicin (low concentration) for chronic neuropathic pain in adults. *Cochrane Database Syst Rev* 2012;9:CD010111. doi: 10.1002/14651858.CD010111. Accessed at http://www.thecochranelibrary.com/view/0/index.html.

43. Qutenza [product information]. NeurogesX, Inc., San Mateo, CA; November 2009. Accessed at www.qutenza.com, August 5, 2013.

44. Matthews P, Derry S, Moore RA, et al. Topical rubefacients for acute and chronic pain in adults. *Cochrane Database Syst Rev.* 2009;3:CD007403. doi: 10.1002/14651858.CD007403.pub2. Accessed at http://www.thecochranelibrary.com/view/0/index.html.

45. Higashi Y, Kiuchi T, Furuta K. Efficacy and safety profile of a topical methyl salicylate and menthol patch in adult patients with mild to moderate muscle strain: a randomized, double-blind, parallel-group, placebo-controlled, multicenter study. *Clin Ther.* 2010;32(1):34–43.

46. National Institute for Health and Clinical Excellence. Osteoarthritis: the care and management of osteoarthritis in adults. Clinical Guideline 59. 2008. Accessed at http://www.nice.org.uk/nicemedia/live/11926/39557/39557.pdf, April 18, 2013.

47. Massey T, Derry S, Moore RA, et al. Topical NSAIDs for acute pain in adults. *Cochrane Database Syst Rev.* 2010;(6):CD007402. doi: 10.1002/14651858.CD007402.pub2. Accesssed at http://www.thecochranelibrary.com/view/0/index.html.

48. Derry S, Moore RA, Rabbie R. Topical NSAIDs for chronic musculoskeletal pain in adults. *Cochrane Database Syst Rev.* 2012;9:CD007400. doi: 10.1002/14651858.CD007400.pub2. Accesssed at http://www.thecochranelibrary.com/view/0/index.html.

49. Bermas B. Musculoskeletal changes and pain during pregnancy and postpartum. Up to Date. St. Louis, MO: Wolters Kluwer Health. Updated June 2013. Accessed at http://www.uptodate.com, August 16, 2013.

50. Capsaicin. Facts and Comparisons eAnswers. St. Louis, MO: Wolters Kluwer Health. Updated January 2010. Accessed at http://online.factsandcomparisons.com, April 3, 2013.

51. Briggs G, Freeman R, Yaffe S. Camphor. *Drugs in Pregnancy and Lactation.* 9th ed. Philadelphia, PA: Lippincott, Williams and Wilkins; 2013:189.

52. Clegg DO, Reda DJ, Harris CL, et al. Glucosamine, chondroitin sulfate, and the two in combination for painful knee osteoarthritis. *N Engl J Med.* 2006;354(8):795–808.

53. Sawitzke AD, Shi H, Finco MF, et al. Clinical efficacy and safety of glucosamine, chondroitin sulphate, their combination, celecoxib or placebo taken to treat osteoarthritis of the knee: 2-year results from GAIT. *Ann Rheum Dis.* 2010;69(8):1459–64.

54. Sawitzke AD, Shi H, Finco MF, et al. The effect of glucosamine and/or chondroitin sulfate on the progression of knee osteoarthritis: a report from the glucosamine/chondroitin arthritis intervention trial. *Arthritis Rheum.* 2008;58(10):3183–91.

REPRODUCTIVE AND GENITAL DISORDERS

VAGINAL AND VULVOVAGINAL DISORDERS

Nicole M. Lodise

Vaginal symptoms are among the most common health concerns of both reproductive age and older women. Vaginal symptoms may be experienced by all women whether married or single, sexually active or abstinent, homosexual or heterosexual, and premenopausal or postmenopausal.[1] About 65% of women experiencing vaginal symptoms will have one of three common vaginal infections: bacterial vaginosis (BV), vulvovaginal candidiasis (VVC), and trichomoniasis.[1] Infections may also be mixed, with more than one causative organism.

In general, vaginal infections are perceived as minor health problems and patients may consider self-treatment. Women may also self-treat noninfectious vaginal symptoms such as vaginal dryness, atrophic vaginitis, and allergic or chemical dermatologic reactions.[1,2] However, BV and trichomoniasis have been linked to significant health problems such as pelvic inflammatory disease (PID), preterm birth, and facilitation of the transmission of human immunodeficiency virus (HIV).[2,3] Given the number of women with vaginal infections and the approval of nonprescription vaginal antifungal products, health care providers should manage these infections carefully and provide patient education for VVC. Patients need to understand vaginal health to make appropriate decisions about self-care for vaginal symptoms.

The vagina is an elastic fibromuscular tube that extends 8–10 cm from the vulva to the uterus. The upper end of the vagina is closed except for the cervical os, the opening to the cervix. Anatomically, the vagina lies between the urinary bladder and the rectum. At the lower (vulvar) end of the vagina are the Bartholin's glands, which produce secretions in response to sexual stimulation. At puberty, under the influence of estrogen, the vaginal lining changes to stratified squamous epithelium, which contains glycogen. *Lactobacillus* bacteria convert glycogen to lactic acid, which creates an acidic pH of 4–4.5. This acidic pH and the production of hydrogen peroxide by these bacteria help protect the vagina from infection with other bacteria. After menopause, thinning of the vaginal lining occurs, concentrations of lactobacilli decline, and pH rises.[4]

The mature vagina is colonized by many organisms. *Lactobacillus* species predominate, accounting for 90%–95% of the vaginal flora. Another 5–10 species of bacteria, including *Corynebacterium, Streptococcus, Staphylococcus epidermidis, Gardnerella vaginalis, Peptostreptococcus,* and *Bacteroides,* are present in small quantities, with anaerobes being more common than aerobes.[2,5] *Candida albicans* and *Escherichia coli* may also be isolated in the absence of active infection in about 20% of women.[5,6]

The vaginal ecosystem is affected by the number and types of endogenous organisms, vaginal pH, and glycogen concentration. Hormonal fluctuations during the menstrual cycle can also influence the vaginal ecosystem in addition to drug therapy, douching, and number of sex partners.

The healthy vagina is cleansed daily by secretions that lubricate the vaginal tract. Normal vaginal discharge, also known as leukorrhea, consists of about 1.5 grams of vaginal fluid daily, which is odorless, clear or white, and viscous or sticky.[6] This discharge consists of endocervical mucus, serum transudate from vaginal capillary beds, endogenous vaginal flora, and epithelial cells.[5,6] An increase in vaginal secretions is normal during ovulation, during pregnancy, following menses, and with sexual excitement or emotional flares. An alteration in vaginal secretions may also occur in response to vaginal irritants such as feminine hygiene deodorant products and vaginal douches, as well as contraceptive products or use of tampons.

Differentiation of Common Vaginal Infections

The signs and symptoms for different vaginal infections may be similar, and the characteristic symptoms that often help distinguish infections may be absent (Table 8–1). Both patients and providers may have difficulty accurately determining the type of infection solely on the basis of symptoms.[7,8]

Accurately distinguishing VVC from BV and trichomoniasis is especially important because of the availability of nonprescription vaginal antifungal therapy.

Given the availability of nonprescription vaginal antifungal products and the cost and inconvenience of an office evaluation, many patients prefer to self-treat empirically for presumed VVC, which may lead to a potential for inappropriate therapy.[9] Women should be encouraged to ask their pharmacists, who can educate and advise patients on appropriate self-care treatment.

Many women have trouble identifying VVC on the basis of the symptoms alone.[7,10,11] One study found that when women who had previously been diagnosed with VVC read a description of the classic symptoms of the infection, only 35% could accurately recognize it.[12] Similarly, another study reported that many women who purchased nonprescription antifungal products to treat vaginal symptoms actually did not have VVC infections.[11] The symptom most likely to differentiate a *Candida* vaginal infection from that of BV and trichomoniasis is the absence of an offensive odor of the vaginal discharge.[13]

table
8–1

table 8–1 Differentiation of Common Vaginal Infections

Classic Symptoms[1]	Differentiating Signs and Symptoms	Etiology and Epidemiology[1]
Bacterial Vaginosis		
Thin (watery), off-white or discolored (green, gray, tan), sometimes foamy discharge; unpleasant "fishy" odor that increases after sexual intercourse or with elevated vaginal pH (e.g., menses)	Vaginal irritation, dysuria, and itching are less frequent with BV than with VVC or trichomoniasis.[18] A foul odor is strongly associated with BV; absence of the odor virtually rules out BV. Increased vaginal discharge ("wetness") is more common with BV than with VVC or trichomoniasis.	Polymicrobial infection resulting from imbalance in normal vaginal flora with increase in *Gardnerella vaginalis* and anaerobes (*Peptostreptococcus, Mobiluncus, Prevotella,* and *Mycoplasma hominis*) and decrease in lactobacilli. Risk factors: new sexual partner, African American race, use of IUD, douching, receptive oral sex, tobacco use, and prior pregnancy. Possible protective factors: use of female hormones, including OC, and condoms. Responsible for 33% of vaginal symptoms. Predominately affects young, sexually active women but can arise spontaneously regardless of sexual activity; found in 12% of virginal adolescents; lower prevalence in postmenopausal women, even with use of hormones
Trichomoniasis		
Copious, malodorous, yellow-green (or discolored), frothy discharge; pruritus; vaginal irritation; dysuria. No symptoms initially in ~50% of affected women. Most men are asymptomatic and serve as reservoirs of the infection	Erythema and vulvar edema can occur with this infection.[7] Yellow discharge increases likelihood of trichomoniasis.	STI caused by *Trichomonas vaginalis*. Risk factors: multiple sex partners, new sexual partner, nonuse of barrier contraceptives, and presence of other STIs. Responsible for 15%–20% of vaginal infections
Vulvovaginal Candidiasis		
Thick, white ("cottage cheese") discharge with no odor; normal pH (see text for detailed information; also referred to as "yeast infection" or "moniliasis")	Presence of erythema, itching, and/or vulvar edema, and absence of malodor increase likelihood of VVC; thick, "cheesy" discharge is strongly predictive of VVC.[7,19]	Organisms: *Candida albicans, Candida glabrata, Candida tropicalis,* and *Saccharomyces*. Risk factors: medications such as antibiotics and immunosuppressants. No identifiable cause for most infections. Responsible for 20%–25% of vaginal infections

Key: BV = Bacterial vaginosis; VVC = vulvovaginal candidiasis; IUD = intrauterine device; OC = oral contraceptive; STI = sexually transmitted infection.

Noninfectious conditions that may be confused with vaginal infections are vulvovaginal irritation or pruritus caused by allergic or hypersensitivity reactions. These reactions may be due to an allergy to latex, spermicides, vaginal lubricants containing propylene glycol, or anesthetics used by men to delay ejaculation.[2] Irritation secondary to douches, feminine hygiene products, soaps and detergents, or frequent use of panty liners or sanitary napkins may also cause these reactions.[2] In addition, urethral irritation and dysuria resulting from vulvovaginitis may be mistaken for a urinary tract infection.

Inappropriate use of vaginal antifungal products has several risks, including unnecessary drug use and a delay in effective treatment for the actual condition. The risks of exposure to the vaginal antifungal products, in the absence of VVC, include local irritation and the cost of therapy.[14] Labeling instructions advise patients to seek help for persistent symptoms, and if these guidelines are followed, the delay in treatment from misdiagnosis will likely present few serious consequences.

One method to assist in appropriate self-care treatment is the use of pH devices. One study evaluated the use of pH devices in symptomatic women. Nearly 57% of women who believed they had a yeast infection did not, which was confirmed by self-testing with the pH device and an examination by a health care provider.[15] The use of pH self-testing devices may be beneficial in reducing inappropriate self-treatment with antifungal products.

Table 8–1 describes the classic symptoms of the three common vaginal infections as well as the symptoms that women typically experience.[1,3,7,16–20]

Vulvovaginal Candidiasis

Vulvovaginal candidiasis is also referred to as a yeast infection and moniliasis. This condition is second only to BV as the most common vaginal infection, and nearly 75% of women will report at least one VVC infection over their lifetime.[5,21] African American women report three times the number of VVC episodes (17.4% of women) compared with white women (5.8%) or women of other races or ethnic groups (4.8%).[22] Recurrent infections occur in fewer than 5% of women.[3] About 20% of women may be colonized with *Candida albicans* without experiencing vaginal symptoms.[7]

Pathophysiology of Vulvovaginal Candidiasis

Candida fungi are the causative organisms, with about 80%–92% of cases caused by *C. albicans*.[3] The incidence of non–*C. albicans* infections has increased in the past two decades. *Candida glabrata, Candida tropicalis,* and *Saccharomyces cerevisiae* now account for about 10% of *Candida* vaginal infections.[3,6] This increase may be a result of the widespread use of nonprescription antifungals, short courses of topical imidazole therapy, and long-term suppressive therapy with imidazole antifungals.[3]

No single causative factor has been identified for most episodes of VVC. Pregnancy, high-dose combined oral contraceptives, and estrogen therapy may increase vaginal susceptibility to *Candida* vaginal infections by increasing the glycogen content of the vagina, although studies are inconsistent. Vaginal pH increases during menstruation, predisposing women to cyclic fungal vaginal infections. During the reproductive years, the vaginal epithelium cells are thick and contain an abundance of glycogen.[23] These cells exfoliate and continually provide the lactobacilli with the glycogen to produce lactic acid.[23] During and after the menopausal transition, the amount of glycogen declines, leading to decreased lactic acid production and an increased vaginal pH, and predisposes patients to vaginal infections. Women with diabetes mellitus are at increased risk for *Candida* vaginal infections, particularly if the glycemic control is poor. Antibiotics may also increase risk of these infections. Between 25% and 70% of women in studies reported developing *Candida* vaginal infections during or just after treatment with antibiotics such as tetracycline, ampicillin/amoxicillin, and cephalosporins.[24,25] The proposed mechanism is a decrease in normal vaginal flora, especially lactobacilli, allowing an overgrowth of *Candida* organisms. However, neither an increase in vaginal *Candida* organisms nor a decrease in lactobacilli occurs in all women who take these antibiotics. In addition, patients who have received an organ transplant or have HIV infection or who are taking systemic corticosteroid, antineoplastic, or immunosuppressant drugs may also be at increased risk for developing *Candida* vaginal infections.

An increased frequency of VVC is associated with the onset of regular sexual activity. However, neither the number of sexual partners nor the frequency of sexual intercourse is related to the occurrence of VVC episodes.[3] Evidence has suggested an increased risk of VVC associated with receptive oral sex.[1] In addition, use of an intrauterine or vaginal sponge contraceptive has increased the risk for VVC.[3]

A consistent association between tight-fitting, nonabsorbent clothing or pantyhose and the development of VVC has not been demonstrated. However, clothing of this type may increase risk by creating a warm and moist environment. Foods that increase the excretion of urinary glucose such as dietary sugars, refined carbohydrates, milk, and artificial sweeteners may increase the risk for *Candida* vaginal infections.[1,16] The consumption of yogurt has been proposed to provide a potential prophylactic benefit against VVC, although further research is needed.[26]

The treatment of *Candida* vaginal infections does not typically include treatment of the male partner. Treatment of male partners has not been shown to prevent recurrence of *Candida* vaginal infections in women. With recurrent infections, male partners may be treated with a topical imidazole. If treatment is necessary, topical imidazoles may be applied to the infected area twice a day for 2–4 weeks.

Clinical Presentation of Vulvovaginal Candidiasis

The characteristic signs and symptoms of VVC are described in Table 8–1. *Candida* vaginal infections typically do not alter vaginal pH, so a pH greater than 4.5 indicates a bacterial or trichomonal vaginal infection. Vaginal pH testing devices use pH to assist consumers in distinguishing *Candida* vaginal infections that can be self-treated from infections that require medical evaluation and prescription drug therapy. The Vagisil Screening Kit for Vaginal Infections (vaginal swab) uses a color test to determine vaginal pH and is easy for patients to use. Limitations with the product include the fact that testing cannot occur until 72 hours after the use of any vaginal preparation, such as a contraceptive spermicide or antifungal product, and 48 hours after sexual intercourse or douching. In addition, the product cannot be used until 5 days after a menstrual period. This screening kit costs about $5 per test.

Treatment of Vulvovaginal Candidiasis

The treatment of VVC is determined by the severity of symptoms and the frequency of episodes. VVC can be categorized as uncomplicated or complicated, with recurrent VVC considered a complicated infection.[13] Complicated infections are reported in about 5% of women and may occur because of host factors such as an inability of normal flora to prevent *Candida* colonization or the presence of fungal organisms that are more resistant to imidazole antifungal therapy.

Treatment Goals

The goals of therapy for vaginal fungal infections are relief of symptoms, eradication of the infection, and reestablishment of normal vaginal flora. A single course of drug therapy is effective in achieving these goals for most women. However, some women will experience persistent or recurrent infections and will require prolonged therapy or higher dosages of medication.

General Treatment Approach

Self-treatment of VVC with nonprescription antifungal therapy is appropriate for women with uncomplicated disease with infrequent episodes and mild-moderate symptoms. Women with more severe symptoms, predisposing illnesses or medications, or recurrent infections should be referred for assessment and treatment by their primary care provider.

Recurrent VVC occurs when a woman experiences at least four documented infections in a 1-year period.[3] Patients should be evaluated for the possibility of a mixed infection or a strain other than *C. albicans*. In addition, frequent or recurrent episodes of VVC may be an early sign of HIV infection or diabetes. The

Food and Drug Administration (FDA) now requires labels of nonprescription drug products to include a warning similar to the following[27]:

> Symptoms that return within 2 months or infections that do not clear up easily with proper treatment require medical evaluation. Possible causes of the infection include pregnancy or a serious underlying medical disorder, such as diabetes or a damaged immune system including damage from infection with HIV, the virus that causes acquired immunodeficiency syndrome.

Preventive measures are not a standard part of therapy for *Candida* vaginal infections.

Women with frequent or unresponsive infections may try dietary changes, as well as other nondrug measures such as the avoidance of nonabsorbent clothing. A 3- to 4-month trial of these approaches is sufficient to determine if they are useful for individual patients.[1] Figure 8–1 outlines the approach to treating the patient with vaginal symptoms.

Nonpharmacologic Therapy

Decreased consumption of sucrose and refined carbohydrates, as well as consumption of yogurt containing live cultures may potentially decrease VVC, particularly for women who experience recurrent infections.[1,16,26]

Discontinuing a drug known to increase susceptibility to *Candida* vaginal infections might be effective in decreasing the incidence. Low-dose oral contraceptives are unlikely to contribute to the occurrence of VVC, but they might be discontinued to determine whether the frequency of infection is altered. Another form of contraception should be recommended before discontinuing the oral contraceptive. Patients taking antibiotics or immunosuppressants should consult their primary care provider regarding these medications.

Pharmacologic Therapy

Vaginal Antifungals

A nonprescription FDA-approved imidazole product is the recommended initial therapy for uncomplicated VVC and relief of external vulvar itching and irritation associated with the infection. Approved drugs include butoconazole, clotrimazole, miconazole, or tioconazole, and they are available as vaginal creams, suppositories, and tablets. Tables 8–2 and 8–3 provide proper dosing and administration guidelines, respectively.

The major antifungal effect is through altering the membrane permeability of the fungi. These antifungal agents inhibit cytochrome P450 enzymes in the fungal cell membrane, thereby decreasing synthesis of the fungal sterol ergosterol. The reduced membrane ergosterol content is accompanied by a corresponding increase in lanosterol-like methylated sterols. These sterols cause structural damage to fungal membranes, resulting in the loss of normal membrane function.

Systemic absorption of butoconazole, clotrimazole, miconazole, and tioconazole is about 1.7%, 3%–10%, 1.4%, and a negligible amount of a vaginal dose, respectively.[28] Fungicidal clotrimazole concentrations are detectable in the vaginal fluid for up to 3 days after a single vaginal 500 mg dose.

Adverse effects from topical imidazoles are minimal and include vulvovaginal burning, itching, and irritation in 3%–7%

of patients.[29] These adverse effects are more likely to occur with the initial application of the vaginal preparation and are similar to symptoms of the vaginal infection. Abdominal cramps (3%), penile irritation, and allergic reactions (3%–7%) are uncommon, and headache may occur in up to 9% of women.[1]

Because of the limited absorption of topical imidazoles, drug interactions are unlikely. However, a case report documented an interaction between miconazole vaginal suppositories (100–200 mg) and warfarin.[30] In this patient, the international normalized ratio (INR) was significantly increased on two occasions when vaginal miconazole was used. Miconazole and warfarin are both metabolized by CYP2C9; concurrent use may decrease the clearance of warfarin and increase unbound drug. The prescriber should be contacted to consider reducing the dosage of warfarin during concurrent therapy to avoid an increase in INR. The product information warns women using warfarin in combination with these products that bleeding or bruising might occur. Aside from an allergy to imidazoles, contraindications do not exist to the use of topical imidazoles.

Pharmacotherapeutic Comparison

Studies have shown the imidazoles to be equally effective, with effectiveness rates of about 80%–90%.[3,5] Miconazole single-dose and 7-day treatments have been compared, resulting in similar overall cure rates with significantly faster rates of symptom relief by day 3 in the single-dose group compared with the 7-day treatment group.[31] Butoconazole nitrate 2% single-dose cream has also been compared with miconazole 7-day treatment, resulting in nonsignificant differences in cure rates.[32] Seven-day regimens of clotrimazole and miconazole; 3-day regimens of butoconazole, clotrimazole, and miconazole; and 1-day regimens of clotrimazole, miconazole, and tioconazole are available without a prescription. Monistat 1 has also been approved for insertion in the morning or at bedtime, allowing flexibility for patients. A similar cure rate exists for the daytime and bedtime treatments.[33]

Several other nonprescription vaginal preparations, including Vagisil and Yeast-Gard, containing benzocaine and resorcinol are also available. These agents provide relief of itching, although the underlying cause is not addressed. The use of these agents is rarely, if ever, appropriate given the benefits of the imidazole antifungals, including superior efficacy, improved patient adherence, less frequent local reactions, and shorter treatment durations. These products and medicated douches may be reserved for vaginal and vulvar irritation and itching and should be used for a limited time only or on the advice of a primary care provider (Table 8–4).

Product Selection Guidelines

Special Populations

Self-treatment of VVC is not appropriate for girls younger than 12 years. This condition is rare in premenarchal girls. Vaginal symptoms in this age group warrant a medical referral to determine the cause because infections in prepubertal children may indicate potential sexual abuse.[34]

Self-care treatment in pregnancy is not appropriate. However, when treatment of VVC is indicated, treatment should consist of butoconazole, clotrimazole, or miconazole. When possible, treatment should be withheld during the first trimester.[34] The health care provider should evaluate for complications such as hyperglycemia and assess for other organisms, given that

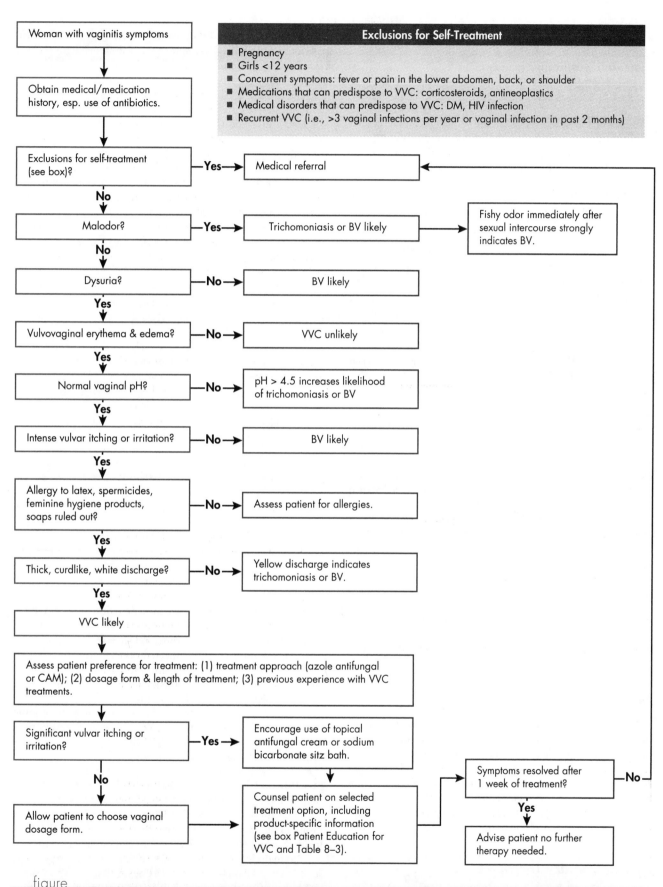

figure

8–1   Self-care of vulvovaginal candidiasis. Key: CAM = Complementary and alternative medicine; DM = diabetes mellitus; HIV = human immunodeficiency virus; VVC = vulvovaginal candidiasis. (*Source:* References 7, 18, and 19.)

table
8-2 Selected Nonprescription Vaginal Antifungal Products and Their Dosages

Trade Name	Primary Ingredient	Dosage
Butoconazole Nitrate Products		
Gynazole 1	Butoconazole nitrate 2%	Insert cream into vagina daily for 1 day.
Clotrimazole Products		
Gyne-Lotrimin 7 Cream Mycelex-7 Cream	Clotrimazole 1%	Insert cream into vagina daily for 7 days; apply to vulva twice daily as needed for itching.
Mycelex-7 Combination Pack	Tablet: clotrimazole 100 mg Cream: clotrimazole 1%	Insert tablet into vagina daily for 7 days; apply cream to vulva twice daily for itching.
Gyne-Lotrimin 3 Cream	Clotrimazole 2%	Insert cream into vagina daily for 3 days; apply to vulva twice daily for itching.
Miconazole Nitrate Products		
Monistat 1 Combination Pack Day or Night Monistat 1 Daytime Ovule	Cream: miconazole nitrate 2% Suppository: miconazole nitrate 1200 mg	Apply cream to vulva twice daily as needed for itching up to 7 days; insert suppository into vagina daily (morning or at bedtime) for 1 day.
Monistat 3 Combination Pack[a]	Cream: miconazole nitrate 2% Suppository: miconazole nitrate 200 mg	Apply cream to vulva twice daily as needed for itching up to 7 days; insert suppository into vagina daily for 3 days.
Monistat 3 Cream[a]	Miconazole nitrate 4%	Insert cream into vagina daily for 3 days; apply to vulva twice daily as needed for itching.
Monistat 7 Suppository	Miconazole nitrate 100 mg	Insert suppository into vagina daily for 7 days at bedtime.
Monistat 7 Cream Femizol-M Cream	Miconazole nitrate 2%	Insert cream into vagina daily for 7 days; apply to vulva twice daily as needed for itching.
Monistat 7 Combination Pack	Cream: miconazole nitrate 2% Suppository: miconazole nitrate 100 mg	Apply cream to vulva twice daily as needed for itching; insert suppository into vagina daily for 7 days.
Tioconazole Products		
Vagistat-1 Ointment 1-Day Ointment	Tioconazole 6.5%	Insert ointment into vagina daily for 1 day.

[a] Prefilled applicators are available for this product.

bacterial vaginosis and trichomoniasis have the potential for adverse pregnancy outcomes. Breast-feeding women can use any of the nonprescription vaginal antifungals.[29]

No special considerations are necessary to treat older women presenting with a VVC infection.

Patient Preferences

Selection of cream, tablet, or suppository formulations can be left to patient preference because some women may prefer the convenience of prefilled applicators. Women who have previously experienced VVC prefer shorter courses of therapy than do those who have not had a prior infection.[1] If vulvar symptoms are significant, a cream preparation or the combination of a cream with vaginal suppositories or tablets is preferred. Morning or bedtime dosing is available to provide flexibility for patients.

Complementary Therapies

An alternative approach to treating VVC is the use of *Lactobacillus* preparations. The rationale for their use is to reestablish normal vaginal flora and inhibit overgrowth of *Candida* organisms. Data on the effectiveness of this approach are limited and

inconsistent. One study of five women with positive vaginal cultures for *C. albicans* found four women had negative cultures after administration of *Lactobacillus rhamnosus* GG suppositories for 7 days.[26] Another study examining the usefulness of *Lactobacillus* and other probiotic bacteria administered orally, vaginally, and by both routes found that none of the regimens protected against the development of postantibiotic VVC.[35] However, eating 8 ounces of yogurt with live cultures daily may be of some benefit in preventing recurrent VVC.[26] Nonprescription probiotic feminine supplements may be used to reestablish *Lactobacillus*. RepHresh Pro-B feminine supplement is a product that is easy to use but expensive (about $25–$30 for a 30-day supply). Patients take one capsule by mouth daily. (For information on probiotics, see Chapter 23 [Table 23–9] and Chapter 51.)

The use of a sodium bicarbonate sitz bath may provide prompt relief of vulvar irritation associated with a *Candida* vaginal infection before antifungal agents can provide benefit.[36]

To manage VVC, some women may prefer natural products such as a vaginal preparation of tea tree oil, which has antibacterial and antifungal properties.[37,38] A 200 mg vaginal suppository containing tea tree oil is available commercially and is used for 6 nights. Allergic dermatitis may occur. (For information on tea tree oil, see Chapter 51.)

<table>
<tr><td colspan="2">table
8–3   **Guidelines for Applying Vaginal Antifungal Products**</td></tr>
</table>

1. Start treatment at night before going to bed. Lying down will reduce leakage of the product from the vagina.
2. Wash the entire vaginal area with mild soap and water, and dry completely before applying the product.
3. *Vaginal cream:* (If prefilled applicators are being used, skip to step 4.) Unscrew the cap; place the cap upside down on the end of the tube. Push down firmly until the seal is broken. Attach the applicator to the tube by turning the applicator clockwise. Squeeze the tube from the bottom to force the cream into the applicator. Squeeze until the inside piece of the applicator is pushed out as far as possible and the applicator is completely filled with cream. Remove the applicator from the tube. *Vaginal tablets or suppositories:* Remove the wrapper and place the product into the end of the applicator barrel.
4. While standing with feet slightly apart and knees bent, as shown in drawing A, or while lying on your back with knees bent, as shown in drawing B, gently insert the applicator into the vagina as far as it will go comfortably.
5. Push the inside piece of the applicator in and place the cream as far back in the vagina as possible. To deposit vaginal tablets or suppositories, insert the applicator into the vagina and press the plunger until it stops.
6. Remove the applicator from the vagina.
7. After use, recap the tube (if using cream). Then clean the applicator by pulling the two pieces apart and washing them with soap and warm water.
8. If desired, wear a sanitary pad to absorb leakage of the vaginal antifungal. Do not use a tampon to absorb leakage.
9. Continue using the product for the length of time specified in the product instructions. Use the product every day without skipping any days, even during menstrual flow.

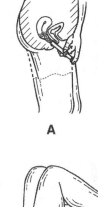

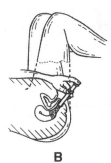

<table>
<tr><td colspan="2">table
8–4   **Selected Nonprescription Drug Products for Vaginal Itching and Irritation (Note: List is not all-inclusive.)**</td></tr>
<tr><th>Trade Name</th><th>Primary Ingredients</th></tr>
<tr><td colspan="2">**Benzocaine Products**[a]</td></tr>
<tr><td>Vagi-Gard Advanced Sensitive Cream
Vagisil Anti-Itch Original Formula</td><td>Benzocaine 5%; resorcinol 2%</td></tr>
<tr><td>Vagisil Maximum Strength</td><td>Benzocaine 20%; resorcinol 3%</td></tr>
<tr><td>Vagi-Gard Maximum Strength Cream</td><td>Benzocaine 20%; benzalkonium chloride 0.13%</td></tr>
<tr><td>Vagi-Gard Cream
VH Essentials</td><td>Benzocaine 5%; benzalkonium chloride 0.13%</td></tr>
<tr><td colspan="2">**Hydrocortisone Products**[b]</td></tr>
<tr><td>Vagisil Satin Anti-Itch Crème</td><td>Hydrocortisone 1%</td></tr>
<tr><td colspan="2">**Povidone/Iodine Products**</td></tr>
<tr><td>Betadine Medicated Suppository[c]</td><td>Povidone/iodine 10%</td></tr>
<tr><td>Betadine Premixed Medicated Disposable Douche
Summer's Eve Special Care Medicated Douche</td><td>Povidone/iodine 0.3% (in disposable bottles)</td></tr>
<tr><td colspan="2">**Homeopathic Products**</td></tr>
<tr><td>Yeast-Gard Suppository[d]</td><td>*Pulsatilla* (28×); *Candida albicans* (28×)
Candida parapsilosis (28×)</td></tr>
<tr><td>Yeast-X Suppository[e]</td><td>*Pulsatilla* (28×)</td></tr>
<tr><td colspan="2">**Other Products**</td></tr>
<tr><td>Summer's Eve Feminine Powder[f]
Vagisil Feminine Powder[f]</td><td>Cornstarch; aloe; mineral oil</td></tr>
</table>

[a] Apply benzocaine products externally.
[b] Apply hydrocortisone products externally; avoid prolonged use; may use concomitantly with antifungal products.
[c] Use 1 povidone/iodine suppository nightly for 7 days.
[d] Use 1 Yeast-Gard suppository daily for 7 days.
[e] Use 1 Yeast-X suppository daily as needed.
[f] Apply feminine powders externally to absorb moisture.

Gentian violet, a dye available in community pharmacies, is an old treatment for VVC. Today, topical gentian violet is used for resistant *Candida* vaginal infections.[39] A tampon may be soaked in gentian violet and inserted into the vagina for several hours or overnight. Often a single application is adequate, but tampons saturated with gentian violet can be used once or twice a day for up to 5 consecutive days. The major disadvantage of using gentian violet is the possible staining of fabrics and skin.[29]

Another option for the treatment of VVC is boric acid 600 mg in a size 0 gelatin capsule inserted vaginally once or twice daily for 14 days. Boric acid 5% in lanolin can be applied topically for vulvar irritation.[3,16,40] Boric acid therapy is useful for non–*C. albicans* infections, which are more likely to be resistant to the imidazole antifungals. Short-term cure rates have been reported to be between 85% and 95% when boric acid is used in women whose infection did not respond to vaginal antifungals.[11,40] For resistant infections, the therapy is used twice weekly for longer durations. Boric acid can be toxic and teratogenic, and human fatalities have been reported from oral ingestion.[40] Boric acid capsules may be compounded

in community pharmacies, and patient counseling should be provided to explain that the capsule should not be ingested. In addition, pregnant women should not use boric acid.

Assessment of Vulvovaginal Candidiasis: A Case-Based Approach

Many episodes of VVC are uncomplicated and can be effectively treated by topical imidazole agents.[3] In particular, otherwise healthy women who experience episodes that are sporadic and uncomplicated and women who predictably experience

VVC following a course of antibiotic therapy are the best candidates for self-treatment.[25]

Determining the appropriateness of self-care and the likelihood of a *Candida* vaginal infection are important initial steps in advising the woman about the management of vaginal symptoms with nonprescription drug therapy.

Health care providers may advise patients when it is appropriate to self-treat for vaginal symptoms consistent with VVC and when medical evaluation, including pelvic examination and laboratory examination of vaginal secretions, is indicated. Self-treatment is most appropriate when the woman meets the following four criteria:

1. Vaginal symptoms are infrequent (i.e., no more than 3 vaginal infections per year and no vaginal infection within the past 2 months).
2. A medical professional diagnosed at least 1 previous episode of VVC.
3. Current symptoms are mild to moderate and consistent with the characteristic signs and symptoms of VVC, particularly in that the discharge does not have a foul odor.
4. If measured, vaginal pH is 4.5 or lower.

Case 8–1 provides an example of the assessment of a patient presenting with a vaginal infection.

Patient Counseling for Vulvovaginal Candidiasis

Health care providers counseling patients who are considering self-treatment with vaginal antifungals should emphasize limiting self-treatment to the presence of mild-moderate classic symptoms, infrequent vaginal symptoms, and predictable antibiotic-associated VVC. A medical evaluation should be obtained if symptoms persist beyond 1 week after treatment or if they recur within 2 months. Also, if vaginal symptoms occur more than 3 times in a 12-month interval, further evaluation is needed. Women taking warfarin should be referred to their provider.

Patients should be informed that a short course of a nonprescription vaginal antifungal product will kill the "yeast" organisms that caused the infection. Label instructions should be reviewed with the patient, stressing that the antifungal is to be used only once a day for the specified length of time. Patients should be advised that symptomatic relief will likely begin within 2–3 days but that it may take a week for complete resolution of symptoms. The patient should also be advised of signs and symptoms that indicate medical attention is needed. The box Patient Education for Vulvovaginal Candidiasis lists specific information to provide patients.

case
8–1

Relevant Evaluation Criteria	Scenario/Model Outcome
Information Gathering	
1. Gather essential information about the patient's symptoms and medical history, including:	
a. description of symptom(s) (i.e., nature, onset, duration, severity, associated symptoms)	Patient is experiencing vulvovaginal intense itching with a white discharge but no malodor. She also reports that symptoms began yesterday.
b. description of any factors that seem to precipitate, exacerbate, and/or relieve the patient's symptom(s)	Patient reports experiencing symptoms throughout the day.
c. description of the patient's efforts to relieve the symptoms	Patient reports that she did try nonprescription VH essentials for the itching but had only minimal relief.
d. patient's identity	Amelia Loddy, travel agent
e. age, weight, sex, and height	31 years old, female, 5 ft 5 in., 135 lb
f. concurrent medical conditions, prescription and nonprescription medications, and dietary supplements	Lo Loestrin Fe 1 daily; daily multivitamin; acetaminophen 325 mg occasionally
g. allergies/other adverse reactions to medications	Sulfa: rash
h. other (describe)	Amelia was diagnosed with a VVC infection twice before per her medical history. Her last vaginal infection was 2 years ago. Her current symptoms are similar to her previous VVC infections.
Assessment and Triage	
2. Differentiate patient's signs/symptoms and correctly identify the patient's primary problem(s) (Table 8–1).	Amelia has itching and a white discharge without malodor, which are symptoms consistent with a *Candida* vaginal infection.
3. Identify exclusions for self-treatment (Figure 8–1).	None
4. Formulate a comprehensive list of therapeutic alternatives for the primary problem to determine if triage to a medical practitioner is required, and share this information with the patient or caregiver.	Options include: (1) Refer Amelia for medical evaluation with her PCP. (2) Recommend self-treatment with an OTC vaginal antifungal product. (3) Take no action.

case

8–1 *continued*

Relevant Evaluation Criteria	Scenario/Model Outcome

Plan

5. Select an optimal therapeutic alternative to address the patient's problem, taking into account patient preferences.

Amelia has classic symptoms associated with VVC. She has had two previous VVC infections. She has no chronic medical problems. She is also a good candidate for self-treatment because she is in a monogamous relationship and is not at risk for STIs. (See Figure 8–1.)

6. Describe the recommended therapeutic approach to the patient or caregiver.

"Several choices of nonprescription vaginal antifungal products are available. Because you have vulvar itching, a cream preparation or a combination pack will provide the best relief of your symptoms." (See the box Patient Education for Vulvovaginal Candidiasis for instructions on proper use.)

7. Explain to the patient or caregiver the rationale for selecting the recommended therapeutic approach from the considered therapeutic alternatives.

"This treatment is appropriate because you have the characteristic symptoms of vulvovaginal candidiasis, your symptoms are mild to moderate, you have no contraindications to self-treatment, and you have infrequent vaginal infections. See your primary care provider if your symptoms do not improve within 3 days or are not gone within 1 week, if the vaginal discharge changes (particularly if it becomes malodorous), or if symptoms return within the next 2 months."

Patient Education

8. When recommending self-care with nonprescription medications and/or nondrug therapy, convey accurate information to the patient or caregiver:

   a. appropriate dose and frequency of administration

   "Insert the clotrimazole cream vaginally once daily for 3 days; apply externally to the vulva as needed for itching."

   b. maximum number of days the therapy should be employed

   "Apply the cream for 3 days."

   c. product administration procedures

   See Table 8–3.

   d. expected time to onset of relief

   "Relief should occur in 2–3 days; often some relief occurs within hours of the first application."

   e. degree of relief that can be reasonably expected

   "All symptoms should be resolved within 1 week after beginning treatment."

   f. most common side effects

   "Vulvovaginal burning and itching are the most common side effects."

   g. side effects that warrant medical intervention should they occur

   "Significant stinging, burning, or itching that persists beyond the first 48 hours of treatment should be medically evaluated."

   h. patient options in the event that condition worsens or persists

   "See your primary care provider if symptoms do not improve in 3 days or worsen."

   i. product storage requirements

   "The product should be stored in a cool area; storage in the bathroom or bedside is appropriate for ease of use."

   j. specific nondrug measures

   None

   Solicit follow-up questions from patient or caregiver.

   (1) "Are any of the nonprescription vaginal antifungal products better than any others? Are some regimens more effective than others?"

   (2) "Is yogurt consumption helpful in reducing VVC infections?"

   Answer patient's or caregiver's questions.

   (1) "No, all of the products and regimens are equally effective."

   (2) "Daily intake of yogurt may provide a prophylactic benefit against VVC infections."

9. Assess patient outcome.

   Ask the patient to call and update you on her treatment outcome. Or you could call her in a week to evaluate the outcome.

Key: VVC = Vulvovaginal candidiasis; PCP = primary care provider; OTC = over-the-counter; STI = sexually transmitted infection.

patient education for
Vulvovaginal Candidiasis

The goals of self-treatment are to cure the vaginal fungal infection and reestablish normal vaginal flora. Carefully following the product instructions and the self-care measures will help ensure optimal therapeutic outcomes.

Nondrug Measures

- If significant irritation of the vulva is present, use a sodium bicarbonate sitz bath to provide relief and give the antifungal medication time to become effective.
  - Add 1 teaspoon sodium bicarbonate to 1 pint of water.
  - Add 2–4 tablespoons of the solution to 2 inches of bath water.
  - Sit in the sitz bath or bathtub for 15 minutes as needed for symptom control.
- For recurrent infections, try eating yogurt (1 cup per day of live culture yogurt) and decreasing dietary sugar and refined carbohydrates.

Nonprescription Medications

- Insert the antifungal product into the vagina once a day, preferably at bedtime to minimize leakage from the vagina. Use a sanitary pad or panty liner to avoid staining of underwear.
- Table 8–3 provides instructions on administering vaginal antifungals. Significant relief of symptoms should occur within 24–48 hours, and relief is often apparent within hours after the first dose. However, the length of treatment (particularly for 1- to 3-day treatments) does not directly correspond to the time of resolution of symptoms.
- Continue the therapy for the recommended length of time, even if symptoms are gone. Stopping treatment early is a common reason for recurrence of vaginal symptoms and, possibly, occurrence of difficult-to-treat organisms.
- Vaginal antifungals can be used during a menstrual period. If desired, wait and treat the infection after menses ends. Do not interrupt a course of therapy if menses begins.
- Do not use tampons or douche while using a vaginal antifungal and for 3 days after use.

- Although adverse effects are uncommon, the first dose of the antifungal may cause some vaginal burning and irritation, and a few women (about 1 in 10) experience a headache.
- Refrain from sexual intercourse during treatment with the vaginal antifungal. Vaginal lubricants and vaginal spermicides should not be used at the same time as the vaginal antifungal. Vaginal antifungals can damage latex condoms and diaphragms and may result in unreliable contraceptive effects. Do not use these contraceptives during therapy or for 3 days after therapy because the antifungal medication remains in the vagina for several days.

Consult Physician First

- Do not use vaginal antifungals if:
  - You have not been medically diagnosed with VVC at least once.
  - You are younger than 12 years old.
  - You are pregnant.
  - You have diabetes mellitus; are human immunodeficiency virus (HIV)-positive or have acquired immunodeficiency syndrome (AIDS); or have impaired immune function, including use of medications that may impair function of the immune system.
- If you are breast-feeding, consult a primary care provider before using a vaginal antifungal.

When to Seek Medical Attention

- Seek medical attention if symptoms do not improve within 3 days or symptoms persist beyond 7 days.
- Seek medical attention if vaginal symptoms worsen or change, especially if the vaginal secretions begin to smell bad, become frothy, or become discolored, or if other symptoms (e.g., abdominal tenderness) occur. These events may indicate that the *Candida* (yeast) organisms are resistant to the nonprescription therapy or that another type of vaginal infection is present.

Evaluation of Patient Outcomes for Vulvovaginal Candidiasis

Symptoms of VVC should improve within 2 or 3 days of initiation of therapy and resolve within 1 week. The length of treatment, particularly for 1- to 3-day treatments, does not directly correspond to the time of resolution of symptoms.

The health care provider should advise patients to call if the symptoms persist, and women should understand the importance of adherence. Persistent or new symptoms that are not consistent with VVC are reasons for advising the patient to seek a medical referral.

Atrophic Vaginitis

Atrophic vaginitis is inflammation of the vagina related to atrophy of the vaginal mucosa secondary to decreased estrogen levels.

Although up to 45% of postmenopausal women may experience symptomatic atrophic vaginitis, only 25% may seek treatment.[41–43] Dyspareunia, or painful intercourse, is a symptom sometimes related to inadequate vaginal lubrication or atrophic vaginitis.

Pathophysiology of Atrophic Vaginitis

During menopause, the postpartum period, and breast-feeding, the vaginal epithelium becomes thin, and vaginal lubrication declines secondary to a decrease in estrogen levels. Women may experience atrophic vaginitis and dyspareunia during these intervals.[43] Atrophic vaginitis may also occur among women with decreased ovarian estrogen production such as after radiation or chemotherapy. Women taking antiestrogenic drugs such as clomiphene, tamoxifen, raloxifene, danazol, leuprolide, and nafarelin may also develop atrophic vaginitis.[29,44] Low–estrogen oral contraceptives may also cause atrophic vaginitis on rare occasions.[8]

Clinical Presentation of Atrophic Vaginitis

An early symptom of atrophic vaginitis is a decrease in vaginal lubrication.[44] Other symptoms include vaginal irritation, dryness, burning, itching, leukorrhea, and dyspareunia. A thin, watery (occasionally bloody), or yellow malodorous vaginal discharge or "spotting" may also be present.[3,6,44] Sexual activity may result in vaginal bleeding or spotting. Any new episode of postmenopausal vaginal bleeding should have a medical referral to rule out endometrial cancer.

Treatment of Atrophic Vaginitis

Self-treatment of atrophic vaginitis is limited to alleviating the primary symptom, vaginal dryness, with lubricant products. Preventing vaginal dryness may necessitate prescription estrogen therapy, a measure that may be considered for women at menopause. Women who are breast-feeding or have recently given birth often have temporary declines in estrogen levels. Vaginal lubricants may be needed only until estrogen levels return to normal.

Treatment Goals

The goals of therapy are to reduce or eliminate the symptoms of vaginal dryness, burning, and itching, and eliminate dyspareunia if vaginal dryness is the cause of painful sexual intercourse.

General Treatment Approach

Vaginal dryness can often be treated with lubricants such as those listed in Table 8–5. Sexual arousal and intercourse may also improve atrophic vaginitis, and women who are sexually active have fewer symptoms of atrophic vaginitis.[44]

Self-treatment is appropriate when the symptoms are mild-moderate and confined to the vaginal area and when no bleeding is present. Women with severe vaginal dryness, dyspareunia, or bleeding should be referred for medical evaluation. In addition, products that may aggravate vaginal symptoms such as irritants and allergens such as powders, perfumes, spermicides, and panty liners should be avoided.[44]

Figure 8–2 outlines the approach to treating vaginal dryness associated with atrophic vaginitis.

table **8–5**	Selected Nonprescription Vaginal Lubricants	
Trade Names	**Primary Ingredients**
Astroglide; K-Y Personal Lubricant Liquid; Vagisil Intimate Moisturizer Lotion*a*	Glycerin; propylene glycol
H-R Lubricating Jelly	Hydroxypropyl methylcellulose
K-Y Jelly	Glycerin; hydroxyethylcellulose
K-Y Warming Liquid Personal Lubricant	Propylene glycol; glycerin; acacia honey type O
Replens Gel	Glycerin; mineral oil

a Fragrance-free formulation.

Pharmacologic Therapy
Vaginal Lubricants

Multiple water-soluble products are available for vaginal lubrication including Astroglide, K-Y Jelly, and Replens. Personal lubricant products temporarily moisten vaginal tissues. These products provide short-term improvement in symptoms such as burning and itching. Personal lubricants can also provide vaginal lubrication to facilitate sexual intercourse.

Petroleum jelly should not be used because it is difficult to remove from the vagina. If the patient is using a latex condom or diaphragm, only water-soluble lubricants should be used because other products may damage the latex and impair the efficacy of these contraceptive methods. Water-soluble lubricant gels can be applied both externally and internally. Initially, the patient should be instructed to use a liberal quantity of lubricant (up to 2 teaspoons) and then to tailor the quantity and frequency of use to her specific needs. Most lubricant products provide an improvement in symptoms for less than 24 hours.[44] If the patient is treating dyspareunia, the lubricant should be applied to both the vaginal opening and the penis. If the use of lubricants does not produce adequate benefit or is esthetically unappealing to the patient, she should be referred for medical evaluation.

Assessment of Atrophic Vaginitis: A Case-Based Approach

When discussing symptoms of vaginal dryness during the patient assessment, the health care provider should obtain a description of symptoms, including their association with sexual intercourse and their severity. Information should also be obtained as to whether the woman has recently given birth, is lactating, or is perimenopausal or postmenopausal. The health care provider should ask patients about the use of any vaginal or feminine hygiene products that may cause or worsen vaginal irritation and dyspareunia.

Case 8–2 provides an example of the assessment of a patient presenting with atrophic vaginitis.

Patient Counseling for Atrophic Vaginitis

The health care provider should stress the short-term nature of atrophic vaginitis to women who are breast-feeding or who recently gave birth. Women who are perimenopausal or postmenopausal should know that long-term treatment with vaginal lubricants may be necessary. In either case, the health care provider should explain the proper use of the lubricants for treatment of vaginal dryness or dyspareunia. The box Patient Education for Atrophic Vaginitis lists specific information.

Evaluation of Patient Outcomes for Atrophic Vaginitis

Symptoms of atrophic vaginitis should improve within a week. The provider should advise the patient to call to discuss treatment effectiveness, if she has any concerns, and to call after 1 week of

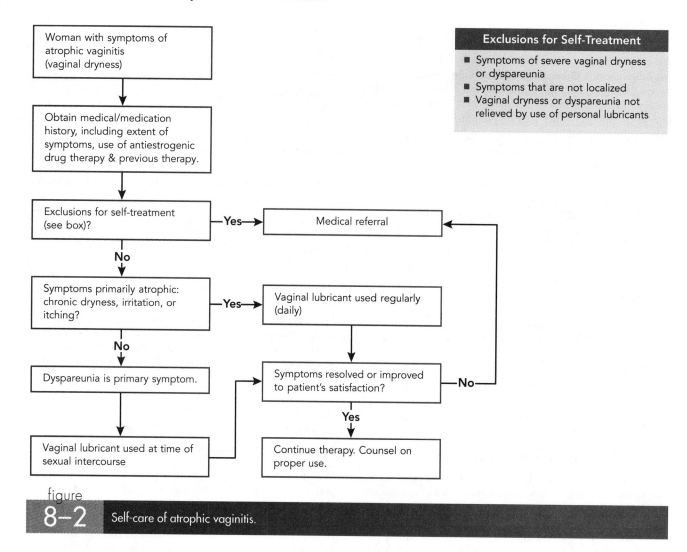

figure

8-2

Self-care of atrophic vaginitis.

case

8-2

Relevant Evaluation Criteria	Scenario/Model Outcome

Information Gathering

1. Gather essential information about the patient's symptoms and medical history, including:

   a. description of symptom(s) (i.e., nature, onset, duration, severity, associated symptoms)

      Patient is experiencing vaginal dryness and significant dyspareunia.

   b. description of any factors that seem to precipitate, exacerbate, and/or relieve the patient's symptom(s)

      She reports experiencing these symptoms for a few weeks.

   c. description of the patient's efforts to relieve the symptoms.

      Patient reports that she has not tried any products.

   d. patient's identity

      Linda Lewis, yoga instructor

   e. age, sex, height, and weight

      50 years old, female, 5 ft 4 in., 132 lb

   f. concurrent medical conditions, prescription and non-prescription medications, and dietary supplements

      Metoprolol 100 mg twice daily; daily multivitamin

   g. allergies/other adverse reactions to medications

      NKDA

   h. other (describe) _____

      Linda is postmenopausal and experiencing vaginal dryness and significant dyspareunia. She reports that she has not tried OTC lubricants, and per her medical history, she has no prior use of estrogen therapy. She also reports a history of a hysterectomy 1 year ago.

Relevant Evaluation Criteria	Scenario/Model Outcome
Assessment and Triage	
2. Differentiate patient's signs/symptoms and correctly identify the patient's primary problem(s).	Linda is postmenopausal. She has vaginal dryness with significant dyspareunia but no symptoms indicative of other vaginal infections. These symptoms are consistent with atrophic vaginitis.
3. Identify exclusions for self-treatment (Figure 8–2).	She has vaginal dryness with significant dyspareunia as a primary symptom.
4. Formulate a comprehensive list of therapeutic alternatives for the primary problem to determine if triage to a medical practitioner is required and share this information with the patient or caregiver.	Options include: (1) Suggest that Linda consider using vaginal lubricants for symptom improvement until she can see her PCP. (2) Refer Linda to her PCP for possible vaginal estrogen therapy. (3) Take no action.
Plan	
5. Select an optimal therapeutic alternative to address the patient's problem, taking into account patient preferences.	Because Linda has significant and bothersome dyspareunia as a primary symptom, this would qualify as exclusion for self-care. The recommended option for this patient would be to see her PCP to further assess her dyspareunia and explore topical estrogen therapy to relieve her symptoms.
6. Describe the recommended therapeutic approach to the patient or caregiver.	See the box Patient Education for Atrophic Vaginitis.
7. Explain to the patient or caregiver the rationale for selecting the recommended therapeutic approach from the considered therapeutic alternatives.	"Given your significant dyspareunia symptoms and vaginal dryness, I recommend that you follow up with your primary care provider to consider the use of a topical (vaginal) estrogen product, such as tablets. However, OTC lubricants may be used to assist in symptom relief until you see your provider."
Patient Education	
8. When recommending self-care with nonprescription medications and/or nondrug therapy, convey accurate information to the patient or caregiver.	Criterion does not apply in this case.
Solicit follow-up questions from patient or caregiver.	(1) "How much and how often may I use OTC lubricants?" (2) "Will I have to take oral estrogen or will topical estrogen work?"
Answer patient's or caregiver's questions.	(1) "A liberal quantity (2 teaspoons) of OTC lubricants may be used and may be used as frequently, as needed." (2) "Oral estrogen therapy is usually not necessary for the treatment of atrophic vaginitis; vaginal estrogen products (creams or tablets) are options."
9. Assess patient outcome.	Contact the patient in a day or two to ensure she made an appointment for further evaluation and medical care.

Key: NKDA = No known drug allergy; OTC = over-the-counter; PCP = primary care provider.

patient education for
Atrophic Vaginitis

The objective of self-treatment with vaginal lubricants is to relieve vaginal dryness and pain during sexual intercourse related to atrophic vaginitis. Carefully following product instructions and the self-care measures listed here will help ensure optimal therapeutic outcomes.

- Apply the vaginal lubricant as frequently as needed for relief of vaginal dryness, irritation, burning, itching, or inadequate vaginal lubrication.
- Begin treatment of atrophic symptoms with a liberal quantity of lubricant (2 teaspoons); tailor subsequent doses to the quantity and frequency of use needed to provide relief.
- If using lubricants at the time of sexual intercourse, apply the lubricant to the vagina, particularly at the vaginal opening, and to the penis.

- Some leakage of product will occur. If desired, use a sanitary napkin or panty liner to avoid staining of underwear.
- Relief of symptoms may be apparent within hours after the first dose. Regular application of a lubricant can reverse atrophic symptoms to some extent.
- If no improvement is noticeable within a week, or if symptoms worsen or there is any vaginal bleeding, see your primary care provider.

treatment to report progress in symptom resolution. Symptoms that persist or the presence of bleeding requires medical evaluation.

Vaginal Douching

Prevalence of Douching

The 2002 National Survey of Family Growth reported that 32% of U.S. women practiced douching in the previous 12 months.[45] Douching rates are influenced by race, geographic region, socioeconomic status, and education.[46] Most women who report douching state they began the practice as adolescents.

The most frequently stated reason for douching is to achieve good vaginal hygiene. Because vaginal douches mechanically irrigate the vagina, clearing away mucus and other accumulated debris, they may be used as cosmetic cleansing agents. Among the women in a focus group study, most considered douching part of normal feminine hygiene, and most reported douching after menstruation and sexual intercourse.[47]

Potential Adverse Effects of Douching

Douching may lead to adverse health outcomes. Frequent douching has been associated with an increased risk for PID, reduced fertility, ectopic pregnancy, vaginal infections such as BV, sexually transmitted infections, low birth weight, and cervical cancer.[46,47] Additional problems include irritation or sensitization from douche ingredients and disruption of normal vaginal flora and pH. Local irritation, sensitization, and contact dermatitis are also possible with many antimicrobial agents found in douches.

The effect of douches on vaginal flora varies depending on the douche ingredients and douching frequency. Water/vinegar (acetic acid) douches have minimal effect on lactobacilli but do inhibit some vaginal pathogens, whereas douches containing antiseptics inhibit all vaginal flora.[48,49] Povidone/iodine has a greater potential than water/vinegar douches to reduce total bacteria, but it may allow pathogenic species to proliferate, increasing the risk for vaginal infection.[50] Allergic reactions have been reported with intravaginal povidone/iodine because systemic absorption is possible. This product should not be used by women who are allergic to iodine. Table 8–4 lists examples of douche products that contain povidone/iodine.

Proper Use of Douche Equipment

Two types of syringes are available for douching purposes: douche bags and bulb douche syringes. The douche bag, or fountain syringe or folding feminine syringe, holds 1–2 quarts of fluid and comes with tubing and a shutoff valve. Two types of tips are supplied: one for enema use (the shorter rectal nozzle) and one for douching. The two tips are not interchangeable; vaginal infections may occur if a single tip is used for both douching and enemas.

Bulb douche syringes are available as both disposable and nondisposable products. The nondisposable units hold 8–16 ounces of fluid, whereas the disposable units contain 3–9 ounces. The flow rate is regulated by the amount of hand pressure exerted when the bulb is squeezed. Gentle pressure is recommended because excess pressure may force fluid through the cervix, causing uterine inflammation. Instructions on proper use of the device are found in Table 8–6.

---

table 8–6   Administration Guidelines for Douches

Bulb Douche Syringe Method

- Choose a comfortable douching position. Two positions are recommended: (1) sitting on the toilet or (2) standing in the shower. Whichever position is chosen, remember that douching is easier when relaxed.
- Gently insert the nozzle about 3 inches into the vagina. Avoid closing the lips of the vagina.
- Squeeze bottle gently, letting solution cleanse the vagina and then flow freely from the body.
- After douching, throw away bottle and nozzle, if disposable.

Douche Bag Method

- Fill the douche bag with the prescribed solution or with a warm water and vinegar solution.
- Lie back in the tub with knees bent. Place the douche bag about 1 foot above the height of hips. Do not place or hang the bag any higher because such height will cause the pressure of fluid entering the vagina to be too high.
- Insert the nozzle several inches into the vagina. Aim the nozzle up and back toward the small of the back. While holding the labia closed around the nozzle, release the clamp slowly to allow fluid to enter the vagina. Rotate the tip and allow fluid to enter the vagina until the vagina feels full. Stop the flow of fluid; then hold the fluid in the vagina for about 30–60 seconds. Release and allow the fluid to flow out; repeat until the douche bag is empty.
- Wash the nozzle with mild soap and water.

Patient Counseling for Douching

Health care providers should discuss a woman's reasons for douching. Women should be informed that douching is not necessary to cleanse the vagina and that douching has potential adverse consequences. Douching for routine hygienic purposes should be discouraged, and douching is contraindicated during pregnancy. Douching should be delayed at least 6–8 hours after sexual intercourse if a vaginal spermicide was used as a contraceptive agent.

An alternative cleansing method for vaginal and perineal areas should be suggested, such as gently washing the vagina and the vulvar, perineal, and anal regions with the fingers using lukewarm water and mild soap. If a woman is douching to prevent or treat symptoms of a vaginal infection such as an abnormal vaginal discharge, she should be counseled about more effective therapy or referred for medical evaluation, as appropriate.

Patients for whom douches have been prescribed or those who insist on douching for other reasons should be instructed on how to use these products safely, appropriately, and effectively. The box Patient Education for Douching lists specific information to provide these patients.

Women should be informed that douching is not necessary for cleansing of the vagina. An alternative cleansing method for vaginal and perineal areas should be suggested, such as gently washing the vagina and the vulvar, perineal, and anal regions with the fingers using lukewarm water and mild soap. Improper methods of douching or too frequent douching can cause vaginal irritation. Douching can also increase the risk for pelvic inflammatory disease and sterility. Strictly following the product instructions and the self-care measures listed here will help avoid these problems.

- Keep all douche equipment clean.
- Use lukewarm water to dilute products.
- Follow the appropriate instructions in Table 8–6 for the method of douching being used.
- Never insert a douche with forceful pressure.
- Do not use these products for birth control.
- Do not douche until at least 8 hours after intercourse during which a diaphragm, cervical cap, or contraceptive jelly, cream, or foam was used.

- Do not douche for at least 3 days after the last dose of vaginal antifungal medication.
- Do not douche for 48 hours before any gynecologic examination.
- Do not douche during pregnancy unless under the supervision of a health care provider.
- Use douches only as directed for routine cleansing.
- Do not douche more often than twice a week, except on the advice of a health care provider.
- If vaginal dryness or irritation occurs, discontinue use of the douche.

Key Points for Vaginal and Vulvovaginal Disorders

➤ Vaginal symptoms are often nonspecific, and may be difficult to distinguish between the three common vaginal infections. The symptom most likely to differentiate a *Candida* vaginal infection from BV and trichomoniasis is the absence of an offensive odor to the vaginal secretions. Measurement of vaginal pH (pH > 4.5 indicates a non-*Candida* infection) may also help to distinguish *Candida* and reduce inappropriate use of nonprescription vaginal antifungals.

➤ *Candida* vaginal infections are typically caused by *C. albicans,* but recently non–*C. albicans* infections have increased. The latter may be more resistant to nonprescription vaginal antifungals.

➤ Self-treatment for a *Candida* vaginal infection is most appropriate when the symptoms are mild-moderate, when she does not have predisposing illnesses or medications, when she has had one previously diagnosed infection, and when her symptoms are not recurrent. Recurrent infections are defined as more than 3 infections within a 12-month period and symptoms occurring within 2 months of previous vaginal symptoms.

➤ All of the nonprescription vaginal antifungals are equally effective. Selection of length of regimen or time of day for administration can be determined by patient preference. A medical referral should be made for women taking warfarin. Patients should be informed that symptoms typically improve shortly after application of the nonprescription vaginal antifungals. Symptoms should improve within 2–3 days after initiation of therapy and resolve within a week. The length of the treatment regimen does not directly correspond to resolution of symptoms.

➤ Use of a sodium bicarbonate sitz bath may provide relief of itching and irritation prior to onset of benefit from the antifungal.

➤ Eating yogurt with live cultures (8 ounces daily) may benefit some patients in preventing recurrent VVC infections.

➤ Atrophic vaginitis can occur after menopause, after giving birth, during breast-feeding, or as a result of antiestrogenic medications. Vaginal dryness and dyspareunia can be relieved by use of topical personal lubricant products. If symptoms do not improve within a week, medical evaluation is needed.

➤ Atrophic vaginitis may cause vaginal bleeding. Any reports of postmenopausal bleeding should have a medical referral to rule out endometrial cancer.

➤ Douching is not necessary for vaginal cleansing, and adverse consequences of douching can occur. Douching is contraindicated during pregnancy and should be postponed until at least 8 hours after sexual intercourse if a vaginal spermicide was used for contraception.

REFERENCES

1. Reed BD. Vaginitis. In: Sloane PD, Slatt LM, Ebell MH, et al., eds. *Essentials of Family Medicine.* 6th ed. Philadelphia: Lippincott Williams & Williams; 2011.
2. Cullins V, Dominguez L, Guberski T, et. al. Treating vaginitis. *Nurse Pract.* 1999;24(10):46–58.
3. Mashburn J. Etiology, diagnosis and management of vaginitis. *J Midwifery Womens Health.* 2006;51(6):423–30.
4. Benjamin F. Anatomy, physiology, growth and development. In: Seltzer V, Pearse WH, eds. *Women's Primary Health Care.* 2nd ed. New York: McGraw-Hill; 1999.
5. Cleveland A. Vaginitis: finding the cause prevents treatment failure. *Cleve Clin J Med.* 2000;67(9):634–46.
6. Quan M. Vaginitis: diagnosis and management. *Postgrad Med.* 2010;122(6): 117–27.
7. Anderson M, Klink K, Cohrssen A, et al. Evaluation of vaginal complaints. *JAMA.* 2004;291(11):1368–79.
8. Ledger W, Monif G. A growing concern: inability to diagnose vulvovaginal infections correctly. *Obstet Gynecol.* 2004;103(4):782–4.
9. Nyirjesy P, Sobel JD. Advances in diagnosing vaginitis: development of a new algorithm. *Curr Infect Dis Rep.* 2005;7(6):458–62.
10. Hainer BL, Gibson MV. Vaginitis: diagnosis and treatment. *Am Fam Physician.* 2011;83(7):807–15.
11. Ferris D, Nyirjesy P, Sobel JD, et al. Over-the-counter antifungal drug misuse associated with patient-diagnosed vulvovaginal candidiasis. *Obstet Gynecol.* 2002;99(3):419–25.
12. Moraes P, Taketomi EA. Allergic vulvovaginitis. *Ann Allergy Asthma Immunol.* 2000;85(4):253–67.
13. Coco A, Vandenbosche M. Infectious vaginitis: an accurate diagnosis is essential and attainable. *Postgrad Med.* 2000;107(4):63–74.
14. Fidler BD. Diagnosis and treatment of vulvovaginal candidiasis. Retail Clinician CE Lesson. 2007:34–42. Accessed at http://www.4healtheducation.com/pdf/RetailClinicianSpring2007.pdf, August 25, 2013.
15. Roy S, Caillouette JC, Faden JS, et al. Improving use of antifungal medications: the role of an over-the-counter vaginal pH self-test device. *Infect Dis Obstet Gynecol.* 2003;11(4):209–16.
16. Haefner H. Current evaluation and management of vulvovaginitis. *Clin Obstet Gynecol.* 1999;42(2):184–95.

17. Holzman C, Leventhal JM, Qui H, et al. Factors linked to bacterial vaginosis in nonpregnant women. *Am J Public Health.* 2001;91(10):1661–70.

18. Klebanoff M, Schwebke J, Zhang, J. Vulvovaginal symptoms in women with bacterial vaginosis. *Obstet Gynecol.* 2004;104(2):267–72.

19. Owen M, Clenney TL. Management of vaginitis. *Am Fam Physician.* 2004;70(11):2125–32.

20. Soper D. Trichomoniasis: under control or undercontrolled? *Am J Obstet Gynecol.* 2004;190(1):281–90.

21. Corsello S, Spinello A, Osnengo G, et. al. An epidemiological survey of vulvovaginal candidiasis in Italy. *Eur J Obstet Gynecol Reprod Biol.* 2003; 110(1):66–72.

22. Foxman B, Barlow R, D'Arcy H, et al. Candida vaginitis: self-reported incidence and associated costs. *Sex Transm Dis.* 2000;27(4):230–5.

23. Castelo-Branco C, Cancelo MJ, Villero J, et al. Management of postmenopausal vaginal atrophy and atrophic vaginitis. *Maturitas.* 2005;52S: S46–52.

24. American College of Obstetricians and Gynecology. Vaginitis. ACOG (American College of Obstetricians and Gynecology) Clinical Management Guidelines Number 72. *Obstet Gynecol.* 2006;107(5):1195–206.

25. Samra-Latif OM. Vulvovaginitis. *Medscape (eMedicine).* Updated August 23, 2013. Accessed at http://emedicine.medscape.com/article/2188931-overview, August 25, 2013.

26. Falagas M, Betsi GI, Athanasiou S. Probiotics for prevention of recurrent vulvovaginal candidiasis: a review. *J Antimicrob Chemother.* 2006;58(2): 266–72.

27. U.S. Food and Drug Administration. Vaginal candidiasis may sometimes be an early warning of HIV infection [press release]. November 16, 1992. Accessed at http://aidsinfo.nih.gov/news/260/vaginal-candidiasis-may-sometimes-be-an-early-warning-of-hiv-infection, July 16, 2014.

28. Singh S. Treatment of vulvovaginal candidiasis. *CPJ.* 2003;136:26–30.

29. Suess J, Holzman C. Vulvar and vaginal disease. In: Smith M, Shimp LA, eds. *Common Problems in Women's Health Care.* New York: McGraw-Hill, Inc.; 2000.

30. Elmer G, Surawicz CM, McFarland LV. Biotherapeutic agents: a neglected modality for the treatment and prevention of selected intestinal and vaginal infections. *JAMA.* 1996;275(11):870–6.

31. Upmalis D, Cone FL, Lamia CA, et al. Single-dose miconazole nitrate vaginal ovule in the treatment of vulvovaginal candidiasis: two single-blind, controlled studies versus miconazole nitrate 100 mg cream for 7 days. *J Womens Health Gend Based Med.* 2000;9(4):421–9.

32. Brown D, Henzl MR, Kaufman RH, Gynazole Study Group. Butoconazole nitrate 2% for vulvovaginal candidiasis: new, single-dosed vaginal cream formulation vs. seven-day treatment with miconazole nitrate. *J Reprod Med.* 1999;44:933–8.

33. Barnhart K. Safety and efficacy of bedtime versus daytime administration of the miconazole nitrate 1200 mg vaginal ovule insert to treat vulvovaginal candidiasis. *Curr Med Res Opin.* 2005;21(1):127–34.

34. Kohlberger P, Bancher-Todesca D. Bacterial colonization in suspected sexually abused children. *J Pediatr Adolesc Gynecol.* 2007;20(5):289–92.

35. Pirotta M, Gunn J, Chondros P, et al. Effect of lactobacillus in preventing post-antibiotic vulvovaginal candidiasis: a randomized controlled trial. *BMJ.* 2004;329(7465):548–51.

36. Korenek P, Britt R, Hawkins C. Differentiation of the vaginosis-bacterial vaginosis, lactobacillosis, and cytolytic vaginosis. *Internet J Adv Nurs Pract.* 2003;6(1). Accessed at http://ispub.com/IJANP/6/1/12743, June 2014.

37. Reid G, Bocking A. The potential for probiotics to prevent bacterial vaginosis and preterm labor. *Am J Obstet Gynecol.* 2003;189(4):1202–8.

38. Van Kessel K, Assefi N, Marrazzo J, et al. Common complementary and alternative therapies for yeast vaginitis and bacterial vaginosis: a systematic review. *Obstet Gynecol Surv.* 2003;58(5):351–8.

39. Watson C, Calabretto H. Comprehensive review of conventional and non-conventional methods of management of recurrent vulvovaginal candidiasis. *Aust N Z J Obstet Gynaecol.* 2007;47(4):262–72.

40. Allen-Davis J, Beck A, Parker R, et al. Assessment of vulvovaginal complaints: accuracy of telephone triage and in-office diagnosis. *Obstet Gynecol.* 2002;99(1):18–22.

41. Santoro N, Komi J. Prevalence and impact of vaginal symptoms among postmenopausal women. *J Sex Med.* 2009;6(8):2133–42.

42. Nappi R, Kokot-Kierepa M. Women's voices in the menopause: results from an international survey on vaginal atrophy. *Maturitas.* 2010;67(3): 233–8.

43. The North American Menopause Society. The role of local vaginal estrogen for treatment of vaginal atrophy in postmenopausal women: 2007 position statement of the North American Menopause Society. *Menopause.* 2007;14(3 pt 1):357–69.

44. Bachman G, Nevadunsky N. Diagnosis and treatment of atrophic vaginitis. *Am Fam Physician.* 2000;61(10):3090–6.

45. Chandra A, Martinez G, Mosher W, et al. Fertility, family planning, and reproductive health of US women: data from the 2002 National Survey of Family Growth. *Vital Health Stat.* 2005;23(25):1–160.

46. Lichtenstein B, Nansel TR. Women's douching practices and related attitudes: findings from four focus groups. *Women Health.* 2000;31 (2–3):117–31.

47. Schwebke J, Desmond RA, Oh MK. Predictors of bacterial vaginosis in adolescent women who douche. *Sex Transm Dis.* 2004;31(7):433–6.

48. Pavlova S, Tao L. In vitro inhibition of commercial douche products against vaginal microflora. *Infect Dis Obstet Gynecol.* 2000;8(2):99–104.

49. Zhang J, Hatch M, Zhang D, et al. Frequency of douching and risk of bacterial vaginosis in African American women. *Obstet Gynecol.* 2004; 104(4):756–60.

50. Martino JL, Vermund SH. Vaginal douching: evidence for risks or benefits to women's health. *Epidemiol Rev.* 2002;24(2):109–24.

chapter 9

DISORDERS RELATED TO MENSTRUATION

Leslie A. Shimp

The menstrual cycle is a regular physiologic event for women that begins in adolescence and usually continues through late middle age. Women are able to self-treat for two common menstrual disorders: primary dysmenorrhea and premenstrual syndrome. Many women use nonprescription products and seek advice from health care providers on how best to manage symptoms of these disorders, including abdominal pain and cramping, irritability, and fluid retention. An understanding of the menstrual cycle will help both patients and health care providers make informed and appropriate decisions about self-care. Health care providers should also be familiar with common menstrual symptoms and disorders, as well as the risks for toxic shock syndrome.

Menstruation results from the monthly cycling of female reproductive hormones. A single menstrual cycle is the time between the onset of one menstrual flow (menstruation or menses) and the onset of the next. The average age of menarche (the initial menstrual cycle) in U.S. women is 12 years, although normal menarche may occur as early as age 11 or as late as age 14.5.[1] The onset of menstruation is influenced by factors such as race, genetics, nutritional status, and body mass. The median menstrual cycle length is 28 days, ranging from 24 to 38 days for adult women; adolescents have a wider cycle length of 20–45 days.[2] Menses lasts 3–7 days, with most blood loss occurring during days 1 and 2.[1,3] The major components of menstrual fluid are blood and endometrial cellular debris; the average blood loss per cycle is 30 mL (10–84 mL).[3] A loss of more than 80 mL per cycle or bleeding lasting longer than 7 days is considered abnormal and may be associated with anemia.

The menstrual cycle (Figure 9–1) results from the hormonal activity of the hypothalamus, pituitary gland, and ovaries; this is known as the hypothalamic-pituitary-ovarian axis. The hypothalamus plays the key role in regulating the menstrual cycle by producing gonadotropin-releasing hormone (GnRH). Low levels of both estradiol and progesterone, present at the end of the previous menstrual cycle, stimulate the hypothalamus to release GnRH, which stimulates pituitary gonadotroph cells to synthesize and secrete luteinizing hormone (LH) and follicle-stimulating hormone (FSH).

Two principal reproductive events, both of which are hormonally controlled, occur during each menstrual cycle. The first event is the maturation and release of an ovum (egg) from the ovaries; the second is the preparation of the endometrial lining of the uterus for the implantation of a fertilized ovum. The events of the menstrual cycle can be described in phases that reflect changes in either the ovary (follicular/ovulatory and luteal phases) or the uterine endometrium (menstrual/proliferative and secretory phases). The follicular/ovulatory phase correlates with the menstrual/proliferative phase, and the luteal phase correlates with the secretory phase.

Cycle day 1 is the first day of menstrual flow and is the beginning of the follicular and menstrual/proliferative phases. The follicular phase can range in length from several days to several weeks, but it lasts an average of 14 days. During the follicular phase, FSH stimulates the maturation of a group of ovarian follicles. These maturing follicles secrete estradiol, which promotes growth of the uterine endometrium.

By about cycle day 8, a single ovarian follicle usually becomes dominant, which typically results in the release or ovulation of only one mature egg. The ovulatory phase of the cycle is about 3 days in length. During this phase, the pituitary gland secretes high levels of LH for a 48-hour period, which is known as the LH surge. The LH surge catalyzes the final steps in the maturation of the ovum and stimulates production of prostaglandins and proteolytic enzymes necessary for ovulation. Estradiol levels also decrease during the LH surge, sometimes resulting in midcycle endometrial bleeding. Ovulation typically occurs 12 hours after the LH surge. Ovulation releases 5–10 mL of follicular fluid, which contains the oocyte mass and prostaglandins; this event may cause abdominal pain (*mittelschmerz,* German for "middle pain") for some women. In adolescents, the LH surge does not occur until 2–5 years after menarche. As a result, 50%–80% of cycles are anovulatory (i.e., no ovulation occurs) and are irregular during the initial years after menarche.

The luteal phase is the time between ovulation and the beginning of menstrual blood flow. After the follicle ruptures, it is referred to as the corpus luteum. The luteal phase is typically consistent in length (about 14 ±2 days) and reflects the 10- to 12-day functional period of the corpus luteum. The corpus luteum secretes progesterone, estradiol, and androgens. The increased levels of estrogen and progesterone alter the uterine endometrial lining. Glands mature, proliferate, and become secretory as the uterus prepares for the implantation of a fertilized egg. Progesterone and estrogen levels increase in the middle of the luteal phase, but LH and FSH levels decline in response to the increased hormone levels. If pregnancy occurs, human chorionic gonadotropin released by the developing placenta supports the function of the corpus luteum until the placenta develops enough to begin secreting estrogen and progesterone. If pregnancy does not occur, the corpus luteum ceases to function. Estrogen and progesterone levels then decline, causing the endometrial lining of the uterus to become edematous and necrotic. The decrease

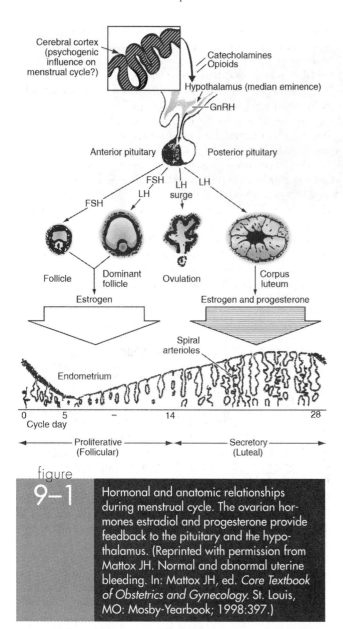

figure
9–1
Hormonal and anatomic relationships during menstrual cycle. The ovarian hormones estradiol and progesterone provide feedback to the pituitary and the hypothalamus. (Reprinted with permission from Mattox JH. Normal and abnormal uterine bleeding. In: Mattox JH, ed. *Core Textbook of Obstetrics and Gynecology.* St. Louis, MO: Mosby-Yearbook; 1998:397.)

in progesterone also leads to prostaglandin synthesis. Following prostaglandin-initiated vasoconstriction and uterine contractions, sloughing of the outer two endometrial layers occurs. The decline in estrogen and progesterone results in an increase in GnRH and in the renewed production of LH and FSH, which begins a new menstrual cycle.

Dysmenorrhea

Dysmenorrhea (difficult or painful menstruation) is the most common gynecologic problem among adolescents and young adult women. Dysmenorrhea is divided into primary and secondary disorders by etiology. Primary dysmenorrhea is associated with cramp-like lower abdominal pain at the time of menstruation in the absence of pelvic disease. Secondary dysmenorrhea is typically associated with pelvic pathology. The prevalence of dysmenorrhea is highest in adolescence, with up to 93% of young women being affected.[4-6] Primary dysmenorrhea usually

develops within 6–12 months after menarche, generally affecting women during their teens and early 20s.[7] Primary dysmenorrhea occurs only during ovulatory cycles. Its prevalence increases between early and older adolescence as the regularity of ovulation increases[4] and decreases after age 24.[7,8]

Severe menstrual pain is reported by 14%–23% of teens.[9] Dysmenorrhea is the leading cause of school absenteeism and lost working hours among adolescent girls and young women. About 26% of adolescent girls report dysmenorrhea-related school absenteeism, which increases to 50% in girls who report severe pain.[6,9] In addition, adolescents with severe menstrual pain reported that the pain interfered with other life activities such as social activities, sports, work, and relationships with friends and family.[4,9] Similarly, an estimated 600 million work hours are lost annually because of dysmenorrhea.[8]

The decreased prevalence and severity of dysmenorrhea in women in their mid-20s and older may be partially explained by oral contraceptive (OC) use (an effective therapy for dysmenorrhea) and pregnancy. The use of OCs decreases the amount of endometrium, resulting in lower prostaglandin production. During the last trimester of pregnancy, uterine adrenergic nerves virtually disappear, and only a portion of the nerves regenerate after childbirth. For many women, this phenomenon results in a decreased prevalence of dysmenorrhea following childbirth.

Factors other than young age and nulliparity can increase the risk for or severity of dysmenorrhea. These include early menarche (prior to age 12); heavy menstrual flow; tobacco smoking; low fish consumption; a body mass index of less than 20 kg/m² or greater than 30 kg/m²; premenstrual symptoms; and stress, anxiety, and depression.[5,6] Obesity is linked to early menarche and can predispose to primary dysmenorrhea.[8] In addition, factors such as attempting to lose weight and stress related to social, emotional, or family issues can all make dysmenorrhea pain more bothersome.[6,8,10]

Pathophysiology of Primary Dysmenorrhea

The cause of primary dysmenorrhea is not fully understood. However, prostaglandins and leukotrienes contribute substantially to the occurrence and severity of dysmenorrhea.[4,5,8] Nitric oxide and vasopressin may also be involved.[5,8] Ovulation increases serum progesterone, which leads to increases in arachidonic acid. During menstruation, arachidonic acid is converted to prostaglandins and leukotrienes, which are then released. Prostaglandin levels are two to four times greater in women with dysmenorrhea than in women without dysmenorrhea; the severity of dysmenorrhea is proportional to the endometrial concentration of the prostaglandin $F_2\alpha$ ($PGF_2\alpha$).[7] Leukotrienes (inflammatory mediators known to cause vasoconstriction and uterine contractions) are elevated in women with dysmenorrhea; levels are correlated with both occurrence and severity. Leukotrienes may contribute significantly to dysmenorrhea in women who do not respond to nonsteroidal anti-inflammatory drugs (NSAIDs).[8] Nitric oxide has also been linked to dysmenorrhea because transdermal nitroglycerine patches increase nitric oxide and decrease dysmenorrhea-related pain. Nitric oxide is the substance that promotes uterine quiescence during pregnancy, and use of nitric oxide during premature labor can stop uterine contractility.[8] Circulating levels of vasopressin (a substance that can produce dysrhythmic uterine contractions) are higher in women with dysmenorrhea than in asymptomatic individuals. However, the role of vasopressin in the etiology of primary dysmenorrhea remains controversial.[4,5]

Prostaglandins stimulate uterine contractions. Normal contractions and vasoconstriction help expel menstrual fluids and control bleeding as the endometrium sloughs. However, the increased levels of prostaglandins and leukotrienes present with dysmenorrhea can lead to strong uterine contractions similar to those experienced during labor and excessive vasoconstriction, resulting in uterine ischemia and pain. In women without dysmenorrhea, uterine contractions are rhythmic, and contraction pressure reaches 120 mm Hg. In contrast, women with dysmenorrhea have more frequent contractions, with pressures up to 180 mm Hg that contribute to ischemia and tissue hypoxia and, thus, pain.[11]

Clinical Presentation of Primary Dysmenorrhea

The pain with primary dysmenorrhea is cyclic in nature and is directly related to the onset of menstruation (Table 9–1). Pain is typically experienced as a continuous dull ache with spasmodic cramping in the lower midabdominal or suprapubic region that may radiate to the lower back and upper thighs. The uterine contractions can force prostaglandins and leukotrienes into the systemic circulation, causing additional symptoms such as nausea, vomiting, fatigue, dizziness, bloating, diarrhea, and headache.[4] A large study of adolescents found that 78% reported fatigue, 71% cramping, 64% headaches, 58% lower back pain, and 37% nausea at the time of menstruation.[9] The onset of pain is several hours prior to or coincident with the onset of menses and usually lasts 1–3 days, typically peaking in the first 24–48 hours.[6,10] For this reason, women with regular periods

may wish to begin treatment before the onset of menses to prevent dysmenorrhea. This clinical presentation can be adequate for the diagnosis of primary dysmenorrhea, if the pain is mild-moderate and the patient responds to NSAID therapy.[4,6,7]

Secondary dysmenorrhea is suggested if the symptoms initially begin years after menarche (at age 25 or older), if pelvic pain occurs at times other than during menses, if the woman has irregular menstrual cycles or has menorrhagia (excessively prolonged or profuse menses), metrorrhagia (irregular uterine bleeding usually between menstrual periods), or a history of pelvic inflammatory disease (PID), dyspareunia, or infertility.[4,5,9] Endometriosis (growth of cells similar to endometrial cells in locations outside the uterus) is the most common cause of secondary dysmenorrhea. Adolescents are being diagnosed increasingly with secondary dysmenorrhea, which accounts for symptoms in 47%–73% of teens with severe menstrual pain and no response to NSAIDs or OCs.[2,9] Secondary dysmenorrhea may also be caused by the presence of an intrauterine contraceptive (IUC).

Treatment of Primary Dysmenorrhea

Many women self-treat for dysmenorrhea using nonprescription products. In a study of adolescents, 66% self-treated with NSAIDs; fewer used acetaminophen or aspirin.[9] Among those who self-treated, 85% reported moderate-to-high effectiveness from the analgesic. Other studies have found that self-care may result in use of low or mistimed doses or use of less effective medications, thus increasing the likelihood of school absence and other activity limitations.[4] Inadequate management of dysmenorrhea pain can lead to increased pain sensitivity at times other than during menses and to increased sensitivity to non-uterine pain, thus having important implications for pain perception and quality of life throughout life.[12]

table
9–1   Differentiation of Primary and Secondary Dysmenorrhea

	Primary Dysmenorrhea	Secondary Dysmenorrhea
Age at onset of dysmenorrhea symptoms	As soon as 6–12 months after menarche but typically several years after menarche; age 13–17 years for most girls	Mid- to late-20s or older; usually 30s and 40s for women with secondary dysmenorrhea
Menses	More likely to be regular with normal blood loss	More likely to be irregular; menorrhagia and metrorrhagia more common
Pattern and duration of dysmenorrhea pain	Onset just prior to or coincident with onset of menses; pain with each or most menses, lasting only 2–3 days	Pattern and duration vary with cause; change in pain pattern or intensity may also indicate secondary disease
Pain at other times of menstrual cycle	No	Yes; may occur before, during, or after menses
Response to NSAIDs and/or OCs	Yes	No
Other symptoms	Fatigue, headache, nausea, change in appetite, backache, dizziness, irritability, and depression may occur at same time as dysmenorrhea pain	Vary according to cause of the secondary dysmenorrhea; may include dyspareunia, pelvic tenderness

Key: NSAID = Nonsteroidal anti-inflammatory drug; OC = oral contraceptive.
Source: References 4 and 9.

Treatment Goals

The goals of treating primary dysmenorrhea are to provide relief or a significant improvement in symptoms and minimize the disruption of usual activities.

General Treatment Approach

An important initial step in managing dysmenorrhea is distinguishing between primary and secondary dysmenorrhea. Self-care is appropriate for an otherwise healthy young woman who has a history consistent with primary dysmenorrhea and who is not sexually active or for a woman who has been diagnosed with primary dysmenorrhea.[4] Adolescents with pelvic pain who are sexually active and thus at risk for PID and women with characteristics indicating secondary dysmenorrhea should be referred for medical evaluation. Table 9–1 compares primary and secondary dysmenorrhea. An estimated 80%-90% of women with primary dysmenorrhea can be successfully treated with NSAIDs, OCs, or both. Other treatment options include nonpharmacologic measures (e.g., use of topical heat; dietary supplementation with omega-3 fatty acids). These fatty acids are found in fish and fish oil and compete with arachidonic acid in the cyclooxygenase and lipoxygenase pathways, leading to a decrease in the production of the proinflammatory cytokines. Increased consumption of fish rich in omega-3 fatty acids (e.g., tuna, salmon, and sardines) or use of fish oil may reduce symptoms.[10] Cholecalciferol, also known as vitamin D_3, is known to decrease the production of prostaglandins and increase prostaglandin inactivation.[13] One small study found a reduction in dysmenorrhea pain among women with low serum vitamin D levels who were given a single 300,000 IU dose of cholecalciferol 5 days prior to menses.[14] Women should be counseled to ingest vitamin D_3 600 IU daily. These measures often serve as adjuncts to drug therapy, although topical heat may be adequate as a sole therapy for some women. Figure 9–2 presents an algorithm for managing primary dysmenorrhea.

A patient with more severe dysmenorrhea, a change in the pattern or intensity of pain, or inadequate response or intolerance to NSAIDs should be referred to her primary care provider. An estimated 10%-25% of women do not respond to NSAIDs, cannot tolerate therapy, or prefer not to use medication for dysmenorrhea.[10] Figure 9–2 lists exclusions for self-care.

Nonpharmacologic Therapy

Many women use nonpharmacologic measures to help manage dysmenorrhea and menstrual discomfort. A study of adolescents found that common nonpharmacologic measures included sleep, hot baths or a heating pad, and exercise.[4] The use of heat is a commonly recommended nondrug therapy. An abdominal heat patch has been tested for the treatment of dysmenorrhea.[15] The heat patch was significantly better and provided 14% greater pain relief than placebo or acetaminophen. The analgesic effect of the heat patch had a faster onset than drug therapy and was additive to the relief provided by ibuprofen. Evidence regarding the benefit of exercise is conflicting; however, participation in regular exercise may lessen the symptoms of primary dysmenorrhea for some women.[4,5] Nonpharmacologic therapy may be especially useful for women who cannot tolerate or do not respond to nonprescription medications.

Smoking and exposure to secondhand smoke have been associated with more severe dysmenorrhea.[4] The severity of dysmenorrhea symptoms reportedly increases with the number of cigarettes smoked per day. The basis for this effect is unknown, but nicotine-induced vasoconstriction may be involved. Discontinuing tobacco smoking or avoiding exposure to tobacco smoke may improve symptoms.

Pharmacologic Therapy

Unfortunately, many women and adolescents with dysmenorrhea remain untreated or are inadequately treated. They continue to experience pain and limitations in their daily activity. The following sections outline the uses and properties of the four nonprescription analgesic medications commonly used by women to treat dysmenorrhea: acetaminophen, aspirin, ibuprofen, and naproxen sodium. Table 9–2 lists their dosages for dysmenorrhea. Chapter 5 provides further discussion of their adverse effects, contraindications, and drug interactions.

Aspirin

Aspirin may be adequate for treating mild symptoms of dysmenorrhea. In low dosages, aspirin has only a limited effect on prostaglandin synthesis and is only moderately effective in treating more than minimal symptoms of dysmenorrhea. Aspirin may also increase menstrual flow.

Acetaminophen

Acetaminophen may also be adequate for treating mild symptoms of dysmenorrhea. Acetaminophen is a weak inhibitor of prostaglandin synthesis; the reduction of $PGF_2\alpha$ levels is much greater with nonsalicylate NSAIDs than with acetaminophen.[16] Even in dosages of 4 grams daily, acetaminophen is less effective than ibuprofen; lower dosages are less likely to be effective.[16]

Nonsalicylate NSAIDs

Nonsalicylate NSAIDs, the first-line treatment for primary dysmenorrhea, include ibuprofen 200 mg and naproxen sodium 220 mg. In clinical trials, these NSAIDs were effective in 66%-90% of patients. Relief of dysmenorrhea typically occurs within the first cycle of use.[10] However, dosages used in clinical trials and dosages of prescription drugs for the treatment of dysmenorrhea are often higher than the labeled nonprescription dosages. Therefore, providers may recommend prescription therapy, or they may recommend that a patient use a prescription dosage of an NSAID using nonprescription products if the lower dosage does not provide adequate symptom relief.

Therapy with nonsalicylate NSAIDs should begin at the onset of menses or pain. If inadequate pain relief occurs, treatment beginning 1–2 days before expected menses may improve symptomatic relief.[5] If the possibility of pregnancy exists, therapy should be initiated only after menses begins. Patients should be instructed that the NSAID is used to prevent cramps and to relieve pain. Optimal pain relief is achieved when these agents are taken on a schedule, rather than on an as-needed basis. Therefore, ibuprofen should be taken every 4–6 hours and naproxen sodium every 8–12 hours for the first 48–72 hours of menstrual flow because that time frame correlates with maximum prostaglandin release (Table 9–2). The therapeutic effect is usually apparent within 30–60 minutes, and benefit will be optimal with continued regular use.

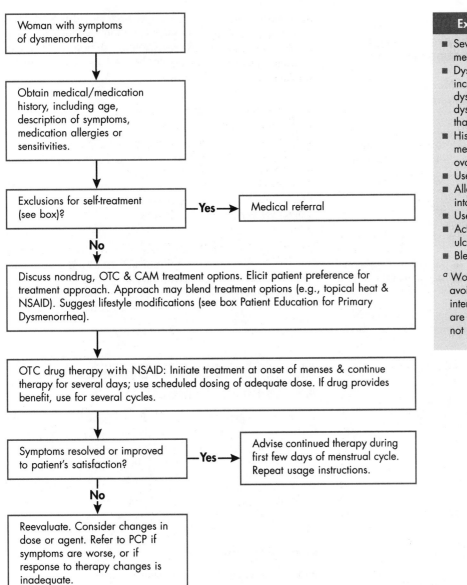

Exclusions for Self-Treatment[a]

- Severe dysmenorrhea and/or menorrhagia
- Dysmenorrhea symptoms inconsistent with primary dysmenorrhea (e.g., onset after age 25, dysmenorrhea pain at times other than onset of menses)
- History of PID, infertility, irregular menstrual cycles, endometriosis, ovarian cysts
- Use of IUC
- Allergy to aspirin or NSAIDs; intolerance for NSAIDs
- Use of warfarin, heparin, or lithium
- Active GI disease (PUD, GERD, ulcerative colitis)
- Bleeding disorder

[a] Women who are lactating should avoid use of herbs. Selected drug interactions and disease interactions are listed in Figure 9–3, but this list is not comprehensive.

Woman with symptoms of dysmenorrhea

Obtain medical/medication history, including age, description of symptoms, medication allergies or sensitivities.

Exclusions for self-treatment (see box)? —Yes→ Medical referral

No

Discuss nondrug, OTC & CAM treatment options. Elicit patient preference for treatment approach. Approach may blend treatment options (e.g., topical heat & NSAID). Suggest lifestyle modifications (see box Patient Education for Primary Dysmenorrhea).

OTC drug therapy with NSAID: Initiate treatment at onset of menses & continue therapy for several days; use scheduled dosing of adequate dose. If drug provides benefit, use for several cycles.

Symptoms resolved or improved to patient's satisfaction? —Yes→ Advise continued therapy during first few days of menstrual cycle. Repeat usage instructions.

No

Reevaluate. Consider changes in dose or agent. Refer to PCP if symptoms are worse, or if response to therapy changes is inadequate.

figure 9–2 Self-care of primary dysmenorrhea. Key: CAM = Complementary and alternative medicine; GERD = gastroesophageal reflux disease; GI = gastrointestinal; IUC = intrauterine contraceptive; NSAID = nonsteroidal anti-inflammatory drug; OTC = over-the-counter; PID = pelvic inflammatory disease; PCP = primary care provider; PUD = peptic ulcer disease.

A patient with dysmenorrhea may respond better to one NSAID than to another. If the maximum nonprescription dosage of one agent does not provide adequate benefit, then switching to another agent is recommended. The analgesic effect for most of these NSAIDs plateaus, so further dosage increases may increase the risk of adverse effects rather than provide additional benefit. Therapy with NSAIDs should be undertaken for three to six menstrual cycles, with changes made in the agent, dosage, or both before judging the effectiveness of these agents for a particular patient. If nonprescription NSAID therapy does not provide an adequate therapeutic effect, alternative therapies that may provide relief from primary dysmenorrhea include prescription NSAIDs; prescription dosages of nonprescription NSAIDs; or use of a combined OC or a progestin implant (Implanon, Nexplanon), estrogen plus progestin vaginal ring (NuvaRing), or the levonorgestrel IUC (Mirena, Skyla).[17]

Adverse effects from a few days of intermittent use usually include gastrointestinal (GI) symptoms such as upset stomach, vomiting, heartburn, abdominal pain, diarrhea, constipation, and anorexia. Adverse effects may also include headache and dizziness. Some GI adverse effects may be decreased by taking the drugs with food.

Pharmacotherapeutic Comparison

A Cochrane review indicated that ibuprofen and naproxen are considered first-line agents for dysmenorrhea because of their effectiveness and tolerability.[18] Cost and patient preference as to

table

9-2 Treatment of Dysmenorrhea with Nonprescription Medications

Agent	Recommended Nonprescription Dosage (maximum daily dosage)
Acetaminophen	650–1000 mg every 4–6 hours (4000 mg)[a]
Aspirin	650–1000 mg every 4–6 hours (4000 mg)
Ibuprofen	200–400 mg every 4–6 hours[b] (1200 mg)
Naproxen sodium	220–440 mg initially; then 220 mg every 8–12 hours (660 mg)

[a] See Table 5–3 for information on the manufacturer's voluntary reduction of maximum daily dosages of Tylenol products sold in the United States.

[b] If 200 mg every 4–6 hours is ineffective, the recommended dosage for dysmenorrhea (400 mg every 6 hours while awake) should be taken.

the number of doses and tablets to take should guide agent selection. Because of restrictions on taking medications to school, adolescents may benefit from naproxen's longer duration of action. Women at risk of GI ulceration should consider the use of a gastroprotective agent or another therapeutic option (e.g., an oral contraceptive). Acetaminophen may provide some relief for patients with hypersensitivity or intolerance to aspirin and for patients with intolerance to the GI and platelet-inhibition adverse effects of aspirin and NSAIDs.

Product Selection Guidelines

Special Populations

The Food and Drug Administration (FDA) recommends that aspirin and combination products containing aspirin not be given to children and adolescents under 19 years of age during episodes of febrile illnesses because of the association between aspirin use and Reye's syndrome in this age group. Pregnant or menopausal women will not experience dysmenorrhea. Women attempting to become pregnant should avoid use of NSAIDs in the periconception time, as these agents may impair implantation of the blastocyct.[19] Acetaminophen and ibuprofen can safely be taken by breast-feeding women, as the amounts of both medications are low in breast milk.[20] Women who are breast-feeding should avoid use of aspirin; if a dose of aspirin is taken, a woman should wait 1–2 hours before breast-feeding.[20] Naproxen sodium is a less optimal choice for breast-feeding women; although levels in breast milk are low, this medication has a long half-life, and a report of a serious adverse reaction in a neonate has been published.[20] A nonpharmacologic approach (e.g., topical heat) may also be a good choice for breast-feeding women.

Patient Factors

Given that NSAIDs are used only temporarily and intermittently, the risk for GI toxicity (e.g., irritation, bleeding, or ulceration) is limited. However, patients who have active peptic ulcer disease, those at risk for GI bleeding, or those with a history of GI ulcers should discuss use of NSAIDs with their primary care provider. They may attempt to treat dysmenorrhea with acetaminophen, nonpharmacologic therapy, or an OC. NSAIDs can also inhibit platelet activity and increase bleeding time. Women on anticoagulants should avoid NSAID use, and women on

other agents that may increase bleeding should use NSAIDs cautiously. Women who consume 3 or more alcohol-containing beverages daily should discuss use of acetaminophen or aspirin with their primary care provider because additive liver or GI toxicity, respectively, may occur.

Patient Preferences

Women may prefer to use an NSAID that they are familiar with, or they may prefer to try another agent if adverse effects were experienced previously. Preferences may also be based on tablet/capsule preferences or cost of products.

Complementary Therapies

Small studies have suggested that intake of several vitamins or minerals (e.g., vitamin B$_1$, vitamin E, or magnesium) may decrease dysmenorrhea.[10] Additionally, data from several randomized controlled trials have found acupressure to be an easily teachable, effective nonpharmacologic therapy for relieving primary dysmenorrhea.[21] All of these potential therapies need further study and verification.

Assessment of Primary Dysmenorrhea: A Case-Based Approach

Before recommending any product to a patient experiencing symptoms of dysmenorrhea, the health care provider should ascertain that the symptoms (particularly the onset and duration of pain in relation to the onset of menses) are consistent with primary dysmenorrhea (Table 9–1).

Case 9–1 illustrates the assessment of a patient with dysmenorrhea.

Patient Counseling for Primary Dysmenorrhea

Adolescents and young women who experience primary dysmenorrhea symptoms should be educated about this condition so they (1) realize primary dysmenorrhea is normal, (2) recognize typical symptoms and symptoms that are inconsistent with primary dysmenorrhea and when to seek medical evaluation, (3) understand that NSAIDs are preferred therapy because of their efficacy, and (4) know how to use these agents for greatest benefit. Patients should also be advised that nonprescription NSAIDs can be appropriate for initial therapy, but that not all women will respond. If response to the first agent is not adequate, another NSAID and/or nondrug intervention can be tried. The health care provider should explain the proper use of these agents and their potential adverse effects. The Patient Education for Primary Dysmenorrhea box lists specific information to provide patients.

Evaluation of Patient Outcomes for Primary Dysmenorrhea

Patient monitoring is accomplished by having the patient report whether her symptoms are improved or resolved. Symptoms should improve within an hour or so of taking an NSAID. The optimal effect of drug therapy may not be seen until the woman

case
9–1

Relevant Evaluation Criteria	Scenario/Model Outcome
Information Gathering	
1. Gather essential information about the patient's symptoms and medical history, including:	
a. description of symptom(s) (i.e., nature, onset, duration, severity, associated symptoms)	Patient is experiencing very painful menstrual cramps. She has had bad menstrual cramps for years. The cramps occur during menses but can also occur at other times of the month. She also has heavy bleeding during her periods.
b. description of any factors that seem to precipitate, exacerbate, and/or relieve the patient's symptom(s)	A hot bath can help sometimes, but even NSAIDs do not always relieve her pain.
c. description of the patient's efforts to relieve the symptoms	She has tried ibuprofen 400 mg three times daily; she has even tried 600 mg doses. She also tried naproxen sodium. She has some left-over acetaminophen with codeine from a dental procedure that she takes when the pain is really bad.
d. patient's identity	Marion Chandler
e. age, sex, height, and weight	27 years old, female, 5 ft 7 in., 140 lb
f. patient's occupation	Elementary school teacher
g. patient's dietary habits	She reports she eats a good diet overall, but will eat pizza or fast-food when busy. Also, she likes chocolate.
h. patient's sleep habits	She sleeps about 8 hours a night; sleep is only a problem if the pain is really bad.
i. concurrent medical conditions, prescription and nonprescription medications, and dietary supplements	Migraine headache: Excedrin, 2 tablets as needed Contraception: Loestrin 1.5/30, 1 daily for 3 weeks monthly Multiple vitamin, 1 daily Calcium/vitamin D 500 mg/400 IU, 1 daily
j. allergies	None
k. history of other adverse reactions to medications	None
l. other (describe) _____	NA
Assessment and Triage	
2. Differentiate patient's signs/symptoms and correctly identify the patient's primary problem(s).	Ms. Chandler has symptoms that are not consistent with primary dysmenorrhea; they are more consistent with secondary dysmenorrhea.
3. Identify exclusions for self-treatment (Figure 9–2).	Abdominal pain at times other than at the onset of menses; menorrhagia; severity of cramps; lack of alleviation or improvement in symptoms by NSAIDs and oral contraceptive
4. Formulate a comprehensive list of therapeutic alternatives for the primary problem to determine if triage to a health care provider is required, and share this information with the patient or caregiver.	Options include: (1) Refer patient to an appropriate health care provider. (2) Recommend self-care with nonprescription and nondrug measures. (3) Recommend self-care until patient can see an appropriate health care provider. (4) Take no action.
Plan	
5. Select an optimal therapeutic alternative to address the patient's problem, taking into account patient preferences.	She should be referred for medical evaluation.
6. Describe the recommended therapeutic approach to the patient or caregiver.	"Your symptoms are not consistent with primary dysmenorrhea. Therefore, there is not a nonprescription drug therapy that will address your symptoms. I advise you to see your primary care provider for a medical evaluation."
7. Explain to the patient or caregiver the rationale for selecting the recommended therapeutic approach from the considered therapeutic alternatives.	"You have tried both nonprescription NSAIDs, and neither has relieved your pain adequately. Also, you are taking an oral contraceptive; OCs typically improve primary dysmenorrhea. But you are still experiencing pain while taking the OC. Because you have had very bad cramps for a long time and neither NSAIDs nor your OC have relieved your pain, I recommend you have this pain evaluated."

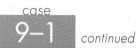

case

9–1   *continued*

Relevant Evaluation Criteria	Scenario/Model Outcome
Patient Education	
8. When recommending self-care with nonprescription medications and/or nondrug therapy, convey accurate information to the patient or caregiver.	Criterion does not apply in this case.
Solicit follow-up questions from the patient or caregiver.	"My mother has had menstrual problems—could this be genetic?"
Answer the patient's or caregiver's questions.	"It is possible—some gynecologic conditions are known to have genetic causes. Tell your primary care provider about your mother's history. Once your primary care provider determines the cause of your symptoms, he or she will be able to tell you if a genetic effect is possible."
Evaluation of Patient Outcome	
9. Assess patient outcome.	NA

Key: NA = Not applicable; NSAID = nonsteroidal anti-inflammatory drug; OC = oral contraceptive.

has used the medication on a scheduled basis. If inadequate pain relief occurs, treatment beginning 1–2 days before expected menses may improve symptomatic relief. The patient with persistent symptoms should be advised to try another nonprescription NSAID, to add adjunct therapy, or to see a primary care provider for evaluation.

Premenstrual Syndrome

Premenstrual syndrome (PMS) is defined as a cyclic disorder composed of a combination of physical, emotional/mood, and behavioral symptoms that occur during the luteal phase of the menstrual cycle. Symptoms improve significantly or disappear by the end of menses and are absent during the first week following menses. The diagnosis of PMS can be made on the basis of symptoms that occur cyclically. Premenstrual dysphoric disorder (PMDD) is a severe form of PMS. The diagnosis of PMDD requires that a specific constellation of symptoms occurs on a cyclical basis and that symptoms are severe enough to interfere with social and/or occupational functioning.[22,23] In addition, the American Congress of Obstetricians and Gynecologists has defined moderate-severe PMS as a condition having at least one psychological or physical symptom resulting in significant impairment and substantiated by prospective symptom ratings.[23]

Almost all women experience some mild physical or mood changes before the onset of menses, and these are normal signs of ovulatory cycles.[4,23] The changes may include physical symptoms; food cravings; and emotional lability, irritability, or lowered mood.

patient education for
Primary Dysmenorrhea

The objective of self-treatment is to relieve or significantly improve symptoms of dysmenorrhea so as to limit discomfort and disruption of usual activities. For most patients, carefully following product instructions and the self-care measures listed here will help ensure optimal therapeutic outcomes.

Nonpharmacologic Measures

- If effective, apply topical heat to the abdomen, lower back, or other painful area.
- Stop smoking cigarettes and avoid second-hand smoke.
- Consider eating more fish high in omega-3 fatty acids or taking a fish oil supplement.
- Participate in regular exercise if it lessens the symptoms.

Nonprescription Medications

- Ibuprofen and naproxen sodium are the best type of nonprescription medication for primary dysmenorrhea. The medications stop or prevent strong uterine contractions (cramping).
- Start taking the medication when the menstrual period begins or when menstrual pain or other symptoms begin. Then take the medication at regular intervals following the product

instructions, rather than just when the symptoms are present. See Table 9–2 for recommended NSAID dosages.
- Take the NSAID with food to limit upset stomach and heartburn.
- Do not take NSAIDs if you are allergic to aspirin or any NSAID, or if you have peptic ulcer disease, gastroesophageal reflux disease, colitis, or any bleeding disorder.
- If you have hypertension, asthma, or heart failure, watch for early symptoms that the NSAID is causing fluid retention.
- Do not take a nonsalicylate NSAID if you are also taking anticoagulants or lithium.
- If abdominal pain occurs at times other than just before or during the first few days of menses, seek medical attention.

When to Seek Medical Attention

- Seek medical attention if the pain intensity increases or if new symptoms occur.

In addition, some women report positive changes (e.g., increased energy, creativity, work productivity, and sexual desire).[22]

The number and severity of symptoms and the extent to which they interfere with functioning distinguish typical premenstrual symptoms, PMS, moderate-severe PMS, and PMDD[24] (Table 9–3). Sixty percent to 80% of women with premenstrual symptoms experience only mild (primarily physical) symptoms that do not interfere with their lives.[25] An estimated 20%–25% of women experience clinically significant symptoms, and 3%–8% report symptoms that cause significant impairment that interferes with relationships, lifestyle, or work.[24]

PMS can occur any time after menarche. Symptoms usually originate when women are in their teens to early 20s; typically, women wait about a decade to seek care.[4,25,26] PMS symptoms occur only during ovulatory cycles. Symptoms disappear during events that interrupt ovulation (e.g., pregnancy and breast-feeding); PMS symptoms disappear at menopause. The use of OCs can cause or exacerbate PMS symptoms, and use of hormone therapy in postmenopausal women may result in recurrence of PMS symptoms.[26]

Many factors contribute to the development of PMS and PMDD. Genetic factors likely play a role. Twin studies have shown that PMS is inherited, with women whose mothers had PMS being more likely to develop PMS.[26,27] In addition, genetic differences exist in the serotonergic 5-HT$_{1A}$ receptor and the estrogen alpha-receptor gene in women with and without PMS symptoms.[23,27] Stress and prior traumatic events (including sexual abuse) are risk factors for PMS/PMDD. Different coping strategies for handling stress, as well as altered psychological and physiologic responses to stress, have been shown in individuals with a history of life stress and abuse.[23,27] Sociocultural factors can also influence the experience of premenstrual symptoms. Exposure to negative expectations about premenstrual symptoms can lead women to interpret normal symptoms more negatively.[27]

Pathophysiology of PMS

The etiology of PMS is not fully understood. The current consensus is that the fluctuations of estrogen and progesterone caused by normal ovarian function are the cyclic trigger for PMS/PMDD symptoms. Although triggered by hormonal fluctuations, no known hormonal imbalances are present in women with PMS. Some women are biologically vulnerable or predisposed to experience PMS because of a neurotransmitter sensitivity to physiologic changes in hormone levels.[4,23,25,27] Serotonin, which is involved in mood and behavior regulation, is affected by estrogen and progesterone levels. Reduced levels of serotonin and serotonin effect in the brain may be linked to certain PMS symptoms (e.g., poor impulse control, irritability, carbohydrate craving, and dysphoria).[4,26] Other neurotransmitters and systems that may be important are allopregnanolone and gamma-aminobutyric acid (GABA) receptors. Allopregnanolone is a progesterone metabolite that binds the GABA receptor, leading to an anxiolytic action.[25] Women with PMS may be less sensitive to the sedating effects of allopregnanolone during the luteal phase and may have different GABA receptor sensitivity.[23,25,27] These alterations may result in luteal phase symptoms (e.g., anxiety and irritability).[26] In addition, selective serotonin reuptake inhibitors (SSRIs), which are known to relieve PMS/PMDD, affect the synthesis of allopregnanolone. Therefore, for symptoms severe enough to warrant prescription drug therapy, treatment is based on medications that affect the levels of serotonin or suppress ovulation and interrupt hormonal cycling.

The pathophysiology of physical symptoms of PMS (e.g., breast tenderness, bloating, and joint/muscle pain) is not as well studied. Women with PMDD have lower beta-endorphin levels, leading to a lower tolerance for discomfort and pain.[23] Studies of fluid retention and breast enlargement have not found tissue changes; abdominal bloating often occurs without weight gain.[23]

table 9–3	Differentiation of PMS and PMDD from Other Conditions with Luteal Phase Symptoms
Typical premenstrual symptoms	Mild physical (breast tenderness, bloating, lower backache, food cravings) or mood (irritability, emotional lability, lowered mood, increased energy or creativity) changes before the onset of menses that do not interfere with normal life functions
Premenstrual syndrome	At least one mood (depression, irritability, anger, anxiety) or physical (breast tenderness, abdominal bloating) symptom during the 5 days prior to menses. Symptoms are virtually absent during cycle days 5–10. The symptom or symptoms have a negative effect on social functioning or lifestyle, but the severity is mild-moderate.
Moderate-severe premenstrual syndrome	At least one mood or physical symptom that results in significant impairment of daily activities or relationships.
Premenstrual dysphoric disorder	Five or more symptoms (mood or physical) are present the last week of the luteal phase of the menstrual cycle, with at least one symptom being significant depression, anxiety, affective lability, or anger. The intensity of the symptoms interferes with work, school, social activities, and social relationships. Symptoms should be absent the week after menses and must not be an exacerbation of the symptoms of another disorder such as depression, panic disorder, or personality disorder.
Premenstrual exacerbation	A worsening of the symptoms of other, typically psychiatric disorders such as depression and anxiety or panic disorders. Conditions such as asthma, endometriosis, hypothyroidism, irritable bowel syndrome, attention-deficit disorder, diabetes mellitus, rheumatoid arthritis, migraine headaches, seizure disorders, and perimenopause can also worsen premenstrually. However, symptoms do not occur only during the luteal phase of the menstrual cycle; there is no symptom-free interval.

Source: References 4, 23, and 30.

Exogenous hormones may influence premenstrual symptoms. Women taking either OCs or postmenopausal hormone therapy may experience adverse effects similar to PMS symptoms as a result of altered hormone levels.[22,26] Conversely, 71% of women reported that the use of their OC had no effect on their PMS symptoms.[4] Certain OCs have been found useful in reducing the symptoms of PMS/PMDD: OCs containing the progestin drospirenone; those with a lower estrogen dose; those with a shortened hormone-free interval between pill packs; and those with continuous or extended cycles.[4,17]

Clinical Presentation of PMS

The symptoms of PMS or PMDD are not unique to these conditions; however, the occurrence of specific symptoms and their fluctuation with the phases of the menstrual cycle are diagnostic. Premenstrual symptoms typically begin or intensify about a week prior to the onset of menses, peak near the onset of menses, and resolve within several days after the beginning of menses.[23,26] Symptoms typically are consistent from month to month.[23] A woman with PMS or PMDD should experience essentially a symptom-free interval during days 5–10 of her menstrual cycle.

Common symptoms of PMS are listed in Table 9–4. Women seeking symptom relief typically report multiple emotional, physical, and behavioral symptoms. Mood and behavioral symptoms are the most upsetting.[26] Most women rate their symptoms as mild-moderate and do not feel that they interfere with their life. Mood symptoms tend to cause more distress than physical symptoms because of their impact on relationships. A large cross-sectional study conducted in multiple countries found that the most common PMS symptoms reported by women included abdominal bloating, cramps or abdominal pain, irritability, breast tenderness, and joint or back pain.[28] These symptoms may be the ones most often reported to providers and may blur the distinction between dysmenorrhea and PMS. In addition, the presence of dysmenorrhea may be associated with a greater severity of PMS.[29]

Symptoms of PMDD are similar to those of PMS. Compared with PMS, women with moderate-severe PMS and PMDD experience more symptoms, more severe symptoms, and symptoms that impair personal relationships and the ability to function well at work to a greater extent. Among women with PMDD, the most common symptoms are affective in nature. The diagnosis of PMDD requires that a patient experiences marked anger or irritability, or depressed mood, anxiety, or emotional lability.[30] Other symptoms of PMDD include difficulty concentrating, lethargy, hypersomnia or insomnia, and physical symptoms such as breast tenderness and bloating. The severity of symptoms must cause significant impairment in the ability to function socially or at work during the week prior to menses.[30] A daily rating of symptoms for several cycles establishes a diagnosis of moderate-severe PMS or PMDD, and these types of symptoms should have occurred during most menstrual cycles over the past year. PMDD symptoms during the last 7 days of the cycle should be at least 30% worse than those experienced during the mid-follicular phase (days 3–9 of the menstrual cycle).

PMS/PMDD should be distinguished from typical premenstrual symptoms and also from premenstrual exacerbations of other disorders, particularly mood disorders. Some medical conditions can be aggravated during the premenstrual phase.[26,30] In addition, mood disorders not occurring solely during the luteal phase must be distinguished from cyclic mood symptoms (Table 9–3).

Lack of a symptom-free interval suggests that the patient has a psychiatric disorder (e.g., anxiety or panic disorder) or another health condition (e.g., the perimenopause or menopausal transition), rather than PMS.

table
9–4 Common Premenstrual Syndrome Symptoms

Most Common Negative Symptoms

Fatigue, lack of energy

Irritability

Labile mood with alternating sadness and anger

Depression

Anxiety, feeling stressed

Crying spells, oversensitivity

Difficulty concentrating

Abdominal bloating, edema of extremities

Breast tenderness

Appetite changes and food cravings

Headache

Gastrointestinal upset

Most Common Positive Symptoms

Increased energy, more efficient at work

Increased libido, more affectionate

Increased sense of control, more self-assured

Source: Adapted from Reference 22.

Treatment of PMS

PMS is a multisymptom disorder involving emotional, behavioral, and physical symptoms. A single therapeutic agent is unlikely to address all symptoms. Thus, treatment should be selected to address the patient's most bothersome symptoms. A symptom log/calendar is a useful tool for documenting the most bothersome symptom(s) and the cyclic nature of this disorder. This information will also be useful in evaluating the efficacy of treatment. Women with severe symptoms are less likely to have symptoms alleviated solely by use of nonprescription therapies. In addition, PMS symptoms are chronic and, in most cases, will continue until menopause. Therefore, the cost of therapy, the possibility that a woman may become pregnant, and the likelihood of adverse effects are important considerations in selecting therapy.

Treatment Goals

The two intended outcomes for women with PMS or PMDD are patient education to better understand PMS and to improve or resolve symptoms to reduce the impact on activities and interpersonal relationships. Typically, therapy is considered effective if symptoms are reduced by 50% or more.

General Treatment Approach

Women with mild-moderate PMS symptoms often do not require pharmacologic therapy. In these cases, initial treatment is generally conservative, consisting of education and nondrug measures (e.g., dietary modifications, physical exercise, and stress management). Women should be educated about the syndrome and encouraged to identify techniques for coping with PMS symptoms and stress. Many women are engaged in multiple social roles, which can increase stress. Knowledge of this disorder can allow a woman to exert some control over her symptoms by anticipating and planning. For example, she might schedule more challenging tasks during the first half of the cycle, thus limiting the influence of this condition on her social and work functioning.

In addition to education, treatment options include lifestyle modifications (e.g., diet and exercise). Nonpharmacologic approaches that can be considered include light therapy, cognitive–behavioral therapy, and acupuncture.[26] Supplements with evidence of potential benefit include calcium, pyridoxine, and chastetree berry (*Vitex agnus-castus*).[26,27] Preliminary data suggest a potential benefit from ginkgo, magnesium pyrrolidone, St. John's wort, and saffron.[31]

Prescription drug therapy should be considered if the treatments outlined in Figure 9–3 are ineffective or if the patient suffers from moderate-severe PMS or PMDD. SSRIs used daily or only during the luteal phase of the menstrual cycle are considered first-line prescription therapy. Agents that suppress ovulation (e.g., OCs and GnRH agonists such as leuprolide) are also used. Newer OCs containing drospirenone, shortened hormone-free intervals, or extended cycling may also be considered first-line therapy for women who prefer a gynecologic approach rather than a psychological approach.[32] Finally, hysterectomy with bilateral oophorectomy is effective for refractory severe symptoms.[33] Surgery may be appealing for women experiencing significant adverse drug reactions and/or costs.[33]

Nonpharmacologic Therapy

Several nonpharmacologic therapies may improve PMS symptoms. These include aerobic exercise, dietary modifications, and cognitive–behavioral therapy.[26] Exercise can increase endorphin levels and may help decrease PMS symptoms.[23,26] Although the benefit of dietary changes is unproven, many health care providers recommend eating a balanced diet while also avoiding salty foods and simple sugars (which may cause fluid retention) and avoiding caffeine and alcohol (which can increase irritability).[26,27] Cravings for foods high in carbohydrates, which contain the serotonin precursor tryptophan, are common in women with PMS. Two studies of a carbohydrate-rich beverage that increased tryptophan levels demonstrated an improvement in emotional symptoms in women with PMS.[27] Consuming foods rich in complex carbohydrates (e.g., whole-grain foods) during the premenstrual interval may reduce symptoms.[23,27]

Stress is reported to increase PMS symptoms. Cognitive–behavioral therapy, which emphasizes relaxation techniques and coping skills, may help reduce symptoms.[26,27] These approaches may be helpful used singly or as adjuncts to other therapies. Data also exist suggesting a possible benefit with light therapy, acupuncture, and massage.[26]

Pharmacologic Therapy

A survey of women with PMS found that 80% use some non-prescription therapy, including vitamins, minerals, and herbs; a number of products have claims for the management of PMS yet little supporting evidence.[31]

Pyridoxine

Pyridoxine has been suggested as a therapy for PMS. Trials have reported mixed results with no dose–response relationship shown, and no trials were performed in women with PMDD.[27,31] One double-blind, placebo-controlled trial found pyridoxine 80 mg daily improved mood symptoms to a greater extent than placebo.[27] The dosage of pyridoxine should be limited to 100 mg daily because of the risk for peripheral neuropathy with higher dosages.[26]

Calcium and Vitamin D

Several randomized trials have evaluated the effect of calcium supplementation on PMS symptoms. The largest trial studied the effect of calcium in a dosage of 600 mg twice daily in 466 women with moderate-severe PMS.[34] Symptoms were significantly reduced by the second month of therapy, and by the third month, calcium had reduced overall symptoms by 48%. Emotional symptoms such as mood swings, depression, and anger, as well as food cravings and physical symptoms, were all reduced. More than 50% of the women taking calcium had a greater than 50% improvement in symptoms; 29% had a greater than 75% improvement in symptoms. Few women experienced adverse effects from calcium; 5 withdrew from the study because of nausea, and 1 woman each in the calcium and placebo groups developed kidney stones. The dosage of calcium used in the trial is consistent with the recommended daily calcium intake for women of reproductive age, which is between 1000 and 1300 mg daily. Similar improvements were noted in smaller studies.[24,31,35] An additional study reported that high dietary intake of both calcium and vitamin D may prevent the development of PMS symptoms.[36] Reduced levels of vitamin D secondary to alterations in calcium and vitamin D metabolism during the luteal phase may trigger PMDD symptoms.[23] Data show an inverse relationship between both milk consumption and a high intake of vitamin D, and PMS.[4] Additionally, all health care providers should be reinforcing adequate calcium and vitamin D intake in women to help prevent osteoporosis.

Magnesium

Magnesium deficiency may lead to some PMS-type symptoms (e.g., irritability), and low magnesium levels in red blood cells have been found in women with PMS. Affective symptoms associated with PMS were reduced by magnesium pyrrolidone carboxylic acid in a dosage of 360 mg daily administered during the luteal phase.[31,37] In contrast, two trials of magnesium oxide found no benefit. The dosage of magnesium pyrrolidone used in the trial was similar to the recommended dietary allowance of magnesium for women (310–360 mg). About 50% of women regularly consume less than that amount, and obtaining adequate magnesium from food sources may be difficult. Food sources of magnesium include spinach, Swiss chard, nuts, legumes (e.g., beans and peas), and whole-grain cereals. Adverse effects other than diarrhea are uncommon.

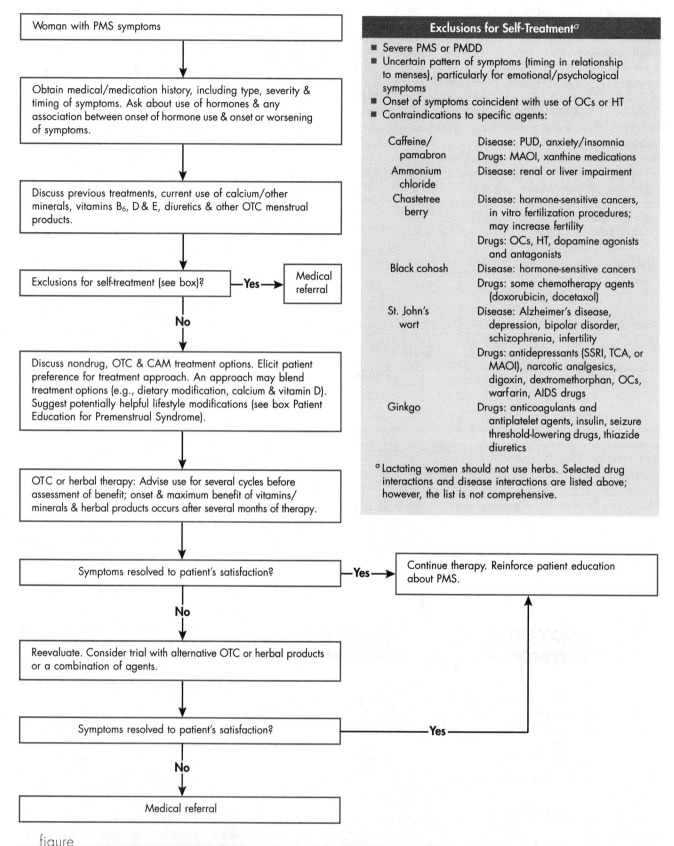

Woman with PMS symptoms

↓

Obtain medical/medication history, including type, severity & timing of symptoms. Ask about use of hormones & any association between onset of hormone use & onset or worsening of symptoms.

↓

Discuss previous treatments, current use of calcium/other minerals, vitamins B₆, D & E, diuretics & other OTC menstrual products.

↓

Exclusions for self-treatment (see box)? —Yes→ Medical referral

↓ No

Discuss nondrug, OTC & CAM treatment options. Elicit patient preference for treatment approach. An approach may blend treatment options (e.g., dietary modification, calcium & vitamin D). Suggest potentially helpful lifestyle modifications (see box Patient Education for Premenstrual Syndrome).

↓

OTC or herbal therapy: Advise use for several cycles before assessment of benefit; onset & maximum benefit of vitamins/minerals & herbal products occurs after several months of therapy.

↓

Symptoms resolved to patient's satisfaction? —Yes→ Continue therapy. Reinforce patient education about PMS.

↓ No

Reevaluate. Consider trial with alternative OTC or herbal products or a combination of agents.

↓

Symptoms resolved to patient's satisfaction? —Yes→ (Continue therapy. Reinforce patient education about PMS.)

↓ No

Medical referral

Exclusions for Self-Treatment[a]

- Severe PMS or PMDD
- Uncertain pattern of symptoms (timing in relationship to menses), particularly for emotional/psychological symptoms
- Onset of symptoms coincident with use of OCs or HT
- Contraindications to specific agents:

Caffeine/ pamabron	Disease: PUD, anxiety/insomnia
	Drugs: MAOI, xanthine medications
Ammonium chloride	Disease: renal or liver impairment
Chastetree berry	Disease: hormone-sensitive cancers, in vitro fertilization procedures; may increase fertility
	Drugs: OCs, HT, dopamine agonists and antagonists
Black cohosh	Disease: hormone-sensitive cancers
	Drugs: some chemotherapy agents (doxorubicin, docetaxol)
St. John's wort	Disease: Alzheimer's disease, depression, bipolar disorder, schizophrenia, infertility
	Drugs: antidepressants (SSRI, TCA, or MAOI), narcotic analgesics, digoxin, dextromethorphan, OCs, warfarin, AIDS drugs
Ginkgo	Drugs: anticoagulants and antiplatelet agents, insulin, seizure threshold-lowering drugs, thiazide diuretics

[a] Lactating women should not use herbs. Selected drug interactions and disease interactions are listed above; however, the list is not comprehensive.

figure 9–3 Self-care of premenstrual syndrome. Key: AIDS = Acquired immunodeficiency syndrome; CAM = complementary and alternative medicine; HT = hormone therapy; MAOI = monoamine oxidase inhibitor; OC = oral contraceptive; OTC = over-the-counter; PMDD = premenstrual dysphoric disorder; PMS = premenstrual syndrome; PUD = peptic ulcer disease; SSRI = selective serotonin reuptake inhibitor; TCA = tricyclic antidepressant.

Nonsteroidal Anti-Inflammatory Drugs

NSAIDs have been shown to reduce some of the physical symptoms (e.g., headache and muscle/joint pains) and mood symptoms associated with PMS when taken for several days prior to the onset of and during the first several days of menses.[26] The benefit from these agents may be a result of the coexistence of dysmenorrhea and PMS or PMS manifesting primarily as physical symptoms.

Diuretics

A common premenstrual complaint is the subjective sensation of fluid accumulation, particularly abdominal bloating. However, most women do not experience any true sodium or water retention and do not experience weight gain.[38] Two factors may explain the sense of abdominal bloating. First, a distinction must be made between fluid redistribution (where weight does not change) and fluid retention (which can be detected by weight gain). The abdominal bloating and swelling observed with PMS are primarily caused by a fluid shift to this area. As a result, diuretics that are indicated for relieving fluid retention are unlikely to be helpful for most women with PMS. Second, abdominal distension may occur secondary to relaxation of the gut muscle caused by progesterone.[38] For women who have true water retention and the resultant weight gain, a diuretic may be useful.

FDA has approved three nonprescription diuretics as useful for relieving water retention, weight gain, bloating, swelling, and the feeling of fullness: ammonium chloride, caffeine, and pamabrom. The latter agent is the most common diuretic in nonprescription menstrual products (Table 9–5).

Ammonium chloride is an acid-forming salt with a short duration of effect. The drug is taken in oral dosages of up to 3 g/day, divided into three doses, for no more than 6 consecutive days. Larger dosages of ammonium chloride can produce significant gastrointestinal and central nervous system adverse effects. Ammonium chloride is contraindicated in patients with renal or liver impairment because metabolic acidosis may result. Ammonium chloride is no longer available as a nonprescription drug but can be obtained as a dietary supplement.

Caffeine promotes diuresis by inhibiting the renal tubular reabsorption of sodium and water. In doses of 100–200 mg every 3–4 hours, caffeine is safe and effective, although patients may develop tolerance to its diuretic effect. Caffeine may also cause anxiety, restlessness, or insomnia, and it may worsen PMS by causing irritability. Additive adverse effects (e.g., nervousness, irritability, or tachycardia) might occur if other caffeine-containing medications, foods, or beverages (especially "energy drinks") are consumed concurrently. Caffeine may also cause GI irritation; thus, it can cause or worsen dyspepsia. Patients taking monoamine oxidase inhibitors (MAOIs) or theophylline should also avoid diuretics that contain caffeine.

Pamabrom, a derivative of theophylline, is used in combination products (along with analgesics and antihistamines) marketed for the treatment of PMS. Pamabrom may be taken in dosages of up to 50 mg 4 times daily.

Combination Products

Multi-ingredient nonprescription products are marketed for women with PMS-type symptoms. Two of the most commonly used product brand names are Midol and Pamprin. Some of these products contain acetaminophen, caffeine/pamabrom, and pyrilamine, whereas others contain only an NSAID or a combination of an analgesic with a diuretic or an antihistamine (Table 9–5). Pain is a relatively uncommon symptom of PMS, and no evidence exists that the sedative effect of an antihistamine such as pyrilamine will provide benefit to women experiencing the emotional symptoms of PMS. Therefore, these types of nonprescription products should not be recommended. More appropriate recommendations are the use of more definitive agents, such as those previously discussed, or referral for prescription drug therapy.

Pharmacotherapeutic Comparison

Calcium can be suggested for the initial treatment of PMS symptoms. If this agent provides inadequate relief, another agent or a combination of two or more agents may be tried. Women

table 9–5	**Selected Combination Nonprescription Menstrual Products**	
Trade Name	**Diuretic (per tablet/capsule)**	**Analgesic and/or Antihistamine (per tablet/capsule)**
Aqua-Ban Diuretic Maximum Strength Tablets; Diurex Water Caplets	Pamabrom 50 mg	
Diurex Original Formula Water Pills	Caffeine 50 mg	Magnesium salicylate 162.5 mg
Pamprin Multisymptom; Premsyn PMS	Pamabrom 25 mg	Acetaminophen 500 mg; pyrilamine maleate 15 mg
Pamprin Max	Caffeine 65 mg	Acetaminophen 250 mg; aspirin 250 mg
Pamprin All Day; Midol Extended Relief	None	Naproxen sodium 220 mg
Pamprin Cramp	Pamabrom 25 mg	Acetaminophen 250 mg; magnesium salicylate 250 mg
Midol Complete	Caffeine 60 mg	Acetaminophen 500 mg; pyrilamine maleate 15 mg
Midol Liquid Gel	None	Ibuprofen 200 mg
Midol Teen	Pamabrom 25 mg	Acetaminophen 500 mg
Midol PM	None	Acetaminophen 500 mg; diphenhydramine 38 mg

who experience bloating with documented weight gain might try pamabrom or caffeine. Caffeine and pamabrom may not be an appropriate choice for women who experience irritability as a PMS symptom. Both caffeine and pamabrom should be used cautiously in patients who have a history of peptic ulcer disease or who are taking MAOIs or other xanthine medications. NSAIDs should be reserved for women who experience both PMS and dysmenorrhea or other pain. Use of combination products containing antihistamines should be discouraged because drowsiness may impair job performance, schoolwork, and driving.

Product Selection Guidelines

Special Populations

PMS does not occur during pregnancy or after menopause. Adolescents and adult women can be treated similarly; they should initially attempt to manage their symptoms with lifestyle changes and with therapies such as calcium supplementation. Adolescents should avoid combination products containing aspirin (see Dysmenorrhea, Special Populations). Women who are breast-feeding should avoid all herbal products because information about their safety for nursing infants is limited. Vitamins and minerals in the dosages used for PMS are generally compatible with breast-feeding, and magnesium use is unlikely to cause diarrhea in infants.[20] Diuretics should be avoided during breast-feeding, as caffeine appears in breast milk about 1 hour after maternal ingestion. Caffeine may cause fussiness and poor sleep in infants, especially if consumed in high dosages or if the infant is preterm or younger than 3 weeks of age.[20]

Patient Factors

Patients using proton pump inhibitors and H_2-receptor antagonists should use calcium citrate rather than calcium carbonate products because the carbonate products are less soluble with a higher gastric pH.

Patient Preferences

Patient preferences for PMS treatment can be accommodated. Women preferring to use dietary supplements should discuss their use with a health care provider to ensure that drug–drug or drug–disease interactions do not exist.

Complementary Therapies

Trials have been conducted with botanical therapies, including chastetree berry (*Vitex agnus-castus*), St. John's wort (*Hypericum perforatum*), ginkgo (*Ginkgo biloba*), and saffron (*Crocus sativus*).[31] The first three dietary supplements are discussed in depth in Chapter 51.

Chastetree berry has shown efficacy in improving mild-moderate PMS symptoms, but trials have used different formulations of chastetree berry. Two trials using a standardized fruit extract ZE 440 of chastetree berry found a significant reduction in PMS symptoms (including mood, irritability/anger, pain/headache, breast tenderness, and fluid retention).[39] Two randomized, double-blind, placebo-controlled trials found that chastetree berry extract reduced many common PMS symptoms and did not cause any serious adverse effects.[40–42] Symptoms were significantly lower by the end of the third cycle of use. In a trial in women diagnosed with PMDD, chastetree

berry was compared with fluoxetine; a similar percentage of patients improved on both agents. Chastetree berry was shown to decrease irritability, breast tenderness, swelling, food cravings, and cramps. In contrast, fluoxetine improved more mood symptoms; symptoms with a 50% reduction included depression, irritability, insomnia, nervous tension, feeling out of control, breast tenderness, and aches. Chastetree berry was well tolerated; nausea and headache were the most common adverse effects. Chastetree berry may offer more benefit for patients with mild-moderate PMS and for women experiencing breast pain.[39,43] Chastetree berry may affect estrogen receptors and inhibit prolactin.[39] Women who are pregnant or lactating should avoid chastetree berry, and it should be used cautiously by women taking hormones or who have hormone-sensitive cancers.

One randomized trial of St. John's wort reported a reduction in anxiety-related symptoms in women with PMS, although its effect was not different from placebo.[31] St. John's wort may improve mild-moderate depression. St. John's wort has many clinically significant drug interactions, including reducing the effectiveness of OCs.

A placebo-controlled randomized trial evaluated ginkgo in a dosage of 160–320 mg daily in 165 women with PMS. Symptoms of anxiety, irritability, and depression associated with PMS were improved with ginkgo, although statistical significance was not demonstrated. However, ginkgo provided a statistically significant reduction in breast pain.[31] Ginkgo has antiplatelet effects and may increase the risk of bleeding.

In one randomized trial, 30 mg saffron extract daily was found to significantly reduce PMS symptoms and depression symptoms compared with placebo.[31]

Assessment of PMS: A Case-Based Approach

The health care provider should obtain a complete description of the patient's symptoms and their timing to determine whether the patient has PMS/PMDD or another disorder with PMS-type symptoms. The severity of PMS symptoms is another factor in self-treatment. As with any disorder, the health care provider should explore the use of medications that might be causing the symptoms or that might potentially interact with nonprescription agents used to treat PMS. Previous treatments for the symptoms should also be explored.

Case 9–2 illustrates the assessment of a patient with PMS.

Patient Counseling for PMS

Educating women with PMS about the timing of symptoms using a symptom log and calendar and educating women about what might control those symptoms may increase compliance with recommended therapies. Health care providers should be prepared to discuss the treatment of behavioral and physical symptoms of mild-moderate PMS. If the patient wants to use nonprescription medications or vitamins, the proper use and potential adverse effects of these agents should be explained. The patient should also be advised that treatment measures must be implemented during every menstrual cycle because it may take several cycles for symptomatic relief to occur. The Patient Education for Premenstrual Syndrome box lists specific information to provide patients.

case

9–2

Relevant Evaluation Criteria	Scenario/Model Outcome

Information Gathering

1. Gather essential information about the patient's symptoms and medical history, including:

   a. description of symptom(s) (i.e., nature, onset, duration, severity, associated symptoms)

   The patient reports that she experiences moodiness (irritability) along with breast tenderness every month. Symptoms occur every month during the week prior to her period.

   b. description of any factors that seem to precipitate, exacerbate, and/or relieve the patient's symptom(s)

   "It seems worse if I am feeling stressed—like around the holidays, or if there is something going on at work that is stressful."

   c. description of the patient's efforts to relieve the symptoms

   "Usually, I just try not to act too grumpy, even if I feel that way. I have not tried anything to address my breast tenderness."

   d. patient's identity

   Ruby Wilcox

   e. age, sex, height, and weight

   22 years old, female, 5 ft 4 in., 118 lb

   f. patient's occupation

   Team leader, cable TV/Internet/phone company

   g. patient's dietary habits

   Vegetarian

   h. patient's sleep habits

   She estimates she gets about 7 hours of sleep nightly; she has no problem falling asleep.

   i. concurrent medical conditions, prescription and nonprescription medications, and dietary supplements

   No chronic health problems

   Tension headaches: ibuprofen 400 mg

   Colds: *Echinacea* extract and zinc lozenges

   Contraception: NuvaRing

   Dietary supplements: vitamin B-complex, B_{12}, flaxseed oil, probiotic blend (all taken once daily)

   j. allergies

   Allergic to cats (sneezes, itchy eyes)

   k. history of other adverse reactions to medications

   NKDA

   l. other (describe) _____

   None

Assessment and Triage

2. Differentiate patient's signs/symptoms and correctly identify the patient's primary problem(s).

   The symptoms she describes are consistent with mild PMS. The time frame for the occurrence of symptoms is also consistent with PMS.

3. Identify exclusions for self-treatment (Figure 9–3).

   Patient does not have any exclusions for self-treatment. Her symptoms are mild, she likely is not pregnant (using contraceptive), and she has no major medical conditions.

4. Formulate a comprehensive list of therapeutic alternatives for the primary problem to determine if triage to a health care provider is required, and share this information with the patient or caregiver.

   Options include:

   (1) Refer patient to an appropriate health care provider.

   (2) Recommend self-care with nonprescription and nondrug measures.

   (3) Recommend self-care until patient can see an appropriate health care provider.

   (4) Take no action.

Plan

5. Select an optimal therapeutic alternative to address the patient's problem, taking into account patient preferences.

   Recommend self-care with nonprescription and nondrug measures.

6. Describe the recommended therapeutic approach to the patient or caregiver.

   "The symptoms you describe are consistent with PMS. Your symptoms are mild, and there are several nonprescription vitamins and minerals that might provide improvement in your symptoms. The best studied approach is the use of calcium in a dose of 1200 mg daily. I suggest you try taking calcium 500–600 mg twice daily." [Assuming that the patient is obtaining some calcium from foods, you could also ask explicitly about calcium-containing foods in her diet.]

   "Also, you should consume vitamin D daily through foods or a supplement—it will help with the absorption of calcium and also has some additive benefits with calcium in the management of PMS. The dose of vitamin D I recommend for you is 600 IU daily."

Relevant Evaluation Criteria	Scenario/Model Outcome
7. Explain to the patient or caregiver the rationale for selecting the recommended therapeutic approach from the considered therapeutic alternatives.	"This approach is recommended because there is evidence for its benefit, it is a safe supplement, and women need calcium to protect against osteoporosis."

Patient Education	
8. When recommending self-care with nonprescription medications and/or nondrug therapy, convey accurate information to the patient or caregiver.	"Calcium should be taken in a dose of 600 mg or less at one time, as that is the highest dose the body can absorb at one time. You are not likely to experience side effects from calcium, but some women experience gastrointestinal distress or constipation. Let me know if that occurs, and I can suggest how to manage those side effects. If you add vitamin D to your regimen also, I suggest a daily dose of 600 IU."
Solicit follow-up questions from the patient or caregiver.	"How long will it take for the calcium to be effective?"
Answer the patient's or caregiver's questions.	"You should take calcium for at least 3 months to determine if it will be beneficial for you. Clinical studies found that some symptoms were improved by the second month of calcium use, but the best effect in reducing symptoms was seen after 3 months of use."

Evaluation of Patient Outcome	
9. Assess patient outcome.	"Try calcium therapy for 3 months; if you still have bothersome symptoms, let me know. There are other nonprescription therapies that may be helpful."

Key: NKDA = No known drug allergies.

patient education for
Premenstrual Syndrome

The objective of self-treatment is to achieve relief from or significant improvement in PMS symptoms to limit discomfort, distress, and the disruption of personal relationships or usual activities. For most patients, carefully following product instructions and the self-care measures listed here will help ensure optimal therapeutic outcomes.

Nondrug Measures

- Try to avoid stress, develop effective coping mechanisms for managing stress, and learn relaxation techniques.
- If possible, participate in regular aerobic exercise.
- During the 7–14 days before your menstrual period, reduce intake of salt, caffeine, chocolate, and alcoholic beverages. Eating foods rich in carbohydrates and low in protein during the premenstrual interval may also reduce symptoms.

Nonprescription Medications

- Nonprescription medications and lifestyle modifications may not improve symptoms for all women, and it may take several months to determine whether these therapies are working.
- Therapy with one nonprescription medication may improve only some of the symptoms; several medications may be needed for optimal symptom control. However, only add one agent at a time so that it is possible to determine which agent causes benefit or adverse effects.

- Follow the guidelines here for the agents that best control your symptoms:
  - Take 1200 mg of elemental calcium daily in divided doses. Calcium can be obtained from food or from supplements. Take no more than 500–600 mg at one time. Calcium may cause stomach upset (if this occurs, take with food) or constipation.
  - Take at least 600 IU of vitamin D daily.
  - Take 300–360 mg of magnesium pyrrolidone daily during the premenstrual interval only. Magnesium may cause diarrhea.
  - Take up to 100 mg of pyridoxine daily. Do not exceed this dosage, or neurologic symptoms caused by vitamin B_6 toxicity may occur.

When to Seek Medical Attention

- If you are taking vitamin B_6 and develop neurologic symptoms (e.g., a sensation of pricking, tingling, or creeping on the skin; bone pain; muscle weakness; or stinging, burning, or itching sensations), stop taking the vitamin and seek medical attention.
- If the PMS symptoms do not improve, or if they worsen, a medical evaluation is suggested.

Evaluation of Patient Outcomes for PMS

Monitoring is accomplished by having the patient report whether the symptoms are resolved. It may take several menstrual cycles to ascertain whether lifestyle changes or nonprescription therapies are reducing the symptoms of PMS. Comparing the occurrence of symptoms before and after vitamin or medication use can help determine the value of a therapy. Women should be encouraged to contact their health care provider to discuss treatment effectiveness and to clarify information or answer any questions. Reasons for advising the patient to see a provider include persistent symptoms, symptoms that the patient reports are disruptive to personal relationships, or symptoms that affect the patient's ability to engage in usual activities or function productively at work.

Toxic Shock Syndrome

Toxic shock syndrome (TSS) is a term originally coined in 1978 to describe a severe multisystem illness characterized by high fever, profound hypotension, severe diarrhea, mental confusion, renal failure, erythroderma, and skin desquamation. In 1980, these symptoms were recognized as affecting a relatively large number of young, previously healthy, menstruating women. TSS is commonly divided into menstrual and nonmenstrual cases.

Menstrual TSS affects primarily young women between 13 and 19 years of age.[44] Almost all cases of menstrual TSS have been associated with menstruation and tampon use (especially the use of high-absorbency tampons).[44]

The decrease in cases of menstrual TSS has been attributed to several factors, including removal of superabsorbent tampons from the market; a change in the composition of tampons; an increased awareness of the recommendations to change tampons frequently and to alternate tampon and pad use; and FDA-required standardized labeling of tampons.[44]

The strongest predictor of risk for menstrual TSS is the use of tampons. Women who currently use tampons still have a 33-fold greater risk for TSS than nonusers. The greatest risk is associated with the use of higher absorbency tampons; for every 1 gram increase in absorbency, the risk for TSS increases 34%–37%. Continuous uninterrupted use of tampons for at least 1 day during menses has also been shown to correlate with an increased risk for menstrual TSS. In addition, using tampons between menstrual periods (to manage vaginal discharge or nonmenstrual bleeding) can increase the likelihood of vaginal ulcers and the risk of TSS.[45] Besides tampons, TSS has been associated with the use of barrier contraceptives, including diaphragms, cervical caps and cervical sponges, and IUCs.

Pathophysiology of Menstrual TSS

Menstrual TSS is caused by the toxin-producing strains of *Staphylococcus aureus*.[46] TSS is an inflammatory immune response to the enterotoxins produced by these bacteria. Toxin-producing strains of *S. aureus* produce the superantigen toxin TSST-1. Most adults have a protective level of antibodies against the TSST-1 toxin. Younger people who lack this antibody protection and

who become infected with a toxin-producing strain of *S. aureus* may develop TSS.[46]

TSS develops in three phases: proliferation of toxin-producing bacteria, production of toxin, and engagement of the immune system. Menstrual blood can serve as a medium for bacterial growth, and the retention of blood in the vagina by the tampon can increase bacterial proliferation. Also, some tampons contain fibers that inhibit lactobacilli, thereby diminishing their ability to limit the proliferation of *S. aureus*.

Four conditions promote toxin production: elevated protein levels, neutral pH, elevated carbon dioxide levels, and elevated oxygen levels.[44] During menses, menstrual blood provides an increase in protein and also increases vaginal pH to 7, or neutral pH. Tampon use may create the environment for TSS by introducing oxygen into the vagina; oxygen is trapped within the tampon, and higher-absorbency tampons carry more oxygen into the vagina.[44,46] Oxygen is a critical factor for the production of TSST-1.[47] After the introduction of a tampon, the vagina takes hours to return to its anaerobic state, with elevated carbon dioxide levels. In addition, tampons, IUCs, and contraceptive sponges create microtrauma, which increases exposure of the toxins to the circulatory and immune systems. Exposure of immune cells to TSST-1 initiates the inflammatory cascade involving interleukin-1 and tumor necrosis factor. This inflammatory response results in the signs and symptoms of TSS.

Clinical Presentation of Menstrual TSS

By definition, menstrual TSS occurs within 2 days of the onset of menses, during menses, or within 2 days after menses. Prodromal symptoms (including malaise, myalgias, and chills) occur for 2–3 days prior to TSS.[46] GI symptoms (e.g., vomiting, diarrhea, and abdominal pain) typically occur early in the illness and affect almost all patients. After that period of time, TSS evolves rapidly into high fever, myalgias, vomiting and diarrhea, erythroderma, decreased urine output, severe hypotension, and shock. Neurologic manifestations (e.g., headache, confusion, agitation, lethargy, and seizures) also occur in almost all cases. Acute renal failure, cardiac involvement, and adult respiratory distress syndrome are also common.

Dermatologic manifestations are characteristic of TSS; both early rash and subsequent skin desquamation are required for a definite diagnosis. The early rash is often described as a sunburn-like, diffuse, macular erythroderma that is not pruritic. About 5–12 days after the onset of TSS, desquamation of the skin on the patient's face, trunk, and extremities (including the soles of the feet and the palms of the hands) occurs.

Prevention of Menstrual TSS

Women can almost entirely prevent menstrual TSS by using sanitary pads instead of tampons during their menstrual cycle. Women who use tampons can reduce the risk of developing TSS by following the guidelines in the box Patient Education for Toxic Shock Syndrome. The addition of substances to tampons that will inhibit production of the TSST-1 exotoxin is being explored.[47]

Women who have had TSS are at risk for recurrence; TSS recurs in about 28%–64% of women with menstrual TSS.[46]

patient education for
Toxic Shock Syndrome

The objective of self-treatment is to reduce the risk of developing toxic shock syndrome (TSS) associated with the use of tampons or contraceptive devices. For most patients, carefully following product instructions and the self-care measures listed here will help ensure optimal therapeutic outcomes.

- To reduce the risk of TSS to almost zero, use sanitary pads instead of tampons during your period.
- To lower the risk of TSS while using tampons, use the lowest-absorbency tampons compatible with your needs. Also, alternate the use of menstrual pads with the use of tampons (e.g., use pads at night) so that tampons are not used continuously for 24 hours.
- Change tampons four to six times a day and at least every 6 hours; overnight use should be no longer than 8 hours.
- Wash your hands with soap before inserting anything into the vagina (e.g., tampon, diaphragm, contraceptive sponge, or vaginal medication). The bacteria causing TSS are usually found on the skin.
- Do not leave a contraceptive sponge, diaphragm, or cervical cap in place in the vagina longer than recommended; do not use any of them during menstruation.

- Do not use tampons, contraceptive sponges, or a cervical cap during the first 12 weeks after childbirth. It may also be best to avoid using a diaphragm.
- Read the insert on TSS enclosed in the tampon package, and become familiar with the early symptoms of this disorder.

When to Seek Medical Attention

- If you develop symptoms of TSS (high fever, muscle aches, a sunburn-like rash appearing after a day or two, weakness, fatigue, nausea, vomiting, and diarrhea), remove the tampon or contraceptive device immediately and seek emergency medical treatment. If left untreated, TSS can cause shock and even death.

Recurrence rates are lower for women who are treated with antibiotics during TSS. Prevention of TSS for these patients includes avoiding tampons, IUCs, diaphragms, cervical caps, and contraceptive sponges.

Assessment of Menstrual TSS: A Case-Based Approach

Obtaining prompt medical attention is a very important aspect of care for patients with symptoms consistent with TSS. A health care provider can be alert to symptoms of TSS when patients seek nonprescription therapy for a severe "flu" with symptoms such as fever, vomiting, diarrhea, and dizziness, or when patients seek help for an unusual skin rash that occurs in conjunction with the previously described symptoms. If TSS is suspected, the patient should be advised to seek medical care immediately; additionally, the patient should be advised to avoid use of NSAIDs for fever and myalgias because these agents may increase the progression of TSS by increasing the production of tumor necrosis factor.

Patient Counseling for Menstrual TSS

Tampons are used by women of all ages during the reproductive years. Health care providers should counsel patients about the prevention of TSS as outlined in the box Patient Education for Toxic Shock Syndrome. In particular, health care providers should emphasize the importance of washing the hands before inserting a tampon, which removes organisms causing TSS from the skin. Similarly, about 18%–36% of women report that they do not always change a tampon at least every 6 hours; health care providers should counsel patients to change tampons frequently, according to product instructions; to alternate the use of tampons with the use of sanitary pads over a 24-hour period; and to use the lowest-absorbency tampons compatible with their needs. The health care provider should emphasize, however, that the risk for this condition is quite small. If a patient presents with early symptoms of TSS, she should be advised to

remove the tampon or any barrier contraceptive device and to seek emergency medical treatment.

Key Points for Disorders Related To Menstruation

➤ Self-care is appropriate for an otherwise healthy young woman whose history is consistent with primary dysmenorrhea and who is not sexually active, or for a woman diagnosed with primary dysmenorrhea. Adolescents with pelvic pain who are sexually active and thus at risk for PID and women with characteristics indicating secondary dysmenorrhea should be referred for medical evaluation.

➤ NSAIDs are the drugs of choice for the management of primary dysmenorrhea. These medications should be taken at the onset of or just prior to menses and should be used in scheduled doses for several days for optimum reduction in pain and cramping.

➤ The use of local topical heat can also provide relief from dysmenorrhea. Its analgesic effect has a faster onset than drug therapy, and it can add to the relief provided by an NSAID. Nonpharmacologic therapy may be especially useful for women who cannot tolerate or who prefer not to use drug therapy or who do not respond to nonprescription NSAIDs.

➤ PMS/PMDD should be distinguished from typical premenstrual symptoms and also from premenstrual exacerbations of other disorders, particularly mood disorders.

➤ PMS/PMDD symptoms typically begin or intensify about a week prior to the onset of menses, peak the 2 days before menses, and resolve within several days to a week after the beginning of menses. A woman with PMS or PMDD experiences a symptom-free interval during days 4–12 of her menstrual cycle.

➤ PMS symptoms are chronic and, in most cases, will continue until menopause. Therefore, the cost of therapy, the possibility that a woman may become pregnant, and the likelihood of adverse effects from therapy are important considerations in selecting therapy.

> Several dietary supplements (particularly calcium, pyridoxine, and chastetree berry) might be suggested to reduce the symptoms of PMS. Moderate-severe PMS and PMDD symptoms warrant prescription drug therapy.

> TSS has been linked to tampon use. To lower the risk for TSS while using tampons, women should use the lowest-absorbency tampons compatible with their needs and should alternate the use of sanitary pads with the use of tampons over a 24-hour period.

REFERENCES

1. Fothergill DJ. Common menstrual problems in adolescence. *Arch Dis Child Educ Pract Ed.* 2010;95:199–203.

2. Peacock A, Alvi NS, Mushtaq T. Period problems: disorders of menstruation in adolescents. *Arch Dis Child.* 2012;97:554–60.

3. Mihm M, Gangooly S, Muttukrishna S. The normal menstrual cycle in women. *Anim Reprod Sci.* 2011;124:229–36.

4. Allen LM, Lam ACN. Premenstrual syndrome and dysmenorrhea in adolescents. *Adolesc Med.* 2012;23:139–63.

5. Harel Z. Dysmenorrhea in adolescents and young adults: an update on pharmacological treatments and management strategies. *Expert Opin Pharmacother.* 2012;13(15):2157–70.

6. French L. Dysmenorrhea in adolescents: diagnosis and treatment. *Paediatr Drugs.* 2008;10:1–7.

7. Mannix LK. Menstrual-related pain conditions: dysmenorrhea and migraine. *J Womens Health.* 2008;17:879–91.

8. Zahradnik HP, Hanjalic-Beck A, Groth K. Nonsteroidal anti-inflammatory drugs and hormonal contraceptives for pain relief from dysmenorrhea: a review. *Contraception.* 2012;81:185–96.

9. Parker A, Sneddon AE, Arbon P. The Menstrual Disorder of Teenagers (MDOT) study: determining typical menstrual patterns and menstrual disturbance in a large population-based study of Australian teenagers. *BJOG.* 2010;117:185–92.

10. Morrow C, Naumburg EH. Dysmenorrhea. *Prim Care.* 2009;36:19–32.

11. Daywood MY. Primary dysmenorrhea advances in pathogenesis and management. *Obstet Gynecol.* 2006;108:428–41.

12. Berkley KJ, McAllister SL. Don't dismiss dysmenorrhea! *Pain.* 2011; 152:1940–1.

13. Bertone-Johnson ER, Manson JE. Vitamin D for menstrual and pain-related disorders in women (Comment on "Improvement of primary dysmenorrhea caused by single oral dose of vitamin D"). *Arch Intern Med.* 2012;172(4):367–9.

14. Lasco A, Catalano A, Benvenga S. Improvement of primary dysmenorrhea caused by single oral dose of vitamin D: results of a randomized, double-blind, placebo-controlled study. *Arch Intern Med.* 2012;172(4):366–7.

15. Akin M, Price W, Rodriguez G Jr, et al. Continuous, low-level, topical heat wrap therapy as compared to acetaminophen for primary dysmenorrhea. *J Reprod Med.* 2004;49:739–45.

16. Dawood MY, Khan-Dawood FS. Clinical efficacy and differential inhibition of menstrual fluid prostaglandin F2alpha in a randomized, double-blind, crossover treatment with placebo, acetaminophen, and ibuprofen in primary dysmenorrhea. *Am J Obstet Gynecol.* 2007;196:35e1–5.

17. American College of Obstetricians and Gynecologists. Noncontraceptive uses of hormonal contraceptives. (Practice Bulletin) 2010;115(1):206–14.

18. Marjoribanks J, Proctor ML, Farquhar C, et al. Nonsteroidal anti-inflammatory drugs for dysmenorrhea. *Cochrane Database Syst Rev.* 2010;1:CD001751. doi: 10.1002/14651858.CD001751. Accessed at http://www.thecochranelibrary.com/view/0/index.html.

19. Avery AJ, Brent SL. Treatment of common, minor and self-limiting conditions. In: Lubin P, Ramsay M, eds. *Prescribing in Pregnancy.* 4th ed. New York, NY: Wiley; 2008.

20. National Institutes of Health. LactMed. Accessed at http://toxnet.nlm.nih.gov/cgi-bin/sis/htmlgen?LACT, May 31, 2013.

21. Cho SH, Hwang EW. Acupressure for primary dysmenorrhea: a systematic review. *Complement Ther Med.* 2010;18:49–56.

22. Campagne DM, Campagne G. The premenstrual syndrome revisited. *Eur J Obstet Gynecol Reprod Biol.* 2007;130:4–17.

23. Cunningham J, Yonkers KA, O'Brien S, et al. Update on research and treatment of premenstrual dysphoric disorder. *Harv Rev Psychiatry.* 2009;17:120–37.

24. Freeman EW. Therapeutic management of premenstrual syndrome. *Expert Opin Pharmacother.* 2010;11(7):2879–89.

25. Jarvis CI, Lynch AM, Morin AK. Management strategies for premenstrual syndrome/premenstrual dysphoric disorder. *Ann Pharmacother.* 2008;42:967–78.

26. Rapkin A, Mikacich JA. Premenstrual syndrome and premenstrual dysphoric disorder in adolescents. *Curr Opin Obstet Gynecol.* 2008;20:455–63.

27. Vigod SN, Ross LE, Steiner M. Understanding and treating premenstrual disorder: an update for the women's health practitioner. *Obstet Gynecol Clin North Am.* 2009;36:907–24.

28. Dennerstein L, Lehert P, Heinemann K. Epidemiology of premenstrual symptoms and disorders. *Menopause International.* 2012;18:48–51.

29. Kitamura M, Takeda T, Koga S, et al. Relationship between premenstrual symptoms and dysmenorrhea in Japanese high school students. *Arch Womens Ment Health.* 2012;15:131–133.

30. American Psychiatric Association. *Diagnostic and Statistical Manual of Mental Disorders: DSM-5.* 5th ed. Arlington, VA: American Psychiatric Association; 2013.

31. Whelan AM, Jurgens TM, Naylor H. Herbs, vitamins and minerals in the treatment of premenstrual syndrome: a systematic review. *Can J Pharmacol.* 2009;16:e407–29.

32. Panay N. Treatment of premenstrual syndrome: a decision-making algorithm. *Menopause Int.* 2012;18(2):90–2.

33. Reid RL. When should surgical treatment be considered for premenstrual dysphoric disorder? *Menopause International.* 2012;18(2):77–81.

34. Thys-Jacobs S, Starkey P, Bernstein D, et al. Calcium carbonate and the premenstrual syndrome: effect on premenstrual and menstrual symptoms. *Am J Obstet Gynecol.* 1998;179:444–52.

35. Ghanbari Z, Haghollahi F, Shariat M, et al. Effects of calcium supplement therapy in women with premenstrual syndrome. *Taiwan J Obstet Gynecol.* 2009;48:124–9.

36. Bertone-Johnson ER, Hankinson SE, Bendich A, et al. Calcium and vitamin D intake and risk of incident premenstrual syndrome. *Arch Intern Med.* 2005;165:1246–52.

37. Panay N. Management of premenstrual syndrome. *J Fam Plann Reprod Health Care* 2009;35(3):187–94.

38. O'Brien PMS, Ismail KMK, Dimmock P. Premenstrual syndrome. In: Shaw RW, Soutter WP, Stanton SL, eds. *Gynecology.* 3rd ed. Edinburgh, UK: Churchill Livingstone; 2003.

39. *Vitex agnus-castus.* Monograph. *Altern Med Rev.* 2009;14:67–71.

40. Ma L, Lin S, Chen R, et al. Treatment of moderate to severe premenstrual syndrome with *Vitex agnus castus* (BNO 1095) in Chinese women. *Gynecol Endocrinol.* 2010;26:612–6.

41. Ma L, Chen R, Zhang Y, et al. Evaluating therapeutic effect in symptoms of moderate-to-severe premenstrual syndrome with *Vitex agnus castus* (BNO 1095) in Chinese women. *Aust N Z J Obstet Gynaecol.* 2010;50:189–93.

42. He Z, Chen R, Zhou Y, et al. Treatment for premenstrual syndrome with *Vitex agnus castus*: a prospective, randomized, multi-center placebo controlled study in China. *Maturitas.* 2009;63:99–103.

43. Atmaca M, Kumru S, Tezcan E. Fluoxetine versus *Vitex agnus castus* extract in the treatment of premenstrual dysphoric disorder. *Hum Psychopharmacol Clin Exp.* 2003;18:191–5.

44. McCormick JK, Yarwood JM, Schlievert PM. Toxic shock syndrome and bacterial superantigens: an update. *Annu Rev Microbiol.* 2001;55: 77–104.

45. U.S. Food and Drug Administration. Tampons and asbestos, dioxin, & toxic shock syndrome. Accessed at http://www.fda.gov/MedicalDevices/Safety/AlertsandNotices/PatientAlerts/ucm070003.htm, June 2, 2013.

46. Reiss MA. Toxic shock syndrome. *Prim Care Update Obstet Gynecol.* 2000;7:85–90.

47. Strandberg KL, Perterson ML, Schaefers MM, et al. Reduction in *Staphylococcus aureus* growth and exotoxin production and in vaginal interleukin 8 levels due to glycerol monolaurate in tampons. *Clin Infect Dis.* 2009;49:1711–7.

PREVENTION OF PREGNANCY AND SEXUALLY TRANSMITTED INFECTIONS

Shareen Y. El-Ibiary and Erin C. Raney

Unprotected sexual activity can result in unintended pregnancy and sexually transmitted infections (STIs), either of which can exact high physical, psychological, and financial tolls on those affected. This chapter discusses how vaccines and properly used nonprescription contraceptive products or methods can reduce the risks of such adverse outcomes.

An estimated 49% of pregnancies in the United States are unintended.[1] The National Survey of Family Growth (NSFG) found that among U.S. women with unintended pregnancies, about half had used a method of contraception during the month they conceived, a result that is indicative of a high level of inconsistent or incorrect use.[1]

In the United States alone, the Centers for Disease Control and Prevention (CDC) estimate that more than 19.7 million persons are infected annually with new STIs, with medical costs estimated at $16 billion a year.[2] Of particular concern is the high risk of pregnancy and STIs in adolescents. The NSFG found that about 40% of teenagers had experienced sexual intercourse.[3] Among sexually active female teenagers, about one-fifth of those at risk for an unintended pregnancy did not use contraception.[4] Low levels of contraceptive use in this population may be due to lack of knowledge and planning, denial, and infrequent or unpredictable intercourse. The teenage pregnancy rate in the United States is one of the highest among developed countries.[3] However, as of 2011, birth rates for U.S. teenagers had reached historic lows for all age and ethnic groups.[5]

Repeat pregnancies are common and are often associated with inadequate contraceptive use after the first pregnancy.[6] Adolescents are particularly vulnerable to STIs, with one in four teenage girls infected with one or more STIs.[7] Reasons for infections include having multiple sexual partners, unprotected intercourse, an inherent biological susceptibility to infection, and barriers to health care utilization.[8]

Perimenopausal women are also at risk of unintended pregnancies. The NSFG found that among women age 40 years or older, 38% of pregnancies were unplanned.[1] Postmenopausal women and older men in sexual relationships that are not mutually monogamous are also at increased risk of STIs.[9]

The availability and relatively low cost of nonprescription methods of contraception for pregnancy and STI prevention are important, especially for those who are unwilling or unable to access family planning services or use prescription contraceptives.

Even if a prescription product is chosen as the primary contraceptive method, low-cost and low-risk nonprescription methods may be appropriate at different times during a person's life. The widespread accessibility of pharmacist-administered immunizations offers another opportunity for STI prevention.

Pathophysiology of Pregnancy and STIs

Pregnancy can result only when a viable egg is available for fertilization by a sperm. (See Chapter 9 for discussion of the reproductive process.) Conception may occur during a 6-day window that begins 5 days before ovulation through the day of ovulation. The estimated risk of pregnancy from unprotected sexual intercourse during this period ranges from 5% to 45%, with peak risk occurring the day before ovulation.[10] Pregnancy can occur despite contraceptive use if the product is used incorrectly or it fails (e.g., condom breakage).

STIs are contracted through contact with infected genital tissues, mucous membranes, and/or body fluids. Table 10–1 summarizes the major infections.[8] Although STIs affect both sexes, women are more likely to develop reproductive consequences, including pelvic inflammatory disease, chronic pelvic pain, ectopic pregnancy, malignancies, and infertility. This likelihood is possibly related to difficulties in diagnosis, lack of patient recognition of symptoms, and a higher probability of asymptomatic infection.[11] Pregnancy-related complications also increase as a consequence of STIs.[11] Transmission rates also differ between sexes. For example, about 50% of women become infected with gonorrhea after a single exposure with an infected man, whereas only about 25% of men contract gonorrhea from a single exposure with an infected woman.[11]

Prevention of STIs and Pregnancy
Vaccines for STI Prevention

Human Papillomavirus Vaccine

Human papillomavirus (HPV) is a virus that may be transmitted by sexual contact and is a major cause of cervical cancer and genital warts.[8,12] With more than 100 different types of HPV identified, HPV types 16 and 18 are responsible for 70% of cervical cancers, and types 6 and 11 are responsible for 90% of genital warts.[13] HPV is also responsible for a subset of vaginal, vulvar, penile, anal, and some head and neck cancers and is the

Editor's Note: This chapter is based on the 17th edition chapter of the same title, which was written by Louise Parent-Stevens and Mitzi Wasik.

table

10–1 Sexually Transmitted Infections

Disease [Scientific Name] (Type)	Incubation Period	Symptoms	Diagnosis/ Treatment	Complications	Congenital Transmission/ Neonatal Complications
Noncurable but Vaccine-Preventable STIs					
Genital warts [Human papillomavirus⁰] (DNA virus)	2–4 months (average)	Asx infections common; warts on external genitalia, rectum, anus, perineum, mouth, larynx, vagina, urethra, cervix	Colposcopy; serology; molecular-based assays/ cytoablation (chemical or physical); antivirals; antimetabolites; immunomodulators	Cervical dysplasia/ neoplasia, anogenital cancers, oropharyngeal cancer	Yes/respiratory papillomatosis
Hepatitis B [Hepatitis B virus] (virus)	6 weeks– 6 months	Acute, self-limited, mild	Serology/antivirals	Cirrhosis, hepatocellular cancer	Yes
Curable STIs					
Genital chlamydia [*Chlamydia trachomatis*] (bacterium)	7–35 days	M: range from asx to urethritis, proctitis, urogenital discharge, itching, dysuria F: range from asx to vaginal discharge, postcoital bleeding, cervicitis	EIA, NAAT/ antibiotics	PID, ectopic pregnancy, infertility	Yes/neonatal conjunctivitis, pneumonia
Gonorrhea [*Neisseria gonorrhoeae*] (bacterium)	Up to 14 days	Urethritis, cervicitis, proctitis, pharyngitis M: mucopurulent urethral discharge F: often asx	Gram stain; EIA; culture; NAAT/ antibiotics	Septic arthritis, perihepatitis, endocarditis, meningitis, PID, infertility, ectopic pregnancy	Yes/sepsis, meningitis, arthritis, ophthalmia neonatorum
Nongonococcal urethritis (men) [Various, including *Chlamydia trachomatis, Ureaplasma urealyticum, Mycoplasma* sp.] (bacteria)	1–2 weeks	M: nonspecific urethritis, discharge, dysuria, pruritus	NAAT; culture/ antibiotics	Epididymitis, proctitis, proctocolitis, Reiter's syndrome	—
Syphilis [*Treponema pallidum*] (spirochete)	3 weeks	Primary syphilis: chancre	Darkfield microscopy; direct fluorescent antibody test; treponemal and nontreponemal serologic tests/antibiotics	Secondary syphilis: rash, lymphadenopathy Tertiary syphilis: cardiovascular, gummatous lesions Neurosyphilis: CNS infection	Yes/fetal death, prematurity, congenital syphilis
Trichomoniasis [*Trichomonas vaginalis*] (protozoan)	Unknown	M: commonly asx F: ~50% asx, malodorous, frothy green vaginal discharge, itching, dyspareunia, postcoital bleeding	Microscopic exam of vaginal fluids; nucleic acid probe test; PCR/ antibiotics	Pregnancy: preterm labor, low birth weight	Yes
Noncurable STIs					
AIDS [HIV] (virus)	Up to 10 years	After initial flu-like illness, asx until OIs occur	Serologic antibody testing, NAAT/ antivirals; prophylaxis for OIs	OIs, malignancies, death	Yes, also transmitted via breast milk

| table | **Sexually Transmitted Infections** *(continued)* | | | | |

Disease [Scientific Name] (Type)	Incubation Period	Symptoms	Diagnosis/ Treatment	Complications	Congenital Transmission/ Neonatal Complications
Genital herpes [HSV-1, HSV-2] (virus)	2–14 days	Asx or vesicular/ ulcerative lesions on mucous membranes	Culture; serology; PCR assay/ antivirals	Disseminated infection, pneumonitis, hepatitis, meningitis/encephalitis	Yes
Hepatitis C [hepatitis C virus] (virus)*b*	8–9 weeks	Asx or mild clinical illness	Serology/antivirals	Cirrhosis, hepatocellular cancer	Yes

Key: AIDS = Acquired immunodeficiency syndrome; Asx = asymptomatic; CNS = central nervous system; EIA = enzyme immunoassay; F = female; HIV = human immunodeficiency virus; HPV = human papillomavirus; HSV = herpes simplex virus; M = male; NAAT = nucleic acid amplification test; OI = opportunistic infection; PCR = polymerase chain reaction; PID = pelvic inflammatory disease.

a Self-clearance of HPV virus may occur.

b Compared with transmission through blood exposure, sexual transmission of hepatitis C is inefficient but may still occur.

Source: Reference 8.

most common STI in this country.[13] In 2008, about 14 million new cases of HPV were reported in the United States.[2,14] At least 80% of all sexually active men and women will be infected with genital HPV at some point in their lives, with the highest risk of infection occurring during the first few years after they become sexually active.[12]

The available vaccines may decrease the risk of HPV. Two vaccines, Gardasil (quadrivalent HPV vaccine) and Cervarix (bivalent HPV vaccine), target the oncogenic strains 16 and 18, with the quadrivalent HPV vaccine also providing protection against genital wart strains 6 and 11 of HPV. The quadrivalent HPV vaccine is indicated for girls and boys ages 9–26 years to prevent cervical, vaginal, vulvar, and anal cancers, with an administration schedule of 0, 2, and 6 months. The bivalent vaccine is indicated for girls and women ages 9–25 years to prevent cervical cancer, with an administration schedule of 0, 1, and 6 months. Completion of the entire series is essential for the individual to obtain the highest immunity. One study found that girls ages 9–13 years who received two doses of the HPV vaccine had less immunity at 18 months after administration compared with those who had received the full three doses within 6 months.[15] The current age range for both vaccines is wide. This wide range is due to the "catch up" series which may be used in women up to 25 or 26 years of age (depending on the agent used) and in men up to 21 years of age (may be up to 26 years of age in men having sex with men). The vaccines work best prior to HPV exposure from sexual contact but previous sexual intercourse does not preclude an individual from receiving the vaccine.[13] The current recommendation of the Advisory Committee on Immunization Practices (ACIP) is for all girls 11–12 years of age (and boys, if receiving the quadrivalent HPV vaccine) to receive the HPV vaccine. If appropriate, vaccines can be given as early as 9 years of age.[13]

The adverse effects of the Gardasil and Cervarix vaccines are similar and may include irritation at the site of administration, malaise, and syncope. Because of the risk of syncope, particularly in younger girls, patients should be monitored for at least 15 minutes after administration of the vaccine.[13]

Hepatitis B Vaccine

Infection with the hepatitis B virus is associated with long-term complications such as hepatitis, cirrhosis, hepatic carcinoma, and death. The virus can be transmitted through contact with blood and other body fluids, and sexual transmission is estimated to cause 19,000 new infections annually.[2]

The hepatitis B vaccine is an inactivated injectable formulation with an administration schedule of 0, 1, and 6 months.[13] Recommended as a routine vaccination for all infants starting at birth, the vaccine is also provided to children and adolescents who did not receive the vaccine as an infant or did not complete the series. Adults who meet risk criteria and who were not previously vaccinated should also receive the three-dose series. Potential candidates for the vaccine include patients with multiple sexual partners; injection drug users; health care and emergency response personnel; patients with diabetes, end-stage renal disease, human immunodeficiency virus (HIV) infection, or liver disease; international travelers; and residents of correctional, drug abuse, or HIV treatment facilities.[13]

Pharmacist-administered vaccination has become more common. Depending on state laws and regulations, those vaccines are available for administration in the pharmacy for the entire series. States may limit the age range to which a pharmacist may administer vaccines, but if no barriers exist, pharmacists should offer their services to increase the number of vaccinated individuals.

Contraception for Pregnancy and STI Prevention

The goal of contraceptive use is to prevent unintended pregnancy and STIs with minimal adverse effects. No method of birth control except abstinence is perfect, and contraceptive choices may change during a person's life.

The effectiveness of a contraceptive method in preventing pregnancy is reported in two ways: the accidental pregnancy

table
10-2 Failure and Use Rates of Various Contraceptive Methods

Method	Accidental Pregnancy in the First Year of Use (%)		% of Women Using Method[c]
	Typical Use[a]	Perfect Use[b]	
No method	85	85	37.8
Withdrawal	22	4	3.2
Fertility awareness–based methods	24		0.7
Calendar method	13	5	
Cervical mucus method	22	3	
Symptothermal method	13–20	0.4	
Lactational amenorrhea method (first 6 months postpartum)	2	0.5	
Standard days method	12	5	
TwoDay method	14	3.5	
Spermicides (foam, creams, gels, vaginal suppositories, vaginal film)	28	18	<0.3
Contraceptive sponge	24 (parous women) 12 (nulliparous women)	20 (parous women) 9 (nulliparous women)	<0.3
Male condom (without spermicide)	18	2	10.2
Female condom (without spermicide)	21	5	<0.3
Prescription methods	0.05–9	≤0.6	29.6
Sterilization (male/female)	≤0.5	≤0.5	22.7

[a] Among typical couples who initiate use of a method (not necessarily for the first time), the percentage who experience an accidental pregnancy during the first year if they do not stop use for any other reason.

[b] Among typical couples who initiate use of a method (not necessarily for the first time) and who use it consistently and correctly, the percentage who experience an accidental pregnancy during the first year if they do not stop use for any other reason.

[c] Percentage of women ages 15–44 years.

Source: References 4 and 16–19.

rate in the first year of *perfect* use (method-related failure rate) and the rate in the first year of *typical* use (use-related failure rate; Table 10–2).[4,16–19] The pregnancy rate with perfect use is difficult to measure and indicates the method's theoretical effectiveness. Perfect use assumes accurate and consistent use of the method every time intercourse occurs. The more realistic rate of typical use includes pregnancies that may have occurred because of inconsistent or incorrect use of the method. Reported use-related failure rates vary, depending on the population studied. Effectiveness increases the longer a particular method is used. Decreased coital frequency and declining fertility in older users may contribute to increased effectiveness rates in this population.[17]

The most effective way for an individual to avoid contracting an STI is either to abstain from risky sexual activity or to be involved in a long-term mutually monogamous sexual relationship with an uninfected partner.[8] In the absence of those options, preventive strategies in conjunction with use of selected contraceptives may provide the best method for reducing risk of infection (Table 10–3[8,11] and Figure 10–1).[8,11,20–23]

Selection of a Contraceptive Method

The acceptability of any given contraceptive method is vital for correct and consistent use of the method. Factors that affect acceptability include the user's religious beliefs and

table
10-3 Prevention Strategies for STIs

- Abstain from sexual activity.
- Avoid intercourse with a known infected partner.
- Avoid intercourse with an individual having multiple sex partners.
- Use a new condom with each episode of anal, oral, or vaginal intercourse.
- Seek a mutually monogamous relationship with an uninfected partner.
- Discuss partner's past sexual experiences.
- Examine partner for genital lesions.
- Practice genital self-examination.
- Avoid sexual activity involving direct contact with blood, semen, or other body fluids.
- Avoid sharing sexual devices that come in contact with semen or other body fluids.
- Choose safe and effective methods (e.g., mechanical barriers) to reduce the risk of STIs (consider adding more effective methods of pregnancy prevention when necessary).
- Avoid sexual activity if signs/symptoms of an STI are present.
- Consider vaccination if at high risk of a vaccine-preventable STI (e.g., HBV and HPV).

Key: HBV = Hepatitis B virus; HPV = human papillomavirus; STI = sexually transmitted infection.

Source: References 8 and 11.

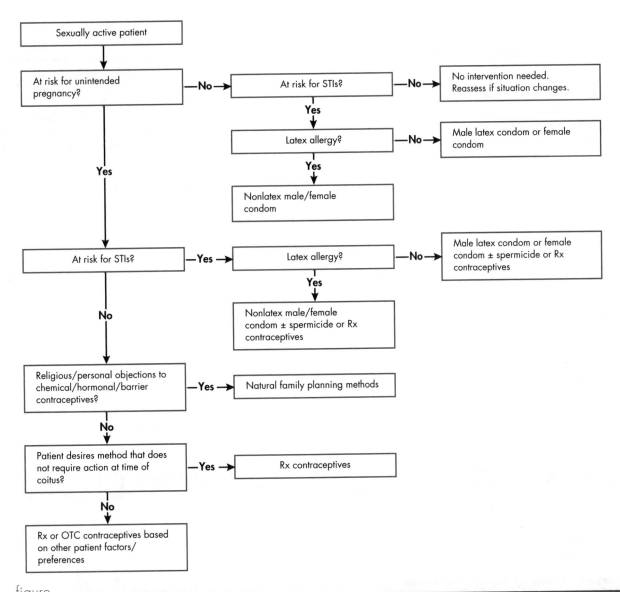

figure

10–1   Prevention of unintended pregnancy and sexually transmitted infections. Key: OTC = Over-the-counter; Rx = prescription; STI = sexually transmitted infection.

future reproductive plans, product effectiveness, partner's preference and support, degree of interruption of spontaneity, ease of use, product accessibility, and cost. To help patients make informed decisions, health care providers should be aware of each method's safety, including potential adverse effects on future fertility and on the fetus, if unintended conception does occur, and the effectiveness, accessibility, and relative cost of different contraceptive methods. The algorithm in Figure 10–1 can assist the provider in making appropriate contraceptive recommendations.

Nonprescription Contraceptive Products

Male Condoms

Condoms, also known as rubbers, sheaths, prophylactics, safes, skins, or pros, are the most important barrier contraceptive device that helps protect against STIs.[17] Male condoms are available in latex, polyurethane, polyisoprene, and lamb cecum (natural membrane or skin) (Table 10–4).

Latex condoms come in various sizes, colors, styles, shapes, and thicknesses and are degraded by oil-based lubricants. Other features include reservoir tips, ribs, studs, spermicide coating with nonoxynol-9, and lubrication. Latex condoms range in price from $0.25 to $1.50 each.[24]

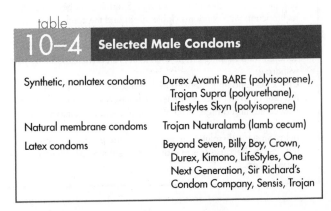

table

10–4   **Selected Male Condoms**

Synthetic, nonlatex condoms	Durex Avanti BARE (polyisoprene), Trojan Supra (polyurethane), Lifestyles Skyn (polyisoprene)
Natural membrane condoms	Trojan Naturalamb (lamb cecum)
Latex condoms	Beyond Seven, Billy Boy, Crown, Durex, Kimono, LifeStyles, One Next Generation, Sir Richard's Condom Company, Sensis, Trojan

Polyurethane condoms conduct heat well, are available pre-lubricated, and are not subject to degradation by oil-based products, but are not as elastic as latex condoms.[25] Another form of condoms include those made of polyisoprene which are more elastic than those made of polyurethane but can be damaged by oil-based lubricants. At a cost of $1.50–$2.50 each, polyurethane and poly-isoprene condoms are more expensive than latex condoms.[24]

Lamb cecum condoms are labeled only for pregnancy prevention because the presence of pores in the membrane may allow passage of viral organisms, including HIV and hepatitis B virus.[20] These condoms conduct heat well, are very strong, and are not degraded by oil-based lubricants. With a price of about $3.00 each, these condoms are also more expensive than latex condoms.[24]

Condoms are regulated by the Food and Drug Administration (FDA) as medical devices and must meet performance standards for strength and integrity. The true incidence of condom breakage is unknown, and breakage rates from studies vary widely, ranging from 0% to 22%.[26] In some studies, a limited group of patients reported multiple instances of breakage, indicating that breakage may be related as much to the individual user as it is to manufacturing defects. Behaviors that have been associated with an increased risk of condom breakage are (1) incorrect placement of the condom/failure to squeeze air from the receptacle tip; (2) use of an oil-based lubricant with latex condoms; (3) reuse of condoms; (4) increased duration, intensity, or frequency of coitus; (5) prior history of condom breakage or slippage; (6) history of STI; (7) contact with sharp objects; and (8) self-reported problems with fit of a condom.[20, 26–28] One study found a decreased incidence of breakage with continued use, indicating that correct use may improve with experience.[26] The benefit of using additional lubrication with lubricated condoms is unclear. One study found that use of additional lubricant increased the risk of condom slippage. However, another study found that use of an additional water-based lubricant was associated with decreased breakage rates but caused no increase in condom slippage rates.[28] A review of comparative studies found that nonlatex synthetic condoms had a significantly higher breakage rate compared with latex condoms.[25,29,30] Two studies also reported a significantly higher pregnancy rate with nonlatex condoms compared with latex condoms.[30,31] Because of these reports, nonlatex condoms should be reserved for use by individuals with intolerance to latex condoms.

The use-related failure rate for condoms is about 15 pregnancies per 100 women during the first year of use, but that rate improves with increasing duration of use (Table 10–2).

Studies support the finding that consistent use of condoms protects against trichomoniasis, bacterial vaginosis, and gonorrhea infections in women, and syphilis, chlamydia, HPV, and herpes simplex virus infections in both men and women.[20] Nonoxynol-9-coated (spermicide-coated) male condoms are no more effective than untreated condoms at preventing STIs. Use of nonoxynol-9-treated condoms is discouraged because of the potential risk of irritation from the spermicide in both men and women, resulting in possible increased risk of infection.[20]

Proper use of condoms is essential to their preventing pregnancy and STIs (Table 10–5). A man using a polyurethane

---

table

10–5 Usage Guidelines for Male Condoms

- Use only condoms that are fresh (not previously opened), that are within their expiration date, and that have been stored in a dry, cool place (not a wallet or car glove compartment).
- Do not attempt to test the condom for leaks before using; this step weakens the condom.
- Be aware that long fingernails or jewelry may easily tear condoms.
- As shown in drawing A, unroll the condom onto the erect penis before the penis comes into any contact with the vagina. If you start to put the condom on backward, discard that condom and use a fresh one. (*Note:* Preejaculate secretions may contain sperm.)
- If you are not using a reservoir-tipped condom, leave one-half inch of space between the end of the condom and the tip of the penis by pinching the top of the condom as you unroll it (drawing B). This method leaves space for the ejaculate (drawing C) and decreases the risk of breakage.
- If your partner has vaginal dryness, use additional lubrication, if desired. This step will help decrease the risk of tears and breakage. Use only water-based lubricants; oil-based lubricants weaken latex condoms and increase the chance of breakage. Spermicidal agents may be used as lubricants with condoms (Table 10–8) and the combination may increase contraceptive effectiveness.
- After ejaculation, withdraw the penis immediately. To prevent the condom from slipping off, hold on to the rim of the condom as you withdraw.
- Check the condom for tears and then discard in a trash can, not a toilet.
- If a tear or break occurs, immediately insert spermicidal foam or jelly containing a high concentration of spermicide into the vagina. Do not use suppositories or a vaginal film in these cases because the delay time for dissolution may decrease the product's efficacy. Do not douche because sperm that are present may be forced into the cervical canal.

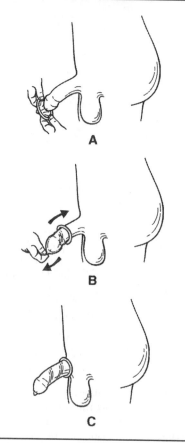

A

B

C

condom should be advised that it is not as elastic as the latex condom and will not fit as snugly. A space must be left at the tip when using condoms without a reservoir.

Prelubricated condoms are a good choice when lubrication is desired. Additional lubrication for use with any latex condom should be selected from products that do not harm or weaken the strength and integrity of the condom (Table 10–6).

Packaged condoms should be kept in their sealed packages until time of use and protected from light and excessive heat, which can rapidly decrease the integrity of the latex. FDA requires that latex condoms be labeled with an expiration date or date of manufacture. The shelf life of packaged condoms under optimal conditions is 3–5 years. Condoms showing signs of discoloration, brittleness, or stickiness should be discarded, even if they are within their expiration date.

The most frequent complaint about condoms is decreased sensitivity of the glans penis, resulting in decreased sexual pleasure for the man. Contact dermatitis caused by latex allergy can occur in the male or female partner, and may be characterized by immediate localized itching and swelling (urticarial reaction) or by a delayed eczematous reaction. In individuals with severe sensitivity, the reaction may include systemic symptoms. Spermicide-treated condoms may enhance latex allergy or cause the sensitivity reactions itself.[32]

For most people, condoms are an effective, acceptable, inexpensive, safe, and nontoxic method of birth control. Given the range of condoms available, men should be encouraged to try a different style or brand if they are dissatisfied with a condom used previously. Before recommending a latex condom, providers should assess for latex allergy. The sensitizers in latex condoms are usually antioxidants or accelerators used in processing the rubber. Some men may be sensitized to components of the lubricant or spermicide. Because manufacturers use different processes, changing brands or using a condom without spermicide may resolve the problem.[20] If switching brands does not eliminate the irritation, the man may use nonlatex synthetic condoms. Natural skin condoms may also be used if the individual recognizes the limitations of the product in preventing STIs.

table		
10–6	**Selected Lubricants/Products That Are Safe or Unsafe to Use with Latex Condoms**	

Safe	Unsafe
Contraceptive foams/gels	Topical oils (e.g., baby oil, mineral oil, massage oil)
Water-based personal lubricants, such as K-Y Jelly	Edible oils/fats (e.g., olive, peanut, corn, canola, and safflower oils; butter; margarine)
Egg white	Hemorrhoidal ointments
Glycerin (USP)	Petroleum jelly (e.g., Vaseline)
Replens Inserts	Vaginal creams (e.g., Monistat, Estrace, Vagisil, Premarin)
Saliva	
Water	

Source: Reference 20.

The use of very thin or ridged condoms, nonlatex synthetic condoms, or natural membrane condoms in a monogamous relationship with a partner screened for STI exposure may alleviate complaints of decreased sensitivity.

Female Condoms

A female condom is another nonprescription contraceptive product. The first female condom, known as the polyurethane F.C. Female Condom (FC1), was approved by FDA in 1993.[33] The FC1 was prelubricated, came with additional lubricant, and resisted degradation by oil-based lubricants. A second-generation female condom, the FC2, made of nitrile, a synthetic latex, was approved in 2009 and replaced the polyurethane condom as supplies of FC1 were exhausted.[34] Although production of the FC1 stopped in 2009, the product has a shelf life of 5 years so existing supplies may still be available. The female condom consists of an outer ring, a sheath or pouch that fits over the vaginal mucosa, and an inner ring that secures the sheath by fitting like a diaphragm over the cervix. The female condom is designed for onetime use only and, at a cost of $2.00 each, is more expensive than the latex male condom.[24]

The breakage rate of the female condom has been shown to be lower than that of latex male condoms, but slippage rates of female condoms may be higher, especially with initial use.[27] The 6-month pregnancy failure rate among all users of the FC1 is 12.4%, similar to that for users of diaphragms and cervical caps. Among perfect users, however, 6-month pregnancy failure rates of 0.8%–2.5% have been documented. The extrapolated annual pregnancy failure rate for the FC1 is 21% for all users and 5% for perfect users (Table 10–2).[1,21,33,34] Although specific data regarding failure rates for the FC2 are not available, it is considered non-inferior to the FC1.[34]

The female condom is an effective barrier to sexually transmitted bacteria and viruses, and appears to be similar in efficacy to latex male condoms in decreasing the risk of STIs.[22]

Table 10–7 provides instructions for proper use of the female condom.[35] Skills in correctly using the female condom improve with practice and continued use.[36] The condom may be inserted up to 8 hours before intercourse, but it is effective immediately on insertion.

Fresh condoms can be stored at room temperature in their unopened packages. Before inserting the female condom, the woman should ensure that the product is within its expiration date.

The most common complaints about the female condom are vaginal irritation and increased noise ("squeaking"). Additional lubrication may resolve those problems. Some women may complain of decreased sensation or discomfort caused by the outer ring during intercourse.

The female condom provides a method for women to protect themselves against pregnancy. It is thinner than many latex condoms and has a lower breakage rate than the male condom.[22] Compared with vaginal spermicides, the female condom can be inserted much earlier before intercourse and is less messy to use. However, some women may find the female condom cumbersome and unattractive. The female condom should not be used together with the male condom. Use of the two products together may cause friction and increase the risk of breakage for either product.[35]

table

10–7 Usage Guidelines for Female Condoms

- Remove the condom from the package. One end of the condom is closed to form a pouch, as shown in drawing A.
- Gently rub the sides together to evenly distribute the lubricant. If needed, add additional lubrication at this point.
- Add a drop of lubricant on the outside of the pouch to improve the ease of insertion if needed. Oil- or water-based lubricants can be used with this condom.
- To place the pouch properly, grasp the inner ring between the thumb and middle finger of one hand. Place the index finger on the sheath between the other two fingers. (See drawing B.)
- Be careful that sharp fingernails or jewelry does not tear the condom.
- Squeeze the inner ring and with your other hand, spread the lips of the vagina. Then insert the squeezed condom into the vagina as far as possible. (See drawing C.)
- Be sure that the inner ring is placed beyond the pubic (pelvic) bone, that the pouch is not twisted, and that the outer ring is outside the vagina, as shown in drawing D.
- During intercourse, make sure that the penis enters the vagina inside the pouch and that the outer ring remains outside the vagina.
- If desired, add more lubricant during intercourse, without removing the condom.
- If you notice the female condom slipping out of the vagina during intercourse or the outer ring is going into the vagina, stop intercourse. Remove the female condom and insert a new condom.
- Remove the pouch before standing by twisting the outer ring and pulling gently. (See drawing E.)
- Discard the used condom in a trash can, not a toilet.
- Insert a new condom for each act of intercourse.
- Do not use a male condom with the female condom. The increased friction could cause displacement of the female condom.

A B C D E

Source: Reference 35.

Vaginal Spermicides

Vaginal spermicides use surface-active agents to immobilize and kill sperm. For gels and foams, the spermicide vehicle also acts as a physical barrier against sperm. The effective spermicides include nonoxynol-9, octoxynol-9, and menfegol, but in the United States, all products contain nonoxynol-9 (Table 10–8). Vaginal spermicide products differ in application method and onset and duration of action (Table 10–9). The cost of vaginal spermicides ranges from $1.00 to $3.00 per dose.[24]

Vaginal gels (jellies) provide additional lubrication and are safe to use with latex condoms. For convenience, applicators may be prefilled before use. Prefilled unit-dose applicators are also available for some products. When selecting an agent to use without a diaphragm or cervical cap, a product with a higher concentration of spermicide, rather than one with a lower concentration labeled for use with barrier methods, should be chosen. Products with a higher concentration of spermicide may be used alone or with a diaphragm or cervical cap.

Vaginal foams distribute more evenly and adhere better to the cervical area and vaginal walls but provide less lubrication than jellies. A new canister should always be available because it is difficult to know when the canister is nearly empty.

Vaginal suppositories are solid or semisolid dosage forms that are activated by moisture in the vaginal tract. Incomplete dissolution of the suppository may result in an unpleasant, gritty sensation. Although vaginal suppositories do not require refrigeration, in warmer climates, refrigeration may be desirable to prevent softening.

Vaginal contraceptive film contains nonoxynol-9 in paper-thin, 2-inch-square sheets. The film is activated by vaginal secretions. One film is used for each act of intercourse. The practice of inserting the film by placing it over the penis should be avoided because this method does not ensure proper placement and does not allow adequate time for dissolution. In one comparison of spermicide dosage formulations, the film was rated the most difficult to use but the least messy.[37] Similarly designed

table

10–8 Selected Nonprescription Vaginal Spermicides Containing Nonoxynol-9

Spermicidal foams	VCF Vaginal Contraceptive Foam 12.5%, 85 mg
Spermicidal gels/jellies	Conceptrol Gel 4%, 100 mg Ortho Options Gynol II Vaginal Contraceptive Jelly[a] 2%, 100 mg Ortho Options Gynol II Extra Strength Vaginal Contraceptive Jelly 3%, 150 mg
Spermicidal suppositories	Encare Vaginal Contraceptive Inserts 100 mg
Spermicidal film	VCF Vaginal Contraceptive Film 28%, 72 mg
Spermicidal sponge	Today Contraceptive Sponge 1000 mg

[a] Product formulated for use with a diaphragm or cervical cap; it should not be used alone.

table
10–9 Administration Guidelines for Vaginal Spermicides

Dosage Form	Application Method	Onset/Duration of Action	Application Time before Intercourse	Reapplication Requirements
Vaginal gel alone	Insert full dose near cervix.	Immediate/1 hour	Up to 30–60 minutes	Reapply for each coital act.
Vaginal gel used with diaphragm/ cervical cap	Fill barrier device one-third full with gel and place it near cervix. Leave barrier in place for at least 6 hours after intercourse.	Immediate/diaphragm: 6 hours; cervical cap: 48 hours	Up to 1 hour	Diaphragm: for each coital act that occurs within 6 hours of initial insertion of device, reapply spermicide without removing device; for coitus after 6 hours of initial insertion, remove and wash device, fill with new spermicide, and re-insert device. Cervical cap: remove and wash device; then reapply spermicide for each coital act that occurs 48 hours after initial insertion of device.
Vaginal foam	Insert full dose near cervix.	Immediate/1 hour	Up to 1 hour	Reapply for each coital act.
Vaginal suppository	Insert suppository near cervix.	10–15 minutes/1 hour	10–15 minutes	Reapply for each coital act.
Vaginal contraceptive film	Drape film over fingertip; place film near cervix.	15 minutes/1–3 hours (brand-dependent)	15 minutes	Reapply for each coital act.
Vaginal contraceptive sponge	Moisten with tap water, insert convex side against cervix.	Immediate/24 hours	Can be inserted up to 24 hours before intercourse.	Leave in for >6 hours after intercourse, but no longer than 30 hours total; polyester loop to facilitate removal.

vaginal films for cleansing or lubrication do not contain spermicide and should not be used for contraception. Patients should be advised to verify that they are using the correct vaginal film product if they desire contraception.

Spermicides used alone have a relatively high typical rate of usage failure among first-year users (Table 10–2). A review of clinical trials found a similar pregnancy rate between dosage forms containing 100–150 mg nonoxynol-9 per dose.[38] A gel containing 52.5 mg nonoxynol-9 per dose, which is not available in the United States, was significantly less effective at preventing pregnancy than the higher-dose formulations.[38] Efficacy improves greatly if spermicides are used with barrier methods, such as diaphragms, cervical caps, or condoms.

Although nonoxynol-9 can inactivate many sexually transmitted pathogens in vitro, clinical studies do not support a protective effect of vaginal spermicides against STI transmission.[21,39] Higher rates of genital lesions, especially in frequent users, have been reported, raising concerns about an increased risk of STI transmission.[21,39] In 2007, FDA ruled that vaginal spermicide products must carry a label stating that the product does not protect against HIV and other STIs.[39] If a risk of STIs exists, spermicides should only be recommended in conjunction with condom use.

Table 10–9 provides guidelines for the proper administration of vaginal spermicides. When using any vaginal spermicide, a woman should delay douching for at least 6 hours after intercourse. Although allergic reactions are rare, either partner may experience such reactions to spermicides. Couples having oral–genital sex may find the taste of some products unpleasant. Frequent use or use of high-concentration products may irritate or damage vaginal and cervical epithelium,[39] which may be associated with an increased risk for STIs. Despite initial

concerns about a possible association between spermicide use and birth defects or miscarriage should an unintended pregnancy occur, current data do not support an increased risk of either attributable to spermicides.[40]

The relatively low effectiveness of spermicides when used alone is their major disadvantage. However, studies suggest that simultaneous use of condoms and spermicides provides efficacy rates similar to those of oral contraceptives and intrauterine contraceptives (IUCs).[17] Their availability and ease of use make spermicides a good choice for women who need a backup method. Spermicides are not recommended for women with anatomic abnormalities that would prevent the proper placement of the spermicide near the cervical opening. Product selection can be based on patient preference and specific product characteristics.

Contraceptive Sponge

The contraceptive sponge marketed as the Today Sponge is a small, circular, disposable sponge made of polyurethane permeated with the spermicide nonoxynol-9. The sponge is believed to act as a contraceptive by serving as a mechanical barrier, providing a spermicide, and absorbing semen. The contraceptive sponge ranges in price from $5 to $8 per sponge.[24]

In two large trials, the failure rate for the contraceptive sponge ranged from 17.4 to 24.5 pregnancies per 100 women in the first year of use.[41] Women who had given birth previously (parous women) had a significantly higher pregnancy rate while using the sponge, compared with women who had never given birth (nulliparous women). That finding may be related to poor fit in women who have delivered vaginally. If the sponge becomes dislodged during intercourse, its efficacy may be decreased.

The contraceptive sponge does not protect against STIs. One study found an increased risk of HIV infection in women with frequent sponge use, possibly because of an increased incidence of vaginal ulceration from the spermicide.[23]

A woman must be able to locate her cervix and must be comfortable in doing so to place the sponge correctly. Table 10–9 provides instructions for proper use. The sponge has a loop attached to the convex side to facilitate removal. Some women have difficulty removing the sponge, and it has been known to fragment on removal. The sponge may be inserted up to 24 hours prior to intercourse but must remain in place for 6 hours after intercourse. The sponge should be stored in its unopened package in a cool place and used before its expiration date.

Vaginal dryness is reported among sponge users. Although the incidence is rare, the contraceptive sponge has been associated with an increased risk of toxic shock syndrome (TSS).[21] Women should take special care to wash their hands before inserting the sponge. The sponge should not be used during menstruation, less than 6 weeks postpartum, or in women with a history of TSS. Use should not exceed the maximum recommended retention time of 30 hours. Women should also be advised to make sure the entire sponge is removed because fragments left in the vagina may serve as a source for infection.

The contraceptive sponge is convenient, safe, and portable. Contraindications for use include spermicide sensitivity, anatomic abnormalities of the vagina, and a history of TSS. The contraceptive sponge should not be routinely recommended to parous women because possible problems with adequate cervical coverage may lead to increased risk of pregnancy.

Emergency Contraception

Emergency contraception (EC) involves the use of hormones in the form of oral tablets or a non-hormonal copper IUC to prevent pregnancy within 3–5 days after unprotected sexual intercourse. Hormones used in EC may include only progestin (synthetic progesterone), estrogen in combination with a progestin, or a selective progesterone receptor modulator. Currently OTC and prescription oral tablet formulations are available. The prescription product, ella, contains 30 mg of ulipristal acetate and is a selective progesterone-receptor modulator that can be taken up to 120 hours after unprotected intercourse. Ulipristal will not be discussed in this chapter because of its prescription-only status, but it follows counseling points similar to those used for progestin-only products. Nonprescription EC products that contain estrogen and progestin together are not available; therefore, this chapter will focus on progestin-only products.

Emergency contraceptive products should be recommended for girls and women of reproductive age who have had recent unprotected intercourse or experienced method failure, such as condom breakage.[16,42,43] Some women may be seeking EC in the case of sexual assault. In addition to providing EC for immediate use, pharmacy staff should refer the individual to health care providers who can evaluate the individual for STIs and report the incident to the authorities as required by state law.

EC products reduce the expected number of pregnancies by at least 89% for levonorgestrel users and 74% for combination oral contraceptive users.[43] The efficacy of EC is due primarily to the suppression of ovulation. Other possible mechanisms of action include interference with transport of sperm or egg, including thickening of cervical mucus.[16,42,43]

Current options on the market include levonorgestrel-containing tablets, available as one-tablet formulations in the generic branded products Next Choice One Dose and My Way or the branded product Plan B One-Step and two-tablet formulations as an unbranded generic product. Progestin-only products cost between $40 and $50 for single incident use.[24] Levonorgestrel-containing EC products were made available OTC to women 18 years of age or older in 2006 and in 2009 to women 17 years of age or older. In 2011, FDA recommended EC to be available OTC to all women. Concerns about the lack of safety data in young girls and political pressure led to the limitation of its use to girls ages 17 years or older.[44] In April 2013, a U.S. district judge reversed the age limitations of levonorgestrel-containing EC products, making them OTC for all ages.[45] In July 2013, FDA granted Teva, the manufacturer of Plan B One-Step, exclusivity to market the one-tablet formulation OTC for 3 years to all ages.[45,46] Thus, other formulations are available OTC to those 17 years of age or older and by prescription to those younger than 17 years.

Next Choice One Dose, My Way, and Plan B One-Step each contain one tablet of levonorgestrel 1.5 mg labeled to be taken as a single dose within 72 hours after unprotected intercourse or contraceptive failure, but studies have shown effectiveness up to 120 hours after intercourse, though efficacy declines with more time post coitus.[43] Therefore, women presenting within 120 hours of unprotected sex should be offered EC. Various generic formulations may contain two pills, each containing 0.75 mg of levonorgestrel, taken 12 hours apart or together within the same time frame after unprotected intercourse. Both methods of administration have equal effectiveness, although taking the full dose of 1.5 mg immediately is preferred because of simplicity and adherence.[43]

Oral contraceptives containing levonorgestrel or D,L-norgestrel may also be used but are not the preferred regimen because of the availability of the dedicated products for EC.[42] EC using combined oral contraceptive tablets is given in two doses.[43] For optimal efficacy, the first dose of the combined regimen should be given as soon as possible after unprotected intercourse, and the second dose 12 hours later. Only certain combined hormonal contraceptive products are appropriate for EC use. Women should check with their providers to determine which combined hormonal product could be used if needed. Because of the increased access to Next Choice One Dose, My Way, and Plan B One-Step as nonprescription products, using progestin-only EC is preferred to using combined oral contraceptives as EC.

The most common adverse effects reported with EC use are nausea and vomiting.[16,43] Nausea occurs in about 50% of women using combination oral contraceptives for EC and about 25% of women using progestin-only products. Vomiting occurs in about 20% and 5% of combination oral contraceptive and progestin-only EC users, respectively. An antiemetic is usually not necessary for progestin-only EC but may be recommended 60 minutes before each dose when using combination oral contraceptive regimen.[16,43] However, if a woman vomits within 1 to 2 hours of taking the dose, she should repeat the dose.[16,43] Headaches, breast tenderness, and dizziness have also been reported by users of both products. Progestin-only EC has been found to be more effective and better tolerated than combination oral contraceptives.

Patients presenting between 5 and 7 days after unprotected intercourse should be referred to a physician for possible insertion of a copper IUC.[16] Although a copper IUC is usually placed up to 5 days after unprotected intercourse, the IUC can be inserted up to 8 days after intercourse if ovulation is known to have occurred more than 72 hours after intercourse.[16] Therefore,

table
10–10 Counseling Points for Emergency Contraception

- Identify whether patient has had recent unprotected sex within the past 120 hours or is at risk for unprotected sex and does not want to get pregnant.
- Identify whether patient is appropriate for EC available as nonprescription products.
- Explain how to take EC: Both doses of generic levonorgestrel EC may be given at the same time or as 2 doses taken 12 hours apart. Plan B One-Step, My Way, or Next Choice One Dose is given as a single dose and should be taken as soon as possible. EC is most effective when taken as soon as possible after unprotected intercourse. The method is effective when taken up to 120 hours after unprotected intercourse though package labeling states within 72 hours.
- Recommend an antiemetic for women using combination oral contraceptive pills for EC.
- Discuss adverse effects of EC, which may include a change in menstrual cycle depending on when emergency contraception is used. Patients may experience their next menstrual cycles early or late or have no change. If a menstrual cycle has not occurred more than 21 days after use of ECPs, the patient should take a pregnancy test.
- Emphasize that EC is not to be used as a regular contraceptive method.
- Recommend that a sexually active woman begin using regular contraception after taking EC. Barrier methods should be used with each subsequent act of intercourse. Hormonal contraceptive methods may be started with the next menses or may be started the day after taking EC, including 7 days of a backup method.
- Explain that EC does not protect against STIs.
- Explain that EC is not 100% effective. Recommend using a pregnancy test if menses is more than 21 days late.
- Provide written instructions.

Key: EC = Emergency contraception; ECP = emergency contraceptive pill; STI = sexually transmitted infection.
Source: References 16 and 42.

if intercourse occurred 3 days prior to ovulation, the patient could potentially still have an IUC placed up to 120 hours after ovulation, though in practice it is usually placed up to 5 days after unprotected intercourse.[16] Table 10–10 provides patient counseling points and information about EC products.

Fertility Awareness–Based Methods

Examples of contraceptive methods that do not use a chemical or barrier to prevent conception include calendar methods, cervical mucus methods, symptothermal method, and the lactational amenorrhea method (LAM). These fertility awareness–based (FAB) methods use various techniques to determine a woman's fertile phase of the menstrual cycle. The techniques are typically chosen because they pose no health risks to the couple or to the fetus should pregnancy occur or because of decreased cost or religious reasons. In some cases, FAB methods are used because of a lack of access to or knowledge of other methods of contraception. Disadvantages of FAB methods include lack of STI protection, lower efficacy than with some other contraceptive methods, and the need for periods of abstinence or the use of another method of contraception, such as condoms, during fertile days.[18]

Calendar Methods

Calendar methods use a woman's monthly menstrual cycle length to calculate the fertile period. These methods factor in the viabilities of ovum (up to 24 hours) and sperm (up to 6 days).[10,18] Menstrual cycles may vary, and therefore, cycle lengths should be recorded for 6–12 cycles to predict the likely range of fertile days. The Calendar Rhythm Method calculates the first fertile day in a woman's menstrual cycle by subtracting 18 from the number of days in her shortest cycle. The last fertile day is calculated by subtracting 11 from the number of days in her longest cycle. Women who have irregular cycles are not optimal candidates for this method as an overestimation of unsafe fertile days could occur.[18] The Standard Days Method is a calendar method recommended only for women with cycles between 26 and 32 days

in length. Counting the first day of menstruation as day 1, a woman should avoid intercourse on days 8 through 19 of her menstrual cycle or use another method of contraception, such as condoms, during this time. Software applications are available to facilitate the tracking of cycle days.[18]

Cervical Mucus Methods

Cervical mucus methods rely on rather consistent changes in cervical mucus that take place during a normal menstrual cycle.[18] Individuals should be encouraged to work with trained instructors to ensure proper interpretation of mucus as well as to avoid intercourse during the first cycle. Examples of cervical mucus methods include the Billings Ovulation Method, the Creighton Model, and the TwoDay Method.

With the Billings Ovulation Method, the woman observes the cervical mucus on a daily basis and charts its character and quantity. After menstruation, most women notice a sensation of vaginal dryness. About 5–6 days before ovulation, estrogen levels rise, causing the cervical mucus to increase in quantity and elasticity and to become clear, resembling raw egg white. The peak symptom, the last day of the clear, stretchy, estrogenic mucus, has been shown to occur within a day of ovulation for most women. With the postovulatory rise in progesterone, the mucus becomes thick and sticky or is absent. The woman is considered fertile from the first day after menstruation on which mucus is detected until 4 days after appearance of the peak symptom, during which time intercourse should be avoided.[18,47] With experience and assistance, a woman learns to differentiate other vaginal secretions, such as seminal fluid or an infectious discharge, from normal mucus, enabling her to seek early treatment for an infection. Women should be informed that vaginal foams, gels, creams, and douches will interfere with cervical mucus. The Creighton Model involves similar principles, but uses more standardized definitions of cervical secretions, involves the male partner, and requires extensive patient training from certified instructors.[47]

Another method of monitoring cervical secretions is called the TwoDay Method.[18,47] The woman should monitor for secretions on a daily basis, and if she notes any secretions that day or the day before, she is likely to be fertile. If she does not note any secretions, she is unlikely to be fertile. The Two-Day Method is a simple method that does not require keeping records or logs. However, training the woman to identify cervical secretions correctly is still important.[47]

Symptothermal Method

The symptothermal method combines methods of fertility awareness to determine the fertile period. Tracking changes in cervical mucus is combined with basal body temperature (BBT) monitoring.[10,18] Observation of the cervical mucus is used to identify the onset of the fertile period, and BBT charting is used to identify the end of the fertile period.[18] Monitoring of BBT can also be used to predict ovulation for conception, which is discussed further in Chapter 48.

To monitor BBT, the woman measures and charts her body temperature every morning, preferably with a digital thermometer calibrated in increments of 0.1°F (0.05°C), to detect small changes in body temperature.[18] The temperature must be obtained before getting out of bed at the same time every day and is recorded on a chart (Figure 10–2). At least 3 hours of uninterrupted sleep are required for a reliable reading. The temperature may be taken orally, vaginally, or rectally, but the same site must be used each day.

In some women, the onset of ovulation may be detected by a drop in BBT 12–24 hours before ovulation. At the time of ovulation, BBT rises by at least 0.4°F (0.2°C) above the lowest point (the nadir).[18] The safe (infertile) period begins once there have been 3 consecutive days of rising temperature and lasts until the end of menses.

Some women do not have a definite or significant temperature dip or rise with ovulation. Stress, inadequate sleep, travel, fever, lactation, or perimenopause may affect BBT.[18] For women who work rotating shifts, an accurate record of BBT may be difficult to maintain. At such times, couples should use an alternative method of contraception.

Home Tests for Ovulation Prediction

Ovulation prediction tests are designed to aid couples in conceiving by detecting the surge in luteinizing hormone that occurs shortly before ovulation (see Chapter 48). These kits detect an increase in urinary excretion of the hormone, which usually occurs 8–40 hours before actual ovulation. These ovulation predictors do

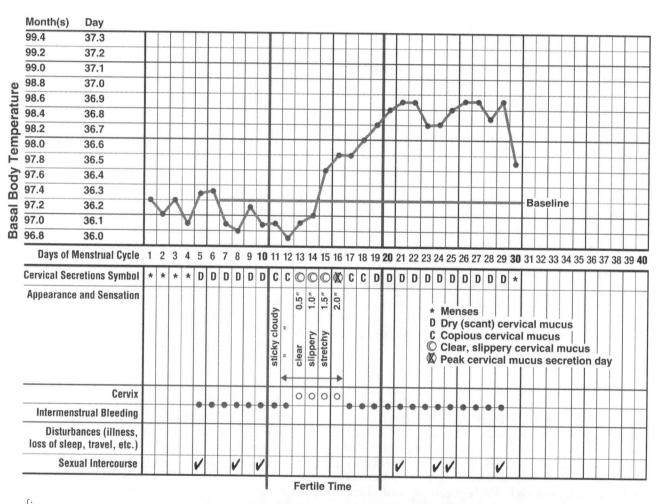

figure

10–2

Symptothermal variations during a model menstrual cycle. (*Source:* Reprinted with permission from Jennings VH, Arevalo M, Kowal D. Fertility awareness-based methods. In: Hatcher RA, Trussell J, Stewart F, et al., eds. *Contraceptive Technology.* 18th rev ed. New York, NY: Ardent Media; 2004:327.)

not give warning of impending ovulation with enough accuracy to be effective contraceptive agents and are not recommended for use other than as an aid for couples desiring pregnancy.[18]

Lactational Amenorrhea Method

In many developing countries, the LAM is used as a contraceptive method for spacing the birth of children. When an infant younger than 6 months of age receives at least 90% of his nutrition from breastfeeding, and the mother is amenorrheic, the LAM offers more than 98% protection against pregnancy.[16,19] Because the suckling action of the infant on the breast at frequent intervals is necessary for the LAM to be effective, milk extraction through a breast pump does not offer the same protection against pregnancy.[19] Although menstrual periods in lactating women may be anovulatory, ovulation may occur before the return of menses. With the LAM, the risk of pregnancy increases after the initial 6 months postpartum as supplementation becomes more commonplace in older infants. In general, if a breastfeeding woman is having menstrual periods, is supplementing her infant's diet, or is more than 6 months postpartum, she should use an additional method of contraception.[16,19] For a woman who is breastfeeding an infant almost exclusively, studies have reported pregnancy rates of 0.5%–2% for the 6-month period after delivery. Once supplemental feedings begin, the efficacy rate decreases significantly.[19]

Effectiveness of Fertility Awareness–Based Methods

Overall, the pregnancy rate for typical use of FAB methods is about 24% (Table 10–2).[17] Compared with condoms, hormonal methods, or the nonhormonal IUC, the risk of pregnancy is higher with any of the FAB methods alone. Consequently, family planners do not recommend using a single method; instead, they suggest using a combination of methods. FAB methods that specifically identify preovulatory and postovulatory changes, such as the sympto-thermal method, have much better outcomes; with perfect use, the annual failure rate is less than 5%.[17] FAB methods also do not provide any protection against STIs and should be recommended solely for couples in mutually monogamous relationships.

Coitus Interruptus

Coitus interruptus (withdrawal) involves coital activity until ejaculation is imminent, followed by withdrawal of the stimulated penis and ejaculation away from the vagina or vulva. Method failures (pregnancy even when the method is used correctly and consistently) occur in part because involuntary preejaculation secretions may contain millions of sperm. Disadvantages of this method include the requirement of considerable self-control by the man, the potential for diminished pleasure for the couple because of interrupted lovemaking, and no STI protection. This method has failure rates of 4% with perfect use and 22% with typical use, comparable to those of other barrier methods.[48]

Assessment of the Prevention of Pregnancy and STIs: A Case-Based Approach

Before advising a couple on contraception and STI prevention, the health care provider must first identify their level of knowledge about these issues because they must understand their risk of pregnancy and STIs to select an appropriate product or method. Individuals who prefer FAB methods must understand the reproductive cycle before they can use these methods effectively. Those who prefer nonprescription contraceptive products must know how to use them properly and be prepared to use them with every act of intercourse. The provider should identify individual preferences for products or methods on the basis of the timing of use or religious or cultural practices.

Case 10–1 illustrates the assessment of a woman who is seeking advice on contraception, whereas Case 10–2 deals with the use of emergency contraception.

Patient Counseling for Prevention of Pregnancy and STIs

As the most accessible health care provider, pharmacists are in a unique position to lower the incidence and consequences of unintended pregnancy and STIs in their communities. The

---

case
10–1

Relevant Evaluation Criteria	Scenario/Model Outcome
Information Gathering	

1. Gather essential information about the patient's symptoms and medical history, including:

    a. description of symptom(s) (i.e., nature, onset, duration, severity, associated symptoms) — Patient is asking for a recommendation for a contraceptive method. She has not used contraception in the past as she has not been sexually active. However, she plans to begin having intercourse with her current boyfriend. She is not sure of his sexual history but expresses interest in a method whose use she can control. She does not have access to a physician at this time because of insurance issues.

    b. patient's identity — Jennifer Grayson

    c. age, sex, height, and weight — 23 years old, woman, 5 ft 3 in., 115 lb

    d. concurrent medical conditions, prescription and nonprescription medications, and dietary supplements — None; no history of sexual partners

    e. allergies — NKA

case
10–1 *continued*

Relevant Evaluation Criteria	Scenario/Model Outcome

Assessment and Triage

2. Differentiate patient's signs/symptoms and correctly identify the patient's primary problem(s).

Risk of undesired pregnancy and STI

3. Identify exclusions for self-treatment.

None

Options include:

4. Formulate a comprehensive list of therapeutic alternatives for the primary problem to determine if triage to a medical provider is required, and share this information with the patient or caregiver.

(1) Recommend use of a male or female condom to provide STI protection in addition to contraception.

(2) Refer patient for a prescription hormonal method of contraception to be used in combination with a male or female condom.

Plan

5. Select an optimal therapeutic alternative to address the patient's problem, taking into account patient preferences.

Nonlatex female condom because patient prefers female-controlled method and does not have medical insurance at this time.

6. Describe the recommended therapeutic approach to the patient or caregiver.

"Use the nonlatex female condom with each act of sexual intercourse."

7. Explain to the patient or caregiver the rationale for selecting the recommended therapeutic approach from the considered therapeutic alternatives.

"There are various OTC contraceptive options whose use are controlled by the woman, including the female condom, contraceptive sponge, and various forms of spermicides. In addition, many prescription hormonal contraceptive products are available. They are more effective than the OTC methods for pregnancy prevention, and I can provide you information on low-cost clinics in the area that may better fit your financial needs for medical care. In the meantime, of the OTC methods, only the female condom provides protection from STIs, which is important to consider when beginning a sexual relationship. This method would be important to continue using even if you started a hormonal method in the future for this reason."

Patient Education

8. When recommending self-care with nonprescription medications and/or nondrug therapy, convey accurate information to the patient or caregiver:

a. appropriate dose and frequency of administration

"Use a fresh condom with each act of sexual intercourse."

b. product administration procedures

See Table 10–7.

c. expected time to onset of relief

"Female condoms are effective immediately once correctly inserted. Although most women insert them between 2 and 20 minutes prior to intercourse, they can be inserted up to 8 hours prior to intercourse."

d. degree of relief that can be reasonably expected

See Table 10–2 for efficacy rates.

e. most common side effects

"Vaginal irritation and increased noise (possible squeaking) are the most common side effects."

f. patient options in the event that condition worsens or persists

"Consult your primary care provider."

g. product storage requirements

See Table 10–7.

Solicit follow-up questions from the patient or caregiver.

"May I use lubricants or vaginal spermicides with the female condom?"

Answer the patient's or caregiver's questions.

"Yes. The female condom comes with its own lubricant, but additional lubrication can also be used. Nitrile and/or the previously marketed polyurethane female condoms are not affected by oil-based lubricants."

Evaluation of Patient Outcome

9. Assess patient outcome.

Ask the patient to call the pharmacy if she has further questions.

Key: NKA = No known allergies; OTC = over-the-counter; PCP = primary care provider; STI = sexually transmitted infection.

case

10–2

Relevant Evaluation Criteria	Scenario/Model Outcome
Information Gathering	

1. Gather essential information about the patient's symptoms and medical history, including:

   a. description of symptom(s) (i.e., nature, onset, duration, severity, associated symptoms)

   Patient had unprotected intercourse with a partner 3 days ago. This is her third time in 6 weeks requesting EC, involving two sexual partners.

   b. patient's identity

   Cindy Smith

   c. age, sex, height, and weight

   22 years old, woman, 5 ft 3 in., 120 lb

   d. patient's occupation

   College student

   e. concurrent medical conditions, prescription and nonprescription medications, and dietary supplements

   Occasional tension headaches: naproxen 220 mg 1 tablet orally as needed for headache; multivitamin 1 tablet daily

   f. allergies

   None

   g. history of other adverse effects to medications

   None

Assessment and Triage

2. Differentiate patient's signs/symptoms and correctly identify the patient's primary problem(s).

   Elevated risk of pregnancy and STI due to unprotected intercourse with multiple partners

3. Identify exclusions for self-treatment.

   Patient has no exclusions for self-treatment with EC but should see her health care provider for STI screening and for possible longer-term prescription contraceptive method.

4. Formulate a comprehensive list of therapeutic alternatives for the primary problem to determine whether triage to a medical provider is required, and share this information with the patient or caregiver.

   Options include:

   (1) Recommend that the patient purchase OTC EC at her local pharmacy.

   (2) Recommend that the patient purchase OTC EC at her local pharmacy. Also refer patient to see her provider for selection of a longer-term prescription contraceptive method and STI screening.

   (3) Recommend that the patient obtain a prescription for ella (ulipristal acetate).

   (4) Recommend that the patient obtain a prescription for an oral contraceptive pill that can be used as EC.

   (5) Recommend that the patient see her provider for evaluation and possible insertion of a copper intrauterine contraceptive.

   (6) Recommend against use of OTC EC because of overuse.

Plan

5. Select an optimal therapeutic alternative to address the patient's problem, taking into account patient preferences.

   The patient prefers to purchase EC at her local pharmacy and considers obtaining a prescription for a regular method of contraception. OTC EC should not be denied to the patient because of multiple uses.

6. Describe the recommended therapeutic approach to the patient or caregiver.

   "You should take Next Choice One Dose, My Way, or Plan B One-Step (levonorgestrel 1.5 mg), 1 tablet by mouth. It is recommended to take the product as soon as possible within 72 hours of unprotected intercourse, but the product can still be effective up to 120 hours after intercourse."

7. Explain to the patient or caregiver the rationale for selecting the recommended therapeutic approach from the considered therapeutic alternatives.

   "Over-the-counter emergency contraception is up to 89% effective in preventing pregnancy and works better the sooner it is taken. It is not intended to be a regular form of birth control. For more effective and less expensive ways of contraception, you should see your provider to obtain a prescription for a more regular form of contraception. Emergency contraception does not protect against sexually transmitted infections. Because you have had unprotected intercourse, you should be screened."

Patient Education

8. When recommending self-care with nonprescription medications and/or nondrug therapy, convey accurate information to the patient or caregiver.

   See Table 10–10.

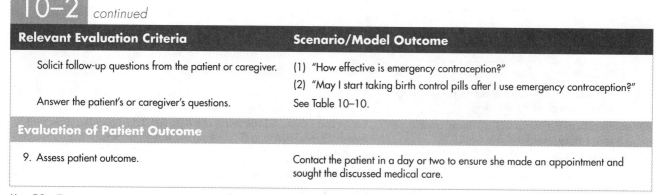

case

10-2 *continued*

Relevant Evaluation Criteria	Scenario/Model Outcome
Solicit follow-up questions from the patient or caregiver.	(1) "How effective is emergency contraception?"
	(2) "May I start taking birth control pills after I use emergency contraception?"
Answer the patient's or caregiver's questions.	See Table 10–10.
Evaluation of Patient Outcome	
9. Assess patient outcome.	Contact the patient in a day or two to ensure she made an appointment and sought the discussed medical care.

Key: EC = Emergency contraception; OTC = over-the-counter; PCP = primary care provider; STIs = sexually transmitted infections.

pharmacist should seek opportunities to discuss specific diseases or prevention strategies with individuals who may be at high risk of unintended pregnancy and STIs. If possible, consultation involving both partners can improve the understanding and acceptance of selected contraceptive methods.

Providers must be familiar with the proper use of available nonprescription contraceptive products and provide opportunities for consultation by removing barriers that may prevent open conversations. Contraceptive products and information as well as STI-related patient information should be available in an area where the individual can browse and the pharmacist can easily interact with the individual, such as near the prescription counter.

In addition to an educational role, the provider may be able to assist an individual in gaining access to other needed medical and social supportive services. In cases of suspected domestic violence or sexual abuse, pharmacists should act on their role as mandatory reporters. A private area for education and counseling is important if adequate discussion is to take place.

Special efforts should be made to offer contraceptive information and services to adolescents. Providers who are uncomfortable discussing reproductive health in a nonjudgmental manner with young people should refer adolescents to a clinic that specializes in services to young people. Adolescents need clear, accurate information on all aspects of reproductive health. The provider should keep in mind that misconceptions about STI and pregnancy risk and proper contraceptive use are common, especially among adolescents; therefore, adequate education is very important. FAB methods are recommended for couples in a stable relationship. These methods, especially the symptothermal and cervical mucus methods, require extensive training and support from health care professionals who have experience with FAB methods. In addition to stocking spermicidal products, BBT thermometers, and monitoring charts, the pharmacist may serve as a referral for individuals who want to use these methods of family planning. A pharmacist with the proper training might consider counseling patients on FAB methods as a unique practice possibility.

Evaluation of Patient Outcomes for Prevention of Pregnancy and STIs

Many sexually active persons are at risk of unintended pregnancy or STIs. The most important factor affecting the ability of a contraceptive to prevent pregnancy and STIs is correct

and consistent use with each sexual encounter. Although any of the methods can be used for pregnancy prevention, male condoms (except for lamb cecum) and the female condom are the preferred methods for prevention of STIs. Individuals who experience an adverse effect after use of a nonprescription contraceptive should switch to an alternative brand or agent. If the symptoms do not resolve or if they recur with the use of other agents, the individuals should seek medical attention. A sexually active woman who misses a menstrual period should be encouraged to perform a home pregnancy test or seek medical attention. Symptoms of an STI in a sexually active individual require medical referral (Table 10–1).

Key Points for Prevention of Pregnancy and STIs

➤ No method of contraception except abstinence is completely effective at preventing unintended pregnancy and STIs.

➤ The HPV vaccine is an effective method of preventing HPV-related consequences, including genital warts and cervical, vaginal, vulvar, penile, and anal cancers.

➤ Selection of a contraceptive product or method must be based on individual risk of undesired outcomes (pregnancy and STI) and efficacy, safety, and acceptability.

➤ Efficacy of nonprescription contraceptives is significantly increased by correct and consistent use of the product/method with each sexual encounter (Tables 10–5 through 10–9).

➤ Male condoms (latex) and female condoms are the preferred contraceptive products for individuals at risk for STIs. Nonlatex condoms other than lamb cecum may be used in persons with latex hypersensitivity for STI prevention.

➤ Spermicides decrease risk of unintended pregnancy but may increase risk of STIs.

➤ Vaginal spermicides are available in different dosage forms to improve patient acceptability.

➤ EC is an effective method of postcoital contraception that can decrease risk of unintended pregnancy, but the risk of STIs is not decreased. EC should not be used as routine contraception.

➤ FAB methods are an inexpensive, modestly effective method of contraception that can be used by couples in a mutually monogamous relationship.

REFERENCES

1. Finer LB, Henshaw SK. Disparities in rates of unintended pregnancy in the United States, 1994 and 2001. *Perspect Sex Reprod Health*. 2006;38(2):90–6.

2. Centers for Disease Control and Prevention. Incidence, prevalence, and cost of sexually transmitted infections in the United States. Accessed at http://www.cdc.gov/std/stats/STI-Estimates-Fact-Sheet-Feb-2013.pdf, April 7, 2013.

3. Martinez G, Copen CE, Abma JC. Teenagers in the United States: Sexual activity, contraceptive use, and childbearing, 2006–2010 National Survey of Family Growth. National Center for Health Statistics. *Vital Health Stat*. 2011;23(31):1–35.

4. Jones J, Mosher W, Daniels K. Current contraceptive use in the United States, 2006–2010, and changes in patterns of use since 1995. National Health Statistics Reports; No. 60. Hyattsville, MD: National Center for Health Statistics; 2012.

5. Hamilton BE, Ventura SJ. Birth rates for U.S. teenagers reach historic lows for all age and ethnic groups. NCHS data brief, no 89. Hyattsville, MD: National Center for Health Statistics; 2012.

6. Paukku M, Quan J, Barney P, et al. Adolescents' contraceptive use and pregnancy history: is there a pattern? *Obstet Gynecol*. 2003;101(3):534–8.

7. Centers for Disease Control and Prevention. Nationally representative CDC study finds 1 in 4 teenage girls has a sexually transmitted disease. Accessed at http://www.cdc.gov/stdconference/2008/press/release-11march2008.htm, April 7, 2013.

8. Workowski KA, Berman S; Centers for Disease Control and Prevention. Sexually transmitted diseases treatment guidelines 2010. *MMWR Recomm Rep*. 2010;59(RR–12):1–110.

9. Sherman AC, Harvey SM, Noell J. "Are they still having sex?" STIs and unintended pregnancy among mid-life women. *J Women Aging*. 2005;17(3):41–55.

10. Sanford JB, White GL Jr, Hatasaka H. Timing intercourse to achieve pregnancy: current evidence. *Obstet Gynecol*. 2002;100(6):1333–41.

11. Marrazo JM, Cates W. Reproductive tract infections including HIV and other sexually transmitted infections. In: Hatcher RA, Trussell J, Nelson A, et al., eds. *Contraceptive Technology*. 20th ed. New York, NY: Ardent Media; 2011:571–620.

12. Cox J, Mahoney M, Saslow D, et al. ACS releases guidelines for HPV vaccination. *Am Fam Physician*. 2008;77:853–6.

13. Centers for Disease Control and Prevention. Epidemiology and prevention of vaccine-preventable diseases: the pink book. 12th ed. Second printing. 2012. Accessed at www.cdc.gov/vaccines/pubs/pinkbook/index.html, August 6, 2013.

14. Satterwhite CL, Torrone E, Meites E, et al. Sexually transmitted infections among U.S. women and men: prevalence and incidence estimates, 2008. *Sex Transm Dis*. 2013;40(3):187–93.

15. Dobson SR, McNeil S, Dionne M, et al. Immunogenicity of 2 doses of HPV vaccine in younger adolescents vs 3 doses in young women: a randomized clinical trial. *JAMA*. 2013;309(17):1793–802.

16. Zieman M, Hatcher RA. *Managing Contraception*. Tiger, GA: Bridging the Gap Foundation; 2012.

17. Trussell J, Guthrie K. Choosing a contraceptive: efficacy, safety, and personal considerations. In: Hatcher RA, Trussell J, Stewart F, et al., eds. *Contraceptive Technology*. 20th rev ed. New York, NY: Ardent Media; 2011:45–74.

18. Jennings VH, Burke A. Fertility awareness-based methods. In: Hatcher RA, Trussell J, Nelson A, et al., eds. *Contraceptive Technology*. 20th rev ed. New York, NY: Ardent Media; 2011:417–34.

19. Kennedy KI, Trussell J. Postpartum contraception and lactation. In: Hatcher RA, Trussell J, Nelson A, et al., eds. *Contraceptive Technology*. 20th rev ed. New York, NY: Ardent Media; 2011:483–511.

20. Warner DL, Steiner MJ. Male condoms. In: Hatcher RA, Trussell J, Stewart F, et al., eds. *Contraceptive Technology*. 20th rev ed. New York, NY: Ardent Media; 2011:371–86.

21. Cates W Jr, Harwood B. Vaginal barriers and spermicides. In: Hatcher RA, Trussell J, Nelson AL, et al., eds. *Contraceptive Technology*. 20th rev ed. New York, NY: Ardent Media; 2011:392–408.

22. Vijayakumar G, Mabude Z, Smit J, et al. A review of female-condom effectiveness: patterns of use and impact on protected sex acts and STI incidence. *Int J STD AIDS*. 2006;17(10):652–9.

23. Kreiss J, Ngugi E, Holmes K, et al. Efficacy of nonoxynol 9 contraceptive sponge use in the prevention of heterosexual acquisition of HIV in Nairobi prostitutes. *JAMA*. 1992;268(4):477–82.

24. Drugstore.com Web site. Accessed at http://www.drugstore.com, August 6, 2013.

25. Gallo MF, Grimes DA, Lopez LM, et al. Non-latex versus latex condoms for contraception (review). *Cochrane Database Syst Rev*. 2006;1:CD003550. doi: 10.1002/14651858.CD003550.pub2. Accessed at http://www.thecochranelibrary.com/view/0/index.html.

26. Crosby RA, Yarber WL, Sanders SA, et al. Men with broken condoms: who and why? *Sex Transm Infect*. 2007;83(1):71–5.

27. Crosby RA, Yarber WL, Graham CS, et al. Does it fit okay? Problems with condom use as a function of self-reported poor fit. *Sex Transm Infect*. 2010;86(1):36–8.

28. Gabbay MB, Thomas J, Gibbs A, et al. A randomized crossover trial of the impact of additional spermicide on condom failure rates. *Sex Transm Dis*. 2008;35(10):862–8.

29. Potter WD, de Villemeur M. Clinical breakage, slippage and acceptability of a new commercial polyurethane condom: a randomized, controlled study. *Contraception*. 2003;68(1):39–45.

30. Walsh TL, Frezieres RG, Peacock K, et al. Evaluation of the efficacy of a nonlatex condom: results from a randomized, controlled clinical trial. *Perspect Sex Reprod Health*. 2003;35(2):79–86.

31. Steiner MJ, Dominik R, Rountree W, et al. Contraceptive effectiveness of a polyurethane condom and a latex condom. *Obstet Gynecol*. 2003; 101(3):539–47.

32. Liccardi G, Senna G, Rotiroti G, et al. Intimate behavior and allergy: a narrative review. *Ann Allergy Asthma Immunol*. 2007;99(5):394–400.

33. Beksinska M, Smit J, Joanis C, et al. Female condom technology: new products and regulatory issues. *Contraception*. 2011;83(4):316–21.

34. New female condom clears FDA committee. *AIDS Alert*. 2009;24(4):42–4.

35. FC2 Female Condom FAQs. Accessed at http://www.fc2femalecondom.com/faqs, August 6, 2013.

36. Beksinska M, Smit J, Joanis C, et al. Practice makes perfect: reduction in female condom failures and user problems with short-term experience in a randomized trial. *Contraception*. 2012; 86(2):127–31.

37. Raymond EG, Chen PL, Condon P, et al. Acceptability of five nonoxynol-9 spermicides. *Contraception*. 2005;71(6):438–42.

38. Grimes DA, Lopez LM, Raymond EG, et al. Spermicide used alone for contraception. *Cochrane Database Syst Rev*. 2005;4:CD005218. doi: 10.1002/14651858.CD005218.pub4. Accessed at http://www.thecochranelibrary.com/view/0/index.html.

39. Over-the-counter vaginal contraceptive and spermicide drug products containing nonoxynol-9; required labeling. Final rule. *Federal Register*. 2007;72(243):71769–85.

40. Briggs G, Freeman RK, Yaffe SJ. *Drugs in Pregnancy and Lactation*. 9th ed. Philadelphia, PA: Lippincott Williams & Wilkins; 2011:1049–52.

41. Kuyoh MA, Toroitich-Ruto C, Grimes DA, et al. Sponge versus diaphragm for contraception: a Cochrane review. *Contraception*. 2003;67(1):15–8.

42. American College of Obstetricians and Gynecologists. ACOG Practice Bulletin No 112: Emergency contraception. *Obstet Gynecol*. 2010;115(5): 1100–9.

43. Trussell J, Bimla Schwarz E. Emergency contraception. In: Hatcher RA, Trussell J, Nelson A, et al., eds. *Contraceptive Technology*. 20th rev ed. New York, NY: Ardent Media; 2011: 113–46.

44. U.S. Food and Drug Administration. FDA News and Events. Statement from FDA Commissioner Margaret Hamburg, M.D. on Plan B One-Step, Dec. 7, 2011. Accessed at http://www.fda.gov/NewsEvents/Newsroom/ucm282805.htm, August 6, 2013.

45. U.S. Food and Drug Administration. FDA News and Events. FDA approves Plan B One-Step emergency contraceptive for use without a prescription for all women of child-bearing potential, June 20, 2013. Accessed at http://www.fda.gov/NewsEvents/Newsroom/PressAnnouncements/ucm358082.htm, August 6, 2013.

46. U.S. Food and Drug Administration. Letter determining exclusivity of Plan B One-Step. Accessed at http://www.hpm.com/pdf/blog/PLAN%20B%20-%20FDA%20Exclusivity%20&%20Carve-Out%20Determination.pdf, March 31, 2014.

47. Pallone SR, Bergus GR. Fertility awareness-based methods: another option for family planning. *J Am Board Fam Med*. 2009;22(2):147–57.

48. Kowal D. Coitus interruptus (withdrawal). In: Hatcher RA, Trussell J, Nelson A, et al., eds. *Contraceptive Technology*. 20th rev ed. New York, NY: Ardent Media; 2011:409–15.

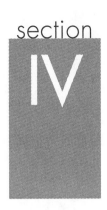

RESPIRATORY DISORDERS

COLDS AND ALLERGY

Kelly L. Scolaro

Colds and allergic rhinitis are two of the most common conditions for which patients access the health care system. This chapter reviews the role of the plethora of non-prescription products that patients may use to self-treat symptoms associated with those two disorders.

Colds

A cold, also known as the common cold, is a viral infection of the upper respiratory tract. According to some estimates, one billion cases of colds occur annually, making this illness one of the top five diagnosed in the United States.[1] Children usually have 6–10 colds per year.[1] Adults younger than 60 years typically have 2–4 colds per year, whereas adults older than 60 years usually have 1 cold per year.[1] Colds may occur at any time, but in the United States, the cold season occurs from late August through early April.[1]

Colds are the leading cause of work and school absenteeism. Colds are usually self-limiting; however, because symptoms are bothersome, patients frequently self-medicate and spend an estimated $7 billion annually on nonprescription cold and cough products.[2]

Pathophysiology of Colds

Colds are limited to the upper respiratory tract and primarily affect the following respiratory structures: pharynx, nasopharynx, nose, cavernous sinusoids, and paranasal sinuses. The respiratory tract's intricate host–defense system usually protects the body from infectious and foreign particles. The respiratory tract, especially the nose, is well perfused and innervated. The nose contains sensory, cholinergic, and sympathetic nerves. When stimulated by an infectious (i.e., a cold) or allergic (i.e., allergic rhinitis) process, those nerves play a role in the resulting symptoms and are also targets for some nonprescription therapies. Stimulation of sensory fibers by mechanical and thermal stimuli or by mediators such as histamine and bradykinin results in sneezing. Cholinergic and sympathetic nerves are involved in congestion because they innervate glands and arteries that supply the glands. Cholinergic stimulation dilates arterial blood flow, whereas sympathetic stimulation constricts arterial blood flow. The sensory, cholinergic, and sympathetic nerves also respond to a variety of neuropeptide neurotransmitters.

More than 200 viruses cause colds. The majority of colds in children and adults are caused by rhinoviruses.[1] Other viruses known to cause colds include coronaviruses, parainfluenza, adenoviruses, echoviruses, respiratory syncytial viruses, and coxsackieviruses. Viral and bacterial coinfection (usually with group A beta-hemolytic streptococci) occurs but is rare. Rhinoviruses bind to intercellular adhesion molecule-1 receptors on respiratory epithelial cells in the nose and nasopharynx.[3] Once inside the epithelial cells, the virus replicates and infection spreads to other cells.[3] Peak viral concentrations occur 2–4 days after initial inoculation, and viruses are present in the nasopharynx for 16–18 days.[3] Infected cells release chemokine "distress signals," and cytokines then activate inflammatory mediators and neurogenic reflexes. These activation processes result in recruitment of additional inflammatory mediators, vasodilatation, transudation of plasma, glandular secretion, and stimulation of pain nerve fibers and sneeze and cough reflexes. Inflammatory mediators and parasympathetic nervous system reflex mechanisms cause hypersecretion of watery nasal fluid. Viral infection ends once enough neutralizing antibody (secretory immunoglobulin A [IgA] or serum IgG) leaks into the mucosa to end viral replication.

The most efficient mode of viral transmission is self-inoculation of the nasal mucosa or conjunctiva after contact with viral-laden secretions on animate (e.g., hands) or inanimate (e.g., doorknobs and telephones) objects. Aerosol transmission is also common. Increased susceptibility to colds has been linked to higher exposure rates (e.g., increased population density in classrooms or day care centers); allergic disorders affecting the nose or pharynx; less diverse social networks; and a weakened immune system due to smoking, a sedentary lifestyle, chronic (i.e., ≥1 month) psychological stress, or sleep deprivation (e.g., poor sleep quality or <7 hours of sleep per night).[1,4,5] There is conflicting information about increased susceptibility due to cold environments, sudden chilling, or exposure to central heating (i.e., low humidity).[1,6] Walking outside barefoot, teething, or suffering from enlarged tonsils or adenoids has not been shown to increase susceptibility to viral upper respiratory infections.[1]

Clinical Presentation of Colds

A predictable sequence of symptoms appears 1–3 days after infection.[7] Sore throat is the first symptom to appear, followed by nasal symptoms, which dominate 2–3 days later. Cough, although an infrequent symptom (<20%), appears by day 4 or 5. Physical assessment of a patient with a cold may yield the following

11–1 Differentiation of Colds and Other Respiratory Disorders

Illness	Signs and Symptoms
Allergic rhinitis	Watery eyes; itchy nose, eyes, or throat; repetitive sneezing; nasal congestion; watery rhinorrhea; red, irritated eyes with conjunctival injection
Asthma	Cough, dyspnea, wheezing
Bacterial throat infection	Sore throat (moderate-severe pain), fever, exudate, tender anterior cervical adenopathy
Colds	Sore throat (mild-moderate pain), nasal congestion, rhinorrhea, sneezing common; low-grade fever, chills, headache, malaise, myalgia, and cough possible
Croup	Fever, rhinitis, and pharyngitis initially, progressing to cough (may be "barking" cough), stridor, and dyspnea
Influenza	Myalgia, arthralgia, fever ≥ 100°F–102°F (37.8°C–38.9°C), sore throat, nonproductive cough, moderate-severe fatigue
Otitis media	Ear popping, ear fullness, otalgia, otorrhea, hearing loss, dizziness
Pneumonia or bronchitis	Chest tightness, wheezing, dyspnea, productive cough, changes in sputum color, persistent fever
Sinusitis	Tenderness over the sinuses, facial pain aggravated by Valsalva's maneuver or postural changes, fever >101.5°F (38.6°C), tooth pain, halitosis, upper respiratory tract symptoms for >7 days with poor response to decongestants
West Nile virus infection	Fever, headache, fatigue, rash, swollen lymph glands, and eye pain initially, possibly progressing to GI distress, CNS changes, seizures, or paralysis
Whooping cough	Initial catarrhal phase (rhinorrhea, mild cough, sneezing) of 1–2 weeks, followed by 1–6 weeks of paroxysmal coughing

Key: CNS = Central nervous system; GI = gastrointestinal.

findings: slightly red pharynx with evidence of postnasal drainage, nasal obstruction, and mildly to moderately tender sinuses on palpation. During the first 2 days of a cold, patients may report clear, thin, and/or watery nasal secretions. As the cold progresses, the secretions become thicker and the color may change to yellow or green. When the cold begins to resolve, the secretions again become clear, thin, and/or watery. Patients may have low-grade fever, but colds are rarely associated with a fever above 100°F (37.8°C). Rhinovirus cold symptoms persist for about 7–14 days.[7] Signs and symptoms of a cold may be confused with symptoms of influenza and other respiratory illnesses (Table 11–1).

Most people do not have complications from colds. However, complications of colds may be severe and, rarely, life-threatening. Complications include sinusitis, middle ear infections, bronchitis, pneumonia, and exacerbations of asthma or chronic obstructive pulmonary disease.

Treatment of Colds

Treatment Goals

Because there is no known cure for colds, the goal of therapy is to reduce bothersome symptoms and prevent transmission of cold viruses to others.

General Treatment Approach

Antibiotics are ineffective against viral infections and the mainstay of treatment is nonpharmacologic therapy. If a patient desires to self-treat, a stepwise approach using single-entity products targeting specific symptoms is preferred over the use of combination products (Figure 11–1) because symptoms appear, peak, and resolve at different times.[7] Patient education regarding the

administration of intranasal drugs (Table 11–2) and ocular drugs (see Chapter 27) is important. Not all patients should self-treat colds (see the exclusions for self-treatment listed in Figure 11–1).

Nonpharmacologic Therapy

Although evidence of efficacy is lacking, popular therapies include increased fluid intake, adequate rest, a nutritious diet as tolerated, and increased humidification with steamy showers, vaporizers, or humidifiers. Vaporizers superheat water to produce steam and can accommodate medications such as Vicks Vapo Steam (camphor 6.2%). In contrast, humidifiers use fans or ultrasonic technology to produce a cool mist and cannot accommodate additives. Saline nasal sprays or drops moisten irritated mucosal membranes and loosen encrusted mucus; salt gargles may ease sore throats. Food products such as tea with lemon and honey, chicken soup, and hot broths are soothing. Limited evidence suggests that a number of substances in chicken soup could have anti-inflammatory activity.[8] Milk products should not be withheld given the lack of evidence that milk increases cough or congestion. Medical devices, such as Breathe Right nasal strips, are marketed for temporary relief from nasal congestion and stuffiness resulting from colds and allergies. Those devices lift the nares open, thus enlarging the anterior nasal passages. Aromatic oil (camphor, menthol, and eucalyptus) products such as Theraflu Vapor Patch (ages ≥ 12 years) and Vicks VapoRub (ages ≥ 2 years) ease nasal congestion and improve sleep by producing a soothing sensation.[9] Children should be supervised closely when these products are used because aromatic oils can irritate the eyes and skin and ingesting large quantities can be toxic.

Nondrug therapy for infants includes upright positioning to enhance nasal drainage. Because children typically cannot blow their own noses until about 4 years of age, carefully clearing

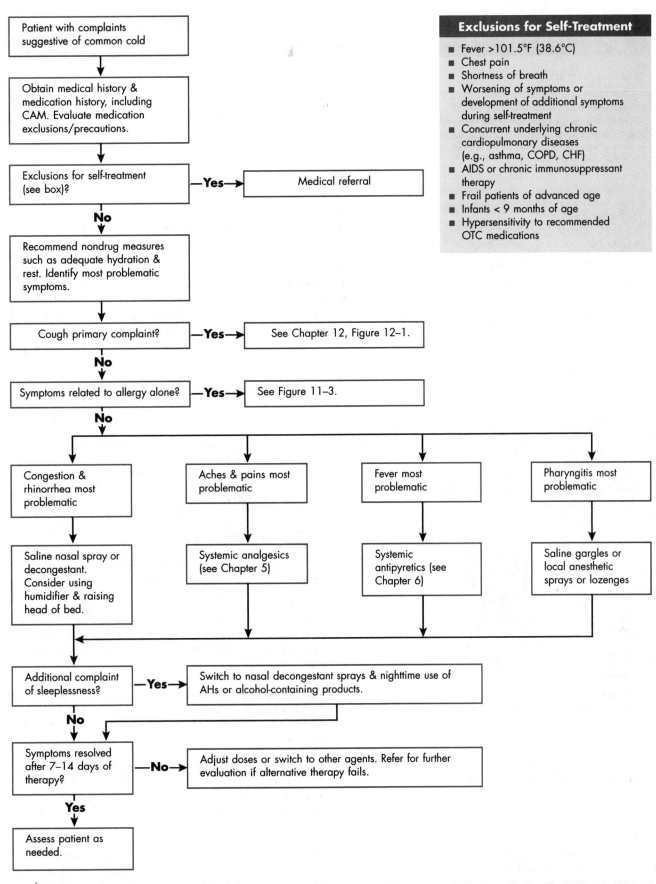

figure

11–1

Self-care of the common cold. Key: AH = Antihistamine; AIDS = acquired immunodeficiency syndrome; CAM = complementary and alternative medicine; CHF = congestive heart failure; COPD = chronic obstructive pulmonary disorder; OTC = over-the-counter. (*Source:* Adapted from Reference 7.)

table
11–2 Administration Guidelines for Nasal Dosage Formulations

General Instructions

- Clear nasal passages before administering the product.
- Wash your hands before and after use.
- Gently depress the other side of the nose with finger to close off the nostril not receiving the medication.
- Aim tip of product away from nasal septum to avoid accidental damage to the septum.
- Breathe through mouth and wait a few minutes after using the medication before blowing the nose.

Nasal Sprays

- Gently insert the bottle tip into one nostril, as shown in drawing A.
- Keep head upright. Sniff deeply while squeezing the bottle. Repeat with other nostril.

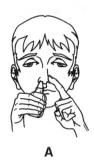

A

Nasal Inhalers

- Warm the inhaler in hand just before use.
- Gently insert the inhaler tip into one nostril, as shown in drawing C. Sniff deeply while inhaling.
- Wipe the inhaler after each use. Discard after 2–3 months even if the inhaler still smells medicinal.

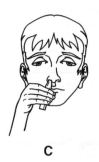

C

Pump Nasal Sprays

- Prime the pump before using it the first time. Hold the bottle with the nozzle placed between the first two fingers and the thumb placed on the bottom of the bottle.
- Tilt the head forward.
- Gently insert the nozzle tip into one nostril (see drawing B). Sniff deeply while depressing the pump once.
- Repeat with other nostril.

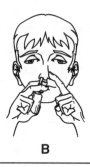

B

Nasal Drops

- Lie on bed with head tilted back and over the side of the bed, as shown in drawing D.
- Squeeze the bulb to withdraw medication from the bottle.
- Place the recommended number of drops into one nostril. Gently tilt head from side to side.
- Repeat with other nostril. Lie on bed for a couple of minutes after placing drops in the nose.
- Do not rinse the dropper.

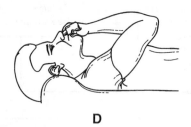

D

Note: Do not share the drug with anyone. Discard solutions if discolored or if contamination is suspected. Remove caps before use and replace tightly after each use. Do not use expired products.

the nasal passageways with a bulb syringe may be necessary if accumulation of mucus interferes with sleeping or eating. To use the syringe and avoid harm to the child, the caregiver should squeeze the large end of the bulb *before* inserting it, continue to squeeze the bulb while gently inserting the tip into the infant's nose, and then slowly release the squeezing pressure to draw out fluid. After the pressure is completely released, the syringe is removed from the infant's nose and the fluid expelled from the syringe by again compressing the bulb.

Proper hand hygiene reduces the transmission of cold viruses. The Centers for Disease Control and Prevention (CDC) encourages frequent hand cleansing with soap or soap substitutes

(e.g., hand sanitizers).[1] Not all hand sanitizers are effective at eradicating rhinoviruses from hands. Alcohol-based products containing isopropanol or ethanol (60%–80% concentration) are preferred but are short-acting and require frequent reapplication.[10] Chlorhexidine, povidone–iodine, and quaternary ammonium compounds are also effective alone or in combination with alcohol-based products.[10] Alcohol-based nasal sanitizers (e.g., Nozin) are also available but lack evidence of efficacy and safety. Use of antiviral disinfectants such as Lysol (kills >99% of rhinoviruses after 1 minute) and antiviral tissues such as Kleenex Anti-Viral (tissue layer containing citric acid and sodium lauryl sulphate) may also help prevent transmission to others.

Pharmacologic Therapy

Decongestants

Decongestants specifically treat sinus and nasal congestion. Decongestants are adrenergic agonists (sympathomimetics). Stimulation of alpha-adrenergic receptors constricts blood vessels, thereby decreasing sinusoid vessel engorgement and mucosal edema. There are three types of decongestants. Direct-acting decongestants (e.g., phenylephrine, oxymetazoline, and tetrahydrozoline) bind directly to adrenergic receptors. Indirect-acting decongestants (e.g., ephedrine) displace norepinephrine from storage vesicles in prejunctional nerve terminals and tachyphylaxis can develop as stored neurotransmitter is depleted. Mixed decongestants (e.g., pseudoephedrine) have both direct and indirect activity.

Systemic nonprescription decongestants include pseudoephedrine and phenylephrine. Intranasal nonprescription decongestants include the short-acting decongestants ephedrine, levmetamfetamine (L-desoxyephedrine), naphazoline, phenylephrine, and propylhexedrine, and the long-acting decongestants xylometazoline (8–10 hours) and oxymetazoline (12 hours). Ophthalmic nonprescription decongestants are also available (see Chapter 27).

Systemic decongestants are rapidly metabolized by monoamine oxidase (MAO) and catechol-O-methyltransferase in the gastrointestinal (GI) mucosa, liver, and other tissues. Pseudoephedrine is well absorbed after oral administration; phenylephrine has a low oral bioavailability (about 38%). Both pseudoephedrine and phenylephrine have short half-lives (pseudoephedrine, 6 hours; phenylephrine, 2.5 hours), and peak concentrations for both drugs occur at 0.5–2 hours after oral administration.

Decongestants are indicated for temporary relief of nasal and eustachian tube congestion and for cough associated with postnasal drip. Nonprescription decongestants are not approved by the Food and Drug Administration (FDA) to self-treat nasal congestion associated with sinusitis.

FDA-approved dosages for decongestants are listed in Tables 11–3[11,12] and 11–4.[11] Nonprescription decongestants are marketed in a variety of dosage formulations, and many combination products are available (Table 11–5).

Adhering to FDA-approved doses of decongestant products is very important, given that acute overdose can be life-threatening, especially in children. Systemic decongestant overdoses cause excessive central nervous system (CNS) stimulation, paradoxical CNS depression, cardiovascular collapse, shock, and coma. Treatment of decongestant overdoses is supportive.

Adverse effects associated with decongestants include cardiovascular stimulation (e.g., elevated blood pressure, tachycardia, palpitation, or arrhythmias) and CNS stimulation (e.g., restlessness, insomnia, anxiety, tremors, fear, or hallucinations). Children and older adults are more likely than other age groups to experience adverse effects. Adverse effects are more common with systemic decongestants because topical decongestants are minimally absorbed. However, accidental ingestion of nasal or ocular decongestants can cause serious adverse effects such as nausea, vomiting, drooling, hypotension, hyperthermia, lethargy, sedation, and coma. Adverse effects specifically related to topical decongestants include propellant- or vehicle-associated effects (e.g., burning, stinging, sneezing, or local dryness) and trauma from the tip of the administration device. Rhinitis medicamentosa (RM; i.e., rebound congestion) has been associated with topical decongestants. The exact cause is unknown, but short-acting products, preservative agents (e.g., benzalkonium chloride), and long duration of therapy have been suspected to contribute to the problem.[13] Currently, therapy of 3–5 days is the accepted duration to avoid RM. However, controversy exists and some studies show that durations of 10 days to 8 weeks appear to be safe and do not cause RM.[13] Further investigation is needed to determine the optimal duration of treatment. Treatment of RM consists of slowly withdrawing the topical decongestant (one nostril at a time); replacing the decongestant with topical normal saline, which soothes the irritated nasal mucosa; and, if needed, using topical corticosteroids and systemic decongestants. Two to 6 weeks of withdrawal measures may be necessary before mucous membranes return to normal. A nonprescription kit, RhinoStat, has been advertised to assist health care providers and patients with management of RM. The product creates a patient-specific mixture of the patient's topical decongestant product and a diluent; however, the kit is not FDA approved.

table 11–3	Dosage Guidelines for Nonprescription Systemic Nasal Decongestants		
	Dosage (maximum daily dosage)		
Drug	**Adults/Children ≥12 Years**	**Children 6 to <12 Years**	**Children 2 to <6 Years[a]**
Phenylephrine HCl	10 mg every 4 hours (60 mg)	5 mg every 4 hours (30 mg)	2.5 mg every 4 hours (15 mg)
Phenylephrine bitartrate	15.6 mg every 4 hours (62.4 mg)	7.8 mg every 4 hours (31.2 mg)	Not recommended for children < 6 years except under advice of PCP
Pseudoephedrine	60 mg every 4–6 hours (240 mg)	30 mg every 4–6 hours (120 mg)	15 mg every 4–6 hours (60 mg)

[a] FDA has advised that cough and cold medications not be used in children under 2 years of age.[12] Manufacturers have voluntarily updated cough and cold product labels to state "do not use" in children under 4 years of age.[26] These actions have not changed the official monograph for cold, cough, allergy, bronchodilator, and antiasthmatic drug products.[12]

Source: Reference 11.

Key: PCP = Primary care provider.

table

11–4 Dosage Guidelines for Nonprescription Topical Nasal Decongestants

Drug	Concentration (%)	Adults/Children ≥12 Years	Children 6 to <12 Years	Children 2 to <6 Years[a]
Sprays/Drops				
Ephedrine[b]	0.5	2–3 drops/sprays in each nostril not more often than every 4 hours	1–2 drops/sprays in each nostril not more often than every 4 hours	Not recommended for children < 6 years except under advice of PCP
Naphazoline	0.05	1–2 drops/sprays in each nostril not more often than every 6 hours	Not recommended for children < 12 years except under advice of PCP	Not recommended for children < 6 years except under advice of PCP
	0.025	—	1–2 drops/sprays in each nostril not more often than every 6 hours	Not recommended for children < 6 years except under advice of PCP
Oxymetazoline	0.05	2–3 drops/sprays in each nostril not more often than every 10–12 hours (max: 2 doses/24 hours)	2–3 drops/sprays in each nostril not more often than every 10–12 hours (max: 2 doses/24 hours)	Not recommended for children < 6 years except under advice of PCP
	0.025	—	—	2–3 drops/sprays in each nostril not more often than every 10–12 hours (max: 2 doses/24 hours)
Phenylephrine	1.0	2–3 drops/sprays in each nostril not more often than every 4 hours	Not recommended for children < 12 years except under advice of PCP	Not recommended for children < 6 years except under advice of PCP
	0.5	2–3 drops/sprays in each nostril not more often than every 4 hours	Not recommended for children < 12 years except under advice of PCP	Not recommended for children < 6 years except under advice of PCP
	0.25	2–3 drops/sprays in each nostril not more often than every 4 hours	2–3 drops/sprays in each nostril not more often than every 4 hours	Not recommended for children < 6 years except under advice of PCP
	0.125	—	—	2–3 drops/sprays in each nostril not more often than every 4 hours
Xylometazoline[b]	0.1	2–3 drops/sprays in each nostril not more often than every 8–10 hours	Not recommended for children < 12 years except under advice of PCP	Not recommended for children < 6 years except under advice of PCP
	0.05	—	2–3 drops/sprays in each nostril not more often than every 8–10 hours	2–3 drops/sprays in each nostril not more often than every 8–10 hours (max: 3 doses/24 hours)

Key: Max = Maximum; PCP = primary care provider.

[a] No recommended dosages exist for children < 2 years, except under the advice and supervision of a PCP.

[b] Products approved by FDA but not currently marketed in the United States

Source: Reference 11.

Decongestants interact with numerous drugs, as summarized in Table 11–6. Decongestants are contraindicated in patients receiving concomitant MAO inhibitors (MAOIs).

Decongestants may exacerbate diseases sensitive to adrenergic stimulation, such as hypertension, coronary heart disease, ischemic heart disease, diabetes mellitus, hyperthyroidism, elevated intraocular pressure, and prostatic hypertrophy. Patients with hypertension should use decongestants only with medical advice. No clear evidence exists that any one agent is safer than other agents in patients with hypertension. Products specifically marketed for patients with hypertension (e.g., Coricidin HBP)

do not contain decongestants. Those products usually contain a combination of ingredients that may or may not be appropriate depending on a patient's symptoms.

Health care providers should be aware of patients wishing to purchase large quantities of pseudoephedrine that may be used illegally to produce methamphetamine. In 2005, passage of the Combat Methamphetamine Epidemic Act changed the classification of pseudoephedrine to "scheduled listed chemical products."[14] That change in classification allowed limits to be placed on sales. All pseudoephedrine products must now be kept in secure areas (e.g., behind a pharmacy counter or in a locked cabinet),

table
11-5   **Selected Nonprescription Products for Nasal Decongestion**

Trade Name	Primary Ingredients
Topical Decongestants	
Afrin Original Nasal Spray	Oxymetazoline HCl 0.05%
Vicks Sinex Nasal Spray	Oxymetazoline HCl 0.05%
Zicam Extreme Congestion Relief Nasal Gel	Oxymetazoline HCl 0.05%
4-Way Fast Acting	Phenylephrine HCl 1%
Neo-Synephrine Regular Strength Nasal Spray	Phenylephrine HCl 0.5%
Little Noses Decongestant Nose Drops	Phenylephrine HCl 0.125%
Otrivin Nasal Spray (Canada)	Xylometazoline 0.1%
Nasal Decongestant Inhalers	
Benzedrex Inhaler	Propylhexedrine 250 mg
Vicks Vapo Inhaler	Levmetamfetamine (l-desoxyephedrine) 50 mg/inhaler
Systemic Decongestants	
Sudafed PE Congestion	Phenylephrine HCl 10 mg
Sudafed 24 Hour Long Acting	Pseudoephedrine HCl 240 mg
Sudafed 12 Hour	Pseudoephedrine HCl 120 mg
Nexafed[a]	Pseudoephedrine HCl 30 mg
Zephrex-D[b]	Pseudoephedrine HCl 30 mg
Combination Products	
Sudafed PE Pressure + Pain	Phenylephrine HCl 5 mg; acetaminophen 325 mg
Alka-Seltzer Plus Sinus	Phenylephrine bitartrate 7.8 mg; aspirin 325 mg
Vicks Dayquil Liquicaps	Phenylephrine HCl 5 mg; acetaminophen 325 mg; dextromethorphan hydrobromide 10 mg
Tylenol Cold Multi-Symptom Nighttime Cool Burst Liquid	Phenylephrine HCl 5 mg/15 mL; acetaminophen 325 mg/15 mL; dextromethorphan hydrobromide 10 mg/15 mL; doxylamine succinate 6.25 mg/15 mL
Triaminic Chest & Nasal Congestion Liquid	Phenylephrine HCl 2.5 mg/5 mL; guaifenesin 50 mg/5 mL
Aleve-D Sinus & Cold	Pseudoephedrine HCl 120 mg; naproxen sodium 220 mg
Mucinex D	Pseudoephedrine HCl 60 mg; guaifenesin 600 mg
Other Products	
Ocean Premium Saline Nasal Spray	Sodium chloride 0.65%
Vicks VapoRub	Camphor (4.8%); eucalyptus (1.2%); menthol (2.6%)

[a] Meth-deterring technology (Impede).
[b] Meth-deterring technology (Tarex).

and purchases are limited to 3.6 grams per day and 9 grams per month per patient.[14] The following information from each sale must be entered into a written or electronic logbook: product name, quantity sold, patient's name and address, and time and date of sale.[14] Patients must show valid identification to purchase pseudoephedrine and then sign the logbook. Some states and corporations have enacted stricter guidelines regarding the sale of pseudoephedrine.

Antihistamines

Reviews have shown that monotherapy with nonprescription antihistamines is not effective in reducing rhinorrhea and sneezing due to colds.[15,16] However, a combination of first-generation (sedating) antihistamines and decongestants showed some benefit in adults, but the significance of the data is questionable.[15,16] Apart from questions of efficacy, an important issue is whether potential benefits of sedating antihistamines outweigh known risks associated with these drugs. (See the discussion of antihistamines in the Allergic Rhinitis section.)

Local Anesthetics

A variety of products containing local anesthetics (e.g., benzocaine or dyclonine hydrochloride) is available for the temporary relief of sore throats (Table 11–7). Local anesthetic products may

table

11–6 Decongestant and Antihistamine Drug Interactions

Drug/Drug Class	Effect (drug-specific data)
Decongestants	
Antacids	Decreased elimination (pseudoephedrine)
Furazolidone; linezolid; MAOIs (e.g., phenelzine, selegiline); procarbazine	Severe hypertension; headache; hyperpyrexia
TCAs (amitriptyline, nortriptyline, imipramine)	Increased blood pressure (direct-acting decongestants); decreased decongestant activity (indirect-acting decongestants)
Antihistamines	
Amiodarone	Increased risk of QT interval prolongation (loratadine)
Antacids (aluminum and magnesium salts); rifampin	Decreased efficacy (fexofenadine)
CNS depressants (alcohol, sedatives)	Increased sedation (sedating antihistamines; cetirizine)
Cholinesterase inhibitors (e.g., donepezil, rivastigmine)	Worsened symptoms of Alzheimer's disease (sedating antihistamines)
Erythromycin; ketoconazole	Increased fexofenadine plasma concentration
Phenytoin	Decreased phenytoin elimination (chlorpheniramine)

Key: CNS = Central nervous system; MAOI = monoamine oxidase inhibitor; TCA = tricyclic antidepressant.

be used every 2–4 hours. Health care providers should counsel patients with a history of allergic reactions to anesthetics to avoid products containing benzocaine. Benzocaine has also been associated with methemoglobinemia, especially in children younger than 2 years, and should be avoided in this age group. Some products contain local antiseptics (e.g., cetylpyridinium chloride or hexylresorcinol) and/or menthol or camphor. Local

antiseptics are not effective for viral infections. Emerging evidence suggests that menthol and camphor may provide pain relief via stimulation of the TRPM8 or "menthol" receptor.[17]

Systemic Analgesics

Systemic analgesics (e.g., aspirin, acetaminophen, ibuprofen, or naproxen) are effective for aches or fever sometimes associated with colds. Concerns that use of aspirin and acetaminophen may increase viral shedding and prolong illness have not been proved.[18] Aspirin–containing products should not be used in children with viral illnesses because of the risk of Reye's syndrome. (See Chapter 5 for a complete discussion of those products, including the manufacturer's voluntary reduction of maximum daily dosages of Tylenol products sold in the United States [see section Acetaminophen and Table 5–3] and developments in liquid infant acetaminophen products [see section Patient Factors].)

table

11–7 Selected Nonprescription Products for Sore Throat

Trade Name	Primary Ingredients
Lozenges	
Cepacol Sore Throat Sugar Free	Benzocaine 15 mg
Chloraseptic Sore Throat	Benzocaine 6 mg; menthol 10 mg
Halls Fruit Breezers	Pectin 7 mg
Sucrets Classic	Dyclonine HCl 2 mg
Vicks VapoDrops	Menthol 1.7 mg (cherry) Menthol 3.3 mg (menthol)
Throat Sprays	
Cepacol Ultra Sore Throat Spray	Benzocaine 5%; glycerin 33%
Chloraseptic Sore Throat	Phenol 1.4%
Alternative Formulations	
Chloraseptic Sore Throat Lollipops[a]	Benzocaine 6 mg

[a] Indicated for children ≥ 3 years of age.

Antitussives and Protussives (Expectorants)

When present, cough associated with colds is usually nonproductive. The use of antitussives (codeine or dextromethorphan) has questionable efficacy in colds and is not recommended.[19] Guaifenesin, an expectorant, has not been proved effective in natural colds.[20] (See Chapter 12 for a complete discussion of those products).

Combination Products

Decongestants and antihistamines are marketed in many combinations, including combinations with analgesics, expectorants, and antitussives. Products are also marketed for daytime or nighttime use. Products for nighttime use usually contain a sedating antihistamine, whereas daytime products do not. Combination products are convenient, but the convenience must be weighed against the risks of taking unnecessary drugs.

Pharmacotherapeutic Comparison

As stated earlier, evidence does not support the use of antihistamines, antitussives, and expectorants for treatment of symptoms related to colds. Local anesthetics and systemic analgesics have good evidence for treatment of pain related to sore throat or fever related to colds.

Topical decongestants are convenient dosage forms and are effective in relieving nasal congestion; however, their use is limited to 3–5 days owing to concerns about RM. The major differences in topical decongestants are duration of action, dosage formulation (e.g., mist versus spray versus drops), moisture content, and preservative content.

Although many manufacturers have reformulated products with phenylephrine as a response to pseudoephedrine regulations, controversy exists with regard to comparison of the safety and efficacy of the systemic decongestants. Clear evidence that oral phenylephrine is safer than pseudoephedrine has yet to be presented.[21,22] Strong evidence supports the efficacy of oral dosage forms of pseudoephedrine, whereas efficacy of the current FDA-approved dose of phenylephrine has been highly debated.[21,23]

Product Selection Guidelines

Special Populations

Drug use during pregnancy and lactation is a balance between risk and benefit. Because most colds are self-limiting with bothersome rather than life-threatening symptoms, many health care providers recommend nondrug therapy. When drugs are considered, those with a long record of safety in animals and humans are preferred. To minimize possible adverse effects on the fetus or newborn, pregnant or lactating women should be advised to avoid products labeled as "extra strength," "maximum strength," or "long-acting," as well as combination products. Systemic decongestants should be avoided as human data suggest risk based on theoretically decreased fetal blood flow.[24,25] Also, pseudoephedrine has been linked to abdominal wall defects (gastroschisis) in newborns.[24,25] There is no clear association between birth defects and the use of intranasal decongestants during pregnancy.[24,25] Oxymetazoline is poorly absorbed after intranasal administration and is the preferred topical decongestant during pregnancy.

The American Academy of Pediatrics has found pseudoephedrine to be compatible with breast-feeding and to be the preferred decongestant for lactating mothers.[25] No human data are available for intranasal phenylephrine and oxymetazoline, so they are considered "probably compatible" in lactating mothers.[25] Because decongestants may decrease milk production, lactating mothers should monitor their milk production and drink extra fluids as needed. Dextromethorphan, guaifenesin, benzocaine, camphor (topical), and menthol (topical) have low risks of birth defects and have been found to be compatible with breast-feeding.[25]

Using nonprescription cold products in children is controversial owing to the lack of clinical evidence of safety and efficacy in this age group. Currently, FDA does not recommend nonprescription cold medications for children younger than 2 years because of the lack of efficacy and risk of misuse or overuse leading to adverse events and death.[12] Manufacturers have voluntarily updated product labeling to include the statement "Do not use in children under four years of age" and added warnings to antihistamine-containing products against their use for sedation purposes.[26] FDA continues to monitor and review the use of nonprescription cold medications in children between the ages of 2 and 11 years.[12] Health care providers should emphasize nondrug measures in children and, if pharmacotherapy is deemed necessary, parents should follow dosing instructions carefully and avoid combination products to avoid overdosage. To address the issue of inaccurate dosing, FDA released guidelines in May 2011 for liquid nonprescription drug products that include any type of dispensing device (dropper, cup, syringe, or spoon).[27,28] These products include liquid analgesics, liquid cough and cold products, and lactase replacement drops. The key points of the guidelines are as follows:

- A dosing device should be included with all oral liquid nonprescription products.
- The device should be calibrated to the dose recommended in the product directions.
- The device should be used only with the product in which it is packaged.
- The markings remain visible even when the liquid is in the device.

Patient Factors

As discussed earlier, it may be difficult to differentiate cold symptoms from some acute and chronic disorders (Table 11–1). If duration of symptoms is longer than 7–14 days or a chronic condition is suspected, patients should not self-treat. Patients with chronic conditions exacerbated by, or those overly sensitive to, adrenergic stimulation should avoid decongestants. Health care providers should educate patients who participate in organized sports that oral decongestants are considered "doping" products and should be used only in accordance with sport regulations.

Patient Preferences

Lozenges, soft chews, and nasal drug delivery forms may be preferred by patients who have difficulty swallowing or when access to water is not convenient. However, nasal delivery forms may be difficult to use for patients with severe arthritis or coordination problems.

For patients who prefer a nasal delivery form, each form has distinct advantages and disadvantages. Nasal sprays are simple to use, cover a large surface area, are relatively inexpensive, and have a fast onset of action. The disadvantages include imprecise dosage, a tendency for the tip to become clogged with repeated use, and a high risk of contamination from aspiration of nasal mucus into the bottle. Metered pump sprays deliver a more precise dose. Nasal drops are preferred for small children but can be difficult to use, cover a limited surface area, and pass easily into the larynx. There is also a high risk of contamination because of the tendency to touch the dropper to the nose during administration. Nasal inhalers are small and unobtrusive, but they require an unobstructed airway and sufficient airflow to distribute the drug to the nasal mucosa. Nasal inhalers lose efficacy after 2–3 months even when tightly capped because of dissipation of the active ingredient. Nasal polyps, enlarged turbinates, and abnormalities such as septal deviation may reduce the efficacy of topical dosage forms.

table

11-8   Selected Complementary Therapies for Colds and Allergies

Agent	Risks	Effectiveness
Botanical Natural Products (Scientific Name)		
African geranium [umckaloabo, active ingredient in Umcka ColdCare products] (*Pelargonium sidoides*)	Allergic reactions or GI disturbances	Some evidence for alleviating symptoms of acute rhinosinusitis associated with colds in adults
Ephedra [ma huang] (*Ephedra sinica*)	Tachycardia, hypertension, heart attack, stroke, seizure	Effective decongestant
Goldenseal (*Hydrastis canadensis*)	Potentially toxic, especially in patients with gluocose-6-dehydrogenase deficiency	Some evidence of anti-inflammatory effects of active ingredient berberine for treatment of pulmonary inflammation

Key: GI = Gastrointestinal.

Complementary Therapies

Numerous complementary therapies are marketed for the treatment of colds (Table 11–8; see also Chapter 51).[29–32] Zinc and high-dose vitamin C are popular therapies.

High local concentrations of zinc ions purportedly block the adhesion of human rhinovirus to the nasal epithelium and are also thought to inhibit viral replication by disrupting viral capsid formation. However, in vitro studies have shown only a modest antiviral effect. Formulations include tablets, capsules, chews, lozenges, syrups, and oral sprays. Nasal formulations were removed from the market because of anosmia (loss of smell).[33] Oral formulations may be associated with GI adverse effects (e.g., nausea, upset stomach, and bitter taste). Since the 1980s, the effectiveness of zinc has been highly debated. A meta-analysis of 17 trials concluded that oral zinc (lozenges or syrup) was effective in reducing cold symptoms or duration of the cold if started within 24 hours of symptom onset and administered every 2 hours while patient is awake. The study also reported prophylaxis with zinc for at least 5 months reduced the incidence of colds in healthy patients.[34]

The efficacy and safety of high-dose (e.g., ≥2 g/day) vitamin C (ascorbic acid) supplementation for prophylaxis and treatment of colds have been debated for more than 70 years. An analysis of 29 trials showed that, although routine use of high-dose vitamin C does not appear to prevent colds in the general population, it did reduce the duration by about 8% in adults and 14% in children.[35] In contrast, high-dose vitamin C prophylaxis was effective in preventing colds in a subgroup of patients subjected to severe physical stress (e.g., marathon runners).[35] Using vitamin C as treatment after the onset of a cold was not effective at reducing severity or duration of symptoms.[35] Regular use of high doses may increase the risk of kidney stones in men.[36] The clinical significance and risk–benefit ratio of these results are debatable. Doses of 4 g/day or greater are associated with diarrhea and other GI symptoms and, therefore, should not be recommended.

Products that claim to strengthen the immune system such as Airborne, Emergen-C Immune+, vitamin D, etc. are available but have not been proved to be effective in preventing colds. Various probiotic products are available and emerging research suggests that they may help support the immune system and prevent colds.[37] (See Chapters 23 and 51 for a complete discussion of those products.)

Assessment of Colds: A Case-Based Approach

After asking questions about the patient's symptoms, medical history, medication use (current and past), and the efficacy of past self-treatment of colds, the health care provider should conduct a brief physical assessment (Table 11–9). If the assessment and patient's answers do not reveal exclusions for self-treatment, the provider should recommend medications that target the patient's most troublesome symptoms.

Case 11–1 is an example of assessment of a patient with a cold.

Patient Counseling for Colds

Nondrug measures may be effective in relieving the discomfort of cold symptoms. The provider should explain the appropriate nondrug measures for the patient's particular symptoms. For patients who prefer to use nonprescription medications, the purpose of each medication should be described, and the patient should be counseled to use only medications that target his or

table

11-9   Physical Assessment of Patient Presenting with Cold Symptoms

1. Observe patient (look and listen for signs of chronic conditions, such as red, watery eyes; wheezing; productive cough; barrel chest; poorly perfused areas; enlarged lymph nodes; rash).

If equipment and privacy allow, conduct the following:

2. Obtain vitals (temperature, respiratory rate, pulse, and blood pressure).
3. Palpate sinuses and neck, and observe any pain/tenderness.
4. Visually examine throat for redness or exudates. If bacterial pharyngitis is suspected, run rapid strep test.
5. Auscultate chest to detect wheezing, crackles, and rapid or irregular heartbeat.

case

Relevant Evaluation Criteria	Scenario/Model Outcome

Information Gathering

1. Gather essential information about the patient's symptoms and medical history, including:

a. description of symptom(s) (i.e., nature, onset, duration, severity, associated symptoms)

Patient complains of nasal congestion and fatigue. Patient had sore throat 3 days ago; then congestion started and has progressively worsened.

b. description of any factors that seem to precipitate, exacerbate, and/or relieve the patient's symptom(s)

Congestion is worse in the morning when patient wakes up, then improves during the day. Congestion worsens again at night.

c. description of the patient's efforts to relieve the symptoms

Patient has tried hot showers, warm compresses, and a Neti pot rinse.

d. patient's identity

Toby Lewis

e. age, sex, height, and weight

19 years old, male, 6 ft, 200 lb

f. patient's occupation

College student

g. patient's dietary habits

Patient has a healthy, low-carbohydrate, low-fat diet. Occasionally patient consumes junk food and alcohol on weekends.

h. patient's sleep habits

Erratic because of studying late at night and social engagements

i. concurrent medical conditions, prescription and nonprescription medications, and dietary supplements

Type 1 diabetes; Lantus 40 units at bedtime; Humalog 5 units with meals; Men's One A Day multivitamin once a day; creatine-protein shake every morning

j. allergies

None

k. history of other adverse reactions to medications

None

l. other (describe) _____

Patient's temperature currently is 100°F (37.8°C), and blood pressure is 118/78 mm Hg. Patient's fasting blood glucose was 100 mg/dL this morning.

Assessment and Triage

2. Differentiate patient's signs/symptoms and correctly identify the patient's primary problem(s).

Onset of congestion after sore throat resolution, lack of high fever, indicative of a cold

3. Identify exclusions for self-treatment (Figure 11–1).

None

4. Formulate a comprehensive list of therapeutic alternatives for the primary problem to determine whether triage to a medical provider is required, and share this information with the patient or caregiver.

Options include:

(1) Recommend separate OTC products for each symptom: nasal saline or decongestant (topical or systemic) for congestion.

(2) Recommend that patient see his PCP for further evaluation and treatment.

(3) Recommend self-care until patient can consult his PCP.

(4) Take no action.

Plan

5. Select an optimal therapeutic alternative to address the patient's problem, taking into account patient preferences.

Recommend that patient use a nasal decongestant to relieve his congestion. Recommend oxymetazoline spray 0.05% 2–3 sprays in each nostril every 10–12 hours (max two doses in 24 hours). Do not use for more than 5 days.

6. Describe the recommended therapeutic approach to the patient or caregiver.

There are no exclusions for self-care. Because congestion is the only symptom, monotherapy with a decongestant is indicated.

7. Explain to the patient or caregiver the rationale for selecting the recommended therapeutic approach from the considered therapeutic alternatives.

"Decongestants may raise your blood glucose. Nasal formulations are not absorbed as much as oral formulations and may reduce the risk."

Relevant Evaluation Criteria	Scenario/Model Outcome
Patient Education	
8. When recommending self-care with nonprescription medications and/or nondrug therapy, convey accurate information to the patient or caregiver.	"Use 2–3 sprays of oxymetazoline in each nostril every 10–12 hours. Nasal congestion should significantly diminish in 10 minutes, and relief should last 10–12 hours after each administration. Nasal congestion will be temporarily relieved but may persist for 7–14 days. Do not use the nasal spray longer than 5 days. Most common adverse effects are nasal stinging or burning, sneezing, dryness. Monitor your blood glucose closely as this medication may raise it. A PCP should be consulted if congestion worsens or if headache or fever develops with treatment or lasts longer than 7–14 days. Store at room temperature with the cap tightly closed."
Solicit follow-up questions from the patient or caregiver.	"Is it OK for me to drink alcohol?"
Answer the patient's or caregiver's questions.	"Alcohol may worsen your congestion, so you should avoid drinking alcohol while you are sick."
Evaluation of Patient Outcome	
9. Assess patient outcome.	Follow up with a phone call in 7 days.

Key: OTC = Over-the-counter; PCP = primary care provider.

her specific symptoms. Patients need an explanation of possible adverse effects, drug interactions, and precautions or warnings. Finally, the provider should explain the signs and symptoms that indicate the disorder is worsening and that medical care should be sought. (See the box Patient Education for Colds.)

Evaluation of Patient Outcomes for Colds

Given that most colds are self-limiting, symptoms will usually resolve on their own in 7–14 days. For the majority of patients, targeted nonprescription therapy will relieve their cold symptoms. Patients should be monitored for worsening symptoms and progression of complications by measuring their temperature, assessing nasal secretions, assessing respirations for wheezing or shortness of breath, identifying productive cough, and asking about facial or neck pain. If complications are suspected, medical referral is necessary. Referral to a primary care provider (PCP) is also required for patients who meet the exclusions for self-treatment in Figure 11–1 or the warnings listed in the box Patient Education for Colds. Follow-up usually is not necessary for patients with uncomplicated colds, but telephone follow-up in 7–14 days may be deemed appropriate.

Allergic Rhinitis

Allergic rhinitis, a systemic disease with prominent nasal symptoms, is a worldwide problem that affects adults and children. An estimated 20% of adults and 40% of children in the United States have this disease, and the number of newly diagnosed cases in the

country has been steadily increasing over the past 3 decades.[38] An estimated 8% of adults and 11% of children in the United States are newly diagnosed with allergic rhinitis annually.[38] Annual direct costs (e.g., medications and office visits) are estimated to be $3.4 billion.[39] Addition of indirect costs (e.g., lost school- and workdays) increases this estimate to $11 billion.[39] Impaired quality of life creates additional significant, but yet to be quantified, intangible costs.

Symptoms of allergic rhinitis generally begin after the second year of life, and the disease is prevalent in children and adults ages 18–64 years.[40] After age 65 years, the number of cases decreases. The prevalence of allergic rhinitis is higher in the southern United States.[40]

Pathophysiology of Allergic Rhinitis

Allergic rhinitis affects the upper respiratory system. (The section Colds provides a detailed discussion of the respiratory anatomy and physiology.) Risk factors for developing allergic rhinitis include family history of atopy (allergic disorders) in one or both parents; filaggrin (skin barrier protein) gene mutation; elevated serum IgE greater than 100 IU/mL before age 6 years; higher socioeconomic class; eczema; and positive reaction to allergy skin tests.[41] Emerging evidence also suggests that diet may be a risk factor in children and adolescents. Children who consume three or more fast-food meals per week showed an increased incidence of allergic disorders.[42] The exact mechanism for that increase is not known but is thought to be related to higher content of fatty acids, especially trans-fatty acids, which trigger an immune response.[42] Allergic rhinitis is triggered by indoor and outdoor environmental allergens. Common outdoor aeroallergens (airborne environmental allergens) include pollen and mold spores. Other nonairborne pollens have also been

patient education for
Colds

The objectives of self-treatment are to (1) reduce symptoms, (2) improve functioning and sense of well-being, and (3) prevent spread of the disease. For most patients, carefully following product instructions and the self-care measures listed here will help ensure optimal therapeutic outcomes.

Nondrug Measures

- To prevent spreading a cold to others, follow these steps:
  - Frequently wash your hands with soap for at least 20 seconds.
  - Use facial tissues to cover your mouth and nose when coughing or sneezing, and then promptly throw the tissues away.
  - Use antiviral products such as Lysol to clean surfaces (e.g., doorknobs or telephones) that you may have touched.
- The following measures may provide relief or speed up recovery from a cold:
  - Getting adequate rest may help you recover more quickly.
  - Drinking fluids and using a humidifier or vaporizer may loosen mucus and promote sinus drainage.
  - Sucking on hard candy, gargling with salt water (½ to 1 teaspoon of salt per 8 ounces of warm water), or drinking fruit juices or hot tea with lemon may soothe a sore throat.

Nonprescription Medications

- Ask a health care provider to help you select medications that target the most bothersome symptoms.

Sore Throat and Cough

- Sore throat may be treated with anesthetic products and/or systemic pain relievers:
  - Allow lozenges, troches, and orally disintegrating strips to dissolve slowly in the mouth; do not chew or bite these products.
  - Benzocaine and dyclonine may numb the mouth and tongue. If these effects occur, do not eat or drink until they go away.
  - Seek medical attention if any of the following occur after using benzocaine products: pale, gray- or blue-colored skin, lips, and nail beds; headache; lightheadedness; shortness of breath; fatigue; and rapid heart rate.
- Cough related to a runny nose (postnasal drip) may be treated with a sedating antihistamine and decongestant combination.

Rhinorrhea (Runny Nose) and Sneezing

- See the box Patient Education for Allergic Rhinitis for treatment of rhinorrhea (runny nose) and sneezing.

Nasal Congestion

- Nasal congestion may be treated with topical or systemic decongestants, which constrict blood vessels in the nose to reduce congestion.
  - Systemic decongestants include pseudoephedrine and phenylephrine. Dosages are listed in Table 11–3.
  - Topical decongestants include ephedrine, naphazoline, oxymetazoline, phenylephrine, and xylometazoline. Dosages are listed in Table 11–4.
- Decongestants have the following adverse effects:
  - The most common adverse effects caused by systemic decongestants are cardiovascular stimulation (e.g., elevated blood pressure, rapid heart rate, palpitations, arrhythmias) and central nervous system stimulation (e.g., restlessness, insomnia, anxiety, tremors, fear, hallucinations).
  - Topical decongestants may cause any of the adverse effects listed for systemic decongestants. However, less of the topical medication gets into the body, so adverse effects are less common.
  - Topical decongestants may irritate the nose, or the bottle tip can injure the nose if used forcefully.
  - Topical decongestants may cause rebound congestion if used longer than 3–5 days.
- Note the following precautions for use of decongestants in persons with other medical conditions:
  - Persons with high blood pressure should use decongestants only with medical advice.
  - Persons with thyroid disorders, heart disease, glaucoma, or an enlarged prostate may experience worsening symptoms of their underlying disease if they take decongestants.
  - Persons with diabetes need to closely monitor their blood glucose concentrations and may need to adjust their dose of insulin if they take decongestants.
- Note the following drug interactions for decongestants:
  - Persons taking MAOIs (e.g., selegiline or phenelzine), certain antibiotics (linezolid and furazolidone), and the anticancer drug procarbazine should not take decongestants.
  - Persons taking tricyclic antidepressants should use decongestants with caution as these medications may increase or decrease blood pressure, depending on the specific decongestant.
  - Large amounts of some antacids or medicines that increase pH decrease the elimination of pseudoephedrine.
- Store all medications according to the manufacturer's recommendations. Do not use expired medications.

When to Seek Medical Attention

- Seek medical attention for the following situations:
  - Sore throat persists more than several days, is severe, or is associated with persistent fever, headache, or nausea or vomiting.
  - Cough does not improve within 7–14 days.
  - Symptoms worsen while nonprescription medications are being taken.
  - Signs and symptoms of bacterial infections develop (e.g., thick nasal or respiratory secretions that are not clear; temperature higher than 101.5°F [38.6°C]; shortness of breath; chest congestion; wheezing, rash, or significant ear pain).

Note about Pediatric Dosing

- Manufacturers of cough and cold medications have revised the labeling to state that these products should not be used in children younger than 4 years. Health care providers should stress this information to caregivers of infants and young children.

---

implicated. Pollutants (e.g., ozone and diesel exhaust particles) are considered environmental triggers and are becoming more of a concern in highly populated areas. Common indoor aeroallergens include house-dust mites, cockroaches, mold spores, cigarette smoke, and pet dander. Occupational aeroallergens include the following: wool dust, latex, resins, biologic enzymes, organic dusts (e.g., flour), and various chemicals (e.g., isocyanate and glutaraldehyde).

The pathogenesis of allergic rhinitis is complex, involving numerous cells and mediators, and consists of four phases.[43] First is the sensitization phase, which occurs on initial allergen exposure. The allergen stimulates beta-lymphocyte–mediated IgE production. Second is the early phase, occurring within minutes of subsequent allergen exposure. The early phase consists of rapid release of preformed mast cell mediators (e.g., histamine and proteases), as well as the production of additional mediators

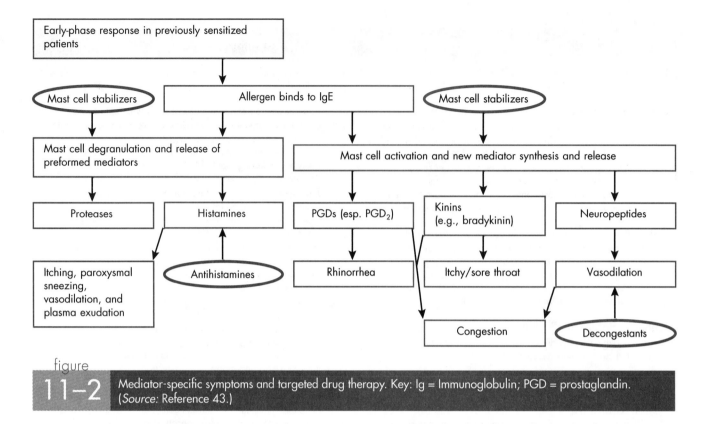

11–2

Mediator-specific symptoms and targeted drug therapy. Key: Ig = Immunoglobulin; PGD = prostaglandin. (*Source:* Reference 43.)

(e.g., prostaglandins, kinins, leukotrienes, and neuropeptides). Figure 11–2 shows mediator-specific symptoms. The third phase is cellular recruitment. Circulating leukocytes, especially eosinophils, are attracted to the nasal mucosa and release more inflammatory mediators. Fourth is the late phase, which begins 2–4 hours after allergen exposure; symptoms include mucus hypersecretion secondary to submucosal gland hypertrophy and congestion. Continued persistent inflammation "primes" the tissue, resulting in a lower threshold for allergic- and nonallergic-mediated triggers (e.g., cold air and strong odors).

Clinical Presentation of Allergic Rhinitis

Allergic rhinitis has been classified as seasonal allergic rhinitis ("hay fever") and perennial allergic rhinitis. New classifications, intermittent allergic rhinitis (IAR) and persistent allergic rhinitis (PER), were proposed in the late 1990s and are now the more accepted terminology.[41,44] Classification depends on the timing and duration of symptoms. Symptoms can be further classified as mild or moderate-severe (Table 11–10).[41] Symptoms of allergic rhinitis and common physical findings in these patients are summarized in Table 11–11[41,43] and can be used to differentiate allergic from nonallergic rhinitis. Table 11–12 lists causes of nonallergic rhinitis.[41,43] Systemic symptoms include fatigue, irritability, malaise, and cognitive impairment.

Acute complications of allergic rhinitis include sinusitis and otitis media with effusion. Chronic complications include nasal polyps, sleep apnea, sinusitis, and hyposmia (diminished sense of smell).[39,41] Allergic rhinitis and asthma share a common pathology, and allergic rhinitis has been implicated in the development of asthma and exacerbations of preexisting asthma in children and adults. Depression, anxiety, delayed speech development, and facial or dental abnormalities have also been linked to allergic rhinitis.[39,41]

Treatment of Allergic Rhinitis
Treatment Goals

Allergic rhinitis cannot be cured. The goals of therapy are to reduce symptoms and improve the patient's functional status and sense of well-being. Treatment is individualized to provide optimal symptomatic relief and/or control.

11–10 | Classification of Allergic Rhinitis

Duration	Severity
Intermittent Symptoms occur ≤4 days per week OR ≤4 weeks.	**Mild** Symptoms do not impair sleep or daily activities[a]; no troublesome symptoms.
	Moderate-Severe One or more of the following occurs: impairment of sleep; impairment of daily activities[a]; troublesome symptoms.
Persistent Symptoms occur >4 days per week AND >4 weeks.	**Mild** Symptoms do not impair sleep or daily activities[a]; no troublesome symptoms.
	Moderate-Severe One or more of the following occurs: impairment of sleep; impairment of daily activities[a]; troublesome symptoms.

[a] Daily activities include work, school, sports, and leisure.
Source: Reference 41.

table

11–11   Differentiation of Allergic Rhinitis from Nonallergic Rhinitis

Symptoms/Findings	Allergic Rhinitis	Nonallergic Rhinitis[a]
Symptom presentation	Bilateral symptoms that are worst upon awakening, improve during the day, then may worsen at night	Unilateral symptoms common but can be bilateral; constant day and night
Sneezing	Frequent, paroxysmal	Little or none
Rhinorrhea	Anterior, watery	Posterior, watery or thick and/or muco-purulent (associated with an infection)
Pruritus (itching) of eyes, nose, and/or palate	Frequent	Not present
Nasal obstruction	Variable	Usually present and often severe
Conjunctivitis (red, irritated eyes with prominent conjunctival blood vessels)	Frequent	Not present
Pain	Sinus pain due to congestion may be present; throat pain due to postnasal drip irritation may be present.	Variable depending on cause
Anosmia	Rare	Frequent
Epistaxis	Rare	Recurrent
Facial, nasal, or throat features	"Allergic shiners" (periorbital darkening secondary to venous congestion) "Dennie's lines" (wrinkles beneath the lower eyelids) "Allergic crease" (horizontal crease just about bulbar portion of the nose secondary to the "allergic salute") "Allergic salute" (patient will rub the tip of the nose upward with the palm of the hand) "Allergic gape" (open-mouth breathing secondary to nasal obstruction) Nonexudative cobblestone appearance of posterior oropharynx	Nasal polyps Nasal septal deviation Enlarged tonsils and/or adenoids

[a] Depending on the cause of the nonallergic rhinitis, not all symptoms may be exhibited.

Source: References 41 and 43.

General Treatment Approach

Allergic rhinitis is treated in three steps: allergen avoidance, pharmacotherapy, and immunotherapy.[41,43] Health care providers should maximize each step before going on to the next intervention. Patient education is an important part of all three steps, especially regarding the administration of nonprescription medications (for instructions, see Table 11–2 for intranasal preparations and Chapter 27 for ocular drugs). The algorithm in Figure 11–3 outlines the self-treatment of IAR and PER and lists exclusions for self-treatment.[41,44] Because allergen avoidance is usually not sufficient to provide complete relief of allergic rhinitis, targeted therapy with single-entity drugs is usually initiated. Nonprescription therapy with intranasal corticosteroids, antihistamines, or decongestants usually treats most symptoms. Drugs with different mechanisms of action or delivery systems may be added if single-drug therapy does not provide adequate relief, or if symptoms are already moderately severe, particularly intense, or long-lasting.

Nonpharmacologic Therapy

Allergen avoidance is the primary nonpharmacologic measure for allergic rhinitis. Avoidance strategies depend on the specific allergen. House-dust mites (*Dermatophagoides* spp.), found in all but the driest regions of the United States, thrive in warm, humid environments. The main allergen is a fecal glycoprotein, but other mite proteins and proteases are also allergenic. Avoidance strategies, targeted at reducing the mite population, include lowering the household humidity to less than 40%, applying acaricides, and reducing mite-harboring dust by removing carpets, upholstered furniture, stuffed animals, and bookshelves from the patient's bedroom and other rooms if possible. Mite populations in bedding are reduced by encasing the mattress, box springs, and pillows with mite-impermeable materials. Bedding that cannot be encased should be washed at least weekly in hot (130°F [54.4°C]) water. Bedding that cannot be encased or laundered should be discarded.

Outdoor mold spores are prevalent in late summer and fall, especially on calm, clear, dry days. *Alternaria* and *Cladosporium* are common outdoor mold allergens; *Penicillium* and *Aspergillus* are common indoor molds. Avoiding activities that disturb decaying plant material (e.g., raking leaves) lessens exposure to outdoor mold. Indoor mold exposure is minimized by lowering household humidity, removing houseplants, venting food preparation areas and bathrooms, repairing damp basements or crawl spaces, and frequently applying fungicide to obviously moldy areas.

Cat-derived allergens (Fel d1; proteins secreted through sebaceous glands in the skin) are small and light, and they stay airborne for several hours. Cat allergens can be found in the house months after the cat is removed. Although unproved, weekly cat baths may reduce the allergen load.

table	
11–12	**Causes of Nonallergic Rhinitis**

Hormonal

Pregnancy, puberty, thyroid disorders

Structural

Septal deviation, adenoid hypertrophy

Drug-Induced

Cocaine, beta-blockers, ACEIs, chlorpromazine, clonidine, reserpine, hydralazine, oral contraceptives, aspirin or other NSAIDs, overuse of topical decongestants

Systemic Inflammatory

Eosinophilic nonallergic rhinitis (NARES)

Lesions

Nasal polyps, neoplasms

Traumatic

Recent facial or head trauma

Autonomic (Vasomotor)

Age-related; physical or chemical agent causes parasympathetic hyperactivity

Key: ACEI = Angiotensin-converting enzyme inhibitor; NSAID = nonsteroidal anti-inflammatory drug.
Source: References 41 and 43.

Cockroaches are major urban allergens. To eliminate cockroaches, patients should be encouraged to keep kitchen areas clean, keep food stored tightly sealed, and treat infested areas with baits or pesticides.

Pollutants (e.g., ozone and diesel fumes) are an additional concern in urban environments. Pollutants such as diesel exhaust particles are especially irritating to the respiratory tract and have been shown to increase the severity of allergic rhinitis.[41] Patients whose allergies are triggered by air pollutants should be aware of the air quality index (AQI; a measure of five major air pollutants per 24 hours) and plan outdoor activities when the AQI is low.

In general, trees pollinate in spring, grasses in early summer, and ragweed from mid-August to the first fall frost. Knowledge of pollen counts (the number of pollen grains per cubic meter per 24 hours) helps patients plan outdoor activities. Most patients are symptomatic when pollen counts are very high, and only very sensitive patients have symptoms when pollen counts are low. Pollen counts are highest early in the morning and lowest after rainstorms clear the air. Avoiding outdoor activities when pollen counts are high and closing house and car windows reduce pollen exposure.

Ventilation systems with high-efficiency particulate air (HEPA) filters remove pollen, mold spores, and cat allergens from household air but not fecal particles from house–dust mites, which settle to the floor too quickly to be filtered. Filters need to be changed regularly to maintain effectiveness. The systems are expensive and not effective for all patients. HEPA filters are also found in some vacuum cleaners. Weekly vacuuming of carpets, drapes, and upholstery with a HEPA filter-equipped vacuum cleaner may help reduce household allergens, including house-dust mites.[43]

Nasal wetting agents (e.g., saline, propylene, and polyethylene glycol sprays or gels) or nasal irrigation with warm saline (isotonic or hypertonic) delivered via a syringe or Neti pot may relieve nasal mucosal irritation and dryness, thus decreasing nasal stuffiness, rhinorrhea, and sneezing. That process also aids in the removal of dried, encrusted, or thick mucus from the nose. No significant adverse effects have been noted with nasal wetting agents. Mild stinging or burning has been noted with saline irrigation. Only distilled, sterile, or boiled tap water should be used to prepare nasal irrigation solutions because of the risk of rare but serious infections.

Pharmacologic Therapy

Intranasal corticosteroids (INCS) have been shown to be the most effective treatment for most symptoms of allergic rhinitis.[43,44] However, until October 2013, INCS were only available by prescription.[45] Other nonprescription options include ocular and oral antihistamines, topical and oral decongestants, and mast cell stabilizers. INCS, antihistamines, and mast cell stabilizers should be used regularly rather than episodically. Patients should start taking those products at least 1 week before symptoms typically appear or as soon as possible before expected allergen exposures. Length of therapy with those medications should be individualized according to duration and severity of symptoms, pattern of allergen exposure (episodic or continuous), and geographical location.

Intranasal corticosteroids

INCS, also known as glucocorticoids, are very effective treatments for nasal symptoms such as itching, rhinitis, sneezing, and congestion as they inhibit multiple cell types and mediators, including histamine, and effectively stop the "allergic cascade."[44] Triamcinolone acetonide (Nasacort Allergy 24 HR) and fluticasone propionate (Flonase Allergy Relief) are currently the only two INCS approved for nonprescription use.[45]

Intranasal triamcinolone acetonide and fluticasone propionate have minimal systemic absorption. However, patients who are sensitive to INCS or use higher-than-recommended doses may experience systemic effects.

Both triamcinolone acetonide and fluticasone propionate are approved for nonprescription use to treat nasal allergy symptoms (nasal congestion, runny nose, sneezing, and itchy nose). Triamcinolone acetonide is approved for use in adults and children ages 2 years and older, whereas fluticasone propionate is approved for use in adults and children ages 4 years and older.[45]

The dosage of triamcinolone acetonide for children ages 2–5 years is 1 spray in each nostril daily (110 mcg/day). Children ages 6–12 years should be started on the same dosage; if symptoms are not relieved, 2 sprays in each nostril daily (220 mcg/day) may be used. The approved adult dosage is 220 mcg/day; once symptom control is achieved, some adults may be able to titrate down to 110 mcg/day. The dosage of fluticasone propionate for children ages 4–11 years is 1 spray in each nostril daily (100 mcg/day). Adults and children ages 12 years and older should use 2 sprays in each nostril daily (200 mcg/day) for 1 week; if complete symptom control is achieved, they can titrate down to 1 spray in each nostril daily. Complete symptom control may not be seen for up to 1 week. Patients should be instructed to shake the bottle well before each use and discard the product

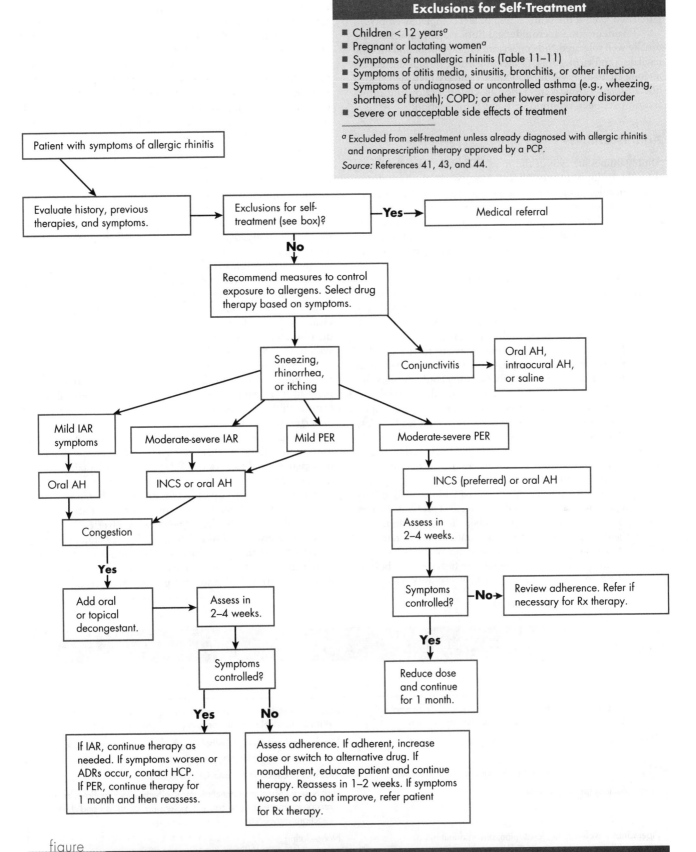

figure
11–3

Self-care of allergic rhinitis. Key: ADR = Adverse drug reaction; AH = antihistamine; COPD = chronic obstructive pulmonary disorder; HCP = health care provider; IAR = intermittent allergic rhinitis; INCS = intranasal corticosteroids; PER = persistent allergic rhinitis; PCP = primary care provider; Rx = prescription. (*Source:* References 41, 43, and 44.)

after a total of 60 or 120 doses, depending on which size was purchased, even if the bottle does not feel completely empty.

Triamcinolone acetonide and fluticasone propionate are usually well tolerated. Side effects are usually minor and include nasal discomfort, bleeding, or sneezing. More serious side effects include changes in vision, glaucoma, cataracts, increased risk of infection, and growth inhibition in children. No drug interactions have been reported with either medication.

Antihistamines

Antihistamines are one of the most frequently prescribed drug classes in the United States.[46] These drugs are classified as sedating (first-generation, nonselective) or nonsedating (second-generation, peripherally selective). The role of sedating antihistamines in treating allergic rhinitis is controversial. Sedating antihistamines are effective, readily available without a prescription, and relatively inexpensive. However, these antihistamines expose patients to risks of anticholinergic effects and should be used with caution.

Antihistamines compete with histamine at central and peripheral histamine$_1$ (H$_1$)-receptor sites, preventing the histamine–receptor interaction and subsequent mediator release. In addition, second-generation antihistamines inhibit the release of mast cell mediators and may decrease cellular recruitment.

Differences among antihistamines relate to the rapidity and degree to which they penetrate the blood–brain barrier as well as to their receptor specificity. Sedating antihistamines are highly lipophilic molecules that readily cross the blood–brain barrier. Nonsedating antihistamines, large protein-bound lipophobic molecules with charged side chains, do not readily cross the blood–brain barrier. Both types of antihistamines are highly selective for H$_1$ receptors but have little effect on H$_2$, H$_3$, or H$_4$ receptors. The sedating antihistamines have anticholinergic, antiserotonin, and anti-alpha-adrenergic effects.

Each antihistamine chemical class (Table 11–13) differs slightly in terms of its activity and adverse effect profile.[47,48] Most sedating antihistamines are well absorbed after oral administration with time to peak plasma concentrations in the range of 1.5–3 hours. Protein binding is in the range of 78%–99%, and sedating antihistamines undergo significant first-pass metabolism through the cytochrome P450 system. Half-lives vary widely, for example, 2–10 hours for diphenhydramine versus 20–24 hours for chlorpheniramine.

The nonsedating antihistamines are also rapidly absorbed after oral administration, with time to peak plasma concentrations in the range of 1–3 hours. Loratadine has the highest protein binding at 97% and is extensively metabolized by the liver to an active metabolite (descarboethoxyloratadine), whereas cetirizine and fexofenadine are minimally metabolized. Half-lives range from 8 hours (loratadine and cetirizine) to 14 hours (fexofenadine).

Antihistamines are indicated for relief of symptoms of allergic rhinitis (e.g., itching, sneezing, and rhinorrhea) and other types of immediate hypersensitivity reactions. FDA-approved dosages for systemic antihistamines are listed in Table 11–14.[11] Nonprescription antihistamines are marketed as immediate- and sustained-release tablets and capsules, chewable tablets, oral disintegrating tablets, solutions, and syrups. Alcohol-, sucrose-, and dye-free formulations are available. (See Chapter 27 for ocular antihistamines.)

Sedating antihistamine overdoses are characterized by excessive H$_1$-receptor and cholinergic-receptor blockade and by alpha-adrenergic and serotonergic activity.[47] Overdoses also cause excessive blockade of fast sodium channels and potassium channels, thus leading to cardiac symptoms (tachycardia and conduction abnormalities, including torsades de pointes).[47] CNS symptoms include toxic psychosis, hallucinations, agitation, lethargy, tremor, insomnia, or tonic-clonic seizures. Children tend to be more sensitive to CNS excitatory effects and adults are more likely to experience CNS depression.[47] Peripheral symptoms include hyperpyrexia, mydriasis, vasodilation, decreased exocrine secretion, urinary retention, decreased GI motility, dystonic reactions, and rhabdomyolysis. Overdoses of nonsedating antihistamines are characterized by drowsiness, restlessness/hyperactivity, and tachycardia. Treatment of antihistamine overdoses is supportive.

The adverse effect profile of systemic antihistamines varies widely and depends on the receptor activity, chemical structure, and lipophilicity of the drug. The primary adverse effects, CNS effects (depression and stimulation) and anticholinergic effects, are common with first-generation antihistamines but are rarely seen with second-generation agents. CNS-depressive effects include sedation and impaired performance (e.g., impaired

table

11–13 Antihistamine Classes

Class (specific drug entities)	Properties
Alkylamines (brompheniramine, chlorpheniramine, dexbrompheniramine, dexchlorpheniramine, pheniramine, triprolidine)	Moderately sedating; strong anticholinergic effects; higher risk of paradoxical CNS stimulation compared with other classes
Ethanolamines (clemastine, diphenhydramine, doxylamine)	Highly sedating; strong anticholinergic effects; large doses cause seizures and arrhythmias
Ethylenediamines (pyrilamine, tripelennamine, thonzylamine)	Weak CNS effects; increased GI effects
Phenothiazines (promethazine)	Highly sedating; strong anticholinergic effects; block alpha-adrenergic receptors; more likely to cause hypotension; akathisia and dystonic reactions may occur
Piperidines (fexofenadine, loratadine, phenindamine)	Nonsedating
Piperazines (cetirizine, chlorcyclizine, hydroxyzine, levocetirizine, meclizine)	Minimally to moderately sedating

Source: References 46 and 47.
Key: CNS = Central nervous system; GI = gastrointestinal.

table

11–14 Dosage Guidelines for Systemic Nonprescription Antihistamines

Drug	Dosage (maximum daily dosage)		
	Adults/Children ≥12 Years	**Children 6 to <12 Years**	**Children 2 to <6 Years**[a]
Brompheniramine maleate	4 mg every 4–6 hours (24 mg)	2 mg every 4–6 hours (12 mg)	1 mg every 4–6 hours (6 mg)
Cetirizine HCl[b]	10 mg every 24 hours	5–10 mg every 24 hours (10 mg)	2.5 mg every 12 hours or 2.5–5.0 mg every 24 hours (5 mg)
Chlorcyclizine HCl[c]	25 mg every 6–8 hours (75 mg)	Not recommended for children < 12 years except under advice of PCP	—
Chlorpheniramine maleate	4 mg every 4–6 hours (24 mg)	2 mg every 4–6 hours (12 mg)	1 mg every 4–6 hours (6 mg)
Clemastine fumarate	1.34 mg every 12 hours (2.68 mg)	Not recommended for children < 12 years except under advice of PCP	—
Dexbrompheniramine maleate	2 mg every 4–6 hours (12 mg)	1 mg every 4–6 hours (6 mg)	0.5 mg every 4–6 hours (3 mg)
Dexchlorpheniramine maleate	2 mg every 4–6 hours (12 mg)	1 mg every 4–6 hours (6 mg)	—
Diphenhydramine citrate	38–76 mg every 4–6 hours (456 mg)	19–38 mg every 4–6 hours (228 mg)	9.5 mg every 4–6 hours (57 mg)
Diphenhydramine HCl	25–50 mg every 4–6 hours (300 mg)	12.5–25 mg every 4–6 hours (150 mg)	6.25 mg every 4–6 hours (37.5 mg)
Doxylamine succinate	7.5–12.5 mg every 4–6 hours (75 mg)	3.75–6.25 mg every 4–6 hours (37.5 mg)	1.9–3.125 mg every 4–6 hours (18.75 mg)
Fexofenadine[d]	60 mg every 12 hours or 180 mg every 24 hours (180 mg)	30 mg every 12 hours (60 mg)	30 mg every 12 hours (60 mg)
Loratadine	10 mg every 24 hours (10 mg)	10 mg every 24 hours (10 mg)	5 mg every 24 hours (5 mg)
Phenindamine tartrate[c]	25 mg every 4–6 hours (150 mg)	12.5 mg every 4–6 hours (75 mg)	6.25 mg every 4–6 hours (37.5 mg)
Pheniramine maleate	12.5–25 mg every 4–6 hours (150 mg)	6.25–12.5 mg every 4–6 hours (75 mg)	3.125–6.25 mg every 4–6 hours (37.5 mg)
Pyrilamine maleate	25–50 mg every 6–8 hours (200 mg)	12.5–25 mg every 6–8 hours (100 mg)	6.25–12.5 mg every 6–8 hours (50 mg)
Thonzylamine HCl[c]	50–100 mg every 4–6 hours (600 mg)	25–50 mg every 4–6 hours (300 mg)	12.5–25.0 mg every 4–6 hours (150 mg)
Triprolidine HCl[c]	2.5 mg every 4–6 hours (10 mg)	1.25 mg every 4–6 hours (5 mg)	Age 4–6 years: 0.938 mg every 4–6 hours (3.744 mg) Age 2 to <4 years: 0.625 mg every 4–6 hours (2.5 mg) 4 months to <2 years: 0.313 mg every 4–6 hours (1.25 mg)

Key: PCP = Primary care provider.

[a] With the exception of cetirizine, fexofenadine, and loratadine, these products are not recommended for children younger than 6 years, except with the advice and supervision of a PCP. FDA recommends that the labels on nonprescription products not provide dosing information for children younger than 6 years.

[b] For adults older than 65 years, 10 mg cetirizine is not recommended, except with the advice and supervision of a PCP.

[c] Drug is FDA approved but not currently marketed in the United States.

[d] For adults older than 65 years, fexofenadine is not recommended, except with the advice and supervision of a PCP.

Source: Reference 11.

driving performance, poor work performance, incoordination, reduced motor skills, and impaired information processing).[48] CNS-stimulatory effects include anxiety, hallucinations, appetite stimulation, muscle dyskinesias, and activation of epileptogenic foci. Adverse effects associated with cholinergic blockage include dryness of the eyes and mucous membranes (mouth, nose, vagina); blurred vision; urinary hesitancy and retention; constipation; and reflex tachycardia.

Antihistamines interact with numerous drugs (Table 11–6). All antihistamines decrease or prevent immediate dermal reactivity and should be discontinued at least 4 days before scheduled allergy skin testing. Fexofenadine should not be taken with any fruit juices (e.g., grapefruit, apple, or orange). Fruit juice is thought to reduce absorption of fexofenadine by directly inhibiting intestinal organic anion transporting polypeptides (OATPs), specifically OATP1A2.[49] Separating fexofenadine dose and fruit juice consumption by at least 2 hours will avoid this interaction.[49]

Sedating antihistamines are contraindicated in newborns or premature infants, lactating women, and patients with narrow-angle glaucoma. Additional contraindications include acute asthma exacerbation, stenosing peptic ulcer, symptomatic prostatic hypertrophy, bladder–neck and pyloroduodenal obstruction, and concomitant use of MAOIs. Formulations of 12- and 24-hour sustained-release loratadine/pseudoephedrine combination products are contraindicated in patients with esophageal narrowing, abnormal esophageal peristalsis, or a history of difficulty swallowing tablets.

Patients with lower respiratory tract diseases (e.g., emphysema and chronic bronchitis) should use sedating antihistamines with caution. Patients requiring mental alertness should not use sedating antihistamines and should use cetirizine with caution. Patients may be impaired even if they do not feel drowsy or if they have taken the dose the evening before. The sedating antihistamines are photosensitizing drugs. Patients should be advised to use sunscreens and wear protective clothing.

Combination Products

Antihistamines are marketed in combination with decongestants and analgesics. Those combinations are also available in sustained-release formulations, allowing convenient dosage regimens. However, these combination products should be used with caution because of the increased risk of adverse effects, especially insomnia, which compounds daytime fatigue already associated with this disease.

Decongestants

Congestion is a common allergic rhinitis symptom controllable with systemic decongestants or short-term (≤5 days) topical nasal decongestants. (See discussion of decongestants in the section Colds.)

Cromolyn Sodium

Cromolyn is a mast cell stabilizer indicated for preventing and treating the symptoms of allergic rhinitis. Cromolyn is thought to work by blocking the influx of calcium into mast cells thereby preventing mediator release. Less than 7% of an intranasal cromolyn dose is absorbed systemically, and what little is absorbed has no systemic activity. The absorbed drug is rapidly excreted unchanged in the feces and urine, with a half-life of 1–2 hours.

Cromolyn is approved for patients ages 2 years or older; the recommended dosage is 1 spray in each nostril 3–6 times daily at regular intervals.[11] Treatment is more effective if started before symptoms begin. It may take 3–7 days for initial treatment efficacy to become apparent and 2–4 weeks of continued therapy to achieve maximal therapeutic benefit. Sneezing is the most common side effect reported for intranasal cromolyn. Other adverse effects include nasal stinging and burning. No drug interactions have been reported with intranasal cromolyn.

Pharmacotherapeutic Comparison

INCS have been shown to be the most effective treatment for moderate-severe IAR and both types of PER. Monotherapy with INCS is considered first-line.[41,43,44] If additional symptom control is needed, combination therapy with antihistamines, decongestants, or mast cell stabilizers can be initiated. Sedating antihistamines are effective, and some evidence does suggest that this group of drugs may be more effective than nonsedating antihistamines in treating symptoms of allergic rhinitis.[50] However, this evidence is based on trials using the maximum daily dosage (50 mg) of diphenhydramine.[50] Sedating antihistamines have a quick onset of action but also have shorter duration of action and require multiple daily doses. The risks of cognition impairment and sedation have been well established with this class of drugs.[48] The World Health Organization and numerous health care providers now recommend nonsedating antihistamines as the nonprescription therapy of choice on the basis of their efficacy and safety profile, quick onset of action, and long duration, which allows once-daily dosing.[41,49]

Cetirizine has been shown to be a more potent antihistamine than loratadine or fexofenadine.[49] However, unlike loratadine and fexofenadine, cetirizine causes sedation (in about 10% of patients).

Product Selection Guidelines

Special Populations

Because pregnancy is a common cause of nonallergic rhinitis, pregnant women should be referred for differential diagnosis. If allergic rhinitis is confirmed and nonprescription therapy is approved by a PCP, several treatment choices are available.[24,25] Intranasal cromolyn is considered compatible with pregnancy and is a first-line option.[24,25] Diphenhydramine and chlorpheniramine are considered compatible with pregnancy.[25] Chlorpheniramine is the first-generation antihistamine of choice in pregnancy because of its long history of safety.[24] If chlorpheniramine is not tolerated, loratadine and cetirizine are considered to have low risk and are preferred alternatives.[24,49] Fexofenadine is considered to have moderate risk.[25] Intranasal fluticasone propionate is considered compatible with pregnancy.[25] Systemic use of triamcinolone acetonide has been linked to cleft palate and low birth weight; however, intranasal use is considered probably compatible with pregnancy because of minimal systemic absorption.[25]

Lactating women diagnosed with allergic rhinitis and approved for self-treatment by a PCP have fewer options. Because of its limited systemic absorption, intranasal cromolyn is a good choice, and there are no reports of adverse effects on nursing infants.[25] Triamcinolone acetonide has a low molecular weight and is thought to be excreted in breast milk. However, there are no reports of intranasal triamcinolone acetonide or fluticasone propionate causing harm in nursing infants.[25] Antihistamines are contraindicated during lactation because of their ability to pass into breast milk. There have been reports of drowsiness and irritability in infants after mothers took clemastine.[25] Short-acting chlorpheniramine, fexofenadine, or loratadine seems to be the best option if an oral antihistamine is needed, but the antihistamine should be used with caution and under the supervision of a PCP. If an oral antihistamine is used during lactation, the mother should avoid long-acting and high-dose antihistamines and should take the dose at bedtime after the last feeding of the day.[25]

Because of concerns of undiagnosed asthma, children younger than 12 years should be referred to a PCP for differential diagnosis.[41] If nonprescription therapy is approved by a PCP, several treatment choices are available for children.[41,49] Intranasal cromolyn and triamcinolone acetonide are safe for children ages 2 years and older, and intranasal fluticasone propionate is safe for children 4 years and older. However, these products may be difficult for children to self-administer. In addition, triamcinolone acetonide and fluticasone propionate have been linked to growth inhibition in children; FDA-mandated labeling for the nonprescription products encourages parents to speak to a health care provider if they plan to use these products in children longer than 2 months per year.[45] Loratadine is the nonprescription antihistamine of choice,

followed by fexofenadine and cetirizine. Sedating antihistamines should be avoided in children because of paradoxical excitation and risk for serious adverse events with misuse.[49]

Sedating antihistamines should be avoided in elderly patients as they are more likely than younger adults to be taking concomitant medications with anticholinergic properties and have increased risk of CNS-depressive adverse effects, including confusion as well as hypotension.[51] Those adverse effects contribute to a higher risk of falling in the elderly.[51] Loratadine and intranasal cromolyn are drugs of choice in the older population. Dosages of fexofenadine should be adjusted in patients with renal impairment, whereas loratadine and cetirizine should be adjusted in patients with renal and/or hepatic impairment.

Patient Factors and Preferences

The duration of treatment and the presence of concomitant symptoms will determine which product is selected (Table 11–15). Product selection may also be based on side effect profiles and cost. For example, all first-generation antihistamines are sedating, but

table 11–15 Selected Nonprescription Products for Allergic Rhinitis

Trade Name	Primary Ingredients
Systemic First-Generation Antihistamine Products	
Chlor-Trimeton Allergy (4, 8, or 12 Hour) Tablets	Chlorpheniramine 4, 8, or 12 mg, respectively
Dayhist Allergy Tablets	Clemastine fumarate 1.34 mg
Benadryl Allergy Tablets	Diphenhydramine HCl 25 mg
Children's Benadryl Allergy Relief Syrup	Diphenhydramine HCl 12.5 mg/5 mL
Kids-EEZE Allergy Soft Chews	Diphenhydramine HCl 12.5 mg
Systemic Second-Generation Antihistamine Products	
Zyrtec Tablets	Cetirizine 10 mg
Children's Zyrtec Syrup	Cetirizine 5 mg/5 mL
Allegra Allergy 24 hour Tablets	Fexofenadine 180 mg
Children's Allegra Orally Disintegrating Tablets[a]	Fexofenadine 30 mg
Claritin Non-Drowsy Tablets	Loratadine 10 mg
Alavert Orally Disintegrating Tablets	Loratadine 10 mg
Combination Systemic Products	
Dimetapp Cold and Allergy Syrup	Brompheniramine 1 mg/5 mL; phenylephrine 2.5 mg/5 mL
Zyrtec D Tablets	Cetirizine 5 mg; pseudoephedrine HCl 120 mg
Actifed Cold and Allergy Tablets	Chlorpheniramine 4 mg; phenylephrine 10 mg
Advil Allergy Sinus Caplets	Chlorpheniramine 2 mg; pseudoephedrine HCl 30 mg; ibuprofen 200 mg
Allegra D 12-Hour Tablets	Fexofenadine 60 mg; pseudoephedrine HCl 120 mg
Claritin-D 24 Hour Tablets	Loratadine 10 mg; pseudoephedrine sulfate 240 mg
Nasal Products	
Nasacort Allergy 24 HR	Triamcinolone acetonide 55 mcg/spray
Ayr Saline Nasal Gel	Sodium chloride; aloe; propylene glycol; glycerin
NasalCrom Spray	Cromolyn sodium 5.2 mg/spray
Ocean Spray	Sodium chloride 0.65%

[a] Contains phenylalanine.

the degree of sedation depends on chemical class (Table 11–13). Nonsedating antihistamines are more expensive but have less risk of sedation and impairment, which may justify the additional cost. Some patients report that antihistamines are less effective after prolonged use. This decline is most likely not indicative of true tolerance but rather stems from several factors, including patient nonadherence, an increase in antigen exposure, worsening of disease, limited effectiveness of antihistamines in severe disease, or the development of similar symptoms from unrelated diseases. Chemical class differences make it reasonable to suggest switching to a different class of antihistamine if a patient has a less-than-optimal response to one class of antihistamine.

Complementary Therapies

Ephedra (ma huang) and feverfew are commonly suggested herbal remedies for allergic rhinitis. Ephedra-containing products are banned by FDA owing to their serious adverse effects (e.g., stroke). Parthenolide, feverfew's biologically active component, may have anti-inflammatory properties, but its safety and efficacy in allergic rhinitis are unproved. (For further discussion of these types of products, see Chapter 51.) Capsaicin-based nasal sprays (e.g., Allergy Buster) are marketed for allergy sufferers, but despite these products being studied since the 1990s, many questions remain about their safety and efficacy. Using local honey or homeopathic products containing known allergens (e.g., bioAllers Animal Hair and Dander Allergy Relief Liquid contains cat, cattle, dog, horse, and sheep wool extracts) to induce long-term resistance by repeated exposure to controlled amounts of allergen has not been proven safe or effective. Safety and efficacy data are also lacking for symptom-specific homeopathic remedies such as sabadilla for nasal and ocular symptoms (red, watery eyes) and wyethia for itching.

Assessment of Allergic Rhinitis: A Case-Based Approach

Asking the patient for a detailed description of symptoms and obtaining the patient's medical and medication use (previous and current) history are essential to determining whether the patient has allergic rhinitis or rhinitis related to other causes and is eligible for self-care (Tables 11–11 and 11–12).

The medical history may uncover other respiratory illnesses that complicate treatment of allergic rhinitis. The patient's current medication use will also alert the health care provider to possible interactions with nonprescription allergy medications. The provider should also ask the patient whether nonprescription products used to treat IAR or PER were effective and without adverse effects.

Case 11–2 presents an example of the assessment of a patient with allergic rhinitis.

Patient Counseling for Allergic Rhinitis

The provider should stress that the best method of treating allergic rhinitis is to avoid allergens. Many patients, however, have no control over their work environment or are unable to implement all the preventive measures at home. These patients usually rely on allergy medications for symptom control. The patient should be advised about proper use of recommended medication(s) and about possible adverse effects, drug–drug and drug–disease interactions, and other precautions and warnings. Patients should also know the signs and symptoms that indicate the disorder has progressed to the point where medical care is needed. The box Patient Education for Allergic Rhinitis lists specific information to provide patients.

case

11–2

Relevant Evaluation Criteria	Scenario/Model Outcome
Information Gathering	

1. Gather essential information about the patient's symptoms, including:

a. description of symptom(s) (i.e., nature, onset, duration, severity, associated symptoms)	Patient has had postnasal drip and moderate congestion for 7 days.
b. description of any factors that seem to precipitate, exacerbate, and/or relieve the patient's symptom(s)	Symptoms are constant day and night, but congestion seems worse at night. Symptoms started one week into second trimester.
c. description of the patient's efforts to relieve the symptoms	Patient has not tried anything.
d. patient's identity	Sarah Connor
e. age, sex, height, and weight	28 years old, female, 5 ft 7 in., 180 lb
f. patient's occupation	Teacher
g. patient's dietary habits	Vegetarian
h. patient's sleep habits	Patient usually sleeps 7–8 hours at night, but congestion has been disrupting sleep.
i. concurrent medical conditions, prescription and nonprescription medications, and dietary supplements	Prenatal vitamin 1 tablet every morning
j. allergies	Penicillin
k. history of other adverse reactions to medications	None

Relevant Evaluation Criteria	Scenario/Model Outcome
Assessment and Triage	
2. Differentiate patient's signs/symptoms and correctly identify the patient's primary problem(s).	Allergic rhinitis symptoms tend to include sneezing, itchy nose or eyes, and anterior runny nose. Patient's symptoms (postnasal drip and congestion) are more indicative of nonallergic rhinitis. Also, because her symptoms started in second trimester, she may have hormonal nonallergic rhinitis.
3. Identify exclusions for self-treatment (Figure 11–3).	Pregnancy, nonallergic rhinitis symptoms
4. Formulate a comprehensive list of therapeutic alternatives for the primary problem to determine if triage to a medical provider is required, and share this information with the patient or caregiver.	Options include:
	(1) Recommend a separate OTC product for each symptom: nonsedating or sedating antihistamine for postnasal drip and topical or systemic decongestant for congestion. Or because the patient has multiple symptoms, a combination product may be appropriate.
	(2) Refer patient to her PCP for evaluation and treatment.
	(3) Recommend self-care until patient can consult her PCP.
	(4) Take no action.
Plan	
5. Select an optimal therapeutic alternative to address the patient's problem, taking into account patient preferences.	Patient should consult a health care provider for evaluation and treatment.
6. Describe the recommended therapeutic approach to the patient or caregiver.	Patient should consult a health care provider for evaluation and treatment.
7. Explain to the patient or caregiver the rationale for selecting the recommended therapeutic approach from the considered therapeutic alternatives.	Because patient's symptoms seem to be related to her pregnancy and not allergies, patient needs to consult a health care provider.
Patient Education	
8. When recommending self-care with nonprescription medications and/or nondrug therapy, convey accurate information to the patient or caregiver.	Criterion does not apply in this case.
Solicit follow-up questions from the patient or caregiver.	"Can I use a Neti pot to help with the congestion?"
Answer the patient's or caregiver's questions.	"Yes. The Neti pot may help wash away some of the mucus in your nose. Be sure to use distilled, sterile, or boiled tap water in the Neti pot to avoid rare but serious infections."
Evaluation of Patient Outcome	
9. Assess patient outcome.	Contact patient in 1 week to ensure that she made an appointment and sought medical care.

Key: OTC = Over-the-counter; PCP = primary care provider.

Evaluation of Patient Outcomes for Allergic Rhinitis

Many patients achieve symptomatic relief with initial nonprescription drug therapy in 3–4 days, but complete relief of symptoms may take 2–4 weeks. After this time frame, the health care provider should follow up with a telephone call or a scheduled appointment to determine whether symptom control has been achieved or the patient is encountering any adverse effects or problems. Patients who respond poorly to treatment should be assessed to determine whether they are complying with allergen avoidance strategies and medication regimens. Options for patients who do not achieve relief include increasing current medications to maximally effective dosages or changing to a different medication or dosage formulation. Patients who do not respond to nonprescription therapy should be referred back to their PCPs for prescription medications such as systemic corticosteroids, leukotriene inhibitors, anticholinergics, or immunotherapy. Patients should also be reassessed, and the diagnosis of allergic rhinitis may need to be reconsidered. Patients who develop any of the warning signs or symptoms listed in the box Patient Education for Allergic Rhinitis should be referred to a PCP.

The primary objective of self-treatment is to prevent or reduce symptoms, which in turn will improve functioning and a sense of well-being. For some patients, prescription therapy such as short-course oral corticosteroids may help control symptoms, whereas other therapy is initiated when symptoms are especially severe. For most patients, carefully following instructions for nonprescription allergy medications and the self-care measures listed here will help ensure optimal therapeutic outcomes.

Nondrug Measures

- Avoidance of allergens is important regardless of whether allergy medications are being taken.
- For symptoms that develop mainly when outdoors:
  - Frequently check local pollen counts and air quality index.
  - Keep house and car windows shut; avoid yard work and outdoor sports on days with high levels of pollen (spring/summer), mold (late summer/fall), or pollution.
- For symptoms that occur mainly when indoors:
  - Try to remove the symptom trigger(s) (e.g., cats, house-dust mites, tobacco smoke, and molds) from rooms.
  - Lower the humidity in the home to reduce molds. Use lower settings on humidifiers, repair damp basements and crawl spaces, vent kitchens and bathrooms, and remove house plants.
  - Wash bedding in hot water (130°F [54.4°C]) every week, and encase mattresses and pillows in coverings resistant to house-dust mites.
- Nasal saline solutions may relieve nasal irritation and dryness, and aid in the removal of dried, encrusted, or thick mucus from the nose.

Nonprescription Medications

- Ask a health care provider for help in selecting an allergy medication that treats the most bothersome symptoms. If needed, additional medications can be added for other symptoms:
  - Intranasal steroids (triamcinolone acetonide) are effective for itchy eyes and noses, sneezing, runny nose, and congestion.
  - Antihistamines are effective for itching, sneezing, and runny nose but, with the exception of newer agents (fexofenadine), have little effect on nasal congestion.
  - Decongestants are effective for nasal congestion but have little effect on other symptoms.
  - Combination therapy with an antihistamine and a decongestant is common.
  - Intranasal and ocular preparations are available to reduce nasal and eye symptoms, respectively.
  - Intranasal cromolyn is the preferred initial drug of choice during pregnancy and lactation. This medication is not absorbed into the body.
  - For intranasal products, follow the dosing and administration directions carefully. See Table 11-2.
  - The most common adverse effects of nasal preparations include nasal stinging and burning.
- Allergy medications are more effective if they are used regularly rather than episodically:
  - If you have intermittent allergies, start allergy medications as soon as possible, before exposure to allergen.
  - If you have persistent allergies, take allergy medications on a regular basis

Nasal Congestion

- See the box Patient Education for Colds for information about relieving nasal congestion.

Rhinorrhea (Runny Nose) and Sneezing

- Many factors cause a runny nose and depending on the factors, nonprescription steroids or antihistamines may only partially treat this symptom. Because some nonprescription antihistamines may make you very drowsy, the potential benefits of the medication must be weighed against the potential risks.
- Sneezing is a common and sometimes bothersome symptom. Sneezing may be reduced with nonprescription intranasal steroids or antihistamines. The potential benefits of using antihistamines must be weighed against the potential risks.

- Intranasal steroids and oral antihistamines are the preferred initial treatment for runny nose and sneezing in persons who are eligible for self-care (see exclusions in Figure 11-3).
- There are two types of antihistamines, sedating and nonsedating. Cetirizine, fexofenadine, and loratadine are nonsedating antihistamines and usually do not cause significant drowsiness.
- Note the following adverse effects for antihistamines:
  - The sedating antihistamines cause drowsiness and impair mental alertness. Mental alertness is impaired even if you do not feel drowsy or if you took the dose the prior evening. While taking these medications, do not drive a vehicle, operate machinery, or engage in other activities that require alertness.
  - Sedating antihistamines may cause sensitivity to sunlight. Use sunscreens and wear protective clothing when outdoors.
  - Use of sedating antihistamines may cause dryness in your mouth, nose, and other areas of your body.
  - Children and elderly persons may experience unexpected excitement with sedating antihistamines.
  - Elderly persons should avoid sedating antihistamines and may need lower doses of nonsedating antihistamines because they are more sensitive to the effects of these medications and take other medications that interact.
- Do not use antihistamines:
  - If you are allergic to antihistamines or similar medications.
  - If you are breast-feeding.
- Do not give antihistamines to newborns or premature infants unless directed to do so by a primary care provider.
- Note the following precautions for use of nonprescription antihistamines:
  - Persons with glaucoma, stenosing peptic ulcer, symptomatic enlarged prostate, bladder-neck obstruction, or stomach-intestinal blockage should not use sedating (first-generation) antihistamines.
  - Persons with lower respiratory tract disease (e.g., emphysema or chronic bronchitis) should use sedating antihistamines with caution.
  - Persons with esophageal narrowing, abnormal esophageal peristalsis, or problems swallowing tablets should not take the 12- or 24-hour sustained-release dosage forms of loratadine combined with pseudoephedrine. There have been reports of esophageal obstruction and perforation with these sustained-release dosage forms.
- Sedating antihistamines interact with the following drugs:
  - Alcohol, sedatives, and other central nervous system depressants may cause additive depressive effects when taken with sedating antihistamines.
  - Sedating antihistamines may block the effects of some drugs used to treat Alzheimer's disease (e.g., donepezil).
  - Chlorpheniramine may increase the adverse effects of phenytoin.
- Nonsedating antihistamines interact with the following drugs:
  - Fexofenadine interacts with ketoconazole, erythromycin, rifampin, and antacids. Also avoid taking with fruit juice.
  - Loratadine interacts with amiodarone.
  - Avoid taking cetirizine with alcohol.
- Store all medications according to the manufacturer's instructions.

When to Seek Medical Attention

- Seek medical attention in the following situations:
  - Your allergy symptoms worsen while you are taking nonprescription medications or do not improve after 2-4 weeks of treatment.
  - You develop signs or symptoms of secondary bacterial infections (e.g., thick nasal or respiratory secretions that are not clear, temperature higher than 101.5°F [38.6°C], shortness of breath, chest congestion, wheezing, significant ear pain, rash).

Key Points for Disorders Related to Colds and Allergic Rhinitis

➤ Colds are self-limiting, viral infections characterized by initial sore throat followed by nasal symptoms and nonproductive cough.

➤ Medical referral is appropriate for patients with suspected colds who are immunocompromised, have underlying cardiopulmonary diseases, or have alarm symptoms (high fever, chest pain, shortness of breath, or wheezing).

➤ Treatment for colds is symptomatic and targeted at the most bothersome symptoms.

➤ Decongestants are the most common nonprescription treatment for congestion related to colds and allergic rhinitis, but they should be used cautiously in patients with hypertension, diabetes, and other chronic diseases.

➤ Therapy for allergic rhinitis is sequential and consists of allergen avoidance, pharmacotherapy, and allergen immunotherapy.

➤ Medical referral is appropriate for patients with symptoms suggestive of nonallergic rhinitis, otitis media, sinusitis, or lower respiratory tract problems such as pneumonia, asthma, or bronchitis, and for those patients who fail to respond to nonprescription medications.

➤ Antihistamines are commonly used to control allergic rhinitis symptoms. Nonsedating (second-generation) antihistamines are preferred over sedating (first-generation) antihistamines on the basis of safety and efficacy data.

REFERENCES

1. National Institute of Allergy and Infectious Diseases. Common cold. August 2012. Accessed at http://www.niaid.nih.gov/topics/common Cold/Pages/default.aspx, March 25, 2013.
2. Consumer Healthcare Products Association. OTC sales by category 2010–2013. Accessed at http://www.chpa.org/OTCsCategory.aspx, April 23, 2014.
3. Patrick A. Rhinovirus chemotherapy. *Antiviral Res.* 2006;71(2–3):391–6.
4. Cohen S, Doyle WJ, Turner R, et al. Sociability and susceptibility to the common cold. *Psychol Sci.* 2003;14(5):389–95.
5. Cohen S, Doyle WJ, Alper CM, et al. Sleep habits and susceptibility to the common cold. *Arch Int Med.* 2009;169(1):62–7.
6. Mäukinen TM, Juvonen R, Jokelainen J, et al. Cold temperature and low humidity are associated with increased occurrence of respiratory tract infections. *Respir Med.* 2009;103(3):456–62.
7. Rajnik M, Tolan Jr RW. Rhinovirus infection. 2014. Accessed at http://emedicine.medscape.com/article/227820-overview, April 23, 2014.
8. Rennard BO, Ertl RF, Gossman GL, et al. Chicken soup inhibits neutrophil chemotaxis *in vitro*. *Chest.* 2000;118(4):1150–7.
9. Paul IM, Beiler J, King TS, et al. Vapor Rub, petrolatum, and no treatment for children with nocturnal cough and cold symptoms. *Pediatrics.* 2010; 126(6):1092–9.
10. World Health Organization. Guidelines on hand hygiene in health care. 2009. Accessed at http://whqlibdoc.who.int/publications/2009/9789241597906_eng.pdf, April 23, 2014.
11. U.S. Food and Drug Administration. Cold, cough, allergy, bronchodilator, and antiasthmatic drug products for over-the counter human use. CFR: Code of Federal Regulations. Title 21, Part 341. Updated June 1, 2013. Accessed at http://www.accessdata.fda.gov/scripts/cdrh/cfdocs/cfCFR/CFRSearch.cfm?CFRPart=341., April 23, 2014.
12. U.S. Food and Drug Administration Web site. Public Health Advisory: FDA recommends that over-the-counter (OTC) cough and cold products not be used for infants and children under 2 years of age. Updated August 20, 2013. Accessed at http://www.fda.gov/ForConsumers/ConsumerUpdates/ucm051137.htm, September 15, 2014.
13. Mortuaire G, de Gabory L, Francois M, et al. Rebound congestion and rhinitis medicamentosa: nasal decongestants in clinic practice. Critical review of the literature by a medical panel. *Eur Ann Otorhinolaryngol Head Neck Dis.* 2013 Feb 1 [Epub ahead of print].
14. U.S. Department of Justice Drug Enforcement Administration. Combat Methamphetamine Epidemic Act 2005. Title VII of USA Patriot Improvement Reauthorization Act of 2005. Pub L No. 109-177. 109th Congress. March 9, 2006. Accessed at http://www.deadiversion.usdoj.gov/meth/index.html, April 23, 2014.
15. Arroll B. Clinical evidence: common cold. *Clin Evid.* 2008;06:1510.
16. De Sutter AI, van Driel ML, Kumar AA, et al. Oral antihistamine-decongestant-analgesic combinations for the common cold. *Cochrane Database Syst Rev.* 2012;2:CD004976. doi: 10.1002/14651858.CD004976.pub3. Accessed at http://www.thecochranelibrary.com/view/0/index.html.
17. Knowlton WM, McKemy DD. TRPM8: from cold to cancer, peppermint to pain. *Curr Pharm Biotechnol.* 2010 Nov 8 [Epub ahead of print].
18. Eccles R. Efficacy and safety of over-the-counter analgesics in the treatment of common cold and flu. *J Clin Pharm Ther.* 2006;31(4):309–19.
19. Irwin RS, Baumann MH, Bolser DC, et al. Diagnosis and management of cough. ACCP evidence-based clinical practice guidelines. *Chest.* 2006; 129(1 suppl 1):1S–292S.
20. Bosler DC. Cough suppressant and pharmacologic protussive therapy: ACCP evidence-based clinical practice guidelines. *Chest.* 2006;129(1 suppl 1): 238S–49S.
21. Hatton RC, Winterstein AG, McKelvey RP, et al. Efficacy and safety of oral phenylephrine: systematic review and meta-analysis. *Ann Pharmacother.* 2007;41(3):381–90.
22. Guthrie EW. The decongestant shuffle. *Pharm Today OTC Suppl.* April 2007;13(4 suppl 1):12–3.
23. Horak F, Zieglmayer P, Zieglmayer R, et al. A placebo-controlled study of the nasal decongestant effect of phenylephrine and pseudoephedrine in the Vienna challenge chamber. *Ann Allergy Asthma Immunol.* 2009;102(2): 116–20.
24. Gilbert C, Mazzotta P, Loebstein R, et al. Fetal safety of drugs used in the treatment of allergic rhinitis. *Drug Saf.* 2005;28(8):707–19.
25. Briggs GG, Freeman RK, Yaffe SJ. *Drugs in pregnancy and lactation: a reference guide to fetal and neonatal risk.* 9th ed. Philadelphia, PA: Lippincott Williams & Wilkins; 2011.
26. Consumer Healthcare Products Association. CHPA announces voluntary labeling updates for oral OTC children's cough and cold medications. CHPA Executive Newsletter. 2008; Issue No. 21-8. Accessed at http://www.chpa.org/workarea/downloadasset.aspx?id=911, April 23, 2014.
27. U.S. Food and Drug Administration. FDA issues final guidance for liquid OTC drug products with dispensing devices [news release]. May 4, 2011. Accessed at http://www.fda.gov/NewsEvents/Newsroom/PressAnnouncements/ucm254029.htm, April 23, 2014.
28. U.S. Food and Drug Administration. Guidance for industry: dosage delivery devices for orally ingested OTC liquid drug products. May 2011. Accessed at http://www.fda.gov/downloads/Drugs/GuidanceComplianceRegulatoryInformation/Guidances/UCM188992.pdf, April 23, 2014.
29. Roxas M, Jurenka J. Colds and influenza: a review of diagnosis and conventional, botanical and nutritional considerations. *Alt Med Rev.* 2007; 12(1):25–48.
30. National Center for Complementary and Alternative Medicine. Herbs at a glance. Accessed at http://nccam.nih.gov/health/herbsataglance.htm, April 23, 2014.
31. Guo R, Pittler MH, Ernst E. Herbal medicines for the treatment of allergic rhinitis: a systematic review. *Ann Allergy Asthma Immunol.* 2007; 99(6):483–95.
32. Timmer A, Gunther J, Rucker G, et al. Pelargonium sidoides extract for acute respiratory tract infections. *Cochrane Database Syst Rev.* 2008;3: CD006323. doi: 10.1002/14651858.CD006323.pub3. Accessed at http://www.thecochranelibrary.com/view/0/index.html.
33. U.S. Food and Drug Administration. Public health advisory: loss of sense of smell with intranasal cold remedies containing zinc. June 16, 2009. Accessed at http://www.fda.gov/drugs/drugsafety/postmarketdrugsafetyinformationforpatientsandproviders/ucm166834.htm, September 15, 2014.

34. Singh M, Das RR. Zinc for the common cold. *Cochrane Database Syst Rev.* 2011;3:CD001364. doi: 10.1002/14651858.CD001364.pub3. Accessed at http://www.thecochranelibrary.com/view/0/index.html.

35. Hemila H, Chalker E. Vitamin C for preventing and treating the common cold. *Cochrane Database Syst Rev.* 2013;1:CD000980. doi:10.1002/14651858. CD000980. pub4. Accessed at http://www.thecochranelibrary.com/view/0/index.html.

36. Thomas LD, Elinder CG, Tiselius HG, et al. Ascorbic acid supplements and kidney stone incidence among men: a prospective study. *JAMA Intern Med.* 2013;173(5):386–8.

37. Kang EJ, Kim SY, Hwang IH, et al. The effect of probiotics on prevention of common cold: a meta-analysis of randomized controlled trial studied. *Korean J Fam Med.* 2013;34(1):2–10.

38. National Center for Health Statistics. *Fastats—Allergies and Hay Fever.* January 2013. Accessed at http://www.cdc.gov/nchs/fastats/allergies.htm, April 23, 2014.

39. Meltzer EO, Bukstein DA. The economic impact of allergic rhinitis and current guidelines for treatment. *Ann Allergy Asthma Immunol.* 2011;106 (2 suppl):S12–6.

40. National Center for Health Statistics. Summary health statistics for U.S. adults: national health interview survey, 2011. *Vital Health Stat.* 2012;10(256):22–3, Table 3. Accessed at http://www.cdc.gov/nchs/data/series/sr_10/sr10_256.pdf, April 23, 2014.

41. Bousquet J, Khaltev N, Cruz AA, et al. Allergic rhinitis and its impact on asthma (ARIA) 2008. *Allergy.* 2008;63(suppl 86):8–160.

42. Ellwood P, Asher MI, Garcia-Marcos L, et al. Do fast foods cause asthma, rhinoconjunctivitis and eczema? Global findings from the international study of asthma and allergies in childhood (ISAAC) phase three. *Thorax.* 2013;68(4):351–60.

43. Tran NP, Vickery J, Blaiss MS. Management of rhinitis: allergic and non-allergic. *Allergy Asthma Immunol Res.* 2011;3(3):148–56.

44. Bousquet J, Schunemann HJ, Samolinski B, et al. Allergic rhinitis and its impact on asthma (ARIA): achievements in 10 years and future needs. *J Allergy Clin Immunol.* 2012;130:1049–62.

45. U.S. Food and Drug Administration. Drugs@FDA. Accessed at http://www.accessdata.fda.gov/scripts/cder/drugsatfda, August 11, 2014.

46. National Center for Health Statistics. National Ambulatory Medical Care Survey: 2010 Summary. Table 23. Accessed at http://www.cdc.gov/nchs/data/ahcd/namcs_summary/2010_namcs_web_tables.pdf, April 23, 2014.

47. Gharahbaghian L, Lopez N. Cough, cold, and allergy preparation toxicity clinical presentation. September 16, 2013. Accessed at http://emedicine.medscape.com/article/1010513-clinical, April 23, 2014.

48. Simons FER, Simons KJ. Histamine and H$_1$-antihistamines: celebrating a century of progress. *J Allergy Clin Immunol.* 2011;128(6):1139–50.

49. Golightly LK, Greos LS. Second generation antihistamines. *Drugs.* 2005; 65(3):341–84.

50. Raphael GD, Angello JT, Wu MM, et al. Efficacy of diphenhydramine vs desloratadine and placebo in patients with moderate-to-severe seasonal allergic rhinitis. *Ann Allergy Asthma Immunol.* 2006;96(4):606–14.

51. American Geriatrics Society 2012 Beers Criteria Update Expert Panel. American Geriatrics Society updated Beers Criteria for potentially inappropriate medication use in older adults. *J Am Geriatr Soc.* 2012; 60(4):616–31.

chapter 12

COUGH

Karen J. Tietze

Cough is an important defensive respiratory reflex with potentially significant adverse physical and psychological consequences and economic impact. Cough is the most common symptom for which patients seek medical care.[1] Cough is also a common reason for emergency department visits. In 2010, cough was the second most common reason for children younger than 15 years to visit emergency departments and the seventh most common reason for adults.[2] Americans spend more than $4 billion annually on nonprescription cough/cold and related medications, more than any other nonprescription sales category.[3]

Pathophysiology of Cough

Cough is initiated by stimulation of chemically and mechanically sensitive, vagally mediated sensory pathways in laryngeal, esophageal, and tracheobronchial airway epithelium.[4,5] The number of afferent nerves activated and the intensity of activation may influence the cough threshold.[6] Receptors in the larynx and proximal large airways are more sensitive to mechanical stimulation, whereas laryngeal receptors are more sensitive to chemical stimulation.[7] A complex medullary brainstem network ("cough control center") processes the sensory input and stimulates the motor efferents. Voluntary cough is controlled by the cerebral cortex.[8] Viruses promote cough by a different though not well-understood mechanism.[9]

A cough starts with a deep inspiration followed by closure of the glottis and forceful contraction of the chest wall, abdominal wall, and diaphragmatic muscles against the closed glottis; pressure within the thoracic cavity may reach 300 mm Hg.[4] When the glottis opens, air is expelled with a velocity of about 11–15 m/s, propelling mucus, cellular debris, and foreign material out of the respiratory system.[10] Cough may occur in epochs ("coughing fits").

Cough, classified as acute (duration of less than 3 weeks), subacute (duration of 3–8 weeks), or chronic (duration of more than 8 weeks), is a symptom of diverse infectious and noninfectious disorders (Table 12–1).[11] In children, cough may also be a symptom of aspiration caused by poor coordination of sucking and swallowing or esophageal motility disorders.[12] Angiotensin-converting enzyme inhibitors cause dry cough in approximately 20% of treated patients.[13] Systemic and ophthalmic beta-adrenergic blockers may cause cough in patients with obstructive airway diseases (e.g., asthma or chronic obstructive pulmonary disease [COPD]).

Clinical Presentation of Cough

Coughs are described as productive or nonproductive. A productive cough (a wet or "chesty" cough) expels secretions from the lower respiratory tract that, if retained, could impair ventilation and the lungs' ability to resist infection. Productive coughs may be effective (secretions easily expelled) or ineffective (secretions present but difficult to expel). The appearance of the secretions is not always a reliable diagnostic indicator, but secretions are typically clear with bronchitis and purulent with bacterial infection. Anaerobic bacterial infections are associated with a distinct malodor. Nonproductive coughs (a dry or "hacking" cough), which are associated with viral and atypical bacterial infections, gastroesophageal reflux disease (GERD), cardiac disease, and some medications, serve no useful physiologic purpose.

Common complications of cough include exhaustion, insomnia, musculoskeletal pain, hoarseness, excessive perspiration, and urinary incontinence. Less common complications include cardiac dysrhythmias, syncope, stroke, and rib fractures. Mechanical irritation from coughing may cause sore throat. Cough may cause prolonged absence from work or school, withdrawal from social activities, and fear that the cough is a symptom of a serious illness, such as cancer or tuberculosis.

Treatment of Cough
Treatment Goals

The primary goal of self-treatment of cough is to reduce the number and severity of cough episodes. The second goal is to prevent complications. Cough treatment is symptomatic; the underlying disorder must be treated to stop the cough.

General Treatment Approach

Selection of a medication for self-care of cough depends on the nature and etiology of the cough. Figure 12–1 lists exclusions for self-care. These exclusions are based on the presence of signs and symptoms of potentially serious medical conditions associated with cough that require medical evaluation.[14,15] Antitussives (cough suppressants) control or eliminate cough and are the drugs of choice for nonproductive coughs. Antitussives should not be used to treat productive cough unless the

table

12–1 Etiology of Cough

Classification	Etiology
Acute	Viral URTI, pneumonia, acute left ventricular failure, asthma, foreign body aspiration
Subacute	Postinfectious cough, bacterial sinusitis, asthma
Chronic	UACS, asthma, GERD, COPD (chronic bronchitis), ACEIs, bronchogenic carcinoma, carcinomatosis, sarcoidosis, left ventricular failure, aspiration secondary to pharyngeal dysfunction

Key: ACEI = Angiotensin-converting enzyme inhibitor; COPD = chronic obstructive pulmonary disease; GERD = gastroesophageal reflux disease; UACS = upper airway cough syndrome; URTI = upper respiratory tract infection.
Source: Reference 11.

potential benefit outweighs the risk (e.g., significant nocturnal cough). Suppression of productive coughs may lead to retention of lower respiratory tract secretions, increasing the risk of airway obstruction and secondary bacterial infection. Protussives (expectorants) change the consistency of mucus and increase the volume of expectorated sputum and may provide some relief for coughs that expel thick, tenacious secretions from the lungs with difficulty.

Cough medications are marketed in a variety of dosage forms (syrups, liquids, solutions, suspensions, tablets, capsules, lozenges, oral granules, topical ointments and creams, topical patches, and vaporizer solutions). Generic formulations are widely available. The Food and Drug Administration (FDA) allows various combinations of antitussives, protussives, analgesics, decongestants, and antihistamines. However, combinations of antitussives and protussives are potentially counterproductive.

Nonpharmacologic Therapy

Nonpharmacologic therapy includes nonmedicated lozenges, humidification, interventions to promote nasal drainage, and hydration. Nonmedicated lozenges may reduce cough by decreasing throat irritation. Humidifiers (ultrasonic, impeller, and evaporative) increase the amount of moisture in inspired air, which may soothe irritated airways. However, high humidity may increase environmental mold, dust mites, minerals, and microorganisms. Vaporizers (humidifiers with a medication well or cup for volatile inhalants) produce a medicated vapor. Cool-mist humidifiers and vaporizers are preferred because fewer bacteria grow at the cooler temperatures and there is less risk of scalding if they are tipped over. Humidifiers and vaporizers must be cleaned daily and disinfected weekly. Babies and young children up to about 2 years of age cannot blow their noses; a rubber bulb nasal syringe may be used to clear the nasal passages and reduce cough if postnasal drip causes cough. Propping infants upright when they sleep and raising the head of the bed at night promotes drainage of nasal secretions. Less viscous and thus easier-to-expel secretions are formed when a person is well hydrated. Cautious hydration is recommended for patients with lower respiratory tract infections, heart failure, renal failure, or other conditions potentially exacerbated by overhydration.

Pharmacologic Therapy

Table 12–2 lists examples of antitussive and expectorant products.

Oral Antitussives

FDA-approved nonprescription oral antitussives include codeine (codeine, codeine phosphate, codeine sulfate), dextromethorphan (dextromethorphan, dextromethorphan hydrobromide), diphenhydramine (diphenhydramine citrate, diphenhydramine hydrochloride), and chlophedianol hydrochloride.[16]

Codeine

At antitussive dosages, codeine is a Schedule C-V narcotic available without a prescription in 30 states (9 of the 30 states limit sales to products sold by a pharmacist in a pharmacy).[17] Codeine-containing Schedule C-V products must contain one or more noncodeine active ingredients and no more than 200 mg of codeine per 100 milliliters.[18] Abuse of the combination of codeine and promethazine hydrochloride, known by the street names of "purple drank" and "lean," is a common problem.[19]

Codeine acts centrally on the medulla to increase the cough threshold. Codeine is methylmorphine; morphine may be the active antitussive. Codeine is well absorbed orally with a 15- to 30-minute onset of action and a 4- to 6-hour duration of effect. The elimination half-life is 2.5–3 hours. Ten percent of a codeine dose is demethylated in the liver to form morphine. Approximately 3%–16% of codeine is eliminated unchanged in the urine.

Codeine is indicated for the suppression of nonproductive cough caused by chemical or mechanical respiratory tract irritation. Codeine's efficacy and safety as an antitussive drug in children are not established; pediatric dosage guidelines are extrapolated from the adult literature. Table 12–3 lists FDA-approved codeine dosages.[16] Reduced doses are appropriate for patients of advanced age and the debilitated. Codeine is available as oral solutions, liquids, suspensions, and syrups in combination with other active ingredients, including guaifenesin, antihistamines, and decongestants. Alcohol-, dye-, gluten-, and sucrose-free formulations are available.

Usual antitussive codeine dosages have low toxicity and little risk of addiction. The most common side effects associated with antitussive codeine dosages are nausea, vomiting, sedation, dizziness, and constipation. The lethal dose of codeine in adults is 0.5–1 gram, with death from marked respiratory depression and cardiopulmonary collapse. Concomitant use of codeine and central nervous system (CNS) depressants (e.g., barbiturates, sedatives, or alcohol) causes additive CNS depression. Codeine is contraindicated in patients with known codeine hypersensitivity and during labor when a premature birth is anticipated. Patients with impaired respiratory reserve (e.g., asthma or COPD) or preexisting respiratory depression, drug addicts, and individuals who take other respiratory depressants or sedatives, including alcohol, should use codeine with caution.

Dextromethorphan

Considered approximately equipotent with codeine, dextromethorphan is a nonopioid with no analgesic, sedative, respiratory depressant, or addictive properties at usual antitussive doses. Dextromethorphan, the methylated dextrorotatory analogue of levorphanol (a codeine analogue), acts centrally in the medulla

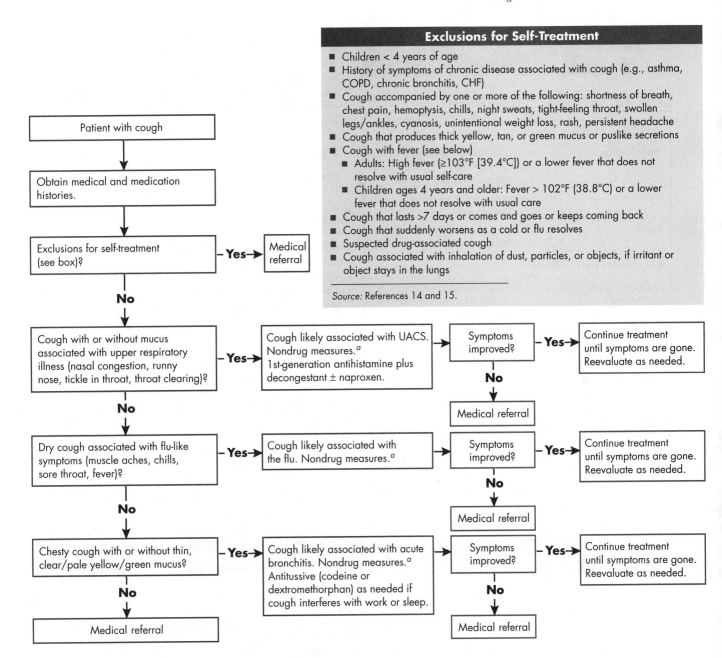

a Nondrug measures: rest, fluids, vaporizer, and reassurance.

figure 12–1 Self-care of cough. Key: CHF = Congestive heart failure; COPD = chronic obstructive pulmonary disease; UACS = upper airway cough syndrome.

to increase the cough threshold. It is well absorbed orally with a 15- to 30-minute onset of action and a 3- to 6-hour duration of effect. Dextromethorphan exhibits polymorphic metabolism, with a usual elimination half-life of 1.2–2.2 hours. However, the half-life may be as long as 45 hours in people with a poor metabolism phenotype.

Dextromethorphan is indicated for the suppression of nonproductive cough caused by chemical or mechanical respiratory tract irritation. The efficacy and safety of dextromethorphan as an antitussive drug in children have not been established.[20] Table 12–3 lists FDA-approved dextromethorphan dosages.[16] Dextromethorphan is marketed in the form of syrups, liquids,

solutions, extended-release oral suspensions, liquid-filled gelcaps, tablets, capsules, powders, and lozenges. Alcohol-, sucrose-, gluten-, and dye-free formulations are available.

Dextromethorphan has a wide margin of safety. Side effects with usual doses are uncommon but may include drowsiness, nausea or vomiting, stomach discomfort, or constipation. Dextromethorphan overdoses cause confusion, excitation, nervousness, irritability, restlessness, drowsiness, as well as severe nausea and vomiting; respiratory depression may occur with very high doses. Additive CNS depression occurs with alcohol, antihistamines, and psychotropic medications. The combination of monoamine oxidase inhibitors (MAOIs) and dextromethorphan may cause

table 12-2 Selected Nonprescription Products for Cough

Primary Ingredients	Trade Name
Single-Ingredient Products	
Dextromethorphan	DayQuil Cough, Delsym Adult 12 Hour Cough, Robitussin Long-Acting CoughGels, Hold DM
Guaifenesin	Mucinex, Robitussin Mucus + Chest Congestion
Menthol	Vicks VapoDrops, Hall's Ice Blue Drops
Combination Products	
Dextromethorphan and guaifenesin	Robitussin Cough + Chest Congestion DM, Mucinex-DM, DayQuil Mucus Control
Codeine and guaifenesin	Guaiatussin AC, Cheratussin AC
Camphor, menthol, and eucalyptus oil	Vicks VapoRub, Mentholatum for Kids

phencyclidine-like euphoric effect ("robo-tripping")[21,22]; abuse may be associated with psychosis and mania. Dextromethorphan abuse is especially common among male adolescents.[23] In 2010, at the request of the Drug Enforcement Administration, FDA's Drug Safety and Risk Management Advisory Committee considered, but voted against, recommending that dextromethorphan be scheduled in the Controlled Substances Act.[24]

Diphenhydramine

Diphenhydramine, a nonselective (first-generation) antihistamine with significant sedating and anticholinergic properties, acts centrally in the medulla to increase the cough threshold. Second-generation antihistamines (e.g., loratadine and fexofenadine) lack antitussive activity. Diphenhydramine is well absorbed following oral administration, with a bioavailability of 40%–70%, an onset of action of about 15 minutes, and a duration of action of about 4–6 hours. The volume of distribution is 3.3–4.5 L/kg. Diphenhydramine is hepatically metabolized to N-dealkylated urine and acidic metabolites with a clearance of 0.4–0.7 L/kg per hour. Less than 4% is excreted unchanged in the urine.

Diphenhydramine is indicated for the suppression of nonproductive cough caused by chemical or mechanical respiratory tract irritation. Table 12–3 lists FDA-approved diphenhydramine dosages.[16] A common ingredient in cold and allergy products, diphenhydramine is available in multiple dosage formulations, including an alcohol-free syrup specifically indicated for cough. Symptoms of diphenhydramine overdose include mild to severe CNS depression (e.g., mental confusion, sedation, or respiratory depression), hypotension, and CNS stimulation (e.g., hallucinations or convulsions).

Side effects of diphenhydramine include drowsiness, disturbed coordination, respiratory depression, blurred vision, urinary

serotonergic syndrome (e.g., increased blood pressure, hyperpyrexia, arrhythmias, and myoclonus). Dextromethorphan should not be taken for at least 14 days after the MAOI is discontinued. Patients who have known hypersensitivity to dextromethorphan or who have a prior history of dextromethorphan dependence should not take it. Dextromethorphan is abused for its

table 12-3 Dosage Guidelines for Nonprescription Oral Antitussives and Expectorants

Drug	Dosage (maximum daily dosage)		
	Adults/Children ≥12 Years	**Children 6 to <12 Years**	**Children 2 to <6 Years[a]**
Chlophedianol[b,c]	25 mg every 6–8 hours (100 mg)	12.5 mg every 6–8 hours (50 mg)	12.5 mg every 6–8 hours (50 mg)
Codeine[b–d]	10–20 mg every 4–6 hours (120 mg)	5–10 mg every 4–6 hours (60 mg)	1 mg/kg/day in 4 equal divided dosages or by average body weight
Dextromethorphan hydrobromide[b]	10–20 mg every 4 hours or 30 mg every 6–8 hours (120 mg)	5–10 mg every 4 hours or 15 mg every 6–8 hours (60 mg)	2.5–5 mg every 4 hours or 7.5 mg every 6–8 hours (30 mg)
Diphenhydramine citrate[b,c]	38 mg every 4 hours (228 mg)	19 mg every 4 hours (114 mg)	9.5 mg every 4 hours (57 mg)
Diphenhydramine HCl[b,c]	25 mg every 4 hours (150 mg)	12.5 mg every 4 hours (75 mg)	6.25 mg every 4 hours (37.5 mg)
Guaifenesin[b]	200–400 mg every 4 hours (2.4 g)	100–200 mg every 4 hours (1.2 g)	50–100 mg every 4 hours (600 mg)

[a] The Consumer Health Care Products Association announced in October 2008 that manufacturers were voluntarily updating cough and cold product labels to state "do not use" in children under 4 years of age.[41] FDA announced that it would not object to the more restrictive labeling.[42] These actions have not changed the official monograph for cold, cough, allergy, bronchodilator, and antiasthmatic drug products.[16]

[b] Not recommended for use in children younger than 2 years; no FDA-approved dosing recommendations.

[c] FDA recommends that the labels on nonprescription products not provide dosage information for children younger than 6 years.

[d] Codeine may be dosed by average body weight: 2 years of age (average body weight of 12 kg) = 3 mg every 4–6 hours (maximum in 24 hours: 12 mg); 3 years of age (average body weight of 14 kg) = 3.5 mg every 4–6 hours (maximum in 24 hours: 14 mg); 4 years of age (average body weight of 16 kg) = 4 mg every 4–6 hours (maximum in 24 hours: 16 mg); 5 years of age (average body weight of 18 kg) = 4.5 mg every 4–6 hours (maximum in 24 hours: 18 mg). A dispensing device such as a dropper calibrated for age or weight should be dispensed along with the product when it is intended for use in children 2 to <6 years of age to prevent possible overdose from an improperly measured dose.

Source: Reference 16.

retention, dry mouth, and dry respiratory secretions. Uncommon side effects reported with diphenhydramine include acute dystonic reactions such as oculogyric crisis (rotation of the eyeballs), torticollis (contraction of neck muscles), and catatonia-like states, as well as allergic and photoallergic reactions. Diphenhydramine may cause excitability, especially in children. Diphenhydramine potentiates the depressant effects of narcotics, nonnarcotic analgesics, benzodiazepines, tranquilizers, and alcohol on the CNS, and it intensifies the anticholinergic effect of MAOIs and other anticholinergics. Diphenhydramine is contraindicated in patients with known hypersensitivity to diphenhydramine or structurally similar antihistamines. Diphenhydramine should be used with caution in patients with diseases potentially exacerbated by drugs with anticholinergic activity, including narrow-angle glaucoma, stenosing peptic ulcer, pyloroduodenal obstruction, symptomatic prostatic hypertrophy, bladder-neck obstruction, asthma and other lower respiratory tract disease, elevated intraocular pressure, hyperthyroidism, cardiovascular disease, or hypertension. Because of the increased risk of toxicity, diphenhydramine-containing antitussives should not be used with any other diphenhydramine-containing product, including topical products.

Chlophedianol

Chlophedianol is a centrally acting oral antitussive originally marketed in 1960 as a prescription antitussive. Reintroduced as a nonprescription product in late 2009, chlophedianol is an alkylamine antihistamine derivative with antitussive, moderate local anesthetic, and mild anticholinergic effects. Chlophedianol is indicated for the suppression of nonproductive cough caused by chemical or mechanical respiratory tract irritation. Table 12–3 lists the FDA-approved chlophedianol dosage.[16] Chlophedianol is marketed in the form of oral liquids, solutions, and syrups. Sugar-, alcohol-, dye-, and gluten-free products are available.

Published data for chlophedianol are limited. It has a slower onset of maximal effect (4 hours vs. 30 minutes) and a longer duration of action than does codeine.[25] Chlophedianol is metabolized hepatically and eliminated renally. Side effects include excitation, hyperirritability, nightmares, hallucinations, hypersensitivity, and urticaria. Dry mouth, vertigo, visual disturbances, nausea, vomiting, and drowsiness have been associated with large doses. If the patient takes MAOIs, chlophedianol should not be administered for at least 14 days after the MAOIs are halted. Chlophedianol is contraindicated in patients with known chlophedianol hypersensitivity.

Protussives (Expectorants)

Guaifenesin (glyceryl guaiacolate), the only FDA-approved expectorant, is indicated for the symptomatic relief of acute, ineffective productive cough.[16] Guaifenesin is not indicated for chronic cough associated with chronic lower respiratory tract diseases such as asthma, COPD, emphysema, or smoker's cough. Guaifenesin loosens and thins lower respiratory tract secretions, making minimally productive coughs more productive. However, few data support its efficacy, especially at nonprescription dosages. Although the pharmacokinetics of guaifenesin is not well described, guaifenesin appears to be well absorbed after oral administration, with a half-life of about 1 hour.

Table 12–3 lists FDA-approved dosages of guaifenesin.[16] Guaifenesin is marketed as oral liquids, syrups, caplets, granules, and immediate-release and extended-release tablets. Alcohol-, sucrose-, and dye-free formulations are also available. Most reports of guaifenesin overdosages involve combinations of drugs and therefore are difficult to assess. However, signs and symptoms of overdosages appear to be extensions of the side effects.

Guaifenesin is generally well tolerated. Side effects include nausea, vomiting, dizziness, headache, rash, diarrhea, drowsiness, and stomach pain. Large doses, either singly or in combination with ephedrine or pseudoephedrine, have been associated with renal calculi.[26] Guaifenesin is contraindicated in patients with a known hypersensitivity to guaifenesin.

Topical Antitussives

Camphor and menthol are the only FDA-approved topical antitussives.[16] Other volatile oils (e.g., eucalyptus), common in many cough and cold preparations, impart a strong medicinal odor to products but are not FDA-approved antitussives. At subtherapeutic doses, menthol is a common flavoring agent. Although the mechanism of action is not well described, inhaled camphor and menthol vapors stimulate sensory nerve endings within the nose and mucosa, creating a local anesthetic sensation and a sense of improved airflow. However, there is little objective evidence of clinical efficacy. A possible drug interaction with menthol cough drops and warfarin resulting in reduced warfarin response has been reported.[27] Table 12–4 provides administration guidelines for these agents.

table **12–4**	**Administration Guidelines for Nonprescription Topical Antitussives (Adults and Children ≥ 2 Years[a])**
Formulation	**Administration**
Ointments[b]	Rub on the throat and chest in a thick layer; application may be repeated up to 3 times daily or as directed by primary care provider; loosen clothing around throat and chest so vapors reach the nose and mouth; cover with a warm, dry cloth (optional). Do not use in the nostrils, under the nose, by the mouth, on damaged skin, or with tight bandages.
Lozenges[c]	Allow lozenge to dissolve slowly in mouth; repeat hourly or as needed or as directed by a primary care provider.
Inhalation[d]	For products intended to be added directly to cold water for use in a steam vaporizer: add measured solution to cold water; place the mixture in the vaporizer; breathe in the medicated vapors up to 3 times daily. For products to be placed in the medication chamber of a hot steam vaporizer: place water in vaporizer; place solution in medication chamber; breathe in the medicated vapors up to 3 times daily.

[a] For children ages < 2 years, consult a primary care provider.
[b] Camphor 4.7%–5.3%; menthol 2.6%–2.8%.
[c] Menthol lozenges, 5–10 mg lozenge; repeat hourly as needed.
[d] Camphor 6.2%; menthol 3.2%.
Source: Reference 16.

Camphor- and menthol-containing ointments, creams, and solutions may splatter and cause serious burns if used near an open flame or placed in hot water or in a microwave oven. Camphor and menthol vapors may be ciliotoxic and pro-inflammatory, especially in young children.[28] These products are also toxic if ingested. Toxicities include burning sensations in the mouth, nausea and vomiting, epigastric distress, restlessness, excitation, delirium, seizures, and death. Ingestion of as little as 4 teaspoons of products containing 5% camphor may be lethal for children.[29]

Product Selection Guidelines

Efficacy

Although antitussives and expectorants have been marketed for decades, efficacy has been difficult to prove and may depend on the etiology of the cough. There is no good evidence that dextromethorphan, codeine, diphenhydramine, or guaifenesin are effective treatments of acute cough in adults or children[30–33]; there is even less evidence for the efficacy of menthol, camphor, and chlophedianol. There is also a lack of evidence for or against the efficacy of nonprescription antitussives as adjuncts to antibiotics for the treatment of acute pneumonia.[34] Factors such as taste, smell, color, viscosity, sugar content, and personal expectation may contribute to a large placebo response (up to 85%).[35] Proof of efficacy will require data from well-designed trials of subjects with natural disease who are assessed with standardized objective outcome parameters.

The American College of Chest Physicians (ACCP) published updated evidence-based diagnosis and management of cough guidelines in 2006[36]; similar international guidelines are available.[37,38] The ACCP guidelines state that central cough suppressants are ineffective in cough associated with the common cold, and they recommend a combination of a first-generation antihistamine plus a decongestant to treat the virus-induced postnasal drip that is most likely the cause of the cough (see Chapter 11).[39] Also, because viral infection increases upper airway afferent nerve sensitivity, the guidelines suggest that the antiinflammatory naproxen may reduce viral-associated cough.[39] The guidelines also recommend empiric treatment of cough associated with chronic upper airway cough syndrome, for which the etiology is unclear, with a first-generation antihistamine/decongestant combination (see Chapter 11).[40] The guidelines recommend codeine or dextromethorphan for the short-term symptomatic relief of cough associated with acute and chronic bronchitis and postinfectious subacute cough. Guaifenesin is not recommended for any indication. The guidelines do not address chlophedianol.

Dosage Formulations

Cough products are marketed in a variety of dosage formulations. Efficacy appears to be the same for all dosage formulations; patients may select a dosage formulation on the basis of preference and convenience. Most products are formulated for dosage intervals of 4–6 hours, but some liquid dosage forms are specifically formulated for an extended dosage interval. For example, some dextromethorphan products are formulated with polymer complexes (e.g., sulfonated styrene-divinylbenzene copolymer; polistirex), conferring an extended dosage interval (8–12 hours). Patients treating nocturnal cough may prefer a product with an extended dosage interval.

Special Populations

In January 2008, FDA issued a public health advisory recommending that nonprescription cough and cold medicines "…not be used to treat infants and children under 2 years of age because several serious and potentially life-threatening side effects can occur."[41] In October 2008, the Consumer Healthcare Products Association (CHPA) announced that manufacturers were voluntarily updating cough and cold product labels to state "do not use" in children under 4 years of age.[42] FDA announced that it would not object to the more restrictive labeling.[43] To address the issue of inaccurate dosing, FDA released guidelines in May 2011 for liquid nonprescription drug products that include any type of dispensing device (dropper, cup, syringe, or spoon).[44,45] These products include liquid analgesics, liquid cough and cold products, and lactase replacement drops. The key points of the guidance are recommendations that

- A dosing device be included with all oral liquid nonprescription products.
- The device be calibrated to the dose recommended in the product directions.
- The device be used only with the product in which it is packaged.
- The markings remain visible even when the liquid is in the device.

The agency continues to assess the safety and efficacy of nonprescription cough and cold medications in children.

Codeine (Pregnancy Category C) should be used during pregnancy only if the potential benefits outweigh the risks. Nonteratogenic concerns include the risk of neonatal respiratory depression if codeine is taken close to the time of delivery and neonatal withdrawal if codeine is used regularly during the pregnancy. Codeine is excreted in breast milk and is associated with drowsiness in nursing infants.[46,47] Because the elderly may be more susceptible to the sedating effects of codeine, the dose should be started at the lower end of the dosage range and titrated as tolerated, with careful monitoring.

Dextromethorphan (Pregnancy Category C) is viewed as probably safe for use during pregnancy.[48] It is not known whether dextromethorphan is excreted in breast milk. Because the elderly may be more susceptible to the sedating effects of dextromethorphan, the dose should be started at the lower end of the dosage range and titrated as tolerated, with careful monitoring.

Diphenhydramine (Pregnancy Category B) is excreted in breast milk and may cause unusual excitation and irritability in the infant; it may also decrease the flow of milk. Compared with the general population, the elderly are more likely to experience dizziness, excessive sedation, syncope, confusion, and hypotension with diphenhydramine. The 2012 American Geriatrics Society Beers Criteria identify diphenhydramine, along with four other nonprescription first-generation H_1-antihistamines and seven prescription first-generation H_1-antihistamines, as potentially inappropriate medications in older adults.[49] Children and the elderly may experience paradoxical excitation, restlessness, and irritability with diphenhydramine. Dosing for the latter group should be started at the lower end of the dosage range and titrated as tolerated, with careful monitoring.

There are no controlled data regarding the use of guaifenesin (Pregnancy Category C) or chlophedianol (Pregnancy Category N) during pregnancy or breast-feeding. There are no special considerations for use of guaifenesin by the elderly.

Chlophedianol should be used with caution in sedated or debilitated patients.

Patient Factors

Cough is a symptom of many acute and chronic diseases. Patients with identified exclusions for self-care (Figure 12–1) should be referred for further evaluation. Patients with known, or signs and symptoms of, chronic diseases associated with cough (Table 12–5) should not attempt to self-treat cough, even cough caused by an acute viral upper respiratory tract infection (URTI) because the acute infection may exacerbate the underlying disease. Patients with smoker's cough should be counseled regarding smoking cessation options; antitussives and expectorants are not indicated (see Chapter 47).

Dextromethorphan, diphenhydramine, and chlophedianol should not be taken concurrently with MAOIs. Diphenhydramine is highly sedating and should be avoided by patients at risk from the anticholinergic properties of the drug. First-generation antihistamines and decongestants should be used only if the potential benefit outweighs the risk (see Chapter 11).

Complementary Therapies

Hundreds of herbal and other complementary therapies are marketed for cough. However, evidence does not support the use of complementary therapies for treating cough, and some products have potential safety issues. (See Chapter 51 for information on those therapies.) For example, honey, a common but unproven home remedy, should not be given to children younger than 1 year owing to the risk of botulism from ingestion of honey contaminated with *Clostridium botulinum*.[50]

Assessment of Cough: A Case-Based Approach

Before recommending any treatment, the health care provider needs to inquire about the duration of the cough, whether the cough is productive, and whether it is associated with a chronic illness (Table 12–5). The provider should also obtain a list of all the patient's current medications to identify possible drug–drug or drug–disease interactions. In addition, the provider should find out how the patient has treated the current cough, as well as previous coughs, and whether these treatments were satisfactory or effective.

Cases 12–1 and 12–2 provide examples of the assessment of patients with cough.

Patient Counseling for Cough

The provider should explain the appropriate drug and nondrug measures for treating the patient's type of cough. After a product is recommended, the dosage guidelines; drug administration techniques (for topical drugs); and possible side effects, drug–drug interactions, and precautions or warnings should be fully explained. The provider should ensure that the patient understands when self-care of the cough should be discontinued and medical care sought. For patients with underlying medical disorders, the provider should explain which nonprescription medications are contraindicated and what symptoms indicate the need to seek medical care. The box Patient Education for Cough lists specific information for patients.

Evaluation of Patient Outcomes for Cough

For most patients, 7 days of nonprescription drug therapy should relieve cough. If the cough persists but has improved at follow-up, the patient should continue the therapy until the cough is resolved. Cough associated with viral URTIs usually resolves within 2 weeks; postviral coughs may persist for 3 weeks or longer. Coughs associated with other respiratory infections typically resolve in 3–4 weeks. In all cases, the patient should be referred for further medical evaluation if the cough worsens or if the patient develops other exclusions for self-treatment (Figure 12–1).

table 12–5	Signs and Symptoms of Diseases Associated with Cough
Disease	**Signs and Symptoms**
Acute bronchitis	Purulent sputum; cough that lasts 1–3 weeks; mild dyspnea, mild bronchospasm and wheezing; usually afebrile though may have a low-grade fever
Asthma	Wheezing or chest tightness; shortness of breath, coughing predominantly at night; cough in response to specific irritants, such as dust, smoke, or pollen
CHF	Fatigue; dependent edema, breathlessness
Chronic bronchitis	Productive cough most days of the month at least 3 months of the year for at least 2 consecutive years
COPD	Persistent, progressive dyspnea; chronic cough (may be intermittent or unproductive), chronic sputum production
GERD	Heartburn; sour taste in mouth; worsening of symptoms when supine; improvement with acid-lowering drugs
Lower respiratory tract infection	Fever (mild to high); thick, purulent, discolored phlegm; tachypnea, tachycardia
UACS	Mucus drainage from nose; frequent throat clearing
Viral URTI	Sneezing; sore throat; rhinorrhea; low-grade temperature

Key: CHF = Congestive heart failure; COPD = chronic obstructive pulmonary disease; GERD = gastroesophageal reflux disease; UACS = upper airway cough syndrome; URTI = upper respiratory tract infection.

Key Points for Cough

➤ Cough is an important respiratory defensive reflex.
➤ Antitussives (cough suppressants) are the drugs of choice for nonproductive coughs.
➤ Protussives (expectorants) are the drugs of choice for coughs that expel thick, tenacious secretions from the lungs with difficulty.

case

12-1

Relevant Evaluation Criteria	Scenario/Model Outcome

Information Gathering

1. Gather essential information about the patient's symptoms and medical history, including:

   a. description of symptom(s) (i.e., nature, onset, duration, severity, associated symptoms)

   The patient has been coughing for about a week. The cough started about 3 days after she got a cold. Her cold symptoms (sore throat, nasal congestion, rhinorrhea) are mostly resolved, but the dry, hacking, nonproductive cough persists.

   b. description of any factors that seem to precipitate, exacerbate, and/or relieve the patient's symptom(s)

   The cough is worse at night or when she lies down.

   c. description of the patient's efforts to relieve the symptoms

   The patient tried menthol cough drops and a combination of dextro-methorphan and guaifenesin cough syrup without relief.

   d. patient's identity

   Janet Carter

   e. age, sex, height, and weight

   25 years old, female, 5 ft 5 in., 125 lb

   f. patient's occupation

   High school math teacher

   g. patient's dietary habits

   Generally eats a well-balanced diet with lots of fresh fruits and vegetables.

   h. patient's sleep habits

   Sleeps 8–9 hours a night.

   i. concurrent medical conditions, prescription and nonprescription medications, and dietary supplements

   No concurrent medical conditions. No routine nonprescription medications or dietary supplements. Is currently taking Yasmin (ethinyl estradiol 30 mcg, drospirenone 3 mg) for oral contraception; started about 5 years ago.

   j. allergies

   NKA

   k. history of other adverse reactions to medications

   None

   l. other (describe) _____

   None

Assessment and Triage

2. Differentiate patient's signs/symptoms and correctly identify the patient's primary problem(s).

   Janet is likely experiencing UACS secondary to the upper respiratory tract viral infection.

3. Identify exclusions for self-treatment (Figure 12–1).

   None

4. Formulate a comprehensive list of therapeutic alternatives for the primary problem to determine if triage to a health care provider is required, and share this information with the patient or caregiver.

   Options include:

   (1) Take no action.

   (2) Recommend that the patient see her PCP for further evaluation and treatment.

   (3) Recommend nondrug treatment (inhale warm steamy vapors, elevate head of bed at night to promote nasal and sinus drainage).

   (4) Recommend self-care with a first-generation antihistamine and decongestant combination product.

Plan

5. Select an optimal therapeutic alternative to address the patient's problem, taking into account patient preferences.

   Janet should treat her cough with a first-generation oral antihistamine (e.g., diphenhydramine) and decongestant (e.g., pseudoephedrine, phenylephrine) combination product; elevating the head of the bed at night or inhaling warm steamy vapors may provide some nondrug symptomatic relief.

6. Describe the recommended therapeutic approach to the patient or caregiver.

   "The upper airway cough syndrome is treated by a combination of the drying effects of an oral first-generation antihistamine and decongestant action of an oral decongestant."

7. Explain to the patient or caregiver the rationale for selecting the recommended therapeutic approach from the considered therapeutic alternatives.

   "Centrally active antitussives such as dextromethorphan and codeine and the expectorant guaifenesin have little efficacy in cough associated with viral infections such as the common cold."

Relevant Evaluation Criteria	Scenario/Model Outcome
Patient Education	
8. When recommending self-care with nonprescription medications and/or nondrug therapy, convey accurate information to the patient or caregiver.	See the box Patient Education for Cough.
Solicit follow-up questions from the patient or caregiver.	"How long can I take the antihistamine/decongestant medication?"
Answer the patient's or caregiver's questions.	"You may take the antihistamine/decongestant medication as needed for relief of symptoms until the cough resolves. Contact your PCP if the cough persists for longer than 7 days; if you develop a high fever 103°F (39.4°C); or if you cough up blood, develop chest pain, or have trouble breathing."
Evaluation of Patient Outcome	
9. Assess patient outcome.	Ask Janet to call to update you on her response to treatment.

Key: NKA = No known allergies; UACS = upper airway cough syndrome; PCP = primary care provider.

case
12–2

Relevant Evaluation Criteria	Scenario/Model Outcome
Information Gathering	
1. Gather essential information about the patient's symptoms and medical history, including:	
a. description of symptom(s) (i.e., nature, onset, duration, severity, associated symptoms)	The patient has a cough that is slowly getting worse. He states that he has had a cough for "years." Initially the cough was a dry morning cough, but over the past few months it has become productive of clear phlegm and persists throughout the day and night.
b. description of any factors that seem to precipitate, exacerbate, and/or relieve the patient's symptom(s)	The cough is worse in the morning when he gets up and persists throughout the day and night. The patient thinks it may be a smoker's cough.
c. description of the patient's efforts to relieve the symptoms	The patient has tried hard candy, menthol cough drops, Echinacea cough drops, and horehound drops, but nothing stops the cough.
d. patient's identity	Martin Lansford
e. age, sex, height, and weight	45 years old, male, 5 ft 11 in., 75 kg
f. patient's occupation	Accountant
g. patient's dietary habits	Mostly eats a meat and potatoes diet with little fresh fruit or vegetables.
h. patient's sleep habits	Sleeps 9 hours a night.
i. concurrent medical conditions, prescription and nonprescription medications, and dietary supplements	Intermittent heartburn and/or sour taste in mouth; has symptoms 3–4 times per year. The patient takes Prilosec (omeprazole) 20 mg once a day for 3–5 days 3–4 times per year. He has no other known medical condition and is not taking any routine nonprescription or dietary supplements.
j. allergies	None
k. history of other adverse reactions to medications	None
l. other (describe) _____	The patient started smoking at age 16 years. He currently smokes 2 ppd.

case

12-2 *continued*

Relevant Evaluation Criteria	Scenario/Model Outcome
Assessment and Triage	
2. Differentiate patient's signs/symptoms and correctly identify the patient's primary problem(s).	The cough appears to be a smoker's cough, but may be a symptom of chronic bronchitis or COPD. Heartburn and dyspepsia may be symptoms of GERD; GERD may cause chronic cough.
3. Identify exclusions for self-treatment (Figure 12-1).	None
4. Formulate a comprehensive list of therapeutic alternatives for the primary problem to determine if triage to a health care provider is required, and share this information with the patient or caregiver.	Options include: (1) Take no action. (2) Recommend that the patient see his PCP for further evaluation and treatment. (3) Recommend nondrug treatment (nonmedicated lozenges, inhale warm steamy vapors). (4) Recommend self-care with a nonprescription centrally acting antitussive or expectorant. (5) Recommend that the patient stop smoking.
Plan	
5. Select an optimal therapeutic alternative to address the patient's problem, taking into account patient preferences.	Martin should be referred to his PCP for further evaluation and treatment of his chronic cough. Centrally acting antitussives (e.g., codeine, dextromethorphan) and expectorants (e.g., guaifenesin) are not effective for the management of smoker's cough, COPD, or chronic obstructive pulmonary disease. Recommend smoking cessation.
6. Describe the recommended therapeutic approach to the patient or caregiver.	"You should consult with your primary care provider about your chronic cough."
7. Explain to the patient or caregiver the rationale for selecting the recommended therapeutic approach from the considered therapeutic alternatives.	"Chronic productive cough is a symptom associated with smoking but also with several chronic medical conditions such as chronic bronchitis and COPD. Chronic cough is also a symptom of lung cancer. Heartburn may trigger cough." (See Chapter 13 for information on the assessment and self-care of heartburn and dyspepsia.)
Patient Education	
8. When recommending self-care with nonprescription medications and/or nondrug therapy, convey accurate information to the patient or caregiver.	Criterion does not apply in this case.
Solicit follow-up questions from the patient or caregiver.	"What are my choices if I decide to stop smoking?"
Answer the patient's or caregiver's questions.	"Nonprescription nicotine replacement choices include nicotine-containing patches, gums, and lozenges. Prescription medications include nicotine-containing nasal sprays and inhalers and medications that reduce nicotine cravings such as bupropion and varenicline. Individual or group counseling are also available to help you quit smoking." (See Chapter 47 for information on self-care assessment of and medications for smoking cessation.)
Evaluation of Patient Outcome	
9. Assess patient outcome.	Ask Martin to call you after he is evaluated by his PCP to update you on his medical condition and decision regarding smoking cessation.

Key: COPD = Chronic obstructive pulmonary disease; GERD = gastroesophageal reflux disease; PCP = primary care provider; ppd = packs of cigarettes smoked per day.

➤ Neither codeine nor dextromethorphan has been shown to be effective for acute coughs associated with viral URTIs in either adults or children.

➤ In 2008, manufacturers voluntarily updated labels for cough and cold products to state "do not use" in children younger than 4 years.

➤ Combination products are convenient but are generally more expensive per dose and increase the risk of undesirable side effects.

➤ Refer patients to their primary care provider if they have cough with thick yellow or green sputum or pus-like secretions, or cough accompanied by one or more of the

patient education for
Cough

The goal of self-treatment is to reduce the number and severity of cough episodes and prevent complications. For most patients, carefully following product instructions and the self-care measures listed here will help ensure optimal therapeutic outcomes.

Nondrug Measures

- Stay well hydrated.
- Reduce throat irritation by slowly dissolving nonmedicated lozenges and candies in the mouth.
- Use humidifiers and vaporizers to increase the moisture in the air and possibly soothe irritated airways.
- Treat the underlying cause of cough (e.g., nasal congestion).

Nonprescription Medications

- Cough is a symptom of an underlying disorder. Contact your primary care provider if you have any of the exclusions for self-care listed in Figure 12–1.
- Select a product on the basis of the active ingredients and dosage formulation. Brand names frequently change and may not clearly represent the active ingredients.
- Slowly dissolve medicated lozenges in your mouth; do not chew.
- Swallow tablets and capsules whole; do not crush or chew.
- Follow the recommended dosing guidelines for each medication.
- Store all these medications according to the manufacturer's recommendations. Do not use any expired drug.

Cough Suppressants (Antitussives)

- Cough suppressants control or eliminate cough and are the drugs of choice for nonproductive coughs.
- Oral nonprescription cough suppressants include codeine (available without a prescription in some states), dextromethorphan, diphenhydramine, and chlophedianol.
- Topical nonprescription antitussives include camphor and menthol.
- Do not heat, microwave, or add topical antitussives to hot water. Do not use topical antitussives near an open flame. Topical antitussive ointments and liquids are toxic if ingested.
- The most common side effects of codeine include nausea, vomiting, sedation, dizziness, and constipation.
- Dextromethorphan's side effects are uncommon but may include drowsiness, nausea, vomiting, stomach discomfort, and constipation.
- The most common diphenhydramine side effects include drowsiness, disturbed coordination, decreased respiration, blurred vision, difficult urination, and dry mouth.
- The most common chlophedianol side effects include nausea, dizziness, and drowsiness.

- Codeine, dextromethorphan, diphenhydramine, and chlophedianol interact with drugs that cause drowsiness (e.g., narcotics, sedatives, some antihistamines, and alcohol).
- Dextromethorphan and chlophedianol also interact with monoamine oxidase inhibitors (e.g., phenelzine, tranylcypromine, and isocarboxazid). Do not take dextromethorphan or chlophedianol within 14 days of taking one of these medications.
- Diphenhydramine and chlophedianol also interact with drugs that have anticholinergic activity.
- Patients with impaired respiratory reserve (e.g., asthma or chronic obstructive pulmonary disease) should use codeine and diphenhydramine with caution.
- Patients with narrow-angle glaucoma, stenosing peptic ulcer, pyloroduodenal obstruction, symptomatic prostatic hypertrophy, bladder-neck obstruction, elevated intraocular pressure, hyperthyroidism, heart disease, or hypertension should use diphenhydramine with caution.
- Talk with your doctor before using any medication while pregnant.
- Codeine and diphenhydramine are excreted in breast milk and may cause side effects in the child.
- Older adults and children may have paradoxical excitation, restlessness, and irritability with diphenhydramine or chlophedianol. Older adults are more likely than the general population to have side effects from diphenhydramine.

Expectorants (Protussives)

- Guaifenesin is the only available nonprescription protussive.
- Guaifenesin is generally well tolerated, but side effects may include nausea, vomiting, dizziness, headache, rash, diarrhea, drowsiness, and stomach pain.
- There are no reported drug interactions with guaifenesin.
- Guaifenesin is contraindicated in patients with a known hypersensitivity to the medication.
- Guaifenesin is not indicated for chronic cough associated with chronic lower respiratory tract diseases such as asthma, chronic obstructive pulmonary disease, emphysema, or smoker's cough.

Note about Pediatric Dosing

- Manufacturers of cough and cold medications have revised product labeling to state that these products should not be used in children younger than 4 years. Health care providers should stress this information to caregivers of infants and young children.

---

following: high fever (adults, ≥103°F; children, >102°F), shortness of breath, chest pain, hemoptysis, chills, night sweats, tight-feeling throat, swollen legs/ankles, cyanosis, unintentional weight loss, rash, or persistent headache.
➤ Refer patients with cough and a history of or symptoms of chronic underlying disease associated with cough (e.g., asthma, COPD, chronic bronchitis, or heart failure) to their primary care provider.

REFERENCES

1. Hsiao C-J, Cherry DK, Beatty PC, et al. *National Ambulatory Medical Care Survey: 2007 Summary.* Hyattsville, MD: National Center for Health Statistics; 2010. National Health Statistics Reports; No. 27. Accessed at http://www.cdc.gov/nchs/data/nhsr/nhsr027.pdf, January 22, 2013.
2. *National Hospital Ambulatory Medical Care Survey: 2010 Emergency Department Summary Tables.* Hyattsville, MD: National Center for Health Statistics. Accessed at http://www.cdc.gov/nchs/data/ahcd/nhames_emergency/2010_ed_web_tables.pdf, March 5, 2013.
3. Joint Committee on Taxation. Present Law and Background Relating to the Tax Treatment of the Cost of Over-the-Counter Medicine as a Medical Care Expense (JCX-37-12), April 23, 2012. Accessed at https://www.jct.gov/publications.html?func=startdown&id=4423, January 22, 2013.
4. Polverino M, Polverino F, Fasolino M, et al. Anatomy and neuropathophysiology of the cough reflex arc. *Multidiscip Resp Med.* 2012;7:5–12.
5. Nasra J, Belvisi MG. Modulation of sensory nerve function and the cough reflex: understanding disease pathogenesis. *Pharmacol Ther.* 2009; 124(3):354–75.
6. Canning BJ. Encoding of the cough reflex. *Pulm Pharmacol Ther.* 2007; 20(4):396–401.
7. Chang AB. The physiology of cough. *Paediatric Respir Rev.* 2006;7(1):2–8.
8. Chung KF, Bolser D, Davenport P, et al. Semantics and types of cough. *Pulm Pharmacol Ther.* 2009;22(2):139–42.
9. Footitt J, Johnston SL. Cough and viruses in airways disease: mechanisms. *Pulm Pharmacol Ther.* 2009;22(2):108–13.

10. Kwon S-B, Park J, Jang J, et al. Study on the initial velocity distribution of exhaled air from coughing and speaking. *Chemosphere.* 2012; 87(11):1260–4.

11. Irwin RS. Introduction to the diagnosis and management of cough. *Chest.* 2006;129(1):25S–7S.

12. Chang AB. Pediatric cough: children are not miniature adults. *Lung.* 2010;188(suppl 1):S33–40.

13. Tumanan-Mendoza BA, Dans AL, et al. Dechallenge and rechallenge method showed different incidences of cough among four ACE-Is. *J Clin Epidemiol.* 2007;60(6):547–53.

14. Snellman L, Adams W, Anderson G, et al. Diagnosis and treatment of respiratory illness in children and adults. Bloomington, MN: Institute for Clinical Systems Improvement. Updated January 2013. Accessed at https://www.icsi.org/_asset/1wp8x2/RespIllness.pdf, September 15, 2014.

15. American College of Emergency Physicians Clinical Policies Committee and the Clinical Subcommittee on Pediatric Fever. Clinical policy for children younger than three years presenting to the emergency department with fever. *Annals Emerg Med.* 2003;42(4):530–45.

16. U.S. Food and Drug Administration. Cold, cough, allergy, bronchodilator, and antiasthmatic drug products for over-the-counter human use. CFR: Code of Federal Regulations, Title 21, Part 341. Updated April 1, 2012. Accessed at http://www.accessdata.fda.gov/scripts/cdrh/cfdocs/cfcfr/CFRSearch.cfm?CFRPart=341&showFR=1, January 15, 2013.

17. National Association of Boards of Pharmacy. 2013 Survey of Pharmacy Law. Mount Prospect, IL: National Association of Boards of Pharmacy; 2012:70–3.

18. U.S. Food and Drug Administration. Controlled Substances Act. Title 21–Food and Drugs, Chapter 13–Drug Abuse Prevention and Control, Subchapter 1–Control and Enforcement, Part B–Authority to Control; Standards and Schedules. Accessed at http://www.fda.gov/regulatory information/legislation/ucm148726.htm, March 8, 2013.

19. Peters R Jr, Yacoubian GS Jr, Rhodes W, et al. Beliefs and social norms about codeine and promethazine hydrochloride cough syrup (CPHCS) use and addiction among multi-ethnic college students. *J Psychoactive Drugs.* 2007;39(3):277–82.

20. Sharfstein JM, North M, Serwint JR. Over the counter but no longer under the radar—pediatric cough and cold medications. *N Engl J Med.* 2007;357(23):2321–4.

21. Reissig CJ, Carter LP, Johnson MW, et al. High doses of dextromethorphan, an NMDA antagonist, produce effects similar to hallucinogens. *Psychopharmacology.* 2012;223:1–15.

22. Bryner JK, Wang UK, Hui JW, et al. Dextromethorphan abuse in adolescence. *Arch Pediatr Adolesc Med.* 2006;160:1217–22.

23. Wilson MD, Ferguson RW, Mazer ME, et al. Monitoring trends in dextromethorphan abuse using the National Poison Data System: 2000–2010. *Clin Toxicol.* 2011;49(5):409–15.

24. U.S. Food and Drug Administration. Summary Minutes of the Drug Safety and Risk Management Advisory Committee, September 14, 2010. Accessed at http://www.fda.gov/downloads/AdvisoryCommittees/CommitteesMeetingMaterials/Drugs/DrugSafetyandRiskManagementAdvisoryCommittee/UCM235010.pdf, July 31, 2013.

25. Chen JYP, Biller HF, Montgomery EG Jr. Pharmacologic studies of a new antitussive, *alpha* (dimethylaminoethyl)-*ortho*-chlorobenzhydrol hydrochloride (SL-501, Bayer B-186). *J Pharmacol Exp Ther.* 1960;128(4):384–91.

26. Song GY, Lockhart ME, Smith JK, et al. Pseudoephedrine and guaifenesin urolithiasis: widening the differential diagnosis of radiolucent calculi on abdominal radiograph. *Abdom Imaging.* 2005;30(5):644–6.

27. Coderre K, Faria C, Dyer E. Probable warfarin interaction with menthol cough drops. *Pharmacotherapy.* 2010;30(1):110.

28. Abanses JC, Arima S, Rubin BK. Vicks VapoRub induces mucin secretion, decreases ciliary beat frequency, and increases tracheal mucus transport in the ferret trachea. *Chest.* 2009;135(1):143–8.

29. American Academy of Pediatrics. Committee on Drugs. Camphor revisited: focus on toxicity. *Pediatrics.* 1994;94(1):127–8.

30. Smith SM, Schroeder K, Fahey T. Over-the-counter (OTC) medications for acute cough in children and adults in ambulatory settings. *Cochrane Database Syst Rev.* 2012;8:CD001831. doi:10.1002/14651858.

CD001831. Accessed at http://www.thecochranelibrary.com/view/0/index.html.

31. Chang AB, Peake J, McElrea MS. Anti-histamines for prolonged non-specific cough in children. *Cochrane Database Syst Rev.* 2010;2:CD005604. doi:10.1002/14651858.CD005604. Accessed at http://www.thecochrane library.com/view/0/index.html.

32. Bolser DC, Davenport PW. Codeine and cough: an ineffective gold standard. *Curr Opin Allergy Clin Immunol.* 2007;7(1):32–6.

33. Paul IM. Therapeutic options for acute cough due to upper respiratory infections in children. *Lung.* 2012;190(1):41–4.

34. Chang CC, Cheng AC, Chang AB. Over-the-counter (OTC) medications to reduce cough as an adjunct to antibiotics for acute pneumonia in children and adults. *Cochrane Database Syst Rev.* 2012;2:CD006088. doi:10.1002/14651858.CD006088. Accessed at http://www.thecochrane library.com/view/0/index.html.

35. Eccles R. Mechanisms of the placebo effect of sweet cough syrups. *Respir Physiol Neurobiol.* 2006;152(3):340–8.

36. Irwin RS, Baumann MH, Bolser DC, et al. Diagnosis and management of cough. Executive summary. *Chest.* 2006;129(1):1S–23S.

37. Morice AH, McGarvey L, Pavord I. Recommendations for the management of cough in adults. *Thorax.* 2006;61(suppl 1):i1–24.

38. Shields MD, Bush A, Everard ML, et al. Recommendation for the assessment and management of cough in children. *Thorax.* 2008;63(suppl 3):iii1–15.

39. Pratter MR. Cough and the common cold. *Chest.* 2006;129(1 suppl):72S–4S.

40. Pratter MR. Chronic upper airway cough syndrome secondary to rhinosinus diseases (previously referred to as postnasal drip syndrome). *Chest.* 2006;129(1 suppl):63S–71S.

41. U.S. Food and Drug Administration. Public Health Advisory: FDA recommends that over-the-counter (OTC) cough and cold products not be used for infants and children under 2 years of age. Updated August 20, 2013. Accessed at http://www.fda.gov/ForConsumers/ConsumerUpdates/ucm051137.htm, September 15, 2014.

42. Consumer Healthcare Products Association. CHPA announces voluntary labeling updates for oral OTC children's cough and cold medications. CHPA Executive Newsletter. 2008;Issue No. 21-08. Accessed at http://www.chpa.org/workarea/downloadasset.aspx?id=911, September 15, 2014.

43. U.S. Food and Drug Administration. FDA statement following CHPA's announcement on nonprescription over-the-counter cough and cold medicines in children [news release]. October 8, 2008. Accessed at http://www.fda.gov/NewsEvents/Newsroom/PressAnnouncements/2008/ucm116964.htm, March 8, 2013.

44. U.S. Food and Drug Administration. FDA issues final guidance for liquid OTC drug products with dispensing devices [news release]. May 4, 2011. Accessed at http://www.fda.gov/NewsEvents/Newsroom/PressAnnouncements/ucm254029.htm, March 8, 2013.

45. U.S. Food and Drug Administration. Guidance for Industry: Dosage Delivery Devices for Orally Ingested OTC Liquid Drug Products. Rockville, MD: U.S. Department of Health and Human Services, Food and Drug Administration, Center for Drug Evaluation and Research; May 2011. Accessed at http://www.fda.gov/downloads/Drugs/Guidance ComplianceRegulatoryInformation/Guidances/UCM188992.pdf, March 8, 2013.

46. Berlin CM, Briggs GG. Drugs and chemicals in human milk. *Sem Fetal Neonatal Med.* 2005;10(2):149–59.

47. Berlin CM Jr, Paul IM, Vesell ES. Safety issues of maternal drug therapy during breastfeeding. *Nature.* 2009;85(1):20–2.

48. Einarson A, Lyszkiewicz D, Koren G. The safety of dextromethorphan in pregnancy. *Chest.* 2001;119(2):466–9.

49. The American Geriatrics Society 2012 Beers Criteria Update Expert Panel. American Geriatrics Society updated Beers criteria for potentially inappropriate medication use in older adults. *J Am Geriatr Soc.* 2012; doi:10.111/j.1532-5415.2012.03923.x.

50. Oduwole O, Meremikwu MM, Oyo-Ita A, et al. Honey for acute cough in children. *Cochrane Database Syst Rev.* 2012;3:CD007094. doi:10.1002/14651858.CD007094.

GASTROINTESTINAL DISORDERS

HEARTBURN AND DYSPEPSIA

Tara Whetsel and Ann Zweber

Heartburn (pyrosis) is one of the most common gastro-intestinal complaints. It is often described as a burning sensation in the stomach or lower chest that rises up toward the neck and occasionally to the back.[1] Patients may also describe it as indigestion, acid regurgitation, sour stomach, or bitter belching. Heartburn is a common symptom of gastroesophageal reflux disease (GERD), but similar symptoms may also occur in patients with peptic ulcer disease (PUD), delayed gastric emptying, gallbladder disease, and numerous other gastrointestinal disorders. Dyspepsia is defined as symptoms originating from the gastroduodenal region and includes bothersome postprandial fullness, early satiation, epigastric pain, and epigastric burning.[2] Patients with dyspepsia may report many of these symptoms, as well as anorexia, belching, nausea and vomiting, and upper abdominal bloating. Heartburn can also occur with dyspepsia. Dyspepsia can be organic, meaning it has an identifiable cause, or functional. Patients with functional dyspepsia have no identifiable organic, systemic, or metabolic disease that is likely to explain the dyspeptic symptoms.

Although rarely a cause of mortality, dyspepsia, heartburn, and GERD are associated with considerable morbidity and cost. Patients with heartburn may limit their activities and restrict their food choices to reduce symptom frequency and severity. Compared with the general population, patients with heartburn have an impaired quality of life, with symptoms affecting activity and work.[3] Nocturnal symptoms of heartburn were reported in 24.9% of the general population and in 74%–79% of patients with heartburn that occurs at least once a week.[4] Nocturnal symptoms are associated with interrupted sleep, decreased health-related quality of life, decreased work productivity, increased daytime sleepiness, and increased complications such as erosive esophagitis and stricture.[4] Patients with dyspepsia report a diminished quality of life similar to patients with mild heart failure or menopause.[5] A retrospective analysis of health insurance claims showed that patients with functional dyspepsia incurred $5138 more in annual costs than people without dyspepsia.[5] The total direct and indirect costs for GERD were over $12.6 billion per year; a large percentage of the costs were for prescription medications.[1]

The prevalence of heartburn and acid regurgitation in the past year in a healthy, predominantly white population were 42% and 45%, respectively.[1] Weekly symptoms were reported by 20% of the population, with an equal gender distribution.[1] Most subjects reported their heartburn to be moderately severe. In a cross-sectional study, the prevalence of heartburn was similar among African Americans, Hispanics, Asians, and whites (23%–27%).[1] However, whites had significantly more esophagitis.

Although men and women are almost equally affected by GERD, males have a higher rate of esophagitis and Barrett's esophagus (a precancerous condition). Older patients have a higher prevalence of GERD complications, but they may experience fewer symptoms because of decreased sensitivity to refluxed acid. The prevalence of GERD has been increasing in Western countries over the past 30 years, while remaining relatively low among residents of Africa and Asia. The rise in Western countries is speculated to be a result of increasing obesity and decreasing prevalence of *Helicobacter pylori* infection.[1] Heartburn is common during pregnancy, with 30%–80% of women complaining of heartburn, especially in the first trimester.[1]

Prevalence of dyspepsia has been estimated to range between 10% and 45%.[2] Much of this variation is influenced by criteria used to define dyspepsia. When heartburn is excluded, the prevalence of uninvestigated dyspepsia is 5%–15%. Women have a slightly higher prevalence compared with men. The incidence of dyspepsia has been estimated to be 2.8% per year.[5] Among patients with dyspepsia, 5%–10% have a peptic ulcer and approximately 20% have erosive esophagitis.

Pathophysiology

Esophageal defense mechanisms (antireflux barriers, esophageal acid clearance, and tissue resistance) help protect the esophageal mucosa from acid damage. Antireflux barriers include the intrinsic lower esophageal sphincter (LES), the diaphragmatic crura, the intra-abdominal location of the LES, the phrenoesophageal ligaments, and the acute angle of His (Figure 13–1). These anatomic structures work together to provide a physical barrier against gastric contents being refluxed into the esophagus. The major component is the LES, the distal 3–4 cm of the esophagus that is contracted at rest. The LES relaxes on swallowing to permit the flow of food, liquids, and saliva into the stomach. Transient relaxations occur when there is no swallowing or esophageal peristalsis, allowing retrograde movement of stomach contents into the esophagus. The crural diaphragm provides an extrinsic squeeze to the LES, contributing to resting pressure and augmenting LES pressure during periods of increased abdominal pressure, such as with coughing, sneezing, or bending over. The angle of His creates a flap valve effect that contributes to the antireflux barrier.

When reflux of acidic gastric material does occur, physiologic mechanisms help protect the esophageal mucosa from

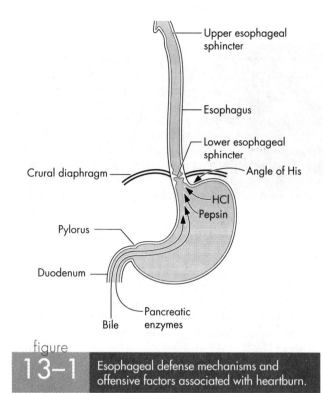

Upper esophageal
sphincter

Esophagus

Lower esophageal
sphincter

Crural diaphragm

Angle of His

HCl
Pepsin

Pylorus

Duodenum

Bile

Pancreatic
enzymes

damage. Esophageal acid clearance occurs when peristalsis moves refluxed material into the stomach, and saliva and esophageal gland secretions neutralize residual acid. Gravity also helps clear the esophagus. Tight junctions and the matrix of lipid-rich glycoconjugates in the intercellular space reduce epithelial damage from hydrogen ions. Epithelial cells are also capable of buffering and extruding hydrogen ions that do penetrate the cell membrane. Tissue resistance is further aided by the esophageal blood supply that delivers oxygen, nutrients, and bicarbonate and removes hydrogen and carbon dioxide, maintaining normal tissue acid–base balance. Even though gastroesophageal reflux is common, particularly postprandially, symptoms and esophageal damage are uncommon because of these esophageal defense mechanisms.

Heartburn is likely related to stimulation of esophageal mucosal chemoreceptors. Heartburn symptoms can arise from acid reflux, weakly acidic reflux, bile reflux, and mechanical stimulation of the esophagus. It is unclear why some reflux episodes produce symptoms whereas most do not. Possible contributing factors include mucosal disruption, decreased acid clearance, inflammation, reduced salivary bicarbonate concentration, volume of refluxate, frequency of heartburn, and interaction of pepsin with acid. One theory is that the esophagus becomes hypersensitive from repeated acid exposure, causing symptoms to occur from smaller boluses of acid.[6] Any disruption in the esophageal defense mechanisms can lead to increased acid exposure. Distension of the proximal stomach by either food or gas is a major stimulus for transient LES relaxations. Some patients may have a relatively hypotensive LES that can be overcome by an abrupt increase in intra-abdominal pressure from coughing, straining, or bending over. A hiatal hernia impairs LES function and esophageal acid clearance. A hiatal hernia displaces the LES from the crural diaphragm, reduces LES pressure, and results in more frequent transient relaxations of the LES, all of which contribute to increased reflux. Prolonged exposure of

the esophagus to the refluxed material can occur when lying down or sleeping and with decreased salivation or with peristaltic dysfunction. Large refluxate volumes from overeating or delayed gastric emptying can also increase esophageal acid exposure. As a result, damage to the tight intercellular junctions of the esophageal mucosa can lead to increased cellular permeability to hydrogen ions, with subsequent cellular injury. This increased permeability partly explains the development of heartburn in the absence of overt esophagitis.[1] The composition of the refluxate is an important contributor to the degree of esophageal damage. Pepsin and/or bile salts combined with acid produce greater injury than acid alone. *Helicobacter pylori* infection lowers gastric acidity, thereby possibly protecting against heartburn, GERD, and related complications.[1]

A number of risk factors are weakly associated with the development of heartburn (Table 13–1).[1,6,7,8] Foods (e.g., fat, chocolate, peppermint) and drugs (e.g., theophylline, morphine,

table **13–1**	**Risk Factors That May Contribute to Heartburn**
Dietary	**Medications**
Alcohol (ethanol)	Alpha-adrenergic antagonists
Caffeinated beverages	Anticholinergic agents
Carbonated beverages	Aspirin/NSAIDs
Chocolate	Barbiturates
Citrus fruit or juices	Benzodiazepines
Coffee	Beta$_2$-adrenergic agonists
Fatty foods	Bisphosphonates
Garlic or onions	Calcium channel blockers
Mint (e.g., spearmint, peppermint)	Chemotherapy
Salt and salt substitutes	Clindamycin
Spicy foods	Dopamine
Tomatoes/tomato juice	Doxycycline
Lifestyle	Estrogen
Exercise (isometric, running)	Iron
Obesity	Narcotic analgesics
Smoking (tobacco)	Nitrates
Stress	Potassium
Supine body position	Progesterone
Tight-fitting clothing	Prostaglandins
Diseases	Quinidine
Motility disorders (e.g., gastroparesis)	TCAs
PUD	Tetracycline
Scleroderma	Theophylline
Zollinger–Ellison syndrome	Zidovudine
	Other
	Genetics
	Pregnancy

Key: NSAID = Nonsteroidal anti-inflammatory drug; PUD = peptic ulcer disease; TCA = tricyclic antidepressant.

Source: References 1, and 6–8.

calcium channel blockers, diazepam) can decrease LES pressure, leading to increased reflux. Foods such as citrus, tomato-based foods, and spicy foods can irritate inflamed esophageal mucosa. Smoking contributes by relaxing LES pressure and decreasing salivation. Anxiety, fear, and worry may lower visceral sensitivity thresholds, leading to increased pain perception. Bending over, straining to defecate, lifting heavy objects, and performing isometric exercises may increase intra-abdominal pressure above the LES pressure, leading to reflux. Obesity increases intra-abdominal pressure, and epidemiologic studies suggest that the prevalence of GERD is considerably higher in obese patients than in those with a normal body mass index.[1]

Dyspepsia may be caused by PUD, GERD, celiac disease, gastric or esophageal malignancy (rarely), or other gastrointestinal (GI) disorders. Specific foods, such as spicy food, coffee, or alcohol, or excessive food intake have not been established as causing dyspepsia. Medications, including iron, antibiotics, narcotics, digoxin, estrogens, theophylline, and nonsteroidal anti-inflammatory drugs (NSAIDs), commonly cause dyspepsia through direct gastric mucosal injury, changes to GI function, exacerbation of reflux, or some other mechanism.[2] The pathophysiology of functional dyspepsia is unclear but may include delayed gastric emptying, impaired gastric accommodation to a meal, hypersensitivity to gastric distension, altered duodenal sensitivity, abnormal intestinal motility, and central nervous system dysfunction.[2] One or more of these disturbances can occur in individual patients. The cause of symptoms in patients with functional dyspepsia has not been established. Population studies have suggested a genetic predisposition. *H. pylori* may play a role in functional dyspepsia, as evidenced by the small improvement in symptoms following eradication. Patients who have recovered from gastroenteritis may suffer from postinfection functional dyspepsia. Psychosocial factors are an important contributor to symptom severity. Patients with functional dyspepsia may also have anxiety disorders, depression, somatoform disorders, and a recent or remote history of physical or sexual abuse. The exact mechanism is unknown, but some studies have suggested a relationship between psychosocial factors and visceral hypersensitivity.[2]

Clinical Presentation

Heartburn may occur alone or be associated with other GI disorders such as GERD and PUD (Table 13–2). Heartburn is most frequently noted within 1 hour after eating, especially after a large meal or ingestion of offending foods and/or beverages. Lying down or bending over may exacerbate heartburn. Regurgitation and, less commonly, water brash may also occur. Regurgitation is characterized by a bitter acidic fluid in the back of the throat. It is more common at night or when bending over. It differs from vomiting: nausea, retching, or abdominal contractions do not occur. Water brash is the sudden filling of the mouth with clear, slightly salty fluid secreted from the salivary glands. Severity of any of these symptoms is subjective, and no standard definitions exist for classifying symptoms as mild, moderate, or severe. Symptoms may be considered mild if they bother the patient a little but do not interfere with normal activities. Symptoms that are somewhat bothersome or annoying and/or interfere with normal activities may be considered moderate. Heartburn occurring two or more times a week is suggestive of GERD.[1] GERD can be complicated by erosive esophagitis, hemorrhage, esophageal ulcers, strictures, Barrett's esophagus, and esophageal adenocarcinoma. Heartburn severity is poorly correlated with esophageal damage, especially in older patients who may have no or mild symptoms despite severe erosive esophagitis or other complications on presentation.[1] Upper endoscopy is the standard for determining the presence and extent of esophageal damage.

Alarm symptoms include dysphagia, odynophagia, upper GI bleeding, and unexplained weight loss, and they can indicate more severe disease and/or complications. Dysphagia (difficulty swallowing) is slowly progressive for solid food and is usually associated with long-standing heartburn. The most common causes are peptic stricture or Schatzki's ring, but severe esophagitis, peristaltic dysfunction, and esophageal cancer are other potential etiologies.[1] Odynophagia (painful swallowing) is less common and may indicate severe ulcerative esophagitis, pill injury (e.g., tetracycline, potassium chloride, vitamin C, NSAIDs, aspirin, or bisphosphonates), or infection. Signs of upper GI bleeding include hematemesis, melena, occult bleeding, and anemia. Patients may

table 13–2	Differentiation of Simple Heartburn from Other Acid-Related Disorders			
	Simple Heartburn	**GERD**	**Dyspepsia**	**PUD**
Etiology	See Table 13–1	See Table 13–1	Possible contributing factors: food, alcohol, caffeine, stress, and medications Chronic dyspepsia: associated with PUD, GERD, celiac disease, and gastric cancer; or may lack an identifiable cause (functional dyspepsia)	Gastric or duodenal ulcer caused most commonly by *Helicobacter pylori* infection and/or NSAIDs
Typical symptoms	Burning sensation behind the breastbone that may radiate toward the neck, throat, and occasionally the back	Heartburn, acid regurgitation	Primary: postprandial fullness, early satiation, epigastric pain, epigastric burning Other: belching, bloating, nausea, vomiting	Gnawing or burning epigastric pain, occurring during day and frequently at night; may be accompanied by heartburn and dyspepsia

Key: GERD = Gastroesophageal reflux disease; GI = gastrointestinal; NSAID = nonsteroidal anti-inflammatory drug; PUD = peptic ulcer disease.

also present with atypical or extraesophageal symptoms related to gastroesophageal reflux. These include noncardiac chest pain, asthma, laryngitis, hoarseness, globus sensation (sensation of a lump in the throat), chronic cough, recurrent pneumonitis, and dental erosion.[1,9] Patients presenting with any alarm symptoms or atypical symptoms should be referred to their primary care provider for further evaluation.

Dyspepsia can present with one or more of four main symptoms. Postprandial fullness is an unpleasant sensation perceived as the prolonged persistence of food in the stomach. Early satiation is the feeling of fullness soon after starting to eat that is out of proportion to the amount of food ingested. Early satiety was the term previously used, but satiation is the correct term according to the most recent diagnostic criteria.[2] Epigastric pain is an unpleasant sensation between the umbilicus and lower end of the sternum. Epigastric burning refers to an unpleasant subjective sensation of heat. Less specific symptoms may include bloating, nausea, vomiting, and belching. Symptoms are mostly intermittent and may or may not be related to meals. Weight loss is considered an alarm symptom that should prompt referral for further investigation. Other alarm symptoms include anemia, blood loss, and dysphagia.

Treatment of Heartburn and Dyspepsia

Treatment Goals

The goals of self-treatment of heartburn and dyspepsia are to (1) provide complete relief of symptoms, (2) reduce recurrence of symptoms, and (3) prevent and manage unwanted effects of medications.

General Treatment Approach

The approach to self-treatment of heartburn and dyspepsia requires an initial assessment to determine whether the patient is a candidate for self-care (Figure 13–2). Individuals with exclusions for self-treatment should be referred for further medical evaluation. If the individual is a candidate for self-treatment, specific nondrug measures should be recommended and continued throughout treatment (see Patient Counseling for Heartburn and Dyspepsia). If appropriate, a recommendation should also be made for a nonprescription medication. The selection of the medication should be based on the frequency, duration, and severity of symptoms; the cost of the medication; potential drug–drug interactions and adverse effects; and the patient's preference. Antacids and nonprescription histamine type 2 receptor antagonists (H₂RAs) should be recommended for individuals with mild, infrequent heartburn and dyspepsia. Antacids are advantageous because they provide rapid relief of symptoms, but relief is brief when taken on an empty stomach (Table 13–3). When used in recommended dosages, the antacids are interchangeable despite differences in antacid salts and potency. Antacid/alginic acid combinations have a comparable onset of action to that of antacids alone and may provide better relief and a slightly longer duration of action.[10,11]

A nonprescription H₂RA is preferred to an antacid when individuals with mild-moderate episodic heartburn require more prolonged relief of symptoms. H₂RAs do not relieve heartburn or dyspepsia as rapidly as an antacid (Table 13–3) but may be used with an antacid if quick relief is desired along with a longer duration of action. The H₂RAs may also be used to prevent heartburn and acid indigestion when given 30 minutes to 1 hour prior to situations in which heartburn is anticipated. Nonprescription H₂RA products containing the lower doses (e.g., famotidine 10 mg up to twice daily) should be recommended for patients with mild, infrequent heartburn, whereas higher nonprescription dosages (e.g., famotidine 20 mg up to twice daily) should be reserved for moderate symptoms. Patients should not exceed 14 days of self-treatment with an H₂RA without consulting their primary care provider.

Nonprescription proton pump inhibitors (PPIs) can be used for treating frequent heartburn (2 or more days per week) or when patients do not respond to nonprescription H₂RAs.[12] The onset of symptomatic relief following a PPI dose is slower than that of an H₂RA (Table 13–3), and complete relief of symptoms may take several days after initiation of therapy. However, PPIs provide better symptomatic relief and a prolonged duration of action compared with the H₂RAs. When used to self-treat, the PPI should be limited to a duration of 14 days and retreatment to every 4 months.

Nonpharmacologic Therapy

Nonpharmacologic measures may benefit some individuals, but these changes alone are unlikely to completely relieve symptoms in the majority of patients. Dietary and lifestyle modifications recommended for heartburn are aimed at avoiding foods and beverages that precipitate heartburn and adopting behaviors that reduce esophageal acid exposure. Nonpharmacologic measures should be recommended for all patients with heartburn and dyspepsia despite the fact that evidence supporting their effectiveness is either lacking or equivocal.[5,7,8] A complete and accurate history will assist in identifying contributing factors (Table 13–1). Individuals should be asked to keep a diary to track dietary, lifestyle, and medication "triggers." Recommendations should be tailored to the individual's specific history. Weight loss should be advised for overweight patients with heartburn. Elevating the head of the bed by placing 6- to 8-inch blocks underneath the legs at the head of the bed or placing a foam wedge (e.g., GERD pillow) beneath the patient's upper torso and head should be recommended for patients troubled with heartburn when recumbent. Use of traditional pillows may worsen symptoms because they cause the individual to bend at the waist, which contributes to an increase in intragastric pressure.

Individuals should be educated about factors that contribute to heartburn and be advised how to manage them (see the box Patient Education for Heartburn and Dyspepsia). Most important, heartburn sufferers should be counseled to eat smaller meals, to reduce intake of dietary fat, and to refrain from eating within 3 hours of going to bed or lying down. Prescription and nonprescription medications should be evaluated for their potential to cause or exacerbate heartburn and dyspepsia (Table 13–1). When possible, individuals should be advised to switch to less troublesome nonprescription medications or to consult their prescriber about prescription drugs that may be exacerbating their symptoms. Use of tobacco products should be discouraged. If alcohol or caffeine consumption is a contributing factor, individuals should be advised to limit or discontinue use.

Pharmacologic Therapy
Antacids

Antacids relieve heartburn and dyspepsia by neutralizing gastric acid. Nonprescription antacid products contain at least one of the following salts: magnesium (hydroxide, carbonate, or trisilicate); aluminum (hydroxide or phosphate); calcium carbonate;

Exclusions for Self-Treatment

- Frequent heartburn for more than 3 months
- Heartburn while taking recommended dosages of nonprescription H2RA or PPI
- Heartburn that continues after 2 weeks of treatment with a nonprescription H2RA or PPI
- Heartburn and dyspepsia that occur when taking a prescription H2RA or PPI[8]
- Severe heartburn and dyspepsia
- Nocturnal heartburn[8]
- Difficulty or pain on swallowing solid foods[1,8]

- Vomiting up blood or black material or passing black tarry stools[1,8]
- Chronic hoarseness, wheezing, coughing, or choking[8]
- Unexplained weight loss[1,8]
- Continuous nausea, vomiting, or diarrhea
- Chest pain accompanied by sweating, pain radiating to shoulder, arm, neck, or jaw, and shortness of breath[8]
- Children < 2 years (for antacids), 12 years (for H2RAs), or 18 years (for PPIs)
- Adults > 45 years with new-onset dyspepsia[2]

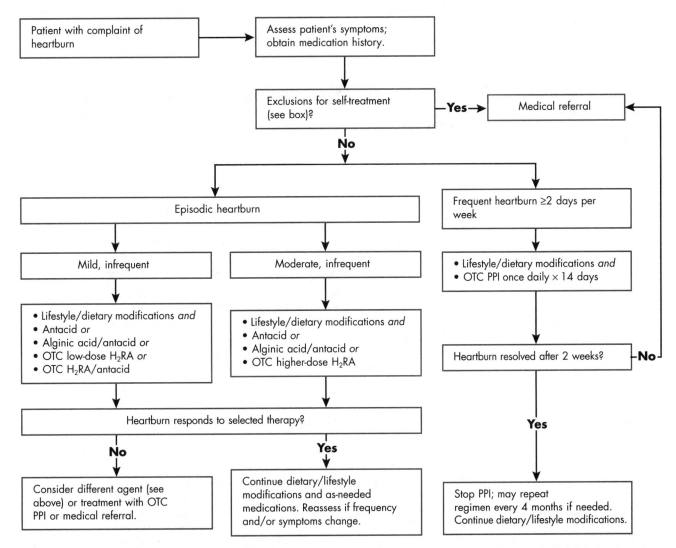

figure

13–2

Self-care of heartburn. Key: H2RA = Histamine type 2 receptor antagonist; OTC = over-the-counter; PPI = proton pump inhibitor.

table 13-3 Onset and Duration of Symptomatic Relief with Nonprescription Medications in Relieving Heartburn

Medication	Onset of Relief	Duration of Relief
Antacids	<5 minutes	20–30 minutes[a]
H$_2$RAs	30–45 minutes	4–10 hours
H$_2$RA + antacid	<5 minutes	8–10 hours
PPIs	2–3 hours	12–24 hours

Key: H$_2$RA = Histamine type 2 receptor antagonist; PPI = proton pump inhibitor.

[a] Food prolongs duration of relief.

or sodium bicarbonate (Table 13–4). Most antacids are relatively inexpensive, making them affordable products for the temporary relief of mild and infrequent heartburn and dyspepsia.

Antacids act as buffering agents in the lower esophagus, gastric lumen, and duodenal bulb. The cations react with chloride, but the anionic portion of the molecule reacts with hydrogen ions to form water and other compounds. Sodium bicarbonate rapidly reacts with gastric acid to form sodium chloride, carbon dioxide, and water. Its duration of action is shortened by its quick elimination from the stomach.[13] Of the magnesium salts, magnesium hydroxide is used most often. Magnesium hydroxide rapidly reacts with gastric acid to form magnesium chloride and water. This agent has a shorter duration of action than that of calcium carbonate and aluminum hydroxide. Calcium carbonate is a potent antacid that dissolves slowly in gastric acid to form calcium chloride, carbon dioxide, and water. This agent's onset of action is slower, but its duration of effect is longer than that of magnesium hydroxide or sodium bicarbonate. Aluminum hydroxide reacts with hydrochloric acid to form aluminum chloride and water.

table 13-4 Selected Nonprescription Antacid and Bismuth Products and Dosage Regimens

Trade Name	Primary Ingredients	Dosage (maximum daily dosage)
Adults/Children ≥ 12 Years		
Alka-Seltzer Heartburn Relief	Sodium bicarbonate 1940 mg; citric acid 1000 mg	Dissolve 2 tablets in 4 ounces of water every 4 hours as needed (8 tablets)
Alka-Seltzer Original	Sodium bicarbonate 1916 mg; citric acid 1000 mg; aspirin 325 mg	Dissolve 2 tablets in 4 ounces of water every 4 hours as needed (8 tablets)
Gaviscon Regular Strength Liquid	Each 15 mL contains[a] aluminum hydroxide 95 mg; magnesium carbonate 358 mg	1–4 tablespoons 4 times a day, after meals and at bedtime (16 tablespoons)
Gelusil Tablets	Aluminum hydroxide 200 mg; magnesium hydroxide 200 mg; simethicone 25 mg	Chew 2–4 tablets; repeat hourly if symptoms return (12 tablets)
Mylanta Ultimate Strength Liquid	Each 5 mL contains aluminum hydroxide 500 mg; magnesium hydroxide 500 mg	2–4 teaspoons between meals and at bedtime (9 teaspoons)
Mylanta Supreme Liquid	Each 5 mL contains calcium carbonate 400 mg; magnesium hydroxide 135 mg	2–4 teaspoons between meals and at bedtime (18 teaspoons)
Pepto-Bismol Maximum Strength Liquid	Each 15 mL contains bismuth subsalicylate 525 mg	2 tablespoons every 1 hour as required (4 doses or 8 tablespoons)
Pepto-Bismol Original Liquid	Each 15 mL contains bismuth subsalicylate 262 mg	2 tablespoons every 30 minutes to 1 hour as required (8 doses or 16 tablespoons)
Rolaids Regular Strength Antacid Tablets	Calcium carbonate 550 mg; magnesium hydroxide 110 mg	Chew 2–4 tablets hourly as needed (12 tablets)
Tums Extra 750 Tablets	Calcium carbonate 750 mg	Chew 2–4 tablets as needed for symptoms (10 tablets)
Tums Regular Strength Tablets	Calcium carbonate 500 mg	Chew 2–4 tablets as needed for symptoms (15 tablets)
Children ≤ 12 Years		
Maalox Children's Relief Chewable	Calcium carbonate 400 mg	Age 2–5 years: 1 tablet (3 tablets) Age 6–11 years: 2 tablets (6 tablets)
Children's Pepto	Calcium carbonate 400 mg	Age 2–5 years: 1 tablet (3 tablets) Age 6–11 years: 2 tablets (6 tablets)

[a] Sodium alginate (alginic acid) is listed as an inactive ingredient.

This agent has a slower onset and a longer duration than those of magnesium hydroxide. As a result of these reactions, a small but noticeable increase in intragastric pH occurs. Increasing the intragastric pH above 5 blocks the conversion of pepsin to pepsinogen.[13] Antacids also increase LES pressure.[1]

Liquid antacids usually have a faster onset than tablets because they are already dissolved or suspended and provide a maximal surface area for action. Of the tablet dosage forms, the quick-dissolving antacid tablets may provide the most rapid relief of symptoms. The duration of action for all antacids is transient, lasting only as long as the antacid remains in the stomach. The presence of food affects the duration of action of antacids. When administered within 1 hour after a meal, antacids may remain in the stomach for up to 3 hours.[13]

Differences in antacids are determined primarily by the cation, specific salt, and potency. Antacid potency is based on the number of milliequivalents of acid neutralizing capacity (ANC), which is defined as the amount of acid buffered per dose over a specified period of time. Factors that contribute to the ANC include product formulation, ingredients, and concentration.[13] As a result, the ANC is product specific; the same number of antacid tablets or equal volumes of different liquid antacids are not necessarily equal in potency.

Most antacids are minimally absorbed into the systemic circulation.[13] Approximately 90% of calcium is converted to insoluble calcium salts; the remaining 10% is absorbed systemically. About 15%–30% of magnesium and 17%–30% of aluminum may be absorbed and then excreted renally; therefore, accumulation may occur in patients with renal insufficiency. Sodium bicarbonate is readily absorbed and is eliminated renally.

Antacids are indicated for the treatment of mild, infrequent heartburn, sour stomach, and acid indigestion. Combination products containing aspirin or acetaminophen are FDA approved for overindulgence in food and drink and for hangover, although effectiveness has not been demonstrated. Individuals with mild dyspepsia may experience some relief with antacids, but no studies demonstrate their effectiveness.[2]

Antacids are administered orally. The effective dose of an antacid varies depending on product ingredients, milliequivalents of ANC, formulation, and the frequency and severity of symptoms. Individuals should be instructed to take product-specific recommended doses at the onset of symptoms. Dosing may be repeated in 1–2 hours, if needed, but should not exceed the maximum daily dosage for a particular product (Table 13–4). Individuals should be reevaluated if antacids are used more than twice a week or regularly for more than 2 weeks. Frequent antacid users may need to be switched to a longer-acting product such as an H$_2$RA, an H$_2$RA plus an antacid, or a PPI.

Antacids are usually well tolerated. Side effects are generally associated with the cation. The most common side effect associated with magnesium-containing antacids is dose-related diarrhea. Diarrhea may be reduced by combining magnesium-containing antacids with aluminum hydroxide. However, when higher dosages are used, the predominating effect is diarrhea. Magnesium excretion is impaired in patients with renal disease and may result in systemic accumulation of magnesium. Magnesium-containing antacids should not be used in patients with a creatinine clearance of less than 30 mL/minute.[13]

Aluminum-containing antacids are associated with dose-related constipation. Aluminum hydroxide binds dietary phosphate in the GI tract, increasing phosphate excretion in the feces. Frequent and prolonged use of aluminum hydroxide may lead to hypophosphatemia.[13] Chronic use of aluminum-containing antacids in patients with renal failure may lead to aluminum toxicity and should be avoided.

Calcium carbonate may cause belching and flatulence as a result of carbon dioxide production. Constipation when taking calcium antacids has been reported, but there is little evidence to support this side effect.[14] Calcium stimulates gastric acid secretion and is hypothesized to cause acid rebound when calcium-containing antacids are used to treat acid-related disorders. The clinical importance of this finding, however, remains uncertain.[13] If renal elimination is impaired, hypercalcemia may occur, and accumulation of calcium may result in the formation of renal calculi. Because many antacids have been reformulated to contain calcium, there is a risk of hypercalcemia when high and frequent dosages of calcium-containing antacids are taken with other calcium supplements or foods such as milk or orange juice with added calcium. Up to 2500 mg/day of elemental calcium can be ingested safely in individuals with normal renal function.[15] (See Chapter 22 for a discussion of calcium supplementation.)

Sodium bicarbonate frequently causes belching and flatulence that result from the production of carbon dioxide.[13] The high sodium content (274 mg sodium/gram sodium bicarbonate) may cause fluid overload in patients with congestive heart failure, renal failure, cirrhosis, or pregnancy, and in those on sodium-restricted diets. Individuals with normal renal function excrete additional bicarbonate, whereas patients with impaired renal function retain bicarbonate, which may cause systemic alkalosis. A high intake of calcium along with an alkalinizing agent (e.g., sodium bicarbonate or calcium carbonate) may lead to hypercalcemia, alkalosis, irritability, headache, nausea, vomiting, weakness, and malaise (milk–alkali syndrome).[13] Individuals who take calcium supplements should avoid using sodium bicarbonate as an antacid.

When given concomitantly with other oral medications, all antacids may potentially increase or decrease the absorption of the other medications by adsorbing or chelating the other drugs or by increasing intragastric pH.[16] Medications such as tetracyclines, azithromycin, and fluoroquinolones bind to divalent and trivalent cations, potentially decreasing antibiotic absorption. Absorption of levothyroxine may be decreased in the presence of an antacid; therefore, it is recommended to separate doses by 4 hours. The absorption of medications such as itraconazole, ketoconazole, and iron, which depend on a low intragastric pH for disintegration, dissolution, or ionization, may also be decreased. Specific antacids, such as aluminum hydroxide, may decrease the absorption of isoniazid. Premature breakdown of enteric-coated products may be increased with concurrent administration of antacids. The intraluminal interactions of antacids with other oral medications can usually be avoided when potentially interacting drugs are separated by at least 2 hours. Antacid-induced alkalization of the urine may increase urinary excretion of salicylates and decrease blood concentrations.[16] In contrast, an increase in urine pH may decrease urinary excretion and increase blood concentrations of amphetamines and quinidine.[13]

Alginic acid reacts with sodium bicarbonate in saliva to form a viscous layer of sodium alginate that floats on the surface of gastric contents, forming a protective barrier against esophageal irritation. Although alginic acid does not neutralize acid, the combination of alginic acid and antacid may provide better symptomatic relief than the antacid alone.[11] Because there is insufficient evidence supporting its efficacy as a single agent, the

Food and Drug Administration (FDA) has not granted alginic acid Category I status. However, alginic acid may be found as an inactive ingredient in several antacid products (Table 13–4). Some antacid products contain simethicone to decrease discomfort related to intestinal gas. (See Chapter 14 for a more detailed description of simethicone.)

Histamine Type 2 Receptor Antagonists

Cimetidine, ranitidine, famotidine, and nizatidine are approved for nonprescription use (Table 13–5) at one-half of the prescription dose and at the lower prescription dose. Products containing nizatidine are not currently available in the United States. When used in recommended dosages, the H$_2$RAs are considered interchangeable despite minor differences in potency, onset, duration of symptomatic relief, and side effects. The H$_2$RAs decrease fasting and food-stimulated gastric acid secretion and gastric volume by inhibiting histamine on the histamine type 2 receptor of the parietal cell. Therefore, the H$_2$RAs are effective in relieving fasting and nocturnal symptoms.[17] Their bioavailability is not affected by food but may be reduced modestly by antacids. Onset of symptomatic relief is not as rapid as with antacids, but the duration of effect is longer (Table 13–3). Cimetidine is the shortest acting (4–8 hours); ranitidine, famotidine, and nizatidine have a somewhat longer duration. Tolerance to the gastric antisecretory effect may develop when H$_2$RAs are taken daily (versus as needed) and may be responsible for diminished efficacy.[18] Therefore, it is preferable to take an H$_2$RA on an as-needed basis rather than regularly every day. All four H$_2$RAs are eliminated by

a combination of renal and hepatic metabolism, with renal elimination being the most important. A reduced daily H$_2$RA dose should be considered in patients with impaired renal function (creatinine clearance of less than 50 mL/minute) and patients of advanced age.[17]

Nonprescription H$_2$RAs are indicated for the treatment of mild-moderate, infrequent, or episodic heartburn and for the prevention of heartburn associated with acid indigestion and sour stomach. H$_2$RAs are more effective than placebo for relief of mild-moderate heartburn and provide moderate improvement in patients with mild, infrequent uninvestigated dyspepsia.[5] H$_2$RAs may be used at the onset of symptoms or 30 minutes to 1 hour prior to an event (e.g., meal or exercise) in which heartburn is anticipated. The combined H$_2$RA and antacid product (famotidine plus magnesium hydroxide and calcium carbonate; see Table 13–5) is indicated for individuals with postprandial heartburn who have not premedicated with an H$_2$RA. This combined product provides immediate relief and a longer duration of effect. Self-treatment dosing should be limited to no more than 2 times a day. If self-treatment with an H$_2$RA is needed for more than 2 weeks, a medical referral is recommended.

H$_2$RAs are well tolerated and have a low incidence of side effects. The most common side effects reported with all four H$_2$RAs include headache, diarrhea, constipation, dizziness, and drowsiness. Thrombocytopenia is a rare but serious adverse event with all four H$_2$RAs, but this effect is reversible upon discontinuation of the drug. Cimetidine is associated with a weak antiandrogenic effect that, when taken in high doses, may result in decreased libido, impotence, or gynecomastia in men.

table
13–5 Selected Nonprescription H₂RA and PPI Products and Dosage Regimens

Trade Name	Primary Ingredients	Dosage (maximum daily dosage)
H$_2$RA Products (Adults/Children ≥ 12 Years)		
Tagamet HB, various generic	Cimetidine 200 mg	1 tablet with a glass of water (2 tablets)
Pepcid AC, various generic	Famotidine 10 mg	1 tablet with a glass of water (2 tablets)
Pepcid AC Maximum Strength, various generic	Famotidine 20 mg	1 tablet with a glass of water (2 tablets)
Pepcid Complete	Famotidine 10 mg; calcium carbonate 800 mg; magnesium hydroxide 165 mg	Chew and swallow 1 tablet (2 tablets)
Tums Dual Action	Famotidine 10 mg; calcium carbonate 800 mg; magnesium hydroxide 165 mg	Chew and swallow 1 tablet (2 tablets)
Zantac 75, various generic	Ranitidine 75 mg	1 tablet with a glass of water (2 tablets)
Zantac 150, various generic	Ranitidine 150 mg	1 tablet with a glass of water (2 tablets)
PPI Products (Adults ≥ 18 Years)		
Prilosec OTC, various generic	Omeprazole magnesium 20.6 mg	1 tablet with a glass of water 30 minutes before morning meal; take daily for 14 days (1 tablet)
Zegerid	Omeprazole 20 mg; sodium bicarbonate 1100 mg	1 capsule with a glass of water 1 hour before morning meal; take daily for 14 days (1 capsule)
Prevacid 24HR, various generic	Lansoprazole 15 mg	1 capsule with a glass of water 30 minutes before morning meal; take daily for 14 days (1 capsule)
Nexium 24HR	Esomeprazole 20 mg	1 capsule with a glass of water 30 minutes before morning meal; take daily for 14 days (1 capsule)

Cimetidine inhibits several hepatic cytochrome P450 (CYP450) isoenzymes (3A4, 2D6, 1A2, and 2C9), resulting in drug interactions with numerous medications (e.g., phenytoin, warfarin, theophylline, tricyclic antidepressants, and amiodarone).[16] Cimetidine also inhibits CYP2C19 and blocks the conversion of clopidogrel to its active form, thus possibly reducing the effectiveness of clopidogrel.[20] CYP450 drug interactions with ranitidine, nizatidine, and famotidine are uncommon at nonprescription doses. Medications such as ketoconazole, itraconazole, indinavir and atazanavir, and iron salts require an acidic environment for absorption.[16,21] When administered with an acid-reducing drug, their absorption may be reduced. Cimetidine may inhibit the renal tubular secretion of drugs such as procainamide, metformin, and dofetilide.

Proton Pump Inhibitors

PPIs are potent antisecretory drugs that relieve heartburn and dyspepsia by decreasing gastric acid secretion. They inhibit hydrogen potassium ATPase (the proton pump), irreversibly blocking the final step in gastric acid secretion, thus providing a more potent and prolonged antisecretory effect than that of the H_2RAs (Table 13–3).[17] The relative bioavailability of PPIs increases with continued daily dosing. Onset of symptomatic relief following an oral dose may occur in 2–3 hours, but complete relief may take 1–4 days.[22] The PPIs are almost completely absorbed after oral administration, regardless of the presence of food.[17]

Omeprazole magnesium 20.6 mg (Prilosec OTC), the first PPI to become available for nonprescription use in the United States (Table 13–5), is available as a delayed-release tablet containing enteric-coated pellets (protection against intragastric degradation) and is converted in the body to omeprazole 20 mg.[17] Nonprescription omeprazole is also available as specific pharmacy-branded products. Immediate-release omeprazole (Zegerid) is formulated with omeprazole 20 mg and sodium bicarbonate 1100 mg. The sodium bicarbonate in Zegerid raises intragastric pH, permitting rapid absorption of omeprazole from the duodenum, but there is insufficient evidence to confirm that this results in a quicker onset of symptomatic relief. Esomeprazole magnesium 22.3 mg (Nexium 24HR) is the S-isomer of omeprazole and is available as a delayed-release capsule. Lansoprazole 15 mg (Prevacid 24HR) is available as a capsule formulation containing enteric-coated granules. Differences in efficacy among the PPIs have not been established. PPI tablets and capsules should not be chewed or crushed because the enteric coating will be compromised, thus decreasing the effectiveness of the drug.[17]

Nonprescription PPIs are indicated for the treatment of frequent heartburn in patients who have symptoms 2 or more days a week. They are not intended for immediate relief of occasional or acute episodes of heartburn and dyspepsia. Because PPIs inhibit only those proton pumps that are actively secreting acid, they are most effective when taken 30–60 minutes before a meal, preferably before breakfast.[23] Self-treatment should be limited to 14 days and no more frequently than every 4 months. If heartburn continues while taking a nonprescription PPI, persists for more than 2 weeks, or recurs within 4 months, a medical evaluation is recommended.

The safety of nonprescription antisecretory medications, when used appropriately, is well established. The most common short-term side effects of PPIs are similar to those reported for the H_2RAs (i.e., diarrhea, constipation, and headache).[18] Chronic acid suppression has the potential to impair natural defenses and

to increase the risk of infection.[24–28] Some studies indicate PPI users may have increased susceptibility to community-acquired pneumonia.[8,25] An association of PPI use with enteric infections, such as *Clostridium difficile* and bacterial gastroenteritis, has been shown to be statistically significant in a number of cohort and case control studies. Patients developing diarrhea or symptoms of gastroenteritis while on a PPI should stop use and contact a health care provider.

An increased risk for hip, spine, and wrist fractures in older patients (>50 years) has been associated with high-dose, long-term (>1 year) PPI therapy.[29] Although reduced gastric acid secretion may decrease calcium absorption, longitudinal studies have not found any evidence of a direct effect of PPIs on bone turnover.[30] FDA released a warning concerning the potential for increased risk of fractures with prescription PPIs but subsequently determined that the risk is low with appropriate nonprescription PPI use.[31]

Rebound acid hypersecretion upon discontinuation of long-term use of PPIs has been reported, but its clinical importance is uncertain.[32] Vitamin B_{12} deficiency, hypomagnesemia, and iron malabsorption have also been described in patients taking PPIs long term (usually >1 year) but not in ambulatory patients taking recommended dosages of nonprescription PPIs short term.[24,26,33] Self-treatment with PPIs should be limited to short-term use at nonprescription doses. Nonprescription PPIs should be used to treat only conditions approved by FDA and listed on the product label. Long-term use and ingestion of high doses of acid-suppressing medications should take place only under medical supervision.

Omeprazole, esomeprazole, and lansoprazole may inhibit the metabolism of medications that depend on hepatic CYP2C19 for metabolism.[34] Although clinically important drug interactions are uncommon, given the widespread use of PPIs, patients taking medications such as diazepam, phenytoin, warfarin, theophylline, or tacrolimus should be warned about the potential for a drug interaction. Omeprazole and esomeprazole appear to have the greatest potential of the nonprescription PPIs to reduce the antiplatelet effect of clopidogrel by inhibiting variants of CYP2C19, thus reducing the conversion of clopidogrel to its active form.[34,35] Patients taking clopidogrel should contact their cardiologist or primary care provider before taking a nonprescription PPI (especially omeprazole or esomeprazole). Omeprazole and esomeprazole have been shown to inhibit the metabolism of cilostazol, resulting in increased serum concentrations of cilostazol and its active metabolites.[36] Lansoprazole may be a safer option for self-treatment of frequent heartburn in patients taking cilostazol. Similar to the action of antacids and H_2RAs, PPIs increase intragastric pH and may decrease the absorption of pH-dependent drugs (see previous discussion of drug–drug interactions for antacids and H_2RAs). PPIs can interfere with elimination of methotrexate and its metabolite, hydroxymethotrexate, leading to increased risk for toxicity. Patients taking methotrexate should check with their primary care provider before using a PPI.[37,38] In addition, PPIs may increase the bioavailability of digoxin, but the clinical importance of this effect is unknown. Calcium citrate is the preferred calcium supplement form for patients taking acid-reducing medications such as PPIs, given that citrate salts do not require an acid environment for dissolution.

Bismuth Subsalicylate

Bismuth subsalicylate (BSS) is indicated for heartburn, upset stomach, indigestion, nausea, and diarrhea. FDA has tentatively determined that BSS is safe and effective for the relief of upset stomach associated with belching and for gas associated with overindulgence in food and drink.[39] It is uncertain how BSS relieves heartburn, but for upset stomach, it is believed to have a topical effect on the stomach mucosa. When used to treat acid-related symptoms, the adult dose of BSS is 262–525 mg every 30 minutes to 1 hour as needed (Table 13–4). BSS is generally not recommended for children and should be avoided in patients with renal failure. In the past, some nonprescription antacid product line extensions with common trade names were reformulated to contain BSS in place of an antacid, or vice versa. Patients and health care providers should examine the ingredients in an antacid product to determine whether it contains BSS because these products are periodically reformulated with different antacids and other ingredients. Individuals taking bismuth salts should know that bismuth may cause the stool and tongue to turn black. Dark-colored stools may be interpreted as an upper GI bleed, prompting needless medical procedures. (For a complete discussion of BSS, see Chapter 16.)

Product Selection Guidelines

Special Populations

Careful consideration should be given to the elderly before recommending self-treatment for new-onset heartburn or dyspepsia. Older patients are more likely to take medications that can contribute to heartburn and dyspepsia. In addition, they are at higher risk for developing complications and may have a more severe underlying disorder. If self-treatment is appropriate, an assessment should be performed to determine whether the individual has renal impairment and to identify potentially problematic medications. Patients with decreased renal function should be cautioned about using aluminum- and magnesium-containing antacids, and if an H$_2$RA is appropriate, the lower dose should be selected. Omeprazole, esomeprazole, and lansoprazole may be used in patients with renal impairment. Sodium bicarbonate should be avoided in patients taking cardiovascular medications.

Antacid selection for eligible patients should be based, in part, on potential side effects. For example, if a patient has a tendency toward constipation, a less-constipating antacid, such as magnesium hydroxide, may be more appropriate, whereas constipating antacids, such as aluminum hydroxide, should be avoided.

Children older than 2 years with mild, transient, and infrequent heartburn; acid indigestion; or sour stomach may try children's formulas of calcium carbonate–containing antacids. If symptoms recur or are not resolved quickly, the child should be referred to his or her primary care provider for further evaluation.[40] Nonprescription antacids containing calcium carbonate are labeled for children ages 2 years and older. If antacids are recommended, an assessment of the child's average daily intake of calcium may help guide the recommendation. The recommended daily intake of calcium for children ages 2–3 years is 700 mg, 4–8 years is 1000 mg, and 9–18 years is 1300 mg.[15] Nonprescription H$_2$RAs are labeled for patients ages 12 years and older, and nonprescription PPIs are indicated for patients ages 18 years or older.

Infrequent and mild heartburn in pregnant women should be treated initially with dietary and lifestyle modifications.[41] Calcium- and magnesium-containing antacids may be used safely if the recommended daily dosages are not exceeded. Special attention should be given to the recommended intake of calcium during pregnancy (1000–1300 mg/day).[15] If a woman is meeting this recommendation, the addition of a calcium-containing antacid may cause her to exceed the upper limit of 2500 mg of calcium per day. Cimetidine, ranitidine, and nizatidine are listed as compatible with pregnancy. Human data for omeprazole and esomeprazole suggest low risk with pregnancy. Famotidine and esomeprazole have limited or no human data to support use in pregnancy; however, animal data suggest low risk.[32] Pregnant women with frequent and moderate-severe heartburn should be referred for medical evaluation.

Aluminum-, calcium-, or magnesium-containing antacids are considered safe in women who are breast-feeding.[42] The American Academy of Pediatrics considers cimetidine to be compatible with breast-feeding. However, famotidine is less concentrated in the breast milk and may be preferable to cimetidine or ranitidine.[43] There is insufficient information regarding the use of omeprazole, esomeprazole, and lansoprazole in women who are breast-feeding; these medications are best avoided during lactation.[43]

Patient Preferences

Antacids and antisecretory drugs are available in a wide range of prices, flavors, and dosage forms. Once the most appropriate nonprescription medication is determined, the individual should be involved in selecting a product that is affordable, palatable, and practical to administer. Inactive ingredients such as dyes, sodium, and sugar should be considered for individuals with allergies, sensitivities, certain medical conditions, or dietary restrictions.

Complementary Therapies

No evidence has shown that any botanical products increase intragastric pH and relieve heartburn. However, peppermint, alone or in combination with other herbs, has been shown in some studies to be useful for dyspepsia. A study of the efficacy of artichoke leaf extract (ALE) for dyspepsia also showed greater improvement of symptoms in the ALE group compared with placebo.[5] (See Chapter 51 for a more thorough discussion of complementary therapies.)

Assessment of Heartburn and Dyspepsia: A Case-Based Approach

Cases 13–1 and 13–2 illustrate the assessment of patients with heartburn and dyspepsia.

Patient Counseling for Heartburn and Dyspepsia

Many cases of uncomplicated heartburn and dyspepsia are self-treatable. For optimal outcomes, individuals need to understand how to treat symptoms appropriately and when to seek additional care. This information is provided in the box Patient Education for Heartburn and Dyspepsia. Health care providers should screen patients for use of a prescription H$_2$RA or PPI and counsel patients to avoid duplication of therapies.

Relevant Evaluation Criteria	Scenario/Model Outcome

Information Gathering

1. Gather essential information about the patient's symptoms and medical history, including:

   a. description of symptom(s) (i.e., nature, onset, duration, severity, associated symptoms)

   Patient complains of recurring substernal burning sensation after eating large meals. It occurs one to two times a week. The discomfort is rated a 4 on a scale of 1–10. It is associated with a feeling of fullness and occasional burping. Symptoms typically last 3–4 hours after eating.

   b. description of any factors that seem to precipitate, exacerbate, and/or relieve the patient's symptom(s)

   Symptoms occur after eating dinner and are often associated with large meals at restaurants.

   c. description of the patient's efforts to relieve the symptoms

   Patient has tried Tums (calcium carbonate 500 mg) after meals to help relieve the symptoms. It works initially, but wears off after an hour and the discomfort returns.

   d. patient's identity

   Steve Lee

   e. age, sex, height, and weight

   55 years old, male, 5 ft 11 in., 215 lb

   f. patient's occupation

   Teacher

   g. patient's dietary habits

   Normal balanced diet; drinks one cup of caffeinated coffee every morning, and 1 ounce of whiskey most evenings with dinner.

   h. patient's sleep habits

   Sleeps 7–8 hours a night.

   i. concurrent medical conditions, prescription and non-prescription medications, and dietary supplements

   Hyperlipidemia: atorvastatin 20 mg every morning; post–myocardial infarction (2 years ago): atenolol 25 mg every morning, clopidogrel 75 mg every morning

   j. allergies

   Sulfamethoxazole

   k. history of other adverse reactions to medications

   None

Assessment Triage

2. Differentiate patient's signs/symptoms and correctly identify the patient's primary problem(s).

   Infrequent postprandial substernal burning is consistent with uncomplicated heartburn.

3. Identify exclusions for self-treatment (Figure 13–2).

   None

4. Formulate a comprehensive list of therapeutic alternatives for the primary problem to determine if triage to a medical provider is required, and share this information with the patient or caregiver.

   Options include:

   (1) Refer Steve to his PCP.

   (2) Recommend lifestyle modifications.

   (3) Recommend an OTC antacid or acid-reducing product.

   (4) Take no action.

Plan

5. Select an optimal therapeutic alternative to address the patient's problem, taking into account patient preferences.

   An OTC acid-reducing product should be effective. Patient will consider lifestyle modifications.

6. Describe the recommended therapeutic approach to the patient or caregiver.

   "Take 20 mg of famotidine 30 minutes prior to meals that may cause heartburn, or when symptoms occur." See directions in Table 13–5.

7. Explain to the patient or caregiver the rationale for selecting the recommended therapeutic approach from the considered therapeutic alternatives.

   "Seeing a PCP may not be necessary if adequate relief is experienced and symptoms do not become more severe or frequent. An antacid will not provide long-lasting relief. You should not use a PPI without consulting your primary care provider because of a possible interaction with your clopidogrel."

Patient Education

8. When recommending self-care with nonprescription medications and/or nondrug therapy, convey accurate information to the patient or caregiver:

   a. appropriate dose and frequency of administration

   See Table 13–5.

   b. maximum number of days the therapy should be employed

   See the box Patient Education for Heartburn and Dyspepsia

   c. product administration procedures

   See Table 13–5.

   d. expected time to onset of relief

   30 minutes to 1 hour if used after symptoms occur.

case
13-1 continued

Relevant Evaluation Criteria	Scenario/Model Outcome
e. degree of relief that can be reasonably expected	Complete prevention of symptoms if used prior to meals or complete relief of symptoms if used after symptom onset.
f. most common side effects	Side effects are uncommon. Some patients report headache, diarrhea, or constipation.
g. side effects that warrant medical intervention should they occur	Moderate-severe diarrhea or symptoms of gastroenteritis
h. patient options in the event that condition worsens or persists	A PCP should be consulted if symptoms are not resolved satisfactorily, if they increase in frequency or severity, or if alarm symptoms occur (Figure 13–2).
i. product storage requirements	See the box Patient Education for Heartburn and Dyspepsia.
j. specific nondrug measures	Eat smaller meals, reduce alcohol intake, and avoid problematic foods. Consider ways to reduce weight. (See the box Patient Education for Heartburn and Dyspepsia for other measures.)
Solicit follow-up questions from the patient or caregiver.	"May I take an antacid for immediate relief of symptoms?"
Answer the patient's or caregiver's questions.	"Yes. Taking a product that contains calcium carbonate or magnesium hydroxide after symptoms occur will provide quick, short-term relief. These can be taken with famotidine if needed. An alternative would be to take a combination product that contains both an antacid and an acid reducer."

Evaluation of Patient Outcome

9. Assess patient response.	Ask Steve to call or update you on his response to the famotidine, or call Steve in a week to evaluate his response.

Key: H$_2$RA = Histamine type 2 receptor antagonist; OTC = over-the-counter; PCP = primary care provider; PPI = proton pump inhibitor.

case
13-2

Relevant Evaluation Criteria	Scenario/Model Outcome
Information Gathering	
1. Gather essential information about the patient's symptoms and medical history, including:	
a. description of symptom(s) (i.e., nature, onset, duration, severity, associated symptoms)	Patient suffers from ongoing upper abdominal discomfort. Patient describes a gnawing pain that causes nausea and fluctuates throughout the day. Pain rating varies from 4–7 on a scale of 10. Symptoms started 3 days ago. Some difficulty breathing.
b. description of any factors that seem to precipitate, exacerbate, and/or relieve the patient's symptom(s)	Discomfort worsens when she walks, especially up and down stairs. Somewhat better at rest.
c. description of the patient's efforts to relieve the symptoms	Patient has tried Pepcid Complete (famotidine 10 mg, calcium carbonate 800 mg, and magnesium hydroxide 165 mg) as well as Zantac 150 (ranitidine 150 mg) with no relief.
d. patient's identity	Angelica Mousa
e. age, sex, height, and weight	62 years old, female, 5 ft 5 in., 165 lb
f. patient's occupation	Retired
g. patient's dietary habits	Eats small meals throughout the day.
h. patient's sleep habits	Averages 6 hours per night.
i. concurrent medical conditions, prescription and non-prescription medications, and dietary supplements	Hyperlipidemia: stopped taking atorvastatin 1 year ago because she couldn't afford it. Takes calcium carbonate 1000 mg with vitamin D 400 IU twice daily.
j. allergies	NKDA
k. history of other adverse reactions to medications	None
l. other (describe) _____	Smokes 15–20 cigarettes/day for the past 40 years. Drinks 2–4 cups of caffeinated coffee daily. Stopped drinking alcohol 5 years ago.

case

13–2 *continued*

Relevant Evaluation Criteria	Scenario/Model Outcome
Assessment and Triage	
2. Differentiate patient's signs/symptoms and correctly identify the patient's primary problem(s).	Late-onset and ongoing GI symptoms; worsening upon exertion. No response to antacid and H₂RAs.
3. Identify exclusions for self-treatment (Figure 13–2).	May be an indication of cardiac problems, or other non-GI issues. Alarm symptoms indicate medical referral.
4. Formulate a comprehensive list of therapeutic alternatives for the primary problem to determine if triage to a medical provider is required, and share this information with the patient or caregiver.	Options include: (1) Refer Angelica to a PCP immediately for a differential diagnosis. (2) Recommend an OTC product with lifestyle modifications. (3) Take no action.
Plan	
5. Select an optimal therapeutic alternative to address the patient's problem, taking into account patient preferences.	Refer the patient to a PCP for a differential diagnosis.
6. Describe the recommended therapeutic approach to the patient or caregiver.	"Call your primary care provider immediately or go to urgent care for a medical evaluation."
7. Explain to the patient or caregiver the rationale for selecting the recommended therapeutic approach from the considered therapeutic alternatives.	"You need to see your primary care provider because your symptoms indicate a more serious medical condition that needs prompt evaluation. OTC therapy is unlikely to be effective or appropriate."
8. When recommending self-care with nonprescription medications and/or nondrug therapy, convey accurate information to the patient or caregiver.	Criterion does not apply in this case.
Solicit follow-up questions from the patient or caregiver.	"I thought heart attacks involved a crushing chest pain, so I am not having a heart attack, right?"
Answer the patient's or caregiver's questions.	"In women heart attacks often present with upper abdominal pain, nausea, shortness of breath, and other symptoms such as jaw, arm or shoulder pain. Your symptoms could be from heart disease and should be medically evaluated as soon as possible."
Evaluation of Patient Outcome	
9. Assess patient response.	Contact Angelica in a day or two to ensure that she sought medical care.

Key: H₂RA = Histamine type 2 receptor antagonist; NKDA = no known drug allergies; OTC = over-the-counter; PCP = primary care provider.

patient education for

Heartburn and Dyspepsia

Heartburn and dyspepsia (indigestion) are often self-treatable conditions. Heartburn is characterized by a burning sensation in the chest, usually occurring after meals. Dyspepsia is characterized by discomfort in the upper abdomen. The goals of self-treatment are to (1) provide complete relief of symptoms, (2) reduce recurrence of symptoms, and (3) prevent and manage unwanted effects of medications.

Nondrug Measures

▪ Avoid food, beverages, and activities that may precipitate or increase the frequency and severity of symptoms.
▪ If possible, avoid the use of medications that may aggravate heartburn or dyspepsia.
▪ Avoid eating large meals.
▪ Stop or reduce smoking.
▪ Lose weight if overweight and not pregnant.
▪ Wear loose-fitting clothing.
▪ If nocturnal symptoms are present:
  – Avoid lying down within 3 hours of a meal.
  – Elevate the head of the bed using 6- to 8-inch blocks, or use a foam pillow wedge.

Nonprescription Medications

▪ Store all medications at 68°F–77°F (20°C–25°C), and protect them from heat, humidity, and moisture. Discard after expiration date.

Antacids

▪ Antacids (sodium bicarbonate, calcium carbonate, magnesium hydroxide, and aluminum hydroxide) are available alone and in combination with each other and other ingredients.
▪ Antacids work by neutralizing acid in the stomach.
▪ Antacids may be used for relief of mild, infrequent heartburn or dyspepsia (indigestion).

patient education for

Heartburn and Dyspepsia *(continued)*

- Antacids are usually taken at the onset of symptoms. Relief of symptoms typically begins within 5 minutes.
- Because antacids come in a variety of strengths and concentrations, it is essential to consult the label of an individual product for the correct dose and frequency of administration. Generally antacids should not be used more than 4 times a day, or regularly for more than 2 weeks.
- If symptoms are not relieved with recommended dosages, consult a health care provider.
- Diarrhea may occur with magnesium- or magnesium/aluminum–containing antacids; constipation may occur with aluminum- or calcium-containing antacids. Consult a health care provider if these effects are troublesome or do not resolve in a few days.
- In children older than 2 years, mild transient and infrequent heartburn; acid indigestion; or sour stomach may be treated with children's products containing calcium carbonate if they are used according to package directions.
- Pregnant women with mild and infrequent heartburn may use calcium- and magnesium-containing antacids safely if recommended daily dosages are not exceeded.
- Patients with kidney dysfunction should consult their primary care provider prior to self-treatment with antacids.
- Patients taking tetracyclines, fluoroquinolones, azithromycin, digoxin, ketoconazole, itraconazole, and iron supplements should not take antacids within 2 hours of taking any of these medications.

Histamine Type 2 Receptor Antagonists (H$_2$RAs)

- H$_2$RAs (cimetidine, famotidine, and ranitidine) may be used to relieve symptoms of or prevent heartburn and indigestion associated with meals.
- H$_2$RAs work by decreasing acid production in the stomach.
- H$_2$RAs are usually taken at the onset of symptoms or 30 minutes to 1 hour before symptoms are expected. Relief of symptoms can be expected to begin within 30–45 minutes. A combination product that contains both an antacid and an H$_2$RA provides faster relief of symptoms.
- H$_2$RAs generally relieve symptoms for 4–10 hours. H$_2$RAs can be taken when needed up to twice daily for 2 weeks.
- H$_2$RAs should be used for relief of mild-moderate, infrequent, and episodic heartburn and indigestion when a longer effect is needed. Use lower dosages for mild infrequent heartburn and higher dosages for moderate infrequent symptoms.
- If symptoms are not relieved with recommended doses, worsen, or persist after 2 weeks of treatment, consult a primary care provider.
- Side effects are uncommon. Consult a primary care provider if side effects are troublesome or do not resolve within a few days.
- Cimetidine may interact with many medications. Consult your primary care provider if you are also taking other medications, including a blood thinner such as warfarin or clopidogrel, an

antifungal such as ketoconazole, an anticonvulsant such as phenytoin, an antianxiety medication such as diazepam, or theophylline and amiodarone.

Proton Pump Inhibitors (PPIs)

- Nonprescription PPIs are indicated for mild-moderate frequent heartburn that occurs 2 or more days a week. They are not intended for the relief of mild, occasional heartburn.
- PPIs (omeprazole, esomeprazole, and lansoprazole) work by decreasing acid production in the stomach.
- PPIs should be taken with a glass of water every morning 30 minutes before breakfast for 14 days. Make sure that you take the full 14-day course of treatment.
- Do not take more than 1 tablet a day.
- Complete resolution of symptoms should be noted within 4 days of initiating treatment.
- If symptoms persist, worsen, are not adequately relieved after 2 weeks of treatment, or recur before 4 months has elapsed since treatment, consult your primary care provider.
- Do not crush or chew tablets or capsules because this may decrease the effectiveness of the PPI.
- Side effects are uncommon. Consult a health care provider if side effects are troublesome or do not resolve within a few days.
- Consult a health care provider if you are also taking other medications, including a blood thinner such as warfarin or clopidogrel, an antifungal such as ketoconazole, an anticonvulsant such as phenytoin, an antianxiety medication such as diazepam, antiretroviral medications, methotrexate, theophylline, tacrolimus, digoxin, or cilostazol.

When to Seek Medical Attention

Consult your primary care provider if you experience any of the following:

- Heartburn or dyspepsia (indigestion) for more than 3 months
- Heartburn or dyspepsia (indigestion) while taking recommended dosages of nonprescription medications
- Heartburn or dyspepsia (indigestion) after 2 weeks of continuous treatment with a nonprescription medication
- Heartburn that awakens you during the night.
- Difficulty or pain on swallowing foods.
- Light-headedness, sweating, and dizziness accompanied by vomiting of blood or black material or black tarry bowel movements.
- Chest pain or shoulder, arm, or neck pain, with shortness of breath.
- Chronic hoarseness, cough, choking, or wheezing.
- Unexplained weight loss.
- Continuous nausea, vomiting, or diarrhea.
- Severe stomach pain.

Evaluation of Patient Outcomes for Heartburn and Dyspepsia

Individuals taking antacids or an H$_2$RA for infrequent heartburn and dyspepsia should obtain symptomatic relief within 30 minutes to 1 hour. Patients taking PPIs may require up to 4 days for complete relief of symptoms, but most individuals are asymptomatic within 1 or 2 days. Self-treating individuals should be encouraged to contact their primary care provider

to report on the effectiveness of therapy and on any problems, such as side effects, that may arise during treatment. In some cases, the provider may make a follow-up contact to assess therapeutic outcomes. Patients should be asked to describe the change in frequency and severity of symptoms following initiation of therapy. Patients should be questioned regarding side effects and any new symptoms that may have developed. If the patient reports an inadequate response to therapy, the individual should be reevaluated to determine whether a different therapy is suitable or whether medical referral is necessary. Side effects may be managed by adjusting the dose or switching to another product. Patients who develop atypical or alarm symptoms (Figure 13–2) should be referred to their primary care provider.

Key Points for Heartburn and Dyspepsia

➤ The self-treatment of heartburn and dyspepsia should be limited to mild or moderate symptoms, including postprandial burning in the upper abdomen or centralized abdominal discomfort.

➤ Patients with atypical or alarm symptoms (Figure 13–2) should be referred for further evaluation.

➤ In children older than 2 years, treatment of mild transient and infrequent heartburn, acid indigestion, or sour stomach symptoms with calcium carbonate–containing antacids should be limited; prompt referral should be made if symptoms recur or persist.

➤ Pregnant women may self-treat mild and infrequent heartburn with calcium- and magnesium-containing antacids.

➤ Patients with heartburn should be counseled on nondrug measures such as dietary and lifestyle modifications (see the box Patient Education for Heartburn and Dyspepsia).

➤ Self-treating individuals should be advised about the advantages and disadvantages of various antacids and acid-reducing products so they can select a product that is best suited to them.

➤ Antacids provide temporary relief for mild and infrequent heartburn and dyspepsia. Dosages are product specific because of variability in antacid ingredients and concentrations.

➤ H_2RAs are indicated for mild and infrequent heartburn or dyspepsia. They may be taken at the onset of symptoms or 1 hour prior to an event (e.g., meal or exercise) that may cause symptoms.

➤ Combining an antacid with an H_2RA provides immediate relief of heartburn and a longer duration of action.

➤ PPIs are indicated for the treatment of frequent heartburn (heartburn that occurs ≥ 2 days a week). PPIs should be used a maximum of 14 days at a time and no more than every 4 months, and they are not intended for immediate relief of infrequent symptoms.

➤ Individuals with self-treatable symptoms should be advised to contact their primary care provider if symptoms worsen or recur after 14 days of effective self-treatment.

REFERENCES

1. Richter JE, Friedenberg FK. Gastroesophageal reflux disease. In: Feldman M, Friedman LS, Brandt LJ, eds. *Sleisenger and Fordtran's Gastrointestinal and Liver Disease.* 9th ed. Philadelphia, PA: Saunders; 2010:705–26.

2. Tack J. Dyspepsia. In: Feldman M, Friedman LS, Brandt LJ, eds. *Sleisenger and Fordtran's Gastrointestinal and Liver Disease.* 9th ed. Philadelphia, PA: Saunders; 2010:183–95.

3. Peery AF, Dellon ES, Lund J, et al. Burden of gastrointestinal disease in the United States: 2012 update. *Gastroenterology.* 2012;143(5):1179–87.

4. Fujiwara Y, Arakawa T, Fass R. Gastroesophageal reflux disease and sleep disturbances. *J Gastroenterol.* 2012;47(7):760–9.

5. Lacy BE, Talley NJ, Locke GR, et al. Review article: current treatment options and management of functional dyspepsia. *Aliment Pharmacol Ther.* 2012;36(1):3–15.

6. DeVault KR. Symptoms of esophageal disease. In: Feldman M, Friedman LS, Brandt LJ, eds. *Sleisenger and Fordtran's Gastrointestinal and Liver Disease.* 9th ed. Philadelphia, PA: Saunders; 2010:173–81.

7. Vemulapalli R. Diet and lifestyle modifications in the management of gastroesophageal reflux disease. *Nutr Clin Pract.* 2008;23(3):293–8.

8. Katz PO, Gerson LB, Vela MF. Guidelines for the diagnosis and management of gastroesophageal reflux disease. *Am J Gastroenterol.* 2013;108(3):308–28.

9. Hom C, Vaezi M. Extraesophageal manifestations of gastroesophageal reflux disease. *Gastroenterol Clin N Am.* 2013;42(1):71–91.

10. Giannini EG, Zentilin P, Dulbecco P, et al. A comparison between sodium alginate and magaldrate anhydrous in the treatment of patients with gastroesophageal reflux symptoms. *Dig Dis Sci.* 2006;51(11):1904–9.

11. Kwiatek MA, Roman S, Fareeduddin A, et al. An alginate formulation can eliminate or displace the postprandial "acid pocket" in symptomatic GERD patients. *Aliment Pharmacol Ther.* 2011;34(1):59–66.

12. Haag S, Andrews JM, Katelaris PH, et al. Management of reflux symptoms with over-the-counter proton pump inhibitors: issues and proposed guidelines. *Digestion.* 2009;80(4):226–34.

13. Maton PN, Burton ME. Antacids revisited: a review of their clinical pharmacology and recommended therapeutic use. *Drugs.* 1999;57(6):855–70.

14. Richter JE. Review article: the management of heartburn in pregnancy. *Aliment Pharmacol Ther.* 2005;22(9):749–57.

15. National Institutes of Health, Office of Dietary Supplements. Dietary supplement fact sheet: calcium. March 14, 2013. Accessed at http://dietary-supplements.info.nih.gov/factsheets/calcium.asp, April 24, 2013.

16. Ogawa R, Echizen H. Clinically significant drug interactions with antacids. *Drugs.* 2011;71(14):1839–64.

17. Berardi RR, Fugit RV. Peptic ulcer disease. In: DiPiro JT, Talbert RL, Yee GC, et al., eds. *Pharmacotherapy: A Pathophysiologic Approach.* 8th ed. New York, NY: McGraw-Hill, Inc.; 2011:563–85.

18. Furuta K, Adachi K, Komazawa Y, et al. Tolerance to H2-receptor antagonist correlates well with the decline in efficacy against gastro esophageal reflux in patients with gastroesophageal reflux disease. *J Gastroenterol Hepatol.* 2006;21:1581–5.

19. U.S. Food and Drug Administration. Information for healthcare professionals: update to the labeling of clopidogrel bisulfate (marketed as Plavix) to alert healthcare professionals about a drug interaction with omeprazole (marketed as Prilosec and Prilosec OTC). November 17, 2009. Accessed at http://www.fda.gov/Drugs/DrugSafety/PostmarketDrugSafetyInformationforPatientsandProviders/ucm190836.htm, April 24, 2013.

20. Plavix® (clopidogrel bisulfate tablets) [package insert]. Bridgewater, NJ: Bristol-Myers Squibb/Sanofi Pharmaceuticals Partnership. December 2011. Accessed at http://products.sanofi-aventis.us/PLAVIX/plavix.html, April 24, 2013.

21. Fulco PP, Vora UB, Bearman GM. Acid suppressive therapy and the effects on protease inhibitors. *Ann Pharmacother.* 2006;40(11):1974–83.

22. Mossner J, Caca K. Developments in the inhibition of gastric acid suppression. *Eur J Clin Invest.* 2005;35(8):469–75.

23. Hatlebakk JG, Katz PO, Camacho-Lobato L, et al. Proton pump inhibitors: better acid suppression when taken before a meal than without a meal. *Aliment Pharmacol Ther.* 2000;14(10):1267–72.

24. Ali T, Roberts DN, Tierney WM. Long-term safety concerns with proton pump inhibitors. *Am J Med.* 2009;122(10):896–903.

25. Heidelbaugh JJ, Goldberg KL, Inadomi JM. Overutilization of proton pump inhibitors: a review of cost-effectiveness and risk. *Am J Gastroenterol.* 2009;104(suppl 2):S27–32.

26. Parikh N, Howden CW. The safety of drugs used in acid-related disorders and functional gastrointestinal disorders. *Gastroenterol Clin North Am.* 2010;39(3):529–42.

27. Janarthanan S, Ditah I, Adler DG, et al. *Clostridium difficile* associated diarrhea and proton pump inhibitor therapy: a meta-analysis. *Am J Gastroenterol.* 2012;107(7):1001–10.

28. Kwok CS, Arthur AK, Anibueze CI, et al. Risk of *Clostridium difficile* infection with acid suppressing drugs and antibiotics: meta-analysis. *Am J Gastroenterol.* 2012;107(7):1011–9.

29. Gray SL, LaCroix AZ, Larson J, et al. Proton pump inhibitor use, hip fracture, and change in bone mineral density in postmenopausal women results from the Women's Health Initiative. *Arch Intern Med.* 2010;170(9):765–71.

30. Targownik LI, Lix LM, Leung S, et al. Proton pump inhibitor use is not associated with osteoporosis or accelerated bone mineral density loss. *Gastroenterology.* 2010;138(3):896–904.

31. U.S. Food and Drug Administration. FDA drug safety communication: possible increased risk of fractures of the hip, wrist and spine with use of proton pump inhibitors. Updated March 23, 2011. Accessed at http://www.fda.gov/Drugs/DrugSafety/PostmarketDrugSafetyInformationforPatientsandProviders/ucm213206.htm, April 24, 2013.

32. Reimer C, Sondergaard B, Hilsted L, et al. Proton-pump inhibitor therapy induces acid-related symptoms in healthy volunteers after withdrawal of therapy. *Gastroenterology.* 2009;137(1):80–7.

33. U.S. Food and Drug Administration. FDA drug safety communication: low magnesium levels can be associated with long-term use of proton pump inhibitor drugs (PPIs). March 2, 2011. Accessed at http://www.fda.gov/Drugs/DrugSafety/ucm245011.htm, April 24, 2013.

34. U.S. Food and Drug Administration. Interaction between esomeprazole/omeprazole and clopidogrel label change. November 2012. Accessed at http://www.fda.gov/Safety/MedWatch/SafetyInformation/ucm327922.htm, April 24, 2013.

35. Frelinger AL 3rd, Lee RD, Mulford DJ, et al. A randomized, 2-period, crossover design study to assess the effects of dexlansoprazole, lansoprazole, esomeprazole, and omeprazole on the steady-state pharmacokinetics and pharmacodynamics of clopidogrel in healthy volunteers. *J Am Coll Cardiol.* 2012;59(14):1304–11.

36. Suri A, Bramer SL. Effect of omeprazole on the metabolism of cilostazol. *Clin Pharmacokinet.* 1999;37(suppl 2):53–9.

37. Bezabeh S, Mackey AC, Kluetz P, et al. Accumulating evidence for a drug–drug interaction between methotrexate and proton pump inhibitors. *Oncologist.* 2012;17(4):550–4.

38. Santucci R, Leveque D, Lescoute A, et al. Delayed elimination of methotrexate associated with co-administration of proton pump inhibitors. *Anticancer Research.* 2010;30(9):3807–10.

39. U.S. Food and Drug Administration. Orally administered drug products for relief of symptoms associated with overindulgence in food and drink for over-the-counter human use. Proposed amendment of the tentative final monograph. *Federal Register.* 2005;70:741–2.

40. Hegeland H, Flagstad G, Grotta J, et al. Diagnosing pediatric functional abdominal pain in children (4–15 years old) according to the Rome III Criteria: results from a Norwegian prospective study. *J Pediatr Gastroenterol Nutr.* 2009;49(3):309–15.

41. Neilson JP. Interventions for heartburn in pregnancy. *Cochrane Database Syst Rev.* 2008;4:CD007065. doi:10.1002/14651858.CD007065. Accessed at http://www.thecochranelibrary.com.

42. Antacids, oral. LactMed. Bethesda, MD: U.S. National Library of Medicine. Updated February 5, 2008. Accessed at http://toxnet.nlm.nih.gov/cgi-bin/sis/htmlgen?LACT, May 1, 2013.

43. Briggs GG, Freeman RK, Yaffe SJ. *Drugs in Pregnancy and Lactation.* 9th ed. Philadelphia, PA: Lippincott Williams & Wilkins; 2011.

chapter

INTESTINAL GAS

14

Jennifer Robinson

Intestinal gas symptoms and conditions that predispose patients to intestinal gas are common, and they may cause considerable discomfort and lifestyle impairment. The most frequent symptoms are eructation (belching of swallowed air), bloating (excessive gas, particularly after eating), and flatulence (excessive passage of air from the stomach or intestines through the anus). Differentiation of healthy individuals with temporary symptoms from those with a chronic gastrointestinal (GI) condition such as irritable bowel syndrome (IBS), lactose intolerance, or celiac disease is important in recommending appropriate nonprescription treatment.

The primary categories of nonprescription pharmacologic therapies for intestinal gas symptoms are antiflatulent medications (simethicone and activated charcoal), digestive enzymes (lactase replacement and alpha-galactosidase products), and probiotic products (*Bifidobacterium, Lactobacillus, Saccharomyces,* and *Streptococcus* species). Sales of antiflatulent and probiotic products account for a significant portion of the nonprescription drug and dietary supplement markets.[1]

A significant portion of the U.S. population is affected by conditions that may cause intestinal gas symptoms. Intestinal gas can be caused by lactose malabsorption (29% of the population), IBS (7%–10%), and other less common medical conditions, such as celiac disease (1%–3% of the general population and 10% of first-degree relatives of the celiac disease population) and pancreatic insufficiency (<1%).[2–4] In the general population, abdominal distention and bloating are reported by approximately 10% and 20% of individuals in the United States, respectively.[5] More than half of symptomatic respondents rated symptoms as moderate-severe; most indicated that symptoms resulted in some limitation in their ability to conduct usual activities, with 10% reporting that their activities were reduced by half or more.

Pathophysiology of Intestinal Gas

The pathophysiology of gas-related complaints in the GI tract (hereafter referred to as intestinal gas) is poorly understood; however, minor disruptions of normal physiologic processes of the GI tract appear to play a role. Each time food, liquid, or saliva is swallowed, a small amount of air passes into the

stomach. Once in the stomach, the swallowed food and air are mixed with gastric acid, pepsin, and other substances; churned into small fragments; and then emptied into the small intestine, where most of the absorption of vitamins, minerals, and digestion products (e.g., food-derived monosaccharides, such as glucose) occurs.[6] The rate at which the stomach empties varies but generally takes about 1–2 hours. Smooth muscle contractions in the small intestine move the liquid food fragments and air downstream toward the large intestine, where the indigestible liquid waste is mixed with the bacterial flora of the colon. In the colon, most of the remaining liquid is absorbed from the mixture of liquid waste, bacteria, and intestinal gas as it is transported toward the rectum and temporarily stored as stool prior to a bowel movement. During a bowel movement, stool is eliminated, and intestinal gas is expelled from the rectum as flatus.

Diet, underlying medical conditions, alterations in intestinal flora, and drugs may precipitate or aggravate symptoms attributed to intestinal gas. Although the exact mechanisms are not fully known, the origin of gas retention and symptoms appears to be affected by alterations in visceral sensitivity and intestinal transit that vary at different physiologic locations along the GI tract.[6]

Certain foods can increase intestinal gas production and lead to bothersome symptoms (Tables 14–1 and 14–2).[7–9] Dietary sugars (e.g., lactose in dairy products and prepared foods; fructose in fruits, vegetables, candies, and soft drinks; sucrose from "table sugar"; and glucose from the breakdown of starches) may be incompletely absorbed in the healthy human small intestine.[7] These sugars are the principal substrates for hydrogen gas (H_2) production in the colon. Similarly, other foods also are malabsorbed, including fatty foods; foods rich in complex carbohydrates (e.g., wheat germ, brown rice, bran, and corn); and indigestible oligosaccharides (e.g., raffinose, found in asparagus, broccoli, Brussels sprouts, and cabbage; and stachyose, found in black-eyed peas, lima beans, and soy beans). These substances remain in the intestinal lumen, are passed into the colon, and provide a substrate for bacterial fermentation and colonic production of H_2 and carbon dioxide (CO_2).[6] Fermentation in the colon is the primary process for generating intestinal gas and is influenced by the quantity of foods ingested.

Diets high in fiber also may lead to bloating and flatulence. Terminology, recommended intake, and potential benefits associated with fiber are discussed in Chapter 23. Fiber is a valuable component of a balanced diet and may be beneficial in the treatment of constipation (see Chapter 15). Soluble fiber absorbs water and stabilizes intestinal contractions; however, soluble fiber supplementation does not appear to decrease IBS

Editor's Note: This chapter is based on the 17th edition chapter of the same title, written by Patrick D. Meek.

table
14-1 Gas-Producing Foods

Foods That Produce Minimal Amounts of Gas

- Meats: fowl, fish
- Vegetables: lettuce, peppers, avocado, tomato, asparagus, zucchini, okra, olives
- Fruit: cantaloupe, grapes, berries
- Carbohydrates: white rice, chips, popcorn, graham crackers
- All nuts, eggs, gelatin, fruit juice

Foods That Cause Moderate Amounts of Gas

- Potatoes
- Eggplant
- Citrus fruits, apples
- Carbohydrates: pastries, bread

Foods That Cause Major Amounts of Gas

- Vegetables: onions, celery, carrots, Brussels sprouts, cucumbers, cabbage, cauliflower, radishes
- Beans
- Fruit: raisins, bananas, apricots, prunes, dried fruit
- Carbohydrates: bagels, wheat germ, pretzels
- Peas
- Green salads
- Bran cereal, food high in bran
- Brown rice
- Leeks, parsnips
- Dairy products: milk, ice cream, cheese (in patients who have trouble digesting lactose; check food labels of processed foods for added lactose or milk-derived ingredients)
- Fatty foods: pan-fried or deep-fried foods, fatty meats; rich cream sauces and gravies (although fatty foods are not carbohydrates, these foods also can contribute to intestinal gas)
- Foods with high sugar content or with high fructose corn syrup (e.g., soft drinks)
- Products containing sorbitol and mannitol (e.g., sugar-free candies, sugar-free brownie and cake mixes, diet foods, chewing gum)

Source: References 7 and 9.

table
14-2 Oligosaccharide-Containing Foods That Alpha-Galactosidase Might Affect

Vegetables	Grains	Beans
Beets	Bagels	Black-eyed peas
Broccoli	Barley	Bog beans
Brussels sprouts	Breakfast cereal	Broad beans
Cabbage	Granola	Chickpeas
Cauliflower	Pasta	Lima beans
Corn	Rice bran	Mung beans
Cucumbers	Rye	Peanuts and peanut butter
Leeks	Sorghum, grain	Pinto beans
Lettuce	Wheat bran	Red kidney beans
Onions	Whole wheat flour	Seed flour (sesame, sunflower)
Parsley	Whole-grain breads	Soy products (including lentils, soy milk, and tofu)
Peppers, sweet		

Source: Reference 8.

symptoms.[10] Patients who experience gas-related symptoms (bloating and flatulence) from natural fiber forms (e.g., psyllium) may prefer a soluble semisynthetic fiber supplement (e.g., calcium polycarbophil). However, fiber may increase intestinal gas symptoms in patients with IBS, slow intestinal transit, and/or diverticulosis.[11] Slowly increasing the intake of fiber or using a variety of fiber-containing foods may help reduce symptoms in patients with these conditions.

The odor attributed to flatulence may be worsened by the ingestion of sulfate-containing foods, such as cruciferous vegetables (e.g., broccoli and cabbage); breads and beers containing sulfate additives; and proteins with a high content of the sulfur-containing amino acids methionine and cysteine (e.g., eggs, macadamia nuts, peanuts, pistachio nuts, and red meats). Sulfur-based gases (e.g., hydrogen sulfide [H_2S]), methanethiol, and dimethyl sulfide are produced through the action of sulfate-reducing bacteria on sulfate.[12] Rating foods by their potential to cause intestinal gas symptoms is difficult, but clinical experience suggests that certain foods are generally more problematic than others (Table 14–1).

Gas-related symptoms also may be associated with the amount of air that enters the upper GI tract upon swallowing. Smoking, chewing gum, sucking on hard candies, drinking carbonated beverages, wearing poor-fitting dentures, hyperventilating, or being overly anxious may cause individuals to swallow larger amounts of air than is normal.[12] Poor eating habits (e.g., gulping food or drinking beverages too rapidly) also may cause larger amounts of air to enter the stomach.

A number of medical conditions cause or predispose patients to the formation of intestinal gas. Some conditions (e.g., carbohydrate malabsorption and pancreatic insufficiency) lead to an increased amount of gas produced from bacterial fermentation in the colon. The most common cause of carbohydrate malabsorption is lactase deficiency. Lactase is the enzyme that normally breaks down lactose in the intestinal lumen so that it can be absorbed. Approximately 50 million people in the United States are lactose maldigesters and experience symptoms of lactose intolerance when eating dairy products. The condition is more common in black (90%) and Asian populations (75%) than in eastern Europeans (6%).

In patients with lactase deficiency, the lactase enzyme is not available in sufficient quantities to break down lactose in dairy products before it reaches the colon. Patients who experience symptoms of lactose intolerance with even small amounts of lactose may inquire about the lactose content of their medications. Reviewing the list of excipients in the package insert with the patients and/or contacting the manufacturer can help to determine the lactose content of individual products. Lactose-free formulations of these medications may be available from the manufacturer. If a lactose-free product is unavailable, a compounded product may be considered.

In the colon, the malabsorbed lactose remains in the intestinal lumen, where it is available to colonic bacteria for fermentation to H_2 and other substances. Individuals with lactase deficiency experience GI symptoms (e.g., gas pains, bloating, nausea, and diarrhea) upon exposure to dairy and other products containing milk or milk-derived carbohydrates (e.g., caramel).[13] Milk-derived protein (e.g., whey powder, caseinate, and other lactoproteins) does not cause lactose-associated GI symptoms unless the product is contaminated with a milk-derived carbohydrate (i.e., lactose).

Bacterial fermentation in the small intestine resulting from bacterial overgrowth also may lead to excessive amounts of intestinal gas. The effects of probiotics on bloating symptoms associated with small bowel bacterial overgrowth and lactose intolerance are uncertain (see Chapter 23). Research suggests that probiotics improve bloating associated with lactose intolerance by producing lactic acid, which in turn improves lactose digestion.[13] Patients with lactose intolerance are at risk for the development of low bone density and osteoporosis because of reduced dietary intake; they should be counseled to supplement their diets to achieve the recommended daily intake of 1000–1200 mg of elemental calcium per day.

Other conditions such as IBS may predispose patients to intestinal gas symptoms. Gas pains and bloating are very common in patients with IBS and may be caused by a number of interrelated factors, including heightened sensation of the GI tract to intestinal stretch (or visceral hypersensitivity), altered intestinal motility, activated intestinal immunity, altered brain-gut interaction, and autonomic dysfunction.[14] Small bowel bacterial overgrowth has been proposed as a unifying theory linking each of these factors, which has stimulated exciting research that aims to further define the relationship between intestinal bacterial overgrowth and the onset of IBS symptoms.[14] Probiotics (e.g., lactobacilli, saccharomyces, and bifidobacteria) are part of the normal "healthy" flora of the intestinal tract. They are thought to maintain intestinal health through a variety of mechanisms, including by shifting the intestinal bacterial content in favor of nonpathologic organisms; by producing beneficial substances (e.g., short-chain fatty acids); and by acting primarily as carbohydrate-fermenting bacteria, thereby reducing intestinal gas production (see Chapter 23). Substances such as oligofructose (a "prebiotic") are used as nutrients by the normal intestinal bacterial flora and by probiotic organisms; however, the normal flora produces greater amounts of CO_2 and H_2, which may result in increased symptoms of intestinal gas.[5,15]

Intestinal gas symptoms also may result from other less common medical conditions (e.g., celiac disease or diabetic gastroparesis). Patients with celiac disease have an intolerance to gluten (a protein contained in wheat, rye, barley, and oats). Once a diagnosis of celiac disease has been made, and once gluten intolerance has been confirmed with an accurate test, patients should follow a gluten-free diet, preferably under the supervision of an experienced dietitian.[2,15] Intestinal gas symptoms may result from the inflammatory response that occurs in the GI tract after exposure to gluten. The most common sources of gluten are baked goods containing the causative grains (wheat and oat cereals, noodles, and pastas); however, many other food products (especially any processed foods containing thickeners) and some medications contain gluten. Successful adherence to a gluten-free diet requires rigorous label reading and close scrutiny of the gluten content of foods and nonprescription medications. A number of valuable resources exist for individuals seeking information about celiac disease.[16,17] In addition, referral to a registered dietitian may be beneficial because *all* gluten must be removed from the diet to avoid symptoms.

A variety of drugs may cause intestinal gas symptoms. These drugs can be categorized broadly by the mechanisms that cause symptoms: drugs that affect intestinal flora (lactulose and antibiotics); drugs that affect metabolism of glucose and other dietary substances (alpha-glucosidase inhibitors, including acarbose and miglitol; and the biguanides, including metformin); and GI lipase inhibitors (orlistat). Drugs that affect GI motility (narcotics, anticholinergics, and calcium channel blockers); drugs that are high in fiber (psyllium) or nonabsorbable polymers (cholestyramine); and drugs that contain or release gas (effervescent solutions such as Alka-Seltzer) also may cause intestinal gas symptoms.

Clinical Presentation of Intestinal Gas

Patients with symptoms of intestinal gas complain most commonly of excessive belching, abdominal discomfort or cramping, bloating, and flatulence. Complaints of gas pains and belching are more common than are complaints of flatulence. Other less common symptoms associated with "gaseousness" include nausea; audible bowel sounds (called borborygmi); and dyspepsia or indigestion.

Everyone experiences belching, especially after eating and drinking. Belching is the easiest way for air to leave the stomach after it is swallowed. Some people have excessive belching, which may be annoying or embarrassing because of its frequency and/or unexpected occurrence. The more frequently a person swallows, the greater the potential for air to enter the stomach. Drinking carbonated beverages or eating food too quickly is an easy way to increase the amount of air that is swallowed inadvertently, which may then cause excessive belching.

Gas pains often are described as a generalized, crampy discomfort associated with gaseousness. Passing gas or having a bowel movement may relieve gas pains. In some patients, symptoms may be brought on by stress or anxiety. In others, the size of a meal may be associated with the onset and severity of gas pains, with larger meals causing more bothersome symptoms. Patients who complain of recurrent gas pains (occurring at least 3 days per month in the last 3 months) that are associated with either diarrhea or constipation may have IBS. Because gas pains can mimic other conditions (e.g., biliary colic [and other diseases of the gallbladder and biliary tract], diabetic gastroparesis, peptic ulcer disease, intestinal obstruction, neoplastic disease, pancreatic insufficiency, or heart disease), a qualified health care provider (pharmacist, physician, nurse practitioner, etc.) should be consulted prior to initiating self-management. Patients should be referred to a primary care provider if they are experiencing new-onset, persistent, or frequent and/or severe symptoms. These symptoms may be related to an undiagnosed condition and should not be self-managed. In addition, patients should be referred to a primary care provider for medical evaluation if any of the criteria for exclusions for self-management are met (Figure 14–1).

Bloating may be characterized as a sensation of tension in the abdominal area after eating or as a subjective sensation

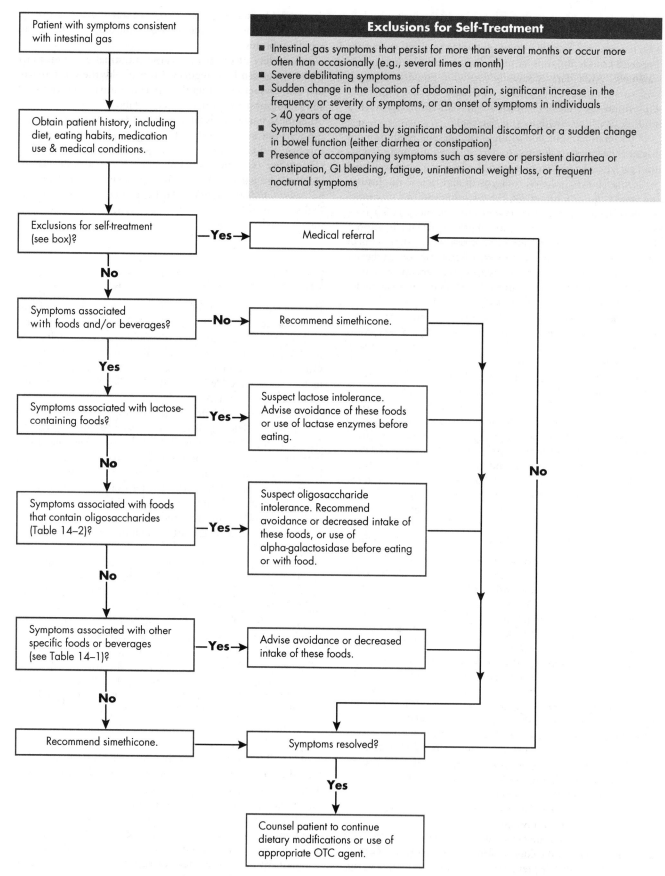

Exclusions for Self-Treatment

- Intestinal gas symptoms that persist for more than several months or occur more often than occasionally (e.g., several times a month)
- Severe debilitating symptoms
- Sudden change in the location of abdominal pain, significant increase in the frequency or severity of symptoms, or an onset of symptoms in individuals > 40 years of age
- Symptoms accompanied by significant abdominal discomfort or a sudden change in bowel function (either diarrhea or constipation)
- Presence of accompanying symptoms such as severe or persistent diarrhea or constipation, GI bleeding, fatigue, unintentional weight loss, or frequent nocturnal symptoms

Patient with symptoms consistent with intestinal gas

Obtain patient history, including diet, eating habits, medication use & medical conditions.

Exclusions for self-treatment (see box)? —**Yes**→ Medical referral

No

Symptoms associated with foods and/or beverages? —**No**→ Recommend simethicone.

Yes

Symptoms associated with lactose-containing foods? —**Yes**→ Suspect lactose intolerance. Advise avoidance of these foods or use of lactase enzymes before eating.

No

Symptoms associated with foods that contain oligosaccharides (Table 14–2)? —**Yes**→ Suspect oligosaccharide intolerance. Recommend avoidance or decreased intake of these foods, or use of alpha-galactosidase before eating or with food.

No

Symptoms associated with other specific foods or beverages (see Table 14–1)? —**Yes**→ Advise avoidance or decreased intake of these foods.

No

Recommend simethicone. → Symptoms resolved? —**No**→ (Medical referral)

Yes

Counsel patient to continue dietary modifications or use of appropriate OTC agent.

figure

14–1 Self-care of intestinal gas symptoms. Key: GI = Gastrointestinal; OTC = over-the-counter.

that the abdomen is larger than normal. Patients with bloating may observe that clothes fit more tightly or are difficult to fit into comfortably. Eating certain foods (Tables 14–1 and 14–2) (especially foods high in fiber), eating too rapidly, or eating too much may contribute to bloating. Similar to chronic gas pains, chronic bloating accompanied by a change in bowel function is suggestive of IBS. Patients with diabetes who complain that their bloating symptoms are accompanied by a sensation of early satiety or fullness after the ingestion of only a small amount of food may be experiencing diabetic gastroparesis and should be referred to a primary care provider.

Most patients who complain of flatulence are referring to the unpleasant, uncontrollable, or frequent passage of intestinal gas through the rectum. Passing gas is normal and occurs either consciously or unconsciously between 20 and 40 times a day, even while sleeping. Certain foods (Tables 14–1 and 14–2) (especially those that contain fiber, fructose, lactose, or oligosaccharides) are more likely to cause gas and therefore can contribute to flatulence. Sorbitol or mannitol from commonly used sweeteners in low-calorie foods and liquid medications also can contribute to flatulence.

Treatment of Intestinal Gas

Treatment Goals

The goals of therapy are to (1) reduce the frequency, intensity, and duration of intestinal gas symptoms and (2) reduce the impact of intestinal gas symptoms on the patient's lifestyle. Because a certain amount of intestinal gas production is normal and necessary for normal GI function, the complete elimination of intestinal gas is not a realistic or attainable goal.

General Treatment Approach

Self-treatment of intestinal gas symptoms should begin with an assessment of the patient's history of symptoms, diet, eating habits, medication use, and relevant medical conditions. Most patients will be able to control their symptoms if they understand how the symptoms occur, follow steps to reduce predisposing factors, and make informed decisions regarding the use of nonprescription medications. Identification of the underlying cause of intestinal gas will guide treatment decisions (Figure 14–1). Inquiry into the patient's diet (including a review of the patient's eating habits and rate of food ingestion) often can lead to appropriate suggestions for reducing the problem. Symptoms that are related to eating habits or diet often will subside quickly, once the source of the problem is identified and the necessary changes are made.

Patients who associate symptoms with foods containing lactose or oligosaccharides and who do not meet the criteria for exclusions for self-treatment (Figure 14–1) may use digestive enzymes (e.g., lactase replacement or alpha-galactosidase products). Although several nonprescription antiflatulent products are available (e.g., activated charcoal and simethicone), their use is largely empiric, and evidence supporting their benefit is limited. Probiotics (see Chapter 23) maintain gastrointestinal health by protecting against pathologic GI flora; they may be useful for some individuals with intestinal gas.[18] No consensus exists on whether probiotics or prebiotics are beneficial in patients with lactose intolerance or chronic abdominal bloating; however,

increasing evidence suggests that probiotics may be beneficial for treatment of intestinal gas symptoms in patients with IBS because the probiotics have favorable effects on the bacterial content of the small intestine and colon.[14,18,19] The benefit of probiotic products may potentially be linked to specific bacterial strains. More research is needed to identify the true value of individual probiotics.[18,19]

Exclusions for self-treatment (Figure 14–1) should be reviewed with the patient prior to recommending therapy. Referral of the patient to a primary care provider for further evaluation should be considered for patients with exclusions for self-treatment and for patients whose symptoms persist after initiating simple treatment options (e.g., dietary modification and nonprescription medications).

Nonpharmacologic Therapy

General information for controlling intestinal gas symptoms is provided in Table 14–3.[20] Patients may benefit from changes in eating habits and changes in diet. Reducing the consumption of gas-producing foods (Tables 14–1 and 14–2) may be appropriate, depending on the patient's history. Some people are unable to tolerate gas-producing foods and need to completely avoid these foods in their diet. Patients with lactose intolerance either should avoid milk and dairy products or should use lactase replacement products. Low-lactose milk products (e.g., Lactaid Milk or Dairy Ease Milk), fortified soy milk, almond milk, or rice milk products also may be used as milk substitutes. Low-lactose milk is a prehydrolyzed milk product (i.e., lactose is already hydrolyzed) and contains the same nutrients as regular milk, but the product is not entirely lactose free. Soy milk, almond milk, and rice milk products are palatable lactose-free milk alternatives that are low in fat and may be fortified to include calcium and vitamin D. Similarly, patients who are unable to tolerate foods with high oligosaccharide content should attempt to reduce or remove these foods from their diet.

Understanding the food values of people from different cultures, ethnicities, and socioeconomic backgrounds may lead to improved identification of dietary patterns known to contribute to intestinal gas symptoms. This knowledge may allow health care providers to identify and explain, in a culturally sensitive manner, why problematic gas-forming foods are not appropriate options for all patients. Addressing dietary issues with family members may be a better approach for developing healthy eating habits over time, especially for children experiencing intestinal gas symptoms.

Pharmacologic Therapy

Simethicone and activated charcoal may relieve symptoms after intestinal gas has formed. Alpha-galactosidase and lactase enzymes are taken with foods to prevent gas from forming. Lactase replacement products may be beneficial for the treatment of intestinal gas and diarrhea associated with lactose intolerance; they also are used as digestive aids, allowing individuals with lactose intolerance to incorporate dairy foods into their diet without producing intolerable symptoms. Most lactose maldigesters can tolerate some milk (up to 1 cup), so use of these products should be individualized according to the patient's report of symptoms.

table 14–3 Useful Information to Help Patients Decrease Symptoms of Intestinal Gas

Eating Habits

- Relax a bit before eating. Follow this simple breathing technique to enhance relaxation and release tension:
  - Sit straight in a comfortable position with your arms and legs uncrossed.
  - Breathe in comfortably, using your abdomen. Pause briefly before exhaling.
  - Each time you exhale, count silently to yourself, "One . . . two . . . three . . . four."
  - Repeat this cycle for 5–10 minutes.
  - Notice your breathing gradually slowing, your body relaxing, and your mind calming as you practice this breathing technique.
- Avoid the temptation to rush through a meal. Eat and drink slowly in a calm environment.
- Chew food thoroughly.
- Avoid washing down solids with a beverage.
- Avoid gulping and sipping liquids, drinking out of small-mouthed bottles or straws, or drinking from water fountains.
- Eliminate pipe, cigar, and cigarette smoking.
- Avoid chewing gum and sucking hard candy, especially those that contain artificial sweeteners (e.g., sorbitol or mannitol).
- Check dentures for proper fit.
- Attempt to be aware of and avoid deep sighing.
- Do not attempt to induce belching or strain to pass gas.
- Do not overload the stomach at any one meal.

Diet

- Keep a dietary diary for a few days while tracking intestinal gas symptoms.
- Avoid gas-producing foods (Table 14–1).
- Avoid foods with air whipped into them (e.g., whipped cream, soufflés, sponge cake, milk shakes).
- Avoid carbonated beverages (e.g., sodas, beer).
- Avoid caffeinated beverages (e.g., coffee, energy drinks).

Medication Use and Lifestyle Habits

- Avoid long-term or frequent intermittent use of medications intended for relief of cold and allergy symptoms (e.g., anticholinergic antihistamines such as brompheniramine, carbinoxamine, chlorpheniramine, clemastine, and diphenhydramine).
- Avoid or minimize the use of drugs affecting GI motility (narcotics and calcium channel blockers).
- Avoid or minimize the use of drugs affecting glucose metabolism (orlistat; alpha-glucosidase inhibitors, including acarbose and miglitol; and the biguanides, including metformin).
- Avoid or minimize the use of drugs that affect the intestinal flora (lactulose and antibiotics).
- Avoid drugs high in fiber (psyllium).
- Avoid nonabsorbable polymers (cholestyramine).
- Avoid drugs that contain or release gas (e.g., Alka-Seltzer).
- Avoid tight-fitting garments, girdles, and belts.
- Do not lie down or sit in a slumped position immediately after eating.
- Develop a regular routine of exercise and rest.

Source: References 9 and 20.

Simethicone

Simethicone (a mixture of inert silicon polymers) is used as a defoaming agent to relieve gas. Simethicone acts in the stomach and intestine to reduce the surface tension of gas bubbles that are embedded in the mucus of the GI tract. As surface tension changes, the gas bubbles are broken or coalesced and then eliminated more easily by belching or passing gas through the rectum.[21]

The Food and Drug Administration (FDA) considers simethicone safe and effective as an antiflatulent agent. In patients with acute, nonspecific diarrhea, the combination of simethicone with loperamide produced quicker relief from gas-related discomfort than either agent alone.[22] However, simethicone's ability to reduce intestinal gas symptoms for all patients with symptoms is questionable.[23] The use of simethicone may be encouraged on a trial basis because some patients report benefit. The usual adult and pediatric dosages for simethicone are provided in Table 14–4.

Many antacid products contain a combination of simethicone and antacids; therefore, patients should follow the label instructions for dosages of these products. However, use of both agents often is unnecessary, and the efficacy of such combination products has not been well-studied. Furthermore, single-ingredient antiflatulent products (Table 14–5) usually contain a higher concentration of simethicone than the combination products. Because simethicone is not absorbed from the GI tract, it has no known systemic side effects; its safety has been well-documented. Simethicone is contraindicated in patients with a known hypersensitivity to simethicone products or suspected intestinal perforation and obstruction.

Activated Charcoal

Activated charcoal also is promoted for relief of intestinal gas; however, it is neither approved nor shown to be effective for this indication.[24] The usual adult dosages for this agent are provided in Table 14–4. The proposed antiflatulent properties of activated charcoal are related to the adsorbent effects of the substance and its potential to facilitate the elimination of intestinal gas from the GI tract. Activated charcoal has been purported to be beneficial for the elimination of malodorous, sulfur-based gases.[24] Activated charcoal also has poor palatability. External devices containing activated charcoal also are available to reduce the odor of flatus in patients with ostomies (see Chapter 21).

Combination Products

Combination products containing simethicone and activated charcoal also are available; these products aim to provide relief from intestinal gas symptoms by combining the gas-reducing activity of each of the individual components. Table 14–5 lists examples of commercially available products, including products containing activated charcoal and simethicone.

Alpha-Galactosidase

Another FDA-approved product for use as an antiflatulent is the enzyme alpha-galactosidase. This enzyme, which is derived from the *Aspergillus niger* mold and is classified as a food, hydrolyzes oligosaccharides into their component parts before they can be metabolized by colonic bacteria. The usual adult and pediatric dosages for alpha-galactosidase are provided in Table 14–4.[21]

table

14–4 Dosage Guideline for Intestinal Gas Products

Agent	Dosage			
	Adults	Children > 12 Years	Children 2 to ≤ 12 Years	Children < 2 Years
Simethicone	40–360 mg after meals and at bedtime, as needed	40–360 mg 4 times daily	40 mg 4 times daily	20 mg 4 times daily, as needed
Activated charcoal	520 mg (2 capsules) orally after meals, as needed; may repeat hourly	Specific guidelines not available		
Alpha-galactosidase	300–450 units per serving of food	Not recommended		
Lactase enzyme	3000–9000 units at first bite of food or drink containing lactose	Specific guidelines not available		
Probiotics	Specific guidelines not available	Specific guidelines not available		

Because high-fiber foods contain large amounts of oligosaccharides, alpha-galactosidase is recommended as a prophylactic treatment of intestinal gas symptoms produced by high-fiber diets or foods that contain oligosaccharides (Table 14–2). Two controlled trials of alpha-galactosidase demonstrated that the agent significantly reduced symptoms of intestinal gas in healthy individuals fed oligosaccharide-containing foods.[25,26]

The safety of alpha-galactosidase remains to be determined. Although this enzyme has been used in food processing for years and is regarded as safe by FDA, the amount contained in available pharmacologic products is probably much greater than that in processed foods. Because the enzyme produces galactose, this product should not be used by patients with galactosemia (an inherited metabolic disorder in which galactose accumulates in the blood because of the deficiency of an enzyme that catalyzes galactose's conversion to glucose). Similarly, patients with diabetes should be cautioned about the use of the enzyme, which may produce 2–6 grams of carbohydrates per 100 grams of food.[25] Because alpha-galactosidase is derived from mold, allergic reactions are possible in patients allergic to molds.

Lactase Replacement Products

Lactase replacement products are used in patients with lactose intolerance (see Chapter 16). Lactase enzymes break down lactose, a disaccharide, into the monosaccharides glucose and galactose, which are absorbed. Lactase replacement products should be used in patients with lactose intolerance to aid in the digestion of dairy products. There are no adverse effects listed for lactase replacement products. The usual adult dose for lactase enzymes is provided in Table 14–4.

Product Selection Guidelines

Special Populations

Several pediatric formulations of simethicone are indicated for the relief of intestinal gas. These products, which contain simethicone 40 mg per 0.6 mL suspension, often are promoted and used to relieve gas associated with colic. However, simethicone has not been found to be superior to placebo for intestinal gas and/or infantile colic.[27] Although its efficacy is questionable, simethicone is not absorbed from the GI tract,

and it is considered safe for use in infants and children. There are no reports linking simethicone to congenital defects.[27] Simethicone is a Pregnancy Category C drug and is considered to be safe for use by nursing mothers.

For alpha-galactosidase products, safety and efficacy have not been evaluated in infants and children. Therefore, this product should not be used in pediatric patients until data are available to support such use. Manufacturers recommend that pregnant or nursing patients first consult with a primary care provider before using alpha-galactosidase.

No special population considerations are listed for lactase replacement products. Patients should consult a primary care provider if symptoms continue after using a lactase replacement product, or if symptoms are unusual and seem unrelated to eating dairy products.

Patient Factors

Alpha-galactosidase and lactase replacement products are used to prevent the onset of symptoms in patients unable to tolerate problematic foods. Patients with gas symptoms who need immediate relief and patients who cannot associate their symptoms with certain foods should use simethicone. Activated charcoal may be an alternative to simethicone for patients with gas symptoms, and also it may be beneficial for patients who experience malodorous gas production. Because alpha-galactosidase produces carbohydrates, patients with galactosemia or diabetes mellitus should avoid this product and use simethicone instead. Patients with lactase maldigestion who experience symptoms of lactose intolerance should consider taking lactase replacement products at the time of exposure to dairy products.

Patient Preferences

Most products for intestinal gas are available in a variety of strengths and dosage forms. A liquid formulation of simethicone is available for infants. Simethicone also is available as chewable tablets, softgels, and an edible filmstrip. Liquid dosage forms and alternative solid dosage forms are generally more expensive than standard solid oral dosage forms (e.g., tablets and capsules) but may be more palatable. Activated charcoal is available in two solid oral dosage forms (tablets and capsules) and in a combination product with simethicone.

table

14–5 Selected Antiflatulent Products

Trade Name	Primary Ingredients
Single-Entity Simethicone Products	
Gas-X Regular Strength Chewable Tablets	Simethicone 80 mg
Gas-X Extra Strength Chewable Tablets	Simethicone 125 mg
Mylanta Gas Chewable Tablets	Simethicone 125 mg
Phazyme Chewable Tablets	Simethicone 125 mg
Gas-X Children's Tongue Twisters	Simethicone 40 mg per edible film strip
Gas-X Thin Strips	Simethicone 62.5 mg per edible film strip
Mylicon Infant's Drops	Simethicone 40 mg/0.6 mL
Activated Charcoal Products	
Charcoal Tablets	Activated charcoal 260 mg
CharcoCaps Capsules	Activated charcoal 260 mg
Combination Charcoal Product	
Charcoal Plus Tablets	Activated charcoal 250 mg; simethicone 80 mg
Alpha-Galactosidase Replacement Products	
Beano Chewable Tablets	Alpha-galactosidase 150 units (1 tablet)
Beano Meltaway Tablets	Alpha-galactosidase 300 units (1 tablet)
Lactase Replacement Products	
Lactaid Original Strength Caplets	Lactase enzyme 3000 units
Lactaid Chewable Tablets	Lactase enzyme 4500 units
Lactase Fast Act Chewable Tablets	Lactase enzyme 9000 units
Lac-Dose Tablets	Lactase enzyme 3000 units
Lactrase Capsules	Lactase enzyme 250 mg (3750 lactase enzyme units)
Lacteeze Drops	Lactase enzyme 5 drops (80 lactase enzyme units)
Probiotic Products	
Activia Probiotic Yogurt	*Lactobacillus bulgaricus; Streptococcus thermophilus; Bifidobacterium animalis* DN173010 (1×10^8 live bacteria per gram[a])
Align Digestive Care Probiotic Supplement Capsules	*Bifidobacterium infantis* 35624 (4 mg = 1×10^9 live bacteria)
Culturelle Probiotic Digestive Health Capsules	*Lactobacillus GG* (1×10^{10} live bacteria per capsule)
DanActive Probiotic Dairy Drink	*Lactobacillus bulgaricus; Streptococcus thermophilus; Lactobacillus casei* DN-114 001
Danimals Yogurt Smoothie Drinks	*Lactobacillus bulgaricus; Streptococcus thermophilus; Lactobacillus rhamnosus GG* (1×10^8 live bacteria per gram[a])
FloraQ	*Lactobacillus acidophilus; Bifidobacterium; Lactobacillus paracasei; Streptococcus thermophilus* 230 mg (an aggregate of a minimum of 8×10^9 freeze-dried bacteria)
Florastor	*Saccharomyces boulardi* freeze-dried capsules 250 mg

[a] Meets National Yogurt Association criteria for live and active culture yogurt.

Alpha–galactosidase is available as tablets, caplets, and meltaway tablets. There is no difference in onset of symptomatic relief between these dosage forms, so the choice between dosage forms is left entirely to personal preference and convenience.

A variety of products also is available for patients with lactose intolerance. Lactase replacement products can be added to milk or dairy products to reduce the amount of lactose in the product, or they can be ingested along with dairy products in an effort to reduce the amount of lactose in the food. Additionally, patients may elect to use one of the available milk alternatives (e.g., low-lactose milk, fortified soy milk, almond milk, or rice milk).

Complementary Therapies

A variety of probiotic dietary supplements (see Chapter 23) is widely used for GI complaints, including intestinal gas and bloating.[18] The most common formulations for intestinal gas (Table 14–5) are capsules with one bacterium (e.g., *Bifidobacterium infantis*) or multiple bacteria (e.g., *Lactobacillus acidophilus, Lactobacillus paracasei, Bifidobacterium,* and *Streptococcus thermophilus*). Functional fermented food products with live active cultures of probiotic species (e.g., kombucha tea and kefir products) also are available. In patients with IBS and those with lactose intolerance, increasing but limited evidence suggests that specific probiotics provide temporary relief from GI symptoms.[18,19] Probiotic bacteria leave the intestine soon after therapy is discontinued. When using probiotic therapy, daily administration is required to maintain bacterial populations in the intestinal flora. An adequate trial of 14 days is generally recommended for patients interested in using probiotic therapy. Research shows that probiotics are effective in reducing the incidence of antibiotic-associated diarrhea. More studies are required to identify which probiotic strains are most efficacious for patients receiving specific antibiotics.[27]

Carminatives (e.g., fennel, Japanese mint, peppermint, and spearmint) are other natural products commonly used for intestinal gas.[28] Despite insufficient evidence, these agents are widely used for the management of intestinal gas and IBS.[28,29] Carminatives may reduce the tone of the lower esophageal sphincter and should be minimized or avoided by patients with gastroesophageal reflux disease (see Chapter 13); however, the effect of carminatives on lower esophageal sphincter tone in healthy individuals with intestinal gas symptoms may be less

problematic.[30] Fennel can cause photodermatitis, is contraindicated during pregnancy, and enters breast milk in lactating women. If fennel is used, patients should be advised to avoid excessive sunlight and to avoid use during pregnancy and lactation. In addition, coadministration of fennel with ciprofloxacin may lead to reduced ciprofloxacin levels through a chelation mechanism, so doses should be spaced appropriately in patients using both agents.[31]

Assessment of Intestinal Gas: A Case-Based Approach

When a patient complains of intestinal gas, it is important to try to discern the causes, duration, and frequency of the symptoms (Table 14–6). Items that produce relief may provide clues as to the cause. A thorough review of dietary habits, medical problems, and use of prescription and nonprescription medications may provide other clues.

Cases 14–1 and 14–2 are examples of the assessment of patients with intestinal gas.

Patient Counseling for Intestinal Gas

Patient counseling is important to ensure the appropriate selection and use of nonprescription medications for intestinal gas. Patients should be encouraged to keep a diary of foods in an effort to identify those that are problematic. Avoidance of foods

---

table

14–6 Differentiation of Intestinal Gas Discomfort and Irritable Bowel Syndrome

Criterion	Intestinal Gas Discomfort	Irritable Bowel Syndrome
Location	Generalized discomfort in the upper, mid, or lower abdomen	Generalized discomfort, bloating, and/or pain in the lower abdomen or colon
Signs	Eructation (upper abdomen): belching of air; bloating (mid abdomen): increased abdominal girth; flatulence (lower abdomen, colon): excessive air or other gas in the stomach and intestines	No physical signs of disease; no fever, melena, hematochezia, or signs of other gastrointestinal conditions
Symptoms	Sensation of accumulated intestinal gas; may present as minimal physical discomfort but with significant negative psychosocial effects	Vary widely but are commonly described as abdominal pain that is relieved after a bowel movement, is accompanied by either diarrhea or constipation, and usually lasts at least 3 months
Onset	May occur at any age	Begins in early adulthood; rarely occurs after the age of 60
Etiology	Symptoms commonly believed to be caused by an excessive amount of gas in the stomach (eructation) and intestines (bloating, flatulence); other causes include lactase deficiency, overgrowth of intestinal bacteria, and excessive air swallowing (aerophagia)	Unknown May result from altered gastrointestinal motility, heightened visceral sensitivity, and/or overgrowth of intestinal bacteria
Exacerbating factors	Diet; underlying medical conditions; and certain drugs (e.g., lactulose, antibiotics, alpha-glucosidase inhibitors, orlistat, narcotics, anticholinergics, calcium channel blockers, psyllium or cholestyramine, and effervescent solutions)	Stress; overeating; problem foods (e.g., alcohol, chocolate, caffeinated beverages, dairy products, and sugar-free products that contain sorbitol or mannitol); foods high in fat
Modifying factors	Minimization of exacerbating factors	Minimization of exacerbating factors; primary care provider evaluation and treatment

case

14–1

Relevant Evaluation Criteria	Scenario/Model Outcome
Information Gathering	

1. Gather essential information about the patient's symptoms and medical history, including:

   a. description of symptom(s) (i.e., nature, onset, duration, severity, associated symptoms)

   The patient complains of occasional stomach pain, bloating, and flatulence. She states the symptoms started about 4–5 months ago and have progressively been getting worse. Symptoms now include diarrhea, nausea, and fatigue.

   b. description of any factors that seem to precipitate, exacerbate, and/or relieve the patient's symptom(s)

   The patient states that the symptoms seem to get worse when she drinks her sugar-free vanilla lattes or eats fast food. There are times when the pain is present in the lower abdomen, and the patient cannot identify a cause. Having a bowel movement tends to relieve some of the pain some of the time.

   c. description of the patient's efforts to relieve the symptoms

   She has tried several OTC products without much success. The products include simethicone 125 mg 4 times a day and Tums 500 mg 3 times daily.

   d. patient's identity

   Ellie Dawn

   e. age, sex, height, and weight

   28 years old, female, 5 ft 6 in., 145 lb

   f. patient's occupation

   Social worker

   g. patient's dietary habits

   Skips breakfast unless she stops at a coffee stand for a latte and whole wheat muffin. Eats sporadically during the day as her schedule allows. Frequently eats at fast food restaurants or consumes prepackaged meals.

   h. patient's sleep habits

   7–8 hours nightly

   i. concurrent medical conditions, prescription and nonprescription medications, and dietary supplements

   Depression: citalopram 10 mg once daily; hypertension: lisinopril 20 mg once daily

   j. allergies

   None

   k. history of other adverse reactions to medications

   None

   l. other (describe) _____

   Over the past several months, the patient reports losing 10 pounds without changing her diet or increasing exercise.

| **Assessment and Triage** | |

2. Differentiate patient's signs/symptoms and correctly identify the patient's primary problem(s) (Table 14–6).

   Abdominal symptoms are consistent with intolerance to multiple foods, which suggests the possibility of a lactose intolerance, oligosaccharide intolerance, and glucose sensitivity (celiac disease). Fatigue and weight loss also support a disorder with a nutritional deficiency component, possibly IBS.

3. Identify exclusions for self-treatment (Figure 14–1).

   Unintended weight loss; length of time symptoms have been present.

4. Formulate a comprehensive list of therapeutic alternatives for the primary problem to determine if triage to a health care provider is required, and share this information with the patient or caregiver.

   Options include:

   (1) Refer to a primary care provider or gastroenterologist for a differential diagnosis.

   (2) Recommend patient keep a food, stress, and symptom diary

   (3) Take no action.

| **Plan** | |

5. Select an optimal therapeutic alternative to address the patient's problem, taking into account patient preferences.

   Ellie should be referred to a primary care provider or gastroenterologist for a differential diagnosis.

6. Describe the recommended therapeutic approach to the patient or caregiver.

   "You should immediately follow up with your primary care provider or gastroenterologist."

7. Explain to the patient or caregiver the rationale for selecting the recommended therapeutic approach from the considered therapeutic alternatives.

   "Current treatment available OTC will not adequately address the severity of the current symptoms you have. It is important that you follow up with your primary care provider to identify the cause of your complaints and associated weight loss."

case

14–1 *continued*

Relevant Evaluation Criteria	Scenario/Model Outcome
Patient Education	
8. When recommending self-care with nonprescription medications and/or nondrug therapy, convey accurate information to the patient or caregiver.	Criterion does not apply in this case.
Solicit follow-up questions from the patient or caregiver.	"Is there anything that I can do right now to address my symptoms prior to getting in to see the doctor?"
Answer the patient's or caregiver's questions.	"Immediately following up with your primary care provider is the best course of action."
Evaluation of Patient Outcome	
9. Assess patient outcome.	Contact the patient in 1–2 days to ensure she sought medical care and made an appointment.

Key: IBS = Irritable bowel syndrome; OTC = over-the-counter.

case

14–2

Relevant Evaluation Criteria	Scenario/Model Outcome
Information Gathering	
1. Gather essential information about the patient's symptoms and medical history, including:	
a. description of symptom(s) (i.e., nature, onset, duration, severity, associated symptoms)	Patient presents with complaints of bloating with an increased amount of burping and flatulence. The symptoms are mild in nature but uncomfortable and embarrassing.
b. description of any factors that seem to precipitate, exacerbate, and/or relieve the patient's symptom(s)	Symptoms seem to be worse after eating large meals, especially when ice cream or milk is consumed. The bloating seems to decrease after episodes of burping or flatulence.
c. description of the patient's efforts to relieve the symptoms	The patient has tried including 1 serving of Activia yogurt into his diet over the past few weeks with no relief.
d. patient's identity	Francis Welker
e. age, sex, height, and weight	44 years old, male, 6 ft, 240 lb
f. patient's occupation	Publicist
g. patient's dietary habits	Never misses a meal and enjoys eating fried southern comfort food, ice cream, and soda.
h. patient's sleep habits	5–7 hours a night
i. concurrent medical conditions, prescription and nonprescription medications, and dietary supplements	Hypertension: losartan 50 mg, 1 tablet every morning GERD: omeprazole 20 mg, 1 capsule every morning with breakfast
j. allergies	Penicillin (rash)
k. history of adverse reactions to medications	None
Assessment and Triage	
2. Differentiate patient's signs/symptoms and correctly identify the patient's primary problem(s).	Patient is currently experiencing intestinal gas and bloating due to dietary intolerances.
3. Identify exclusions for self-treatment (Figure 14–1).	None

case

14-2 continued

Relevant Evaluation Criteria	Scenario/Model Outcome
4. Formulate a comprehensive list of therapeutic alternatives for the primary problem to determine if triage to a health care provider is required, and share this information with the patient or caregiver.	Options include: (1) Refer patient to an appropriate health care provider. (2) Recommend self-care with lactose intolerance product (e.g., Lactaid) in addition to simethicone and a reduction in meal size. (3) Recommend self-care until patient can see an appropriate provider. (4) Take no action.

Plan

5. Select an optimal therapeutic alternative to address the patient's problem, taking into account patient preferences.	Francis should take a lactase enzyme whenever he eats more than 4 ounces of dairy. Gas or bloating can be treated with simethicone. He should avoid large meals and carbonated beverages.
6. Describe the recommended therapeutic approach to the patient or caregiver.	"You should take Lactaid Original Strength Capsules whenever you eat more than 4 ounces of dairy. The Gas-X Extra Strength tablets can be taken with meals or snacks. You should avoid large meals and carbonated beverages."
7. Explain to the patient or caregiver the rationale for selecting the recommended therapeutic approach from the considered therapeutic alternatives.	"The Lactaid will help with the digestion of dairy products—including yogurt, milk, and ice cream—which should decrease the amount of gas produced. If you do experience an increase in belching, flatulence, or bloating, you can use Gas-X, which helps expel gas bubbles formed within your stomach and intestine. By reducing your meal size and avoiding carbonated beverages, you should notice some relief from the bloating you have been experiencing."

Patient Education

8. When recommending self-care with nonprescription medications and/or nondrug therapy, convey accurate information to the patient or caregiver.	
a. appropriate dose and frequency of administration	See Table 14–4.
b. maximum number of days the therapy should be employed	No maximum, as long as the symptoms are relieved and do not worsen.
c. product administration procedures	Take the product by mouth.
d. expected time to onset of relief	Soon after administration.
e. degree of relief that can be reasonably expected	"If your bloating and gas are being caused by lactose intolerance, then the Lactaid should give you mild to moderate relief."
f. most common side effects	None
g. side effects that warrant medical intervention should they occur	None
h. patient options in the event that condition worsens or persists	See Figure 14–1.
i. product storage requirements	"Store in a cool, dry place out of children's reach."
j. specific nondrug measures	See Table 14–3.
Solicit follow-up questions from the patient or caregiver.	"Can I double the dose of any of the medications for quicker relief?"
Answer the patient's or caregiver's questions.	"No, follow the manufacturer's directions. Additional doses will not provide added benefit."

Evaluation of Patient Outcome

9. Assess patient outcome.	Ask the patient to call and update you on his response to your recommended treatment; alternatively, you could call him in a week to evaluate his response to the treatment. If the latter, be sure you have the patient's current telephone number.

Key: GERD = Gastroesophageal reflux disease.

---

patient education for
Intestinal Gas

The objectives of self-treatment are to (1) reduce the symptoms of intestinal gas and (2) reduce the chance of its recurrence. For most patients, carefully following product instructions and the self-care measures listed below will help ensure optimal therapeutic outcomes.

Nondrug Measures

- If possible, avoid foods known to cause intestinal gas.
- Avoid activities known to introduce gas into the digestive system, such as drinking carbonated beverages.

Nonprescription Medications

- Lactase replacement products and alpha-galactosidase should be taken with foods to prevent intestinal gas from forming.
- Simethicone is used to treat intestinal gas after it has occurred.

Alpha-Galactosidase

- Do not cook with this product. Add to food after it has cooled because food temperatures higher than 130°F may inactivate the enzyme.
- If using drops, add drops to the first bite of problem foods.
- If using tablets, swallow, chew, or crumble tablets with the first bite of problem foods.
- An average meal may contain three servings of a problem food. If needed, use more tablets for larger meals, up to the maximum recommended dose.

Lactase Replacement Products

- Take at first bite of dairy or lactose-containing food.
- Dosing may vary according to the amount of lactase in the product and the level of lactose intolerance.
- Do not take more than the recommended maximum daily dose.
- Low-lactose milk or fortified soy milk products also may be used to supplement dietary intake of calcium.

Simethicone

- For infants, to ease administration, mix the suspension with 1 ounce of cool water, infant formula, or other liquid.
- Discontinue simethicone if adequate relief is not obtained within 24 hours.

When to Seek Medical Attention

- Seek medical attention if symptoms do not improve or they worsen.

---

or other substances that cause intestinal gas is the best advice to give patients. The health care provider should explain the proper use of medications for intestinal gas and should warn the patient of possible adverse effects. The box Patient Education for Intestinal Gas contains specific information to provide patients.

Evaluation of Patient Outcomes for Intestinal Gas

Many patients with intestinal gas have mild-moderate distress, and the discomfort is generally self-limiting within 24 hours. Mild-moderate gas and bloating are managed primarily with diet modification, and some relief may occur with symptomatic drug therapy. With effective treatment, the patient can expect reduced intensity and duration of gas-related symptoms such as belching, abdominal pain, bloating, and flatulence. Patients who achieve symptomatic relief should be advised to continue the self-care measures as needed. The provider should ask the patient to return or call after 1 week of self-treatment with dietary measures, nonprescription antiflatulents, or digestive enzymes so outcomes can be assessed. Medical referral is necessary if any of the following occurs before or during treatment:

- Intestinal gas symptoms that persist for more than several days or occur more often than occasionally (e.g., several times a month) and are associated with diarrhea or constipation.
- Sudden change in the location of abdominal pain.
- Significant increase in the severity or frequency of symptoms.
- Sudden change in bowel function.
- Presence of accompanying symptoms such as severe or persistent diarrhea/constipation; greasy or malodorous stools; GI bleeding (e.g., hematemesis, melena, or hematochezia); fatigue; unintentional weight loss; or frequent nocturnal symptoms.

Key Points for Intestinal Gas Complaints

➤ Limit the self-treatment of intestinal gas symptoms to minor symptoms and to cases in which exclusions for self-treatment (Figure 14–1) do not exist.

➤ Counsel patients on dietary measures that may reduce the amount of intestinal gas. Certain foods (Tables 14–1 and 14–2) are more likely to cause gas and contribute to symptoms.

➤ Patients who associate symptoms with lactose- or oligosaccharide-containing foods and who do not meet criteria for exclusions for self-treatment may use digestive enzymes (lactase replacement or alpha-galactosidase products).

➤ Probiotics may be helpful for patients with lactose intolerance who experience bloating or for patients with bloating associated with irritable bowel syndrome.

➤ Antiflatulents such as activated charcoal and simethicone also may be used, although there is contradictory evidence supporting the ability of these agents to reduce the amount of intestinal gas formed.

➤ Referral to a primary care provider for further evaluation should be considered for patients with exclusions for self-treatment and for patients whose symptoms persist after initiating simple treatment options (e.g., dietary modification and nonprescription medications).

REFERENCES

1. Top 200 OTC/HBC brands of 2007. *Drug Top.* Accessed at http://drug topics.modernmedicine.com/drugtopics, May 22, 2011.
2. World Gastroenterology Organization Global Guidelines on Celiac Disease. *J Clin Gastroenterol.* 2013;47(2):121–6.
3. Montalto M, Curigliano V, Santoro L, et al. Management and treatment of lactose malabsorption. *World J Gastroenterol.* 2006;12(2):187–91.
4. Brandt LJ, Chey WD, Foxx-Orenstein AE, et al. An evidence-based systematic review on the management of irritable bowel syndrome. *Am J Gastroenterol.* 2009;104(suppl 1):S1–35.
5. Ringel Y, Williams RE, Kalilani L, et al. Prevalence, characteristics, and impact of bloating symptoms in patients with irritable bowel syndrome. *Clin Gastroenterol Hepatol.* 2009;7(1):68–72.

6. Johnson LR. *Gastrointestinal Physiology: Regulation.* 7th ed. Philadelphia, PA: Mosby; 2007:107–26.

7. Choi YK, Kraft N, Zimmerman B, et al. Fructose intolerance in IBS and utility of fructose-restricted diet. *J Clin Gastroenterol.* 2008;42(3):233–8.

8. Problem foods. Research Triangle Park, NC: GlaxoSmithKline; 2010. Accessed at http://www.beanogas.com/about-beano/problem-foods, February 18, 2013.

9. Helpful hints for controlling gas (flatus). University of Michigan Health Systems Michigan Bowel Control Program. Accessed at http://www.med.umich.edu/fbd/docs/Gas%20reduction%20diet.pdf, September 16, 2013.

10. Ford AC. In irritable bowel syndrome, antispasmodics and antidepressants improve abdominal pain and global assessment and symptoms scores, but there is no evidence for the effectiveness of bulking agents. *Evid Based Med* 2012;17(4):114–5.

11. Korzenik JR. Case closed? Diverticulitis: epidemiology and fiber. *J Clin Gastroenterol.* 2006;40(suppl 3):S112–6.

12. Azpiroz F, Malagelada JR. The pathogenesis of bloating and visible distension in irritable bowel syndrome. *Gastroenterol Clin North Am.* 2005;34(2):257–69.

13. Shaukat A, Levitt MD, Taylor BC, et al. Systematic review: effective management strategies for lactose intolerance. *Ann Intern Med.* 2010; 152(12):797–803.

14. Lin HC. Small intestinal bacterial overgrowth: a framework for understanding irritable bowel syndrome. *JAMA.* 2004;292(7):852–8.

15. Bizzaro N, Tozzoli R, Villalta D, et al. Cutting-edge issues in celiac disease and in gluten intolerance. *Clin Rev Allergy Immunol.* 2012;42(3):279–87.

16. Gluten free drugs. Accessed at http://www.glutenfreedrugs.com, September 16, 2013.

17. Celiac Sprue Association (CSA/USA). Accessed at http://www.csaceliacs.info, September 16, 2013.

18. Whelan K. Probiotics and prebiotics in the management of irritable bowel syndrome: a review of recent clinical trials and systematic reviews. *Curr Opin Clin Nutr Metab Care.* 2011;14(6):581–7.

19. Whelan K, Quigley MM. Probiotics in the management of irritable bowel syndrome and inflammatory bowel disease. *Curr Opin Gastroenterol.* 2013;29(2):184–9.

20. Mayer EA. The neurobiology of stress and emotions. *Participate* [quarterly publication of the International Foundation of Functional Gastrointestinal Disorders]. 2010;10(4):2–5.

21. McEvoy GK, ed. *AHFS Drug Information.* Bethesda, MD: American Society of Health-System Pharmacists; 2013:2944.

22. Hanauer SB, DuPont HL, Cooper KM, et al. Randomized, double-blind, placebo-controlled clinical trial of loperamide plus simethicone versus loperamide alone and simethicone alone in the treatment of acute diarrhea with gas-related abdominal discomfort. *Curr Med Res Opin.* 2007; 23(5):1033–43.

23. Hall B, Chesters J, Robinson A. Infantile colic: A systematic review of medical and conventional therapies. *J Paediatr Child Health.* 2012;48 (2):128–37.

24. Suarez FL, Furne J, Springfield J, et al. Failure of activated charcoal to reduce the release of gases produced by the colonic flora. *Am J Gastroenterol.* 1999;94(1):208–12.

25. Ganiats TG, Norcross WA, Halverson AL, et al. Does Beano prevent gas? A double-blind crossover study of oral alpha-galactosidase to treat dietary oligosaccharide intolerance. *J Fam Pract.* 1994;39(5):441–5.

26. Di Stefano M, Miceli E, Gotti S, et al. The effect of oral alpha-galactosidase on intestinal gas production and gas-related symptoms. *Dig Dis Sci.* 2007; 52(1):78–83.

27. Hempel S, Newberry SJ, Maher AR, et al. Probiotics for the prevention and treatment of antibiotic-associated diarrhea: a systematic review and meta-analysis. *JAMA.* 2012;307(18):1959–69.

28. Merat S, Khalili S, Mostajabi P, et al. The effect of enteric-coated, delayed-release peppermint oil on irritable bowel syndrome. *Dig Dis Sci.* 2010;55:1385–90.

29. Alam MS, Roy PK, Miah AR, et al. Efficacy of peppermint oil in diarrhea-predominant IBS—a double-blind randomized placebo-controlled study. *Mymensingh Med J.* 2013;22(1):27–30.

30. Bulat R, Fachnie E, Chauhan U, et al. Lack of effect of spearmint on lower oesophageal sphincter function and acid reflux in healthy volunteers. *Aliment Pharmacol Ther.* 1999;13(6):805–12.

31. Brinker FJ. *Herb Contraindications & Drug Interactions: Plus Herbal Adjuncts With Medicines.* 4th ed. Sandy, OR: Eclectic Medical Publications; 2010: 227–50.

CONSTIPATION

Kristin W. Weitzel and Jean-Venable "Kelly" R. Goode

Constipation is a common gastrointestinal (GI) complaint. Although individual bowel frequency varies, health care providers generally define constipation in adults as having fewer than 3 bowel movements per week that are characterized by straining and the difficult passage of hard, dry stools.[1,2] Patients' perceptions of and definitions of normal bowel frequency and constipation vary widely. Patients may describe constipation as (1) straining to have a bowel movement; (2) passing hard, dry stools; (3) passing small stools; (4) feeling as though bowel evacuation is not complete; or (5) experiencing decreased stool frequency. Constipation usually results from the abnormally slow movement of feces through the colon, resulting in accumulation in the descending colon.[2,3]

Constipation is a common symptom that occurs in males and females of all ages. The prevalence in the general population ranges from 2% to 28%.[1,4–6] Constipation leads to 2.5 million physician visits per year in the United States, with direct costs of diagnosis and treatment estimated at billions of dollars annually.[7] It is reported more often in women, nonwhites, children, and older individuals.[1,4,8] Older adults (>65 years) are 5 times more likely to develop constipation than younger adults, and women are more than 3 times as likely to experience constipation than are men.[2] Constipation also is a frequent complaint in late pregnancy and after childbirth.[8] If untreated, constipation can lead to hemorrhoids, anal fissures, rectal prolapse, fecal impaction, or other complications.[9]

Pathophysiology of Constipation

All structures shown in Figure 15–1 contribute to the process of digestion. With normal functioning gastric motility, food is retained in the stomach for approximately 3 hours and in the small intestine for the same amount of time. Tonic contractions of the stomach churn and knead food, and large peristaltic waves move food toward the duodenum.[10]

Once ingestible matter has passed through the stomach, it enters the small intestine and passes through the large intestine before defecation. After ingestion of food, contractions occur in the small intestine to promote movement of nondigestible materials into the large intestines. Fecal matter is stored in the sigmoid colon until defecation occurs.[10]

The process of defecation begins with a peristaltic movement that propels fecal matter into the rectum. This movement results in a desire to defecate, relaxation of the internal anal sphincter, and tightening of the abdominal wall muscles. A Valsalva maneuver forces the stool down. Defecation is either voluntarily inhibited (by keeping the external anal sphincter contracted) or facilitated (by relaxing the sphincter and contracting the abdominal muscles).[10]

Causes of constipation include various medical conditions and medications; psychological and physiologic conditions (e.g., menopause and dehydration); and lifestyle characteristics. Constipation can stem from either primary or secondary causes. Primary constipation is often characterized by slower-than–normal movement of fecal matter through the GI tract (slow transit time) or by defecatory disorders (e.g., pelvic floor dysfunction, anal sphincter abnormalities, rectal prolapse, etc.).[2,6,8] Secondary causes of constipation include systemic, neurological, or psychological disorders, as well as structural abnormalities that result in obstruction (Table 15–1).[1–3,5,6]

Dietary fiber dissolves or swells in the intestinal fluid, which increases the bulk of fecal mass and, in turn, aids in stimulating peristalsis and eliminating stools. A diet that is low in calories, carbohydrates, or fiber may contribute to diet-related constipation. Inadequate intake of fluids may also promote constipation in patients who are dehydrated. Intestinal fluids are essential for eliminating stools and therefore must be replenished.[1] Gravity and good abdominal muscle tone also aid in proper bowel function. Exercise increases muscle tone and promotes bowel motility.

Avoiding the urge to empty the bowel can eventually lead to constipation. When the urge is ignored or suppressed, rectal muscles can lose tonicity and become less effective in eliminating stool. Nerve pathways may degenerate and stop sending the signal to defecate. In these cases, bowel retraining often is necessary to establish a pattern of regular bowel movements.

Medications can also contribute to constipation (Table 15–2).[2,3,11,12] Constipation is of particular concern in patients taking multiple medications and in those who also have conditions that can induce constipation. Opioid-induced constipation is a common reason for self-care laxative use.

Clinical Presentation of Constipation

Patients will often present with a complaint of constipation. In addition to the patient's report of decreased frequency or difficulty passing stools, other presenting symptoms may include anorexia, dull headache, lassitude, low back pain, abdominal discomfort, bloating, flatulence, and psychosocial distress.[1] Occasional bouts

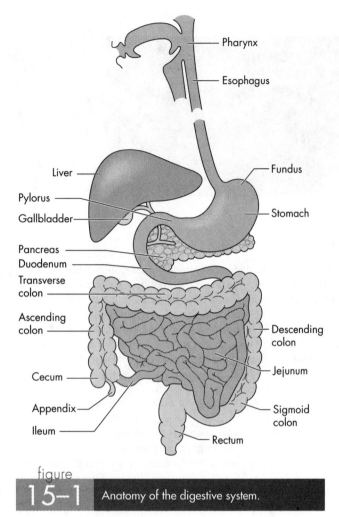

15–1 | Selected Conditions Associated with Constipation

Structural

Colorectal or anorectal injury, inflammation, or damage (e.g., anal fissure)

Pelvic floor disorders

Structural abnormalities (e.g., tumors, hernias, strictures) leading to bowel obstruction

Systemic

Electrolyte imbalances

Thyroid disorders

Diabetes mellitus

Irritable bowel syndrome

Uremia

Pituitary disorders

Neurological

Autonomic neuropathy

Multiple sclerosis

Parkinsonism

Cerebrovascular accidents

Dementia

Psychological

Depression

Eating disorders

Situational stress

Source: References 1–3, 5, and 6.

figure

15–1 | Anatomy of the digestive system.

---

of temporary constipation usually are treatable with self-care measures. Constipation continuing over several weeks to months is considered to be chronic and may require more sustained and aggressive therapy directed by a health care provider.[13,14] The Rome criteria are a set of guidelines developed primarily to aid researchers in classifying chronic constipation.[1] These criteria are used to some extent in routine practice, but providers generally rely on patient history and clinical presentation to characterize constipation and assist in treatment decisions.

Longstanding or untreated constipation can lead to complications. Acutely, straining to pass hard stool can lead to hemorrhoids, anal fissures with rectal bleeding, or rectal prolapse. If hard stool is packed very tightly in the rectum or intestine, fecal impaction or rectal ulcers may occur. Because defecation has been found to alter hemodynamics, straining to defecate may result in blood pressure surges or cardiac rhythm disturbances.[9]

Treatment of Constipation

Treatment Goals

The primary goals of treatment are to (1) relieve constipation and reestablish normal bowel function, (2) establish dietary and exercise habits that aid in preventing recurrences, and (3) promote the safe and effective use of laxative products.

General Treatment Approach

Initial management of constipation involves adjusting the diet to include foods high in fiber, increasing fluid intake, and engaging in some form of exercise. Pharmacologic intervention can be used in conjunction with lifestyle modifications if more immediate relief is desired. Laxatives should be selected according to the age and health status of the patient, as well as the mechanism of action of the individual product. Food and Drug Administration (FDA) labeling for nonprescription products limits patients to short-term (<7 days) treatment duration without medical referral, which is consistent with the need for medical supervision of chronic constipation treatment.[13,14] Accordingly, patients should not use any nonprescription laxative product for more than 7 days unless the therapy is directed by a health care provider. If rectal bleeding occurs at any time during the use of a laxative, or if constipation persists in spite of laxative therapy, patients should stop use of the laxative and receive medical referral.[1,15]

Self-care is inappropriate and medical referral is also necessary in other instances, including the presence of marked or severe abdominal pain, significant abdominal distention or cramping, marked or unexplained flatulence, fever, nausea and/or vomiting with constipation, or a sudden change in bowel habits that persists for 2 weeks.[1–3] Abdominal pain, nausea,

table

15-2 Selected Drugs That May Induce Constipation

Analgesics (including nonsteroidal anti-inflammatory drugs)

Antacids (e.g., calcium and aluminum compounds, bismuth)

Anticholinergics (e.g., benztropine, glycopyrrolate)

Anticonvulsants (e.g., carbamazepine, divalproate)

Antidepressants (specifically tricyclics such as amitriptyline)

Antihistamines (e.g., diphenhydramine, loratadine)

Antimotility (e.g., diphenoxylate, loperamide)

Antimuscarinics (e.g., oxybutynin, tolterodine)

Barium sulfate

Benzodiazepines (especially alprazolam and estazolam)

Calcium channel blockers (e.g., verapamil, diltiazem)

Calcium supplements (e.g., calcium carbonate)

Clonidine

Diuretics (e.g., hydrochlorothiazide, furosemide)

Gastrointestinal antispasmodics (e.g., dicyclomine, hyoscyamine)

Hematinics (especially iron)

Hyperlipidemia agents (e.g., cholestyramine, pravastatin, simvastatin)

Hypotensives (e.g., angiotensin-converting enzyme inhibitors, beta-blockers)

Memantine

Muscle relaxants (e.g., cyclobenzaprine, metaxalone)

Opiates (e.g., morphine, codeine)

Parasympatholytics (e.g., atropine)

Parkinsonism agents (e.g., bromocriptine)

Polystyrene sodium sulfonate

Psychotherapeutic drugs (e.g., phenothiazines, butyrophenones)

Sedative hypnotics (e.g., zolpidem, benzodiazepines, phenobarbital)

Sucralfate

Source: References 2, 3, 11, and 12.

vomiting, or marked cramping or distention may indicate the presence of fecal impaction or bowel obstruction.[15] A sudden change in bowel habits that persists for 2 weeks may indicate an underlying disease process such as inflammatory bowel disease or colorectal cancer.[1] Similarly, patients with underlying disorders (e.g., inflammatory bowel disease) or constipation presenting with symptoms of a potential underlying disorder (e.g., dark or tarry stool) should also be referred for medical care.[8] A treatment algorithm (Figure 15–2) provides a systematic approach to the self-care of constipation and lists exclusions for self-treatment.[1–3,8]

Nonpharmacologic Therapy

To prevent constipation, patients should adhere to a balanced diet that incorporates recommendations from the Dietary Guidelines for Americans, 2010, including increasing fruit and vegetable intake and consuming at least half of all grains as whole grain. The American Dietetic Association recommends an adult daily dietary fiber intake of 14 grams per 1000 kcal, or 25 grams for adult women and 38 grams for adult men.[16,17] (See Chapter 23 for information on dietary fiber types, sources, intake, and benefits.)

Added fiber increases stool weight and also tends to normalize frequency of bowel movements to 1 movement per day and GI transit time to 2–4 days. This normalization of bowel movement frequency is important; the longer stool is retained in the bowel, the more water is absorbed out of the bowel and into the intestinal cells, leading to hard stools and difficulty in passing stool.[17] Patients complaining of constipation should gradually increase their intake of insoluble fiber (e.g., whole grains, wheat bran, and vegetables), which is associated with laxation.[8,17] Patients should also limit intake of foods with little or no fiber (e.g., cheese, meat, and processed foods) to promote normal bowel function.

If dietary modifications are not effective, patients may choose to supplement their diet with a commercially available fiber supplement. Many newer flavorless and texture-free fiber supplements (e.g., inulin) are classified as dietary supplements (Table 15–3).[8] Others (e.g., psyllium and methylcellulose) are bulk-forming laxatives approved as FDA drug products. The pharmacologic effects of FDA-approved fiber supplements have been studied more extensively than dietary supplement products (see Pharmacologic Therapy). The onset of laxation from a high-fiber diet or fiber supplement usually is not immediate. Individual benefits will vary and may take 3–5 days or longer. Patients should be encouraged to find the fiber supplement that provides the best balance of tolerability, desirable dosage form, effectiveness at promoting laxation, and cost (see Chapter 23 and www.nationalfibercouncil.org for more information).

Significantly increasing dietary fiber from any source may lead to erratic bowel habits, flatulence, and abdominal discomfort during the first few weeks. Some fiber-supplemented foods contain approximately 10 grams of fiber per serving and can cause significant side effects if added to the diet too quickly. Recommend that patients gradually increase fiber intake over a period of 1–2 weeks to improve tolerance.[1,8,17] Advise patients to increase their fluid intake when increasing dietary fiber. In general, 2 liters of fluid per day is recommended. Fluid requirements increase for pregnant and lactating women; an additional 300 mL and 750–1000 mL of fluid, respectively, should be added to daily requirements.[17]

Behavior modifications (or "bowel training") can also be beneficial for promoting regular bowel movements. Promptly heeding the urge to pass the stool and allowing sufficient time for toileting are important. Gastrocolic reflexes are greatest first thing in the morning and 30 minutes after a meal, so attempting a bowel movement at these times can help promote defecation consistent with the body's normal physiologic response.[1,18]

Although there is no consistent evidence that exercise relieves constipation, low levels of physical activity have been associated with an increased risk of constipation.[1,18] Encourage regular physical activity consistent with a healthy lifestyle to decrease the risk of constipation.

Pharmacologic Therapy

The ideal laxative (1) would be nonirritating and nontoxic, (2) would act only on the descending and sigmoid colons, and

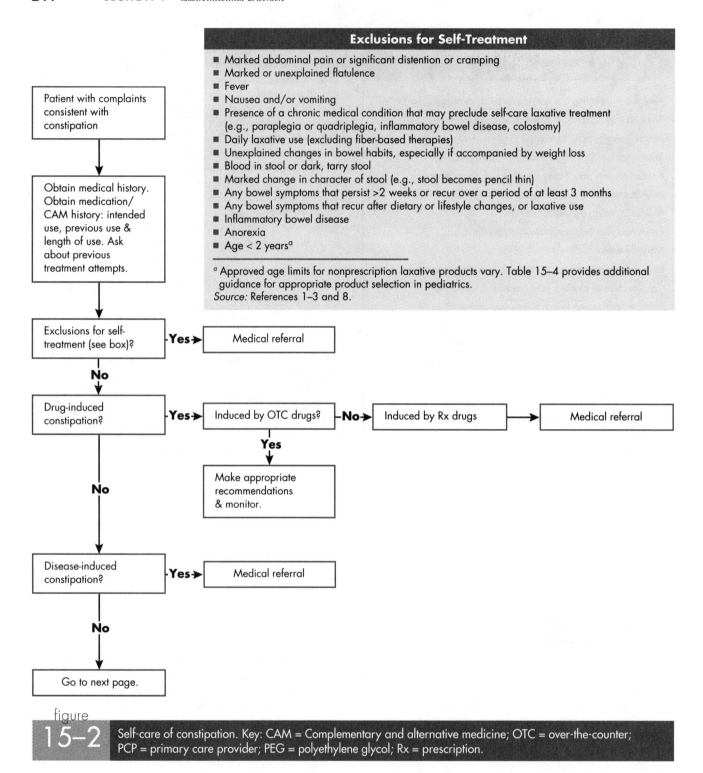

Exclusions for Self-Treatment

- Marked abdominal pain or significant distention or cramping
- Marked or unexplained flatulence
- Fever
- Nausea and/or vomiting
- Presence of a chronic medical condition that may preclude self-care laxative treatment (e.g., paraplegia or quadriplegia, inflammatory bowel disease, colostomy)
- Daily laxative use (excluding fiber-based therapies)
- Unexplained changes in bowel habits, especially if accompanied by weight loss
- Blood in stool or dark, tarry stool
- Marked change in character of stool (e.g., stool becomes pencil thin)
- Any bowel symptoms that persist >2 weeks or recur over a period of at least 3 months
- Any bowel symptoms that recur after dietary or lifestyle changes, or laxative use
- Inflammatory bowel disease
- Anorexia
- Age < 2 years[a]

[a] Approved age limits for nonprescription laxative products vary. Table 15–4 provides additional guidance for appropriate product selection in pediatrics.
Source: References 1–3 and 8.

figure 15–2 Self-care of constipation. Key: CAM = Complementary and alternative medicine; OTC = over-the-counter; PCP = primary care provider; PEG = polyethylene glycol; Rx = prescription.

(3) would produce a normally formed stool within a few hours, after which time the laxative's action would cease and normal bowel activity would resume. Because no currently available laxative precisely meets these criteria, proper selection of a laxative depends on the etiology of the constipation and individual patient factors and preferences.

Agents used to treat constipation are classified by mechanism of action and include bulk-forming, hyperosmotic, emollient, lubricant, saline, and stimulant agents (Table 15–4).

Bulk-Forming Agents

Products classified as bulk-forming laxatives include those containing methylcellulose, polycarbophil, and psyllium. Bulk-forming products are the recommended choice for the treatment of most instances of constipation because they most closely approximate the physiologic mechanism in promoting evacuation.[1,5,8] These agents dissolve or swell in the intestinal fluid of the small and large intestines, forming emollient gels that stimulate peristalsis

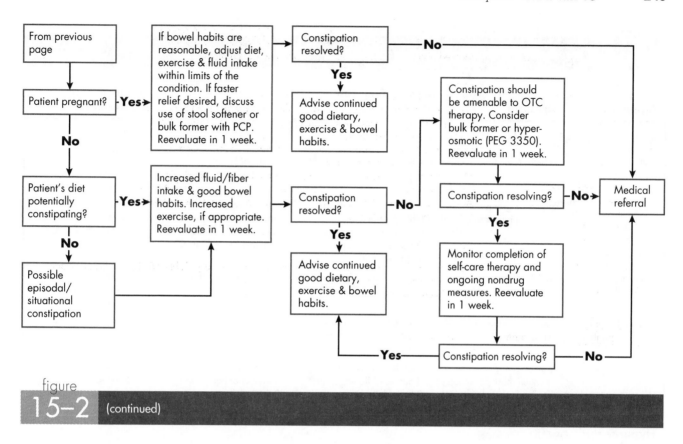

figure

15–2 (continued)

and facilitate passage of the intestinal contents. Available dosage forms include tablets or capsules; powders to be mixed with water or other liquids; and fiber chews, wafers, or gummies.

Bulk-forming agents are not absorbed systemically; the usual onset of action is from 12 to 24 hours, but onset may be delayed as long as 72 hours. They are indicated as short-term therapy to relieve constipation and may be useful for (1) patients on low-fiber diets; (2) postpartum women; (3) older adults; and (4) patients with colostomies, irritable bowel syndrome, or diverticular disease. They are also indicated prophylactically in patients who should refrain from straining during a bowel movement. Dosages vary according to the type of product (Table 15-4). Exceeding the recommended doses for a bulk-forming agent could lead to increased flatulence or obstruction if appropriate fluid intake is not maintained.

When taken as directed, bulk-forming agents have few systemic side effects. The most common adverse effects include abdominal cramping and flatulence. If not taken with adequate fluid, bulk-forming laxatives may swell in the throat or esophagus and cause choking. Bulk-forming products should be avoided in patients who have swallowing difficulties or esophageal strictures; additionally, bulk-forming agents may be inappropriate for patients who must restrict fluid intake (e.g., those with heart failure). Obstruction is a particular risk for palliative care patients and those patients suffering from opiate-induced constipation who have inadequate fluid intake.[19] Patients experiencing chest pain, vomiting, difficulty swallowing, or difficulty breathing after use should seek immediate medical attention. Granular psyllium products have been taken off the market because of reports of esophageal obstruction.[20]

Acute bronchospasm has been associated with inhalation of dry hydrophilic mucilloid, as well as hypersensitivity reactions to psyllium characterized by anaphylaxis.[21] Individuals who are sensitive to inhaled or ingested psyllium should avoid these products.

Bulk-forming laxatives are not systemically absorbed, but they may interfere with the absorption of oral medications because of physical binding in the GI tract or other mechanisms. Additionally, calcium polycarbophil may decrease the absorption

table

15–3 Types of Fiber Supplements

Type of Fiber	Examples of Common Brands
Products Classified as Bulk-Forming Laxatives[a]	
Methylcellulose	Citrucel
Calcium polycarbophil	FiberCon
Psyllium	Metamucil, Konsyl
Products Classified as Dietary Supplements	
Inulin	FiberChoice, Metamucil Clear & Natural
Partially hydrolyzed guar gum	Sunfiber
Powdered cellulose	Unifiber
Wheat dextrin	Benefiber

[a] Products classified as bulk-forming laxatives are FDA-labeled to treat constipation.

Source: Adapted with permission from reference 8.

table

15–4 Dosage Guidelines for Nonprescription Laxative Products[a]

Agent	Dosage Form/ Strength	Adults/Children ≥ 12 Years	Children 6 to < 12 Years[b]	Children 2 to < 6 Years[b,c]
Bulk-Forming Agents				
Methylcellulose	Caplet: 500 mg	2 caplets up to 6 times daily	1 caplet up to 6 times daily	Not recommended for children < 6 years, except under advice of a PCP
	Powder: 2 grams per heaping tablespoon	Starting dose: 1 rounded tablespoon; increase as needed, 1 rounded tablespoon at a time, up to 3 times daily	Starting dose: 2 level teaspoons; increase as needed, 2 level teaspoons at a time, up to 3 times daily	Not recommended for children < 6 years except under advice of a PCP
Calcium polycarbophil	Caplet: 625 mg	2 caplets 1–4 times daily	1 caplet 1–4 times daily	Not recommended for children < 6 years, except under advice of a PCP
Psyllium (plantago seeds, ispaghula)	Capsule: psyllium husk, 0.52 gram	5 capsules with 8 ounces of liquid (swallow 1 capsule at a time), up to 3 times daily	Not recommended for children < 12 years except under advice of a PCP	Not recommended for children < 6 years except under advice of a PCP
	Powder: 3.4 grams psyllium husk per scoop or per packet of "fiber singles" product	1 rounded tablespoon in 8 ounces of liquid, up to 3 times daily	1/2 of adult dose in 8 ounces of liquid, up to 3 times daily	Not recommended for children < 6 years except under advice of a PCP
Hyperosmotic Agents				
Polyethylene glycol 3350	Powder: 17 grams per capful	17 grams in 4–8 ounces of beverage once daily in adults and children ≥ 17 years	Not recommended for children < 17 years, except under advice of a PCP	Not recommended for children < 17 years, except under advice of a PCP
Glycerin	Rectal solid suppository: 2 grams	1 suppository, or as directed by a PCP	1 suppository, or as directed by a PCP	Not recommended for children < 6 years except under advice of a PCP
	Rectal solid suppository: 1 gram (pediatric formulation)	—	—	1 suppository, or as directed by a PCP
	Rectal liquid suppository: 5.6 grams glycerin per 5.5 mL	1 suppository, or as directed by a PCP	1 suppository, or as directed by a PCP	Not recommended for children < 6 years, except under advice of a PCP
	Rectal liquid suppository: 2.8 grams glycerin per 2.7 mL (pediatric formulation)	—	—	1 suppository, or as directed by a PCP
Emollient Agents				
Docusate sodium	Capsules: 50 mg and 100 mg	50–300 mg daily in single or divided doses	50–150 mg daily in single or divided doses	50–150 mg daily in single or divided doses
	Syrup: 60 mg per 15 mL	1–6 tablespoons daily, or as directed by a PCP, in single or divided doses (doses must be given in 6–8 ounces of milk or juice to prevent throat irritation)	1–2 1/2 tablespoons daily, or as directed by a PCP, in single or divided doses (doses must be given in 6–8 ounces of milk or juice to prevent throat irritation)	1–2 1/2 tablespoons daily, or as directed by a PCP, in single or divided doses (doses must be given in 6–8 ounces of milk or juice to prevent throat irritation)
	Syrup: 50 mg/15 mL (pediatric formulation)	—	1–3 tablespoons daily, in single or divided doses (doses must be given in 6–8 ounces of milk or juice to prevent throat irritation)	1–3 tablespoons daily, in single or divided doses (doses must be given in 6–8 ounces of milk or juice to prevent throat irritation)

table

15–4 | Dosage Guidelines for Nonprescription Laxative Products[a] *(continued)*

Agent	Dosage Form/ Strength	Adults/Children ≥ 12 Years	Children 6 to < 12 Years[b]	Children 2 to < 6 Years[b,c]
Docusate calcium	Capsule: 240 mg	1 capsule daily for several days, or until bowel movements are normal	Not recommended for children < 12 years, except under advice of a PCP	Not recommended for children < 6 years, except under advice of a PCP
Lubricant Agent				
Mineral oil[d]	Oral liquid	1–3 tablespoons (15– 45 mL); maximum 3 tablespoons (45 mL) in 24 hours	1–3 teaspoons (5–15 mL); maximum 3 teaspoons (15 mL) in 24 hours	Not recommended for children < 6 years except under advice of a PCP
	Oral liquid emulsion: 2.5 mL mineral oil/5 mL	6–15 teaspoons (30–75 mL) per day, or as directed by a PCP	2–5 teaspoons (10–25 mL) per day, or as directed by a PCP	Not recommended for children < 6 years except under advice of a PCP
	Rectal liquid enema: 118 mL	1 bottle as directed	1/2 bottle as directed	1/2 bottle as directed
Saline Laxative Agents				
Magnesium citrate	Liquid: 10 fluid ounces; 300 mL	1/2–1 bottle (150–300 mL)	1/3–1/2 bottle (100–150 mL)	Not recommended for children < 6 years except under advice of a PCP
Magnesium hydroxide	Liquid: 400 mg/5 mL	2–4 tablespoons daily as single or divided doses	1–2 tablespoons daily as single or divided doses	Not recommended for children < 6 years except under advice of a PCP
	Concentrated liquid: 2400 mg/15 mL	1–2 tablespoons daily as single or divided doses	1/2–1 tablespoon daily as single or divided doses	Not recommended for children < 6 years except under advice of a PCP
	Chewable tablet: 311 mg per tablet	8 tablets once in a 24-hour period, preferably at bedtime, in divided doses or as directed by a PCP	4 tablets once in a 24-hour period, preferably at bedtime, in divided doses or as directed by a PCP	Children 3–5 years: chew 2 tablets once in a 24-hour period, preferably at bedtime, in divided doses or as directed by a PCP Not recommended for children < 3 years except under advice of a PCP
	Chewable tablet: 400 mg per tablet (pediatric formulation)	—	3–6 tablets daily in single or divided doses	1–3 tablets daily in single or divided doses
Monobasic sodium phosphate/ dibasic sodium phosphate	Rectal liquid enema: 118 mL	1 bottle, as directed	Not recommended for children < 12 years, except under advice of a PCP	Not recommended for children < 6 years, except under advice of a PCP
	Rectal liquid enema: 197 mL	1 bottle, as directed	Not recommended for children < 12 years, except under advice of a PCP	Not recommended for children < 6 years, except under advice of a PCP
	Rectal liquid enema: 59 mL (pediatric formulation)	—	Children 5–11 years: 1 bottle or as directed by a PCP	Children 2–5 years: 1/2 bottle
Magnesium sulfate (Epsom salt)[d]	Solid: magnesium sulfate USP	2–6 level teaspoons (10–30 grams) daily[d]	1–2 level teaspoons (5–10 grams) daily[d]	Not recommended for children < 6 years except under advice of a PCP

table

15–4 Dosage Guidelines for Nonprescription Laxative Products[a] *(continued)*

Agent	Dosage Form/ Strength	Adults/Children ≥ 12 Years	Children 6 to < 12 Years[b]	Children 2 to < 6 Years[b,c]
Stimulant Agents				
Senna	Tablets: 8.6 mg sennosides	Starting dose: 2 tablets once daily	Starting dose: 1 tablet once daily	Starting dose: 1/2 tablet once daily
		Maximum dose: 4 tablets twice daily	Maximum dose: 2 tablets twice daily	Maximum dose: 1 tablet twice daily
	Tablets or chocolate pieces: 15 mg sennosides	2 tablets or chocolate pieces 1–2 times daily	1 tablet or chocolate piece 1–2 times daily	Not recommended for children < 6 years, except under advice of a PCP
	Tablets: 17.2 mg sennosides	Starting dose: 1 tablet once daily	Starting dose: 1/2 tablet once daily	Not recommended for children < 6 years, except under advice of a PCP
		Maximum dose: 2 tablets twice daily	Maximum dose: 1 tablet twice daily	
	Pills: 25 mg sennosides	2 pills 1–2 times daily	1 pill 1–2 times daily	Not recommended for children < 6 years, except under advice of a PCP
	Liquid[e]: senna concentrate 33.3 mg senna pod concentrate/mL (pediatric formulation [i.e., Fletcher's Laxative for Kids])	—	Age 6–15 years: 2–3 teaspoons 1–2 times daily	1–2 teaspoons 1–2 times daily
	Liquid[e]: sennosides 1.8 mg sennosides/mL	2–3 teaspoons once a day	1–1 1/2 teaspoons once a day	1/2–3/4 teaspoon once a day
Bisacodyl	Tablets: 5 mg	1–3 tablets (usually 2) once daily	1 tablet daily	Not recommended for children < 6 years except under advice of a PCP
	Rectal solid suppository: 10 mg	1 suppository in a single daily dose	1/2 suppository in a single daily dose	Not recommended for children < 6 years except under advice of a PCP
Castor oil[d]	Liquid	1 to a maximum of 4 tablespoons (15–60 mL) in a single daily dose[d]	1 to a maximum of 3 teaspoons (5–15 mL) in a single daily dose[d]	Not recommended for children < 6 years except under advice of a PCP

Key: FDA = Food and Drug Administration; OTC = over-the-counter; PCP = primary care provider.

[a] All doses are based on FDA-labeled instructions and are for oral products, unless indicated otherwise.

[b] All doses for children are listed as those for ages 2 to < 6 years or ages 6 to < 12 years, unless otherwise indicated in FDA-labeled dosing instructions. In these cases, FDA-labeled age ranges are provided within the table.

[c] No recommended dosages exist for children < 2 years of age, except under the advice and supervision of a PCP.

[d] Although magnesium sulfate (Epsom salt) and castor oil are approved as nonprescription laxatives, they are not recommended because safer, better tolerated, and well-studied alternatives are available. Self-care use of mineral oil is also discouraged in most cases. See Pharmacologic Therapy for specific recommendations on appropriate use of each agent.

[e] Liquid senna products vary in product concentration and dosing, depending on the form of senna. Take care to ensure that patients are following FDA-labeled dosing instructions with use of these products, especially in pediatric patients.

of oral tetracyclines and quinolones secondary to calcium chelation. Patients should separate doses of bulk-forming laxatives from other medications by at least 2 hours to avoid potential drug interactions.

Because of the danger of fecal impaction or intestinal obstruction, individuals with intestinal ulcerations, stenosis, or disabling adhesions should not take bulk-forming products. Diarrhea, abdominal discomfort, flatulence, and excessive loss of fluid can also occur.

The maximum calcium content of calcium polycarbophil is approximately 150 mg (7.6 mEq) per tablet. Certain patients (e.g., older adults; individuals with malignancy, renal disease, or AIDS) may be at risk for hypercalcemia with recommended doses of calcium polycarbophil.

The sugar content of bulk-forming agents should be evaluated before use by patients with diabetes or those with restricted caloric intake. Sugar-free agents that contain aspartame should be avoided by patients with phenylketonuria.

Hyperosmotic Agents

Hyperosmotic agents include polyethylene glycol 3350 (PEG 3350) and glycerin (Table 15–4). These products contain large, poorly absorbed ions or molecules that draw water into the colon or rectum through osmosis to stimulate a bowel movement.[22] Other commonly used agents in this class are prescription-only products, including lactulose, sorbitol, and PEG solutions with electrolytes (e.g., Colyte and GoLYTELY).

PEG 3350 is available for self-care use in individuals ages 17 years or older; it comes in a powder for oral administration and is usually taken as 17 grams of powder (approximately 1 capful or 1 packet) per day mixed into 4–8 ounces of water. After oral administration, the PEG 3350 dose remains almost entirely within the GI tract and is not subject to degradation by intestinal enzymes or bacterial metabolism. The very small amount that is systemically absorbed (0.2%) is rapidly excreted in the urine. PEG 3350 usually produces a bowel movement in 12–72 hours, but onset may take as long as 96 hours in some patients.

PEG 3350 is safe and effective for the short-term treatment of occasional constipation, with few side effects.[23] PEG 3350 is generally well-tolerated because very little drug is absorbed systemically. Adverse effects may include bloating, abdominal discomfort, cramping, and flatulence. Higher doses (e.g., 34 g/day) might lead to diarrhea and excessive stool frequency. FDA-approved labeling indicates that patients who have renal disease or irritable bowel syndrome should be cautioned to consult with their primary care provider before using PEG 3350. No clinically significant drug–drug interactions have been reported with PEG 3350.

Glycerin has been available for many years in suppository form for lower bowel evacuation (Table 15–4). It works primarily in the colon and is poorly absorbed after rectal administration. Glycerin suppositories usually produce a bowel movement within 15–30 minutes of administration. They are considered to be safe for occasional use in all approved age groups but may cause rectal irritation with overdosage. Use of liquid glycerin as an enema is not recommended because of rectal irritation.

Other than potential rectal irritation, adverse reactions with glycerin suppositories are minimal. Interactions between glycerin and other drugs are not clinically important. Use of glycerin may be inappropriate in patients who have an existing condition that involves rectal irritation. Chronic use or overuse may lead to reduced serum potassium concentrations.

Emollient Agents

Emollients (stool softeners) are anionic surfactants that act in the small and large intestines to increase the wetting efficiency of intestinal fluid, facilitating a mixture of aqueous and fatty substances to soften the fecal mass (Table 15–4). They are used primarily to prevent straining and painful defecation with anorectal disorders or in patients who should avoid straining (e.g., those with severe hypertension or cardiovascular disease, recent abdominal or rectal surgery, or recent myocardial infarction; or women who are immediately postpartum). Although emollients can be used to treat occasional constipation, they are more often used in combination with a stimulant (e.g., senna or bisacodyl) as a long-term treatment for opioid-induced constipation.[19,24] (See the box A Word about Opioid-Induced Constipation.)

Docusate, available as a sodium and calcium salt, has an onset of action of 12–72 hours. Effectiveness is usually achieved within 48 hours, but some patients may require as long as 3–5 days. Docusate sodium is supplied in capsule or syrup form in multiple strengths; docusate calcium is available as a 240 mg capsule. Although no therapeutic differences exist between these salt forms, docusate sodium's availability in multiple strengths and dosage forms results in more frequent use.

Docusate is generally well tolerated but can potentially cause diarrhea and mild abdominal cramping. Emollients can increase systemic absorption of mineral oil and should not be used in combination with products containing mineral oil. Doses above those recommended by the manufacturer may result in weakness, sweating, muscle cramps, and an irregular heartbeat in some patients. These agents are not believed to be appreciably absorbed from the GI tract and do not hamper absorption of nutrients from the intestinal tract.

Lubricant Agent

Mineral oil (liquid petrolatum) is the only nonprescription lubricant. Mineral oil acts in the colon to soften fecal contents by coating the stool and preventing colonic absorption of fecal water. It is available in liquid forms for oral or rectal administration (Table 15–4). Mineral oil's onset of action is about 6–8 hours after oral administration and 5–15 minutes after rectal administration.

Mineral oil can help maintain a soft stool, and its uses are similar to those of emollient laxatives for preventing straining or painful defecation. However, because of safety concerns with mineral oil, docusate forms are preferred if a stool softener is needed.[8] Although patients may use mineral oil for an occasional bout of constipation, its use in self-care is strongly discouraged because of the availability of safer agents.

The most significant acute safety concern with mineral oil is lipid pneumonia resulting from aspiration into the lungs after an oral dose. Patients most at risk for aspiration include young children, older patients, debilitated or bedridden patients, and those with swallowing difficulties or dysphagia. Mineral oil should not be used in these patients or given to any patients before they lie down. FDA-approved labeling for mineral oil products includes a warning against its use in patients younger than 6 years, pregnant women, bedridden or older adults, and those with difficulty swallowing.

Opioid use is common in the treatment of non-cancer and cancer pain. Constipation is experienced by approximately 40% of patients and is the most common adverse effect with opioid use. Opioid-induced constipation may prevent patients from receiving appropriate pain-relieving dosages or may cause discontinuation of therapy despite the need for pain relief. Opioids cause constipation by binding to bowel and central nervous system receptors to decrease GI motility and intestinal secretions, leading to longer retention time of fecal matter in the intestines and drying of the stool. Unlike other opioid-induced side effects, patients generally do not develop tolerance to constipation over time. Constipating effects of opioids are dependent on the opioid dose and duration of use.[19,24]

Some forms of opioids are more likely to cause constipation. Oral opioids generally are more constipating than parenteral agents. Transdermal fentanyl patches have fewer constipating effects than oral opioids and may be an option for outpatients requiring chronic opioid therapy.[11,24]

Patients on chronic opioids will require a long-term laxative regimen to prevent and/or treat constipation. Stimulant laxatives (e.g., senna or bisacodyl, with or without docusate) are most commonly recommended.[24] The stimulant helps to propel the stool through the colon, whereas the emollient (docusate) increases wetting of the stool and softens the fecal mass. Typically, a stool softener alone is not effective. Polyethylene glycol preparations or other osmotic agents may also be used for prevention and treatment of opioid-induced constipation. Saline laxatives or rectal preparations may be needed intermittently for acute evacuation. Bulk-forming laxatives are unlikely to be adequately effective if used alone and may not be tolerated because of fluid restrictions or immobility in some chronic opioid patients (e.g., palliative care).[19,24]

Identify patients at risk for opioid-induced constipation to help prevent problems, including patients with cancer- and non-cancer–related pain. Educate patients on the role of nondrug measures to help prevent constipation (e.g., increasing fluid intake, fiber intake, and physical activity as tolerated). For patients on chronic opioid therapy, emphasize the importance of bowel regimen adherence, and explain the need for long-term use of laxatives with chronic opioids. If appropriate, suggest alternative opioids (e.g., transdermal fentanyl) that may be less constipating than oral agents. Inform patients on short-term opioid therapy about constipating effects of opioids, and help individuals take steps to prevent constipation. This is especially true in patients who have other risk factors for constipation, such as those taking opioids immediately after abdominal surgery or childbirth.

Patients can also experience adverse effects related to high doses or long-term use. Taking larger than recommended doses can cause leakage of oil through the anal sphincter, resulting in anal pruritus (pruritus ani), cryptitis, or other perianal conditions. Patients can avoid this by reducing or dividing the dose, or by using a stable emulsion of mineral oil. FDA-approved labeling for mineral oil products directs patients to stop its use and consult their primary care provider if leakage of oil occurs. With repeated and prolonged use of mineral oil, the droplets may reach the mesenteric lymph nodes and may also be present in the intestinal mucosa, liver, and spleen, where they elicit a typical foreign-body reaction.

Mineral oil may impair the absorption of the fat-soluble vitamins A, D, E, and K, as well as many oral medications (including oral contraceptives and digitalis glycosides). Mineral oil's effects on vitamin K may increase blood-thinning properties of some oral anticoagulants. To minimize any interactions, patients should not take mineral oil with food. Concomitant use of mineral oil with docusate emollients should be avoided because of potential increased absorption of mineral oil.

Saline Laxative Agents

Saline laxative agents include magnesium citrate, magnesium hydroxide, dibasic sodium phosphate, monobasic sodium phosphate, and magnesium sulfate. They are available in liquid or solid form for oral administration and in liquid form for rectal administration (Table 15–4). Saline laxatives act primarily by osmosis in the small and large intestines (oral products) or in the colon (rectal forms). After administration, ions are retained in the intestinal wall and draw water in by osmosis, thereby increasing intraluminal pressure and intestinal motility. Saline laxatives are used for occasional relief of constipation or for acute bowel evacuation that is required before a procedure (e.g., colonoscopy preparation).

Oral magnesium hydroxide is appropriate for treatment of occasional constipation in otherwise healthy patients. When administered at standard doses, magnesium hydroxide produces a bowel movement within 30 minutes to 6 hours of administration.[8]

Other saline agents (magnesium citrate and sodium phosphate preparations) are more commonly used orally or rectally for acute catharsis (e.g., prior to a colonoscopy; only the prescription version of the oral formulation should be used for this indication). When used for these purposes, the onset of action is generally 30 minutes to 3 hours for oral doses and 2–15 minutes for rectal doses. Magnesium sulfate (Epsom salt) is labeled for nonprescription use, but it is not recommended because safer and better-studied laxatives are available.

Adverse effects related to saline laxatives most often include abdominal cramping, nausea, vomiting, or dehydration. Patients who cannot tolerate fluid loss should not use saline laxatives. In patients who are not fluid restricted, oral doses of magnesium salts should be followed by at least 1 full glass of water to prevent dehydration. When used for treatment of occasional constipation, doses should be administered at bedtime, if possible.

Saline laxatives can cause serious electrolyte imbalances if used long term or at higher-than-recommended doses. As much as 20% of the administered magnesium ion may be absorbed from magnesium salts, potentially leading to hypermagnesemia.[8] FDA-approved labeling for these products recommends against their use in patients on sodium-, phosphate-, or magnesium-restricted diets. Although some health care providers continue to recommend regular use of oral magnesium hydroxide to promote regularity, alternative treatment options with more favorable adverse effect profiles exist. Toxicity risk is increased in newborns, older adults, and patients with renal impairment; therefore, magnesium-containing laxatives should be avoided in those populations. Symptoms of magnesium toxicity include hypotension, muscle weakness, and fatigue.

Products containing sodium phosphate can cause hyperphosphatemia, hypocalcemia, and hypernatremia; therefore, they should be used cautiously in patients with renal impairment, in cardiac patients on sodium-restricted diets, and in those taking medications that may affect serum electrolyte levels (e.g., diuretics).[8] Sodium phosphate products are contraindicated in patients with congestive heart failure. Additionally, rectally administered sodium phosphate should be avoided in patients with megacolon, gastrointestinal obstruction, imperforate anus, or colostomy.

Acute phosphate nephropathy leading to renal function impairment has also been reported with the use of oral sodium phosphate products for bowel cleansing prior to colonoscopy or other procedures. A 2008 FDA warning restricted nonprescription oral sodium phosphate solutions to treatment of constipation only (i.e., not for use as bowel preparations) and required prescription products to carry a boxed warning and MedGuide. In 2014, FDA noted continued reports of acute phosphate nephropathy occurring with these agents and provided further guidance to ensure their safe use for bowel preparation, including the development of a risk evaluation and mitigation strategy (REMS) for prescription products. Although nonprescription oral sodium phosphate products are indicated only for treatment of constipation, FDA also announced at that time that additional labeling changes would be made for these agents to support their appropriate and safe use as self-care laxatives.[25] Of note, at the time of this writing (July 2014), no nonprescription oral sodium phosphate solution products were available.

Saline laxatives can interact with oral anticoagulants, digitalis glycosides, and some phenothiazines (especially chlorpromazine). Magnesium-containing laxatives may interfere with the absorption of oral tetracycline products. If used concurrently with a magnesium salt, sodium polystyrene sulfonate may bind with magnesium and lead to systemic alkalosis.

Stimulant Agents

Stimulant laxatives are classified according to their chemical structure and pharmacologic activity as anthraquinones (e.g., senna) or diphenylmethanes (e.g., bisacodyl). FDA has deemed formerly available products containing cascara sagrada, casanthranol, and phenolphthalein as "not safe and effective."[26,27] Because some of these unapproved agents are marketed as dietary supplements, they may be available in some pharmacies and health food stores; however, unapproved supplement products should not be recommended (see Complementary Therapies). Although rhubarb and aloe were not included in FDA rulings, providers should not recommend the use of those very irritating substances.

Stimulant laxatives (Table 15–4) work primarily in the colon to increase intestinal motility either by local irritation of the mucosa or by a more selective action on the intramural nerve plexus of intestinal smooth muscle. They also increase secretion of water and electrolytes in the intestine.[5]

The onset of senna and bisacodyl is usually 6–10 hours after oral use but may require up to 24 hours. Bisacodyl suppositories usually take effect 15–60 minutes after administration.

Bisacodyl, administered orally or rectally, is also a component of bowel preparation regimens before colonoscopy or other bowel procedures. Stimulant laxatives are often used in combination with docusate to prevent or treat constipation in patients taking chronic opioids.[19,24] (See the box A Word about Opioid-Induced Constipation.) Overdoses of stimulants may lead to sudden vomiting, nausea, diarrhea, or severe abdominal cramping and require prompt medical attention.

Major hazards of stimulant laxative use are severe cramping, electrolyte and fluid deficiencies, enteric loss of protein, malabsorption caused by excessive hypermotility and catharsis, and hypokalemia. All stimulants may produce cramping, colic, increased mucus secretion, and (in some people) excessive evacuation of fluid at excess doses. Stimulants can be effective but should be recommended cautiously. Nevertheless, these laxatives are frequently used for constipation by those who self-medicate or by patients who perceive a benefit to frequent or thorough "cleansing" of the colon. Consequently, stimulant laxatives may be subject to overuse.[28–31] (See the box A Word about Laxative Overuse.)

Prolonged use of senna can also cause a harmless, reversible melanotic pigmentation of the colonic mucosa (melanosis coli), which may be seen on sigmoidoscopy, colonoscopy, or rectal biopsy. Senna may color urine pink to red, red to violet, or red to brown, and its presence may affect interpretation of the phenolsulfonphthalein test.

Enteric-coated bisacodyl tablets prevent irritation of the gastric mucosa. These should not be broken, crushed, chewed, or given with agents that increase gastric pH. The administration of bisacodyl tablets within 1 hour of antacids, histamine$_2$-receptor antagonists, proton pump inhibitors, or milk results in rapid erosion of the bisacodyl's enteric coating, which may lead to gastric or duodenal irritation.

Although castor oil historically has been viewed as a stimulant laxative, its exact mechanism is unknown.[31] Castor oil acts quickly and has significant laxative effects with accompanying abdominal cramping. Prolonged use of castor oil may result in excessive loss of fluid, electrolytes, and nutrients. Its use in the self-care setting is discouraged because safer and better-tolerated alternatives are available.[8,19]

Combination Products

Combination laxative products are also available (Table 15–5). Companies attempt to take advantage of multiple mechanisms of action to create a product that better meets the criteria for an ideal laxative. For example, several combination products contain both a stimulant and an emollient (e.g., senna with docusate sodium). Emollients do not stimulate bowel movements when used alone, but they support bowel movements when combined with stimulant laxatives.

In cases of fecal impaction, a solution of docusate is often added to the enema fluid. Some products incorporate senna with psyllium. The desired effect is for the senna to act quickly, whereas the bulk-forming agent aids in producing easier stools after the initial movement. Other available combination oral products include psyllium, bisacodyl, docusate, or another agent as the principal ingredient, with glycerin as an adjunctive agent; glycerin's contributing effect likely is insignificant to the overall laxative action of these products.

Patients should be counseled that combining laxatives can have the potential for greater adverse effects because a common ingredient in most combination products is a stimulant. If a stimulant and a stool softener are combined, the potential for adversity depends largely on the stimulant. However, if a stimulant and a saline are combined, the potential for adverse effects is enhanced, given that both agents have significant effects on the intestine.

Laxative Overuse

Health care providers should stay alert for patients who may be at risk for laxative overuse. Some patients perceive that a daily bowel movement is normal and routinely take stimulant or other laxatives to achieve this bowel pattern. Older adults may perceive that natural changes in bowel habits as a result of declining physical mobility or dietary changes are actually "constipation." Other patients are looking to "cleanse" their system of toxins through the use of colon-cleansing regimens marketed for this purpose; such regimens often contain high doses of laxatives.[28] Individuals may also have comorbid conditions that contribute to laxative overuse. For example, patients with anorexia or bulimia nervosa may abuse laxatives to "purge" unwanted food, or as a form of self-harm.[29] Factors that contribute to laxative overuse include older age, misconceptions about normal bowel movement frequency, fear of constipation, and widespread availability of laxatives.[30]

Excessive use of laxatives can acutely cause diarrhea and vomiting, fluid and electrolyte losses (especially hypokalemia), and dehydration. Concerns about long-term consequences of chronic stimulant laxative use have been disproved in the literature. Although previous cases of potential adverse effects of chronic use of stimulant laxatives have been reported, well-designed recent clinical trials do not support an increased risk of colonic muscle or nerve damage or colorectal cancer with the use of these laxatives.[30,31]

Acute adverse effects are concerning in patients who take large doses of laxatives for purging, colon-cleansing, or detoxification effects. Colon-cleansing preparations are available in many pharmacies and are promoted for a wide range of potential benefits, including removing toxins, losing weight, or preventing disease. These products often contain a combination of stimulant laxatives, probiotics, herbals, or other ingredients. No literature supports a medical benefit of colon cleansing for "detoxification." In fact, acute overuse of laxatives or colon-cleansing regimens can cause serious dehydration, electrolyte imbalances, or other adverse effects and should be avoided. Also inform patients that enemas, colonic irrigation, and "colon hydrotherapy" carry additional risks (e.g., bowel perforation or infection) and are not recommended.[28] If laxative overuse for purging related to anorexia or bulimia is suspected, medical referral for appropriate care is needed.

Educate patients whose misperceptions about the need for a daily bowel movement contribute to unnecessary laxative use. Older adults may be especially susceptible to this pattern of behavior. Discuss laxative use with patients if concerns arise about unnecessary use or overuse. Explain that normal bowel patterns vary and that daily bowel movements are not a physical necessity. Encourage lifestyle changes that can promote regularity, such as increased fluid intake, fiber intake, and physical activity.[30]

Note that chronic laxative use may be appropriate in some patients (e.g., patients who require chronic opioid therapy or who have certain medical conditions). A thorough medical history can help determine if laxative use and choice are appropriate for individual patients and if medical referral for further evaluation is necessary.

Pharmacotherapeutic Comparison

Head-to-head comparison studies of solely nonprescription laxatives are largely unavailable because most nonprescription laxative ingredients became available prior to the current emphasis on comparative evidence. With many products, much of what is practiced has been learned through observation and a common-sense approach. For example, a bulk-forming product should soften the stool by its normal action. Because both a stool softener and a bulk-forming agent take about the same length of time to work, a bulk-forming agent may be the correct choice for some patients who require stool softening. Although stimulants and saline-type laxatives have been used widely for self-care, health care providers should recommend a product with the lowest likelihood of untoward effects.

PEG 3350 was approved as a nonprescription product relatively recently and therefore has been the subject of more clinical trials. In a 2012 Cochrane review of osmotic and stimulant laxatives, PEG 3350 was found to be likely superior to placebo, lactulose, and milk of magnesia, although the overall quality of evidence was poor.[32] PEG 3350 has also been compared with psyllium (ispaghula husk) and has been demonstrated to be superior in terms of efficacy, with similar rates of adverse effects.[33] Of the available nonprescription agents, many professional groups and practitioners consider PEG 3350 to have the strongest support for efficacy and safety; this conclusion is based on the relatively large body of clinical evidence supporting its effectiveness.[34]

Product Selection Guidelines

When considering the use of any laxative to treat simple constipation, the provider should remember that normal defecation empties only the rectum and the descending and sigmoid branches of the colon. A bulk-forming laxative most closely duplicates this normal physiologic process and is often recommended as the initial treatment choice for patients needing self-care for acute constipation. However, bulk-forming laxatives may take up to 72 hours or longer for effectiveness. If faster onset is desired, or if a bulk-forming agent is ineffective or inappropriate, the hyperosmotic PEG 3350 is also considered a first-line agent, given its effectiveness and favorable adverse effect profile. If PEG 3350 is unable to produce a satisfactory response, a stimulant (e.g., bisacodyl) should be considered.[6,8,9] In each case, the lowest effective dose should be used, and the dose should be reduced once symptoms improve. Patients not achieving a therapeutic response after 7 days of self-treatment warrant medical referral.

Special Populations

Children. Constipation in children is generally defined as a delay or difficulty in bowel movements for 2 weeks or longer.[35,36] Constipation affects 16%–37% of children and is the most common cause of abdominal pain in children.[15,37] A number of factors can alter a child's bowel habits, including unavailable toilet facilities; emotional distress; febrile illness; chronic medical conditions (e.g., cystic fibrosis and hypothyroidism); family conflict; dietary changes (e.g., switching from human to cow milk); fear of defecation; or a change in daily routine or environment.[35]

Although parents often focus on regular bowel movements as a sign of good health in their child, constipation associated with underlying disease is uncommon in children.[15,35] Bowel movement patterns vary widely among children and at different ages; therefore, constipation can be a complex problem that is

table 15–5 Selected Nonprescription Laxative Products

Trade Name	Primary Ingredients
Bulk-Forming Laxatives	
Citrucel Powder	Methylcellulose 2 g/heaping tablespoon
Citrucel Sugar Free Powder	Methylcellulose 2 g/heaping tablespoon
FiberCon Caplets	Calcium polycarbophil 625 mg/caplet
Metamucil Smooth Texture, Sugar Free Orange Flavor Powder/Individual Packets	Psyllium fiber 3 g/packet
Emollient Laxatives	
Colace Capsules	Docusate sodium 100 mg/capsule
Lubricant Laxatives	
Fleet Mineral Oil Enema	Mineral oil 100%
Kondremul Emulsion	Mineral oil 55%
Saline Laxatives	
Magnesium Citrate Oral Solution	Magnesium citrate 1.745 g/30 mL
Fleet Enema	Monobasic sodium phosphate 19 g/118 mL; dibasic sodium phosphate 7 g/118 mL
Pedia-Lax Enema	Monobasic sodium phosphate 9.5 g/59 mL; dibasic sodium phosphate 3.5 g/59 mL
Phillips' Milk of Magnesia Suspension	Magnesium hydroxide 400 mg/5 mL
Hyperosmotic Laxatives	
Fleet Glycerin Suppository (adult size)	Glycerin 2 g/suppository
MiraLAX	Polyethylene glycol 3350 17 g/capful
Stimulant Laxatives	
Dulcolax Tablets	Bisacodyl 5 mg/tablet
Senokot Tablets	Sennosides 8.6 mg/tablet
Fletcher's Laxative for Kids	Senna concentrate 33.3 mg/mL
Combination Laxatives	
Senokot-S Tablets	Sennosides 8.6 mg/tablet; docusate sodium 50 mg/tablet

often difficult to detect and manage. Children typically describe constipation as difficulty in passing stools; parents or caregivers are usually concerned that a child's stool is too large, too hard, too infrequent, or painful.[35] If a child experiences pain from straining to pass large or hard stools, the child may then avoid or withhold bowel movements, resulting in worsening symptoms and a fear of toileting.

Before a laxative product is recommended, the possible causes for constipation should be assessed thoroughly, with consideration of the child's age and any previous laxative use. The route of administration and the taste of oral products are especially significant in children. Laxative use can often be avoided in older children by encouraging them to adhere to suggested dietary guidelines to improve stool regularity.

Evaluation of constipation in children should begin with determination of exclusions for nonprescription therapy (Figure 15–2). Constipation in children often presents with fecal impaction.[15] Children with suspected symptoms of impaction (abdominal cramping; rectal bleeding; small, semi-formed stools; fecal soiling; and/or constipation symptoms alternating with or accompanied by watery diarrhea) should be referred for further evaluation and/or disimpaction.[15,35]

Mild constipation in children can often be relieved with dietary or behavioral modifications, such as increasing intake of fluids and fruit juices containing sorbitol (e.g., prune, apple, or grape), or adding small amounts of barley malt extract or corn syrup to juice or milk.[15,35] Once solid foods are introduced, adding or increasing the amount of high-fiber cereals or grains, vegetables, and fruits to the diet may relieve symptoms of constipation. The recommended dietary fiber intake (in grams) for children older than 2 years should equal or exceed their age plus 5 g/day.[17] Parents should also be encouraged to establish a regular stooling time for toilet-trained children (usually after a morning meal) and to develop a supportive system (e.g., charts or stickers) for positively reinforcing bowel movements. Children should be encouraged to promptly heed the urge to pass a bowel movement to avoid negative consequences of retaining stool in the rectum (e.g., increased hardening, pain, and abdominal distention).[35,36]

If dietary or behavior modifications are insufficient or inappropriate, pharmacologic therapy is indicated (Table 15–4). Nonprescription laxative therapy should be administered to children younger than 2 years only under the direction of a medical provider.

Nonprescription laxatives approved for self-care in children ages 2 to younger than 6 years include oral docusate sodium, magnesium hydroxide, or senna. Rectal use of glycerin, mineral oil, or sodium phosphate products is also approved in this age group. Oral products approved for children ages 6 to younger than 12 years include methylcellulose, calcium polycarbophil, psyllium powder, docusate sodium, mineral oil, magnesium citrate, magnesium hydroxide, magnesium sulfate, senna, bisacodyl, and castor oil (see Pharmacologic Therapy for recommendations about use of individual agents). Oral use of PEG 3350 is FDA approved in patients ages 17 years or older, but its use in children is increasing. Health care providers may be called on to assist parents and caregivers in appropriate use of PEG 3350 in cooperation with prescribers.[15,34–38] Rectal products approved for children ages 6 to younger than 12 years include glycerin suppositories, mineral oil, sodium phosphate, and bisacodyl.

If medication is needed for the occasional relief of temporary constipation in children ages 2 to younger than 6 years, oral docusate sodium or magnesium hydroxide can be recommended first.[15,35] Docusate sodium may be especially helpful if the primary complaint is difficulty passing dry, hard stools. If faster relief is needed, providers can recommend pediatric glycerin suppositories, taking care to ensure that caregivers select the pediatric size suppositories for this age group (1 gram) and understand proper administration technique. Oral senna or magnesium citrate and rectal mineral oil or sodium phosphate enemas should be reserved for use when other treatments fail or should be used under the supervision of a health care provider.[15,35–38]

In children ages 6 to younger than 12 years, bulk-forming agents, docusate sodium, or magnesium hydroxide can be recommended for the occasional relief of temporary constipation, with oral stimulants reserved for when other treatments fail.[15,33–36] If faster relief is needed, glycerin or bisacodyl suppositories can be recommended, with mineral oil or sodium phosphate enemas reserved for when other treatments fail, or at the direction of a health care provider.[15] Magnesium sulfate (Epsom salt) and castor oil are not recommended because safer, better-tolerated, and well-studied laxatives are available.

Patients of Advanced Age. Compared with the general adult population, the prevalence of constipation in older adults is higher, with 15%–20% of community-dwelling older patients and up to 50% of nursing home residents reporting constipation.[5] Older adults report passing fewer stools per week and often describe constipation as straining to move bowels. Although aging itself does not cause constipation, older adults are at greater risk for constipation because of dietary changes (e.g., reduced caloric, fiber, and/or fluid intake); decreased physical activity; presence of comorbid conditions (e.g., parkinsonism, diabetes, or depression); and increased use of medications that can cause constipation (e.g., opioids and anticholinergics).[5,18]

Laxative recommendations should be patient specific. Older individuals can have complicating pathology and multiple medical complaints, and they are vulnerable to medication effects. With older patients, one of the first interventions should be a complete medication review to identify agents that may contribute to constipation and where necessary, discussion of suggestions for appropriate alternatives.[5] As with other age groups, lifestyle modifications are an important initial step, including increased fiber and fluid intake, physical activity as tolerated, and bowel training.[5,19] Notably, recent data support the use of prunes or prune juice as an effective dietary alternative to medications in some patients.[5] Consideration should be given to fluid or other restrictions that may be associated with comorbid conditions (e.g., congestive heart failure or renal failure). Often, constipation is an indication of dehydration in older individuals; therefore, fluid status should be monitored closely. Frail, older patients may also have activity restrictions or limitations secondary to arthritis, cardiovascular, or other chronic conditions.[5]

If medication adjustments and lifestyle changes do not provide adequate relief, laxative therapy is needed. Similar to other populations, treatment of constipation in older adults is often based on experience rather than scientific evidence. Bulk-forming laxatives can be considered a first step. Sugar-free products are recommended for patients with diabetes. Patients who are dehydrated, very frail, bedridden, or unable to drink adequate fluid to prevent mechanical obstruction or fecal impaction should not use bulk-forming laxatives. If these laxatives cannot be used or do not provide sufficient relief, or if faster onset is desired, PEG 3350 is also used as a first-line option because of its efficacy and tolerability.[5,39] Stool softeners (e.g., docusate) may be helpful in older adults with anal fissures or with hemorrhoids that cause painful defecation.[18]

A number of nonprescription laxatives should be avoided or used very cautiously in this population. Mineral oil is not recommended because of the increased risk of aspiration and depletion of fat-soluble vitamins. Saline laxatives such as magnesium hydroxide should be avoided in older individuals, given

the potential for magnesium toxicity in those with reduced renal function and given the potential for drug interactions with medications such as digoxin.[5] Older patients are particularly sensitive to shifts in fluid and electrolytes. Use of any laxative that alters the fluid and electrolyte balance (particularly saline and stimulant laxatives) may be inappropriate in certain patients of advanced age. These laxatives can place older patients at risk for adverse effects (particularly those who are on diuretics or who have decreased fluid intake).[5,18] Although regular use of stimulant laxatives is sometimes recommended, these products have limited evidence in older adults.[40]

Older adults may also require rectal therapy with a suppository or enema, especially if fecal impaction is suspected. Rectal preparations are generally considered to be safe in older adults, although there is limited comparative evidence of safety and effectiveness among individual preparations.[5,40] Sodium phosphate enemas are effective, but they can result in hyperphosphatemia in patients with renal disease.[5] Additionally, older adults may be more susceptible to water and electrolyte imbalances with sodium phosphate enemas.[40]

Chronic laxative use is common among older adults, but it may not always be indicated. Health care providers should counsel older adults about appropriate use of medications with lifestyle and dietary changes. Laxative overuse may predispose patients to dehydration, electrolyte imbalances, and pharmacokinetic drug interactions. Laxatives can also increase GI motility and decrease absorption and effectiveness of concurrent medications.

Pregnancy and Lactation. Constipation is common during pregnancy and after childbirth. It affects up to one-third of women throughout pregnancy and the postpartum period.[41] The increasing size of the growing uterus compresses the colon, affecting the emptying of fecal material. Other contributing factors during pregnancy include increasing progesterone levels, low fluid and fiber intake, and iron and calcium in prenatal vitamin and mineral supplements.[41] Constipation in pregnancy can lead to backaches, hemorrhoids, and fecal impaction.

The main goal of treatment in pregnancy is to achieve soft stools without the use of laxatives. Dietary measures (e.g., increasing fiber and fluid intake or adding prunes or prune juice to the diet) should be attempted as an initial measure.[41] If dietary measures are insufficient, a laxative may be indicated. Bulk-forming laxatives are recommended initially (taken with plenty of fluid to prevent worsening constipation).[41–44] Docusate may also be used for patients who have primarily dry, hard stools, and it is a component of some prenatal vitamins.[44] If needed, short-term use of senna or bisacodyl is considered low-risk in pregnancy.[42–44] Some experts also consider PEG 3350 to be a first-line choice in pregnancy because very little is absorbed systemically.[44] However, short-term use of senna or bisacodyl is preferred by some practitioners because more data are available for use of these agents in pregnancy than for use of PEG 3350.[41,42] In more severe cases, or when the safety of a laxative product is questionable, consultation with a woman's health care provider is recommended prior to laxative use.

Some laxatives should be used very cautiously or avoided altogether in pregnancy. Castor oil is associated with uterine contraction and rupture, and it should be avoided. Mineral oil may impair maternal fat-soluble vitamin absorption and should not be recommended. Saline laxatives (e.g., magnesium hydroxide, etc.) used long-term or at high doses may cause dehydration or electrolyte imbalances and generally should be avoided, given that better options exist.[42–44]

Laxatives may also be necessary postpartum to reestablish normal bowel function. Senna, bisacodyl, PEG 3350, and docusate are considered compatible or low risk with breast-feeding.[43,45,46] Research has shown that, at usual doses, these agents are minimally absorbed or are not present in significant concentrations in breast milk; no data are available to suggest that infants may experience any potential toxicity.[42,45,46] Castor oil and mineral oil should not be used during breast-feeding.[42]

Patient Factors

Laxative products are available in a wide array of oral dosage forms. This variety yields the most benefits for pediatric and geriatric patients. Many of the dosage forms (e.g., thin film strip formulations for children) enhance patient acceptability. However, laxatives available as chewing gum, wafers, effervescent granules, gummy candy, or chocolate tablets may be more likely to be misused or abused. Additionally, the glucose and calorie contents of these dosage forms should be considered for patients with diabetes or calorie restrictions.

Patient factors may also limit the use of some laxatives. For example, patients with fluid restrictions should avoid bulk-forming laxatives that require significant fluid intake. Patients on sodium-restricted diets should examine the sodium content of laxative products (especially saline laxatives). FDA requires manufacturers of laxative products to list sodium content on the product labeling.[47] Patients with severely limited mobility (e.g., postoperative patients or older adults) are at increased risk

for constipation and may require regular use of stool softeners or laxative products to promote laxation.

Enemas and suppositories may be required for some patients with constipation. Enemas are routinely used in preparing patients for surgery, child delivery, and GI radiologic or endoscopic examinations. The enema fluid determines the mechanism by which evacuation is produced. Vegetable oils lubricate, soften, and facilitate the passage of hardened fecal matter, whereas tap water, normal saline, and sodium phosphate enemas create bulk through an osmotic volume effect. Sodium phosphate enemas are more efficient and effective than tap water, soapsuds, saline, or vegetable oil enemas. However, chronic use is not recommended because sodium phosphate enemas can significantly alter fluid and electrolyte balance.

A properly administered enema cleans only the distal colon, most nearly approximating a normal bowel movement. However, improper use or administration may result in adverse effects (e.g., fluid and electrolyte imbalances, mucosal changes or spasm of the intestinal wall, abrasion of the anal canal, or colonic perforation). Advise patients to follow all directions carefully when using these products (Table 15–6).

Suppositories containing bisacodyl are used for postoperative, antepartum, and postpartum care and are adequate in preparing for proctosigmoidoscopy. Although bisacodyl suppositories are prescribed and used more often than other suppositories, some providers still prefer enemas as agents for cleaning the lower bowel. Glycerin suppositories are useful in initiating the defecation reflex in children and in promoting rectal emptying in adults.

---

table 15–6 Administration of Enemas and Rectal Suppositories

Enemas

1. If someone else is administering the enema, lie on your left side with knees bent or in the knee-to-chest position (see drawings A and B). Position A is preferred for children younger than 2 years. If self-administering the enema, lie on your back with your knees bent and buttocks raised (see drawing C). A pillow may be placed under the buttocks.
2. If using a concentrated enema solution, dilute solution according to the product instructions. Prepare 1 pint (500 mL) for adults and ½ pint (250 mL) for children.
3. Lubricate the enema tip with petroleum jelly or other non-medicated ointment/cream. Apply the lubricant to the anal area, as well.
4. Gently insert the enema tip 2 inches (recommended depth for children) to 3 inches into the rectum.
5. Allow the solution to flow into the rectum slowly. If you experience discomfort, the flow is probably too fast.
6. Retain the enema solution until definite lower abdominal cramping is felt. (The parent/caregiver may have to gently hold a child's buttocks closed to prevent the solution from being expelled too soon.)

Suppositories

1. Gently squeeze the suppository to determine if it is firm enough to insert. Chill a soft suppository by placing it in the refrigerator for a few minutes, or by holding it under cool running water.
2. Remove the suppository from its wrapping.
3. Dip the suppository in lukewarm water for a few seconds to soften the exterior.
4. Lie on your left side with knees bent or in the knee-to-chest position (see drawings A and B). Position A is best for self-administration of a suppository. Small children can be held in a crawling position.
5. To ease insertion, relax the buttocks just before inserting the suppository. Gently insert the tapered end of the suppository high into the rectum. If the suppository slips out, it was not inserted past the anal sphincter (the muscle that keeps the rectum closed). In this case, reinsert the suppository correctly.
6. Continue to lie down for a few minutes, and hold the buttocks together to allow the suppository to dissolve in the rectum. (The parent/caregiver may have to gently hold a child's buttocks closed.)
7. Remember that the medication is most effective when the bowel is empty. Try to avoid a bowel movement for up to 1 hour after insertion of the suppository so that the intended action can occur.

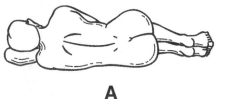

A

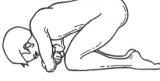

B

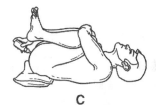

C

Patient Preferences

Palatability and convenience are important considerations with laxative products, especially for patients needing products on a regular basis. Liquid formulations of emollients may be made more palatable if mixed with juices or milk. Mixing gritty, bulk-forming laxative powders (e.g., psyllium) with orange juice instead of water may increase their taste and texture palatability. Patients may also prefer wafer or single-use packets of bulk-forming laxative powders for convenience and ease of use. Patients should be reminded that many fiber products marketed as grit-free, flavor-free, or taste-free may contain ingredients that have not been studied as bulk-forming laxatives and are approved only as dietary supplements (e.g., inulin).

Cost is also an important consideration in patient preference. Most laxative ingredients are available in some form as a generic. However, patients with a specific dosage form or other preference may need to choose a brand-name product. It is important to help patients choose the laxative product with the optimal balance of cost, effectiveness, tolerability, and palatability, depending on their individual needs.

Complementary Therapies

Dietary supplements commonly used to treat constipation include flaxseed, aloe, cascara, and probiotics.[48] Evidence supporting the safety and efficacy of these products varies. A single double-blind trial demonstrated the superiority of flaxseed over psyllium in decreasing constipation, bloating, and abdominal pain over a 3-month period in patients with irritable bowel syndrome. However, a much larger body of evidence supports psyllium's effectiveness, and practitioners should not recommend flaxseed on the basis of limited efficacy and safety data.[48]

Although many commercially available stimulant laxatives are derived from plants, patients should be advised to choose FDA-approved products if a stimulant laxative is indicated. FDA has banned the use of aloe and cascara in nonprescription stimulant laxatives, and both agents are classified as generally unsafe and not effective. Senna is available in dietary supplement form, but use of standardized, FDA-approved senna drug products is preferred.

Probiotics are thought to work in constipation through alteration of GI flora, stimulation of motility and peristalsis, and/or acceleration of gut transit.[5,49] However, from a mechanistic or clinical efficacy standpoint, little available evidence consistently supports these agents. A systematic review conducted by Chmielewska and colleagues[50] identified five randomized controlled trials (n = 377) of probiotic supplementation for constipation management. Study results suggested there may be a potential benefit, but authors questioned the overall efficacy and clinical relevance of specific study outcomes. Probiotics should be considered investigational for constipation until more efficacy and safety evidence are available.[5,49,50]

Assessment of Constipation: A Case-Based Approach

The health care provider should obtain as much lifestyle and medical information as possible before making any recommendations for preventing or treating constipation. Appropriate information allows the provider to make rational recommendations that are based on knowledge of the patient, the problem, and available products, as well as on the provider's own judgment and experience. A patient who presents with constipation should initially be evaluated for any signs of significant GI problems that may warrant medical evaluation or in which laxative use is inappropriate (Figure 15–2). Health care providers should initially ask questions related to diet, fluid intake, physical activity, and any underlying pathology that may produce constipation as a symptom.

Patients should then be questioned regarding the characteristics of bowel movements, including the caliber, color, and texture of stools, as well as the frequency of elimination. Additional assessment should include questions about use of medications (both prescription and nonprescription), natural products, and previous laxative use. For patients without a history of constipation, a thorough investigation should be conducted to determine whether acute cases of constipation have resulted from new or old diseases or from the use of medications. When information is insufficient to assess the cause of the symptoms, or if any doubt exists regarding the patient's disease status, medical referral is appropriate. Cases 15–1 and 15–2 provide sample assessments for patients presenting with constipation.

case

15–1

Relevant Evaluation Criteria	Scenario/Model Outcome
Information Gathering	

1. Gather essential information about the patient's symptoms and medical history, including:

   a. description of symptom(s) (i.e., nature, onset, duration, severity, associated symptoms) — Patient indicates he has not had a bowel movement over the past week because he has been studying for exams, eating fast food, and not exercising or playing sports. It is really bothersome because he has exams looming and wants fast relief.

   b. description of any factors that seem to precipitate, exacerbate, and/or relieve the patient's symptom(s) — Patient does not recall having problems with constipation in the past.

   c. description of the patient's efforts to relieve the symptoms — Patient has been taking docusate sodium capsules daily for the past 3 days.

   d. patient's identity — Jake Richardson

   e. age, sex, height, and weight — 19 years old, male, 6 ft, 190 lbs

case

15–1 *continued*

Relevant Evaluation Criteria	Scenario/Model Outcome
f. patient's occupation	Freshman in college
g. patient's dietary habits	Diet usually consists of no breakfast, sandwiches for lunch, and a meat or pasta dish with vegetables or salad for dinner.
h. patient's sleep habits	Sleeps 4–5 hours a night.
i. concurrent medical conditions, prescription and nonprescription medications, and dietary supplements	Perennial allergies: loratadine 10 mg daily
j. allergies	Pollen and dust mites
k. history of other adverse reactions to medications	None
l. other (describe) _____	He typically has 1 bowel movement every day. Patient is active in intramural sports and exercises regularly.

Assessment and Triage

2. Differentiate patient's signs/symptoms and correctly identify the patient's primary problem(s).	The patient is experiencing constipation most likely precipitated by his change in routine, eating fast food, and not exercising. Constipation during periods of change in routine and stress is common.
3. Identify exclusions for self-treatment (Figure 15–2).	None
4. Formulate a comprehensive list of therapeutic alternatives for the primary problem to determine if triage to a health care provider is required, and share this information with the patient or caregiver.	Options include:

(1) Refer patient to an appropriate health care provider.

(2) Recommend nondrug measures:

    a. Resume a balanced diet with adequate fiber, fruits, and vegetables.

    b. Drink at least 2 liters of fluid daily.

    c. Resume a regular exercise routine, and get more sleep to decrease the effect of stress.

    d. Recommend strategies to prevent future recurrences.

(3) Recommend continuing docusate sodium and adding a bulk-forming laxative to help facilitate resolution of symptoms.

(4) Recommend a hyperosmotic (e.g., an adult glycerin suppository or PEG 3350). The glycerin suppository will offer the fastest resolution, if the patient is willing to use that dosage form.

(5) Recommend a stimulant laxative once daily for resolution of symptoms. A stimulant laxative will also offer fast relief from symptoms.

(6) Recommend self-care until patient can see an appropriate health care provider.

(7) Refer patient to an appropriate health care provider if therapeutic option and lifestyle changes do not alleviate symptoms within a week.

(8) Take no action.

Plan

5. Select an optimal therapeutic alternative to address the patient's problem, taking into account patient preferences.	Patient would like some help resolving his symptoms quickly given that final exams are coming soon. Because he has tried docusate sodium for the past 3 days, and because a bulk-forming laxative has a similar onset of action, it may be helpful to consider an alternative. If the patient is willing, a glycerin suppository could be used for a quick resolution. If the patient prefers an oral medication, PEG 3350 is also an option, but it will take longer to work. To prevent similar recurrences in the future, the patient should be encouraged to increase fiber and fluid intake while studying. If he is unable to modify his diet during study periods, discuss a fiber supplement to eat during this time, (e.g., a fiber-enriched granola bar, psyllium wafer, or fiber packet added to beverage).
6. Describe the recommended therapeutic approach to the patient or caregiver.	"You should resume a proper diet that includes more fiber, fruits, and vegetables, and increase your fluid intake. You should restart your regular exercise routine. A stronger laxative medication can be tried for quick relief of symptoms, including a glycerin suppository or oral polyethylene glycol 3350, also called PEG 3350."

case

15–1 *continued*

Relevant Evaluation Criteria	Scenario/Model Outcome
7. Explain to the patient or caregiver the rationale for selecting the recommended therapeutic approach from the considered therapeutic alternatives.	"Because you have been experiencing constipation for 1 week and have been taking docusate sodium for 3 days, perhaps you should try another agent with a quicker onset of action. If you are willing to use a suppository, a glycerin suppository will provide quick relief. If you prefer taking a medication by mouth, PEG 3350 will take longer to work than the suppository, but it usually works very well to relieve constipation. If the glycerin suppository or oral PEG 3350, along with changes in your diet and exercise routine, do not successfully relieve your constipation, or if your symptoms get worse, you should make an appointment with your primary care provider to discuss other treatment options and ways to prevent constipation."

Patient Education

8. When recommending self-care with nonprescription medications and/or nondrug therapy, convey accurate information to the patient or caregiver.	
a. appropriate dose and frequency of administration	See the box Patient Education for Constipation.
b. maximum number of days the therapy should be employed	See the box Patient Education for Constipation.
c. product administration procedures	See Table 15–6 for patient education for administering a suppository. "If you opt for PEG 3350, measure a 17 gram dose of PEG 3350 powder (1 capful or packet of the OTC product), stir and dissolve powder in 4–8 ounces of any beverage, and then drink."
d. expected time to onset of relief	"The glycerin suppository will work in about 15–30 minutes. PEG 3350 usually produces a bowel movement in 12–72 hours, but the onset of action may take as long as 96 hours in some patients."
e. degree of relief that can be reasonably expected	"Your constipation symptoms should be relieved with the use of either of these drugs."
f. most common side effects	"You may experience cramping or stomach pain, diarrhea or loose stools, or rectal irritation from the glycerin suppository."
g. side effects that warrant medical intervention should they occur	"Contact your primary care provider if you experience rectal bleeding; nausea, bloating, cramping, or abdominal pain persist or worsen; a bowel movement does not occur; diarrhea occurs; or symptoms are not relieved within a week."
h. patient options in the event that the condition worsens or persists	"Contact your primary care provider."
i. product storage requirements	"Store glycerin suppositories in the tightly closed container in a cool, dry location. Protect from heat."
j. specific nondrug measures	See the box Patient Education for Constipation.
Solicit follow-up questions from the patient or caregiver.	"I'd prefer not to use the suppository; I will try the PEG 3350 instead. Is there any difference between the brand-name and generic PEG 3350 products? What type of beverage can be used to dissolve the powder?"
Answer the patient's or caregiver's questions.	"There's no difference in the brand-name versus the generic product except for the cost. Whichever product you prefer is fine, and the generic will save a little bit of money. It doesn't matter what beverage you dissolve the powder in, and the beverage can be hot, cold, or at room temperature."

Evaluation of Patient Outcome

9. Assess patient outcome.	Ask the patient to call to update you on his response to your recommendations; alternatively, you could call him in a few days to evaluate his response.

Key: OTC = Over-the-counter; PEG = polyethylene glycol.

case
15–2

Relevant Evaluation Criteria	**Scenario/Model Outcome**

Information Gathering

1. Gather essential information about the patient's symptoms and medical history, including:

   a. description of symptom(s) (i.e., nature, onset, duration, severity, associated symptoms)

   Patient says that she is having a very difficult time passing her stools. She admits to straining to pass "normal looking" but hard stools, and she is experiencing severe abdominal pain. She has only about one bowel movement per week. She has been experiencing these symptoms over the past 3 months.

   b. description of any factors that seem to precipitate, exacerbate, and/or relieve the patient's symptom(s)

   Patient notes that her problems really started when her primary care provider added an additional medication to help control her chronic back pain.

   c. description of the patient's efforts to relieve the symptoms

   The patient has occasionally used a stool softener.

   d. patient's identity

   Ann Holcomb

   e. age, sex, height, and weight

   45 years old, female, 5 ft 5 in., 150 lb

   f. patient's occupation

   Teacher

   g. patient's dietary habits

   Usual diet consists of some vegetables, occasional fruit, pastas, occasional whole-grain breads, meat and fish, caffeinated coffee, diet sodas, and desserts.

   h. patient's sleep habits

   Sleeps about 4 hours per night.

   i. concurrent medical conditions, prescription and nonprescription medications, and dietary supplements

   Chronic back pain: Celebrex 200 mg daily, Lortab every 4–6 hours as needed for pain; Osteoporosis prevention: calcium 600 mg plus vitamin D 600 IU twice daily

   j. allergies

   Penicillin

   k. history of other adverse reactions to medications

   None

   l. other (describe) _____

   She typically has 3–4 bowel movements every week. She takes about 3–4 Lortab tablets per day.

Assessment and Triage

2. Differentiate patient's signs/symptoms and correctly identify the patient's primary problem(s).

   The patient recently started an opioid medication, Lortab, which can cause constipation. The patient's constipation appears to be correlated with the start of this medication. The patient takes calcium plus vitamin D, which can also contribute to constipation.

3. Identify exclusions for self-treatment (Figure 15–2).

   Presence of marked abdominal pain, unexplained changes in bowel habits, bowel symptoms that persist for more than 2 weeks.

4. Formulate a comprehensive list of therapeutic alternatives for the primary problem to determine if triage to a health care provider is required, and share this information with the patient or caregiver.

   Options include:

   (1) Refer patient to an appropriate health care provider.

   (2) Recommend self-care with a nonprescription laxative and nondrug measures.

   (3) Recommend self-care until patient can see an appropriate health care provider.

   (4) Refer patient to an appropriate health care provider if therapeutic option and lifestyle changes do not alleviate symptoms within a week.

   (5) Take no action.

Plan

5. Select an optimal therapeutic alternative to address the patient's problem, taking into account patient preferences.

   Patient has experienced constipation secondary to the initiation of an opioid medication. She has been experiencing these symptoms for 3 months with abdominal pain. She should consult a health care provider. However, she should also implement nondrug measures to help prevent constipation and promote a healthy lifestyle.

case
15-2 *continued*

Relevant Evaluation Criteria	Scenario/Model Outcome
6. Describe the recommended therapeutic approach to the patient or caregiver.	"You should consult a health care provider. You should also modify your diet to include more fiber, fruits, and vegetables. You should add a fiber supplement to your diet, and you should increase your fluid intake. Also, you should establish a regular exercise routine."
7. Explain to the patient or caregiver the rationale for selecting the recommended therapeutic approach from the considered therapeutic alternatives.	"This option is best because your constipation began after you started your new pain medication, and it has been occurring for 3 months. Additionally, you have been experiencing marked abdominal pain. Under these conditions, nonprescription laxative therapy may not be the best choice right now. You should be evaluated by your health care provider."

Patient Education	
8. When recommending self-care with nonprescription medications and/or nondrug therapy, convey accurate information to the patient or caregiver.	"Even though you need to see your health care provider, you can still implement nondrug measures that promote a healthy lifestyle, such as eating more fiber, fruits, and vegetables, and beginning a regular exercise routine. You should consult your health care provider about these measures as well."
Solicit follow-up questions from the patient or caregiver.	"Can you suggest some high-fiber foods that I could add to my diet?"
Answer the patient's or caregiver's questions.	"I would start by adding more fruits and vegetables to your diet, as well as eating a high-fiber cereal like Bran Buds, All Bran, or Kashi GoLean for breakfast each morning. Be sure to increase your dietary fiber gradually to avoid side effects such as gas, bloating, or diarrhea during the first few weeks following these dietary changes."

Evaluation of Patient Outcome	
9. Assess patient outcome.	Contact the patient in a day or two to ensure that she made an appointment and sought medical care.

Patient Counseling for Constipation

Patient education about laxative products is important for all patients (particularly for children, their caregivers, and older adults). Before recommending a laxative product, the health care provider should first inform the patient of the nondrug measures available for treating constipation. Pregnant women and children, especially, should be counseled on proper diet, adequate fluid intake, and reasonable exercise. If a laxative is needed, explain why a particular type of laxative is appropriate for the present situation, how to use the laxative, when to expect to see results, what adverse effects could occur, and what precautions to take. The box Patient Education for Constipation lists specific information to provide patients.

Evaluation of Patient Outcomes for Constipation

Constipation often presents with a great degree of variability among individuals. Although a decrease in frequency of bowel movements is typically associated with constipation, difficulty passing stools and a decrease in the amount passed are also common complaints. The type, severity, and chronicity of symptoms are important determinants in selecting the most appropriate treatment modality. Once therapy has been selected, effectiveness is determined by how rapidly constipation is relieved and to what

degree normal bowel habits have been restored. For acute constipation, dietary changes, exercise, or the use of bulk-forming laxatives may take several days to weeks to provide relief. Most hyperosmotic, saline, or stimulant laxatives will provide relief within 3–72 hours. Enemas can produce evacuation within minutes. If initial treatment of constipation is ineffective, therapy should be repeated according to product-specific directions.

If an adequate response is not achieved after a short period of laxative use (usually within 7 days) follow-up should assess whether the patient needs medical referral. If a laxative must be continued for an extended period of time, the patient should be referred for further evaluation, as frequent use may be a sign of (1) a more severe form of constipation, (2) a medication side effect, or (3) an underlying medical problem. Adhering to a high fiber diet and drinking plenty of fluids can aid in preventing constipation and should be continued even during periods when bowel habits are normal.

Key Points for Constipation

➤ Nonprescription laxative treatment should not be recommended if exclusion criteria for self-treatment are met (Figure 15–2). Patients meeting these criteria should receive medical referral.

➤ Special circumstances and patient characteristics (e.g., pregnancy or age) should be considered when assessing the need for self-medication.

Constipation

The goals of self-treatment are to relieve constipation and restore "normal" bowel functions through (1) dietary and lifestyle measures and/or (2) the safe use of laxative products. For most patients, carefully following the product instructions and the self-care measures listed here will help achieve this.

Nondrug Measures

- To promote regular bowel movements, use nondrug strategies such as a high-fiber diet (slowly increase intake to 25–35 grams per day), plenty of fluid intake, and regular exercise.
- Increase dietary fiber by eating foods with whole grains, oats, fruits, and vegetables.
- Avoid constipating foods, such as processed cheeses and concentrated sweets.
- Drink plenty of fluids (six to eight 8-ounce glasses a day) to help soften your stool and move food through your gastrointestinal tract.
- Develop and maintain a routine exercise program. Walking can be helpful if your heart is healthy and if you have no other apparent health risks.
- Establish a regular pattern for bathroom visits. Do not delay in responding to the urge to use the bathroom; allow adequate time for elimination in a relaxed, unhurried atmosphere.
- Maintain general emotional well-being and avoid stressful situations.

Nonprescription Medications

- Bulk-forming laxatives (e.g., methylcellulose, psyllium)
- Hyperosmotic laxatives (e.g., polyethylene glycol [PEG] 3350, glycerin)
- Emollient laxatives, or "stool softeners" (e.g., docusate sodium)
- Lubricant laxative (mineral oil)
- Saline laxatives (e.g., magnesium citrate, magnesium hydroxide)
- Stimulant laxatives (e.g., bisacodyl, senna)

Complementary Therapies

- Not routinely recommended for self-treatment of constipation.

Disease Information

- Constipation is usually defined as having fewer than 3 bowel movements per week that involve straining and the difficult passage of dry, hard stools. In most cases, constipation is temporary. Self-treatment of constipation is safe for short-term symptoms in patients without other underlying disorders or conditions.
- You do not need to take laxatives routinely because your bowel habits are interrupted for 1 or 2 days, nor do you need to routinely "clean your system."

Drug Information
Bulk-Forming Laxatives

- Unless a rapid effect is needed (e.g., to clean out the bowel for a diagnostic procedure or x-ray), take a bulk-forming laxative. Be sure to drink at least 8 ounces of fluid with each dose to prevent an intestinal blockage. If you have swallowing difficulties, alert your health care provider before taking a bulk-forming laxative.
- If you have diabetes or are on a carbohydrate- or calorie-restricted diet, choose sugar-free bulk-forming agents, if possible. Many bulk-forming agents contain sugar and have a high caloric content per dose.
- Do not give sugar-free bulk-forming products to patients with phenylketonuria.

Hyperosmotic Laxatives

- If you have irritable bowel syndrome, do not take PEG 3350 without the supervision of your primary care provider.

- When using PEG 3350, use the provided cap to measure the dose, or use 1 packet of powder. Mix the powder with 4–8 ounces of a hot, cold, or room temperature beverage (e.g., water, juice, soda, coffee, or tea).
- Consult a primary care provider before using glycerin suppositories if you have previously had a condition that caused rectal irritation.

Emollient Laxatives

- Do not take docusate if you are taking mineral oil unless told to do so by a primary care provider. Taking these together can increase the amount of mineral oil that gets into your body.

Lubricant Laxative

- Although some patients use mineral oil for occasional bouts of constipation, its use in self-care is strongly discouraged because safer agents that work just as well are available.
- Do not give mineral oil to children younger than 6 years, pregnant women, older adults, or bedridden patients without the supervision of a primary care provider. These patients are at a higher risk for adverse effects from mineral oil.
- Do not take mineral oil with emollient laxatives (e.g., docusate). Taking these together can increase the amount of mineral oil that gets into your body.
- To avoid delaying the absorption of foods, nutrients, and vitamins, do not take mineral oil within 2 hours of eating.
- Stop use and consult your health care provider if anal leakage of oil occurs. This may indicate your dose is too high.

Saline Laxatives

- Take doses with an 8-ounce glass of water, if possible, to prevent dehydration.
- Consult your health care provider before using a saline laxative if you are taking a diuretic ("water pill") for high blood pressure (e.g., hydrochlorothiazide or furosemide); if you are taking other drugs that can cause electrolyte changes; or if you are on a sodium-, phosphate-, or magnesium-restricted diet.
- If you are an older adult, you may be at increased risk for dehydration or electrolyte imbalances with saline laxatives. Consult a health care provider before using these agents.
- Do not use magnesium sulfate (Epsom salt) to treat constipation except under the advice of a primary care provider.

Stimulant Laxatives

- Do not use castor oil to treat constipation except under the advice of a health care provider.
- Do not chew or crush bisacodyl tablets, which may cause stomach discomfort, faintness, and cramps. Do not use bisacodyl within 1 hour after taking an antacid or milk. Doing so can cause the tablet's coating to break down too quickly.

Administration of Medication/Safe Usage

- Read and carefully follow labeled dosage and administration instructions for all laxative products.
- Oral laxatives are available as tablets, capsules, thin-film strips, chewing gum, wafers, effervescent granules, gummy candy, chocolate tablets, and other forms. Choose the best form for you, and consider glucose and caloric content if you have diabetes or calorie restrictions.

- Rectal laxatives (enemas, suppositories) should be used according to administration instructions (Table 15–6).
- If constipation symptoms continue after 7 days of laxative treatment, contact your health care provider.
- Do not give laxatives to children younger than 2 years unless the use is recommended by a primary care provider.
- Take most laxatives at bedtime, especially if more than 6–8 hours will be needed to produce results.
- Do not take any laxatives at doses higher than the recommended amounts.

Warning Signs/Symptoms

- Do not take laxatives if you have marked abdominal pain, nausea, vomiting, significant abdominal distention, cramping, or fever. These may be symptoms of a more serious condition (e.g., appendicitis).
- Do not take laxatives if you have a sudden change in bowel habits that persists more than 2 weeks because that can be a sign of a more serious condition. See your primary care provider for treatment recommendations.
- If rectal bleeding, blood in your stool, or black, tarry stools occur, see your health care provider. These may be symptoms of an underlying medical condition.
- If you have kidney or liver disease, heart failure, hypertension, or other conditions requiring sodium, potassium, magnesium, or calcium restriction, do not use laxative products with a maximum daily dose of more than 345 mg (15 mEq) sodium, 975 mg

(25 mEq) potassium, 600 mg (50 mEq) magnesium, or 1800 mg (90 mEq) calcium.

- Consult your health care provider before using laxatives if you currently have or have a history of any condition that may affect self-treatment of constipation (e.g., paraplegia or quadriplegia, inflammatory bowel disease, colostomy, megacolon, or ileostomy).
- Some laxatives require you to drink a lot of water with each dose. Patients with fluid restrictions should avoid bulk-forming or other laxatives that require fluid intake.

Adverse Effects

- The most common adverse effects of laxatives are abdominal cramping, gas, bloating, or diarrhea.

Interactions

- Avoid taking laxatives within 2 hours of other medications.
- To make sure you avoid any potential drug–drug interactions, alert your health care provider if you are taking anticoagulants (blood thinners), digoxin (a heart medicine), sodium polystyrene sulfonate (a treatment for high potassium levels), or other drugs that need to be maintained at precise levels.

Storage of Medications/Expiration Date/ Signs of Instability

- Discard any medications that are outdated, that appear to have been tampered with, or that have an unusual appearance.

- For most cases of simple constipation, a balanced diet, exercise, and adequate fluid intake are helpful.
- Bulk-forming laxatives and PEG 3350 as directed are first-line laxative choices in most adults, but they may take up to 72 hours to work. Glycerin suppositories or stimulant laxatives provide faster relief, if needed.
- Therapy with any laxative product should be limited to 7 days, unless supervised by a health care provider.
- If rectal bleeding occurs at any time during use of a laxative, or if constipation persists in spite of therapy, patients should stop using the laxative and consult their health care provider.[15]
- To reduce the potential for drug interactions, patients should avoid taking most laxatives within 2 hours of other medications.

REFERENCES

1. Leung L, Riutta T, Kotecha J, Rosser M. Chronic constipation: an evidence-based review. *J Am Fam Board Med.* 2011;24(4):436–51.
2. World Gastroenterology Organisation. Practice guideline – constipation – updated with Cascades; 2010. Accessed at http://www.worldgastroenterology.org/constipation.html, May 10, 2013.
3. Bleser S, Brunton S, Carmichael B, et al. Management of chronic constipation: recommendations from a consensus panel. *J Fam Pract.* 2005;54(8):691–8.
4. American Gastroenterological Association. Technical review on constipation. *Gastroenterology.* 2013;144(1):219–38.
5. Gallegos-Orozco JF, Foxx-Orenstein AE, Sterler SM, et al. Chronic constipation in the elderly. *Am J Gastroenterol* 2012;107(1):18–25.
6. American Gastroenterological Association. Medical position statement on constipation. *Gastroenterology.* 2013;144(1):211–7.
7. Mugie SM, Benninga MA, Di Lorenzo C. Epidemiology of constipation in children and adults: a systematic review. *Best Practice & Research Clinical Gastroenterology.* 2011;25(1):3–18.
8. Berardi R, Chan J. *OTC Advisor: Self-Care for Gastrointestinal Disorders, Module 2.* Washington, DC: American Pharmacists Association; 2010. Accessed at http://www.pharmacist.com, May 10, 2013.
9. National Digestive Diseases Information Clearinghouse (NDDIC). Constipation. 2007. Accessed at http://digestive.niddk.nih.gov/ddiseases/pubs/constipation, May 10, 2013.
10. Camilleri M, Murray JA. Diarrhea and constipation. In: Longo DL, Fauci AS, Kasper DL, et al., eds. *Harrison's Principles of Internal Medicine.* 18th ed. New York, NY: McGraw-Hill Professional; 2012:245.
11. Fabel PH, Shealy KM. Diarrhea, constipation, and irritable bowel syndrome. In: DiPiro JT, Talbert RL, Yee GC, et al., eds. *Pharmacotherapy: A Pathophysiologic Approach.* 9th ed. New York, NY: McGraw-Hill Professional; 2014.
12. Wald A. Chronic constipation: advances in management. *Neurogastroenterol Motil.* 2007;19(1):4–10.
13. Jamshed N, Lee ZE, Olden KW. Diagnostic approach to chronic constipation in adults. *Am Fam Physician.* 2011;84(3):299–306.
14. Johanson JF. Review of the treatment options for chronic constipation. *MedGenMed.* 2007;9(2):25.
15. Felt B, Brown P, Coran A, et al. Functional constipation and soiling in children. University of Michigan Health System Guidelines for Clinical Care; 2008. Accessed at http://www.med.umich.edu/1info/fhp/practiceguides/newconstipation.html, May 10, 2013.
16. U.S. Department of Health and Human Services, U.S. Department of Agriculture. Dietary Guidelines for Americans; 2010. Accessed at http://www.health.gov/dietaryguidelines/dga2010/DietaryGuidelines2010.pdf, May 13, 2013.
17. Slavin JL. Position of the American Dietetic Association: health implications of dietary fiber. *J Am Diet Assoc.* 2008;108(10):1716–31.
18. Hsieh C. Treatment of constipation in older adults. *Am Fam Physician.* 2005;72(11):2277–84.

19. Ford AC, Talley NJ. Laxatives for chronic constipation in adults. *BMJ.* 2012;345:e6168.

20. U.S. Food and Drug Administration. Laxative drug products for over-the-counter human use; psyllium ingredients in granular dosage forms. *Federal Register.* 2007;72:14669–74.

21. Hoffman D. Psyllium: keeping this boon for patients from becoming a bane for providers. *J Fam Pract.* 2006;55(9):770–2.

22. Seinela L, Sairanen U, Laine T, et al. Comparison of polyethylene glycol with and without electrolytes in the treatment of constipation in elderly institutionalized patients. *Drugs Aging.* 2009;26(8):703–13.

23. Ramkumar D, Rao SSC. Efficacy and safety of traditional medical therapies for chronic constipation: systematic review. *Am J Gastroenterol.* 2005;100(4):936–71.

24. Swegle JM, Logemann C. Management of common opioid-induced adverse effects. *Am Fam Phys.* 2006;74(8):1347–54.

25. U.S. Food and Drug Administration. Oral Sodium Phosphate (OSP) Products for Bowel Cleansing (marketed as Visicol and OsmoPrep, and oral sodium phosphate products available without a prescription); 2014. Accessed at http://www.fda.gov/Drugs/DrugSafety/PostmarketDrug SafetyInformationforPatientsandProviders/ucm103354.htm, July 17, 2014.

26. U.S. Food and Drug Administration. Status of certain additional over-the-counter drug category II and III active ingredients. *Federal Register.* 2002;67:31125–7.

27. U.S. Food and Drug Administration. Laxative drug products for over-the-counter human use. *Federal Register.* 1999;64:4535–40.

28. Acosta RD, Case BD. Clinical effects of colonic cleansing for general health promotion: a systematic review. *Am J Gastroenterol.* 2009;104(11):2830–6.

29. Tozzi F, Thornton LM, Mitchell J, et al. Features associated with laxative abuse in individuals with eating disorders. *Psychosom Med.* 2006;68(3):470–7.

30. Muller-Lissner SA, Kamm MA, Scarpignato C, et al. Myths and misconceptions about chronic constipation. *Am J Gastroenterol.* 2005;100(1):232–42.

31. Kamm MA, Mueller-Lissner S, Wald A, et al. Oral bisacodyl is effective and well-tolerated in patients with chronic constipation. *Clin Gastroenterol Hepatol.* 2011;9(7):577–83.

32. Gordon M, Naidoo K, Akobeng AK, et al. Osmotic and stimulant laxatives for the management of childhood constipation. *Cochrane Database Syst Rev.* 2012;7:CD009118. doi: 10.1002/14651858.CD009118.pub2. Accessed at http://www.thecochranelibrary.com/view/0/index.html.

33. Zurad EG, Johanson JF. Over-the-counter laxative polyethylene glycol 3350: an evidence-based appraisal. *Curr Med Res Opin.* 2011;27(7):1439–52.

34. Horn JR, Mantione MM, Johanson JF. OTC polyethylene glycol 3350 and pharmacists' role in managing constipation. *J Am Pharm Assoc.* 2012;52(3):372–80.

35. Constipation Guideline Committee of the North American Society for Pediatric Gastroenterology, Hepatology and Nutrition. Clinical Practice Guidelines: evaluation and treatment of constipation in infants and children. *J Pediatr Gastroenterol Nutr.* 2006;43(3):e1–13.

36. Auth MK, Vora R, Farrelly P, et al. Childhood constipation. *BMJ.* 2012;345:e7309.

37. Alper A, Pashankar DS. Polyethylene glycol: a game-changer laxative for children. *J Pediatr Gastroenterol Nutr.* 2013;57(2):134–40.

38. Pijpers MA, Tabbers MM, Benninga MA, et al. Currently recommended treatments of childhood constipation are not evidence based: a systematic literature review on the effect of laxative treatment and dietary measures. *Arch Dis Child.* 2009;94(2):117–31.

39. Cash BD, Chang L, Sabesin S, et al. Update on the management of adults with chronic idiopathic constipation. *J Fam Pract.* 2007;56(6): S13–20.

40. Fleming V, Wade WE. A review of laxative therapies for treatment of chronic constipation in older adults. *Am J Geriatr Pharmacother.* 2010; 8(6):514–50.

41. Vazquez JC. Constipation, haemorrhoids, and heartburn in pregnancy. *Clin Evid.* February 20, 2008;pii:1411. Accessed at http://www.ncbi. nlm.nih.gov/pmc/articles/PMC2907947/pdf/2008-1411.pdf, May 10, 2013.

42. Mahadevan U, Kane S. Technical review on the use of gastrointestinal medications in pregnancy. *Gastroenterology.* 2006;131(1):283–311.

43. Mahadevan U, Kane S. Medical position statement on the use of gastrointestinal medications in pregnancy. *Gastroenterology.* 2006;131(1):278–82.

44. Trottier M, Erebara A, Bozza P. Treating constipation during pregnancy. *Can Fam Physician.* 2012;58(8):836–8.

45. Drug and Lactation Database. National Library of Medicine. Accessed at http://toxnet.nlm.nih.gov/cgi-bin/sis/htmlgen?LACT, May 10, 2013.

46. American Academy of Pediatrics Committee on Drugs. Transfer of drugs and other chemicals into human milk. *Pediatrics.* 2001(3);108:776–89.

47. U.S. Food and Drug Administration. Drug labeling: sodium labeling for over-the-counter drugs. Final rule. *Federal Register.* 2001;76:7743–57.

48. Natural Standard: the Authority on Integrative Medicine [database online]. Cambridge, MA: Natural Standard; 2012. Accessed at http:// www.naturalstandard.com, May 10, 2013.

49. Quigley EMM. Probiotics in the management of functional bowel disorders: promise fulfilled? *Gastroenterol Clin N Am.* 2012;41:805–19.

50. Chmielewska A, Szajewska H. Systematic review of randomized controlled trials: probiotics for functional constipation. *World J Gastroenterol.* 2010;16:69–75.

chapter 16

DIARRHEA

Paul C. Walker

Diarrhea is a symptom characterized by an abnormal increase in stool frequency, liquidity, or weight. Although the normal frequency of bowel movements varies with each individual, having more than 3 bowel movements per day is considered abnormal.

Diarrhea may be acute, persistent, or chronic. Acute diarrhea, defined as symptoms lasting less than 14 days, can generally be managed with fluid and electrolyte replacement, dietary interventions, and nonprescription drug treatment. In persistent diarrhea, symptoms last 14 days to 4 weeks. Chronic diarrhea, by definition, lasts more than 4 weeks. Chronic and persistent diarrheal illnesses are often secondary to other chronic medical conditions or treatments and need medical care; therefore, these illnesses are outside the scope of this chapter.

Diarrhea is a common cause of morbidity. Worldwide, approximately 2.5 billion episodes of acute diarrhea occur each year, causing significant morbidity and mortality among all age groups, especially children under 5 years of age, in whom it causes 1.9 million deaths annually.[1] Approximately 179 million cases of acute gastroenteritis (irritation of the gastrointestinal tract commonly caused by viruses or bacteria) occur in the Unites States each year.[2] The overall prevalence of acute diarrhea is estimated to be 5.1%; the incidence rate is 0.6 episodes per person per year.[3] The prevalence of diarrheal disease is highest in children younger than 5 years and lowest in older adults (ages 65 years and older); prevalence rates are estimated to be 7%–10% for children younger than 5 and 2%–3% for older adults.[3] Most patients experience illness without seeking medical attention; however, in the United States more than 500,000 patients are hospitalized each year and approximately 5000 deaths result from acute gastroenteritis and its complications.[2]

Pathophysiology of Diarrhea

Table 16–1 highlights some of the common viral, bacterial, and protozoal diarrheas and their treatment. Epidemiologic factors that increase the risk for particular infectious diarrheal diseases or their spread include attendance or employment at day care centers, occupation as a food handler or caregiver, congregate living conditions (e.g., nursing homes, prisons, and multifamily dwellings), consumption of unsafe foods (e.g., raw or undercooked meat, eggs, and shellfish), and presence of medical conditions, such as acquired immunodeficiency syndrome (AIDS) or diverticulitis. Acute diarrhea may also be caused by poisoning, medications, intolerance of certain foods, or various non-gastrointestinal (GI) acute or chronic illnesses.

Viral Gastroenteritis

Noroviruses are the most common cause of diarrhea in adults and the second most common cause in children. They cause more than 90% of epidemic viral gastroenteritis and approximately 50% of all-cause epidemic gastroenteritis worldwide.[4] In addition, noroviruses play a major role in sporadic acute gastroenteritis, accounting for up to 36% of cases.[5] The symptoms, clinical course and treatment are described in Table 16–1. Although the virus is most often transmitted by contaminated water or food, it can also be transmitted from person to person and through contact with contaminated environmental surfaces. Outbreaks of norovirus gastroenteritis frequently occur in certain populations, such as restaurant patrons, cruise ship passengers, students on college campuses, residents of long-term care facilities and hospitals, military personnel, and immunocompromised patients.

Rotavirus is the most common cause of severe gastroenteritis in infants and young children worldwide. In the United States, prior to widespread rotavirus vaccine administration, approximately 80% of children developed rotavirus gastroenteritis before reaching 5 years of age.[6] Rotavirus accounted for 30%–50% of all hospitalizations for gastroenteritis in those patients.[6] Two oral vaccines are available to prevent rotavirus gastroenteritis and are recommended for routine use in healthy infants. These vaccines prevent 75%–85% of all rotavirus gastroenteritis and 95%–98% of severe infections, and they have substantially reduced the health care burden of rotavirus disease.[6–8] Rotavirus also causes diarrheal disease in adults, although specific epidemiological data are lacking.[9] The virus has been found in 18% of stool specimens of adults presenting to emergency departments with acute gastroenteritis and may account for 3%–5% of adult hospitalizations due to diarrheal disease.[10,11]

Rotavirus tends to be a seasonal infection, with peaks of gastroenteritis occurring between November and February. It is spread by the fecal–oral route, can cause severe dehydration and electrolyte disturbances, and may result in death. Clinical features are presented in Table 16–1. Other, less frequent viral causes of gastroenteritis include adenoviruses, astroviruses, and hepatitis A virus.

table

16–1   Common Infectious Diarrheas and Their Treatment

Type	Epidemiologic/ Etiologic Factors	Symptoms	Treatment	Usual Prognosis
Viral				
Rotavirus	Infects infants; oral–fecal spread	Onset of 24–48 hours; vomiting, fever, nausea, acute watery diarrhea	Vigorous fluid and electrolyte replacement	Self-limiting, usually lasts 5–8 days
Norovirus	Infects all ages; frequently spread person to person by the fecal–oral route; causes "24-hour stomach flu"	Onset of 24–48 hours; sudden-onset vomiting, nausea, headache, myalgia, fever, watery diarrhea	Fluid and electrolytes	Self-limiting, usually lasts 12–60 hours
Bacterial				
Campylobacter jejuni	Ingestion of contaminated food or water; oral–fecal spread; immuno-compromised host	Onset of 24–72 hours; nausea, vomiting, headache, malaise, fever, watery diarrhea	Fluid and electrolytes; in severe or persistent diarrhea, antibiotics may be required[a]	Self-limiting, usually lasts <7 days
Salmonella	Ingestion of improperly cooked or refrigerated poultry and dairy products; immuno-compromised host	Onset of 12–24 hours; diarrhea, fever, chills, malaise, myalgia, epigastric pain, anorexia	Fluid and electrolytes for mild cases; antibiotics reserved for compli-cated cases[b]	Self-limiting
Shigella	Ingestion of contaminated vegetables or water; frequently spread person to person; immuno-compromised host	Onset of 24–48 hours; nausea, vomiting, diarrhea	Fluid and electrolytes; antibiotics	Self-limiting
Escherichia coli (entero-toxigenic *E. coli* [ETEC], enteroaggregative *E. coli* [EAEC])	Ingestion of contaminated food or water; recent travel outside the United States or to a U.S. border area	Onset of 8–72 hours; watery diarrhea, fever, abdominal cramps, bloating, malaise, occasional vomiting	Fluid and electrolytes; antibiotics[c]	Self-limiting, usually within 3–5 days
Shiga toxin–producing *E. coli* (STEC), including *E. coli* O157:H7 and non-O157 strains	Ingestion of contaminated food or water; direct person-to-person spread	Onset of 8–72 hours; watery and often bloody diarrhea, abdominal cramps, hemolytic uremic syndrome	Fluid and electrolytes	Self-limiting, usually within 5–10 days
Clostridium difficile	Antibiotic-associated diarrhea leading to pseudomembranous colitis	Onset during or up to several weeks after anti-biotic therapy; watery or mucoid diarrhea, high fever, cramping	Fluid and electrolytes; discontinuation of offending agent; antibiotics	Self-limiting
Clostridium perfringens	Ingestion of contaminated food, especially meat and poultry	Onset of 8–14 hours; watery diarrhea without vomiting, cramping, mid-epigastric pain	Fluid and electrolytes	Self-limiting; usually resolves within 24 hours
Staphylococcus aureus	Ingestion of improperly cooked or stored food	Onset of 1–6 hours; nausea, vomiting, watery diarrhea	Fluid and electrolytes	Self-limiting
Yersinia enterocolitica	Ingestion of contaminated food	Onset within 16–48 hours; fever, abdominal pain, diarrhea, vomiting	Fluid and electrolytes; antibiotics may be needed in severe cases	Self-limiting, although diarrhea may persist for up to 3 weeks
Vibrio cholerae	Ingestion of contaminated food, including under-cooked or raw seafood; recent travel outside the United States	Onset within 24–48 hours; painless, watery, and often voluminous diarrhea, vomiting	Fluid and electrolytes; antibiotics needed in moderate-severe cases	Self-limiting, although severe, fatal illness may occur

table
16–1 Common Infectious Diarrheas and Their Treatment *(continued)*

Type	Epidemiologic/ Etiologic Factors	Symptoms	Treatment	Usual Prognosis
Bacillus cereus	Ingestion of contaminated food	Onset within 10–12 hours; abdominal pain, watery diarrhea, tenesmus, nausea, vomiting	Fluid and electrolytes	Self-limiting
Protozoal				
Giardia lamblia	Ingestion of water contaminated with human or animal feces; frequently spread person to person; immunocompromised host	Onset of 1–3 weeks; acute or chronic watery diarrhea, nausea, vomiting, anorexia, flatulence, abdominal bloating, epigastric pain	Fluids and electrolytes; antimicrobial therapy[d]	Resolves with treatment
Cryptosporidium spp.	Frequently spread person to person; travel outside the United States; AIDS, immunocompromised host	Onset of 2–14 days; acute or chronic watery diarrhea, abdominal pain, flatulence, malaise	Fluid and electrolytes; antimicrobial therapy[e]	Self-limiting, lasting up to 3 weeks, except in patients with AIDS or other immunosuppressive diseases
Entamoeba histolytica	Travel outside the United States; fecal-soiled food or water; immunocompromised host	Chronic watery diarrhea, abdominal pain, cramps	Fluid and electrolytes; antibiotics[f]	Good, except for immunocompromised host
Isospora belli	Ingestion of contaminated food or water; immunocompromised host	Onset of approximately 1 week; profuse watery diarrhea, malaise, anorexia, weight loss, abdominal cramps	Fluid and electrolytes; antibiotics	Self-limited, remitting in 2–3 weeks

Key: AIDS = Acquired immunodeficiency syndrome.

[a] Empirical therapy with prescription antibiotics (e.g., azithromycin or erythromycin) should be considered for patients with febrile diarrheal illness, especially if moderate-severe invasive disease is suspected, and for patients in whom supportive therapy fails to manage symptoms. Ciprofloxacin has been recommended, but it is no longer considered a first-line agent because many *Campylobacter* strains are resistant to fluoroquinolones.

[b] Antibiotics are not indicated routinely for *Salmonella* gastroenteritis; antibiotic therapy is used in infants and young children who fail to respond to supportive treatment, who do not spontaneously remit, or who are at increased risk of disseminated disease. Antibiotic therapy is also indicated for suspected bacteremia in patients at high risk for this complication. These include patients who appear to be toxic with high fever (>102.2°F [39°C]); infants (<3 months); older adult patients (>65 years); patients with cancer, immunodeficiency (e.g., AIDS), or hemoglobinopathy (e.g., sickle cell disease); patients receiving corticosteroids or who are on hemodialysis; and patients with vascular grafts or prosthetic joints. Fluoroquinolones are used for adults; ceftriaxone is used for children. Duration of antimicrobial therapy is usually 7–10 days.

[c] Antibiotic treatment with fluoroquinolones, azithromycin, or rifaximin (prescription antibiotics) is given for travelers' diarrhea caused by *E. coli*. Trimethoprim/sulfamethoxazole is no longer an optimal choice because of increasing worldwide resistance. Antibiotic treatment is not recommended for gastroenteritis caused by *E. coli* 0157:H7 because the treatment is likely to enhance toxin release and may increase risk for hemolytic uremic syndrome.

[d] Self-treatment of giardiasis is not appropriate; metronidazole, nitazoxanide, and tinidazole are effective prescription alternatives for treating giardiasis.[42,43]

[e] Self-treatment of cryptosporidiosis is not appropriate. Symptomatic relief of cryptosporidiosis may be achieved in patients with AIDS by adding paromomycin and azithromycin (both prescription antimicrobial agents) to patients' antiretroviral therapy.[42]

[f] Self-treatment of amebiasis is not appropriate; prescription therapy with metronidazole followed by either paromomycin or iodoquinol is preferred.[42]

Source: Adapted from Sanford Guide to Antimicrobial Therapy. Sanford Guide Web Edition 2. Antimicrobial Therapy, Inc. 2013. Accessed at http://webedition.sanfordguide.com/, March 11, 2013; and American Academy of Pediatrics. *AAP 2012 Red Book Online: Report of the Committee on Infectious Diseases.* Accessed at http://aapredbook.aappublications.org/, March 11, 2013.

Bacterial Gastroenteritis

Bacterial pathogens cause approximately 10% of acute diarrheal illnesses each year; most cases result from food-borne transmission. Pathogens most commonly responsible, in order of decreasing causality, are *Campylobacter* spp.; *Salmonella* spp.; *Shigella* spp.; *Escherichia coli* (including O157:H7, non–O157:H7 Shiga toxin–producing *E. coli* [STEC], enterotoxigenic *E. coli* [ETEC], diffusely adherent *E. coli* [DAEC], and other diarrheagenic strains); *Staphylococcus* spp.; *Clostridium* spp.; *Yersinia enterocolitica;* and *Bacillus cereus.* In addition, *Aeromonas* spp., *Arcobacter* spp., enterotoxigenic *Bacteroides fragilis, Klebsiella oxytoca, Laribacter hongkongensis,* and *Plesiomonas shigelloides* cause acute diarrhea.[12,13]

Bacteria cause diarrhea through elaboration of enterotoxin (e.g., ETEC and *Staphylococcus aureus*), by attachment and production of localized inflammatory changes in the gut (e.g., enteroaggregative *E. coli* [EAEC], enteropathogenic *E. coli*, STEC, and *Clostridium difficile*), or by directly invading the mucosal epithelial cells (e.g., *Shigella, Salmonella, Yersinia, Campylobacter jejuni,* and invasive *E. coli*).[14,15] Patients with diarrhea caused by toxin-producing pathogens have a watery diarrhea, which primarily involves the small intestine. If the large intestine is the primary site of infection, invasive organisms produce a dysentery-like (bloody diarrhea) syndrome characterized by fever, abdominal cramps, tenesmus (straining), and the frequent passage of small-volume stools that may contain blood and mucus. Clinical features of common bacterial diarrheas are presented in Table 16–1.

Enteric infection, most notably bacterial infection caused by *Campylobacter, Shigella, Salmonella,* and diarrheagenic *E. coli,* can cause prolonged bowel dysfunction, including irritable bowel syndrome (IBS), a functional bowel disorder characterized by abdominal pain and discomfort following resolution of the infection. Norovirus may also cause postinfectious IBS. IBS develops in 2%–30% of patients following enteric infection, depending on the causative agent, and is usually diagnosed 1–2 years after an episode of acute bacterial gastroenteritis.[16] The prognosis is favorable for most patients, and symptoms of IBS resolve 4–8 years after diagnosis. Acute gastroenteritis may also unmask or exacerbate underlying chronic gastrointestinal diseases, such as celiac disease, Crohn's disease, or ulcerative colitis.

Protozoal Diarrhea

Diarrhea may also be caused by protozoa, including *Giardia lamblia, Entamoeba histolytica, Isospora belli,* and *Cryptosporidium* spp. No nonprescription therapies are available to manage diarrhea caused by these pathogens, and self-management is inappropriate.

Food-Borne Gastroenteritis

Food-borne transmission of pathogens causes 47.8 million episodes of acute gastroenteritis that lead to 135,000 hospitalizations and approximately 3000 deaths in the United States each year.[2,17] When pathogens are identified, 59% of those infections are caused by viruses (predominantly noroviruses), 39% by bacteria, and 2% by protozoa.[17] Recent surveillance statistics on the incidence of food-borne illnesses confirm that *Salmonella* and *Campylobacter,* which caused 16.47 and 14.31 cases of illness per 100,000 population in 2011, respectively, are the most

frequently diagnosed bacterial pathogens. These are followed by *Shigella* (3.21 cases per 100,000 population), STEC O157:H7 (0.98 cases per 100,000 population), *Listeria* (0.34 cases per 100,000 population), *Vibrio* (0.33 cases per 100,000 population), and *Yersinia* (0.32 cases per 100,000 population).[18]

Outbreaks of food-borne bacterial infection have been traced to poor sanitation and manufacturing practices in food production facilities, including meat-processing plants, and contamination of foods in various retail locations such as grocery stores and restaurants. Outbreaks of infection have also been associated with specific foods (Table 16–2).[18] Therefore, taking a thorough history regarding the patient's food intake 48–72 hours before the onset of diarrhea is essential in identifying a possible cause.

Outbreaks of acute food-borne illness caused by *E. coli* O157:H7 and other STECs are a major public health issue. Toxins produced by these organisms cause an acute bloody diarrhea and may also be associated with serious, potentially fatal systemic complications such as hemolytic uremic syndrome or thrombotic thrombocytopenic purpura. Other causes of food-borne gastroenteritis include *Listeria monocytogenes, Cyclospora cayetanensis,* and rotovirus.

table

16–2   Specific Foods Associated with Food-Borne Gastroenteritis

Organism	Associated Foods	
Shiga toxin–producing *E. coli* (STEC), including *E. coli* O157:H7 and non-O157 strains	Apple cider, unpasteurized	Lettuce
	Bologna	Milk, raw
	Clover sprouts, raw	Cookie dough, raw, refrigerated prepackaged
	Eggs	
	Gouda cheese	Spinach
	Ground beef (undercooked)	
Salmonella	Chicken	Papayas
	Dry dog food[a]	Peanut butter
	Eggs	Pine nuts
	Ground beef	Pistachio nuts
	Ground turkey	Red and black pepper spice
	Jalapeno peppers	
	Mangoes	Yellowfin tuna, raw, scraped, ground
	Melons (e.g., cantaloupe)	
Campylobacter	Milk	
	Chicken	
Listeria	Hummus	
	Melons	
	Ricotta cheese	
Cyclospora	Raspberries	

[a] *Salmonella* infection is a zoonotic disease, i.e., the infection can be transmitted from animals to people, and people have developed *Salmonella* infections after contact with contaminated dry pet food or with an animal that has eaten contaminated dry pet food. Spread is by the fecal–oral route.

Source: Adapted from reference 17.

Travelers' Diarrhea

Travelers' diarrhea is an acute, secretory diarrhea acquired mainly through ingestion of contaminated food or water. It is usually caused by bacterial enteropathogens; however, a cause may not be identifiable in as many as 40% of cases. Enterotoxigenic *E. coli* (ETEC), enteroaggregative *E. coli* (EAEC), and diffusely adherent *E. coli* (DAEC) are responsible for most cases of travelers' diarrhea.[19-21] ETEC is found in 50%–76% of travelers with diarrhea in various areas around the world.[21] Other important pathogens that cause travelers' diarrhea include *Shigella* spp., *Salmonella* spp., *C. jejuni, Aeromonas* spp., *Plesiomonas* spp., and noncholera *Vibrio;* noroviruses cause 12%–17% of cases.[21] The causative organisms are found most often on foods such as fruits, vegetables, raw meat, seafood, and even hot sauces. Less commonly, pathogens are found in the local water, including ice cubes. After ingestion, ETEC produces two plasmid-mediated enterotoxins that cause symptoms; one of these enterotoxins is closely related structurally, functionally, and immunologically to cholera toxin. The pathogenic mechanisms underlying diarrhea caused by EAEC are not well understood. These organisms may produce disease through elaboration of an enterotoxin or a cytotoxin, or by some other means. The diarrheal disorder caused by these organisms is characterized in Table 16–1. Patients may experience between three and eight (or more) watery stools per day, with symptoms usually subsiding over 3–5 days.

Food-Induced Diarrhea

Food intolerance can provoke diarrhea and may result from a food allergy or ingestion of foods that are excessively fatty or spicy or contain a high amount of dietary fiber or many seeds. Dietary carbohydrates (e.g., lactose and sucrose) are normally hydrolyzed to monosaccharides by the enzyme lactase. If not hydrolyzed, these carbohydrates pool in the lumen of the intestine and produce an osmotic imbalance. The resulting hyperosmolarity draws fluid into the intestinal lumen, causing diarrhea. Lactase

activity may be reduced by infectious diarrhea; thus, acute viral diarrhea may cause temporary milk intolerance in patients of all ages. Lactase deficiency resulting from viral gastroenteritis is short-lived, but it is particularly problematic during the first few days of the disease. Infants born with lactase deficiency and adults who develop lactase deficiency are intolerant of cow milk and milk-based products. Lactase enzyme products are effective treatments for some patients (see Treatment of Diarrhea).

Clinical Presentation of Diarrhea

The most common signs and symptoms of acute infectious diarrheal illnesses are shown in Table 16–1. Variability in the causes of diarrhea makes identification of the pathophysiologic mechanisms difficult. The etiology, and subsequently the pathophysiology, can be determined by conducting a thorough medical history in most cases. However, a complete medical assessment, including clinical laboratory evaluation, may be required to identify the cause in a subset of patients with severe or persistent diarrhea.

Diarrhea can be classified as osmotic, secretory, inflammatory, or motor, depending on the underlying pathophysiologic mechanisms that disrupt normal intestinal function. The common mechanisms of acute diarrhea are osmotic and secretory, whereas motor and inflammatory mechanisms commonly underlie chronic diarrheal illnesses. Table 16–3 correlates the clinical groups and mechanisms with their most common causes.

Bacterial enterotoxins play a role in the pathophysiology of secretory diarrheas. Enterotoxins elaborated by *E. coli* and *Vibrio cholerae* evoke the release of endogenous secretagogues that mediate secretory reflexes, including serotonin, substance P, and vasoactive intestinal peptide. Some enterotoxins, such as cholera toxin, can directly stimulate GI secretomotor neurons to increase intestinal secretion. *Clostridium difficile* enterotoxin A also injures enterocytes and evokes a necroinflammatory response that causes a secretory diarrhea. Although viruses such as rotavirus also

table 16–3	Clinical Classification of Diarrhea	
Type	**Mechanism**	**Common Causes**
Osmotic	▪ Unabsorbed solutes in intestines increase luminal osmotic load, retarding fluid absorption. ▪ Decreased absorption of solutes and fluid can be secondary to brush border damage caused by lactase deficiency or infection. ▪ Viral-induced damage to epithelial cells accelerates migration of immature crypt cells to the tip of the villus; altered epithelial turnover also decreases absorption.	Noroviruses, rotaviruses, *Escherichia coli, Campylobacter jejuni,* lactase deficiency, excess magnesium antacid intake
Secretory	▪ Stimulation of crypt cells produces net flow of electrolytes and fluids into intestinal lumen. ▪ Tumors can secrete GI hormones and peptides that act as secretagogues.	*C. jejuni, Clostridium difficile, E. coli, Salmonella, Shigella, Vibrio,* rotaviruses, *Giardia lamblia, Cryptosporidium* spp., *Isospora,* ileal resection, thyroid cancer
Inflammatory	▪ Impaired fluid absorption and leaking of mucus, blood, and pus into lumen caused by inflammation of intestinal mucosa (e.g., IBD) or bacterial infection (i.e., dysentery).	*C. jejuni, E. coli, Salmonella, Shigella, Yersinia, Entamoeba histolytica,* ulcerative colitis, Crohn's disease
Motor	▪ Abnormally rapid intestinal transit time reduces contact time between luminal contents and absorptive areas of intestinal wall.	IBS, diabetic neuropathy

Key: GI = Gastrointestinal; IBD = inflammatory bowel disease; IBS = irritable bowel syndrome.

produce enterotoxins, the role of viral enterotoxins in the disease pathophysiology is uncertain. In addition, inflammatory mediators (e.g., interleukins 1 and 6, prostaglandins, substance P, tissue necrosis factor-alpha, and platelet-activating factor) evoked by enteric infection stimulate a characteristic GI motility pattern that leads to the urgent defecation associated with diarrhea. This altered motility also causes abdominal cramps.

Stool characteristics give valuable information about the diarrhea's pathophysiology. For example, undigested food particles in the stool suggest disease of the small intestine. Black, tarry stools may indicate upper GI bleeding, and red stools suggest possible lower bowel or hemorrhoidal bleeding or simply recent ingestion of red food (e.g., beets) or drug products (e.g., rifampin). In secretory diarrhea of the small bowel, chloride secretion and inhibition of sodium absorption appear to be the major events; thus, stools will be high in sodium.[14] Passage of many small-volume stools suggests a colonic disorder. Yellowish stools may suggest the presence of bilirubin and a potentially serious pathology of the liver. A whitish tint to the stool suggests a fat malabsorption disease.

Fluid and electrolyte imbalance is the major complication of diarrheal illness. Therefore, assessment of the patient's risk for dehydration and the degree of dehydration present is a key factor in determining the appropriateness of self-care and the need for medical referral. The specific signs and symptoms of dehydration are associated with the severity of the diarrhea, as well as the etiology and degree of fluid and electrolyte losses (Table 16–4).[22]

table

16–4 Assessment of Dehydration and Severity of Acute Diarrhea

	Self-Treatable		Not Self-Treatable
	Minimal or No Dehydration	**Mild-Moderate Dehydration/Diarrhea**	**Severe Dehydration/ Diarrhea**
Degree of dehydration (% loss of body weight)	<3%	3%–9%	>9%
Signs of dehydration[a]			
Mental status	Good, alert	Normal, fatigued or restless, irritable	Apathetic, lethargic, unconscious
Thirst	Drinks normally, might refuse liquids	Thirsty, eager to drink	Drinks poorly, unable to drink
Heart rate	Normal	Normal to increased	Tachycardia, bradycardia in most severe cases
Quality of pulses	Normal	Normal to decreased	Weak, thready, impalpable
Breathing	Normal	Normal, fast	Deep
Eyes	Normal	Slightly sunken[b]	Deeply sunken[b]
Tears	Present	Decreased[b]	Absent
Mouth and tongue	Moist	Dry	Parched
Skin fold	Instant recoil	Recoil in <2 seconds	Recoil in >2 seconds
Capillary refill	Normal	Prolonged	Prolonged, minimal
Extremities	Warm	Cool	Cold, mottled, cyanotic
Urine output	Normal to decreased	Decreased[b]	Minimal[b]
Number of unformed stools/day	<3	3–5	6–9
Other signs/symptoms	Afebrile, normal blood pressure, no orthostatic changes in blood pressure/pulse	May be afebrile or may develop fever >102.2°F (39°C); normal blood pressure; possible mild orthostatic blood pressure/pulse changes with or without mild orthostatic-related symptoms[c]; sunken fontanelle[d]	Fever > 102.2°F (39°C), low blood pressure, dizziness, severe abdominal pain

[a] If signs of dehydration are absent, rehydration therapy is not required. Maintenance therapy and replacement of stool losses should be undertaken.

[b] Signs and symptoms experienced especially by young children.

[c] Postural (orthostatic) hypotension is defined as a drop in the systolic and/or diastolic pressure of greater than 15–20 mm Hg on movement from a supine to an upright position and may cause lightheadedness, dizziness, or fainting. On rising, the diastolic pressure normally remains the same or increases slightly, and the systolic pressure drops slightly. If the blood pressure drops, the pulse should be checked simultaneously; the pulse rate should increase as blood pressure drops. Failure of the pulse to rise suggests the problem is neurogenic (e.g., diabetic patients with peripheral neuropathy) or that the patient may be taking a beta-blocker. The presence of orthostatic hypotension suggests that the patient has lost ≥1 liter of vascular volume, and referral for medical care is necessary.

[d] Signs and symptoms of concern for young infants.

Source: Adapted from reference 22.

Children younger than 5 years and adults older than 65 years are at greater risk for complications than other age groups. In the United States, most children recover completely from diarrhea; however, approximately 300–450 children (mostly infants) die annually from complications of acute gastroenteritis.[3,22] Children 2 years of age and younger are more likely to suffer complications that require hospitalization. In newborns, water may make up 75% of total body weight; severe diarrhea may cause water loss equal to 10% or more of body weight. After 8–10 bowel movements within a 24-hour period, a 2-month-old infant could lose enough fluid to cause circulatory collapse and renal failure.

In recent years, deaths from viral and bacterial GI infection have increased most sharply among people 65 years of age and older. Diarrhea in this population is likely to be more severe than in other adults; older adults experience the highest rate of death from enteric infections.

Treatment of Diarrhea

Treatment Goals

The goals of self-treatment of diarrhea are to (1) prevent or correct fluid and electrolyte loss and acid–base disturbance, (2) control symptoms, (3) identify and treat the cause, and (4) prevent acute morbidity and mortality.

General Treatment Approach

Infectious diarrhea is often self-limiting. Initial self-management for adults and children with mild-moderate, uncomplicated diarrhea should focus on fluid and electrolyte replacement by administering commercially available oral rehydration solutions (ORS) in adequate doses (Table 16–5). Simultaneous implementation of oral rehydration and specific dietary measures is appropriate for treating mild-moderate diarrheal illness. Symptomatic control can also be achieved by using nonprescription antidiarrheal drugs, such as loperamide, in carefully selected patients. Normal function of the alimentary tract is often restored in 24–72 hours without additional treatment.

Diarrhea of any severity in infants younger than 6 months of age and moderate diarrhea in children 2 years of age and younger who have unusually high fluid output or mental status changes require evaluation by a primary care provider, a pediatrician, or a health care provider in an emergency department. Severe diarrhea constitutes a medical emergency, especially in young children, and requires immediate referral for medical evaluation and treatment with intravenous (IV) fluid therapy. Specific exclusions for self-treatment that require referral for medical evaluation are listed in Figure 16–1.

Patients with uncomplicated acute diarrhea who are otherwise healthy usually improve clinically within 24–48 hours. If the condition remains the same or worsens after 48 hours of onset, medical referral is necessary to prevent complications. Patients who have stool that contains blood or mucus need medical evaluation. Certain medical conditions can increase the risk for dehydration. Referral for medical care should be considered for patients with diabetes mellitus, severe cardiovascular or renal diseases, or multiple unstable chronic medical conditions. Patients with severe abdominal pain (particularly those >50 years of age) may have a complicating illness such as ischemic bowel disease and should be referred for medical evaluation. Immunocompromised patients, such as those receiving cancer treatment, organ transplant recipients, and patients with AIDS, also need medical evaluation because their diarrhea will often be complicated and difficult to manage. Self-care during pregnancy is not appropriate; pregnant women who develop diarrhea should consult with a primary care provider or an obstetrician.

table
16–5   Selected Oral Rehydration Products

Trade Name	Osmolarity	Calories	Carbohydrate	Electrolytes
CeraLyte 50 Powder Packets	<200 mOsm/L	160 cal/L	Rice starch polymers 40 g/L; sucrose 10 g/L	Sodium 50 mEq/L; chloride 40 mEq/L; citrate 30 mEq/L; potassium 20 mEq/L
CeraLyte 70 Powder Packets	<260 mOsm/L	160 cal/L	Rice starch polymers 40 g/L	Sodium 70 mEq/L; chloride 60 mEq/L; citrate 30 mEq/L; potassium 20 mEq/L
CeraLyte 75 Powder Packets	<250 mOsm/L	160 cal/L	Rice starch polymers 40 g/L	Sodium 75 mEq/L; chloride 80 mEq/L; citrate 30 mEq/L; potassium 20 mEq/L
CeraLyte 90 Powder Packets	<260 mOsm/L	160 cal/L	Rice starch polymers 40 g/L	Sodium 90 mEq/L; chloride 80 mEq/L; citrate 30 mEq/L; potassium 20 mEq/L
Enfamil Enfalyte Solution	160 mOsm/L	126 cal/L	Corn syrup solids 30 g/L	Sodium 50 mEq/L; chloride 45 mEq/L; citrate 33 mEq/L; potassium 25 mEq/L
Pedialyte[a]	249 mOsm/L	100 cal/L	Dextrose 20 g/L; fructose 5 g/L	Sodium 45 mEq/L; chloride 35 mEq/L; citrate 30 mEq/L; potassium 20 mEq/L
Pedialyte Freezer Pops[b]	270 mOsm/L	6.25 cal/L	Dextrose 25 g/L	Sodium 45 mEq/L; chloride 35 mEq/L; citrate 30 mEq/L; potassium 20 mEq/L

Key: ORS = Oral rehydration solution; WHO = World Health Organization.

[a] Many generic products (e.g., store brands) are available.

[b] Product to be used with appropriate maintenance ORS.

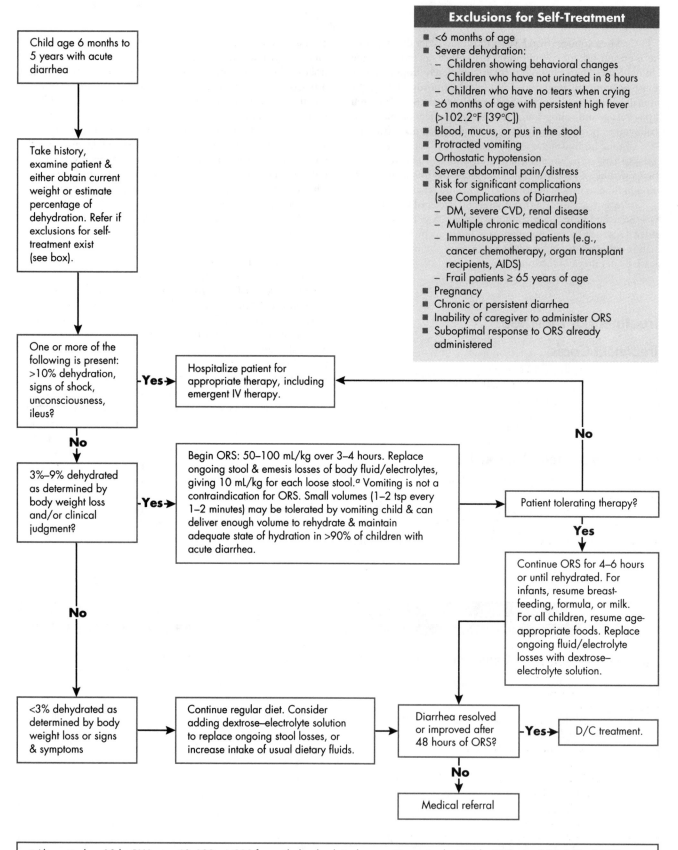

Child age 6 months to 5 years with acute diarrhea

Take history, examine patient & either obtain current weight or estimate percentage of dehydration. Refer if exclusions for self-treatment exist (see box).

Exclusions for Self-Treatment

- <6 months of age
- Severe dehydration:
  - Children showing behavioral changes
  - Children who have not urinated in 8 hours
  - Children who have no tears when crying
- ≥6 months of age with persistent high fever (>102.2°F [39°C])
- Blood, mucus, or pus in the stool
- Protracted vomiting
- Orthostatic hypotension
- Severe abdominal pain/distress
- Risk for significant complications (see Complications of Diarrhea)
  - DM, severe CVD, renal disease
  - Multiple chronic medical conditions
  - Immunosuppressed patients (e.g., cancer chemotherapy, organ transplant recipients, AIDS)
  - Frail patients ≥ 65 years of age
- Pregnancy
- Chronic or persistent diarrhea
- Inability of caregiver to administer ORS
- Suboptimal response to ORS already administered

One or more of the following is present: >10% dehydration, signs of shock, unconsciousness, ileus?

—Yes→ Hospitalize patient for appropriate therapy, including emergent IV therapy.

No

3%–9% dehydrated as determined by body weight loss and/or clinical judgment?

—Yes→ Begin ORS: 50–100 mL/kg over 3–4 hours. Replace ongoing stool & emesis losses of body fluid/electrolytes, giving 10 mL/kg for each loose stool.ᵃ Vomiting is not a contraindication for ORS. Small volumes (1–2 tsp every 1–2 minutes) may be tolerated by vomiting child & can deliver enough volume to rehydrate & maintain adequate state of hydration in >90% of children with acute diarrhea.

Patient tolerating therapy?

No

Yes

Continue ORS for 4–6 hours or until rehydrated. For infants, resume breast-feeding, formula, or milk. For all children, resume age-appropriate foods. Replace ongoing fluid/electrolyte losses with dextrose–electrolyte solution.

No

<3% dehydrated as determined by body weight loss or signs & symptoms

Continue regular diet. Consider adding dextrose–electrolyte solution to replace ongoing stool losses, or increase intake of usual dietary fluids.

Diarrhea resolved or improved after 48 hours of ORS?

—Yes→ D/C treatment.

No

Medical referral

ᵃ Alternatively: <10 kg BW, give 60–120 mL ORS for each diarrheal stool or vomiting episode; ≥10 kg BW, give 120–240 mL ORS.

figure

16–1 Self-care of acute diarrhea in children 6 months to 5 years. Key: AIDS = Acquired immunodeficiency syndrome; BW = body weight; CVD = cardiovascular disease; D/C = discontinue; DM = diabetes mellitus; IV = intravenous; ORS = oral rehydration solution.

Nonpharmacologic Therapy

Fluid and Electrolyte Management

Rehydration using ORS is the preferred treatment for mild-moderate diarrhea. This approach is as effective as IV therapy in managing fluid and electrolytes in children with mild-moderate dehydration secondary to diarrhea.

Water absorption in the small intestine is passive and depends on the absorption of electrolytes and selected solutes such as sodium, chloride, glucose, small peptides, and amino acids. As these substances are absorbed, water accompanies their movement to maintain an isotonic state. Sodium ion transport is the primary mechanism controlling water movement. An active sodium–potassium adenosine triphosphatase pump present in enterocytes moves sodium into the cell in exchange for potassium ions. Other transport mechanisms include the sodium–glucose and sodium–amino acid co-transport processes (each of which transports these substances into the enterocytes) and the sodium luminal exchange mechanism. The sodium–glucose co-transport mechanism, in which glucose absorption is coupled with active transport of sodium, is important in the management of diarrhea. Unlike other sodium transport systems, the sodium–glucose co-transport mechanism is not adversely affected by most diarrheal diseases, and hypotonic ORS containing low concentrations of glucose or dextrose (2%–2.5%) can be useful in managing fluid and electrolyte balance. The sugar molecules provide little caloric support but facilitate intestinal sodium and water absorption. Maximal sodium absorption occurs at a molar glucose-to-sodium ratio close to 1. Health care providers can safely recommend an ORS for mild-moderate diarrhea.

Depending on the patient's fluid and electrolyte status, oral treatment may be carried out in two phases: rehydration therapy and maintenance therapy. Rehydration over 3–4 hours quickly replaces water and electrolyte deficits to restore normal body composition. In the maintenance phase, electrolyte solutions are given to maintain normal body composition until adequate dietary intake is reestablished. Figures 16–1 and 16–2 outline rehydration and maintenance therapies, including fluid and electrolyte recommendations for children and adults. Although ORS is generally recommended for adults with diarrhea, little evidence supports this use, and ORS may not provide any real benefit to otherwise healthy adults with mild diarrhea who can maintain an adequate fluid intake during the episode of diarrhea. For these patients, fluid and electrolyte status can be maintained by increasing intake of fluids such as clear juices, soups, or sports drinks.

A variety of oral rehydration products are available (Table 16–5). Most products are premixed solutions; a few are available as dry powders of glucose and electrolytes that require the addition of water. The premixed products are preferred for use in children because they are safe and convenient, and improper mixing of dry powders by caregivers has led to fluid and electrolyte complications and injury. All available premixed solutions are equally safe and effective; there is no evidence that one product is clinically superior to another for rehydration. The World Health Organization (WHO) and United Nations Children's Fund (UNICEF) recommend use of an ORS containing 75 mEq/L of sodium.[23] Compared with the standard WHO ORS (which contains 90 mEq/L of sodium), this ORS significantly reduces the need for unscheduled IV therapy, the duration of diarrhea, stool output, and the incidence of vomiting in children with noncholera diarrhea. This ORS is also effective in children and adults with cholera,

although transient, asymptomatic hyponatremia may develop in adults. Rehydration solutions available in the United States contain 70–90 mEq/L of sodium; maintenance ORSs contain 45–50 mEq/L of sodium.

Some cereal-based products use complex carbohydrates (e.g., rice syrup solids) instead of glucose. Complex carbohydrates are converted into glucose at the intestinal brush border and provide more co-transport molecules while reducing the osmotic load of the ORS. Cereal-based ORS therapy potentially reduces stool volume by 20%–30% in children with cholera, but this therapy may not significantly alter stool volume in children with noncholera acute diarrhea.

A variety of common household oral solutions have also been used for oral rehydration and maintenance (Table 16–6). These solutions may be sufficient to manage mild, self-limiting diarrhea in some patients, but they should be avoided if dehydration or moderate-severe diarrhea is present. Unlike commercial ORS, these remedies are not formulated on the basis of the physiology of acute diarrhea. The inappropriately high carbohydrate content and osmolality of these solutions can worsen diarrhea, and their low sodium content can contribute to the development of hyponatremia. Sports drinks may be used in children older than 5 years and adults if additional sources of sodium, such as crackers or pretzels, are used concomitantly. Colas, ginger ale, apple juice, sports drinks, and similar products are not recommended for infants and young children (6 months to 5 years of age) with diarrhea. Tea, another popular household remedy, is also inappropriate for children because of its low sodium content. Chicken broth is not recommended because of its inappropriately high sodium content.

Dietary Management

Oral intake does not worsen diarrhea, and clinically significant nutrient malabsorption is uncommon in acute diarrhea. In fact, during acute diarrhea, patients are able to absorb 80%–95% of dietary carbohydrates, 70% of fat, and 75% of the nitrogen from protein. Furthermore, early refeeding, in combination with maintenance oral rehydration, improves outcomes in children by reducing the duration of the diarrhea, reducing stool output, and improving weight gain. Current guidelines recommend withholding food no longer than 24 hours and encourage the reintroduction of a normal, age-appropriate diet once the patient has been rehydrated, which should take no longer than 3–4 hours to accomplish.[22] Most infants and children with acute diarrhea can tolerate full-strength breast milk and cow milk. The BRAT diet (bananas, rice, applesauce, and toast) is not recommended; it provides insufficient calories, protein, and fat, especially in situations of strict or prolonged use.[22] Patients (or their parents) should be advised to avoid fatty foods, foods rich in simple sugars (e.g., carbonated soft drinks, juice, gelatin desserts) that can cause osmotic diarrhea, spicy foods that may cause GI upset, and caffeine-containing beverages, which can promote fluid secretion and may worsen diarrhea.

There is no evidence that fasting or dietary modification influence outcomes of acute diarrhea in adults; however, the previous recommendations about foods to avoid can be applied if a normal diet is not tolerated.[22]

Preventive Measures

Infectious diarrhea, especially acute viral gastroenteritis, often occurs in congregate living conditions such as day care centers

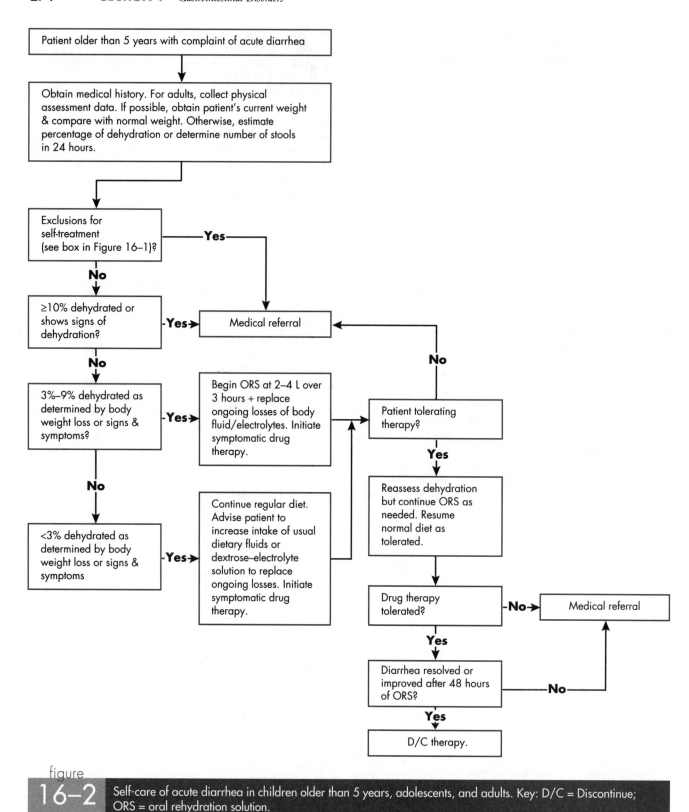

figure

16–2   Self-care of acute diarrhea in children older than 5 years, adolescents, and adults. Key: D/C = Discontinue; ORS = oral rehydration solution.

and nursing homes through person-to-person transmission. Isolating the individual with diarrhea, washing hands, and using sterile techniques are basic preventive measures that reduce the risk of transmission among such populations and their caregivers. Strict food handling, sanitation, and other hygienic practices help control transmission of bacteria and other infectious agents.

Short-term bismuth subsalicylate (BSS) prophylaxis is frequently recommended to provide protection against travelers' diarrhea; however, the Food and Drug Administration (FDA) has deemed that available data are insufficient to support prophylactic use of BSS.[24] Antibiotics with reliable activity against endemic enteropathogens (e.g., fluoroquinolones, rifaximin)

table 16–6	**Comparison of Electrolyte and Dextrose Concentrations of Household Fluids**				
Clear Liquids	**Sodium (mEq/L)**	**Potassium (mEq/L)**	**Bicarbonate (mEq/L)**	**Dextrose (g/L)**	**Osmolarity (mOsm/L)**
Cola	2	0.1	13	50–150 dextrose and fructose	550
Ginger ale	3	1	4	50–150 dextrose and fructose	540
Apple juice	3	20	0	10–150 dextrose and fructose	700
Chicken broth	250	5	0	0	450
Tea	0	0	0	0	5
Gatorade	20	3	3	45 dextrose and other sugars	330
Seven Up	7.5	0.2	0	80 dextrose and fructose	564

provide effective prophylaxis. However, prophylactic antimicrobial agents are not currently recommended for most travelers.[24] Prophylactic antibiotics may be considered for short-term travelers who are high-risk hosts (e.g., immunosuppressed patients) or travelers with underlying conditions that may be complicated by diarrheal illness, or for critical trips during which even a short bout of diarrhea could adversely affect the purpose of the trip.[25]

Pharmacologic Therapy

Although most acute, nonspecific diarrhea in the United States is self-limiting, nonprescription antidiarrheal products may provide symptom control and will usually do no harm when used according to label instructions. Table 16–7 lists dosage and administration guidelines for these agents. However, evidence is lacking to show that pharmacologic agents other than loperamide and BSS reduce stool frequency or duration of disease in adults. Table 16–8 lists available trade-name products that contain loperamide and BSS. No antidiarrheal drugs have been shown to significantly improve clinical outcomes of acute, nonspecific diarrhea in infants and children ages 5 years and younger.

Loperamide

Loperamide is a popular, effective, and safe nonprescription antidiarrheal agent. It is a synthetic opioid agonist that lacks central nervous system (CNS) effects because it is a substrate for P-glycoprotein. P-glycoprotein is an efflux transporter found in many tissues, including the blood–brain barrier. Loperamide is so efficiently removed from the CNS by this efflux transporter that pharmacologically effective concentrations in the CNS are not normally achieved and the risk of CNS adverse effects is minimized.[26] Loperamide produces antidiarrheal effects by stimulating peripheral micro-opioid receptors on the intestinal circular muscles to slow intestinal motility and allow absorption of electrolytes and water. Disruption of cholinergic and non-cholinergic mechanisms involved in the regulation of peristalsis may also contribute to this effect. Loperamide also has anti-secretory effects that may be mediated through stimulation of GI micro-opioid receptors, inhibition of calmodulin function, and inhibition of voltage-dependent calcium channels.

Loperamide provides symptomatic relief of acute, non-specific diarrhea. Its therapeutic effects include reduced daily fecal volume, increased viscosity and bulk volume, and reduced fluid and electrolyte loss. It may be used when the patient is afebrile or has a low-grade fever and does not have bloody stools. Nonprescription loperamide is labeled for use in children 6 years of age and older; the product information for prescription loperamide provides directions for use in children as young as 2 years of age. However, use of loperamide in children younger than 6 years is not recommended because it produces only modest, clinically insignificant effects on stool volume and duration of illness, with an unacceptably high risk of side effects, including life-threatening ileus and toxic megacolon.[23]

Loperamide is also indicated for treatment of travelers' diarrhea (in combination with antibiotics) and chronic diarrhea associated with IBS and inflammatory bowel disease, as well as to reduce the volume of discharge from high-output ileostomies. Off-label uses include control of chronic diarrhea secondary to diabetic neuropathy and other conditions, and control of toddler diarrhea (defined as diarrhea of at least 1 month in duration in an otherwise healthy, active, well-nourished child in whom stool examination has revealed no bacterial, viral, or protozoal pathogens). Off-label uses require medical supervision.

At usual doses (Table 16–7), loperamide has few side effects other than occasional dizziness and constipation. Infrequently occurring adverse effects include abdominal pain, abdominal distension, nausea, vomiting, dry mouth, fatigue, and hypersensitivity reactions. Loperamide is generally not recommended for use in patients with invasive bacterial diarrhea (enteroinvasive *E. coli, Salmonella, Shigella,* or *C. jejuni*) or antibiotic-associated diarrhea (*C. difficile*) because it may worsen diarrhea or cause toxic megacolon or paralytic ileus. However, there is no evidence that these complications occur in actual practice when loperamide is used with appropriate antimicrobial therapy. Patients with symptoms suggestive of infection with invasive organisms or antibiotic-associated diarrhea (i.e., fecal leukocytes, high fever, or blood or mucus in the stool) require medical evaluation for proper management. If abdominal distension, constipation, or ileus occurs, loperamide should be discontinued.

Very few clinically significant drug–drug interactions are reported for loperamide. Although loperamide is a substrate for P-glycoprotein, interactions with P-glycoprotein inhibitors (e.g., quinidine, ketoconazole, and ritonavir) do not appear to result in clinically significant CNS depression or opioid toxicity when loperamide is used in the recommended doses.[26] Loperamide is metabolized primarily by CYP3A4 and CYP2C8.

table

16–7 Recommended Dosages of Nonprescription Antidiarrheal Agents for Acute Diarrhea

Medication	Dosage Forms	Adult Dosages (maximum daily dosage)	Pediatric Dosages	Duration of Use
Loperamide	Caplets (2 mg), liquid (1 mg/7.5 mL)	4 mg initially, then 2 mg after each loose stool (not to exceed 8 mg/day)	Consult product instructions; not recommended for children <6 years except under medical supervision 6–8 years (48–59 lb): Caplets: 2 mg initially, then 1 mg after each loose stool (not to exceed 4 mg/day) Liquid: 1.3 mg (2 teaspoonfuls) initially, followed by 1 mg (1.5 teaspoonfuls) after each loose stool. Do not give more than 2.7 mg (4 teaspoonfuls) in 24 hours. 9–11 years (60–95 lb): Caplets: 2 mg initially, then 1 mg after each loose stool (not to exceed 6 mg/day) Liquid: 1.3 mg (2 teaspoonfuls) initially followed by 1 mg (1.5 teaspoonfuls) after each loose stool. Do not give more than 4 mg (6 teaspoonfuls) in 24 hours.	48 hours
Bismuth subsalicylate	Tablets (262 mg), caplets (262 mg), liquids (262 mg/15 mL, 525 mg/15 mL)	525 mg every 30–60 minutes up to 4200 mg/day (8 doses/day)	Not recommended for children <12 years except under medical supervision	48 hours
Digestive enzymes (lactase)	Chewable tablets, caplets, liquids	5–15 drops placed in or taken with dairy product; 1–3 tablets or 1–2 capsules with first bite of dairy product	Same as adult dosage	Taken with each consumption of dairy product

Concurrent administration of loperamide with other substrates for these enzymes (e.g., protease inhibitors, cyclosporine, erythromycin, or clarithromycin) may elevate loperamide concentrations, but the effect on loperamide disposition does not appear to be associated with clinically relevant outcomes when taken in the recommended doses.[26,27] However, loperamide may significantly decrease saquinavir concentrations, and patients receiving saquinavir should be advised not to use loperamide, especially for long periods of time.[28]

Bismuth Subsalicylate

BSS is effective in the treatment of acute diarrhea. BSS reacts with hydrochloric acid in the stomach to form bismuth oxychloride and salicylic acid. Bismuth oxychloride is insoluble and poorly absorbed from the GI tract; less than 1% of the administered dose is absorbed systemically. The salicylate is readily and efficiently absorbed. Both moieties are pharmacologically active. The bismuth moiety exerts direct antimicrobial effects against ETEC and EAEC, *C. jejuni,* and other diarrheal pathogens, whereas the salicylate moiety exerts antisecretory effects

that reduce fluid and electrolyte losses. These effects reduce the frequency of unformed stools, increase stool consistency, relieve abdominal cramping, and decrease nausea and vomiting. In travelers' diarrhea, the salicylate appears to be the active moiety. Its antisecretory effects may be mediated by several mechanisms, including inhibition of prostaglandin synthesis, inhibition of intestinal secretion through stimulation of sodium and chloride reabsorption, or disruption of calcium-mediated processes that regulate intestinal ion transport. The antimicrobial effects of the bismuth moiety have not been shown to be important in the treatment of travelers' diarrhea, although they may play a role in the prophylactic use of this drug. BSS also directly binds to enterotoxins produced by *E. coli* and other diarrheal pathogens; however, the clinical significance of this effect in the treatment of diarrhea is not clear.

BSS is FDA approved for management of acute diarrhea, including travelers' diarrhea, in adults and children 12 years of age and older; it is not recommended for use in young children. BSS is also indicated for indigestion and as an adjuvant to antibiotics for treating *Helicobacter pylori*—associated peptic ulcer disease. Table 16–7 provides dosing information for BSS.

table
16–8 Selected Antidiarrheal Products

Loperamide Products	Primary Ingredients
Imodium A-D Caplets	Loperamide HCl 2 mg
Imodium EZ Chews (Tablets)	Loperamide HCl 2 mg
Imodium Advanced Caplets	Loperamide HCl 2 mg; simethicone 125 mg
Imodium Advanced Chewable Tablets	Loperamide HCl 2 mg; simethicone 125 mg
Imodium A-D Liquid	Loperamide HCl 1 mg/7.5 mL
Bismuth Subsalicylate Products	
Kaopectate Vanilla Flavor Liquid	Bismuth subsalicylate 262 mg/15 mL (contains 130 mg of salicylate)
Kaopectate Extra Strength Peppermint Flavor Liquid	Bismuth subsalicylate 525 mg/15 mL (contains 236 mg of salicylate)
Kaopectate Peppermint Flavor Liquid	Bismuth subsalicylate 262 mg/15 mL (contains 130 mg of salicylate)
Kaopectate Cherry Flavor Liquid	Bismuth subsalicylate 262 mg/15 mL (contains 130 mg of salicylate)
Kaopectate Antidiarrheal Caplets	Bismuth subsalicylate 262 mg (contains 99 mg of salicylate)
Maalox Total Relief Peppermint Flavor Liquid	Bismuth subsalicylate 525 mg/15 mL (contains 232 mg of salicylate)
Maalox Total Relief Strawberry Flavor Liquid	Bismuth subsalicylate 525 mg/15 mL (contains 232 mg of salicylate)
Pepto-Bismol Caplets	Bismuth subsalicylate 262 mg (contains 99 mg of salicylate)
Pepto-Bismol Cherry Liquid	Bismuth subsalicylate 262 mg/15 mL (contains 130 mg of salicylate)
Pepto-Bismol Cherry Chewable Tablets	Bismuth subsalicylate 262 mg (contains 99 mg of salicylate)
Pepto-Bismol Chewable Tablets	Bismuth subsalicylate 262 mg (contains 102 mg of salicylate)
Pepto-Bismol Original Liquid	Bismuth subsalicylate 262 mg/15 mL (contains 130 mg of salicylate)
Pepto-Bismol Maximum Strength Liquid	Bismuth subsalicylate 525 mg/15 mL (contains 236 mg of salicylate)
Pepto-Bismol With Instacool Peppermint Chewable Tablets	Bismuth subsalicylate 262 mg (contains 102 mg of salicylate)

Note: Pepto-Bismol adult formulations contain bismuth subsalicylate, but the products for children that contain calcium carbonate as the active ingredient are not listed.

BSS is available in several dosage forms; each contains various amounts of salicylate (Table 16–8). If a patient is taking aspirin or other salicylate-containing drugs, toxic levels of salicylate may be reached even if the patient follows dosing directions on the label for each medication.

Mild tinnitus, a dose-related side effect, may be associated with moderate-severe salicylate toxicity. If tinnitus occurs, the product should be discontinued and the patient referred for medical evaluation. Salicylates may cause adverse effects that are independent of the dose. Children and adolescents who have or are recovering from chicken pox or influenza are at risk of Reye's syndrome, a rare but serious illness associated with salicylates. These patients should not use BSS. However, Children's Pepto has been reformulated to contain calcium carbonate as the active ingredient. Unlike other forms of Pepto-Bismol, Children's Pepto Antacid is not associated with Reye's syndrome, but it is not labeled for treatment of diarrhea. In susceptible patients, salicylate-induced gout attacks have occurred. Patients who are sensitive to aspirin (i.e., experience asthmatic bronchospasm) should not use BSS.

Although the oral bioavailability of bismuth from BSS is poor (<1%), BSS has rarely been associated with bismuth-related neurotoxicity. Encephalopathy characterized by slow onset of tremors, postural instability, ataxia, myoclonus, poor concentration, confusion, memory impairment, seizures, visual and auditory hallucinations, psychosis, delirium, depression, and death can occur when bismuth concentrations in the blood exceed

50 mcg/L. Use of BSS in the recommended doses, even for several weeks, such as in prophylaxis for travelers' diarrhea, produces mean blood concentrations well below 50 mcg/L and does not result in bismuth-related neurotoxicity. However, AIDS patients with acute diarrhea may be at particular risk for bismuth encephalopathy, perhaps resulting from altered GI absorption; BSS should not be used in patients with AIDS.

Harmless black staining of stool (which should not be confused with melena) and darkening of the tongue occur in more than 10% of patients treated with BSS. Bismuth salts react with hydrogen sulfide produced by bacteria in the mouth and colon. The resulting compound, bismuth sulfide, imparts the black discoloration. It is easily removed from the surface of the tongue by brushing the tongue with a soft-bristled brush. It may also be treated by discontinuing the bismuth product.

Bismuth is radiopaque and may interfere with radiographic intestinal studies. BSS may interact adversely with a number of other drugs, particularly those that potentially interact with aspirin. The salicylate moiety can increase the risk of toxicity with warfarin, valproic acid, and methotrexate by significantly decreasing plasma protein binding of these drugs in vivo. Salicylate can also increase the plasma concentration of methotrexate by decreasing its renal clearance. The uricosuric effects of probenecid may be inhibited by the salicylate moiety. The bismuth moiety is a trivalent cation and may decrease absorption of other medications, such as tetracycline and quinolone antibiotics, by forming complexes with them in the GI tract. Solid dosage forms of BSS contain calcium carbonate, which may enhance this interaction. When fluoroquinolones are used to treat travelers' diarrhea, the patient should be instructed to discontinue BSS.

Digestive Enzymes

For patients with lactase deficiency who are intolerant of milk products, lactase enzyme preparations (Table 16–9) may be taken with milk or other dairy products to prevent osmotic diarrhea.

Product Selection Guidelines

Table 16–7 provides a quick reference for recommended dosages and durations of therapy for selected antidiarrheal agents. Tables 16–8 and 16–9 list dosage forms and primary ingredients of selected trade-name products.

In May 2011, FDA released final guidance on nonprescription liquid products that include any type of measuring device, such as the dropper packaged with lactase drops.[29] Other devices mentioned include cups, syringes, and spoons. The key points of the guidance are the recommendations that:

- A dosing device be included with all oral liquid nonprescription products
- The device be calibrated to the dose recommended in the product directions
- The device be used only with the product in which it is packaged
- The markings remain visible even when the liquid is in the device

Special Populations

For young children (5 years and younger), self-treatment is limited to treating dehydration with ORS; antidiarrheal medications are not recommended. If diarrhea persists despite oral rehydration therapy, a primary care provider or pediatrician must be consulted.

table

16–9 Selected Lactase Enzyme Products

Trade Name	Primary Ingredient
Lactaid Caplets	Lactase enzyme 3000 FCC units[a]/caplet
Lactaid Fast Act Caplets	Lactase enzyme 9000 FCC units[a]/caplet
Lactaid Fast Act Chewable Tablets	Lactase enzyme 9000 FCC units[a]/tablet
Lacteez Drops	Lactase enzyme 80 FCCLU[b]/5 drops
Lactrase Capsules	Lactase enzyme 250 mg/capsule

[a] FCC units are standardized units established by the Food Chemicals Codex (FCC), a compendium of internationally recognized standards for purity and identity of food ingredients published by the United States Pharmacopeia.

[b] FCCLU = FCC lactase units.

Elderly patients (65 years and older) should be strongly cautioned against self-treatment with antidiarrheal medications. Diarrhea in these patients is more likely to be severe or possibly fatal; therefore, these patients should be referred for medical evaluation.

Use of nonprescription antidiarrheals may be inappropriate during pregnancy; therefore, pregnant women should also be referred for medical evaluation before self-treating. Both loperamide and BSS are classified as Pregnancy Category C drugs. BSS-containing products are contraindicated during pregnancy because of concerns that the salicylate component may inhibit platelet function and, in the third trimester, cause premature closure of the fetal ductus arteriosus. Nursing women should generally avoid BSS.

Patient Factors and Preferences

Selection of antidiarrheal products for older children and adults should be based on factors such as the etiology of the diarrhea (if known), prominent symptoms, potential interactions with prescribed medications, and applicable contraindications. For example, BSS is suggested to be the preferred agent when vomiting is the predominant clinical symptom of acute gastroenteritis. BSS should not be used to treat diarrhea in immunocompromised patients (e.g., AIDS and transplant recipients) because they are at increased risk for bismuth encephalopathy. A patient's preference for a particular dosage form and products requiring fewer doses should also be considered.

Complementary Therapies

Convincing evidence suggests that probiotics, including several *Lactobacillus* species, *Bifidobacterium lactis,* and *Saccharomyces boulardii,* are effective in preventing and treating mild acute, uncomplicated diarrhea, especially rotavirus diarrhea in children.[30–32] (See Chapter 23 for discussion of probiotics.) Although the exact mechanisms underlying their effects are not clear, probiotics produce acids (e.g., lactic acid) that lower intestinal pH and suppress growth of pathogenic bacteria, enhance immune responses, produce antimicrobial substances, and compete with pathogenic bacteria for intestinal mucosal binding sites. Their role in moderate-severe diarrhea is not supported conclusively by available evidence.

Probiotics appear to be safe for most patients. Major side effects, such as *Lactobacillus* or *Saccharomyces* sepsis, occur only rarely. Elderly, critically ill, and immunocompromised patients and patients with severe bowel diseases are at risk for systemic infection from probiotic use. The Food and Agriculture Organization of the United Nations and WHO have recognized the benefits of probiotics in the prevention and treatment of acute diarrhea, and recent European evidence-based guidelines for management of acute gastroenteritis in children support the use of selected probiotics.[33,34] However, probiotics are not recognized as medications by FDA. Their classification as dietary supplements or components of functional foods limits the health claims that can be made, and they cannot be recommended for treatment or prevention of acute, uncomplicated diarrhea.

Compelling evidence also demonstrates that daily zinc supplementation reduces the duration, severity, and persistence of acute diarrhea in children younger than 5 years of age.[35–41] Most of the studies showing a benefit were conducted in malnourished children in developing countries where zinc deficiency is prevalent. Few studies have been conducted in developed countries; thus, the role of zinc supplementation in young children with diarrhea in developed countries is not yet defined. Zinc produces antidiarrheal effects by stimulating intestinal water and electrolyte absorption, preventing villous atrophy, and enhancing overall immunity, perhaps in part, through upregulation of T helper (Th1) immune responses, including macrophage activation and cell-mediated immunity. WHO and UNICEF recommend that children with acute diarrhea receive zinc (10 mg of elemental zinc/day for infants younger than 6 months; 20 mg of elemental zinc/day for older infants and children) for 10–14 days in addition to ORS.[23] Zinc supplementation in children with diarrhea is associated with an increased risk for vomiting.[37–40]

There is no evidence to substantiate the safety and effectiveness of herbal products and homeopathic remedies in the management of acute diarrheal diseases. Therefore, their use cannot be recommended.

Assessment of Diarrhea: A Case-Based Approach

To evaluate a patient with diarrhea, the health care provider differentiates symptoms and makes clinical judgments. This triage function is based on the patient's responses to questions designed to help determine the cause of the specific signs and symptoms, their characteristics, and their severity (Tables 16–1 and 16–3). The provider should therefore ask the patient about vomiting, high and/or prolonged fever, and other symptoms to determine the patient's susceptibility to complications. Persistent or chronic diarrhea precludes self-treatment and requires immediate medical referral, as does the presence of high fever (greater than 102.2°F [39°C]), protracted vomiting, abdominal pain in patients older than 50 years, or blood or mucus in the stool. If none of these significant findings is present, the degree of dehydration should be assessed (Table 16–3); the provider should ask about the nature and amount of fluid intake. Severity of dehydration can be accurately assessed by evaluating changes in body weight. For example, in children, mild dehydration is associated with a 3%–5% loss of body weight, whereas severe dehydration is associated with a loss of more than 9%. However, the patient (or the parent) seldom knows the exact premorbid weight for comparison, and distinguishing between mild and moderate dehydration may be difficult.

The initial assessment of a pediatric patient should also seek to determine plausible causes of the symptoms. The common symptoms of acute gastroenteritis (e.g., vomiting, loose stools, and fever) are nonspecific findings associated with many other childhood diseases (e.g., acute otitis media, bacterial sepsis, meningitis, pneumonia, and urinary tract infections). This information is a key factor in recommending a proper course of action, which may include self-treatment or referral for medical evaluation. A complete medication history must be assessed before a product is selected.

Physical assessment of a patient with complaints of diarrhea can provide information useful in assessing the severity of the diarrhea (Table 16–3). Checking skin turgor and moistness of oral mucous membranes will help determine the degree of dehydration. Vital signs (e.g., pulse, temperature, respiration, and blood pressure) are important indicators of illness severity and should be routinely measured. Symptoms of moderate-severe dehydration may include postural (orthostatic) hypotension, defined as a drop in the systolic and/or diastolic pressure of greater than 15–20 mm Hg when a patient moves from a supine to an upright position. Normally, the diastolic pressure remains the same or increases slightly and the systolic pressure drops slightly on rising. If the blood pressure drops, the pulse should be checked simultaneously; the pulse rate should increase as blood pressure drops. Failure of the pulse to rise suggests that the problem is neurogenic (e.g., diabetic patients with peripheral neuropathy) or that the patient may be taking a beta blocker. The presence of orthostatic hypotension suggests that the patient has lost 1 liter or more of vascular volume, and referral for medical care is necessary.

Cases 16–1 and 16–2 provide examples of assessment of patients with diarrhea.

Patient Counseling for Diarrhea

Patients with diarrhea may focus on the need for a nonprescription medication to stop the frequent bowel movements. The health care provider should remind them that most episodes of acute diarrhea stop after 48 hours and that preventing dehydration is the most important component of treatment. Counseling on the two-step treatment of dehydration and the need for dietary management should follow. For infants and children, educating parents and caregivers on the appropriate use of an ORS (including appropriate volumes to administer, rates of administration, and use in vomiting) and of dietary management is very important. For patient safety reasons, premixed solutions are preferred. If dry powder ORS is selected, however, the provider should give parents (or caregivers) explicit directions for mixing and verify that they understand the directions. For families with infants, the Centers for Disease Control and Prevention recommends a home supply of ORS because its early administration at home is vital if hospitalization is to be avoided. If travelers are using ORS dry powder in developing countries, potable water should be used to reconstitute the powder.

If an antidiarrheal product is recommended:

- Review label instructions with the patient or caregiver.
- Calculate an appropriate dosage on the basis of the patient's age and weight, and emphasize the maximum number of doses that can be taken in 24 hours.
- Explain potential drug interactions, side effects, contraindications, and the maximum duration of treatment before the patient should seek medical help.

The box Patient Education for Diarrhea contains specific information to provide patients.

Evaluation of Patient Outcomes for Diarrhea

Many patients have mild-moderate diarrhea that is generally self-limiting within 48 hours. Mild-moderate diarrhea is managed with oral rehydration therapy, symptomatic drug therapy, and dietary measures. The patient should be monitored for dehydration by measuring body weight, vital signs, and mental alertness. With effective symptomatic treatment, the patient can expect reduced stool frequency and normal consistency of stools, as well as a reduction in generalized symptoms such as lethargy and abdominal pain. As the diarrhea resolves, the patient's appetite will return to normal and the patient can return to a regular diet.

case

16-1

Relevant Evaluation Criteria	Scenario/Model Outcome

Information Gathering

1. Gather essential information about the patient's symptoms and medical history, including:

   a. description of symptom(s) (i.e., nature, onset, duration, severity, associated symptoms)

The patient describes acute onset diarrhea that started about 36 hours ago. Since it started, she has had 3–4 loose stools per day. She complains of mild-moderate abdominal cramping and 1 episode of vomiting, but has no other relevant signs or symptoms. She remarks, "This diarrhea is exhausting. I feel like it's taken a lot out of me."

   b. description of any factors that seem to precipitate, exacerbate, and/or relieve the patient's symptom(s)

None noted.

   c. description of the patient's efforts to relieve the symptoms

None. She tells you, "I thought it would get better by itself, but it hasn't."

   d. patient's identity

Marjorie Lewis

   e. age, sex, height, and weight

36 years old, female, 5 ft 2 in., 180 lb

   f. patient's occupation

Social worker

   g. patient's dietary habits

She eats a well-balanced diet, although she likes dessert; drinks wine and beer several times weekly.

   h. patient's sleep habits

Sleeps 5–6 hours nightly.

   i. concurrent medical conditions, prescription and nonprescription medications, and dietary supplements

Migraine headaches: sumatriptan 25 mg as needed; back pain: ibuprofen 400 mg as needed

   j. allergies

NKA

   k. history of other adverse reactions to medications

None

   l. other (describe) _____

Assessment and Triage

2. Differentiate patient's signs/symptoms and correctly identify the patient's primary problem(s) (Table 16–1).

Patient appears to have acute diarrhea, most likely of viral etiology.

3. Identify exclusions for self-treatment (Figure 16–1).

None

4. Formulate a comprehensive list of therapeutic alternatives for the primary problem to determine if triage to a health care provider is required, and share this information with the patient or caregiver.

Options include:

(1) Refer Marjorie to an appropriate health care provider.

(2) Recommend self-care with a nonprescription antidiarrheal product, such as loperamide, and nondrug measures, such as ORS.

(3) Recommend self-care with a nonprescription antidiarrheal product, such as loperamide, and nondrug measures, like ORS, until patient can see an appropriate health care provider.

(4) Take no action.

Plan

5. Select an optimal therapeutic alternative to address the patient's problem, taking into account patient preferences.

Patient has minimal to no dehydration and no exclusions for self-care. It is appropriate to recommend self-care with a nonprescription antidiarrheal product.

6. Describe the recommended therapeutic approach to the patient or caregiver.

"Loperamide is the preferred treatment for symptomatic relief of your diarrhea. You may continue your regular diet during treatment, but you should increase your intake of your usual fluids to prevent dehydration."

7. Explain to the patient or caregiver the rationale for selecting the recommended therapeutic approach from the considered therapeutic alternatives.

"Nonprescription antidiarrheal products are safe and effective in managing symptoms of acute diarrhea when no fever or signs of serious infection are present."

Relevant Evaluation Criteria	Scenario/Model Outcome
Patient Education	
8. When recommending self-care with nonprescription medications and/or nondrug therapy, convey accurate information to the patient or caregiver.	
a. appropriate dose and frequency of administration	See the box Patient Education for Diarrhea.
b. maximum number of days the therapy should be employed	See the box Patient Education for Diarrhea.
c. product administration procedures	See the box Patient Education for Diarrhea.
d. expected time to onset of relief	Onset of effect is 1–3 hours.
e. degree of relief that can be reasonably expected	No unformed stools within 48–72 hours of starting loperamide
f. most common side effects	See the box Patient Education for Diarrhea.
g. side effects that warrant medical intervention should they occur	See the box Patient Education for Diarrhea.
h. patient options in the event that condition worsens or persists	See the box Patient Education for Diarrhea.
i. product storage requirements	Store in a cool, dry place out of children's reach.
j. specific nondrug measures	See the box Patient Education for Diarrhea.
Solicit follow-up questions from the patient or caregiver.	"May I use a sports drink to keep from getting dehydrated?"
Answer the patient's or caregiver's questions.	"Yes, sports drinks can be used to help prevent dehydration in mild diarrhea, as long as you also eat something salty, like pretzels, along with them to help maintain your sodium levels, too. You could also use Pedialyte or a similar product."
Evaluation of Patient Outcome	
9. Assess patient outcome.	Contact the patient in a day or two to evaluate the response to your recommendations.

Relevant Evaluation Criteria	Scenario/Model Outcome
Information Gathering	
1. Gather essential information about the patient's symptoms and medical history, including:	
a. description of symptom(s) (i.e., nature, onset, duration, severity, associated symptoms)	The patient describes sudden onset of diarrhea with severe abdominal cramps that awakened him from sleep at about 3 am this morning. Since then, he has experienced 3 episodes of loose, watery stools in the last 6 hours and notes that his last stool looked as if it contained some blood. He also complains of lightheadedness and becomes somewhat dizzy on standing. He denies fever, but says that at times, he feels his heart beating faster.
b. description of any factors that seem to precipitate, exacerbate, and/or relieve the patient's symptom(s)	None noted.
c. description of the patient's efforts to relieve the symptoms	The patient has not tried anything to relieve his symptoms.
d. patient's identity	Andrew Mitchell
e. age, sex, height, and weight	37 years old, male, 5 ft 11 in., 195 lb
f. patient's occupation	Businessman/sales executive
g. patient's dietary habits	Eats a well-balanced diet.
h. patient's sleep habits	Sleeps 6–7 hours nightly.

case
16–2 *continued*

Relevant Evaluation Criteria	Scenario/Model Outcome
i. concurrent medical conditions, prescription and nonprescription medications, and dietary supplements	Hypertension: atenolol 50 mg daily, amlodipine 10 mg daily, hydrochlorothiazide 25 mg daily. Hyperlipidemia: simvastatin 20 mg daily. Cardiac prophylaxis: aspirin 81 mg daily.
j. allergies	Penicillin: anaphylaxis
k. history of other adverse reactions to medications	None
l. other (describe) _____	Not applicable

Assessment and Triage

2. Differentiate patient's signs/symptoms and correctly identify the patient's primary problem(s) (Table 16–1).	Patient is experiencing acute infectious diarrhea, most likely of bacterial etiology.
3. Identify exclusions for self-treatment (see Figure 16–1).	Severe abdominal cramps, blood in the stool
4. Formulate a comprehensive list of therapeutic alternatives for the primary problem to determine if triage to a health care provider is required, and share this information with the patient or caregiver.	Options include: (1) Refer patient to an appropriate health care provider. (2) Recommend self-care with a nonprescription antidiarrheal product, such as bismuth subsalicylate, and nondrug measures, like ORS. (3) Recommend self-care with a nonprescription antidiarrheal product, such as bismuth subsalicylate, and nondrug measures, such as ORS, until patient can see an appropriate health care provider. (4) Take no action.

Plan

5. Select an optimal therapeutic alternative to address the patient's problem, taking into account patient preferences.	Refer patient to an appropriate health care provider, urgent care center, or emergency department for evaluation and treatment.
6. Describe the recommended therapeutic approach to the patient or caregiver.	"You need to seek urgent medical care from your primary care provider, urgent care center, or emergency department right away."
7. Explain to the patient or caregiver the rationale for selecting the recommended therapeutic approach from the considered therapeutic alternatives.	"Your symptoms suggest that your condition is serious. You probably have a bacterial infection that requires prescription antibiotics. No nonprescription remedies are available to treat bloody diarrhea."

Patient Education

8. When recommending self-care with nonprescription medications and/or nondrug therapy, convey accurate information to the patient or caregiver.	Criterion does not apply in this case.
Solicit follow-up questions from the patient or caregiver.	"Can I take some Pepto-Bismol before I go to the emergency department?"
Answer the patient's or caregiver's questions.	"No. If you have a bacterial infection, Pepto-Bismol may actually make your condition worse. You should not take any nonprescription medicine while seeking medical attention."

Evaluation of Patient Outcome

9. Assess patient outcome.	Ask patient to call after seeking medical attention to update you on his condition, or obtain his phone number and call him in a few days.

Key: ORS = Oral rehydration solution.

The primary objective of self-treatment is to prevent excessive fluid and electrolyte losses. For most patients, carefully following product instructions and the self-care measures listed here will help ensure optimal outcomes.

Nondrug Measures

Infants and Children 6 Months to 5 Years

- For mild-moderate diarrhea, indicated by three to five unformed bowel movements per day, give the child or infant an oral rehydration solution (ORS) at a volume of 50–100 mL/kg of body weight over 2–4 hours to replace the fluid deficit. Give additional ORS to replace ongoing losses. Continue to give the solution for the next 4–6 hours or until the child is rehydrated.
- If the child is vomiting, give 1 teaspoon of ORS every few minutes.
- If the child is not dehydrated, give 10 mL/kg or ½–1 cup of the ORS for each bowel movement, or 2 mL/kg for each episode of vomiting. As an alternative, to replace ongoing fluid losses, children weighing less than 10 kg should be given 60–120 mL of ORS for each episode of vomiting or diarrheal stool, and children weighing more than 10 kg should be given 120–240 mL for each episode of vomiting or diarrheal stool.
- After the child is rehydrated, reintroduce food appropriate for the child's age, while also administering an ORS as maintenance therapy.
- If breast-feeding an infant with diarrhea, continue the breast-feeding. If the infant is bottle-fed, consult your primary care provider or pediatrician about replacing a milk-based formula with a lactose-free formula.
- Give children complex carbohydrate–rich foods, yogurt, lean meats, fruits, and vegetables. Do not give them fatty foods or sugary foods. Sugary foods can cause osmotic diarrhea.
- Do not withhold food for more than 24 hours.

Adults and Children Older Than 5 Years

- For mild-moderate dehydration, indicated by a 3%–9% drop in body weight or three to five unformed stools per day, drink 2–4 liters of an ORS over 4 hours.
- If not dehydrated, drink ½–1 cup of ORS or fluids after each unformed bowel movement.
- If no medical conditions exist, sports drinks (with salty crackers, etc.), diluted juices, soups, and broths may be consumed until the diarrhea stops.
- Do not withhold food for more than 24 hours.

Nonprescription Medications

- See Table 16–7 for dosages of loperamide and bismuth subsalicylate.

Loperamide

- Note that loperamide can cause dizziness and constipation.
- Do not give this agent to children 2 years of age and younger. Loperamide is not recommended for children younger than 6 years, except under the supervision of a primary care provider or pediatrician.
- If loperamide is not effective in treating your diarrhea (if no clinical improvement is observed in 48 hours), check with your primary care provider or pharmacist about using a different nonprescription medication. You may have a bacterial diarrhea or pseudomembranous colitis; these conditions require specific antibiotic therapy that loperamide cannot treat.

Bismuth Subsalicylate

- Note that bismuth subsalicylate can cause a dark discoloration of the tongue and stool.
- Do not take this medication if you are taking tetracyclines, quinolones, or medicines for gout (uricosurics).
- Do not give this medication to children younger than 12 years.
- Do not give this medication to children or adolescents who have or are recovering from influenza or chicken pox. Reye's syndrome, a rare but serious condition, could occur.
- Do not give this medication to patients with AIDS.
- Do not take this medication if you are sensitive to aspirin, have a history of gastrointestinal bleeding, or have a history of problems with blood coagulation.

When to Seek Medical Attention

- If the diarrhea has not resolved after 72 hours of initial treatment, see your primary care provider.
- Monitor for excessive number of bowel movements, signs of dehydration, high fever, or blood in the stool. If any of these complications are present, discontinue bismuth subsalicylate and consult your primary care provider.

Medical referral is necessary if any of the following signs and symptoms occur before or during treatment: high fever, worsening illness, bloody or mucoid stools, diarrhea continuing beyond 48 hours, or signs of worsening dehydration (e.g., low blood pressure, rapid pulse, or mental confusion). Also, medical referral is advised for infants, young children, frail patients of advanced age, pregnant patients, and patients with chronic illness at risk from secondary complications (e.g., diabetes mellitus).

Key Points for Diarrhea

➤ Self-treatment of diarrhea should be limited to patients with mild-moderate acute diarrhea who have minimal, mild, or moderate dehydration. Patients who appear volume depleted, weak, dizzy, febrile (temperature > 102.2°F), or hypotensive should be referred for evaluation.

➤ ORS is the mainstay of therapy and should be used to rehydrate patients with minimal or mild-moderate dehydration.

➤ Rehydration should be performed rapidly (i.e., within 3–4 hours). Additional ORS should be given to maintain hydration and replace ongoing fluid losses resulting from diarrheal stools and/or vomiting (Figures 16–1 and 16–2).

➤ Patients or their caregivers should be instructed how to prepare and administer an ORS.

➤ Older children and adults may use sports drinks instead of an ORS if additional sources of sodium (e.g., crackers and pretzels) are used concomitantly.

➤ An age-appropriate, unrestricted diet should be initiated as soon as the patient is rehydrated. Food should be withheld for no more than 24 hours.

➤ Loperamide and BSS may be used to help control acute diarrhea in carefully selected patients.

➤ Antibiotic therapy is generally not indicated for patients with acute diarrhea unless it is travelers' diarrhea.

REFERENCES

1. Farthing M, Salam MA, Lindberg G, et al. Acute diarrhea in adults and children: a global perspective. *J Clin Gastroenterol.* 2013;47(1): 12–20.

2. Scallan E, Griccin PM, Angulo FJ, et al. Foodborne illness acquired in the United States—unspecified agents. *Emerg Infect Dis.* 2011;17(1):16–22.

3. Jones TF, McMillian MB, Scallan E, et al. A population-based estimate of the substantial burden of diarrhoeal disease in the United States; Food-Net, 1996–2003. *Epidemiol Infect.* 2007;135(2):293–301.

4. Patel MM, Hall AJ, Vinje J, et al. Noroviruses: a comprehensive review. *J Clin Virol.* 2009;44(1):1–8.

5. Patel MM, Widdowson M, Glass RI, et al. Systematic literature review of role of noroviruses in sporadic gastroenteritis. *Emerg Infect Dis.* 2008; 14(8):1224–231.

6. Cortese MM, Parashar UD. Prevention of rotavirus gastroenteritis among infants and children: recommendations of the Advisory Committee on Immunization Practices (ACIP). *MMWR Recomm Rep.* 2009; 58(RR-2):1–25.

7. Cortese MM, Tate JE, Simonsen L, et al. Reduction in gastroenteritis in United States children and correlation with early rotavirus vaccine uptake from national medical claims databases. *Pediatr Infect Dis J.* 2010; 29(6):489–94.

8. Flores AR, Szilagyi PG, Auinger P, et al. Estimated burden of rotavirus-associated diarrhea in ambulatory settings in the United States. *Pediatrics.* 2010;125(2):e191–8.

9. Cardemil CV, Cortese MM, Medina-Marion A, et al. Two rotavirus outbreaks caused by genotype G2P[4] at large retirement communities. *Ann Intern Med.* 2012;157(9):621–31.

10. Breese JS, Marcys R, Venezia RA, et al. The etiology of severe acute gastroenteritis among adults visiting emergency departments in the United States. *J Infect Dis.* 2012;205(9):1374–81.

11. Anderson EJ, Katz BZ, Polin JA, et al. Rotavirus in adults requiring hospitalization. *J Infect.* 2012;64(1):89–95.

12. Marcos LA, DuPont HL. Advances in defining etiology and new therapeutic approaches in acute diarrhea. *J Infect.* 2007;55(5):385–93.

13. Kayman T, Abay S, Hizlisoy H, et al. Emerging pathogen *Arcobacter* spp. in acute gastroenteritis: molecular identification, antibiotic susceptibilities and genotyping of the isolated arcobacters. *J Medical Microbiol.* 2012; 61:1439–44.

14. Venkatasubramanian J, Rao MC, Sellin JH. Intestinal electrolyte absorption and secretion. In: Feldman M, Friedman LS, Brandt LJ, eds. *Sleisenger and Fordtran's Gastrointestinal and Liver Disease.* 9th ed. Vol. 2. New York, NY: Elsevier; 2010:1675–1694.

15. Hodges K, Gill R. Infectious diarrhea: cellular and molecular mechanisms. *Gut Microbes.* 2010;1(1):4–21.

16. DuPont HL. Gastrointestinal infections and the development of irritable bowel syndrome. *Curr Opin Infect Dis.* 2011;24(5):503–8.

17. Scallan E, Hoekstra RM, Angulo FJ, et al. Foodborne illness acquired in the United States—major pathogens. *Emerg Infect Dis.* 2011;17(1):7–15.

18. Centers for Disease Control and Prevention. CDC Estimates of foodborne illness in the United States. Accessed at http://www.cdc.gov/foodborneburden/2011-foodborne-estimates.html, July 11, 2014.

19. Shah N, DuPont HL, Ramsey DJ. Global etiology of travelers' diarrhea: systematic review from 1973 to the present. *Am J Trop Med Hyg.* 2009; 80(4):609–14.

20. DuPont HL. Systematic review: the epidemiology and clinical features of travellers' diarrhoea. *Alimen Pharmacol Ther.* 2009;30(3):187–96.

21. Pareded-Paredes M, Flores-Figueroa J, DuPont HL. Advances in the treatment of travelers' diarrhea. *Curr Gastroenterol Rep.* 2011;13(5):402–7.

22. King CK, Glass R, Bresee JS, et al. Managing acute gastroenteritis among children: oral rehydration, maintenance, and nutritional therapy. *MMWR Morb Mortal Wkly Rep.* 2003;52(RR-16):1–16.

23. World Health Organization, United Nations Children's Fund. WHO/UNICEF joint statement: clinical management of acute diarrhoea. Accessed at http://www.unicef.org/publications/files/ENAcute_Diarrhoea_reprint.pdf, February 6, 2013.

24. Centers for Disease Control and Prevention. Traveler's diarrhea. Accessed at http://www.cdc.gov/nczved/divisions/dfbmd/diseases/travelers_diarrhea/, February 6, 2013.

25. DuPont HL, Ericsson CD, Farthing MJG, et al. Expert review of the evidence base for prevention of travelers' diarrhea. *J Travel Med.* 2009; 16(3):149–60.

26. Vandenbossche J, Huisman M, Xu Y, et al. Loperamide and P-glycoprotein inhibition: assessment of the clinical relevance. *J Pharm Pharmacol.* 2010; 62(4):401–12.

27. Regnard C, Twycross R, Mihalyo M, et al. Loperamide. *J Pain Symptom Manage.* 2011;42(2):319–23.

28. Mikus G, Schmidt L, Burhenne J, et al. Reduction of saquinavir exposure by coadministration of loperamide. *Clin Pharmacokinet.* 2004;43(14): 1015–24.

29. U.S. Food and Drug Administration. FDA issues final guidance for liquid OTC drug products with dispensing devices [press release]. May 4, 2011. Accessed at http://www.fda.gov/NewsEvents/Newsroom/Press Announcements/ucm254029.htm, February 6, 2013.

30. Goldin BR, Gorbach SL. Clinical indications for probiotics: an overview. *Clin Infect Dis.* 2008;46(suppl 2):S96–100.

31. Gaundalini S. Probiotics for children with diarrhea: an update. *J Clin Gastroenterol.* 2008;42(suppl 2):S53–7.

32. Szajewska H, Skorka A, Dylag M. Meta-analysis: *Saccharomyces boulardii* for treating acute diarrhea in children. *Aliment Pharmacol Ther.* 2007;25(3): 257–64.

33. Food and Agriculture Organization of the United Nations, World Health Organization. Health and nutritional properties of probiotics in food including powder milk with live lactic acid bacteria, a joint FAO/WHO expert consultation. Cordoba, Argentina, 1 - 4 October 2001. Accessed at http://www.fao.org/documents/pub_dett.asp?lang=en&pub_id=61756, September 13, 2014.

34. Guarino A, Albano F, Ashkenazi S, et al. European Society for Paediatric Gastroenterology, Hepatology, and Nutrition/European Society for Paediatric Infectious Diseases evidence-based guidelines for the management of acute gastroenteritis in children in Europe. *J Pediatr Gastroenterol Nutr.* 2008;46(suppl 2):S81–122.

35. Patel A, Mamtani M, Dibley MJ, et al. Therapeutic value of zinc supplementation in acute and persistent diarrhea: a systematic review. *PLoS One.* 2010;5(4):e10386.

36. Patro B, Golicki D, Szajewska H. Meta-analysis: zinc supplementation for acute gastroenteritis in children. *Aliment Pharmacol Ther.* 2008;28(6):713–23.

37. Lukacik M, Thomas RL, Aranda JV. A meta-analysis of the effects of oral zinc in the treatment of acute and persistent diarrhea. *Pediatrics.* 2008; 121(2):326–36.

38. Aggarwal R, Sentz J, Miller MA. Role of zinc administration in prevention of childhood diarrhea and respiratory illnesses: a meta-analysis. *Pediatrics.* 2007;119(6):1120–30.

39. Haider BA, Bhutta ZA. The effect of therapeutic zinc supplementation among young children with selected infections: a review of the evidence. *Food Nutr Bull.* 2009;30(suppl 1):S41–59.

40. Lazzerini M, Ronfani L. Oral zinc for treating diarrhea in children. *Cochrane Database Syst Rev.* June 13, 2012; 6:CD005436. doi: 10.1002/14651858. CD005436.pub3.

41. Passariello A, Terrin G, De Marco G, et al. Efficacy of a new hypotonic oral rehydration solution containing zinc and prebiotics in the treatment of childhood acute diarrhea: a randomized controlled trial. *J Pediatr.* 2011;158(2)288–92.

42. Sanford Guide to Antimicrobial Therapy. Sanford Guide Web Edition 2. Antimicrobial Therapy, Inc. 2013. Accessed at http://webedition.sanford guide.com/, March 11, 2013.

43. American Academy of Pediatrics. AAP 2012 Red Book Online: Report of the Committee on Infectious Diseases. Accessed at http://aapredbook. aappublications.org/, March 11, 2013.

ANORECTAL DISORDERS

Juliana Chan

Anorectal disorders involve the perianal area, anal canal, and lower rectum. Many signs and symptoms associated with hemorrhoids may be related to nonhemorrhoidal anorectal disorders.[1] Hemorrhoids often are self-treated, whereas other anorectal disorders may require immediate medical attention. A number of products are available for the symptomatic treatment of anorectal disorders. Hemorrhoidal complaints are a medical burden for the health care system, with an estimated 1 million ambulatory care visits and nearly 2 million prescriptions filled for anorectal products.[2–4] Despite a significant decrease in hospitalizations over the past several decades, anorectal disorders ranked as the 13th most common digestive disease for ambulatory care visits.[4] More than 10 million people in the United States are estimated to have hemorrhoids, and 75% of those individuals are estimated to be older than 45 years.[2,5] However, the true prevalence of hemorrhoids is unknown because people often do not seek medical attention.[2,4] The diagnosis of hemorrhoids is equal in men and women and increases with advancing age.[2] In the United States, age-adjusted hospitalization rates are higher in blacks when compared to whites.[2] Although epidemiologic data are lacking, approximately 25%–35% of the general population (and up to 85% of women of childbearing age) have some degree of pain and discomfort that is associated with hemorrhoids.[6]

Pathophysiology of Anorectal Area

Anorectal disorders occur in the perianal area (the portion of the skin immediately surrounding the anus), the anal canal, and the lower portion of the rectum (Figure 17–1). The anal canal is about 2.5–5 cm long and connects the rectum with the outside of the body.[7] Two different types of epithelium line the anal canal; their junction is defined by the dentate line (also known as the pectinate line). The dentate line divides squamous epithelium from columnar epithelium, thus delineating where sensory pain fibers are located in the anal canal. Anorectal disorders occurring below the dentate line may be associated with pain, whereas disorders above the line rarely cause any discomfort.[7] The area proximal to the dentate line contains several longitudinal folds known as the columns of Morgagni. In between and next to these columns are small pockets or crypts containing ducts and glands that may become obstructed and cause infections (e.g., abscesses and fistulas).[8]

The external anal sphincter is a voluntary muscle located at the bottom of the anal canal that remains closed under normal conditions to prevent involuntary passage of feces. The internal sphincter is an involuntary muscle innervated by the autonomic nervous system. When the sphincters are relaxed, defecation occurs. In healthy individuals, skin covering the anal canal serves as a barrier against absorption of substances into the body. If that protective barrier breaks, then the absorptive character of the anal skin may be altered, diminishing the skin's protective capabilities.

The rectum, which lies above the anal canal, is about 12–18 cm long and is the terminal portion of the large intestine.[7] The highly vascular rectal mucosa is lined with a semipermeable membrane to protect the body from fecal bacteria. Three hemorrhoidal arteries and their accompanying veins are the most prominent parts of the vasculature. The arteries and veins lying above the dentate line are referred to as internal and those below as external. Blood returns to the heart through the hemorrhoidal veins; therefore, rectal medications may be absorbed and enter the systemic circulation without passing through the liver.[7]

Hemorrhoids are large, bulging, symptomatic conglomerates of hemorrhoidal vessels, supporting tissues, and overlying mucous membranes in the anorectal region.[9] Hemorrhoids are believed to develop as a result of inflammation of vascular cushions. The cushions (located circumferentially around the anal canal, above the dentate line) contain blood vessels, smooth muscle, and supportive connective tissue that project into the lumen and cause a downward pressure during defecation. With increasing age or poor bowel habits (e.g., prolonged sitting and straining at defecation), muscle fibers may weaken and cause vascular cushions to slide, become congested, bleed, and eventually protrude.[9,10] Downward pressure during defecation and a high resting anal pressure are common in the development of hemorrhoids.

Internal hemorrhoids originate from the superior hemorrhoidal vein and are located above the dentate line, an area that is covered with columnar epithelium and lacks sensory fibers (Figure 17–1).[9,10] Hemorrhoids are graded by severity of prolapse into the anal canal using a degree system[10]:

■ First-degree hemorrhoids are enlarged but do not prolapse into the anal canal.
■ Second-degree hemorrhoids protrude into the anal canal and return spontaneously on defecation.
■ Third-degree hemorrhoids protrude into the anal canal on defecation but can be returned to their original position manually.
■ Fourth-degree hemorrhoids are permanently prolapsed and cannot be reintroduced into the anus.

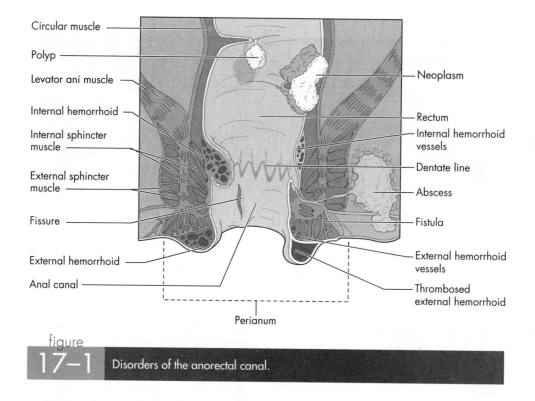

Circular muscle

Polyp

Levator ani muscle

Internal hemorrhoid

Internal sphincter muscle

External sphincter muscle

Fissure

External hemorrhoid

Anal canal

Neoplasm

Rectum

Internal hemorrhoid vessels

Dentate line

Abscess

Fistula

External hemorrhoid vessels

Thrombosed external hemorrhoid

Perianum

figure

17–1   Disorders of the anorectal canal.

External hemorrhoids develop from the inferior hemorrhoidal vein and originate below the dentate line, which is covered with squamous epithelium (Figure 17–1).[9,10] These hemorrhoids are visible as bluish lumps at the external or distal boundary of the anal canal (known as the anal verge). The blue color may be caused by thrombosed blood vessels, which cause symptoms ranging from minimal discomfort to severe pain.[10]

Nonhemorrhoidal Anorectal Disorders

Potentially serious nonhemorrhoidal anorectal disorders (e.g., abscesses, fistulas, fissures, neoplasms, polyps, and pruritus ani) may present as hemorrhoid-like symptoms; these disorders should not be self-treated but referred for immediate medical evaluation (Table 17–1).[8,11]

Clinical Presentation of Anorectal Disorders

The Food and Drug Administration (FDA) Advisory Review Panel identified signs and symptoms for which a nonprescription anorectal product is indicated.[12] These symptoms include itching, discomfort, irritation, burning, soreness, inflammation, pain, dry anal tissue, and swelling in the perianal area.[12] In contrast, abdominal pain, bleeding, seepage, change in bowel patterns, prolapse, and thrombosis may indicate a more serious condition requiring immediate medical attention (Table 17–2).[9,11,13]

Treatment of Anorectal Disorders
Treatment Goals

The primary goal of treatment is to maintain soft stools to prevent straining while having a bowel movement.[9,14] Additional goals for patients with symptoms associated with anorectal disorders are to (1) alleviate and maintain remission of anorectal symptoms and (2) prevent complications.

General Treatment Approach

Figure 17–2 presents an algorithm for treating minor anorectal symptoms and lists exclusions for self-treatment. If the complaint is self-treatable, the clinician may recommend nonpharmacologic measures and an OTC agent to treat the symptoms. Patients should be advised to maintain adequate fluid intake and a well-balanced high-fiber diet. Practicing good perianal hygiene and avoiding prolonged sitting on the toilet may also minimize anorectal symptoms. Table 17–3 outlines guidelines for applying anorectal products.[8,9,15]

Nonpharmacologic Therapy

Nondrug measures for treating anorectal disorders include dietary modifications, surgical interventions, and nonoperative methods.[3,9] Patients diagnosed with or suspected of having hemorrhoids should avoid lifting heavy objects, discontinue foods that aggravate symptoms (e.g., alcohol, caffeinated beverages, citrus, and spicy foods), and increase dietary fiber.[14] Nonsteroidal anti-inflammatory drugs or aspirin may promote bleeding and therefore should be avoided.

Dietary fiber softens stool and may prevent further irritation of symptomatic hemorrhoids and anorectal complaints.

table
17–1 Nonhemorrhoidal Anorectal Disorders

Disorder	Definition	Common Signs and Symptoms	Comments
Anal abscess	Collection of pus causing an obstruction of the anal glands, resulting in a bacterial infection	Pain, perirectal swelling, discharge, fever, or chills; pain worsens with sitting and defecation	Possible life-threatening sepsis if not identified and treated promptly
Anal fistula (or groove)	Abnormal internal opening that connects with an external opening (i.e., tube-like appearance between the rectum and anus)	Chronic, persistent drainage; pain; possible bleeding on defecation; perianal itching; stool seeping through external opening	Surgical repair required
Anal fissure	Slit-like ulcer in anal canal resulting from a traumatic tear during passage of stool or explosive diarrhea	Severe or burning pain during and after defecation, lasting several minutes to hours; anal spasms; blood may be seen on toilet tissue	Young, middle-aged individuals; equal in women and men
Anal neoplasms	Include a variety of histologic types classified as epidermoid carcinomas	Rare and usually asymptomatic in 25% of patients; bleeding; changes in bowel habits; anal discharge; anal mass; pain; pruritus; rash	Relatively uncommon, accounting for 1%–2% of all GI malignancies; most are curable, but poor prognosis with anorectal melanomas
Pruritus ani	Itching sensation localized in anorectal area	Persistent itching, scratching in perianal region; more bothersome at bedtime or when patient is not preoccupied	More common in men

Source: References 7, 8, 11, and 17.

A meta-analysis confirmed that initiating fiber therapy in subjects with first- or second-degree hemorrhoids improves bleeding and overall symptomatic relief.[14,16] Increasing fiber intake to at least 20–30 grams daily may permit the passage of softer stools, thus reducing or preventing irritation and straining at defecation.[8,17] Increased fiber intake should be introduced slowly and accompanied by increased fluid intake. If the amount of dietary fiber intake cannot be increased, fiber supplements such as psyllium or methylcellulose may be added (see Chapter 15).

Proper bowel habits should be encouraged, and avoiding urges to defecate should be discouraged because doing so may lead to constipation resulting in anorectal discomfort. Avoidance of sitting on the toilet for long periods of time reduces strain and decreases pressure on the hemorrhoidal vessels.[3,10,17] Proper hygiene of the anal area (e.g., cleaning the area regularly and after each bowel movement using mild, unscented soap and water, or using commercially available hygienic and lubricated wipes or pads) may relieve anorectal symptoms. Excessive scrubbing should be discouraged to minimize aggravation.[1] A measure often recommended to promote good anal hygiene is sitting in warm water (≤120°F [48.89°C]) in a bath tub or sitz bath (a small bath tub that fits over the toilet rim, available at pharmacies and medical supply vendors) for 10–20 minutes 2–4 times a day[3,8,9,18]; however, the exact therapeutic usefulness of this measure is still in question. A systematic review of randomized controlled trials found no evidence to support the use of sitz baths to relieve pain or assist in wound healing associated with anorectal disease.[18] Additionally, in a systematic review of four randomized controlled trials, evidence to support the use of sitz baths to relieve pain or assist in wound healing associated with anorectal disease was lacking.[19]

Large and prolapsed hemorrhoids often are treated surgically. The surgical procedure that involves excising one or more of the three hemorrhoidal masses is called a hemorrhoidectomy. Nonsurgical procedures treating hemorrhoids include injection of sclerosing agents, rubber band ligation, cryosurgery, electrocoagulation, infrared photocoagulation, and local anal hypothermia.[3,9,17]

Pharmacologic Therapy

Local anesthetics, vasoconstrictors, protectants, astringents, keratolytics, analgesics, anesthetics, antipruritics, and corticosteroids are commonly used to relieve anorectal symptoms.[12,15] Certain astringents, protectants, and vasoconstrictors may be used only intrarectally and should be administered with an applicator (i.e., "pile pipe") so that the product may reach the affected area.[12] Suppositories may be considered another way of administering drug to the anal area; however, their effectiveness is in question, as suppositories may not "stay in place" after insertion.[20] The remaining agents are for external use only and are not indicated for the relief of anorectal pain, bleeding, seepage, prolapse, or thrombosis.[12] Table 17–4 provides FDA-approved dosages for anorectal drug products.[12]

table
17-2   Signs and Symptoms of Anorectal Disorders

Sign/Symptom	Definition/Etiology
Usually Self-Treatable	
Itching (pruritus)	Mild stimulation of sensory nerve fibers; associated with many anorectal disorders, including hemorrhoids (typically with a mucoid discharge from prolapsing internal hemorrhoids). Common causes include poor hygiene (e.g., incomplete wiping/cleaning after defecation); diarrhea; parasitic or fungal infections; allergies (e.g., sensitivity to fabrics, soaps, laundry detergents, dyes, perfumes in toilet tissue); anorectal lesions; moisture in anal area. May be secondary to swelling; diet (e.g., caffeinated beverages, chocolate, citrus fruits); oral broad-spectrum antibiotics. Rare cause includes psychogenic origins.
Discomfort	May result from burning, itching, pain, irritation, inflammation, and swelling.
Irritation	Uncomfortable feeling associated with stimulation of sensory nerve fibers.
Burning	Greater degree of irritation of sensory nerve fibers than seen in anal itching; often associated with hemorrhoids; sensation of warmth or intense heat. May be constant or occur only at defecation.
Inflammation	Tissue reaction characterized by heat, redness or discoloration, pain, and swelling; often associated with trauma, allergy, or infection.
Swelling	Temporary enlargement of cells and/or tissue resulting from excess fluid; may be accompanied by pain, burning, and itching.
Requires Medical Referral	
Pain	Intense stimulation of sensory nerve fibers caused by inflammation or irritation. Internal hemorrhoids usually are painless; external hemorrhoids often cause mild pain; acute, severe perianal pain may be from a thrombosed external hemorrhoid. Pain from anal fissure during bowel movement often described as "being cut with sharp glass." Other possible causes of pain include abscess, fistula, or anorectal neoplasm.
Bleeding	Hemorrhoids are most common cause of minor anorectal disorders (e.g., from straining or passage of hard stool, or ulceration of perianal skin overlying thrombosed external hemorrhoid). Often appears as bright red spots or streaks on toilet tissue, or bright red blood around stool or in toilet. Black or tarry stools (melena) may indicate a possible upper GI bleed (e.g., PUD, erosive esophagitis, or gastric varices). Large amounts of red blood (hematochezia) in toilet bowl indicative of lower GI bleeding (e.g., fissure, IBD, polyps, malignant disease of the colon or rectum). Possible indications of large-volume blood loss include shortness of breath, dizziness, fatigue, or light-headedness, especially upon standing (orthostatic hypotension).
Seepage	Involuntary passage of fecal material or mucus caused by an incompletely closed anal sphincter; may include discharge of pus or feces from a fistula connecting the rectum to the anal canal.
Change in bowel pattern	Unexplained change in bowel frequency or in stool form; may signal serious underlying GI disorder (e.g., IBD) or colorectal cancer.
Prolapse (protrusion)	Protrusion of hemorrhoidal or rectal tissue of variable size into anal canal; usually appears after defecation, prolonged standing, unusual physical exertion, or swelling of hemorrhoidal tissue with loss of muscular support; painless except when accompanied by thrombosis, infection, or ulceration.
Thrombosis	Strangulation of protruded (external) hemorrhoid by anal sphincter, possibly leading to thrombosis; pain is most acute during first 48–72 hours but usually resolves after 7–10 days. Minimal pain with thrombosed internal hemorrhoids; patient likely to be unaware of condition unless sudden change in bowel habits occurs. If a thrombosed hemorrhoid persists, ulcers or gangrene may develop and cause bleeding, especially during defecation.

Key: GI = Gastrointestinal; IBD = inflammatory bowel disease; PUD = peptic ulcer disease.
Source: References 7, 8, and 17.

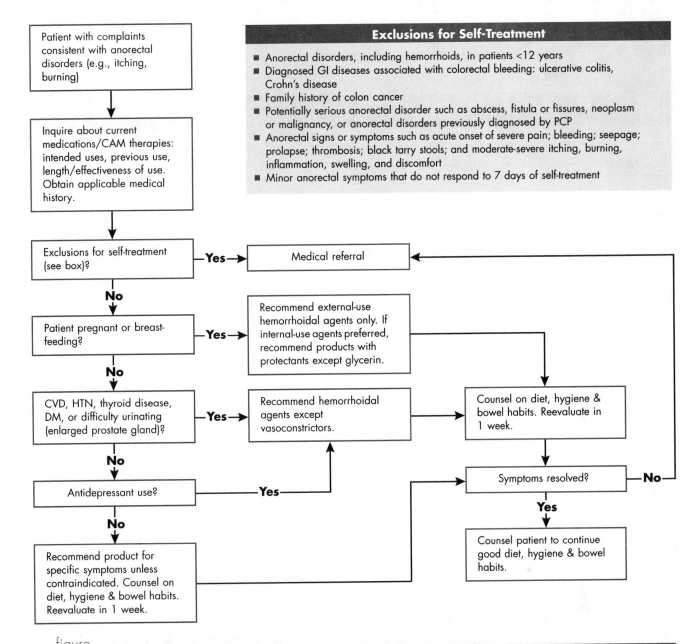

figure 17-2 Self-care of hemorrhoids. Key: CAM = Complementary and alternative medicine; CVD = cardiovascular disease; DM = diabetes mellitus; GI = gastrointestinal; HTN = hypertension; PCP = primary care provider.

table 17-3 Guidelines for Applying or Inserting Anorectal Products

- Clean affected anorectal area after bowel movement with mild, nonmedicated, unscented soap and warm water; rinse thoroughly.
- Clean anorectal area prior to applying products containing aluminum hydroxide gel or kaolin. Be sure to remove any previously used petrolatum-containing or greasy ointment.[a]
- Dry anorectal area gently by patting or blotting with unscented and uncolored toilet tissue or a soft cloth prior to applying product.
- Apply a thin layer to the perianal area and anal canal when using an external anorectal product.
- Insert anorectal products indicated for intrarectal use by using an intrarectal applicator or a finger. Intrarectal applicators are preferred to digital application because an applicator enables the drug product to be applied to the rectal mucosa (which cannot be reached with a finger).
- Ensure intrarectal applicators have lateral openings and holes in the tip to facilitate anorectal application and coverage of the rectal mucosa.
- Lubricate intrarectal applicator by spreading product around the applicator tip prior to inserting into the anorectal area.
- Avoid using the intrarectal applicator in the anorectal area if it causes additional pain.
- Do not exceed the recommended daily dosage unless directed by a primary care provider.

[a] *Ointment* refers to all semisolid preparations.
Source: References 1, 8, 20, 34.

table

17–4   Dosage Guidelines for Anorectal Products

Ingredient	Concentration per Dosage Unit (%)	Frequency of Use (maximum daily dosage)
Local Anesthetics		
Benzocaine	5–20	Up to 6 times/day (2.4 g)
Benzyl alcohol	1–4	Up to 6 times/day (480 mg)
Dibucaine, dibucaine hydrochloride	0.25–1	Up to 3–4 times/day (80 mg)
Dyclonine hydrochloride	0.5–1	Up to 6 times/day (100 mg)
Lidocaine	2–5	Up to 6 times/day (500 mg)
Pramoxine hydrochloride[a]	1	Up to 5 times/day (100 mg)
Tetracaine, tetracaine hydrochloride	0.5–1	Up to 6 times/day (100 mg)
Vasoconstrictors		
Ephedrine sulfate	0.1–1.25	Up to 4 times/day (100 mg)
Epinephrine hydrochloride/epinephrine	0.005–0.01	Up to 4 times/day (800 mg)
Phenylephrine hydrochloride	0.25	Up to 4 times/day (2 mg)
Protectants		
Aluminum hydroxide gel, cocoa butter, glycerin, hard fat, kaolin, lanolin, mineral oil, white petrolatum, calamine,[c] petrolatum, shark liver oil,[d] zinc oxide,[e] topical starch, cod liver oil[d]	See footnote b.	Petrolatum/white petrolatum as often as needed; other protectants up to 6 times/day or after each bowel movement
Astringents		
Calamine[c]	5–25	Up to 6 times/day or after each bowel movement
Zinc oxide	5–25	Up to 6 times/day or after each bowel movement
Witch hazel	10–50	Up to 6 times/day or after each bowel movement
Keratolytics		
Alcloxa	0.2–2	Up to 6 times/day
Resorcinol	1–3	Up to 6 times/day
Analgesics, Anesthetics, Antipruritics		
Menthol	0.1–1	Up to 6 times/day
Juniper tar	1–5	Up to 6 times/day
Camphor	0.1–3	Up to 6 times/day
Corticosteroids		
Hydrocortisone	0.25–1	Up to 3–4 times/day

[a] External dosage forms may include aerosol foams, ointments, creams, and jellies (water-miscible base).

[b] Any two, three, or four protectants may be combined, provided that the combined percentage by weight of all protectants in the combination is at least 50% of the final product (e.g., 1 gram of a 2-gram dosage unit). Any protectant ingredient included in the combination must be present at a level that contributes at least 12.5% by weight (e.g., 0.25 gram of a 2-gram dosage unit), except cod liver oil and shark liver oil. If cocoa butter is included in the combination, it must not exceed the concentration limit for calamine,[c] cod liver oil,[d] or shark liver oil.[d]

[c] Calamine not to exceed 25% by weight per dosage unit (based on the zinc oxide content of calamine).

[d] Provided that the product is labeled so that the amount of the product that is used in a 24-hour period represents a quantity that provides 10,000 USP units of vitamin A and 400 USP units of cholecalciferol.

[e] Any product containing calamine or zinc oxide for use as a protectant and/or as an astringent may not have a total weight of zinc oxide exceeding 25% by weight per dosage unit.

Key: USP = United States Pharmacopeia.

Source: Reference 12.

Local Anesthetics

Local anesthetics are approved for the temporary relief of external anal symptoms (e.g., itching, irritation, burning, discomfort, and pain); they provide relief by reversibly blocking transmission of nerve impulses (Table 17–4).[12] These products should be used with caution, as they may mask the pain of more severe anorectal disorders.[7,15]

Local anesthetics may produce allergic reactions (e.g., burning and itching) that are indistinguishable from the anorectal symptoms. Several cases of contact dermatitis have been reported with hemorrhoidal anesthetics, including benzocaine, dibucaine, and lidocaine.[21–23] Patients who have an allergic reaction to a local anesthetic should use agents with different chemical structures (e.g., pramoxine) or avoid use of these agents completely. Local anesthetic preparations must carry a warning stating that allergic reactions may occur.[12] These agents should be avoided on open sores because they are rapidly absorbed through abraded skin and may cause cardiovascular and central nervous systemic effects. Accidental oral ingestion of dibucaine-containing anorectal products has been reported in children, resulting in lethargy, seizures, and cardiorespiratory arrest.[15] All anorectal products containing any local anesthetic should be kept out of children's reach.[12,24]

Vasoconstrictors

Vasoconstrictors are structurally related to the endogenous catecholamines epinephrine and norepinephrine. When ephedrine or epinephrine is applied to the anorectal area, stimulation of alpha-adrenergic receptors in the vascular beds constricts arterioles, producing a modest and transient reduction of swelling. These agents are indicated (Table 17–4) for relief of itching, discomfort, and irritation and to shrink and decrease swelling of the hemorrhoidal tissues.[14] Ephedrine sulfate and phenylephrine hydrochloride are safe and effective for external and intrarectal use, and epinephrine hydrochloride is approved for external use.[12]

Adverse effects of ephedrine and epinephrine include increased cardiac rate and contractility, as well as bronchodilation if absorbed systemically. In contrast, because phenylephrine HCl is structurally related to norepinephrine, effects on the central nervous system and cardiac rhythm are minimal. When used in recommended dosages, vasoconstrictors may cause nervousness, tremors, sleeplessness, nausea, and loss of appetite.[15] Serious adverse effects (e.g., elevation of blood pressure, aggravation of hyperthyroidism, cardiac arrhythmias, and irregular heart rate) are less likely to occur with topical than with oral administration.[15] Prolonged use may lead to rebound vasodilatation, anxiety, and (rarely) paranoia. Contact dermatitis may also occur.

Rectally administered vasoconstrictors may attenuate the effects of oral antihypertensive agents and increase blood pressure. Alternatively, the hypertensive effects of vasoconstrictors may be potentiated by monoamine oxidase inhibitors and tricyclic antidepressants. Concomitant use may lead to serious and even lethal outcomes, including cerebral hemorrhage or stroke.[12,15] Patients with diabetes, thyroid disease, heart disease, hypertension, or enlarged prostate, as well as those taking antidepressants, antihypertensive agents, or cardiac medications, should not use hemorrhoidal agents with vasoconstrictors without first consulting their primary care provider.[12,25,26]

Protectants

Protectants are ingredients that provide a physical protective barrier and soften the anal canal by preventing fecal matter from irritating the perianal mucosa.[12,15] This drug class includes absorbents, adsorbents, demulcents, and emollients. Approved indications for most protectants include the temporary relief of discomfort, irritation, and burning with external and internal hemorrhoids (one exception is glycerin, which is for external use only) (Table 17–4).[12] Kaolin or aluminum hydroxide gel is indicated for the temporary relief of itching associated with moist anorectal conditions.[12]

Systemic absorption of protectants is minimal; therefore, adverse reactions as a class are uncommon. Lanolin is a natural product obtained from the fleece of sheep, and it may cause allergic reactions.[17] Chemically modified lanolin is available and may be less sensitizing.

A warning statement for anorectal products says that, because of their greasy properties, petrolatum or greasy ointments should be removed prior to applying products containing aluminum hydroxide gel or kaolin.[12]

Astringents

Astringents are products that promote coagulation of surface protein in the anorectal skin cells to protect the underlying tissue. Astringents also act to decrease cell volume, making the affected environment drier. To prevent further irritation, astringents form a thin protective layer over the injured mucosal membrane.[12,15] Astringents listed in Table 17–4 are approved for the temporary relief of itching, irritation, and burning symptoms associated with anorectal disorders.[15] Witch hazel (known as hamamelis water prior to January 1, 1995) is indicated for external use, whereas calamine and zinc oxide may be used for external and internal anorectal disorders.[12]

Adverse effects with the topical use of astringents are uncommon. Upon application, witch hazel may cause a slight stinging sensation from the alcohol used to prepare the compound. Contact dermatitis may occur with witch hazel because it contains a small amount of volatile oil.[27] If calamine or zinc oxide is used for prolonged periods of time (especially for internal anorectal disorders), systemic zinc toxicity (nausea, vomiting, lethargy, and/or severe pain) may develop.[15]

Keratolytics

Keratolytics are agents that cause desquamation and debridement (or sloughing) of epidermal surface cells. By fostering cell turnover and loosening surface cells, low concentrations of keratolytics may expose the underlying tissue. When other anorectal ingredients are used in combination with keratolytics, they reduce itching and inflammation (Table 17–4).[12,15] Because mucous membranes do not contain a keratin layer, intrarectal use is not justified and may be harmful.[15]

With repeated dosing, the absorption of the keratolytic resorcinol has led to methemoglobinemia, exfoliative dermatitis, death in infants, and myxedema in adults.[15] Other adverse effects range from tinnitus, increased pulse rate, diaphoresis, and shortness of breath to circulatory collapse, unconsciousness, and convulsions. Products containing resorcinol must list the following warnings to minimize absorption through abraded mucosal lining and to decrease the potential for systemic toxicity:

(1) "Certain persons can develop allergic reactions to ingredients in this product. If the symptoms being treated do not subside, or if redness, irritation, swelling, pain, or other symptoms develop or increase, discontinue use and consult a doctor." (2) "Do not use on open wounds near the anus."[15] Although keratolytics are available in selected anorectal preparations, their use must be weighed against their potentially serious adverse effects.

Analgesics, Anesthetics, and Antipruritics

Formerly classified as "counterirritants," menthol, juniper tar, and camphor are safe and effective when used for external perianal disorders. These agents (Table 17–4) are approved for the temporary relief of itching and inflammation by producing a cool, warm, or tingling sensation.[12,15] The agents should not be used internally because the rectum has no identifiable nerve fibers. Menthol-containing products must have the following warning: "Certain persons can develop allergic reactions to ingredients in this product. If the symptoms being treated do not subside, or if redness, irritation, swelling, pain, or other symptoms develop or increase, discontinue use and consult a doctor."[12] Extensive application of menthol to the trunk of the body has caused laryngospasm, dyspnea, and cyanosis; therefore, menthol should be used only sparingly.[15] Juniper tar, which contains phenol, also should be used only sparingly; it should not be ingested orally because organ failure and cardiac rhythm abnormalities may result.[28] Camphor is readily absorbed through mucous membranes, and it stimulates the central nervous system, which may cause convulsions or death. The latter is seen mostly with accidental oral ingestion, especially in children.[29]

Corticosteroids

Approximately 60% of the topical anorectal agents contain corticosteroids, which act as a vasoconstrictor and antipruritic by producing lysosomal membrane stabilization and antimitotic activity.[30] The onset of action may take up to 12 hours, but the effect has a longer duration than that of most other agents (e.g., local anesthetics). Hydrocortisone, in concentrations of no more than 1%, is the only corticosteroid approved for nonprescription use in anorectal preparations for the temporary relief of minor external anal itching caused by minor irritation or rash.[31] Local adverse effects include rare skin reactions and skin atrophy with prolonged use. Hydrocortisone may mask the symptoms of bacterial and fungal infections.

Combination Products

Federal regulations state that a nonprescription anorectal product may combine two or more active ingredients; combination products generally are recognized as safe and effective when (1) each active ingredient contributes to the claimed effect; (2) the combination of active ingredients does not decrease the safety or effectiveness of any individual active ingredient; and (3) the combination, when listing adequate directions for use and warning against unsafe use, provides rational, concurrent therapy for a significant proportion of the target population.[12,15] FDA restrictions on combination anorectal products can be found by accessing the *Federal Register*.[15] Use of combination products is reasonable, given that some self-treatable anorectal disorders may have concurrent symptoms. However, a combination of active ingredients has not been shown to be any more effective than a preparation

containing a therapeutic amount of a single agent.[15,30] Theoretically, restricting the number of ingredients should decrease the risk of interactions and adverse drug reactions, while also lessening the likelihood of altering the product's effectiveness.[30]

Product Selection Guidelines

Table 17–5 contains examples of products that can be recommended for hemorrhoids.

table **17–5**	Selected Nonprescription Products for Hemorrhoids
Trade Name	**Primary Ingredients**
Local Anesthetics	
Americaine Ointment[a]	Benzocaine 20%
Tronolane Anesthetic Hemorrhoid Cream[b]	Pramoxine HCl 1%; zinc oxide 5%
TUCKS Hemorrhoidal Ointment[c]	Pramoxine HCl 1%; zinc oxide 12.5%; mineral oil 46.6%
TUCKS Fast Relief Spray[c]	Pramoxine HCl 1%
Vasoconstrictors	
Preparation H Cooling Gel[d]	Witch hazel 50%; phenylephrine HCl 0.25%
Preparation H Suppositories[d]	Phenylephrine HCl 0.25%; cocoa butter 88.4%
Skin Protectants	
Preparation H Ointment[d]	Mineral oil 14%; petrolatum 74.9%; phenylephrine HCl 0.25%
TUCKS Internal Soothers Suppositories[c]	Topical starch 51%
Hydrocortisone Products	
Preparation H Anti-Itch Cream Hydrocortisone 1%[d]	Hydrocortisone 1%
Miscellaneous Combination Products	
Preparation H Maximum Strength Pain Relief Cream[d]	Glycerin 14.4%; phenylephrine HCl 0.25%; pramoxine HCl 1%; white petrolatum 15%
Preparation H Medicated Wipes[d]	Witch hazel 50%
TUCKS Medicated Cooling Pads[c]	Witch hazel 50%

[a] *Source:* Insight Pharmaceuticals Web site. Accessed at http://www.insightpharma.com/products/americaine/americaine-ointment, March 25, 2014.

[b] *Source:* Monticello Drug Company Web site. Accessed at http://www.monticellodrug.com/products/tronolane-cream/, March 25, 2014.

[c] *Source:* TUCKS Web site. Accessed at http://www.tucksbrand.com/, March 25, 2014.

[d] *Source:* Preparation H Web site. Accessed at http://www.preparationh.com/, March 25, 2014.

Knowledge of a patient's medical history, medication profile, and relevant socioeconomic factors is necessary to determine how an individual may respond to self-treatment. Selection of a product should be based on (1) the type, location, and severity of the anorectal disorder; (2) diseases or significant past medical history; (3) medications; (4) allergies; (5) ability to apply or insert the medication (considering physical, mental, and emotional limitations); and (6) any other factors that may affect treatment (e.g., diet, daily activities, and the cost of the product).

Special Populations

Pregnant and breast-feeding women should use products recommended for external use; exceptions include the recommended protectants, which may be used internally. Recommending nonpharmacologic interventions, including increasing dietary fiber and fluid intake to minimize constipation, may be of benefit throughout the trimesters.[32] Children younger than 12 years who have hemorrhoids or any other anorectal disorder should be referred for further medical evaluation.[15] Because constipation is more common in the older population, these patients may be more prone to hemorrhoids and anal fissures.[32] Treatment for this population is similar to treatment of young patients. Patients who have a positive family history of colon cancer should be referred for further medical evaluation.[32,33]

Patient Factors

FDA does not require comparison trials between combination and individual products; therefore, therapeutic differences are unknown. However, when used to treat indicated anorectal symptoms, combination products containing approved ingredients in appropriate dosages are most likely therapeutically similar to individual drug products.[12,15] Any perceived differences most likely are related to personal preference for a specific product or dosage form. Using more than one product or products containing multiple ingredients is reasonable because patients may have multiple different symptoms that may not be completely treated by one product alone.[10,12,15,30]

Medications used to treat anorectal disorders are available in many dosage forms, including ointments, creams, suppositories, and gels. Applicators, intrarectal applicators, or the patient's fingers are used to facilitate applying and instilling the anorectal preparations. Creams, gels, ointments, pastes, liquids, and foams are used externally. Although considerable pharmaceutical differences exist among these dosage forms, therapeutic differences do not appear to be clinically different.[15] This discussion uses the term *ointment* to refer to all semisolid preparations designed for intrarectal or external use in the anorectal area. The primary function of an ointment is to provide a vehicle for the safe and efficient delivery of the active ingredients, yet some ointments also possess inherent protectant and emollient properties.

Suppositories are solid dosage forms that deliver drugs into body orifices, typically in the anorectal area.[34] Suppositories should not be recommended as an initial dosage form because they may leave the affected anal region and ascend into the rectum and lower colon when the patient is in an upright position.[15,34] If the patient remains in an upright position after inserting a suppository or ointment, the active ingredients may not distribute evenly over the anal mucosa. Therefore, when inserting the suppository, patients should lie on their left side with knees bent so that the drug remains in the affected area for at least 15–20 minutes.[20] Suppositories have a relatively slower onset of action than other formulations because the solid dosage form must dissolve to release the active ingredients (see Chapter 15). To prolong retention rates in the anorectal area, some health care providers recommend introducing the base of the suppository first, rather than the tapered end.[34] Also, a suppository that is too soft to administer can be hardened in the refrigerator for at least 30 minutes before use.[34]

Foam products theoretically should provide more rapid release of active ingredients compared with ointments.[15] However, foams are more expensive than ointments and do not offer any advantage. Also, foams may not remain in the affected area, and differences in the size of the foam bubbles may result in different concentrations of the active ingredient.[15]

Complementary Therapies

Dietary supplements used to treat hemorrhoids have been researched poorly, although several have evidence of efficacy to support their use.[35] The combination of diosmin and hesperidin (a micronized purified flavonoid fraction) has been used to stop acute bleeding and decrease symptoms associated with hemorrhoids.[36] The mechanism of action is still in question, but animal models suggest this product inhibits prostaglandin and thromboxane mediators, thereby decreasing the inflammatory processes. The combination appears safe when both are taken orally for less than 6 months, with the most common adverse effects being abdominal pain, diarrhea, and gastritis.[36,37] Purified diosmin without hesperidin administered orally or topically has been shown as effective in reducing pain, bleeding, and swelling with hemorrhoids.[38] Butcher's broom combined with other dietary supplements (e.g., flavonoids) may be effective in reducing pain associated with hemorrhoids.[36,37] Horse chestnut seed extract (HCSE) has been used to reduce bleeding and decrease swelling associated with hemorrhoids.[37] When the herbal agent is processed properly, it is considered relatively safe; the most commonly reported side effects include itching, nausea, and vomiting.[39] Improperly prepared HCSE preparations may be poisonous and may lead to death. (See Chapter 51 for further discussion of HCSE.)

Assessment of Anorectal Disorders: A Case-Based Approach

To accurately assess whether the anorectal disorder is self-treatable, a health care provider should obtain a thorough description of the patient's signs and symptoms. For self-treatable disorders, the provider should ask questions about the presence of specific diseases (e.g., hypertension, diabetes mellitus, benign prostatic hyperplasia, and psychiatric illness); prescription and nonprescription medications; complementary and alternative medicines; and diet, lifestyle, and exercise before recommending self-treatment.

Cases 17–1 and 17–2 illustrate assessment of patients with anorectal disorders.

Patient Counseling for Anorectal Disorders

The most appropriate drug and nondrug measures for treating patient-specific anorectal signs and symptoms should be explained to each patient. Counseling should include dosage

case
17-1

Relevant Evaluation Criteria	Scenario/Model Outcome

Information Gathering

1. Gather essential information about the patient's symptoms and medical history, including:

a. description of symptom(s) (i.e., nature, onset, duration, severity, associated symptoms)

> Pregnant patient complains of heartburn for 2 weeks. Over the past 5 days, she has experienced symptoms of burning discomfort in the anal area and occasional pain with bowel movements. Blood was seen in the stools and on the toilet paper.

b. description of any factors that seem to precipitate, exacerbate, and/or relieve the patient's symptom(s)

> Straining during defecation causes discomfort. Bowel movement causes anal pain. Stool has become harder over the past few months, more so as she goes through her pregnancy. Drinking water seems to help her symptoms.

c. description of the patient's efforts to relieve the symptoms

> When able to, scratching the anal area seems to relieve symptoms. She notices that her symptoms are less problematic on days she drinks more water.

d. patient's identity

> Victoria Mills

e. age, sex, height, and weight

> 35 years old, female, 5 ft 4 in., 144 lb

f. patient's occupation

> Stay-at-home mom

g. patient's dietary habits

> Eats meat, ice cream, sweets, and pickles. Used to eat vegetables but now avoids them. Will occasionally eat some fruits, mostly pineapple.

h. patient's sleep habits

> 5–8 hours nightly

i. concurrent medical conditions, prescription and nonprescription medications, and dietary supplements

> Pregnant, early third trimester; MVI daily, folate daily, iron twice daily; docusate sodium as needed (few times weekly)

j. allergies

> NKA

k. history of other adverse reactions to medications

> None

l. other (describe) _____

> Patient does water exercises every other day, but she admits exercising is becoming difficult as she approaches giving birth.

Assessment and Triage

2. Differentiate patient's signs/symptoms and correctly identify the patient's primary problem(s) (Tables 17–1 and 17–2).

> Patient is suffering from constipation, which may be causing the patient to have anorectal symptoms.

3. Identify exclusions for self-treatment (Figure 17–2).

> None

4. Formulate a comprehensive list of therapeutic alternatives for the primary problem to determine if triage to a health care provider is required, and share this information with the patient or caregiver.

> Options include:
>
> (1) Recommend self-care with an appropriate OTC anorectal product, and advise on nondrug measures.
>
> (2) Recommend self-care with an appropriate OTC anorectal product, and advise on nondrug measures until patient contacts her primary care provider.
>
> (3) Refer patient to her primary care provider for medical evaluation of her symptoms.
>
> (4) Take no action.

Plan

5. Select an optimal therapeutic alternative to address the patient's problem, taking into account patient preferences.

> The best option is #2: self-care and nondrug measures until patient can contact PCP. Recommend an external-hemorrhoidal agent only. If internal-use agents preferred, recommend products with protectants (except glycerin). Recommend patient increase fluid intake (water), dietary fibers (fruits, vegetables), and, if possible, exercise. Sitz baths used 3 times a day may resolve anorectal symptoms.

case

17–1 *continued*

Relevant Evaluation Criteria	Scenario/Model Outcome
6. Describe the recommended therapeutic approach to the patient or caregiver.	"Your symptoms, including blood in the stools, may be related to hemorrhoids. The hemorrhoids may have developed because you are in your third trimester and have a baby growing in your uterus. These changes in your body cause you to have a lot of pressure, especially when you are having a bowel movement, which may produce hemorrhoids. Although your symptoms are infrequent, I'm concerned about the blood in your stools. Even though I'm recommending you use a self-care product, you should contact your PCP for further evaluation in a few days, if your symptoms do not improve."
7. Explain to the patient or caregiver the rationale for selecting the recommended therapeutic approach from the considered therapeutic alternatives.	"Although your symptoms, including blood in the stools, may be related to hemorrhoids, you should contact your PCP for further evaluation because other conditions may also cause similar symptoms, including rectal bleeding."

Patient Education

8. When recommending self-care with nonprescription medications and/or nondrug therapy, convey accurate information to the patient or caregiver.	
a. appropriate dose and frequency of administration	See Table 17–4.
b. maximum number of days the therapy should be employed	"Contact your PCP as soon as possible, even if your symptoms resolve with treatment. Be sure to let your primary care provider know what self-care measures you have taken. Ask your PCP whether you should continue with your self-treatment if your symptoms do not resolve after 7 days."
c. product administration procedures	See Table 17–3.
d. expected time to onset of relief	"The irritation, burning, and discomfort may be relieved within a few days of applying the topical agent as directed. Straining may be relieved with adequate fluids and a healthy diet that is high in dietary fibers. If required, keep using the stool softener, or add a fiber supplement, as needed. Although the rectal bleeding may stop with treatment, still contact your PCP."
e. degree of relief that can be reasonably expected	"Complete relief of your anorectal symptoms may be possible, but you should expect to continue to have these symptoms until the birth of your child."
f. most common side effects	"Most products applied to the anal area are usually well-tolerated."
g. side effects that warrant medical intervention should they occur	"If you develop an allergic reaction to the product (redness, swelling, increased irritation, or pain), discontinue use, and contact your PCP as soon as possible."
h. patient options in the event that condition worsens or persists	"If your symptoms worsen, contact your PCP as soon as possible."
i. product storage requirements	"Store medication out of the reach of children and at a controlled room temperature."
j. specific nondrug measures	"Practice good anal hygiene, take sitz baths, and consider modifying your diet to increase fluids and fiber to soften stools and decrease straining."
Solicit follow-up questions from the patient or caregiver.	"Will this affect my newborn baby?"
Answer the patient's or caregiver's questions.	"Probably not. The anorectal complaints usually affect the mother. The newborn should not have anorectal problems at such a young age. Anorectal problems usually are not hereditary."

Evaluation of Patient Outcome

9. Assess patient outcome.	Ask the patient to call to update you on her response to your recommendations; alternatively, you could call her in a week to evaluate her response and make sure that she touched base with her PCP.

Key: MVI = Multiple vitamin; NKA = no known allergies; OTC = over-the-counter; PCP: primary care provider.

case

17–2

Relevant Evaluation Criteria	**Scenario/Model Outcome**

Information Gathering

1. Gather essential information about the patient's symptoms and medical history, including:

  a. description of symptom(s) (i.e., nature, onset, duration, severity, associated symptoms)

Patient complains of bleeding in the anal area for the past 3 days. Patient experiences burning, pain, and blood on the toilet paper with each wiping. He has had these symptoms before but says there is more blood this time than he has seen in the past. He describes his stool as being more "pencil-like" over the past few months.

  b. description of any factors that seem to precipitate, exacerbate, and/or relieve the patient's symptom(s)

Symptoms are worst at night, especially after eating and before going to bed. This time is also when he has his bowel movements. He has not changed his soaps or detergents, and he has not changed his diet or exercise.

  c. description of the patient's efforts to relieve the symptoms

The patient has tried topical hydrocortisone cream in the anorectal area without relief for the last 2 days.

  d. patient's identity

Simon Jabor

  e. age, sex, height, and weight

42 years old, male, 5 ft 11 in., 193 lb

  f. patient's occupation

Attorney

  g. patient's dietary habits

Eats healthy meals, including meat, fruits, and vegetables. Occasionally eats sweets. Drinks alcohol at social events, which is about once every few months.

  h. patient's sleep habits

8–9 hours nightly

  i. concurrent medical conditions, prescription and nonprescription medications, and dietary supplements

Hypertension diagnosed at age 38: felodipine 5 mg daily

  j. allergies

Sulfa (anaphylactic reaction)

  k. history of other adverse reactions to medications

None

  l. other (describe) _____

Simon's dad died 20 years ago secondary to colon cancer at the age of 45. His mom is alive and diagnosed with diabetes. He has no siblings. He is happily married and has two children.

Assessment and Triage

2. Differentiate patient's signs/symptoms and correctly identify the patient's primary problem(s) (Tables 17–1 and 17–2).

Patient noticed burning, pain, and blood on the toilet paper with each wiping. He states that this is not uncommon but that lately there is a lot more blood than he has seen in the past. He states that his diet, fluid, and exercise regimens have not changed. He is 42. Considering that Simon is in his 40s and has a family history of colon cancer, there may be a genetic relationship; therefore, there is a probability that he has an oncologic condition.

3. Identify exclusions for self-treatment (Figure 17–2).

Bleeding in the anal area; change in stool consistency to "pencil-like." Strong family history of colon cancer.

4. Formulate a comprehensive list of therapeutic alternatives for the primary problem to determine if triage to a health care provider is required, and share this information with the patient or caregiver.

Options include:

(1) Recommend self-care with an appropriate OTC anorectal product, and advise on nondrug measures.

(2) Recommend self-care with an appropriate OTC anorectal product, and advise on nondrug measures until patient contacts his PCP.

(3) Refer patient to his PCP for medical evaluation of his symptoms immediately.

(4) Take no action.

case
17–2 *continued*

Relevant Evaluation Criteria	Scenario/Model Outcome
Plan	
5. Select an optimal therapeutic alternative to address the patient's problem, taking into account patient preferences.	Patient should consult a health care provider immediately for medical evaluation to rule out bleeding from a source other than a hemorrhoid. He is young and has had a change in stool consistency over the past few months. Patient may have colon cancer because there is a strong family history of cancer (Figure 17–2).
6. Describe the recommended therapeutic approach to the patient or caregiver.	"You should consult a health care provider for immediate medical evaluation. I'm concerned about a few things, including your symptoms and your family history."
7. Explain to the patient or caregiver the rationale for selecting the recommended therapeutic approach from the considered therapeutic alternatives.	"Because you tried using the hydrocortisone cream for 2 days with no relief, the best option is for you to see your primary care provider immediately. You have a strong family history of colon cancer. The signs and symptoms you are complaining about may be symptoms of colon cancer. Please see your primary care provider to have your symptoms evaluated and testing done as soon as possible."
Patient Education	
8. When recommending self-care with nonprescription medications and/or nondrug therapy, convey accurate information to the patient or caregiver.	Criterion does not apply in this case.
Solicit follow-up questions from the patient or caregiver.	"Is my wife at risk of acquiring colon cancer?"
Answer the patient's or caregiver's questions.	"No. Colon cancer is not transmitted via blood. Your wife may have other colon cancer risk factors (e.g., a low-fiber diet), but she cannot contract it from you."
Evaluation of Patient Outcome	
9. Assess patient outcome.	Contact the patient in a day or two to ensure he made an appointment and sought immediate and appropriate medical care.

Key: NKA = No known allergies; OTC = over-the-counter; PCP = primary care provider.

and frequency of administration, administration technique, possible adverse effects, precautions or warnings, and product storage. Patients should understand when self-care should be discontinued and when to consult a primary care provider. If the topical nonprescription agents do not resolve the anorectal symptoms within 7 days, medical referral is appropriate.[12] The box Patient Education for Anorectal Disorders lists specific information to provide patients.

Evaluation of Patient Outcomes for Anorectal Disorders

Self-treatment of anorectal disorders should be limited to minor symptoms. If serious or severe symptoms are present, or if symptoms become progressively worse, advise the patient to contact his or her primary care provider. In addition, if alarm signs or symptoms are present, including blood in the stool or severe anal pain, or if symptoms persist beyond 7 days of self-treatment, the patient should be counseled to seek immediate medical attention.[12] If symptoms

resolve, the patient should be encouraged to maintain a well-balanced diet, good personal hygiene, and good bowel habits.[20]

Key Points for Anorectal Disorders

➤ Limit self-treatment to burning, itching, discomfort, swelling, and irritation.
➤ Refer patients to their primary care provider when symptoms include anorectal seepage, bleeding, thrombosis, severe pain, fevers, or a change in bowel patterns.
➤ Advise patients with self-treatable symptoms to contact their primary care provider if symptoms worsen or do not improve after 7 days.
➤ Advise pregnant and breast-feeding women to use only products for external use (except for protectants that do not contain glycerin, which can be used internally).
➤ Refer parents and caregivers of children younger than 12 years to seek medical attention from a primary care provider.

patient education for
Anorectal Disorders

The objectives of self-treatment are to (1) relieve specific signs and symptoms and (2) prevent complications leading to serious problems. For most patients, carefully following product instructions and the self-care measures listed here will help ensure relief of symptoms.

Nondrug Measures

- Maintain hydration and a healthy diet. If experiencing hard stools, straining, or constipation, increase amount of fiber and fluids in the diet to reduce or prevent straining during bowel movements (see Chapter 15).
- Avoid medications that cause constipation, if possible (see Chapter 15).
- Clean anorectal area after each bowel movement with a moistened, unscented, white toilet tissue or wipe.
- Use a sitz bath, or soak in a bathtub two to four times a day, which may help mild anal itching, burning, irritation, and discomfort. Avoid use of soaps, salts, and oils.

Nonprescription Medications

- Select products containing only the ingredients needed to relieve specific anorectal symptoms.
- See Table 17–3 for guidelines for applying anorectal products.
- See Table 17–4 for recommended dosages of these products.
- Use only selected vasoconstrictors (ephedrine and phenylephrine), protectants (not glycerin), and astringents (calamine and zinc oxide) intrarectally.
- (If patient is pregnant) Use only products approved for external use. If internal use is required, protectants, with the exception of glycerin, may be used.
- (If patient has a history of cardiovascular disease, diabetes, hyperthyroidism, hypertension, depression, or difficulty urinating

because of prostate problems) Avoid topical products that contain vasoconstrictors.
- (If taking medications for hypertension or depression) Avoid using any anorectal product containing vasoconstrictors without first consulting your primary care provider.
- Monitor for nervousness, tremor, sleeplessness, nausea, and possible loss of appetite when using an anorectal product containing ephedrine sulfate or phenylephrine.
- Explain that a reduction or relief of symptoms should occur within a few days of self-treatment.
- Review patient's preferences, especially when the patient may choose from an ointment, cream, or suppository, and when generic products are available.

When to Seek Medical Attention

- Stop using the anorectal product and contact a primary care provider as soon as possible if insertion of a product into the anorectal area causes pain.
- Contact a primary care provider if symptoms worsen, if new symptoms (e.g., bleeding) develop, or if symptoms do not improve after 7 days of self-treatment.
- Discontinue using product and contact a primary care provider at the first occurrence of side effects (e.g., a rash; increased itching, redness, burning, or swelling in the anorectal area).
- Discontinue product and contact a primary care provider immediately if allergic or hypersensitivity reactions to the anorectal product develop.

- ➤ To minimize undesirable effects, advise patients to select an anorectal product containing the fewest number of ingredients necessary to treat specific symptoms.
- ➤ Instruct patients on the proper use or application of specific anorectal products (Table 17–3).
- ➤ Counsel patients on nondrug measures (e.g., dietary measures and perianal hygiene) (see the box Patient Education for Anorectal Disorders).
- ➤ Do not use vasoconstrictors in patients with conditions such as diabetes, hypertension, and cardiac disease because of the possibility of systemic adverse effects.
- ➤ Advise patients on the advantages and disadvantages of various anorectal dosage forms so the best product can be selected for their needs.

REFERENCES

1. Lacy BE, Weiser K. Common anorectal disorders: diagnosis and treatment. *Curr Gastroenterol Rep.* 2009;11:413–19.
2. National Digestive Diseases Information Clearinghouse. Digestive Diseases Statistics for the United States. Bethesda, MD: National Digestive Diseases Information Clearinghouse; 2010. NIH Publication No. 10–3873. Accessed at http://digestive.niddk.nih.gov/statistics/statistics.aspx, March 17, 2013.
3. Rivadeneira DE, Steele SR, Ternent C, et al. Practice parameters for the management of hemorrhoids (revised 2010). *Dis Colon Rectum.* 2011;54(9):1059–64.
4. Peery AF, Dellon ES, Lund J, et al. Burden of gastrointestinal disease in the United States: 2012 update. *Gastroenterology.* 2012;143(5):1179–87.
5. Riss S, Weiser FA, Schwameis K, et al. The prevalence of hemorrhoids in adults. *Int J Colorectal Dis.* 2012;27(2):215–20.
6. Ebrahimi N, Vohra-Miller S, Koren G. Anorectal symptom management in pregnancy: development of a severity scale. *J Popul Ther Clin Pharmacol.* 2011;18:e99–e105.
7. Barleben A, Mills S. Anorectal anatomy and physiology. *Surg Clin North Am.* 2010;90:1–15.
8. Schubert MC, Sridhar S, Schade RR, et al. What every gastroenterologist needs to know about common anorectal disorders. *World J Gastroenterol.* 2009;15:3201–9.
9. Madoff RD, Fleshman JW, and Clinical Practice Committee, American Gastroenterological Association. American Gastroenterological Association technical review on the diagnosis and treatment of hemorrhoids. *Gastroenterology.* 2004;126:1463–73.
10. Sneider EB, Maykel JA. Diagnosis and management of symptomatic hemorrhoids. *Surg Clin North Am.* 2010;90:17–32.
11. Daram SR, Lahr C, Tang SJ. Anorectal bleeding: etiology, evaluation, and management (with videos) *Gastrointest Endosc.* 2012;76(2):406–17.
12. U.S. Food and Drug Administration. Anorectal drug products for over-the-counter human use. *Federal Register.* 2012;276–81. Accessed at http://www.accessdata.fda.gov/scripts/cdrh/cfdocs/cfcfr/CFRSearch.cfm?CFRPart=346, March 18, 2013.
13. Daniel WJ. Anorectal pain, bleeding and lumps. *Aust Fam Physician.* 2010;39(6):376–81.
14. Lohsiriwat V. Hemorrhoids: from basic pathophysiology to clinical management. *World J Gastroenterol.* 2012;18(17):2009–17.
15. U.S. Food and Drug Administration. Anorectal drug products for over-the-counter human use: establishment of a monograph. *Federal Register.* 1980; 45:35576–7.
16. Alonso-Coello P, Mills E, Heels-Ansdell D, et al. Fiber for the treatment of hemorrhoids complications: a systematic review and meta-analysis. *Am J Gastroenterol.* 2006;101:181–8.
17. Abramowitz L, Weyandt GH, Havlickova B, et al. The diagnosis and management of haemorrhoidal disease from a global perspective. *Aliment Pharmacol Ther.* 2010 May;31(suppl 1):1–58.

18. Tejirian T, Abbas MA. Sitz bath: where is the evidence? Scientific basis of a common practice. *Dis Colon Rectum.* 2005;48:2336–40.

19. Lang DS, Tho PC, Ang EN. Effectiveness of the Sitz bath in managing adult patients with anorectal disorders. *Jpn J Nurs Sci.* 2011;8(2):115–28.

20. Gupta PJ. Supportive therapies in ano-rectal diseases—are they really useful? *Acta Chir Iugosl.* 2010;57(3):83–7.

21. Lodi A, Ambonati M, Coassini A, et al. Contact allergy to 'caines' by anti-hemorrhoidal ointments. *Contact Dermat.* 1999;41:221–2.

22. Ramirez P, Sendagorta E, Floristan U, et al. Allergic contact dermatitis from antihemorrhoidal ointments: concomitant sensitization to both amide and ester local anesthetics. *Dermatitis.* 2010;21:176–7.

23. Jovanović M, Karadaglić D, Brkić S. Contact urticaria and allergic contact dermatitis to lidocaine in a patient sensitive to benzocaine and propolis. *Contact Dermat.* 2006;54:124–6.

24. U.S. Food and Drug Administration. Requirements for child-resistant packaging; requirements for products containing lidocaine or dibucaine. *Federal Register.* 1995;60:17992–8005. Accessed at http://www.cpsc.gov/PageFiles/77793/007.txt, March 22, 2013.

25. Pray WS, Pray GE. Nonprescription products and heart warnings. *US Pharm.* 2011;36(2):12–5.

26. Pray WS. Nonprescription products to avoid with hypertension. *US Pharm.* 2010;35(2):12–5.

27. Acheson AG, Scholefield JH. Management of haemorrhoids. *BMJ.* 2008;336:380–3.

28. Koruk ST, Ozyilkan E, Kaya P, et al. Juniper tar poisoning. *Clin Toxicol.* 2005;43:47–9.

29. U.S. Food and Drug Administration. Anorectal drug products for over-the-counter human use; reopening of the administrative record. *Federal Register.* 1980;45:63876–8. Accessed at http://www.fda.gov/downloads/Drugs/DevelopmentApprovalProcess/DevelopmentResources/Over-the-CounterOTCDrugs/StatusofOTCRulemakings/ucm078691.pdf, March 23, 2013.

30. Havlickova B. Topical corticosteroid therapy in proctology indications. *Aliment Pharmacol Ther.* 2010:31:19–32.

31. U.S. Food and Drug Administration. External analgesic drug products for over-the-counter human use; amendment of tentative final monograph. *Federal Register.* 1990;55:6932–51. Accessed at http://www.fda.gov/downloads/Drugs/DevelopmentApprovalProcess/DevelopmentResources/Over-the-CounterOTCDrugs/StatusofOTCRulemakings/UCM077992.pdf, March 23, 2013.

32. Gupta PJ. Ano-rectal pathologies encountered under special circumstances. *Acta Chir Iugosl.* 2010;57(3):77–82.

33. Jones R, Charlton J, Latinovic R, et al. Alarm symptoms and identification of non-cancer diagnoses in primary care: cohort study. *BMJ.* 2009;339:b3094.

34. Gupta PJ. Suppositories in anal disorders: a review. *Eur Rev Med Pharmacol Sci.* 2007;11(3):165–70.

35. Chauhan R, Ruby K, Dwivedi J. Golden herbs used in piles treatment: a concise report. *Int. J. Drug Dev Res.* 2012, 4(4):50–68.

36. Misra MC, Parshad R. Randomized clinical trial of micronized flavonoids in the early control of bleeding from acute internal haemorrhoids. *Br J Surg.* 2000;87:868–72.

37. Gami B. Hemorrhoids—a common ailment among adults, causes & treatment: a review. *Int J Pharm Pharm Sci.* 2011;3(suppl 5):5–12.

38. Misra MC, Imlitemus. Drug treatment of haemorrhoids. *Drugs.* 2005;65(11):1481–91.

39. National Center for Complementary and Alternative Medicine. Herbs at a glance: horse chestnut. Modified March 24, 2011. Accessed at http://nccam.nih.gov/health/horsechestnut, May 13, 2011.

PINWORM INFECTION

Jeffery A. Goad and Edith Mirzaian

*E*nterobius vermicularis, commonly referred to as "pinworm," "seatworm," "threadworm," or oxyuriasis, is an intestinal nematode and the primary agent that causes human enterobiasis. This chapter will focus on the detection and management of pinworm infection because it is the most common worm infestation in the United States, and it is the only helminthic infection for which a nonprescription medication has been approved for treatment. This infection is most common in temperate regions of the world; in the United States, pinworms are found with a high prevalence in day care settings and urban areas.[1,2] Although pinworms are a nuisance, the pinworm infection presents little risk to the infected individual or the public.

Pinworm infection may be the most common helminth infection in the United States, with the greatest infection rate in children ages 5–14 years.[3] Enterobiasis is associated with all socioeconomic levels and, in contrast to other helminthic infections, does not affect any particular race or culture. Nearly 50% of all *E. vermicularis* cases occur among individuals who are institutionalized (e.g., in child care facilities or hospitals) and among family members.[3,4,6]

Pathophysiology of Pinworm Infection

Humans are the only hosts of *E. vermicularis*. Unlike most other worm infections, pinworms do not live in the soil or water and are not transmitted through animal feces. However, animal fur of household dogs and cats may be a carrier of infective eggs.[4] The most common pinworm transmission route is through ingestion of infective eggs by direct anus-to-mouth transfer by fingers or fomites. Reinfection may occur readily. because eggs often are found under fingernails of infected children who have scratched the anal area. Finger sucking may be considered a source of infection, particularly in children with recurring symptoms.[4] Nail biting and nose picking have not been associated with the initial infection; however, they certainly can contribute to reinfection.[5] Embryonated eggs also can be transferred from the perianal region to clothes, bedding, or bathroom fixtures; because of their small size, pinworm eggs sometimes can become airborne in dust and reach the intestinal tract through the nose during breathing.[1,6] The eggs can remain viable outside the intestinal tract for 20 days (especially under humid conditions) and can spread within a microcommunity (e.g., a household or school).[7]

After 1–2 months of molting, the adult pinworm emerges as small, white, thread-like worm with a pin-shaped, pointed tail (from which the name is derived; see Color Plates, photograph 1A); its lifespan is about 2 months.[3,7] Adult male and female worms inhabit the first portion of the large intestine, or ileocecum, and seldom cause damage to the intestinal wall. The mature female, approximately 8–13 mm in length, usually stores approximately 11,000 eggs in her body (see Color Plates, photograph 1B). After her nocturnal migration down the colon and out the anus, she deposits her sticky eggs in the perianal region and dies shortly afterward. Males are smaller (2.5 mm), live approximately 2 weeks, and do not migrate. If eggs are not washed off, they hatch within a few hours, and larvae may return to the large intestine through the anus (retroinfection). Within 2–6 weeks of egg ingestion, larvae are released and mature into gravid females, thus continuing the cycle indefinitely unless appropriate behavioral and pharmacotherapeutic interventions are instituted.

Rarely, extraintestinal infestations, typically involving the genitourinary tract, may occur. As many as 36% of young girls with urinary tract infections may be infected with pinworms because the pinworms have mistakenly crawled into the urogenital tract.[1] Genitourinary pinworm infections are harder to treat because of the low systemic absorption of antiparasitic agents.[7]

Clinical Presentation of Pinworm Infection

Patients with minor pinworm infections often are asymptomatic. Nocturnal pruritus ani, a perianal or perineal itch, is the most common symptom of enterobiasis.[1] Perianal itching occurs predominantly at night and is caused by an inflammatory reaction to the presence of adult worms and eggs on the perianal skin.[2] Major infestations may produce symptoms ranging from abdominal pain, insomnia, and restlessness, to anorexia, diarrhea, and intractable localized itching.[4,5] Patients with severe symptoms of major infestations and extraintestinal disease should be referred to a primary care provider (PCP) for further evaluation. Before recommending treatment or referral, the pharmacist should ask appropriate assessment questions to rule out diaper dermatitis in children, as well as constipation and hemorrhoids in older patients because these conditions also can cause inflammation in the rectal region, leading to itching and discomfort.

In addition to physical signs and symptoms, psychological trauma (i.e., pinworm neurosis) to patients and parents also can occur when worms are found near a child's anus. Patients and parents need to be assured that pinworms are common and curable and that no social stigma is attached to their occurrence.[5]

Scratching to relieve itching from pinworm infection may lead to secondary bacterial infection of the perianal and perineal regions.[7] Helminthic infections in the genital tract may lead to endometritis, salpingitis, tubo-ovarian abscess, pelvic inflammatory disease, vulvovaginitis, and possibly infertility.[7-9] Pinworms also may migrate into the peritoneal cavity and form granulomas. Rarely, they may cause appendicitis in children.[10]

Treatment of Pinworm Infection

Treatment Goals

The goals of self-treatment are to relieve symptoms of pinworm infection and to eradicate pinworms from the patient and the household, thereby preventing reinfection.

General Treatment Approach

The management of pinworm infection and prevention of reinfection includes drug treatment with pyrantel pamoate for the patient and for every household member. Strict hygiene (e.g., washing linens and disinfecting toilet seats) is an integral part of the treatment. Figure 18–1 outlines self-care of this infection and lists exclusions for self-treatment.

Nonpharmacologic Therapy

Once pinworm infection is suspected, the patient or caregiver should follow the nondrug measures in Table 18–1 to minimize family and household infections and reinfections. Children can usually return to school after the first dose of an appropriate antihelminthic agent and after their fingernails are cut and cleaned. Health care providers are in an ideal position to inform patients of behaviors that may increase their risk of helminthic infections.

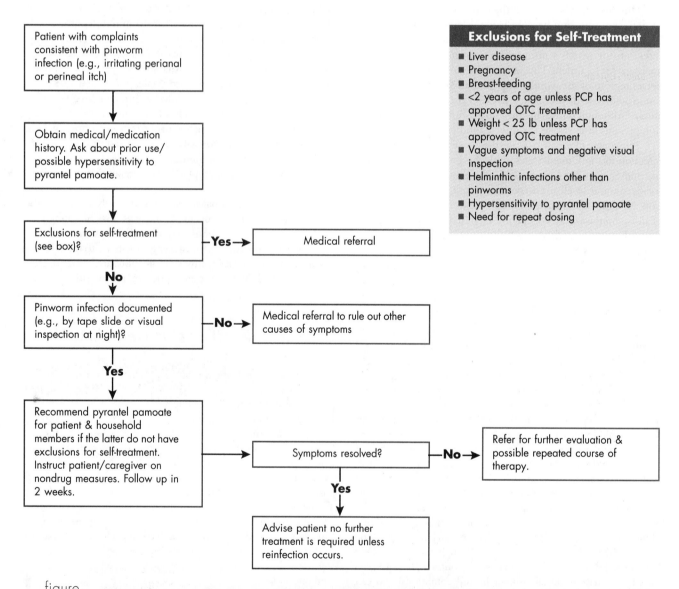

Exclusions for Self-Treatment

- Liver disease
- Pregnancy
- Breast-feeding
- <2 years of age unless PCP has approved OTC treatment
- Weight < 25 lb unless PCP has approved OTC treatment
- Vague symptoms and negative visual inspection
- Helminthic infections other than pinworms
- Hypersensitivity to pyrantel pamoate
- Need for repeat dosing

Patient with complaints consistent with pinworm infection (e.g., irritating perianal or perineal itch)

Obtain medical/medication history. Ask about prior use/possible hypersensitivity to pyrantel pamoate.

Exclusions for self-treatment (see box)? → **Yes** → Medical referral

No

Pinworm infection documented (e.g., by tape slide or visual inspection at night)? → **No** → Medical referral to rule out other causes of symptoms

Yes

Recommend pyrantel pamoate for patient & household members if the latter do not have exclusions for self-treatment. Instruct patient/caregiver on nondrug measures. Follow up in 2 weeks. → Symptoms resolved? → **No** → Refer for further evaluation & possible repeated course of therapy.

Yes

Advise patient no further treatment is required unless reinfection occurs.

figure
18–1   Self-care of pinworm infection. Key: OTC = Over-the-counter; PCP = primary care provider.

table

18–1   Nondrug and Preventive Measures for Treating Pinworm Infection

- Educate the public in personal hygiene, particularly the need to wash hands before eating or preparing food and after using the toilet. Encourage keeping fingernails short to prevent harboring of eggs and autoinoculation (hand-to-mouth reinfection); discourage biting nails and scratching anal area.
- Eggs are destroyed by sunlight and ultraviolet rays, so ensure blinds or curtains are open in the affected room to enhance cleaning of the environment.
- Wash bed linens, underwear, bedclothes, and towels of the infected individual and the entire family in hot water daily during treatment. Pinworm eggs are killed by exposure to temperatures of 131°F (55°C) for a few seconds; therefore, the "hot" cycle should be used while washing and drying.
- Bathe daily in the morning; showers (stand-up baths) are preferred over tub baths.
- Change underwear, nightclothes, and bed sheets daily for several days after treatment.
- Clean and vacuum (do not sweep) house daily for several days after treatment of cases. Wet mopping before or instead of vacuuming may limit spread of pinworm eggs into the air.
- Reduce overcrowding in living accommodations.

Source: Heymann D. *Control of Communicable Diseases Manual.* 19th ed. Washington, DC: American Public Health Association; 2008.

Pharmacologic Therapy

Pyrantel Pamoate

Pyrantel pamoate is the only nonprescription medication approved for treatment of pinworm infection. Pyrantel pamoate was first used in veterinary practice as a broad-spectrum drug for pinworms, roundworms, and hookworms. It has become an important drug for treating certain helminthic infections in humans. Pyrantel pamoate has a cure rate of 90%–100% when used for treatment of enterobiasis.[11] This variable cure rate may be a result of the medication's lack of effect on eggs and larvae as well as the eggs' viability for up to 20 days, which may lead to reinfection.

Although this product is readily available in a nonprescription form, helminthic infections other than those caused by pinworms require a medical referral and should be diagnosed and treated by a PCP.

Pyrantel pamoate is a depolarizing neuromuscular agent that paralyzes adult worms, causing them to loosen their hold on the intestinal wall and subsequently be passed out in the stool before they can lay eggs. The drug is poorly absorbed, with 50% excreted unchanged in the feces and about 7% excreted in the urine as unchanged drug and metabolites.[11]

A single oral dose of pyrantel pamoate (liquid, caplet, or chewable tablet) is based on the adult or child patient's body weight (11 mg/kg of the pyrantel base). The maximum single dose is 1 gram. The recommended dosage is the same for children younger than 2 years or weighing less than 25 pounds; however, they should not be treated without first consulting a PCP. The product includes a schedule of recommended dosages that is based on a range of body weights. The dose can be repeated in 2 weeks if symptoms do not resolve because reinfection can

occur; however, the repeat dose should be administered only after consultation with a PCP. Pyrantel pamoate may be taken at any time of the day without regard to meals, and it may be taken or mixed with milk or fruit juice.[11] A special diet or fasting before or after administration is not necessary. The liquid formulation (containing 50 mg/mL of the pyrantel base) should be shaken well before the dose is measured.

Side effects usually are mild, infrequent, and transient. The most common adverse effects involve the gastrointestinal (GI) tract and include nausea, vomiting, tenesmus, anorexia, diarrhea, and abdominal cramps.[12] These adverse effects are typically related to expulsion of the helminths from the GI tract. However, a patient who experiences severe or persistent abdominal symptoms or other side effects after taking the first or second dose of this medication should be referred to a PCP for further evaluation. Less common side effects such as headache, dizziness, drowsiness, insomnia, rash, fever, and weakness may occur. In very rare circumstances, transient increases in aspartate aminotransferase, ototoxicity, optic neuritis, and hallucinations with confusion and paresthesia have been reported.[11]

Patients who do not respond to the recommended doses of pyrantel pamoate should be evaluated further, and the use of prescription products should be considered. Mebendazole (Vermox) once was considered by experts to be the drug of choice to treat pinworm infection,[13,14] but it has since been discontinued by the manufacturer. The currently available prescription agent for treatment of pinworm infection is albendazole. Albendazole is approved to treat other helminthic infections, but FDA considers its use off label when used to treat pinworms. Albendazole is given as a single oral dose (400 mg for patients ages 2 years and older; 200 mg for patients younger than 2 years).

Product Selection Guidelines

Pyrantel pamoate is a safe and effective treatment for pinworms. The brands listed in Table 18–2 are comparatively priced and generally less expensive than prescription treatment (e.g., albendazole). Pyrantel pamoate is contraindicated in patients with

table

18–2   Selected Nonprescription Pyrantel Pamoate Products

Trade Name	Primary Ingredient
Pin-X Liquid/Chewable Tablet	Pyrantel 50 mg/mL (base) and 250 mg/tablet (base)
Pyrantel Suspension	Pyrantel 50 mg/mL (base)
Reese's Pinworm Caplet	Pyrantel 180 mg (equals 62.5 mg base)
Reese's Pinworm Medicine Liquid	Pyrantel 144 mg/mL (equals 50 mg/mL base)
Reese's Pinworm Medicine Family Pack	Pyrantel 144 mg/mL (equals 50 mg/mL base); contains two 1-fl oz bottles to treat the entire family

hypersensitivity to the drug. Patients with preexisting liver dysfunction or severe malnutrition should not self-medicate without first consulting a PCP. Pyrantel pamoate is Pregnancy Category C and has not been studied in pregnant women; therefore, it should be used during pregnancy only when the benefits clearly outweigh the risks, and only under the direction of a PCP.[15] The World Health Organization does not recommend the use of pyrantel pamoate during the second and third trimesters for high-risk patients.[6] Pyrantel pamoate also should not be used in patients younger than 2 years or those weighing less than 25 pounds, unless under the direction of a PCP.

Complementary Therapies

Various home remedies (e.g., applying a combination of garlic paste and Vaseline to the anus, or ingesting coconut oil and castor oil) and complementary therapies (e.g., white willow bark, green tea, or turmeric) have been used to treat pinworm infection. These remedies should not be recommended because insufficient efficacy and safety evidence exists to support their use for the treatment of pinworm infections. Because of the high risk of transmission of this infection, patients instead should take nonprescription medications such as pyrantel pamoate or prescription medications that are approved by the Food and Drug Administration (FDA) for pinworm infection.

Assessment of Pinworm Infection: A Case-Based Approach

Before recommending treatment, the provider should explain how to confirm a pinworm infection by any of the following methods: (1) nighttime perianal or perineal itching in a child, (2) visual inspection of the perianal or perineal area for the adult worm, or (3) a cellophane tape or an adhesive paddle test. Adult pinworms and eggs are seldom found in the feces; therefore, looking for worms in the stool is not a reliable way to diagnose enterobiasis.[16] When symptoms of pinworms (e.g., nocturnal perianal or perineal itching) are present in children, nonprescription therapy may be initiated. Other more vague symptoms (e.g., sleep disturbances and GI complaints) should be evaluated medically before initiating nonprescription therapy. However, asymptomatic disease is common in enterobiasis, and visual inspection may be necessary. To conduct a visual inspection, the parent should inspect the anal area during the night with a flashlight while the child is sleeping or in the very early morning before the child arises. White, thread-like, wriggling worms between 3 and 7 mm in length (about the size of a staple) may be seen. If pinworms are present, treatment should be initiated. Finally, if pinworms are suspected but symptoms are vague and/or visual inspection is negative, a PCP may instruct the patient to obtain a cellophane tape sample. The parent should apply the sticky side of the tape to the perianal area (usually with a tongue depressor) and affix it sticky side down on a glass slide. Commercially available kits, such as the Falcon SWUBE paddles, use a sticky paddle instead of tape to affix to a slide (see Color Plates, photograph 1C). These pinworm paddles usually are supplied by laboratories to conduct the test. Samples should be taken over 3 consecutive days upon the child's awakening, which may increase the likelihood of detection to around 90%.[5] The samples should then be taken to a PCP for microscopic

examination. If the test is positive, treatment of the pinworm infection should be initiated.

Cases 18–1 and 18–2 illustrate the assessment of patients with pinworm infections.

Patient Counseling for Pinworm Infection

Once the decision to treat the pinworm infection with pyrantel pamoate is made, the package insert material should be reviewed with the patient or caregiver. The insert explains the pinworm life cycle, symptoms of pinworm infection, and methods of transmitting the infection. Doses should be calculated for the patient and all family members, and the need to treat the whole family should be emphasized. The patient or caregiver should be advised to implement strict hygienic measures to prevent reinfection or transmission of the infection to other family members (Table 18–1). In addition, it should be explained that the side effects of pyrantel pamoate usually are mild and infrequent, but that medical referral may be necessary if more severe effects occur. Patients who experience severe or persistent symptoms after taking this medication should be referred for medical evaluation. Finally, patients should be advised that pinworm infection symptoms (e.g., nocturnal perianal itching) should improve within 2 weeks of treatment and that if symptoms persist or worsen to include systemic complaints (e.g., abdominal discomfort, insomnia, and/or nervousness), medical referral may be necessary. The box Patient Education for Pinworm Infection lists specific information to provide patients.

Evaluation of Patient Outcomes for Pinworm Infection

The patient or caregiver should be instructed to contact a PCP if anal itching persists beyond 2 weeks, if the itching recurs, or if new symptoms develop. Because of pyrantel pamoate's variable cure rate, a second dose may be required. It should be given 2 weeks after the first dose and only under the care of a PCP. In addition, the patient or caregiver should be asked about the implementation of hygienic measures. If these measures are not being followed, their importance for preventing reinfection should be stressed again.

Key Points for Pinworm Infection

➤ Pinworms are common in the United States and rarely cause significant morbidity.
➤ Health care providers should be familiar with common helminthic infections, their symptoms, and their treatment.
➤ A medical referral may be necessary when helminths other than pinworms are suspected.
➤ Although pyrantel pamoate is used in treating other helminthic infections, only pinworm infection should be evaluated for self-treatment with this nonprescription agent.
➤ Health care providers can aid patients and caregivers in the self-diagnosis, counseling, and self-treatment with nonprescription pinworm medication.

case

18-1

Relevant Evaluation Criteria	Scenario/Model Outcome

Information Gathering

1. Gather essential information about the patients' symptoms, including:

   a. description of symptom(s) (i.e., nature, onset, duration, severity, associated symptoms)

   A man presents to the pharmacy requesting assistance in selecting an OTC product for his family. He reports that his daughter was diagnosed with pinworms by the pediatrician, who recommended an OTC medication to treat the daughter as well as mom and dad. The father says his daughter has been complaining about perianal itching that is most intense at night. He and his wife have no current symptoms. He needs a liquid formulation because his daughter cannot swallow tablets or capsules.

   b. description of any factors that seem to precipitate, exacerbate, and/or relieve the patients' symptom(s)

   No precipitating factors

   c. description of the patients' efforts to relieve the symptoms

   The parents applied hydrocortisone cream to the child's perianal region for itching, with no relief.

   d. patients' identity

   Daughter: Bella Turner; mother: Karen Turner; Father: Ray Turner

   e. age, sex, height, and weight

   Daughter: 5 years old, female, 3 ft 6 in., 39 lb; mother: 32 years old, female, 5 ft. 6 in., 143 lb; father: 36 years old, male, 5 ft 11 in., 190 lb

   f. patients' occupation

   The father is an attorney, and his wife is a real estate agent.

   g. patients' dietary habits

   Normal diet

   h. patients' sleep habits

   Daughter: frequent awakenings at night caused by perianal itching; parents: normal sleep habits

   i. concurrent medical conditions, prescription and non-prescription medications, and dietary supplements

   Daughter: daily children's chewable multivitamin; mother: oral contraceptive pills, daily multivitamin; father: fish oil capsules daily

   j. allergies

   Daughter: NKDA, mother: NKDA, father: penicillin allergy

   k. history of other adverse reactions to medications

   None

   l. other (describe) _____

   The father does cardio and weight training at the gym 3 days a week.

Assessment and Triage

2. Differentiate patients' signs/symptoms and correctly identify the patient's primary problem(s).

   Bella is experiencing perianal itching because of a pinworm infection, which results in restless sleep at nights.

3. Identify exclusions for self-treatment (Figure 18–1).

   Patients should be excluded for self-treatment if they (1) are allergic to the OTC product, (2) are younger than 2 years (unless treatment is approved by PCP), (3) weigh less than 25 lb (unless treatment is approved by PCP), or (4) have liver disease.

   The patients do not have exclusions for self-treatment.

4. Formulate a comprehensive list of therapeutic alternatives for the primary problem to determine if triage to a medical provider is required, and share this information with the patients or caregiver.

   Options include:

   (1) Recommend an appropriate OTC product (e.g., pyrantel pamoate) at appropriate doses for each member of the family, along with nondrug therapies.

   (2) Recommend that mother and father see their PCP for a prescription medication.

   (3) Counsel only on environmental control measures.

   (4) Take no action.

Plan

5. Select an optimal therapeutic alternative to address the patients' problem, taking into account patient preferences.

   OTC treatment with pyrantel pamoate is appropriate for all three patients. The child is not comfortable swallowing tablets or caplets, but she can take chewable tablets or liquid formulations; therefore, pyrantel pamoate is a good choice.

6. Describe the recommended therapeutic approach to the patients or caregiver.

   "Both albendazole and pyrantel pamoate are effective in the treatment of pinworms. However, pyrantel pamoate is available without a prescription, and albendazole requires a prescription. Because one of your family members was recently diagnosed with pinworm infection and the medical provider instructed that other family members be treated, pyrantel pamoate is a reasonable option."

case

18-1 *continued*

Relevant Evaluation Criteria	Scenario/Model Outcome
7. Explain to the patients or caregiver the rationale for selecting the recommended therapeutic approach from the considered therapeutic alternatives.	"Pinworms are not life threatening and may resolve on their own. However, if the infection is untreated, the infected person (in this case, your daughter) may reinfect herself or infect other family members. She also may experience some complications of infection if she is not treated. Therefore, treatment is recommended. Pyrantel pamoate is a reasonable option because it is available without a prescription; therefore, the other family members do not need to visit a primary care provider, which could have increased the cost of treatment and delay its initiation. Pyrantel pamoate also is available as a chewable tablet or an oral suspension, which offers flexible dosing that is based on weight for multiple family members. Other formulations (e.g., tablets and caplets) are available, if preferred."

Patient Education

8. When recommending self-care with nonprescription medications and/or nondrug therapy, convey accurate information to the patients or caregiver:

a. appropriate dose and frequency of administration

Bella (daughter) weighs 17.7 kg (39 lb); the dose of pyrantel is 11 mg/kg, so she should receive about 195 mg. She can take 4 mL of the liquid formulation (144 mg/mL equivalent to 50 mg/mL pyrantel base).

Karen (mom) weighs 65.0 kg, so she should receive at least 715 mg of pyrantel pamoate (which would be approximately 3 chewable tablets or 15 mL of the liquid formulation).

Ray (dad) weighs 86.4 kg, so he should receive 950 mg of pyrantel pamoate (4 chewable tablets or about 25 mL of the liquid formulation).

b. maximum number of days the therapy should be employed

"A single dose usually is required. If symptoms persist after 2 weeks, contact your primary care provider for evaluation and, if needed, recommendation for a second dose."

c. product administration procedures

"Pyrantel pamoate may be taken at any time of day without regard to meals. It may be mixed with milk or fruit juice. If using the oral suspension, shake well before administering."

[*Note:* Prior to administering medication, the practitioner should verify that other family members who need to be treated do not meet criteria for exclusion for self-treatment. Doses will need to be calculated for the other family members.]

d. expected time to onset of relief

"Relief of symptoms may take several days. The repeat dose should not be administered until 2 weeks have elapsed and should be administered only if recommended by your primary care provider."

e. degree of relief that can be reasonably expected

"Perianal itching should decrease after several days, with complete pinworm eradication after at least 2 weeks."

f. most common side effects

"Adverse effects are usually mild and may consist of nausea, vomiting, loss of appetite, diarrhea, or abdominal cramps."

g. side effects that warrant medical intervention should they occur

"Severe or persistent abdominal symptoms require medical attention."

h. patient options in the event that condition worsens or persists

"Contact the appropriate health care provider if any family member's condition worsens, or if any family member experiences any severe adverse effects, such as severe or persistent abdominal symptoms, after taking the medication."

[*Note:* The practitioner should reinforce to the parents that pinworms are very common and rarely cause serious problems, but that the condition will continue and potentially spread to others if not treated.]

i. product storage requirements

"Store at room temperature away from direct light with container sealed tightly."

j. specific nondrug measures

See Table 18-1.

case
18–1 *continued*

Relevant Evaluation Criteria	Scenario/Model Outcome
Solicit follow-up questions from the patient or caregiver.	"Should my daughter receive a prescription medication instead because she has an active infection?"
Answer the patient's or caregiver's questions.	"Both the prescription and nonprescription medications are equally effective in treating pinworms. You can use either the prescription medication or the non-prescription pyrantel pamoate, depending on your preferences (such as cost)."
Evaluation of Patient Outcomes	
9. Assess patient outcome	You can call the parents in 1–2 weeks to assess the child's response to the medication. If symptoms have resolved, reinforce the importance of hygienic measures. If symptoms persist, another single dose of pyrantel pamoate can be administered but only after reevaluation by the child's pediatrician.

Key: NA = NKDA = No known drug allergies; OTC = over-the-counter; PCP = primary care provider.

case
18–2

Relevant Evaluation Criteria	Scenario/Model Outcome
Information Gathering	
1. Gather essential information about the patient's symptoms, including:	
a. description of symptom(s) (i.e., nature, onset, duration, severity, associated symptoms)	A woman presents to the pharmacy requesting assistance choosing a product to help "tie up her stomach" and a product to help her with intense itching. She says she's had loose stool and generalized abdominal pain for about 2 weeks. She mentions that her stool has been watery most of the time and that she's noticed little white squiggly things on the tissue after wiping. The itching, which began approximately 10 days before the diarrhea started, is mostly in her perineal and vaginal area and is worse at night.
b. description of any factors that seem to precipitate, exacerbate, and/or relieve the patient's symptom(s)	No precipitating factors
c. description of the patient's efforts to relieve the symptoms	She tried bismuth subsalicylate for 3 days without much relief. She took 3 doses of loperamide, which helped the diarrhea temporarily but did not help the itching. She's tried applying hemorrhoidal ointment and hydrocortisone ointment to the region to help with the itching.
d. patient's identity	Letty Whitaker
e. age, sex, height, and weight	46 years old, female, 5 ft 2 in., 140 lb
f. patient's occupation	Dance instructor
g. patient's dietary habits	Normal diet, high in fruits and vegetables
h. patient's sleep habits	Frequent awakenings at night caused by perineal itching
i. concurrent medical conditions, prescription and non-prescription medications, and dietary supplements	Daily multivitamin; occasional ibuprofen or acetaminophen for pain
j. allergies	NKDA
k. history of other adverse reactions to medications	None

case
18–2 *continued*

Relevant Evaluation Criteria	Scenario/Model Outcome

Assessment and Triage

2. Differentiate patient's signs/symptoms and correctly identify the patient's primary problem(s).

Patient's symptoms, such as perianal itching at night, are consistent with pinworms, but prolonged diarrhea and abdominal pain are unusual symptoms and should be evaluated medically. The appearance of "white squiggly things" on the tissue may indicate the presence of pinworms, but a tape test or a slide test must be done to confirm infection.

3. Identify exclusions for self-treatment (Figure 18-1).

Consider the patient to be excluded from self-treatment if she (1) is allergic to the OTC product, (2) is younger than 2 years (unless treatment approved by PCP), (3) weighs less than 25 lb (unless treatment approved by PCP), (4) has liver disease, (5) is pregnant, (6) is breast-feeding, or (7) has vague symptoms and negative visual inspection.

4. Formulate a comprehensive list of therapeutic alternatives for the primary problem to determine if triage to a medical provider is required, and share this information with the patient or caregiver.

Options include:

(1) Recommend an appropriate OTC product at appropriate doses for the patient, along with nondrug therapies.

(2) Refer the patient to a PCP for further evaluation, diagnosis, and recommended treatment.

(3) Counsel on only environmental control measures.

(4) Take no action.

Plan

5. Select an optimal therapeutic alternative to address the patient's problem, taking into account patient preferences.

Medical evaluation by a PCP is warranted for the perineal, gastrointestinal, and vaginal symptoms and subsequent treatment.

6. Describe the recommended therapeutic approach to the patient or caregiver.

"You should see your primary care provider for further evaluation of your symptoms, appropriate diagnosis, and recommended treatment."

7. Explain to the patient or caregiver the rationale for selecting the recommended therapeutic approach from the considered therapeutic alternatives.

"Because you have no documented pinworm infection, either by visual inspection or by tape slide, and because you have other symptoms that may be complications of a pinworm infection, self-treatment is not appropriate. Your symptoms may be consistent with pinworm infection, but other possibilities need to be ruled out."

Patient Education

8. When recommending self-care with nonprescription medications and/or nondrug therapy, convey accurate information to the patient or caregiver.

Self-treatment is not appropriate, but you should institute environmental control measures shown in Table 18–1 and seek medical care.

Solicit follow-up questions from the patient or caregiver.

(1) "What are some of the complications associated with pinworms?"

(2) "How are pinworms normally treated?"

Answer the patient's or caregiver's questions.

(1) "If untreated, pinworms may possibly lead to secondary bacterial infections in the perianal and perineal regions. Pinworms also can lead to pelvic inflammatory disease, endometritis, and urinary tract infections. In addition, other possible symptoms associated with pinworm infection include insomnia, restlessness, and anorexia."

(2) "Patients may be treated with a single dose of various nonprescription (pyrantel pamoate) or prescription (albendazole) medications. Along with medications, patients also must follow specific nondrug measures to prevent reinfection."

Evaluation of Patient Outcome

9. Assess patient outcome

Ask the patient to call you in 1 week, or initiate a follow-up call to the patient to assess whether she was evaluated by a physician and whether her symptoms are improving.

Key: OTC = Over-the-counter; PCP = primary care provider.

patient education for
Pinworm Infection

The objectives of self-treatment are to (1) eradicate pinworms in the infected patient, (2) prevent reinfection, and (3) prevent transmission of the infection to others. For most patients, carefully following product instructions and the self-care measures listed here will help ensure optimal therapeutic outcomes.

Nondrug Measures
- See Table 18–1 for nondrug/preventive measures.

Nonprescription Medications
- Read package insert for pyrantel pamoate information carefully; this information will help prevent reinfection or transmission of the infection.
- Consult a primary care provider before giving the medication to a person with liver disease or severe malnutrition, a child who is younger than 2 years and/or weighs less than 25 pounds, or a woman who is pregnant or breast-feeding.
- Treat all household members to ensure elimination of the infection. Medical referral may be necessary if household members meet criteria for exclusion for self-treatment (e.g., malnutrition, pregnancy, liver disease, anemia, or age younger than 2 years).
- Take only one dose as shown on the dosing schedule included with the product. For adults and children older than 2 years, dosing is the same: 11 mg/kg taken orally. The maximum dose is 1 gram.

- Shake the liquid formulation well, and use a measuring spoon to ensure an accurate dose.
- If desired, pyrantel pamoate may be taken with food, milk, or fruit juices on an empty stomach any time during the day. The liquid formulation may be mixed with milk or fruit juice.
- Note that fasting, laxatives, and special diets are not necessary to aid treatment.

When to Seek Medical Attention
- Seek medical attention if you experience any of the following:
  - Abdominal cramps, nausea, vomiting, anorexia, rash, diarrhea, headache, drowsiness, or dizziness occurs and persists after taking the medication.
  - Symptoms of the pinworm infection persist beyond 2 weeks after the initial dose of pyrantel pamoate. A second dose of pyrantel pamoate can be given if symptoms are present beyond 2 weeks, but only if directed to do so by a primary care provider.
  - Rare symptoms such as vaginal itching or bleeding, pain upon urination, urinary tract infection, and hives are present.

REFERENCES

1. Wang L, Hwang K, Chen E. *Enterobius vermicularis* infection in schoolchildren: a large-scale survey 6 years after a population-based control. *Epidemiol Infect.* 2010;138(1):28–36.
2. Stermer E, Sukhotnic I, Shaoul R. Pruritus ani: an approach to an itching condition. *J Pediatr Gastroenterol Nutr.* 2009;48(5):513–6.
3. Cappello M, Hotez P. Intestinal nematodes. In: Long S, ed. *Principles and Practice of Pediatric Infectious Diseases* [subscription electronic library]. 4th ed. New York, NY: Churchill Livingstone; 2012. Accessed December 4, 2013.
4. St Georgiev V. Chemotherapy of enterobiasis (oxyuriasis). *Expert Opin Pharmacother.* 2001;2(2):267–75.
5. Kucik CJ, Martin GL, Sortor BV. Common intestinal parasites. *Am Fam Physician.* 2004;69(5):1161–8.
6. Centers for Disease Control and Prevention. Parasites—enterobiasis. 2013. Accessed at http://www.cdc.gov/parasites/pinworm, April 18, 2013.
7. Burkhart CN, Burkhart CG. Assessment of frequency, transmission, and genitourinary complications of enterobiasis (pinworms). *Int J Dermatol.* 2005;44(10):837–40.
8. Young C, Tataryn I, Kowalewska-Grochowska KT, et al. *Enterobius vermicularis* infection of the fallopian tube in an infertile female. *Pathology Research and Practice.* 2010;206(6):405–7.

9. Swaim L, Zietz B, Qu Z. An uncommon cause of vaginal bleeding in a child. *Obstet Gynecol.* 2007;110(2 pt 1):416–20.
10. Arca MJ, Gates RL, Groner JI, et al. Clinical manifestations of appendiceal pinworms in children: an institutional experience and a review of the literature. *Pediatr Surg Int.* 2004;20(5):372–5.
11. Anthelmintics. In: McEvoy GK, Snow KE, eds. *AHFS Drug Handbook.* STAT!Ref Online Electronic Medical Library. Bethesda, MD: American Society of Health-System Pharmacists; 2010. Accessed November 2, 2010.
12. Bagheri H, Simiand E, Montastruc J-L, et al. Adverse drug reactions to anthelmintics. *Ann Pharmacother.* 2004;38(3):383–8.
13. Jacobson CC, Abel EA. Parasitic infestations. *J Am Acad Dermatol.* 2007;56(6):1026–43.
14. Drugs for parasitic infections. *Med Lett Drugs Ther* [online version]. 2007;5 (suppl):e1–15. Accessed November 20, 2010.
15. Briggs G, Freeman R, Yaffe S. Pyrantel pamoate. In: Briggs G, Freeman R, Yaffe S, eds. *Drugs in Pregnancy and Lactation: A Reference Guide to Fetal and Neonatal Risk.* 8th ed. Philadelphia, PA: Lippincott Williams & Wilkins; 2008.
16. Maguire J. Intestinal nematodes (roundworms). In: Mandell GL, Bennett JE, Dolin R, eds. *Mandell, Douglas, and Bennett's Principles and Practice of Infectious Diseases.* Expert Consult Online Electronic Medical Library. Philadelphia, PA: Churchill Livingston Elsevier; 2010.

chapter 19

NAUSEA AND VOMITING

Stefanie P. Ferreri and Adam C. Welch

Nausea and vomiting (N/V) symptoms can occur in both adults and children from a variety of circumstances associated with several medical disorders. Common self-care disorders that involve N/V are motion sickness, pregnancy (NVP), acute viral gastroenteritis, and "upset stomach" (overeating or indigestion). Nonprescription antiemetics can be used to prevent or treat the symptoms of N/V for these disorders. Vomiting accounts for 2.3% of all emergency department visits in the United States.[1] Accurate data on the epidemiology of N/V are not available because these symptoms occur in many medical disorders and many individuals do not report these disturbances to a health care provider.

The severity of N/V related to motion sickness is difficult to quantify because of interindividual variability and susceptibility to the condition. Motion sickness rarely occurs in children younger than 2 years. Women are more susceptible than men to motion sickness (1.7:1), and symptoms of nausea occur more often during menstruation and pregnancy.[2]

The incidence of N/V in early pregnancy is quoted as between 50% and 80%. Typically these symptoms subside by the 20th week of pregnancy, but they may persist throughout the pregnancy in 20% of women.[3] Half of all pregnant women have both nausea and vomiting, one-fourth have nausea only, and it is rare for only vomiting to occur.[4] A very severe form of pregnancy-related vomiting, hyperemesis gravidarum, occurs in less than 1% of women and may require rehydration and hospitalization.[5]

The third typically self-treatable cause of N/V is acute viral gastroenteritis. Viral gastroenteritis is an inflammation of the stomach and small intestines that commonly presents with acute vomiting and diarrhea.[6] This illness may affect any age group and is usually self-limiting, but pediatric patients may experience serious consequences from dehydration.[7] Gastroenteritis is most commonly caused by rotavirus and norovirus and occurs most often in autumn and winter[8] (see Chapter 16). The Centers for Disease Control and Prevention (CDC) reports that in children, rotavirus infections result in approximately 400,000 physician visits, up to 272,000 emergency room visits, and 55,000–70,000 annual hospitalizations, with total costs approximating $1 billion.[9] The rotavirus vaccine is included in the childhood immunization schedule.[10] CDC estimates that 19–21 million cases of acute gastroenteritis each year are due to norovirus infection, and that norovirus is the most common cause of foodborne disease outbreaks.[11]

The last self-care disorder that involves N/V is indigestion or distension associated with overeating. Limited treatment options for this disorder are discussed in this chapter. A more comprehensive discussion occurs in Chapter 13.

Pathophysiology of Nausea and Vomiting

The pathophysiology of N/V involves both the central nervous system (CNS) and the gastrointestinal (GI) tract. Figure 19–1 shows four different areas of the body that provide input to a complex system of neurons in the medulla oblongata in the brain stem, known as the vomiting center (VC): the chemoreceptor trigger zone (CTZ), vestibular apparatus, cerebral cortex, and visceral GI tract afferent nerves.[12–14]

The neurons in the CTZ are outside the blood–brain barrier, therefore the CTZ responds to stimuli from either the bloodstream or the cerebral spinal fluid.[13,14] The vestibular apparatus is located in the bony labyrinth of the temporal lobe. It detects motion and body position, including changes in equilibrium; direct input to the VC is through cholinergic pathways. The cerebral cortex system provides input to the VC through higher cortical centers; this pathway for initiating emesis is the least understood. Sensory input, including sight, smell, anticipation, or memory, may elicit a strong sensation of nausea through the cerebral cortex.[14] Finally, visceral afferent nerve pathways from the GI tract have numerous neurotransmitters that provide input to the VC. Major neurotransmitters and receptors involved in vomiting include serotonin, dopamine, histamine type 1, acetylcholine, opioid, and neurokinin receptors.[12,13]

The VC is triggered by different stimuli in the CNS and GI tract, sending impulses to the salivation center, vasomotor center, respiratory center, and cranial nerves, and then to the pharynx and GI tract, after which nausea and/or vomiting may occur.[14] Table 19–1 lists several stimuli that may elicit N/V; however, many of these are not self-limiting and require medical evaluation and treatment.[12–16] Causes discussed in this chapter (motion sickness, pregnancy, viral gastroenteritis, and overeating) may be self-treatable or prevented with proper patient education.

Emesis, or vomiting, is thought to be a complicated defense response secondary to a variety of different mechanisms. Retching may occur after subjective feelings of nausea. The abdominal and diaphragmatic musculature may contract or relax, and the associated coordinating circuitry involves other areas such as the laryngeal or pharyngeal muscles. The epiglottis closes to prevent aspiration, the soft palate is elevated, a retrograde contraction occurs while the gastric fundus relaxes, and the stomach contents move into the esophagus and are expelled as vomiting begins.[14]

Nausea and vomiting of motion sickness are produced by overstimulation of the labyrinth (inner ear) apparatus.[2] The three semicircular canals in the labyrinth on each side of the head are

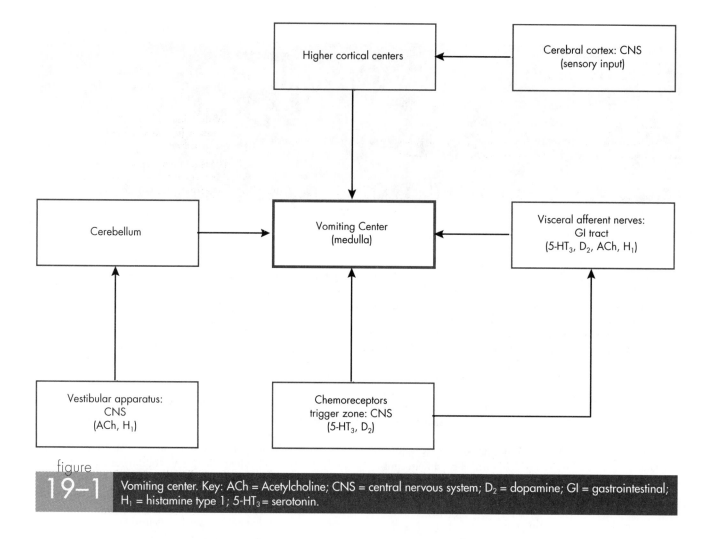

figure
19-1 Vomiting center. Key: ACh = Acetylcholine; CNS = central nervous system; D₂ = dopamine; GI = gastrointestinal; H₁ = histamine type 1; 5-HT₃ = serotonin.

responsible for maintaining equilibrium. Postural adjustments are made when the brain receives nerve impulses initiated by the movement of fluid in the canals. When the head is rotated on two axes simultaneously, unusual motion patterns may produce motion sickness. Inaccurate interpretation of visual stimuli while standing or sitting motionless may also produce motion sickness. For instance, a person may experience motion sickness when watching a film taken from a roller coaster, watching an airplane performing aerobatics, or extending the head upward while standing on a rotating platform.[2] Individuals differ in their response to motion sickness stimuli, such as flying and boating, but no one is immune. Regardless of the type of stimulus-producing event, motion sickness is easier to prevent than to treat with antiemetics that target the primary neurotransmitters acetylcholine and histamine type 1 in the vestibular apparatus.[17] In pregnancy, it is unclear which neurotransmitters are the cause of N/V, as it is thought to be multifactorial.[17] A Cochrane review published in 2010 found that certain nonprescription antiemetics, such as doxylamine and dimenhydrinate, are generally effective in NVP, but little information exists on fetal outcomes.[3] Approximately 10% of women with NVP will require treatment with medication,[18] but providers may avoid antiemetics until dehydration, weight loss, or electrolyte imbalances occur.[16]

Nausea and vomiting secondary to acute gastroenteritis are caused by intestinal irritation. The visceral afferent nerves are

mediated primarily through dopamine, serotonin, acetylcholine, and histamine type 1 receptors; therefore, therapy is targeted at those neurotransmitters.[12,14,16,17]

Gut distension and decreased GI emptying may stimulate mechanoreceptors and may be responsible for eliciting N/V related to overeating.[8]

Clinical Presentation of Nausea and Vomiting

Nausea and vomiting consist of three different processes: (1) nausea (characterized by a person's subjective feeling of a need to vomit); (2) retching (involuntary rhythmic diaphragmatic and abdominal contractions); and (3) vomiting (rapid, forceful expulsion of the GI tract contents).[12,13,16] Although most cases of N/V are self-limiting, a patient may show signs and symptoms that warrant medical referral. Possible acute complications of vomiting include dehydration, esophageal tears manifested by blood in the vomitus, aspiration, malnutrition, electrolyte and/or acid–base abnormalities, diaphragmatic herniation, and Mallory–Weiss syndrome.[16] Dehydration and electrolyte imbalances are the major concerns associated with vomiting. Signs and symptoms of dehydration include dry mouth, decreased skin turgor, excessive thirst, little or no urination,

table
19–1   Primary Causes of Nausea and Vomiting

GI Tract (visceral afferent nerves)	CNS Disorders	Other Disorders
Mechanical Obstruction GI obstruction (e.g., PUD, gastric carcinoma, pancreatic disease); small intestine obstruction **Motility Disorders** Gastroparesis (e.g., DM, drug-induced, post-viral); chronic intestinal pseudo-obstruction; IBS; anorexia nervosa; idiopathic gastric stasis **Peritoneal Irritation** Appendicitis; bacterial peritonitis; pancreatitis **Infections** Viral gastroenteritis[a] (e.g., norovirus, rotavirus); food poisoning (e.g., toxins from *Bacillus cereus, Staphylococcus aureus, Clostridium perfringens*); hepatitis A or B; acute systemic infections **Topical Gastrointestinal Irritants** Alcohol; NSAIDs; antibiotics, iron	**Vestibular Disorders** Labyrinthitis; Ménière's syndrome; motion sickness[a] **Increased Intracranial Pressure** CNS tumor; subdural or subarachnoid hemorrhage; pseudotumor cerebri **Infections** Meningitis; encephalitis **Psychogenic** Anticipatory vomiting; bulimia; psychiatric disorders (anxiety) **Other CNS Disorders** Migraine headache **Irritation of CTZ (medication-induced)** Chemotherapy; opiates; theophylline or digoxin toxicity; antibiotics; radiation therapy; drug withdrawal (e.g., opiates, BDZs)	Cardiac disease (e.g., MI, HF); urologic disease (e.g., stones, pyelonephritis); overeating[a] DM (e.g., DKA); renal disease (e.g., uremia); adrenocortical crisis (e.g., Addison's disease); pregnancy[a]

Key: BDZ = Benzodiazepine; CNS = central nervous system; CTZ = chemotrigger receptor zone; DKA = diabetic ketoacidosis; DM = diabetes mellitus; GI = gastrointestinal; HF = heart failure; IBS = irritable bowel syndrome; MI = myocardial infarction; NSAIDs = nonsteroidal anti-inflammatory drugs; PUD = peptic ulcer disease.

[a] Self-treatable or preventable disorders.

Source: References 8, 9, 11, 12, 14, and 15.

dizziness, lightheadedness, fainting, and reduced blood pressure.[16] These symptoms warrant medical referral for further evaluation.

In infants and small children, recurrent or protracted N/V (with accompanying diarrhea) may lead to marked dehydration and electrolyte imbalance that should not be ignored. Parents should be educated to recognize signs and symptoms of dehydration, such as dry mucous membranes, decreased skin turgor, irritability, altered mental status, and weight loss (Table 19–2).[19–21] The child should be referred for further evaluation if there are any exclusions for self-care of N/V.[6,19]

Treatment of Nausea and Vomiting

Treatment Goals

The goals of treating N/V are to (1) provide symptomatic relief, (2) identify and correct the underlying cause, (3) prevent and correct complications, and (4) prevent future occurrences.

General Treatment Approach

Most acute cases of N/V are self-limiting and will resolve spontaneously. A clear evaluation should be made to determine whether a patient is a candidate for self-treatment. The algorithms in Figures 19–2 and 19–3 outline the self-care treatment

table
19–2   Signs and Symptoms of Dehydration in Children

- Dry mouth and tongue
- Sunken and/or dry eyes
- Sunken fontanelle
- Decreased urine output (dry diapers for several hours)
- Dark urine
- Fast heartbeat
- Thirst (drinks extremely eagerly)
- Absence of tears when crying
- Decreased skin turgor
- Unusual lethargy, sleepiness, decreased alertness, or irritability
  - Body is "floppy"
  - Lightheadedness when sitting or standing up (in older children)
  - Difficulty in waking up the child (may indicate severe dehydration)
- Weight loss
  - Noticeable decrease in abdominal ("tummy") size
  - Clothes or diaper fits loosely
  - <3% body weight loss, indicating minimal or no dehydration
  - 3%–9% body weight loss, indicating mild-moderate dehydration
  - >9% body weight loss, indicating severe dehydration

Source: References 18–20 and 23.

Exclusions for Self-Treatment

- Urine ketones and/or high BG with signs of dehydration in patients with DM (may indicate DKA or HHS)
- Suspected food poisoning that does not clear up after 24 hours
- Severe abdominal pain in the middle or right lower quadrant (may indicate appendicitis or bowel obstruction)
- N/V with fever and/or diarrhea (may indicate infectious disease)
- Severe right upper quadrant pain, especially after eating fatty foods (may indicate cholecystitis or pancreatitis)
- Blood in the vomitus (may indicate ulcers, esophageal tears, or severe nosebleed)
- Yellow skin or eye discoloration and dark urine (may indicate hepatitis)
- Stiff neck with or without headache and sensitivity to brightness of normal light (may indicate meningitis)

- Head injury with N/V, blurry vision, or numbness and tingling
- Persons with glaucoma, BPH, chronic bronchitis, emphysema, or asthma (may react adversely to OTC antiemetics)
- Pregnancy (severe symptoms) or breastfeeding
- N/V caused by cancer chemotherapy; radiation therapy; serious metabolic disorders; CNS, GI, or endocrine disorders
- Drug-induced N/V: adverse effects of drugs used therapeutically (e.g., opioids, NSAIDs, antibiotics, estrogens); toxic doses of drugs used therapeutically (e.g., digoxin, theophylline, lithium); ethanol
- Psychogenic-induced N/V: bulimia, anorexia
- Chronic disease-induced N/V: gastroparesis with DM; DKA or HHS with DM; GERD

Source: References 11, 20, and 21.

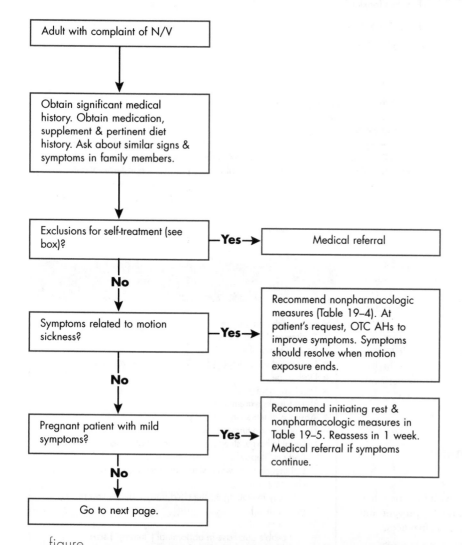

figure

19–2

Self-care of N/V in adults. Key: AH = Antihistamine; BG = blood glucose; BPH = benign prostatic hyperplasia; CNS = central nervous system; DKA = diabetic ketoacidosis; DM = diabetes mellitus; GERD = gastroesophageal reflux disease; GI = gastrointestinal; HHS = hyperosmolar hyperglycemic syndrome; H₂RA = histamine type 2 receptor antagonist; NSAID = nonsteroidal anti-inflammatory drug; ORS = oral rehydration salt; OTC = over-the-counter; PCP = primary care provider.

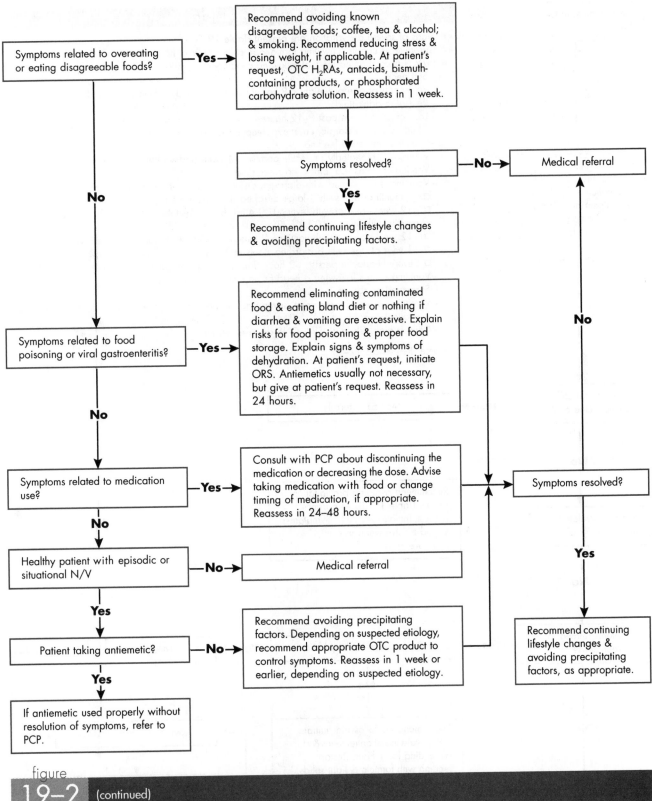

figure
19-2 (continued)

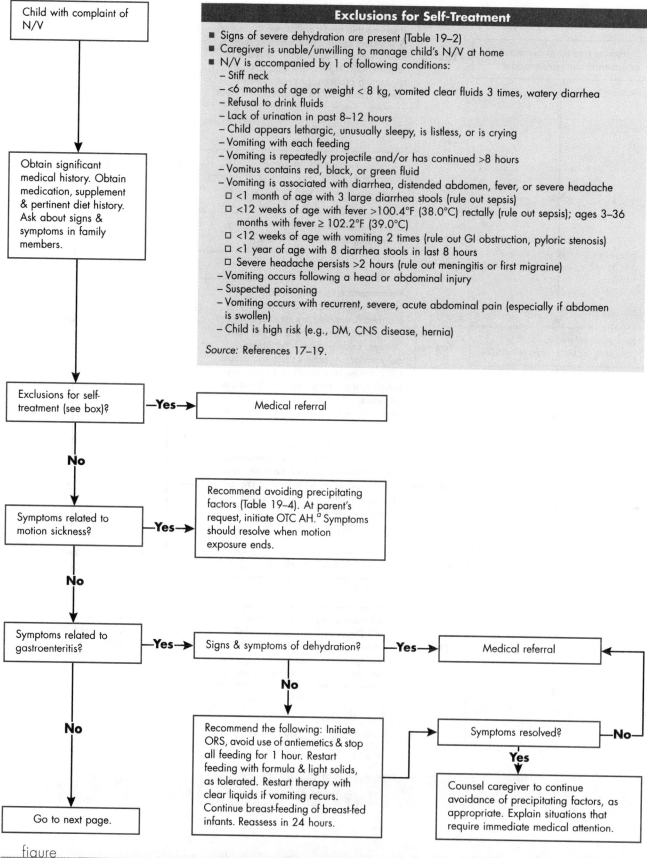

Exclusions for Self-Treatment

- Signs of severe dehydration are present (Table 19–2)
- Caregiver is unable/unwilling to manage child's N/V at home
- N/V is accompanied by 1 of following conditions:
  – Stiff neck
  – <6 months of age or weight < 8 kg, vomited clear fluids 3 times, watery diarrhea
  – Refusal to drink fluids
  – Lack of urination in past 8–12 hours
  – Child appears lethargic, unusually sleepy, is listless, or is crying
  – Vomiting with each feeding
  – Vomiting is repeatedly projectile and/or has continued >8 hours
  – Vomitus contains red, black, or green fluid
  – Vomiting is associated with diarrhea, distended abdomen, fever, or severe headache
    ☐ <1 month of age with 3 large diarrhea stools (rule out sepsis)
    ☐ <12 weeks of age with fever >100.4°F (38.0°C) rectally (rule out sepsis); ages 3–36 months with fever ≥ 102.2°F (39.0°C)
    ☐ <12 weeks of age with vomiting 2 times (rule out GI obstruction, pyloric stenosis)
    ☐ <1 year of age with 8 diarrhea stools in last 8 hours
    ☐ Severe headache persists >2 hours (rule out meningitis or first migraine)
  – Vomiting occurs following a head or abdominal injury
  – Suspected poisoning
  – Vomiting occurs with recurrent, severe, acute abdominal pain (especially if abdomen is swollen)
  – Child is high risk (e.g., DM, CNS disease, hernia)

Source: References 17–19.

figure 19–3 Self-care of N/V in children. Key: AH = Antihistamine; CNS = central nervous system; DM = diabetes mellitus; FDA = Food and Drug Administration; GI = gastrointestinal; ORS = oral rehydration salt; OTC = over-the-counter; PCP = primary care provider.

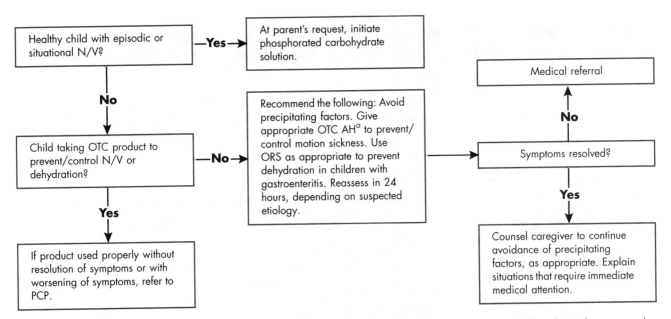

^a Do not use meclizine in children younger than 12 years. Do not use cyclizine in children younger than 6 years. Although FDA has approved dosages of diphenhydramine and dimenhydrinate for children ages 2–6 years, be extremely cautious in recommending these products for young children.

figure

19–3 (continued)

options and exclusions for self-care of N/V in adults[16,22–24] and children,[19–21] respectively. Severe cases of vomiting can result in dehydration or electrolyte imbalances. This may necessitate further evaluation or hospitalization. Treatment of nausea and vomiting can involve pharmacologic prescription and nonprescription therapies, as well as nonpharmacologic options. Pharmacologic nonprescription options are limited and include antihistamines. Because most cases of N/V are acute, the nonpharmacologic treatment is primarily directed to correct dehydration and electrolyte imbalances. Commercial oral rehydration salt (ORS) solutions should be recommended to prevent these complications. These products contain sodium, chloride, potassium, and a carbohydrate such as glucose or dextrose to restore loss of electrolytes and also restore loss of fluids.

Nonpharmacologic Therapy

ORS can be used for dehydration associated with vomiting or diarrhea.[25] In cases of vomiting, absorption of fluids may be compromised by continuous emesis in some patients. The World Health Organization (WHO) in conjunction with the United Nations Children's Fund (UNICEF) developed a solution for the treatment of dehydration.[26] The WHO/UNICEF ORS has a total osmolarity of 245 mOsm/L and includes 13.5 g/L of carbohydrates, 75 mmol/L of sodium, 20 mmol/L of potassium, 65 mmol/L chloride, and 30 mmol/L of a base. A simple, glucose-based ORS solution can be made by mixing one-half teaspoon of salt and 6 teaspoons of sugar in 1 liter of clean water.[27] In third world countries with low health literacy, this formula is roughly explained as a pinch of salt and a handful of sugar. Although glucose-based ORS solution does not contain potassium, supplementation with bananas or orange juice could

be given. The glucose-based ORS solution is more isomolar and therefore more effective at rehydrating than water alone. Commercially available products and common examples can be found in Table 19–3.

Sports drinks such as Gatorade or Powerade often do not contain the recommended balance of electrolytes. The preferred ratio of sugar to sodium is 3:1. Original formula Gatorade contains a sugar-to-sodium ratio of 15:1. Dilution of sports drinks with water by the patient may be an option, but it is difficult to achieve accurate sugar-to-sodium ratios, plus sports drinks are often available in multiple formulations. Too much sugar may draw water into the gastrointestinal tract and facilitate further dehydration. Likewise, sodas such as ginger ale or cola and fruit juices such as apple may also contain too much sugar.[28]

The typical dosing of ORS solution varies according to the level of dehydration and the age and weight of the patient. For minimal dehydration, children weighing less than 10 kg should be given 60–120 mL of solution after each vomiting episode; children weighing 10 kg or over should be given 120–240 mL per episode. Mild-moderate dehydration should be treated with 50–100 mL/kg over 3–4 hours. Severe dehydration should be referred to emergency care for intravenous rehydration.[28] Adults should also be rehydrated but may gauge their need according to thirst. Replacing 30%–50% of the fluid loss in the first 24 hours is preferred.[16]

Oral rehydration should be offered 10 minutes after the last episode of vomiting and should be offered in small increments. In general, 5 mL of ORS solution may be given to children every 5 minutes, and 15 mL may be given to older children and adults every 5 minutes.[28] Dosage forms such as Pedialyte Freezer Pops may offer the slow administration desired in active vomiting.

table
19–3 Selected ORS Solution Therapy

Solution	Carbohydrate (g/L)	Sodium (mmol/L)	Potassium (mmol/L)	Chloride (mmol/L)	Base (mmol/L)	Total Osmolarity (mOsm/L)
WHO/UNICEF ORS	13.5	75	20	65	30	245
Enfalyte	30	50	25	45	34	200
Pedialyte	25	45	20	35	30	250
Rehydralyte	25	75	20	65	30	305
CeraLyte	40	50–90	20	NA	30	220

Key: NA = Not applicable; ORS = oral rehydration salt.
Source: Reference 27.

Other nonpharmacologic measures such as those listed in Table 19–4 can also be tried to minimize and prevent motion sickness.[2] Because teratogenicity is a major consideration, many providers are reluctant to prescribe medications for pregnant women. Similarly, many of the medications are excreted in breast milk of lactating women, so nonpharmacologic approaches may be recommended in these populations, although such measures are not evidence based (Table 19–5).[29]

Pharmacologic Therapy

Selection of a nonprescription medication for N/V is largely determined by the potential cause.

Nausea Associated with Motion Sickness

Antihistamines are effective and generally safe and well tolerated for nausea and vomiting related to motion sickness. A detailed description of antihistamines can be found in Chapter 11. Meclizine is the only FDA-approved nonprescription agent for the prevention of nausea, vomiting, or dizziness associated with motion sickness. Both doxylamine and diphenhydramine have been used as off-label treatments for nausea. Table 19–6 lists age-specific dosages and maximum daily limits for these antiemetics.[30] Because of their anticholinergic effects, antihistamines may thicken bronchial secretions and should be used with caution in patients with respiratory conditions such as asthma, chronic bronchitis, and emphysema. In addition, the mydriatic

effects of antihistamines may exacerbate angle-closure glaucoma. The urinary retention effects of antihistamines may also exacerbate symptoms of benign prostatic hypertrophy. Other side effects of nonprescription antihistamines include dry mouth, confusion, dizziness, tremors, and constipation.[17] Drowsiness is also a common adverse effect of antihistamines. Patients should avoid concomitant use with other CNS depressants, such as alcohol, hypnotics, and sedatives. This drowsiness, coupled with the potential for blurred vision, may inhibit the ability to safely drive or operate heavy machinery. Meclizine may be less sedating than doxylamine and diphenhydramine. Paradoxical stimulatory reactions such as insomnia, nervousness, and irritability may occur in some patients. Diphenhydramine is a mild-moderate inhibitor of the cytochrome P450 (CYP) 2D6 enzyme. Therefore, it should be used with caution with other medications metabolized by CYP2D6, such as certain opiates, psychiatric medications, beta blockers, and antiarrhythmics. Some case reports have noted that ultrarapid metabolizers of CYP2D6 may be

table
19–4 Nonpharmacologic Measures to Prevent Motion Sickness

- Avoid reading during travel.
- Focus the line of vision fairly straight ahead (e.g., seat the patient in a position that allows vision out of the car window).
- Avoid excess food or alcohol before and during extended travel.
- Stay where motion is least experienced (e.g., front of the car; near the wings of an airplane; or midship [midway between bow and stern], preferably on deck).
- Avoid strong odors, particularly from food or tobacco smoke.
- Drive the vehicle if possible.

Source: Reference 2.

table
19–5 Nonpharmacologic Measures to Prevent NVP

- Make sure you have fresh air in the room where you sleep.
- Before getting out of bed, eat several dry crackers and relax in bed for 10–15 minutes.
- Get out of bed very slowly, and do not make any sudden movements.
- Before eating breakfast, nibble on dry toast or crackers.
- Make sure there is plenty of fresh air in the area where meals are prepared and eaten.
- Eat four to five small meals per day instead of three large meals. Do not overeat at meals.
- Do not drink fluids or eat soups at mealtime. Instead, drink small sips of liquid between meals.
- When nauseated, try small sips of carbonated beverages or fruit juices.
- Avoid greasy or fatty foods such as fried foods, gravy, mayonnaise, and salad dressing, as well as spicy or acidic foods (citrus fruits and beverages, tomatoes).
- If necessary, eat food that is chilled rather than warm or hot (cold foods tend to be less nauseating).
- Eat dry, bland, and high-protein foods.

Source: References 17 and 35.

table 19-6 Dosage Guidelines for Nonprescription Antiemetic Antihistamines[a]

Agent	Dosage (maximum daily dosage)		
	Adults and Children ≥12 Years	**Children 6 to <12 Years**	**Children 2 to <6 Years**
Cyclizine	50 mg 30 minutes before travel, then 50 mg every 4–6 hours (200 mg)	25 mg every 6–8 hours (75 mg)	Not recommended
Dimenhydrinate	50–100 mg every 4–6 hours (400 mg)	25–50 mg every 6–8 hours (150 mg)	12.5–25 mg every 6–8 hours (75 mg)
Diphenhydramine	25–50 mg every 4 hours (300 mg)	12.5–25 mg every 4 hours (150 mg)	6.25 mg every 4 hours (25 mg)
Meclizine	25–50 mg 1 hour before travel (50 mg)	Not recommended	Not recommended

[a] Take antihistamines at least 30–60 minutes before travel; then take continuously for the duration of travel.

Source: Reference 41.

at a higher risk for this paradoxical excitation. In the United States, approximately 1–2% of the population are estimated to be ultrarapid metabolizers.[31]

Nausea Associated with Food or Beverages

Nausea and vomiting may be associated with overindulgence in food or beverage or consumption of disagreeable foods, and it may present as heartburn, indigestion, and upset stomach. Antacids and histamine type 2–receptor antagonists (H2RAs) are approved to relieve symptoms associated with acid indigestion and sour stomach. However, antacids have marginal efficacy for the treatment of N/V secondary to nonulcer dyspepsia. Prolonged and predominant nausea and bloating may be a sign of gastrointestinal motility dysfunction and may require prescription pro-motility agents.[32]

Bismuth subsalicylate may have some benefits for nausea associated with consumption or nonulcer dyspepsia.[33] Bismuth subsalicylate is approved to treat various GI complaints, including nausea, heartburn, and fullness. An in-depth discussion of bismuth subsalicylate can be found in Chapters 13 and 16.

Phosphorated carbohydrate solution (PCS) may also be useful in nausea associated with a food or beverage. This solution is a mixture of dextrose (glucose), levulose (fructose), and phosphoric acid.[34] The hyperosmolar solution is believed to relieve N/V by direct local action on the GI tract wall that may decrease smooth muscle contraction and delay gastric emptying time.[35]

Alternatively, concentrated cola syrup has been used, which also contains the sugars and phosphoric acid that are in PCS. Because commercially available soda is often at a 5:1 water-to-syrup ratio, substituting soda is not recommended, even if flattened. PCS should be given in adults at 15–30 mL every 15 minutes until distress subsides. Taking more than 5 doses in 1 hour is not recommended. Children 2–12 years can take 5–10 mL every 15 minutes. Dosing should not be diluted, and other fluids should be avoided immediately before or after taking PCS.[34]

Possible adverse effects of PCS are stomach pain and diarrhea. Each 5 mL of PCS contains 3.74 grams of total sugar,[36] so caution should be used in patients with diabetes. Likewise, patients with hereditary fructose intolerance should avoid using PCS.

Product Selection Guidelines

Several factors that should be considered in the choice of antiemetic products include whether the patient is pregnant or lactating, the patient is a child or of advanced age, and the patient has any limitations such as hepatic or renal impairment. These factors may affect drug selection and dosing. Furthermore, the product should also be compatible with the patient's lifestyle, concurrent medication use, sensitivity to certain product ingredients such as dyes or fructose, and preference for frequency of dosing. Hence, product selection guidelines should be compatible with special populations and patient factors and should consider patient preferences such as whether the product is chewable or contains alcohol (Table 19–7).

table 19-7 Selected Nonprescription Antiemetic Products

Trade Name	Primary Ingredients/ Features
Bonine Chewable Tablets	Meclizine HCl 25 mg
Dramamine Less Drowsy Tablets	Meclizine HCl 25 mg
Bonine Kids Chewable Tablets	Cyclizine HCl 25 mg
Marezine Tablets	Cyclizine HCl 50 mg
Dramamine Orange Chewable Tablets	Dimenhydrinate 50 mg
Emetrol Cherry Flavor Liquid	Phosphoric acid 21.5 g/5 mL; dextrose 1.87 g/5 mL; fructose 1.87 g/5 mL
Pepto-Bismol Tablets, Suspension, Chewable Tablets	Bismuth subsalicylate 262 mg
BioBand[a]	Acupressure band worn on one wrist
ReliefBand NST (Nerve Stimulation Model)	Acupressure band worn on one wrist
Sea-Band	Acupressure band worn on both wrists

[a] See http://www.biobands.com/instructions.htm for guidelines on using this product.

Source: References 4, 17, and 41.

Special Populations

Pregnancy

Several nonpharmacologic recommendations can be made to help control NVP. For prevention of mild nausea, frequent small meals and avoidance of spicy or fatty foods or sensory stimuli that may provoke symptoms can be used. Bland carbohydrates, such as crackers, and high-protein snacks may be beneficial, especially in the morning. However, there is little published evidence supporting dietary changes for prevention of N/V. The American College of Obstetricians and Gynecologists (ACOG) recommends taking a multivitamin at the time of conception to decrease the severity of NVP in patients with a history of NVP.[29] This may not be useful if pregnant patients are presenting with nausea, but it may be an option for future preconception counseling.

Pyridoxine is pregnancy category A at recommended daily allowance (RDA) doses of 1.9 mg/day. It is Pregnancy Category C at doses above the RDA.[37] Pyridoxine is also excreted in breast milk. Extremely high doses of pyridoxine (600 mg/day) may inhibit prolactin secretion. The ACOG recommends pyridoxine with or without doxylamine as first-line pharmacotherapy for NVP.[29] From 1957 to 1983 a combination product of pyridoxine and doxylamine was available on the U.S. market. It has since been voluntarily removed because of lawsuits associated with congenital anomalies; however, current evidence does not support these claims.[38] Today, the combination product may be compounded by pharmacists.[29] Ginger may be as effective as pyridoxine for treating NVP. See the complementary therapies section in this chapter for further discussion.

Patients of Advanced Age

Antihistamines should be used with caution in patients of advanced age because of the increased risk of adverse effects. The anticholinergic and sedative effects may not be tolerable in this patient population. The American Geriatrics Society treats these medications as potentially inappropriate and strongly recommends avoiding antihistamines in patients of advanced age.[39] In addition, a comprehensive medication review may be necessary in this population to identify and resolve any potential drug-related problems, including drug interactions.

PCS may be used if the patient does not have uncontrolled blood glucose levels or hereditary fructose intolerance. Acupressure, or any acustimulation products such as acupressure bands, should not be used in patients with pacemakers. Other nonpharmacologic options such as avoiding trigger foods and scents could also be considered.

Lactation

Antihistamines may adversely affect the mother's milk supply and should be avoided in nursing mothers. Bismuth subsalicylate should also be used cautiously according to the American Academy of Pediatrics. Although the bismuth is poorly absorbed, the salicylate is excreted and eliminated slowly in the milk.[40] There is little evidence on the safety of ginger use in lactating women.

Children

In newborns and infants, vomiting may rapidly lead to dehydration and acid–base disturbances. Vomiting is different from simple regurgitation, which is common in infants. Vomiting is distinguished as being more forceful and containing larger amounts of emesis. In newborns, vomiting may be caused by GI tract obstruction. In infants, vomiting may be a sign of gastro-esophageal reflux disease (GERD). Nausea and vomiting can occur in children for a variety of reasons, including GI obstruction, central nervous system abnormalities, and infection.[41]

The Centers for Disease Control and Prevention (CDC) classifies dehydration in children as mild if less than 3% of body weight is lost, moderate if 3%–9% is lost, and severe if greater than 9% of body weight is lost.[28] Moderate-severe cases of dehydration should be referred for treatment. Mild-moderate cases of dehydration should be treated with oral rehydration therapy as described in this chapter and in Chapter 16. Antihistamines may diminish mental alertness and occasionally produce paradoxical excitation in young children.[30] Bismuth subsalicylate is not recommended in children because of the potential risk of Reye's syndrome, especially in children exposed to viral illness.[40]

Complementary Therapies

Some evidence supports the use of complementary therapies such as ginger, pyridoxine (vitamin B₆), and acupressure bands in nausea.

Ginger

Ginger (*Zingiber officinale*) has been used for nausea related to pregnancy, motion sickness, and surgery.[42] A 2010 Cochrane review suggested that ginger may be superior to placebo in preventing NVP. The review reported no difference in spontaneous abortion, congenital abnormalities, or other fetal adverse outcomes, although the included studies may not have had sufficient power.[3] Other data are limited regarding the safety of ginger in pregnancy. Larger doses of ginger may lead to mild adverse GI effects including heartburn, diarrhea, and mouth irritation.[43] Some evidence suggests that ginger may have anticoagulant and hypotensive effects. In some countries, such as Finland and Denmark, ginger carries cautionary warnings for its use in pregnancy.[44]

Ginger can be dosed at 250 mg of the root given orally four times daily for nausea. The total daily dose of 1 gram has also been given in 2–3 divided doses. Caution should be used in formulations that exceed the 1 gram daily recommended dose. Ginger may be as effective as pyridoxine for treating N/V. Compared with dimenhydrinate, ginger may cause fewer adverse effects.[45] (See Chapter 51 for an in-depth discussion of ginger.)

Most ginger ale products are often artificially flavored or contain amounts of ginger that are too insignificant to be therapeutic.

Pyridoxine (Vitamin B₆)

Pyridoxine is a water-soluble B vitamin that is important in various metabolic functions, including protein metabolism, hemoglobin synthesis, and neurotransmitter function.[37] The RDA of pyridoxine in healthy adults is 1.3–2 mg/day. Pyridoxine may be used in NVP. Typical dosing of pyridoxine for nausea is 10–25 mg three times a day.

Pyridoxine is generally well tolerated. Large doses (>200 mg/day) of pyridoxine over longer periods of time (>2 months) may result in adverse effects such as peripheral neuropathy, weakness, lethargy, and nystagmus.

Pyridoxine has had mixed results for efficacy in treating N/V. Overall data suggest that pyridoxine is effective.[29] Pregnancy-related nausea and vomiting is an off-label indication for pyridoxine. Some evidence suggests that pyridoxine may be more effective in severe cases of N/V.[46]

Acupressure

The use of acupressure involves direct pressure on the pericardium-6 (P6) point on either wrist. The P6 point is located approximately two thumb widths from the middle crease of the wrist (see acupuncture-points.org). Pressure can be applied either with the finger or a wristband. Data suggest that both the finger and a wristband are effective in reducing the rate of nausea and vomiting in pregnancy and motion sickness.[47,48] In some studies, a high placebo rate is seen (i.e., pressure at a different anatomical site). The "dosing" of acupressure can vary from as needed, to 10 minutes three times a day, to continuous pressure. There are mixed results on the efficacy of each of the dosing regimens.[48]

Aromatherapy

The use of peppermint oil for the treatment of N/V does not have reliable evidence to support its efficacy. In addition, the use of isopropyl alcohol may be more effective than a saline placebo but less effective than other standard antiemetic medications (both prescription and nonprescription). This lack of efficacy was found in studies that looked at the use of rescue antiemetics for postoperative nausea and vomiting. Evidence is lacking to support aromatherapy for self-treatment of N/V.[49]

Summary of Treatment Options

Nonprescription antihistamines may be appropriate to prevent or control N/V associated with motion sickness. In general, antihistamines may cause drowsiness and anticholinergic adverse effects that can limit their use in young children, persons of advanced age, and lactating women.

PCS may be used in N/V associated with overeating. Other agents, such as antacids, H2RAs, and bismuth subsalicylate, have also been used. PCS should be avoided in patients with hereditary fructose intolerance. Bismuth subsalicylate should be avoided in children and patients sensitive to salicylates.

ORS is important in patients with dehydration secondary to vomiting. It provides a more balanced electrolyte distribution during rehydration. Smaller but more frequent doses of ORS solution are given to patients who are actively vomiting and may have trouble holding down fluids. All age groups, including pregnant and lactating women, may safely use ORS solution.

Complementary agents such as ginger, vitamin B_6 (pyridoxine), acupressure, and aromatherapy have also been used for N/V. There is mixed data for safety and efficacy of these treatment options. According to the American College of Obstetricians and Gynecologists, pyridoxine is a first-line agent for pregnancy-related nausea and vomiting. Acupressure and ginger have better efficacy data than aromatherapy.

Assessment of Nausea and Vomiting: A Case-Based Approach

Vomiting is a symptom produced not only by benign processes but also by serious illnesses, and it may cause various complications. Physical assessment of the patient may help to determine whether some of the complications of N/V listed in the section Clinical Presentation of Nausea and Vomiting have occurred. Physical assessment should include the patient's general appearance, mental status, and volume status, and the presence of any abdominal pain. Evaluation of vital signs such as blood pressure, heart rate, temperature, and weight is also pertinent. Evaluation of concurrent signs and symptoms is useful in determining the potential cause of vomiting. It is also vital to determine whether a toxin could be the cause of the acute onset of vomiting. Therefore, asking about possible ingestion of a toxin, especially in preschoolers and adolescents, is necessary. Detailed information about the patient's medical history related to the GI tract is especially helpful in determining potential causes.

A major concern with vomiting is the loss of fluids and the inability to eat or drink. This situation may result in dehydration and electrolyte disturbances. Self-care is inappropriate for patients with dehydration, severe anorexia, weight loss, or poor nutritional status. Medical evaluation for dehydration should be provided when severe vomiting or diarrhea persists for more than several hours in children or for 48 hours in adults.[23,24]

Providers should be aware that some patients might use nonprescription antiemetics to self-treat the early stages of a serious illness. Therefore, to avoid potential additive toxicity, providers should ask patients what they have already used to treat the symptoms. Many patients choose to self-medicate with various nonprescription products to avoid a medical office visit. However, providers should be cautious about recommending self-medication for N/V symptoms and should ask appropriate questions to determine whether medical referral is indicated.

Cases 19–1 and 19–2 are examples of the assessment of patients presenting with vomiting.

Patient Counseling for Nausea and Vomiting

Providers should stress that treatment of N/V must focus on identifying and, if possible, correcting the underlying cause. Patients prone to overeating, eating disorders, or motion sickness should try to avoid behaviors or situations that cause N/V. Patients should be advised that acute vomiting typically requires only symptomatic treatment because it is usually self-limiting and will resolve spontaneously. If the cause of the symptoms is known and self-treatment is appropriate, proper use of the recommended product should be explained. Patient education should also include information about possible adverse effects, as well as signs and symptoms that indicate further medical attention is warranted. The box Patient Education for Nausea and Vomiting lists specific information to provide patients.

Evaluation of Patient Outcomes for Nausea and Vomiting

After a provider has provided information or suggestions for self-management and treatment of N/V, a follow-up assessment of the patient should occur within 24 hours of the initial encounter. This evaluation may best be accomplished by a follow-up phone call and then, if desired by the patient, a scheduled appointment. The follow-up should include an assessment of whether the N/V has diminished or abated; whether the patient

case
19–1

Relevant Evaluation Criteria	Scenario/Model Outcome

Information Gathering

1. Gather essential information about the patient's symptoms and medical history, including:

a. description of symptom(s) (i.e., nature, onset, duration, severity, associated symptoms)

Patient has had frequent episodes of nausea and occasional vomiting; this has been going on for 3–4 days. The episodes last a few hours during the main part of the day. She has maintained her appetite.

b. description of any factors that seem to precipitate, exacerbate, and/or relieve the patient's symptom(s)

Symptoms seem to worsen when the patient smells coffee brewing and when she wakes up in the morning. Her husband now buys coffee instead of brewing it at home, but she still gets nauseated at work.

c. description of the patient's efforts to relieve the symptoms

The patient eats some dry toast and takes a few sips of ginger ale or water. She does not like the idea of taking "drugs" for her nausea.

d. patient's identity

Annabelle Grace

e. age, sex, height, and weight

28 years old, female, 5 ft 5 in., 135 lb

f. patient's occupation

Loan officer

g. patient's dietary habits

Balanced diet with plenty of fruits and vegetables

h. patient's sleep habits

Averages 7–8 hours per night.

i. concurrent medical conditions, prescription and nonprescription medications, and dietary supplements

Patient found out she is 7 weeks pregnant, has started taking a prenatal vitamin, and denies use of dietary supplements.

j. allergies

Penicillin: rash

k. history of other adverse reactions to medications

Stomach upset with codeine

l. other (describe) _____

NA

Assessment and Triage

2. Differentiate patient's signs/symptoms and correctly identify the patient's primary problem(s).

Nausea lasting a few hours during the main part of the day; occasional vomiting. She does not like the smell of certain foods; NVP is likely.

3. Identify exclusions for self-treatment (Figure 19–2).

None

4. Formulate a comprehensive list of therapeutic alternatives for the primary problem to determine if triage to a health care provider is required, and share this information with the patient or caregiver.

Options include:

(1) Recommend self-care with:
   – Nondrug strategies (dietary and environmental changes [Table 19–5]).
   – Acupressure or acustimulation bands.
   – OTC pyridoxine.
   – OTC doxylamine.
   – OTC phosphorated carbohydrate solution.
   – Ginger.

(2) Recommend lifestyle modifications until health care provider may be consulted.

(3) Make a medical referral.

(4) Take no action.

Plan

5. Select an optimal therapeutic alternative to address the patient's problem, taking into account patient preferences.

Because the patient does not appear dehydrated and can drink small amounts of ginger ale and water, and she can tolerate dry toast, you encourage her to continue to take sips of liquids and eat toast. She does not have signs/symptoms of dehydration, such as fast heartbeat, decreased skin turgor, noticeable weight loss, or clothes that fit loosely. A therapeutic alternative is the use of acupressure bands because the patient has stated that she would prefer not to use "drugs" if possible. If symptoms persist, then she can try doxylamine 12.5 mg 3–4 times a day and vitamin B_6 10 mg 3–4 times a day. Other nonpharmacologic suggestions in Table 19–5 should be followed. If symptoms persist, she should consult her provider.

Relevant Evaluation Criteria	Scenario/Model Outcome
6. Describe the recommended therapeutic approach to the patient or caregiver.	"You probably have nausea and vomiting of pregnancy, or NVP. The acupressure bands may work, but if they do not, a combination of the antihistamine doxylamine and vitamin B_6 may help. These products should be taken 3–4 times a day. You may also benefit from other nonpharmacologic techniques (Table 19–5), such as continuing the dry toast or eating bland foods and crackers in the morning before arising, sleeping in a well-ventilated room, and avoiding strong odors. If you do not feel better, you may want to contact your provider."
7. Explain to the patient or caregiver the rationale for selecting the recommended therapeutic approach from the considered therapeutic alternatives.	"Published information regarding acupressure bands has shown that they may help with NVP. However, the evidence-based guidelines of the American College of Obstetricians and Gynecologists state that doxylamine and vitamin B_6, up to 4 tablets daily, may help your symptoms. Because you are able to drink fluids and are not dehydrated, seeking medical care may not be necessary at this time. However, if nausea or vomiting worsens, medical attention for further evaluation is necessary."

Patient Education

8. When recommending self-care with nonprescription medications and/or nondrug therapy, convey accurate information to the patient or caregiver.	
a. appropriate dose and frequency of administration	(1) "Wear acupressure bands." (2) "Add vitamin B_6 10 mg combined with 12.5 mg of doxylamine (one-half of a 25 mg tablet). Doxylamine is available in the United States as an OTC sleep aid (Unisom Sleeptabs 25 mg)."
b. maximum number of days the therapy should be employed	(1) "Wear acupressure bands continually." (2) "There are no limits to the number of days that vitamin B_6 and doxylamine can be taken."
c. product administration procedures	(1) "Wear the band on each wrist, 2 finger widths up from the first wrist crease." (2) "Take vitamin B_6 and doxylamine with a small glass of water 3–4 times a day."
d. expected time to onset of relief/degree of relief that can be reasonably expected	"Expected time to onset of relief and degree of relief are variable for all products and measures."
e. most common side effects	(1) "Acupressure bands are not likely to cause side effects." (2) "Vitamin B_6 is not likely to cause any side effects. Drowsiness is the most common side effect of doxylamine; therefore, it is important not to drive or operate machinery while taking doxylamine. Other possible side effects include dry mouth, dry eyes, nasal congestion, urinary retention, and constipation."
f. patient options in the event that condition worsens or persists	"Medical attention is necessary if the NVP does not improve or if side effects from the OTC product occur."
g. product storage requirements	"Store at 59°F–86°F."
h. specific nondrug measures	See Table 19–5 for dietary and other measures.
Solicit follow-up questions from the patient or caregiver.	(1) "Will any of these products hurt my baby?" (2) "What other products could I use instead?"
Answer the patient's or caregiver's questions.	(1) "These products have been used by many other pregnant women and have not caused harm to the mother or baby. They are considered Pregnancy Category A, which is the safest class." (2) "Another product used for nausea during pregnancy is an acustimulation device that is worn as a wristwatch on a single wrist, but this product is expensive. Ginger can also be considered. It has comparable efficacy to pyridoxine. Phosphorated carbohydrate solution may also be tried. If these products do not work, then medical attention is necessary to consider a prescription product for your nausea."

Evaluation of Patient Outcome

9. Assess patient outcome.	Monitor for episodes of nausea and vomiting.

Key: NA = Not applicable; NKDA = no known drug allergies; NVP = nausea and vomiting of pregnancy; OTC = over-the-counter.

case
19–2

Relevant Evaluation Criteria	Scenario/Model Outcome

Information Gathering

1. Gather essential information about the patient's symptoms and medical history, including:

a. description of symptom(s) (i.e., nature, onset, duration, severity, associated symptoms)

Patient has had six episodes of nausea, vomiting, and diarrhea in the past 10 hours. The patient seems somnolent and quiet except for violent episodes of vomiting or diarrhea.

b. description of any factors that seem to precipitate, exacerbate, and/or relieve the patient's symptom(s)

Symptoms worsen when the patient's mother attempts to provide small sips of Gatorade.

c. description of the patient's efforts to relieve the symptoms

Patient's mother tried to get the child to eat a few bites of soda crackers or drink sips of fluid.

d. patient's identity

Ryan John

e. age, sex, height, and weight

18 months old, male, 25 inches, 23 lb (26 lb on previous day)

f. patient's occupation

NA

g. patient's dietary habits

Normal healthy diet, consisting of cereals, mashed vegetables, pasta, rice, chicken, yogurt, milk, and juice

h. patient's sleep habits

Up at 7:00 am; in bed at 7:30 pm; naps for 2 hours from 1–3 pm.

i. concurrent medical conditions, prescription and non-prescription medications, and dietary supplements

Children's multivitamin

j. allergies

NKDA

k. history of other adverse reactions to medications

None

l. other (describe) _____

NA

Assessment and Triage

2. Differentiate patient's signs/symptoms and correctly identify the patient's primary problem(s).

Patient has had several episodes of nausea, vomiting, and diarrhea. The patient appears drowsy and unusually lethargic, and his body appears floppy. The child appears dizzy when he stands up and his abdomen seems somewhat flat. He has had a dry diaper for several hours. Although the child appears to cry, few tears are noted.

Patient appears dehydrated and may have viral gastroenteritis.

3. Identify exclusions for self-treatment (Figure 19–3).

On the basis of his signs/symptoms, patient appears severely dehydrated (Table 19–2).

4. Formulate a comprehensive list of therapeutic alternatives for the primary problem to determine if triage to a health care provider is required, and share this information with the patient or caregiver.

Options include:

(1) Recommend that patient's mother administer:
 – OTC oral rehydration salt (ORS) solution.
 – OTC phosphorated carbohydrate solution.
 – An acupressure band.

(2) Recommend that patient's mother administer self-care modalities until a health care provider can be consulted.

(3) Refer patient for further medical evaluation.

(4) Take no action.

Plan

5. Select an optimal therapeutic alternative to address the patient's problem, taking into account patient preferences.

Ryan is unable to drink small amounts of fluid or eat small bites of crackers. He also has signs/symptoms of dehydration (appears drowsy and lethargic; has a floppy body, dizziness, flat abdomen; has lost 3 pounds since the previous day; has a dry diaper and sheds few tears). On the basis of these signs/symptoms, the patient's mother should immediately take the child for medical evaluation and attempt to administer small sips of ORS on the way to the emergency department.

6. Describe the recommended therapeutic approach to the patient or caregiver.

"Your child needs to be seen by a health care provider because he appears dehydrated. Please have someone drive you and your child to the emergency room at the hospital. On the way, administer 1 teaspoonful of ORS every 1–2 minutes."

7. Explain to the patient or caregiver the rationale for selecting the recommended therapeutic approach from the considered therapeutic alternatives.

"Your child's symptoms (floppy body, flat abdomen, weight loss, dry diaper, few tears) indicate that he is dehydrated. Because he has been unable to drink sufficient fluids or eat anything to counter the dehydration, he needs medical attention."

case

19-2 *continued*

Relevant Evaluation Criteria	Scenario/Model Outcome

Patient Education

8. When recommending self-care with nonprescription medications and/or nondrug therapy, convey accurate information to the patient or caregiver.

Criterion does not apply in this case.

Solicit follow-up questions from the patient or caregiver.

Is there a nonprescription medication that might work so that I don't have to take him to the emergency room?

Answer the patient's or caregiver's questions.

No. Your child is dehydrated; he needs urgent medical care so that he can feel better and get well.

Evaluation of Patient Outcome

9. Assess patient outcome.

Monitor for signs of dehydration, including weight. Look for normal behaviors and activities.

Key: NA = Not applicable; NKDA = no known drug allergies; ORS = oral rehydration solution; OTC = over-the-counter.

patient education for
Nausea and Vomiting

The objectives of self-treatment are to (1) improve the symptoms of occasional, self-limited nausea and vomiting (N/V), (2) identify and correct the underlying cause, (3) prevent and correct complications of vomiting, and (4) prevent future occurrences. For most patients, carefully following product instructions and the self-care measures listed here will help ensure optimal therapeutic outcomes.

Nondrug Measures

- To prevent NVP, eat small, frequent meals that are low in fat content. Sleep in a room with fresh air. Also, try eating crackers before getting up in the morning. Try lying down to relieve the symptoms once they occur (Table 19–5.)
- To prevent motion sickness in young children, place them in a car seat that allows them to look out the windows (Table 19–4.) Try acupressure wristbands to prevent motion sickness in adults or older children.
- To prevent nausea associated with overeating, avoid foods or beverages known to cause nausea; consume foods and beverages in moderation.

Nonprescription Medications
Antacids, Histamine Type 2 Receptor Antagonists (H₂RAs), and Bismuth Subsalicylate

- Take antacids, H₂RAs (e.g., ranitidine or famotidine), or bismuth subsalicylate for nausea caused by overeating. Follow product instructions for dosages. (See Chapters 13 and 16 for additional information on these medications.)

Phosphorated Carbohydrate Solution

- Take phosphorated carbohydrate solutions for nausea and vomiting associated with upset stomach caused by viral gastroenteritis, food indiscretions, and pregnancy. (Table 19–6 lists selected brand-name products.)
- Give 1–2 tablespoonful (15–30 mL) of the solution to adults at 15-minute intervals until vomiting stops. For children ages 2–12 years old, give 1–2 teaspoonful (5–10 mL). Do not give more than 5 doses in 1 hour.
- Do not dilute the solution, and do not allow the patient to consume other liquids for 15 minutes after taking a dose.
- Patients with hereditary fructose intolerance should not take this product.

- Patients with diabetes should consult their medical provider before taking this product.

Antihistamines

- Take antihistamines for self-treatment of N/V caused by motion sickness.
- To prevent motion sickness, take antihistamines at least 30–60 minutes before departure. Continue taking the medication during travel. Follow the dosage guidelines in Table19–6.
- While using antihistamines, avoid driving or operating hazardous machinery or engaging in tasks that require a high degree of mental alertness. Drowsiness is the most common adverse effect of these medications.
- Patients with asthma, narrow-angle glaucoma, obstructive disease of the GI or genitourinary tract, or benign prostatic hypertrophy should consult a health care provider before using antihistamines.
- Caution patients that antihistamines may increase the sedative effects of alcohol, tranquilizers, hypnotics, and sedatives. Antihistamines may produce excitability in children or mental confusion in persons of advanced age.
- Do not take oral diphenhydramine products if topical (external) diphenhydramine preparations are being used.

Oral Rehydration Salt (ORS) Solution

- If needed, take an ORS to prevent dehydration secondary to vomiting and diarrhea.
- Consider placing ORS solution in the refrigerator to improve taste. Alternatively, the patient can use freezer pops or another dosage form to improve palatability.

When to Seek Medical Attention

- Seek medical attention if there are signs and symptoms of serious dehydration associated with N/V.
- Seek medical attention if vomiting does not stop after 5 doses of a phosphorated carbohydrate solution.

has any residual related symptoms, such as signs or symptoms of dehydration; whether abnormal vital signs such as tachycardia have returned to normal; and whether the patient is afebrile. If the patient had prolonged N/V (>24–48 hours) or a change in or worsening of symptoms that required immediate referral for medical evaluation, the provider should follow up to determine whether the patient sought medical help and what type of treatment was administered. It is also important for the provider to assess whether he or she needs to provide any further counseling or answer additional questions. The provider should also use this opportunity to provide reassurance and support.

Key Points for Nausea and Vomiting

➤ N/V are symptoms of an underlying disorder; therefore, treatment should focus on identifying and correcting the underlying cause.

➤ Nonprescription antiemetic medications are suitable for preventing and controlling the symptoms of occasional self-limiting N/V.

➤ Overeating, food poisoning, viral gastroenteritis, and motion sickness may cause self-limiting N/V.

➤ Antacids, nonprescription H_2RAs, or PCS may improve symptoms associated with indigestion from overeating.

➤ Antihistamines are the agents of choice to treat N/V secondary to motion sickness.

➤ Agents that may be used safely to treat N/V in all persons 2 years of age and older, as well as NVP, include acupressure/acustimulation devices and PCS.

➤ Uncomplicated NVP may be treated with pyridoxine, doxylamine, PCS, ginger, or acupressure/acustimulation devices.

➤ Loss of fluids and the inability to eat or drink because of N/V may result in dehydration and electrolyte disturbances. This primary complication of N/V should be treated with ORS.

➤ A patient who presents with complications related to N/V may not be a candidate for self-treatment but instead should be referred for medical evaluation.

REFERENCES

1. Adekoya N. Reasons for visits to emergency departments for Medicaid and State Children's Health Insurance Program patients: United States, 2004. *N C Med J.* Mar/Apr 2010;71(2):123–30.

2. Gibson N, Ward B, Birk H, et al. An Advisory Committee Statement: Committee to Advise on Tropical Medicine and Travel (CATMAT). Statement on motion sickness. *Can Commun Dis Rep.* 200315;29:1–12.

3. Matthews A, Dowswell T, Haas DM, et al. Interventions for nausea and vomiting in early pregnancy. *Cochrane Database Syst Rev.* 2010;9:CD007575. doi:10.1002/14651858.CD007575. Accessed at http://www.thecochrane library.com/view/0/index.html.

4. Badell ML, Ramin SM, Smith JA. Treatment options for nausea and vomiting during pregnancy. *Pharmacotherapy.* 2006;26(9):1273–87.

5. Einarson A, Maltepe C, Boskovic R, et al. Treatment of nausea and vomiting in pregnancy—an updated algorithm. *Can Fam Physician.* 2007; 53(12):2109–11.

6. Allen K. The vomiting child: What to do and when to consult. *Aust Fam Physician.* 2007;36(9):684–7.

7. Colletti JE, Brown KM, Sharieff GQ, et al. The management of children with gastroenteritis and dehydration in the emergency department. *J Emerg Med.* 2010;38(5):686–98.

8. Metz A. Nausea and vomiting in adults: a diagnostic approach. *Aust Fam Physician.* 2007;36(9):688–92.

9. Centers for Disease Control and Prevention. Prevention of rotavirus gastroenteritis among infants and children. Recommendations of the Advisory Committee on Immunization Practices (ACIP). *MMWR Morb Mortal Wkly Rep.* 2009;58(RR02):1–25.

10. Committee on Infectious Disease. Prevention of rotavirus disease: updated guidelines for use of rotavirus vaccine. *Pediatrics.* 2009;123:1412–20.

11. Centers for Disease Control and Prevention. Norovirus: Overview. Updated July 26, 2013. Accessed at http://www.cdc.gov/norovirus/ about/overview.html, July 16, 2014.

12. Wilhelm SM, Dehoorne-Smith ML, Kale-Pradhan PB. Prevention of postoperative nausea and vomiting. *Ann Pharmacother.* 2007;41(1):68–78.

13. DiPiro CV, Ignoffo RJ. Nausea and vomiting. In: Dipiro JT, Talbert RL, Yee GC, et al., eds. *Pharmacotherapy: A Pathophysiologic Approach.* 8th ed. New York, NY: McGraw-Hill Professional; 2011:607–19.

14. Sharkey KA, Wallace JL. Treatment of disorders of bowel motility and water flux; antiemetics; agents used in biliary and pancreatic disease. In: Brunton LL, Chabner BA, Knollmann BC, eds. *Goodman and Gilman's The Pharmacological Basis of Therapeutics.* 12th ed. New York, NY: McGraw-Hill, Inc.; 2011:1323–49.

15. Scorza K, Williams A, Phillips D, et al. Evaluation of nausea and vomiting. *Am Fam Physician.* 2007;76(1):76–84.

16. Quigley EM, Hasler WL, Parkman HP. AGA technical review on nausea and vomiting. *Gastroenterology.* 2001;120(1):263–86.

17. Flake ZA, Scalley RD, Bailey AG. Practical selection of antiemetics. *Am Fam Physician.* 2004;69(5):1169–74,1176.

18. Niebyl JR. Nausea and vomiting in pregnancy. *N Engl J Med.* 2010; 363(16):1544–50.

19. King CB, Glass R, Bresee JS, et al. Managing acute gastroenteritis among children: oral rehydration, maintenance, and nutritional therapy. *MMWR Recomm Rep.* 2003;52(RR16):1–16. Accessed at http://www.cdc.gov/ mmwr/PDF/RR/RR5216.pdf, June 7, 2011.

20. Khanna R, Lakhanpaul M, Burman-Roy S, et al. Diarrhea and vomiting caused by gastroenteritis: diagnosis, assessment and management in children younger than 5 years: summary of NICE guidance. *BMJ.* 2009;338:b1350.

21. Acute Gastroenteritis Guideline Team, Cincinnati Children's Hospital Medical Center. Evidence-based care guideline: prevention and management of acute gastroenteritis (AGE) in children ages 2 months to 18 years. Guideline 5 [pages 1–20]. December 21, 2011. Accessed at http://www. cincinnatichildrens.org/workarea/linkit.aspx?linkidentifier=id&itemid= 94774&libid=94464, August 11, 2014.

22. American Medical Directors Association (AMDA). *Dehydration and Fluid Maintenance in the Long-Term Care Setting.* Columbia, MD: American Medical Directors Association. 2009. Accessed at http://www.guideline. gov/content.aspx?id=15590, October 2, 2013.

23. Jueckstock J, Kaestner R, Mylonas I. Managing hyperemesis gravidarum: a multimodal challenge. *BMC Med.* 2010;8:46–57.

24. World Gastroenterology Organisation (WGO). WGO Practice Guideline: Acute Diarrhea. Munich, Germany: World Gastroenterology Organisation; March 28, 2008. Accessed at http://www.guideline.gov/ content.aspx?id=12679, August 11, 2014.

25. American Academy of Family Physicians (AAFP). Vomiting and diarrhea, treatment. November 2010. Accessed at http://familydoctor.org/family doctor/en/diseases-conditions/vomiting-and-diarrhea/treatment.html, March 7, 2013.

26. World Health Organization. WHO position paper on oral rehydration salts to reduce mortality from cholera. 2013. Accessed at http://www. guideline.gov/content.aspx?id=47569, September 14, 2014.

27. Rehydration Project. Oral rehydration therapy. November 10, 2012. Accessed at http://rehydrate.org/rehydration/index.html#10, March 7, 2013.

28. Centers for Disease Control and Prevention (CDC). Managing acute gastroenteritis among children: oral rehydration, maintenance, and nutritional therapy. *MMWR Morbidity and Mortal Wkly Rep.* November 21, 2003;52(RR16):1–13.

29. American College of Obstetricians and Gynecology. Nausea and vomiting in pregnancy. ACOG Practice Bulletin No. 52. *Obstet Gynecol.* 2004;103(4):803–14.

30. Antihistamines. Drug Facts and Comparisons eAnswers. Facts & Comparisons [database online]. St. Louis, MO: Wolters Kluwer Health, Inc.; 2013. Accessed at http://online.factsandcomparisons.com/, April 12, 2013.

31. deLeon J, Nikoloff DM. Paradoxical excitation on diphenhydramine may be associated with being a CYP2D6 ultrarapid metabolizer: three case reports. *CNS Spectr.* 2008;13(2):133–5.

32. American Gastroenterological Association. Medical position statement: evaluation of dyspepsia. *Gastroenterology.* 2005;129(5):1753–5.

33. Moayyedi P. Pharmacological interventions for non-ulcer dyspepsia. *Cochrane Database Syst Rev.* 2006;18:CD001960 doi:10.1002/14651858. CD001960. Accessed at http://www.thecochranelibrary.com/view/0/index.html.

34. U.S. National Library of Medicine, National Institutes of Health. Daily Med: Formula EM. July 2012. Accessed at http://dailymed.nlm.nih.gov/dailymed/drugInfo.cfm?id=72079#nlm34068-7, March 28, 2013.

35. Phosphorated carbohydrate solution. Drug Facts and Comparisons. Facts & Comparisons [database online]. St. Louis, MO: Wolters Kluwer Health, Inc.; February 2013. Accessed at http://online.factsandcomparisons.com, April 3, 2013.

36. Wellspring Pharmaceuticals. Emetrol. 2012. Accessed at http://www.emetrol.com, March 28, 2013.

37. Pyridoxine hydrochloride (B6). Drug Facts and Comparisons. Facts & Comparisons [database online]. St. Louis, MO: Wolters Kluwer Health, Inc.; January 2008. Accessed at http://online.factsandcomparisons.com/, April 3, 2013.

38. Nausea and vomiting in pregnancy. DynaMed [subscription database online]. EBSCO Publishing. Updated February 28, 2013. Accessed at http://search.ebscohost.com/login.aspx?direct=true&site=DynaMed&id=113862, April 4, 2013.

39. The American Geriatrics Society 2012 Beers Criteria Update Expert Panel. American Geriatrics Society updated beers criteria for potentially inappropriate medication use in older adults. *J Am Geriatr Soc.* April 2012;60(4):616–30.

40. Bismuth subsalicylate. Drug Facts and Comparisons eAnswers. Facts & Comparisons [database online]. St. Louis, MO: Wolters Kluwer Health, Inc.; Jul 2011. Accessed at http://online.factsandcomparisons.com, April 12, 2013.

41. Nausea and vomiting in infants and children. DynaMed [subscription database online]. EBSCO Publishing. Updated January 31, 2013. Accessed at https://dynamed.ebscohost.com/, September 14, 2014.

42. National Center for Complementary and Alternative Medicine (NCCAM). Herbs at a glance—ginger. Accessed at http://www.nccam.nih.gov/health/ginger, February 20, 2013.

43. Ginger. Drug Facts and Comparisons. Facts & Comparisons [database online]. St. Louis, MO: Wolters Kluwer Health, Inc.; March 2008. Accessed at http://online.factsandcomparisons.com/, April 3, 2013.

44. Tiran D. Ginger to reduce nausea and vomiting during pregnancy: evidence of effectiveness is not the same as proof of safety. *Complement Ther Clin Pract.* February 2012;18(1):22–5. Accessed at http://www.sciencedirect.com/science/article/pii/S1744388111000739, April 12, 2013.

45. Holst L, Wright D, Haavik S, et al. Safety and efficacy of herbal remedies in obstetrics—review and clinical implications. *Midwifery.* February 2011;27(1):80–86. Accessed at http://www.sciencedirect.com/science/article/pii/S0266613809000722, April 12, 2013.

46. Sahakian V, Rouse D, Sipes S, et al. Vitamin B6 is effective therapy for nausea and vomiting of pregnancy: a randomized, double-blind placebo-controlled study. *Obstet Gynecol.* 1991;78(1):33–6.

47. Helmreich RJ, Shiao SPK, Dune LS. Meta-analysis of acustimulation effects on nausea and vomiting in pregnant women. *Journal of Science and Healing.* September 2006;2(5):412–21.

48. Ezzo J, Streitberger K, Schneider A. Cochrane Systematic Reviews Examine P6 Acupuncture-Point Stimulation for Nausea and Vomiting. *J Altern Complem Med.* 2006;12(5):489–95.

49. Hines S, Steels E, Chang A, et al. Aromatherapy for treatment of postoperative nausea and vomiting. *Cochrane Database System Rev.* 2012;4:007598. doi:10.1002/14651858.CD007598. Accessed at http://www.thecochranelibrary.com/view/0/index.html.

POISONING

Wendy Klein-Schwartz and Barbara Insley Crouch

Poisoning is the leading cause of injury death, surpassing motor vehicle traffic deaths and deaths from firearms, and it is a major public health problem.[1] Deaths involving opioid analgesics have increased exponentially since 1999 along with sales of opioid pain relievers and admissions for opioid pain reliever treatment; deaths from opioid analgesics have far exceeded the deaths from heroin and cocaine.[2] Emergency department visits for nonmedical use of certain prescription medications increased dramatically between 2004 and 2008.[3] The most dramatic increase involved opioid analgesics (111% increase), but significant increases also were noted with certain benzodiazepines, zolpidem, and carisoprodol.

Older adults may be especially vulnerable to adverse effects and poisoning from nonprescription medication given their comorbid conditions and the potential for interactions with chronic medications. Acetaminophen is one of the leading nonprescription pain relievers. It also is a leading cause of poisoning reported to U.S. poison control centers for both unintentional and intentional poisonings. More than 600 products containing acetaminophen are on the market; thus misunderstanding their use and unintended misuse are common for all ages.[4,5] The Acetaminophen Awareness Coalition, whose members include the American Pharmacists Association, the National Association of Boards of Pharmacy, and the National Community Pharmacists Association, launched a Web site (www.knowyourdose.org) to educate patients and consumers about how to use acetaminophen correctly. Several initiatives to promote safe acetaminophen use include converting pediatric liquid acetaminophen preparations to one strength and highlighting the ingredient acetaminophen on nonprescription labels.

Nonmedical use of prescription medications and abuse of nonprescription medications by adolescents are concerns, according to data from the National Survey on Drug Use and Health.[6] Abuse of attention-deficit/hyperactivity disorder medications in adolescents reported to poison control centers rose 76% over an 8-year period.[7]

Most poisonings in young children are unintentional, whereas poisonings in other age groups may be unintentional or intentional (e.g., suicide attempts, substance abuse, or medication misuse). The majority of poisonings are a result of ingestion of a substance, but poisonings also may occur after a toxin is inhaled or comes in contact with the skin and eyes. Bites and envenomations are other potential sources of toxin exposures. First aid for poisonings focuses on minimizing the extent of the exposure and stemming the progression or development of toxicity.

Poison control centers are 24-hour resources for poison information, clinical toxicology consultation, and poison prevention education. They are staffed around the clock with pharmacists, nurses, physicians, and physician's assistants with additional training in clinical toxicology. They are available for consultation with health care professionals as well as with the public. The entire United States and its territories are covered by a network of poison control centers. A poison control center should be contacted for assessment and treatment of poisonings, as well as for educational materials on poison prevention. Figure 20–1 shows the nationwide poison control center number and logo.

In 2011, a total of 57 poison control centers serving the United States and territories reported 2,334,004 cases to the National Poison Data System of the American Association of Poison Control Centers.[8] The majority of poison exposures (49.05%) occur in children younger than 6 years, of which 89% involve children 3 years of age and younger.[8] Nonprescription and prescription medications are frequently responsible for potentially toxic exposures reported to poison control centers. Nonprescription products, such as analgesics, cough and cold preparations, topical preparations, vitamins, and antihistamines, are among the most common substances ingested by young children. The large number of nonprescription medications involved in pediatric exposures reflects the common use and availability of these products in the home. Other common substances involved in poison exposures in children younger than 6 years include cosmetics and personal care products, cleaning substances, foreign bodies or toys, pesticides, and antimicrobials.

Nearly 70% of poison exposures reported to poison control centers are managed onsite, usually in a residence. Only 11.3% of children younger than 6 years are managed in a health care facility, and major effects or fatal outcomes occur in less than 1%.[8] Poison control centers are cost effective and have a favorable cost-benefit ratio.[9] A significant portion of the cost savings results from home observation, as well as from the reduction of unnecessary emergency medical transport and treatment costs. Poison control center consultation results in shorter length of hospital stay and lower charges for those patients who require hospitalization.[10,11] A policy analysis group reviewed the existing literature on the cost savings associated with use of a poison control center and estimated medical care savings and reduced productivity loss of $13.39 per year per dollar of poison control center funding.[12] A recent study of pediatric poison exposures treated in a tertiary children's hospital found that 18.6% of visits were for nontoxic exposures that could have been managed on site by the poison control center. Children with nontoxic exposures were more likely to be covered by Medicaid or no insurance (73%) and had a mean charge of $286 per patient.[13] Health care professionals are encouraged to work closely with their local poison control centers to ensure the most appropriate, cost-effective care of the poisoned patient.

Unintentional childhood poisonings remain a common cause of injury-related morbidity, requiring significant expenditures of health care dollars for inpatient and outpatient care. Unintentional poisonings are one of the leading causes of injury-related hospitalizations in preschool children; however, fatalities among preschoolers have declined significantly since the early 1970s. According to a recent analysis of the National Electronic Injury Surveillance System–All Injury Program (NEISS–AIP), an estimated 58,000 children younger than 6 years are evaluated in emergency departments annually for unintentional medication-related exposures.[14] Hospitalization or specialized medical care was required in nearly 16% of cases. The most common categories of medications were acetaminophen, cough and cold medications, antidepressants, and nonsteroidal anti-inflammatory drugs (NSAIDs).

The National Safety Council reported 50 deaths caused by unintentional poisoning in children younger than 5 years in 2011.[15] Only 26 of the 1158 fatalities reported by poison control centers in 2011 involved children younger than 6 years.[8] Medications and illicit drugs (excluding ethanol) were the primary substances responsible for fatalities. Child-resistant closures (CRCs) legislated through the Poison Prevention Packaging Act (PPPA) of 1970 help prevent unintentional poisonings. These closures have been responsible for a decline in pediatric fatalities associated with prescription and nonprescription medications.[16] Although CRCs have improved child safety, exemptions to the law allow dispensing medications without CRCs.[17] A recent analysis of NEISS data revealed that an estimated 55% of nonfatal poisonings in children younger than 5 years treated in an emergency department involved a product regulated by the PPPA.[18] Whereas child-resistant closures may reduce unintentional pediatric poisoning, use of nonstandard liquid measuring devices and caregiver misinterpretation of nonprescription medication labels increase the risk for pediatric poisoning. Further work is needed to improve the format and content of nonprescription labels to improve caregiver understanding of the medication and dosing instructions.[19–21]

Clinical Presentation of Poisoning

Poisons can affect every organ system. Signs and symptoms of poisoning can range in severity from mild to life threatening. For some drugs, toxicity after overdose is similar to the drug's adverse effect profile with therapeutic use. For example, ibuprofen overdose is characterized primarily by nausea, vomiting, and abdominal pain. Patients with diphenhydramine overdose may exhibit sedation or stimulation (e.g., agitation or hallucinations), tachycardia, hypertension, dry mouth, and dilated pupils from the drug's antimuscarinic properties. Overdoses of other drugs, such as aspirin, result in multiorgan system effects including gastrointestinal (GI), central nervous system (CNS), metabolic, cardiovascular, pulmonary, and hematologic toxicity. A lack of symptoms immediately after a poison exposure does not preclude toxicity. Patients may be asymptomatic initially, but they can develop severe toxicity hours after ingestion of some sustained-released or enteric-coated products or products that delay gastric emptying or slow GI motility (e.g., antihistamines). For other drugs (e.g., acetaminophen) and some chemicals (e.g., methanol and acetonitrile), clinical effects are delayed while the substance is metabolized to active or toxic metabolites. The time course of acetaminophen overdose is related to formation and covalent binding of a toxic metabolite to hepatic cells. As a result, a relatively mild initial clinical course characterized by nausea, vomiting, anorexia, and malaise can be followed by severe hepatic and renal toxicity 3–5 days later. Keep in mind that symptoms may be due to causes other than poisoning. Regardless of the cause of symptoms, if symptoms are serious enough, they warrant medical attention.

Treatment of Poisoning

Most unintentional poison exposures in small children result in minimal, if any, adverse effects and require no treatment other than observation. Although self-treatment may be appropriate, health care providers, caregivers, and patients are encouraged to seek counsel from the nearest poison control center before attempting any treatment.

Treatment Goals

The primary goal of home or prehospital therapy is to prevent absorption of toxins or stem the progression of toxicity, thus minimizing morbidity and mortality.

General Treatment Approach

The first step in assessing a potential poison exposure is to determine whether the patient has symptoms and whether the exposure puts the patient at risk of toxicity. Many exposures are, in fact, nontoxic or minimally toxic because either the substance has a very low inherent toxicity or the amount consumed is too low to cause toxicity. A decision regarding the option for self-treatment depends on the reason or circumstance of the poison exposure, toxicity of the agent, and general health status of the patient. Self-treatment should be considered only if the ingestion is unintentional and the potential for toxicity is assessed as minor. Any inadvertent exposure to a toxin that can potentially result in moderate-severe toxicity, as well as all intentional exposures, should be referred immediately to a hospital. If the patient exhibits

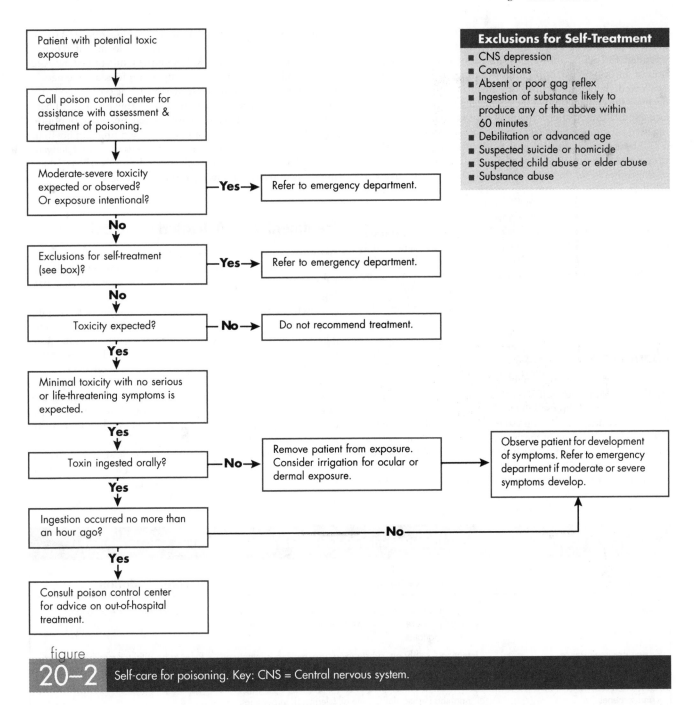

figure

20–2 Self-care for poisoning. Key: CNS = Central nervous system.

potentially life-threatening clinical effects (e.g., coma, convulsions, or syncope), transportation to an emergency department should be arranged immediately through the emergency 911 system. Additional exclusions for self-treatment can be found in Figure 20–2. Hospital care includes observing the patient, supporting vital functions (e.g., airway, breathing, and circulation), preventing absorption, enhancing elimination, and using antidotes.

The majority of individuals who do not require immediate hospital referral are managed with on-site observation only and no specific treatment.[8] In some instances, the approach is to attenuate the exposure by irrigating or preventing further absorption. The nonprescription drug activated charcoal may prevent or reduce the absorption of some ingested substances. However, its routine use is not recommended without consultation with a poison control center. In the past, ipecac syrup,

nonprescription cathartics, or both were recommended to induce vomiting or decrease absorption of substances by facilitating their elimination through the GI tract. However, ipecac syrup is no longer available, and cathartics by themselves are not beneficial in the treatment of a poisoned patient. Figure 20–2 outlines self-care of exposure to poisons.

Nonpharmacologic Therapy

Inhalation exposures are managed by removing the patient from the toxic fumes to fresh air. Irrigation may be beneficial to decrease the contact time of a chemical with the skin or mucosal surface. Skin surfaces should be washed with soap and water (usually twice) to decrease the contact time of a chemical exposure, taking care to include nail beds and hair when appropriate. Irrigation of the eye with water should be initiated immediately after an ocular exposure to a chemical or drug not intended for ocular use (e.g., inadvertent ocular administration of an otic preparation). If an irritating chemical has been swallowed, the administration of a small amount of fluids may decrease the contact time of the chemical with the mucosal surface. Neutralization after a chemical contacts skin or eyes or for ingested substances is not recommended.

The administration of oral fluids after an ingestion of a drug is not recommended. The administration of a large amount of fluids should be discouraged because the fluids are likely to result in spontaneous vomiting, which is risky in some situations. The fluids theoretically may facilitate dissolution of a solid dosage form, thereby enhancing its absorption. Administering fluids after ingestions of drugs should be considered for drugs that are known to have a high risk of esophageal impaction, such as bisphosphonates, or those that may cause renal injury owing to dehydration, such as ibuprofen or other NSAIDs. Manually stimulating the gag reflex at the back of the throat with either a blunt object or a finger may induce vomiting, but this practice is not recommended and can lead to soft palate injury.

Pharmacologic Therapy

Activated charcoal, an adsorbent, and ipecac syrup, an emetic, are the only approved self-treatments for ingested poisons. In 2011, ipecac syrup was used in less than 0.01% of cases reported to poison control centers, and activated charcoal was used in 2.9% of cases.[8] In some of these cases, it is likely that ipecac was administered by parents or caregivers before consulting the poison control center. The American Academy of Pediatrics Committee on Injury, Violence, and Poison Prevention and other organizations recommend that ipecac no longer be used or that its use be strictly limited because of lack of documented benefit and potential for misuse.[22] Although the Code of Federal Regulations still states that ipecac syrup is considered the emetic of choice for certain poisoning scenarios, ipecac syrup is no longer commercially available as a nonhomeopathic product.[23] Therefore, it is no longer a viable option for self-treatment of poisoning. Pharmacists should recommend that existing supplies in the home be discarded. Controversy surrounds the use of activated charcoal as a self-treatment, given the lack of evidence that it improves outcome and its poor tolerability.

Treatment with Activated Charcoal

Activated charcoal is a tasteless, gritty, fine, black insoluble powder made from the pyrolysis of various organic materials.[24] Its large surface area of 950–2000 m²/g makes activated charcoal a highly effective adsorbent.[24]

Activated charcoal has been shown to adsorb a large number of commonly ingested drugs and many other toxic agents. These substances are bound in the internal surface of the pores of the charcoal molecule, thereby preventing their absorption. Activated charcoal is not absorbed from the GI tract. As the ratio of activated charcoal to toxin increases, the proportion of bound toxin increases.[24] Highly ionized substances, such as potassium and lithium, are poorly adsorbed by activated charcoal. Activated charcoal does not bind well to alcohols or glycols (e.g., ethanol, methanol, or ethylene glycol), hydrocarbons, mineral acids and alkali, heavy metals (e.g., iron, lead, and arsenic), or cyanide (Table 20–1). The presence of food in the GI tract may reduce the efficacy of activated charcoal.

table

20–1 Contraindications to GI Decontamination with Activated Charcoal as Self-Treatment

Category	Inclusion Criteria	Recommendation
Patient condition	Coma, seizures, syncope, airway or breathing problems, blood pressure or pulse irregularities, hallucinations, and severe agitation	Refer to hospital for evaluation.
Reason or circumstance	Intentional self-harm, substance abuse, malicious intent	Refer to hospital for medical and psychiatric or social service evaluation.
Ingestion of low-viscosity hydrocarbons and terpenes	Gasoline; kerosene; mineral seal oil (furniture polish); naphtha (lighter fluid); pine oil (cleaners); turpentine (paint removers); mineral oil	Contact poison control center.
Ingestion of caustic substances	Methacrylic acid (artificial nail primers); sodium silicate and carbonate (automatic dishwashing detergents); sulfuric acid (automotive battery, drain cleaners, toilet bowl cleaners); sodium hydroxide (Clinitest tablets, drain cleaners, oven cleaners, hair relaxers); hypochlorites (bleach, pool chlorine); thioglycolates (hair relaxers); hydrofluoric acid (rust removers); hydrochloric acid (toilet bowl cleaner)	Contact poison control center.
Ingestion of substances not adsorbed by charcoal	Ethanol (alcoholic beverages, colognes, mouthwashes, aftershaves); isopropyl alcohol (rubbing alcohol); methanol (windshield washer fluid); ethylene glycol (antifreeze); ionized substances (potassium); metals (iron, lithium, lead, arsenic); cyanide (potassium cyanide, acetonitrile artificial nail remover, laetrile)	Contact poison control center.

Key: GI = Gastrointestinal.

Activated charcoal is approved by the Food and Drug Administration for use as an emergency antidote in the treatment of an ingested poison. The usual dose of activated charcoal is approximately 1 g/kg (Table 20–2).[24] This dose provides an estimate of the amount of activated charcoal to administer, rounding to the nearest full or half-full bottle. Activated charcoal is available premixed with water, sorbitol (for catharsis), or water and carboxymethylcellulose. Examples of nonprescription activated charcoal products are Actidose-Aqua or Liqui-Char with or without sorbitol generally available at concentrations of 15 or 25 g/120 mL and 50 g/240 mL. Activated charcoal slurries are prone to settling, so they should be vigorously shaken before administration. Activated charcoal also is available as a powder for reconstitution into an oral suspension just before use; this product should be stirred thoroughly or vigorously shaken after water is added. Flavoring agents have been used to try to increase the palatability of activated charcoal. Activated charcoal is most effective if given within 1 hour after ingestion. Repeat doses of activated charcoal (given in a health care facility setting only) may enhance the elimination of some drugs (e.g., phenobarbital and theophylline) after they are absorbed into the systemic circulation.

Activated charcoal combined with sorbitol also is available to improve palatability and act as a cathartic, shortening transit time of the activated charcoal complex through the GI tract and preventing constipation. Sorbitol-containing activated charcoal products are not recommended in children younger than 1 year or when multiple doses of activated charcoal are administered. In these situations, the risk of fluid and electrolyte disturbances and hypotension is higher. Most activated charcoal products marketed specifically for home use do not contain sorbitol. Activated charcoal capsules marketed as a dietary supplement for GI complaints or other ailments should not be used to manage poisonings because the surface area of charcoal in these products is too small to effectively adsorb toxins.

Activated charcoal is used primarily for patients managed in a health care facility. Although this agent is available as a nonprescription drug, it is not available in most homes, nor is it routinely recommended for home use by poison control centers. Health care providers should consult their poison control center to determine whether to promote routine availability of activated charcoal in the home.

The most common adverse effects of activated charcoal are vomiting and black stools. Vomiting occurs in 12%–20% of patients receiving activated charcoal.[24] One-fifth of children younger than 18 years who were given activated charcoal for poisoning vomited a median time of 10 minutes after initiation of charcoal administration. More serious complications, such as pulmonary aspiration and GI obstruction, are associated more often with administration of multiple doses of activated charcoal.

Activated charcoal is contraindicated in patients in whom the GI tract is not anatomically (e.g., following caustic injury) or functionally (e.g., ileus) intact. Following bariatric surgery patients may not tolerate charcoal or may need smaller, more frequent doses. Activated charcoal also is contraindicated in patients at high risk for aspiration without airway protection (Table 20–1). Activated charcoal should not be administered after ingestion of substances that it does not adsorb, unless the presence of other ingestants that are adsorbed by charcoal is suspected.

Pharmacotherapeutic Considerations for Activated Charcoal

Studies have demonstrated that the effectiveness of GI decontamination decreases significantly with increasing time interval since ingestion. For most overdoses, GI decontamination with activated charcoal should be performed early, usually within an hour of the ingestion.[25]

There is no convincing evidence that activated charcoal improves patient outcomes, and its utility in adults with intentional overdoses has been questioned, particularly in patients with mild-moderate poisoning.[26,27] A position statement by the American Academy of Clinical Toxicology and the European Association of Poison Control Centers and Clinical Toxicologists concluded that activated charcoal may be considered for a potentially toxic amount of a poison ingested up to 1 hour before treatment. There are insufficient data to support or exclude use of charcoal when poison ingestion occurred more than 1 hour previously.[24] The majority of studies upon which the position statement was based were conducted in a controlled research or hospital environment.

Poison control centers vary in recommending home use of activated charcoal. Home administration of activated charcoal is usually intended for patient management outside a health care facility, but sometimes the agent is given to provide early prehospital GI decontamination in patients who subsequently are transported to an emergency department. Data on prehospital administration provide insight into the potential difficulty in administering activated charcoal in the home. A study of prehospital emergency medical technicians or paramedics reported that charcoal was not given to 15.4% of patients in whom administration was attempted; in 71% of these cases the reason was patient refusal.[28]

Consideration of home use of activated charcoal requires addressing the following questions: What are the benefits? Will children drink it at home? Does home administration shorten the interval between the overdose and charcoal administration? Is it safe to give at home?[29] Eldridge et al.[29] cited two studies (21 children total) that questioned whether activated charcoal can be successfully administered at home after researchers found that most children did not drink a full dose administered by parents. Three other studies (217 children total) reported that a full dose was administered in 64% of children and a partial dose was ingested in 16% of 157 children.[29] Problems with these studies include reliance on parent reports and lack of validation of the accuracy of the amount of charcoal administered.

table 20–2	Activated Charcoal Dosing Information	
Age	**Dose**
0–12 months[a]	10–25 grams
1–12 years	25–50 grams
>12 years	25–100 grams

[a] Used primarily in a health care setting in this age group.
Source: Reference 24.

Home administration shortens time to charcoal administration.[29, 30] When administered at home, charcoal is generally given within the desired 1 hour. Consideration should be given to the relative benefit of parents administering charcoal to children before arrival at the emergency department compared to the risk associated with possible delay in emergency department treatment if charcoal was administered earlier.

To date, experience with home administration of activated charcoal has shown that it is relatively safe. GI effects have been reported, with the main adverse effect being vomiting. There is concern that if home use of activated charcoal becomes more prevalent and parents administer charcoal when it is contraindicated (e.g., hydrocarbon ingestion or altered mental status with compromised airway), serious adverse effects such as aspiration may increase.[29] Before a health care provider recommends use of activated charcoal, a poison control center should be consulted.

Assessment of Poisoning: A Case-Based Approach

After obtaining the history of the exposure to a poison and performing an initial assessment of the patient's condition, the health care provider must decide whether to refer the patient directly to an emergency treatment facility, to manage him or her at home, or not to recommend any specific treatment. Clearly patients with serious clinical effects including altered mental status (e.g., stupor, coma, seizures, agitation, or hallucinations), respiratory distress, or changes in cardiovascular status (e.g., syncope or hypotension) are not candidates for self-care and should be transported immediately to the emergency treatment facility. Alternatively, recognizing nontoxic or minimally toxic exposures that can be managed outside a health care facility is an essential component of self-treatment of poisoning. Involving the poison control center in this triage and treatment decision is important because poison control centers have considerable experience managing poisoned patients and specialized resources that are not usually available to providers. The nationwide toll-free poison control center number, 800-222-1222, connects callers to the center near them (Figure 20–1).

Self-treatment at home is primarily intended for unintentional poison exposures in children younger than 6 years in whom no or, at most, minimal toxicity is expected. In addition, unintentional inhalation or skin or eye exposures in any age group, with possible minimal toxicity, often can be self-treated.

If an individual inquires about purchasing activated charcoal, the pharmacist must determine whether these drugs are being purchased for an acute situation, in which case the poison control center should be contacted to assess the appropriateness of self-treatment. The poison control center will need information about the patient (age, weight, medical history, and whether the patient is currently experiencing clinical effects), the toxin (name of the toxin, dose, route of exposure, and time since exposure), and what treatment, if any, has already been administered.

Cases 20–1 and 20–2 provide examples of assessment of patients who have been poisoned.

Patient Counseling for Poisoning

After patients are removed from toxic fumes, they should be counseled about when to seek medical attention (e.g., difficulty breathing, or worsening or persistent symptoms). In the home or other nonindustrial setting, fumes often are soluble, irritant gases (e.g., chlorine), so clinical effects are evident immediately and usually resolve soon after exposure stops. Patients also should be counseled about ventilating the room to disperse the vapor. If the exposure resulted from mixing products such as bleach and ammonia, the patient should be warned not to mix household products in the future. If carbon monoxide is suspected, the patient should be instructed to have the source turned off or removed (e.g., malfunctioning furnace, stove, or vehicle). The poison control center should be contacted to assess the severity and expected duration of clinical effects in symptomatic patients and the possibility of delayed onset in asymptomatic patients. Home carbon monoxide detectors are important home safety devices, and homeowners should be encouraged to install them to prevent or minimize carbon monoxide exposures.

Patients with eye exposures should be counseled on how to irrigate the eye at home under the faucet. Contact lenses should be removed before irrigation. Instructions should include running the water at room temperature and at a low pressure. Irrigating the eyes in the shower or using a clean cup to pour water into the eyes may be an easier alternative in children. Placing a damp washcloth on the eye or irrigating with small-volume nonprescription eyewashes is ineffective. Finally, eye drops, including topical vasoconstrictors, should not be used after irrigation. Patients with skin exposures should be counseled to remove clothing, if necessary, and wash affected areas thoroughly. For eye and skin exposures, counseling should stress the importance of immediate irrigation or washing.

If the poison control center in a region recommends activated charcoal for home use, pharmacies in that area should stock the appropriate product, and pharmacists should educate parents that activated charcoal should never be used without first consulting a poison control center staff member. Patients who purchase activated charcoal for immediate use following the recommendation of a poison control center should be counseled to ensure appropriate drug use, including provision of instructions on preparation (depending on the formulation). The pharmacist also should explain potential adverse effects, as well as signs and symptoms that indicate medical attention should be sought.

Counseling older adults on self-managing their medications can prevent poisonings and adverse drug reactions. Polypharmacy means that older adults are at risk for errors relating to dose, dosage regimen, and possibly administration techniques. Educating them about the potential for interactions, including drug–drug, drug–food and drug–alcohol, is important. Remind them that they should seek advice before mixing nonprescription or herbal products with prescription medications. Counseling older adults should emphasize the importance of ongoing communication with their health care providers to assure both efficacy and safety of their medication regimen.

Patients who are taking multiple prescriptions and using a regular pill minder should be advised to purchase a locking pill minder if they are around young children. When loading the device, they should place a paper or cardboard underneath the

case

20-1

Relevant Evaluation Criteria	Scenario/Model Outcome
Information Gathering	

1. Gather essential information about the patient's symptoms and medical history, including:

   a. description of symptom(s) (i.e., nature, onset, duration, severity, associated symptoms)

   A man asks the pharmacist for a recommendation for a single product that can treat his cold and flu symptoms but won't make him drowsy during the day. For the past week he has been taking a multisymptom product marketed for cold, flu, and sinus congestion, a product marketed for head congestion on occasion, and several doses a day of acetaminophen for his sinus headache. He states he sometimes feels drowsy and jittery.

   b. description of any factors that seem to precipitate, exacerbate, and/or relieve the patient's symptom(s)

   Symptoms are exacerbated when both products are taken together.

   c. description of the patient's efforts to relieve the symptoms

   On occasion he has taken a nighttime nonprescription sleep aid to help him sleep.

   d. patient's identity

   Sam Silver

   e. age, sex, height, and weight

   35 years old, male, 6 ft 1 in., 175 lb

   f. patient's occupation

   Marketing representative

   g. patient's dietary habits

   2 cups of coffee in the morning with several caffeinated soft drinks in the afternoon

   h. patient's sleep habits

   5 hours nightly

   i. concurrent medical conditions, prescription and nonprescription medications, and dietary supplements

   Cold, flu, and sinus product contains phenylephrine 5 mg, chlorpheniramine 2 mg, and acetaminophen 325 mg. The head congestion product contains dextromethorphan 10 mg, phenylephrine 5 mg, and acetaminophen 325 mg. He estimates he has taken 1–2 of each of these products for the past 3 days. He also has taken 1–2 extra-strength acetaminophen tablets at least 3 times daily for a sinus headache over the same 3-day period.

   j. allergies

   Medications—none, but he has bad seasonal allergies.

   k. history of other adverse reactions to medications

   None

   l. other (describe) _____

   NA

| **Assessment and Triage** | |

2. Differentiate patient's signs/symptoms and correctly identify the patient's primary problem(s).

   Sam's jitteriness is likely related to taking two products with phenylephrine in addition to caffeine. His drowsiness is likely related to the chlorpheniramine and dextromethorphan. In addition, all three products contain acetaminophen. His total daily acetaminophen dose is 1650 mg, which is below the recommended maximum daily dose.

3. Identify exclusions for self-treatment (Figure 20–2).

   None

4. Formulate a comprehensive list of therapeutic alternatives for the primary problem to determine if triage to a health care provider is required, and share this information with the patient or caregiver.

   Options include:

   (1) Counsel Sam to avoid taking multiple cough and cold products together because they often contain the same or similar ingredients.

   (2) Counsel Sam to check all prescription and nonprescription medications and to avoid taking more than one product that contains acetaminophen at the same time.

   (3) Take no action.

| **Plan** | |

5. Select an optimal therapeutic alternative to address the patient's problem, taking into account patient preferences.

   Help Sam choose a nonprescription product that meets his needs.

6. Describe the recommended therapeutic approach to the patient or caregiver.

   "Sam should be counseled about the use of more than one cough and cold product at the same time and about products with acetaminophen."

7. Explain to the patient or caregiver the rationale for selecting the recommended therapeutic approach from the considered therapeutic alternatives.

   "Sam experienced adverse effects from his therapeutic regimen, but they were not significant enough to warrant further treatment."

case

20–1 *continued*

Relevant Evaluation Criteria	Scenario/Model Outcome
Patient Education	
8. When recommending self-care with nonprescription medications and/or nondrug therapy, convey accurate information to the patient or caregiver.	Criterion does not apply in this case.
Solicit follow-up questions from the patient or caregiver.	"Is it okay to take a sleep aid as well as acetaminophen for a headache to help me sleep?"
Answer the patient's or caregiver's questions.	"Some nonprescription sleep aids also contain acetaminophen."
Evaluation of Patient Outcome	
9. Assess patient outcome.	Ask the patient to call to update you on his response to your recommendations, or you could call him in a week to evaluate the response.

Key: NA = Not applicable.

case

20–2

Relevant Evaluation Criteria	Scenario/Model Outcome
Information Gathering	
1. Gather essential information about the patient's symptoms and medical history, including:	
a. description of symptom(s) (i.e., nature, onset, duration, severity, associated symptoms)	A mother asks the pharmacist about treatment options for her previously healthy 2-year-old daughter, who was found with an open aspirin bottle. The now empty bottle of 325 mg aspirin originally contained 50 tablets and 42 had been used previously. The ingestion happened 1 hour ago. The child vomited once and is sleepy.
	Mom states that child vomited 15 minutes ago, and mom saw one partially dissolved tablet in the vomit. The child is sleepy and looks a little pale. When asked if child is breathing faster than normal, mom nods "yes."
b. description of any factors that seem to precipitate, exacerbate, and/or relieve the patient's symptom(s)	NA
c. description of the patient's efforts to relieve the symptoms	Mom gave the child some juice to drink after she vomited.
d. patient's identity	Emily Gold
e. age, sex, height, and weight	2 years old, female, 32 in., 22 lb
f. patient's occupation	NA
g. patient's dietary habits	She ate lunch 2 hours before the exposure.
h. patient's sleep habits	It is close to her nap time.
i. concurrent medical conditions, prescription and nonprescription medications, and dietary supplements	Healthy; takes no medications.
j. allergies	NKDA
k. history of other adverse reactions to medications	None
l. other (describe) _____	NA

case
20–2 *continued*

Relevant Evaluation Criteria	Scenario/Model Outcome
Assessment and Triage	
2. Differentiate patient's signs/symptoms and correctly identify the patient's primary problem(s).	Acute unintentional overdose of aspirin. Although mom saw a partially dissolved tablet, one should assume that close to 8 tablets were ingested. Therefore, she ingested 8 aspirin 325 mg; total dose of 2.6 grams or 260 mg/kg.
3. Identify exclusions for self-treatment (Figure 20–2).	Emily is sleepy. She has taken a toxic dose of aspirin.
4. Formulate a comprehensive list of therapeutic alternatives for the primary problem to determine if triage to a health care provider is required, and share this information with the patient or caregiver.	Options include: (1) Contact the poison control center for recommendations regarding whether to refer Emily to an emergency department for possible GI decontamination and evaluation. (2) Have her mother administer an OTC treatment to decrease absorption at home. (3) Have her mother administer oral fluids to dilute the aspirin. (4) Take no action.
Plan	
5. Select an optimal therapeutic alternative to address the patient's problem, taking into account patient preferences.	The poison control center should be contacted immediately. The center will determine whether it is safe to manage the child at home.
6. Describe the recommended therapeutic approach to the patient or caregiver.	No treatment should be provided at home because the child has ingested a toxic dose, has vomited and may continue to vomit, and needs medical management. Doses above 150 mg/kg cannot be managed at home. The poison control center recommends that Emily be treated at the hospital.
7. Explain to the patient or caregiver the rationale for selecting the recommended therapeutic approach from the considered therapeutic alternatives.	"Emily has ingested a large dose of aspirin that can cause her to become even sleepier and can affect her breathing and heart. It can cause abnormal blood values that could become dangerous. There are specific blood tests and therapies that can only be done in the hospital. If the hospital is near, you can transport her in your private vehicle, but she must be taken immediately. If you live farther away from a hospital or feel uncomfortable taking her by yourself, call 911."
Patient Education	
8. When recommending self-care with nonprescription medications and/or nondrug therapy, convey accurate information to the patient or caregiver.	Criterion does not apply in this case.
Solicit follow-up questions from the patient or caregiver.	"I have ipecac syrup at home. Can I give it instead of taking her to the hospital?"
Answer the patient's or caregiver's questions.	"No, ipecac syrup is no longer recommended and should be discarded. Also, Emily needs to be treated in a hospital."
Evaluation of Patient Outcome	
9. Assess patient outcome.	Determine which hospital Emily will be transported to. The poison control center will call ahead to make them aware that Emily is on her way in, provide information on the situation, and provide recommendations on laboratory evaluation and treatment. The poison control center will follow up to check on how Emily is doing and to provide additional recommendations if needed.

Key: GI = Gastrointestinal; NA = not applicable; NKDA = no known drug allergies; OTC = over-the-counter.

The objectives of self-treatment are to (1) minimize exposure and reduce development of toxicity by removing the patient to fresh air, irrigating the skin or eyes, or preventing absorption of potentially toxic agents in the GI tract and (2) treat patients with minimally toxic ingestions at home under the supervision of a poison control center. For most patients, carefully following the self-care measures listed here will help ensure optimal therapeutic outcomes.

Treatment

- For eye exposures, immediately irrigate with water for 10–15 minutes.
- For skin exposures, immediately wash with soap and water.
- For inhalation exposures, immediately remove the patient to fresh air.

When to Seek Medical Attention

Referral to an emergency department by contacting 911 directly is appropriate if the patient:

- Is lethargic or comatose or is having convulsions or hallucinations.
- Has decreased respirations or is having difficulty breathing.
- Has abnormal blood pressure or pulse.
- Has taken medications that may produce a rapid decline in consciousness or convulsions.

---

pill minder to catch stray pills that might fall on the floor. Pharmacists also can prevent therapeutic 10-fold error types of poisonings by always dispensing 1 mL oral syringes for prescription medications that are dosed in infants at less than 1 mL, such as metoclopramide. The box Patient Education for Toxic Exposures lists specific information to provide parents, caregivers, or patients.

Counseling should include providing the nationwide toll-free number for the poison control center (Figure 20–1) and promoting poison prevention practices, including purchase of nonprescription drugs and household products with child-resistant packaging. However, caregivers should be reminded that child-resistant closures are not child proof; regardless of whether a product has a child-resistant closure, it should be stored up and out of reach of small children and preferably in a locked cabinet. The Up and Away campaign (www.upandaway.org) is a new initiative developed by PROTECT, a public–private initiative (Preventing Overdoses and Treatment Errors in Children Taskforce) in partnership with the Centers for Disease Control.

Evaluation of Patient Outcomes for Poisoning

Patients who have inhaled potentially toxic fumes or spilled or splashed a substance on their skin or in their eye should be reassessed for symptoms after removal to fresh air or irrigation. If clinical effects are minimal and resolve within a relatively short period of time (e.g., under 30 minutes), the patient may be observed at home. If symptoms persist or worsen, the patient should be referred to a primary care provider or the emergency department, depending on the severity of symptoms and immediacy of need for medical evaluation. The poison control center can facilitate the referral to the appropriate health care facility and provide treatment recommendations to the health care provider.

Patients who receive activated charcoal should be contacted afterward at least once to determine whether any symptoms related to the exposure develop. The time of the call depends on what substance was ingested, how rapidly it is absorbed, and

when symptoms would be anticipated. If clinical effects develop and are minor, the patient may be observed at home. If more significant effects develop, the patient should be referred to an emergency department for treatment. If the poison control center recommended self-treatment with activated charcoal, the center staff should remain involved in subsequent decisions regarding the appropriateness of continued home treatment of these patients.

Key Points for Poisoning

➤ Poison exposures are a common cause of pediatric and adult injury.

➤ Medication errors are a common cause of drug-related toxicity, especially in older adults.

➤ Minimizing the duration or limiting the extent of the exposure is the rationale for most self-treatment practices.

➤ There are no data demonstrating that self-treatment for poisoning with activated charcoal improves patient outcomes. Use only upon recommendation of a poison control center.

➤ Self-treatment should be considered only for unintentional poison exposures that are likely to cause no or minimal toxicity (i.e., no serious or life-threatening symptoms; Figure 20–2).

➤ Health care providers should consult with the poison control center for guidance on patient assessment and on decisions for the appropriateness of self-treatment.

➤ Referral directly to the poison control center should be considered for complicated cases, including those with unclear patient histories or lacking specific product or toxin information, and to ensure case follow-up.

➤ All patients who exhibit potentially life-threatening clinical effects (e.g., seizures or coma) should be referred to an emergency department through the emergency 911 system.

REFERENCES

1. Warner M, Chen LH, Makuc DM, et al. Drug poisoning deaths in the United States, 1980–2008. Hyattsville, MD: National Center for Health Statistics; 2011. NCHS Data Brief No. 81.

2. Centers for Disease Control and Prevention. Vital signs: Overdoses of prescription opioid pain relievers—United States, 1999–2008. *MMWR Morb Mortal Wkly Rep.* 2011;60(43):1487–92.

3. Centers for Disease Control and Prevention. Emergency department visits involving nonmedical use of selected prescription drugs—United States, 2004–2008. *MMWR Morb Mortal Wkly Rep.* 2010;59(23):705–9.

4. Shone LP, King JP, Doane C, et al. Misunderstanding and potential unintended misuse of acetaminophen among adolescents and young adults. *J Health Comm.* 2011;16:256–67.

5. King JP, Davis TC, Bailey SC, et al. Developing consumer-centered, non-prescription drug labeling. A study in acetaminophen. *Am J Prev Med.* 2011;40(6):593–8.

6. Substance Abuse and Mental Health Services Administration, Office of Applied Studies. The NSDUH report: Misuse of over-the-counter cough and cold medications among persons aged 12 to 25. January 10, 2008. Accessed at http://www.oas.samhsa.gov/2k8/cough/cough.htm, May 12, 2011.

7. Setlik J, Bond GR, Ho M. Adolescent prescription ADHD medication abuse is rising along with prescriptions for these medications. *Pediatrics.* 2009;124(3):875–80.

8. Bronstein AC, Spyker DA, Cantilena LR, et al. 2011 annual report of the American Association of Poison Control Centers' National Poison Data System (NPDS): 29th annual report. *Clin Toxicol.* 2012;50(10):911–1164.

9. Galvao TF, Silva EN, Silva MT, et al. Economic evaluation of poison centers: a systematic review. *Int J Technol Assess Health Care.* 2012;28(2):86–92.

10. Vassilev ZP, Marcus SM. The impact of a poison control center on the length of hospital stay for patients with poisoning. *J Toxicol Environ Health A.* 2007;70(2):107–10.

11. Kostic MA, Oswald J, Gummin DD, et al. Poison center consultation decreases hospital length of stay and inpatient charges. *Clin Toxicol.* 2010;48:605.

12. The Lewin Group Inc. *Final Report on the Value of the Poison Control System.* Alexandria, VA: American Association of Poison Control Centers; 2012. Accessed at https://aapcc.s3.amazonaws.com/files/library/Value_of_the_Poison_Center_System_FINAL_9_26_2012_--_FINAL_FINAL_FINAL.pdf, March 16, 2013.

13. Polivka BJ, Casavant M, Baker SD. Factors associated with healthcare visits by young children for nontoxic poisoning exposures. *J Community Health.* 2010;35(6):572–8.

14. Schillie SF, Shehab NE, Thomas KE, et al. Medication overdoses leading to emergency department visits among children. *Am J Prev Med.* 2009;37(3):181–7.

15. National Safety Council. *Injury Facts 2013 Edition.* Itasca, IL: National Safety Council; 2013.

16. Rodgers GB. The safety effects of child-resistant packaging for oral prescription drugs. Two decades of experience. *JAMA.* 1996;275(21):1661–5

17. U.S. Consumer Product Safety Commission. *Poison Prevention Packaging: A Guide for Healthcare Professionals.* Washington, DC: U.S. Consumer Product Safety Commission; 2005. Publication 384. Accessed at http://www.cpsc.gov/cpscpub/pubs/384.pdf, April 12, 2011.

18. Franklin RL, Rodgers GB. Unintentional childhood poisonings treated in United States hospital emergency departments: national estimates of incident cases, population-based poisoning rates, and product involvement. *Pediatrics.* 2008;122:1244–51.

19. Yin HS, Parker RM, Wolf MS, et al. Health literacy assessment of labeling of pediatric non-prescription medications: examination of characteristics that may impair parent understanding. *Academ Pediatrics.* 2012;12(4):288–96.

20. Wallace LS, Keenum AJ, DeVoe JE, et al. Women's understanding of different dosing instructions for a liquid pediatric medication. *J Ped Health Care.* 2012;26 (6):443–50.

21. Lokker NL, Sanders L, Perrin EM, et.al. Parental misinterpretations of over-the-counter pediatric cough and cold medication labels. *Pediatrics.* 2009;123:1464–71.

22. Committee on Injury, Violence, and Poison Prevention. Poison treatment in the home. *Pediatrics.* 2003;112:1182–5.

23. Ipecac syrup; warnings and directions for use for over-the-counter sale. CFR: Code of Federal Regulations. Title 21. Part 201, Section 201.308. Updated April 1, 2013. Accessed at http://www.gpo.gov/fdsys/search/pagedetails.action?collectionCode=CFR&searchPath=Title+21%2FChapter+I%2FSubchapter+C%2FPart+201%2FSubpart+G&granuleId=CFR-2013-title21-vol4-sec201-308&packageId=CFR-2013-title21-vol4&oldPath=Title+21%2FChapter+I%2FSubchapter+C%2FPart+201&fromPageDetails=true&collapse=true&ycord=339&browsePath=Title+21%2FChapter+I%2FSubchapter+C%2FPart+201%2FSubpart+G%2FSection+201.308&fromBrowse=true, October 14, 2013.

24. Chyka PA, Seger D, Krenzelok EP, et al.; American Academy of Clinical Toxicology; European Association of Poisons Centers and Clinical Toxicologists. Position paper: Single-dose activated charcoal. *Clin Toxicol.* 2005;43:61–87.

25. Albertson TE, Owen KP, Sutter ME, et al. Gastrointestinal decontamination in the acutely poisoned patient. *Int J Emerg Med.* 2011;4:65. doi: 10.1186/1865-1380-4-65

26. Olson KR. Activated charcoal for acute poisoning: One toxicologist's journey. *J Med Toxicol.* 2010;6(2):190–8.

27. Isbister GK, Kumar VV. Indications for single-dose activated charcoal administration in acute overdose. *Curr Opin Crit Care.* 2011;17(4):351–7.

28. Alaspaa AO, Kuisma MJ, Hoppu K, et al. Out-of-hospital administration of activated charcoal by emergency medical services. *Ann Emerg Med.* 2005;45(2):207–12.

29. Eldridge DL, Van Eyk J, Kornegay C. Pediatric toxicology. *Emerg Med Clin North Am.* 2007;15(2):283–308.

30. Lapus RM. Activated charcoal for pediatric poisonings: The universal antidote? *Curr Opin Pediatr.* 2007;19(2):216–22.

OSTOMY CARE AND SUPPLIES

chapter 21

Joan Lerner Selekof and Sharon Wilson

An ostomy is an opening or outlet through the abdominal wall created surgically for the purpose of eliminating waste. The opening is usually made by bringing a portion of the bladder, colon, small intestine, or ureters through the abdominal wall. The opening of the ostomy is called the *stoma* (from the Latin word for mouth).

The creation of an ostomy may be a dramatic, life-changing event. Therefore, it is important for health care providers to provide reassurance, support, and education for the patient and family. An understanding of improvements in surgical procedures, ostomy supplies, and outcomes can allay much of a patient's fear and anxiety. The goal in ostomy care is to enable the individual to resume his or her lifestyle—to be a person, not a patient. A person with an ostomy carefully notes the reactions of providers to the disorder; any negative response may reinforce the patient's negative feelings about the ostomy.

More than 700,000 Americans are currently living with an ostomy.[1] Ostomy surgery is performed on individuals of all ages and for many conditions, both acquired and congenital. When medically advisable, the current surgical trend in ostomy surgery is laparoscopic surgery. Patients report experiencing less pain, quicker recovery, and less scarring compared to traditional ostomy surgery.

Indications for Ostomies

Ostomies may be permanent or temporary, and they are performed in individuals ranging from neonates to the elderly. Reasons for performing ostomies include congenital anomalies (e.g., imperforate anus and Hirschsprung's disease), inflammatory bowel disease, familial polyposis, cancer, radiation damage, pressure ulcers, trauma, and any other need to divert the urinary or fecal stream.[2,3] The type of ostomy depends on the condition being treated.

The two most common disorders leading to ileostomy surgery are (1) ulcerative colitis, which affects the large intestine and rectum, and (2) Crohn's disease, which may involve any part of the gastrointestinal (GI) tract. Other conditions that may result in an ileostomy include traumatic injury, cancer, familial polyposis, and necrotizing enterocolitis.

The most common reasons for colostomy surgery are (1) cancer of the colon or rectum, (2) diverticulitis, and (3) trauma. Other indications include obstruction of the colon or rectum, genetic malformation, radiation colitis, and loss of

anal muscular control. In some cases, a temporary colostomy may be performed to protect areas of the colon that have been surgically repaired. Healing of a diseased or damaged bowel may take several weeks, months, or years, but eventually the colon and rectum are reconnected and bowel continuity is restored. Figure 21–1 shows the location of various types of colostomies.

Urinary diversions are created to correct bladder loss or dysfunction, which can be caused by cancer, neurogenic bladder, genetic malformation, or interstitial cystitis.

Types of Ostomies

The three basic types of ostomies are (1) ileostomy, (2) colostomy (the most common type), and (3) urinary diversion (see Color Plates, photographs 2A–I). Each type of ostomy has several variations depending on the location of the stoma, the reason for the surgical procedure, or whether the procedure renders a patient continent.

Ileostomy

An ileostomy is surgically created by bringing a portion of the ileum through the abdominal wall (see Color Plates, photograph 2A). Initially, the discharge is liquid, but as the ileum adapts, it assumes some of the absorptive functions of the colon and the discharge may become semisoft. The discharge is continuous and contains intestinal enzymes that may irritate the peristomal skin.

Several types of continent ileostomies exist (see Color Plates, photograph 2B). An internal pouch is created from the ileum, and an intussusception (a slipping of a length of intestine into an adjacent portion) of the bowel is used to create a "nipple" that renders the patient continent for stool and flatus. The pouch is periodically emptied by inserting a catheter through the nipple, which is attached to the skin usually in the right lower quadrant, into the pouch. At first, the pouch holds about 75 mL, but it stretches with use so that, at 6 months postoperatively, it may hold 600–800 mL and can be drained three to five times daily. Patients do not need to wear an external pouching system, but they often wear a gauze pad or stoma cap.

The restorative proctocolectomy (S pouch or J pouch) ileoanal reservoir spares the rectum of patients with ulcerative colitis or familial polyposis. The colon is removed and the diseased

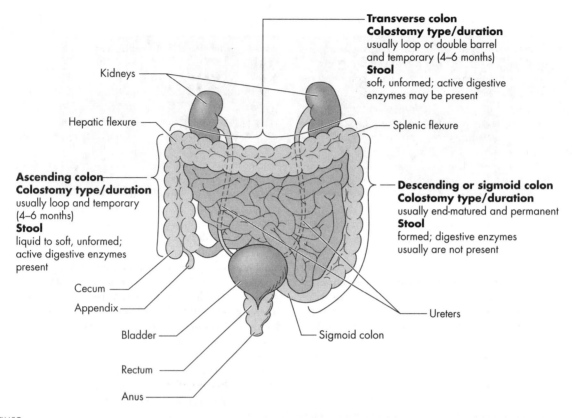

Kidneys

Hepatic flexure

Transverse colon
Colostomy type/duration
usually loop or double barrel
and temporary (4–6 months)
Stool
soft, unformed; active digestive
enzymes may be present

Splenic flexure

Ascending colon
Colostomy type/duration
usually loop and temporary
(4–6 months)
Stool
liquid to soft, unformed;
active digestive enzymes
present

Descending or sigmoid colon
Colostomy type/duration
usually end-matured and permanent
Stool
formed; digestive enzymes
usually are not present

Cecum

Appendix

Bladder

Rectum

Anus

Ureters

Sigmoid colon

figure
21–1
Anatomic drawing of the lower digestive and urinary tracts depicting location and permanence of colostomies.
(*Source:* Adapted with permission from *Am J Nurs.* 1977;77:443.)

mucosa is stripped from the rectum, and an internal pouch is created from the ileum. The distal end of the small intestine is stapled or hand sewn to the remaining rectal tissue. The sphincter is preserved and ostomy pouching systems are unnecessary. However, a patient undergoing this procedure may have a temporary (about 3–6 months) stoma to protect the healing pouch. Patients will have more frequent bowel movements and may experience perianal skin irritation.

Colostomy

A colostomy is created by bringing a portion of the colon through the abdominal wall. The discharge may be semisoft, paste-like, or formed depending on the portion of bowel used (Figure 21–1).

Ascending colostomies are uncommon. The ascending colon is retained, but the rest of the large bowel is removed or bypassed (see Color Plates, photograph 2C). The stoma is usually on the right side of the abdomen. The discharge is semisoft and a pouch must be worn at all times.

The transverse colon is the site of most temporary colostomies (Figure 21–1). A loop of the transverse colon is lifted through the abdominal incision, and a rod or bridge (which is removed within 1–2 weeks) is placed under the loop to give it support while the stoma heals. The discharge is usually semiliquid or very soft.

Loop colostomies have one large opening but two tracts (see Color Plates, photograph 2D). The proximal tract discharges fecal material, and the distal tract secretes small amounts of mucus. A

pouching system must be worn at all times. A person with a loop colostomy may also pass a minimal amount of stool or mucus through the rectum. This is a normal occurrence.

For a *double-barrel transverse colostomy,* the bowel is completely divided by bringing both the proximal end and the distal end through the abdominal wall, and then suturing them to the skin (see Color Plates, photograph 2E). The distal stoma may also be called the mucous fistula.

Descending and sigmoid colostomies are fairly common; generally the stoma is on the left side of the abdomen (see Color Plates, photograph 2F). The fecal discharge has a paste-like consistency and at times may consist of formed stool. This type of colostomy may be regulated by irrigation; therefore, a pouching system may not be needed. However, many patients prefer a pouch to irrigation. Not everyone with a descending or sigmoid colostomy is a good candidate for irrigation or prefers irrigation. Factors to consider in making the decision to irrigate include the presence or absence of stomal complications and the patient's normal stooling pattern, psychomotor ability, and willingness to commit the time required to properly irrigate the ostomy.

Urinary Diversions

Urinary diversion surgery diverts the urine through an opening in the abdominal wall. Urinary stomas should function immediately after surgery. The broad term for a urinary diversion is *urostomy.*

The *ileal conduit* is the most common type of urinary diversion (see Color Plates, photograph 2G). After the bladder is removed, ileal and colon conduits are created by implanting the ureters into an isolated loop of bowel; one end of the bowel loop is sutured, and the distal end is brought to the surface of the abdomen. The stoma looks similar to the stoma in an ileostomy or colostomy. A pouching system must be worn continuously. Mucous shreds will be present in the urine if both the small intestine and the large intestine are used to create the diversion (see Color Plates, photograph 2H). Because the ileum is used to create an ileal conduit, some people incorrectly refer to the ileal conduit as an ileostomy. Clarification of the type of effluent (stool or urine) will help in selecting the correct type of pouch.

In a *ureterostomy,* one or both ureters are detached from the bladder and brought to the outside of the abdominal wall, where a stoma is created. This procedure is used less frequently because the ureters tend to narrow unless they have been dilated permanently because of previous disease (see Color Plates, photograph 2I).

A *cystostomy* is performed when blockage or narrowing of the urethra occurs. Urine is diverted from the bladder to the abdominal wall. A pouch must be worn continuously. An infant may use diapers instead of a pouch.

The *continent urinary diversion* is available for selected patients, but its use requires that certain criteria be met. An Indiana pouch is a type of continent urostomy in which a pouch is created from part of the cecum and ileum, with a portion of the ileum brought through the abdominal wall to create a stoma. The ureters are attached to the cecum pouch. The remaining ileum is reattached to the colon for normal digestive flow. The ileocecal valve is left intact and becomes part of the continence mechanism, preventing urine from exiting the pouch. The internal pouch is emptied by inserting a catheter into the stoma to drain the urine. Patients are usually placed on a strict schedule and will catheterize the stoma often enough to avoid leakage. The new pouch may hold up to 600 mL of urine. An external pouching system is not necessary. Most patients wear a gauze pad or stoma cap. The orthotopic neobladder is a rebuilt bladder. The small intestine is used to create a pouch, and the pouch is then attached to the native urethra. This procedure allows patients to void using their urethra, but voiding relies on the patients using their abdominal muscles to empty the neobladder.

Management of Ostomies
Management Goals

The ideal ostomy pouching system should be leak-proof, odor-proof, comfortable, easily manipulated, inconspicuous, safe, and as inexpensive as possible. Because the patient has lost a normal body function, the pouching system assists the patient in managing that loss, and it becomes almost a part of the body. It is common for patients and their families to find discussing ostomy needs difficult or embarrassing, especially during the first several weeks or months after surgery.

The ostomy industry is highly specialized and rapidly changing as it tries to improve designs, resulting in a wide range of choices. Pouch selection is extremely personal and is based on the patient's specific needs and abilities and on the cost of the system.

General Management Approach

Adult and adolescent patients must be taught self-care skills to manage the ostomy, including (1) sizing the stoma, (2) cutting a pouch or skin barrier to fit the stoma (or selecting a precut pouch or barrier), (3) cleaning the skin, (4) applying paste (caulking) or powder if necessary, (5) applying the pouch, (6) removing the pouch, and (7) emptying the pouch. Patients must be prepared for effluent from the stoma at any time.

Patients are most likely to achieve optimal outcomes if a pouching system is properly fitted (Figure 21–2) and if the stoma is cared for appropriately. The provider should always be aware of the sensitive nature of the topic and ensure that privacy is respected during all discussions. Failure to provide a comfortable environment in which to discuss problems, concerns, and alternatives may cause patients to avoid such discussions and may result in less-than-optimal outcomes. Follow-up assessment and care may be accomplished through a telephone call or scheduled appointment or during the patient's routine visits to purchase supplies or medications.

Frequent changes in the pouching system and accessories should signal a potential problem, as should the use of multiple products intended for the same purpose. In many cases, patients may be referred to a primary care provider or wound, ostomy, and continence (WOC) nurse for follow-up of problems identified by a health care provider. Complications such as impotence; peristomal hernia; and stenosis, prolapse, retraction, or peristomal skin injury require medical referral. In some cases, however, self-care is appropriate, particularly by experienced ostomy patients.

The presence of an ostomy and its location in the gastrointestinal or urinary system should always be noted on the patient's profile to minimize medication-related risks. It is helpful to maintain a record of current and past ostomy products that the patient has used and any problems that the patient has experienced. This information can be useful in making future recommendations.

Types of Ostomy Pouches

The surgical technique used to create the stoma influences the pouching system required, the complexity of the pouching procedure, and the risks of stomal and peristomal complications (e.g., necrosis, stenosis, or hernia). In the past, most ostomy pouches were reusable. The advantages of reusable pouching systems were their durability, availability in numerous configurations, and relatively low cost. Their disadvantages were that they required cleaning before each use, were heavy, tended to retain odor, and often required a separate skin barrier.

Ostomy patients are now fitted with odor-proof, lightweight, disposable pouching systems. The health care provider measuring the stoma should ensure a clearance of $1/16$–$1/8$ inch between the barrier opening and stoma, whether the barrier is precut or cut to fit. Most pouches incorporate a solid skin barrier in each flange or one-piece pouch, which eliminates the need for a separate skin barrier. Disposable equipment is available in one- and two-piece systems (Figure 21–3). The one-piece system, in which the skin barrier and the pouch are available in one piece, is easy to apply, especially for patients with impaired manual dexterity. In the two-piece system, the skin barrier is separate from the pouch. This allows patients to access the flange easily and change the pouch, if desired, without removal of the flange from the skin. The flange is easy to apply and is generally more pliable and adaptable to different abdominal contours.

One- and two-piece pouching systems are also available for young children. Although pouches are available for infants, some ostomies are managed with a diaper instead. If a diaper is used,

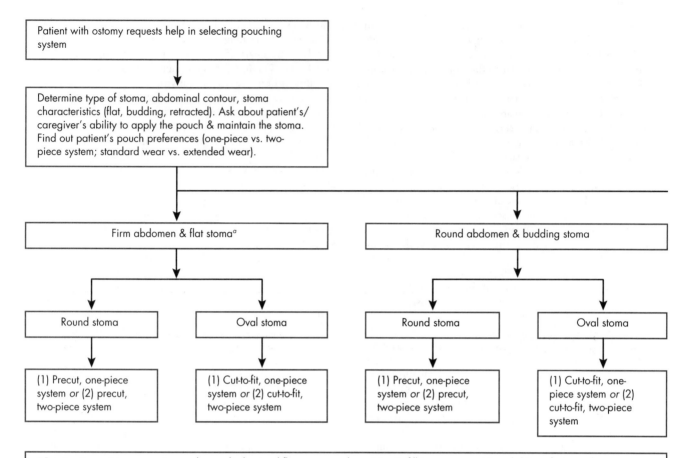

^a Barrier rings, strips, or paste may be applied around flange or pouch opening to fill in uneven peristomal skin surfaces and increase wear time.

Notes for convex systems:

When pouch flange presses into peristomal skin, it increases the degree of stomal protrusion and reduces risk of leakage. The flange also mirrors the peristomal skin surface.

Barriers, strips, or pastes may be used to fill in uneven surfaces.

Binders or belts are frequently used with convex pouching systems to provide additional support.

If not fitted correctly, convex flanges may cause ulcers under barrier. Patient should notify WOC nurse to assess changes in body contour.

figure

21–2   Selection of ostomy pouching system. Key: WOC = Wound, ostomy, and continence.

care must be taken to avoid skin irritation from a caustic effluent. Moisture barrier ointments and creams are required for neonates and infants who are only diapered. The decision to diaper or pouch is based on the location of the stoma, the type and amount of effluent, and the child's activity. Once a child is crawling or exploring, it is difficult to keep stool contained in a diaper.

Both one- and two-piece pouch systems are available in drainable, high-output, closed-end, and urostomy styles. Drainable styles are used when bowel regulation cannot be established; they allow for easy and frequent emptying. A closed-end system requires the wearer to remove and discard the pouch when it is almost full. Closed-end systems are used by patients who have regulated colostomies, have one or two formed bowel movements within 24 hours, or routinely irrigate the ostomy to remove output. The goal is to avoid output between irrigations; however, this outcome may not occur immediately, and

output can also be affected by the patient's diet, activity, and illness. Urostomy systems allow a constant output of urine and easy emptying throughout the day through a narrow valve opening. At night, most urostomy patients connect their pouch to dependent drainage to prevent overfilling of the pouch.

Fitting and Application

Reusable and disposable pouches are available in transparent and opaque styles and in various sizes. The pouch opening may be cut to fit or presized. Other options in skin barriers include a flat or convex skin barrier. When convex barriers are indicated, they are available with round, oval, or moldable openings.

Measuring the stoma to determine the proper fit of a pouch is an important part of ostomy care. The diameter of the round stoma is measured at the base, where the mucosa

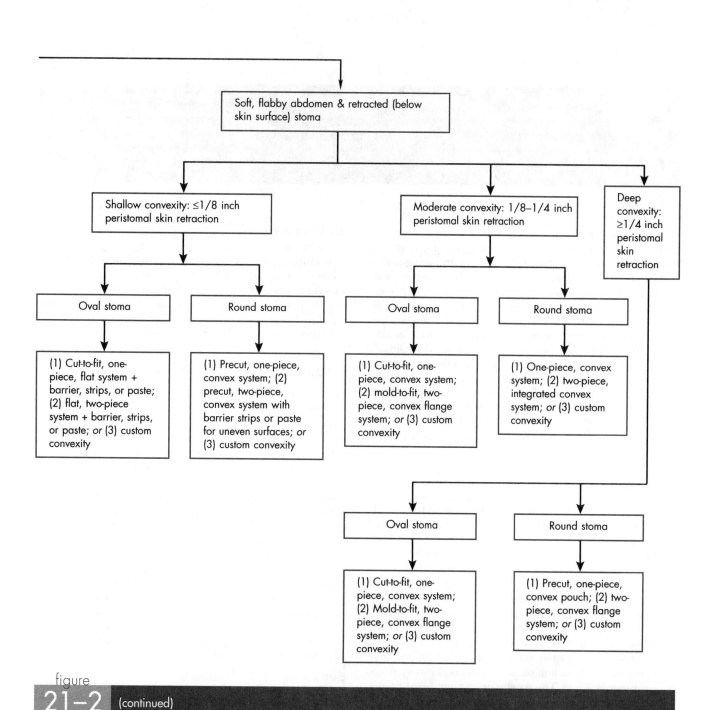

figure
21–2 (continued)

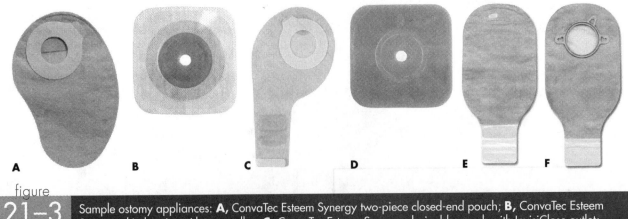

figure
21-3

Sample ostomy appliances: **A,** ConvaTec Esteem Synergy two-piece closed-end pouch; **B,** ConvaTec Esteem Synergy skin barrier with tape collar; **C,** ConvaTec Esteem Synergy drainable pouch with InvisiClose outlet; **D,** ConvaTec Esteem Synergy skin barrier without tape collar; **E** and **F,** Hollister New Image two-piece pouching system with Lock'n Roll closure: pouch and flange views, respectively. (A–D reprinted with permission from ConvaTec, a Bristol Myers Squibb Company, Skillman, NJ; E and F reprinted with permission from Hollister Incorporated, Libertyville, Illinois.)

meets the skin; this area is considered the widest measurement. Oval stomas should be measured at their widest and narrowest diameters. A stoma may swell if the adhesive fits too tightly or slips, or if the patient falls or experiences a hard blow to the stoma. It is important to periodically reassess the size for proper fitting.

Other considerations in fitting the pouch include body contour, stoma location, skin creases and scars, and ostomy type. The lack of uniformity in types of ostomies and ostomy equipment makes it difficult to give standard instructions for application. In addition, the stoma and the contour of the surrounding area change over time, necessitating continuous adjustments to pouches and accessories. In general, when a rigid faceplate or flange is used, the opening should provide a clearance of 1/16–1/8 inch around the stoma. Less clearance (0–1 mm) is required with a flexible barrier. A WOC nurse is an excellent source of assistance in custom fitting these pouching systems.

Wearing Time

The pouch should be emptied when it is one-third to one-half full to prevent leakage. With a two-piece system, the closed-end pouch is simply removed from the flange and thrown away. Patients who want to save on pouch costs may use the two-piece drainable system and alternate the use of two pouches. The full pouch is removed and replaced by a second pouch; the first pouch is then emptied, washed, and reused when the second pouch is changed. One-piece, closed-end systems are removed and disposed of once or twice daily; those that can be drained can be left in place as long as they are comfortable and there is no leakage. The flange and skin barrier may be left in place for 3–7 days depending on the condition of the skin and skin barrier. Average wear time is 4 days. The skin barrier is constructed from a material called a hydrocolloid. The hydrocolloid softens in the presence of moisture. As the hydrocolloid softens, less adhesive is present to secure the seal. Therefore, a person with a high liquid output or very moist skin (heavy perspiration) may find that the skin barrier must be changed in 3–4 days. A person with solid to semisolid stool may be able to wear the skin barrier longer than 4 days. Although activities such as swimming or playing tennis may decrease the wear time of the pouch, this decreased time

should not discourage participation in physical activities. New pouch adhesives can effectively keep the system in place during these activities. Because water will not enter the stoma, it is not necessary to cover it while bathing or showering. The patient doesn't need to cover a continent stoma when swimming. However, the pouching system can be secured with waterproof tape (e.g., Hy-Tape and Pink Tape) by taping around the edges of the wafer/flange to prevent leakage of output from the stoma.

Product Selection Guidelines

The selection of products must be tailored to the patient's activity level and, if present, specific disabilities. Some systems require manipulation that a patient with arthritis may not be able to perform. Special products are also available to assist patients who have poor vision. In general, patients with visual or physical impairments will do best with one-piece systems because these systems have precut pouches and require minimal manipulation. Waterproof materials or a stoma cover should be included with the system. Table 21–1 lists ostomy manufacturers. Their Web sites list all available products and product information. No particular device will prevent patients who are confused from reaching and dislodging the pouching system (e.g., patients with Alzheimer's disease). It may be helpful to dress these patients in garments that make it difficult for them to reach the pouch. Dressing infants in one-piece clothing will help prevent them from exploring and pulling off their pouches.

Ostomy Accessories

Belts

Special elastic belts that attach to various pouching systems provide additional support. However, not all ostomy patients need to wear belts. Indications for their use are a deeply convex flange, short pouch-wearing time, high activity level (especially in children), heavy perspiration, and personal preference. Some patients may find that wearing a belt for just a few hours after changing their pouch helps the adhesive adhere, thereby increasing wear time and decreasing the risk of leakage. Belts that are too tight may

table
21-1 Sources of Ostomy Support and Information

Organization/Manufacturer	Telephone Number	Web Site
American Cancer Society	800-ACS-2345	www.cancer.org
Colo-majic Liners	866-611-6028	www.colomajic.com
Coloplast	800-533-0464	www.coloplast.com
ConvaTec	800-422-8811	www.convatec.com
Crohn's and Colitis Foundation of America, Inc.	800-343-3637	www.ccfa.org
Cymed Ostomy Company	800-582-0707	www.cymed-ostomy.com
C&S Ostomy Pouch Covers	877-754-9913	www.cspouchcovers.com
Dansac (Incutech, Inc., is the importer)	800-699-4232	www.incutech.com; www.dansac.dk
Hollister, Inc.	800-323-4060	www.hollister.com
Hy-Tape Corporation	800-248-0101	www.hytape.com
International Ostomy Association	N/A	www.ostomyinternational.org
Kem-Osto EZ-Vent	888-562-8802	www.kemOnline.com
Marlen Manufacturing	276-292-9196	www.marlenmfg.com
Nu-Hope Laboratories, Inc.	800-899-5017	www.nu-hope.com
Options Ostomy Support/Barrier, Inc.	800-736-6555	www.options-ostomy.com
Ostomysecrets	877-613-6246	www.ostomysecrets.com
Rally 4 Youth		www.rally4youth.org
Schena Ostomy Technologies	239-263-9957	www.ostomyezclean.com
Safe n' Simple	248-214-4877	www.SnS-medical.com
Stealth Belt	800-237-4491	www.stealthbelt.com
Stoma Guard	800-814-4195	www.sto-med.com
The Parthenon Company, Inc.	800-453-8898	www.parthenonInc.com
Torbot Group, Inc.	800-545-4254	www.torbot.com
United Ostomy Associations of America, Inc.	800-826-0826	www.uoaa.org
▪ Continent Diversion Network		▪ www.uoaa.org/forum/viewforum.php?f=8
▪ GLO Network—Gay/Lesbian/Bisexual Ostomates and their partners		▪ www.glo-uoaa.org
▪ Pull-Thru Network		▪ www.pullthrunetwork.org
United Ostomy Association of Canada, Inc.	416-595-5452; 888-969-9698 (Canadian residents only)	www.ostomycanada.ca
Wound, Ostomy and Continence Nurses Society (WOCN)	888-224-WOCN (9626)	www.wocn.org

cause skin ulcers. To be effective, the belt must be kept even with the belt hooks. If the belt slips up around the waist, it may cause poor adherence and, possibly, cut the stoma. Women may find that pantyhose and a panty girdle are excellent alternatives to a belt.

Many belts contain latex, so the patient should be asked about a latex allergy before a belt is recommended.

Skin Barriers, Powders, and Pastes

Skin barriers, powders, and pastes are available for special skin problems (Table 21–2). Skin barriers are intended to protect the skin immediately adjacent to the stoma from stoma discharge and to serve as a means of attaching a pouching system. They correct imperfections in the skin surface, allowing the pouching system to fit securely. Powders are used on weeping skin to absorb excessive moisture and support healing, but excessive powder must be dusted off or sealed with a no–sting liquid skin preparation before pouch application. Pastes (which are not a glue but have a paste–like consistency) are used to seal the area around the stoma and fill creases in the skin. Pastes produce a flat surface for application of other skin barriers and can be used to caulk the edge of the skin barrier.

table

21–2 Selected Ostomy Skin Barriers, Adhesives, Adhesive Removers, Belts, Powders, Cleaners, and Air Vent System

Hollister Adapt Lubricating Deodorant	Available in 8 ounce bottle or 8 mL packs. Facilitates emptying of pouch by providing lubrication
Coloplast Brava: rings, strips, strip paste	Moldable strips/paste to fill in uneven surfaces
ConvaTec AllKare Adhesive Remover Wipes	Helps prevent skin damage by easing removal of all adhesives; has oily residue; skin should be washed after use
ConvaTec AllKare Protective Barrier Wipes	Thin film protects against skin stripping; excellent liquid skin barrier for adhesives, tapes, and self-adhesive dressings
ConvaTec Eakin Cohesive Seals	Moldable, double-sided adhesive seals designed to help prevent skin damage; absorbs moisture and forms a gel to further protect skin; adheres to moist, sore skin; suitable for all types of ostomies (especially hard-to-fit stomas); can be used with pastes and all skin barriers and pouching systems
ConvaTec Stomahesive Paste	Pectin product; helps prevent leakage and skin irritation by filling in uneven surfaces; new easy-to-squeeze tube
ConvaTec Stomahesive Powder	Pectin base; light dusting applied to denuded skin to promote healing
Hollister Adapt Barrier Rings, Strips, Paste	Custom (molded, bent, shaped, and stacked) convex barrier rings; barrier strips can mold and stack; paste in easy-to-squeeze tube
Hollister Medical Adhesive	Improves adhesive contact between skin and barrier
Hollister M9 Cleaner/Decrystallizer	Cleans urinary drainage systems; pH balanced and nonacidic
Hollister M9 Odor Eliminator	Available in spray or drops, scented or unscented; is an enzyme that helps to neutralize odor
Hollister Adapt Powder	Light dusting applied to denuded skin to promote healing
Hollister Universal Remover Wipes	Removes adhesives and barriers; available as spray and wipes
KEM Air VENT System (OSTO-EZ-VENT)	Quickly and easily releases gas buildup in ostomy pouches
Nu-Hope Barrier Rings and Strips	Karaya/pectin; moldable rings and strips
Nu-Hope Cement	Natural rubber; hexane; excellent adherence for difficult pouching
Nu-Hope Support Belt	Standard 2⅜-inch opening; 3- to 9-inch widths; customized belts available; provides excellent support to prevent parastomal herniation; prolapse overbelt and custom openings available
Smith & Nephew Adhesive Remover	Helps prevent skin damage by easing removal of all adhesives
Torbot Skin Cement	4 ounce can; natural rubber; hexane; excellent adherence for difficult pouching
3M No Sting Wipes	Does not contain alcohol; thin film protects against skin stripping; excellent liquid skin barrier for adhesives, tapes, and self-adhesive dressings

Solid skin barriers are preattached to the pouch (one-piece system) or provided separately (two-piece system) and may be custom-cut (sizable) or precut (presized). Some manufacturers will custom cut the barriers; however, in most cases, the patient or WOC nurse modifies the barrier to fit the stoma. The opening in the skin barrier should match the size and shape of the patient's stoma. To apply a skin barrier, the patient should place a bead of skin barrier paste either around the stoma or directly to the inside edge of the skin barrier, apply the skin barrier to dry wrinkle-free skin, and then press the skin barrier around the stoma to improve adherence. Newer moldable seals are now available from major manufacturers.

Solid skin barriers may melt if exposed to high temperatures. Therefore, during the summer and especially when traveling, the solid skin barrier should be put in an insulated box (ice is not required) to minimize the risk of melting. Pouches should not be left in the car during the day, unless the car is completely shaded and the outside temperature is not extremely high.

Absorbent Gel Packets and Flakes

Absorbent gel packets and flakes (e.g., Ileosorb and Par-Sorb) dissolve as the pouch fills, turning the liquid effluent into a gel.

They reduce noise caused by sloshing of stomal fluids, control odor, prevent peristomal skin irritation, and prevent leakage, especially at night while the patient sleeps.

Cleansing and Special Skin Care Products

Cleansing of the stoma and surrounding skin is best done with plain water. If soap is used, it should be rinsed off thoroughly and the skin should be dried before a new pouching system is applied. Use of moisturizers and products containing lanolin, petrolatum, or oils should be avoided because they prevent the pouching system from adhering to the skin.

Adhesives

Adhesives, in the form of cements or tapes, may be used by some to keep the pouch in place. Hypoallergenic tape may be used to support the pouch. A strip may be applied across the top, bottom, and sides of the flange, with half on the flange and half on the skin. Waterproof tape may be used during swimming or bathing. Solvents are available to remove adhesive residue; however, solvents or adhesive removers must be removed from the skin prior to application of the new pouching system.

Irrigating Sets

Irrigating sets can be used to maintain control of output without the use of a pouch in patients with colostomies who are candidates for irrigation. Irrigation is similar to performing an enema at the site of the stoma. Approximately 1000 mL of lukewarm tap water is instilled into the bowel through a cone inserted in the stoma. The bowel then expands, causing peristalsis and elimination of waste through the stoma. A good candidate for irrigation is an adult patient who has a colostomy distal to the splenic flexure; does not have a history of irritable bowel syndrome or a disability; has good mentation, manual dexterity, and appropriate bathroom facilities (running water); and is not undergoing chemotherapy or radiation therapy. For the process to be safe and effective, the patient should use a colostomy irrigation set rather than a standard enema set.

Frequency of irrigation depends somewhat on a patient's normal bowel habits. The recommended frequency is to irrigate at the same time every day and eventually to regulate irrigation to every other day. Patients take approximately 6 weeks to become regulated. After achieving control, the patient may wear a security pouch or a piece of gauze, a stoma cover, or a cap over the stoma. Irrigation is not necessary for health; it is merely one method of colostomy management. Patients should use this procedure only if desired and instructed in technique by a WOC nurse or primary care provider.

Deodorizers

If needed, deodorizers are available as liquids or tablets. Liquid concentrates, which are available as companion products with most ostomy pouches, can be placed directly into the pouch to neutralize odor. DevKo external tablets may also be placed into the pouch to decrease odor. Derifil internal deodorant tablets (active ingredient is 100 mg chlorophyllin copper complex sodium) may also be used. The purpose of the deodorizers is to lessen the odor upon emptying; no odor should be detectable when the pouch is on and adequately sealed.

Changes in Diet

Diet does not generally play an important role in ostomy management. Most patients can eat their usual diet, including all the food they ate before surgery if they chew their food well. However, it is wise to remain on a diet low in fiber for the first 6 weeks after surgery to allow the intestine to heal and the swelling to resolve. The usual diet can be resumed after that time.

The effects of various foods on ostomy output are summarized in Table 21–3. Patients with a urostomy may want to avoid foods that cause odor. Patients with colostomies, especially those who irrigate, should avoid foods that cause loose stools. (This problem varies among individuals.) Because they have no control over passage of gas, patients with a fecal ostomy may prefer to reduce their intake of gas-forming foods. Products such as alpha-D-galactosidase may be used to control gas (see Chapter 14). Patients with ileostomies are more prone to intestinal obstruction from high-fiber foods eaten in large quantities or eaten exclusive of other foods (Table 21–4).[4,5] Thoroughly chewing high-fiber foods and eating them in small amounts and with other types of food will help prevent food blockage. The patient should be instructed how to manage a food blockage. Table 21–5 lists signs and symptoms of blockage; Table 21–6 describes its management.

table **21–3** **Effects of Food on Stoma Output**

Foods That Thicken Stool

Applesauce; bananas; bread; buttermilk; cheese; marshmallows; milk; pasta, boiled; peanut butter, creamy; potatoes; pretzels; rice; tapioca; toast; yogurt

Foods That Loosen Stool

Beer and other alcoholic beverages; chocolate; dried or string beans; fried foods; greasy foods; highly spiced foods; leafy green vegetables (lettuce, broccoli, spinach); prune or grape juice; raw fruits (except bananas); raw vegetables, fruit juices, milk

Foods That Cause Stool Odor

Asparagus; beans; cabbage-family vegetables (onions, cabbage, brussels sprouts, broccoli, cauliflower); cheese; eggs; fish; garlic; some spices; turnips

Foods That Cause Urine Odor

Asparagus; seafood; some spices

Foods That Combat Urine Odor

Buttermilk; cranberry juice; yogurt

Foods That Cause Gas

Beans (dried, string, or baked); beer; cabbage-family vegetables (onions, cabbage, brussels sprouts, broccoli, cauliflower); carbonated beverages; corn; cucumbers; dairy products; mushrooms; peas; radishes; spinach; spicy foods

Foods That Color Stool

Beets; berries; chocolate; fats; fish; meat (large amounts of red meat); milk; red gelatin; vegetables

Source: References 4 and 5.

table **21–4** **High-Fiber Foods**[a]

Apple skins	Hot dogs
Apricots	Mushrooms
Asparagus	Nuts
Beans and lentils	Oranges and orange rinds
Bologna	Pineapples
Bran	Popcorn
Celery	Potato peels
Chinese vegetables	Raisins
Coconut	Raw vegetables
Corn	Sausage
Dried figs	Seeds
Grapefruit	Shrimp
Grapes	Tomatoes

[a] To be consumed cautiously by persons with ileostomies.
Source: References 4 and 5.

table

21-5 Signs and Symptoms of Intestinal Obstruction

Partial Obstruction	Complete Obstruction
Cramping abdominal pain	Absence of output (urine and fecal)
Watery output with foul odor	Severe cramping pain
Abdominal distension (possible)	Abdominal distension
Stomal swelling (possible)	Stomal swelling
Nausea and vomiting (possible)	Nausea and vomiting Decreased pulse rate Fever (possible)

Source: Reference 4.

table

21-6 Conservative Management of Food Blockage

1. Sit in warm tub bath to relax abdominal muscles.
2. Massage the peristomal area while in the knee-to-chest position to attempt dislodgement of fibrous mass.
3. If stoma is swollen, remove pouch and replace with a pouch that has a larger stoma opening.
4. If able to tolerate fluids (i.e., not vomiting) and passing stool, increase intake of fluid and electrolytes, but avoid solid foods. Drink one glass of liquid each time pouch is emptied. Juices such as grape juice exert a mild cathartic effect.
5. If vomiting, not passing stool, or both, do not take liquids or solid food orally.
6. Notify a primary care provider or WOC nurse if any of the following develops:
   - Stool output stops (complete blockage).
   - Conservative measures (listed above) fail to resolve symptoms.
   - Signs of partial obstruction persist (Table 21–5).
   - Inability to tolerate fluids or replace fluids and electrolytes develops.
   - Signs and symptoms of fluid and electrolyte imbalance (Table 21–7) develop.

Source: Reference 4.

Complications of Ostomies

Persons with ostomies may experience both psychological and physical complications. The health care provider should be prepared to address these complications or to refer patients to their primary care provider or a WOC nurse. These nurses are often based in hospitals or home health care agencies. The United Ostomy Associations of America is an organization that provides peer support for patients. Before surgery, patients should receive a thorough explanation that describes what procedure will be performed, what to expect during the postsurgical recovery period, and what pouching and supplies will be used. The following information on potential complications can be used to assist patients seeking advice after their surgery.

Psychological Complications

Some patients anticipating ostomy surgery fear that they will not be able to continue their former job, participate in sports, perform sexually, or have children. These patients need reassurance that an ostomy rarely impairs their ability to carry out such activities. Contacting the local United Ostomy Associations of America is of utmost importance in assisting with the rehabilitation of these patients; both providers and patients may contact this organization. Patients may also want to find a local WOC nurse. Patient education and counseling on ostomy care provides information and support before and after ostomy surgery. Literature is available from all of the major ostomy product manufacturers, the United Ostomy Associations of America, and the American College of Surgeons.

Physiologic Complications

The major physiologic consequence of a GI ostomy is fluid and electrolyte imbalance. This is most problematic in patients with a liquid or semisoft stoma discharge, such as ileostomies or ascending and transverse colostomies. Patients with these types of ostomies must maintain adequate fluid intake to compensate for loss of the absorptive function of the colon and loss of ileocecal valve function. Patients with ileostomies lose about 500–1000 mL of fluid daily through the stoma, whereas individuals with a normally functioning colon lose 100–200 mL daily.[3] During illnesses, patients with ileostomies, especially infants, are particularly vulnerable to fluid and electrolyte imbalance caused by vomiting and diarrhea. Caregivers and patients should be counseled regarding common signs and symptoms of imbalance (Table 21–7).[4,5]

Because the GI tract is the site of nutrient absorption, some patients with ostomies may experience deficiencies. For example, iron and vitamins D_2 and D_3 are absorbed in the small intestine; riboflavin is absorbed in the upper GI tract; vitamin B_{12} is absorbed in the terminal ileum; phytonadione is absorbed in the proximal small intestine; menadione is absorbed in the distal small intestine; and calcium, pyridoxine, pantothenic acid, biotin, choline, inositol, carnitine, vitamins C and E, and thiamine (vitamin B_1) are absorbed in various sites within the intestinal tract (specific sites not identified). Vitamin A deficiency may be seen in individuals with disease of the terminal ileum (e.g., Crohn's disease). Hypophosphatemia and hypomagnesemia are present in individuals with calcium deficiency caused by malabsorption. In addition, copper deficiency, which interferes with the absorption of iron, has been reported in individuals who have undergone intestinal bypass surgery. Folic acid absorption requires interaction with enzymes present in the upper part of the jejunum; therefore, most absorption of folic acid takes place in the proximal part of the small intestine.[6–9] The effect of ostomy surgery on absorption of vitamins and minerals has not been well studied; however, patients with ileostomies or colostomies should be monitored for signs and symptoms of deficiencies.

Patients with a urostomy, an ileostomy, or an ascending colostomy must include an adequate amount of fluid in their diets to prevent the precipitation of crystals or kidney stones in the urine. In addition, they may have an increased incidence of gallbladder stone formation. Patients with a urostomy should adjust their diet to produce acidic urine, thereby reducing the risk of infection and crystal formation around the stoma. Cranberry products have been studied in the prevention of recurrent urinary

table

21–7   Signs and Symptoms of Fluid and Electrolyte Imbalance

Adults	Infants
Increased thirst	Depressed fontanel
Dry mouth and mucous membranes	Lethargy
Orthostatic hypotension	Sunken eyes
Decreased urine volume	Weak cry
Increased urine concentration (dark in color)	Decreased frequency of wet diaper
Sunken eyes	Increased urine concentration (dark in color)
Extreme weakness	
Flaccid muscles	
Diminished reflexes	
Muscle cramps (abdominal and leg)	
Lethargy	
Tingling or cramping in feet and hands	
Confusion	
Nausea and vomiting	
Shortness of breath	

Source: References 4 and 5.

tract infections. Evidence does not support the use of cranberry products for the treatment of urinary tract infections.[10-15] (See Chapter 51 for an in-depth discussion of cranberry.)

Systemic Complications

Constipation is caused by the regular use of constipating analgesics or other medications or by a patient's eating habits. Constipation may be a problem in patients with descending and sigmoid colostomies. Treatment depends on the cause and may include dietary changes or medication adjustment. Patients having problems with constipation should be encouraged to avoid the foods listed in Table 21–3 that can thicken the stool.[4,5]

Certain foods can cause diarrhea in ostomy patients (Table 21–3).[4,5] Gut pathology (e.g., ulcerative colitis, Crohn's disease, or *Clostridium difficile* colitis) or obstruction caused by a food bolus can also cause diarrhea. Medications, influenza, and food poisoning are other potential causes. Diarrhea is a special problem in patients with ileostomies and ascending colostomies because they cause impaired fluid and electrolyte reabsorption. Patients with chronically loose stools may want to use an absorptive agent (e.g., Ileosorb or Par-Sorb) designed for use in the pouch. Absorptive agents do not correct the problem; they assist in coping with the problem. Increased fiber (e.g., Metamucil or Citrucel) may be used to help correct diarrhea in patients with a colon. Antidiarrheals may be ordered to slow transit time and decrease output. In addition, an unexpected high or decreased output or no output in a patient with an ileostomy may represent a partial small-bowel obstruction. In this case, the patient needs to seek emergency medical attention.

Intestinal gas may be related to food. Eliminating foods that cause gas from the diet may solve the problem (Table 21–3). Use of simethicone to reduce gas production or pouches with gas filters may be helpful. Odor is not normal except when the pouching system is changed or emptied. Otherwise, odor may be an indication of poor hygiene, leakage, or failure to properly connect the pouch to the skin barrier. The provider should review proper care and connection of the pouching system with patients who are concerned about odor. Oral deodorants that will act in the digestive system to eliminate odors from digested foods are discussed in the section Deodorizers.

Local Complications

The normal stoma is shiny, moist, and either pink or red. The stoma does not contain nerve fibers, so it does not transmit pain or other sensations. In an adult, the stoma size is approximately 1/8–3 inches depending on the portion of the bowel or urinary tract used. The stoma gradually shrinks after surgery and reaches its permanent size within 6 weeks.

Skin irritation around the stoma can result from stoma effluent contacting the skin for a prolonged period of time. Ostomy pouching systems and accessories can also irritate skin because of poor fit or the materials used in their composition. The peristomal skin may look weepy or erythematous and have papules and macules. The Ostomy Skin Tool (OST) is a new standardized peristomal skin assessment tool that was developed by WOC nurses and an ostomy manufacturing company. This tool has three clinical parameters: discoloration, erosion, and tissue overgrowth.[16] The patient may use a skin barrier powder, ostomy cream, or barrier to protect the skin, although a properly fitting pouching system should be the first priority.

Denuded peristomal skin is caused by erosion of the epidermis by digestive enzymes. The eroded or denuded epidermis may bleed, and it is painful when touched and when the pouch is applied. Denuded peristomal skin occurs when an improper pouch is worn, when the pouch opening is too big or too small, or when the pouch has leaked and not been promptly replaced. These problems can allow the output to come in contact with the skin. The output produced by patients with ileostomies is particularly irritating to skin. The patient should be referred to a WOC nurse or primary care provider for treatment. Once the etiology of the denuded skin is determined and corrected, a skin barrier powder may be applied to the peristomal skin before the pouch is applied. A skin barrier powder may be composed of a pectin or karaya powder, which absorbs skin moisture and provides a dry surface. A liquid skin barrier may be used over the powder so the pouching system can adhere. This is called "crusting." The pouch should be changed more often to reduce the risk of further irritation. Treatment should be continued until the skin is intact.

Contact dermatitis is characterized by burning, stinging, itching, and red or denuded skin. This complication usually results from an allergic reaction to the pouching system or an accessory. A patch test will identify the allergen in patients who have a history of allergy, a reaction to adhesive tape, eczema, or psoriasis, as well as in those who have very fair skin. Patients exhibiting sensitivity may need to change products. A fabric pouch cover may be helpful if the allergy is to the pouch itself. Special precautions are necessary in patients with a latex allergy. On request, a manufacturer will provide written information regarding the natural latex rubber content of its products and packaging (see the manufacturer's Web site). In some products, the latex source is a dry, natural latex rubber, which is used to seal blister packs that contain nonlatex products.

Alkaline dermatitis (encrustation) may occur in patients with urinary diversions because of the alkaline nature of the output. The stoma or peristomal skin may feel gritty, like sandpaper. Alkaline dermatitis, which renders the stoma extremely friable, is a common cause of blood in the pouch. A cloth soaked with a solution of one-third white vinegar to two-thirds water should be applied to the involved area for 5 to 10 minutes at least once weekly before the pouching system is put on. Patients who use a two-piece system can apply the solution as often as three to four times daily. The vinegar may cause the stoma to blanch, but blanching is not indicative of damage. The two-piece pouching system allows the wearer to remove the pouch and access the stoma if the stoma is involved in the encrustations.

Treatment for alkaline dermatitis is acidification of the urine. Patients should avoid alkaline ash foods, such as citrus fruits and juices; paradoxically these foods are acidic when consumed but are excreted in alkaline form. Increasing fluid intake to between 2 and 3 quarts daily may reduce alkalinity. Use of a urinary appliance with an antireflux feature is recommended because this feature prevents urine from contacting the skin when the patient is lying down.

Hyperplasia (an overgrowth of skin) occurs when the pouch opening is too large. There is no pain in the early stages, but later the affected skin cells multiply and cause agonizing pain. The condition resembles a mucosal polyp and may also be called *hyperkeratosis* or *pseudoverrucous lesion*. Treatment entails ensuring that the pouch has the correct opening size and that the seal is secure. The seal is achieved with paste, paste strips, or a moldable seal or skin barrier ring that will mold into the irregular surfaces. Other management approaches include cauterization using silver nitrate sticks and/or surgical removal.

Mechanical injury is caused by a poorly fitting appliance or skin barrier, a stoma that is difficult to access, or tight-fitting clothing. A poorly fitting pouching system can be corrected by measuring the stoma before each purchase of supplies, selecting a skin barrier of the proper size, and adjusting the size of the skin barrier opening, if necessary. The opening should be $\frac{1}{16}$–$\frac{1}{8}$ inch larger than the stoma. New "moldable flanges" should fit at the mucocutaneous junction. Patients experiencing mechanical injury should be encouraged to contact a WOC nurse.

Skin stripping refers to inadvertent sloughing or removal of the top layer of skin around the stoma. The skin around the stoma may be irritated from use of a strong adhesive or removal of the skin barrier in a rough manner. The skin barrier should be removed by pushing the skin away from the barrier, not by pulling the barrier away from the skin. Adhesive removers are useful in preventing skin damage if the stoma is new or the peristomal skin is fragile. After use of adhesive removers, the peristomal skin must be cleaned to remove all adhesive remover residue because blistering, irritation, or ineffective adhesion of a new pouching system may occur.

Stenosis of the stoma results from the formation of scar tissue. Excessive scar tissue is usually caused by improper surgical construction, postoperative ischemia, active disease, or alkaline stomatitis or dermatitis. Although dilation of the stoma is often advocated to prevent or palliate this problem, the only cure is revision of the stoma.

Excessive sweating under the pouch can decrease wearing time and cause monilial infection. A skin sealant or cement plus a belt may be necessary to hold the pouching system in place. Purchasing or making a cover or bib to keep the pouch material from touching the skin can alleviate discomfort from perspiration underneath the collection pouch.

Folliculitis, an inflammation of the hair follicles, is characterized by redness at the base of the hair follicles around the stoma. Aggressive removal of any adhesive around the stoma can remove hairs, resulting in irritation and infection. Using an electric razor to shave the areas on which adhesive will be applied may help prevent folliculitis. Because folliculitis is related to an overgrowth of staphylococci on the skin, the use of an antibacterial wash should be considered; in some advanced cases, use of an oral antibiotic may be considered.

Infections are not more frequent in patients with ostomies, with the possible exceptions of patients with Crohn's disease, diabetes, or ruptured diverticulitis, or those undergoing radiation or chemotherapy. In some cases, however, infections under the pouching system can be problematic. Candidal infection may be a problem in patients who wear a pouch continuously. A dark, warm, moist environment promotes the growth of *Candida* species. The primary symptoms are itching and rash. If the infection is allowed to continue unchecked, the skin will become denuded, the pouching system will not stick, and additional skin irritation will result from the output.

If the skin is indurated, swollen, and red, an abscess may be present, which may necessitate incision and draining. Culture and susceptibility testing should be performed, and an appropriate antibiotic should be prescribed for topical use, systemic use, or both. Patients should be encouraged to contact a WOC nurse for assistance. Minor candidal infections may be treated with nystatin powder or 2% miconazole powder. Excessive powder should be brushed off before the pouch is applied. Antifungal preparations are generally used every pouch change for 1 week after the skin has become clear. In treatment of candidal infections, it is important to ascertain whether the patient is taking antibiotics. Any antibiotic, but especially a broad-spectrum agent, changes the flora of the skin, and the entrenched *Candida* can become difficult to eradicate. Therefore, in patients with an ostomy being treated with antibiotics, it is often helpful to continue using nystatin powder or 2% miconazole powder for 1 month after all signs of candidal infection are gone.[17,18]

Peristomal hernia is a protrusion of the colon or ileum through a defect in the fascia in the area around the stoma. It usually occurs if the abdominal wall is weak or the stoma was placed lateral to the rectus muscle. The patient may complain of a bulge when standing or sitting, pain, pouching difficulties, leakage, and peristomal skin irritation. Modification of the pouching system or technique may help to alleviate some of the symptoms of a peristomal hernia. An ostomy support belt or binder may be used to provide comfort and possibly prevent further herniation. The patient should be referred to the WOC nurse for a plan of care. Surgery may be required if the patient has increased pain at the site, has increased herniation, or develops signs of stoma obstruction.

Fistula is the formation of an opening between two internal organs or from inside the body to the skin. Enterocutaneous fistulas can occur in patients with or without an ostomy. This complication is most often a manifestation of Crohn's disease. Other causes include cancer, abscess formation, foreign body retention, radiation, tuberculosis, and trauma. If a fistula has excessive drainage, an ostomy pouching system may be applied to contain the drainage and prevent the skin from becoming denuded.

Prolapse is a telescoping of the bowel through the stoma. This problem results when the opening in the abdominal wall is too large. Women with ileostomies may experience prolapse of the ileostomy during pregnancy. Other causes include inadequate fixation of the bowel to the abdominal wall; poorly developed fascial support; or increased abdominal pressure associated with tumors, coughing, or crying (the latter being of special concern in infants). The danger of prolapse is the resulting decrease in blood supply to the bowel outside the abdominal cavity.

A prolapse may be reduced by having the patient lie on his or her back and apply continuous pressure on the most distal part of the stoma. Once the prolapse is reduced, a rigid pouching system should be avoided because of the risk of strangulation of the stoma. The patient should apply a flexible pouch with a resized opening while lying on his or her back. A support belt may also be used. Surgical correction may be required if the stoma becomes purple or ecchymotic or continues to prolapse.

Retraction, a recession of the stoma to a subnormal length at or below skin level, is caused by several factors. Active Crohn's disease and weight gain may lead to this damage of the skin surface. If the retraction is not severe, use of a convex pouching system and an elastic belt may be adequate. In other cases, surgical correction may be required.

Organic impotence is caused by a radical resection of the rectum or bladder, which results in disruption of nerves and vascular supply. Male patients who are impotent should be referred to a urologist for evaluation and treatment.

Medication Absorption Challenges for Ostomies

An understanding of the absorption characteristics of medications is important to optimize their effectiveness in patients with ostomies. The upper portion of the small intestine is the major absorptive site for many medications. However, certain preparations rely on an intact colon for drug absorption.[18,19] Both prescription and nonprescription medications should be reviewed to assess the best formulation for the patient. Potential drug interactions and side effects should be addressed in the drug therapy plan. Table 21–8 lists some general drug management principles for patients with colostomies, ileostomies, and urostomies.[18,19]

Drug Absorption

Patients with ostomies should be instructed to check the pouch for undissolved tablets or tablet fragments whenever they take solid oral medications. If the absorptive areas of the intestine have been altered, coated or sustained-release preparations may pass through the intestinal tract without being absorbed, potentiating drug failure. In addition, some medications are contained within a wax matrix (e.g., Slow K) from which the active drug leaches as the tablet moves through the GI tract. Table 21–9 lists a broad selection of medications and their potential to cause adverse effects, which vary with different dosage forms.[21–33]

Antibiotics

In general, antibiotics may alter the normal flora of the intestinal tract, causing diarrhea or fungal infection of the skin surrounding the stoma.

table 21–8	General Drug Management Principles
Type of Ostomy	**General Management**
Ileostomy, colostomy	Avoid medications that are sustained release, extended release, or enteric coated or that contain a wax matrix. Liquid, crushed, and chewable preparations are preferred.
Ileostomy, colostomy	Do not crush medications before first consulting an appropriate health care provider.
Ileostomy, colostomy	Check pouch for undissolved tablets.
Ileostomy, colostomy, urostomy	Review medication plans for potential drug interactions and/or adverse effects.
Ileostomy, colostomy, urostomy	Alert patients to medication-induced color changes to urine and/or stool.

Source: References 18 and 19.

Sulfa Drugs

Sulfa drugs should be used with caution, given that crystallization in the kidney may occur more often in patients who have difficulty with fluid balance. To minimize this problem, patients should increase fluid intake.

Diuretics

Diuretics can increase the amount of fluids and electrolytes lost through urostomies and can add to the losses already inherent in patients with ileostomies. Diuretics should be used with caution. Frequent monitoring of fluid balance and serum electrolytes is required.

Laxatives

Because of the risk of electrolyte imbalance and dehydration, ileostomy patients should never use laxatives unless they have been prescribed. Patients with colostomies may use laxatives, but only under close supervision. If the patient is constipated, a prescriber may recommend a stool softener.

Antacids

Products that contain calcium may cause stone formation in patients with a urostomy. Magnesium-based products can cause diarrhea in patients with ileostomies. If patients have problems with constipation, they should avoid aluminum-based antacids, which can also cause constipation.

Urine and Stool Discoloration

Patients with ostomies have to adapt to many challenges in their life. Encouraging them to become involved in their health care and health care plans helps to alleviate much of the fear and

table

21—9   Potential Effects of Selected Prescription Drugs in Patients with Ostomies

Class	Type of Ostomy	Potential Effects
Histamine₁-receptor antagonists	Ileostomy, colostomy, urostomy	No problems have been reported with cetirizine, loratadine, or fexofenadine.
Anti-inflammatories	Ileostomy	NSAIDs are associated with GI irritation and bleeding. Use with caution if history of GI ulceration or bleeding exists (COX-2 inhibitors may have lower risk profile). No problems have been reported with Celecoxib.
Opiates	Colostomy	Tramadol's opiate agonist activity can cause constipation, similar to opiates such as oxycodone. Liquids, IR products, or patches are preferred to avoid erratic absorption associated with ER products.
Selective serotonin reuptake inhibitors	Ileostomy	No problems have been reported with sertraline, citalopram, or fluoxetine. Hyponatremia and diarrhea have been reported with paroxetine, requiring close monitoring of fluid and electrolyte status.
Antipsychotics	Colostomy, ileal conduit	Constipation has been reported with olanzapine and clozapine and can occur with all anticholinergic drugs. Reported delayed lithium toxicity requires close monitoring of serum levels in patients with ileal conduits.
Antidiabetics	Ileostomy	Possible dose-related GI effects are related to variable absorption of metformin, a weak base primarily absorbed in the small intestine. Some patients have experienced increased stoma output, requiring a change in their antidiabetic regimen. No problems have been reported with other antidiabetic agents.
Anticonvulsants	Ileostomy	Erratic absorption has been reported with enteric-coated and SR products. Use of liquids or IR products is generally recommended.
Antilipidemics	Ileostomy, colostomy, urostomy	No problems have been reported with use of HMG-CoA reductase inhibitors.
Cardiac/antihypertensive drugs	Ileostomy	Fluid and electrolyte abnormalities are common with diuretics. Careful monitoring is recommended during use of ACE inhibitors. Hyperkalemia may be a particular problem.
GI medications	Ileostomy, colostomy	Diarrhea is associated with all PPIs, requiring careful monitoring of fluid and electrolyte status. No problems have been reported with H₂RAs. Avoid laxatives in patients with ileostomies owing to risk of severe fluid and electrolyte disturbances.
Antimicrobial agents	Ileostomy, urostomy, colostomy	Altered normal bowel flora and diarrhea related to broad-spectrum antibiotics can be a significant problem for patients with ileostomies. High doses of ciprofloxacin are associated with alkaline urine; if used, urinary acidification to avoid bacterial overgrowth in urostomy patients requires close monitoring.
Other drugs	End jejunostomy, ileostomy	Some reports of drug failure are associated with malabsorption of warfarin in patients with short-bowel syndrome. Length of the functionally intact proximal small bowel is important in cyclosporine dosing; if liquid formulation or IV is required, more frequent monitoring is recommended. Variable volume of distribution and increased clearance of gentamicin have been reported in patients with ileostomies, possibly requiring more frequent monitoring. Highly variable bioavailability of digoxin (depends on length of remaining bowel) requires monitoring for drug failure.

Key: ACE inhibitors = Angiotensin-converting enzyme inhibitors; COX-2 = cyclooxygenase-2; ER = extended release; GI = gastrointestinal; HMG-CoA = hydroxymethyl glutaryl coenzyme A; H₂RAs = histamine type 2 receptor antagonists; IR = immediate release; IV = intravenous; NSAID = nonsteroidal anti-inflammatory drug; PPI = proton pump inhibitor; SR = sustained release.

Source: References 20–33.

anxiety often expressed by these patients. Some medications can cause color changes in the urine and/or feces. These events can be unsettling to an uninformed patient and cause unnecessary anxiety. Table 21–10[34-37] lists common medications that cause color changes. The health care provider should discuss these possible events with their patients.

Dietary Supplements

Herbal products are not regulated by the Food and Drug Administration (FDA) because they are considered dietary supplements. Moreover, not all ingredients contained in a product are listed on the label. Herbal supplements can interact with medications

table
21–10   Selected Drugs That Discolor Feces and Urine

Drugs That Discolor Feces

Black		Blue	Orange-Brown
Acetazolamide	Fluorouracil	Chloramphenicol	Rifabutin
Aluminum hydroxide	Hydralazine	Manganese dioxide	**Pink-Red**
Aminophylline	Iodide-containing drugs	Methylene blue	Anticoagulants[a]
Amphetamine	Iron	**Gray**	Aspirin
Amphotericin B[a]	Levodopa	Colchicine	Barium
Anticoagulants[a]	Melphalan		Cefdinir[b]
Aspirin[a]	Methotrexate	**Green**	Clofazimine
Barium	Nitrates	Indomethacin	Nonsteroidal anti-inflammatory drugs[a]
Bismuth	Nonsteroidal anti-inflammatory drugs[a]	Iron	Tetracycline syrup
Chloramphenicol	Phenylephrine	Medroxyprogesterone	**White or Speckled**
Chlorpropamide	Potassium salts[a]	**Green-Gray**	Aluminum hydroxide
Cholestyramine	Procarbazine	Oral antibiotics	Barium
Corticosteroids	Sulfonamides		Oral antibiotics
Cyclophosphamide	Tetracycline	**Orange-Red**	**Yellow or Yellow-Green**
Cytarabine	Thallium	Phenazopyridine	Senna
Ethacrynic acid	Theophylline	Rifampin	
	Thiotepa[a]	Rifapentine	

Drugs That Discolor Urine

Black	Dark	Purplish Red	Yellow
Ferrous salts	Aminosalicylic acid	Chlorzoxazone	Aloe
Phenacetin	Chloroquine	**Red**	Riboflavin, Tolcapone
Senna	Metronidazole	Carbidopa/levodopa	Sulfasalazine
Blue or Green	Nitrofurantoin	Daunorubicin	Vitamin B_{12}
Amitriptyline	Phenacetin	Dimethylsulfoxide	**Yellow-Brown**
Cimetidine (injection)	Primaquine	Doxorubicin	Cascara
Flutamide	**Orange**	Idarubicin	Nitrofurantoin
Indomethacin	Chlorzoxazone	**Red-Brown**	Primaquine
Magnesium salicylate	Dantrolene	Aloe	Senna
Methocarbamol	Warfarin Entacapone	Levodopa	Sulfonamides
Methylene blue	**Orange-Red**	Phenytoin	**Yellow-Orange**
Mitoxantrone	Phenazopyridine	Quinine	Sulfasalazine
Promethazine (injection)	Rifampin	Warfarin	Vitamin A
Propofol (injection)	**Pink-Red**	**Violet**	**Yellow-Pink**
Triamterene	Phenothiazines	Senna	Cascara
	Phenytoin		Aspirin

[a] Discoloration may be caused by bleeding.
[b] Discoloration caused by nonabsorbable complex between cefdinir or metabolites and iron in the GI tract.
Source: References 34–37.

and cause a variety of adverse effects. Patients with ostomies who desire to use herbal agents should do so only under medical supervision.

Assessment of Patients with Ostomies: A Case-Based Approach

In most cases, ostomy surgery necessitates the use of a pouching system designed to collect the waste material normally eliminated through the bowel or bladder. Because each ostomy patient is different, one patient may benefit from a particular type of pouch or accessory, whereas another may develop problems with the same products. Moreover, a patient's needs may change over time. A pouching system or accessory that previously produced ideal outcomes may no longer be appropriate because of changes in body contour caused by aging, pregnancy, weight change, or concurrent medical conditions. As the rate of obesity continues to rise, so do the challenges for health care providers caring for the special needs of that ostomy population.

Patients who must have an ostomy often are apprehensive about how the surgery will proceed, how to manage the ostomy, and how they will be perceived by others. An ostomy patient's self-esteem may also be affected. Therefore, a special effort should be made to ensure the patient's privacy and to gain the patient's confidence during the assessment. Cases 21–1 and 21–2 illustrate assessment of patients with ostomies.

case
21-1

Relevant Evaluation Criteria	Scenario/Model Outcome
Information Gathering	
1. Gather essential information about the patient's symptoms and medical history, including:	
a. description of symptom(s) (i.e., nature, onset, duration, severity, associated symptoms)	The patient's symptoms began during the summer when she was at the beach and perspired a lot.
b. description of any factors that seem to precipitate, exacerbate, and/or relieve the patient's symptom(s)	She has experienced itching and rash underneath her urostomy for the past week, and now the skin is becoming denuded and weepy. Her pouch has started to leak more often. She usually wears this pouching system for 1 week, but now she can keep it on for only 24 hours.
c. description of the patient's efforts to relieve the symptoms	The patient applied pectin-based powder before appliance changes, but her symptoms have not resolved.
d. patient's identity	Dora Smith
e. age, sex, height, and weight	60 years old, female, 5 ft 6 in., 150 lb
f. patient's occupation	Retired
g. patient's dietary habits	MNT diet for diabetes
h. patient's sleep habits	NA
i. concurrent medical conditions, prescription and nonprescription medications, and dietary supplements	Glucophage 500 mg twice daily, Flovent 220 mg 2 puffs twice daily, albuterol 2 puffs every 6 hours as needed; underwent ileal loop for bladder cancer 2 years earlier
j. allergies	Aspirin
k. history of other adverse reactions to medications	None
l. other (describe) _____	NA
Assessment and Triage	
2. Differentiate patient's signs/symptoms and correctly identify the patient's primary problem(s).	Since the summer, Dora has developed a rash and itching. The rash appears to be caused by infection of denuded skin around the stoma caused by Dora's leaking pouching system and perspiration. Dora's diabetes is another related factor.
3. Identify exclusions for self-treatment.	None
4. Formulate a comprehensive list of therapeutic alternatives for the primary problem to determine if triage to a medical provider is required, and share this information with the patient or caregiver.	Options include:
	(1) Refer Dora to a WOC nurse.
	(2) Recommend application of 2% miconazole powder to affected area with each pouch change.
	(3) If 2% miconazole is not effective, have Dora see her primary care provider for a prescription for nystatin powder to apply to the affected area with each pouch change.
	(4) Take no action.

case

21–1 *continued*

Relevant Evaluation Criteria	Scenario/Model Outcome
Plan	
5. Select an optimal therapeutic alternative to address the patient's problem, taking into account patient preferences.	OTC treatment with a powder containing 2% miconazole is appropriate for Dora. She should also change her pouching system more frequently.
6. Describe the recommended therapeutic approach to the patient or caregiver.	"You can use an OTC powder containing 2% miconazole to treat the rash and itching. You should change your pouching system more often and apply the powder at each change to prevent these symptoms from occurring again."
7. Explain to the patient or caregiver the rationale for selecting the recommended therapeutic approach from the considered therapeutic alternatives.	"Seeing a wound, ostomy, and continence nurse or your primary care provider is very important to treat this situation."
Patient Education	
8. When recommending self-care with nonprescription medications and/or nondrug therapy, convey accurate information to the patient or caregiver.	"Wash peristomal skin per your usual routine. Apply 2% miconazole powder sparingly, and massage it into the peristomal skin. Dust off excess powder. A sealant (3M No Sting Skin Prep, etc.) may be applied to enhance the pouch seal. Apply the pouch. Use the miconazole powder with each pouch change until 1 week after the rash has resolved. You should change the appliance every other day until the rash clears; then you can return to once-a-week appliance changes. If rash and itching continue, consult a WOC nurse or your primary care provider."
Solicit follow-up questions from the patient or caregiver.	"How long should I continue using the 2% miconazole or the nystatin powder?"
Answer the patient's or caregiver's questions.	"Use for 1 week after rash has resolved. You may use it as needed if the rash develops again."
Evaluation of Patient Outcome	
9. Assess patient outcome.	Ask the patient to call and update you within a week. If the itching has not improved, have the patient schedule an appointment with the WOC nurse.

Key: MNT = Medical nutrition therapy; NA = not applicable; OTC = over-the-counter; WOC = wound, ostomy, and continence.

Patient Counseling for Ostomy Care

The pharmaceutical care needs of a patient with an ostomy include procurement and distribution of ostomy supplies and selection of appropriate products. Monitoring a patient's management of the ostomy and counseling the patient on special needs (e.g., skin care, diet, fluid intake, and drug therapy) are other important components of ostomy care for these patients.

Counseling of an ostomy patient should be done in a sensitive and caring manner. An ostomy patient's self-esteem is often damaged; therefore, when assisting a patient with ostomy needs, special care must be taken to avoid verbal or facial expressions that might convey negative feelings regarding the procedure. Peer support can be especially helpful to such patients. Patients should be provided a list of local and national ostomy associations and a list of product manufacturers who can supply information about product use (Table 21–1). Patients can also receive assistance by contacting a WOC nurse in their area (www.wocn.org). The following self-help books should also be recommended to patients with ostomies:

- Barrie B. *Second Act.* New York, NY: Scribner; 1997.
- Benirschke R. *Alive & Kicking.* San Diego, CA: Rolf Benirschke Enterprises; 1999.
- Benirschke R. *Embracing Life.* San Diego, CA: Rolf Benirschke Enterprises; 2009.
- Benirschke R. *Great Comebacks.* San Diego, CA: Rolf Benirschke Enterprises; 2002.
- Elsagher B. *I'd Like to Buy a Bowel Please! Ostomy A to Z.* Andover, MN: Expert Publishing; 2006.
- Elsagher B. *If the Battle Is Over Why Am I Still in Uniform? Humor as a Survival Tactic to Combat Cancer.* Andover, MN: Expert Publishing; 2005.
- Kupfer B, Foley-Bolch K, Kasouf MF, et al. *Yes We Can.* Worchester, MA: Chandler House Press; 2000.
- Ruggieri P. *Colon & Rectal Cancer. A Patient's Guide to Treatment.* Omaha, NE: Addicus Books; 2001.

A patient with an ostomy has to adapt to many challenges in his or her life. Encouraging the patient to become involved in his or her health care and health care plans helps to alleviate much of the fear and anxiety often expressed by ostomy patients. The patient should be encouraged to express problems and concerns so that his or her ability to achieve self-treatment objectives can be better assessed. Health care providers or managers should also consider patients' special needs for conditions unrelated to the ostomy. The box Patient Education for Ostomy Care lists specific information health care providers should give patients with an ostomy.

case
21–2

Relevant Evaluation Criteria	Scenario/Model Outcome

Information Gathering

1. Gather essential information about the patient's symptoms and medical history, including:

a. description of symptom(s) (i.e., nature, onset, duration, severity, associated symptoms)

Patient has developed leakage from his ileostomy pouching system in the past few weeks. He also noticed redness and denuded skin around his ileostomy. Pain at the site is also frustrating the patient.

b. description of any factors that seem to precipitate, exacerbate, and/or relieve the patient's symptom(s)

Since his surgery 1 year ago, the patient has gained 30 pounds. He usually changes his pouch twice a week, but now he has to change it every day and continues to have leakage and redness.

c. description of the patient's efforts to relieve the symptoms

Patient applied skin barrier powder and skin sealant to protect skin, but he continues to have skin irritation and leakage.

d. patient's identity

Kevin Lerner

e. age, sex, height, and weight

31 years old, male, 5 ft 11 in., 175 lb

f. patient's occupation

Graphic designer

g. patient's dietary habits

High-fiber diet with junk food

h. patient's sleep habits

NA

i. concurrent medical conditions, prescription and non-prescription medications, and dietary supplements

Nasonex 2 spray in each nostril once daily or 1 spray in each nostril once daily; Imodium A-D 2 mg taken 30 minutes before each meal or every 6 hours while the stool is liquid or volume is high.

Kevin developed ulcerative colitis 7 years ago. After a major bleeding episode and failure of medical management, he underwent total colectomy and ileostomy.

j. allergies

Latex

k. history of other adverse reactions to medications

None

l. other (describe) _____

Patient has been nervous about family issues and has been constantly eating, which has increased his weight.

Assessment and Triage

2. Differentiate patient's signs/symptoms and correctly identify the patient's primary problem(s).

Leakage, burning sensation, and denuded skin around his ileostomy are caused by abdominal creases from increased weight.

3. Identify exclusions for self-treatment.

None

4. Formulate a comprehensive list of therapeutic alternatives for the primary problem to determine if triage to a medical provider is required, and share this information with the patient or caregiver.

Options include:

(1) Refer Kevin to a WOC nurse for further assessment and treatment.

(2) Recommend use of a skin barrier powder to improve peristomal skin, followed by application of a skin sealant.

(3) Recommend use of a convex pouch and belt for support.

(4) Take no action.

Plan

5. Select an optimal therapeutic alternative to address the patient's problem, taking into account patient preferences.

Assessment of the stoma and skin indicates that a convex pouch with a belt for support is needed. Upon further discussion, Kevin says he prefers a one-piece convex pouch with belt versus a two-piece pouch.

6. Describe the recommended therapeutic approach to the patient or caregiver.

"Because your stoma has retracted to skin level, you will need a convex pouch with a belt for support. Treat skin around the stoma with a skin barrier powder, such as Stomahesive powder, and a skin sealant, such as 3M No Sting Skin Prep, before applying the pouch. Change the pouching system every 2 days until the peristomal skin is free of burning and is no longer denuded; then resume pouch changes twice a week."

"Losing some weight will also decrease the retraction of the stoma."

7. Explain to the patient or caregiver the rationale for selecting the recommended therapeutic approach from the considered therapeutic alternatives.

"Pouch leakage, denuded skin, and pain will decrease with proper follow-up with a WOC nurse to modify your pouching technique.

Refer to the local chapter of the United Ostomy Associations of America for peer support to improve your self-esteem and body image." (See Table 21–1.)

case

21–2 *continued*

Relevant Evaluation Criteria	Scenario/Model Outcome

Patient Education

8. When recommending self-care with nonprescription medications and/or nondrug therapy, convey accurate information to the patient or caregiver:

a. appropriate dose and frequency of administration	See Figure 21–2 for proper assessment of convexity, and Figure 21–3 and Table 21–2 for proper pouching and skin accessories.
b. maximum number of days the therapy should be employed	"Change pouch twice a week."
c. product administration procedures	"Wash peristomal skin as usual. Apply thin layer of powder. Massage powder into skin well and dust off excess powder. Apply skin sealant before applying the pouch."
d. expected time to onset of relief	"With proper convexity and powder application, leakage and excoriation should decrease within 24 hours. You will notice a decrease in the burning sensation."
e. degree of relief that can be reasonably expected	"You should notice a decreased intensity of symptoms within 24–48 hours."
f. most common side effects	"Some ostomates have had an allergic reaction to the powder or pouch adhesive."
g. side effects that warrant medical intervention should they occur	"Consult a WOC nurse if burning, stinging, or local irritation occurs."
h. patient options in the event that condition worsens or persists	"Consult a WOC nurse or your primary care provider if leakage or burning continues after 1 week of treatment."
i. product storage requirements	"Store pouch away from heat."
j. specific nondrug measures	"Change pouch every 2 days until peristomal skin is clear."
Solicit follow-up questions from the patient or caregiver.	"What happens if I can't lose weight, I develop more creases, and my stoma retracts more?"
Answer the patient's or caregiver's questions.	"Consult a WOC nurse; you may need another type of pouching system. In addition, obesity is now epidemic; consult a nutritionist for a proper diet program."

Evaluation of Patient Outcome

9. Assess patient outcome.	Ask the patient to call you at the next pouch change to ensure that no further leakage has occurred and that the skin has improved. If the leakage continues, have the patient call the WOC nurse.

Key: NA = Not applicable; WOC = wound, ostomy, and continence.

Key Points for Ostomy Care

➤ Patients with ostomies may experience both psychological and physical complications after ostomy surgery. Their issues should be addressed, and they should be referred to their primary care provider, WOC nurse, and/or United Ostomy Associations of America.

➤ The objectives of self-care of an ostomy are to understand how the stoma functions, to effectively manage it, to understand the proper use of the pouching system and accessories, to avoid complications that result from improper use, and to reduce the risks of other complications.

➤ Patients should be advised about the effects of food on stomal output and the need to monitor for signs and symptoms of dehydration.

➤ The selection of an appropriate pouching system depends on the patient's body contour, manual dexterity, and type of ostomy.

➤ The ideal ostomy pouching system should be leak-proof, odor-proof, comfortable, and easy to use. Providers can assist the patient in achieving these outcomes.

➤ Patients should be counseled on the effects of medications:
  – Use of liquid, crushed, or chewable medications is preferable.
  – Coated or sustained-release medications should be used with caution because if the GI tract has been shortened, full absorption may not occur. Most tablets should not be crushed or chewed.
  – Caution is warranted with use of antibiotics and diuretics. Antibiotics can cause diarrhea or fungal infections of the skin around the stoma. Diuretics can cause dehydration or electrolyte imbalance in patients with ileostomies.
  – Laxatives, antidiarrheals, or other medications that alter GI motility should be used with caution. Laxatives can increase fecal output in patients with ileostomies, whereas antidiarrheals decrease the fecal output.

The objectives of self-care of ostomies are to (1) understand how the stoma functions and how to manage it; (2) understand the proper use of the pouching system and accessories, and avoid complications that result from improper use; and (3) reduce the risk of other types of complications. For most patients, carefully following the product instructions and the self-care measures listed here will help to ensure optimal therapeutic outcomes.

Pouching System Selection and Use

- Use only the type of pouching system recommended for your type of ostomy.
- If your system no longer fits well, consult your WOC nurse or primary care provider before changing to a different type of pouching system.
- Do not consider skin irritation to be inevitable; identify the cause and correct and treat the irritation as soon as it occurs.
- If possible, identify the cause for leakage around the pouching system and correct the problem immediately. Consult your WOC nurse or primary care provider if you cannot determine the cause.
- Establish a routine for ostomy care. Keep the routine simple; use as few accessories as possible.

Effects of Medication Use

- Sustained- or extended-release medicines may undergo erratic absorption, which makes their effect unpredictable. These medications should be used with caution. Coated medications, as well as sustained- or extended-release medications, should not be crushed or chewed.
- Use caution when taking antibiotics and diuretics. Antibiotics can cause diarrhea or fungal infections of the skin around the stoma. Diuretics can cause dehydration or electrolyte imbalance in individuals with ileostomies.

- Use caution when taking laxatives, antidiarrheals, or other medications that alter gastrointestinal motility. Laxatives can increase fecal output in individuals with ileostomies, whereas antidiarrheals decrease the fecal output.
- Know which medications will discolor the urine or feces (Table 21–10).

When to Seek Medical Attention

- Consult your WOC nurse or primary care provider about using nonprescription medications to treat diarrhea or constipation. Return for reevaluation of the problem after 1 week of treatment.
- See your WOC nurse if you experience any of the following complications:
  - Depression and anxiety
  - Sexual dysfunction
  - Abdominal pain
  - Narrowing of the stoma
  - A bulge near the stoma
  - An extension of the bowel through the stoma
  - Recession of the stoma to a subnormal length
  - Bleeding from or around the stoma
  - Pain when touching the skin around the stoma or when applying the appliance
  - Overgrowth of the skin around the stoma

Key: WOC = Wound, ostomy, and continence.

REFERENCES

1. Increasing Awareness of and Recognizing the Life-Saving Role of Ostomy Care and Prosthetics in the Daily Lives of Hundreds of Thousands of People in the United States. Senate Resolution 95. 112th Congress (2011–2012). March 8, 2011. Accessed at http://thomas.loc.gov/cgi-bin/bdquery/D?d112:95:./list/bss/d112SE.lst::, July 25, 2011.

2. Wise B, McKenna C, Gavin G, et al. *APSNA Nursing Care of the General Pediatric Surgical Patient.* Gaithersburg, MD: Aspen Publishers; 2000.

3. Wound Ostomy and Continence Nurses Society. *WOCN Best Practice for Clinicians Series: Management of the Patient with a Fecal Ostomy.* Mount Laurel, NJ: Wound Ostomy and Continence Nurses Society; 2010.

4. Colwell JC, Goldberg MT, Carmel JE. *Fecal & Urinary Diversions Management Principles.* St. Louis, MO: Mosby, Inc.; 2004.

5. Krenta KS. *Living with Confidence after Ileostomy Surgery.* Princeton, NJ: ConvaTec, a Bristol Myers Squibb Co.; 2003.

6. Hillman RS. Hematopoietic agents: growth factors, minerals, and vitamins. In: Hardman JG, Limbird LE, eds. *Goodman and Gilman's The Pharmacological Basis of Therapeutics.* 10th ed. New York, NY: McGraw-Hill, Inc.; 2001:1487–517.

7. Marcus R. Agents affecting calcification and bone turnover: calcium, phosphate, parathyroid hormone, vitamin D, calcitonin, and other compounds. In: Hardman JG, Limbird LE, eds. *Goodman and Gilman's The Pharmacological Basis of Therapeutics.* 10th ed. New York, NY: McGraw-Hill, Inc.; 2001:1715–43.

8. Marcus R, Coulston AM. Water-soluble vitamins: the vitamin B complex and ascorbic acid. In: Hardman JG, Limbird LE, eds. *Goodman and Gilman's The Pharmacological Basis of Therapeutics.* 10th ed. New York, NY: McGraw-Hill, Inc.; 2001:1753–71.

9. Marcus R, Coulston AM. Fat-soluble vitamins: vitamins A, K, and E. In: Hardman JG, Limbird LE, eds. *Goodman and Gilman's The Pharmacological Basis of Therapeutics.* 10th ed. New York, NY: McGraw-Hill, Inc.; 2001: 1773–91.

10. Wang CH, Fang CC, Chen NC, et al. Cranberry-containing products for prevention of urinary tract infections in susceptible populations: A systemic review and meta-analysis of randomized controlled trials. *Arch Intern Med.* 2012;172(13):988–96.

11. Wang P. The effectiveness of cranberry products to reduce urinary tract infections in females: a literature review. *Urol Nurs.* 2013;33(1):38–45.

12. Bailey DT, Dalton C, Daugherty J, Tempesta MS. Can a concentrated cranberry extract prevent recurrent urinary tract infections in women? A pilot study. *Phytomedicine.* 2007;14(4):237–41.

13. Jepson RG, Williams G, Craig JC. Cranberries for preventing urinary tract infections. *Cochrane Database Syst Rev.* 2012;10:CD001321. doi: 10.1002/14651858.CD001321.pub5. Accessed at http://www.thecochranelibrary.com/view/0/index.html.

14. Wing DA, Rumney PJ, Preslicka CW, et al. Daily cranberry juice for the prevention of asymptomatic bacteriuria in pregnancy: a randomized, controlled pilot study. *J Urol.* 2008;180(3):1367–72.

15. McMurdo ME, Argo I, Phillips G, et al. Cranberry or trimethoprim for the prevention of recurrent urinary tract infections? A randomized controlled trial in older women. *J Antimicrob Chemother.* 2009;63(2):389–95.

16. Haugen V, Ratliff C. Tools for assessing peristomal skin complications. *J Wound Ostomy Continence Nurs.* 2013;40(2):131–4.

17. Aly R, Forney R, Bayes C. Treatment for common superficial fungal infections. *Dermatol Nurs.* 2001;13(2):91–9.

18. Erwin-Toth P. Caring for a stoma. *Nursing. 2001.* 2001;31(5):36–40.

19. Ward N. The impact of intestinal failure on oral drug absorption: a review. *J Gastrointest Surg.* 2010;14(6):1045–51.

20. Severijnen R, Bayat N, Bakker H, et al. Enteral drug absorption in patients with short small bowel. *Clin Pharmacokinet.* 2004;43(14):951–62.

21. McEvoy GK, ed. *AHFS Drug Information 2009.* Bethesda, MD: American Society of Health-System Pharmacists; 2009.

22. Tewari A, Ward RG, Sells RA, et al. Reduced bioavailability of cyclosporine A capsules in a renal transplant patient with partial gastrectomy and ileal resection. *Ann Clin Biochem.* 1993;30(pt 6):587–9.

23. Gaskin TL, Duffull SB. Enhanced gentamicin clearance associated with ileostomy fluid loss. *Aust N Z J Med.* 1997;27(2):196–7.

24. Ritchie HA, Duggull SB. Another case of high gentamicin clearance and volume of distribution in a patient with high output ileostomy. *Aust N Z J Med*. 1998;28(6):212–3.

25. Al-Habet S, Kinsella HC, Rogers HJ, et al. Malabsorption of prednisolone from enteric-coated tablets after ileostomy. *BMJ*. 1980;281(6244):843–4.

26. Owens JP, Mirtallo JM, Murphy CC. Oral anticoagulation in patients with short-bowel syndrome. *DICP*. 1990;24(6):585–9.

27. Lutomski DM, LaFrance RJ, Bower RH, et al. Warfarin absorption after massive small bowel resection. *Am J Gastroenterol*. 1985;80(2):99–102.

28. Chen JP. Ileostomy and ramipril-induced acute renal failure and shock. *Heart Lung*. 2007;36(4):298–9.

29. Brophy DF, Ford SL, Crouch MA. Warfarin resistance in a patient with short bowel syndrome. *Pharmacotherapy*. 1998;18(3):1375–6.

30. Roberts R, Sketris IS, Abraham I, et al. Cyclosporine absorption in two patients with short-bowel syndrome. *DICP*. 1988;22(7–8):570–2.

31. Lavi E, Rivkin L, Carmon M, et al. Clozapine-induced colonic obstruction requiring surgical treatment. *IMAJ*. 2009;11(6):385–6.

32. Knoben JE, Anderson PO. *Handbook of Clinical Drug Data*. 7th ed. Hamilton, IL: Drug Intelligence Publications; 1998.

33. Alhasso A, Bryden AA, Neilson D. Lithium toxicity after urinary diversion with ileal conduit. *BMJ*. 2000;320(7241):1037.

34. Allen J, Burson SC. Drug discoloration of the urine. Document 150907. *Pharm Lett*. 1999;15(9):150907.

35. *Physicians' Desk Reference Electronic Library*. Montvale, NJ: Medical Economics; 2003.

36. Fecal discoloration induced by drugs, chemicals, and disease states. Drug Consults. Micromedex 2.0. Englewood, CO: Thomson Reuters; April 14, 2010.

37. Urine discoloration—drug and disease induced. Drug Consults. Micromedex 2.0. Englewood, CO: Thomson Reuters; November 20, 2007.

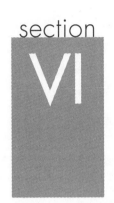
NUTRITION AND NUTRITIONAL SUPPLEMENTATION

ESSENTIAL AND CONDITIONALLY ESSENTIAL NUTRIENTS

Mary M. Bridgeman and Carol J. Rollins

Vitamin and mineral supplements represent one of the largest and most widely used over-the-counter product categories in the United States today. Vitamin- and mineral-containing supplements in combination with multivitamin and multimineral products accounted for 42% of all dietary supplement sales in the United States in 2011, with annual sales of $12.4 billion.[1] Thirty-three percent of the U.S. population uses a multivitamin-multimineral supplement on a routine basis, with use increasing over the past 25 years.[2,3] Although nutrition experts agree that foods are the preferred source of vitamins and minerals and that most individuals can easily meet their daily requirements by eating a balanced diet, experts agree less about the extent to which the U.S. population consumes such a diet. The lack of overt symptoms of nutritional deficiency in this country supports the position that most Americans receive adequate intake of vitamins and minerals from dietary sources; however, concern is growing that subclinical deficiencies may be contributing to chronic diseases. This concern emphasizes the importance of encouraging the selection of nutrient-dense foods throughout the life cycle.

Health-conscious consumers often seek nutritional supplements as a means of prevention and self-treatment for a myriad of actual or perceived health ailments. Marketing claims and natural product enthusiasts encourage these self-care behaviors by promoting use of nutrient supplementation, often in doses well above established tolerable upper limits.[4] However, the issue of who will benefit from or be harmed by the use of nutritional supplements is unresolved. Regular use of supplements can help some people meet their recommended dietary requirements; however, a potential risk exists that some users will exceed the tolerable upper intake levels of some nutrients.[4] Currently, little to no available evidence supports the use of supplements for cancer prevention. In fact, evidence suggests the potential for increased cancer risk with certain nutrients at higher doses when used for prolonged periods of time.[5] The United States Preventive Services Task Force (USPSTF) evaluated randomized trials of vitamin supplementation with beta-carotene, vitamins A, C, and E, folic acid, or antioxidants in the prevention of cancer or cardiovascular disease.[6] The evidence was conflicting and insufficient to support regular supplementation for this purpose, and potential harm was associated with beta-carotene supplementation in certain populations. Current American Cancer Society Guidelines indicate that

dietary supplementation is not associated with a reduction in cancer risk and instead recommend eating whole foods as part of an overall healthy diet.[7] Results from the Women's Health Initiative support the USPSTF and American Cancer Society's positions, having found no benefit of multivitamin supplementation for either postmenopausal women in terms of reduction of cardiovascular disease or cancer risk or overall mortality.[8] Further, the National Institutes of Health–sponsored State-of-the-Science Conference concluded that insufficient evidence exists to support routine use of multivitamin and multimineral supplements for primary prevention of chronic diseases.[9]

Beyond their risk of toxicity, one of the greatest dangers of food fads, use of multiple supplements, and large doses of single vitamins is that some people use them in place of sound medical care. The lure of marketing or the desire to self-treat may attract desperate or uninformed patients who have serious illnesses, thereby placing them at greater risk because they delay seeking appropriate medical attention. Furthermore, drug–nutrient interactions can be significant, yet they are often overlooked as part of the patient's medical history. For these reasons, practitioners should be well aware of the potential use—as well as the benefits and risks—of various nutrient supplements.

Epidemiology/Etiology of Nutritional Deficiencies

Although overt nutrient deficiency is rare in the United States, the prevalence of subclinical nutrient deficiencies is unknown. Specific patient populations may be at higher risk of deficient nutrient intakes because of pathophysiologic, physiologic, behavioral, or economic situations (Table 22–1).[10]

Because foods contain numerous other compounds that are important for health maintenance and disease prevention, health care professionals play an important role in educating patients on nutrient-dense food choices before vitamin and/or mineral supplementation is recommended.

Pathophysiology of Nutritional Deficiencies

A comprehensive discussion of the pathophysiology of vitamin and mineral deficiencies is outside the scope of this chapter. The reader is referred to standard medical and nutrition textbooks for such information.

Editor's Note: This chapter is based on the 17th edition chapter of the same title, written by Yvonne Huckleberry and Carol J. Rollins.

table

22–1 Factors Contributing to Nutritional Deficiency

- Inadequate dietary intake resulting from substance abuse, poverty, eating disorders, dementia, or restrictive diets
- Poor dentition, swallowing difficulty, or xerostomia
- Loss of taste, smell, or sight perception
- Decreased absorption resulting from cystic fibrosis, short bowel syndrome, Roux-en-Y gastric bypass, gastric hypochlorhydria, or chronic diarrhea
- Inability to buy or prepare meals because of tremor, fatigue, or arthritic pain
- Anorexia caused by reduced physical activity, social isolation, pain, disease, or depression
- Lack of knowledge about balanced nutrition
- Increased metabolic requirements resulting from severe injury, infection, trauma, pregnancy, or prolonged physical exercise
- Medications affecting judgment, coordination, memory, appetite, nutrient absorption, gastric pH, or gastrointestinal tract function

Clinical Presentation of Nutritional Deficiencies

A vitamin deficiency may evolve in several stages, and clinical signs may not be present until prolonged and significant deficiency occurs (Table 22–2).[10] Attributing clinical symptoms to a single nutrient deficiency is difficult, as symptoms may overlap and reflect multiple rather than individual nutrient deficiencies. Signs and symptoms of specific vitamin and mineral deficiencies are discussed in the individual micronutrient sections later in the chapter.

Globally speaking, poor nutrition increases the risks of chronic disease, infection, and complications associated with reproduction, acute illness, surgery, and chemotherapy. For the pediatric population, growth, development, and learning may be compromised. For adults, poor nutrition over a lifetime can exacerbate the aging process, causing earlier morbidity and mortality. Balanced nutrition (with varied food choices providing adequate protein, appropriate calories, vitamins, and minerals) is essential for health through all stages of the life cycle.

Nutrient Supplementation

Vitamin and mineral supplements should be used as *adjuncts* to a balanced diet and not as substitutes for nutritious food. Although nutritional supplements can be obtained without a prescription and are typically self-prescribed, they are complex

table

22–2 Stages in Evolution of Vitamin Deficiency

1. Inadequate nutrient delivery, synthesis, or absorption
2. Depletion of nutrient stores
3. Biochemical changes
4. Physical manifestations of deficiency
5. Morbidity and mortality

agents with specific indications. Medical assessment should precede their use, especially if daily intakes exceed the dietary reference intakes (DRIs) for a specific nutrient. Furthermore, patients should be reminded that vitamins and minerals are often better absorbed from food sources than from supplements. Practitioners may refer patients to a registered dietitian for personalized counseling on diet modification as well as nutritional supplementation.

Intent of Use

Nutritional supplement use is intended to prevent nutritional deficiencies, replenish compromised nutrient stores, or maintain the present nutritional status. Nonprescription nutritional supplements are not intended for the self-treatment of vitamin deficiencies.

General Approach to Use

If a patient's diet is not providing the daily required amount of micronutrients necessary for normal growth and function, supplementation with vitamins and minerals may be appropriate, provided the patient has no underlying pathology or contraindication to use. A once-daily multivitamin with minerals providing no more than 100% of the DRIs should suffice in most cases. Patients should be reminded that healthy individuals derive no established benefit from supplementing nutrients in doses above the DRI; also, tolerable upper limits for daily use should not be exceeded without medical supervision.

Practitioners should counsel patients regarding the potential disparity between a product's actual contents and its label. The potential for labeling inaccuracy exists because, despite U.S. regulations requiring that the actual content of a vitamin or mineral supplement be greater than or equal to the product's labeling (to account for shelf-life losses and differences between manufacturer product batches), dietary supplements are not assessed for compliance or standardization by any government agency.[11] Unlike prescription drugs, dietary supplements do not require proof of safety or efficacy before being marketed, and inspection for production under good manufacturing practices has not been required since passage of the Dietary Supplement Health and Education Act (DSHEA) in 1994. However, the United States Pharmacopeia (USP) provides a Dietary Supplement Verification Program that allows product labeling with the USP mark if the tested product meets specific requirements, including verification of the product's ingredients and amounts; effective disintegration and dissolution for absorption; absence of harmful contaminants; and safe, sanitary, well-controlled manufacturing.[12] Practitioners should advise patients to look for the USP mark on vitamin and mineral supplement labels.

Some patients require supplemental macronutrients (e.g., fat, protein, and carbohydrates) in addition to micronutrients because they are unable to consume all required daily nutrients. Liquid nutritional supplements for that purpose (e.g., Ensure and Boost) are discussed in Chapter 23.

Nonpharmacologic Therapy

The best method for avoiding nutritional deficiencies is to consume a balanced diet each day that includes foods from sources high in several essential nutrients. To guide consumers in selecting a balanced diet while allowing for individual preferences,

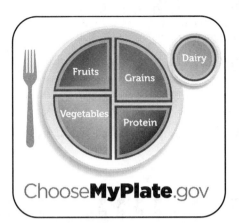

figure

22–1   *MyPlate.* (*Source:* Image from www.choose myplate.gov.)

the U.S. Department of Health and Human Services released the reference Dietary Guidelines for Americans, 2010.[13] In these guidelines, consumers are advised to regularly choose a variety of nutrient-dense foods in moderate portion sizes, as exemplified in the *MyPlate* figure (Figure 22–1). Each food group represented on *MyPlate* provides a significant source of essential nutrients. For example, the dairy group is a major source of calcium, whereas the fruit and vegetable groups are sources of fiber and the primary sources of antioxidant vitamins. By selecting a variety of foods within the various groups and eating the appropriate number of servings from each food group daily, consumers can "balance" their diet relative to essential and conditionally essential nutrients. *MyPlate* is an evidence-based tool that is both user friendly and comprehensive for assessing the need for nutrient supplementation. When performing a nutritional assessment and determining the need for multivitamin supplementation, practitioners should inquire about the patient's intake from these food groups.[13]

Pharmacologic Therapy

Although situations exist in which high doses of specific vitamins and minerals are reported to be of therapeutic benefit, megavitamin enthusiasts' claims have not been confirmed objectively. To the contrary, as noted earlier, some clinical trials have suggested potential harm from supplementation originally claimed to be beneficial. These are described within the individual micronutrient sections.

Vitamins and minerals that have therapeutic value in the treatment of medical conditions (e.g., niacin therapy for hyperlipidemia) are being used as drugs rather than as supplements for disease prevention or health maintenance. Deficiency states should be treated under medical supervision. Furthermore, prolonged ingestion of megadoses of vitamin and mineral supplements has not been evaluated in large-scale clinical trials for safety and efficacy in many cases. Some vitamins (e.g., A, D, niacin, and pyridoxine) and minerals (e.g., iron and fluoride) are known to be toxic in high doses. Therefore, patients should be cautioned against initiating high-dose self-medication with vitamins and minerals. Practitioners should discourage chronic, high-dose ingestion of any nutrient without proper medical supervision.

Vitamins

Vitamins are nutrients that cannot be synthesized in the body in sufficient quantities and must be obtained through the diet. Conditionally essential vitamins have adequate endogenous production in most circumstances, but there are conditions (e.g., cardiovascular disease) in which dietary intake is essential to meet requirements. Vitamins are used as both dietary supplements and therapeutic agents to treat deficiencies or other pathologic conditions.

DRIs have replaced the traditional recommended dietary allowances (RDAs) as reference values of daily nutrient intake recommended by the Food and Nutrition Board of the Institute of Medicine of the National Academies (Tables 22–3 and 22–4).[14,15] The DRIs include four reference categories: estimated average requirements (EARs), RDAs, adequate intakes (AIs), and tolerable upper intake levels (ULs). EARs are values obtained after a careful review of the literature on specific nutrients. The EARs provide nutrient intake values that are estimated to meet the requirements of half of the healthy individuals in a specific gender and age group. The RDA is defined as the amount of a nutrient needed per day for maintenance of good health. This value is set at 2 standard deviations above the EAR as an estimate of daily nutrient intake sufficient to meet the requirements of nearly all (97%–98%) healthy individuals of a specified age group and gender. AIs are used as recommended intakes for nutrients for which inadequate scientific data exist to establish an EAR with confidence. Finally, the ULs are the highest dose of nutrient intake that may be consumed daily without risk of adverse effects in the general population. ULs are based on current literature, but they are not available for all nutrients (Table 22–5).[14,15] DRIs should be used as guidelines for nutritional assessment in healthy individuals; adjustment according to strenuous physical activity or the presence of disease may be necessary. As nutritional supplements, vitamins are usually dosed at 50%–150% of the DRI values. Practitioners should advise caution with high-dose supplements that provide greater than 200% of the DRI. As therapeutic agents, vitamins should be recommended only for specific evidence-based medical indications.

The Food and Drug Administration (FDA) has published a less comprehensive set of values to be used for food and dietary supplement labeling.[16] Nutrients are listed as a percentage of daily value (%DV). These values are based on the recommended intakes for a 2000-calorie diet for adults older than 18 years. The vitamin or mineral supplement label includes a box with the heading Supplement Facts. In addition to information on serving size and servings per container, the label lists all required nutrients that are present in the dietary supplement in significant amounts and the %DV, if a reference has been established. It also lists all other dietary ingredients that are present in the product (including botanicals and amino acids) for which no %DV has been established. The %DV is based on DRI values for adults and for children ages 4 years and older, unless the product is designed for children younger than 4 years or for women who are pregnant or lactating.

Frequently, "natural" vitamin products are supplemented with synthetic vitamins. For example because the amount of vitamin C that can be acquired from rose hips (the fleshy fruit of a rose) is relatively small, synthetic vitamin C is added to prevent too large a tablet size. However, this addition may not be noted on the label, and the price of the partially natural product is often considerably higher than that for the completely synthetic—but equally effective—product. Patients should be

table
22–3

Dietary Reference Intakes (DRIs): Recommended Dietary Allowances and Adequate Intakes, Vitamins Food and Nutrition Board, Institute of Medicine, National Academies

Life Stage Group	Vitamin A (µg/day)a	Vitamin C (mg/day)	Vitamin D (IU/day)b,c	Vitamin E (mg/day)d	Vitamin K (µg/day)	Thiamin (mg/day)	Riboflavin (mg/day)	Niacin (mg/day)e	Vitamin B6 (mg/day)	Folate (µg/day)f	Vitamin B12 (µg/day)	Pantothenic Acid (mg/day)	Biotin (µg/day)	Choline (mg/day)g
Infants														
0–6 mo	400*	40*	400	4*	2.0*	0.2*	0.3*	2*	0.1*	65*	0.4*	1.7*	5*	125*
6–12 mo	500*	50*	400	5*	2.5*	0.3*	0.4*	4*	0.3*	80*	0.5*	1.8*	6*	150*
Children														
1–3 y	300	15	600	6	30*	0.5	0.5	6	0.5	150	0.9	2*	8*	200*
4–8 y	400	25	600	7	55*	0.6	0.6	8	0.6	200	1.2	3*	12*	250*
Males														
9–13 y	600	45	600	11	60*	0.9	0.9	12	1.0	300	1.8	4*	20*	375*
14–18 y	900	75	600	15	75*	1.2	1.3	16	1.3	400	2.4	5*	25*	550*
19–30 y	900	90	600	15	120*	1.2	1.3	16	1.3	400	2.4	5*	30*	550*
31–50 y	900	90	600	15	120*	1.2	1.3	16	1.3	400	2.4	5*	30*	550*
51–70 y	900	90	600	15	120*	1.2	1.3	16	1.7	400	2.4h	5*	30*	550*
>70 y	900	90	800	15	120*	1.2	1.3	16	1.7	400	2.4h	5*	30*	550*
Females														
9–13 y	600	45	600	11	60*	0.9	0.9	12	1.0	300	1.8	4*	20*	375*
14–18 y	700	65	600	15	75*	1.0	1.0	14	1.2	400i	2.4	5*	25*	400*
19–30 y	700	75	600	15	90*	1.1	1.1	14	1.3	400i	2.4	5*	30*	425*
31–50 y	700	75	600	15	90*	1.1	1.1	14	1.3	400i	2.4	5*	30*	425*
51–70 y	700	75	600	15	90*	1.1	1.1	14	1.5	400	2.4h	5*	30*	425*
>70 y	700	75	800	15	90*	1.1	1.1	14	1.5	400	2.4h	5*	30*	425*

Life Stage Group													
Pregnancy													
14–18 y	750	80	600	15	75*	1.4	1.4	18	1.9	600i	2.6	6*	30*	450*
19–30 y	770	85	600	15	90*	1.4	1.4	18	1.9	600i	2.6	6*	30*	450*
31–50 y	770	85	600	15	90*	1.4	1.4	18	1.9	600i	2.6	6*	30*	450*
Lactation													
14–18 y	1200	115	600	19	75*	1.4	1.6	17	2.0	500	2.8	7*	35*	550*
19–30 y	1300	120	600	19	90*	1.4	1.6	17	2.0	500	2.8	7*	35*	550*
31–50 y	1300	120	600	19	90*	1.4	1.6	17	2.0	500	2.8	7*	35*	550*

Note: This table (taken from the DRI reports; see www.nap.edu) presents recommended dietary allowances (RDAs) in **bold type** and adequate intakes (AIs) in regular type followed by a *single asterisk* (*). Both RDAs and AIs may be used as goals for individual intake. RDAs are set to meet the needs of almost all (97%–98%) individuals in a group. For healthy breast-fed infants, AI is the mean intake. AI for other life stage and gender groups is believed to cover the needs of all individuals in the group, but lack of data or uncertainty in the data prevents being able to specify with confidence the percentage of individuals covered by this intake.

a As retinol activity equivalents (RAEs). 1 RAE = retinol 1 mcg, beta-carotene 12 mcg, alpha-carotene 24 mcg, or beta-cryptoxanthin 24 mcg. To calculate RAEs from retinol equivalents (REs) of provitamin A carotenoids in foods, divide REs by 2. For preformed vitamin A in foods or supplements and for provitamin A carotenoids in supplements, 1 RE = 1 RAE.

b Cholecalciferol 1 mcg = vitamin D 40 IU.

c In the absence of adequate exposure to sunlight.

d As alpha-tocopherol. Alpha-tocopherol includes *RRR*-alpha-tocopherol, the only form of alpha-tocopherol that occurs naturally in foods, and the *2R*-stereoisomeric forms of alpha-tocopherol (*RRR*-, *RSR*-, *RSR*-, *RRS*-, and *RSS*-alpha-tocopherol) that occur in fortified foods and supplements. It does not include the *2S*-stereoisomeric forms of alpha-tocopherol (*SRR*-, *SSR*-, *SRS*-, and *SSS*-alpha-tocopherol), also found in fortified foods and supplements.

e As niacin equivalents (NE). Niacin 1 mg = tryptophan 60 mg; 0–6 months = preformed niacin (not NE).

f As dietary folate equivalents (DFE). 1 DFE = food folate 1 mcg = folic acid 0.6 mcg from fortified food or as a supplement consumed with food = supplement 0.5 mcg taken on an empty stomach.

g Although AIs have been set for choline, insufficient data exist to assess whether a dietary supply of choline is needed at all stages of the life cycle; the choline requirement may be met by endogenous synthesis at some of these stages.

h Because 10%–30% of people of advanced age may malabsorb food-bound B₁₂, those older than 50 years should meet their RDA mainly by consuming foods fortified with B₁₂ or a supplement containing B₁₂.

i In view of evidence linking folate intake with neural tube defects in the fetus, all women capable of becoming pregnant should consume folate 400 mcg from supplements or fortified foods, in addition to intake of food folate from a varied diet.

j RDA assumes that women will continue consuming folic acid 400 mcg from supplements or fortified food until their pregnancy is confirmed and they enter prenatal care, which ordinarily occurs after the end of the periconceptional period, the critical time for formation of the neural tube.

Source: Reprinted with permission from reference 14.

table 22–4 Dietary Reference Intakes (DRIs): Recommended Dietary Allowances and Adequate Intakes, Elements Food and Nutrition Board, Institute of Medicine, National Academies

Life Stage Group	Calcium (mg/day)	Chromium (µg/day)	Copper (µg/day)	Fluoride (mg/day)	Iodine (µg/day)	Iron (mg/day)	Magnesium (mg/day)	Manganese (mg/day)	Molybdenum (µg/day)	Phosphorus (mg/day)	Selenium (µg/day)	Zinc (mg/day)
Infants												
0–6 mo	200*	0.2*	200*	0.01*	110*	0.27*	30*	0.003*	2*	100*	15*	2*
6–12 mo	260*	5.5*	220*	0.5*	130*	11	75*	0.6*	3*	275*	20*	3
Children												
1–3 y	700	11*	340	0.7*	90	7	80	1.2*	17	460	20	3
4–8 y	1000	15*	440	1*	90	10	130	1.5*	22	500	30	5
Males												
9–13 y	1300	25*	700	2*	120	8	240	1.9*	34	1250	40	8
14–18 y	1300	35*	890	3*	150	11	410	2.2*	43	1250	55	11
19–30 y	1000	35*	900	4*	150	8	400	2.3*	45	700	55	11
31–50 y	1000	35*	900	4*	150	8	420	2.3*	45	700	55	11
51–70 y	1000	30*	900	4*	150	8	420	2.3*	45	700	55	11
>70 y	1200	30*	900	4*	150	8	420	2.3*	45	700	55	11
Females												
9–13 y	1300	21*	700	2*	120	8	240	1.6*	34	1250	40	8
14–18 y	1300	24*	890	3*	150	15	360	1.6*	43	1250	55	9
19–30 y	1000	25*	900	3*	150	18	310	1.8*	45	700	55	8
31–50 y	1000	25*	900	3*	150	18	320	1.8*	45	700	55	8
51–70 y	1200	20*	900	3*	150	8	320	1.8*	45	700	55	8
>70 y	1200	20*	900	3*	150	8	320	1.8*	45	700	55	8
Pregnancy												
14–18 y	1300*	29*	1000	3*	220	27	400	2.0*	50	1250	60	12
19–30 y	1000*	30*	1000	3*	220	27	350	2.0*	50	700	60	11
31–50 y	1000*	30*	1000	3*	220	27	360	2.0*	50	700	60	11
Lactation												
14–18 y	1300*	44*	1300	3*	290	10	360	2.6*	50	1250	70	13
19–30 y	1000*	45*	1300	3*	290	9	310	2.6*	50	700	70	12
31–50 y	1000*	45*	1300	3*	290	9	320	2.6*	50	700	70	12

Note: This table presents recommended dietary allowances (RDAs) in **bold type** and adequate intakes (AIs) in regular type followed by a *single* asterisk (*). Both RDAs and AIs may be used as goals for individual intake. RDAs are set to meet the needs of almost all (97%–98%) individuals in a group. For healthy breast-fed infants, AI is the mean intake. AI for other life stage and gender groups is believed to cover the needs of all individuals in the group, but lack of data or uncertainty in the data prevents the ability to specify with confidence the percentage of individuals covered by this intake.

Source: Reprinted with permission from reference 14.

table 22–5 Adult Tolerable Upper Intake Levels of Selected Micronutrients

Nutrient	Tolerable UL (mg/day)
Vitamin A	3
Vitamin D	0.1 (4000 IU/day)
Vitamin E	1000
Vitamin C	2000
Folate	1
Niacin	35
Vitamin B$_6$	100
Choline	3500
Calcium	3000 mg/day (9–18 years of age) 2500 mg/day (19–50 years of age) 2000 mg/day (>50 years of age)
Iron	45
Magnesium	350
Phosphorus	4000 (9–70 years of age) 3000 (>70 years of age)
Copper	10
Fluoride	10
Iodine	1.1
Manganese	11
Molybdenum	2
Selenium	0.4
Zinc	40

Source: Reference 14.

informed that the body cannot distinguish between a vitamin molecule derived from a synthetic source and one derived from a natural source, and that most synthetic vitamins are equal to the more expensive "natural" vitamins.

Vitamins are grouped into two broad classifications: fat-soluble and water-soluble. Vitamins A, D, E, and K are fat-soluble vitamins. They are soluble in lipids and are usually absorbed into the lymphatic system of the small intestine before passing into general circulation. Their absorption is facilitated by bile. These vitamins are stored in body tissues, so ingestion of excessive quantities may be toxic. Deficiencies occur when fat intake is limited or fat absorption is compromised. Disease states that may cause malabsorption of fat-soluble vitamins include celiac disease, cystic fibrosis, obstructive jaundice, hepatic cirrhosis, and short-bowel syndrome. These deficiencies may also be precipitated by drugs that affect lipid absorption, such as cholestyramine, which binds bile acids, thereby hindering lipid emulsification; orlistat, which inhibits gastric and pancreatic lipases in the intestinal lumen; and mineral oil, which is an unabsorbed oil that increases fecal loss of fat-soluble vitamins. A daily multivitamin supplement is recommended by the manufacturer for those taking orlistat; refer to Chapter 26 for a more comprehensive discussion on the use of orlistat for weight loss.

Vitamin C and the B-complex vitamins (riboflavin, thiamin, B$_6$, B$_{12}$, niacin, pantothenic acid, biotin, and folic acid) are water-soluble vitamins. These vitamins are generally not stored in the body, and excessive quantities tend to be excreted in the urine. Therefore, daily intake of these vitamins is desirable for optimal health.

Vitamin A

The designation *vitamin A* refers to a large group of compounds that includes the retinoids (e.g., retinol) and the carotenoids (e.g., alpha-carotene and beta-carotene). Biochemical changes occur in some of these compounds during absorption in the intestine to form active vitamin A. Other compounds (e.g., the carotenoids, lutein, and lycopene) are not converted to active vitamin A but have other health-promoting properties. These compounds can be found in dark green vegetables and red, orange, or deep yellow vegetables and fruits.

In healthy adults, more than 90% of the body's supply of vitamin A is stored in the liver. Because of this generous reserve, the risk of deficiency during short-term periods of inadequate intake or fat malabsorption is minimal. Infants and young children, however, are more susceptible to vitamin A deficiency because they have not established the necessary reserves.

Function. Vitamin A is essential for normal growth and reproduction, normal skeletal and tooth development, and proper functioning of most organs of the body (notably, the specialized functions of the eye involving the conjunctiva, retina, and cornea). Vitamin A is thus indicated in preventing and treating symptoms of vitamin A deficiency, such as xerophthalmia (dry eye) and nyctalopia (night blindness). Synthesis of the glycoproteins necessary to maintain normal epithelial cell mucous secretions also requires vitamin A. This mucosal barrier is vital to the body's defense against bacterial infections in the upper respiratory system.

Dietary Sources. See Table 22–6.[13,17]

Deficiency. Vitamin A deficiency is rare in well-nourished populations. However, approximately 500,000 children worldwide develop blindness each year because of vitamin A deficiency.[18] Conditions such as celiac or Crohn's disease, pancreatic disorders, cancer, tuberculosis, pneumonia, and prostate disease, as well as therapy with corticosteroids, may cause excessive excretion of vitamin A. Fat malabsorption may impair vitamin A absorption. Neomycin, cholestyramine, or orlistat may cause significant malabsorption of vitamin A as well as other fat-soluble vitamins; long-term use may precipitate fat-soluble vitamin deficiencies. In the United States, vitamin A deficiency occurs more often from diseases of fat malabsorption than from malnutrition.

One of the earliest symptoms of vitamin A deficiency is night blindness.[18] Other characteristic clinical findings include follicular hyperkeratosis, loss of appetite, impaired taste and smell, and impaired equilibrium. Some of these findings may be masked by concurrent deficiencies of other nutrients. The drying and hyperkeratinization of the skin caused by the disruption of vitamin A–dependent epithelial integrity predisposes patients to infections.

Dose/DRI. Vitamin A is indicated for use in the treatment and prevention of vitamin A deficiency.[19] To avoid toxicity, the patient's dietary intake of vitamin A should be estimated when determining a dose for supplementation.

The DRI values for vitamin A are measured in micrograms of retinol activity equivalents (RAEs). The Food and Nutrition

table
22–6 Food Sources Rich in Selected Nutrients

Vitamin	Food Sources
Vitamin A	Liver, milk fat, egg yolk, yellow and dark green leafy vegetables, apricots, cantaloupe, peaches, carrots
Vitamin D	Vitamin D–supplemented milk, egg yolk, liver, salmon, tuna, sardines, milk fat
Vitamin E	Wheat germ, vegetable oils, margarine, green leafy vegetables, milk fat, egg yolks, nuts
Vitamin K	Liver, vegetable oil, spinach, kale, cabbage, cauliflower
Vitamin C	Green and red peppers, broccoli, spinach, tomatoes, potatoes, strawberries, citrus fruit, kiwi
Vitamin B_{12}	Liver, meat, poultry, oysters, clams, dairy products
Folate	Liver, lean beef, wheat, whole-grain cereals, eggs, fish, dry beans, lentils, green leafy vegetables
Niacin	Lean meats, fish, liver, poultry, many grains, eggs, peanuts, milk, legumes
Pantothenic acid	Eggs, kidney, liver, salmon, yeast, some present in all foods
Vitamin B_6	Meats, cereals, lentils, legumes, nuts, egg yolk, milk
Riboflavin	Meats, poultry, fish, dairy products, green leafy vegetables, enriched cereals and breads, eggs
Thiamin	Legumes, whole-grain and enriched cereals and breads, wheat germ, pork, beef
Biotin	Liver, egg yolk, mushrooms, peanuts, milk, most vegetables, bananas, yeast
L-Carnitine	Dairy products, meat
Choline	Egg yolk, cereal, fish, meats
Calcium	Dairy products, sardines, clams, oysters, turnip greens, mustard greens
Iron	Liver, meat, egg yolk, legumes, whole or enriched grains, dark green vegetables, shrimp
Magnesium	Whole-grain cereals, tofu, nuts, legumes, green vegetables
Phosphorus	Milk, meat, poultry, fish, seeds, nuts, egg yolk
Chromium	Liver, fish, clams, meats, whole-grain cereals, milk, corn oil
Cobalt	Organ meats, oysters, clams, poultry, milk, cream, cheese
Copper	Liver, shellfish, whole grains, cherries, legumes, poultry, oysters, chocolate
Manganese	Vegetables, fruits, nuts, legumes, whole-grain cereals
Molybdenum	Legumes, cereals, dark green leafy vegetables, organ meats, milk
Selenium	Meat, grains, onions, milk
Silicon	Cereal products, root vegetables
Vanadium	Shellfish, mushrooms, parsley, dill seed, black pepper
Zinc	Oysters, shellfish, liver, beef, lamb, pork, legumes, milk, wheat bran

Source: References 13 and 17.

Board recommends RAEs as a way to determine the amount of absorption of carotenoids, as well as their degree of conversion to vitamin A in the body. These RAEs are listed in Table 22–7. RAEs replace the former designation of retinol equivalents (REs) used to calculate total vitamin A values from various dietary sources.

The DRI values for vitamin A are listed in Table 22–3. The UL of 3 mg vitamin A daily in adults has been established on the basis of congenital birth defect risks and liver abnormalities associated with vitamin A toxicity.[14] Evidence suggests that high-dose vitamin A intake, even if below the established UL, may be associated with an increased risk of bone fractures.[20]

Clearly, if the practitioner determines that vitamin A supplementation is appropriate, a nonprescription multivitamin containing no more than the DRI value of vitamin A should be recommended. Preferably, a significant percentage of total vitamin A content should be contributed by beta-carotene because beta-carotene intake is not associated with the risk of fractures

or vitamin A toxicity. Beta-carotene's improved safety profile may be related to limitations in absorption and conversion to retinol.[20] However, the increased cancer risk associated with beta-carotene supplementation in those who smoke should be kept in mind (see Safety Considerations, below). High-dose vitamin A or beta-carotene therapy should never be undertaken without close medical supervision.

Safety Considerations. Because vitamin A is stored in the body, high doses of it can lead to a toxic syndrome known as hypervitaminosis A. The incidence of hypervitaminosis A is increasing because of publicity regarding the potential therapeutic benefits of vitamin A in cancer, skin disorders, and wound healing. Long-term administration of vitamin A is unlikely to cause toxicity when administered at doses less than 10,000 IU per day of retinol or equivalents; however, the risk for toxicity may increase in individuals with chronic renal or liver disease, and in those with low body weight, protein malnutrition,

table	
22–7	**Retinol Activity Equivalents**

1 retinol activity equivalent	= 1 retinol equivalent
	= 1 mcg retinol
	= 12 mcg beta-carotene
	= 24 mcg alpha-carotene
	= 24 mcg beta-cryptoxanthin
	= 3.33 IU vitamin A activity from retinol
	= 10 IU vitamin A activity from beta-carotene

alcohol consumption, or vitamin C deficiency.[19] Headache is a predominant symptom, but it may be accompanied by diplopia (double vision), nausea, vomiting, vertigo, fatigue, or drowsiness. Treatment consists of discontinuing vitamin A supplementation, which should result in complete recovery. Although beta-carotene toxicity is not likely, eating large amounts of carrots in the daily diet may result in carotenemia, which can produce a yellow skin hue. Pregnant women or women of childbearing age should avoid vitamin A doses above the DRI because of the teratogenic risk. For this reason, women of childbearing age should carefully evaluate the total vitamin A content of all dietary supplements and fortified foods consumed regularly. These patients should be reminded not to take other dietary supplements when a prescription prenatal vitamin is dispensed.

The potential role of vitamin A as a cancer-preventing antioxidant prompted large randomized controlled trials evaluating supplementation for patients at risk of lung cancer. In the Alpha-Tocopherol, Beta Carotene (ATBC) Cancer Prevention Study, more than 29,000 male smokers were randomized to receive 50 mg alpha-tocopherol, 20 mg beta-carotene, both supplements, or placebo. After 8 years of study, findings suggested no benefit to supplementation.[21] Furthermore, those who received beta-carotene supplementation appeared to be at greater risk of lung cancer.

Similar results were shown in a subsequent study, the Beta-Carotene and Retinol Efficacy Trial (CARET).[22] This study included more than 18,000 participants randomized to receive either 30 mg beta-carotene and 25,000 IU retinyl palmitate or placebo. Enrollees were either smokers, previous smokers, or those exposed to asbestos. After an average of 4 years of participant enrollment, the CARET trial was prematurely ended because of the association of higher rates of lung cancer, cardiovascular disease, and death in those receiving supplementation. Furthermore, these effects were observed for years after the exposure to supplementation, although the increased risks of disease were not statistically significant. Such trials confirm that vitamin supplementation cannot provide the same health benefits as a diet rich in fruits and vegetables.

Potential Drug–Nutrient Interactions. See Table 22–8.

Vitamin D (Calciferol)

A number of chemical compounds are associated with vitamin D activity. Cholecalciferol (vitamin D₃) is the naturally occurring form of vitamin D that is synthesized in the skin from endogenous or dietary cholesterol on exposure to ultraviolet radiation (sunlight). Ergocalciferol (vitamin D₂), which is used as a food additive, differs only slightly in structure from cholecalciferol.

Metabolic activation of vitamin D requires hydroxylation by both the liver and the kidneys. The metabolite, 25-hydroxycholecalciferol (calcidiol), is formed by the liver and then hydroxylated by the kidneys to its active form, 1,25-dihydroxycholecalciferol (calcitriol). Therefore, either renal or hepatic dysfunction may result in clinical manifestations of vitamin D deficiency, including hypocalcemia unresponsive to over-the-counter vitamin D supplementation. These patients require a hydroxylated vitamin D preparation available only by prescription.

Function. Vitamin D, which has properties of both a hormone and a vitamin, is necessary for the proper formation of bone and for mineral homeostasis. It is closely involved with the activity of parathyroid hormone, phosphate, and calcitonin in maintaining homeostasis of serum calcium levels. Adequate vitamin D intake and supplementation used in conjunction with sufficient calcium, not vitamin D alone, may reduce the risk of bone fractures and falls in postmenopausal women with osteoporosis when dosed according to clinical evidence.[23,24] Other non-skeletal effects (e.g., reduced overall mortality and risk of diabetes, cancer, multiple sclerosis, and risk of allergies and asthma) have been evaluated in controlled clinical trials with varying results.[25] Recent clinical data suggest that vitamin D deficiency may be associated with increased risk of cardiovascular diseases, including hypertension, coronary artery disease, and cardiomyopathy.[26] Vitamin D supplementation may be associated with reduced mortality in heart failure patients, although much of this literature is derived from retrospective database review rather than prospective clinical investigation.[27] Regarding cancer risks, practitioners should advise individuals to avoid excess supplementation because some people may show greater risk of breast, esophageal, prostate, and pancreatic cancers.[25,28] Additional controlled trials are needed to confirm the health benefits, risks, and role of vitamin D supplementation for specific patient populations. Further, as data on vitamin D supplementation and the role of serum level monitoring continue to evolve, dosing recommendations for prescription-only vitamin D formulations that are based on serum monitoring may be considerably higher.

Dietary Sources. Milk and milk products are the major sources of preformed vitamin D in the United States, given that milk is routinely supplemented with 100 IU (2.5 mcg) of vitamin D per cup. Other sources of vitamin D are listed in Table 22–6.

Deficiency. Vitamin D deficiency may result from inadequate intake; gastrointestinal (GI) diseases (e.g., hepatobiliary disease, malabsorption, or chronic pancreatitis); chronic renal failure; inadequate sunlight exposure or dark skin pigment; hereditary disorders of vitamin D metabolism; obesity or gastric bypass therapy; or long-term therapy with antiepileptic medications (e.g., phenytoin, carbamazepine, and primidone). Older patients' aging skin may not synthesize vitamin D efficiently, and the converting process that takes place in the liver and kidneys may also be compromised. The altered physiologic actions—in addition to older patients' reduced sun exposure, absorption, and dietary intake of vitamin D—leave the elderly at increased risk of vitamin D deficiency.

The signs and symptoms of vitamin D deficiency are reflected as calcium abnormalities, specifically those involved with bone formation. Vitamin D deficiency has also been associated with muscle weakness, an increased risk of falls, and an increased risk of cardiovascular disease and certain cancers.[28]

table
22–8 Micronutrient–Drug and Micronutrient–Micronutrient Interactions

Micronutrient	Drug/Micronutrient	Effect	Precautionary Measures
Vitamins			
Vitamins A, E (large doses)	Warfarin	Increased anticoagulation and risk of bleeding	Take only recommended U.S. DRIs.
Vitamins A, E, D, K, C	Cholestyramine, colestipol, orlistat, or mineral oil	Decreased vitamin absorption	Avoid prolonged use of cholestyramine, colestipol, orlistat, or mineral oil.
Vitamin D	Phenytoin, carbamazepine, barbiturates	Increased metabolism of vitamin D	Ensure adequate dietary intake of vitamin D.
	Corticosteroids	May impair metabolism of vitamin D	Ensure adequate dietary intake of vitamin D.
Vitamin K	Broad-spectrum antibiotics (long-term therapy)	Vitamin K deficiency induced by decreased gut flora	Ensure adequate dietary intake of vitamin K.
	Warfarin	Decreased anticoagulation	Keep daily intake of vitamin K consistent.
	Vitamin E (large doses)	Antagonizes function of vitamin K	Avoid chronic supplementation with high-dose vitamin E.
	Vitamin A (large doses)	May interfere with vitamin K absorption	Avoid chronic supplementation with high-dose vitamin A.
Vitamin B_{12}	Metformin, colchicine, anticonvulsants, ascorbic acid supplements, gastric acid lowering agents, tetracyclines, and long-term use of antibiotics	Potential decreased absorption of cyanocobalamin	Clinical significance is unknown.
Folic acid	Phenytoin and possibly other related anticonvulsants (chronic use)	Possible inhibition of folic acid absorption, leading to megaloblastic anemia; subsequent increased folic acid supplementation may decrease serum phenytoin levels and complicate seizure control	Monitor for megaloblastic anemia. Consult with neurologist regarding supplementation, if possible.
	Trimethoprim	Weak folic acid antagonism; decreased activity/effectiveness; rare occurrence of megaloblastic anemia in patients with low folic acid level at onset of trimethoprim therapy	Monitor for megaloblastic anemia.
	Pyrimethamine (large doses)	Possible megaloblastic anemia	Monitor for megaloblastic anemia.
	Methotrexate	Folic acid antagonism; decreased activity/effectiveness	Monitor use of folic acid in patients on maintenance regimens for psoriasis or rheumatoid arthritis.
	Sulfasalazine	Decreased folic acid absorption when these agents are administered together	Separate dosing of these agents.
Niacin	Oral hypoglycemic agents; Sulfinpyrazone and probenecid	Decreased hypoglycemic effects; possible inhibited uricosuric effects	Monitor blood glucose with regular finger sticks.
Vitamin B_6	Isoniazid	Pyridoxine antagonism, manifested as perioral numbness resulting from peripheral neuropathy	Routinely take 50 mg/day of pyridoxine hydrochloride with isoniazid, or 10 mg of pyridoxine for each 100 mg of isoniazid.
	Phenobarbital and phenytoin	Decreased serum drug levels	Consider monitoring levels in patients taking high-dose pyridoxine.
	Levodopa	Levodopa antagonism; decreased effectiveness	Avoid supplemental pyridoxine or, if possible, substitute levodopa-carbidopa for levodopa.

table

22–8 Micronutrient–Drug and Micronutrient–Micronutrient Interactions *(continued)*

Micronutrient	Drug/Micronutrient	Effect	Precautionary Measures
Minerals			
Calcium	Iron, zinc, magnesium	Inhibited nutrient absorption caused by high calcium intake	Separate dosing by at least 2 hours.
	Corticosteroids	Inhibited calcium absorption from gut; increased bone fractures and osteoporosis	Consider calcium supplementation.
	Aluminum-containing antacids, phosphates, cholestyramine	Decreased calcium absorption	Separate dosing by at least 2 hours.
	H_2-blockers, proton pump inhibitors	Decreased absorption of calcium carbonate, which requires an acidic environment	Consider calcium citrate supplementation.
	Levothyroxine	Reduced drug absorption	Separate dosing by 4 hours.
	Tetracyclines, fluoroquinolones	Decreased antibiotic absorption	Separate dosing by 2 hours before or 6 hours after the antibiotic.
	Phenytoin, carbamazepine, phenobarbital	Decreased calcium absorption by increasing metabolism of vitamin D	Consider calcium and vitamin D supplementation.
Magnesium	Tetracyclines, fluoroquinolones	Decreased antibiotic absorption	Separate dosing by 2 hours before or 6 hours after the antibiotic.
	Levothyroxine	Reduced drug absorption	Separate dosing by 4 hours.
Phosphorus	Sucralfate or antacids containing magnesium, calcium, or aluminum	Decreased absorption of phosphorus	Ensure adequate intake of dietary phosphorus.
Iron	Antacids	Decreased iron solubility and absorption	Separate dosing by at least 2 hours.
	Tetracyclines, fluoroquinolones	Decreased antibiotic and iron absorption	If concurrent administration is medically necessary, take tetracycline or fluoroquinolone 2 hours before or 6 hours after taking iron.
	Levothyroxine	Decreased drug absorption	Separate dosing by 4 hours.
Trace Elements			
Copper	Zinc, high-dose vitamin C	Copper antagonism	Micronutrients may compete for absorption and utilization; ensure supplements are administered in balanced doses, or monitor for signs of deficiency.
Fluoride	Magnesium, aluminum, calcium	Decreased effect and absorption of fluoride	Separate supplementation by at least 2 hours.
Iodine (potassium iodide)	Lithium salts	Possible additive hypothyroid effects	Monitor thyroid function tests.
Zinc	Copper	Possible decreased copper levels	High-dose, prolonged zinc supplementation may require copper supplementation.
	Tetracyclines, fluoroquinolones	Possible decreased antibiotic absorption	Separate dosing by 2 hours before or 6 hours after the antibiotic.

Key: DRI = Dietary reference intake.

The classic vitamin D deficiency state is rickets; osteoporosis with increased risk of fractures also occurs. Vitamin D increases calcium and phosphate absorption from the small intestine, mobilizes calcium from bone, permits normal bone mineralization, improves renal reabsorption of calcium, and maintains serum calcium and phosphorus levels. As serum calcium levels fall, compensatory mechanisms (e.g., increased secretion of parathyroid hormone) become activated in an attempt to restore serum calcium homeostasis. Long-term increases in parathyroid hormone secretion ultimately lead to secondary hyperparathyroidism. If physiologic mechanisms fail to make the appropriate adjustments in calcium and phosphorus levels, demineralization of bone ensues to maintain essential plasma calcium levels. During growth, demineralization leads to a failure of bone matrix mineralization, widening of the epiphyseal plate from weight load on softened bone structures, and deformed joints. In adults, such demineralization may lead to severe osteomalacia.

The incidence of rickets in the United States is low but not absent. Rickets is most likely to occur in children who abstain from milk and in infants breast-fed by mothers who receive an inadequate intake of vitamin D.

Dose/DRI. Most people obtain the AI for vitamin D from dietary sources and from exposure to sunlight (Table 22–3). People regularly exposed to sunlight will generally have no dietary requirement for vitamin D. However, substantial segments of the U.S. population receive limited sunlight exposure, especially during the winter months. Regular use of sunscreen is broadly encouraged to prevent skin cancer, but that protection limits vitamin D synthesis in the skin and warrants careful consideration of vitamin D intake from dietary sources.

Vitamin D is FDA approved for the treatment of hypocalcemia and hypophosphatemia associated with hypoparathyroidism. Prescription vitamin D analogues (e.g., calcitriol) are FDA-approved for the treatment of secondary hyperparathyroidism in patients with chronic renal failure.[19]

If the practitioner determines that vitamin D supplementation is appropriate on the basis of poor dietary intake or inadequate exposure to sunlight, a multivitamin supplement containing cholecalciferol (vitamin D$_3$) 15–20 mcg (600–800 IU) taken daily should be recommended. Some evidence suggests that vitamin D intake of up to 25 mcg (1000 IU) daily may have health benefits. The current UL for vitamin D is 100 mcg (4000 IU) daily, although this value may be increased in the future. Data gathered from the recent upswing in use of prescription-only high-dose (50,000 IU weekly) vitamin D supplements suggests such doses are safe and necessary to achieve adequate serum concentrations.

Safety Considerations. Taking more than the UL of vitamin D daily may lead to adverse effects, including anorexia, hypercalcemia, soft tissue calcification, kidney stones, renal failure, and increased risk of certain types of cancer.[15] Patients receiving doses above the UL (e.g., doses used for treatment of rickets or based on low serum concentrations) should be under medical supervision and closely monitored for these adverse effects.

Potential Drug–Nutrient Interactions. See Table 22–8.

Vitamin E (Tocopherol)

The term *vitamin E* refers to the tocopherols and the tocotrienols, which are compounds naturally occurring in plants.

Function. Vitamin E functions primarily as an antioxidant, protecting cellular membranes from oxidative damage or destruction. This process may be aided by selenium and vitamin C. Vitamin E may also have a role in heme biosynthesis, steroid metabolism, and collagen formation.

Vitamin E supplements, often combined with other antioxidants, have been promoted for treatment of numerous diseases (e.g., atherosclerosis, diabetes, cancer, Parkinson's disease, and Alzheimer's disease). These recommendations are often based on observational studies in which regular intake of fruits and vegetables rich in antioxidants have shown beneficial effects in health maintenance and prevention of disease. However, clinical trials have suggested a lack of benefit with vitamin E supplementation in reducing risks of cardiovascular events or mortality, stroke, cancer prevention, diabetes, or Alzheimer's disease.[29–31] On the contrary, antioxidant supplementation that includes vitamin E may be associated with an increased risk of congestive heart failure in certain populations, increased risk of hemorrhagic stroke in adults, and an increased risk of fetal loss when given to prevent preeclampsia.[31–33]

Practitioners should keep in mind that vitamin supplementation is not necessarily benign and has not shown benefit over a well-balanced diet, especially when taken in excess of the DRI.

Dietary Sources. See Table 22–6.

Deficiency. Vitamin E deficiency is extremely rare but may occur in two groups: premature infants with very low birth weight and patients who do not absorb fat normally. For example, neurologic abnormalities responsive to supplemental vitamin E have been reported in some patients with biliary disease and cystic fibrosis. Vitamin E deficiency has also been associated with symptoms of peripheral neuropathy, intermittent claudication, muscle weakness, and hemolytic anemia.

Dose/DRI. The recommended dietary allowance for vitamin E is reported as milligrams of alpha-tocopherol. However, most food and nutrient supplement labels list vitamin E content in international units. Note that 1 mg of alpha-tocopherol vitamin E is equivalent to 1.49 IU.

The average diet contains approximately 3–15 mg/day of vitamin E; therefore, large doses in excess of the DRI are not necessary unless the patient is experiencing fat malabsorption. The FDA-approved use of vitamin E is for prevention and treatment of hemolytic anemia associated with deficiency.[19]

Vitamin E requirements may vary in proportion to the amount of polyunsaturated fatty acids in the diet. The polyunsaturated fatty acid content of the U.S. diet has increased, and the plant oils responsible for the increase are rich in tocopherol. The lack of evidence of deficiency at the present intake supports the current adult RDA of 15 mg/day. The UL for vitamin E is 1000 mg daily.

Safety Considerations. Potential risks associated with vitamin E supplementation are described in the preceding section.

Potential Drug–Nutrient Interactions. Vitamin E has been reported to enhance warfarin anticoagulation, possibly by inducing vitamin K deficiency.[19] This and other potential drug–nutrient interactions are listed in Table 22–8.

Vitamin K

Phytonadione (vitamin K$_1$) is present in many vegetables. Menaquinone (vitamin K$_2$) is a product of colonic bacterial metabolism. Menadione (vitamin K_3) is a synthetic compound that is 2–3 times as potent as the natural vitamin K.

Function. Vitamin K has important roles in normal physiology. First, it promotes the synthesis of clotting factors II, VII, IX, and X in the liver. Second, it activates these factors, along with the anticoagulation proteins C and S. The clotting factors remain inactive in the liver in the presence of warfarin or in the absence of vitamin K. When vitamin K is administered, normal activity of the clotting factors resumes. Third, vitamin K is key in the activation of osteocalcin, which appears to play a role in bone mineralization and the prevention of osteoporosis.[34]

Dietary Sources. See Table 22–6.

Deficiency. The DRI value for vitamin K is 90–120 mcg/day for adults, depending on age and sex.[14] The microbiologic flora of the normal gut synthesizes enough menaquinone to supply a significant part of the body's requirement for vitamin K. Therefore, the incidence of deficiency among healthy, well-nourished individuals is low. Interference with bile production or secretion may contribute to vitamin K deficiency because vitamin K absorption in the small intestine requires bile. Malabsorption syndromes and bowel resections may decrease vitamin K absorption. Liver disease may also cause symptoms of vitamin K deficiency if hepatic production of the prothrombin clotting factor is decreased. Other potential causes of deficiency include intestinal disease or resection and chronic, broad-spectrum antibiotic therapy. A deficiency may be evidenced by unusual bleeding and demonstrated by a prolonged prothrombin time (PT). Lower dietary intake of vitamin K compared to higher intake may also be associated with increased risk of osteoporotic fractures. However, well-designed trials are needed to confirm this association.[34]

Dose/DRI. The DRI values for vitamin K are listed in Table 22–3. Vitamin K_1 (phytonadione) is FDA-approved for use in neonates at birth (1 dose of 1 mg) to prevent hemorrhage. This dose is necessary because placental transport of vitamin K is low, and the neonate has yet to acquire the intestinal microflora that produce the vitamin. Other approved uses include the prevention and treatment of hypoprothrombinemia caused by drug-induced deficiency and the treatment of hemorrhage.[19] A UL for vitamin K has not been established.

Safety Considerations. Even in large amounts over an extended period, vitamin K does not produce toxic manifestations.

Potential Drug–Nutrient Interactions. Consistent dietary intake of vitamin K (70–140 mcg/day) does not usually interfere with warfarin anticoagulant activity. However, sudden changes in the dietary or supplemental intake of vitamin K can significantly alter the patient's PT and international normalized ratio (INR). Other potential drug interactions with this vitamin are listed in Table 22–8.

Vitamin C (Ascorbic Acid)

Vitamin C is the most easily destroyed of all the vitamins because of its sensitivity to heat, oxygen, and alkaline environments. Although it is a relatively simple compound, vitamin C is a powerful antioxidant that serves to protect the capillary basement membrane.

Function. Vitamin C is necessary for the biosynthesis of hydroxyproline, a precursor of collagen, osteoid, and dentin. It also assists in the absorption of nonheme iron from food by reducing the ferric iron in the stomach to ferrous iron. However, use of vitamin C supplementation with iron is generally not necessary for patients with normal gastric acidity who are taking adequate iron supplementation.

Large doses of vitamin C (500–1000 mg/day) have been promoted to prevent and treat the common cold. However, such claims are largely unsupported by well-designed controlled clinical studies.[18,35] Consumption of 5 servings or more of fruits and vegetables daily ($\geq$200 mg vitamin C) has been associated with a lower incidence of cancer, heart disease, stroke, and certain eye diseases.[36] However, currently available data supporting vitamin C supplementation above the DRI for the prevention or treatment of these chronic conditions are inadequate.[35]

Dietary Sources. Vitamin C has been called the "fresh food" vitamin, and most of the daily intake is derived from vegetables and fruit sources (Table 22–6).

Deficiency. Characteristics of vitamin C deficiency include fatigue, capillary hemorrhages and petechiae, swollen hemorrhagic gums, and bone changes. A deficiency may also impair wound healing. A profound dietary deficiency can eventually lead to scurvy, producing widespread capillary hemorrhaging and a weakening of collagenous structures.

Scurvy is rare in the United States because it develops only with chronically inadequate consumption of vitamin C. Infants who are fed artificial formulas without vitamin supplements may develop symptoms of scurvy. In adults, however, scurvy occurs after 3–5 months of a diet free of vitamin C.

Dose/DRI. Practitioners are rarely confronted with overt symptoms of vitamin C deficiency. Only 10 mg/day of vitamin C prevents scurvy; a normal diet containing fresh fruits and vegetables contains many times this amount. The DRI values for vitamin C are listed in Table 22–3. Supplementation of 100–125 mg/day has been recommended for smokers, on the basis of higher daily ascorbic acid losses observed in these individuals.[35] The UL for vitamin C is 2 g/day.

Most adult multivitamin supplements contain 60–100 mg of vitamin C, an appropriate amount to consume if supplements are required. A daily dose greater than 400 mg is rarely indicated, and excess intake is excreted in the urine. In patients with a severe vitamin C deficiency as evidenced by clinical signs of scurvy, 100–300 mg/day of vitamin C for at least 2 weeks is recommended to replenish body stores.[19] Infants who do not have vitamin C supplements in their formula should receive 40–50 mg/day; infants who are breast-fed by well-nourished mothers will receive a sufficient amount. If a supplement is warranted for an adult, practitioners may recommend a multivitamin product containing 60–200 mg of vitamin C to be taken once a day. Vitamin C is FDA approved for use in the prevention and treatment of scurvy and to acidify the urine.[19]

Safety Considerations. The practitioner is urged to weigh the relative risks and benefits of ascorbic acid therapy. Short-term use to promote wound healing in potentially deficient patients may warrant a trial of ascorbic acid with medical supervision. Megadoses, however, may cause nausea, stomach cramps, diarrhea, and nephrolithiasis. Ascorbic acid toxicity can also lead to hemolysis in patients deficient in glucose 6-phosphate dehydrogenase. Rebound scurvy in infants whose mothers took megadoses of vitamin C during pregnancy has occurred on sudden withdrawal of ascorbic acid. Vitamin C in doses of 1 g/day with 400 IU of vitamin E resulted in an increased risk of fetal loss or perinatal death when given as prenatal supplementation.[33] Patients with diabetes mellitus, recurrent renal calculi, or renal dysfunction should also avoid prolonged use of high-dose vitamin C supplementation.

Potential Drug–Nutrient Interactions. See Table 22–8.

Vitamin B₁₂ (Cyanocobalamin)

Vitamin B_{12} is the most complex vitamin molecule, and it exists in several forms, all of which contain the element cobalt. The term *vitamin B_{12}* refers to all cobalamins that have vitamin activity in humans. Cyanocobalamin, the common pharmaceutical form of the vitamin, is the most stable of the cobalamins.

Function. Vitamin B_{12} is active in all cells, especially those in the bone marrow, the central nervous system (CNS), and the GI tract. It is also involved in fat, protein, and carbohydrate metabolism. A cobalamin coenzyme functions in the synthesis of DNA and in the synthesis and transfer of single-carbon units (e.g., the methyl group in the synthesis of methionine and choline). Vitamin B_{12} participates in methylation reactions and cell division, usually in concert with folic acid. Vitamin B_{12} is necessary for the metabolism of folates; therefore, a folate deficiency may be observed as a feature of vitamin B_{12} deficiency. Vitamin B_{12} is also necessary for the metabolism of lipids and the formation of myelin.

Vitamin B_{12} has been studied in relation to elevated levels of homocysteine, an amino acid that requires vitamins B_{12}, B_6, and folate as cofactors for metabolism. Hyperhomocysteinemia has been identified as an independent risk factor for cardiovascular disease. Supplementation with folate, vitamin B_6, and vitamin B_{12} has been shown to reduce plasma homocysteine levels. However, this has not been proven to lower the risk of major coronary or major vascular events in individuals at increased risk for cardiovascular disease.[37]

Dietary Sources. Vitamin B_{12} is found almost exclusively in animal protein (Table 22–6).

Deficiency. In healthy individuals who have no dietary restrictions, vitamin B_{12} deficiency is rare because the body stores so much vitamin B_{12} in the liver that a deficiency would take approximately 3 years to develop. Vitamin B_{12} deficiency may be caused by poor absorption or utilization, or by an increased requirement or excretion of this vitamin. In patients with conditions that affect absorption (e.g., those with ileal diseases, intestinal resection, or gastrectomy), the reabsorption phase of the enterohepatic cycle is affected, and deficiency may occur. Patients older than 50 years are at increased risk of vitamin B_{12} deficiency resulting from the inability to absorb food-bound vitamin B_{12}. Reduced intestinal motility, achlorhydria, and use of gastric acid–lowering agents in this patient population contribute to bacterial overgrowth in the small intestine, resulting in more microorganisms utilizing available vitamin B_{12}.[38] In addition, atrophic gastritis is a condition that affects 10%–30% of older adults, and it can result in pernicious anemia as a result of inadequate production of gastric intrinsic factor, which is necessary for vitamin B_{12} absorption. For these reasons, vitamin B_{12} supplementation from either fortified foods or a dietary supplement is recommended for this age group; prescription-only vitamin B_{12} injections may be necessary for the treatment of pernicious anemia.[39] ,

Long-term treatment with metformin can induce malabsorption of vitamin B_{12}, thereby contributing to the development of vitamin B_{12} deficiency.[40] In fact, vitamin B_{12} deficiency has been reported after as little as 3 months of metformin therapy.[38]

Vegetarians who do not consume any animal products (including infants breast-fed by vegetarian mothers) are also at risk for developing vitamin B_{12} deficiency. Vitamin B_{12} supplementation should be encouraged for these patients.

The symptoms of vitamin B_{12} deficiency mimic those of folate deficiency and are manifested in organ systems with rapidly duplicating cells. One such organ system is the hematopoietic system resulting in macrocytic anemia. The GI tract is also affected, with glossitis and epithelial changes occurring along the entire digestive tract. Because vitamin B_{12} is necessary for the maintenance of myelin, deficiency states produce many neurologic symptoms (e.g., paresthesia, peripheral neuropathy, unsteadiness, poor muscular coordination, mental confusion, agitation, hallucinations, and overt psychosis).

Practitioners should caution patients that an accurate diagnosis of a suspected anemia via laboratory assessment of the complete blood cell count and differential is essential in selecting effective treatment. For example, anemia resulting from a folic acid deficiency should be treated with folic acid; pernicious anemia should be treated with vitamin B_{12}; and iron-deficiency anemia should be treated with iron. Practitioners should avoid use of a "shotgun" antianemia preparation that contains multiple hematinic factors.

Dose/DRI. The DRI values for vitamin B_{12} are listed in Table 22–3. Oral forms can be used if the deficiency is caused by inadequate intake; high-dose oral supplementation may be appropriate for deficiencies caused by malabsorption, although intramuscular or deep subcutaneous administration is sometimes used given poor oral bioavailability. Vitamin B_{12} is FDA approved for use in the treatment of pernicious anemia and vitamin B_{12} deficiency. Other approved uses include supplementation during periods of increased requirements (e.g., pregnancy, thyrotoxicosis, hemorrhage, malignancy, liver disease, or kidney disease).[19] Patients who have undergone bariatric surgery (e.g., gastric bypass) require lifelong vitamin B_{12} supplementation to prevent deficiency. A UL has not been established for vitamin B_{12}.

Hydroxocobalamin, a prescription-only product equal in hematopoietic effect to cyanocobalamin, may be appropriate for some patients. It is more extensively bound to proteins at the site of injection and in plasma, making renal excretion slower and prolonging the duration of action.

Safety Considerations. Excessive doses have not resulted in toxicity; however, nondeficient patients taking large quantities of the vitamin have reported no benefit.

Potential Drug–Nutrient Interactions. See Table 22–8.

Folic Acid (Pteroylglutamic Acid, Folate)

Function. Folate is an important nutrient that is essential for cell division, DNA production, and brain and spinal cord development. It is also used in the metabolism of various amino acids. Folic acid refers to the synthetic version of this vitamin found in nutritional supplements and in fortified foods; folate is the naturally occurring form found only in food sources.

Folic acid, whether contained in a nutritional supplement or consumed through dietary sources, is not biologically active and must undergo *in vivo* enzymatic conversion to the usable form. Following consumption, folic acid is converted to dihydrofolate, which is then converted to tetrahydrofolate by the enzyme dihydrofolate reductase. Tetrahydrofolate is then converted by methylenetetrahydrofolate reductase (MTHFR) to the biologically active form, l-methylfolate.[41] A significant percentage of the population may have a genetic polymorphism of MTHFR that results in inadequate enzyme activity.[42] Patients with this polymorphism cannot convert folic acid to its active form. This has major implications for pregnant women because folic acid supplementation in patients with this polymorphism is not effective at reducing the risk of neural tube defects.[41] Other genetic defects in folate metabolism may lead to abnormalities in homocysteine metabolism (leading to elevated homocysteine levels), which has been associated with neural tube defects.[43] Folate deficiency is closely linked with deficiency of other water-soluble vitamins; low plasma concentrations of folate, vitamin B_6, and vitamin B_{12} have been associated with elevated concentrations of homocysteine, which may increase the risk of cardiovascular disease. Folate supplementation may reduce elevated serum homocysteine concentrations, although this effect has not translated into improved cardiovascular outcomes.[39]

Dietary Sources. Folates are present in a wide variety of food sources. Primary food sources are listed in Table 22–6. Folates are heat labile, so the folic acid content of food depends on how the food is processed. Many commercially prepared carbohydrate foods (e.g., breads and pasta) are now fortified with folic acid.

Deficiency. The requirements for folic acid are related to metabolic rate and cell turnover, and increased amounts of folic acid are needed during pregnancy, lactation, and infancy. Infection, hemolytic anemia, blood loss (in which red blood cell production must be increased to replenish blood supply), and hypermetabolic states (e.g., hyperthyroidism) also increase folic acid requirements. Because folic acid deficiency has been associated with an increased risk of neural tube defects in newborns, supplementation for all women of child-bearing age is recommended.

Causes of folic acid deficiency include alcoholism, malabsorption, food faddism, and liver disease. Iatrogenic causes are associated with administration of certain medications, including dihydrofolate reductase inhibitors (e.g., methotrexate or trimethoprim), anticonvulsants, and sulfasalazine.[19]

A deficiency of folic acid results in impaired cell division and protein synthesis. Symptoms of folic acid deficiency are similar to those of vitamin B_{12} deficiency, including sore mouth, diarrhea, and CNS symptoms (e.g., irritability and forgetfulness). The most common laboratory-identified feature of folic acid deficiency is megaloblastic anemia (an anemia characterized by large erythroblasts circulating in the blood).

Because vitamin B_{12} is essential for the metabolism of folates, a megaloblastic anemia responsive to folic acid administration is a feature of vitamin B_{12} deficiency. Folic acid given without vitamin B_{12} to patients with inadequate intrinsic factor (pernicious anemia) or vitamin B_{12} deficiency would correct the anemia but would not stop the damage to the CNS (characterized by lack of coordination, impaired sense of position, and various behavioral disturbances). Because of the potential for folic acid to mask the signs—but not the progression—of

vitamin B_{12} deficiency, patients should receive an appropriate medical evaluation for the cause of anemia rather than an empiric vitamin supplement.

Dose/DRI. The DRI values for folic acid are listed in Table 22–3. Folate is FDA-approved for use in the treatment of megaloblastic anemias caused by folate deficiency. Folate also is approved for prevention of neural tube defects of the newborn.[19]

All women of childbearing age should consume synthetic folic acid at a dose of 400 mcg/day from fortified foods and/ or dietary supplementation in addition to the folate obtained from food sources.[14]

Individuals known to have a polymorphism in MTHFR should receive a prescription vitamin containing biologically active derivatives of folic acid, available in forms such as l-methylfolate, 5-methyltetrahydrofolate calcium salt, and (6S)-5-methyltetrahydrofolate glucosamine salt.[41]

The supplemental dose of folic acid for correction of a deficiency in adults is usually 1 mg/day, particularly if the deficiency occurs with conditions that may increase the folate requirement or suppress red blood cell formation (e.g., pregnancy, hypermetabolic states, alcoholism, or hemolytic anemia). Doses larger than the UL of 1 mg/day are not necessary, except in some life-threatening hematologic diseases. Maintenance therapy for deficiencies may be stopped after 1–4 months if the diet contains at least one fresh fruit or vegetable daily. For chronic malabsorption diseases, folic acid treatment may be lifelong, and parenteral doses may be required.

Safety Considerations. Folic acid toxicity is virtually nonexistent because of its water solubility and rapid excretion. Doses up to 15 mg/day have been given without toxic effect. The UL is set to minimize the risk of masking vitamin B_{12} deficiency. Several drugs, when taken chronically, may increase the need for folic acid (Table 22–8).

Niacin (Nicotinic Acid)

The physiologically active form of niacin is niacinamide. Niacin and niacinamide are constituents of the coenzymes nicotinamide adenine dinucleotide and nicotinamide adenine dinucleotide phosphate.

Function. The niacin coenzymes are electron transfer agents; that is, they accept or donate hydrogen in the aerobic respiration of all body cells. Niacin is a unique vitamin because humans can synthesize it from dietary tryptophan, with about 60 mg of tryptophan being equivalent to 1 mg of niacin. Most individuals receive about 50% of their niacin requirement from tryptophan-containing proteins and the rest as preformed niacin or niacinamide.

Dietary Sources. See Table 22–6.

Deficiency. The classic and only described niacin deficiency state is pellagra. Pellagra is rare, occurring most often in alcoholics, poorly nourished persons of advanced age, and individuals on diets that severely restrict sources of niacin. It may also occur in areas where large quantities of corn are consumed, as some of the niacin found in corn is bound to undigestible constituents, making it unavailable for absorption. Other causes of pellagra include isoniazid therapy and decreased tryptophan conversion, as in Hartnup disease and carcinoid tumors.

Clinical findings of niacin deficiency include the "three D's" of <u>d</u>ermatitis, <u>d</u>iarrhea, and <u>d</u>ementia, often accompanied by neuropathy, glossitis (beefy red tongue), stomatitis, and proctitis. Patients manifest a characteristic rash with well-demarcated lesions of hard, cracked skin with blackish pigmentation that is crusty and scaly. Lesions occur primarily on sun-exposed areas, including dorsal surfaces of the hands, arms and feet, on the neck (Casal necklace), and face. Secondary infections may occur in such lesions. The entire GI tract is generally affected, with atrophy of the epithelium. Inflammation of the small intestine may be associated with episodes of occult bleeding and/or diarrhea.

Dose/DRI. The DRI values for niacin are listed in Table 22–3. The recommended UL for this vitamin in adults is 35 mg/day.[14]

Niacin requirements are increased after a severe injury, infection, or burn, or when the patient has an acute illness; has substantially increased caloric expenditure or dietary caloric intake; or has a low tryptophan intake (e.g., a low-protein diet or a high intake of corn as a staple in the diet). The FDA-approved use of both niacin and niacinamide is the prevention and treatment of pellagra. Niacin, but not niacinamide, is also approved for adjunctive treatment of hyperlipidemia and hypercholesterolemia.[19]

Niacin or niacinamide, 150–500 mg daily in divided doses, is used for treatment of pellagra. Daily dosages of 1–2 grams 3 times per day, up to 8 g/day, of niacin (*not* niacinamide) are used to treat hypercholesterolemia and hyperlipidemia. Niacin increases beneficial high-density lipoprotein cholesterol and decreases concentrations of potentially harmful triglycerides, total cholesterol, and low-density lipoprotein cholesterol by mechanisms unrelated to its function as an essential micronutrient. However, such high dose niacin therapy should not be undertaken as self-care; close medical supervision is required because of potentially serious drug-induced toxicity.

Safety Considerations. Niacinamide is associated with little toxicity; conversely, niacin toxicity can involve GI symptoms (e.g., nausea, vomiting, and diarrhea), hepatotoxicity, skin lesions, tachycardia, and hypertension. Patients should be forewarned that therapeutic doses of niacin may cause flushing and a sensation of warmth, especially around the face, neck, and ears. This reaction, which is prevalent upon initiation of therapy, may be diminished with aspirin 325 mg or ibuprofen 200 mg taken 30–60 minutes before the niacin dose, provided no contraindications exist. Alternatively, the extended-release formulation may cause less flushing but has a greater risk of gastric and hepatic side effects. Itching or tingling and headache may also occur with niacin supplementation. These effects will usually subside or decrease in intensity within 2 weeks of continued therapy. If niacin causes GI upset, it should be taken with meals.

Because of the adverse effects on the GI tract, high doses of niacin are contraindicated in patients with gastritis or peptic ulcer disease. Niacin can provoke the release of histamine, so its use in patients with asthma should be undertaken carefully. Niacin may also impair liver function, disturb glucose tolerance, and cause hyperuricemia. Patients prescribed therapeutic doses of this nutrient must be monitored regularly for potential adverse effects.

Potential Drug–Nutrient Interactions. See Table 22–8.

Pantothenic Acid

Pantothenic acid is a water-soluble vitamin of the B-complex family.

Function. Pantothenic acid is a precursor of coenzyme A (CoA), a product that is active in many biological reactions and plays a primary role in cholesterol, steroid, and fatty acid synthesis. Pantothenic acid is important for acetylation reactions and the formation of citric acid for the Krebs cycle, and it is crucial in the intraneuronal synthesis of acetylcholine. It also is important in gluconeogenesis; synthesis and degradation of fatty acids; synthesis of sterols, steroid hormones, and porphyrins; and in the release of energy from carbohydrates.

Dietary Sources. Pantothenic acid is widely distributed in foods (Table 22–6).

Deficiency. Because pantothenic acid is contained in many foods, deficiency states are rare and hard to detect. In malabsorption syndromes, it is difficult to distinguish pantothenic acid deficiency symptoms from those of other deficiencies. Symptoms of pantothenic acid deficiency include somnolence, fatigue, cardiovascular instability, abdominal pain, and paresthesia of hands and/or feet followed by hyperreflexia and muscular weakness in the legs. Administration of pharmacologic doses of pantothenic acid reverses these symptoms and has even been used to eliminate burning feet syndrome.

Dose/DRI. AI values for this vitamin are listed in Table 22–3. There is no established UL for pantothenic acid.

Safety Considerations. Pantothenic acid generally is considered nontoxic, even in large doses. Doses as high as 10 g/day of calcium pantothenate have been given to young men for 6 weeks with no toxic symptoms. However, ingestion of more than 20 grams has been reported to result in diarrhea and water retention.

Potential Drug–Nutrient Interactions. Significant drug–nutrient interactions with pantothenic acid have not been reported.

Vitamin B₆ (Pyridoxine)

This water-soluble vitamin exists in three forms: pyridoxine (vitamin B₆), pyridoxal, and pyridoxamine. Although all three forms are equally effective in nutrition, pyridoxine hydrochloride is the form most often used in vitamin formulations.

Function. Vitamin B₆ serves as a cofactor for more than 60 enzymes, including decarboxylases, synthetases, transaminases, and hydroxylases. It is important in heme production and in the metabolism of homocysteine. As previously stated, hyperhomocysteinemia is a potential risk factor for cardiovascular disease, and it has been shown to respond particularly to folic acid supplementation but also to vitamin B₆. Whether the impact of these nutrients on homocysteine levels results in improved clinical outcomes has yet to be determined.[37] Vitamin B₆ has also been suggested as a potential treatment of carpal tunnel syndrome, premenstrual syndrome (PMS), depression, and migraine. Unfortunately, no clinical research evidence supports use of vitamin B₆ for these ailments.[44]

Dietary Sources. See Table 22–6. Cooking destroys some vitamin B₆.

Deficiency. Causes of vitamin B₆ deficiency include alcoholism, severe diarrhea, food faddism, malabsorptive syndromes, drugs (isoniazid and penicillamine), and genetic diseases (cystathioninuria and xanthurenic aciduria).

The symptoms of severe vitamin B_6 deficiency in infants include irritability and convulsive disorders. Medical referral is indicated, and treatment with vitamin B_6 hydrochloride generally normalizes the electroencephalogram and resolves clinical symptoms. Symptoms in adults whose diets are deficient in vitamin B_6 or who have been given a vitamin B_6 antagonist are difficult to distinguish from symptoms of niacin and riboflavin deficiencies. These symptoms include pellagra-like dermatitis; oral lesions; peripheral neuropathy; scaliness around the nose, mouth, and eyes; and dulling of mentation. Serious deficiency symptoms include convulsions, peripheral neuritis, and sideroblastic anemia.

Dose/DRI. DRI values for vitamin B_6 are listed in Table 22–3. The FDA-approved use of this vitamin is for treatment of vitamin B_6 deficiency, including drug-induced deficiency as seen with isoniazid.[19] Daily doses up to 250 mg of vitamin B_6 have been used in the treatment of hyperhomocysteinemia.[37] However, the UL for this vitamin is 100 mg daily for adults.[14]

Treatment of sideroblastic anemia requires 50–200 mg/day of pyridoxine hydrochloride to aid production of hemoglobin and erythrocytes. Several vitamin B_6–dependent inborn errors of metabolism have been shown to respond to large doses of vitamin B_6.

Safety Considerations. Vitamin B_6 may be toxic in high doses. A severe sensory neuropathy similar to that observed with the deficiency state has been reported when gram quantities were taken to relieve symptoms of PMS. Similar symptoms have been reported in women taking doses as small as 50 mg/day for PMS. Recovery occurred slowly upon withdrawal of vitamin B_6.

High daily doses of vitamin B_6 (200–600 mg) inhibit prolactin. Prenatal vitamins, which contain 1–10 mg per dosage unit, do not appear to have a significant antiprolactin effect.

Potential Drug–Nutrient Interactions. See Table 22–8.

Riboflavin (Vitamin B₂)

Riboflavin is a water-soluble vitamin essential for cellular growth and maintenance of vision, mucous membranes, skin, nails, and hair.

Function. Riboflavin is a constituent of two coenzymes: flavin adenine dinucleotide and flavin mononucleotide. It is involved in numerous oxidation and reduction reactions, including the cytochrome P450 reductase enzyme system involved in drug metabolism.

Dietary Sources. See Table 22–6.

Deficiency. Riboflavin deficiency, although rare, may be caused by inadequate intake, alcoholism, or malabsorptive syndromes. Deficiency of this vitamin may occur in association with other vitamin B-complex deficiency states (e.g., pellagra) or during pregnancy. Early signs of riboflavin deficiency may involve ocular symptoms, as the eyes become light sensitive and easily fatigued. The patient may develop blurred vision; itching, watering, sore eyes; and corneal vascularization, which causes a bloodshot appearance of the eye. Clinical findings of more advanced deficiency include stomatitis, seborrheic dermatitis, and magenta tongue.

Dose/DRI. The DRI values for riboflavin are listed in Table 22–3. The need for riboflavin appears to increase during periods of increased cell growth, such as during pregnancy and wound healing. Absorption is enhanced when taken with food. The FDA-approved use of riboflavin is in the prevention and treatment of riboflavin deficiency.[19] No UL has been determined for this vitamin.

Limited data suggest high-dose riboflavin (400 mg daily) may be effective in the prevention of migraine. An open-label study of 23 patients suggested reduced incidence of migraine, but no effect on duration or intensity.[45] Further study on riboflavin therapy for migraine prevention is warranted.

Safety Considerations. The use of riboflavin typically causes a yellow-orange fluorescence or discoloration of the urine. Patients who report this effect should be reassured that this color is normal. There is no known toxic concentration.

Potential Drug–Nutrient Interactions. No significant drug interactions have been reported for riboflavin.

Thiamin (Vitamin B₁)

Thiamin is a water-soluble, B-complex vitamin available in oral tablet and injectable dosage forms.

Function. Thiamin's active form, thiamin pyrophosphate (formerly known as cocarboxylase), plays a vital role in the oxidative decarboxylation of pyruvic acid; in the formation of acetyl CoA, which enters the Krebs cycle; and in other important biochemical conversion cycles. Thiamin is necessary for myocardial function, nerve cell function, and carbohydrate metabolism. The amount of thiamin required increases with increased carbohydrate consumption.

Dietary Sources. Dietary sources highest in thiamin are listed in Table 22–6. The thiamin content of food can be destroyed by heat, oxidation, and an alkaline environment but is stable through frozen storage.

Deficiency. The primary causes of thiamin deficiency are generally inadequate diet, alcoholism, malabsorptive syndromes, prolonged diarrhea, chronic furosemide therapy, increased requirements (e.g., pregnancy), and food faddism.

Thiamin deficiency in the United States is found primarily in alcoholics. Not only is their diet often nutritionally deficient, but alcohol ingestion also impairs thiamin absorption and transport across the intestine, and it also increases the rate of destruction of thiamin diphosphate. Thiamin deficiency, also known as beriberi, may present with neuromuscular symptoms such as peripheral neuritis, weakness, and Wernicke's encephalopathy. Cardiac dysfunction may also be observed, possibly accompanied by edema, tachycardia on minimal exertion, enlarged heart, and electrocardiographic abnormalities. Because of these risks, a vitamin supplement containing thiamin should be prescribed for alcoholic patients.

Dose/DRI. The DRI values for thiamin are listed in Table 22–3. Signs and symptoms of thiamin deficiency are preferably treated with intravenous thiamin. However, long-term supplementation may be recommended for patients at risk of continued losses, such as those prescribed high-dose furosemide therapy. The FDA-approved use of thiamin is for the treatment of thiamin deficiency.[19]

Safety Considerations. The kidney easily clears excessive thiamin intake, and oral doses of 500 mg have been found to be nontoxic.

Potential Drug–Nutrient Interactions. Diuretics have been shown to increase the urinary excretion of thiamin. Therefore, patients on chronic diuretic therapy (e.g., those with congestive heart failure or hypertension) may be at risk of subclinical thiamin deficiency and associated cardiovascular complications. Recommending supplementation with 100% of the DRI for this vitamin is reasonable.[46]

Biotin (Vitamin H)

Biotin is included in several multivitamin preparations.

Function. Biotin, a member of the B-complex group of vitamins, is required for various metabolic functions, including carbohydrate, fat, and amino acid metabolism. Several biotin-dependent enzymes are known to exist.

Dietary Sources. Food sources of biotin are listed in Table 22–6. In addition to food sources, colonic flora probably synthesizes a considerable amount of biotin, which is then absorbed from the large intestine into the bloodstream.

Deficiency. Deficiency states of biotin are rare but appear to result in symptoms of nausea, vomiting, lassitude, muscle pain, anorexia, anemia, and depression. Dermatitis, a grayish color of the skin, and glossitis may be among the physical findings; hypercholesterolemia and cardiac abnormalities may also occur.

Biotin deficiency in humans can be caused by ingesting a large number of raw egg whites. Raw egg whites contain avidin, a protein that binds biotin, thereby preventing its absorption. Individuals undergoing a rapid weight-loss program with intense caloric restriction and those with chronic malabsorption may not obtain adequate biotin and should receive supplementation.

Dose/DRI. See Table 22–3.

Safety Considerations. Adverse effects have not been reported with biotin therapy.

Vitamin-Like Compounds and Pseudovitamins

Vitamin-like compounds, or pseudovitamins, are substances that have a chemical structure very similar to that of vitamins but lack the usual physiologic or biochemical actions. That is, they are not essential for specific body functions of growth, maintenance, and reproduction.

Choline

Choline is contained in most living cells and in foods. It is usually present in the form of phosphatidylcholine, commonly known as lecithin, and in several other phospholipids found in cell membranes. Intestinal mucosal cells and pancreatic secretions contain enzymes capable of splitting phospholipids to release choline. Choline is also found in sphingomyelin and is highly concentrated in nervous tissue.

Function. Choline, a precursor in the biosynthesis of acetylcholine, is an important donor of methyl groups used in the biochemical formation of other substances in vivo. It can be biosynthesized in humans. Furthermore, choline and inositol are considered to be lipotropic agents (i.e., agents involved in the mobilization of lipids). They have been used to treat fatty liver and abnormal fat metabolism, but their efficacy has not been established.

Dietary Sources. Although choline is found in food sources, it is also synthesized in the body. Therefore, choline most likely is not a vitamin. Choline is obtained from the diet as either choline or lecithin. Food sources are listed in Table 22–6.

Deficiency. A deficiency state has not been identified in humans, possibly because choline is readily available in the diet and is synthesized in the body.

Dose/DRI. See Table 22–3 for DRI values. An average diet furnishes ample choline daily. The recommended UL for choline is 3.5 g/day.[14]

Safety Considerations. The administration of large doses of lecithin has been associated with sweating, GI distress, vomiting, and diarrhea.

Potential Drug–Nutrient Interactions. No drug interactions have been reported.

Minerals

Minerals constitute about 4% of body weight. These micronutrients are present in the body in a diverse array of organic compounds (e.g., phosphoproteins, phospholipids, hemoglobin, and thyroxine). They function as constituents of many enzymes, hormones, vitamins, and inorganic compounds (e.g., sodium chloride, potassium chloride, calcium, and phosphorus) that are present as free ions. Different body tissues contain various quantities of different minerals. For example, bone has a high content of calcium, phosphorus, and magnesium, whereas soft tissue has a high quantity of potassium. Minerals are involved in regulating cell membrane permeability, osmotic pressure, and acid–base and water balance. In addition, certain ions act as the mediators of action potential conduction and neurotransmitter action.

A well-balanced diet is required to maintain proper mineral balance. Optimal mineral intake values for humans are still imprecise; only AIs are available for trace element minerals such as chromium, fluoride, and manganese. Similarly, the possible adverse effects of long-term ingestion of high-dose mineral supplements are often unknown, and high doses of one mineral can decrease the bioavailability of other minerals and vitamins.

Calcium

The most abundant cation in the body is calcium (about 1200 grams). Approximately 99% of calcium is present in the skeleton, and the remaining 1% is present in the extracellular fluid, intracellular structures, and cell membranes. Calcium is a major component of bones and teeth. The calcium content in bone is continuously undergoing a process of resorption and formation. In people of advanced age, the resorption process predominates over formation, and a decrease in calcium absorption efficiency results in a gradual loss of bone density that leads to osteoporosis. This effect can be minimized by encouraging optimal calcium and vitamin D intake throughout the life cycle and by encouraging regular participation in weight-bearing exercise.

Function. Calcium is important for several reasons, as it activates a number of enzymes and is required for acetylcholine synthesis. Calcium increases cell membrane permeability, aids in vitamin B_{12} absorption, regulates muscle contraction and relaxation, and catalyzes several steps in the activation of plasma-clotting factors. Calcium is also necessary for the functional integrity of many cells, especially those of the neuromuscular and cardiovascular system.

Dietary Sources. Dietary sources of calcium are listed in Table 22–6. Teenagers experiencing rapid growth and bone maturation need to consume adequate calcium through dairy products (especially milk) or through a nutritional supplement. Most adults can easily meet calcium RDAs by incorporating dairy products into their diets daily. Each 8-ounce serving of nonfat milk contains about 300 mg of calcium. As an alternative, calcium supplements are usually well tolerated in daily doses of less than 2 grams. Table 22–9 lists selected calcium supplements.

Practitioners should evaluate the dietary intake of calcium (including calcium-fortified foods) before recommending daily calcium supplementation. Calcium fortification is found in numerous nontraditional sources (e.g., juices, breads, and breakfast bars). To optimize calcium absorption, patients should avoid co-ingestion with bran, whole-grain cereals, or high-oxalate foods (e.g., cocoa, soybeans, or spinach); for those using a supplement, a product co-formulated with vitamin D should be recommended.

Deficiency. Decreased calcium concentrations may have profound and diverse consequences, including convulsions, tetany, behavioral and personality disorders, mental and growth retardation, and bone deformities (the most common being rickets in children and osteomalacia in adults). Changes that occur in osteomalacia include softening of bones, rheumatic-type pain in the bones of the legs and lower back, general weakness with difficulty walking, and spontaneous fractures. Common causes of hypocalcemia and associated skeletal disorders include malabsorptive syndromes; hypoparathyroidism; vitamin D deficiency; renal failure with impaired activation of vitamin D; long-term anticonvulsant therapy (with increased breakdown of vitamin D); and decreased dietary intake of calcium, particularly during periods of growth, pregnancy and lactation, and among people of advanced age.

Dose/DRI. The RDAs for calcium are listed in Table 22–4. Oral calcium supplements are FDA approved for use in the treatment and prevention of calcium deficiency, which may result in rickets, osteomalacia, or osteoporosis. Other FDA-approved uses include treatment of acid indigestion and hyperphosphatemia associated with end-stage renal disease.[19] The recommended UL for calcium is 2–3 g/day for individuals older than 1 year.[15]

Recommendations for calcium intake are based on elemental calcium content, not the calcium salt. Because labels can be misleading, practitioners should be familiar with the many salt forms and the different percentages of calcium in each, including carbonate (40%), citrate (21%), lactate (13%), gluconate (9%), and phosphate salts (23%–39%).[47] Calcium carbonate and calcium phosphate salts are insoluble in water and should be taken with meals to enhance absorption, which is optimal in a low pH. Patients requiring supplementation who have achlorhydria or who are on chronic therapy with histamine₂ antagonists or proton pump inhibitors may benefit most from taking one of the water-soluble salt formulations (e.g., calcium citrate), which are absorbed more readily in basic environments.

The small intestine controls calcium absorption. Patients ingesting relatively low amounts of calcium absorb proportionately more calcium than those with adequate intake; patients taking large amounts of calcium excrete more as fecal calcium. Optimal absorption occurs with individual doses of 500 mg or less; therefore, patients taking more than 500 mg of supplemental calcium should be encouraged to take calcium in divided doses.[15] In conjunction with adequate calcium and vitamin D intake, weight-bearing exercise is essential in maintaining bone mass.

High intake of calcium and vitamin D may be effective in the prevention of premenstrual syndrome.[48] Numerous studies have evaluated the relationship between calcium intake and the risk of colon cancer; however, the results of these studies have been inconsistent. Further research to better define this relationship is needed.

Claims have also been made in relation to calcium intake and weight loss or maintenance. However, randomized controlled trials have found no relationship between higher calcium intakes and body weight.[49]

Safety Considerations. Calcium in doses greater than 3 g/day can be harmful. Large amounts taken as dietary supplements or antacids can lead to high levels of calcium in the urine and to the formation of renal stones; development of the latter may result in permanent renal damage. Development of hypercalcemia is possible (particularly in patients taking concomitant high-dose vitamin D preparations) and is associated with anorexia, nausea, vomiting, constipation, and polyuria. Increased deposition of calcium in soft tissue can also occur with hypercalcemia. The USPSTF is more conservative regarding calcium intake and recommends that daily calcium intake not exceed 1000 mg.[50] USPSTF's recommendation is based on the fact that insufficient evidence exists to determine whether calcium supplementation can reduce fractures in community-dwelling adults and on concerns that high-dose supplementation may increase the risk of adverse effects.

The relationship between dietary and supplemental calcium intake and increased cardiovascular disease risk has caused much controversy and uncertainty in the medical community over the past several years. According to results of a prospective study conducted in 388,229 men and women ages 50–71 years designed to evaluate the effects of both dietary and supplemental calcium intake on mortality from cardiovascular disease, heart disease, and stroke, supplemental calcium intake at a dose more than 1000 mg/day was associated with an increased risk of death from heart disease in men.[51] Supplemental calcium intake at any dose in women, on the other hand, was not found to correlate with increased risk of cardiovascular disease, heart disease, or cerebrovascular death in this trial. Moreover, dietary

table

22–9 Selected Nonprescription Calcium Supplements

Trade Name	Primary Ingredients Per Serving
Caltrate 600+D Tablets	Elemental calcium 600 mg (as carbonate); vitamin D 200–800 IU (depending on formulation)
Citracal Maximum Caplets	Elemental calcium 630 mg (as citrate); vitamin D 500 IU
Os-Cal Calcium+D3 Chewable Tablets	Elemental calcium 500 mg (as carbonate); vitamin D 600 IU
Tums Regular Strength Chewable Tablets	Elemental calcium 400 mg (as carbonate)
Viactiv Calcium Soft Chews plus D	Elemental calcium 500 mg (as carbonate); vitamin D 500 IU; vitamin K 40 mcg

calcium intake was found to be unrelated to increased risk of cardiovascular death in either men or women, underscoring the importance of dietary calcium intake over supplemental calcium use. Results from a post-hoc analysis of the Women's Health Initiative dataset also identified no increased risks of myocardial infarction, coronary heart disease, total heart disease, stroke, or overall cardiovascular disease in postmenopausal women receiving 1000 mg/day elemental calcium carbonate plus 400 IU/day of vitamin D_3.[52] Clearly, more information is necessary to further elucidate the correlations between calcium supplementation and cardiovascular disease risk. Patients considering calcium supplementation should undergo a complete dietary and lifestyle evaluation to determine the possible risks and benefits of supplementation with this mineral.

Calcium intake has also been suggested to influence risk of prostate cancer. In fact, three trials have found an increased risk for prostate cancer with calcium intakes greater than 1500 mg daily from either supplements or dietary sources.[49] Recommending calcium intakes closer to the DRI/RDA for those at risk of prostate cancer is reasonable until further evidence clarifies this association.

Practitioners should counsel patients regarding potential constipation associated with calcium supplementation and the importance of adequate hydration, dietary fiber, and physical activity in preventing this side effect.

Potential Drug–Nutrient Interactions. See Table 22–8.

Iron

Iron is widely available in the U.S. diet. Iron absorption from the intestinal tract is controlled by the body's need for iron, the intestinal lumen conditions, the food source of iron, and the other components of the meal (e.g., the meal's vitamin C content).

Function. Iron plays an important role in oxygen and electron transport. In the body, it is either functional or stored. Functional iron is found in hemoglobin, myoglobin, heme-containing enzymes, and transferrin, which is the transport form of iron. Stored iron is primarily found in the hemoglobin of red blood cells, which contain 60%–70% of total body iron. The remainder is stored primarily in the forms of ferritin and hemosiderin in the intestinal mucosa, liver, spleen, and bone marrow.

Dietary Sources. Dietary iron is available in two forms: heme and nonheme iron. Heme iron is found in meats and is reasonably well absorbed. Nonheme iron (e.g., that found in enriched grains and dark green vegetables) constitutes most of the dietary iron but is poorly absorbed. Therefore, the published values of iron content in foods are misleading because the amount absorbed depends on the nature of the iron. Although specific ways to calculate the iron absorption from a given meal exist, the available iron content of foods is often estimated by assuming that about 10% of the total iron (heme plus nonheme) is absorbed if no iron deficiency exists. In the iron-deficient state, iron absorption improves, so as much as 20% may be absorbed and utilized from an average diet. However, this estimate is not valid in the absence of heme iron. Less iron is absorbed from vegetarian diets.

Ingested nonheme iron (which is mostly in the form of ferric hydroxide) is solubilized in gastric juice to ferric chloride, then reduced to the ferrous form, and finally chelated to substances such as ascorbic acid, sugars, and amino acids. Chelates have a low molecular weight and can be solubilized and absorbed before they reach the alkaline medium of the distal small intestine, where precipitation may occur. When released at the spleen, liver, bone marrow, intestinal mucosa, and other iron storage sites, the iron is combined with apoferritin to form ferritin or hemosiderin. As needed, ferritin is released into the plasma, where it is oxidized to the ferric state and bound to a beta-globulin to form transferrin. Iron is used in all cells of the body; however, most of it is incorporated into the hemoglobin of red blood cells.

Deficiency. The major source of iron loss is through blood loss (e.g., hemorrhagic loss and menstruation). Iron is also lost from the body by the sloughing of skin cells and GI mucosal cells, and by excretion in urine, sweat, and feces. Excess iron loss may result in iron deficiency. Early symptoms of iron deficiency are vague. Although pallor and easy fatigability may be associated with iron deficiency, they can be attributed to other causes and are nonspecific findings. Other signs and symptoms of iron-deficiency anemia include split or "spoon-shaped" nails, sore tongue, angular stomatitis, and dyspnea on exertion. Coldness and numbness of the extremities may also be reported. Hypochromic microcytosis, as evidenced by a decreased mean corpuscular volume and low hemoglobin concentration (decreased mean corpuscular hemoglobin concentration), characterizes iron deficiency on laboratory assessment.

Iron-deficiency anemia is a widespread clinical problem and the most common form of anemia in the United States. Although it causes few deaths, it does contribute to poor health and suboptimal performance. Iron deficiency results from inadequate intake (e.g., inadequate diet or malabsorption) or increased demands (e.g., pregnancy and lactation, growth, blood loss, or treatment with erythropoietic stimulating agents). Because normal iron losses through the urine, feces, and skin are minimal, and because the majority of total body iron is efficiently stored and conserved (recycled), iron deficiency caused by poor diet or malabsorption develops very slowly over the course of several months.

Despite fortification of flour and educational efforts regarding proper nutrition, iron deficiency remains a problem, especially during the following four life periods:

■ During childhood (younger than 2 years): Children obtain low iron content from cow's milk.
■ During adolescence: In addition to blood loss during menses, young women experience rapid growth, which entails an expanding red cell mass and the need for iron in myoglobin.
■ During and after pregnancy: Women face the expanding blood volume of pregnancy, the demands of the fetus and placenta, and the blood loss of childbirth.
■ During later years: Persons of advanced age (i.e., 65 years or older) often consume inadequate dietary iron, demonstrate compromised absorption caused by achlorhydria, and experience an increased incidence of GI tract blood loss resulting from malignancy, gastric ulceration, or use of nonsteroidal anti-inflammatory drugs. However, the prevalence of elevated iron stores may be significantly greater than the prevalence of iron deficiency in this age group. Therefore, absent a confirmed diagnosis of iron-deficiency anemia, routine supplementation is not recommended for this age group.

Supplemental iron may be warranted for women with heavy or prolonged menstrual blood loss or for individuals who frequently donate blood. Iron may also be indicated during recovery from disease- and injury-associated blood loss (e.g., peptic ulcer disease, esophageal varices, cancer, and traumatic injury such as motor vehicle accidents). In addition, infants being fed human milk may need supplemental iron beginning between the ages of 4–6 months if iron-rich foods are not introduced into the diet.

Chronic use of drugs such as salicylates, nonsteroidal anti-inflammatory drugs, corticosteroids, or anticoagulants may cause drug-induced blood loss. This effect may be the result of direct irritation of the gastric mucosa or the increased bleeding tendency these medications cause. Iron supplementation should be used cautiously, if at all, in patients at high risk for GI bleeding.

Dose/DRI. The DRI values for iron are listed in Table 22–4. Because of the GI side effects associated with oral iron supplementation, the UL for elemental iron has been set at 45 mg/day for adults.[14] Oral iron supplements are FDA approved for the prevention and treatment of iron-deficiency anemia.[19]

When iron supplementation is appropriate, the practitioner will need to evaluate which iron product is best. The choice should be based on how well the iron preparation is absorbed and tolerated, on the amount of elemental iron per dose, and on its price. Because ferrous salts are absorbed 3 times more efficiently than ferric salts, an iron product of the ferrous group is usually appropriate. Ferrous sulfate is the standard against which other iron salts are compared.

Ferrous sulfate contains 20% elemental iron, or about 65 mg in a 325 mg tablet. In patients with iron deficiency, 20% of the elemental iron (12 mg) may be absorbed. Maximum incorporation of iron into red blood cells and replacement of stores is supported by 36–48 mg of elemental iron daily; thus, the usual therapeutic dose for treating iron deficiency is 2–4 (325 mg) ferrous sulfate tablets daily for 3 months. Inadequate response or worsening symptoms during this time indicate the patient should consult a primary care provider. In cases of severe or chronic iron deficiency, when serious medical conditions have been ruled out, continuous maintenance doses of 3–4 (325 mg) ferrous sulfate tablets daily for 3–6 months should normalize hemoglobin and replace iron stores (in the absence of ongoing bleeding).

Table 22–10 lists comparison data on various iron salts.[53]

Ferrous salts may be given in combination with ascorbic acid to improve iron absorption. The practitioner can encourage the consumption of fruit or juice high in ascorbic acid or a vitamin C supplement to be taken with the iron, if necessary.

Combination products with iron and ascorbic acid are also available, but these products can be expensive, and the dose of vitamin C is often inadequate. Chemicals that may decrease iron absorption include phosphates in eggs and milk, carbonates, oxalates, tannins, and phytates in cereals.

Safety Considerations. All iron products tend to irritate the GI mucosa and may produce nausea, abdominal pain, constipation, and (less frequently) diarrhea. These adverse effects may be minimized by reducing the dose or by giving iron with meals; however, food may decrease the amount of iron absorbed by as much as 50%. Practitioners may want to recommend that iron be initiated on an empty stomach; they should instruct the patient to change this routine and take the iron with food, if GI side effects occur.

A frequent side effect of iron therapy is constipation. This adverse effect has prompted the formulation of iron products that also contain a stool softener (e.g., docusate). During iron therapy, stools commonly have a black, tarry appearance because of the presence of unabsorbed iron in the feces. Unfortunately, this symptom may also indicate GI blood loss and a serious medical problem. Medical evaluation is indicated if an underlying GI condition is suspected, or if a history of GI disease exists. If the stool does not darken somewhat during iron therapy, however, the iron product may not have disintegrated properly or released the iron.

Iron must be dispensed and stored in a child-resistant container. Accidental poisonings with iron occur most often in children, who are attracted to the sugar-coated, colored tablets or who may accidentally overdose on chewable multivitamins containing iron. Such poisoning is considered a medical emergency, and any accidental ingestion of iron should be referred for evaluation by a medical provider or to a Poison Control Center. The clinical outcome depends on the speed and adequacy of treatment.

Symptoms of acute iron poisoning include abdominal pain, vomiting, diarrhea, electrolyte imbalances, and shock. In later stages, cardiovascular collapse may occur, especially if the cause has not been properly recognized and treated as a medical emergency. Treatment of iron toxicity may begin immediately at home after consultation with a Poison Control Center or local emergency department.

Potential Drug–Nutrient Interactions. See Table 22–8.

table

22–10 Common Nonprescription Oral Iron Formulations

Iron Formulation	Typical Dose	Percent Elemental Iron	Comparison Data
Ferrous sulfate	325 mg/tablet	20% (65 mg/tablet)	The gold standard for supplementation; available in multiple dosage forms; extensive history of use; proven effective; and economical. Delayed-release and enteric-coated products may improve tolerability, but iron absorption may be reduced.
Ferrous fumarate	60 mg/tablet	33% (20 mg/tablet)	No advantage over ferrous sulfate; however, may be better tolerated for some individuals.
Ferrous gluconate	225 mg/tablet	12% (27 mg/tablet)	No advantage over ferrous sulfate; however, may be better tolerated for some individuals.

Source: Reference 55.

Magnesium

Magnesium is essential for all living cells. It is the second most plentiful cation of intracellular fluids and the fourth most abundant cation in the body. About 2000 mEq magnesium are present in an average 70 kg adult, with about 50% of this amount in the bone, about 45% as an intracellular cation, and about 1%–5% in the extracellular fluid.

Function. Magnesium is required for normal bone structure formation and the proper function of more than 300 enzymes, including those involved with adenosine triphosphatase (ATP)–dependent phosphorylation, protein synthesis, and carbohydrate metabolism. Extracellular magnesium is critical to both the maintenance of nerve and muscle electrical potentials and the transmission of impulses across neuromuscular junctions.

Magnesium tends to mimic calcium in its effects on the CNS and skeletal muscle. Magnesium deficiency blunts the normal response of the parathyroid glands to hypocalcemia. Therefore, tetany, caused by a lack of calcium, cannot be corrected with calcium unless hypomagnesemia is also corrected. Similarly, magnesium deficiency impairs the transport of potassium into cells; therefore, hypokalemia cannot be corrected in the presence of magnesium deficiency.

Dietary Sources. Individuals who consume fresh foods regularly should not develop magnesium deficiency because all unprocessed foods contain magnesium (albeit in widely varying amounts). Food sources highest in magnesium are listed in Table 22–6. Processing (during which the germ and outer layers of cereal grains are removed) results in significant loss of available magnesium.

Deficiency. Deficiency states are usually caused by GI or renal losses. Examples include malabsorptive syndromes, acute or chronic diarrhea, steatorrhea, and drug-induced magnesium wasting in the urine, as seen with alcohol abuse, diuretic therapy, long-term use of proton pump inhibitors, and nephrotoxins (e.g., amphotericin B). Symptoms of magnesium deficiency may include neuromuscular irritability, increased CNS stimulation, delirium, and convulsions.

Dose/DRI. The DRI values for magnesium are listed in Table 22–4. Oral magnesium supplements are FDA approved for use in the treatment and prevention of hypomagnesemia.[19] The recommended UL for magnesium is 350 mg/day for older children and adults.[14]

Safety Considerations. No evidence is available to suggest that oral intake of magnesium is harmful to individuals with normal renal function, although diarrhea may occur with large doses. Hypermagnesemia can occur with overzealous use of magnesium sulfate (Epsom salts) or magnesium hydroxide (milk of magnesia) as a laxative, or with use of magnesium-containing antacids in patients with severe renal failure. Hypermagnesemia may cause diminished deep tendon reflexes and varying degrees of muscle weakness, lethargy, and sedation. These effects may progress to stupor and coma, especially at high serum concentrations. Cardiovascular symptoms may include hypotension and dysrhythmia.

Potential Drug–Nutrient Interactions. See Table 22–8.

Phosphorus

Phosphorus is present throughout the body, but approximately 85% of the body's store is located in bone.

Function. Phosphorus is essential for many metabolic processes. It serves as an integral structural component of the bone matrix as calcium phosphate, and it is a functional component of phospholipids, carbohydrates, nucleoproteins, and high-energy nucleotides. Plasma phosphate levels are under the tight biologic control of parathyroid hormone, calcitonin, and vitamin D. DNA and RNA structures contain sugar-phosphate linkages. Cell membranes contain phospholipids, which regulate the transport of solutes into and out of the cell. Many metabolic processes depend on phosphorylation. The adenosine diphosphate (ADP)–ATP system (which provides a mechanism for the storage and release of energy for use in all of the body's metabolic processes) involves phosphorus compounds. Additionally, an important buffer system of the body consists of inorganic phosphates.

Calcium and phosphorus have a reciprocal relationship. Both minerals are regulated partially by parathyroid hormone. Secretion of parathyroid hormone stimulates an increase in serum calcium levels through increased bone resorption, gut absorption, and reabsorption in renal tubules. Parathyroid hormone also causes a decrease in the reabsorption of phosphate by the kidney. Therefore, when serum calcium is high, serum phosphate is generally low, and vice versa.

Dietary Sources. Phosphorus is present in nearly all foods, especially protein-rich foods and cereal grains (Table 22–6).

Deficiency. Because nearly all foods contain phosphorus, deficiency states usually do not occur unless induced. For example, patients receiving aluminum hydroxide as an antacid for prolonged periods may exhibit hypophosphatemia, characterized by weakness, anorexia, malaise, pain, and bone loss. Aluminum binds dietary phosphorus, forming insoluble and poorly absorbed complexes.

Dose/DRI. The DRI values for phosphorus are listed in Table 22–4. The FDA-approved use for phosphorus is to alleviate signs and symptoms of deficiency. The recommended UL for phosphorus is 4 grams/day for older children and most adults.[14]

Safety Considerations. GI side effects (e.g., diarrhea and stomach pain) have been reported with oral supplementation of phosphate salts.

Potential Drug–Nutrient Interactions. See Table 22–8.

Trace Elements

Trace elements, which are present in minute quantities in plant and animal tissue, are considered essential for numerous physiologic processes. Zinc and manganese are trace elements. "Ultratrace" minerals have been defined as those elements with an estimated dietary requirement of less than 1 mg/day. The essential ultratrace minerals include arsenic, boron, cobalt, copper, chromium, iodine, molybdenum, nickel, selenium, and silicon. Lithium and vanadium possibly are essential minerals, but further study is required. Bromine, cadmium, fluorine, lead, and tin are not considered essential.

Chromium

Approximately 5 mg chromium is present in the normal adult, and levels are known to decline with age.

Function. Chromium is a component of glucose tolerance factor. This dietary organic chromium complex potentiates the activity of insulin.

Chromium combines with picolinic acid (a metabolite of tryptophan) to form chromium picolinate (a form of chromium with enhanced bioavailability). Chromium picolinate in doses of 200 mcg/day, has been promoted for the general population as an aid in controlling diabetes, lowering cholesterol, producing weight loss, and increasing muscle mass. However, reliable data are insufficient to support any therapeutic value of chromium supplementation in the absence of a diagnosed deficiency.

Dietary Sources. See Table 22–6.

Deficiency. Deficiency of trivalent chromium (the chemical form present in the diet) is manifested by glucose intolerance, elevated circulating insulin, glycosuria, fasting hyperglycemia, elevated serum cholesterol and triglycerides, neuropathy, and encephalopathy.

Dose/DRI. Chromium intake in the United States is low (about 50 mcg/day) compared with that of other countries. The estimated DRI values for chromium are listed in Table 22–4. Oral administration of trivalent chromium has a relatively high margin of safety, and no UL for chromium has been set.[14]

Safety Considerations. Oral chromium has not been reported to be toxic. However, the hexavalent forms of chromium can be toxic and carcinogenic. These forms are encountered through industrial exposure and may enter the body through inhalation or cutaneous absorption.

Potential Drug–Nutrient Interactions. Drug interactions have not been reported for chromium.

Cobalt

Cobalt is an essential component of vitamin B_{12}.

Function. Cobalt's nutritional functions are the same as those for cyanocobalamin and are discussed in the section(see Cyanocobalamin [Vitamin B_{12}]).

Dietary Sources. Cobalt is an integral part of vitamin B_{12}; therefore, the normal dietary sources of cobalt are the same as for vitamin B_{12} (Table 22–6).

Deficiency. No deficiency state for cobalt is reported to exist in humans.

Dose/DRI. No DRI values exist for cobalt.

Safety Considerations. Large doses of cobalt may result in goiter, congestive heart failure, and myxedema. Cardiomyopathy has also been described. Cyanosis and coma may result from accidental ingestion by children.

Potential Drug–Nutrient Interactions. No interactions have been reported with cobalt.

Copper

Copper ions exist in two states: the cuprous ion and the cupric ion (a potent oxidizing agent). Copper is similar to zinc in the complexes it forms with a number of the same chelating agents. Copper is found in virtually all tissues of the body, but concentrations are highest in the liver, brain, heart, and kidney.

Function. Copper is essential for the proper structure and function of the CNS, and it plays a major role in iron metabolism. Ceruloplasmin, one of the copper metalloenzymes, is especially important in converting absorbed ferrous iron to transported ferric iron. Other copper-containing enzymes are cytochrome oxidase, dopamine beta-hydroxylase, and superoxide dismutase.

Dietary Sources. See Table 22–6.

Deficiency. Copper deficiency is uncommon in humans, with a few notable exceptions. Deficiencies have been observed in premature infants; in severely malnourished infants that are fed milk-based, low-copper diets; following Roux-En-Y gastric bypass in individuals who do not consume a supplement; and in patients receiving parenteral nutrition with inadequate copper.

One of the prominent features of copper deficiency is impaired iron absorption, which results in hypochromic anemia. Spontaneous rupture of major vessels may also be observed in deficiency states.

Dose/DRI. The DRI values for copper are listed in Table 22–4. For protection against possible hepatotoxicity, the recommended UL for copper is 10 mg/day for adults.[14]

Safety Considerations. Copper sulfate doses in excess of 250 mg produce vomiting.

Wilson's disease is an inborn error of metabolism resulting in copper retention. These individuals must avoid any copper supplementation. Wilson's disease results in CNS, kidney, and liver damage. Acute symptoms of copper toxicity include nausea, vomiting, diarrhea, hemolysis, convulsions, and GI bleeding. Symptoms respond to treatment with penicillamine.

Supplementation should be avoided in patients with severe hepatic dysfunction or cholestasis, as biliary clearance of copper may be compromised.

Potential Drug–Nutrient Interactions. See Table 22–8.

Fluoride

Available therapeutic forms of fluoride include sodium fluoride, acidulated phosphate fluoride, and stannous fluoride. Sodium fluoride contains about 45% fluoride ion, whereas stannous fluoride contains about 24% fluoride ion.

Function. Fluoride occurs normally in bones and tooth enamel as a calcium salt. Intake of small amounts has been shown to reduce tooth decay markedly, presumably by making the enamel more resistant to the erosive action of acids produced by bacteria in the oral cavity.

Dietary Sources. Fluoride is present in soil and water, but the content varies widely from region to region. Most municipal water supplies are fluoridated to 1 ppm of fluoride, a level that has been shown to be safe and to reduce dental caries in children by nearly 50%. Estimates of fluoride intake from food, beverages, and water vary greatly, depending on the presence of fluoridated drinking water.

Deficiency. Fluoride deficiency states in humans, other than potential dental decay, have not been described.

Dose/DRI. The DRI values for fluoride are listed in Table 22–4. The recommended UL for this trace element is 10 mg/day for older children and adults.[14]

Fluoride is FDA approved for use in the prevention of dental caries.[19] Fluoride is a normal constituent of the diet, given that it occurs in soils, water supplies, plants, and animals. All sources of fluoride should be evaluated before supplementation is recommended for children whose home water supply is low in fluoride. Children may obtain fluoride from other water sources (e.g., day care or school) or from other beverages (e.g., soft drinks, juices, and bottled water that may contain varying amounts of fluoride).[54]

Sodium fluoride is available by prescription as oral tablets and solutions, topical solutions, and gels, as well as in combination products. Nonprescription topical rinses containing fluoride 0.01%–0.02% (e.g., sodium fluoride) and gels containing 0.4% stannous fluoride (e.g., Gel-Kam) are rinsed or brushed onto the teeth to reduce sensitivity and prevent dental cavities.

Safety Considerations. Excessive fluoride can be toxic. Acute toxicity should not result from the low levels present in drinking water but may result from the administration of excessive doses of fluoride supplements. Because acute toxicity affects the GI system and the CNS, it can be life threatening. Symptoms include salivation, GI distress, muscle weakness, tremors, and (rarely) seizures. Because fluoride binds calcium, symptoms of calcium deficiency (including tetany) may also be seen. Eventually, respiratory and cardiac failure may occur. All accidental ingestions of fluoride in children should be referred for evaluation by a medical practitioner or Poison Control Center, as fluoride intoxication may be fatal. Treatment includes precipitation of the fluoride by using gastric lavage with calcium hydroxide 0.15% solution, intravenous administration of dextrose and saline for hydration, and treatment with calcium to prevent tetany.

Chronic fluoride toxicity is manifested as changes in the structure of bones and teeth. Tooth enamel, if still under development, acquires a mottled appearance consisting of white, patchy plaques occurring with pitting brown stains. Prolonged ingestion of water that contains more than 2 ppm of fluoride has resulted in a significant incidence of mottling. Extremely large doses (e.g., 20–80 mg/day) have resulted in chalky, brittle bones that tend to fracture easily, a condition known as crippling skeletal fluorosis.

Potential Drug–Nutrient Interactions. See Table 22–8.

Iodine

The thyroid gland contains about one-third of the iodine in the body, stored in the form of a complex glycoprotein, thyroglobulin. The only known function of thyroglobulin is to provide thyroxine and triiodothyronine, which are hormones that regulate the metabolic rate of cells, thereby influencing physical and mental growth, nervous and muscle tissue function, circulatory activity, and nutrient utilization.

Function. Iodine is an essential micronutrient required to synthesize thyroxine and triiodothyronine. High concentrations of iodine inhibit the release of these hormones.

Dietary Sources. The primary dietary source of iodine is iodized salt, which contains 1 part of sodium or potassium iodide per 10,000 parts (0.01%) of salt. A dose of about 95 mcg of iodine can be obtained from about one-fourth teaspoon of salt (1.25 grams). In the United States, most of the table salt sold is iodized; however, salt used in food processing and for institutional use is not. Additional dietary sources of iodine include saltwater fish and shellfish. Produce may also be a source of iodine; the iodine content of produce reflects that of the soil in which it was grown.

Deficiency. A moderate iodine deficiency can lead to thyroid hypertrophy, resulting in goiter; severe deficiency results in

hypothyroidism. The consumption of foods from diverse locations and the addition of iodide to table salt have essentially eliminated goiter as a health problem in the United States.

Dose/DRI. Because of the fortification of salt, the iodine content of typical diets in the United States is still well above the DRI values for adults (Table 22–4). Iodine supplements are unwarranted for most individuals. Potassium iodide is available as a tablet, syrup, and solution, and it is included in various combination products.

Safety Considerations. Some individuals are allergic to iodine or organic preparations containing iodine and may develop a rash. Symptoms of chronic iodism (iodine intoxication) may include an unpleasant taste and burning in the mouth or throat, along with soreness of the teeth or gums. Increased salivation, sneezing, eye irritation, and eyelid swelling can occur. In addition, prolonged use of iodine supplementation can result in hypothyroidism.[18] A UL of 1.1 mg/day in adults has been recommended.[14]

Potential Drug–Nutrient Interactions. See Table 22–8.

Manganese

The body concentrates its stores of manganese in the liver, pancreas, kidney, muscle, and bone.

Function. Manganese is required for the utilization of glucose; the synthesis of mucopolysaccharides of cartilage; the biosynthesis of steroids, cholesterol, and fatty acids; and the biological activity of pyruvate carboxylase.

Dietary Sources. Manganese is widely available in foods; primary dietary sources are listed in Table 22–6.

Deficiency. Manganese deficiency is extremely rare, and the only theorized method of manganese deficiency is insufficient dietary intake.

Dose/DRI. Manganese is poorly absorbed after oral administration; however, sufficient quantities are present in the average diet to maintain appropriate levels. A supplemental dose or dietary intake of 2 to 5 mg/day is considered safe and adequate. The estimated RDAs for manganese are listed in Table 22–4. The recommended UL of 11 mg/day in adults is based on data that showed no adverse effects with long-term consumption at this level.[14]

Safety Considerations. Toxicity is rare for orally administered manganese. Toxicity has been observed, however, from inhalation of dust and industrial fumes containing manganese. Intravenous administration has resulted in toxicity from accumulation of manganese in the brain. Because of the reduced biliary clearance of manganese in patients with severe liver dysfunction or cholestasis, supplementation should be avoided under those conditions.

Potential Drug–Nutrient Interactions. Drug–manganese interactions have not been reported.

Molybdenum

Molybdenum is an ultratrace mineral that only rarely has been associated with deficiency. Practitioners monitoring patients on long-term parenteral nutrition must be aware of the potential for deficiency in this population.

Function. Molybdenum readily changes its oxidation state and acts as an electron transfer agent in oxidation-reduction reactions. It may also function as an enzyme cofactor and is involved in the metabolism of sulfur and purines.

Dietary Sources. The molybdenum content of food varies depending on its growth environment and/or food source. Dietary sources of molybdenum are listed in Table 22–6.

Deficiency. Molybdenum is a cofactor for several flavoprotein enzymes and is found in xanthine oxidase. Because xanthine oxidase is involved in the oxidation of xanthine to uric acid, high molybdenum intake has been associated with gout-like symptoms. Symptoms of molybdenum deficiency may include tachycardia, tachypnea, headache, lethargy, and disorientation. Congenital deficiency of specific molybdenum cofactors results in severe neurologic dysfunction and mental retardation.

Dose/DRI/Safety Considerations. The human molybdenum requirement is low and is easily furnished by the average diet (Table 22–4). Supplements are rarely warranted. On the basis of animal studies showing impaired reproduction and growth with prolonged intake of excessive molybdenum, a UL of 2 mg/day in adults is recommended.[14]

Potential Drug–Nutrient Interactions. No significant drug interactions have been reported with molybdenum.

Selenium

Selenium is present in all tissues and is generally incorporated into organic compounds involving amino acids (e.g., methionine or cysteine). Selenium compounds are about 80% absorbed. The highest concentrations are in the kidneys and liver; the lowest are in the lungs and brain. The kidney is the primary route of excretion, although losses can also occur through the GI tract.

Function. Selenium is an antioxidant that serves as part of glutathione peroxidase. This enzyme protects cells from the peroxidase-induced oxidative damage that occurs with cellular metabolism. The antioxidant properties of selenium have prompted evaluation for its use in cancer prevention. Numerous animal and in vitro studies indicate selenium may have anticarcinogenic effects, although human studies to-date indicate mixed results and inconsistent findings as to which individuals may benefit from selenium supplementation.[55]

Additional trials evaluating the role of selenium in cancer risk reduction are warranted.

Dietary Sources. See Table 22–6. The selenium content of food depends on the soil in which the plants are grown.

Deficiency. Selenium is an essential trace element in humans, but deficiencies are not common in the general population. Selenium deficiency has been reported in patients with alcoholic cirrhosis, likely resulting from dietary insufficiency or altered selenium metabolism. Deficiency has been rarely reported in patients on long-term parenteral nutrition. Limited evidence in humans suggests that deficiency results in cardiomyopathy, musculoskeletal pain, bleaching of the hair and skin, and abnormal nail beds. Epidemiologic studies suggest that cancer and heart disease may be common in areas of low selenium availability. Keshan disease (a cardiomyopathy that occurs almost exclusively in children) has been shown to respond to selenium.

Dose/DRI. The DRI values for selenium are listed in Table 22–4. The UL for this mineral in adolescents and adults is 400 mcg/day.[14]

Safety Considerations. Toxic effects of selenium may include loss of hair and nails, skin lesions, muscular weakness, fatigue, and CNS abnormalities.

Potential Drug–Nutrient Interactions. No significant drug interactions with selenium have been reported.

Zinc

Zinc is an integral part of at least 70 metalloenzymes, including carbonic anhydrase, lactic dehydrogenase, alkaline phosphatase, carboxypeptidase, aminopeptidase, and alcohol dehydrogenase.

Function. Zinc is a cofactor in the synthesis of DNA and RNA. It is involved in the mobilization of vitamin A from the liver and in the enhancement of follicle-stimulating hormone and luteinizing hormone. Zinc is essential for normal cellular immune functions, as well as for spermatogenesis and normal testicular function. It is also important in the stabilization of membrane structure.

The divalent ion is most commonly found and used in the body. Zinc has a relatively rapid turnover rate. The balance between zinc absorption from the small intestine and excretion through the feces is efficiently regulated by the body. Vegetarians may require higher amounts of zinc because diets high in fiber and phytates hinder zinc absorption.

Dietary Sources. Most dietary zinc (about 70%) is derived from animal products (Table 22–6).

Deficiency. Zinc deficiency is not widespread in the United States. Marginally low zinc values have been associated with birth defects, growth retardation in children, and slow wound healing in adults. Additional symptoms include immunologic abnormalities, impaired taste and smell, delayed sexual maturation, hypogonadism, hypospermia, and dermatitis.

Malabsorptive syndromes, infection, major surgery, alcoholism, pregnancy, lactation, and high-fiber diets rich in phytates predispose individuals to zinc deficiency. Zinc depletion is relatively rare but may be seen in patients on long-term parenteral nutrition and in patients with GI tract abnormalities (e.g., fistulas and prolonged, severe diarrhea).

Zinc deficiencies adversely affect DNA, RNA, carbohydrate, and protein catabolism. Iron supplements decrease zinc absorption just as zinc supplements decrease iron absorption, likely resulting from competition for the same transport system. If these minerals are taken with a meal, the adverse interaction is less pronounced. In patients with impaired wound healing, zinc supplementation may be marginally beneficial.

Dose/DRI. The DRI values for zinc are listed in Table 22–4. Typical Western diets supply 10–15 mg of zinc per day. Because only 10%–40% of zinc is absorbed from the GI tract, ingestion of zinc sulfate 220 mg (50 mg of elemental zinc) will supply 5–20 mg of zinc. Treatment of suspected deficiencies usually involves short-term administration of elemental zinc. Patients with large GI losses through fistulas, ostomies, or stool require larger supplemental doses of zinc. At doses above 40 mg elemental zinc per day, copper deficiency may be induced. On the basis of this interaction, the UL for elemental zinc is 40 mg daily in adults if therapy with zinc is going to be long term.[14] Absorption of zinc supplements may be reduced if taken with foods high in calcium or phosphorus.

Zinc has been evaluated in numerous studies as a potential treatment for the common cold. However, zinc formulations and doses have varied, and trial results have been conflicting. Insufficient evidence exists at this time to recommend zinc supplementation for the treatment or prevention of the common cold.[56]

Safety Considerations. Because ingestion of 2 grams or more of zinc sulfate has resulted in GI irritation and vomiting, zinc should be taken with food. Zinc is also toxic; however, the emetic effect that occurs after consumption of large amounts may minimize problems with accidental overdose. Reported signs of zinc toxicity in humans include vomiting, dehydration, poor muscle coordination, dizziness, and abdominal pain.

Potential Drug–Nutrient Interactions.   See Table 22–8.

Multivitamin and Multimineral Supplements

Multivitamin and multimineral supplements, as previously described, are not intended to supplant a healthy, balanced diet but rather to augment dietary sources and support general health. Specific nutrients of concern for inadequate intake specified by the *2010 Dietary Guidelines for Americans* include dietary calcium, vitamin D, and potassium.[13] However, multivitamin and multimineral supplements do not target these or any specific nutrients, but rather provide a broad range of micronutrients. When such a product is being evaluated for an individual, the practitioner should consider recommending a preparation that contains the basic and essential vitamins and minerals, including the following: vitamins C, B_1 (thiamin), B_2 (riboflavin), B_3 (niacin), B_6 (pyridoxine), B_9 (folic acid), B_5 (pantothenic acid), A, E, D_2 or D_3 (cholecalciferol), and K, as well as biotin, potassium, iodine, selenium, borate, zinc, calcium, magnesium, manganese, molybdenum, and beta carotene. The multitude of different multivitamin products available over-the-counter warrant further consideration of an individual's age and sex to assure selection of a formulation that is most likely to meet individual nutritional needs. Most multivitamins formulated for women ages 18–50 years contain increased amounts of iron and folic acid to prevent anemia related to menstrual blood loss and neural tube defects in those of child-bearing age. Multivitamins formulated for men younger than 50 generally contain higher amounts of certain vitamins and less iron. Finally, senior multivitamins formulated for individuals older than age 50 may contain more calcium and certain B vitamins (like B_6 and B_{12}) but do not contain iron. Individuals should be reminded to refer to the product labeling for directions for use and not to exceed the recommended intake.

Assessment of Nutritional Adequacy: A Case-Based Approach

Assessing an individual's nutritional status is difficult in the ambulatory environment. Clinical impressions are often erroneous, given that the stages between well-nourished and poorly nourished states are not readily evident. However, guidelines may help provide a more objective assessment of an individual's nutritional status. Practitioners should exercise good observational skills, know which questions yield helpful information (see cases for examples of questions), and know which population groups tend to be at risk for particular deficiencies. By asking key questions, the practitioner may detect cultural, physical, environmental, and social conditions that suggest inadequate

vitamin intake. The more specific the information obtained from the individual, the more helpful the practitioner can be in determining the need for nutritional supplementation. Questions about the absence of food-types in the diet and about previous treatment of similar symptoms may also be important.

Although most nutritional assessment measures are beyond the scope of routine pharmacy practice, the pharmacist can observe the physical status of the patient. For example, an individual's fingernails may indicate malnutrition if the nails are not lustrous and are dark at the upper ends. The texture, amount, and appearance of hair may indicate the patient's nutritional status. The eyes (particularly the conjunctiva) may indicate vitamin A and iron deficiencies. The mouth may show stomatitis, glossitis, or hypertrophic or pale gums. Poor dentition may limit the foods that an individual is able to eat, thereby compromising intake from certain food groups, such as protein. Visible goiter, poor skin color and texture, obesity or thinness relative to bone structure, and the presence of edema may also indicate malnutrition. The pharmacist should be able to recognize overt but nonspecific symptoms of vitamin and mineral deficiencies for which prompt referral to a primary care provider may be crucial. Additionally, pharmacists should refer individuals at risk for nutritional deficiency or with increased metabolic demands (e.g., the elderly, chronic alcohol abusers, and pregnant and lactating women) for appropriate medical evaluation as necessary.

Checking a patient's medication history is important because of the number of potential drug–micronutrient interactions (Table 22–8). Practitioners are also responsible for referring patients with a suspected serious illness to a primary care provider. Just as nutritional deficiencies may lead to disease, disease may lead to nutritional deficiencies. Patients may present with one or more deficiencies, which may be very difficult to identify. Rarely in the United States do practitioners encounter patients with severe deficiencies resulting in diseases such as scurvy, pellagra, or beriberi. However, milder forms of malnutrition may be seen.

Cases 22–1 and 22–2 are examples of the assessment of patients with nutritional inadequacy.

Patient Counseling for Nutrient Supplementation

The public is often exposed to exaggerated and fraudulent claims concerning vitamin products. The practitioner should keep up with medical and pharmaceutical literature and should not support or appear to support claims until they are substantiated by reliable clinical studies. Patients inquiring about such claims should be educated regarding increased potential risk with nontraditional use of vitamins.

Patients purchasing a nonprescription liquid dietary supplement should be instructed on its proper use and storage, including dilution and preparation techniques. In addition, the practitioner should counsel the patient on possible adverse effects (e.g., diarrhea or constipation).

The box Patient Education for Nutritional Deficiencies lists specific information to provide patients. The practitioner could also refer the consumer to Web sites and printed literature with evidence-based recommendations for vitamin and mineral supplementation, such as those listed in the reference section of this chapter.

case

22–1

Relevant Evaluation Criteria	Scenario/Model Outcome
Information Gathering	

1. Gather essential information about the patient's symptoms and medical history, including:

   a. description of symptom(s) (i.e., nature, onset, duration, severity, associated symptoms)

   Patient inquires about information found in a magazine that touted supplementation with various vitamins to help prevent cancer. He indicates that he currently takes Centrum Silver each day along with his other prescription medications.

   b. description of any factors that seem to precipitate, exacerbate, and/or relieve the patient's symptom(s)

   NA

   c. description of the patient's efforts to relieve the symptoms

   NA

   d. patient's identity

   Patrick McLaughlin

   e. age, sex, height, and weight

   68 years old, male, 6 ft 3 in., 190 lb

   f. patient's occupation

   Retired school teacher; widowed

   g. patient's dietary habits

   Eats alone: typically cereal, milk, and juice or fruit for breakfast; soup or sandwich for lunch; easy meals for dinner (e.g., frozen dinners with protein, starch, vegetable).

   h. patient's sleep habits

   NA

   i. concurrent medical conditions, prescription and non-prescription medications, and dietary supplements

   Patient has a history of heartburn, high cholesterol, and high blood pressure. Every morning he takes pantoprazole 40 mg; the combination hydrochlorothiazide/lisinopril 12.5/20 mg; 2 omega-3 fish oil capsules; and 1 Centrum Silver multivitamin. After dinner, he takes atorvastatin 40 mg. When he has a migraine, he takes acetaminophen 1000 mg plus aspirin 650 mg.[a]

   j. allergies

   Sulfa

   k. history of other adverse reactions to medications

   NA

| **Assessment and Triage** | |

2. Differentiate patient's signs/symptoms and correctly identify the patient's primary problem(s).

   The patient's age and dietary habits may warrant consideration of a multivitamin supplement. Evidence from a recent large-scale study indicated men taking a daily senior multivitamin experienced a reduction in cancer risk; however, cancer is a multifactorial disease. No evidence to date supports the use of multivitamins to completely negate cancer risk.[57]

3. Identify exclusions for self-treatment.

   None

4. Formulate a comprehensive list of therapeutic alternatives for the primary problem to determine if triage to a medical provider is required, and share this information with the patient or caregiver.

   Options include:

   (1) Assess the client's perceived need for the nutrient supplements.

   (2) Evaluate dietary intake from food groups, encouraging at least 5 servings of produce, 3 servings of low-fat dairy products, 2 servings of protein, and 6 servings of whole-grain food sources daily.

   (3) Discuss which nutrients may need supplementation on the basis of the patient's patterns of dietary intake, age, and special requirements. Evaluate Centrum Silver for adequacy, while avoiding intakes above the UL.

   (4) Discuss the lack of data and potential harm associated with mega doses of vitamins.

   (5) Take no action.

case
22-1 continued

Relevant Evaluation Criteria	Scenario/Model Outcome

Plan

5. Select an optimal therapeutic alternative to address the patient's problem, taking into account patient preferences.

Regular intake of a well-balanced diet that includes fruit, vegetables, whole grains, and low fat dairy and lean protein sources is recommended for patients with high blood pressure. A multivitamin and mineral supplement that includes vitamin B_{12} and a balance of other nutrients would be reasonable for this elderly patient who needs simple, easy meals and is on chronic acid suppression therapy. He should also be evaluated for adequate calcium and vitamin D intake.

6. Describe the recommended therapeutic approach to the patient or caregiver.

"A nutrient-rich diet, as described, has been shown to be beneficial in the prevention of many diseases, including hypertension and cancer. This could be done by adding a fruit or vegetable to your mid-day meal or as a snack. Choose whole grain breads and cereals. Look for healthy frozen meals and soups as opposed to those with much hidden fat and salt. It would be reasonable to continue your daily multivitamin supplement to ensure you are meeting daily nutritional needs. If you are not regularly consuming dairy products, calcium and vitamin D supplementation is recommended. Check your intake from supplemented products, such as some orange juice brands, and the multivitamin as well."

7. Explain to the patient or caregiver the rationale for selecting the recommended therapeutic approach from the considered therapeutic alternatives.

"There is no evidence that vitamin supplements, in the absence of deficiency, can completely reduce cancer risk. In the recent study alluded to, the effect of the multivitamin on cancer risk reduction was observed only in those men without a family history of cancer; men having a family history of cancer did not experience the same benefit. Furthermore, authors found no difference on the incidence of a specific type of cancer or on the incidence of cancer-related mortality between the treatment and placebo groups.[57] When selecting a multivitamin, be sure to compare the level of supplementation of each nutrient, including calcium and vitamin D, compared with the DRI. Additional supplementation in excess of the DRI is often unnecessary unless specifically recommended by your doctor."

Patient Education

8. When recommending self-care with nonprescription medications and/or nondrug therapy, convey accurate information to the patient or caregiver:

   a. appropriate dose and frequency of administration

"Consider one USP-approved senior multivitamin daily that contains no more than 100% of DRI for nutrients."

   b. maximum number of days the therapy should be employed

NA

   c. product administration procedures

"You may take your multivitamin with your current medications in the morning. However, check with your pharmacist about taking your vitamin with any newly prescribed medications."

Solicit follow-up questions from the patient or caregiver.

"What about antioxidant vitamins? Do they prevent cancer?"

Answer the patient's or caregiver's questions.

"Data from well-designed trials do not support antioxidant supplementation for the prevention or treatment of cancer. In fact, some trials have suggested potential harm is associated with supplementation of vitamins A, E, and C, selenium, and other nutrients in relation to cancer risk. Therefore, dosing of these nutrients above the DRI cannot be recommended at this time."

Evaluation of Patient Outcome

9. Assess patient outcome

Enquire about patient's compliance with multivitamin recommendations and dietary modification. If necessary, reinforce the recommendations.

Key: DRI = Dietary reference intake; NA = not applicable; UL = upper intake level; USP = United States Pharmacopeia.
[a] See Chapter 5, Acetaminophen and Table 5–3, for information on the manufacturer's voluntary reduction of maximum daily dosages of Tylenol products sold in the United States.

case
22–2

Relevant Evaluation Criteria	Scenario/Model Outcome

Information Gathering

1. Gather essential information about the patient's symptoms and medical history, including:

a. description of symptom(s) (i.e., nature, onset, duration, severity, associated symptoms)

Patient's daughter approaches the pharmacy counter seeking a recommendation. She reports her elderly mother recently fell at home; she believes that if her mother falls again, her mother may fracture her hip. She wants her mother to start a calcium and vitamin D supplement after reading that such supplements can reduce fracture risk.

b. description of any factors that seem to precipitate, exacerbate, and/or relieve the patient's symptom(s)

NA

c. description of the patient's efforts to relieve the symptoms

NA

d. patient's identity

Elizabeth Small

e. age, sex, height, and weight

84 years old, female, 5 ft 4 in., 110 lb

f. patient's occupation

Homemaker; grandmother

g. patient's dietary habits

Eggs, juice, and tea with milk for breakfast; soup or a sandwich for lunch; easy-to-prepare microwavable meals for dinner

h. patient's sleep habits

NA

i. concurrent medical conditions, prescription and nonprescription medications, and dietary supplements

Suffers from high blood pressure, gastroesophageal reflux disease, insomnia, and depression.

Each morning, Mrs. Small takes enalapril 2.5 mg and omeprazole 40 mg. At bedtime, she takes mirtazapine 30 mg and zolpidem 5 mg as needed.

j. allergies

NKA

k. other (describe)

Family history of glaucoma and osteoporosis

Assessment and Triage

2. Differentiate patient's signs/symptoms and correctly identify the patient's primary problem(s).

According to recent warnings, use of chronic acid suppressive medications can reduce dietary calcium intake and potentially increase fracture risk. Furthermore, given Mrs. Small's history of a fall and family history of osteoporosis, she may warrant further medical evaluation.

3. Identify exclusions for self-treatment.

None

4. Formulate a comprehensive list of therapeutic alternatives for the primary problem to determine if triage to a medical provider is required, and share this information with the patient or caregiver.

Options include:

(1) Focus on potential drug–nutrient interactions in counseling her daughter about need for calcium supplementation.

(2) Discuss the role of balanced nutrition as the ideal route of taking vitamins and minerals. Identify nutritional needs unique to this client and where supplementation may be recommended.

(3) Refer Mrs. Small for medical evaluation and osteoporosis screening. Given her age, body habitus, and family history of osteoporosis, coupled with her recent history of non-traumatic fall and chronic use of acid suppressive therapy, she may be at an increased risk of osteoporosis and bone fracture.

(4) Take no action.

Plan

5. Select an optimal therapeutic alternative to address the patient's problem, taking into account patient preferences.

Assess the client's perceived need for the nutrient supplements.

Evaluate dietary intake from food groups, encouraging at least 5 servings of produce, 3 servings of low-fat dairy products, 2 servings of protein, and 6 servings of whole-grain food sources daily.

case
22-2 *continued*

Relevant Evaluation Criteria	Scenario/Model Outcome
6. Describe the recommended therapeutic approach to the patient or caregiver.	Discuss the vitamin and mineral content of the various supplements and the total intake in comparison with the DRIs.
	"For a woman of your mother's age, a daily calcium and vitamin D intake of 1200 mg and 800 IU, respectively, is indicated. Speak with a health care provider about your mother's potential risk for osteoporosis and fracture."
7. Explain to the patient or caregiver the rationale for selecting the recommended therapeutic approach from the considered therapeutic alternatives.	"Calcium and vitamin D supplementation alone may not be sufficient intervention to reduce your mother's risk of fracture from a fall if she has underlying osteoporosis. Further, her need for chronic acid suppressive therapy may further increase this risk and complicate her management. Calcium absorption from both dietary and supplement forms may be affected by stomach acid production; suppression of acid with medications like omeprazole may result in impaired calcium absorption. Alternate forms of calcium are available for supplementation; however, asking your mother's PCP whether continued use of acid suppressive therapy is also warranted."
Patient Education	
8. When recommending self-care with nonprescription medications and/or nondrug therapy, convey accurate information to the patient or caregiver.	Criterion does not apply in this case.
Evaluation of Patient Outcome	
9. Assess patient outcome	Enquire about the patient's compliance with multivitamin recommendations and dietary modifications. If necessary, reinforce the recommendations

Key: DRI = Dietary reference intake; NA = not applicable; NKA = no known allergies; PCP = primary care provider; UL = upper intake level; USP = United States Pharmacopeia.

patient education for
Nutritional Deficiencies

The objective of self-treatment is to prevent nutritional deficiencies or maintain present nutritional status. For most patients, carefully following product instructions and the self-care measures listed here will help ensure optimal therapeutic outcomes.

Vitamins, Minerals, and Trace Elements

- To ensure proper nutrition, eat a varied diet as recommended in *MyPlate* (Figure 22–1). Vitamin supplements are not a substitute for a well-balanced diet.
- Read labels on all vitamin and mineral preparations carefully before taking them. Note the quantity of vitamins and minerals required to meet the DRI, or dietary reference intake, values.
- Do not take doses of vitamins and minerals higher than the recommended DRIs. High doses of vitamins or minerals may be dangerous and should not be taken indiscriminately.
- Take vitamin and mineral supplements with meals if you experience gastrointestinal symptoms.
- Women of childbearing age should take 400 mcg of supplemental folic acid in addition to a well-balanced diet. This has been shown to reduce the risk of neural tube defects in the fetus.

- Be aware that iron supplements or vitamins with iron may turn the stool black. This occurrence is not a cause for alarm, unless it is associated with other symptoms consistent with a gastrointestinal bleed.
- As with any medicine, store vitamin and combination vitamin/mineral supplements out of the reach of children, especially if the product contains iron. Teach children that vitamins are drugs and potential poisons and therefore cannot be taken indiscriminately.
- Be aware that therapeutic use of niacin-containing products (but not niacinamide) may cause a flushing, itching, or tingling sensation, which should decrease in intensity with continued therapy. Taking an aspirin or nonsteroidal anti-inflammatory agent 30–60 minutes before taking niacin may help decrease these effects.
- Do not self-medicate if you suspect a vitamin deficiency; consult a health care practitioner instead.

Evaluation of Patient Outcomes for Nutritional Adequacy

Nutritional therapy should involve a diet that is based on *MyPlate* and possibly the use of nutritional supplements. The practitioner should advise patients to return 30 days after implementing nutritional therapy (or sooner, if symptoms worsen). Patients whose symptoms have worsened should be referred to a primary care provider. Patients whose symptoms have improved while taking nutritional supplements should be encouraged to eat a healthful diet and not to rely on supplements as the primary source for vitamins and minerals.

Key Points for Nutritional Adequacy

➤ The benefits of a varied, balanced diet in terms of health maintenance and disease prevention have been demonstrated repeatedly. However, the same benefits have not been observed when suboptimal dietary intake is augmented with vitamin and mineral supplementation.

➤ Practitioners can assess the variety of a patient's food choices by comparing the patient's typical food pattern to that recommended in *MyPlate*. The practitioner may refer patients to a registered dietitian for personalized and more complete counseling on diet modification as well as nutritional supplementation.

➤ Overt vitamin or mineral deficiencies are rare in this country; however, subclinical deficiencies may be contributing to chronic disease.

➤ Vitamin, mineral, or multivitamin/multimineral supplementation may be appropriate on the basis of the practitioner's assessment of the patient's dietary intake, metabolic requirements, absorptive capability, and potential drug–micronutrient interactions. However, supplementation should rarely exceed 100% of the DRI. Clinical trials continue to reveal unanticipated health risks with megadoses of various micronutrients.

REFERENCES

1. National Institutes of Health, Office of Dietary Supplements. Dietary supplement fact sheet: multivitamin/multimineral supplements. Accessed at http://ods.od.nih.gov/factsheets/MVMS-HealthProfessional/, September 27, 2013.
2. Gahche J, Bailey R, Burt V, et al. Dietary supplement use among U.S. adults has increased since NHANES III (1988–1994). *NCHS Data Brief.* 2011(61);61:1–8.
3. Bailey RL, Gahche JJ, Lentino CV, et al. Dietary supplement use in the United States, 2003–2006. *J Nutr.* 2011;141(2):261–6.
4. Troppmann L, Gray-Donald K, Johns T. Supplement use: is there any nutritional benefit? *J Am Diet Assoc.* 2002;102(6):818–25.
5. Martínez ME, Jacobs ET, Baron JA, et al. Dietary supplements and cancer prevention: balancing potential benefits against proven harms. *J Natl Cancer Inst.* 2012;104(10):732–9.
6. U.S. Preventive Services Task Force. *Routine Vitamin Supplementation to Prevent Cancer and Cardiovascular Disease: Recommendations and Rationale.* Rockville, MD: Agency for Healthcare Research and Quality; June 2003. Accessed at http://www.uspreventiveservicestaskforce.org/uspstf/uspsvita.htm, July 25, 2013.
7. Kushi LH, Doyle C, McCullough M, et al. American Cancer Society Guidelines on nutrition and physical activity for cancer prevention: reducing the risk of cancer with healthy food choices and physical activity. *CA Cancer J Clin.* 2012;62(1):30–67.
8. Neuhouser ML, Wassertheil-Smoller S, Thomson C, et al. Multivitamin use and risk of cancer and cardiovascular disease in the Women's Health Initiative cohorts. *Arch Intern Med.* 2009;169(3):294–304.
9. Coates PM, Dwyer JT, Thurn AL. Introduction to State-of-the-Science Conference: multivitamin/mineral supplements and chronic disease prevention. *Am J Clin Nutr.* 2007;85(1):255S–6S.
10. Wells JL, Dumbrell AC. Nutrition and aging: assessment and treatment of compromised nutritional status in frail elderly patients. *Clin Intervent Aging.* 2006;1(1):67–79.
11. Yetley EA. Multivitamin and multimineral dietary supplements: definitions, characterization, bioavailability, and drug interactions. *Am J Clin Nutr.* 2007;85(suppl):269S–76S.
12. U.S. Pharmacopeial Convention. USP verified dietary supplements. Accessed at http://www.usp.org/usp-verification-services/usp-verified-dietary-supplements, July 25, 2013.
13. U.S. Department of Agriculture, U.S. Department of Health and Human Services. *Dietary Guidelines for Americans, 2010.* 7th ed. Washington, DC: U.S. Government Printing Office; December 2010. Accessed at http://www.cnpp.usda.gov/dgas2010-policydocument.htm, July 25, 2013.
14. National Agricultural Library, United States Department of Agriculture. Dietary reference intakes tables. Accessed at http://fnic.nal.usda.gov/dietary-guidance/dietary-reference-intakes/dri-tables, July 26, 2013.
15. Institute of Medicine of the National Academies. Dietary reference intakes for calcium and vitamin D. Accessed at http://www.iom.edu/Reports/2010/Dietary-Reference-Intakes-for-Calcium-and-Vitamin-D.aspx, July 25, 2013.
16. U.S. Food and Drug Administration, Guidance for industry: a food labeling guide. Accessed at http://www.fda.gov/Food/GuidanceRegulation/GuidanceDocumentsRegulatoryInformation/LabelingNutrition/ucm064928.htm, August 1, 2013.
17. Centers for Disease Control and Prevention, National Center for Environmental Health, Division of Laboratory Sciences. Second National Report on Biochemical Indicators of Diet and Nutrition in the U.S. population, 2012. Accessed at http://www.cdc.gov/nutritionreport/, July 26, 2013.
18. Balint JP. Physical findings in nutritional deficiencies. *Pediatr Clin North Am.* 1998;45(1):245–60.
19. DRUGDEX® System (electronic version). Truven Health Analytics, Greenwood Village, Colorado, USA. Accessed at: http://www.micromedexsolutions.com/, July 26, 2013.
20. Feskanich D, Singh V, Willett W, et al. Vitamin A intake and hip fractures among postmenopausal women. *JAMA.* 2002;287(1):47–54.
21. The Alpha-Tocopherol, Beta Carotene Cancer Prevention Study Group. The effect of vitamin E and beta carotene on the incidence of lung cancer and other cancers in male smokers. *N Engl J Med.* 1994;330(15):1029–35.
22. Goodman GE, Thornquist MD, Balmes J, et al. The Beta-Carotene and Retinol Efficacy Trial: incidence of lung cancer and cardiovascular disease mortality during 6-year follow-up after stopping beta-carotene and retinol supplements. *J Natl Cancer Inst.* 2004;96(23):1743–50.
23. Avenell A, Gillespie WJ, Gillespie LD, et al. Vitamin D and vitamin D analogues for preventing fractures associated with involutional and postmenopausal osteoporosis. *Cochrane Database System Rev.* 2009;2:CD000227. DOI: 10.1002/14651858.CD000227.pub3. Accessed at http://www.thecochranelibrary.com/view/0/index.html.
24. Fosnight S, Zafirau W, Hazelett S. Vitamin D supplementation to prevent falls in the elderly: evidence and practical considerations. *Pharmacotherapy.* 2008;28(2):225–34.
25. Thacher TD, Clarke BL. Vitamin D insufficiency. *Mayo Clin Proc.* 2011; 86(1):50–60.
26. Vacek JL, Vanga SR, Good M, et al. Vitamin D deficiency and supplementation and relation to cardiovascular health. *Am J Cardiol.* 2012;109(3):359–63.
27. Gotsman I, Shauer A, Zwas DR, et al. Vitamin D deficiency is a predictor of reduced survival in patients with heart failure; vitamin D supplementation improves outcomes. *Eur J Heart Fail.* 2012;14(4):357–66.
28. Toner C, Davis C, Milner J. The vitamin D and cancer conundrum: aiming at a moving target. *J Am Diet Assoc.* 2010;110:1492–500.
29. Lee IM, Cook NR, Gaziano JM, et al. Vitamin E in the primary prevention of cardiovascular disease and cancer: the Women's Health Study: a randomized controlled trial. *JAMA.* 2005;294:56–65.

30. Issac MG, Quinn R, Tabet N. Vitamin E for Alzheimer's disease and mild cognitive impairment. *Cochrane Database Syst Rev.* 2008;3:CD002854. doi: 10.1002/14651858.CD002854.pub3. Accessed at http://www.the cochranelibrary.com/view/0/index.html.

31. Schurks M, Glynn RJ, Rist PM, et al. Effects of vitamin E on stroke subtypes: meta-analysis of randomized controlled trials. *BMJ.* 2010;341:c5702.

32. Bjelakovic G, Nikolova D, Gluud LL, et al. Antioxidant supplements for prevention of mortality in healthy participants and patients with various diseases. *Cochrane Database Syst Rev.* 2008;2:CD007176. doi: 10.1002/14651858.CD007176. Accessed at http://www.thecochraneli brary.com/view/0/index.html.

33. Xu H, Perez-Cuevas R, Xiong X, et al. An international trial of antioxidants in the prevention of preeclampsia (INTAPP). *Am J Obstet Gynecol.* 2010;202(3):239.e1–10.

34. Pearson DA. Bone health and osteoporosis: the role of vitamin K and potential antagonism by anticoagulants. *Nutr Clin Pract.* 2007;22(5):517–44.

35. Lykkesfelt J, Poulsen HE. Is vitamin C supplementation beneficial? Lessons learned from randomized controlled trials. *Br J Nutr.* 2010;103(9):1251–9.

36. Jacob RA, Sotoudeh G. Vitamin C function and status in chronic disease. *Nutr Clin Care.* 2002;5(2):47–9.

37. Clarke R, Halsey J, Lewington S, et al. Effects of lowering homocysteine levels with B vitamins on cardiovascular disease, cancer, and cause-specific mortality: meta-analysis of 8 randomized trials involving 37,485 individuals. *Arch Intern Med.* 2010;170(18):1622–31.

38. Dharmarajan TS, Adiga GU, Norkus EP. Vitamin B12 deficiency: recognizing subtle symptoms in older adults. *Geriatrics.* 2003;58(3):30–8.

39. Fuhrman MP. Identifying your patient's risk for a vitamin deficiency. *Nutr Clin Pract.* 2001;16:S8–11.

40. de Jager J, Kooy A, Lehert P, et al. Long term treatment with metformin in patients with type 2 diabetes and risk of vitamin B-12 deficiency: randomized placebo controlled trial. *BMJ.* 2010;340:c2181.

41. Greenberg JA, Bell SJ, Guan Y, et al. Folic acid supplementation and pregnancy: more than just neural tube defect prevention. *Rev Obstet Gynecol.* 2011;4(2):52–9.

42. Greenberg JA, Bell SJ. Multivitamin supplementation during pregnancy: emphasis on folic acid and L-methylfolate. *Rev Obstet Gynecol.* 2011; 4(3/4):126–7.

43. Whitehead AS, Gallagher P, Mills JL. A genetic defect in 5,10 methylenetetrahydrofolate reductase in neural tube defects. *QJM.* 1995;88(11):763–6.

44. Bender DA. Non-nutritional uses of vitamin B6. *Br J Nutr.* 1999;81(1):7–20.

45. Boehnke C, Reuter U, Flach U, et al. High-dose riboflavin treatment is efficacious in migraine prophylaxis: an open study in a tertiary care centre. *Eur J Neurol.* 2004;11(7):475–7.

46. Suter PM, Vetter W. Diuretics and vitamin B1: are diuretics a risk factor for thiamin malnutrition? *Nutr Rev.* 2001;58:319–23.

47. Straub DA. Calcium supplementation in clinical practice: a review of forms, doses, and indications. *Nutr Clin Prac.* 2007;22(3):286–96.

48. Bertone-Johnson ER, Hankinson SE, Bendich A, et al. Calcium and vitamin D intake and risk of incident premenstrual syndrome. *Arch Intern Med.* 2005;165(11):1246–52.

49. U.S. Department of Health and Human Services, Agency for Healthcare and Research Quality. Vitamin D and calcium: systemic review of health outcomes. Accessed at http://ahrq.gov/downloads/pub/evidence/pdf/vitadcal/vitadcal.pdf, July 29, 2013.

50. U.S. Preventive Health Task Force, Understanding Task Force Recommendations: Vitamin D and Calcium Supplementation to Prevent Fractures. Accessed at http://www.uspreventiveservicestaskforce.org/uspstf12/vitamind/vitdfact.pdf, July 29, 2013.

51. Xiao Q, Murphy RA, Houston DK, et al. Dietary and supplemental calcium intake and cardiovascular disease mortality: The National Institutes of Health-AARP Diet and Health Study. *JAMA.* 2013;173(8):639–46.

52. Prentice RL, Pettinger MB, Jackson RD, et al. Health risks and benefits from calcium and vitamin D supplementation: Women's Health Initiative clinical trial and cohort study. *Osteoporos Int.* 2013;24(5):567–80.

53. National Institutes of Health, Office of Dietary Supplements. Dietary supplement fact sheet: iron. Accessed at http://ods.od.nih.gov/fact sheets/Iron-HealthProfessional/, July 29, 2013.

54. Centers for Disease Control and Prevention. FAQs for dental fluorosis. Accessed at http://www.cdc.gov/fluoridation/safety/dental_fluorosis.htm, July 30, 2013.

55. Steinbrenner H, Speckmann B, Sies H. Toward understanding success and failures in the use of selenium for cancer prevention. *Antioxid Redox Signal.* 2013;19(2):181–91.

56. Singh M, Das RR. Zinc for the common cold. *Cochrane Database Syst Rev.* 2011;2:CD001364. doi: 10.1002/14651858.CD001364.pub3. Accessed at http://www.thecochranelibrary.com/view/0/index.html.

57. Gaziano JM, Sesso HD, Christen WG, et al. Multivitamins in the prevention of cancer in men: the Physicians' Health Study II randomized controlled trial. *JAMA.* 2012;308(18):1871–80.

FUNCTIONAL AND MEAL REPLACEMENT FOODS

Carol J. Rollins and Cedric B. Baker

Foods serve many purposes in our lives. Foremost is their role in survival; foods provide us with sustenance to maintain metabolism and be physically active. Scientific research suggests that foods also affect health and wellness, and consumers are aware of these findings. In a 2013 survey of 1005 adults selected to reflect the American population, 90% believed health benefits other than basic nutrition are associated with certain foods.[1] Americans also report making changes to improve the healthfulness of their diet, including making an effort to eat more fruits and vegetables (87%) and more foods with whole grains (75%).[2] Decisions about purchasing foods and beverages are influenced by healthfulness (61%) slightly more than convenience (53%); however, taste (87%) continues to dominate purchasing decisions, followed by price (73%). Lack of time to plan and prepare meals leads health-conscious consumers to seek convenient methods to optimize nutrition for wellness and health promotion, including fast yet healthy alternatives to traditional "sit-down" meals. In addition, more individuals are living independently with conditions or impairments that affect their ability to obtain adequate nutrients through a regular diet, and they may seek convenient methods to supplement or replace conventional meals. Although dietitians are the recognized food and nutrition experts, all health care providers should be aware of the role that foods may play in an overall plan to improve or maintain health, especially foods that have benefits beyond their basic nutrients or that help patients reach nutrient goals when healthy meals are not readily available or cannot be ingested. (Chapter 22 reviews basic nutrition.) This chapter provides an introduction to foods used for their potential health benefits (functional foods), as well as foods intended to replace regular meals (meal replacement foods).

Drugs, Dietary Supplements, and Foods

The Food and Drug Administration (FDA) is charged with regulating drugs, dietary supplements, and foods (Chapter 4 discusses regulatory issues). *Foods* are defined as articles used for food or drink or components of any such article, or substances providing taste, aroma, or nutritive value.[3] Specific FDA regulations pertain to food safety and labeling. FDA requires that all regulated foods provide assurance in advance (premarket) that ingredients are safe and that claims are substantiated, truthful, and not misleading. Particular forms or uses of foods, such as infant formulas (see Chapter 25) and medical foods, are required

to meet additional criteria to ensure the safety of somewhat vulnerable groups.

Functional Foods

Functional foods (FF) blur the distinction between drugs and foods, as defined by FDA, much as dietary supplements did until 1994, when the Dietary Supplement Health and Education Act (DSHEA) established a distinct regulatory scheme for dietary supplements.[3] The term *functional food* is not officially sanctioned by FDA, and there is no legal definition or regulatory category for FF. A specific FF may be regulated as a drug or in one of several subcategories of food depending on its intended use and labeling.[3,4] This lack of validation of products makes it difficult to determine sales figures and market estimates; however, the global market of FF has recently been estimated at $50 billion annually.[5] Probiotics represent a $15 billion share. Projections of annual growth in FF vary widely, from 5% to 30% depending on country and product type.[5] Contemporary U.S. health care reforms that mandate preventive care, along with the emerging field of nutrition economics, will likely fuel the growth of FF as their role in dietary recommendations and public health policy increases, including as a primary care option.[6]

Health care providers should be familiar with FF to fully evaluate their patients' diets in relation to preventive and proactive lifestyle changes that modify risks for chronic diseases. Unfortunately, making evidence-based decisions related to the use of FF can be difficult because few randomized controlled trials have been conducted, and for many studies, only a small number of subjects are enrolled. Epidemiologic studies generally rely on people recalling their food intake, which obscures true associations between selected food components and disease risk. If researchers are to translate the epidemiology of dietary patterns into clinical interventions, they need a detailed look at specific diets from certain geographic regions that have low and very low incidence of the major chronic diseases, along with detailed quantification and qualification of dietary phytochemical content.[7] Other factors to consider include the use of biomarkers and nutrigenomic and epigenomic effects of dietary phytochemicals in whole foods as bioactive food components in individuals.[8] This daunting complexity makes clinical trials aimed at prevention challenging to design and conduct.

Isolating the food component and administering it as a dietary supplement rather than as a FF, as is done in many clinical studies, simplifies study design and reduces interactions among food components. Unfortunately, available data do not support this approach because multiple-constituent dietary phytochemicals in the matrix of plant-based whole foods appear to be safer and more effective than single and multiple constituent high-dose dietary supplements.[9–11] Associations between FF or bioactive food components and health maintenance or disease prevention usually show a relative risk of less than 2.[12] In a traditional medical toxicology model, where exposures are generally large doses of a single component, a relative risk of less than 2 is considered weak. In contrast, nutritional exposures are broad based and occur in small doses of multiple-component mixtures within whole foods over a prolonged time. Relative risk of 1.5 should be ranked as strong for such exposures. Given the limitations of available data and the potential for complex interactions between FF and bioactive food components, lifestyle factors, and genetics, the evaluation of FF requires examination of the totality of evidence, including that from biological models and multiple types of research (preclinical, epidemiologic, clinical, and translational).[12] Dietary phytochemical patterns in whole foods and functional dietary patterns have become leading areas for FF science and functional nutrition in current research programs and will become more important in future research as understanding of this area evolves.[11,12] To compare results or combine results for analysis, researchers must include preparation methods and sources of FF (whole food, isolated component, or dietary supplement) in study reports.

"Health benefits beyond those of basic nutrition" is a broad definition of FF, encompassing unmodified whole foods (fruits, vegetables, and whole-grain products) and designer foods such as purple carrots.[3,4] A somewhat narrower definition used by the International Life Sciences Institute restricts FF to unmodified foods with naturally occurring bioactive components.[4] Examples include tomatoes, for their lycopene content, and soybeans, which provide isoflavones. The Institute of Medicine (IOM) Food and Nutrition Board restricts the definition of FF to those foods in which the concentration of one or more ingredients has been altered to enhance the food's contribution to a healthful diet.[3,4] This definition includes foods enriched or fortified with nutrients, phytochemicals, or botanical products, including foods such as orange juice with added calcium. Elements isolated from nontraditional food sources and added to traditional foods, such as stanol esters added to margarine-type spreads, also fit this definition of FF. From the viewpoint in current biomedical paradigms, plant-based foods are considered functional because of synergy in dietary phytochemicals.[6,11]

Categories of Foods Classified as Functional Foods

FF typically fit into one of five categories on the basis of statutory definitions and regulatory guidelines for health claims on food labels:

1. Foods associated with health claims recognized by FDA
2. Foods that carry structure or function claims
3. Foods for special dietary use
4. Medical foods
5. Certain conventional foods

Providers should have a basic understanding of these categories because the need for medical supervision varies by category. All labeling claims require prior approval by FDA; however, the required level of supporting science varies depending on the category under which the FF are marketed (i.e., greater supporting science is required for medical foods than for structure–function claims).

Foods with Health Claims

Health claims characterize the relationship between a substance (food, food component, dietary ingredient, or dietary supplement) and a disease or health-related condition.[3,4,13] (See Chapters 50 and 51 for discussion of dietary supplements.) Only claims about reduction of disease risk are allowed; no claim about "diagnosis, cure, mitigation, or treatment of disease" can be made. Three types of health claims can be made for conventional foods: authorized, authoritative, and qualified. Each type of claim is associated with specific levels of supportive data and specified labeling criteria. *Authorized* health claims require publication of an FDA regulation after an extensive review of the scientific literature, along with significant scientific agreement that the food/nutrient and disease relationship is well established. Of the health claims allowed for foods, authorized claims undergo the most thorough FDA review. The exact wording of the claim statement is not specified, although the statement appearing on the food label must meet specific criteria.

Statements for authorized health claims cannot quantify the degree of risk reduction, and the terms *may* or *might* must be used to qualify the relationship between a food or dietary component and disease. The label must state that the disease or health-related condition depends on many factors, implying that diet is not the only consideration in disease management. It also must indicate that the benefit related to a disease or health-related condition is part of a total dietary pattern; thus, the need for an overall healthy diet is reinforced. No health claims are permitted for foods containing more than 13 grams of fat, 4 grams of saturated fat, 60 mg of cholesterol, or 480 mg of sodium per reference amount customarily consumed (RACC); up to double these amounts are allowed for main dishes and meal products.[13] The RACC is typically one serving as defined on the product label. Health claims cannot be indicated for children younger than 2 years. Table 23–1 lists authorized health claims, requirements for foods listing these health claims, and sample statements that might be used on a food label.[3,4,13]

Certain health claims for foods, food components, or dietary ingredients (but not dietary supplements) can be made through notification of FDA by the manufacturer after the agency receives a statement from an authoritative scientific body of the U.S. government with responsibility to protect public health or to conduct research related to human nutrition (an *authoritative* claim).[3,13] The National Institutes of Health, the Centers for Disease Control and Prevention, and the National Academy of Sciences are sources for authoritative claims. Significant scientific evidence supports such health claims, although FDA itself does not complete an extensive review of the data. Authoritative health claims currently recognized by the FDA and required wording for the claims statement are listed in Table 23–1.[3,13]

The third type of health claim is a *qualified* claim. Qualified health claims are appropriate for use when evidence of health benefits of a food, food component, or dietary supplement is

table
23–1 Authorized and Authoritative Health Claims

Authorized Health Claims

Health Claim	Requirements for Foods	Sample Claim Statement Containing Required Components	Selected Foods Meeting Claim Requirements
Calcium—osteoporosis [Calcium and vitamin D—osteoporosis]	High in calcium [High in calcium and vitamin D] Bioavailable Phosphorus content no more than calcium content	Regular exercise and healthy diet with enough calcium [and vitamin D] helps teens and white and Asian women maintain good bone health, and may reduce their high risk of osteoporosis later in life.	Milk Orange juice with added calcium
Sodium—hypertension	Low sodium content	Diets low in sodium may reduce the risk of high blood pressure, a disease associated with many factors.	Fruits and vegetables, canned or frozen with no added salt, fresh
Dietary fat—cancer	Low fat "Extra lean" fish and game meat	Development of cancer depends on many factors. A diet low in total fat may reduce the risk of some cancers.	Fruits and vegetables, fresh, frozen, or canned Most cereals Nonfat and low-fat milk and dairy products
Dietary saturated fat and cholesterol—risk of coronary heart disease	Low saturated fat Low cholesterol Low fat "Extra lean" fish and game meat	While many factors affect heart disease, diets low in saturated fat and cholesterol may reduce the risk of this disease.	Fruits and vegetables, fresh, frozen, or canned Most cereals Nonfat and low-fat milk and dairy products
Fiber-containing grain products, fruits, and vegetables—cancer	Grain product, fruit, or vegetable containing dietary fiber Low fat Good source of fiber without fortification	Low-fat diets rich in fiber-containing grain products, fruits, and vegetables may reduce the risk of some types of cancer, a disease associated with many factors.	Fruits and vegetables, fresh, frozen, or canned Whole-grain breads, cereals, and pasta Brown rice
Fruits, vegetables, and grain products that contain fiber, particularly soluble fiber—risk of coronary heart disease	Fruit, vegetable, or grain product containing fiber Low saturated fat Low cholesterol Low fat Minimum of 0.6 gram soluble fiber per RACC without fortification Soluble fiber content provided on the label	Diets low in saturated fat and cholesterol and rich in fruits, vegetables, and grain products that contain some types of dietary fiber, particularly soluble fiber, may reduce the risk of heart disease, a disease associated with many factors.	Fruits and vegetables, fresh, frozen, or canned Whole-grain breads, cereals, and pasta Brown rice
Fruits and vegetables—cancer	Fruit or vegetable Low fat Good source of vitamin A or C, or dietary fiber without fortification	Low-fat diets rich in fruits and vegetables (foods that are low in fat and may contain dietary fiber, vitamin A, or vitamin C) may reduce the risk of some types of cancer, a disease associated with many factors. [X food is high in vitamin A, vitamin C, and/or is a good source of fiber.]	Broccoli Berries Green beans Carrots Cantaloupe Citrus fruits Most dark green leafy vegetables

table
23–1 Authorized and Authoritative Health Claims *(continued)*

Health Claim	Requirements for Foods	Sample Claim Statement Containing Required Components	Selected Foods Meeting Claim Requirements
Folate—neural tube defects	Contains at least 40 mcg folate per serving Foods in conventional form that are a good source without fortification Contains not more than the RDI for vitamin A as retinol, or preformed vitamin A or D Amount of folate must be in the nutrition label	Healthful diets with adequate folate may reduce a woman's risk of having a child with a brain or spinal cord defect.	Most dark green leafy vegetables (see Chapter 22)
Dietary noncarcinogenic carbohydrate sweeteners—dental caries	Sugar-free Eligible substances listed in 21 CFR 101.80; examples include xylitol, sorbitol, mannitol, erythritol, d-tagatose, and sucralose Does not lower plaque pH below 5.7 when fermentable carbohydrate is present	Frequent between-meal consumption of foods high in sugars and starches promotes tooth decay. The sugar alcohols in [name of food] do not promote tooth decay. Short claim for small packages: Does not promote tooth decay.	Many "dietetic" sugar-free products marketed for people with diabetes Many low-calorie products marketed for weight loss
Soluble fiber from certain foods—risk of coronary heart disease	Low saturated fat Low cholesterol Low fat Includes one or more: (1) an eligible source of whole oat or barley with ≥0.75 gram soluble fiber per RACC, (2) Oatrim containing ≥0.75 gram beta-glucan per RACC, (3) psyllium husk containing ≥1.7 gram soluble fiber per RACC Amount of soluble fiber per RACC must be declared in the nutrition label	Soluble fiber from foods such as [name of soluble fiber source (optional—name of food product)], as part of a diet low in saturated fat and cholesterol, may reduce the risk of heart disease. A serving of [name of food product] supplies [X] grams of the [necessary daily dietary intake for the benefit] soluble fiber from [name of soluble fiber source] necessary per day to have this effect.	Rolled oats, oatmeal Whole oats cold cereals Barley Cereals with added psyllium
Soy protein—risk of coronary heart disease[a]	Contains ≥6.25 grams soy protein per RACC Low saturated fat Low cholesterol Low fat, unless fat is from whole soybeans	Example 1: Foods containing 25 grams of soy protein a day, as part of a diet low in saturated fat and cholesterol, may reduce the risk of heart disease. A serving of [name of food] supplies [X] grams of soy protein. Example 2: Diets low in saturated fat and cholesterol that include 25 grams of soy protein a day may reduce the risk of heart disease. One serving of [name of food] provides [X] grams of soy protein.	

Claim	Criteria	Model claim statement	Food sources
Plant sterol/stanol esters—risk of coronary heart disease[b]	Spreads and salad dressings must contain ≥0.65 gram plant sterol esters per RACC Spreads, salad dressings, and snack bars must contain ≥1.7 grams plant stanol esters per RACC Low saturated fat Low cholesterol	Example 1: Foods containing at least 0.65 gram per serving of vegetable oil sterol esters, eaten twice a day with meals for a total intake of at least 1.3 grams, as part of a diet low in saturated fat and cholesterol, may reduce the risk of heart disease. A serving of [name of food] supplies [X] grams of vegetable oil sterol esters. Example 2: Diets low in saturated fat and cholesterol that include two servings of foods that provide a daily total of at least 3.4 grams of plant stanol esters in two meals may reduce the risk of heart disease. A serving of [name of food] supplies [X] grams of plant stanol esters.	Margarine spreads with added sterol/stanol esters Orange juice with added sterol/stanol esters Nonfat milk with added sterol/stanol esters

Authoritative Health Claims[c]

Claim	Criteria	Model claim statement	Food sources
Whole-grain foods—risk of heart disease and certain cancers	Must contain ≥51% whole-grain ingredients by weight per RACC Low fat Must meet specified dietary fiber content: 3 grams/RACC of 55 grams; 2.8 grams/RACC of 50 grams; 2.5 grams/RACC of 45 grams; 1.7 grams/RACC of 35 grams	Diets rich in whole-grain foods and other plant foods and low in total fat, saturated fat, and cholesterol may reduce the risk of heart disease and some types of cancer.	Low-fat whole-grain breads and cereals Whole-grain cereals and pasta Brown rice
Potassium—risk of high blood pressure and stroke	Good source of potassium Low sodium Low total fat Low saturated fat Low cholesterol	Diets containing foods that are a good source of potassium and that are low in sodium may reduce the risk of high blood pressure and stroke.	Many fruits and vegetables (see Chapter 22)
Fluoridated water—reduced risk of dental caries	Total fluoride > 0.6–1 mg/L Bottled water must meet standards of identity and quality Excludes bottled water for infants	Drinking fluoridated water may reduce the risk of dental caries or tooth decay.	Bottled water containing fluoride
Saturated fat, cholesterol, and trans fat—reduced risk of heart disease	Low saturated fat Low cholesterol Quantity of trans fat on label and <0.5 gram trans fat per RACC Total fat < 6.5 grams	Diets low in saturated fat and cholesterol, and as low as possible in trans fat, may reduce the risk of heart disease.	Fruits and vegetables, fresh, frozen, or canned Most cereals Nonfat and low-fat milk and dairy products

Key: CFR = Code of Federal Regulations; RACC = reference amount customarily consumed (usually one serving as listed on label); RDI = recommended dietary intake.

[a] Soy protein content of foods is available from the Agricultural Research Service, U.S. Department of Agriculture (USDA). Nutrient Data Laboratory [database online]. [Search for "standard reference."] Accessed at http://www.nal.usda.gov/fnic/foodcomp/search, May 16, 2013.

[b] A proposed rule amending the health claim for phytosterols and risk of coronary heart disease has been published. The claim would include use of nonesterified (free) phytosterols, broaden the range of foods to which the claim could apply, modify the dietary intake for the claimed benefit, and adjust the minimum content for a claim. Department of Health and Human Services, Food and Drug Administration. Food labeling; health claim; phytosterols and risk of coronary heart disease; proposed rule. 21 CFR Part 101. *Federal Register.* 2010;75:76526-71. Accessed at http://edocket.access.gpo.gov/2010/pdf/2010-30386.pdf, May 16, 2013.

[c] Wording in the sample claim statement for authoritative claims is required by the Food and Drug Administration.

Source: References 3, 13, and 14.

still emerging; scientific research supporting the claim tends to be limited or preliminary; and the "significant scientific agreement" level of evidence required for authorized and authoritative health claims cannot be met. Table 23–2 lists qualified claims and specific "qualifying" terms required by FDA to indicate that evidence for the claim is limited.[3,4,14] Labeling guidance issued by FDA for qualified health claims intermixes information regarding labeling of dietary supplements and conventional foods.[14] Chapter 50 provides further discussion of qualified health claims and labeling.

Foods with Structure–Function Claims

Structure–function claims are commonly associated with dietary supplements but can also appear on food labels. These claims indicate the effect of consuming the product on a body structure or function. They differ from health claims in that FDA validation or authorization is not required before use, although prior notification of FDA regarding the claim is required. These claims cannot make reference regarding reduced risk of disease because such a reference would place the product under regulation as a drug.[3,4,13] For example, a probiotic yogurt marketed as preventing or treating diarrhea is considered a drug; however, if the label instead claims to "improve digestion," it is considered an acceptable structure–function claim. Other examples of structure–function claims include statements that the product builds strong bones, supports the immune system, improves memory, maintains intestinal flora, improves strength,

and promotes urinary tract health. Foods carrying a structure–function claim are considered FF; they are not dietary supplements when represented as a conventional food. For instance, margarine-type spreads with added stanol esters are a food, with the stanol ester considered a food additive. However, dietary supplements in food form (drinks and bars) that are labeled and marketed as dietary supplements are regulated as dietary supplements (see Chapter 50). Distinguishing FF from dietary supplements can therefore be confusing.

Foods for Special Dietary Use

Foods for special dietary use, as defined by FDA, include foods used to supply *particular dietary needs*, or to supplement or fortify the usual diet, and are marketed as such; they do not meet general dietary needs (see Chapter 22).[3,13] Particular dietary needs may exist because of physical, physiologic, pathologic, or other conditions, such as disease, convalescence, pregnancy, lactation, underweight, overweight, infancy, or need for sodium restriction. Foods intended for use as the only nutrient source in the diet and those intended to supplement the diet by increasing total dietary intake of a specific ingredient (vitamin, mineral, or other nutrient) are also considered to meet a particular dietary need. These foods are subject to general labeling requirements for foods, and medical supervision of their use is not required. By some definitions, foods for special dietary use are considered FF; however, this approach to marketing FF is seen in the food supply much less broadly than is structure–function labeling.

table
23–2   Qualified Health Claims for Conventional Foods[a]

Food/Nutrient	Disease/Condition	Level of Evidence	Comments
Claims Related to Cardiovascular Disease			
Omega-3 fatty acids: EPA and DHA	CHD	Supportive but not conclusive research	Total fat, saturated fat, cholesterol, and sodium maximum limits apply
Walnuts	Heart disease	Supportive but not conclusive research	1.5 ounces of whole or chopped walnuts per day
Nuts	Heart disease	Supportive but not conclusive research	Limited to almonds, hazelnuts, peanuts, pecans, some pine nuts, pistachio nuts, walnuts; 1.5 ounces per day
Monounsaturated fat from olive oil	CHD	Limited and not conclusive evidence	Suggested intake of about 2 tablespoons (23 grams) daily; replaces a similar amount of saturated fat and does not increase the total number of calories
Unsaturated fatty acids from canola oil	CHD	Limited and not conclusive evidence	Suggested intake of about 1.5 tablespoons (19 grams) daily; replaces a similar amount of saturated fat and does not increase the total number of calories
Corn oil and corn oil–containing products	Heart disease	Very limited and preliminary evidence	Suggested intake of about 1 tablespoon (16 grams) daily; replaces a similar amount of saturated fat and does not increase the total number of calories
Claims Related to Cancer Risk			
Green tea	Cancer	Highly unlikely to reduce risk	Breast cancer and prostate cancer studies evaluated
Tomatoes, tomato sauce	Prostate, ovarian, gastric, and pancreatic cancers	Unlikely, uncertain, or little scientific evidence	Few studies; major study limitations and conflicting results

Key: CHD = Coronary heart disease; DHA = docosahexaenoic acid; EPA = eicosapentaenoic acid.
[a] Includes only claims related to conventional foods. Claims related to dietary supplements are not included.
Source: References 3, 4, 13, 14, and 20.

Medical Foods

Medical foods were first defined in the *Federal Register* in 1973; they were represented by an infant formula for patients with phenylketonuria, which had previously been regulated as a drug.[3] The Orphan Drug Act Amendments of 1988 also define medical foods and require that specific criteria be met before use and distribution. These foods are to be recommended or prescribed by a physician and used under continued medical supervision; however, many are not prescription-only products in the same manner as prescription drugs since they can be sold without a physician's written order. Medical foods do not occur naturally; rather, they are specially formulated and processed to meet *distinctive nutritional requirements* of the disease or condition for which they are intended.[3] Distinctive requirements for a select medicinal component in the food (or the food product as a whole) must be established by prior medical evaluation on the basis of recognized scientific principles. Providers should be able to distinguish between medical foods that require physician supervision and products that can be safely used as "nutritional self-care" by the public. (See the Medical Foods and Meal Replacement Foods section of this chapter for further discussion of medical foods.)

Conventional Foods

Conventional foods that do not fit into any of the preceding four categories can also be classified as FF. Research on conventional FF comes from contemporary medical ethnobiology and ethnopharmacy, with the foundation being ethnic or traditional foods associated with health benefits in various cultures and supported by epidemiologic studies. For example, long-standing systems of traditional FF use in Asia are linked epidemiologically to some of the lowest cancer rates in the world and to very low incidence of other chronic diseases.[15,16] The strength of evidence supporting a functional role for such foods is typically weak-moderate, and clinical trials tend to be lacking; therefore, even a qualified health claim often cannot be supported at this time.[4] However, other foods are known in which specific compounds have been identified as the functional component, for which molecular functional nutrition and pharmacology studies have been conducted. Studies of dietary phytochemicals and fish oils have revealed a variety of specific phytochemicals and marine zoochemicals (e.g., EGCG, resveratrol, curcumin, EPA, DHA) that modulate several molecular targets at the same time and can serve collectively as agents for chronic disease prevention and health preservation.[10,17-19] Table 23-3 provides examples of conventional foods and the components likely

table 23-3 Examples of Conventional Foods Classified as Functional Foods

Food	Functional Component	Potential Health Benefit	Comments
Apples	Flavonols, phenols, proanthocyanidins, soluble fiber (pectin)	Decreased risk of certain types of cancer; improved glucose and cholesterol concentrations; may contribute to maintenance of heart health	Recommend one a day but amount for health benefit not defined
Banana, ripe	Prebiotics, FOS	Decreased hypertension and hypercholesterolemia	Weak evidence for 3–10 g/day
Berries; cherries	Anthocyanidins	Antioxidant functions; may contribute to healthy immune system	Recommend 1/2–1 cup/day but amount for health benefit not defined
Cinnamon	Proanthocyanidins	May contribute to maintenance of urinary tract and heart health	Weak evidence; amount for health benefit not well researched
Citrus fruits	Ascorbic acid, zeaxanthin, limonene	Decreased risk of age-related macular degeneration; decreased cancer risk	Weak-moderate evidence for decreased macular degeneration with 6 mg/day as lutein; rodent studies with limonene and cancer
Cocoa, chocolate	Flavonols	Antioxidant functions, decreased risk of coronary heart disease	Dark chocolate appears to be best
Corn	Lutein, zeaxanthin, free stanols/sterols	Decreased risk of age-related macular degeneration; may decrease risk of CHD	Weak-moderate evidence for 6 mg/day as lutein; health claim for stanol/sterol esters added to foods
Cranberry juice	Proanthocyanidins	Decreased UTI from decreased adherence of bacteria to cell walls; may also prevent adhesion of plaque-forming bacteria in the mouth	Moderate evidence for 300 mL/day to decrease UTI (58% reduction in bacteriuria in 150 elderly women in the first randomized controlled trial [1994])
Cruciferous vegetables: broccoli, brussels sprouts, cauliflower, cabbage	Glucosinolates, indoles, isothiocyanates (sulphoraphane), organosulfur compounds, thiols	Decreased risk of certain types of cancer	Weak-moderate evidence for greater than 1/2 cup/day

Food	Functional Component	Potential Health Benefit	Comments
Dairy products, including some cheese	Conjugated linoleic acid	Decreased risk of breast cancer; possible role in improved body composition	Weak evidence for breast cancer link; animal studies suggest role in decreased body fat; necessary amount not determined for health effects
Dairy products, fermented (acidophilus milk, buttermilk, kefir, yogurt)	Probiotic organisms (lactobacilli, bifidobacteria)	Maintenance of GI tract health; decreased colon cancer risk; decreased cholesterol	See discussion of probiotics in this chapter
Eggs (yolk)	Lutein, zeaxanthin	Decreased risk of age-related macular degeneration	Weak-moderate evidence for 6 mg/day as lutein
Eggs, enriched with DHA	DHA	Decreased risk of CHD; increased HDL cholesterol	Chickens are fed fish oils or algae as a source of DHA
Fatty fish (wild salmon, herring)	Omega-3 fatty acids	Decreased triglycerides and risk of heart disease, including fatal and nonfatal MI	Recommend 2 meals/week with fatty fish; supportive but not conclusive evidence per qualified health claim
Flax	Phytoestrogens (lignans), alpha-linolenic acid	Decreased risk of CHD by decreasing cholesterol and platelet aggregation; weak estrogenic activity may decrease hormone-related cancers; maintenance of a healthy immune system; alpha-linolenic acid may contribute to maintenance of visual function	Weak evidence for CHD association; very weak evidence for cancer risk; amounts necessary for health benefit from flax are not defined
Garlic	Organosulfur compounds, thiols	Decreased total and LDL cholesterol; may decrease the risk of gastric cancer; promotes healthy immune function	Weak-moderate evidence for about one fresh clove daily for cholesterol; epidemiologic evidence for decreased cancer is equivocal; considerable variation exists in the amount of active compounds for available products
Grapes, red and black	Anthocyanidins, phenolic compounds	Antioxidant functions; decreased cardiovascular risk	Epidemiologic evidence suggesting inverse association with cardiovascular disease risk
Grape juice	Resveratrol	Decreased risk of MI caused by decreased platelet aggregation	Moderate-strong evidence for 8–16 ounces/day
Greens: spinach, kale, collards	Lutein, zeaxanthin	Decreased risk of age-related macular degeneration	Weak-moderate evidence for 6 mg/day as lutein
Jerusalem artichoke	Prebiotics, FOS	Decreased hypertension; decreased hypercholesterolemia	Weak evidence for 3–10 g/day
Meat (beef, lamb, turkey) and milk	Conjugated linoleic acid	Antitumor effect proposed; possible role in improved body composition	Suppression of cancer cell growth in rat studies; animal studies suggest role in decreased body fat; necessary amount not determined for health effects
Onions, leeks, scallions	Organosulfur compounds, thiols	Decreased total and LDL cholesterol	Weak-moderate evidence
Onion powder	Prebiotics, FOS	Decreased hypertension; decreased hypercholesterolemia	Weak evidence for 3–10 g/day
Rye	Phytoestrogens (lignans)	May contribute to maintenance of heart health and healthy immune system	Amounts necessary for health benefit from rye are not defined
Tea, black	Polyphenols, flavonoids	Decreased risk of CHD	Evidence is not conclusive

table
23–3   Examples of Conventional Foods Classified as Functional Foods *(continued)*

Food	Functional Component	Potential Health Benefit	Comments
Tea, green	Catechins (epigallocate-chin-3-gallate, epigallocate-chin, epicatechin-3-gallate, epicatechin)	Decreased risk of certain types of cancer; improved CV health; weight control	Qualified health claim evaluation concluded it is highly unlikely that green tea (not specifically catechins) reduces risk for cancer; prevention of CV and obesity weak (intake estimates of >4 cups/day)
Tomatoes and processed tomato products	Lycopene	Antioxidant that efficiently decreases singlet oxygen in biological systems; possible decreased risk of certain cancers (prostate) and MI	Weak evidence based on inverse associations of tissue lycopene and cancers or MI; qualified health claim evaluation concluded it is unlikely or uncertain that tomatoes or sauce (not specifically lycopene) reduce risks
Tree nuts	Monounsaturated fatty acids, vitamin E	Decreased risk of CHD	Moderate evidence for 1–2 ounces/day; some nuts have qualified health claim

Key: CHD = Coronary heart disease; CV = cardiovascular; DHA = docosahexaenoic acid; FOS = fructooligosaccharides; GI = gastrointestinal; HDL = high-density lipoprotein; LDL = low-density lipoprotein; MI = myocardial infarction; UTI = urinary tract infection.
Source: Adapted from references 4, 20, and 21.

responsible for their role as FF; and Table 23–4 lists examples of functional components and typical food sources.[4,6,8,12,20–23] Figure 23–1 shows the narrowing cascade of knowledge from an extensive array of plants on Earth to the few phytochemicals identified as health modifiers; the figure also serves as an indicator of the extensive research needed to fully understand the potential of FF in health.[9,10,16,19,22]

Functional Foods and Biomarkers: Epigenomics and Chemoprevention

The disposition of dietary phytochemicals is similar to drugs and xenobiotics to the extent that they can be studied with respect to individual pharmacokinetics and pharmacodynamics.[23] Pharmacokinetic studies suggest that variations in disease risk or

table
23–4   Examples of Functional Flavonoid Components in Conventional Foods

Functional Component (Subclass of Flavonoids)	Dietary Phytochemicals	Food Source	Potential Health Benefit
Anthocyanins	Cyanidin Delphinidin Malvidin	Red, blue, and purple berries and grapes; cherries; potatoes; purple sweet potatoes; blue corn; rhubarb; plums	Augment cellular antioxidant defenses; may contribute to maintenance of brain function
Flavones	Hesperetin Naringenin	Citrus fruits and juices	Neutralize free radicals, which may damage cells; augment cellular antioxidant defenses
Flavonols	Isorhamnetin Kaempferol Myricetin Quercetin	Apples, berries, broccoli, kale, tea, onions (scallions, yellow onions; highest flavonol content in onions)	Neutralize free radicals, which may damage cells; augment cellular antioxidant defenses
Flavanols (monomers)	Catechin Epicatechin Epigallocatechin ECG EGCG	Teas (green and white), chocolate, grapes, berries, apples	May contribute to maintenance of heart health
Flavanols (polymers)	Proanthocyanidins Theaflavins Thearubigins	Teas (oolong and black), chocolate, apples, berries, red grapes	May contribute to maintenance of heart health and urinary tract health

Key: ECG = Epicatechin-3-gallate; EGCG = epigallocatechin-3-gallate.
Source: Adapted from references 3, 4, and 20.

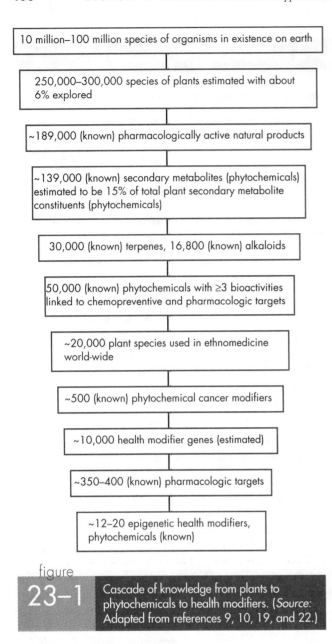

10 million–100 million species of organisms in existence on earth

250,000–300,000 species of plants estimated with about 6% explored

~189,000 (known) pharmacologically active natural products

~139,000 (known) secondary metabolites (phytochemicals) estimated to be 15% of total plant secondary metabolite constituents (phytochemicals)

30,000 (known) terpenes, 16,800 (known) alkaloids

50,000 (known) phytochemicals with ≥3 bioactivities linked to chemopreventive and pharmacologic targets

~20,000 plant species used in ethnomedicine world-wide

~500 (known) phytochemical cancer modifiers

~10,000 health modifier genes (estimated)

~350–400 (known) pharmacologic targets

~12–20 epigenetic health modifiers, phytochemicals (known)

figure 23–1 Cascade of knowledge from plants to phytochemicals to health modifiers. (*Source:* Adapted from references 9, 10, 19, and 22.)

preventive efficacy of certain dietary phytochemicals may be at least partially related to genetic polymorphisms in metabolism that result in altered enzyme activity; thus, the same phytochemical may have different pharmacodynamic effects with different individuals. Because of such complexities, common biomarkers used to monitor a condition or health risk may be inadequate to establish a link between a phytochemical and clinical endpoints. The IOM developed a framework for the qualification of risk biomarkers that recommends evaluation of the relationship between the clinical endpoint and the risk biomarker as well as of evidence that the intervention affecting the risk biomarker is concomitantly linked to the clinical endpoint.[15,23] Linking biomarkers for health and disease to epigenomics (defined as heritable changes in gene expression that occur without a change in DNA sequence)[19] is a major challenge in FF research.[8]

Fiber

Fiber is a component of FF that has been widely studied for associations with potential health benefits. Fiber consists of dietary components that humans cannot digest, including plant cell walls; nonstarch polysaccharides from seaweed, microorganisms, or seed husks (psyllium); resistant starches; and nondigestible oligosaccharides.[24] The terms *dietary fiber* and *functional fiber* are related to dietary reference intakes (see Chapter 22) and distinguish between sources of fiber.[24,25] Total fiber is the sum of dietary and functional fiber. Dietary fiber is defined as nondigestible carbohydrates and lignin that are naturally occurring (intrinsic and intact) in plants. Functional fiber is defined as isolated nondigestible carbohydrates that have beneficial physiologic effects in humans; it includes fiber extracted or modified from plants or animal sources. Effects of fiber extracted from cell walls may differ from effects of in situ fiber because of altered chemical and physical properties. Viscosity and fermentability may be more important correlates with health effects than solubility; however, the terms *soluble fiber* and *insoluble fiber* remain pervasive in both professional and nonprofessional literature, and these terms are used here.[26,27]

Recommended and Actual Intake

Adequate intakes (AIs) for total fiber published by the IOM range from 21–38 g/day, with amounts for women and elderly people being lower than for men and younger people.[25] (See Chapter 22 for general information on AIs.) AIs are based on usual caloric intake in each age group and 14 grams of dietary fiber per 1000 calories, which appears to be the amount needed to promote heart health.[24,28] Unfortunately, actual mean fiber intake is only about 14–16 g/day, with little progress toward meeting goals over the past two decades.[29]

Soluble and Insoluble Fibers

Soluble fibers typically undergo substantial degradation and fermentation in the colon; negligible degradation and fermentation occur with most insoluble fibers. Table 23–5 outlines food components, food sources, and functional fiber sources typically associated with soluble and insoluble fibers. The food sources listed are good to excellent sources of fiber, as defined by FDA.[30]

Methods of Increasing Fiber Intake

Table 23–6 lists ideas for increasing fiber content in the diet. Caution is advised for the use of fiber-containing products in patients with poor gastrointestinal (GI) motility or underlying GI dysfunction, including narcotic-associated dysmotility. Inadequate fluid intake may also contribute to GI distress from a high-fiber diet. It is advisable to increase fiber intake gradually, because a sudden increase can cause bloating, gas, and occasionally diarrhea. A reasonable approach is to add one or two servings of foods that are abundant in fiber, as listed in Table 23–5, to the diet every few days until the goal for fiber intake is reached. Reading ingredient labels is essential to ensure adequate fiber content, especially for breads and cereals, in which a *whole* grain should be the first ingredient listed.

Benefits of Fiber

The generally accepted benefits of fiber are laxation effects, normalization of blood lipid concentrations, and attenuation of blood glucose response.[26,30] These benefits are the accepted measures of efficacy as required for label claims of fiber content in Canada; only evidence of safety is required in the United States, but appropriate evidence must support any health claim

table
23–5   Components and Sources of Soluble and Insoluble Fiber

	Soluble Fiber	Insoluble Fiber
Food component	Pectins, gums, mucilages, algal substances, and some hemicellulose	Cellulose, lignin, and most hemicellulose
Food sources with ≥2.5 grams of total fiber per serving[a]	Cereals: oat bran (uncooked, ⅔ cup), oatmeal (cooked, 1 cup) Fruits: apples and pears with skin on, oranges (1 medium), figs and prunes (3 small) Vegetables: broccoli, carrots, cauliflower, corn, kale and other greens, dark green or loose leaf lettuce, peas, squash, zucchini (cooked, 3/4–1 cup)	Bran and whole-grain (corn, rye, wheat) products: bran cereals (dry cereal, 1/3–1 cup), brown rice (cooked, 1 cup), whole-wheat bread (2 slices) Dried beans: lima, kidney, pinto, white (cooked, 1/4–1/2 cup) Dried peas: green, split (cooked, 1/4–1/2 cup)
Functional fiber sources	Beet fiber, FOS, guar gum (galactomannan, Benefiber), inulin, karaya gum, konjac mannan, locust bean gum, pectin, psyllium (ispaghula seed husk)	Calcium polycarbophil, methylcellulose, powdered cellulose, soy polysaccharide (also has significant soluble fiber effects)

Key: FOS = Fructooligosaccharides.

[a] Serving size shown in parentheses. The food sources listed are good (2.5–4.9 grams of fiber per serving) to excellent (5 grams or more of fiber per serving) sources of total dietary fiber and are listed under the heading that exemplifies their predominant health effects.[30]

made. Benefits of fiber, such as cancer risk reduction and weight control, have been suggested in humans; however, results are limited and conflicting.

Laxation. Stool characteristics associated with laxation, or improved bowel function, include increased stool bulk, weight, and water content; decreased stool transit time and normalization of stool frequency to once daily; reduced symptoms of constipation; and an overall improvement in ease of defecation. Epidemiologic studies strongly support the positive role of fiber from whole grains, fruits, and vegetables in laxation. Insoluble fiber has been most frequently associated with improved

laxation, although evidence also indicates some soluble fibers have similar effects. The role of functional fibers in laxation is well accepted, and adequate scientific evidence exists to support FDA approval of some fibers as nonprescription bulking agents for treatment of *occasional* constipation, as discussed in Chapter 15. Studies supporting the efficacy of bulk-forming fibers in *chronic* constipation are less certain and tend to be of intermediate to low quality.

Normalization of Blood Lipid Concentrations. Data on reduced risk of coronary heart disease (CHD) are sufficient for certain fibers to support an FDA-authorized health claim

table
23–6   Methods for Increasing Fiber in the Diet

- Eat breads containing whole-wheat grain, whole-wheat flour, or other whole grains as the first ingredient on the label. These products should replace breads from refined flours that do not include whole grains.
- Replace part of refined-grain cereals with whole-grain cereal for individuals who prefer refined cereals; or mix very high fiber cereals into a favorite brand of cereal.
- Eat oatmeal as a hot breakfast cereal, or select a cold cereal with oats or whole grain as the primary ingredient.
- Sprinkle bran on cereal, yogurt, or other foods.
- Eat brown rice, whole-wheat pasta, and whole-grain crackers rather than white rice and products from refined grains.
- Add fruit to breakfast cereals, breads, yogurt, and salads.
- Select recipes that use whole-grain flours, and/or add rolled oats to baked goods.
- Select recipes for baked goods that include apples, applesauce, carrots, pumpkins, or other fruits or vegetables as a significant ingredient.
- Add kidney, garbanzo, navy, or other beans to salads and soups, including canned soups. Rinse and drain canned beans to reduce components prone to cause gas.
- Serve fruit and/or vegetable salads with picnic lunches instead of potato chips.
- Serve canned beans (black, kidney, white, or baked) as an alternative protein source.
- Eat fresh or dried fruit for snacks and desserts; frozen and canned fruits can also be used.
- Use a low-fat refried bean dip or hummus with whole-wheat baked tortilla chips for snacks.
- Eat fruits and vegetables, including potatoes, with the skin on.
- Select snack or meal replacement bars containing at least 2.5 grams of fiber per serving.
- Include "finger food" vegetables (carrots, celery, cauliflower pieces, and broccoli flowerets) in lunch boxes and as snacks.
- For children, make animal or other fun shapes from vegetables pieces.
- Eat nuts and/or seeds for snacks, or add to mixed dishes, salads, breads, and cereals.

(Table 23–1).[3,4,13] Multiple epidemiologic studies have reported a reduced risk of CHD or cardiovascular disease (CVD) with high dietary fiber intake and/or fiber-rich foods. The relationship appears to hold over many years and across ethnic groups. Table 23–7 summarizes data related to risk of CHD from several large, well-designed prospective epidemiologic studies with longer-term follow-up and pooled data studies.[24,28,31–35]

The key to fiber's ability to lower cholesterol and reduce CHD risk appears to be consuming an adequate quantity of highly viscous fiber, primarily from whole-grain cereal (oats, barley, or rye) and beans (legumes), or from guar gum, pectin, and psyllium. Fruit fiber may have a beneficial effect relative to CHD/CVD, but the association is less clear. Vegetable fiber does not appear to be associated with reduced risk of CHD/CVD.

Attenuation of Blood Glucose Response.

Multiple large, well-designed prospective epidemiologic and cohort studies with longer-term follow-up have reported an association between consumption of fiber and attenuation of blood glucose, improved insulin response, and/or reduced risk of diabetes, as summarized in Table 23–7.[24,28,31–36] The overall conclusion from these studies is that an inverse relationship exists between risk of diabetes and intake of dietary fiber. Intake of cereal fiber appears to be most frequently related to improved glucose control and/or reduced risk of diabetes; foods most likely to provide a positive effect include cereal grains such as oats, barley, and rye. Some

legumes (beans), fruits, and vegetables, as well as guar gum and pectin, may also have a beneficial effect on glucose control. Evidence suggests that nonviscous fibers, such as wheat bran, have little effect on glycemic control.

Weight Loss and Maintenance.

Epidemiologic studies show a lower body mass in participants who eat a high-fiber diet and greater incidence of obesity in those with low intake of dietary fiber.[24,28] Interventional studies show mixed results with high-fiber diets and weight loss, although there is an association of less weight gain over time with higher intake of whole grains.[35] Research suggests that fiber intake may influence body weight through various mechanisms, such as delayed gastric emptying, prolonged small bowel transit time and subsequent effects on peptides associated with satiety and gut function, activation of the ileal break, and stimulation of colonic cells, resulting in production of appetite-regulating hormones.[37]

Prebiotics, Probiotics, and the Gut Microbiota

Microflora in the GI tract are known as the enteric microbiota. The GI tract hosts approximately 300–500 species of commensal bacteria, with concentrations up to 10^9 colony-forming units (CFU)/mL in the terminal ileum and 10^{12} CFU/mL in the colon.[38] However, the enteric microbiota may be far more diverse than is currently recognized. Only within the past 15 years or so

table 23–7	Summary of Selected Studies Related to Fiber and Risk of CHD and Improved Glucose Control	
Study Name and Population Characteristics[a]	**Follow-Up Time (years)**	**Results/Conclusions**
Nurse's Health Study[24,31]: cohort design; >65,000 women; ages 37–64 years	10	*CHD:* Inverse relationship between dietary fiber intake and risk of CHD only for dietary fiber from cereal sources, not fruits and vegetables; cereal fiber intake averaging 7.7 g/day reduced risk of CHD by 34%, compared with average intake of 2.2 g/day; RR 0.77 with higher fiber intake; 19% decrease in risk for CHD events per 10 g/day increase in dietary fiber and a 37% decrease per 5-gram increase in cereal fiber. *Glucose:* RR type 2 DM 2.5 for high-GL/low-cereal-fiber diet (<2.5 g/day), compared with low-GL/high-cereal-fiber diet (>5.8 g/day); more frequent intake of dark breads, whole-grain breakfast cereals, and brown rice was associated with decreased likelihood of developing diabetes.
Nurses' Health Study, type 2 DM subgroup[32]: cohort design; 7822 women; ages 37–64 years	Up to 26 (70,102 person-years)	*CVD:* RR CVD-specific mortality 0.65 for highest fifth of bran intake after multivariate adjustment. RR all-cause mortality 0.75 for highest fifth of bran intake.
Health Professionals' Follow-Up Study[24,31]: cohort design; >42,000 men; ages 40–75 years	6–12	*CHD:* RR fatal CHD 0.45 and RR total MI 0.59 in those averaging 28.9 grams dietary fiber/day, compared with those averaging 12.5 g/day; stronger association with cereal fiber than with fruits and vegetables; 19% decrease in risk of MI per 10 g/day increase in dietary fiber and a 29% decrease per 10 g/day increase in cereal fiber. *Glucose:* RR type 2 DM 2.17 for high-GL/low-cereal-fiber diet (<2.5 g/day), compared with low-GL/high-cereal-fiber diet (>5.8 g/day).
Iowa Women's Health Study[24,31]: cohort design; nearly 36,000 women, postmenopause	6	*CHD:* About one-third decrease in risk of fatal CHD with ≥1 serving/day of whole grains, compared with those with little whole-grain intake; risk decreased with fiber from cereals, not fruits and vegetables; decreased likelihood of mortality from ischemic heart disease with more frequent intake of dark (whole-grain) bread and whole-grain breakfast cereals. *Glucose:* Inverse relationship of insoluble fiber intake from cereals and risk of DM; no relationship to fruit, vegetable, legume intake; RR diabetes 0.79 for median intake of 20.5 servings/week of whole-grain products, compared with median of 1 serving/week.

table

23–7 Summary of Selected Studies Related to Fiber and Risk of CHD and Improved Glucose Control *(continued)*

Study Name and Population Characteristics[a]	Follow-Up Time (years)	Results/Conclusions
Iowa Women's Health Study[33]: cohort design; 27,312 women, postmenopause; ages 55–69 years	17	*CVD/CHD:* Inverse relationship between total whole-grain intake and mortality from CVD and CHD. After multivariate adjustment, RR mortality from CVD and CHD 0.73 and 0.72, respectively, for consuming >19 g/week versus rarely to never consuming whole-grain products. Participants were free of CVD at baseline.
Cardiovascular Health Study, fiber intake analysis[28]: cohort design; 3588 men and women; ages ≥65 years (average 72 at baseline)	8.6	*CHD/CVD:* Cereal fiber intake was inversely associated with incident CVD. Hazard ratio 0.79 (21% lower risk) in highest quintile of fiber intake versus lowest quintile. The difference was seen with about 4.6 grams fiber/day (2 slices whole-grain bread). Lower risk predominantly with fiber in dark bread (whole-wheat, rye, pumpernickel). Fruit and vegetable fiber intake was not associated with incident CVD. Participants were free of known CVD at baseline.
Alpha-tocopherol, beta-carotene cancer prevention study[24]: nearly 22,000 men; ages 50–69 years	6	*CHD:* RR CHD 0.84 for those averaging 34.5 grams dietary fiber/day, compared with those averaging 16.1 g/day with fiber intake adjusted to 2000 calories; high-fiber intake: 12.9 g/1000 cal; low-fiber intake: 5.9 g/1000 cal.
Pooled data, prospective cohort studies[28]: total of 91,058 men and 245,186 women in 10 studies; ages 35–98 years	6–10	*CHD:* RR for all coronary events 0.86 (14% decrease) and RR 0.73 (27% decrease) for coronary death for each 10 g/day increment of total dietary fiber. For cereal fiber, RR 0.9 for all coronary events and RR 0.75 for death; for fruit fiber, RR 0.84 and 0.7; for vegetable fiber, RR 1.00 for all coronary events and death. Similar results for men and women.
Japanese Collaborative Cohort Study for Evaluation of Cancer Risks[28,35]: 58,730 men and women; ages 40–79 years	14.3	*CHD:* Fiber intake from fruit and from cereal but not vegetables was inversely related to CHD mortality. Overall CHD risk was 0.79 for highest quintile of fiber versus lowest. The association for insoluble fiber was stronger than for soluble fiber. All participants were Japanese.
Atherosclerosis Risk in Communities (ARIC) Study, subset with retinal vascular caliber measurements[31]: 10,659 men and women; ages 45–64 years	6	*CVD–retinal vascular caliber:* Inverse dose–response relationship between wider retinal arteriolar caliber/narrower venular caliber and fiber from all sources and from cereal fiber but not from vegetable fiber. Wider retinal arteriolar caliber and narrower venular caliber provide an objective measurement associated with lower CVD risk. Participants included whites and African Americans.
Atherosclerosis Risk in Communities (ARIC) Study[31]: 12,251 men and women: 9529 whites and 2722 African Americans; ages 45–64 years	9	*Glucose:* Inverse relationship with 1 g/day of cereal fiber intake and risk of DM in both African American and white subgroups, but statistically significant only in whites; no relationship to fruit and legume intake in either subgroup. Participants were free of DM at baseline.
Insulin Resistance Atherosclerosis Study (IRAS), subgroup with carotid sonograms[34]: 1178 men and women; ages 40–69 years	5	*CVD–carotid artery intimal medial thickness (IMT) and IMT progression:* Inverse relationship between whole-grain intake and common carotid artery IMT and IMT progression. Carotid IMT is an objective measure related to atherosclerosis; IMT progression is associated with subsequent cardiovascular events. Multi-ethnic participants, with a relatively high proportion of ethnic minority at 26%.
Finnish Mobile Clinic Health Examination Survey[28,31]: 2286 men and 2030 women; ages 40–69 years	10	*Glucose:* Inverse relationship of cereal fiber intake and risk of DM (cereal fiber predominantly from rye; little wheat).
Nurses' Health Studies: NHS-I and NHS-II[28]: cohort design; total 161,737 women; NHS-I: 73,327, ages 37–64 years; NHS-II: 88,410, ages 26–46 years	12–18	*Glucose:* For each 40-gram increment in whole-grain intake, multivariate analysis indicated RR for DM of 0.54 (NHS-I) and 0.64 (NHS-II). BMI accounted for 42% and 57% of the association with RR after adjusting for BMI of 0.7 and 0.83, respectively, for NHS-I and NHS-II.
Black Women's Health Study[36]: cohort design; 40,078 black women with no prior history of diabetes or CVD; ages 21–69 years	8	*Glucose:* Inverse relationship between cereal fiber intake and DM (IRR 0.82). Risk of DM was 18% less for highest quintile of cereal fiber intake compared to lowest quintile. GId associated with risk of DM (IRR 1.23) for the highest quartile versus lowest. Stronger associations for BMI < 25.

Key: BMI = Body mass index; CHD = coronary heart disease; CVD = cardiovascular disease; DM = diabetes mellitus; GId = glycemic index; GL = glycemic load; IMT = intimal medial thickness; IRR = incident rate ratio; = MI = myocardial infarction; RR = relative risk.

[a] Number of participants included in the analysis is not always the entire study population; number of trials included in meta-analysis.

Source: References 24, 28, and 31–36.

have the GI microbiome and its role in human health and disease been explored in earnest. The extent of microbiota influence on health maintenance and disease development appears significant. Although understanding of the complex interactions between the GI tract and enteric microbiota remains incomplete, the paradigm of human biology is shifting to embrace the ecology of the individual and the transgenomic and epigenomic co-metabolism of the individual with his or her own unique GI microbiome.[39,40] The microbiome is being viewed by some as a "superorganism" in a symbiotic relationship with the gut mucosa.[41]

Prebiotics

Prebiotics support the enteric microbiota and are typically substances fermented in the colon. Some fibers act as prebiotics. The undigested fiber enters the colon and is fermented by bacteria, primarily bifidobacteria and lactobacilli. Fermentation products, including short-chain fatty acids (acetate, butyrate, and propionate) and lactate, produce an environment favorable to growth of these beneficial bacteria. To be considered a prebiotic, fiber must selectively stimulate the growth and/or activity of one or a limited number of health-promoting bacterial species residing in the colon and benefit the host.[38,41–43]

Sources and Intake. Inulin-type fructans, including their partial hydrolysis product fructooligosaccharides (FOS), are the most common prebiotics. They are found in low amounts in asparagus, bananas, chicory, Jerusalem artichoke, leek, onion, soy, and wheat.[43] Inulin-type fructans are isolated from such sources and added to foods to attain concentrations contributing to prebiotic effects. Average intake for adults in the United States is estimated at 2.6 g/day.[44]

Health Effects. Both inulin-type fructans and FOS significantly increase bifidobacteria in humans. Doses vary greatly in studies; 5–8 g/day is thought to be adequate for prebiotic effects, and up to 20 g/day is considered an amount that should not cause bloating, distension, and flatulence.[44]

Beneficial effects of prebiotics supported by some human data include stool bulking and decreased constipation, better absorption of calcium and magnesium, reduced triglycerides in mildly hypercholesterolemic individuals, and stimulation of bifidobacteria growth.[41,44,45] Studies using prebiotics for diarrhea are conflicting; results may depend on etiology.[45] Improved vaccine response, decreased GI infections, stimulation of intestinal hormonal peptides, improvement of inflammatory bowel disease symptoms, and reduced tumor growth are other possible benefits of prebiotics. Some beneficial effects may be enhanced with synbiotics, a mixture of both prebiotics and probiotics that together improve host welfare.[43]

Probiotics

Probiotics are nonpathogenic, living microorganisms that have a beneficial effect on the host when consumed in adequate amounts.[38,43] Probiotics must withstand processing, storage, and delivery of the product and survive gastric acidity, bile acid lysis, and pancreatic enzyme digestion.[41,42] Lactic acid–producing bacteria, especially of the genuses *Lactobacillus, Bifidobacterium,* and *Streptococcus,* are most often used in foods and studies. Beyond early infancy, these microorganisms do not permanently colonize the GI tract and must be ingested regularly in sufficient quantity to maintain their presence. When a sufficient number of these bacteria are present, colonization by pathogenic bacteria

is reduced and mucosal defenses in the GI tract are enhanced. Table 23–8 lists possible protective effects of probiotics and postulated mechanisms of action.[41,45,46] Health care providers should use caution when interpreting data; multiple species and strains of common probiotic bacteria exist, and effects cannot be extrapolated across species or even across different strains.[43] Dosing may explain variance in treatment response in published studies. The optimum dose for a given probiotic is not known; however, studies showing efficacy typically use a minimum of 10^7 to 10^{10} CFU per dose or 10^8 to 10^{10} CFU daily.[43,47]

Sources. Many traditional foods are fermented by bacteria and contain high concentrations of lactobacilli. Corn, cassava, millet, leafy vegetables (cabbage), and beans commonly serve as the basic food for fermentation. A few fermented foods are occasionally eaten in the United States, such as brined olives, kimchi (Korean fermented cabbage), miso, sauerkraut, and tempeh; however, the major food source of probiotic bacteria is dairy foods. Many major brands of yogurt contain probiotic bacteria, although viable cultures are not required for yogurt in the United States, and labels do not list the number of viable probiotic organisms. Liquid yogurt drinks (kefir) and cultured fluid milk, such as sweet acidophilus milk and buttermilk, can contain variable amounts of viable organisms; however, most provide adequate amounts (10^8 viable organisms per gram). With the interest in probiotics, new products are appearing regularly with added probiotic organisms, sometimes with little or no data on the organisms added or on the efficacy of the combinations used.

Health Effects. Interest in probiotics has increased dramatically in the past decade. Research covers a wide range of disease states and all ages (premature neonate to elderly). A comprehensive review is beyond the scope of this text; only a glimpse into this active area of research can be provided. Clinical data, for the most part, are preliminary; however, moderate-quality evidence supports the use of probiotics to prevent antibiotic-associated diarrhea, including *C. difficile* diarrhea.[48,49] Table 23–9 lists some of the uses of probiotics and associated organisms.[38–40,43,45–53] Results may be influenced by the dose, frequency of dosing, and/or organisms in any individual probiotic product. Most studies have been small and have used isolated bacteria (classified as nutritional supplements) or foods with added probiotics, rather than foods that naturally contain the beneficial bacteria.

Assessment of Functional Food Use: A Case-Based Approach

FF play a role in preventing disease and optimizing health. For patients who have mild signs of or are at risk for CHD, FF may be a viable alternative to pharmacotherapy, as Case 23–1 illustrates.

Medical Foods and Meal Replacement Foods

Traditional medical foods include products developed for patients with inborn errors of metabolism ("metabolics"). Product descriptions are available on manufacturer Web sites

table
23–8 Possible Protective Effects of Probiotics

Effect of Probiotic	Possible Mechanism for the Effect
GI Barrier Function	
Induce production of protective cytokines mediating EC regeneration and inhibiting apoptosis	Action through TLRs; intestinal homeostasis and EC protection requires recognition of commensal bacteria by TLRs Induction of IL-6
Redistribute and increase expression of factors involved in maintaining EC tight junctions	Altered protein kinase C signaling
Counteract effects or inhibit production of inflammatory cytokines associated with increased EC permeability	IL-10 upregulation (regulatory cytokine) Reduced effect of TNF-alpha and INF-gamma Reduce TNF-alpha production Stimulation of IgA secretion
Antimicrobial Activity	
Inhibit growth of potential pathogens	Decreased luminal pH Production of bactericidal proteins (bacteriocins)
Inhibit adhesion of pathogenic bacteria to EC	Increased mucin production Reduced transepithelial resistance associated with binding of some pathogens Competitive exclusion of pathogens from EC surface binding sites due to nonspecific binding associated with the hydrophobic cell surface properties; mucus-binding pili enhance binding to mucosal surface Binding to pathogenic microorganisms, thereby preventing interaction between the microorganism and EC surface
Influence production of cryptdins by Paneth cells Alter virulence	Antibacterial action of cryptdins Altered secretion of molecules influencing expression of genes controlling virulence
EC Inflammatory Responses	
Alter EC cytokine production	Downregulation of bacteria-induced protein kinase C and IL-6 Inhibition of TNF-alpha-induced IL-8 production Downmodulation of genes associated with proinflammatory signal induction Attenuation of nuclear factor-kappa B activation
Lymphoid Cell	
Enhance antiviral activity	Inhibition of T-cell proliferation Induction of macrophages to express increased amounts of inflammatory cytokines and nitric oxide Stimulation of granulocyte colony-stimulating factor release by macrophages Increased natural killer T-cell activity
Activate macrophages	Increased antigen presentation to B lymphocytes
Regulatory T-Cell Induction	
Increase CD4+ (regulatory) T cells with cell-surface TGF-beta (regulatory cytokine)	Monocyte-derived dendritic cells inducing IL-10 production by T cells

Key: EC = Epithelial cell; GI = gastrointestinal; IgA = immunoglobulin A; IL = interleukin; INF = interferon; TGF = transforming growth factor; TLR = toll-like receptor; TNF = tumor necrosis factor.
Source: References 38, 41–43, and 45.

and may be available from the federally funded Special Supplemental Nutrition Program for Women, Infants, and Children (WIC), because this program is often involved in distribution of products and patient monitoring. Enteral nutrition formulas, specialty formulas in particular, may meet the definition of a medical food; however, many are better classified as food for "special dietary use" because they are readily available without medical supervision and are marketed directly to consumers as regular foods, often as meal replacement products. Enteral formulas are typically semisynthetic liquid formulas intended for oral consumption or administration through a feeding tube. Certain liquid diets designed for use in medically supervised

table
23–9 Evidence-Based Uses of Probiotics[a]

Condition/Disease	Probiotics Most Often Associated with Benefit	Comments
Allergy		
Atopic dermatitis, prevention and treatment	L. rhamnosus GG, B. lactis	Conflicting results; several studies show decreased severity; most studies were small limited studies with good design and adequate power to support effectiveness for atopic eczema associated with cow milk allergy. Meta-analysis with 1477 infants indicated reduced eczema with selected probiotics; however, Cochrane review did not find adequate evidence to support addition of probiotics to infant formula. A subset of infants at high risk of atopic dermatitis may benefit from probiotic administration to the mother during pregnancy and to the infant for several months after birth (this should be done under the supervision of a physician and not done as self-care).
Diarrhea		

Acute, non-antibiotic-associated treatment in pediatrics and adult	Pediatrics:
	  L. rhamnosus GG, L. acidophilus + B. infantis,
	  L. reuteri ATTC 55730,
	  L. casei DN-114 001,
	  S. boulardii lyo
	Adult:
	  Enterococcus faecium LAB SF68,
	  L. rhamnosus GG,
	  S. boulardii
		Multiple studies and meta-analyses; duration of diarrhea reduced by about 1 day. Evidence is stronger for viral gastroenteritis than for bacterial infection. Timing of administration may affect efficacy. Evidence is stronger for treatment than for prevention.

Antibiotic-associated, prevention (not *Clostridium difficile*)	Pediatrics:
	  L. rhamnosus GG,
	  B. lactis Bb12 + Strep. thermophilus,
	  S. boulardii lyo
	Adult:
	  B. clausii,
	  Enterococcus faecium LAB SF68,
	  L. rhamnosus GG,
	  L. acidophilus CL1285 + L. casei Lbc80r,
	  L. casei DN-114 001 + L. bulgaricus + Strep. thermophilus,
	  S. boulardii, VSL#3[b]
		Multiple studies in both adults and pediatric patients. Some conflicting results; however, literature supports benefit overall, except in *Clostridium difficile*–associated diarrhea.

Clostridium difficile colitis, prevention and treatment	S. boulardii lyo, L. rhamnosus GG, L. casei DN-114 001 + L. bulgaricus + Strep. thermophilus, L. acidophilus + B. bifidum	Positive results in some controlled studies; however, there are conflicting results from other studies. Meta-analysis shows benefit. Promising role as adjuvant in treatment of recurrent *C. difficile* diarrhea.

Infectious (not invasive bacterial diarrhea) and travelers' diarrhea	Pediatrics:
	  L. rhamnosus GG,
	  L. reuteri
	Adult:
	  S. boulardii,
	  L. rhamnosus GG
		Results in randomized controlled studies are conflicting; modest positive results with some strains.

Lactose intolerance	L. delbrueckii subsp. bulgaricus, Strep. thermophilus; mixed cultures in fermented milk products	Improved symptoms of lactose intolerance. Microbial beta-galactosidase improves lactose hydrolysis.
Radiation enteritis	L. acidophilus NDCO1748, VSL#3	Limited number of studies provide promising results; probiotic may reduce severity of diarrhea or improve consistency without improving the incidence of diarrhea. Overall, data are inadequate to establish effectiveness at this time.
Rotavirus infection	L. rhamnosus GG, L. reuteri, L. casei GG, B. bifidum, B. lactis	Studies in infants/children strongly support beneficial effect for prevention and treatment.

table

23–9 Evidence-Based Uses of Probiotics[a] *(continued)*

Condition/Disease	Probiotics Most Often Associated with Benefit	Comments
Tube-feeding associated	*S. boulardii*	Data from clinical trials are insufficient to recommend probiotic use. Limited studies available; most are small and have design limitations; conflicting results. No benefit with *L. acidophilus* and *L. bulgaricus*.
IBD		
Crohn's disease, induce and maintain remission	*E. coli* Nissle 1917, *S. boulardii*, VSL#3, *L. rhamnosus* GG	Small clinical studies, some with up to 1 year of follow-up; several randomized controlled trials with equivocal results. Some positive studies; however, data are inadequate to establish effectiveness. No evidence of effectiveness in maintaining remission per Cochrane review.
Pouchitis, preventing and maintaining remission	VSL#3	Strong evidence for effectiveness; randomized, double-blind, placebo-controlled studies. Inadequate studies to establish effectiveness for inducing remission.
Ulcerative colitis	VSL#3, *E. coli* Nissle	Randomized controlled trials have not demonstrated benefit for inducing or maintaining remission. Some positive studies with similar efficacy to anti-inflammatory medications; however, data are inadequate to establish effectiveness.
IBS		
Motility disorders	*B. animalis* DN-173 010 + *L. bulgaris* + *Strep. thermophilus*, *L. shirota*, *L. rhamnosus* GG, *L. rhamnosus* LC705, *S. boulardii*, VSL#3, *B. infantis*	May normalize muscle hypercontractility. Decreased bloating and flatulence in multiple studies; reduced abdominal pain or relief of constipation or diarrhea in some studies; however, there are conflicting results from other studies. Most studies are small and open label. Two larger randomized controlled trials with *B. infantis* showed positive results with a decrease in some symptoms.
Immune Response		
Vaccinations	*L. acidophilus*, *L. plantarum*, *L. johnsonii*, *L. rhamnosus* GG, *B. lactis*	Improved immunologic response to oral vaccinations is supported by randomized trials.
Infection		
Helicobacter pylori	*B. clausii*, bifidobacteria strains, *L. salivarious*, *L. johnsonii*, *L. rhamnosus* GG, *S. boulardii* lyo, *L. casei* DN-114 001 + *L. bulgaricus* + *Strep. thermophilus*	Probiotic appears to reduce treatment-related side effects and improve compliance. Meta-analysis of 14 trials indicates certain probiotics may increase eradication when used with antibiotic therapy, especially with previous treatment failure. Probiotic may inhibit colonization.
Vaginosis and vaginitis	*L. acidophilus*, *L. reuteri*, *L. rhamnosus* GG]	Decreased vaginosis was shown in women with recurrent disease in one study; however, there are conflicting results from other studies; evidence is inadequate to support effectiveness.
Intestinal Permeability		
NEC prevention	*L. acidophilus* + *B. infantis*, *B. bifidus* + *B. infantis* + *Strep. thermophilus*	Strong support for effectiveness in preterm infants; Cochrane review supports supplementation of probiotics in reducing risk of severe NEC and mortality in premature infants.

Key: *B.* = Bifidobacterium; *E.* = Escherichia; IBD = inflammatory bowel disease; IBS = irritable bowel syndrome; *L.* = Lactobacillus; NEC = necrotizing enterocolitis; *S.* = Saccharomyces; *Strep.* = Streptococcus.

[a] Supported by at least one well-designed and adequately powered study and/or included in guidelines for probiotic use or disease management.

[b] VSL#3 contains four lactobacilli strains, three bifidobacteria strains, and *Streptomyces thermophilus*. VSL#3 is marketed as a probiotic medical food.

Source: References 38, 41, 43, and 45–52.

case
23–1

Relevant Evaluation Criteria	Scenario/Model Outcome

Information Gathering

1. Gather essential information about the patient's symptoms and medical history, including:

  a. description of symptom(s) (i.e., nature, onset, duration, severity, associated symptoms)

> Patient has no symptoms; she recently had a health assessment at work and was told that she is at risk of coronary heart disease because of her family history. She says she does not feel sick but she does not want to end up taking a "bunch of pills everyday" like her mother and oldest brother. She wants to do what she can to avoid heart disease and is particularly interested in "functional foods" because of a healthy lifestyle program she recently watched.

  b. description of any factors that seem to precipitate, exacerbate, and/or relieve the patient's symptom(s)

> NA

  c. description of the patient's efforts to relieve the symptoms

> NA

  d. patient's identity

> Maria Bracamonte

  e. age, sex, height, and weight

> 28 years old, female, 5 ft 5 in., 195 lb

  f. patient's occupation

> Third-grade teacher

  g. patient's dietary habits

> Eats breakfast most mornings: typically a cup of coffee and cereal bar from home or a fast food English muffin with egg and bacon.
>
> Lunch: most often a sandwich with potato chips and soft drink from the cafeteria.
>
> Afternoon snack: typically has a candy bar or granola bar.
>
> Dinner: meat (beef, pork, or chicken mostly; fish every once in a while when someone has gone fishing); potatoes or pasta most nights; fresh, frozen, or canned vegetable four to five times per week; sweet dessert (cake, pie, baked goods) or ice cream five to six times a week; typically has a soft drink with dinner, occasionally an alcoholic drink.

  h. patient's sleep habits

> Usually sleeps about 8 hours per night

  i. concurrent medical conditions, prescription and nonprescription medications, and dietary supplements

> None; birth control pill and multivitamin with folate

  j. allergies

> NKDA

  k. history of other adverse reactions to medications

> None

  l. other (describe) _____

Assessment and Triage

2. Differentiate patient's signs/symptoms and correctly identify the patient's primary problem(s).

> Mrs. Bracamonte has no signs/symptoms of disease but wants to follow a preventive strategy with diet.

3. Identify exclusions for self-treatment (Table 23–13).

> None

4. Formulate a comprehensive list of therapeutic alternatives for the primary problem to determine if triage to a health care provider is required, and share this information with the patient or caregiver.

> Options include:
>
> (1) Refer Mrs. Bracamonte to her PCP for a more thorough assessment of heart disease and evaluation of her risk.
>
> (2) Refer Mrs. Bracamonte to a registered dietitian for comprehensive nutritional assessment and counseling.
>
> (3) Inform Mrs. Bracamonte of foods that have health claims associated with reduced risk of heart disease.
>
> (4) Take no action.

Plan

5. Select an optimal therapeutic alternative to address the patient's problem, taking into account patient preferences.

> A combination of the options is appropriate.
>
> (1) Provide basic information and counseling related to functional foods with health claims associated with heart disease. Emphasize authorized and authoritative health claims (Table 23–1) because these have strong scientific evidence supporting the claim. The limited evidence for qualified claims and structure–function claims can be presented along with a discussion of where they fit, if at all, in the patient's overall plan.

case

23-1 continued

Relevant Evaluation Criteria	Scenario/Model Outcome
	(2) Refer Mrs. Bracamonte for cholesterol screening (or perform screening in the pharmacy) and assessment for heart disease.
	(3) Refer Mrs. Bracamonte to a dietitian if she wants/needs more than basic counseling on nutrition, or have her request a referral from her PCP (may be necessary for insurance coverage).
	(4) Weight control and heart disease should be discussed with Mrs. Bracamonte, or these issues should be suggested as part of the discussion with her PCP or a dietitian.
6. Describe the recommended therapeutic approach to the patient or caregiver.	"A number of foods with health claims are associated with decreased risk of heart disease. For several foods, there is significant scientific agreement regarding the potential benefits. Using these foods in place of some of your current foods may reduce your risk of heart disease. However, it would also be helpful to know what your risks are, including your cholesterol level."
7. Explain to the patient or caregiver the rationale for selecting the recommended therapeutic approach from the considered therapeutic alternatives.	"Given your family history, you should have your cholesterol checked periodically and be evaluated for other risk factors for heart disease. Your weight is a risk factor for heart disease for you."
	"I can provide you with basic information on foods that have health claims related to heart disease and that may be of benefit in maintaining heart health. Dietitians are the food and nutrition experts; they can do a comprehensive assessment of your diet and provide more in-depth dietary counseling if you want that."

Patient Education

8. When recommending self-care with nonprescription medications and/or nondrug therapy, convey accurate information to the patient or caregiver.	(1) Decreased dietary saturated fat and cholesterol: No more than 10% of your calories should come from saturated fat, and you should keep cholesterol in your diet at no more than 300 mg cholesterol a day, but less is better. When you use milk, you might want to try 1% milk; most people find that to be more acceptable than nonfat (skim) milk, and it is lower in fat than 2% milk, or you could try soy milk. Low-fat yogurt is also another good calcium source and is usually tolerated by people with lactose intolerance.
	(2) Fruits, vegetables, and grain products that contain fiber, particularly soluble fiber: Recommend replacement of white breads and pasta with whole grain. Total dietary fiber should be at least 25 g/day (AI for women 19–50 years of age).
	(3) Soluble fiber from oat bran, rolled oats, or whole oat flour in certain foods, or barley: Incorporate these products into the diet as replacement for breads and cereals that are not whole grain.
	(4) Soy protein: 25 g/day is required in conjunction with a diet low in saturated fat and cholesterol. For many people, the major dietary modifications needed to eat this much soy are very difficult to make, especially if all family members are not committed to the changes.
	(5) Plant sterol and stanol esters: Total intake is at least 1.3 g/day of sterol esters or 3.4 g/day of stanol esters, as part of a diet low in saturated fat and cholesterol. You usually need to eat the products at least twice a day to get the recommended amount. Some margarines and orange juice have added plant sterol/stanol esters.
	(6) Whole-grain foods: This health claim overlaps somewhat with that for "grain products that contain fiber" (#2) but does not specify "particularly soluble fiber." Insoluble fibers are also important in health. Look for whole grains, such as whole wheat, as the first ingredient on labels.

To make these health claims, foods must generally contain a certain amount of the component. Check food labels for these claims and for ingredient amounts.

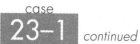

case
23–1 *continued*

Relevant Evaluation Criteria	Scenario/Model Outcome
	There are also health claims with less vigorous supporting data for which evidence suggests a benefit but research is not conclusive (does not prove a benefit); therefore, these claims may not be as effective, or the claims might be changed if new studies are reported. Because the following foods are otherwise healthy foods when used in moderation, they can still be safely incorporated into your diet.
	(1) Walnuts and several other types of nuts: 1.5 ounces a day; remember that nuts are a concentrated source of calories, so use judiciously.
	(2) Omega-3 fatty acids: specifically eicosapentaenoic acid (EPA) and docosahex-aenoic acid (DHA), found in salmon, lake trout, herring, and other oily fish.
	(3) Monounsaturated fats from olive oil: 23 g/day (2 tablespoons) in place of a similar amount of saturated fat. A number of salad dressings and a few soft margarines now include olive oil.
	(4) Canola oil, unsaturated fatty acids: 19 g/day (1.5 tablespoons) in place of a similar amount of saturated fat. Some cooking oil, a number of salad dressings, a few soft margarines, and some baked goods include canola oil.
Solicit follow-up questions from the patient or caregiver.	(1) "Are there any things I need to be aware of as I add these foods into my diet?"
	(2) "Are there any side effects from changing my diet?"
	(3) "Where can I find more information on dietary changes and diet plans to prevent heart disease?"
	(4) "May I use dietary supplements instead of changing to functional foods? Most information on the Internet is advertising for dietary supplements."
Answer the patient's or caregiver's questions.	(1) "These foods should replace other foods in your diet so that the total calories do not increase. The more "healthful" fats must replace saturated fats and not increase the total fat intake. You will need to read food labels carefully to be sure you are getting whole grains, low saturated fats, low cholesterol, and sterol/stanol esters in the product. Also look for the amount of soy or soluble fiber."
	(2) "Rapid increases in fiber content of the diet can cause gas and bloating, so it is best to gradually increase the fiber in your diet. Replace 1–2 servings of white bread and pasta with whole-grain products every few days until the refined foods are totally replaced. Also add extra fiber by gradually replacing the low-fiber cereals with a whole-grain cereal or oatmeal. Fruits and vege-tables can be increased gradually as well to replace snacks and desserts. Be sure to drink plenty of water when eating a high-fiber diet."
	(3) "The FDA Web site (www.fda.gov) includes information on health claims and food labels that you might find helpful. You could consider making an appointment with a registered dietitian, who could help develop some menus that incorporate foods you like and provide more specific plans for substitut-ing healthier foods. Your health insurance plan may contract with a dietitian for coverage. If not, the Academy of Nutrition and Dietetics can provide the name(s) of private consultants and the contact information for a dietitian. The phone number for referrals is on their Web site (www.eatright.org)."
	(4) "In general, foods are better than supplements. Many studies have shown beneficial effects from a diet containing fiber-rich foods and whole grains but not with isolated supplements. Psyllium, found in products like Metamucil, fits criteria for a health claim related to soluble fiber and risk of congestive heart disease, and could be used to increase soluble fiber. It also has the added benefit of reducing constipation, as do fibers from whole grains."

Evaluation of Patient Outcome

9. Assess patient outcome.	"Can we talk about the changes you have made when you pick up your prescrip-tion refills next month?"

Key: AI = Adequate intake; FDA = Food and Drug Administration; NA = not applicable; NKDA = no known drug allergies; PCP = primary care provider.

very-low-calorie diets or bariatric programs are classified as medical foods. Various puddings, shakes, and other solid or semi-solid food forms specially formulated and processed to meet *distinctive* nutritional requirements of the disease or condition for which they are intended can also be classified as medical foods. Both liquid and solid medical foods replace regular meals or enhance nutrient intake to meet the distinctive nutritional requirements of patients. However, these products are also frequently used to meet general nutritional needs.

Providers involved with self-care counseling should determine when a product is used as a medical food to meet truly distinctive nutritional requirements, as determined by scientific studies, and when it is used as meal replacement or enhancement to meet *general* nutritional requirements. Foods intended to meet general nutritional requirements (see Chapter 22) do not need medical oversight and can be used safely for self-care. In contrast, FDA regulations state that medical foods require recommendation or prescription by a physician or authorized prescriber and ongoing medical supervision.[3,13] When enteral formulas are used to meet general nutritional requirements, however, third-party providers may refuse to cover the cost under insurance benefits, leaving patients with self-care responsibility.

Enteral Formula Uses

Tube Feeding

Enteral formulas are best known as complete nutritional replacements for patients requiring a feeding tube to meet their nutritional needs, such as stroke patients with severe dysphagia. Patients who cannot, should not, or will not take adequate nutrients by mouth are candidates for tube feeding and should be under medical care; tube feeding is not a condition conducive to safe and effective self-care. For information related to tube feeding, the reader is referred to one of the many specialized references available, to the American Society for Parenteral and Enteral Nutrition (www.nutritioncare.org), or to the Oley Foundation (www.oley.org), a consumer-oriented organization for support of individuals requiring intravenous or tube feeding.

Many enteral preparations currently are available. Most formulas provide nutritional support consistent with general dietary guidelines and are safe for use in self-care. Formulas intended for patients with impaired digestion and those designed for specific metabolic or clinical conditions require oversight by a health care provider. Characteristics that are likely to result in the use of a formula as a true medical food requiring medical supervision are listed in Table 23–10, along with a few representative products.

Supplementation of Nutrition Intake

Enteral products are frequently used as oral supplements for people of advanced age when effects of chronic disease and impaired mobility decrease nutrient intake. Oral nutritional supplements appear to benefit hospitalized members of this population who are undernourished at baseline; however, routine supplementation at home or for those who are well nourished in any setting is not supported by available evidence.[54] Finally, enteral formulas have been increasingly marketed as "meal replacements." Marketing targets healthy individuals who perceive meal replacement products as healthier alternatives to eating fast foods or skipping a meal or those seeking portion control.

table
23–10 Enteral Formula Characteristics Consistent with Need for Medical Supervision

Characteristic	Examples
Protein as peptides and/or free amino acids	Peptamen, Crucial, Vital
Alteration of the amino acid content by addition of individual amino acids, such as glutamine, arginine, or branch-chain amino acids	Juven, Impact, Perative
Addition of specific fatty acids to alter the inflammatory response	Oxepa
Addition of significant amounts of medium-chain triglycerides to alter absorption	Portagen, Enfaport
High percentage (>50%) of calories from fat	Pulmocare, Nutren Pulmonary
Very high protein content (≥25% of calories as protein)	Impact, Nutren Replete, Promote
Intended for patients with organ failure	Nepro, NutriRenal, NutriHep

Classification of Enteral Nutrition Products

Enteral products are classified as polymeric formulas, oligomeric formulas, and modular components. In addition, a growing segment of meal supplement and meal replacement products, including beverages, bars, and puddings, is designed to assist in meeting nutrient goals within an appropriate caloric intake.

Polymeric Formulas

Polymeric formulas are used most commonly. They are for individuals with normal digestive capability and contain macronutrients in the form of intact (whole) proteins, carbohydrates, and fatty acids or oils. Most individuals requiring alternative nutrition support will tolerate and do well with standard polymeric formulas. The standard formulas usually (1) are 1 kcal/mL unless concentrated to provide less free water; (2) contain a macronutrient composition typical of the American diet (carbohydrate: 45%–70%; protein: 10%–18%; and fat: 20%–40%); and (3) are isotonic to slightly hypertonic (300–450 mOsm/kg); however, flavored products are often in the range of 500 to 700 mOsm/kg. These formulas are generally safe for self-care when taken orally. Formulas listed as being generally safe for self-care are polymeric formulas (Table 23–11).

Oligomeric Formulas

Oligomeric products require minimal digestion and are also known as predigested, peptide, or elemental formulas. They contain free amino acids, hydrolyzed or partially hydrolyzed protein, and less complex carbohydrates. These formulas frequently alter the fat content to improve absorption in patients with impaired absorption. They are rarely consumed orally because of very poor palatability. In general, oligomeric formulas require medical supervision.

table
23–11 **Meal Replacement Products/Liquid Formulas Suitable for Self-Care[a]**

Product Name	Energy (kcal/mL)	Protein grams (% kcal)	CHO grams (% kcal)	Fat grams (% kcal)	Fiber grams	Comments
Routine Formula						
Boost	240 (1.0)	10 (17)	41 (67)	4 (16)	None	Hypertonic
Ensure	250 (1.06)	9 (14)	40 (64)	6 (22)	None	Hypertonic
Jevity 1 Cal	250 (1.06)	10.4 (17)	6.5 (54)	8.2 (29)	3.4	Fiber from soy; isotonic
Routine Formula with Extra Protein						
Boost High Protein Drink	240 (1.0)	15 (24)	33 (55)	6 (21)	None	
Ensure High Protein	230 (0.97)	12 (21)	31 (55)	6 (24)	None	
Routine Concentrated (High-Calorie) Formula						
Boost Plus	350 (1.5)	14 (16)	45 (50)	14 (34)	None	
Ensure Plus	350 (1.5)	13 (15)	51 (57)	11 (28)	None	
Jevity 1.5 Cal	355 (1.5)	15 (17)	51 (54)	11.8 (29)	5.3 (75% I; 25% S; 10 grams FOS)	Osmolite 1.5 Cal has similar nutrient profile without fiber.
Diabetic Formula[b]						
Boost Glucose Control	250 (1.06)	14 (22)	20 (35)	12 (43)	3.5 (I: 0.9; S: 2.6; FOS)	Complex CHO including tapioca starch
Glucerna 1.2 Cal	285 (1.2)	14.2 (20)	27 (35)	14.2 (45)	3.8 (I, S, FOS: 2.4)	Higher omega-3 fat content than many routine formulas; 1 and 1.5 Cal versions are available.
Nutren Glytrol	250 (1.0)	11.3 (18)	25 (40)	11.9 (42)	3.8 (I: 1.3; S: 2.5)	Amylase starch (low glycemic index)

Pulmonary Formula[c]

	Calories (serving)	Protein g (%)	CHO g (%)	Fat g (%)	Fiber	Comments
Pulmocare	355 (1.5)	14.8 (17)	25 (28)	22 (55)	None	High-fat content.
Nutren Pulmonary	375 (1.5)	17 (18)	25 (27)	23.7 (55)	None	High-fat content.

Other Meal Replacements and Supplements

	Calories (serving)	Protein g (%)	CHO g (%)	Fat g (%)	Fiber	Comments
Ensure Clear	200 (0.61)	7 (20)	43 (80)	None		6.7-ounce serving package; clear liquid; not intended as sole source of nutrition.
Carnation Breakfast Essentials (powder for mixing)	220 (0.8)	13 (23)	39 (74)	0.5 (3)	<1	Put 1 packet in 1 cup fat free milk for 9-ounce serving; mixing with 2% or whole milk would increase calories as fat. Can mix with soy milk or reduced lactose milk.
Carnation Ready to Drink	220 (0.8)	14 (24)	31 (57)	5 (19)		
Glucerna Shake	200 (0.84)	10 (20)	26 (48)	7 (32)	3	Fiber from FOS and soy polysaccharide; product not intended as sole source of nutrition.

Modular Components

	Calories (serving)	Protein g (%)	CHO g (%)	Fat g (%)	Fiber	Comments
Beneprotein	25	6 (100)	None	None	None	Listed content per 7-gram packet or 1 scoop.
ProMod Liquid Protein	100	10 (40)	14 (60)	None	None	Listed content per ounce.
Benecalorie	330 (7.5)	7 (9)	None	33 (91)	None	Listed content per 1.5-ounce serving (44 mL). Product is a modular component; add to enteral formula or foods to increase calories.

Key: CHO = Carbohydrate; FOS = fructooligosaccharides; I = insoluble fiber; S = soluble fiber.

[a] Amounts per 8 ounce serving unless otherwise indicated.

[b] Use sparingly for self-care because the fat content is relatively high compared in studies with high-fat/low-carbohydrate diets and is higher than recommended by general dietary guidelines. In accordance with recommendations from the American Diabetes Association (www.ada.org; see American Diabetes Association, Bantle JP, Wylie-Rosett J, et al. Nutrition recommendations and interventions for diabetes: a position statement of the American Diabetes Association. Diabetes Care. 2008;31(suppl 1):S61–78), monounsaturated fatty acid content tends to be higher than in many standard formulas and saturated fat content is low.

[c] Use sparingly for self-care because the fat content is higher than recommended by general dietary guidelines.

Note: The most current and detailed information is available at manufacturer Web sites, including Abbott Nutrition (www.abbottnutrition.com) and Néstle Nutrition (www.ensure.com/products).

Modular Products

Modular products supplement a single macronutrient. Examples include protein powder, medium-chain triglyceride oil, emulsified oils, and powdered, flavorless glucose polymers. These products can be incorporated into food to increase protein and calorie content. For example, a protein powder may benefit a person of advanced age who is having difficulty meeting protein requirements with his or her usual oral diet.

Specialty Formulas

Specialty formulas may be either polymeric or oligomeric. They are designed to optimize the nutrient intake and improve disease management for patients with specific disease states such as renal insufficiency, diabetes mellitus, hepatic dysfunction, and carbon dioxide–retaining pulmonary dysfunction. The use of specialty formulas is controversial because data supporting improved outcomes are minimal. In general, use of specialty formulas requires medical supervision. Consultation with a registered dietitian, certified nutrition support clinician, or board-certified nutrition support pharmacist may be warranted.

Some specialty formulas, such as certain pulmonary and diabetic formulas, alter the ratio of fat and carbohydrate but contain no special dietary components. Although technically such products are medical foods, there would be little concern for most individuals who used them to replace a few meals per week. However, individuals must be encouraged to limit their use of these products unless otherwise advised by their primary care provider or a provider who specializes in nutritional management of their condition. They should advise their primary care provider when they use these products, because management of the underlying disease itself requires medical oversight. Table 23–11 includes a few examples of pulmonary and diabetic formulas.

Product Use for Self-Care

All products recommended for self-care should contain basic nutrition labeling, including serving size, calories, protein, fat, and other components consistent with food labeling so that nutrient intake can be determined in the same manner as with regular foods. Many formulas are available in a variety of flavors to reduce taste fatigue; slight differences in nutrient content may be noted among the flavors.

Administration and Monitoring Guidelines for Enteral Nutrition

For products taken orally, the individual should be encouraged to vary flavors to avoid taste fatigue and to consume the product after an attempt to eat a well-balanced meal or a between-meal snack. Chilling may improve palatability. Once opened, the container should be kept refrigerated to prevent bacterial growth, and all open or prepared products should be discarded after 24 hours.

When products are given as tube feeding, medical supervision is recommended. Enteral nutrition practice recommendations are available at the American Society for Parenteral and Enteral Nutrition Web site (www.nutritioncare.org). Referral to a nutrition support provider may be appropriate. Medical referral is appropriate for individuals who develop diarrhea, nausea, or abdominal distension when taking meal replacement

formulas. Formula-related diarrhea is an osmotic diarrhea that usually stops within 24 hours of discontinuing the formula; diarrhea that persists longer is unlikely to be caused by the formula per se. Lactose intolerance is seldom an issue with enteral formulas because most formulas are lactose-free except powders prepared with milk. High-fat products can delay gastric emptying, resulting in nausea and/or bloating.

Food–Medication Interactions

Interactions between medications and enteral formulas often are complex and poorly understood. Interactions involving a formula component have the potential to occur with either oral administration or feeding tube administration. The provider is advised to consult specialty references for a more complete list and explanation of such interactions. General practice for certain medications (including phenytoin, carbamazepine, and warfarin) is to withhold the formula for 1 or 2 hours before and after administering the medication, especially when therapeutic levels are not achieved with typical doses. It is reasonable to suggest this same precaution of separating the drug by 1 or 2 hours when formula is taken by mouth and to advise supervision of the medication response by a primary care provider. Vitamin K content of the formula should also be checked for individuals on warfarin. Although most formulas provide no more vitamin K than that of a typical diet, a few contain amounts that could interfere with anticoagulation. Manufacturers' Web sites, such as those listed in the footnotes of Table 23–11, provide detailed, up-to-date information on the nutrient content of formulas.

Other Medical Food and Meal Replacement Food

In recent years, several medical foods have become available for a range of common diseases treated in the ambulatory care setting, as shown in Table 23–12. Foods used in weight-loss and bariatric programs are also medical foods requiring medical supervision when used as intended because of significant risks

table
23–12 | **Medical Foods for Common Conditions**

Condition	Product (Manufacturer)
Alzheimer's disease	Axona (Accera Inc.)
Depression	Deplin (Pamlab)
Depression-associated sleep disorders	Sentra PM (Targeted Medical Pharma)
Irritable bowel syndrome	VSL#3 probiotic (Sigma-Tau Pharmaceuticals)
Osteoarthritis	Limbrel (Primus Pharmaceuticals)
Osteopenia/ osteoporosis	Fosteum (Primus Pharmaceuticals)
Pain and inflammation	Theramine (Targeted Medical Pharma)
Ulcerative colitis	VSL#3 probiotic (Sigma-Tau Pharmaceuticals)

table

23–13   Exclusions for Self-Care with Enteral Formulas

Condition	Example/Comment
Organ dysfunction requiring diet modification	Renal insufficiency requiring restriction of protein and electrolytes eliminated through the kidneys (potassium, phosphorus, magnesium).
Gastrointestinal dysfunction	Poor motility: Dietary modification may be required to avoid bowel obstructions; enteral formula may be appropriate under the supervision of a primary care provider or nutrition specialist, but not as self-care. Reduced absorption: Hydrolyzed protein, modified fats, and/or relatively simple carbohydrates may be necessary for adequate absorption; monitoring for nutrient deficiencies is required. Dysphagia: Referral for medical evaluation is required. Bariatric surgery: Medical supervision is required; recommendations of primary care provider or nutrition specialist should be followed.
Significant unintended weight loss	Refer for medical evaluation to determine the etiology. Life-threatening fluid and electrolyte abnormalities can occur when refeeding these individuals; medical supervision and monitoring are required.
Disease state affected by diet, such as diabetes mellitus, chronic obstructive pulmonary disease	Enteral formula may be appropriate to meet nutritional requirements; however, use should be under the supervision of a primary care provider or nutrition specialist, but not as self-care.

associated with rapid weight loss. Meal replacement foods such as Slim Fast, Weight Watchers, and Jenny Craig products are not medical foods. They can be used safely without medical supervision to help control portion size and balance nutrient intake; however, they should be used as part of an overall weight-loss plan (see Chapter 26).

Assessment of Enteral Nutrition and Meal Replacements: A Case-Based Approach

The first step in assessing the type of meal replacement (or supplement) to recommend is to determine whether the individual has any exclusion to self-care as listed in Table 23–13. If self-care is appropriate, the provider should ascertain the reason for a meal replacement or supplement so that the most appropriate product can be selected. For instance, a person of advanced age with early satiety may benefit from a concentrated formula that provides 1.5 or 2 kcal/mL, whereas a young person wanting a meal supplement for use with weight lifting may benefit from a higher-protein formula. The selected formula should be appropriate to meet the individual's specific nutritional needs according to health status while avoiding excessive or contraindicated macronutrients and micronutrients.

Meal replacement products can have efficacy for the treatment of many health concerns. Traditionally, meal replacement has been considered a therapeutic intervention needed to maintain adequate nutrition in malnourished patients, to completely replace nutritional intake in patients with a physical limitation that interferes with nutritional intake such as dysphagia, or to precisely control intake of specific dietary components (calories for obesity and phenylalanine in phenylketonuria). Increasingly, nutrition products are used as lifestyle choices of self-directed therapy. This practice is particularly true of the meal replacement products used by working individuals who are too busy to prepare or eat a proper meal or who perceive these products as healthier alternatives to fast foods.

Case 23–2 illustrates assessment of a patient with dysphagia and weight loss who seeks a liquid meal replacement.

Patient Counseling for Enteral Nutrition and Meal Replacements

Advancements in enteral products and home infusion therapy are allowing more people with serious, even terminal, illnesses to be cared for at home. Enteral products are also appropriate for ambulatory patients with metabolic or digestive diseases and for persons who want to ensure adequate nutrition for their life stage. Providers serve a pivotal role in helping patients to use the product best suited for their nutritional needs and to use it under medical supervision when appropriate. The box Patient Education for Enteral and Meal Replacement Products lists specific information to provide patients and caregivers.

Key Points for Functional and Meal Replacement Foods

➤ The definition of FF typically includes "health benefits beyond those of basic nutrition."

➤ Health claims are statements describing an association between a food, food component, dietary ingredient, or dietary supplement and the risk of a disease or health-related condition.

➤ *Authorized* and *authoritative* health claims meet the significant scientific agreement level of evidence. These claims should routinely be incorporated into counseling for lifestyle changes associated with health benefits and, when appropriate, as part of an overall plan for management of diseases associated with the claim.

➤ *Qualified* health claims do not meet the significant scientific agreement level of evidence; claims statements must

case
23–2

Relevant Evaluation Criteria	Scenario/Model Outcome

Information Gathering

1. Gather essential information about the patient's symptoms and medical history, including:

a. description of symptom(s) (i.e., nature, onset, duration, severity, associated symptoms)

Alzheimer's dementia symptoms, progressive. Patient is easily frustrated and demanding of attention.

Patient's daughter describes him as being very forgetful and showing more signs of Alzheimer's dementia in the past month. At the Alzheimer's family support meeting last week, she heard about a new food/liquid meal that is helpful with slowing Alzheimer's progression and is requesting this product for her father.

b. description of any factors that seem to precipitate, exacerbate, and/or relieve the patient's symptom(s)

NA

c. description of the patient's efforts to relieve the symptoms

Patient is currently taking donepezil. He also takes a multivitamin-mineral supplement.

d. patient's identity

Lambert Jorgenson

e. age, sex, height, and weight

84 years old, male, 5 ft 10 in., 155 lb

f. patient's occupation

Retired truck driver

g. patient's dietary habits

Usually takes two meals daily and a couple snacks. Must be reminded to eat and encouraged to eat more than one food off his plate.

h. patient's sleep habits

Sleeps about 6 hours at night but also naps during the day.

i. concurrent medical conditions, prescription and non-prescription medications, and dietary supplements

Hydrochlorothiazide for hypertension; multivitamin/mineral supplement

j. allergies

Codeine; sulfa (rash)

k. history of other adverse reactions to medications

Ataxia with metronidazole

l. other (describe) _____

Assessment and Triage

2. Differentiate patient's signs/symptoms and correctly identify the patient's primary problem(s).

Patient's daughter is requesting a medical food for use in Alzheimer's dementia.

3. Identify exclusions for self-treatment.

Medical foods require medical supervision.

4. Formulate a comprehensive list of therapeutic alternatives for the primary problem to determine if triage to a health care provider is required, and share this information with the patient or caregiver.

Options include:

(1) Refer patient to his PCP to discuss use of the medical food and obtain a prescription.

(2) Recommend self-care with a general supplement to improve nutrient intake.

(3) Take no action.

Plan

5. Select an optimal therapeutic alternative to address the patient's problem, taking into account patient preferences.

"Patient's daughter should consult with her father's PCP regarding the medical food."

6. Describe the recommended therapeutic approach to the patient or caregiver.

"You are requesting a product that requires medical supervision for use. The pharmacy can order the product for you once you have discussed this with your father's physician and you have a prescription."

7. Explain to the patient or caregiver the rationale for selecting the recommended therapeutic approach from the considered therapeutic alternatives.

"In addition to verifying that your father has medical supervision for using the product, a prescription may make the product eligible for coverage by your father's insurance."

case
23–2 *continued*

Relevant Evaluation Criteria	Scenario/Model Outcome
Patient Education	
8. When recommending self-care with nonprescription medications and/or nondrug therapy, convey accurate information to the patient or caregiver.	Criterion does not apply in this case.
Solicit follow-up questions from the patient or caregiver.	"Do you know how this product works, and could I just change what I cook for my father rather than getting a prescription?"
Answer the patient's or caregiver's questions.	"The product is based on a specific type of fat that is absorbed and metabolized differently than the typical oils found in the grocery store. It must be given in an appropriate amount with a proper balance of other nutrients to achieve the desired effect."
Evaluation of Patient Outcome	
9. Assess patient outcome.	"Let me know when you have the prescription and want me to order the product. If you want more information on the product, you can also check the Web site (www.about-axona.com)."

Key: PCP = Primary care provider.

include language that indicates the qualified nature of the health claim.

➤ *Structure–function* claims lack the significant scientific agreement level of evidence and make no association between the product and risk of a disease or health-related condition; they do not require validation or authorization by FDA.

➤ Health care providers should understand the limitations of qualified health claims and structure–function claims. When counseling for lifestyle changes, the limited scientific evidence for these claims should be clearly delineated so individuals can understand the role, or lack thereof, for these products in a healthy lifestyle.

➤ Foods for special dietary use meet *particular dietary needs* related to physical, physiologic, pathologic, or other conditions, such as disease, convalescence, pregnancy, lactation, underweight, overweight, infancy, or need for sodium restriction, or they supplement or fortify the usual diet; they are subject to general labeling requirements for foods and do not require use under medical supervision.

➤ Medical foods are specially formulated and processed to meet *distinctive nutritional requirements* (established by medical evaluation based on recognized scientific principles) of the disease or condition for which they are intended. These foods are to be recommended and used under medical supervision.

➤ Conventional foods classified as FF are typically associated with health benefits in epidemiologic studies; evidence supporting a functional role for these foods is weak-moderate, with clinical trials often lacking.

➤ Fiber is associated with improved laxation, cholesterol reduction, satiety, and probably glucose control for select fiber sources.

patient education for
Enteral and Meal Replacement Products

The objective of self-treatment is to provide the appropriate amounts and types of specific micronutrients and macronutrients to meet the individual's nutritional needs. For most individuals, the product instructions and self-care measures listed here will help ensure optimal therapeutic outcomes.

- Typical products provide 1 cal/mL; higher-calorie products are available if you must limit your fluid intake or can drink only a small amount at a time.
- When drinking the formula, take about 1/2–1 can at a time. You can drink the formula at room temperature, but it may taste better if chilled or semifrozen as a slush-type drink.
- Varying the flavor of the formula may reduce taste fatigue.
- For tube feeding, the product should be used as directed by your primary care or nutrition care provider. The Oley Foundation (www.oley.org) provides consumer information on tube feeding.
- Keep opened containers refrigerated and covered to prevent bacterial growth; discard all remaining prepared products

after 24 hours. Unopened product can be stored at room temperature.
- Use of meal replacement products as the sole or primary source of nutrition for more than a short time (2–3 weeks) requires medical supervision and should be discussed with your primary care provider. Periodic laboratory testing may be appropriate to detect electrolyte abnormalities in this situation.

When to Seek Medical Attention

- Monitor blood glucose levels if you have diabetes or have had high blood glucose (sugar) levels. Talk to your primary care provider if blood glucose levels are high or low.

➤ Prebiotics are fermentable dietary components that selectively stimulate the growth and/or activity of one or a limited number of bacteria in the colon (bifidobacteria and lactobacilli), thereby benefiting the host.

➤ Probiotics are nonpathogenic, living microorganisms that have a beneficial effect on the host when consumed regularly in adequate amounts. They are often present in fermented products from milk (yogurt and kefir) or plants (sauerkraut and miso).

➤ Probiotics have shown beneficial effects in a number of diseases; however, the particular species and strain and the dose necessary for beneficial effects often remain controversial and may vary from condition to condition.

➤ Enteral nutrition products may be classified as medical foods; however, many polymeric enteral formulas are readily available and can often be used safely as a meal replacement product.

➤ Specialty enteral formulas should be used with medical supervision, not for self-treatment.

REFERENCES

1. International Food Information Council. Functional foods consumer survey results: consumer insights to help Americans step up to the (functional foods) plate. Accessed at http://www.foodinsight.org/blogs/2013-functional-foods-consumer-survey-results-consumer-insights-help-americans-step-functional, September 15, 2014.

2. International Food Information Council. Food and health survey: consumer attitudes toward foods safety, nutrition and health. Accessed at http://www.foodinsight.org/2012_Food_Health_Survey_Consumer_Attitudes_toward_Food_Safety_Nutrition_and_Health, September 15, 2014.

3. Pew Initiative on Food and Biotechnology. Applications of biotechnology for functional foods. Washington, DC: Pew Charitable Trusts; 2007. Accessed at http://www.pewtrusts.org/en/research-and-analysis/reports/0001/01/01/application-of-biotechnology-for-functional-foods, September 15, 2014.

4. Academy of Nutrition and Dietetics. Position of the Academy of Nutrition and Dietetics: functional foods. *J Acad Nutr Diet.* 2013;113(8):1096–103.

5. Caselli M, Cassol F, Calo G, et al. Actual concept of "probiotics": is it more functional to science or business? *World J Gastroenterol.* 2013;19(10):1527–40.

6. Wijnkoop-Lenoir I, Jones PJ, Milner J, et al. Nutrition economics: food as an ally of public health. *Br J Nutr.* 2013;109(5):777–84.

7. Panagiotakos DB, Polychronopoulous E. The role of the Mediterranean diet in the epidemiology of metabolic syndrome: converting epidemiology to clinical practice. *Lipid Health Dis.* 2005;4:7–12.

8. Ong TP, Moreno FS, Ross SA. Targeting the epigenome with bioactive foods components for cancer prevention. *J Nutrigenetics Nutrigenomics.* 2011;4(5):275–92.

9. Liu RH. Health benefits of fruits and vegetables are from additive and synergistic combinations of phytochemicals. *Am J Clin Nutr.* 2003;78 (3 suppl):517s–20s.

10. Baker CB, Rodriquez E. New models in translational phytotherapy: dietary phytochemicals in functional nutrition management and pharmaconutrition. *Pharmaceut Biol.* 2012;5(2):642–9.

11. Son TG, Camandola S, Mattson MP. Hormetic dietary phytochemicals. *Neuromolecular Med.* 2008;10(4):236–46.

12. Navia J, Byers T, Djordjevic D, et al. Integrating the totality of food and nutrition evidence for public health decision making and communication. *Crit Rev Food Sci Nutr.* 2010;50(suppl 1):1–8.

13. U.S. Food and Drug Administration, Center for Food Safety and Applied Nutrition. Food ingredients, packaging, and labeling: labeling and nutrition. Health claims meeting significant scientific agreement (SSA). Updated July 19, 2013. Accessed at http://www.fda.gov/Food/IngredientsPackagingLabeling/LabelingNutrition/ucm2006876.htm, July 26, 2013.

14. U.S. Food and Drug Administration, Office of Nutritional Products, Labeling, and Dietary Supplements. Summary of Qualified Health Claims Subject to Enforcement Discretion. Latest update March 13, 2013. Accessed at http://www.fda.gov/Food/IngredientsPackagingLabeling/LabelingNutrition/ucm073992.htm, June 22, 2013.

15. Combs GF Jr., Trumbo PR, McKinley MG, et al. Biomarkers in nutrition: new frontiers in research and application. *Ann NY Acad Sci.* 2013;1278:1–10.

16. Kato H. Nutrigenomics: the cutting edge and Asian perspectives. *Asian Pacific J Clin Nutr.* 2008;17(1):12–5.

17. Pezzuto JM, Venkatasubramanian V, Hamad M, et al. Unraveling the relationship between grapes and health. *J Nutr.* 2009;139(9):1783S–7S.

18. Lordan S, Ross RP, Stanton C. Marine bioactives as functional food ingredients: potential to reduce the incidence of chronic diseases. *Mar Drugs.* 2011;9(6):1056–100.

19. Reuter S, Gupta S, Park B, et al. Epigenetic changes induced by curcumin and other natural compounds. *Genes Nutr.* 2011;6(2):93–108.

20. International Food Information Council Foundation. Functional foods. July 2011. Accessed at http://www.foodinsight.org/Content/3842/Final%20Functional%20Foods%20Backgrounder.pdf, June 16, 2013.

21. International Food Information Council Foundation. Functional food fact sheet: antioxidants. *Food Insight,* October 15, 2009. Accessed at http://www.foodinsight.org/Resources/Detail.aspx?topic=Functional_Foods_Fact_Sheet_Antioxidants, June 16, 2013.

22. Baker, CB. Traditional functional foods for the chemoprevention of chronic diseases: phytopharmacological concepts in food synergy. In: Martirosyan D, Abate N, eds. *Functional Foods for Chronic Diseases: Diabetes and Related Diseases.* Vol. 5. Richardson, Texas: Food Science Publisher; 2010:343–4.

23. Lampe JW. Interindividual differences in response to plant-based diets: implications for cancer risk. *Am J Clin Nutr.* 2009;89(5):1553S–7S.

24. Food and Nutrition Board, Institute of Medicine, National Academy of Sciences. Dietary, Functional, and Total Fiber. In: *Dietary Reference Intakes for Energy, Carbohydrates, Fiber, Fat, Protein and Amino Acids (Macronutrients).* Washington, DC: National Academies Press; 2005:339–421. Accessed at http://www.nap.edu/openbook.php?record_id=10490&page=339, June 30, 2013.

25. Food and Nutrition Board, Institute of Medicine, National Academy of Sciences. Summary tables, dietary reference intakes. Recommended intakes for individuals, total water and macronutrients. In: *Dietary Reference Intakes for Energy, Carbohydrates, Fiber, Fat, Protein and Amino Acids.* Washington, DC: National Academies Press; 2002:1324. Accessed at http://www.iom.edu/Reports/2002/Dietary-Reference-Intakes-for-Energy-Carbohydrate-Fiber-Fat-Fatty-Acids-Cholesterol-Protein-and-Amino-Acids.aspx, June 15, 2013.

26. Kendall CWC, Esfahani A, Jenkins DJA. The link between dietary fibre and human health. *Food Hydrocolloids.* 2010;24:42–8.

27. Chutkan R, Fahey G, Wright WL, et al. Viscous versus nonviscous fiber supplements: mechanisms and evidence for fiber-specific health benefits. *J Am Acad Nurse Pract.* 2012;24(8):476–87.

28. Bernstein AM, Titgemeier B, Kirkpatrick K, et al. Major cereal grain fibers and psyllium in relation to cardiovascular health. *Nutrients.* 2013;5(5):1471–87.

29. King DE, Mainous AG III, Lambourne CA. Trends in dietary fiber intake in the United States, 1999–2008. *J Acad Nutr Diet.* 2012;112(5):642–8.

30. International Food Information Council Foundation. Fiber fact sheet. Food Insight, November 24, 2008. Accessed at http://www.foodinsight.org/Content/6/FINAL%20IFICFndtnFiberFactSheet%2011%20 21%2008.pdf, September 15, 2014.

31. Parillo M, Riccardi G. Diet composition and the risk of type 2 diabetes: epidemiological and clinical evidence. *Br J Nutr.* 2004;92(1):7–19.

32. He M, van Dam RM, Rimm E, et al. Whole-grain, cereal fiber, bran, and germ intake and the risks of all-cause and cardiovascular disease-specific mortality among women with type 2 diabetes mellitus. *Circulation.* 2010;121(20):2162–8.

33. Jacobs DR, Anderson LF, Blomhoff R. Whole-grain consumption is associated with a reduced risk of noncardiovascular, noncancer death attributed to inflammatory diseases in the Iowa Women's Health Study. *Am J Clin Nutr.* 2007;85:1606–14.

34. Mellen PB, Liese AD, Tooze JA, et al. Whole-grain intake and carotid artery atherosclerosis in a multiethnic cohort: the Insulin Resistance Atherosclerosis Study. *Am J Clin Nutr.* 2007;85(6):1495–502.

35. Ye EQ, Chacko SA, Chou EL, et al. Greater whole-grain intake is associated with lower risk of type 2 diabetes, cardiovascular disease, and weight gain. *J Nutr.* 2012;142(7):1304–13.

36. Krishnan S, Rosenberg L, Singer M, et al. Glycemic index, glycemic load, and fiber intake and risk of type 2 diabetes in US black women. *Arch Intern Med.* 2007;167(21):2304–9.

37. Kristensen M, Jensen MG. Dietary fibres in the regulation of appetite and food intake. Importance of viscosity. *Appetite.* 2011;56(1):65–70.

38. Quigley EM. Prebiotics and probiotics; modifying and mining the microbiota. *Pharmacol Res.* 2010;61(3):213–8.

39. Tang H, Zhao G, Nicholson JK, et al. Symbiotic gut microbes modulate human metabolic phenotypes. *PNAS.* 2008;105(6):2117–22.

40. Mugge BD, Kuczynski J, Knight D, et al. Diet drives convergence in gut microbiome functions across mammalian phylogeny and within humans. *Science.* 2011;332(6032):970–4.

41. Vieira AT, Teixeira MM, Martins FS. The role of probiotics and prebiotics in inducing gut immunity. *Front Immunol.* 2013;4(article 445):1–12.

42. Charalampopoulos D, Rastall RA. Prebiotics in foods. *Curr Opin Biotech.* 2012;23(2):187–91.

43. Guarner F, Khan AG, Garisch J, et al. Probiotics and prebiotics. World Gastroenterology Organisation practice guideline. May 2008. Accessed at http://www.worldgastroenterology.org/probiotics-prebiotics.html, June 21, 2013.

44. Roberfroid MB. Inulin-type fructans: functional food ingredients. *J Nutr.* 2007;137(11 suppl):2493S–502S.

45. Boirivant M, Strober W. The mechanisms of action of probiotics. *Curr Opin Gastroenterol.* 2007;23(6):679–92.

46. Nagpal R, Kumar A, Kumar M, et al. Probiotics, their health benefits and applications for developing healthier foods: a review. *FEMS Microbiol Lett.* 2012;334(1):1–15.

47. Saavedra JM. Use of probiotics in pediatrics: rationale, mechanisms of action, and practical aspects. *Nutr Clin Pract.* 2007;22(3):351–65.

48. Goldenberg JZ, Ma SSY, Martzen MR, et al. Probiotics for the prevention of Clostridium difficile-associated diarrhea in adults and children (review). *Cochrane Database System Rev.* 2013;5:CD006095. doi: 10.1002/14651858. CD006095.pub3. Accessed at http://www.thecochranelibrary.com/view/0/index.html.

49. Kale-Pradhan PB, Jassat HR, Wilhelm SM. Role of Lactobacillus in the prevention of antibiotic-associated diarrhea: a meta-analysis. *Pharmacotherapy.* 2010;30(2):119–26.

50. Farnworth ER. The evidence to support health claims for probiotics. *J Nutr.* 2008;138(6):1250S–4S.

51. Minocha A. Probiotics for preventative health. *Nutr Clin Pract.* 2009; 24(2):227–41.

52. Floch MH, Walker A, Guandalini S, et al. Recommendations for probiotic use–2008. *J Clin Gastroenterol.* 2008;42(suppl 2):S104–8.

53. Diamant M, Blaak EE, de Vos M. Do nutrient-gut-microbiota interactions play a role in human obesity, insulin resistance and type 2 diabetes? *Obes Rev.* 2011;12(4):272–81.

54. Milne AC, Avenell A, Potter J. Meta-analysis: protein and energy supplementation in older people. *Ann Intern Med.* 2006;144(1):37–48.

SPORTS NUTRITION AND PERFORMANCE-ENHANCING NUTRIENTS AND SUPPLEMENTS

Mark Newnham

Competing athletes exercise at various levels. Recreationally active individuals may spend 5–10 hours or more per week in physical activity, and diet alone should meet their nutritional needs. By comparison, high-volume intense training for 10–20 hours or more per week may require specific nutritional intake to maintain or enhance performance.[1] This chapter reviews the effects of products that contain macronutrients and nutritional supplements on physical activity and performance for both the recreational athlete and the more aggressive competitor. Food supplements and natural products are marketed as ergogenic aids to athletes and active people for three primary purposes: (1) to improve strength and power, (2) to prolong the duration of exercise by providing fuel for continued effort, and (3) to replace water and electrolytes lost from sweat to prevent dehydration and to support normal muscle contractions. Readers are referred to two guidelines for detailed discussions on this topic: (1) the International Society of Sports Nutrition (ISSN) Exercise and Sport Nutrition Review[1] and (2) a joint statement of the American Dietetic Association (ADA), the Canadian Dietetic Association, and the American College of Sports Medicine guidelines (ADA guidelines) for Nutrition and Athletic Performance.[2]

Popularity of Sports Nutrition Products

Sports nutrition products and performance-enhancing supplements have gained wide acceptance in both highly trained athletes and mildly to moderately active individuals. Increasing numbers of consumers are choosing sports nutrition products as lifestyle alternatives to traditional beverages and snacks. In 2013, the sports nutrition market was estimated to reach $10 billion in sales.[3] The market segment includes traditional carbohydrate and electrolyte sports drinks along with energy drinks with supplemental caffeine, recovery drinks, and other nutrient-enhanced soft drinks, juices, and waters. The market for solid forms includes meal replacement bars and easy-to-digest carbohydrate gels. Tablets, capsules, and powders that contain macronutrients, electrolytes, and herbal supplements are included in the supplement market.

FDA, NCAA, Antidoping Agencies, and Regulation of Performance-Enhancing Supplements

The Food and Drug Administration (FDA) does not approve dietary supplements or validate claims of performance enhancement. Reports of nutritional supplement misbranding are common.[4,5]

Misbranding occurs when products contain an ingredient not listed on the nutrition facts and ingredients label, or when products contain less than the stated quantity of a labeled ingredient. Unlabeled doping substances including amphetamines and anabolic steroids were found in 19% of vitamin and creatine supplements submitted for voluntary testing by Olympic athletes in 2002.[4] More recently, products purchased over the counter or through the Internet were found to contain the following recombinant hormones: erythropoetin, growth hormone, insulin-like growth factor, and growth-hormone-releasing protein.[5] The antidoping agencies state clearly that athletes are responsible for substances they ingest. A positive test results in a violation regardless of the package label. Nutritional products are tested at independent laboratories such as ConsumerLab. com, which provides reports for a fee. A list of banned substances and antidoping resources is available at these Web sites: www. usantidoping.org, www.wada-ama.org, and www.consumer lab.com. Chapter 50 provides a more detailed discussion of dietary supplement regulation.

Dietary supplements and prescription drugs are used and shared among college and high school athletes, possibly for performance gains. In 2009, the National Collegiate Athletic Association (NCAA) surveyed 20,474 athletes who participated in sports at division I, II, and III levels.[6] The NCAA survey reported high rates of nutritional supplement use, including a 44.5% and 13.9% rate for using an energy drink or an energy booster in the previous 12 months, respectively. Other observations include a 38.4% use of protein supplements and a 13.8% use of creatine. Use of energy drinks and protein supplements was higher than general multivitamin use (20.3%). The NCAA survey also reported that amphetamine, ephedrine, and anabolic steroid use were all reduced from previous surveys. Amphetamine use was reduced from 4.5% in 2005 to 3.7% in 2009, and anabolic steroid use was reduced from 1.7%–0.5%. Ephedrine is no longer available as an nonprescription product and its use is only 0.4%. Friends, teammates, and relatives continue to be a common source of unprescribed amphetamines. Reports of amphetamine swapping are concerning because these activities are illegal and show a willingness to break the law to improve sports or academic performance.

High school athletes are also exposed to nutritional supplements and may have access to prescription medications that affect performance.[7] A survey of American high school athletes in 2007 noted that 5.9% of male seniors reported using an anabolic steroid. This survey also revealed a high rate of nutritional supplement use: 62% used a daily multivitamin, 31% used energy drinks, 22% used protein powders, and 12% used creatine. Among female athletes, 18.6% reported using a "fat burner" to lose weight. High school athletes reported greater use of these substances than college-age students; therefore, education on the safe and effective use of nutritional intervention, supplements, and performance-enhancing products is needed as early as the high school level.

The American Academy of Pediatrics (AAP) has determined that the average child engaged in routine physical activity should drink water. The AAP has taken the position that carbohydrate-containing sports drinks are not necessary and that caffeine-containing "energy drinks" should not be consumed by children and adolescents.[8]

Macronutrient Use for Athletic Performance—Basic Concepts

Macronutrients (carbohydrates, fats, and proteins) play pivotal roles in athletic performance and muscle development, but each type of macronutrient has unique properties and use. Even during competition, the primary drive is to preserve muscle glycogen for "fight or flight" responses. Four primary concepts explain sports nutrition macronutrient intake and its contribution to energy provision for athletic performance. First, when not exercising, macronutrient intake is stored for use later. Second, during exercise stored macronutrients are used slowly according to the exerciser's aerobic capacity to burn fats rather than glycogen, thus preserving glycogen. Fatty-acid oxidation is the primary fuel for aerobically intense activity, thus allowing muscle glycogen to be preserved for periods of higher intensity. Third, when faster intensities are maintained for longer durations, muscle glycogen depletes faster. Finally, at the highest intensities, an anaerobic energy system contributes energy from muscle phosphocreatine directly to depleted adenosine diphosphate (ADP), permitting restoration of muscle adenosine triphosphate (ATP).

Muscles are always seeking a state of optimal muscle glycogen. When the body's muscles are at rest, caloric intake is converted to energy storage for use at a later time. Carbohydrate intake that exceeds current metabolic need is first converted to glycogen, which is stored in muscles and the liver for rapid, immediate use. When glycogen stores are complete, any remaining carbohydrates are converted to fatty acids for storage. Humans are biologically designed to maintain a full reserve of glycogen as an immediate energy source for short-duration, high-intensity activity such as fight or flight. At the lowest level of exercise intensity, a walking state, calorie utilization per minute is minimal, with 80% of the calories obtained from fatty-acid oxidation and the remaining 20% from carbohydrates.[9,10] As exercise intensity increases from walking to aerobic jogging, calorie consumption per minute increases, and fatty-acid oxidation continues to provide about 80% of the fuel.[9,10] Conversion of fatty acids to energy is slow and rate limited, and the conversion rate varies from athlete to athlete. The only known way to improve fatty-acid oxidation is adaptation to exercise.[11] No functional foods or supplements improve the rate of fatty-acid metabolism.[1,2] A detailed discussion on fatty-acid metabolism is beyond the scope of this chapter and can be found elsewhere.[10,11]

Second, calories burned per minute from fat are limited and reach a plateau; therefore, athletic performance is impaired without additional calories from other sources such as carbohydrates.[9,10] At the intensity of a fast run, such as a 10-km running race, fatty-acid oxidation can't meet all of the energy requirement, and carbohydrate utilization is added to the energy derived from fats. At this level of intensity, carbohydrate utilization increases to 50% of total calorie expenditure.[12] The rate reaches 80%–90% for sprint events (200 meters).[12] Progression of exercise intensity from walking to running to sprinting is seen in many sports, and some sports, such as soccer or field hockey, have a combination of extreme high-intensity effort intermixed with efforts at a more aerobic pace. The oxidation of fatty acids is the predominant fuel until exercise intensity requires the faster energy conversion from carbohydrates.

Third, glycogen depletion is an intensity and durational concept. Marathon runners refer to muscle glycogen depletion as "hitting the wall." A similar term, "bonking," references the cognitive and mental attention deficits athletes can experience when glycogen depletion leads to hypoglycemia. Limited storage capacity exists for glucose as glycogen within the liver and skeletal muscle; an average 150-pound individual stores only about 2000 total calories of glycogen. High-intensity exercise over time depletes glycogen stores.[9,10,13] Muscle glycogen is burned initially, and as this resource is depleted, the liver releases glucose from stored glycogen to maintain serum glucose levels. When both muscle and liver glycogen stores are depleted, serum glucose decreases and athletic performance declines. Sudden drops in blood glucose levels affect the athlete's mental acuity, attention, and focus.[9,10] Endurance athletes slow to an aerobic effort in which fatty-acid mobilization predominates, but they are less competitive at that rate of intensity. Athletes participating in sports that require high cognitive skill, such as shooting sports, archery, and automobile racing, experience lower performance and brain activity as their serum glucose levels decrease.[1,2] The rate of glycogen depletion is dependent on the intensity and duration of exercise, as well as the fitness level of the athlete.[9,10] Endurance runners can deplete muscle glycogen in about 2–2.5 hours at a marathon running pace and do not require carbohydrate intake unless exercising that duration or longer.[1,2] The same runners may deplete glycogen in 60 minutes when running at the faster intensity of a 10-kilometer run, but generally do not require carbohydrate supplements because they complete the event in less time (30–40 minutes) than it takes to deplete muscle glycogen.[1,2] Team sports such as football, lacrosse, field hockey, and basketball have official game-time durations of 90 minutes or less, as well as time-outs, half-times, and player substitutions that allow for periods of aerobic recovery. For these sports and durations, glycogen depletion is not expected to occur. Very fit athletes adapt over time to a state of efficient fatty-acid utilization and require less glycogen; their carbohydrate stores are available in later stages of events compared with undertrained athletes.[9,10]

A fourth concept is that the highest-intensity sports, those requiring short bursts of power lasting less than 30 seconds to 1 minute, use the phosphagen system and energy stored primarily as ATP.[14] Examples include track and field events and weight lifting. Energy stored in phosphate bonds is depleted in a matter of seconds and then regenerates with rest. This energy system is discussed further in the section on creatine. Intermittent high-intensity sports such as football, soccer, basketball, tennis, and ice hockey use both very short (phosphagen and ATP) energy systems and intermediate (glycogen) systems over the competition range of 30–60 minutes.

Sports Nutrition Market Basics

The sports nutrition market was developed for well-trained athletes competing at high intensities for long durations. College football players may exercise for 4 hours daily and exceed 20 hours of exercise per week. These athletes may need to provide fuel during exercise to delay or prevent glycogen depletion or may require rapid muscle glycogen restoration between morning and afternoon practices. Sports drinks can be consumed during practice or competition and have replaced the concept of carbohydrate loading prior to long-duration events. Most marathon runners and triathletes consume carbohydrates during the event.[1,2] Sports products also contain electrolytes to prevent deficiencies from sweat loss.

By comparison, moderate physical activity such as daily exercise for health and wellness usually occurs at a lower intensity and typically lasts 60 minutes or less per day.[1,2] Glycogen depletion is unlikely for recreational athletes, even if they exercise 7 hours per week; consequently, calorie-dense sports products are unnecessary for health and wellness athletes or sedentary individuals for whom performance is not an issue.[1,2]

Carbohydrate-Based Products

Sugar content is listed separately from total carbohydrate in the nutrition facts on food labels. Carbohydrate-based sports nutrition products contain monosaccharides (glucose and fructose) as well as the disaccharide sucrose (glucose + fructose); these sugars provide rapid absorption and availability of carbohydrates. Maltodextrin (glucose + glucose as a polymer) is used in endurance formulas and is marketed as having slower absorption. Lactose (glucose + galactose), or milk sugar, can also be used as a recovery fuel after exercise.[1,2]

The ADA guidelines recommend 30–60 grams of carbohydrate intake per hour of continued exercise.[2] This translates to 10–15 grams of carbohydrates, or 4–8 ounces of a sports drink every 15 minutes, given that most sports nutrition drinks contain 6%–8% carbohydrates for optimal absorption and gastrointestinal (GI) tolerance.[1,2] The amount of carbohydrates is small and should be rapidly used during continuing exercise; however, the fluid volume is relatively large. These products should be used in practice and under simulated competition so that the athlete can learn how they tolerate a product. Larger doses of carbohydrates (80 grams) in single doses are not recommended. Limited research suggests that large doses of carbohydrate may result in a larger insulin release, leading to hypoglycemic symptoms and reduced performance.[15] The various carbohydrate forms (i.e., drinks, gels, and bars) do not differ in their effectiveness; however, the amount of water and electrolytes and the specific sugar sources vary. Bars and gels are lighter and easier to carry than an equivalent amount of calories in the form of a sports drink; however, they require a water source for proper dissolution, absorption, and GI tolerance. In addition, compared with sports drinks, the bars tend to contain other macronutrients, such as fats, proteins, and vitamins, making them better suited for recovery after exercise than for glycogen preservation during an event.

Although the original intent of these products was to provide fuel on the go, the market has evolved to provide meal replacements for active people in a hurry. These products are misunderstood by the public as healthier than soft drinks, candy bars, or even regular meals, despite their high sugar and caloric content. The health care provider should be prepared to read and interpret the nutrition label with patients and to calculate total calories if the package offers multiple servings. These products are not required by active adults or children who exercise 60–90 minutes in any one session.[2,8] Recreational athletes and sedentary individuals should be discouraged from using these products before, during, or after exercise that lasts less than 90 minutes.[2,8] The ADA and AAP recommend eating a meal after exercise as a suitable glycogen recovery method.[2,8] Examples of bars, gels, and drinks are presented in Table 24–1.

Fats: Triglyceride-Containing Products

Fats are an important source of energy, fat-soluble vitamins, and essential fatty acids for athletes, and their consumption should not be restricted.[2] The timing of fat intake may be important.[2] Long-chain triglycerides, found in typical fats and oils, should be avoided in sports nutrition products used 1–2 hours before and during exercise because they tend to slow gastric emptying and may cause discomfort, bloating, and GI intolerance during intense exercise. Medium-chain triglycerides (MCTs) are packaged into sports drinks and powders to provide an alternative fuel to glucose and to reduce muscle glycogen utilization.[11] The moderate length (8–12 carbons) of MCTs results in absorption from the GI tract directly into the bloodstream, allowing more rapid utilization than with long-chain triglycerides, which are absorbed through the lymphatic system. Some MCT beverages are marketed to strength and conditioning athletes on low-carbohydrate diets. Clinical data in athletes suggest that MCTs are utilized metabolically within 30 minutes of ingestion, but no data show improved performance or muscle glycogen sparing[11] (Table 24–1.)

Protein Products for Muscle Mass Gain

Athletes commonly train with weights to build muscle and to develop a bigger, stronger, or more toned body. Many athletes believe they need to consume large quantities of protein to provide substrates for muscle development. The dietary source of protein can vary and may include meat and dairy; vegetarian sources such as legumes, beans, and nuts; and prepackaged protein sources, such as protein powders, amino acid supplements, and various protein-containing bars, gels, and drinks.

Most adults who are not active athletes require 0.8–1 gram of protein per kilogram of body weight per day (g/kg/day) to provide enough protein to maintain a neutral nitrogen balance, to fuel the many repair and maintenance functions throughout the body, and to maintain muscle mass.[16] These sedentary adults generally do not require more than 25 kcal/kg/day for weight maintenance. Compared with the general population, active athletes who exercise for 10 or more hours per week have increased protein and calorie requirements.[16] The ADA guidelines recommend protein intake of 1.2–1.7 g/kg/day in highly active adults who participate in endurance exercise and those who are attempting to increase body mass; this recommendation is in addition to an increased overall caloric intake to meet higher metabolic demands.[2] Anecdotal evidence of athletes ingesting 1.8–2.5 g/kg/day of protein has been reported despite lack of data supporting its effectiveness.[2,16] A large number of protein supplement products exist in the marketplace, spurred by manufacturer claims that building muscle requires increased amounts of specific amino acids, the essential amino acids or the branch-chain amino acids, and by the large market demand.

table 24–1 Sports Nutrition Products[a]

Serving Size	Energy (kCal)	Carbohydrate (gram)	Sugars (gram)	Protein (gram)	Fat (gram)	Sodium (mg)	Potassium (mg)
Electrolyte Drinks and Wafers (low calorie)[b]							
Gatorade G2 Low Cal — 8 ounces	20	5	5	0	0	110	30
Nuun Active Hydration Wafer — 16 ounces, 1 wafer	0	0	0	0	0	360	100
Powerade Zero — 12 ounces	0	0	0	0	0	150	35
Propel Zero — 8 ounces	0	0	0	0	0	80	20
Ultima Replenisher (Orange) — 1 scoop (4.4 grams)	15	4	0	0	0	5	75
Zym Endurance Wafer — 16 ounces, 1 wafer	7	1	1	0	0	250	50
Energy Drinks (carbohydrates and electrolytes)[c]							
Accelerade — 31 grams, 1 scoop, 12 ounces water	120	21	20	5	1	210–220	65–95
Cytomax — 25 grams, 1 scoop, 12 ounces water	90	22	12	0	0	120	60
Gatorade Thirst Quencher — 8 ounces	50	14	14	0	0	110	30
Powerade — 12 ounces	80	22	21	0	0	150	35
Recovery Drinks (carbohydrate, protein, electrolytes, hydration)[d]							
Endurox R4 — 74 grams, 2 scoops, 12 ounces water	270–280	52	38–40	13	1	220	170–180
Gu Brew Recovery — 3 scoops, 16 ounces water	250	52	17	8	0	160	70
IsoPure ZeroCarb — 62 grams, 2 scoops	210	0	0	50	0	320	750

Milk, Low Fat, Chocolate Flavor	1/2 pint 236 mL	140	25	24	7	1	190	—
Muscle Milk, Chocolate Flavor	14 ounces 1 serving	230	12	3	25	9	430	1050
Energy Gels (carbohydrate and electrolytes)^e								
Accel Gel	1 packet	100	20	13	5	0	100	20
CarbBoom	1 packet	103–110	26–27	2–3	0	0	50–51	50
Clif Shot	1 packet	100–110	22–24	12	0	0–1	60–90	50–80
E Gel	1 packet	150	37	7	0	0	230	85
Gu	1 packet	100	20–25	5–6	0	0–2	40–65	35–60
Gu Roctane	1 packet	100	25	5	1.22	0	125	55
Hammer Gel	1 packet	80–90	21–22	2–4	0	0	20–35	10–25
Energy/Recovery Bars (carbohydrates, protein, fat, electrolytes)^f								
Balance Bar Original	1 bar	180–210	20–22	14–18	13–15	6–7	110–200	120–320
Cliff Bar	1 bar	230–240	42–44	16–25	9–10	3.5–7	125–240	180–280
Luna Bar	1 bar	180–190	25–28	11–13	8–10	4.5–7	115–210	90–160
Muscle Milk Bar	1 bar	300	28	11	25	11	270	150
Fat (MCT)–Containing Products^g								
MCT Fuel (Twin Lab)	30 mL	130	12	0	0	9	0	0

^a Composition per serving. Slight differences exist within products with multiple flavors or formulations. Please refer to the product nutrition label or the manufacturer's Web site for the most current information.

^b Intended as a healthy, low-calorie alternative to carbohydrate sports drinks. For rehydration and electrolyte replacement following exercise time of an hour or less when glycogen depletion is not a concern. Performance benefits are unproven.

^c Intended for use during exercise to provide carbohydrates for energy and glycogen sparing, as well as electrolytes and water for rehydration.

^d Intended for use after exercise of prolonged duration when glycogen depletion is expected.

^e Intended for use during exercise to provide carbohydrates for energy and glycogen sparing. Require a water source for proper dissolution and absorption. Not intended for rehydration.

^f Intended for use during exercise to provide electrolytes as well as carbohydrates for energy and glycogen sparing. Can serve as a meal replacement product. Often contain added vitamins and minerals.

^f Intended for postexercise recovery after exercise of prolonged duration when glycogen depletion is expected. Can serve as a meal replacement product. Often contain added vitamins and minerals.

^g Intended as fuel for recovery in athletes who choose a low-carbohydrate diet.

However, the ISSN and the ADA guidelines indicate that simple adjustments to the athlete's diet can provide sufficient protein to meet dietary intake goals for increasing muscle mass.[1,2] No evidence supports packaged protein supplements or a specific amino acid mixture as more effective at increasing body mass than eating whole foods with equal amounts of protein.[1,2,16] Free amino acids result in a higher osmotic effect, which can cause GI distress and diarrhea, and specific amino acid supplements can be deficient in one or more of the essential amino acids, which may adversely affect growth and development.[1,2]

Athletes attempting to gain muscle mass may require an increased total calorie intake of 30–35 kcal/kg/day to balance their increased energy needs from exercise and to provide protein for muscle building.[2] Muscle-building athletes should be educated to not exceed reasonable total calorie goals. Any excessive calories, including any additional protein, will be converted to fats for storage, defeating the athlete's goal of a lean physical appearance.

Clinical Evidence of Protein Needs for Muscle Building

Muscle protein is in a constant state of synthesis and breakdown. Resistance exercise induces changes in muscle that effectively stimulate muscle remodeling and growth, provided the diet offers an adequate quality and timing of protein for that growth.[16] The process is slow and requires repeated exercise stimulus, optimal nutrition, and several months to observe weight gain. A net positive protein balance is thought to be evidence of an increase in muscle fiber diameter and in the muscle proteins actin and myosin.[16] Muscle weight gain relies equally on the quality of the protein, the amino acid profile of the protein source, the timing of protein intake relative to exercise, and the exercise experienced by the athlete; quantity of protein consumed has a minimal influence. The athlete must also consider the total calorie consumption per day required to meet the intensity of training and, accordingly, consume adequate calories to allow the protein to be used for building muscle.[2,16] Data from inexperienced athletes beginning a weight-training program suggest that 1.4 g/kg/day of protein provides neutral protein balance, and 1.7 g/kg/day is recommended for muscle accumulation.[16] Well-designed studies of protein intake at 2 g/kg/day and greater have not resulted in consistent increases in lean body mass compared with the control group and indicate only increased protein oxidation for energy.[16] Protein intake up to 2.6 g/kg/day did not influence further lean body mass accumulation or total body weight gain in inexperienced athletes. Similar results have been found in experienced strength-training athletes; therefore, the ADA recommends that strength-training athletes target 1.4–1.7 g/kg/day of protein for muscle accumulation.

Adverse Effects of Diets with High Protein Intake (2 g/kg/day)

Little is known regarding nephrotoxicity risk from high-protein diets, defined here as 2 g/kg/day or greater. In theory, elimination of the amine group, or the nitrogenous waste, from protein intake may affect glomerular filtration. Unfortunately, available data are either anecdotal or retrospective. One retrospective observation used diet and exercise histories to compare groups of experienced athletes claiming to have followed a regular diet or a high-protein diet for up to 3 years.[17] Diet logs indicated average protein intake of 1.4 g/kg/day for the regular-diet group and 2.0 g/kg/day in the high-protein group. No difference was observed between the groups for serum creatinine measurement or estimated creatinine clearance from a 24-hour urine collection. Nitrogen clearance was not measured. Reliability of this study is questionable because a diet high in red meat may increase measured serum creatinine and urine creatinine levels, thereby affecting the accuracy of a calculated creatinine clearance. The available data are not sufficient to prove that high-protein diets over many years are either safe or unsafe.

High dietary protein intake may affect hydration status or increase the risk of dehydration from the increased nitrogenous waste that must be eliminated. Adequate hydration is required to optimize elimination of the waste. A frequent method for predicting dehydration risk is to evaluate urine color, with pale or light yellow urine considered a good sign of adequate hydration. A second method to monitor dehydration is for athletes to weigh themselves every morning, after voiding, for several days to obtain a reliable baseline weight.[18] Subsequently, the athletes can measure body weight before and after exercise. Any significant weight loss from short-duration exercise is likely to reflect dehydration. A similar method could be used before introduction of high-protein intake. Methods to calculate the rate of sweat production are discussed elsewhere.[18] Objective measures of hydration require laboratory analysis of serum and urine osmolality and electrolyte levels. A urine test to measure specific gravity is available to consumers, but further laboratory testing and validation are required to determine hydration status.[18]

Water and Electrolytes

Water and electrolytes are essential to performance. A 2% decrease in total body weight can affect physical and mental performance.[18] Dehydration results in increased physical strain, as measured by elevations in core body temperature, heart rate, and perceived exertion. The greater the body water deficit, the greater is the strain for a given task. Dehydration can also affect cognitive performance such as mental concentration and focus on skilled tasks. Dehydration (3%–5% body weight) does not appear to affect anaerobic performance or muscle strength. Readers are referred to the position statement of the American College of Sports Medicine for guidelines and detailed discussion of this topic.[18]

Dehydration involves both water loss and electrolyte concentrations as separate issues. Athletes generate heat from exercise-related muscle contractions in proportion to the intensity and duration of exercise. This heat generation is transferred to the blood and then to the body core. Blood circulation through peripheral blood vessels and the skin allows radiant heat exchange with the environment. Fluid and electrolyte loss as sweat onto the skin surface facilitates evaporative cooling. Environmental conditions such as temperature, humidity, air motion, helmets, and layers of clothing influence the success of evaporative cooling. If sweat-related water and electrolyte losses are not replaced, the athlete experiences dehydration.

The significance of dehydration depends on environmental conditions, exercise intensity, and its duration. For example, compared with a recreational runner, an elite marathon runner may demonstrate a higher sweat rate, as measured by sweat loss per hour, but both athletes will have similar total sweat losses for the event owing to the prolonged time that the recreational athlete needs to complete the event. By comparison, American football players have significantly greater sweat rates than soccer players practicing in identical conditions owing to the football players' layers of clothing and equipment, which contribute to the greater heat accumulation and greater sweat and electrolyte losses, while preventing evaporative cooling. The risk of dehydration in football players is further influenced by twice-daily practice sessions, which may not allow adequate time between sessions for water replacement.

Health Conditions Related to Dehydration

Hydration can affect health through water loss or water gain (overdrinking) and can affect serum sodium levels sufficiently to endanger health. In general, dehydration is more common, but overhydration resulting in hyponatremia can be equally life threatening. Signs of dehydration include fatigue, confusion, irritability, and increased risk of heat illness with symptoms of muscle cramps, heat exhaustion, heat stroke, and exertional rhabdomyolysis.[18] Rhabdomyolysis has been reported as a result of dehydration, heat stress, and novel training. Novel training involves the introduction of new exercise patterns in athletes who have not been acclimated to the new exercise, such as military recruits at boot camp or high school students attending preseason football camps.

Prevention of Dehydration

Meal consumption is the most important aspect of maintaining optimal hydration status.[2,18] Eating promotes fluid intake and retention. Meals generally contain sufficient electrolytes to replace sweat losses. Consuming a meal and allowing 4–24 hours between workouts is sufficient to return to baseline water status. As mentioned previously, athletes can obtain a first-morning body weight, after voiding, to track day-to-day changes in weight. Sports drinks can provide water and electrolytes after exercise, but when assessed 24 hours after a workout, the drinks have not proven superior to the consumption of a meal.[1,2,18] Water alone is sufficient for rehydration during events lasting 60 minutes or less.[2,8] No evidence supports requiring an electrolyte sports drink to prevent dehydration in recreational events of this duration.

Hyponatremia Risk from Drinking Excessive Free Water

Most laboratory-based studies of dehydration have occurred on stationary treadmills in climate-controlled rooms with little-to-no convective airflow to help sweat evaporation.[18] Because of such studies, athletes have been taught to drink as much water as possible to prevent dehydration. However, liberal water intake has been called into question following clinical observations of weight gain, severe hyponatremia, cerebral edema, and death in athletes who consumed water without added electrolytes during athletic events lasting longer than 4 hours.[18–20] Improved water availability to athletes competing in marathons has not resulted in fewer athletes seeking medical care after races.[19,20] The original research was directed at elite-level athletes competing for 60–150 minutes who consumed small sips of water while running very fast and generating significant body

heat and high sweat rates. Unfortunately, this description does not apply to average athletes, who complete the same marathon races at a much slower pace, generate less heat accumulation, and have lower sweat rates.

Observations under more realistic conditions resulted in an advisory statement from the International Marathon Medical Directors Association (IMMDA).[20] This advisory statement suggests that heat production by athletes is significantly affected by their effort (the combination of duration and intensity or speed of the exercise); therefore, a 10-kilometer race effort will generate more heat than a marathon effort (42.2 kilometers). Average athletes run slower than elite athletes; therefore, average athletes are at less risk of heat illness than elite athletes and have more time to consume water at aid stations. The result is that clinical hyponatremia occurs more frequently in nonelite athletes, particularly women who require more than 4 hours to finish a marathon, and in long-course triathletes who require 13–17 hours to complete their events.[18–20] The IMMDA recommendations suggest that fluid consumption in athletes' drinks be based on the trigger of actual thirst, rather than on a set volume of fluid intake. As the athletes' thirst increases, they can increase fluid intake from sips of water to a calculated sweat rate. The IMMDA strongly recommends that the athlete choose an electrolyte replacement drink instead of free water to avoid the risk of hyponatremia when competing in events that last 4 hours or longer.[20]

Athletes competing for 2 or more hours can determine their individual sweat rates by observing their total body weight before and after prolonged exercise. For example, an athlete who takes a 2-hour run on a hot afternoon may drop 2 kilograms in body weight. Each kilogram change in body weight would be associated with a 1000-mL water deficit, suggesting that the athlete has lost 2000 mL of water. This athlete can target a drinking rate of 1000 mL per hour, or 240 mL (8 ounces) every 15 minutes during prolonged exercise.

Providing athlete education before the event and electrolyte-containing sports drinks during the event reduces hyponatremia cases in triathletes[21] but not in experienced marathon runners.[18–20] Other factors are likely involved. For example, clinical observations indicate exercise-induced hyponatremia may increase with concurrent use of nonsteroidal anti-inflammatory agents (NSAIDs) in marathon runners[20] and long-course triathletes.[21] An exact mechanism is unknown; however, NSAIDs may interfere with normal prostaglandin-mediated regulation of glomerular filtration and renal blood flow. Triathletes with significant hyponatremia were observed to have elevated nitrogen and potassium levels, suggestive of reduced glomerular filtration.[21]

Postural hypotension, rather than heat-related illness or dehydration, has been recognized as a health risk in endurance running that is not directly related to fluid intake. When athletes cross the finish line, the sudden decrease in leg muscle contractions allows pooling of blood in the legs and decreased venous return. The resulting decrease in cardiac output may leave the brain underperfused with oxygenated blood, causing the athlete to black out.[20] Athletes should continue walking past the finish line to prevent this reaction. Only athletes demonstrating a rectal temperature higher than 104°F (40°C) should be treated for heat illness.[20]

Carbonated and Oxygen-Enhanced Water

Carbonation of water is not beneficial to athletes and may be detrimental. Dissolved gases can accumulate and cause GI distress and bloating, resulting in decreased total fluid consumption.[18]

Oxygenated water claims to have 30% or higher dissolved oxygen; however, when packed in plastic bottles, it may contain no more dissolved oxygen than tap water, and 12 ounces of oxygenated water in glass bottles contains less oxygen than a single breath of room air.[22] Available research does not substantiate a performance benefit of oxygenated water in humans.[22]

Electrolytes and Water without Added Carbohydrates

Several sports nutrition drinks have been developed that offer water, electrolytes, and vitamins, often using artificial sweetener to replace the flavoring and calories from carbohydrates. These electrolyte waters have not been evaluated for sports performance. No evidence indicates they are effective at preventing hyponatremia, and they have minimal or no calories for sustained effort. These artificially sweetened electrolyte drinks can be chosen as an alternative to carbohydrate-containing sports drinks but are no different than water, other than the observation that a small amount of added sodium improves the absorption rate of water and the volume of fluid consumed.[2,18]

Electrolytes, Carbohydrates, and Water

Addition of carbohydrates to sports drinks benefits athletes competing longer than an hour by replacing muscle glycogen lost during periods of intense or prolonged effort. Carbohydrate supplementation during exercise provides exercising muscles with fuel for energy while allowing muscles to conserve stored carbohydrate energy as glycogen. This strategy of providing fuel during exercise at a rate of 3060 grams per hour for events lasting longer than 60 minutes has been shown to prolong the time to exhaustion in football and soccer players, as well as in long-distance endurance athletes such as runners and cyclists.[2] Using a 6%–7% carbohydrate sports drink would require the athlete to drink 500–1000 mL per hour to meet this targeted carbohydrate provision. The fluid volume is large and can cause GI side effects that affect performance. Many triathletes and runners use a carbohydrate gel during the event and drink smaller amounts of water to assist in dissolution and absorption of the carbohydrate.

Low-calorie carbohydrate-containing sports drinks provide as little as 3 grams of carbohydrates per 8-ounce serving, or just 10 kilocalories, contrasting with 11–18 grams of carbohydrates and 50–80 kilocalories per 8-ounce serving of most carbohydrate-containing sports drinks. These low-calorie electrolyte waters have not been evaluated for performance benefits.

Electrolytes, Carbohydrates, Protein, and Water

Several sports nutrition drinks combine an electrolyte-carbohydrate solution with added protein. The protein is added to provide an additional metabolic fuel for ATP production.[25] These products are marketed to endurance athletes competing at aerobic intensities for long durations, including marathon runners (2.5–5 hours), long-distance triathletes (2–17 hours), and adventure racers (12 hours to 5 days). The initial studies compared a control group drinking a 6%–8% carbohydrate-electrolyte solution to a second group drinking the same sports drink with the addition of calories from protein. These initial studies showed modest improvements in exercise duration in cyclists; however, these studies could not determine if the improvements were related to the additional calories or to the protein itself. The second round of studies was better designed. These follow-up studies provided equal calories to both groups and resulted in no differences in cycle exercise duration.[23,24] An interesting observation from these studies was a lower rate of muscle soreness the day after the cycle exercise, as reported by the athletes who received protein calories. In theory, muscle soreness could impact performance measurements on subsequent days of exercise. Unfortunately, these studies did not measure cycling performance on subsequent days and can't show an association between performance and the observed muscle soreness.

Although ready-to-drink options exist, some protein-containing drinks are powders that require reconstitution and can release significant amounts of gas when mixed with water. Bubbles and foam appear from the hydrated powder, which can influence GI tolerance in athletes. Protein-containing sports drinks should be introduced as part of the training regimen so that athletes can determine their tolerance and the impact on performance before the drinks are used during an event. Because hydrolysis can affect stability of some proteins once mixed with water, athletes should not hydrate protein-containing dry powder drinks the night before an event. Optimal protein potency and effect may require athletes to carry unmixed powder and add water during the event, a potentially unsafe practice. For example, athletes could lose control of their bicycle when reconstituting powder in triathlon events. Once mixed, all sports drinks should be consumed or stored in the refrigerator within 2 hours to prevent bacterial growth.

Preexercise Nutrition and Hydration

The ADA guidelines recommend that a prehydration fluid of 5–7 mL/kg of body weight be consumed at least 4 hours before exercise. For example, a 59-kilogram athlete would consume 295–413 mL of fluid prior to exercise. This allows excretion of excess fluid in the urine before exercise begins. Hyperhydration with glycerol increases the risk of needing to void during competition, provides no performance advantage, and is discouraged.[18,26] Carbohydrate loads of 200–300 grams (from food and/or fluids) consumed 3 hours or more before exercise may enhance performance. However, the ADA guidelines state that optimal performance depends on individually determined distribution of macronutrient intake prior to exercise because of variations in athlete size, the energy demands of different sports, overall daily calorie needs, and the timing of macronutrient intake prior to the practice or event. Individual athletes should consider nutrition a part of their training regimen and should practice the timing, quality, and quantity of intake to become familiar with their own tolerance and timing. All athletes are discouraged from experimenting with new foods prior to important competitions.

Nutrition and Hydration during Exercise

For competitions lasting longer than an hour, athletes are recommended to determine a sweat rate by measuring their pre- and postexercise body weights. A reasonable goal is to drink 16–24 fluid ounces of a sports drink for every 0.5 kilogram of body weight loss during exercise.[2] The ADA guidelines recommend consuming 30–60 grams of carbohydrate (from food and/or fluids) per hour during exercise to maintain blood glucose levels.[2] These rates are adjustable according to an athlete's tolerance. A carbohydrate drink concentration of 6%–8% is recommended because concentrations greater than 8% are associated with adverse GI effects.[2]

Postexercise Nutrition and Recovery Drinks

Goals of postexercise recovery nutrition are to rehydrate, restore muscle glycogen, and provide protein to repair muscle damage and synthesize new muscle tissue, thereby preparing the athlete for another period of activity. The choice of recovery nutrition is dependent upon how much time is available until the next session of intense activity. Most active adults will exercise once daily and do not require specific sports nutrition supplements for recovery. When recovery time is 4 hours or greater, the ADA recommends that an athlete consume a balanced meal for glycogen restoration, optimal rehydration, and correction of electrolyte imbalances.[2] Several studies have compared a carbohydrate-only sports nutrition drink with consuming a glass of low-fat milk containing an equal number of calories from low concentrations of fat, carbohydrate, and protein. Consumption of low-fat milk was associated with greater hydration, lower urine output, and improved weight replacement after exercise.[27] In addition, low-fat milk was associated with a longer time to exhaustion in subsequent exercise sessions.[28,29] Drinking milk more accurately reflected a postexercise meal and is better for recovery after exercise than a carbohydrate-only sports drink.

When recovery time is less than 4 hours, drinking a carbohydrate sports drink improves muscle glycogen recovery when compared to drinking water. The sooner the carbohydrate is consumed after exercise, the sooner muscle glycogen is replaced. The ADA guidelines recommend carbohydrate consumption of 1.5 grams per kilogram within 30 minutes after exercise.[2] This dose may be repeated at 2 and 4 hours postexercise when total muscle glycogen depletion is suspected.[2] The ADA guidelines state that protein intake may be beneficial for muscle recovery and that this need is optimally met with a balanced meal.[2]

Safety and Efficacy of Specific Ergogenic Supplements

This section discusses the safety and efficacy of specific nutritional supplements and micronutrients for sports performance. Unlike the macronutrients discussed previously, here the evidence supporting the use of herbs, plant extracts, antioxidants, and other supplements purported to improve sports performance is discussed. These nutritional supplements are marketed as "foods" and are not regulated as drugs by the FDA. These foods are not required to provide safety and efficacy data in humans to prove their effectiveness on the playing field, nor do they require testing to prove their labeled contents. Readers are reminded of previous evidence of misbranding and the frequency of substances banned by antidoping agencies appearing in these products.[4,5] They are also referred to Table 24–2 for a list of substances for which evidence is available that does not support claimed effectiveness. Athletes should take extreme caution regarding the use of nutritional supplements and sports performance, as indicated by misbranding that may lead to doping

infractions as well as case reports of serious adverse effects and deaths reported from supplement use. Athletes should focus on training and proper nutrition, and not rely on nutritional supplements or other artificial means for reaching their best performance.

Caffeine and Caffeine-Supplemented Energy Drinks

Several studies suggest an ergogenic benefit from caffeine supplementation.[1,2,30,31] Ordinarily, this effect would result in a no-tolerance testing policy. However, caffeine appears in nutritional products that are unrelated to exercise or performance benefit. Incidental exposure is common, and complete avoidance is unrealistic. The World Anti-Doping Agency does not list caffeine as a problematic substance. Caffeine intake at doses of 2–6 mg/kg, given 1 hour before exercise testing, appears to produce improvement in time to exhaustion on a cycle ergometer and in resistance (weight) training.[30] The addition of caffeine can also improve mental acuity and alertness. This is particularly beneficial in long-duration endurance sports such as 24-hour bicycle races where caffeine counteracts some of the effects of sleep deprivation. The exact mechanism for caffeine's ergogenic effect is unknown, and benefits appear to occur at doses that are common from drinking several cups of coffee or tea. Many questions remain regarding the effective use of caffeine for ergogenic benefit.

The class of products labeled as providing "energy" is broad and increasingly popular, although the vast majority of consumption is recreational and unrelated to sports.[3,31] Energy drinks (EDs) and energy shots (ESs) are similar to sports drinks, but they contain caffeine in addition to water and electrolytes. EDs may contain carbohydrates or be labeled as calorie free. They usually contain a blend of other nutrients and herbal additives such as taurine or guarana that are proposed to effect exercise performance or mental performance during exercise. Most of these additives have not been proven to affect sports performance or weight loss. Readers are referred to an ISSN position paper on EDs for a more detailed assessment.[31] In general, EDs should prolong exercise in a manner consistent with their carbohydrate component, although many contain more carbohydrate than the typical 6%–8% seen in sports drinks and may not be tolerated as well.

EDs are not without a risk for unintended side effects. The additional caloric load may affect blood sugar and insulin levels and promote weight gain.[31] The amount of caffeine present in EDs is not enforced within the United States at this time and may range from 100–286 mg per drink, whereas Canada has limited EDs to 180 mg per drink.[31] The quantity of caffeine is similar to a 16-ounce serving of coffee. Users are cautioned to consider the possible side effects from cumulative daily doses of caffeine. Side effects include insomnia, nervousness, tachycardia, tremors, and anxiety in addition to GI intolerance. A recent clinical observation in healthy college-age adults showed that a single dose of an ES can increase systolic and diastolic blood pressure by 5 mm Hg from baseline.[32] None of the healthy subjects were reported to have reached a level of prehypertension. More severe adverse effects from EDs are prompting emergency department visits and are related to indiscriminate use of EDs, often with other illicit drugs or alcohol.[33] The AAP has concluded that children and school-age athletes should not consume EDs or ESs and that they have no place in sports

table
24–2   Selected Products Marketed as Ergogenic Supplements

Ingredient	Marketed Claim	Conclusion/Evidence
Antioxidants[1,2,44]	Antioxidants claim to be able to reduce oxidative stress from exercise and/or to speed recovery following exercise. Many antioxidants have been included in sports nutrition supplements, including alpha-lipoic acid, carotenoids, glutathione, n-acetylcysteine, ubiquinones (coenzyme Q10), vitamin B complex, vitamin C, and vitamin E.	Evidence does not support an effect on reducing oxidative damage or enhancing performance. Frequent exercise is associated with an enhanced antioxidant system.
Arginine[45]	Arginine has been promoted to improve muscle building and cardiovascular functioning through the production of nitrous oxide, which causes cardiac vasodilatation and increased oxygen delivery to the heart.	Evidence does not support an effect on performance enhancement.
BCAAs[1,2,46] (branch-chain amino acids)	BCAAs are isoleucine, leucine, and valine. Skeletal muscle cells use BCAAs to supply energy during exercise. Supplementation may reduce fatigue and increase exercise time to exhaustion by reducing serum levels of L-tryptophan and its effect on serotonin levels in the brain.	Evidence does not consistently support an effect on endurance performance.
Carnitine[2]	Carnitine is an essential cofactor for the transport of long-chain fatty acids into the mitochondria. Product is proposed to improve fatty acid oxidation, fat burning, and oxygen absorption as well as to reduce lactic acid accumulation.	Evidence does not support an effect on performance.
Chromium[2]	Chromium is marketed to enhance carbohydrate utilization in the body, promoting fat burning and dietary protein sparing for muscle building. Product is marketed to improve endurance and strength.	Evidence does not support an effect on performance.
Citrulline[2]	L-Citrulline is a metabolic precursor to arginine. Citrulline is not affected by first-pass hepatic metabolism and is converted by the kidneys to arginine. Product is proposed to improve oxygen consumption and time to exhaustion in treadmill running.	Evidence does not support an effect on performance.
Conjugated linoleic acid[2] (CLA)	CLA is promoted to endurance athletes as a thermogenic aid, body fat reducer, and ergogenic aid that enhances fat metabolism. CLA may increase cardiac risk by lowering high-density lipoprotein and increasing lipoprotein(a) concentrations.	Evidence does not support an effect on performance or body composition.
Cordyceps sinensis[47,48]	*Cordyceps sinensis* is used in Chinese medicine to treat lung disease and fatigue. Products claim that this mushroom can decrease oxygen consumption and improve endurance. Product is frequently combined with *Rhodiola*. Available research published in English is limited and does not show a performance benefit.	Evidence does not consistently support an effect on performance.
Eleuthero[49]	Extracts of Siberian ginseng have been reported to affect cardiorespiratory performance, fat metabolism, and improved endurance.	Evidence does not support an effect on performance.
Ginseng[50]	Extracts of *Panax ginseng* have been reported to improve lactate clearance and delay the onset of fatigue.	Evidence does not support an effect on performance.
Glycerol[2,51]	Glycerol is reported to act as an osmotic agent to promote hyperhydration prior to exercise, therefore reducing the risk of dehydration from intensive exercise in the heat.	Evidence does not support an effect on performance.
Hydroxy-methylbutyrate[2,45] (HMB)	Beta-HMB is a metabolite of leucine metabolism, purported to decrease muscle protein breakdown after a workout and to increase muscle mass. HMB has also been proposed to improve aerobic performance.	Evidence does not consistently support an effect on performance.
Lecithin[52]	Lecithin is a source of choline and a precursor to acetylcholine. Decreased plasma choline and acetylcholine levels have been reported in marathon runners. Supplementation of lecithin before a marathon does prevent the decline in serum acetylcholine levels but does not affect finishing times.	Evidence does not support an effect on performance.
Rhodiola rosea[48,53,54]	*Rhodiola rosea* is a Chinese herb used to stimulate the nervous system, improve aerobic work performance, and reduce fatigue. *Rhodiola* is reported to improve oxygenation at high altitudes and is thought to be helpful for endurance athletes. Available research published in English is limited and does not show performance benefit.	Evidence does not consistently support an effect on performance.

competition.[8] The ISSN further states that diabetics and individuals with preexisting cardiovascular, neurologic, or metabolic disorders should avoid these products.[31] Avoiding the use of EDs and ESs for sports performance is generally appropriate advice for any age group.

Creatine

Creatine is the most widely used ergogenic aid among athletes, and it has the most consistent data.[14,34] Creatine, a naturally occurring substance, is synthesized in the body by the combining of arginine and glycine, or it is absorbed intact after ingestion of red meats and fish.[14,34] Creatine is found in all skeletal muscle as free creatine or high-energy phosphorylated creatine (PCr). PCr functions as an energy buffer, transferring a phosphate group to ADP, thereby rapidly regenerating ATP during periods of exercise. Skeletal muscle contains limited amounts of energy stored as ATP at rest; exercise depletes this stored ATP energy quickly. The body must oxidize macronutrients through the Krebs cycle to restore ADP to the high-energy ATP state for continuous or repeated efforts. PCr transfers its energy to ADP in seconds, acting as a secondary fuel. However, the total amount of PCr energy in muscles lasts for only 20–30 seconds.[14,34]

Performance gains with creatine are limited to laboratory-based studies of short bursts of anaerobic activity lasting 30 seconds or less. Creatine supplementation attenuates normal decreases in the force associated with repeated work applications.[14,34] For example, a weight lifter performs three sets of a bench press, with a goal of 10 lifts, or repetitions, per set. The lifter takes 30 seconds of rest between each set. Ordinarily, the lifter may be able to move a planned amount of weight for 10 repetitions in the first set, 8 repetitions in the second set, and only 6 repetitions in the third set. The decreasing number of lifts is called attenuation and is related to decreased energy (ATP) in the muscles. Creatine can improve the amount of ATP energy available to lift the weight; the same athlete may complete more repetitions in each subsequent set (e.g., 10, 10, and 8 repetitions rather than 10, 8, and 6).[14,34] Similar improvements in maximum weight lifted in a single lift have also been reported.[14,34] Creatine is useful for athletic events that require repeated, short, explosive bursts of power such as sprinting and jumping seen in American football, soccer, and track and field events. By comparison, creatine does not benefit athletes in sports that require more than 20–30 seconds of high-intensity activity. Aerobic activities as short as 800-meter (2-minute) and 1600-meter (5-minute) runs on a track have not shown performance benefits.[34]

Current evidence does not support that creatine can induce structural changes in muscle fibers. The muscles may be larger and weigh more, owing to the presence of creatine and water in complex with creatine. The athlete may gain mass and appear stronger in the gym, but this change is dependent upon maintenance supplementation. Short-term studies show a return to normal muscle creatine concentrations and depletion of the extra PCr energy upon cessation of creatine supplementation. Creatine itself does not appear to cause permanent alteration of muscle fiber types.[35,36] Poor study design and inappropriate statistical analysis affect interpretation of existing studies. An observation of increased satellite cells after 8 weeks of supplementation was not validated after 12 weeks or confirmed after stopping the supplement.[35] A similar observation of increased myosin heavy chain expression and increased type IIx muscle fibers were not properly compared between groups or confirmed after stopping the supplement.[36]

Loading doses are not required if performance benefits are not desired within 10–14 days.[34,35] A maintenance dose of 5–6 grams daily is adequate to boost muscle creatine levels and is associated with fewer GI side effects. If an immediate improvement in strength is required, benefits can be detected in 5 days following a loading dose of creatine at 20 g/day (or 0.3 g/kg/day).[34] This loading dose is usually divided into 4 doses to reduce GI side effects of stomach upset and nausea. Nausea may be related to osmotic effects or to malabsorption. Other adverse effects reported with creatine include weight gain and muscle cramping. Weight gain may be related to an osmotic gain in water within muscles. Muscle cramping raises concerns of increasing risk of heat-related illness with creatine supplementation. Two reports followed college football players who took creatine supplements for as long as 3 years and compared them with teammates who did not take the supplements.[37,38] The athletes were followed for reports of muscle cramping, heat illness, dehydration, muscle strains, total injury reports, and missed practices. The occurrence of adverse effects did not differ between the groups. Creatine supplements have also been reported to be misbranded and to contain substances banned by antidoping agencies.[4]

All athletes should be discouraged from using creatine supplements until regulated testing is required. They should be encouraged to seek natural creatine sources from food sources rather than supplements. When the athlete insists on using creatine, providers can assist the athlete by recommending that creatine be used only as long as necessary, such as maintaining supplementation only during the competitive season. No reason exists to continue the supplements during the off season. Providers should also recommend appropriate additional hydration during creatine exposure because creatine is a protein that is filtered through the kidneys. If an athlete becomes significantly dehydrated, it is best to temporarily hold creatine until proper fluid balance is restored.

Dimethylamylamine (DMAA), Geranium seeds, and extracts

Dimethylamylamine (DMAA) is also known as methylhexanamine and was previously marketed as a sympathomimetic to treat nasal congestion. It has recently appeared in nutritional supplements claiming to increase muscle mass and reduce body weight, implying that the chemical was derived from a natural source such as geranium stems or extract. These products are associated with multiple cases of cardiac toxicity, acute hepatic failure, liver transplant, and death.[39] One report indicated 29 cases of hepatic failure with 40% of cases requiring hospitalization. Twenty-four of these individuals reported use of a DMAA-containing supplement in the 60 days prior to hepatic injury. Twelve of these individuals reported no other supplement intake besides the DMAA-containing supplement.[39]

Ephedra and Pseudoephedrine

Pseudoephedrine is available without a prescription and may be troublesome for elite athletes even when used temporarily for appropriate medical reasons because of random drug testing. Urine concentrations of pseudoephedrine greater than 150 mcg/mL are flagged as inappropriate use as a stimulant. No evidence supports performance enhancement with pseudoephedrine at nonprescription doses.[40] However, at 2.5 mg/kg, a dose roughly five times the recommended nonprescription dose, one study of seven runners showed an average 6-second improvement in 1500-meter time.[41] Reports that ephedra was associated with hypertension, cardiac arrhythmias, and seizures in otherwise healthy young adults were used to determine that ephedra was unsafe for human consumption, and it was removed from U.S. markets in 2004.[42] No data support ephedra as useful for athletic performance.[40] The data are included here because plant alkaloids related to ephedra may appear in nutritional supplements and because ephedra is available in foreign markets and through Internet sales.

Steroidal Precursors and Aromatization Inhibitors

The Anabolic Steroid Control Act of 2004 defined hormone substances that are pharmacologically related to testosterone as legend, or prescription-only, drugs. Dehydroepiandrosterone (DHEA) and androstenedione, prohormone precursors to testosterone, were sold as nutritional supplements prior to the act, but they have been identified as misbranded ingredients in nutritional supplements sold in the United States after the act. Well-designed studies demonstrate significant elevations in estradiol and estrone in men who take the supplements but no elevations in serum testosterone.[43] Aromatase inhibitors prevent the conversion of testosterone to estrone, and their use is specifically prohibited by the antidoping agencies. Many body-building supplements claim to include substances, such as *Tribulus terrestris,* that act as aromatase inhibitors. No data support these claims. Products that suggest that they boost testosterone or provide aromatase inhibition should not be recommended as performance-enhancing supplements.

Stacking

Sports nutrition products often combine several agents into a single product, a process known as "stacking." Many products include individual vitamins, minerals, metabolites, amino acids, or herbal supplements. They claim to improve endurance and muscle strength or to reduce oxidative stress related to exercise. Products with insufficient data for a clear positive effect on performance are reviewed in Table 24-2.[44-54]

Assessment of Performance-Enhancing Nutrients: A Case-Based Approach

Performance enhancers run the gamut from electrolyte solutions to energy bars to herbal supplements. To help someone select a product, the provider should determine the type of exercise or physical activity in which the individual engages, the intensity and duration of activity, and any products previously tried. The individual should also be asked about any ill effects experienced after physical activity or after using a performance enhancer.

Cases 24-1 and 24-2 illustrate assessment of individuals who wish to use a performance-enhancing product.

Sales of sports nutrition products designed to enhance or improve performance are increasing every year. The most common self-treatments are creatine to improve muscle power

and carbohydrate administration during exercise to preserve muscle glycogen and prolong time to fatigue across all sports. Several herbal supplements claim to enhance performance, but evidence to support these claims is currently lacking. Although these natural herbal products are touted as safe, evidence suggests that some may have detrimental effects on long-term health by altering cardiovascular risk, high-density lipoprotein levels, and natural, sex-determined hormone levels.

Patient Counseling for Performance-Enhancing Nutrients

The quest for enhanced physical performance has resulted in serious health consequences for some athletes. Clinical studies of many botanical and hormonal dietary supplements touted as performance-enhancing products reveal significant adverse effects and little or no enhancement in physical performance. Providers should discourage use of performance-enhancing products because none except creatine has been found to be effective. The box Patient Education for Performance-Enhancing Nutrients lists specific information to provide individuals.

Registered dietitians with national board certification as Certified Specialist in Sports Dietetics are uniquely qualified to assist athletes of all levels in evaluating their nutritional needs and to work with them on their hydration, and the quality, quantity, and timing of foods and supplements for optimal performance. Sports dietitians can be found at the Sports, Cardiovascular and Wellness Nutrition Web site (www.scandpg.org).

Key Points for Sports Nutrition and Performance-Enhancing Nutrients

➤ Training regularly and eating a well-balanced diet are consistently shown to benefit sports performance and activity. Most athletes do not require sports nutrition products.

➤ Despite marketing claims, the benefits of most performance-enhancing nutritional products and ergogenic aids are unproven, and several may be unsafe.

➤ Misbranding of nutritional supplements has occurred and can lead to positive screens from antidoping agencies as well as lead to unintentional safety risks.

➤ Most sports nutrition drinks, gels, and bars are significant sources of carbohydrate calories. The AAP has developed a position that these carbohydrate and energy drinks should not be used in adolescents and children. They should similarly be avoided in adults.

➤ Dehydration can significantly affect performance. However, no evidence supports sports nutrition drinks as beneficial when used during events lasting 60 minutes or less. For activity over 60 minutes, electrolytes in sports drinks are encouraged and may enhance fluid absorption.

➤ Sports nutrition drinks containing carbohydrates and electrolytes can prolong the time to fatigue (glycogen depletion) in events or practice lasting 60–90 minutes or longer and, therefore, may be considered when exercise duration is anticipated to exceed this duration.

case
24–1

Relevant Evaluation Criteria	Scenario/Model Outcome
Information Gathering	
1. Gather essential information about the patient's symptoms and medical history, including:	
a. description of symptom(s) (i.e., nature, onset, duration, severity, associated symptoms)	The individual reports that he competes in the shot put and discus field events in high school. Last year he qualified for the regional meet but not the state meet, and he hopes to improve his chances of qualifying in his senior track season that starts in 3 months. Participation in the shot put and discus events can require up to six attempts, three each in the preliminary and final rounds. He feels that improving his muscle mass will result in a stronger performance and longer distances in his events.
b. description of any factors that seem to precipitate, exacerbate, and/or relieve the patient's symptom(s)	His performance in these events can be affected by the number of attempts that he needs to qualify for the final round and to make his best effort in the final round. In his six attempts, he often fouls one or two attempts, particularly in the discus. He may require multiple attempts to reach his goal distances of a 50-foot shot put and a 155-foot discus throw.
c. description of the patient's efforts to relieve the symptoms	He has made no specific adjustments to his diet to maintain optimal glycogen levels before or during the track season. He does drink up to 12 ounces of a 5% CHO sports drink during the meet as a taste preference over drinking water. He plans to initiate training by lifting weights in September and participating in indoor track events during the winter season.
d. patient's identity	Michael Longtree
e. age, sex, height, and weight	17 years old, male, 6 ft 1 in., 205 lb
f. patient's occupation	High school student
g. patient's dietary habits	Michael has been eating a diet consistent with the *MyPlate* servings shown in Chapter 22.
h. patient's sleep habits	Michael sleeps 7–8 hours on school nights.
i. concurrent medical conditions, prescription and nonprescription medications, and dietary supplements	A preseason medical examination identified no issues. Michael's blood pressure and fasting glucose levels are normal, and he takes no medications or supplements.
j. allergies	NKA
k. history of other adverse reactions to medications	None
l. other (describe) _____	NA
Assessment and Triage	
2. Differentiate patient's signs/symptoms and correctly identify the patient's primary problem(s).	Michael's performance in the meet is not significantly affected by the duration of effort. Each activity lasts for only a few seconds, and the total duration of activity for up to 12 attempts is less than 60 seconds of anaerobic energy utilization; therefore, muscle glycogen depletion is not a cause. Michael may be experiencing a decline in muscle energy from the phosphagen system that is associated with repeated high-intensity activities.
3. Identify exclusions for self-treatment.	None
4. Formulate a comprehensive list of therapeutic alternatives for the primary problem to determine if triage to a medical provider is required, and share this information with the patient or caregiver.	Options include: (1) Michael can choose to take no action other than optimization of training. Regular, intensity-specific exercise can improve oxygen uptake and optimize muscle ATP production during periods of rest. Training to improve his throwing technique can result in improved distances and eliminate the need for multiple attempts in the qualification round. (2) Michael can consider increasing his muscle mass naturally by optimizing his dietary intake of protein with healthy food choices rather than a nutrition supplement.

case
24-1 *continued*

Relevant Evaluation Criteria	Scenario/Model Outcome
Plan	
5. Select an optimal therapeutic alternative to address the patient's problem, taking into account patient preferences.	Michael will adjust his dietary selections to optimize his dietary protein intake.
6. Describe the recommended therapeutic approach to the patient or caregiver.	"You can adjust your food consumption to optimize protein intake and build muscle strength naturally, without having to rely on a packaged nutrition supplement. Keep a record of your protein intake for review and recommendations."
7. Explain to the patient or caregiver the rationale for selecting the recommended therapeutic approach from the considered therapeutic alternatives.	"A diet that is high in protein will provide protein for muscle building and recovery after intensive workouts. It will also provide a natural source of creatine and the amino acids arginine and glutamine from which the body can build creatine. The dietary boost to creatine will provide an increase in the quantity of energy stored in PCr bonds. Although each physical attempt or throw will reduce muscle ATP energy, the energy available in PCr can transfer to muscle ADP and return the ADP to ATP status in seconds, thus restoring your muscle energy."
Patient Education	
8. When recommending self-care with nonprescription medications and/or nondrug therapy, convey accurate information to the patient or caregiver:	
a. appropriate dose and frequency of administration	"The ADA recommends an intake of 1.4–1.7 g/kg/day of protein to optimize muscle building. Michael weighs 93 kg, making his target intake 130–160 grams per day."
b. maximum number of days the therapy should be employed	"An athlete starting a new training program can benefit from an increase in protein intake to help establish a positive nitrogen balance and to build muscle. It is reasonable to boost protein intake to 1.5–1.7 g/kg/day (160 grams/day) for 3–4 months and then reduce to a maintenance level. Athletes who have been training for several months can maintain their muscle mass and a neutral nitrogen balance with 1.4 g/kg/day of protein intake during maintenance training."
c. product administration procedures	"The ADA recommends that the athlete consume a small amount of protein (30 grams) within 30 minutes after the completion of intense physical exercise because protein has been associated with improved muscle building. A simple snack such as 8–12 ounces of skim milk with a 4-ounce serving of chicken or tuna would meet this requirement. Michael should consider maintaining a diet journal of his meals and snacks. This information can be assessed later to determine an estimated protein intake and make further recommendations."
d. expected time to onset of relief	"Performance benefits from intense training can be measured in as little as 2–3 weeks. By comparison, measuring an increase in total body weight may require 2 months or more. The best way for Michael to assess the gains from his dietary plan is to follow his muscle strength gains from training."
e. degree of relief that can be reasonably expected	"How much a gain in muscle mass will help your performance is difficult to measure. Individual performance gains vary and still require good technique to avoid fouling on early attempts."
f. most common side effects	"The side effects from small increases in dietary protein intake are minimal. Gastrointestinal discomfort such bloating, cramping, and diarrhea have been reported. Be sure to drink plenty of fluids to allow the nitrogen waste from the protein to be eliminated through your kidneys."
g. side effects that warrant medical intervention should they occur	"During any period of increased training, you should always tell your coach if you are not feeling well. Any signs of heat illness, muscle cramping, or pain on urination should be reported immediately."
h. patient options in the event that condition worsens or persists	NA

Relevant Evaluation Criteria	Scenario/Model Outcome
i. product storage requirements	"Most food sources of protein require refrigeration to avoid spoiling and possible bacterial growth on the food. Store your lunches or protein snacks in a cooler or refrigerator if you will not be using it all within 2 hours."
Solicit follow-up questions from the patient or caregiver.	"Why isn't a creatine supplement recommended for me when many of my friends are using it?"
Answer the patient's or caregiver's questions.	"The protein available from dietary meat sources will contain a sufficient amount of creatine to meet your needs. As an athlete, you should be aware that many dietary supplements have been mis-branded and actually contain performance-enhancing chemicals that are on banned substances lists. It is important, particularly for the high school athlete, to prepare for competition with appropriate training and experience to reach their personal best effort. Using an artificial substance to enhance athletic potential is not as great a victory as reaching it on your own."

Evaluation of Patient Outcome

9. Assess patient outcome.	Contact the patient within 2–3 weeks to review his diet intake to ensure that he has adjusted his diet appropriately.

Key: ADP = Adenosine diphosphate; ATP = adenosine triphosphate; CHO = carbohydrate; PCr = phosphocreatine; NA = not applicable; NKA = no known allergies.

case

24-2

Relevant Evaluation Criteria	Scenario/Model Outcome
Information Gathering	
1. Gather essential information about the patient's symptoms and medical history, including:	
a. description of symptom(s) (i.e., nature, onset, duration, severity, associated symptoms)	The patient is an enthusiastic weight lifter who enjoys the camaraderie of the gym but does not participate in competitions. He has been lifting for 25 years and has reached a plateau in weight lifting. He has been unable to improve his lifted weight and for the last several years has started to lower the maximum weight he lifts. He does not want to increase his body mass but has been taking supplements that claim he will be stronger to prevent this perceived loss of strength. He has asked for a review of his supplements for safe use, following a recent adverse drug effect that may have been related to interacting medications.
b. description of any factors that seem to precipitate, exacerbate, and/or relieve the patient's symptom(s)	He spends 8 hours a week in the gym, splitting time between upper body and lower body exercise. He reports increasing symptoms of muscle soreness and decreased recoverability between workouts.
c. description of the patient's efforts to relieve the symptoms	He has been taking a number of oral supplements at the recommendation of other gym members and the sales clerks at the nutrition store. He has needed to take ibuprofen 200 mg every afternoon because of muscle soreness that he associates with sitting at a desk during the day.
d. patient's identity	Craig Johnson
e. age, sex, height, and weight	52 years old, male, 5 ft 9 in., 235 lb
f. patient's occupation	Logistics manager for a trucking company
g. patient's dietary habits	Eats well at home and prepares healthy meals for his lunch breaks.

case
24–2 *continued*

Relevant Evaluation Criteria	Scenario/Model Outcome
h. patient's sleep habits	Works the day shift and spends his late afternoon in the gym. Generally asleep by 10 pm. Awakens daily at 6 am to go to work.
i. concurrent medical conditions, prescription and nonprescription medications, and dietary supplements	Amlodipine 10 mg daily for hypertension; simvastatin 40 mg daily for elevated LDL and low HDL; L-arginine 2 grams daily; creatine 5 grams daily; conjugated linoleic acid 9 grams daily
j. allergies	NKA
k. history of other adverse reactions to medications	None reported. His HTN is controlled.
l. other (describe) _____	None

Assessment and Triage

2. Differentiate patient's signs/symptoms and correctly identify the patient's primary problem(s).	Craig has symptoms of myopathic pain that may be the result of statin use or a drug interaction between the simvastatin and amlodipine. Craig is taking a number of supplements that he is not certain are helpful to his hobby of weight lifting. He wants to be assured that they are not adversely affecting his medical condition.
3. Identify exclusions for self-treatment.	Craig should not take supplements that might affect his LDL and HDL cholesterol.
4. Formulate a comprehensive list of therapeutic alternatives for the primary problem to determine if triage to a medical provider is required, and share this information with the patient or caregiver.	Options include: (1) Refer patient to his PCP to review the use of simvastatin and amlodipine. The combination may be contributing to the myopathy that he sees as a performance limitation. A change in his prescription medications may be appropriate. (2) Craig should stop taking conjugated linoleic acid because this supplement has been associated with lower HDL levels and has no proven performance benefits. (3) Craig could consider discontinuation of all of his supplements because he does not require performance benefits for competition and any benefits from these unproven supplements do not outweigh the risk from adverse effects or misbranding.

Plan

5. Select an optimal therapeutic alternative to address the patient's problem, taking into account patient preferences.	The patient should consult his PCP regarding the myopathic pain. He should discontinue conjugated linoleic acid immediately and consider discontinuing the other supplements that have not been proven to affect weight-lifting performance. Craig would prefer to continue taking creatine for strength benefits.
6. Describe the recommended therapeutic approach to the patient or caregiver.	(1) "You are feeling muscle soreness after workouts. This soreness could be related to the hard workouts or may be related to a known medication adverse effect. A change in prescription medication may reduce the amount of myopathic discomfort that you are feeling." (2) "You may choose to continue taking the supplement creatine because it has good evidence for improved strength and has not been associated with affecting HDL or LDL levels."
7. Explain to the patient or caregiver the rationale for selecting the recommended therapeutic approach from the considered therapeutic alternatives.	"A known drug interaction exists between simvastatin and amlodipine. A reduction in the dose of simvastatin, or changing to a non-interacting statin, may improve the muscle soreness."

Patient Education

8. When recommending self-care with nonprescription medications and/or nondrug therapy, convey accurate information to the patient or caregiver:	

case
24–2 *continued*

Relevant Evaluation Criteria	Scenario/Model Outcome
a. appropriate dose and frequency of administration	"Creatine maintenance doses are taken as 5 grams per day. These maintenance doses will increase the quantity of high-energy phosphocreatine (PCr). PCr will transfer its available energy to ADP, restoring ATP. There does not appear to be a benefit from taking more than 5 grams per day. Taking creatine for years has not been prospectively studied; however, short-term studies have consistently been associated with modest gains in many weight-lifting measurements."
b. maximum number of days the therapy should be employed	"Creatine has been taken for years by young football players. However, the effects of long-term supplementation in patients your age have not been determined."
c. product administration procedures	"Creatine is usually taken as a powder and mixed into a smoothie or shake. Taking the creatine supplement within 30 minutes after exercise may improve muscle building."
d. expected time to onset of relief	NA
e. degree of relief that can be reasonably expected	"You should have some mental relief that your medications and creatine have no significant interactions. You should not expect any changes to your weight-lifting abilities from stopping these supplements. Repeat your serum lipid levels on your usual schedule. Your HDL changes will be minimal."
f. most common side effects	"Large doses of creatine can cause gastrointestinal distress and cramping; however, your years of experience indicate that you can tolerate this 5 gram dose without difficulty. Some concern exists that long-term protein loading can affect kidney function, so you should continue your regular physician visits and laboratory monitoring. Be aware that misbranding of creatine supplements can result in an inadvertent exposure to chemicals that are regulated by antidoping agencies."
g. side effects that warrant medical intervention should they occur	"If you observe a urine color that is significantly darker than usual or includes a new foul smell, first assess your hydration status. If the urine changes are persistent with proper hydration, you will want to follow up with your primary care provider."
h. patient options in the event that condition worsens or persists	"Stopping creatine is always a consideration because you are not seeking competition-related performance benefits. Stopping the supplement has little effect other than a small reduction in weight-lifting measures."
i. product storage requirements	"Unmixed creatine powder can be stored at room temperature, but mixed creatine shakes should be refrigerated or consumed within 2 hours."
Solicit follow-up questions from the patient or caregiver.	"Could you provide more information on the other side effects I might experience from the simvistatin–amlodipine interaction. Should I stop these medications before seeing my physician?"
Answer the patient's or caregiver's questions.	"The interaction results in higher-than-normal serum levels of simvastatin. You should call your physician immediately because you are already experiencing muscle pain, tenderness, and weakness. Other symptoms of a more severe reaction include fever, joint swelling, joint pain, unusual bruising and/or yellowing of the skin or eyes. You should not stop taking your medications until you discusses these possible adverse effects with your physician."

Evaluation of Patient Outcome

9. Assess patient outcome.	Contact the patient within 1 week to determine if he has made an appointment with his physician.

Key: ADP = Adenosine diphosphate; ATP = adenosine triphosphate; HDL = high-density lipoprotein; HTN = hypertension; LDL= low-density lipoprotein; NA= not applicable; NKA = no known allergies; PCP = primary care provider.

patient education for

Performance-Enhancing Nutrients

The objective in selecting a performance enhancer is to choose a product that is safe and appropriate for the type, intensity, and duration of the physical activity. Following the recommendations of a primary care provider (PCP) and other health care providers, as well as carefully following product instructions and the self-care measures listed here, will help ensure optimal therapeutic outcomes.

Muscle Glycogen Preservation

▪ Carbohydrate-containing sports drinks contain one or more forms of sugar and the electrolytes sodium and potassium. These drinks are optimal for intermediate sprint activities, such as soccer and football, and for endurance events and practice or training sessions that last longer than 60 minutes. Small doses repeated every 15–20 minutes may be necessary for sustained energy over longer events to maintain glucose levels for performance energy, thereby delaying the time to fatigue.

▪ Athletes with diabetes should seek the advice of a PCP or sports dietitian before beginning an exercise program to ensure that they are prepared to avoid hypoglycemia while exercising.

▪ Note that sports bars often contain other macronutrients, such as fats and proteins. Many of these bars are more appropriate for after-exercise recovery than for use during athletic events. If a well-balanced meal is unavailable within 2 hours of exercise, many of these bars may be an appropriate after-exercise fuel replenishment source. (Table 24–1 lists specific products.)

▪ Long-chain triglycerides can cause discomfort and bloating during intense exercise; therefore, avoid consuming meals that contain large amounts of fat at least 2 hours before exercise.

Enhancement of Muscle Mass

▪ Athletes do not need to exceed the recommended daily intake of 1.7 grams of protein per kilogram of body weight to increase body mass. Available data indicate that higher intakes do not produce additional muscle mass or strength.

▪ Athletes who ingest high amounts of protein, either through their foods or protein supplements, should discuss this practice with their PCP or sports dietitian. Blood urea nitrogen and serum creatinine levels may be monitored to ascertain whether high protein intake is affecting kidney function.

Hydration and Electrolytes

▪ For athletes exercising less than 60 minutes, water intake alone is usually sufficient to complete the exercise.

▪ Athletes exercising longer than 60 minutes may consider incorporating a carbohydrate- and electrolyte-containing sports drink into the exercise program for optimal performance.

▪ Endurance athletes exercising for 4 hours and longer are discouraged from drinking only free (regular) water owing to the risk of dilutional hyponatremia. Exercise of this duration (e.g., marathon running and long-distance triathlons) will require electrolyte and carbohydrate replacement for optimal performance.

▪ Athletes should not target a set quantity of water to consume during exercise; rather, athletes should drink according to the trigger of thirst. Slower runners and walkers exercising in cool conditions can consume water at a lower rate (sips), whereas faster and heavier athletes and those exercising in heat and humidity should be prepared to drink more. Individual calculations of sweat rate for fluid needs during exercise and an additional calculation for recovery fluids can be made to better meet the athlete's needs.

▪ Athletes should consume 6–12 ounces of plain water if exercise lasts less than 60 minutes. If exercise lasts longer than 60 minutes, consider a carbohydrate- and electrolyte-containing sports drink. (See Fluid Tips for Training and Competition, available at: www. extension.arizona.edu/sites/extension.arizona.edu/files/pubs/az1387.pdf)

▪ Carbonated water may cause GI distress and bloating; avoid drinking carbonated water before or during an athletic event.

Ergogenic Supplements

▪ Little or no clinical evidence supports the performance-enhancing claims of most herbal supplements.

▪ Creatine may help increase muscle strength and power in events that require short bursts of power, but GI discomfort may occur. To avoid this problem, do not take loading doses. The same benefits occur within 7–14 days of taking a daily maintenance dose of 5 g/day. Maintain proper hydration to assist in the elimination of metabolic waste and to avoid dehydration.

▪ Long-term use of creatine has no known benefit. The strength improvements of creatine are not maintained and will "wash out" to baseline when the supplement is stopped. Athletes should consider optimizing their nutritional intake rather than using creatine.

Key: GI = Gastrointestinal.

➤ To minimize the risk of dehydration or hyponatremia caused by the intake of salt-free fluids, athletes exercising for very long periods of time should use sports drinks that contain electrolytes and carbohydrates rather than plain water.

➤ Creatine supplementation can increase muscle phosphocreatine concentrations, thus increasing the amount of stored energy in muscles. Phosphocreatine can lend its high-energy phosphate bond to ADP to rapidly restore ATP, allowing increased power for single and repeated activities for 30 seconds or less.

➤ Pseudoephedrine is monitored by the U.S. Anti-Doping Agency, and athletes subject to testing for banned substances should be warned of any product containing pseudoephedrine. A similar warning should be given for any cough and cold product that includes a sympathomimetic amine as a decongestant, such as oxymetazoline nasal spray.

REFERENCES

1. Kreider RB, Wilborn CD, Taylor L, et al. ISSN exercise & sport nutrition review: research & recommendations. *J Int Soc Sports Nutr.* 2010;7:7. Accessed at http://www.ncbi.nlm.nih.gov/pmc/articles/PMC2853497/, June 22, 2011.

2. Rodriguez NR, Di Marco NM, Langley S. Position of the American Dietetic Association, Dieticians of Canada, and the American College of Sports Medicine: nutrition and athletic performance. *J Am Diet Assoc.* 2009;109(3):509–27.

3. Johnson M. Packaged Facts: Sports drinks, nutrition bars a $10 billion business in 2013. July 16, 2013. Accessed at http://www.drugstorenews.com/article/packaged-facts-sports-drinks-nutrition-bars-10-billion-business-2013, September 15, 2014.

4. deHon O, Coumans B. The continuing story of supplements and doping infractions. *Br J Sports Med.* 2007;41(11):800–5.

5. Kohler M, Thomas A, Geyer H, et al. Confiscated black market products and nutrition supplements with non-approved ingredients analyzed in the Cologne doping control laboratory 2009. *Drug Test Anal.* 2010;2(11–12):533–7.

6. National College Athletic Association. *National Study of Substance Use Trends among NCAA College Student-Athletes.* Indianapolis, Indiana: The National Collegiate Athletic Association; January 2012. Accessed at http://www.ncaa.org/sites/default/files/13.%20Substance%20Use%20Report%202009.pdf, July 17, 2014.

7. Hoffman JR, Faigenbaum AD, Ratamess NA, et al. Nutritional supplementation and anabolic steroid use in adolescents. *Med Sci Sport Exerc.* 2008;40(1):15–24.

8. American Academy of Pediatrics Committee on Nutrition and the Council on Sports Medicine and Fitness. Clinical report—sports drinks and energy drinks for children and adolescents: are they appropriate? *Pediatrics.* 2011;127(6):1182–9.

9. Coyle EF. Physical activity as a metabolic stressor. *Am J Clin Nutr.* 2000;72(suppl):512S–20S.

10. Coyle EF. Substrate utilization during exercise in active people. *Am J Clin Nutr.* 1995;61(4 suppl):968S–79S.

11. Howowitz JF, Klein S. Lipid metabolism during endurance exercise. *Am J Clin Nutr.* 2000;72(2 suppl):558S–63S.

12. Spencer MR, Gastin PB. Energy system contribution during 200- to 1500-m running in highly trained athletes. *Med Sci Sport Exerc.* 2001;33(1);157–62.

13. Burke LM, Hawley JA. Fat and carbohydrate for exercise. *Curr Opin Clin Nutr Metab Care.* 2006;9(4):476–81.

14. Bemben MG, Lamont HS. Creatine supplementation and exercise performance. *Sports Med.* 2005;35(2):107–25.

15. Foster C, Costill DL, Fink WJ. Effects of preexercise feedings on endurance performance. *Med Sci Sport Exerc.* 1979;11(1):1–5.

16. Phillips SM, Van Loon LJ. Dietary protein for athletes: from requirements to optimum adaptation. *J Sport Sci.* 2011;29(suppl 1):S29–38.

17. Poortmans JR, Dellalieux O. Do regular high protein diets have potential health risks on kidney function in athletes? *Int J Sport Nutr Exerc Metab.* 2000;10(1):28–38.

18. Sawka MN, Burke LM, Eichner ER, et al. Exercise and fluid replacement: the American College of Sports Medicine position stand. *Med Sci Sport Exerc.* 2007;39(2):377–90.

19. Almond CS, Shin AY, Fortescue EB, et al. Hyponatremia among runners in the Boston marathon. *N Engl J Med.* 2005;325(15):1550–6.

20. Hew-Butler T, Verbalis JG, Noakes TD. Updated fluid recommendation: position statement from the International Marathon Medical Directors Association (IMMDA). *Clin J Sport Med.* 2006;16(4):283–92.

21. Wharham PC, Speedy DB, Noakes TD, et al. NSAID use increases the risk of developing hyponatremia during an ironman triathlon. *Med Sci Sports Exerc.* 2006;38(4):618–22.

22. Hampsom NB, Pollock NW, Piantadosi CA. Oxygenated water and athletic performance. *JAMA.* 2003;290(18):2408–9.

23. Valentine R, Saunders MJ, Todd MK, et al. Influence of carbohydrate-protein beverage on cycling endurance and indices of muscle disruption. *Int J Sport Nutr Exerc Metab.* 2008;18(4):363–78

24. Toone RJ, Betts JA. Isocaloric carbohydrate versus carbohydrate-protein ingestion and cycling time-trial performance. *Int J Sport Nutr Exerc Metab.* 2010;20(1):34–43

25. Kersick C, Harvey T, Stout J, et al. International Society of Sports Nutrition position stand: nutrient timing. *J Int Soc Sports Nutr.* 2008;5:17. Accessed at http://www.jissn.com/content/5/1/17, June 22, 2011.

26. van Rosendal SP, Osborne MA, Fassett RG, et al. Physiological and performance effects of glycerol hyperhydration and rehydration. *Nutr Rev.* 2009;67(12):690–705.

27. Shirreffs SM, Watson P, Maughan RJ. Milk as an effective post-exercise rehydration drink. *Br J Nutr.* 2007;98(1):173–80.

28. Pritchett K, Bishop P, Pritchett R, et al. Acute effects of chocolate milk and a commercial recovery beverage on post exercise recovery indices and endurance cycling performance. *Appl Physiol Nutr Metab.* 2009;34(6):1017–22.

29. Thomas K, Morris P, Stevenson E. Improved endurance capacity following chocolate milk consumption compared with 2 commercially available sport drinks. *Appl Physiol Nutr Metab.* 2009;34(1):78–82.

30. Davis JK. Caffeine and anaerobic performance: ergogenic value and mechanism of action. *Sports Med.* 2009;39(10):813–32.

31. Campbell B, Wilborn C, LaBounty P, et al. International Society of Sports Nutrition position stand: energy drinks. *J Int Soc Sports Nutr.* 2013;10(1):1–16

32. Kurtz AM, Leong J, Anand M, et al. Effects of caffeinated versus decaffeinated energy shots on blood pressure and heart rate in healthy young volunteers. *Pharmacotherapy.* 2013;33(8):779–86.

33. Howland J, Rohsenow JR. Risks of energy drinks mixed with alcohol. *JAMA.* 2013;309(3):245–6.

34. Terjung RL, Clarkson P, Eichner ER, et al. American College of Sports Medicine consensus statement. The physiological and health effects of oral creatine supplementation. *Med Sci Sport Exerc.* 2000;32(3):706–17.

35. Olsen S, Aagaard P, Kadi F, et al. Creatine supplementation augments the increase in satellite cell and myonuclei number in human skeletal muscle induced by strength training. *J Physiol.* 2006;573(pt 2):525–34.

36. Willoughby DS, Rosene J. Effects of oral creatine and resistance training on myosin heavy chain expression. *Med Sci Sport Exerc.* 2001;33(10):1674–81.

37. Greenwood M, Kreider RB, Greenwood L, et al. Cramping and injury incidence in collegiate football players are reduced by creatine supplementation. *J Athlet Train.* 2004;38(3):216–9.

38. Greenwood M, Kreider RB, Melton C, et al. Creatine supplementation during college football training does not increase the incidence of cramping or injury. *Mol Cell Biochem.* 2003;244(1–2):83–8.

39. Centers for Disease Control and Prevention (CDC). Notes from the field: acute hepatitis and liver failure following the use of a dietary supplement intended for weight loss or muscle building, May–October 2013. *MMWR Morb Mortal Wkly Rep.* 2013;62(40):817–9.

40. Shekelle PG, Hardy ML, Morton SC, et al. Efficacy and safety of ephedra and ephedrine for weight loss and athletic performance: a meta analysis. *JAMA.* 2003;289(12):1537–45.

41. Hodges K, Hancock S, Currell K, et al. Pseudoephedrine enhances performance in 1500m runners. *Med Sci Sports Exerc.* 2006;38(2):329–33.

42. Centers for Disease Control and Prevention. Adverse events associated with ephedrine containing products–Texas, December 1993–September 1995. *MMWR Morb Mortal Wkly Rep.* 1996;45(32):689–93.

43. Hoffman JR, Kraemer WJ, Bhasin S, et al. Position stand on androgen and human growth hormone use. *J Strength Cond Res.* 2009;23 (5 suppl):S1–59.

44. Fisher-Wellman K, Bloomer RJ. Acute exercise and oxidative stress: a 30 year history. *Dyn Med.* 2009;8:1–25.

45. Flakoll P, Sharp R, Levenhagen D, et al. Effect of beta-hydroxy-beta-methylbutyrate, arginine and lysine supplementation on strength, functionality, body composition, and protein metabolism in elderly women. *Nutrition.* 2004;20(5):445–51.

46. Cheuvront SN, Carter R, Kolka MA, et al. Branched-chain amino acid supplementation and human performance when hypohydrated in the heat. *J Appl Physiol.* 2004;97(4):1275–82.

47. Parcell AC, Smith JM, Schulthies SS, et al. Cordyceps sinensis (Cordy-Max Cs-4) supplementation does not improve endurance exercise performance. *Int J Sport Nutr Exerc Metab.* 2004;14(2):236–42.

48. Colson SN, Wyatt FB, Johnston DL, et al. Cordyceps sinensis- and Rhodiola rosea-based supplementation in male cyclists and its effect on muscle tissue oxygen saturation. *J Strength Cond Res.* 2005;19(2):358–63.

49. Goulet ED, Dionne IJ. Assessment of the effects of Eleutherococcus senticosus on endurance performance. *Int J Sport Nutr Exerc Metab.* 2005;15(1):75–83.

50. Engels H, Fahlman MM, Wirth JC. Effects of ginseng on secretory IgA, performance and recovery from interval exercise. *Med Sci Sports Exerc.* 2003;35(4):690–6.

51. Nelson JL, Robergs RA. Exploring the potential ergogenic effects of glycerol hyperhydration. *Sports Med.* 2007;37(11):981–1000.

52. Buchman AL, Awal MA, Jenden D, et al. The effect of lecithin supplementation on plasma choline concentrations during a marathon. *J Am Coll Nutr.* 2000;19(6):768–70.

53. De Bock K, Eijnde BO, Ramaekers M, et al. Acute Rhodiola rosea intake can improve endurance exercise performance. *Int J Sport Nutr Exerc Metab.* 2004;14(3):298–307.

54. Earnest CP, Morss GM. Effects of a commercial herbal-based formula on exercise performance in cyclists. *Med Sci Sports Exerc.* 2004;36(3):504–9.

chapter 25

INFANT NUTRITION AND SPECIAL NUTRITIONAL NEEDS OF CHILDREN

M. Petrea Cober

Human milk is most physiologically suited to infants and is the optimal milk source for feeding infants until 12 months of age. The American Academy of Pediatrics (AAP) recommends that human milk be used as the sole source of nutrition for infants during the first 6 months of life. For infants whose mothers choose not to breast-feed, the nutritional quality, safety, and convenience of infant formulas make them an appropriate alternative. Variations among formulas allow for product selection that will meet a specific infant's nutritional needs while offering differences in palatability, digestibility, nutrient sources, convenience, and cost.

A health care provider should be able to provide information to parents or other caregivers to encourage successful breast-feeding. In addition, in consultation with the child's parents and primary care provider, the health care provider should be able to evaluate indications, advise on formula selection, and help ensure its appropriate use. This service requires knowledge of infant and child nutrition needs, breast-feeding, and commercially prepared infant and pediatric formulas, including differences in formula composition and specific uses for therapeutic formulas.

Some children will require enteral formulas after the age of 1 year because of various disease states and conditions. The health care provider needs to be knowledgeable about these products and their appropriate use to be able to answer caregiver questions about them, facilitate their procurement, and do triage for complications associated with these products.

Organ Maturation and Infant Growth

Knowledge of the development of the gastrointestinal (GI) tract and the kidney is crucial to understanding infant nutrition. Monitoring the infant's growth and growth rate using the World Health Organization (WHO) growth charts is important for assessing possible abnormal or unhealthy growth. The WHO growth charts are recommended for children less than 24 months of age, and the Centers for Disease Control and Prevention (CDC) growth charts are recommended for children over the age of 24 months.[1]

Gastrointestinal Maturation

By the end of the second trimester of pregnancy, all segments of the fetus's GI tract are formed and display some physiologic function. The third trimester, however, is the period of maximal

GI tract growth and differentiation. Therefore, premature infants (those born before 37 weeks gestation) often have reduced GI tract function, especially those born prior to 32 weeks gestation. Transition from intrauterine nutrition through the maternal–fetal unit (i.e., the placenta) to extrauterine nutrition through milk requires the maturation of many physiologic processes. These processes include effective sucking, swallowing, gastric emptying, intestinal peristalsis, and defecation; salivary, gastric, pancreatic, and hepatobiliary secretions; and intestinal brush border enzymes and transport systems (Table 25–1).[2]

Nutritive sucking develops at approximately 33–34 weeks gestation. In term infants, a mature, efficient pattern of sucking is seen within a few days after birth. In premature infants, an immature, inefficient pattern may persist for a month or more. Infants born before 34 weeks gestation cannot coordinate sucking, swallowing, and breathing; therefore, they may require tube feedings for several weeks to months until these reflexes mature. Liquid nutrition is appropriate for all infants until complex tongue movements and swallowing reflexes mature. Maturation of these reflexes typically occurs at 4–6 months of age, and it is at this time that solid foods can be safely added to an infant's diet.[2]

Early in life, frequent feedings (every 2–3 hours) are necessary, because the stomach capacity of a term newborn with a birth weight greater than 2500 grams (5 pounds 8 ounces) is only 20–90 mL. Gastric capacity increases to 90–150 mL by 1 month of age, at which time longer periods between feedings are possible. Human milk empties more rapidly from the stomach than infant formula; therefore, human milk–fed infants will typically eat more often than their formula-fed peers.

In term infants, gastric acid and pepsin secretion peak in the first 10 days of life, decrease between 10 and 30 days of life, and then increase to adult levels by 3 months of age. In premature infants, basal acid output is lower than that of a term infant but increases with postnatal age. Milk in the infant's stomach causes a sharp increase in the pH of the gastric contents and a slower return to lower pH values than in older children and adults. Gastric acidity in the newborn is unsuitable for optimal pepsin action. Therefore, little protein digestion occurs in the stomach because of low pepsin activity. The extent of protein absorption, however, is similar to that seen in children and adults. Amino acids and peptides produced by protein digestion are absorbed passively or by active transport mechanisms that reach adult capacity by the age of 14 weeks.

Premature and full-term infants can digest most carbohydrates, because the production of intestinal enzymes such as sucrase, maltase, isomaltase, and glucoamylase is sufficiently

Function	Weeks of Gestation When First Detectable	Comments
Sucking and swallowing	16	16 weeks: swallowing of amniotic fluid 26 weeks: sucking 33–35 weeks: mature, coordinated sucking, swallowing, and breathing
Gastric motility and secretion	20	Gastric emptying delayed in first few days of life; affected by caloric density, carbohydrate concentration, pathologic conditions
Intestinal motility	20	26–30 weeks: disorganized contractile activity 30–34 weeks: repetitive groups of contractions 34–35 weeks: more mature migrating motor complexes

Digestion and Absorption

Examples of Factors Important in Digestion and Absorption	Weeks of Gestation When First Detectable	Proportion of Adult Values
Protein		
Enterokinase	24–26	20% at 30 weeks 10%–25% at term
Hydrochloric acid	At birth	<20% at 30 weeks <30% at term, 50% for first 3 months
Peptidases	<12	15% at 30 weeks Nearly 100% at term
Trypsinogen/chymotrypsinogen	20	10%–60% at term
Amino acid transport	ND	Nearly 100% at term
Macromolecule absorption	ND	Nearly 100% at term
Fat		
Lingual lipase	30	Nearly 100% at term
Pancreatic lipase	16–20	5%–10% at term
Bile acids	22	25% at 32 weeks 50% at term
Medium-chain triglyceride uptake	ND	100% (absorption occurs in the stomach)
Long-chain triglyceride uptake	ND	10%–90% at term
Carbohydrate		
Pancreatic alpha-amylase	22–30	0% at term Secretion begins at 6 months of age
Salivary alpha-amylase	16	0% at 30 weeks 10%–20% at term
Lactase	10	30% at 28–34 weeks Nearly 100% at term
Monosaccharide absorption	11–19	Glucose absorption: 50%–60% at term

Key: ND = Not determined.

Source: Reference 2, and Kleinman RE, Kamin DS. Gastrointestinal development. In: Baker SS, Baker RD, Davis AM, eds. *Pediatric Nutrition Support.* Sudbury, MA: Jones and Bartlett; 2007:15–27.

mature at birth. Lactase activity increases relatively late in fetal life and begins to decline after the age of 3 years, especially in African American and Asian children. By adulthood, approximately 15% of Caucasians, 40% of Asians, and 85% of African Americans are deficient in intestinal lactase.[3] Pancreatic amylase secretion does not reach adult levels until approximately 1 year of age. Salivary amylase may help compensate for this relative lactase and amylase deficiency in early infancy. Despite this relative lactase deficiency, most term and preterm infants tolerate lactose-containing formulas with negligible unabsorbed carbohydrate output in their stools. Unabsorbed lactose that enters the colon undergoes bacterial fermentation (colonic salvage) to short-chain fatty acids, which creates an acidic environment that favors growth of acidophilic bacterial flora (lactobacilli) and suppresses growth of more pathogenic organisms. This acidity also promotes water absorption and prevents osmotic diarrhea. Because of the relative abundance of glucoamylase, compared with lactase, in the premature infant's intestine, glucose polymers are digested and absorbed better than lactose.[2]

Newborns exhibit low pancreatic lipase concentrations and slow rates of bile acid synthesis, both of which are important for fat absorption. The rate of bile acid synthesis increases throughout gestation and with increasing postnatal age. The bile acid pool in a premature infant is one-fourth that of an adult, whereas a term infant's is one-half that of an adult. However, fat malabsorption is not a major problem in preterm or term infants, given that lingual and gastric lipases are present. Infants born earlier than 34 weeks gestation, however, may exhibit steatorrhea.

Intestinal length may also affect nutrient absorption. At birth, a term infant's small intestine is approximately 270 cm (106 inches) long. During the third trimester the intestinal length approximately doubles. Therefore, infants born prematurely will have less small intestine and, subsequently, decreased surface area for absorption. Adult intestinal length of 4–5 meters (13–16.5 feet) is reached by about 4 years of age.

Kidney Maturation

Maturation of the kidney is also important in nutrition, because it determines the ability of the kidney to excrete a solute load. Glomerular filtration begins around the ninth week of fetal life; however, kidney function does not appear to be necessary for normal intrauterine homeostasis, given that the placenta serves as the major excretory organ. After birth, the rate of glomerular filtration increases until growth stops, toward the end of the second decade of life. Even after correction for body surface area, the glomerular filtration rate of a child does not approximate adult values until the third year of life.

Growth

Birth weight is determined primarily by maternal prepregnancy weight and pregnancy weight changes. The average birth weight of a term infant is approximately 3500 grams (7 pounds 8 ounces). Premature infants are categorized on the basis of birth weight: low-birth-weight infants weigh less than 2500 grams (5 pounds 8 ounces); very low-birth-weight infants weigh less than 1500 grams (3 pounds 4 ounces); extremely low-birth-weight infants weigh less than 1000 grams (2 pounds 3 ounces); and micropreemies weigh less than 750 grams (1 pound 10 ounces).

Water weight loss (6%–10% of body weight) occurs immediately after birth over a period of 1–2 weeks and is followed by an average weight gain of 1%–2% of birth weight daily (25–35 g/day in term infants) during the first 4 months, and 15 g/day over the next 8 months. Most term infants double their birth weight by 4 months of age and triple it by 12 months. Premature infants may reach these milestones sooner. From 2 years to approximately 10 years of age, the growth rate is fairly constant at about 2.3 kg (5 pounds) each year. Growth velocity increases and a major growth spurt occurs during adolescence. Height shows a growth pattern similar to that of weight; most infants increase their length by 50% in the first year, 100% in the first 4 years, and 300% by 13 years of age. Changes in body composition accompany height and weight changes. Most notably, total body water decreases as adipose tissue increases. Total body water accounts for approximately 90% of total body weight at 24 weeks gestation, 70% at term, and 60% by 1 year of age.

Normal values of weight, length/height, and head circumference (until 3 years of age) for infants and children are generally expressed in terms of percentile-for-age; the reference standards most commonly used are the WHO growth standards for infants and children less than 2 years of age and the CDC growth charts developed by the National Center for Health Statistics (NCHS) for children greater than 2 years of age. In 2006, the CDC, National Institutes of Health (NIH), and AAP met to discuss the use of the recently released WHO growth standards in the United States. Three primary benefits of the WHO growth standards for infants and children less than 2 years of age were cited as the reason for their use in the United States. These benefits include establishing growth of the breast-fed infant as the norm for growth, providing a better description of physiologic growth in infancy, and basing information on a high-quality study designed explicitly for creating growth charts. For children greater than 2 years of age, the CDC growth charts should still be used, because the methods used to create both the CDC and WHO growth charts were similar for 2- to 5-year-olds, and the WHO growth charts only represent children up to 5 years of age.[1] Charts can be downloaded free of charge at www.cdc.gov/growthcharts. The infant charts are intended for use in term infants. Once premature infants reach 40 weeks gestational age, their growth parameters can be plotted on these charts, but their age must be corrected for gestational age (i.e., chronological age in weeks minus number of weeks premature) until 24 months of age for weight and 36 months for length/height and head circumference. Charts for premature infants less than 40 weeks gestation and children with specific conditions (e.g., cerebral palsy or Turner syndrome) are available and should be used when appropriate. These specialized growth charts can be found on various Web sites, including the Kennedy Krieger Institute for children with disorders of the brain and spinal cord, such as cerebral palsy (www.kennedykrieger.org), and the Turner Syndrome Society of the United States (www.turnersyndrome.org). Specialized growth charts are no longer recommended by AAP for children with Down syndrome (www.ndss.org), and standard charts for age should be used.[4] The most commonly used charts for premature infants are the Babson and Benda charts (charts can be accessed at www.biomedcentral.com/1471-2431/3/13). Most infants' growth parameters will fall between the 2nd and 98th percentiles on the gender-specific weight-for-age, length/height-for-age, weight-for-length, and head circumference-for-age charts. Most children grow along a percentile established shortly after birth, but spurts and plateaus are common. Failure to thrive is defined as a fall of two or more growth percentiles from a previously established percentile in 6 months or less. If growth is not progressing as expected, particularly in the first year of life when growth should be rapid, the infant's diet and other potential contributory factors (e.g., environment, diseases, or syndromes) should be evaluated. Satisfactory growth is the most sensitive indicator of whether nutritional needs are being met.

For children older than 2 years, body mass index (BMI)-for-age charts can be useful in assessing obesity risk. BMI, a measure of body weight adjusted for height, is a useful tool to assess body fat. BMI is calculated as weight in kilograms divided by height in meters squared. According to current CDC guidelines, a child with a BMI at or above the 85th percentile on the gender-specific, BMI-for-age NCHS chart is considered "at risk of overweight," and a child with a BMI at or above the 95th percentile is "overweight." However, in 2005, the American Medical Association, in collaboration with the Health Resources and Services Administration and the CDC, convened an expert committee charged with revising these recommendations. The committee's nomenclature changes were intended to make it easier to discuss children's weight issues with parents and children and to transition to adult assessments. These new recommendations state that a child whose BMI is at or above the 85th percentile but below the 95th percentile or 30 kg/m², whichever is smaller, should be classified as "overweight." A child whose BMI is at or above the 95th percentile or 30 kg/m², whichever is smaller, should be classified as "obese."[5] In 2009–2010, 12.3% of children and adolescents 2–19 years of age were greater than or equal to the 97th percentile, 16.9% were greater than or

equal to the 95th percentile, and 31.8% were greater than or equal to the 85th percentile for BMI-for-age growth.[6] The prevalence of obesity in children has not changed since 2007–2008. However, between 1999–2000 and 2009–2010, a significant increase in the prevalence of obesity was observed in males 2–19 years of age but not in females. Also, a significant increase in BMI was observed in males 12–19 years of age but not in females. A BMI below the 5th percentile is indicative of underweight. The health care provider should realize that, because of the way the growth charts were developed, 5% of normally growing and healthy children will fall below the 5th percentile and 5% will fall above the 95th percentile on the weight-for-age or height-for-age charts. These children should not be branded as "malnourished" or "obese."

Energy Requirements and Growth

Acceptable growth is achievable only with adequate intake; absorption; and utilization of energy, protein, carbohydrates, minerals, and vitamins. The Food and Nutrition Board of the National Research Council has established dietary reference intakes (DRIs). as reference values for nutrient intake sufficiency and safety. The DRIs for micronutrients are discussed in detail in Chapter 22, and tables in that chapter list the current established recommended dietary allowances (RDAs) and adequate intakes (AIs) for healthy infants and children. Table 25–2 provides the

table 25–2 Dietary Reference Intakes of Macronutrients for Full-Term Infants and Children[a,b]

Nutrient	0–6 Months	7–12 Months	1–3 Years	4–8 Years	9–13 Years
Energy[c] (kcal/day)	M: 570 F: 520	M: 743 F: 676	M: 1046 F: 992	M: 1742 F: 1642	M: 2279 F: 2071
Protein[c] (g/kg/day)	1.5	1.5[d]	1.1[d]	0.95[d]	0.95[d]
(g/day)	9.1	13.5[d]	13[d]	19[d]	34[d]
Carbohydrate (g/day)	60	95	130[d]	130[d]	130[d]
Water (L/day)[e]	0.7	0.8	1.3	1.7	M: 2.4 F: 2.1
Fat (g/day)	31	30	ND	ND	ND
Alpha-linolenic acid (g/day)	0.5	0.5	0.7	0.9	M: 1.2 F: 1
Linoleic acid (g/day)	4.4	4.6	7	10	M: 12 F: 10
Fiber (g/day)	ND	ND	19	25	M: 31 F: 26

Key: AI = Adequate intake; DRI = dietary reference intake; F = female; M = male; ND = not determined; RDA = recommended dietary allowance.

[a] Expressed as AIs unless noted otherwise.

[b] DRIs have not been established for premature infants.

[c] Estimated requirements; include needs associated with growth (i.e., energy expenditure plus energy deposition). The assumed normal body weight and length used for the DRIs are 0–6 months: 6 kg, 62 cm; 7–12 months: 9 kg, 71 cm; 1–3 years: 12 kg, 86 cm; 4–8 years: 20 kg, 115 cm; and 9–13 years: 36 kg, 144 cm for males, 37 kg, 144 cm for females.

[d] Expressed as RDA.

[e] Water from all sources including formula, human milk, foods, beverages, and drinking water.

Source: Reference 7.

DRIs of macronutrients for healthy infants and children.[7] Children with various diseases and syndromes may have different needs. One example is the need for "catch-up" calories in infants and children recovering from failure to thrive. Calorie requirements for catch-up growth are often 1.25 times those of age-matched peers, depending on the degree of catch-up growth needed. In patients with fat malabsorption (e.g., patients with cystic fibrosis or other cause of pancreatic insufficiency, bile acid deficiency, and short-bowel syndrome), calories for catch-up growth may be 1.5 times or more those of age-matched peers.

Energy requirements vary with age and clinical condition. Total energy expenditure is a combination of basal energy needs, the energy required to digest food (thermic effect of feeding, also called "specific dynamic action of food"), thermoregulation, and activity. Estimates of energy requirements for infants and children are based on meeting total energy expenditure plus promoting growth. An infant's energy requirement is higher in relation to body mass than that of an adult or older child because of the rapid growth experienced during infancy. Estimated energy requirements for term infants and children are shown in Table 25–2.[7] Although no RDA has been established, premature infants require as much as 120–150 kcal/kg/day or more for adequate growth.

Infant Nutritional Standards

An amendment to the Federal Food, Drug, and Cosmetic Act (Infant Formula Act of 1980; amended 1986) gives the Food and Drug Administration (FDA) the authority to revise nutrient levels for infant formulas, establish quality control, and require adequate labeling. FDA sets specifications for minimum amounts of 29 nutrients and maximum amounts of 9 of those nutrients. All formulas marketed in the United States must meet these requirements. Parents should be cautioned against using any infant formula not manufactured in the United States. FDA alerts have warned of the dangers of using infant formulas from China whose contents fall well below FDA standards. Formulas granted exemption from FDA-established nutrient specifications must be labeled for use by infants who have inborn errors of metabolism, had a low birth weight, or otherwise have unusual medical problems or dietary needs. A list of exempt formulas can be obtained at the FDA Web site (www.fda.gov).

Components of a Healthy Diet

Infants require the same dietary components as adults: fluid, carbohydrates, proteins, fats, and micronutrients. However, the desired proportion of these components in the infant diet differs.

Fluid

Water is an important part of an infant's diet, given that it makes up a larger proportion of the infant's body weight than in older children or adults. The Holliday–Segar method is most often used to estimate maintenance water needs: 100 mL/kg/day for the first 10 kg of body weight, plus 50 mL/kg/day for each kilogram between 10 and 20 kg, and 20 mL/kg/day for each kilogram over 20 kg. Body surface area may also be used to estimate daily fluid requirements; fluid requirements are approximately 1500 mL/m²/day. These methods will underestimate the needs of premature infants, whose requirements are, in general, much higher (i.e., 120–170 mL/kg/day or more). Adequate water intake in the first 6 months of life can be derived from human milk or formula. Both contain sufficient amounts of water, so the normal, healthy infant does not need supplemental water. From 6–12 months of age, when solid foods are introduced, water intake remains high, because most infant foods contain at least 60%–70% more water than other foods, and formula or human milk intake should still be high.

Renal excretion, evaporation from the skin and lungs, and, to a lesser extent, feces are the major routes of fluid loss. Increased water loss caused by diarrhea, fever, or unusually rapid breathing, particularly in concert with decreased water intake, may result in significant dehydration and electrolyte imbalance, and must be offset by fluid intake in excess of maintenance needs.

Carbohydrates

An AI for carbohydrates has been established for infants (Table 25–2).[7] Under normal circumstances, an infant can efficiently use a diet with 40%–50% of total calories from a carbohydrate source. Carbohydrate intake should be balanced with adequate fat intake to allow proper neurologic development. A carbohydrate-free diet is generally undesirable, because it may lead to metabolic modifications favoring fatty acid breakdown, dehydration, and tissue protein and cation loss. However, children with seizures may receive an essentially carbohydrate-free diet, the ketogenic diet, because these metabolic effects may facilitate seizure control. Use of a ketogenic diet should be under the direct, strict supervision of a physician along with a registered dietitian or other qualified health care provider. Lactose, the primary carbohydrate source in human milk and most milk-based formulas, is hydrolyzed to its monosaccharide components, glucose and galactose, by gastric acid and lactase. Congenital lactase deficiency is a rare type of lactose intolerance resulting from an inborn error of metabolism. Infants born prematurely, prior to the maturation of significant lactase activity (before approximately 36 weeks gestation), are relatively lactase deficient. Secondary lactase deficiency is a temporary reduction in intestinal lactase caused by gastroenteritis or significant malnutrition. Because of low lactase activity, infants with congenital lactase deficiency, premature infants, and infants recovering from diarrhea or severe malnutrition may be unable to completely metabolize the quantity of lactose found in human milk or milk-based infant formulas, and may develop lactose intolerance resulting in diarrhea, abdominal pain or distention, bloating, gas, and cramping.

Fiber intake is of considerable interest because, in adults, high-fiber diets have been associated with the prevention of diverticular disease, colon cancer, and coronary heart disease. (See Chapter 23 for further discussion of fiber.) The American Health Foundation has recommended a daily fiber intake calculated by using the following equation: fiber (grams/day) = age (in years) plus 5. Age-plus-10 g/day is also felt to be a safe intake.[8] An AI for fiber for infants 0–12 months of age has not been established. Infants rarely require fiber to maintain normal bowel function. However, from age 6–12 months, whole cereals, green vegetables, and legumes provide a source of fiber in the infant's diet. The fiber AI for older children is shown in Table 25–2. Adult values are reached by the teenage years.

Protein and Amino Acids

The most recent revision of the DRIs established new AIs for protein in term infants and children (Table 25–2).[7] Total body protein increases by an average of 3.5 g/day in the first 4 months of life and by 3.1 g/day over the next 8 months, representing an overall increase in body protein composition from 11%–15% of total body weight.

The protein's amino acid composition (i.e., chemical value) is also important. Amino acids are classified as essential (or indispensable), nonessential, or conditionally essential. The amino acids cysteine, histidine, isoleucine, leucine, lysine, methionine, phenylalanine, threonine, tryptophan, tyrosine, and valine are considered essential for infants because the human body cannot synthesize them from other amino acid and carbohydrate precursors. In the neonate and young infant, immature biochemical pathways for synthesis or conversion of amino acids may prevent adequate synthesis for normal growth and development.

Taurine is an especially important amino acid in infancy. Quantities in human milk are high, and all infant formulas are supplemented during the manufacturing process to provide the same margin of physiologic safety as that provided by human milk.[9] Taurine is not an energy source and is not used for protein synthesis, but it serves as a cell membrane protector by attenuating toxic substances (e.g., oxidants, secondary bile acids, and excess retinoids) and acting as an osmoregulator. Taurine deficiency can result in retinal dysfunction, slow development of auditory brain stem–evoked response in preterm infants, and poor fat absorption in preterm infants and children with cystic fibrosis. These conditions can be improved with taurine supplements.

Despite similar amino acid densities and milk intakes in formula-fed compared with human milk–fed infants, serum concentrations of some amino acids measured in formula–fed infants tend to exceed those measured in human milk–fed infants; however, the growth of these infants is equivalent. The protein content of human milk adjusts to a growing infant's needs, but the high protein needs of preterm infants are not completely met by early human milk. Fortification with commercially available powders or liquids is required for the preterm infant to achieve reasonable amino acid profiles and to meet expected growth rates. In evaluating the adequacy of an infant's protein intake, one must consider not only the absolute amount of protein ingested but also the growth rate, the quantity of nonprotein calories and other nutrients necessary for protein synthesis, and the quality of the protein itself.

Fat and Essential Fatty Acids

Fat is the most calorically dense component in the diet, providing 9 kcal/g compared with 4 kcal/g for both protein and carbohydrates. Fat accounts for approximately 50% of the nonprotein energy in both human milk and infant formula. Infant feeding practices, especially fat and calorie intake, are increasingly being linked to obesity and other diseases (e.g., diabetes and cardiovascular disease) in adulthood. Despite these concerns, children younger than 2 years (the time of most rapid growth and development requiring high-energy intakes) should not receive a fat- or cholesterol-restricted diet unless medically prescribed. Children between 12 months and 2 years who are at increased risk for cardiovascular disease (CVD) because of a family history of obesity, dyslipidemia, or CVD may be candidates for reduced-fat milk products.[10] AAP supports this position because

of the need for adequate fatty acid intake for normal neurologic development and adequate calories for growth.[10] Parents of children between 2 and 5 years of age should be encouraged to adopt a diet that contains 20%–30% of total calories from fat, with less than 10% of calories from saturated fats and less than 1% from trans fatty acids.[10]

The diet must also contain small amounts of the two essential polyunsaturated fatty acids (PUFAs): linoleic acid, an omega-6 (n-6) fatty acid, and linolenic acid, an omega-3 (n-3) fatty acid. These fatty acids are precursors for the n-3 and n-6 long-chain PUFAs: docosahexaenoic acid (DHA) and arachidonic acid (ARA), respectively. Essential fatty acid deficiency, rarely seen in the United States, can manifest as increased metabolic rate, failure to thrive, hair loss, dry flaky skin, thrombocytopenia, and impaired wound healing. Because of substantial fat stores, overt clinical manifestations of essential fatty acid deficiency are generally delayed for weeks to months in older children and adults; however, rapid onset (within days to weeks) may occur in premature infants with inadequate linoleic acid in their diets. Linoleic acid represents the bulk of PUFAs in infant formulas. Generally, an intake of linoleic acid equal to 1%–2% of total dietary calories is adequate to prevent essential fatty acid deficiency; 3%–7% is the amount found in human milk. The AI for the essential PUFAs is shown in Table 25–2.[7]

Historically, infant formulas contained only the precursor PUFAs: linoleic and linolenic acid. Now, most infant formulas are supplemented during manufacturing with DHA and ARA. In fact, more than 60 countries permit the addition of these fatty acids to infant formulas. AAP has not taken an official stand on whether infant formulas should be supplemented with DHA and ARA. These long-chain PUFAs, which are abundant in human milk but not in cow milk, are not considered essential but are thought to provide extra benefits. Increased amounts of DHA beyond what is currently being added to term infant formulas to mimic term human milk levels are being recommend for some preterm infants.[11] DHA is important in both brain and eye development; the direct role of ARA is less clear. However, supplementation of DHA without ARA may lead to ARA deficiency and possible growth suppression.

Whether the addition of DHA and ARA to infant formulas improves visual and cognitive function remains controversial. Some studies have shown benefits to an infant's visual function, cognitive and behavioral development, and growth with DHA and ARA supplementation; other studies have shown no differences in supplemented versus control infants.[12-19] Benefits such as decreasing allergies and the incidence of common respiratory illnesses have also been suggested, but studies have had mixed results.[20,21] No adverse effects have been noted in infants receiving DHA- and ARA-supplemented formulas; however, two studies in which the formula was supplemented with only DHA reported growth suppression, stressing the importance of supplementation with both DHA and ARA.[15] More recent studies have examined the long-term benefits, particularly cognitive, of DHA supplementation and have not found sustained benefits.[22-25] FDA has issued a "generally recognized as safe" (GRAS) notification to Martek Biosciences Corporation for its patented plant-based fatty acid blends DHASCO and ARASCO, which are currently used to supplement infant formulas during manufacturing. There is also evidence that maternal diet can affect fatty acid concentrations in the infant, both in utero and during lactation for human milk–fed infants.[26,27] Many prenatal vitamins, both prescription (e.g., Nexa Plus, Duet DHA

Balanced) and over-the-counter (e.g., Similac Prenatal, various store brands), currently are available with an additional softgel capsule containing either DHA or DHA with eicosapentaenoic acid (EPA). The sources of DHA and EPA range from fish-based products to plant-derived sources. Enfamil Expecta Prenatal, softgel capsules containing 200 mg DHA, is marketed as a non-fish-based supplement for pregnant and lactating women to increase maternal dietary DHA and potentially increase DHA concentrations in their infants. These capsules may have less aftertaste than other sources of DHA and ARA. Routine supplementation during pregnancy and lactation remains controversial and should be discussed with a health care provider.

Micronutrients

DRIs for term infants (given as AIs, if defined, or as RDAs, if AIs are not defined) for vitamins and minerals, including trace elements, are shown in Tables 22–3 and 22–4 in Chapter 22. Precise needs are difficult to define and depend on energy, protein, and fat intakes as well as absorption and nutrient stores. Infant formulas are supplemented with adequate amounts of vitamins and minerals to meet the needs of most term and premature infants when the appropriate formula is chosen. As with protein, human milk must be fortified to meet the micronutrient needs of most premature infants. Appropriate supplementation is included in the discussion of specific milks and formulas.

Infant Food Sources

Human milk– and cow milk–based formulas are the primary food sources for most infants in the United States. Soy protein–based formulas and goat milk are alternatives. A variety of formulas are available to feed infants with special nutritional needs, including those unable to consume a regular oral diet, those with inborn errors of metabolism, and those with various malabsorptive conditions. Most infants and children receive either human milk or an enteral formula orally; however, some children will receive these through feeding tubes such as naso- or orogastric, gastrostomy, or jejunostomy tubes. A discussion of these feeding techniques is beyond the scope of this chapter.

Human Milk

Both WHO and AAP recommend that infants be breast-fed without supplemental foods or liquids for approximately the first 6 months (i.e., exclusive breast-feeding).[28-30] Breast-feeding initiation rates worldwide have increased steadily since 1990, with the rate at hospital discharge increasing from a low of 24.7% in 1971 to 77% in 2010 (provisional rates with final values to be reported in August 2014). However, in 2013, the reported rate of any breast-feeding at 6 and 12 months of age was only 49% and 27%, respectively. Sociodemographic factors affect breast-feeding rates. Black women are less likely than white, Hispanic, and Asian women to breast-feed. For infants born in 2007, approximately 60% of black women ever breast-fed and 30% breast-fed when their infants were 6 months of age, compared with 78% and 45% for white women, 81% and 46% for Hispanic women, and 86% and 59% for Asian women, respectively. At 1 year of age, rates continue to differ, although less so, with 24% of white women, 25% of Hispanic women, and 35% of Asian women still breast-feeding at that time, compared

with 13% of black women.[31-33] Poor, unmarried, and poorly educated women are also less likely to breast-feed their infants.

Because breast-feeding is a major public health concern, breast-feeding goals were included in *Healthy People 2020: National Health Promotion and Disease Prevention Objectives,* the national plan to improve the health of the American people.[34] One objective of *Healthy People 2020* is to have 82% of all infants in the United States breast-fed at birth, with 61% receiving human milk at 6 months of age and 34% receiving human milk at 1 year of age. As of 2008 (the last official reporting of information), the levels of achievement for these three goals were 75% at birth, 44% at 6 months, and 23% at 1 year. *Healthy People 2020* also includes targets for breast-feeding exclusivity, such as a target of 46% for exclusive breast-feeding through 3 months and 25% through 6 months, as well as a decrease in formula supplementation within the first 2 days of life to 14%. As of 2008, the breast-feeding exclusivity goals had current baseline levels of 34% at 3 months, 15% at 6 months, and formula supplementation within the first 2 days of life at 25%. All values showed improvement from the 2006 baseline levels except for formula supplementation within the first 2 days of life, which was previously 24% (www.healthypeople.gov). AAP recommends support for breast-feeding through the first year of life. The AAP policy statement on breast-feeding and the use of human milk was updated in 2012 and includes reinforcement of breast-feeding and human milk as the reference normative standards for infant feeding and nutrition and reaffirmation of the recommendation to exclusively breast-feed for 6 months, followed by continued breast-feeding for 1 year or longer as mutually desired by mother and infant. AAP cautions that medical contraindications to breast-feeding are rare in the United States. Moreover, AAP recommends (1) the use of the WHO growth charts to avoid mislabeling of underweight and failure-to-thrive infants, (2) hospital initiatives to encourage and support the initiation and sustaining of exclusive breast-feeding, (3) support by pediatricians as advocates of breast-feeding, and (4) acknowledgment of the economic benefits to society of breast-feeding.[29]

Breast-feeding not only offers an optimal source of nutrition for the infant, but also provides other benefits, such as improved mother–child bonding, and advantages to the infant's general health, growth, and development. Strong evidence indicates human milk decreases the incidence and severity of various infections (e.g., nonspecific gastrointestinal tract infections, respiratory tract infections, otitis media) in infants, and necrotizing enterocolitis in premature infants.[29] Other proposed benefits of human milk include decreased rates of sudden infant death syndrome, types 1 and 2 diabetes mellitus, leukemia, overweight, obesity, hypercholesterolemia, asthma, atopic dermatitis, eczema, celiac disease, and childhood inflammatory bowel disease. Breast-feeding has also been associated with slightly enhanced performance on tests of cognitive development; however, the effect of genetic and socioenvironmental factors on intelligence is difficult to measure separately from breast-feeding.[29] For premature infants, improvement is also seen in clinical feeding tolerance, quicker attainment of full enteral feeding, and improved neurodevelopmental outcomes. With these benefits in mind, AAP recommends the use of human milk for all preterm infants. If the mother's own milk cannot be provided, pasteurized donor milk should be used.[29]

Besides enhanced mother–child bonding, maternal benefits of breast-feeding include decreased postpartum bleeding, more rapid uterine involution, decreased menstrual blood loss, increased spacing between children, earlier return to prepregnancy weight, decreased risk of breast and ovarian cancer, decreased risk of rheumatoid arthritis, and decreased hip fracture and osteoporosis in the postmenopausal period.

A savings of $13 billion per year ($3.7 billion in direct and indirect pediatric health costs with $10.1 billion in premature death from pediatric diseases) could be saved if 90% of mothers in the United States would exclusively breast-feed for 6 months.[35] For businesses, the case for breast-feeding is an economic one. For every $1 businesses spend on creating and supporting lactation support programs at the business site, they have a $2–$3 return on their investment.[36] An economic analysis of estimated direct health care costs for diarrhea, lower respiratory tract infections, and otitis media in the first year of life found that costs for infants who were never breast-fed were $300 more than for infants exclusively breast-fed for at least 3 months.[37]

Many unanswered questions exist regarding the protective effects of breast-feeding. What is the duration of protection after breast-feeding has been discontinued? What influence does maternal age have on the protective effect? How great is the interactive effect of social and demographic variables? How does the addition of solid foods (complementary feeding) to the diet of a human milk–fed infant influence the protective effect? What consequence does partial formula feeding have on the protective effect? Well-designed studies are needed to answer these questions.

The impact of the use of breast pumps also should be considered. The 2005–2007 Infant Feeding Practices Study II (IFPS II) assessed the use of expressed human milk among breast-feeding mothers of infants between the ages of 1.5 and 4.5 months.[38] Of these mothers, 85% had expressed human milk sometime during the life of their infant, and 5.6% of mothers had exclusively fed their infants expressed human milk. As with breast-feeding rates in general, the use of expressed human milk is more common among women with a higher level of education and a higher household income. The primary reason reported in IFPS II for the use of expressed human milk is the ability to have someone else feed the infant, allowing many mothers to continue to provide breast milk while working outside of the home.

Although this process can provide many of the same benefits to the infant and mother, some concerns should be noted. If an electric breast pump is used improperly, a mother can have mastitis, pain, trauma, and nipple wounds. For the infant, expressed human milk can become contaminated with bacteria if it is stored improperly. Storing human milk in nonglass containers can destroy some key milk components, and storing milk at either refrigeration or freezer temperatures can reduce levels of key milk components (i.e., vitamin C, lipids, and immunologic cells). Finally, the composition of human milk changes throughout a single feeding and with the infant's age. For example, most mothers who express human milk feed the infant and then express the remainder for later use. This method separates the foremilk, which is high in carbohydrate content, from the hindmilk, which is high in fat content. This feeding separation of the macronutrient components within the mother's milk can lead to adverse gastrointestinal effects such as diarrhea. Well-designed research is needed in this area to assess the true impact of the use of breast pumps on maternal health and infant nutrition.[38]

Very few contraindications to the use of human breast milk exist. In developed countries, such as the United States,

one reason for women not breast-feeding is the maternal diagnosis of human immunodeficiency virus (HIV) infection, which can be transmitted through human milk. Women with HIV in underdeveloped countries, however, are encouraged to breast-feed, because the risk of infant morbidity and mortality with formula use (from inadequate sanitation, refrigeration, and illiteracy) is greater than the risk of HIV transmission.[29] Other reasons women in developed countries may not be able to breast-feed, either temporarily or permanently, are classic galactosemia; active, untreated tuberculosis; human T-cell lymphotropic virus types I or II; herpes simplex lesion on the breast (may use other breast); and the use of contraindicated drugs (Table 25–3). Several excellent texts provide information regarding the use of drugs during lactation and pregnancy[39,40] (see also Appendix I of this book). In addition, a comprehensive database of available information regarding drugs in lactation (LactMed) is maintained by the US National Library of Medicine (http://toxnet.nlm.nih.gov/cgi-bin/sis/htmlgen?LACT). Further questions can be directed to the poison control center (800-222-1222) or the National Breastfeeding Helpline at 800-994-9662 (http://www.womenshealth.gov/breastfeeding/). The overall risk of a drug to a breast-fed infant depends on the concentration in the infant's blood and the effects of the drug on the infant. Feeding immediately before the mother's dose may help minimize exposure, because the concentration in milk is likely to be lowest toward the end of the dosing interval. This may not be true for lipid-soluble drugs. Alternating breast- and bottle-feeds or pumping and discarding breast milk is an option, if the need for a particular drug is short term.

In the United States and other countries, human milk donor banks have been established, with 13 member banks in the Human Milk Banking Association of North America (HMBANA) and 7 sites in various stages of development. Human milk donations are taken from carefully screened, unpaid donors; then the milk undergoes Holder pasteurization to eliminate potential viral and bacterial contaminants while maintaining most of the milk's unique immunologic factors.[41] It is estimated that about 50% of the immunoglobulin A (IgA) is lost in processing; however, because cow milk contains no IgA, infants who receive donor human milk still benefit from its presence. The cost is approximately $4 per ounce plus shipping and handling. More information about donor milk banks, including how to be a donor or receive donor milk, can be obtained at HMBANA's Web site (www.hmbana.org).

Cow Milk

Cow milk is the primary nutrient source for commercially prepared milk-based infant formulas. Both human and cow milk contain more than 200 ingredients in the fat- and water-soluble fractions. Estimates of the major nutrients contained in pooled mature human milk and whole cow milk are listed in Table 25–4.

Whole Cow Milk

Whole cow milk is not suitable for providing nutrition to infants younger than 1 year. Because of the low concentration and poor bioavailability of iron, whole cow milk has been associated with iron-deficiency anemia.[42,43] Sensitivity to dietary proteins, most commonly cow or soy milk proteins, can manifest as occult GI bleeding, further increasing the risk of anemia. In the past decade, convincing evidence has accumulated to indicate that iron deficiency impairs psychomotor

table
25-3 | Selected Drugs Contraindicated or to Be Used Cautiously While Breast-Feeding

Prescription Drugs	Drugs of Abuse	Radiopharmaceuticals (time to wait after exposure)
Contraindicated Drugs		
Ciprofloxacin	Amphetamine	Copper 64 (50 hours)
Cyclophosphamide	Cocaine	Gallium 67 (2 weeks)
Cyclosporine	Heroin	Indium 111 (20 hours)
Doxepin	Marijuana	Iodine 123 (36 hours)
Doxorubicin	Phencyclidine	Iodine 125 (12 days)
Ergotamine		Iodine 131 (2–14 days)
Leflunomide		Radioactive sodium (96 hours)
Methotrexate		Technetium 99m (15 hours to 3 days)
Drugs to Be Used Cautiously Because of Significant Potential Adverse Effects		
Acebutolol	Clemastine	Primidone
Amiodarone	Chloramphenicol	Sulfasalazine
5-Aminosalicylic acid	Gold salts	Tetracyclines (long-term)
Atenolol	Lithium	Vitamin D (high-dose)
Aspirin	Phenobarbital	
Bromocriptine	Phenytoin	

Source: American Academy of Pediatrics, Committee on Drugs. Transfer of drugs and other chemicals into human milk. *Pediatrics.* 2001;108(3):776–89. Contains manufacturers' prescribing information and information from the U.K. Drugs in Lactation Advisory Service. Accessed at http://pediatrics.aappublications.org/content/108/3/776.full.pdf+html, June 2, 2013.

table
25-4 | Average Composition of Mature Human Milk and Whole Cow Milk

Component	Mature Human Milk[a]	Whole Cow Milk
Water (mL/100 mL)	87.1	87.2
Energy		
(kcal/100 mL)	65–70	66–68
(kcal/oz)	19.5–21	19–20
Protein (g/100 mL)	0.9–1.3	3.3–3.4
Whey:casein ratio	72:28	18:82
Alpha-lactalbumin (g/100 mL)	0.3	0.1
Alpha-lactoglobulin (g/100 mL)	—	0.4
Lactoferrin (g/100 mL)	0.2	Trace
Secretory IgA (g/100 mL)	0.1	Trace
Albumin (g/100 mL)	0.04	0.04
Fat (g/100 mL)	3.9	3.4–3.8
Carbohydrate (g/100 mL)	6.7–7.2[b]	4.7–4.8[c]
Minerals		
Calcium (mg/L)	200–280	1200
Phosphorus (mg/L)	120–140	980
Calcium:phosphorus ratio	2:1	1.3:1
Sodium (mg/L)	120–250	500

table
25–4 Average Composition of Mature Human Milk and Whole Cow Milk (continued)

Component	Mature Human Milk[a]	Whole Cow Milk
Potassium (mg/L)	400–550	1560
Chloride (mg/L)	400–450	1020
Magnesium (mg/L)	30–35	120
Vitamins		
Vitamin A (international units/L)	2000	1000
Thiamin (mcg/L)	200	300
Riboflavin (mcg/L)	400–600	1750
Niacin (mg/L)	1.8–6	0.8
Pyridoxine (mg/L)	0.1–0.3	0.5
Pantothenate (mg/L)	2–2.5	3.6
Folic acid (mcg/L)	80–140	50
Biotin (mcg/L)	5–9	35
Vitamin B_{12} (mcg/L)	0.5–1	4
Vitamin C (mg/L)	80–100	17
Vitamin D (international units/L)	22	24
Vitamin E (international units/L)	2–8	0.4–0.9
Vitamin K (mcg/L)	2–3	5
Trace Minerals		
Chromium (mcg/L)	45–55	20
Manganese (mcg/L)	3	20–40
Copper (mg/L)	0.2–0.4	100
Zinc (mg/L)	1–3	3.5
Iodine (mcg/L)	150	80
Selenium (mcg/L)	7–33	5–50
Iron (mcg/L)	400	460
Fluoride (mcg/L)	4–15	—

Key: IgA = Immunoglobulin A.

[a] ≥28 days postpartum.

[b] As lactose, glucose, and oligosaccharides.

[c] As lactose.

Source: Picciano MF. Representative values for constituents of human milk. In: Schanler RJ, ed. Breastfeeding 2001, part 1: the evidence for breastfeeding. *Pediatr Clin North Am.* 2001;48:263–4; American Academy of Pediatrics, Committee on Nutrition. Appendix C and Appendix E. In: Kleinman RE, ed. *Pediatric Nutrition Handbook.* 6th ed. Elk Grove Village, IL: American Academy of Pediatrics; 2008:1199–204, 1243–6.

development and cognitive function in infants, even with relatively mild anemia. Milk-protein intolerance and/or allergy can also result in rash, wheezing, diarrhea, vomiting, colic, and anaphylaxis when whole cow milk is used. When whole cow milk is fed with solid food, infants receive unnecessarily high intakes of protein and electrolytes, resulting in a high renal solute load (RSL; Table 25–5).[44,45] The implications of a high RSL will be discussed later in this chapter. The current position of AAP's Committee on Nutrition (CON) is that iron-fortified infant formula is the only acceptable alternative to human milk. The use of cow milk is not recommended during the first year of life.[42]

Reduced-Fat Cow Milk

Reduced-fat cow milk, such as skim milk (0.1% fat), low-fat milk (1% fat), and reduced-fat milk (2% fat), has been advocated to prevent obesity and atherosclerosis as part of a "healthy diet." However, when the low-fat diet recommended for adults is imposed on children younger than 2 years, it puts them at risk for failure to thrive and impaired neurologic development. Infants who receive a major percentage of their caloric intake from reduced-fat milk may receive an exceedingly high protein intake and an inadequate intake of essential fatty acids. The maximum protein concentration allowed by FDA in infant

table
25–5 | Potential Renal Solute Load of Selected Milks and Infant Formulas

	PRSL	
	mOsm/L	mOsm/100 kcal
Human milk	93	14
Milk-based formula	135–260	20–39
Soy protein–based formula	160	24
Whole cow milk	308	46
Skim cow milk	326	93
FDA upper limit	277	41
Beikost[a]	153	23

Key: FDA = Food and Drug Administration; PRSL = potential renal solute load.

[a] Beikost is foods other than milk or formula.

Source: References 44 and 45.

formulas is 4.5 g/100 kcal, but skim milk and 2% milk provide approximately 8–10 g/100 kcal and 7–10 g/100 kcal, respectively. Therefore, using reduced-fat cow milk for infant nutrition provides an unbalanced percentage of calories supplied from protein, fat, and carbohydrates.

Per unit volume, skim milk has a slightly higher potential RSL (PRSL) than does whole cow milk (Table 25–5). The solute concentration is further increased by water loss during processing. Reduced-fat milk is not recommended during episodes of diarrhea because of the possibility of hypertonic dehydration. As stated earlier, AAP does not recommend the use of low-fat diets during the first 2 years of life, except for children between 12 months and 2 years with a family history of CVD.

Evaporated Milk

Evaporated milk is a sterile, convenient source of cow milk with standardized concentrations of protein, fat, and carbohydrate. However, it is not recommended for infant feeding.

Goat Milk

Although goat milk is the primary milk source for more than 50% of the world's population, it is rarely used in the United States for infants intolerant to cow milk. Goat milk is commercially available in powdered and evaporated forms. It contains primarily medium- and short-chain fatty acids; therefore, the fat is more readily digested than the fat in cow milk. Unfortified goat milk is not recommended during infancy because it is deficient in folate and low in iron and vitamin D. The evaporated form of Meyenberg goat milk, however, is supplemented with vitamin D and folic acid. Powdered Meyenberg goat milk is supplemented with only folic acid; therefore, it is recommended only for children older than 1 year. Because the powder formulation is not a complete formula, vitamin supplementation is required if it is used for infant nutrition.

Commercial Infant Formulas

When provision of human milk to an infant is not possible or not desired by the mother, then commercially supplied infant formulas are an acceptable alternative (Table 25–6). Differences in palatability, digestibility, sources of nutrients, convenience of administration, and cost among these formulas allow for individualization to the infant's special nutrient needs and the family's resources.

Formula Properties

The International Formula Council is a voluntary, nonprofit trade association composed of the five companies that manufacture and market infant formulas and adult nutritionals: Abbott Nutrition, Mead Johnson Nutritionals, Nestlé Infant Nutrition, Perrigo Nutritionals, and Pfizer Nutrition. The association has established guidelines requiring liquid formulations to be free of all viable pathogens, their spores, and other organisms that may cause product degradation. In addition, infant formula constituents must meet certain concentrations to ensure optimum nutrition. Guidelines have been established to ensure safety and efficacy of infant formulas.

Microbiologic Safety

Manufacturers sterilize liquid formulas using heat treatment, and the product is free of microbes as long as the container remains intact. Powdered formulas are not required or guaranteed to be sterile; however, coliforms and other pathogens are absent, and contamination with other microorganisms is below acceptable government standards. If clinically significant microbiologic contamination occurs, an infant ingesting the formula could develop diarrhea with subsequent fluid and electrolyte losses. In 2002, FDA issued an alert after the death of an infant in a neonatal intensive care unit because of contamination of powdered formula with *Enterobacter sakazakii* at the manufacturing site.[46]

Risk for infection after exposure to contaminated formula likely depends on a number of factors, including immune status. For that reason, to minimize risk for premature and immunocompromised infants, ready-to-feed or liquid concentrates are recommended unless no suitable alternative to a powdered formula exists.

Physical Characteristics

Infant formulas are emulsions of edible oils in aqueous solutions, but fat separation rarely occurs. If it does, shaking the container will usually redisperse the fat. Redispersion may not happen if stabilizers are lacking or if the formula was stored beyond its shelf life. Liquid infant formulas may contain thickening agents, stabilizers, and emulsifiers to provide uniform consistency and prolong stability. Protein agglomeration may occur, however, if storage time is excessive. This agglomeration ranges from a slight, grainy development through increased viscosity and gel formation to eventual protein precipitation. Agglomeration and separation do not affect a formula's safety or nutritional value; however, the formula's appearance may deter caregivers from using it.

Caloric Density

The standard caloric density for infant formulas is 20 kcal/oz or approximately 67 kcal/100 mL, which mimics the average

table
25–6   **Selected Formulas for Infants and Children**

Infant Formulas
Milk-Based Formulas

Trade Name [form] (Mfr)	Kilocalories[a] (per ounce)	Protein[a] (g/L) (C:W ratio)	Protein Source(s)	Carbohydrate[a] (g/L)	Carbohydrate Source(s)	Fat[a] (g/L)	Fat Source(s)	MCTs (% fat kcal)	Iron[a] (mg/L)
Enfamil Premium Infant[b] [C,P,R] (MJ)	20	14 (40:60)	Nonfat milk, whey protein concentrate	75	Lactose, galactool-igosaccharides, polydextrose	35	Vegetable oil (palm olein, coconut, soy, and high oleic sunflower oils), DHA, ARA, linoleic acid, linolenic acid, soy lecithin	—	12
Enfamil Gentlease[c] [P,R] (MJ)	20	15 (40:60)	Partially hydrolyzed nonfat milk and whey protein concentrate (soy)	72	Corn syrup solids	35	Vegetable oil (palm olein, soy, coconut, and high oleic sunflower oils), DHA, ARA, linoleic acid, linolenic acid	—	12
Gerber Good Start Gentle [C,P,R] (G)	20	14.9 (0:100)	100% whey protein concentrate (milk)	79	Corn maltodextrin (30%), lactose (70%), galactooli-gosaccharides	34.5	Vegetable oil (palm olein, soy, coconut, high oleic safflower or sunflower oils), DHA, ARA, linoleic acid, linolenic acid, soy lecithin	—	10.1
Gerber Good Start Protect [P] (G)	20	14.9 (0:100)	100% whey protein concentrate (milk)	79	Lactose, corn maltodextrin	34.2	Vegetable oil (palm olein, soy, coconut, high oleic safflower or sunflower oils), DHA, ARA, linoleic acid, linolenic acid, soy lecithin	—	10.1
Gerber Good Start Soothe [P] (G)	20	15 (0:100)	100% whey protein concentrate (milk)	75.8	Corn maltodextrin	34.5	Vegetable oil (palm, soy, coconut, high oleic safflower or sunflower oils), DHA, ARA, linoleic acid, linolenic acid, soy lecithin	—	10

Similac Advance [C,P,R] (A)	19	13.3	Nonfat milk, whey protein concentrate	69.2	Lactose, galactooligosaccharides	36.2	Vegetable oil (palm, soy, coconut, high oleic safflower or sunflower oils), DHA, ARA, linoleic acid, linolenic acid, soy lecithin	—	12.2
Similac Advance Organic [P,R] (A)	20	14	Organic nonfat milk	71	Organic maltodextrin, organic sugar, fructooligosaccharides	38	Organic high oleic sunflower, organic soy, and organic coconut oils, DHA, ARA	—	12.2
Soy Protein–Based Therapeutic Formulas									
Enfamil ProSobee [C,P,R] (MJ)	20	16.7	Soy protein isolate, L-methionine, taurine	71	Corn syrup solids	35	Vegetable oils (palm olein, soy, coconut, and high oleic sunflower oils), DHA, ARA, linoleic acid, linolenic acid		12
Gerber Good Start Soy [C,P,R] (G)	20	16.9	Enzymatically hydrolyzed soy protein isolate, L-methionine, taurine	75.1	Corn maltodextrin, sucrose	34.5	Vegetable oils (palm olein, soy coconut, and high oleic safflower or sunflower oils), DHA, ARA, linoleic acid, linolenic acid, soy lecithin	—	12.1
Similac Soy Isomil [C,P,R] (A)	19	15.8	Soy protein isolate, L-methionine	67	Corn syrup solids, sugar, fructooligosaccharides	35.1	High oleic safflower, soy, and coconut oils; DHA, ARA	—	12.2
Similac Expert Care for Diarrhea [R] (A)	20	18	Soy protein isolate, L-methionine	68.3 (6 g/L of dietary fiber)	Corn syrup solids, sugar	36.9	Soy, coconut oils	—	12.2
Other Therapeutic Infant Formulas									
Enfamil A.R. [P,R] (MJ)	20	16.7	Nonfat milk	75	Rice starch, lactose, maltodextrin, galactooligosaccharides, polydextrose	34	Vegetable oils (palm olein, soy, coconut, and high oleic sunflower oils), DHA, ARA, linoleic acid, linolenic acid	—	12
Similac Sensitive [C,P,R]/Similac Sensitive For Spit Up [P,R] (A)	19/20	13.8/14.5	Milk protein isolate	71.4/74.1	Corn syrup, rice starch, sugar	36.5	High oleic safflower, soy, and coconut oils; DHA, ARA	—	12.2
Similac PM 60/40 [P] (A)	20	15 (40:60)	Whey protein caseinate, sodium caseinate	69	Lactose	37.9	High oleic safflower, soy, and coconut oils	—	4.7

table 25-6	Selected Formulas for Infants and Children *(continued)*								
Trade Name [form] (Mfr)	Kilocalories[a] (per ounce)	Protein[a] (g/L) (C:W ratio)	Protein Source(s)	Carbohydrate[a] (g/L)	Carbohydrate Source(s)	Fat[a] (g/L)	Fat Source(s)	MCTs (% fat kcal)	Iron[a] (mg/L)
Nutramigen[d] [C,R]	20	18.7	Casein hydrolysate, L-cystine, L-tyrosine, L-tryptophan, taurine	68.7	Corn syrup solids, modified corn starch	35.4	Vegetable oils (palm olein, soy, coconut, and high oleic sunflower oils), DHA, ARA, linoleic acid, linolenic acid	—	12
Pregestimil [P,R]/ Pregestimil 24 [R] (MJ)	20/24	18.9/23	Casein hydrolysate (milk), L-cystine, L-tyrosine, L-tryptophan, taurine	69/83	Corn syrup solids, modified corn starch	37.8/45	MCT, soy, corn, and high oleic vegetable oils (sunflower/safflower); DHA, ARA, linoleic acid, linolenic acid	55	12/14.3
Similac Expert Care Alimentum [P,R] (A)	20	18.6	Casein hydrolysate, L-cystine, L-tyrosine, L-tryptophan	69	Corn maltodextrin, sugar	37.5	High oleic safflower, MCT, and soy oils; DHA, ARA	33	12.2
EleCare DHA/ ARA [P] (A)	20	20.9	Free amino acids	72	Corn syrup solids	32.4	High oleic safflower, MCT, and soy oils; DHA, ARA	33	9.9
Neocate Infant DHA&ARA [P] (Nut)	20	21	Free L-amino acids	78	Corn syrup solids	30	MCT (palm kernel/ coconut), high oleic sunflower, and soy oils; DHA, ARA	33	12.4
Enfaport [R] (MJ)	30	36	Calcium and sodium caseinates (milk)	103	Corn syrup solids	55	MCT and soy oils, DHA, ARA, linoleic acid, linolenic acid, soy lecithin	84	18.3
RCF[e] [C] (A)	20	20.3	Soy protein isolate, L-methionine, taurine	68.2	None in actual product	35.8	High oleic safflower, soy, and coconut oils; soy lecithin	—	12.2
3232A[e] [P] (MJ)	20	18.7	Casein hydrolysates (milk), L-cystine, L-tyrosine, L-tryptophan, taurine	89	Modified tapioca starch	28	MCT and corn oils, soy lecithin	85	12.5
PurAmino [P] (MJ)	20	18.7	Free L-amino acids	69	Corn syrup solids	35.3	Vegetable oil (palm olein, coconut, soy, and high oleic sunflower oils), DHA, ARA, linoleic acid	—	12

Formulas for Premature Infants: Initial Feeding

Formula			Protein source		Carbohydrate source		Fat source		
Enfamil Premature 20 Cal [R] (MJ)	20	20 (40:60)	Nonfat milk, whey protein concentrate	74	Corn syrup solids, lactose	34	MCT, soy, and high oleic vegetable oils (sunflower/safflower); DHA, ARA, linoleic acid, linolenic acid	40	12.2
Similac Special Care 20 with Iron [R] (A)	20	20.3	Nonfat milk, whey protein concentrate	69.7	Corn syrup solids, lactose	36.7	MCT, soy, coconut oils; DHA, ARA, soy lecithin	50	12.2
Gerber Good Start Premature 20 [R] (G)	20	20 (0:100)	100% enzymatically hydrolyzed whey protein isolate	71	Lactose, maltodextrin	35	MCT, high oleic oils (sunflower or safflower), soy oils; DHA, ARA, linoleic acid, linolenic acid	40	12
Enfamil Premature 24 Cal [R]/Enfamil Premature 24 Cal High Protein [R] (MJ)	20/24	24.8/28 (40:60)	Nonfat milk, whey protein concentrate	89/85	Corn syrup solids, lactose	41	MCT, soy, and high oleic vegetable oils (sunflower or safflower); DHA, ARA, linoleic acid, linolenic acid	40	14.6 (low iron = 4.1)
Similac Special Care 24 with Iron [R]/Similac Special Care 24 High Protein [R] (A)	24	24.3/26.8	Nonfat milk, whey protein concentrate	84/81	Corn syrup solids, lactose	44.1	MCT, soy, coconut oils; DHA, ARA, soy lecithin	50	14.6
Gerber Good Start 24 [R]/Gerber Good Start 24 High Protein [R] (MJ)	24	24/29 (0:100)	100% enzymatically hydrolyzed whey protein isolate	85	Lactose, maltodextrin	42	MCT, high oleic (sunflower or safflower), soy oils; DHA, ARA, linoleic acid, linolenic acid	40	12
Enfamil Premature 30 Cal [R] (MJ)	30	30 (40:60)	Nonfat milk, whey protein concentrate	112	Maltodextrin	52	MCT, soy, and high oleic vegetable oils (sunflower/safflower); DHA, ARA, linoleic acid, linolenic acid, soy lecithin	40	18.3
Similac Special Care 30 with Iron [R] (A)	30	30.4 (50:50)	Nonfat milk, whey protein concentrate	78.4	Corn syrup solids, lactose	67.1	MCT, soy, coconut oils; DHA, ARA, soy lecithin	50	18.3

table
25–6 Selected Formulas for Infants and Children *(continued)*

Trade Name [form] (Mfr)	Kilocalories[a] (per ounce)	Protein[a] (g/L) (C:W ratio)	Protein Source(s)	Carbohydrate[a] (g/L)	Carbohydrate Source(s)	Fat[a] (g/L)	Fat Source(s)	MCTs (% fat kcal)	Iron[a] (mg/L)
Formulas for Premature Infants: Transition or Postdischarge									
Enfamil Enfa-Care [P,R] (MJ)	22	21 (40:60)	Nonfat milk, whey protein concentrate	77	Powder = corn syrup solids, lactose; Liquid = maltodextrin, lactose	39	High oleic vegetable (sunflower or safflower), soy, MCT, and coconut oils; DHA, ARA, linoleic acid, linolenic acid	20	13.3
Gerber Good Start Nourish [R,P] (G)	22	21 (0:100)	100% enzymatically hydrolyzed whey protein isolate (milk)	78	Lactose, maltodextrin	39	High oleic sunflower or safflower, MCT, and soy oils, DHA, ARA, linoleic acid, linolenic acid, soy lecithin	20	13
Similac Expert Care NeoSure [P,R] (A)	22	20.8	Nonfat milk, whey protein concentrate	75.1	Corn syrup solids, lactose	40.9	Soy, high oleic safflower, MCT, and coconut oils; DHA, ARA, soy lecithin	25	13.4
Older Infant/Toddler Milk-Based Formulas									
Gerber Graduates Gentle [P] (G)	20	15 (0:100)	100% whey protein concentrate (milk)	78	Lactose, maltodextrin, galactooligosaccharides	34	Palm olein, soy, coconut, and high oleic safflower or sunflower oils; DHA, ARA, linoleic acid, linolenic acid, soy lecithin	—	14
Gerber Graduates Protect[f] [P] (G)	20	14.9 (0:100)	100% whey protein concentrate (milk)	75.8	Lactose, maltodextrin	34.5	Palm olein, soy, coconut, and high oleic safflower or sunflower oils; DHA, ARA, linoleic acid, linolenic acid, soy lecithin	—	14
Similac Go & Grow Milk-based Formula [P] (A)	20	19.5 (52:48)	Nonfat milk	66	Lactose, galactooligosaccharides	35	High oleic safflower, soy, and coconut oils; DHA, ARA	—	13.5

Product			Protein source		Carbohydrate source		Fat source		
Enfagrow Premium Next Step [P,R] (MJ)	20	17.3 (80:20)	Nonfat milk	70	Corn syrup solids, lactose, galactooligosaccharides	35.4	Vegetable oils (palm, olein, soy, coconut, and high oleic sunflower oils), DHA, ARA, linoleic acid, linolenic acid	—	13.3
Enfagrow Gentlease Next Step [P] (MJ)	20	17.3	Partially hydrolyzed nonfat milk, whey protein concentrate solids (soy)	70	Corn syrup solids, galactooligosaccharides, polydextrose	35	Vegetable oils (palm, olein, soy, coconut, and high oleic sunflower oils), DHA, ARA, linoleic acid, linolenic acid	—	13.3
Soy-Based Products									
Enfagrow™ Soy Toddler [P] (MJ)	20	22	Soy protein isolate, L-methionine, taurine	78.7	Corn syrup solids	29.3	Vegetable oils (palm, olein, soy, coconut, high oleic sunflower oils), DHA, ARA, linoleic acid, linolenic acid, soy lecithin	—	13.3
Gerber Graduates Soy [P] (G)	20	17	Enzymatically hydrolyzed soy protein isolate, L-methionine, taurine	75	Corn maltodextrin, sucrose	34	Vegetable oils (palm, olein, soy, coconut, high oleic safflower or sunflower oils), DHA, ARA, linoleic acid, linolenic acid, soy lecithin	—	12
Similac Go & Grow Soy-based Formula [P] (A)	20	18.9	Soy protein isolate, L-methionine, taurine	69.6	Corn syrup solids, sugar, fructooligosaccharides	37	High oleic safflower, soy, and coconut oils; DHA, ARA	—	13.5
Children's Formulas									
PediaSure/ PediaSure Enteral Formula[g] [R] (A)	30	30	Milk protein concentrate	139	Corn maltodextrin, sugar	38	High oleic safflower, soy, and MCT oils; soy lecithin	16	11
PediaSure 1.5 [R] (A), vanilla	45	59	Milk protein concentrate	160	Corn maltodextrin	68	High oleic safflower, soy, and MCT oils; soy lecithin, DHA	15	11
PediaSure with Fiber[h]/ PediaSure Enteral Formula with Fiber[h] [R] (A)	30	30	Milk protein concentrate	143 (13 grams/L of dietary fiber with 6.5 grams/L of scFOS[h])	Corn maltodextrin, sugar	38	High oleic safflower, soy, and MCT oils; soy lecithin	16	11

table 25–6   Selected Formulas for Infants and Children (continued)

Trade Name [form] (Mfr)	Kilocalories[a] (per ounce)	Protein[a] (g/L) (C:W ratio)	Protein Source(s)	Carbohydrate[a] (g/L)	Carbohydrate Source(s)	Fat[a] (g/L)	Fat Source(s)	MCTs (% fat kcal)	Iron[a] (mg/L)
PediaSure 1.5 with Fiber[h] [R] (A), vanilla	45	59	Milk protein concentrate	165 (13 g/L of dietary fiber with 6.5 g/L of scFOS[h])	Corn maltodextrin	68	High oleic safflower, soy, and MCT oils; soy lecithin, DHA	15	11
Nutren Junior [R]/Nutren Junior with Fiber[i] [R] (Nes)	30	30 (50:50)	Milk protein concentrate, 50% whey protein concentrate	110 (3.8 g/L of insoluble fiber and 2.2 g/L of soluble fiber as PreBio[j])	Maltodextrin, sugar; fiber product also contains pea fiber, fructooligosaccharides, inulin	50	Soybean, canola, and MCT oils (coconut and/or palm kernel oils); soy lecithin	20	14
Boost Kid Essentials [R] (Nes)	30	28	Sodium and calcium caseinates, whey protein concentrate	134	Sugar, maltodextrin	38	High oleic sunflower, soybean, MCT (coconut and/or palm kernel oil), and soy oils; soy lecithin	20	13.9
Boost Kid Essentials 1.5 [R]/Boost Kid Essentials 1.5 with Fiber [R] (Nes)	45	42	Sodium and calcium caseinates, whey protein concentrate	165 (8 g/L of fiber)	Maltodextrin, sugar	75	MCT, soy, and sunflower oils; soy lecithin	10	13.9
Compleat Pediatric [R] (Nes)	30	37.6	Chicken, sodium caseinate, and pea puree	132 (6.8 g/L of Nutrisource Fiber)	Corn syrup, green pea and green bean puree, peach and cranberry juice, maltodextrin	39	Canola and MCT oils (coconut and/or palm kernel); hydroxylated soy lecithin	20	14
Carnation Breakfast Essentials [P,R] (Nes)	24	35	Powder = nonfat milk; liquid = calcium caseinate	103	Sugar, maltodextrin; powder also has lactose; liquid also has sucralose	35	Powder = trace butterfat; liquid = corn oil	—	13.6

Other Therapeutic Formulas—Older Infants, Toddler, and Pediatric

Trade Name [form] (Mfr)	Kilocalories[a] (per ounce)	Protein[a] (g/L) (C:W ratio)	Protein Source(s)	Carbohydrate[a] (g/L)	Carbohydrate Source(s)	Fat[a] (g/L)	Fat Source(s)	MCTs (% fat kcal)	Iron[a] (mg/L)
E028 Splash [R] (Nut), flavored	30	25	Free L-amino acids	146	Maltodextrin, sugar	35	Fractionated coconut, canola, and high oleic sunflower oils	35	7.7
EleCare Jr [P] (A), flavored or unflavored	30	31	Free amino acids	107	Corn syrup solids	49	High oleic safflower, MCT, and soy oils	33	14.9

Product			Protein source		Carbohydrate source		Fat source		
Neocate Junior [P] (Nut), flavored or unflavored	30	33	Free L-amino acids	104	Corn syrup solids	50	MCT, refined vegetable oils (palm kernel and/or coconut, canola, and high oleic safflower oils)	35	16
Pepdite Junior [P] (Nut), flavored or unflavored	30	31	Hydrolyzed pork and soy proteins	106	Corn syrup solids	50	MCT, fractionated coconut, canola, and high oleic safflower oils	35	14
Peptamen Junior [R] (Nes)	30	30 (0:100)	Enzymatically, hydrolyzed whey protein (milk)	136	Maltodextrin, sugar, corn starch, guar gum, sucralose	38	MCT (coconut and/or palm kernel oil), soybean, and canola oils; soy lecithin	60	14
Peptamen Junior 1.5 with PreBio[i] [R] (Nes), flavored or unflavored	45	45	Enzymatically, hydrolyzed whey protein (milk)	180	Maltodextrin, corn starch, fructooligosaccharides, inulin, guar gum	68	MCT (coconut and/or palm kernel oils), soybean, and canola oils; soy lecithin	60	20.8
Peptamen Junior Fiber with PreBio[i] [R] (Nes)	30	30 (0:100)	Enzymatically, hydrolyzed whey protein (milk)	136 (7.4 g/L of fiber[i])	Maltodextrin, sugar, corn starch, pea fiber, fructooligosaccharides, inulin	38.4	MCT (coconut and/or palm kernel oils), soybean, and canola oils; soy lecithin	60	14
Vivonex Pediatric [P] (Nes)	24	24	100% free L-amino acids	130	Maltodextrin, modified corn starch	23	MCT (coconut and/or palm kernel oil), soybean oils	70	10
Portagen [P] (MJ)	30	35	Sodium caseinate	115	75% corn syrup solids, 25% sugar	48	MCT and corn oils, soy lecithin	87	18.8

Key: A = Abbott Nutrition; ARA = arachidonic acid; C = concentrate; C:W = casein:whey ratio; DHA = docosahexaenoic acid; G = Gerber; MCTs = medium-chain triglycerides; mfr = manufacturer; MJ = Mead Johnson Nutritionals; Nes = Nestlé Nutrition; Nut = Nutricia North America; P = powder; R = ready-to-feed; scFOS = short-chain fructooligosaccharides.

Note: Federal regulations require nutrient values to be reported as intakes per 100 kcal. These intakes can be found on the manufacturers' Web sites. Values per liter of formula are provided for ease of calculation. Changes occur periodically in formula composition; for the most up-to-date information, refer to the Web sites.

[a] When powder is prepared to the stated caloric density.

[b] Available as newborn formulation [R,P] with C:W ratio of 20:80. Provides sufficient vitamin D (400 international units) in minimum volume of 27 fl oz.

[c] Has ⅓ of the lactose content of standard milk-based formula.

[d] Powder form available as Nutramigen with Enflora LGG.

[e] When carbohydrate is added as directed to make a 20 kcal/oz concentration. For RCF, 54 grams of carbohydrate + 12 fl oz water + 13 fl oz of RCF to yield 26 fl oz. For 3232A, 81 grams of 3232A + 59 grams carbohydrate per quart prepared.

[f] Contains *Bifidus* BL, *Bifidobacterium lactis*, which is similar to probiotics found in human milk.

[g] Enteral formula contains less sucrose and has a lower osmolality.

[h] Prebiotic Nutraflora scFOS are short-chain fructooligosaccharides that provide fuel for beneficial bacteria in the digestive tract to help support a healthy immune system.

[i] PreBio is a unique blend of fructooligosaccharides and inulin. These compounds may increase colonic mucosal integrity and permeability, promote potentially beneficial bacteria, and improve colonic absorption of water and electrolytes.

Source: Abbott Nutrition (www.abbottnutrition.com); Gerber (www.medical.gerber.com); Mead Johnson Nutritionals (www.mjn.com); Nestlé Nutrition [clinical] (http://www.nestle-nutrition.com/Public/Default.aspx); and Nutricia North America (www.nutricia-na.com). Accessed June 6, 3013.

caloric density of human milk. One recent exception is selected standard infant formulas manufactured by Abbott Nutrition, which, if prepared according to standard preparation instructions, provide 19 kcal/oz or approximately 65 kcal/100 mL (Table 25–6). A healthy, term infant should have no difficulty consuming enough formula to meet both calorie and fluid needs with this caloric density. Premature, malnourished, volume-restricted (i.e., cardiac or liver disease, or poor oral feeding), or severely ill infants may require more calories (130–150 kcal/kg/day or higher) or formulas with higher caloric densities (e.g., 22, 24, or 27 kcal/oz) to meet their calorie needs. Infant formulas with caloric densities significantly lower or higher than 20 kcal/oz are regarded as therapeutic formulas to be used in managing special clinical conditions (Tables 25–6 and 25–7). Concentrated formulas should be used only under close medical supervision, especially with monitoring for dehydration caused by the reduction in free water consumed.

Osmolality and Osmolarity

Osmolality is the preferred term for reporting the osmotic activities of infant formulas. Osmolality represents the number of osmoles of solute per kilogram of solvent (Osm/kg). Any dietary component soluble in water contributes to osmolality. Osmolality is directly related to the concentration of molecular or ionic particles in the solution (i.e., amino acids, small peptides, electrolytes, and simple sugars) and inversely proportional to the concentration of water in the formula. The osmolality of human milk is approximately 295 mOsm/kg; osmolality of standard caloric density formulas is 200–300 mOsm/kg.

The osmolarity of an infant formula may be expressed as the concentration of solute per unit of total volume of solution or as the number of osmoles of solute per liter of solution (Osm/L). The osmolarity of human milk is approximately 273 mOsm/L. Formulas for infants should have osmolarities no higher than 400 mOsm/L. Unless the formula is very concentrated, there is no meaningful difference between osmolality and osmolarity of infant formulas.

The osmolality of a formula increases with increasing caloric density. The relationship between osmolality and caloric density is reasonably linear within the range of caloric concentrations usually fed to infants. Therefore, if the osmolality of a 20 kcal/oz formula is known, the same formula with any other caloric density can be calculated, assuming a direct proportion between osmolality and caloric density. For example, if a 20 kcal/oz formula has an osmolality of 283 mOsm/kg, then the same formula concentrated to 24 kcal/oz would have an osmolality of approximately 340 mOsm/kg.

No clinically meaningful difference exists in the osmolalities of the commonly used 20 kcal/oz, ready-to-use formulas. In addition, when concentrated products are diluted to provide a formula with 20 kcal/oz, there are no meaningful differences in osmolalities compared with the similar ready-to-use product. However, directions for diluting concentrated and powdered formulas must be followed exactly. Soy protein–based formulas have somewhat lower osmolalities than milk-based formulas because of the difference in carbohydrate source.

Potential Renal Solute Load

The PRSL is the solute load derived from the diet that must be excreted by the kidney if the amino acids from protein digestion are not used for growth or eliminated by nonrenal routes. The PRSL of an infant formula can be calculated with the following equation: PRSL (mOsm) = N/28 + sodium + chloride + potassium + phosphorus$_{(available)}$, where N is the total nitrogen in milligrams, and sodium, chloride, potassium, and phosphorus$_{(available)}$ (P$_a$) are expressed as millimoles (or milliosmoles). The P$_a$ is assumed to be the total phosphorus content except in soy-based formulas, in which it is only two-thirds of the total phosphorus. Table 25–5 lists PRSLs for various milks and infant formulas compared with the FDA-recommended upper PRSL limit.[44,45] Excretion of 1 mOsm of ingested solute requires 1 mL of water intake. Standard 20 kcal/oz infant formulas supply approximately 1.5 mL of water per kilocalorie ingested, an adequate amount of water to provide usual needs. Therefore, when the infant is healthy the PRSL is generally not a factor; however, during illnesses associated with water loss, such as vomiting, diarrhea, and fever, or in infants with compromised renal function or diabetes insipidus, the PRSL of the infant's formula becomes a factor in maintaining fluid balance. Feeding a formula with a high PRSL (i.e., high protein content or concentrated to more than 24 kcal/oz) may produce a hypertonic urine, leading to increased renal water losses and dehydration.

Types, Uses, and Selection of Commercial Infant Formulas

Standard formulas for term infants are milk based or milk based with added whey protein (whey-predominant). Other formulas are available for infants and children with specific dietary needs and should be used only under medical supervision.

Milk-Based Formulas

Milk-based formulas (Table 25–6) are prepared from nonfat cow milk, vegetable oils, and added carbohydrate (lactose). The added carbohydrate is necessary, because the ratio of carbohydrate to protein in nonfat cow milk solids is less than desirable for infant formulas. The most widely used vegetable oils are corn, coconut, safflower, sunflower, palm olein, and soy. Replacement of the butterfat with vegetable oils allows for better fat absorption. Although Similac Sensitive is a milk-based formula, it contains sucrose with corn maltodextrin, rather than lactose, as the carbohydrate source and may be used for infants with lactose intolerance. Enfamil Gentlease and Gerber Good Start Soothe contain decreased lactose amounts (20% and 50%, respectively) when compared with their product-line's standard milk-based formulas, and both are marketed for infant colic.

Therapeutic Formulas

Therapeutic infant formulas are used for infants with conditions requiring dietary adjustment and should be used with medical supervision, rather than being self-selected by parents. Table 25–7 lists indications for various therapeutic formulas, including soy protein–based, casein-based, casein hydrolysate–based or whey hydrolysate–based, and low-electrolyte and low-mineral formulas. Formulas intended for use by premature infants and those formulated specifically for children from 1–10 years of age are also considered therapeutic formulas.

Prethickened Milk-Based Formulas. Enfamil A.R. and Similac Sensitive For Spit-Up were developed specifically for infants with gastroesophageal reflux. These iron-fortified formulas contain rice starch. Before ingestion, the viscosity of Enfamil A.R. or Similac Sensitive For Spit-Up is much lower than a standard infant formula thickened with rice cereal. Therefore, these formulas flow better through a nipple than standard infant formula

table
25–7 | Indications for Therapeutic Infant Formulas[a]

Problem	Suggested Therapeutic Formula	Comments
Allergy or sensitivity to cow milk or soy protein	EleCare DHA/ARA, Neocate Infant DHA & ARA, Nutramigen, PurAmino, Pregestimil, Similac Expert Care Alimentum	Protein hydrolysate or free amino acid formula is best. Up to 50% cross-sensitivity between cow milk and soy protein allergies. Powder form of Similac Expert Care Alimentum contains corn, whereas the ready-to-feed form does not.
Biliary atresia, cholestatic liver disease	EleCare DHA/ARA, Enfaport, Pregestimil, Similac Expert Care Alimentum	Impaired digestion and absorption of long-chain fats; higher percentage of MCTs may improve absorption.
Carbohydrate intolerance (severe)	3232A, RCF	Carbohydrate-free; a patient-tolerated carbohydrate source is added gradually (e.g., dextrose, glucose, sucrose, fructose).
Cardiac disease	No therapeutic formula generally necessary	Low electrolyte content (Similac PM 60/40), if renal insufficiency. Electrolyte supplementation may be needed in patients receiving diuretics. Calorically dense, standard formulas often used due to failure to thrive and volume restriction.
Celiac disease	EleCare DHA/ARA, Neocate Infant DHA & ARA, Nutramigen, PurAmino, Pregestimil, Similac Expert Care for Diarrhea	Advance to standard formulas as intestinal epithelium returns to normal; diet must be gluten free.
Chylothorax or chylous ascites	Enfaport	High MCT intake decreases flow through the lymphatic system.
Constipation	No therapeutic formula necessary	Continue routine formula; increase water; refer severe constipation.
Cystic fibrosis	EleCare DHA/ARA, Pregestimil, Similac Expert Care Alimentum	Impaired digestion and absorption of long-chain fats; cow milk–based formula or human milk may be used with appropriate pancreatic enzyme supplementation. Enzyme supplementation may be required even with predigested therapeutic formulas; soy protein–based formulas contraindicated.
Diarrhea, chronic nonspecific	Enfamil ProSobee, Nutramigen, Similac Sensitive, Similac Soy Isomil, Gerber Good Start Soy	Trial of lactose-free cow milk or soy protein–based formula may be needed; avoid fruit juices.
Diarrhea, intractable	3232 A, EleCare DHA/ARA, PurAmino, Pregestimil, RCF, Similac Expert Care Alimentum	Hydrolyzed protein needed because of impaired digestion of intact protein, long-chain fats, and disaccharides. Similac Expert Care Alimentum contains sucrose and may not be appropriate for all cases.
Diarrhea, antibiotic-associated	Similac Expert Care for Diarrhea	Contains added dietary fiber from soy and was specifically formulated for infants with diarrhea secondary to antibiotics; use short term until diarrhea resolves.
Failure to thrive	No therapeutic formula generally necessary; EleCare DHA/ARA, Pregestimil, Similac Expert Care Alimentum	Most cases related to inadequate intake. Start with standard formula; may need more calorically dense formula for catch-up growth; change to predigested formula only if malabsorption present.
Galactosemia	Enfamil ProSobee, Nutramigen, Pregestimil	Formulas without lactose or sucrose; cow and human milk contraindicated.
Gastroesophageal reflux	Enfamil A.R., Similac Sensitive For Spit-Up	In otherwise healthy children, may start with standard formula thickened with rice cereal. (Start with 1–2 teaspoons per ounce of formula and increase to a maximum of 1 tablespoon per ounce as tolerated.) Thickening formula with rice cereal increases the caloric density, may cause constipation, results in delivery of less volume, and usually requires enlarging the nipple. Some infants may have an allergic-type reaction to rice cereal; oatmeal may be used in these cases. Attempt small, frequent feedings; avoid using products like Thick-It and SimplyThick to thicken formula (products are intended for patients with dysphagia or swallowing difficulties); use more calorically dense formula if decreased volume or catch-up growth needed.

table
25–7 Indications for Therapeutic Infant Formulas[a] *(continued)*

Problem	Suggested Therapeutic Formula	Comments
Hepatitis without liver failure	No therapeutic formula necessary	Impaired digestion or absorption of long-chain fats is uncommon.
Hepatitis with liver failure	EleCare DHA/ARA, Enfaport, Pregestimil, Similac Expert Care Alimentum	Impaired digestion or absorption of long-chain fats may occur.
Increased ostomy output	Similac Expert Care for Diarrhea	Improve consistency in term infants without malabsorption (e.g., Hirschsprung's disease, imperforate anus, necrotizing enterocolitis, or intestinal atresias).
Lactose intolerance (primary or secondary)	Enfamil ProSobee, Similac Sensitive, Similac Soy Isomil, Gerber Good Start Soy	Remove lactose from diet; use lactose-free formula.
Necrotizing enterocolitis (during recovery or postresection)	EleCare DHA/ARA, Neocate Infant DHA & ARA, Pregestimil, Similac Expert Care Alimentum	Impaired digestion or absorption requires a hydrolysate or free amino acid formula.
Prematurity	Fortified human milk (preferred); Enfamil Premature 20 Cal, Similac Special Care 20 with Iron, Gerber Good Start Premature 20, or transition infant formula (Enfamil EnfaCare, Similac Expert Care NeoSure, or Gerber Good Start Nourish)	Human milk fortifier needed; transition formula (see formula column) can be added to human milk to increase caloric density after discharge (1 tsp/90 mL milk makes 24 kcal/oz).
Renal insufficiency	Similac PM 60/40	Formula is low phosphate, low PRSL.

Key: MCT = Medium-chain triglyceride; PRSL = potential renal solute load.

[a] Products are listed alphabetically; list is not all-inclusive; other products may be acceptable.

Source: Abbott Nutrition (www.abbottnutrition.com); Mead Johnson Nutritionals (www.mjn.com); Gerber (www.medical.gerber.com); Nestlé Nutrition (www.nestle-nutrition.com/Public/Default.aspx); and Nutricia North America (www.nutricia-na.com). Accessed June 6, 2013.

thickened with rice cereal. Once ingested, however, the viscosity increases dramatically in the stomach's acidic pH, reaching a viscosity equal to the combination of standard infant formula plus rice cereal. This effect may be minimized in infants receiving a histamine$_2$-receptor antagonist (e.g., ranitidine or famotidine) or proton pump inhibitor (e.g., omeprazole, lansoprazole, or esomeprazole) for treatment of their gastroesophageal reflux, if the gastric pH is greater than 5.4. Also, Similac Sensitive For Spit-Up is a lactose-free formula. Neither Enfamil A.R. nor Similac Sensitive For Spit-Up is recommended for use in premature infants because neither will adequately meet their needs, especially for protein, calcium, and phosphorus. In May 2011, the FDA cautioned parents against using, thickening agents such as SimplyThick and Thick-It in premature infants because of reports of necrotizing enterocolitis. This cautionary statement was expanded to infants of all ages in September 2012.[47]

Soy Protein–Based Formulas. Despite relatively few true indications for soy protein–based formulas, approximately 20% of formulas sold in the United States are soy protein based, suggesting that these formulas are being selected by parents rather than being prescribed by health care providers.[34,37] Soy protein–based formulas (Table 25–6) contain a soy isolate fortified with L-methionine; none contain lactose. Soy formulas are a safe and nutritionally sound alternative for normal growth and development in infants who are not fed human milk, who do not tolerate cow milk–based formula, or whose parents choose them for other reasons (e.g., vegetarians). However, because soy formulas have insufficient amounts of calcium, phosphorus, and vitamin D

in relationship to some infants' increased needs, they are not recommended for patients weighing less than 1800 grams.[48]

Food allergy occurs in infants because the immature digestive and metabolic processes may not be completely effective in converting dietary proteins into nonallergenic amino acids. Cow milk protein allergy occurs in 2%–3% of infants and is defined as symptomatology involving the respiratory tract (wheezing), skin (rash), or GI tract (diarrhea and bloody stools) disappearing when cow milk is removed from the diet and reappearing on two separate challenges when cow milk is reintroduced during a symptom-free period. Symptoms of cow milk protein intolerance generally regress within 3–4 years in most children.

Soy protein–based formulas are appropriate for infants with lactose intolerance resulting from lactase deficiency and with documented immunoglobulin E (IgE)–mediated allergy to cow milk protein. However, infants with cow milk protein–induced enteropathy or enterocolitis are also frequently sensitive to soy protein (up to 50% cross-sensitivity); therefore, AAP/CON recommends protein hydrolysate formulas for these infants.[48] Most infants suspected of having adverse reactions to milk-based formulas have not experienced life-threatening manifestations. These infants appear to tolerate soy protein–based formulas that are less expensive and better tasting than the protein hydrolysate formulas. Routine use of soy protein–based formulas has no proven value in prevention of atopic disease.[49] Some infants with moderate–severe gastroenteritis develop intolerance to lactose and sucrose because of a temporary lactase and sucrase deficiency. However, after rehydration, most infants with diarrhea can be managed by continuing their usual nutrition regimen whether milk based or soy protein based.

RCF is a soy protein–based formula that contains no carbohydrates. Use of this formula is limited to infants unable to tolerate the type or amount of carbohydrates in human milk or infant formulas. A carbohydrate source (sucrose, dextrose, fructose, or glucose polymers) is added gradually in increasing amounts to slowly improve carbohydrate tolerance.

In addition, soy protein–based formulas are not recommended for infants with cystic fibrosis, because these children do not use soy protein adequately, will lose substantial nitrogen in their stools, and will develop hypoproteinemia or even anasarca (generalized infiltration of fluid into subcutaneous connective tissue). Formula-fed infants with cystic fibrosis do well nutritionally when given an easily digested formula that contains semi-elemental protein and medium-chain triglycerides (MCTs) (e.g., a casein hydrolysate–based formula). However, studies have shown that infants with cystic fibrosis grow equally well on a regular cow milk–based formula or human milk as long as adequate pancreatic enzyme supplementation is given.[50]

Casein Hydrolysate–Based Formulas. Protein is supplied by enzymatically hydrolyzed, charcoal-treated casein rather than by whole protein in casein hydrolysate–based formulas, which include Pregestimil, Nutramigen, and Similac Expert Care Alimentum (Table 25-6). These formulas are classified as semi-elemental and contain nonantigenic polypeptides with molecular weights less than 1200 daltons; therefore, they can be fed to infants who are sensitive to intact milk protein. Casein hydrolysate–based formulas are supplemented with L-cysteine, L-tyrosine, and L-tryptophan, because the concentrations of these amino acids are reduced during the charcoal treatment.

Carbohydrate sources in casein hydrolysate–based formulas vary and include corn syrup solids, modified corn and tapioca starch, corn maltodextrin, and sucrose (Table 25-6). Glucose polymers found in corn syrup solids, modified corn starch, or corn maltodextrin are particularly useful in infants who have malabsorption disorders and are frequently intolerant to high concentrations of lactose, sucrose, and glucose. In addition, glucose polymers contribute little to the total osmolar load. Low osmolality is an advantage in intestinal disorders in which the osmolar load of disaccharide- or glucose-containing elemental diets may not be tolerated. The formula 3232 A is an extensively hydrolyzed casein-based formula with added amino acids that is intended, like RCF, to be used with small amounts of carbohydrate to gradually improve tolerance. This product contains modified tapioca starch and fat, 85% of which is MCTs.

Hydrolysate formulas usually contain modified fat sources. MCTs are typically included since they do not require emulsification with bile and are more easily digested and absorbed than long-chain fats. Shorter-chain fatty acids and MCTs are directly absorbed into the portal system, not into the lacteals of the lymphatic system. In addition, MCTs enhance the absorption of long-chain triglycerides and do not require carnitine for transport into the mitochondria, where oxidation and energy production occur. However, MCTs cannot be the sole source of dietary fat, given that they do not provide essential fatty acids, increasing the risk of essential fatty acid deficiency. Pregestimil, Nutramigen, and Similac Expert Care Alimentum contain DHA and ARA as long-chain fatty acids. Diarrhea can result from MCT malabsorption caused by overfeeding or intestinal mucosal disease.

Use of casein hydrolysate–based formulas for allergy prophylaxis is controversial. AAP's policy statement on hypoallergenic formulas states that infants with a high risk for developing allergy identified by a strong family history (both parents or one parent and a sibling) may benefit from a hypoallergenic formula, but studies are not conclusive.[48] Currently, no evidence exists to support the use of hydrolysate formulas for treating colic, irritability, or gastroesophageal reflux. Although these symptoms are common in infants, they are rarely a result of an IgE-mediated allergic reaction to cow milk protein.

Extensively hydrolyzed casein formulas are less palatable than standard formulas. If the formula is rejected by the infant when first offered, it should be tried again after a few hours. These products are designed to provide a sole source of nutrition for infants up to 4–6 months of age and a primary source of nutrition through 12 months of age, when indicated. Extended use of hydrolysate formulas as a sole source of nutrition in children older than 6 months requires close medical supervision and monitoring.

Whey Hydrolysate–Based Formulas. Enzymatically hydrolyzed whey protein is another protein source used in infant formulas (Gerber Good Start Gentle). Infants who have GI intolerance to cow milk but are not allergic to it often tolerate whey hydrolysate–based formula. This product is promoted as having a pleasant taste, smell, and appearance. It may be better accepted than casein hydrolysate–based formulas, which parents and infants find differ noticeably from cow milk– and soy protein–based formulas in both appearance and taste. There are no specific indications for these products, so they may be chosen according to parent/patient or program preference.

Amino Acid–Based Formulas. Occasionally, infants are intolerant to even hydrolyzed casein and require a free amino acid–based formula. Neocate Infant DHA & ARA, EleCare DHA/ARA, and PurAmino contain 100% free amino acids and are considered hypoallergenic. They are used for infants with cow milk protein allergy, multiple food protein allergies, or intolerance to casein hydrolysate formulas.

High MCT Formulas. Enfaport and Portagen are unique formulas because of their high MCT content (i.e., 84% and 87% of the fat, respectively). They also contain higher concentrations of both lipid- and water-soluble vitamins than are found in casein hydrolysate–based formulas. The higher concentrations of MCTs and vitamins in these formulas help compensate for the impaired digestion and absorption of long-chain fats in patients with pancreatic insufficiency (e.g., cystic fibrosis), bile acid deficiency (e.g., biliary atresia or cholestatic jaundice), and intestinal resection. Another use is to decrease lymphatic flow in patients with lymphatic anomalies such as chylothorax and chylous ascites. Enfaport can be used as the sole dietary source for infants, whereas Portagen can be used as the sole dietary source for children and adults or as a beverage to be consumed with each meal as a supplement. Children with fat malabsorption who receive Portagen can develop essential fatty acid deficiency. Linoleic acid (e.g., corn or safflower oil, or Microlipid) can be given in the diet, either by mixing with the formula or by syringe through a feeding tube, to prevent essential fatty acid deficiency.

Low PRSL Formulas. Similac PM 60/40 is an infant formula with lower mineral (potassium and phosphorus) and protein (1.5 g/100 mL) content, and therefore lower PRSL than standard infant formulas. It is most appropriately used for infants with renal insufficiency. Similac PM 60/40 also contains less calcium and iron than standard infant formulas; supplementation of these minerals may be necessary.

Premature Infant Formulas. AAP's current recommendation is for all premature infants to receive maternal human milk or donor human milk.[29] However, inadequate nutrient intake can occur in human milk–fed premature infants because unfortified human milk does not meet the needs of this population. Because of their increased nutrient needs and somewhat decreased ability to consume an adequate volume, premature infants (especially those less than 34 weeks gestation) often need feedings providing a higher caloric density, as well as increased protein, calcium, phosphorus, and other nutrients. The nutritional goal for a preterm infant is to achieve a postnatal growth rate approximating the intrauterine growth rate of a normal fetus of the same postconceptional age.

No commercially available formula is completely satisfactory for premature infants. Formulas for premature infants (Table 25–6) share features such as whey-predominant proteins, carbohydrate mixtures of lactose and corn syrup solids, and fat mixtures containing both MCTs and long-chain triglycerides. They differ in electrolyte, vitamin, mineral, protein, and caloric content. When given in sufficient volume, these formulas promote adequate growth in preterm infants. An isotonic osmolality (approximately 300 mOsm/kg of water) is maintained at a caloric density of 24 kcal/oz or 80 kcal/100 mL.

Calcium and phosphorus are crucial to the development and maintenance of the human skeleton. In addition, calcium and phosphorus are integral components of many biochemical reactions. Calcium requirements are affected by protein and phosphorus intake in that these nutrients interact with the renal tubular reabsorption of calcium. Calcium-to-phosphorus weight ratios vary significantly for human milk (2:1) and cow milk (1.2:1). This ratio also varies in commercial infant formulas. Formulas designed for term infants will not meet the calcium and phosphorus needs of premature infants. For these infants, the additional calcium and phosphorus found in premature infant formulas is necessary for normal bone growth and mineralization. Typical amounts of calcium and phosphorus found in 20 kcal/oz infant formulas are 111–121 mg calcium/100 mL and 56–68 mg phosphorus/100 mL for preterm formulas versus 45–53 mg calcium/100 mL and 25–29 mg phosphorus/100 mL for term formulas. Human milk fed to premature infants requires calcium and phosphorus fortification with either a human milk fortifier or a transitional premature formula, which is discussed later in this chapter.

Nutrient-enriched transition or postdischarge formulas are designed specifically to provide for continued catch-up growth in premature infants after hospital discharge. Similac Expert Care NeoSure, Enfamil EnfaCare, and Gerber Good Start Nourish (all milk-based formulas) contain MCTs as part of the fat source. The caloric (22 kcal/oz), protein, vitamin, and mineral content of these formulas exceed those of standard term formulas but are less than those of 24 kcal/oz premature infant formulas. Use of these formulas in preterm infants until 9 months postnatal age results in greater linear growth, weight gain, and bone mineral content than are seen with the use of standard, term infant formulas.[51]

Human Milk Fortifiers. Mothers who deliver prematurely produce milk that is higher in protein, sodium, potassium, and possibly other nutrients than the milk of mothers who deliver at full term. However, these nutrients decline to the amounts found in mature human milk by 4–8 weeks after delivery. During the third trimester, the fetus receives 125–150 mg of calcium and 65–80 mg of phosphorus daily, most of which are deposited in bone. Without supplementation, human milk, whether preterm or mature, cannot supply that amount of calcium and phosphorus, which are needed to prevent osteopenia of prematurity. Therefore, human milk must be fortified for premature infants to achieve adequate growth.[52]

Commercial products have been developed to supplement the nutrient content of human milk so that it meets the needs of most preterm infants. Enfamil Human Milk Fortifier Acidified Liquid, Similac Special Care 30 with Iron, and Prolact+ H2MF are all liquids that add nutrients to human milk without displacing a significant amount of volume. Enfamil Human Milk Fortifier Acidified Liquid and Similac Special Care 30 with Iron are made from cow milk supplemented with whey protein to provide a casein:whey ratio of 40:60 and a fat mixture to provide MCTs. When added to human milk, fortifiers increase the osmolality by only 10–36 mOsm/kg. Prolact+ H2MF is made from concentrated 100% human milk. It provides extra protein, calories, vitamins, and minerals and is specifically indicated for preterm infants weighing less than 1250 grams. Table 25–8 lists the composition of the human milk fortifiers. Studies support adequate weight gain and nutrient retention in infants when either fortified human milk or commercial preterm formulas are ingested.[53,54] However, human milk has been shown to provide various immunologic benefits, as well as improve the IQ of infants born small for gestational age and very low-birth-weight infants.[55] The use of these products will result in weight gain equivalent to intrauterine growth rates in most premature infants. Product selection will therefore be dictated by cost and clinical preference. These products are expensive. Enfamil Human Milk Fortifier Acidified Liquid costs approximately $2.60 per vial, and one vial is generally added to each 25 mL of human milk to yield a 24 kcal/oz concentration. Moreover, this product comes only in cartons of 100–200 vials. Similac Special Care 30 with Iron costs as much as $0.83 per ounce and, when added in equal parts (2 ounces of human milk to 2 ounces of Similac Special Care 30 with Iron), yields a 25 kcal/oz concentration. Prolact+ H2MF is the most expensive, costing approximately $6.25 per milliliter, and requiring the addition of 20 mL of Prolact+4 H2MF with 80 mL of human milk to yield a 24 kcal/oz concentration. The greatest evidence supporting the financial benefit of human milk as a sole source of nutrition is in relation to decreased incidence of necrotizing enterocolitis (NEC).[56,57] Once the infant is ready for discharge from the hospital or has reached a weight of 2.5 kg, one of the transition or postdischarge formulas can be added to human milk to increase the caloric density (1 teaspoon of powder added to 90 mL of formula yields 24 kcal/oz) and delivery of other nutrients.

Metabolic Formulas. Infants with various inherited inborn errors of metabolism require specific formulas tailored to their particular condition and must be under the care of a specialist, usually a pediatric endocrinologist or geneticist. Information about these formulas is available on the various manufacturers' Web sites. These formulas, as well as formulas intended for use in low-birth-weight infants or in patients with specific medical conditions or dietary needs, are classified by FDA as "exempt formulas," which means they are exempt from FDA nutrient content and labeling requirements.[58]

Concentrated Formulas. A child with caloric needs exceeding normal requirements may be given concentrated formula under medical supervision. A few ready-to-use formulas made from cow milk are available in a caloric density of 22 or 24 kcal/oz

table 25–8	Human Milk Fortifiers		
Component	**Enfamil Human Milk Fortifier Acidified Liquid**[a]	**Similac Special Care with Iron 30**[b]	**Prolact+4 H²MF**[c]
Calories	30	60	28
Protein (g)	2.2	1.8	1.2
Fat (g)	2.3	4	1.8
Carbohydrates (g)	<1.2	4.7	1.8
Vitamin A (international units)	1160	750	61
Vitamin D (international units)	188	90	26
Vitamin E (international units)	5.6	2.4	0.4
Vitamin K (mcg)	5.7	7.2	<0.2
Thiamin (mcg)	184	150	4
Riboflavin (mcg)	260	372	15
Vitamin B$_6$ (mcg)	140	150	4.1
Vitamin B$_{12}$ (mcg)	0.64	0.33	0.05
Niacin (mg)	3.7	3	0.0524
Folic acid (mcg)	31	22.2	5.4
Pantothenic acid (mg)	0.92	1.14	0.0748
Biotin (mcg)	3.4	22.2	—
Vitamin C (mg)	15.2	22.2	<0.2
Calcium (mg)	116	110	103
Phosphorus (mg)	64	60.8	53.8
Magnesium (mg)	1.84	7.2	4.7
Iron (mg)	1.76	1.1	0.1
Zinc (mg)	0.96	0.9	0.7
Manganese (mcg)	10	7.2	<12
Copper (mcg)	60	150	64
Selenium (mcg)	—	1.1	—
Sodium (mg)	27	26.2	37
Potassium (mg)	45.2	78.5	50
Chloride (mg)	28	49.3	29

[a] Amount per 4 vials; generally mixed with 100 mL human milk to yield 120 mL with a caloric density of 24 kcal/oz.

[b] Amount per 60 mL; generally mixed with 60 mL human milk to yield 120 mL with a caloric density of 25 kcal/oz.

[c] Amount per 20 mL of Prolact + 4; generally mixed with 80 mL human milk to yield 100 mL with a caloric density of 24 kcal/oz. Nutrient contribution from Prolact + 4 based on target values for macronutrients and minerals and averages of three lots (vitamins).

Source: Abbott Nutrition (www.abbottnutrition.com); Mead Johnson Nutritionals (www.mjn.com); and Prolacta Bioscience (www.prolacta.com). Accessed June 10, 2013.

(Table 25–6). Various concentrations can be prepared from liquid concentrates or powders by varying the amount of water added (Tables 25–9 and 25–10). Increasing caloric density by adding less water also increases delivery of all nutrients, including protein and electrolytes, and decreases free water delivery. Increased concentration of protein and electrolytes (i.e., PRSL) in conjunction with decreased fluid intake may result in dehydration and electrolyte imbalances. Careful monitoring of the infant's fluid intake and output, weight, serum electrolytes, blood urea nitrogen, serum creatinine, and urine specific gravity and osmolality is recommended, especially on initiation of the concentrated formula.

Modular macronutrient components (Table 25–11) can be added to either human milk or infant formula and are available as alternatives to concentrating formulas. Adding carbohydrates as glucose can result in diarrhea. Protein supplementation may increase the PRSL. Fat may be added as MCTs (MCT Oil; Nestlé Nutrition) or Microlipid (Nestlé Nutrition) for infants with fat malabsorption or intolerance. Microlipid is an emulsion made from safflower oil that provides long-chain fatty acids and mixes well with formula. Addition of fat can lead to diarrhea, steatorrhea, delayed gastric emptying, vomiting, and gastroesophageal reflux. Adding modular components is more expensive and time-consuming than simply concentrating the

<table>
<tr><td colspan="3">**table 25–9**   **Dilution of Concentrated Liquid Infant Formulas**[a]</td></tr>
<tr><td>**Caloric Concentration Desired (kcal/oz)**</td><td>**Liquid Formula Concentrate (ounce)**</td><td>**Added Water (ounce)**</td></tr>
<tr><td>20</td><td>1</td><td>1</td></tr>
<tr><td>22 (actual 21.8)</td><td>3</td><td>2.5</td></tr>
<tr><td>24</td><td>3</td><td>2</td></tr>
<tr><td>26–27 (actual 26.7)</td><td>3</td><td>1.5</td></tr>
<tr><td>28–29 (actual 28.6)</td><td>5</td><td>2</td></tr>
</table>

[a] Commercial concentrates of infant formula contain 40 kcal/oz before dilution with water.

<table>
<tr><td colspan="3">**table 25–10**   **Dilution of Powdered Term Infant Formulas**[a]</td></tr>
<tr><td>**Caloric Concentration Desired (kcal/oz)**</td><td>**Formula Powder (scoop)**[b]</td><td>**Added Water (ounce)**</td></tr>
<tr><td>20</td><td>1</td><td>2</td></tr>
<tr><td>24</td><td>3</td><td>5</td></tr>
<tr><td>28</td><td>4</td><td>5.5</td></tr>
<tr><td>28</td><td>7</td><td>10</td></tr>
</table>

[a] Powdered infant formulas generally contain 44 kcal per level, packed scoop before dilution. If a large volume of formula is to be prepared, add powder necessary to supply desired calories; then add water to the final volume desired. Directions for preparation may vary; check manufacturer's information.

[b] Historically, the conversion of 1 scoop = 1 tablespoon of powder has been used. However, this measurement varies between powders. For improved accuracy, parents and caregivers should be instructed to use the manufacturer's provided scoop for all measurements.

formula; these components should be reserved for situations in which a single nutrient is needed or further concentration of the formula is not appropriate.

Toddler Formulas. Toddler formulas (second part of Table 25–6; e.g., Gerber Graduates Gentle, Similac Go & Grow Milk-based Formula, Enfagrow Premium Next Step) are designed for infants and children 9–24 months of age. AAP/CON, however, has stated that these formulas offer no nutritional advantages; standard formulas are appropriate for infants up to 12 months of age.[42]

Formulas for Children 1–13 Years of Age. Nutritionally complete, isotonic, virtually lactose-free enteral formulas designed for young children who cannot tolerate a normal diet or eat solid food are available (second part of Table 25–6; e.g., PediaSure, Nutren Junior, Boost Kid Essentials). Flavored products contain sucrose, have a pleasant taste, and can be used as oral supplements. These formulas are also appropriate to use as tube feedings regardless of tube tip placement. They contain adequate amounts of calcium, phosphorus, iron, and vitamin D for this age group; the amounts contained in adult enteral products are typically inadequate.

<table>
<tr><td colspan="4">**table 25–11**   **Modular Additives**</td></tr>
<tr><td>**Additive[a] (Mfr)**</td><td>**Nutrient(s) Provided**</td><td>**Amount of Nutrient(s)**</td><td>**Calories**</td></tr>
<tr><td>Beneprotein (Nes)</td><td>Whey protein isolate (milk)</td><td>Per 7 gram scoop or packet: protein 6 grams</td><td>25.2 kcal/scoop</td></tr>
<tr><td>Polycose (A)</td><td>Carbohydrate (glucose polymers derived from controlled hydrolysis cornstarch)</td><td>Per tablespoon (6 grams): carbohydrate 5.6 grams</td><td>23 kcal/tablespoon</td></tr>
<tr><td>Microlipid (Nes) (liquid)</td><td>Long-chain fats (safflower oil)</td><td>Per mL: fat 0.5 gram</td><td>4.5 kcal/mL</td></tr>
<tr><td>MCT Oil (Nes) (liquid)</td><td>MCTs (coconut/palm kernel oil)</td><td>Per mL: fat 0.93 gram</td><td>7.7 kcal/mL</td></tr>
<tr><td>Super Soluble Duocal (Nut)</td><td>Carbohydrate, fat (MCT 35%)</td><td>Per tablespoon: carbohydrate 6.3 grams; fat 1.9 grams</td><td>25 kcal/scoop
42 kcal/tablespoon</td></tr>
<tr><td>Benecalorie (Nes) (liquid)</td><td>Calcium caseinate (milk); high oleic sunflower oil</td><td>Per 1.5 ounces: protein 7.2 grams; fat 33.75 grams</td><td>7.5 kcal/mL</td></tr>
<tr><td>ProMod Liquid Protein (A) (liquid)</td><td>Hydrolyzed beef collagen</td><td>0.33 grams protein/mL</td><td>3.3 kcal/mL</td></tr>
<tr><td>Liquid Protein Fortifier (A) (liquid)</td><td>Casein hydrolysate</td><td>0.17 grams protein/mL</td><td>0.67 kcal/mL</td></tr>
</table>

Key: A = Abbott Nutrition; MCT = medium-chain triglycerides; Nes = Nestlé Nutrition; Nut = Nutricia North America.

[a] Products listed are powders unless specified otherwise.

Source: Abbott Nutrition (www.abbottnutrition.com); Nestlé Nutrition (www.nestle-nutrition.com/Public/Default.aspx); and Nutricia North America (www.nutricia-na.com). Accessed May 4, 2013.

Several therapeutic formulas have also been developed for children 1–13 years of age (Table 25–6). Peptamen Junior is a peptide-based, semi-elemental formula. Vivonex Pediatric, Neocate Junior, E028 Splash (a flavored, nutritionally complete drink), and EleCare Jr are amino acid–based elemental formulas, whereas Pepdite Junior is a peptide-based, amino acid–based elemental formula. These products are intended for use in children with altered digestive or absorptive capabilities caused by a number of conditions, including severe protein allergy and eosinophilic esophagitis (Table 25–7).

Nutritional Problems in Infancy

GI problems, especially diarrhea, can occur with the use of infant formulas, as well as with human milk or any food. Tooth decay and nutritional deficiencies are other potential problems.

Diarrhea

Diarrhea can lead to failure to thrive (chronic) and dehydration (acute). Infants are particularly susceptible to dehydration because of their high metabolic rate and ratio of surface area to weight and height. Fluid depletion by diarrhea or vomiting may quickly (within 24 hours) produce severe dehydration with fluid and electrolyte imbalances, shock, and possible death. A potential formula-related cause of diarrhea and vomiting is the improper dilution of a concentrated liquid or powdered formula or the incorrect addition of a modular product.

If diarrhea develops, the health care provider should ascertain the severity and duration, stool frequency, and formula preparation method. If the diarrhea appears severe (i.e., many more stools per day than normal) or has continued for more than 72 hours, or if the infant is clinically ill (fever, lethargy, anorexia, irritability, dry mucous membranes, or decreased urine output), the infant should be referred for medical attention. (Diarrhea is discussed in Chapter 16.)

Mild diarrhea will usually resolve without the need for medical intervention, but the infant should be observed closely for signs of dehydration. Temporarily discontinuing usual dietary intake is not recommended except during a 4- to 6-hour period of oral rehydration if the infant is dehydrated. Oral electrolyte replacement solutions manufactured especially for infants (e.g., Pedialyte, Enfalyte) may be used for short-term replacement of fluid and electrolyte losses in mild-to-moderate dehydration to augment fluid intake, but these solutions should not replace formula or human milk intake.[59] Prevention of dehydration by replacement of ongoing losses with a glucose/electrolyte solution in liquid or frozen form is the best intervention for diarrhea in infants and children.

Lactose-free formulas or a lactose-free diet may be considered for infants and children with moderate-severe diarrheal illness, but full-strength lactose-containing formulas, human milk, or a regular diet can be used in most infants. Parents should be advised that diarrhea is likely to continue for 3–7 days regardless of the type of formula, and seeking medical consultation is advised if a sudden increase in stool output occurs with resumption of feeding.[59]

Other GI Issues

Adverse GI effects of formula include mechanical obstruction (inspissated milk curds) and hypersensitivity to specific milk protein. Cow milk intolerance is associated most often with an inability to digest lactose or milk proteins. Hyperosmolar formulas may adversely affect premature infants during the early neonatal period and may be a contributing factor in the development of necrotizing enterocolitis, a severe inflammation of the intestinal mucous membranes. For this reason, initiation of feedings in these infants is most often done with unfortified human milk or a 20 kcal/oz premature infant formula. Only after the infant has reached 100 mL/kg/day of enteral feedings is the caloric density advanced.[60] Initiation and advancement of formula for premature infants should occur under medical supervision and are not appropriate for self-care.

Tooth Decay

Baby bottle tooth decay can occur in children who are bottle-fed beyond the typical weaning period (1 year) and who go to sleep with their bottles. It can also occur if the infant is allowed to sip on a bottle or training cup frequently during the day. Caries can be seen in children younger than 2 years and may involve the maxillary incisors, maxillary and mandibular first molars, or maxillary and mandibular canines. Restorative dentistry is often required, leading to the potential for difficulty in speech development. Methods for prevention once teeth start to erupt include substituting plain water for carbohydrate-containing formula or other drinks given in a bottle until the infant is weaned from the bottle, encouraging the use of a cup for high-sugar drinks such as juice, using either infant juices that contain a higher portion of water or standard juices diluted with additional water, ensuring adequate fluoride intake, cleaning the baby's mouth at least once daily, and weaning from breast or bottle by 10–12 months of age.[61] Going to sleep with a bottle should be actively discouraged for all infants.

Nutritional Deficiencies or Toxicities

Generally, age- and condition-appropriate commercial infant formulas are nutritionally adequate and safe for most infants and children. Nutritional deficiencies reported historically with commercial infant formulas are unlikely today with appropriate supplementation procedures and technological advances in processing.

Because of a concern about possible aluminum contamination of infant formulas, the Food and Agriculture Organization of the United Nations has set a provisional tolerable aluminum intake of 1 mg/kg/day. Aluminum toxicity can interfere with cellular and metabolic processes in the nervous system as well as negatively affect bone and liver tissues.[62] Aluminum toxicity is primarily a concern in patients with decreased or immature renal function, such as premature infants. If an infant were to ingest as much as 200 mL/kg/day of a formula known to have the highest aluminum content, the amount of aluminum received per day would still be less than 0.5 mg/kg/day. The highest aluminum concentrations in infant formulas (500–2400 mg/L) have been reported in soy protein–based formulas, because plants readily absorb aluminum from soil.

Infant Formula Preparation

Most formulas are available as a ready-to-use liquid or as a liquid concentrate or powder for reconstitution mixed with water. Ready-to-use formulas should *never be diluted.* They are convenient but usually more expensive. In contrast, concentrated liquids *must be diluted,* typically by mixing equal amounts of water and concentrated liquid (e.g., 13-ounce can of formula with 13-ounce can of water) to prepare a 20 kcal/oz formula (Table 25–10). Powdered term and preterm transition or post-discharge formulas provide a measuring scoop in the can and require addition of 1 packed level scoop of powder to each 2 ounces of water for a 20 kcal/oz term formula and a 22 kcal/oz preterm postdischarge formula. Directions for preparation may vary and should always be compared with the manufacturer's or health care professional's directions. If the family is given alternative directions from those printed on the can, these should be given in writing and explained thoroughly to the caregiver. Directions should be provided in the appropriate language for non-English-speaking patients. Before use, infant formula containers should be inspected for the expiration date and damage. Unopened formula containers, cans, or bottles can be stored at room temperature but must not be subjected to extreme temperature changes.

Preparation Techniques

Each infant formula has specific instructions for preparation, and most formulas have symbols on the containers that can be used as guidelines in preparing formula. Because infants may be more susceptible to infection, various sterilization methods have been recommended for infant formula preparation. Table 25–12 reviews sterilization methods for different types of formulas. Studies have shown that the clean method of preparing formula (i.e., not boiling the water) is as safe as terminal sterilization (i.e., boiling the water); therefore, some providers do not recommend boiling water. WHO and AAP currently recommend that all water for formula preparation be boiled because of reports of municipal water supply contamination in some areas. If well or pond water is used or if the area is prone to flooding, the water must be boiled.[63,64] If tap water is used, cold water should be run for at least 2 minutes before use to clear any lead that might be in the pipes and decrease lead exposure. If bottled water is used in infant formula preparation, it should be treated the same as tap or well water (i.e., boil and cool it prior to use) unless the water is labeled as sterile.

Table 25–12 provides handling instructions and recommendations for storage of infant formulas once the original container has been opened. Expressed human milk should be stored in glass or plastic airtight containers, refrigerated, and used within 24–48 hours. Human milk can be frozen, preferably in the rear of the freezer compartment, for up to 2 weeks if the freezer compartment is inside the refrigerator, up to 3–4 months when the freezer has a separate door from the refrigerator, and up to 6 months if in a 0°F (−17.8°C) freezer. Frozen milk should be rapidly thawed by holding the container under tepid running water or placing it in a tepid water bath. Thawed human milk should always be used within 24 hours of thawing and never refrozen.

Adverse Effects of Improperly Prepared and/or Administered Formulas

As stated previously, the failure to properly dilute a concentrated infant formula can result in a hypertonic solution that could result in diarrhea and dehydration. In extreme cases, the ingestion of an overly concentrated formula can lead to hypernatremic dehydration (induced by water deficit), metabolic acidosis, and renal failure. Excessive formula dilution can lead to water intoxication that can result in irritability, hyponatremia, coma, brain damage, or death. Such a situation may occur when a

caregiver misunderstands the instructions for preparing a concentrated formula, dilutes a ready-to-use formula, or tries to make the baby's formula last longer by diluting it.

Parents or other caregivers may have questions about how much infant formula their child should receive. Typically, a health care provider at the hospital will have given parents feeding instructions prior to discharge. However, when a formula change is made after hospital discharge, adequate information may not be provided in some health care settings. Generally, the required daily formula intake depends on an infant's age, weight, and individual considerations such as the need for catch-up growth (Table 25–13). During the first year of life, a normal healthy formula-fed term infant usually eats every 3–5 hours (average of 4 hours). Small or weak infants may eat every 2–3 hours, because they have smaller stomach capacities or shorter gastric emptying times, or tire easily during feedings. Breast-fed infants or those receiving human milk from a bottle also will nurse or eat more often, given that human milk empties from the stomach more rapidly than formula. Most term infants will lengthen the interval between feedings to 4 hours by the age of 3–4 weeks. Premature infants may continue to require frequent feedings past 6–8 weeks of age, depending on the infant's birth weight and growth. Some infants begin to stop nighttime feedings after 1–2 months of age, whereas others take as long as 4–6 months. The process is highly variable and may depend more on the weight of the infant than on his or her age; most infants are able to sleep through the night when they reach approximately 11 pounds.

The amount of formula offered to a bottle-fed infant should be consistent with the DRI for energy according to age and weight (Table 25–2). Table 25–13 lists typical quantities of feedings for various age groups. The infant should be fed on demand and not forced to take more formula than is desired at any one feeding. If the infant finishes a bottle and still seems hungry, more formula should be offered. Parents should also be aware that an infant typically loses weight (mostly water) during the first week of life, but by 2 weeks of age, the child should be gaining weight. Appropriate weight gain usually indicates that an infant is receiving an appropriate amount of formula. The WHO standardized growth charts are used to determine whether an infant is growing appropriately. Weight, length/height, and head circumference should be plotted at each medical visit.

Both underfeeding and overfeeding are potential problems. Infants who like to "graze" all day can take in too much milk and gain too much weight. However, this can also be a sign of inadequate intake in breast-fed infants and lead to failure to thrive. Other problems associated with overfeeding are regurgitation, gastroesophageal reflux, vomiting, loose stools, constipation, and colic. Spitting up a small amount of formula, even if it is after every feeding, is usually not a cause for concern. If an infant is regurgitating or vomiting significant amounts, a primary care provider should be consulted. Bilious (green) emesis is always a reason to immediately consult the child's primary care provider.

Loose stools are normal for some infants, especially those receiving human milk or hydrolyzed formulas. They may also be caused by an improperly concentrated formula, overfeeding, or administration of contaminated formula. Human milk–fed infants may have only 1 stool every 1–3 days; however, some infants will have 10–12 stools each day. Formula-fed infants usually have 1–3 stools per day. Diarrhea, defined as increased stool volume and frequency that differ from the usual volume and frequency, warrants medical attention when it persists for more than 3 days or when the infant appears dehydrated. Constipation is rare in human milk– or formula-fed infants; it most

table 25-12 Sterilization Method for Infant Formula Preparation

General Preparation

- Always wash hands before preparing formula or handling bottles and nipples; repeat washing if interrupted.
- Sterilize bottles and other equipment (e.g., glass measuring cup, spoons, nipples, rings, and disks) separately from the formula.[a] Many pediatricians and other primary care providers now consider the use of a dishwasher with a heated drying cycle as adequate for sterilization of infant feeding supplies.
- Using tongs, place all equipment in a deep pan or sterilizer, cover all equipment with cold tap water, bring to a boil, and continue boiling for 5 minutes.
- Tap and bottled water should be heated until it reaches a rolling boil, allowed to continue to boil for 1–2 minutes, and then allowed to cool to room temperature. Boiling for a longer period of time may concentrate impurities (e.g., lead) in the water.
- Using tongs, remove all items from the pan or sterilizer and place on a clean towel. Place bottles and nipples on the towel with their open ends facing down.

Concentrated Liquid Formula

- For cans, wash top of can with hot water and detergent, rinse in hot running water, and dry. Shake can well and open it with a clean punch-type can opener.
- For bottles, the protective cap must be removed. Shake bottle well and open.
- Mix appropriate amounts of concentrated liquid and sterilized water (according to product label or health care provider instructions). For accuracy, use a measuring cup for all measurements of formula and water.
- Pour formula into sterilized bottles; place nipples, rings, and disks on bottles.
- Tightly cover any unused formula and store in refrigerator. Use formula within 48 hours of preparation or discard.

Powdered Formula

- Wash top of can with hot water and detergent, rinse in hot running water, and dry.
- Open can and mix appropriate amounts of powder and sterilized water (according to product label or health care provider instructions). For accuracy, use the scoop provided or a dry measuring cup for all measurements.
- Pour formula into sterilized bottles; place nipples, rings, and disks on the bottles.
- Tightly cover any unused formula and store in the refrigerator. Use formula within 48 hours of preparation.
- Cover any formula remaining in the can with the plastic top. Write the date on the opened can. Store in a cool, dry place for up to 1 month.

Ready-to-Use Formula

Ready-to-Use Cans

- Wash top of can with hot water and detergent, rinse in hot running water, and dry.
- Shake can well, and open it with a clean punch-type can opener.
- Add the amount of formula needed for a single feeding to one sterilized bottle or to the number of bottles needed for a full day's feedings.
- *Do not add water.*
- Prepared bottles and any formula left in the can should be tightly covered and refrigerated for up to 48 hours after the can was opened.

Ready-to-Use Bottles

- The protective cap must be removed, and a sterile nipple must be screwed onto the bottle before feeding.
- Shake each bottle well to ensure mixing of formula.

All Types of Formulas

- Warm bottle to desired temperature by immersing in hot water bath or running under hot water.
- Heating bottles in the microwave is not recommended.
- Never boil or overheat formula.
- Shake each bottle well before feeding infant.
- Test formula temperature before feeding infant.
- After feeding, discard any formula left in bottle, and immediately rinse bottle and nipple in cool water.

[a] If disposable bottle liners are used, only nipples, rings, and screw tops of bottles need to be sterilized; the manufacturer has sterilized the bottle liners.

often results from inadequate formula intake. Severe or prolonged constipation with straining and blood streaks on the stool warrant a visit to the primary care provider.

Product Selection Guidelines

For healthy, term infants, a milk–based formula with or without added whey protein is indicated, except for those who require a therapeutic formula. Recommendations for a formula should be based on the preparation methods, the parents' or caregiver's ability to follow directions, the parents' attitudes and preferences, sanitary conditions and availability of refrigeration facilities, and cost. Before assisting parents in selecting a therapeutic formula, the health care provider should determine whether a primary care provider recommended the formula.

For many parents, cost may be a critical factor in formula selection. Concentrated liquids and powders are typically less expensive than ready-to-use products. Convenience is also a

table 25–13 Average Age-Appropriate Number of Daily Feedings and Volume per Feeding

Age	Average Number of Daily Feedings	Average Volume per Feeding (ounce)
Birth–2 weeks	6–10	2–3
2 weeks–1 month	6–8	4–5
1–3 months	5–6	5–6
3–4 months	4–5	6–7
4–12 months	3–4	7–8

consideration. The preparation of powdered and concentrated liquid formulas requires more manipulative functions and more attention to clean technique. The formula selected should be one that is well tolerated by the infant, convenient for the parents, and priced to fit the family's budget. To simplify formula preparation away from home, parents can select products available in unit-of-use packaging for ready-to-use liquids, or they can place powder packets or powder in an empty bottle and add water whenever needed.

The federal grant program Special Supplemental Nutrition Program for Women, Infants, and Children (WIC) helps ensure that all infants; children (up to 5 years of age); and pregnant, postpartum, and breast-feeding women have access to adequate nutrition. State health departments and other agencies regulate and allocate funds in the federal grant program (i.e., $6.6 billion in FY2012). Formula and preventive services are free to eligible participants. More than 9 million people received WIC benefits each month in 2011, most of them infants and children.[65]

Vitamin and Mineral Supplementation

Routine multivitamin and mineral supplementation is generally unnecessary for most formula- or human milk–fed term infants. However, some infants may be at risk for deficiency and require supplementation. Cases of vitamin D–deficiency rickets continue to be reported in the United States, and the prevalence of iron-deficiency anemia in children ages 1–3 years is 2.1% in the general population.[43,66] Therefore, particular care should be taken to ensure that children in this age group get adequate dietary iron. AAP does not, however, endorse routine iron supplementation in children ages 1–3 years, unless the child's diet is low in iron-containing foods.[43]

Vitamin and mineral supplementation may be needed for preterm and human milk–fed infants whose nutrition is inadequate (Table 25–14).[67] These infants and those with other

table 25–14 Guidelines for Use of Vitamin and Mineral Supplements in Healthy Infants[a]

	Multivitamin/ Mineral	Vitamin D[b]	Vitamin E	Folate	Iron[c]
Full-Term Infants					
Human milk–fed	0	+	0	0	±
Formula-fed	0	±[d]	0	0	0
Preterm Infants					
Human milk–fed[e]	+	+	0	0	+
Formula-fed[e]	+	+	0	0	+
Older Infants (>6 Months)					
Normal	0	0	0	0	±
High-risk[f]	+	0	0	0	±

Key: + = Supplement usually indicated; ± = supplement sometimes indicated; 0 = supplement not usually indicated.

[a] Not shown is vitamin K for newborn infants and fluoride in areas where there is insufficient fluoride in the water (Table 25–15).

[b] All infants should have a minimal intake of 400 international units of vitamin D per day beginning during the first few days of life; this intake should be continued throughout childhood and adolescence.

[c] Iron-fortified formula and infant cereals are more convenient and reliable sources of iron than a supplement.

[d] Supplement typically indicated if receiving less than 1000 mL/day of infant formula. Exception is Enfamil Premium Newborn, which is indicated from birth to 3 months of age and provides 400 international units of vitamin D in 810 mL (27 fl oz).

[e] Multivitamin supplements (plus added folate) are needed primarily when calorie intake is below approximately 300 kcal/day or when the infant weighs less than 2.5 kg; vitamin D should be supplied at least until 6 months of age in human milk–fed infants. Iron should be started by 2 months of age.

[f] Multivitamin/mineral preparations including iron are preferred to supplements containing iron alone.

Source: References 7 and 67.

nutritional deficiencies, malabsorptive and other chronic diseases, rare vitamin-dependent conditions, inborn errors of vitamin or mineral metabolism, or deficiencies related to the intake of certain medications will need medically supervised vitamin and mineral supplementation.

Human Milk–Fed, Full-Term Infants

The healthy, full-term, human milk–fed infant requires little to no special supplementation for the first 4–6 months of life except for vitamin D and iron. AAP recommends vitamin D supplementation (400 international units per day) for all human milk–fed infants unless they are weaned to at least 1000 mL/day of vitamin D–fortified formula. Risk factors for vitamin D deficiency include higher birth order (third child or later), dark skin, cultural factors that minimize maternal skin exposure to sunlight, and delayed intake of dairy products in the infant or mother because of intolerance or other factors.[68] Mothers should be encouraged to maintain a balanced diet and to drink three to five 8-ounce glasses of milk each day while breast-feeding. If the mother cannot tolerate milk because of lactose intolerance, lactose digestion aids (e.g., Lactaid and Dairy Ease) or lactose-free milk are available. Mothers who do not drink milk should be encouraged to increase vitamin D and calcium intake through other dietary sources or by taking supplements. Furthermore, if the infant is showing signs or symptoms of being excessively colicky, the primary care provider should consider a milk sensitivity. If sensitivity is confirmed, the breast-feeding mother should decrease her diary consumption and seek nondairy sources of calcium and vitamin D.

Human milk–fed infants rarely develop iron-deficiency anemia before 4–6 months of age.[43] Although the iron concentration in human milk averages only 0.3–0.5 mg/L, the form of iron is well absorbed. At 4–6 months of age and beyond, the iron stores in infants fed human milk exclusively may become exhausted, requiring a supplemental source. The addition of iron-enriched foods such as fortified infant cereals will usually meet needs, or alternatively, an iron supplement (elemental iron 2 mg/kg/day) can be given. However, a more recent study indicates an association between increased duration of breast-feeding and decreased iron stores in the body.[69] Term infants who are small for gestational age are likely to have higher requirements, but the necessity of supplementation in this population is unclear.[70]

The first iron-enriched food introduced into the infant's diet is typically infant cereal. Bioavailability of the large-particle, electrolytic iron powder used to fortify dry infant cereals is substantially less than ferrous sulfate iron used in milk- or soy protein–based formulas. Cereals also contain potent inhibitors of iron absorption and are unreliable in preventing iron deficiency when infants receive minimal iron from other sources. Iron-fortified, wet-packed cereal and fruit combinations marketed in jars offer no exposure of the iron sulfate to oxygen until the jar is opened; therefore, iron absorption is improved. Consuming fruit juices and other products containing ascorbic acid along with iron-fortified cereals has been shown to enhance iron absorption.[71]

Formula-Fed, Full-Term Infants

Full-term infants who consume adequate amounts of an iron-fortified, milk-based formula do not need vitamin and mineral supplementation in the first 6 months of life. An iron-fortified formula is preferred to ensure adequate iron stores for growing infants. Infants fed iron-fortified formulas do not demonstrate a difference in stool consistency, fussiness, colic, or regurgitation compared with infants fed low-iron formulas. Vitamin and mineral supplements are not needed for infants older than 6 months who receive a diet consisting of formula and increasing amounts of infant and table foods. A multivitamin with minerals may be needed, however, if the infant is at special nutritional risk.

Preterm Infants

Preterm infants fed with either human milk or formula need vitamin and mineral supplementation. Their nutrient needs are greater than those of full-term infants because of their more rapid growth rate, inability to ingest an adequate volume of formula or human milk, decreased intestinal absorption, and decreased body stores. Until these infants can consume about 300 kcal/day or until they reach a body weight of 2.5 kg, a multivitamin supplement should be administered to provide the equivalent of the recommended intakes for full-term infants.

Premature infants are especially susceptible to iron-deficiency anemia because of marginal iron stores at birth. Without supplementation (e.g., blood transfusions), iron stores will be depleted by 2 months of age, in contrast to depletion at 4–6 months of age in full-term infants.

Original AAP/CON recommendations included iron supplementation at a dosage of 2 mg elemental iron per kilogram daily for premature infants with birth weights between 1500 and 2500 grams once they are 2 months old or have doubled their birth weight.[43,51] AAP now recommends that preterm infants who receive human milk should receive elemental iron supplementation (2 mg/kg/day) earlier, within 1 month through 12 months of age. If these preterm infants are transitioned to formula, they will most likely not require iron supplementation once they are consuming 150 mL/kg/day. However, recent reports have shown that approximately 14% of preterm infants receiving appropriate formula will still need a supplement at 4–8 months of age because of decreased iron stores.[43] To prevent such diminished stores, some advocate even earlier initiation of iron supplementation in preterm infants less than 30 weeks gestational age by starting supplementation as early as 2 weeks of age with elemental iron doses of 2–4 mg/kg/day.[72] Infants receiving erythropoietin should receive 6 mg of elemental iron per kilogram daily. To minimize the possibility of hemolytic anemia in infants with insufficient vitamin E absorption, iron supplements should be withheld until the preterm infant is several weeks old. However, with adequate vitamin E supplementation in the formula, the risk of hemolytic anemia is minimal.

Supplementation of calcium, phosphorus, and vitamin D in preterm infant formulas is necessary to ensure adequate bone mineralization and to prevent osteopenia and rickets. The prevention of severe bone disease in preterm infants appears to depend on both high oral intakes of calcium and phosphorus and the intake of at least 400 international units (12.5 mg) of vitamin D per day.[51] Therefore, preterm infants should receive a special preterm infant formula containing appropriate amounts of calcium, phosphorus, and vitamin D. Depending on the volume of formula consumed, vitamin D supplementation may be necessary along with a premature formula to provide 400–800 international units per day.

table

25-15 Recommended Fluoride Supplementation (mg/day)[a]

Age	Fluoride Concentration of Drinking Water (ppm)		
	<0.3	0.3–0.6	>0.6
Recommended Supplementation			
Birth–6 months	0	0	0
6 months–3 years	0.25	0	0
3–6 years	0.50	0.25	0
6–16 years	1.00	0.50	0

[a] Sodium fluoride 2.2 mg contains fluoride 1 mg.
Source: References 73 and 75.

Fluoride Supplementation

When used appropriately, fluoride is both safe and effective in preventing and controlling dental caries. Fluoride reduces dental decay by reducing the solubility of enamel, reducing the ability of bacteria to produce acid, and promoting remineralization. Systemic fluoride, such as that obtained from fluoridated water, primarily provides a topical benefit to teeth, given that fluoride is secreted from the salivary glands.[73] In 2010, the CDC reported 74% of the U.S. population who receive their water supply from a community water system receive adequate fluoride.[74]

Fluoride supplementation is currently not recommended from birth to 6 months of age. Furthermore, the recommended supplementation for children 6 months to 6 years of age whose drinking water is inadequately fluoridated and who do not receive adequate fluoride from other sources has been decreased from previous recommendations because of an increased incidence of fluorosis.[75] Fluorosis, which affects approximately 22% of children, is a change in the appearance of the teeth, ranging from minor white lines running across the teeth to a very chalky appearance resulting from too much fluoride. Infants who are being fed powdered or concentrated formula should be given fluoride supplements only if the community's drinking water, or bottled water used for making formula, contains less than 0.3 ppm of fluoride. Bottled water is often free of fluoride and supplementation should be administered. Table 25–15 can be used to determine the proper fluoride supplementation for a child, depending on the fluoride level in the drinking water. Ready-to-use formulas are manufactured with defluoridated water and contain less than 0.3 ppm of fluoride. The primary care provider may recommend a fluoride supplement for infants not receiving adequate fluoride.

Assessment of Infant Nutrition: A Case-Based Approach

Body weight, length, and head circumference are the growth standards for determining whether infants are receiving the appropriate nutrients, are digesting and absorbing ingested nutrients, or both. If an infant appears to be underweight or underdeveloped, the health care provider should advise the parent to take the infant to a primary care provider for evaluation.

The provider's primary role is to provide information about breast-feeding and infant formula products, including assistance with product selection and preparation instructions.

Cases 25–1 and 25–2 are examples of assessment of infant nutrition.

Patient Counseling for Infant Nutrition

The number and variety of infant formulas available may bewilder some parents. Once the formula type recommended or prescribed by the baby's primary care provider is known, the parents can be directed to the appropriate product. If the parents need further assistance with product selection, a product to match the parents' preferences can be recommended. At these encounters, the parents should be questioned to make sure they know how to properly prepare their baby's formula and how much formula to give at each feeding. The box Patient Education for Infant Nutrition lists specific information to provide parents. In addition, families who may qualify for WIC but are not enrolled can be advised of its availability and benefits.

Key Points for Infant Nutrition and Special Nutritional Needs of Children

➤ Human milk is the optimal food for infants under 12 months of age, and its use should be encouraged for nearly all infants. When breast-feeding or provision of human milk is not possible or desired, commercial infant formulas provide a safe, nutritionally adequate substitute.

➤ Commercial formulas are available in a variety of types to meet the needs of most infants, as well as children with special nutritional needs, such as those with a feeding tube.

➤ Therapeutic formulas designed for infants and children with alterations in requirements caused by disease or other conditions, including prematurity, vary in content and are not generically equivalent. These formulas should be used under medical supervision and are not self-selected.

➤ Accurate preparation of formula is critical to ensure optimal nutrition outcomes. Parents should be counseled on proper preparation techniques.

➤ Some infants will require vitamin and/or mineral supplementation when their needs are not adequately met by their formula intake.

➤ Parents should be referred to their child's primary care provider if their infant or child has persistent vomiting or if at any time the emesis is bilious (green).

➤ Parents should be referred to their child's primary care provider if their infant or child has diarrhea lasting more than 3 days, especially if dehydration develops, if the child looks clinically ill, or if there is blood in the stool.

case
25–1

Relevant Evaluation Criteria	Scenario/Model Outcome

Information Gathering

1. Gather essential information about the patient's symptoms and medical history, including:

a. description of symptom(s) (i.e., nature, onset, duration, severity, associated symptoms)

Emma Miller's mother is worried about Emma spitting up formula after every feeding, almost always with a little force. Although some emesis has occurred since birth, the amount and frequency have increased over the last week. Emma's mother thinks Emma appears to have more gas, often crying from "gas pains." Emma has always been a "good burper" so her mother feels her "gas pains" are not related to too much air in her stomach. The infant girl appears well hydrated and according to her mother, she has no temperature.

b. description of any factors that seem to precipitate, exacerbate, and/or relieve the patient's symptom(s)

Emesis occurs only after feedings. Emma appears to be more comfortable after each episode of emesis. Irritability associated with gas pains appears to be relieved by simethicone.

c. description of the patient's efforts to relieve the symptoms

Emma's mother has been giving simethicone for gas. Nothing specific has been done for the emesis.

d. patient's identity

Emma Miller

e. patient's age, sex, height, and weight

8 weeks old, girl, 23 in., 11 lb 7 oz (5.2 kg)

f. patient's dietary habits

Emma was receiving breast milk exclusively until 1 week ago when her mother stopped breast-feeding. The infant was changed to Similac Advance. Per the mother's report, the formula is being mixed to a standard 20 kcal/ounce concentration according to the instructions on the container. The infant takes approximately 120 mL (4 ounces) every 3 hours. No extra water or juice is given during the day.

g. patient's sleep habits

Emma has not started sleeping through the night yet.

h. concurrent medical conditions, prescription and non-prescription medications, and dietary supplements

Emma is a healthy, term infant without any significant medical conditions or past medical history. Her mother is currently giving her simethicone 20 mg four times a day as needed for gas pain. Emma's mother reports she usually gives about 2–3 doses per day.

i. allergies

NKA

j. history of other adverse reactions to medications

None

k. other (describe) _____

NA

Assessment and Triage

2. Differentiate patient's signs/symptoms and correctly identify the patient's primary problem(s).

Primary problem: emesis with feedings

Secondary problem: increased intestinal gas

3. Identify exclusions for self-treatment.

Bloody or bilious emesis

Signs of dehydration: sunken fontanelle, dry mucous membranes, decreased wet diapers, dark urine, decreased oral intake

4. Formulate a comprehensive list of therapeutic alternatives for the primary problem to determine if triage to a medical provider is required, and share this information with the patient or caregiver.

Options include:

(1) Refer Emma to immediate medical attention/PCP.

(2) Review preparation of infant formula with Emma's mother.

(3) Monitor Emma's symptoms and recommend nondrug measures only.

(4) Recommend a medication alone or combined with nondrug measures.

(5) Take no action.

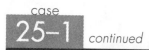

case
25–1 continued

Relevant Evaluation Criteria	Scenario/Model Outcome

Plan

5. Select an optimal therapeutic alternative to address the patient's problem, taking into account patient preferences.

Emma's current feeding schedule, 120 mL of 20 kcal/oz formula every 3 hours, provides 185 mL/kg/day and 123 kcal/kg/day. Both are within the usual recommended intakes for a healthy, term infant (Tables 25–2 and 25–13). Because the emesis and gas pain have increased since Emma was transitioned from breast-feeding to infant formula, Emma most likely does not tolerate the bovine milk proteins found within Similac Advance, but she needs to be seen by her PCP for further assessment. Explain the correlation between the increased emesis and gas pain and the transition to milk protein–containing formula. Recommend Emma see her PCP to discuss changing to either a soy-based formula such as Similac Soy Isomil or to a partially hydrolyzed formula such as Similac Expert Care Alimentum. If Emma continues to have problems after a change in formula, she should follow up with her PCP for further management.

6. Describe the recommended therapeutic approach to the patient or caregiver.

"The increased emesis and gas pain are caused by the transition from breast-feeding to a formula containing cow milk protein. A change in the infant formula type such as soy formula or a partially hydrolyzed formula should improve Emma's symptoms. If the symptoms persist after the change in formulations, Emma should be seen again by her PCP."

7. Explain to the patient or caregiver the rationale for selecting the recommended therapeutic approach from the considered therapeutic alternatives.

"Because the symptoms started (or acutely worsened) with the change from breast milk to infant formula, and both the caloric density and the volume of the infant formula are appropriate for a healthy, term infant, intolerance to cow milk protein is the most likely cause of Emma's emesis and irritability. If cow milk protein intolerance is the major issue, changing the formula should produce relief of symptoms within several days."

Patient Education

8. When recommending self-care with nonprescription medications and/or nondrug therapy, convey accurate information to the patient or caregiver:

   a. product storage requirements

"Infant formula should be used soon after mixing or kept tightly covered in the refrigerator and used within 24 hours of preparation. See product information for any specific storage requirements."

   b. specific nondrug measures

NA

Solicit follow-up questions from the patient or caregiver.

"What if Emma continues to have emesis and gas pain after seeing the PCP and changing formulas?"

Answer the patient's or caregiver's questions.

"From the history, it sounds like Emma might have a cow milk protein intolerance. If she receives a soy or partially hydrolyzed formula, she should have improvement in her emesis and gas pains. If a change in formula does not improve her symptoms, her PCP will further assess her GI intolerance."

Evaluation of Patient Outcome

9. Assess patient outcome.

Ask the patient's mothers to call in 2–3 days to update you on Emma's response to your recommendations; or you could call her in 2–3 days to evaluate the response. If no improvement has been made, ensure that the mother has made an appointment with Emma's PCP to further management.

Key: GI = Gastrointestinal; NA = not applicable; NKA = no known allergies; PCP = primary care provider.

case
25–2

Relevant Evaluation Criteria	Scenario/Model Outcome

Information Gathering

1. Gather essential information about the patient's symptoms and medical history, including:

a. description of symptom(s) (i.e., nature, onset, duration, severity, associated symptoms)

Stephen Shultz is a healthy-appearing 4-month-old, term infant. His mother comes to the pharmacy today because she is wondering if she should start to give Stephen vitamins because he is exclusively breast-fed. Her pediatrician suggested this at his recent well child checkup.

b. description of any factors that seem to precipitate, exacerbate, and/or relieve the patient's symptom(s)

None

c. description of the patient's efforts to relieve the symptoms

NA

d. patient's identity

Stephen Schultz

e. age, sex, length, and weight

4 months old, boy born at 38 weeks gestational age, 25 in., birth weight 15 lb 2 oz (6.9 kg)

f. patient's occupation

NA

g. patient's dietary habits

Stephen's mother is still on maternity leave. Stephen is exclusively breast-fed, eating approximately every 3–4 hours during the day.

h. patient's sleep habits

He sleeps from 10 pm to 6 am.

i. concurrent medical conditions, prescription and nonprescription medications, and dietary supplements

Stephen is a healthy, term infant with no preexisting medical conditions. He currently takes no prescription or nonprescription medications and no dietary supplements.

j. allergies

NKA

k. history of other adverse reactions to medications

None

l. other (describe) _____

NA

Assessment and Triage

2. Differentiate patient's signs/symptoms and correctly identify the patient's primary problem(s).

Potential for vitamin D and iron deficiency due to age and exclusive breast-fed diet.

3. Identify exclusions for self-treatment.

None

4. Formulate a comprehensive list of therapeutic alternatives for the primary problem to determine if triage to a medical provider is required, and share this information with the patient or caregiver.

Options include:

(1) Refer to the PCP.

(2) Recommend an over-the-counter multivitamin with iron.

(3) Take no action.

Plan

5. Select an optimal therapeutic alternative to address the patient's problem, taking into account patient preferences.

Recommend a standard infant multivitamin containing ferrous sulfate.

6. Describe the recommended therapeutic approach to the patient or caregiver.

"Your PCP suggested a multivitamin since Stephen is now 4 months of age and is exclusively breast-fed. I would recommend a standard infant multivitamin containing ferrous sulfate."

7. Explain to the patient or caregiver the rationale for selecting the recommended therapeutic approach from the considered therapeutic alternatives.

"Term infants have approximately a 4- to 6-month store of iron reserves in their bodies. Human milk is very low in iron but meets most infants' needs for the first 4–6 months. Moreover, Stephen's need for adequate vitamin D currently exceeds the amount provided in breast milk. For these reasons, your PCP suggested you start giving a daily multivitamin containing iron."

Patient Education

8. When recommending self-care with nonprescription medications and/or nondrug therapy, convey accurate information to the patient or caregiver:

a. appropriate dose and frequency of administration

"Infant multivitamin with iron (e.g., Enfamil Poly-Vi-Sol with Iron Drops) 1 mL by mouth daily."

b. maximum number of days the therapy should be employed

"Until recommended to discontinue per Stephen's PCP."

case

25-2 *continued*

Relevant Evaluation Criteria	Scenario/Model Outcome
c. product administration procedures	"Measure liquid using the dropper that comes with the medication and have Stephen swallow the liquid."
d. expected time to onset of relief	NA
e. degree of relief that can be reasonably expected	NA
f. Most common side effects	"Side effects are rare but gastrointestinal effects are possible. Give the iron drops with food if these effects occur."
g. Side effects that warrant medical attention	"Contact a health care provider if signs of an allergic reaction, such as a rash or trouble breathing, occur after a dose is given."
h. Patient's options in the event that condition worsens or persists	NA
i. Product storage requirements	"Keep medication in a tightly secured container away from any extreme temperature and out of children's reach."
j. Specific nondrug measures	NA
Solicit follow-up questions from the patient or caregiver.	"What do I do if Stephen spits out a dose of the multivitamin product?"
Answer the patient's or caregiver's questions.	"If Stephen spits out a dose of the multivitamin product, do not try to give the dose again. The medication is not so vital that it must be given each day for a medical condition, and Stephen could potentially receive too much iron if given multiple doses. Be cautious of the potential for the multivitamin product to stain clothing."

Evaluation of Patient Outcome

9. Assess patient outcome.	Ask Stephen's mother to call to update you on his response to your recommendations; or you could call her in a week to evaluate his response.

Key: NA = Not applicable; NKA = no known allergies; PCP = primary care provider.

patient education for

Infant Nutrition

Optimal nutrition is critical in infants and children to ensure normal growth and development. Parents who carefully follow product instructions and the measures listed here will help ensure optimal nutrition-related outcomes.

- Check unopened formula containers for damage. Do not use products if they are significantly dented or if the expiration date has passed.
- When preparing formula from powder or liquid concentrate, carefully follow instructions for diluting the formula to the desired caloric density (Tables 25–9 and 25–10). If the formula is too concentrated, the baby may have diarrhea or become dehydrated. If it is too dilute, the baby can become water intoxicated, which might lead to irritability, seizures, coma, or brain damage.
- When preparing formula from powder or liquid concentrate, follow the technique for aseptic sterilization. Be sure to sterilize the bottles (or use sterile liners) and other equipment, and boil the water used to make the formula (Table 25–12).
- When preparing ready-to-use formulas, do not add water to the formula. Follow the instructions in Table 25–12. Be sure to sterilize the bottles (or use sterile liners) and other equipment.
- Use prepared or opened ready-to-use formula within 48 hours. Keep refrigerated.
- Feed your baby according to the frequency and quantities listed in Table 25–13 unless instructed otherwise by the baby's primary care provider. Paying careful attention to your infant's hunger and fullness cues is important to avoid over- and underfeeding. Discuss any concerns with your infant's primary care provider.
- Heating formula in a microwave is not recommended. However, if formula or human milk is warmed in a microwave, follow the instructions below to prevent exploding containers, scalds, or burns to the baby's mouth:
  - Remove the bottle's lid to allow heat to escape.
  - Heat only 4 ounces or more of refrigerated milk; do not thaw frozen human milk in a microwave. Place frozen human milk in a tepid water bath to thaw.
  - Heat 4 ounces of refrigerated formula on full power for no longer than 30 seconds; heat 8 ounces of refrigerated formula for 45 seconds.
  - After heating the formula, replace the nipple assembly and invert the bottle a minimum of 10 times.
  - Test the formula's temperature by putting a few drops on your tongue or the top part of your hand or the back of the wrist. Do not feed the baby the formula unless it feels cool to the touch.

When to Seek Medical Attention

- Seek medical attention if:
  - Your baby is regurgitating or vomiting significant amounts of formula. A small amount of spitting up is normal. Projectile vomiting or bilious vomiting (i.e., green) always requires immediate medical attention.
  - Your baby has severe diarrhea or diarrhea that persists for more than 3 days.
  - Your baby appears dehydrated (e.g., decreased number of wet diapers, dark urine, limp, no tears, or lethargic).
  - Your baby's stools have blood in them.

REFERENCES

1. Grummer-Strawn LM, Reinold C, Krebs NF; Centers for Disease Control and Prevention (CDC). Use of World Health Organization and CDC growth charts for children aged 0–59 months in the United States. *MMWR Recomm Rep.* 2010;59(RR-9):1–15. Accessed at http://www.cdc.gov/mmwr/pdf/rr/rr5909.pdf, June 11, 2013.

2. Committee on Nutrition, American Academy of Pediatrics. Infant nutrition and the development of gastrointestinal function. In: Kleinman RE, ed. *Pediatric Nutrition Handbook.* 6th ed. Elk Grove Village, IL: American Academy of Pediatrics; 2008:3–28.

3. Branski D. Disorders of malabsorption. In: Kliegman RM, Stanton BF, St. Gene JW, et al., eds. *Nelson Textbook of Pediatrics.* 19th ed. Philadelphia, PA: Elsevier Science; 2011:1304–22.

4. Bull MJ and Committee on Genetics. Health supervision for children with Down syndrome. *Pediatrics.* 2011;128(2):393–406. doi: 10.1542/peds.2011-1605. Accessed at http://pediatrics.aappublications.org/content/128/2/393.full.pdf+html, June 11, 2013.

5. Krebs NF, Himes JH, Jacobson D, et al. Assessment of child and adolescent overweight and obesity. *Pediatrics.* 2007;120(suppl 4):S193–228. Accessed at http://pediatrics.aappublications.org/content/120/Supplement_4/S193.full.pdf+html, June 11, 2013.

6. Ogden CL, Carroll MD, Kit BK, et al. Prevalence of obesity and trends in body mass index among US children and adolescents, 1999–2010. *JAMA.* 2012;307(5):483–90. doi: 10.1001/jama.2012.40. Accessed at http://jama.jamanetwork.com/article.aspx?articleid=1104932, June 11, 2013.

7. Institute of Medicine, Food and Nutrition Board, Standing Committee on the Scientific Evaluation of Dietary Reference Intakes. *Dietary Reference Intakes for Energy, Carbohydrate, Fiber, Fat, Fatty Acids, Cholesterol, Protein, and Amino Acids.* Washington, DC: National Academy Press; 2005. Accessed at http://www.nap.edu, May 19, 2013.

8. Committee on Nutrition, American Academy of Pediatrics. Carbohydrate and dietary fiber. In: Kleinman RE, ed. *Pediatric Nutrition Handbook.* 6th ed. Elk Grove Village, IL: American Academy of Pediatrics; 2008:343–56.

9. Heird WC. Taurine in neonatal nutrition—revisited. *Arch Dis Child Fetal Neonatal.* 2004;89(6):473–4.

10. Daniels SR, Greer FR; Committee on Nutrition, American Academy of Pediatrics. Lipid screening and cardiovascular health in childhood. *Pediatrics.* 2008;122(1):198–208. Accessed at http://pediatrics.aappublications.org/content/122/1/198.full.pdf+html, June 11, 2013.

11. Lapillonne A, Groh-Wargo S, Gonzalez GHL, et al. Lipid needs of preterm infants: updated recommendations. *J Pediatr.* 2013;162(3 suppl):S37–47. doi: 10.1016/j.jpeds.2012.11.052.

12. Koletzko B, Lien E, Agostoni C, et al. The roles of long-chain polyunsaturated fatty acids in pregnancy, lactation and infancy: review of current knowledge and consensus recommendations. *J Perinat Med.* 2008;36(1):5–14. doi: 10.1515/JPM.2008.001.

13. Smithers LG, Gibson RA, McPhee A, et al. Effect of long-chain polyunsaturated fatty acid supplementation of preterm infants on disease risk and neurodevelopment: a systematic review of randomized controlled trials. *Am J Clin Nutr.* 2008;87:912–20. Accessed at http://ajcn.nutrition.org/content/87/4/912.full.pdf+html, June 11, 2013.

14. Simmer K, Patole SK, Rao SC. Long chain polyunsaturated fatty acid supplementation in infants born at term. *Cochrane Database Syst Rev.* 2008;1:CD000376. doi: 10.1002/14651858.CD000376.pub3. Accessed at http://www.thecochranelibrary.com/view/0/index.html.

15. Simmer K, Schulzke SM, Patole S. Long chain polyunsaturated fatty acid supplementation in preterm infants. *Cochrane Database Syst Rev.* 2008;1:CD000375. doi: 10.1002/14651858.CD000375.pub4. Accessed at http://www.thecochranelibrary.com/view/0/index.html.

16. de Jong C, Kikkert HK, Fidler V, et al. The Groningen LCPUFA study: no effect of postnatal long-chain polyunsaturated fatty acids in healthy term infants on neurological condition at 9 years. *Br J Nutr.* 2010;104(4):566–72. doi: 10.1017/S0007114510000863. Accessed at http://journals.cambridge.org/download.php?file=%2FBJN%2FBJN104_04%2FS0007114510000863a.pdf&code=54b9ae47a85e3524be3d4e84592ebdd3, June 11, 2013.

17. Birch EE, Carlson SE, Hoffman DR, et al. The DIAMOND (DHA Intake and Measurement of Neural Development) Study: a double-masked, randomized controlled clinical trial of the maturation of infant visual acuity as a function of the dietary level of docosahexaenoic acid. *Am J Clin Nutr.* 2010;91(4):848–59. doi:10.3945/ajcn.2009.28557. Accessed at http://ajcn.nutrition.org/content/91/4/848.full.pdf+html, June 11, 2013.

18. Beyerlein A, Hadders-Algra M, Kennedy K, et al. Infant formula supplementation with long-chain polyunsaturated fatty acids has no effect on Bayley developmental scores at 18 months of age—IPD meta-analysis of 4 large clinical trials. *J Pediatr Gastroenterol Nutr.* 2010;50(1):79–84. doi: 10.1097/MPG.0b013e3181acae7d. Accessed at http://journals.lww.com/jpgn/pages/articleviewer.aspx?year=2010&issue=01000&article=00020&type=abstract, June 11, 2013.

19. Campoy C, Escolano-Margarit MV, Anjos T, et al. Omega 3 fatty acids on child growth, visual acuity and neurodevelopment. *J Perinatol.* 2012;32(8):598–603. doi: 10.1038/jp.2011.152. Accessed at http://journals.cambridge.org/download.php?file=%2FBJN%2FBJN107_S2%2FS0007114512001493a.pdf&code=8d507567cc6150dcbe3d4e84592ebdd3, June 11, 2013.

20. Atwell K, Collins CT, Sullivan TR, et al. Respiratory hospitalization of infants supplemented with docosahexaenoic acid as preterm neonates. *J Paediatr Child Health.* 2013;49(1):E17–22. doi: 10.1111/jpc.12057. Accessed on http://onlinelibrary.wiley.com/doi/10.1111/jpc.12057/pdf, June 11, 2013.

21. Birch EE, Khoury JC, Berseth CL, et al. The impact of early nutrition on incidence of allergic manifestations and common respiratory illnesses in children. *J Pediatr.* 2010;156(6):902–6, 906.e1. doi: 10.1016/j.peds.2010.01.002. Accessed at http://download.journals.elsevierhealth.com/pdfs/journals/0022-3476/PIIS002234761000003X.pdf, June 11, 2013.

22. Drover JR, Felius J, Hoffman DR, et al. A randomized trial of DHA intake during infancy: school readiness and receptive vocabulary at 2–3.5 years of age. *Early Hum Dev.* 2012;88(11):885–91. doi: 10.1016/j.earlhumdev.2012.07.007.

23. Isaacs EB, Ross S, Kennedy K, et al. 10-year cognition in preterms after random assignment to fatty acid supplementation in infancy. *Pediatrics.* 2011;128(4):e890–8. doi: 10.1542/peds.2010-3153. Accessed at http://pediatrics.aappublications.org/content/128/4/e890.full.pdf+html, June 11, 2013.

24. Campoy C, Escolano-Margarit MV, Ramos R, et al. Effects of prenatal fish-oil and 5-methyltetrahydrofolate supplementation on cognitive development of children at 6.5 y of age. *Am J Clin Nutr.* 2011;94(6 suppl):1880S–8S. doi: 10.3945/ajcn.110.001107. Epub 2011 Aug 17. Accessed at http://ajcn.nutrition.org/content/94/6_Suppl/1880S.full.pdf+html, June 11, 2013.

25. Beyerlein A, Hadders-Algra M, Kennedy K, et al. Infant formula supplementation with long-chain polyunsaturated fatty acids has no effect on Bayley development scores at 18 months of age—IPD meta-analysis of 4 large clinical trials. *J Pediatr Gastroenterol Nutr.* 2010;50(1):79–84. doi: 10.1097/MPG.0b013e3181acae7d. Accessed at http://journals.lww.com/jpgn/pages/articleviewer.aspx?year=2010&issue=01000&article=00020&type=abstract, June 11, 2013.

26. Hadders-Algra M. Prenatal long-chain polyunsaturated fatty acid status: the importance of a balanced intake of docosahexaenoic acid and arachidonic acid. *J Perinat Med.* 2008;36(2):101–9. doi: 10.1515/JPM.2008.029.

27. Muhlhausler BS, Gibson RA, Makrides M. Effect of long-chain polyunsaturated fatty acid supplementation during pregnancy or lactation on infant and child body composition: a systematic review. *Am J Clin Nutr.* 2010;92(4):857–63. doi: 10.3945/ajcn.2010.29495. Accessed at http://ajcn.nutrition.org/content/92/4/857.full.pdf+html, June 11, 2013.

28. World Health Organization. *Global Strategy for Infant and Young Child Feeding.* Geneva, Switzerland: World Health Organization; 2003. Accessed at http://www.who.int/nutrition/publications/gs_infant_feeding_text_eng.pdf, May 19, 2013.

29. Section on Breastfeeding, American Academy of Pediatrics. Breastfeeding and the use of human milk. *Pediatrics.* 2012;129(3):e827–41. doi: 10.1542/peds.2011-3552. Accessed at http://pediatrics.aappublications.org/content/129/3/e827.full.pdf+html, June 11, 2013.

30. Horta BL, Victora CG. Long-term effects of breastfeeding: a systematic review. World Geneva, Switzerland: Health Organization, 2013. Accessed at http://apps.who.int/iris/bitstream/10665/79198/1/9789241505307_eng.pdf, June 11, 2013.

31. McDowell MM, Wang C-Y, Kennedy-Stephensen J. Breastfeeding in the United States: findings from the National Health and Nutrition Examination Surveys, 1999–2006. Hyattsville, MD: National Center for Health Statistics; 2008. NCHS Data Brief, No 5. Accessed at http://www.cdc.gov/nchs/data/databriefs/db05.pdf, May 19, 2013.

32. Centers for Disease Control and Prevention. Breastfeeding among US children born 2000–2010: CDC National Immunization Survey. Centers for Disease Control and Prevention, Atlanta, Georgia, July 2013. Accessed at http://www.cdc.gov/breastfeeding/data/NIS_data/index.htm, January 2, 2014.

33. Centers for Disease Control and Prevention. Breastfeeding report card—United States, 2013. July 2013. Accessed at http://www.cdc.gov/breastfeeding/pdf/2013BreastfeedingReportCard.pdf, January 2, 2014.

34. U.S. Department of Health and Human Services. *Healthy People 2020: National Health Promotion and Disease Prevention Objectives.* Washington, DC: U.S. Government Printing Office; 2010. Accessed at http://www.healthypeople.gov/2020/default.aspx, June 11, 2013.

35. Batrick M. Breastfeeding and the U.S. economy. *Breastfeed Med.* 2011;6:313–8. doi: 10.1089/bfm.2011.0057. Accessed at http://online.liebertpub.com/doi/pdf/10.1089/bfm.2011.0057, June 11, 2013.

36. Tuttle DR, Siavit WI. Establishing the business case for breastfeeding. *Breastfeed Med.* 2009;4(suppl 1):S59–62. doi: 10.1089/bfm.2009.0031.

37. Ball TM, Bennett DM. The economic impact of breastfeeding. *Pediatr Clin North Am.* 2001;48(1):253–62.

38. Rasmussen KM, Geraghty SR. The quiet revolution: breastfeeding transformed with the use of breast pumps. *Am J Public Health.* 2011; 101(8):1356–9. doi: 10.2105/AJPH.2011.300136. Accessed at http://www.ncbi.nlm.nih.gov/pmc/articles/PMC3134520/pdf/1356.pdf, January 2, 2014.

39. Briggs GG, Freeman RK, Yaffee SJ, eds. *Drugs in Pregnancy and Lactation.* 9th ed. Philadelphia, PA: Lippincott Williams & Wilkins; 2011.

40. Hale TW. *Medications & Mothers' Milk 2012.* 15th ed. Amarillo, TX: Hale Publishing; 2012.

41. Jones F. History of North American donor milk banking: one hundred years of progress. *J Hum Lact.* 2003;19(3):313–8. Accessed at http://jhl.sagepub.com/cgi/content/abstract/19/3/313, June 2, 2013.

42. Committee on Nutrition, American Academy of Pediatrics. Formula feeding of term infants. In: Kleinman RE, ed. *Pediatric Nutrition Handbook.* 6th ed. Elk Grove Village, IL: American Academy of Pediatrics; 2008:61–78.

43. Baker RD, Greer FR; Committee on Nutrition American Academy of Pediatrics. Diagnosis and prevention of iron deficiency and iron-deficiency anemia in infants and young children (0–3 years of age). *Pediatrics.* 2010;126(5):1040–50. doi:10.1542/peds.2010-2576. Accessed at http://pediatrics.aappublications.org/content/126/5/1040.full.pdf+html, June 6, 2013.

44. Fomon SJ, Ziegler EE. Renal solute load and potential renal solute load in infancy. *J Pediatr.* 1999;134(1):11–4.

45. Fomon SJ. Potential renal solute load: considerations related to complementary feedings of breastfed infants. *Pediatrics.* 2000;106(5 suppl):1284.

46. Centers for Disease Control and Prevention. Enterobacter sakazakii infections associated with the use of powdered infant formula—Tennessee, 2001. *MMWR Morb Mortal Wkly Rep.* 2002;51(RR-15):297–300. Accessed at http://www.cdc.gov/mmwr/PDF/wk/mm5114.pdf, June 11, 2013.

47. U.S. Food and Drug Administration. FDA expands caution about Simply-Thick. U.S. Food and Drug Administration, Silver Spring, MD, September 18, 2012. Accessed at http://www.fda.gov/ForConsumers/ConsumerUpdates/ucm256250.htm, June 2, 2013.

48. Bhatia J, Greer F; American Academy of Pediatrics Committee on Nutrition. Use of soy protein-based formulas in infant feeding. *Pediatrics.* 2008;121(5):1062–8. doi: 10.1542/peds.2008-0564. Accessed at http://pediatrics.aappublications.org/content/121/5/1062.full.pdf+html, June 11, 2013.

49. Greer FR, Sicherer SH, Burks AW; American Academy of Pediatrics Committee on Nutrition; American Academy of Pediatrics Section on Allergy and Immunology. Effects of early nutritional interventions on the development of atopic disease in infants and children: the role of maternal dietary restriction, breastfeeding, timing of introduction of complementary

foods, and hydrolyzed formulas. *Pediatrics.* 2008;121(1):183–91. doi: 10.1542/peds.2007-3022. Accessed at http://pediatrics.aappublications.org/content/121/1/183.full.pdf+html?sid=c4681050-2e74-4a5e-af02-6855c87e5a86, June 6, 2013.

50. Ellis L, Kalnias D, Corey M, et al. Do infants with cystic fibrosis need a protein hydrolysate formula? A prospective, randomized, comparative study. *J Pediatr.* 1998;132(2):270–6.

51. Committee on Nutrition, American Academy of Pediatrics. Nutritional needs of preterm infants. In: Kleinman RE, ed. *Pediatric Nutrition Handbook.* 6th ed. Elk Grove Village, IL: American Academy of Pediatrics; 2008:79–112.

52. Underwood MA. Human milk for the premature infant. *Pediatr Clin North Am.* 2013;60(1):189–207. doi: 10.1016/j.pcl.2012.09.008.

53. Reis BB, Hall RT, Schanler RJ, et al. Enhanced growth of preterm infants fed a new powdered human milk fortifier: a randomized, controlled trial. *Pediatrics.* 2000;106(3):581–8.

54. Porcelli P, Schanler R, Greer F, et al. Growth in human milk-fed very low birth weight infants receiving a new human milk fortifier. *Ann Nutr Metab.* 2000;44(1):2–10.

55. Slykerman RF, Thompson JM, Becroft DM, et al. Breastfeeding and intelligence of preschool children. *Acta Pediatr.* 2005;94(7):832–7.

56. Sullivan S, Schanler RJ, Kim JH, et al. An exclusively human milk-based diet is associated with a lower rate of necrotizing enterocolitis than a diet of human milk and bovine milk-based products. *J Pediatr.* 2010 Apr;156(4):562–7. e1. doi: 10.1016/j.jpeds.2009.10.040. Accessed at http://ac.els-cdn.com/S0022347609010853/1-s2.0-S0022347609010853-main.pdf?_tid=511a68ae-d21c-11e2-a68f-00000aacb361&acdnat=1370903163_b1643cff6c820b0aaf5dd21c85929554, June 10, 2013.

57. Ganapathy V, Hay JW, Kim JH. Costs of necrotizing enterocolitis and cost-effectiveness of exclusively human milk-based products in feeding extremely premature infants. *Breastfeed Med.* 2012 Feb;7(1):29–37. doi: 10.1089/bfm.2011.0002. Accessed at http://online.liebertpub.com/doi/pdf/10.1089/bfm.2011.0002, June 10, 2013.

58. U.S. Food and Drug Administration, Center for Food Safety and Applied Nutrition. Exempt infant formulas marketed in the United States by manufacturer and category. March 22, 2013. Accessed at http://www.fda.gov/Food/GuidanceRegulation/GuidanceDocumentsRegulatoryInformation/InfantFormula/ucm106456.htm, June 6, 2013.

59. Centers for Disease Control and Prevention. Managing acute gastroenteritis among children: oral rehydration, maintenance, and nutritional therapy. *MMWR Morb Mortal Wkly Rep.* 2003;52(RR-16):1–20. Accessed at http://www.cdc.gov/mmwr/PDF/rr/rr5216.pdf, June 6, 2013.

60. Tudehope D, Fewtrell M, Kashyap S, et al. Nutritional needs of the micropreterm infant. *J Pediatr.* 2013 Mar;162(3 suppl):S72–80. doi: 10.1016/j.jpeds.2012.11.056.

61. Caufield PW, Griffen AL. Dental caries: an infectious and transmissible disease. *Pediatr Clin North Am.* 2000;47(5):1001–20.

62. Committee on Nutrition, American Academy of Pediatrics. Aluminum toxicity in infants and children. *Pediatrics.* 1996;97(3):413–6. Accessed at http://pediatrics.aappublications.org/content/97/3/413.full.pdf+html?sid=35eaebf7-76d7-45b5-8313-a602cc7052f, June 6, 2013. [Guideline reaffirmed by AAP in January 2004.]

63. Committee on Environmental Health and Committee on Infectious Diseases. Drinking water from private wells and risks to children. *Pediatrics.* 2009;123(6);1599–605. doi: 10.1542/peds.2009-0751. Accessed at http://pediatrics.aappublications.org/content/123/6/1599.full.pdf+html, June 11, 2013.

64. World Health Organization; Food and Agriculture Organization of the United Nations. Safe Preparation, Storage and Handling of Powdered Infant Formula: Guidelines. 2007. Geneva, Switzerland: World Health Organization; 2007. Accessed at http://www.who.int/foodsafety/publications/micro/pif_guidelines.pdf, June 10, 2013.

65. U.S. Department of Agriculture, Food and Nutrition Service. WIC: the Special Supplemental Nutrition Program for Women, Infants and Children. Accessed at http://www.fns.usda.gov/wic, June 6, 2013.

66. Abrams SA; Committee on Nutrition. Calcium and vitamin D requirements of enterally fed preterm infants. *Pediatrics.* 2013;131(5):e1676–83. doi: 10.1542/peds.2013-0420. Accessed at http://pediatrics.aappublications.org/content/131/5/e1676.full.pdf+html, June 11, 2013.

67. Committee on Nutrition, American Academy of Pediatrics. Vitamins. In: Kleinman RE, ed. *Pediatric Nutrition Handbook.* 6th ed. Elk Grove Village, IL: American Academy of Pediatrics; 2008:453–96.

68. Wagner CL, Greer FR; American Academy of Pediatrics Section on Breastfeeding; American Academy of Pediatrics Committee on Nutrition. Prevention of rickets and vitamin D deficiency in infants, children, and adolescents. *Pediatrics.* 2008;122(5):1142–52. doi: 10.1542/peds.2008-1862. Accessed at http://pediatrics.aappublications.org/content/122/5/1142.full.pdf+html?sid=519c6127-5422-4dfe-91dd-7f0dc3ff55ab, June 6, 2013.

69. Maguire JL, Salehi L, Birken CS, et al. Association between total duration of breastfeeding and iron deficiency. *Pediatrics.* 2013;131(5);e1530. doi: 10.1542/peds/2012-2465.

70. Griffin IJ, Abrams SA. Iron and breastfeeding. *Pediatr Clin North Am.* 2001;48(2):401–13.

71. Lynch SR, Stoltzfus RJ. Iron and ascorbic acid: proposed fortification levels and recommended iron compounds. *J Nutr.* 2003;133(9):2978S–84S.

Accessed at http://jn.nutrition.org/content/133/9/2978S.full.pdf+html, June 11, 2013.

72. Tudehope D, Fewtrell M, Kashyap S, et al. Nutritional needs of the micropreterm infant. *J Pediatr.* 2013 March;162(3 suppl):S72–80. doi: 10.1016/j.jpeds.2012.11.056.

73. Committee on Nutrition, American Academy of Pediatrics. Nutrition and oral health. In: Kleinman RE, ed. *Pediatric Nutrition Handbook.* 6th ed. Elk Grove Village, IL: American Academy of Pediatrics; 2009:1041–56.

74. Centers for Disease Control and Prevention. 2010 water fluoridation statistics. July 27, 2012. Accessed at http://www.cdc.gov/fluoridation/statistics/2010stats.htm, June 11, 2013.

75. Centers for Disease Control and Prevention. Recommendations for using fluoride to prevent and control dental caries in the United States. *MMWR Morb Mortal Wkly Rep.* 2001;50 (RR-14):1–59. Accessed at http://www.cdc.gov/mmwr/PDF/rr/rr5014.pdf, June 11, 2013.

OVERWEIGHT AND OBESITY

Sarah J. Miller and Cathy L. Bartels

Obesity rates have increased at an alarming rate since the mid-1970s. Overweight and obesity are significant because they are associated with increased morbidity and mortality from various conditions, including cardiovascular diseases (CVD), type 2 diabetes mellitus (type 2 DM), gallbladder disease, osteoarthritis, obstructive sleep apnea, nonalcoholic steatohepatitis, and several cancers.[1] In the United States, increasing concern centers on overweight and obesity in children and adolescents.

The National Health and Nutrition Examination Surveys (NHANES) of the U.S. population have tracked prevalence of overweight and obesity in adults from 1960 to the present. These surveys have demonstrated a marked increase in obesity in both men and women across all age and ethnic groups. More than one-third of U.S. adults are currently obese (Figure 26–1).[2] Increases in obesity prevalence appear to have slowed for both females and males between 1999 and 2010, but the percentage of morbidly obese adults continues to rise.[3] Figure 26–1 also illustrates the changes in prevalence of the overweight population across recent NHANES surveys. These have remained fairly stable at 32%–34%.[2]

Prevalence of obesity during childhood and adolescence, as tracked by the NHANES data, has risen considerably, as shown in Figure 26–2.[2] These increases also appear to have slowed over the period 1999–2010.[4]

The economic impact of overweight and obesity is substantial. The estimated direct medical costs of obesity are as high as $147 billion annually.[5] The Institute of Medicine recently estimated that obesity-related illness costs about $190 billion, accounting for more than 20% of annual health spending in the United States.[6] Quantification of costs that are directly due to obesity is difficult, given that many comorbidities of obesity have other etiologies.

Americans spend billions of dollars on weight-control products and services annually. Use of nonprescription or dietary supplement weight-loss products is very common. Health care providers should be knowledgeable in discussing benefits as well as limitations and potential harm of weight-loss products and should be comfortable in recommending effective nonpharmacologic lifestyle changes such as diet and exercise. If patients need additional strategies, the provider may then refer them for consideration of prescription weight-loss therapies.

Clinical Indicators of Overweight and Obesity

The 2013 American Heart Association/American College of Cardiology/The Obesity Society (AHA/ACC/TOS) "Guideline for the Management of Overweight and Obesity in Adults"

defines overweight and obesity in adults by body mass index (BMI), a parameter that takes into account both height and weight.[7] The U.S. Preventive Services Task Force (USPSTF) on screening for and management of obesity also recommends BMI for screening of obesity.[8] Table 26–1 illustrates BMI values for persons of various heights and weights and gives equations for calculation of the BMI. Overweight is defined in adults as a BMI of 25–29.9 (kg/m²) and obesity as a BMI of 30 or greater.

There are limitations to the exclusive use of BMI as an indicator of overweight and obesity, as it does not take into account extreme variation in body composition. Very muscular persons, for example, may be classified by BMI as overweight or obese when, in fact, they are not carrying excessive adipose tissue. Alternatively, some people with BMI in the desirable range may have less than optimal muscle mass and high body fat. Some of these persons may be classified as "metabolically obese normal weight," with increased insulin resistance, hypertriglyceridemia, and a predisposition to type 2 DM and CVD.[9] Finally, ethnic groups may differ in what BMI range is optimal for minimizing the risk of obesity-related CVD.

The importance of the distribution of body fat to risk of morbidity and mortality has long been recognized. Central fat around the waist and deep visceral adipose surrounding internal organs are associated with greater health risk than inert subcutaneous adipose in regions such as the buttock or thigh. Fat cells in the viscera of the abdomen are associated with chronic inflammation, which in turn can contribute to chronic diseases such as CVD, type 2DM, and cancer.[10] Men with waist circumference greater than 40 inches and women with waist circumference greater than 35 inches are often considered at increased relative risk of type 2 DM and CVD. The USPSTF recommendations suggest that waist circumference may be an alternative to BMI in some populations.[8] In an effort to better identify and address obesity and its related risks, providers are strongly encouraged to take measurements of height, weight, and waist circumference; these physical assessment techniques can be realistically accomplished even in a busy clinical setting.

Metabolic syndrome is characterized by the presence of certain metabolic risk factors and has been associated with increased risk of coronary artery disease, other vascular diseases, and type 2 DM. Patients with three or more of the following are said to have metabolic syndrome:

- Waist circumference greater than 40 inches in men or 35 inches in women (numbers may vary in differing ethnicities)
- Serum triglycerides of 150 mg/dL or greater
- High-density lipoprotein (HDL) cholesterol less than 40 mg/dL in men or less than 50 mg/dL in women

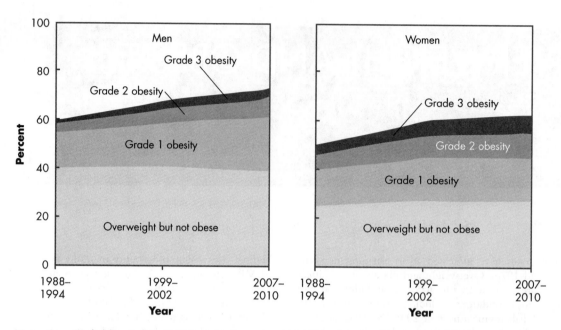

Notes: Overweight but not obese is BMI greater than or equal to 25 but less than 30; grade 1 obesity is BMI greater than or equal to 30 but less than 35; grade 2 obesity is BMI greater than or equal to 35 but less than 40; grade 3 obesity is BMI greater than or equal to 40.

figure

26-1 Overweight and obesity among adults 20 years of age and over. Key: BMI = Body mass index; CDC = Centers for Disease Control and Prevention; NCHS = National Center for Health Statistics. (*Source:* Reference 2.)

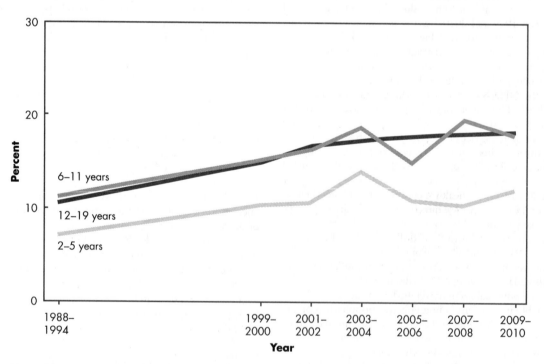

Notes: Obesity is BMI at or above the sex- and age-specific 95th percentile BMI cutoff points from the 2000 CDC Growth Charts.

figure

26-2 Obesity among children. Key: BMI = Body mass index; CDC = Centers for Disease Control and Prevention; NCHS = National Center for Health Statistics. (*Source:* Reference 2.)

table

26-1 BMI Corresponding to Height and Body Weight[a]

Height (inches)	BMI (kg/m²)[b,c]														
	19	20	21	22	23	24	25	26	27	28	29	30	35	40
	Body Weight (pounds)														
58	91	96	100	105	110	115	119	124	129	134	138	143	167	191
59	94	99	104	109	114	119	124	128	133	138	143	148	173	198
60	97	102	107	112	118	123	128	133	138	143	148	153	179	204
61	100	106	111	116	122	127	132	137	143	148	153	158	185	211
62	104	109	115	120	126	131	136	142	147	153	158	164	191	218
63	107	113	118	124	130	135	141	146	152	158	163	169	197	225
64	110	116	122	128	134	140	145	151	157	163	169	174	204	232
65	114	120	126	132	138	144	150	156	162	168	174	180	210	240
66	118	124	130	136	142	148	155	161	167	173	179	186	216	247
67	121	127	134	140	146	153	159	166	172	178	185	191	223	255
68	125	131	138	144	151	158	164	171	177	184	190	197	230	262
69	128	135	142	149	155	162	169	176	182	189	196	203	236	270
70	132	139	146	153	160	167	172	181	188	195	202	207	243	278
71	136	143	150	157	165	172	179	186	193	200	208	215	250	286
72	140	147	154	162	169	177	184	191	199	206	213	221	258	294
73	144	151	159	166	174	182	189	197	204	212	219	227	265	302
74	148	155	163	171	179	186	194	202	210	218	225	233	272	311
75	152	160	168	176	184	192	200	208	216	224	232	240	279	319
76	156	164	172	180	189	197	205	213	221	230	238	246	287	328

Key: BMI = Body mass index.

[a] To determine BMI, find the height in the left-hand column; then move across the row to a given weight. The number above the weight column is the BMI for that height and weight.

[b] BMI calculations: weight (kg)/height (m²) or (weight [lb]/height [in.²]) × 703.

[c] BMI 30–34.9 known as Class I obesity; BMI 35–39.9 known as Class II obesity; BMI ≥ 40 known as Class III obesity.

■ Blood pressure level of 130/85 mm Hg or higher
■ Fasting serum glucose of 100 mg/dL or greater

Individuals with metabolic syndrome are likely to demonstrate insulin resistance and may benefit more from weight loss for reduced morbidity and mortality compared to overweight or obese persons without the syndrome. In addition, increased muscle mass is associated with improved insulin sensitivity. Therefore, physical activity resulting in increased muscle mass may result in improved insulin sensitivity even in the absence of weight loss.

Recent data have challenged the concept that a "normal" BMI of 18.5–25 confers a mortality advantage. A 2013 meta-analysis indicates that although obesity is associated with higher all-cause mortality, overweight is associated with lower all-cause mortality compared with normal weight.[11] Whether these results are related to overweight patients receiving earlier or better health care, reflect some protection by metabolic reserves, or are due to some other mechanism is speculative at this time, and controversy over the results continues. These seemingly puzzling findings emphasize that factors such as blood pressure, lipid levels, fasting blood sugars, and waist circumference as well as BMI are important risk factors.

Some evidence suggests that the correlation between obesity and CVD is not as strong as it once was, perhaps because of improvements in medical care for CVD and its risk factors. However, this reduction in obesity-related CVD mortality has been accompanied by an increase in obesity-associated disability, perhaps because of people becoming overweight or obese at earlier ages or because of their living longer. Some evidence supports cardiorespiratory fitness as an independent determinant of mortality in overweight and obese persons (i.e., the concept that being fat but fit carries significantly lower risk than being fat and unfit).[9]

The Endocrine Society has published guidelines for obesity in children.[12] These guidelines define children and adolescents with a BMI "percentile for age" between the 85th and 95th percentiles as overweight and 95th percentile or greater as obese, based on Centers for Disease Control and Prevention growth charts.

Pathophysiology of Overweight and Obesity

Weight gain is a reflection of energy intake exceeding energy expenditure. A pound of adipose tissue represents about 3500 calories (kcal) of energy. An excessive intake of only 10 kcal/day over the level of energy expenditure could result in a gain of approximately 1 pound of fat in a year's time. The physiology of energy intake and expenditure is complex and involves numerous body systems, including the hypothalamic–pituitary axis, autonomic nervous system, central nervous system, endocrine system, gastrointestinal (GI) tract, and adipose tissue.

Both genetic and environmental factors are important in the etiology of overweight and obesity, and there is a complex interplay between these factors. The rapid increase in obesity over the past few decades argues for a strong environmental role. Increased portion sizes and caloric intakes are undoubtedly contributing to recent trends in obesity rates. Today's lifestyle and environment are likely modulating genetic expression of obesity in many individuals. For example, one recent study showed that persons with higher intakes of sugar-sweetened beverages were likely to express more alleles known to be associated with obesity compared to patients consuming fewer sugar-sweetened beverages.[13] However, consumers should be cautioned about commercial weight management programs offering genetic analysis as part of their packages; such programs may be beneficial, but currently marketing trumps the underlying science.

Researchers studying obesity have identified several different hormones and proteins potentially involved in energy balance.[14] Studies are ongoing to determine whether excesses, deficiencies, or resistance to specific substances are related to weight homeostasis. Leptin is an example of a hormone secreted by adipose tissues where resistance to the hormone may be a factor. Other compounds of research interest include neuropeptide Y, ghrelin, and melanocortins. An in-depth discussion of this topic is beyond the scope of this chapter.

Environmental factors contributing to recent increases in obesity include decreased physical activity coupled with increased food availability and consumption, especially calorie-dense foods. Guidelines for regular moderate physical activity are met by one-half to two-thirds of Americans.[15] Initiation of even modest amounts of exercise by sedentary persons can have multiple health benefits including maintenance of current weight instead of continued weight gain.

Significant increases in portion sizes of food and increased sedentary working hours may be environmental factors contributing to excessive energy intake. Twenty years ago, the typical muffin contained about 200 calories, whereas today it contains closer to 500 calories. Similarly, a typical chocolate chip cookie contained less than 100 calories, whereas today a single serving cookie often contains more than 250 calories. See Chapter 22 for a discussion of a healthy diet and *MyPlate*.

Another factor receiving attention as a possible etiology of overweight and obesity is sleep duration.[16] Several epidemiologic studies have associated high BMI values with shorter sleep duration.

Still another concept in the etiology of obesity relates to the gut microbiome.[17] Obese persons have been found to have different proportions of certain bacteria compared with lean persons. Furthermore, these proportions have been shown to change with weight loss. These findings may lead to investigation of prebiotics, probiotics, and antibiotics as tools for weight maintenance and weight loss.

Some medications can lead to weight gain.[18] There is clear evidence that the majority of the second-generation antipsychotics contribute to significant weight gain and related metabolic disorders. Older antidepressants (tricyclics and monoamine oxidase inhibitors) are associated with modest weight gain. Although some of the selective serotonin reuptake inhibitor antidepressants have been touted as producing weight loss, this loss is usually short lived, and weight gain can eventually occur. Other important groups of medications contributing to significant weight gain are hormonal contraceptives, systemic corticosteroids, certain anticonvulsants, certain sulfonylureas, thiazolidinediones, and insulins. The latter three groups are noteworthy because patients with type 2 DM placed on these medications frequently are already overweight.

Complications of Obesity

Overweight and obesity are associated with myriad chronic health problems.[1] Many of these problems improve with even modest weight loss. Obese persons experience more difficulties in performing activities of daily living such as walking several flights of stairs or bending and kneeling.

Obesity is associated with coronary heart disease (CHD) through its impact on risk factors such as hypertension, dyslipidemia, and type 2 DM. Overweight and obesity have been linked to increased risk for heart failure, arrhythmias, and stroke. Prevalence of hypertension begins to increase at relatively low levels of overweight. Weight loss in obese persons is associated with significant reductions in blood pressure.[19]

The relationship between CHD and obesity is confounded by other risk factors such as blood lipid levels, blood pressure, type 2 DM, and smoking. Despite this, several studies that carefully controlled for confounders have shown BMI and abdominal fat to be independent risk factors for the development of CHD in both genders.[19] As noted previously, central visceral adiposity is more closely associated with cardiovascular disease than is subcutaneous adiposity.

Data from the Physicians' Health Study showed approximately a twofold increase in risk of either ischemic or hemorrhagic stroke in subjects with a BMI of 30 or higher compared with those with a BMI of 23 or lower.[19] This effect appeared to be independent of the presence of hypertension, type 2 DM, or dyslipidemia. BMI may affect stroke risk through an increase in prothrombotic and proinflammatory factors found in obese persons. Venous thromboembolism risk is also increased in obese persons.[19]

There is a correlation between increasing BMI and increasing triglyceride and low-density lipoprotein (LDL) cholesterol levels. Beneficial HDL cholesterol levels tend to be lower in both men and women with higher BMI values. However, it is important to recognize that these correlations do not prove causation. Even modest weight loss of 3–8 kg can have a beneficial effect on blood lipid levels.[7]

The relationship between overweight and obesity and type 2 DM is well documented (see Chapter 45). Visceral adiposity (high waist circumference) has been shown to be a risk factor for development of type 2 DM. Persons who are initially insulin resistant, typically evidenced by high plasma triglycerides and low HDL cholesterol, are most likely to benefit from weight loss for reduced morbidity and mortality. Modest weight loss is effective in improving blood glucose control in patients with type 2 DM and preventing development of type 2 DM in those at risk.[7]

Negative attitudes exist toward obese people, leading to social stigmatization and discrimination. Overweight children may develop psychosocial difficulties stemming from compromised peer relationships.[20]

Obesity appears to increase the risk for a number of other diseases, including gallbladder disease, nonalcoholic fatty liver disease, osteoarthritis, sleep apnea, asthma, certain types of cancer, and disorders of female reproduction.[1] Obesity is a risk factor for hyperuricemia and gout.[1] Overweight is believed to contribute to a significant proportion of certain cancers and increased mortality from cancer.[1] Of particular concern are cancers with a hormonal basis such as cancers of the breast, prostate, or endometrium, as well as cancers of the colon, rectum, and gallbladder. Hypertension and gestational diabetes are more likely in obese women who become pregnant.

Management of Overweight and Obesity

Management Goals and General Management Approach

For many individuals, losing weight or maintaining weight loss is a lifelong challenge. Lifestyle changes, including dietary modification and increased exercise, are cornerstones of management. Successful weight loss and maintenance of loss require significant behavioral modification. Pharmacologic therapy using nonprescription agents should be only a short-term measure unless a primary care provider (PCP) supervises therapy. Long-term use of prescription therapies under the care of a PCP may be an option for patients with a BMI of 30 or higher or a BMI of 27 or higher with comorbid conditions.[7] However, pharmacologic interventions often result in only modest weight loss that is regained after drug discontinuation. Bariatric surgery may be considered for patients with a BMI of 40 or higher or a BMI of 35 or higher with comorbid conditions, including hypertension, hyperlipidemia, and type 2 DM.[7] This surgery is effective for helping achieve weight loss for many patients, although success following surgery also requires lifestyle changes. The procedures carry their own significant risks.

Many chronic diseases and conditions improve with weight loss. However, weight-loss goals set by many individuals are unrealistic and based on cosmetic rather than health benefit. Weight loss (and maintenance of that loss) of 5%–10% of initial weight can have positive benefits in individuals with hypertension and type 2 DM. The AHA/ACC/TOS guidelines state that the initial goal of weight loss is to reduce body weight by about 5%–10% over 6 months.[7] If this goal is achieved and further weight loss is indicated, it can be attempted. The first 10% loss carries the greatest health benefits and is easiest to attain, given that weight loss often plateaus after 6 months because of decreased basal metabolic rate. It is more important to maintain the 10% weight loss than to pursue further weight loss in many patients, and most patients find the weight maintenance to be harder than the initial modest weight loss. An approach often overlooked may be to prevent further weight gain in persons who have slowly but steadily gained weight over a period of years. Figure 26–3 is a guide for the health care provider in recommending weight-loss measures.

Nonpharmacologic Therapy (Lifestyle Intervention)

Dietary modification or restriction is the mainstay of weight-loss therapy. Physical activity is less effective in producing weight loss initially, but becomes extremely important in maintaining weight loss and improving overall fitness. The term *lifestyle intervention* describes a strategy of dietary change, physical activity, and behavior therapy. One major key to weight loss and maintenance of that loss is employment of lifestyle interventions that are sustained over a long period of time. Lifestyle intervention programs should be included in pharmaceutical care services.[21]

Dietary Change

Dietary change is the most commonly used weight-loss strategy. Diet strategies include caloric restriction; changes in dietary proportions of fat, protein, and carbohydrate; use of macronutrient substitutes (i.e., sugar and fat substitutes); and changes in timing or frequency of meals. Short-term success for many methods has been documented; however, data on longer-term effectiveness and safety are limited. Weight loss at the end of relatively short-term programs can exceed 10% of initial body weight. However, there is a strong tendency to regain this weight. A relatively small portion of participants do maintain weight loss over more extended periods, although the actual percentage of these successful participants varies. The National Weight Control Registry tracks individuals who have maintained weight loss of at least 30 pounds for at least 1 year.[22] To initially lose weight, persons in this registry used a variety of methods; about half were self-directed and half used some type of program. Most individuals reported maintaining weight loss through a combination of a low-calorie, low-fat diet and exercise, most commonly walking.

Even small changes in dietary patterns can have a positive effect. Cutting portion sizes, switching to water or diet soda rather than sugar-sweetened beverages, using smaller plates for meals, and keeping healthy snacks such as fruits and vegetables on hand are useful, sustainable strategies. Trying to emphasize foods in the diet with low energy density (i.e., low calories per weight of food) may be helpful because these foods tend to promote satiety. Because these are long-term lifestyle changes, patients should be encouraged to make these realistic, smaller changes rather than opt for the more radical fad diets that are difficult to adhere to long term. (See Chapter 22 for more details about healthy diets.)

Caloric Restriction

Daily caloric allowances for moderately active individuals vary with age, gender, and body weight. The U.S. population suffers from "portion distortion" and needs to relearn appropriate food portion sizes based on age and activity levels. Daily caloric intake allowances for an average 30-year-old man (BMI, 18.5–25; height, 5 ft 11 in.) in a temperate climate range from 2200–3000 kcal/day, depending on activity level. Corresponding figures for an average 30-year-old woman (BMI, 18.5–25; height, 5 ft 5 in.) are 1800–2800 kcal/day.[23] These figures are lower for older persons and higher for younger adults. Caloric requirements for women increase during pregnancy and lactation (see Chapter 22).[23] Self-initiated weight loss during pregnancy is not recommended.

A diet that is individually planned and seeks to create a deficit of ≥500 kcal/day should be an integral part of any weight-loss

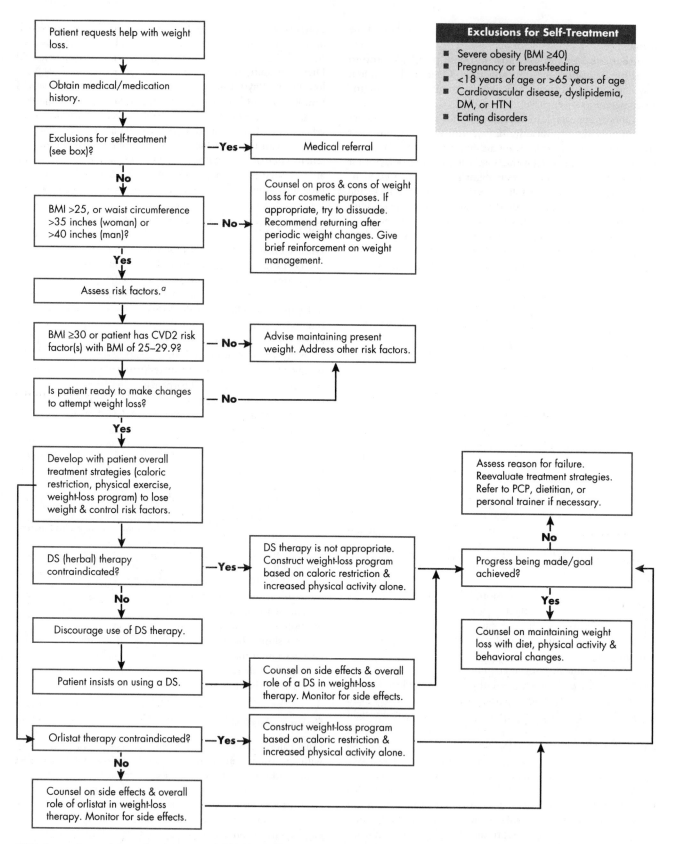

ª Risk factors for cardiovascular disease, as defined by AHA/ACC/TOS, include diabetes, prediabetes, hypertension, dyslipidemia, and waist circumference > 35 inches (88 cm) in women or > 40 inches (102 cm) in men.

figure

26–3   Self-care of overweight and obesity. Key: ACC = American College of Cardiology; AHA = American Heart Association; BMI = body mass index; CVD = cardiovascular disease; DM = diabetes mellitus; DS = dietary supplement; HTN = hypertension; PCP = primary care provider; TOS = The Obesity Society.

program.[7] Two levels of caloric restriction are commonly used. A low-calorie diet (LCD) of about 1200–1800 kcal/day may involve a structured commercial program, or it may involve guidelines for selecting conventional foods, including careful attention to portion sizes. Weight loss on an LCD is typically 1–2 pounds per week. A very-low-calorie diet (VLCD) of 800 or fewer calories per day should be conducted and monitored under medical supervision and accompanied by high-intensity lifestyle intervention. VLCDs are frequently administered as liquid formulas given several times a day. Although weight loss with VLCDs over 12–16 weeks is typically double that of LCDs, long-term results are generally no better. A multivitamin and multimineral preparation should be recommended to patients consuming fewer than 1200 kcal/day for prolonged periods.

Total fasting or semistarvation is sometimes proposed as a means of weight reduction in severely obese persons. However, starvation depletes the body of lean tissue (protein) and essential electrolytes in addition to fat. If total fasting is undertaken, hospitalization and medical supervision are recommended.

Altered Proportions of Food Groups

The most commonly recommended diets for weight loss are reduced-calorie diets emphasizing decreased fat intake, particularly decreased saturated fat. The 2010 Dietary Guidelines for Americans recommends a diet supplying no more than 35% of total calories from fat, of which no more than 10% of total calories come from saturated fat[24] Future guidelines will probably place less emphasis on restricting fat calories and more emphasis on including monounsaturated and polyunsaturated fat while minimizing saturated fat. A low-fat diet alone is inadequate for weight loss; the diet must also reduce total calories.

Very-low-fat vegetarian diets in the context of other lifestyle changes have been advocated. Although such programs can result in regression of coronary atherosclerosis in some patients with moderate-severe CHD, applicability to larger populations remains questionable with regard to compliance.[25] Dietary fat must be carefully chosen when consuming a very-low-fat diet to prevent essential fatty acid deficiency. Such diets increase triglyceride levels and lower HDL cholesterol in the short term because of high carbohydrate content.

There is a spectrum of popular high-protein, higher-fat, low-carbohydrate diets. Some contain very low amounts of carbohydrates (about 5% to 15% of total calories; e.g., Atkins diet) and are ketogenic, whereas others are considered moderate-carbohydrate diets (about 35% to 50% of calories from carbohydrate; e.g., Zone diet). People often start out on the ultralow form of the diet and transition to a more moderate form. Part of the success of low carbohydrate diets may lie in the fact that they simplify food choices, thus facilitating dietary adherence.

The theory behind very low carbohydrate diets is that they prevent elevated insulin levels that promote storage of body fat. Much of the weight loss seen with these diets is a result of decreased caloric intake from avoiding high-carbohydrate foods. Initial weight-loss results partially from a diuretic effect and glycogen depletion. Low carbohydrate diets result in significant weight loss over 6–24 months. Concerns about long-term safety of these diets still exist. Most studies have indicated that serum lipid levels, overall, are not affected deleteriously over the short term in most dieters, mainly because of weight loss. Triglycerides and HDL cholesterol levels are generally affected more favorably with low-carbohydrate diets, whereas low-fat diets have more favorable effects on LDL and total cholesterol.[26]

Potential adverse effects include lack of essential nutrients such as potassium, calcium, and magnesium. High-protein foods consumed in large quantities on these diets could increase uric acid levels and precipitate gout, although this problem has not been common in studies with up to a year of follow-up. High animal protein content promotes calcium excretion in the urine that could be deleterious to bone health. Restriction of fruits, vegetables, whole grains, and milk products could increase a person's risk of various cancers by depleting essential vitamins, minerals, and fiber and could also lead to constipation. A high-protein, low-carbohydrate (HPLC) diet has been shown to alter metabolic profiles in the colon of obese men after as little as four weeks of consumption.[27] Decreases in protective short chain fatty acids and increases in potentially carcinogenic N-nitroso compounds in a HPLC diet could be risk factors for colonic disease if this diet is followed for long periods. Attention to the type of fiber content included in HPLC diets could help offset these effects, but this benefit has not yet been proven.

High-protein content may predispose people to dehydration and hyperfiltration by the kidneys, leading to eventual kidney damage, particularly in diabetic patients. Headache, muscle weakness, and fatigue are other adverse events reported by some persons on low-carbohydrate diets. Several published randomized trials of such diets demonstrated relative safety of the low-carbohydrate, higher-fat, high-protein diets for 6–24 months, with greatest weight loss seen in the first 6 months.[26] In the Women's Health Initiative trial, reduction of total fat intake for 8 years did not reduce risk for CVD.[28] This finding may be related to the observation that carbohydrate-restricted diets have more favorable effects, when compared with fat-restricted diets, not only on triglyceride and HDL cholesterol levels, but also on small dense LDL cholesterol mass.[28]

Low-glycemic-index food products are promoted commercially. Glycemic index refers to the amount of blood glucose rise seen over a set period of time after ingestion of a standardized amount of a food. Many high-carbohydrate, low-fat diets exhibit a high glycemic index. By making carbohydrate choices carefully, a lower glycemic response can be obtained. Low-glycemic-index diets would promote satiety, prevent large fluctuations in insulin concentrations, and might help maintain insulin sensitivity. Studies have not consistently supported the usefulness of low-glycemic-index diets in weight control, and the methods used to classify foods with this system are controversial.

Use of Food Additives

Some patients may use food additives such as artificial sweeteners and fat substitutes to reduce caloric intake. Although theoretically the use of these agents should help decrease caloric intake, the existing data are conflicted as to beneficial effects these products may produce. Table 26–2 outlines information related to sugar and fat substitutes.

Meal Replacement Therapy

Diets that use meal replacements typically involve replacing up to two meals a day with a liquid drink, snack bar, or measured frozen meal, with the dieter encouraged to eat a "reasonable" third meal each day. The main advantage to this approach is portion control. Products typically contain about 200–300 kcal per serving and are low fat, although low-carbohydrate options are also available. The challenge with this approach is that dieters enter their third meal extremely hungry and may consume

table

26–2   Sugar and Fat Substitutes

Substitute (sample trade name)	Comments
Sugar Substitutes	
Monk fruit extract[a] (Nectresse)	Products may contain very small amounts of other natural sweeteners such as erythritol, molasses, and sugar
Saccharin (Sweet 'n Low)[a]	Has bitter taste; has been replaced largely by newer sweeteners
Aspartame (Nutra Sweet)[a]	Contains phenylalanine; therefore, contraindicated in patients with phenylketonuria; not for use in cooking or baking as heat breaks it down into free amino acids, which impart a bitter taste
Fructose	Nutritive sweetener and should not be viewed as sugar free; insulin not required for fructose utilization in the body; contains approximately 10 calories when supplied in an amount providing the equivalent of about 1 teaspoon of sucrose
Sorbitol	Nutritive sweetener and should not be viewed as sugar free; does not cause tooth decay, but can cause osmotic diarrhea when ingested in large quantities; contains approximately 10 calories when supplied in an amount providing the equivalent of about 1 teaspoon of sucrose
Xylitol	Nutritive sweetener and should not be viewed as sugar free; does not cause tooth decay; contains approximately 10 calories when supplied in an amount providing the equivalent of about 1 teaspoon of sucrose
Acesulfame potassium (Sweet One)[a]	May be substituted for sucrose in cooking; may be combined with aspartame, because some people detect a metallic aftertaste with acesulfame potassium alone
Sucralose (Splenda)[a]	May be used in cooking
Neotame[a]	Chemically similar to aspartame; may be used in cooking
Cyclamates[a]	Banned by FDA in 1969 because of association with cancer in animals; applicability of this finding to humans has been challenged; remains available in many countries
Stevia[a]	Approved in United States as of 2008 as a food additive in a specific purified form
Fat Substitutes[b]	
Microparticulated protein (Simplesse)	Used in frozen desserts, salad dressing; unstable to heat
Soluble fiber (Oatrim)	Derived from oats and designed to replace fat in meats, cheeses, baked goods, and frozen desserts
Sucrose polyester (Olean)	Also known as olestra; is not absorbed; can cause malabsorption of fat-soluble vitamins; GI side effects can be seen with ingestion of large quantities; can be used for cooking and frying

Key: FDA = Food and Drug Administration; GI = gastrointestinal.

[a] Can be labeled as noncaloric based on FDA labeling regulations; cyclamates no longer approved by FDA for use as sugar substitute.

[b] Use of these fat substitutes in food products in place of fat typically decreases caloric content of the foods by about half unless extra sugars are added into the products.

excessive calories by overeating at this time. Early weight loss with these products, part of which may be a result of low sodium content leading to water loss, can give a psychological boost to adhere to the program. Meal replacement products are discussed further in Chapter 23.

Commercial Weight-Loss Programs

Structured commercial weight-loss programs such as Weight Watchers, Jenny Craig, and Take Off Pounds Sensibly (TOPS) are very popular in the United States. Women tend to gravitate to these programs more than men. Participation in structured commercial programs may be expensive, because participants are required to purchase program-specific tools as well as specially packaged snacks or meals. The success seen with these programs is likely at least partially due to the social support that develops with periodic meetings. Online tools such as diet and exercise diaries and support groups are increasingly available; these resources may be less expensive than community-based structured commercial programs.

Physical Activity

Encouragement of physical activity for preventing overweight and obesity is an important public health strategy for all age groups, including children. The U.S. Department of Health and

Human Services outlines physical activity recommendations as shown in Table 26–3.[29] For older adults, regular exercise can reduce functional declines that occur with aging.

Increased physical activity is an important component of weight-loss therapy and is even more important in weight maintenance after weight loss. Patients who regularly exercise may, in general, be more committed to a healthy lifestyle. Exercise builds muscle, which has a higher metabolic rate than a corresponding amount of fat. Weight loss that can be achieved by an exercise program is modest; combining a reduced-calorie diet with increased physical activity produces greater weight loss and reduction in abdominal fat than either approach alone. Some patients may have medical conditions restricting the types of exercise in which they should participate. These patients should have a medical evaluation before starting an exercise regimen. Regardless of concomitant diseases, current recommendations call for men older than age 40 and women older than age 50 to undergo a medical evaluation before starting an exercise program.

For sedentary patients, a walking program is often a good place to begin. A pedometer may be an inexpensive aid to increasing activity in some individuals. Patients can start by walking 30 minutes each day for 3 days a week, building up to at least 60 minutes of moderate-intensity physical activity most days of the week. The 60-minute activity periods can be accrued in multiple smaller increments throughout the day with similar benefit. Patients should be encouraged to participate in activities that they enjoy and are therefore more likely to continue.

Behavioral Therapy

Behavioral therapy can improve the outcome of weight-loss programs when used in combination with other strategies such as diet, exercise, and medications. Behavioral interventions are most effective when patients participate in sessions at least once or twice a month.[8] Behavioral therapy may be administered in either an individual or group setting by professionals or lay leaders. Remote coaching and mobile technologies are increasingly being explored as less expensive methods for encouraging adherence to lifestyle modifications.

Behavioral techniques include the following:

- Environmental modification: Do not have high-calorie foods readily available and thus avoid problem foods altogether.
- Thought-pattern modification: Set reasonable, specific, proximate goals; identify and plan for potential obstacles.
- Self-efficacy: Maintain an optimistic and positive approach.
- Social support: Rely on family, friends, and health care providers.[30]

Public Health Initiatives

In an era when federal and state governments bear an increasing percentage of the cost of health care in the United States, interest in public health initiatives to decrease overweight and obesity has increased. Efforts by all levels of government to require dietary information in restaurant menus, to limit portion sizes of sugar-sweetened beverages, to limit trans-fat content in commercial foods, and to levy taxes on certain unhealthy foods are just a few examples of initiatives that have been considered or actually implemented. Many schools have banned the sale of sugar-sweetened beverages and high-fat snacks on their premises. These measures are controversial, and positive benefits on public health are not consistently shown at this time.

Pharmacologic Therapy

Pharmacologic therapy is generally not recommended for weight loss, as exemplified by the fact that more weight-loss products have been removed from the market than approved in recent years because of safety concerns. The ideal drug, which would provide fast and permanent weight loss with no adverse effects, simply does not exist despite the billions of research and consumer dollars spent on weight-loss products every year.

The most current guidelines for weight loss recommend that prescription weight-loss medications approved by the Food and Drug Administration (FDA) for long-term use be reserved as an adjunct to diet and physical activity for patients with BMI of 30 or higher or for patients with BMI of 27 or higher with concomitant diseases or risk factors.[7] The drugs can be used singly and at the lowest effective dose to reduce the likelihood of adverse events. The same guidelines should apply to all weight-loss products, whether prescription or nonprescription drugs or dietary supplements, although nonprescription orlistat (Alli) is recommended for BMI greater than 25 as outlined in the following section. Any of these medications or supplements should be used with concomitant lifestyle intervention and continuous assessment for efficacy, safety, and tolerance.

Status of Nonprescription Weight-Loss Products

Because of the lack of safety and efficacy data, FDA banned 111 weight-control ingredients in nonprescription drug products in 1991.[31] In 2000, FDA requested that all drug companies discontinue marketing phenylpropanolamine-containing products because of safety issues.[32] In addition, nonprescription drugs containing ephedrine and related alkaloids in combination with

table
26–3 Physical Activity Recommendations[a]

Children and Adolescents

Aerobic: ≥60 minutes of moderate or vigorous aerobic activity a day, including vigorous activity at least 3 days a week

Muscle and bone: strengthening physical activity should occur at least 3 times a week

Adults

Aerobic: 150 minutes of moderate aerobic activity or 75 minutes of vigorous physical activity a week, performed in ≥10-minute episodes[b]

Muscle: strengthening activities involving major muscle groups should occur at least twice a week

[a] As proposed by the U.S. Department of Health and Human Services, "2008 Physical Activity Guidelines for Americans."[25]

[b] More activity than is outlined here is necessary to promote weight loss in most persons. Exercise should be used in combination with dietary restriction to promote weight loss.

a stimulant or analgesic could no longer be marketed as of 2001,[33] and the stimulant laxative ingredients aloe and cascara sagrada were banned as ingredients in nonprescription drugs in 2002.[34] In 2004, FDA banned dietary supplements containing ephedrine alkaloids, declaring these supplements adulterated because they present an unreasonable risk of illness or injury.[35] This ban was upheld in 2007.[36] Common names used for the various botanicals that contain ephedrine alkaloids include sea grape, yellow horse, joint fir, popotillo, ma huang, and country mallow. Whereas these products are banned from sale in the United States, similar substances that may pose similar risks are still included in dietary supplements and are often found as components of weight-loss products.

Dietary supplements are distinct entities from nonprescription drugs. They include herbal and other products meant to supplement the diet and are regulated under the Dietary Supplement Health and Education Act of 1994 (see Chapters 50 and 51). They are generally recognized as safe unless proven otherwise by FDA. Nonprescription drugs, conversely, are regulated as drugs by FDA and must adhere to more stringent regulations of safety, efficacy, and quality.

The majority of drugs currently considered safe and efficacious for weight loss are restricted to prescription-only status and include benzphetamine (Didrex), diethylpropion (Tenuate), mazindol (Sanorex), methamphetamine (Desoxyn), orlistat (Xenical), phendimetrazine (Bontril), phentermine (Ionamin), phentermine/topiramate (Qsymia), and lorcaserin (Belviq). Sibutramine (Meridia) was removed from the U.S. market in October 2010. Of note, both phentermine/topiramate and lorcaserin were only recently approved by FDA in an effort to provide practitioners with some additional prescription options to promote weight loss. The reader is directed to standard references for more information about these drugs.

Orlistat was approved by FDA as a prescription weight-loss medication (Xenical) in 1999 and as a nonprescription weight-loss medication (Alli) in 2007.[37] The prescription strength of orlistat is approved for use in patients ages 12 years and older, whereas the nonprescription medication is approved for those ages 18 years and older.

GlaxoSmithKline Consumer Healthcare provides free support to those using Alli through an individually tailored online plan called myalliplan (www.myalli.com). The Alli starter pack provides reference guides to help patients follow the program as well as information for joining the online plan. FDA issued a public warning in 2012 about a counterfeit version of Alli being sold on the Internet that was illegal and unsafe. Tips on how to recognize the counterfeit product and further information can be found at the FDA Web site.[38]

Orlistat aids in weight loss by decreasing absorption of dietary fats. It inhibits gastric and pancreatic lipases and specifically reduces absorption of fat by inhibiting hydrolysis of triglycerides.[39] It is recommended for use along with a reduced-calorie, low-fat diet and exercise program. The labeling for the prescription product states that the drug is indicated for obese patients with a BMI of 30 or higher or for patients with a BMI of 27 or higher who also demonstrate risk factors such as diabetes, hypertension, or dyslipidemia. The labeling for the nonprescription product simply states that the drug is indicated for use in overweight adults, which by the standard definition would be persons with a BMI of 25 or higher.[39]

The recommended dosage of prescription-strength orlistat is 120 mg three times a day before meals containing fat; at this dosage, it inhibits dietary fat absorption by about 30%.[39] The nonprescription form of the drug is recommended at a dosage of 60 mg three times a day before meals containing fat; its inhibition of fat absorption may be less. With either dosage of orlistat, there is increased risk of greasy diarrhea as the amount of fat increases in a meal. Because of its mechanism of action, there is no need to give the drug with a fat-free meal.

Most studies have used the 120 mg dosage in combination with a reduced-calorie diet and have reported modest weight losses, especially during the first 6 months of therapy. This dosage may also be useful for weight-loss maintenance following initial weight loss. In one of the few full-text studies published with the 60 mg nonprescription dose, weight loss after 16 weeks in the active drug group was significantly greater than in patients receiving placebo (3.05 kg versus 1.90 kg; $p < .001$).[40] The nonprescription product labeling notes that most patients lost 5–10 pounds (about 2–5 kg) over 6 months in clinical trials. Patients receiving orlistat have had significantly greater reductions in LDL cholesterol and blood pressure compared with placebo. Effects on lipid levels may be independent of weight loss, whereas the changes in blood pressure are probably largely due to weight loss. Orlistat in the 120 mg dosage has been shown to be effective in preventing and delaying development of type 2 DM over a 4-year period in patients with impaired glucose tolerance,[41] and it resulted in significant weight loss and weight-loss maintenance in obese patients with chronic kidney disease.[42]

Orlistat may decrease absorption of fat-soluble vitamins (A, D, E, and K). It is recommended that patients taking this medication take a multivitamin once daily at bedtime or separated by at least 2 hours from an orlistat dose. Orlistat is minimally absorbed and therefore exhibits little systemic toxicity. Common GI side effects are caused by the increased fat present in the GI tract and include flatulence with oily spotting, loose and frequent stools, fatty stools, and fecal urgency and incontinence. Decreasing the amount of ingested fat can minimize these effects. These side effects are expected to be less common with the nonprescription dosage compared to the prescription dosage, and they generally improve within a few weeks of initiating therapy.

Drug interactions with orlistat are unlikely because of the drug's limited absorption. A theoretical concern exists when a patient is taking both orlistat and warfarin because of the potential for orlistat to decrease vitamin K absorption; close monitoring of the international normalized ratio (INR) is recommended with concomitant use of these medications. Orlistat should be avoided in patients receiving cyclosporine; reductions in cyclosporine plasma concentrations have been noted. Patients with malabsorption disorders should avoid taking orlistat, and patients with a history of thyroid disease, cholelithiasis, nephrolithiasis, or pancreatitis should consult their primary care provider before taking orlistat. In addition, the package label advises patients taking medications to treat diabetes to consult a doctor or pharmacist before using orlistat. In May 2010, FDA required labeling changes of both the prescription and nonprescription strengths of orlistat because of rare cases of severe liver injury. The following statement was added to the package inserts: "Patients should stop use of orlistat and contact their healthcare professional if they develop the signs and symptoms of liver injury, including itching, yellow eyes or skin, dark urine, light-colored stools, or loss of appetite."[43] This action by FDA was based on 13 reported cases of severe liver injury with orlistat, including one case in the United States associated with the nonprescription strength. There has been concern about potential associations between orlistat and development of breast and colon cancers. However, FDA concluded there was not a causal relationship between orlistat and cancer.[44]

Nonprescription orlistat may be useful as an adjunct to lifestyle changes in helping patients lose modest amounts of weight. Results will be more favorable when this agent is combined with a reduced-calorie, low-fat diet and increased physical activity. Orlistat has the ability to help change people's eating habits. Rather than suppressing the appetite, an effect that goes away once the drug in discontinued, orlistat helps people choose food with less fat content, resulting in fewer side effects. Once the drug is discontinued, these people should be able to continue to make these healthier food choices. Patients should be aware that the GI side effects of the medication are likely to be exacerbated by concomitant ingestion of a low-carbohydrate, high-fat diet. There is some concern that this nonprescription agent may be misused, particularly by adolescents; it would be prudent for health care providers to watch for adolescents purchasing this medication.

Orlistat is rated pregnancy category X and is contraindicated in pregnancy because weight loss offers no potential benefit to a pregnant woman and may result in fetal harm. It is not known if orlistat crosses into human milk. Caution should be exercised when orlistat is administered to a nursing mother. The safety and effectiveness of the nonprescription orlistat product have not been established for patients younger than age 12. Clinical studies of orlistat did not include sufficient numbers of patients ages 65 years and older to determine whether they respond differently from younger patients. No dosage adjustment is recommended in patients with renal or hepatic dysfunction.

Use of Inappropriate Medications for Weight Loss

Individuals seeking to lose weight will sometimes turn to inappropriate, potentially dangerous methods to induce loss, such as using laxatives or diuretics. The risks associated with laxatives and diuretics are discussed in Chapters 15 and 9, respectively.

Reformulated Weight-Loss Products

Since FDA ruling on ephedra-containing dietary supplements, many manufacturers are including bitter orange (*Citrus aurantium*) in weight-loss medications, often in combination with sources of caffeine such as cola nut (*Cola acuminata* or *Cola nitida*), guarana (*Paullinia cupana* or *Paullinia sorbilis*), or maté (*Ilex paraguariensis*). Bitter orange contains synephrine, which is structurally similar to epinephrine, and octopamine, which is similar to norepinephrine. Bitter orange is being touted as a safe alternative to ephedra in many herbal weight-loss products. Although adrenergic effects of synephrine and octopamine have the potential for appetite suppression and lipolysis, these products also carry the same potential health risks as ephedra. A randomized, double-blind, placebo-controlled study of single doses of *C. aurantium* in healthy adults reported significant increases in heart rate and blood pressure compared with placebo. The authors state that the effects likely are due to a combination of *C. aurantium*, caffeine, and other stimulants contained in the multicomponent preparation.[45] Clinical trials of *C. aurantium* for weight loss have failed to support efficacy for this indication.

Numerous nonprescription weight-loss products list multiple ingredients, many of which are herbal extracts with varying active ingredients, together with vitamins and minerals. Many of these ingredients lack any scientific evidence for usefulness in weight loss. To confuse matters even more, many of the herbal extracts are listed by their common or not-so-common names (e.g., bitter orange, Seville orange, and sour orange are all common names for *C. aurantium*), and many do not list the botanical name, making it difficult to determine exactly what the herbal product contains. The majority of these products have not been clearly demonstrated to be effective or safe, and many have been associated with serious adverse effects. Health care providers are advised to carefully review the labels of all dietary supplement weight-loss products to determine the risk for adverse reactions and drug–supplement interactions.

Herbal Products

A summary of botanicals commonly used in weight-loss supplements is provided in Table 26–4.[46–49] Many of these supplements also contain vitamins and minerals, presumably to ensure adequate intake of these essential nutrients by patients on low-caloric diets. In addition, the majority of these supplements contain multiple ingredients with several purported actions, although the advertising claims frequently focus on one solitary ingredient or action or both. To further complicate the problem, many of the supplements contain "proprietary blends." Ingredients of proprietary blends must be listed, but their amounts do not have to be specified. It is important to note, however, that none of these ingredients have sufficient scientific evidence to support their usefulness in weight loss. Broadly speaking, the ingredients of weight-loss supplements can be categorized as follows:

- Stimulants and energy boosters and thermogenic aids claim to increase basal metabolism, increase energy, and counteract fatigue (e.g., caffeine and bitter orange).
- Fat and carbohydrate modulators claim to alter fat or carbohydrate metabolism or both, resulting in decreased body fat mass and increased lean muscle mass (e.g., green tea, chromium, and garcinia).
- Appetite suppressants and satiety promoters claim to decrease caloric intake by suppressing appetite or promoting satiety (e.g., guar gum, glucomannan, and psyllium).
- Fat absorption blockers claim to block intestinal absorption of dietary fat (e.g., chitosan).
- Carbohydrate absorption blockers claim to block intestinal absorption of dietary carbohydrates (e.g., kidney bean extract and mung bean extract).
- Cortisol blockers claim to block stress-induced release of cortisol, which is claimed to cause increased appetite and fat storage (e.g., beta-sitosterol, phosphatidylserine, and theanine).
- Laxatives (e.g., cascara sagrada and psyllium) claim to promote weight loss by increasing fecal loss.
- Diuretics (e.g., dandelion and caffeine) claim to promote weight loss by increasing urination.

Herbal laxatives and diuretics are often included in multiple-ingredient dietary supplements marketed for weight loss. For example, "dieter's" or "slimming" teas contain a variety of botanical laxatives and diuretics. Diuretics, whether herbal or

table
26–4   Complementary Therapies Commonly Used for Weight Loss

Agent	Risks
Stimulants, Energy Boosters, and Thermogenic Aids	
Bitter orange (*Citrus aurantium*)	Synephrine may cause hypertension, cardiovascular toxicity, myocardial infarction, stroke, and seizure.
Caffeine: Cola nut (*Cola acuminata, Cola nitida*), green tea (*Camellia sinensis*), guarana (*Paullinia cupana, Paullinia sorbilis*), maté (*Ilex paraguariensis*)	Caffeine may cause GI distress, nausea, dehydration, headaches, insomnia, nervousness, anxiety, muscle tension, heart palpitations, hypertension, addiction, decreased appetite, vertigo, and possible genetic damage; avoid in patients with gastric ulcers. Use with caution in patients with renal disease, panic disorder, hyperthyroidism, anxiety, or susceptibility to spasm; use only under medical supervision in patients with peptic ulcers, cardiovascular disease, or blood-clotting abnormalities; discontinue use at least 24 hours before surgery; may alter effects of anticoagulant medications.
Fat and Carbohydrate Modulators	
Chromium	Chromium is generally well tolerated at low doses. Rhabdomyolysis and renal failure may occur with large doses. May cause mood and sleep changes, headaches, and cognitive and perception dysfunction. Evidence of benefit of chromium picolinate is inconsistent and controversial.
Conjugated linoleic acid (CLA)	CLA causes GI upset.
Garcinia or brindleberry (*Garcinia cambogia*)	Hydroxycitric acid may cause GI distress with high doses; not recommended in patients with diabetes mellitus or dementia.
Green coffee	Green coffee is generally well tolerated. Green coffee extract contains caffeine (see Caffeine, listed above). No long-term, high-quality studies have been published, and available evidence of benefit is conflicting.
Green tea (*Camellia sinensis*)	See Caffeine, listed above.
Licorice (*Glycyrrhiza glabra*)	Pseudoaldosteronism, hypertension, and hypokalemia may occur.
Pyruvate	GI upset may occur.
Appetite Suppressants and Satiety Promoters	
Glucomannan (*Amorphophallus konjac*)	Risks are similar to those of plantain. No large, well-designed studies have been published, and available evidence of benefit is conflicting.
Guar gum (*Cyamopsis tetragonolobus*)	Risks are similar to those of plantain.
Hoodia (*Hoodia gordonii*)	No risks are reported. Although unpublished trials suggest a reduced caloric intake in patients taking hoodia, there is a general lack of well-conducted clinical evidence to support the use of hoodia for weight loss.
Plantain or psyllium (*Plantago lanceolata, Plantago major, Plantago psyllium, Plantago arenatia*)	Flatulence, GI distress, nausea, and vomiting may occur; plantain may interact with lithium or carbamazepine.
Fat Absorption Blockers	
Chitosan	Chitosan is generally well tolerated; may cause GI upset, flatulence, nausea, increased stool bulk, constipation; may exhibit cross-sensitivity in patients with shellfish allergies.
Green coffee	See comments under Fat and Carbohydrate Modulators.
Raspberry ketones extract (*Rubus idaeus*)	No reliable information about adverse effects of raspberry extract is available. The active ingredient is structurally similar to phenylephrine; see Bitter Orange, listed above.
Carbohydrate Absorption Blockers	
Ginseng (*Panax* sp.)	Ginseng may cause nervousness, excitation, inability to concentrate, estrogenic effects, Stevens–Johnson syndrome, allergy, and hypoglycemic effects; may interact with several drugs including warfarin, digoxin, alcohol, and phenelzine.
Laxatives and Diuretics	
Cascara sagrada (*Rhamnus purshiana*)	Abdominal pain, cramps, and diarrhea may occur; chronic use can lead to potassium depletion, disturbed heart function, and muscle weakness; avoid in patients taking digoxin or potassium-depleting diuretics.
Dandelion (*Taraxacum officinale*)	Avoid use in patients with allergies to ragweed, marigolds, etc. (Asteraceae/Compositae family); contraindicated in patients with gallbladder or bile-duct obstruction, or with bowel obstruction or pus in the pleural cavity.

table **26–4**	**Complementary Therapies Commonly Used for Weight Loss** *(continued)*

Agent	Risks
Miscellaneous	
Calcium	Constipation, nausea, and vomiting may occur; possibly effective when ingested as naturally occurring calcium in foods, but not when used as a dietary supplement.
Guggul (*Commiphora mukul*)	GI distress, diarrhea, nausea, and skin rash may occur; use only under medical supervision in patients with hyperthyroidism; may alter effects of thyroid medications, cholesterol-lowering medications, anticoagulants, antiplatelet medications, propranolol, and diltiazem.
Pyruvate	No risks are reported.
Willow bark (*Salix alba*)	Willow bark is a salicin source; no risks reported when taken orally.

Key: GI = Gastrointestinal.

Source: References 46–49. Also see Chapter 51 for additional related information.

drug, may result in an initial transient weight loss, but this effect lasts only a few days. Herbal or drug laxatives typically act in the colon and, therefore, will not decrease caloric absorption in the small intestine, which is the primary site of food absorption. Many of these botanicals are stimulant laxatives that should be used for only 1–2 weeks at a time. Prolonged use may lead to electrolyte imbalances and dependence on the laxative for regular bowel movements (cathartic colon), as discussed in Chapter 15.

Herbal sources of caffeine have often been used in combination with ephedra and willow bark (as a source of salicin) for weight loss because of purported synergistic effects. This combination is often referred to as a "fat-burning stack" or "ECA" (ephedrine-caffeine-aspirin), with claims of additive thermogenic or heat-producing effects.[48,49] However, adverse reactions to these products, either alone or in combination, range from relatively mild symptoms, such as headache, nervousness, and hypertension, to more severe reactions, such as stroke, myocardial infarction, and sudden death. In several cases, significant adverse events occurred in otherwise healthy young or middle-aged adults, and many occurred following consumption of relatively low doses for short periods.[48,49]

Economically Motivated Adulteration

Although adulteration of medications is not a new concept, it is of increasing concern in the dietary supplement industry. A working definition of economically motivated adulteration proposed by FDA is the "fraudulent, intentional substitution or addition of a substance in a product for the purpose of increasing the apparent value of the product or reducing the cost of its production, i.e., for economic gain."[50] For example, a recent examination of a hoodia weight-loss product determined the material was actually derived from cacti and contained no hoodia.[51] FDA tracks tainted supplements; the most common issue related to weight-loss supplements is the undisclosed inclusion of sibutramine, a prescription weight-loss medication that was voluntarily withdrawn from the U.S. and Canadian markets because of an increased risk of heart attack and stroke in patients with concomitant CVD.[52] Economic adulteration, whether intentional or unintentional, is of particular concern in the weight-loss dietary supplement industry because increasing

numbers of cases with the potential for causing serious adverse events are appearing in the literature.

Assessment of Overweight and Obesity: A Case-Based Approach

When health care providers are asked to recommend a weight-loss method or product, they should determine the patient's motivation for weight loss. The reason may be immediately obvious for some patients; others may want to lose a few pounds to improve their appearance or to enhance their perception of good health. The provider should perform a waist circumference test and calculate the BMI to assess the patient. The provider should review current prescription and nonprescription drugs and ask about use of herbal products and other dietary supplements.

The provider should assess what weight-loss strategies were used previously and whether the attempts were successful. Part of this assessment also includes any dietary counseling or physical activity training the patient may have received in the past. The patient's support system should be taken into consideration; support from family and friends is a critical component for success. Likewise, cultural backgrounds should be considered, as cultural and social factors have a strong effect on food decisions. Such factors should not be seen as insurmountable obstacles. The provider can serve an important role to motivate and encourage the patient in weight loss.

Using all information obtained during the assessment, the provider can decide whether weight loss is appropriate and, if warranted, can help select the type, intensity, and length of a weight-loss program. Patients with significant comorbid conditions in addition to obesity should be discouraged from using dietary supplements. Individuals within the normal height and weight range who want to lose weight for other reasons (e.g., improved appearance or sense of well-being) should be advised about the difficulty of the task and the potential adverse physical and psychological effects; often these individuals can be refocused to engage in healthy exercise activities that will attain the results they are seeking.

Cases 26–1 and 26–2 illustrate assessment of patients who seek assistance with weight control.

case
26–1

Relevant Evaluation Criteria	Scenario/Model Outcome

Information Gathering

1. Gather essential information about the patient's symptoms and medical history, including:

   a. description of symptom(s) (i.e., nature, onset, duration, severity, associated symptoms)

   Patient has been overweight since childhood. She has never been severely obese but typically gains a few pounds each year. Her obese status does not significantly affect her ability to perform her activities of daily living.

   b. description of any factors that seem to precipitate, exacerbate, and/or relieve the patient's symptom(s)

   Patient eats when stressed. She snacks while watching television at night as well as at her desk at work.

   c. description of the patient's efforts to relieve the symptoms

   Patient has tried various diet and exercise programs over the past 20 years. These usually result in a 5- to 10-pound weight loss; she then typically gains weight back when she gets bored with the regimen or gets stressed by work.

   d. patient's identity

   Rhonda Price

   e. age, sex, height, and weight

   42 years old, female, 5 ft. 5 in., 185 lb.

   f. patient's occupation

   Secretary

   g. patient's dietary habits

   Usually eats a bagel for breakfast. Sometimes takes leftovers for lunch and sometimes eats out with coworkers. Typically fixes a well-balanced meal for her family for dinner; fixes a rich dessert once or twice a week. Patient states that she has a "weakness" for chips, which she frequently eats while watching television at night.

   h. patient's sleep habits

   Goes to bed late and gets up early; averages about 5.5 hours of sleep per night during the week and 7–8 hours on the weekends.

   i. concurrent medical conditions, prescription and nonprescription medications, and dietary supplements

   No current prescription medications. Takes ibuprofen occasionally for aches and pains and famotidine for heartburn.

   j. allergies

   NKA

   k. history of other adverse reactions to medications

   None

   l. other (describe) _____

   Does not engage in regular exercise. When she goes on a diet, she may make an effort to walk a mile at lunchtime during the work week.

Assessment and Triage

2. Differentiate patient's signs/symptoms and correctly identify the patient's primary problem(s).

   Patient's BMI is 31, placing her in the obese category (Table 26–1). Poor dietary habits, inadequate sleep, and lack of exercise probably contribute.

3. Identify exclusions for self-treatment (Figure 26–3).

   None identified.

4. Formulate a comprehensive list of therapeutic alternatives for the primary problem to determine if triage to a health care provider is required, and share this information with the patient or caregiver.

   Options include:

   (1) Refer Rhonda to a dietitian and personal trainer for diet and exercise advice, respectively.

   (2) Refer Rhonda to reputable Web sites such as choosemyplate.gov for tracking food intake and exercise and for advice on these.

   (3) Refer Rhonda to a support group such as Weight Watchers.

   (4) Counsel Rhonda on diet and exercise.

   (5) Recommend a dietary supplement for weight loss.

   (6) Recommend orlistat.

   (7) Take no action.

Plan

5. Select an optimal therapeutic alternative to address the patient's problem, taking into account patient preferences.

   The patient chooses to try nonprescription orlistat while also trying to lower her caloric intake, mostly by cutting back on bread, pasta, chips, and desserts. She agrees to try to get exercise in sustainable ways throughout the day, such as parking farther away from work and taking a short walk during lunch or after work most days of the week. During inclement weather, she identifies that she could climb the five stories of steps a couple of times a day for exercise. She is encouraged to enlist fellow coworkers or friends who need to lose weight to join her in an informal or formal weight-loss support group.

case
26–1 continued

Relevant Evaluation Criteria	Scenario/Model Outcome
6. Describe the recommended therapeutic approach to the patient or caregiver.	"Take orlistat up to 3 times a day before meals that contain fat. Skip the dose if a meal contains no fat."
7. Explain to the patient or caregiver the rationale for selecting the recommended therapeutic approach from the considered therapeutic alternatives.	"Orlistat should not be used as the sole method for weight loss but should be combined with a lower-calorie diet and increased physical activity."

Patient Education

8. When recommending self-care with nonprescription medications and/or nondrug therapy, convey accurate information to the patient or caregiver.	
a. appropriate dose and frequency of duration	"Take 60 mg up to 3 times a day."
b. maximum number of days the therapy should be employed	"The biggest weight loss is usually seen within the first 6 months of therapy. Decreased serum cholesterol and blood pressure may accompany weight loss."
c. product administration procedures	"Take before meals that contain fatty foods. Spreading dietary fat among 3 meals a day, plus minimizing the amount of dietary fat should help minimize gastrointestinal side effects, such as oily discharge and gas. Taking a multivitamin supplement at bedtime (separated from orlistat) is recommended, as orlistat can cause malabsorption of fat-soluble vitamins."
d. expected time to onset of relief	"Some weight loss should occur within 2 weeks of initiating orlistat therapy, especially if diet and exercise regimens are being followed."
e. degree of relief that can be reasonably expected	"Loss of 5–10 pounds during the first 6 months of therapy is a common outcome."
f. most common side effects	"Flatulence, oily spotting, loose and frequent stools, fatty stools, fecal urgency, and fecal incontinence may be experienced. These can be minimized by decreasing dietary fat and also tend to decrease with time."
g. side effects that warrant medical intervention should they occur	"Because of rare reports of liver toxicity, you should contact your primary care provider immediately if itching, yellow eyes or skin, dark urine, or loss of appetite occurs."
h. patient options in the event that condition worsens or persists	"Consult a dietitian or personal trainer for diet and exercise advice. Consult with primary care provider about prescription therapy for weight loss."
i. product storage requirements	None
j. specific nondrug requirements	"Dietary caloric restriction and exercise are of paramount importance. Find exercise that is enjoyable and sustainable. Try to spend more time standing rather than sitting throughout the day and especially in the evening. Attempt to reduce stress and thus stress eating. Keep healthy snacks such as fruits and vegetables in the house for nighttime snacking instead of eating chips. Consider cutting down on making desserts and serve fresh fruit instead. Too little sleep has been associated with increased body weight, so sleep hygiene measure may be helpful." (See Chapter 46.)
Solicit follow-up questions from the patient or caregiver.	"Can I double the dose of medication if weight loss slows?"
Answer the patient's or caregiver's questions.	"Dosage above 60 mg up to 3 times a day should be attempted only under the supervision of a primary care provider."

Evaluation of Patient Outcome

9. Assess patient outcome.	Ask Rhonda to weigh herself twice a week and record these values. She should return to you in a month to show you her progress and to discuss her diet and exercise regimen. A weight loss of a few pounds over the first month should be considered a success.

Key: BMI = Body mass index; NKA = no known allergies.

case
26–2

Relevant Evaluation Criteria	Scenario/Model Outcome

Information Gathering

1. Gather essential information about the patient's symptoms and medical history, including:

a. description of symptom(s) (i.e., nature, onset, duration, severity, associated symptoms)

Patient is concerned about her weight and overall appearance. She has been considered overweight since kindergarten. She wants to lose around 30 pounds by the time of her eighth-grade semiformal dance, which is in 6 months.

b. description of any factors that seem to precipitate, exacerbate, and/or relieve the patient's symptom(s)

Patient mimics her brothers when it comes to foods: she likes potato chips, nachos, soda, and pizza. She also eats a lot of rice and beans.

c. description of the patient's efforts to relieve the symptoms

Patient has not tried to lose weight in the past because her parents have thought her to be a healthy weight.

d. patient's identity

Angel Marquez

e. age, sex, height, and weight

13 years old, female, 5 ft 3 in., 185 lb

f. patient's occupation

Eighth-grade student

g. patient's dietary habits

She typically eats a hot breakfast with her family, which often includes beans, tortillas, and eggs or burritos with chorizo and beans. She usually eats lunch at the lunch cafeteria. She often gets potato chips and a soda from a snack machine in the afternoon. She has a big dinner every night with her family, often including dessert.

h. patient's sleep habits

Averages about 7–8 hours a night

i. concurrent medical conditions, prescription and nonprescription medications, and dietary supplements

Multivitamin once daily

j. allergies

NKA

k. history of other adverse reactions to medications

None

l. other (describe) _____

Patient participates in physical education classes at school twice a week. She has no other regular exercise activity. Patient is Hispanic, and both of her parents are overweight.

Assessment and Triage

2. Differentiate patient's signs/symptoms and correctly identify the patient's primary problem(s).

Patient's BMI is 32.8 k, placing her in the obesity category (Table 26–1). This places her at increased risk for type 2 DM, high cholesterol, hypertension, sleep apnea, and orthopedic problems during adolescence and adulthood if her weight is not normalized. Having daily sodas, regularly consuming fatty and salty snacks, and eating heavy breakfasts and dinners, together with minimal physical activity, are contributing to her weight problem. Her cafeteria lunches may also be a contributing factor.

3. Identify exclusions for self-treatment (Figure 26–3).

Age younger than 18 years is an exclusion for self-treatment.

4. Formulate a comprehensive list of therapeutic alternatives for the primary problem to determine if triage to a health care provider is required, and share this information with the patient or caregiver.

Options include:

(1) Refer Angel to a PCP for a health screen.

(2) Refer to a dietitian and personal trainer for diet and exercise advice, respectively.

(3) Recommend nonprescription orlistat.

(4) Recommend a dietary supplement weight-loss product.

(5) Take no action.

Plan

5. Select an optimal therapeutic alternative to address the patient's problem, taking into account patient preferences.

Refer the patient to a PCP for a health screen.

6. Describe the recommended therapeutic approach to the patient or caregiver.

"Your primary care provider may refer you for a health screen, or the provider could also offer prescription-strength orlistat."

case
26-2 *continued*

Relevant Evaluation Criteria	Scenario/Model Outcome
7. Explain to the patient or caregiver the rationale for selecting the recommended therapeutic approach from the considered therapeutic alternatives.	"You need to see your provider to determine if a diet and exercise program is appropriate. Healthy eating habits and exercise are the mainstays of successful weight loss, and these should be a lifelong goal."
Patient Education	
8. When recommending self-care with nonprescription medications and/or nondrug therapy, convey accurate information to the patient or caregiver.	Criterion does not apply in this case.
Solicit follow-up questions from the patient or caregiver.	"Is there an OTC medication that might work?"
Answer the patient's or caregiver's questions.	"No OTC medications are approved or appropriate to recommend in a patient younger than age 18 without referral from a primary care provider."
Evaluation of Patient Outcome	
9. Assess patient outcome.	Contact the patient in a day or two to ensure she made an appointment and sought medical care.

Key: BMI = Body mass index; DM = diabetes mellitus; N/A = not applicable; NKA = no known allergies; OTC = over-the-counter; PCP = primary care provider.

Patient Counseling for Overweight and Obesity

The objectives for counseling patients who want to lose weight are to foster realistic goals for weight loss together with promoting a healthy restricted-calorie diet and increased physical activity. The ultimate goal is to achieve a healthy weight and maintain that weight over the long term. For patients unable to lose weight, the objective is to prevent further weight gain. The box Patient Education for Overweight and Obesity lists specific information for patients.

Evaluation of Patient Outcomes for Overweight and Obesity

Successful weight loss generally requires a lifelong approach that combines healthy eating and exercise patterns. Realistic weight-loss goals of 5–10% of the initial weight over 6 months, or 1–2 pounds per week, should be encouraged. During any weight-loss program, the patient should be monitored for healthy eating and exercise patterns, and, at a minimum, blood pressure should be routinely measured. More extensive physical examinations and laboratory measures may be indicated, particularly in patients with comorbid conditions such as hypertension or type 2 DM. Follow-up with patients attempting weight loss should be encouraged, preferably monthly or quarterly. In addition to measuring weight at follow-up visits, the health care provider should explore eating habits and exercise patterns with the patient, especially if weight loss is not being achieved. Goals that were set should

be reexamined and followed up by the provider, with new goals or modifications set as appropriate. Referral to a dietitian or personal trainer may be helpful. Following weight loss, emphasis should be placed on the importance of maintaining the weight loss by continuing healthful dietary and exercise habits. Referral for pharmacologic therapy or consideration of bariatric surgery may be an option for patients with more significant obesity who fail to lose weight through lifestyle interventions.

Key Points for Overweight and Obesity

➤ A reasonable goal for weight loss in most overweight and obese subjects is a 5–10% loss over 6 months.

➤ Although this amount of weight loss may not result in the cosmetic effect desired by the dieter, it is associated with a reduction in risk for chronic disease.

➤ The safest approach to losing weight entails combining a reduced-calorie diet with increased physical activity.

➤ Physical activity typically needs to be something the person enjoys if it is to be sustained over long periods of time.

➤ A key to sustained weight loss is modification of behavior related to eating and exercise.

➤ If nonprescription or dietary supplement products for weight loss are used, they should be continuously assessed for efficacy, safety, and tolerance. All health care providers should be informed of the product(s) used. Labels of nonprescription or dietary supplement weight-loss products should be carefully reviewed to determine the risk for adverse reactions and drug–supplement interactions.

patient education for
Overweight and Obesity

The objectives of self-treatment are to (1) foster realistic weight-loss and exercise goals, (2) maintain a healthy weight, and (3) prevent further weight gain. Carefully following the self-care measures listed here, together with continued adherence to a safe and effective weight-loss program, will help ensure optimal therapeutic outcomes.

Health Risks of Obesity

- Health risks related to overweight and obesity include the following:
  - Coronary heart disease
  - Type 2 diabetes mellitus
  - Sleep apnea
  - Elevated serum triglycerides and dyslipidemia
  - Hypertension
  - Stroke
  - Gallbladder disease
  - Osteoarthritis
  - Certain types of cancers

Nondrug Treatment Guidelines

- Focus on small, gradual changes in eating and exercise patterns.
- Maintain realistic goals for weight loss and increased activity levels.
- Eat a low-calorie balanced diet.
- Eat meals at the table, and do nothing else while eating (no television, etc.).
- Set a regular eating schedule, and avoid skipping meals.
- Eat slowly and enjoy the food.
- Put down your fork or spoon between bites.
- Try to leave some food on your plate each time you eat.
- Wait 5 minutes before going back for extra helpings of food.
- Remove serving dishes from the table after the first servings have been made.
- Leave the table or at least clear food from the table after eating.

- Use smaller plates so moderate servings do not appear too small.
- Start a meal with a broth-based soup (low salt) to help you feel fuller.
- Strive to consume at least five servings a day of fruits and vegetables.
- Keep on hand healthful snacks such as fruits and vegetables, low-fat cheese and yogurt, and frozen fruit juice bars.
- Drink at least eight glasses of noncaloric beverages each day to help you feel full.
- When you experience a craving, try doing something else, such as going for a walk; cravings generally pass within minutes.
- Shop for food immediately after a meal, and use a prepared list.
- Gradually increase your activity level, with the goal of engaging in 60 minutes of moderate-intensity physical activity most days of the week.
- Increase your lifestyle activity: walk and stand more, climb stairs, and park farther from your destination.
- Limit the amount of time spent watching television, playing video games, or using the Internet.
- Keep a diary of your weight, physical activity, and caloric intake so you can see your progress and success.

Drug Management Guidelines

- Avoid taking nonprescription drugs and supplements marketed for weight loss, with the exception of orlistat. They are not proven to work, and they can cause significant side effects.
- If you do decide to take one of these products, make sure to notify your primary care provider and pharmacist so you can be adequately followed for potential side effects and interactions with drugs.

REFERENCES

1. Karam JG, McFarlane SI. Tackling obesity: new therapeutic agents for assisted weight loss. *Diabetes Metab Syndr Obes* 2010;3:95–112.
2. National Center for Health Statistics. *Health, United States, 2011: With Special Feature on Socioeconomic Status and Health.* Hyattsville, MD: U.S Department of Health and Human Services, Centers for Disease Control and Prevention, National Center for Health Statistics; 2012. DHHS Publication No. 2012–1232. Accessed at http://www.cdc.gov/nchs/data/hus/hus11.pdf, June 20, 2014.
3. Flegal KM, Carroll MD, Kit BK, et al. Prevalence of obesity and trends in the distribution of body mass index among US adults, 1999–2010. *JAMA.* 2012;307(5):491–7.
4. Ogden CL, Carroll MD, Kit BK, et al. Prevalence of obesity and trends in body mass index among US children and adolescents, 1999–2010. *JAMA.* 2012;307(5):483–90.
5. Finkelstein EA, Trogden JG, Cohen JW, et al. Annual medical spending attributable to obesity: payer and service-specific estimates. *Health Aff.* September/October 2009;28(5):w822–31.
6. Institute of Medicine, National Academy of Sciences. Accelerating progress in obesity prevention. Solving the weight of the nation. 2012. Accessed at http://www.iom.edu/~/media/Files/Report%20Files/2012/APOP/APOP_rb.pdf, June 20, 2014.
7. Jensen MD, Ryan DH, Apovian CM, et al. 2013 AHA/ACC/TOS Guideline for the management of overweight and obesity in adults: a report of the American College of Cardiology/American Heart Association Task Force on Practice Guidelines and The Obesity Society. *Circulation.* 2014;129(25 suppl 2));S102–38. Accessed at http://circ.ahajournals.org/content/early/2013/11/11/01.cir.0000437739.71477.ee.full.pdf, July 31, 2014.
8. Moyer VA, on behalf of the U.S. Preventive Services Task Force. Screening for and management of obesity in adults: U.S. Preventive Services Task Force recommendation statement. *Ann Intern Med* 2012;157(5):373–8.
9. Florez H, Castillo-Florez S. Beyond the obesity paradox in diabetes: fitness, fatness, and mortality. *JAMA* 2012;308(6):619–20.
10. Heber D. An integrative view of obesity. *Am J Clin Nutr* 2010;91(1):280S–3S
11. Flegal KM, Kit BK, Orpana H, et al. Association of all-cause mortality with overweight and obesity using standard body mass index categories. *JAMA.* 2013;309(1):71–82.
12. August GP, Caprio S, Fennoy I, et al. Prevention and Treatment of Pediatric Obesity. Chevy Chase, MD: Endocrine Society and *Journal of Clinical Endocrinology and Metabolism;* 2008. Accessed at https://www.endocrine.org/~/media/endosociety/Files/Publications/Clinical%20Practice%20Guidelines/FINAL-Standalone-Pediatric-Obesity-Guideline.pdf, June 20, 2014.
13. Qi Q, Chu AY, Kang JH, et al. Sugar-sweetened beverages and genetic risk of obesity. *New Engl J Med* 2012;367(15):1387–96.
14. Panickar KS. Effects of dietary polyphenols on neuroregulatory factors and pathways that mediate food intake and energy regulation in obesity. *Molec Nutr Food Res.* 2013;57(1):34–47.
15. Centers for Disease Control and Prevention. Prevalence of self-reported physically active adults–United States, 2007. *MMWR Morb Mortal Wkly Rep.* 2008;57(48):1297–300.
16. Shlisky JD, Hartman TJ, Kris-Etherton PM, et al. Partial sleep deprivation and energy balance in adults: an emerging issue for consideration by dietetics practitioners. *J Acad Nutr Diet.* 2012;112(11):1785–97.
17. Cani PD, Delzenne NM. Interplay between obesity and associated metabolic disorders: new insights into the gut microbiota. *Curr Opin Pharmacol.* 2009;9(6):737–43.

18. Leslie WS, Hankey CR, Lean ME. Weight gain as an adverse effect of some commonly prescribed drugs: a systematic review. *Q J Med.* 2007;100(7):395–404.

19. Poirier P, Giles TD, Bray GA, et al. Obesity and cardiovascular disease: pathophysiology, evaluation, and effect of weight loss. *Circulation.* 2006;113(6):898–918.

20. Pulgaron E. Childhood obesity: a review of increased risk for physical and psychological comorbidities. *Clin Ther.* 2013;35(1):A18–32.

21. Lloyd KB, Thrower MR, Walters NB, et al. Implementation of a weight management pharmaceutical care service. *Ann Pharmacother.* 2007;41(2): 185–92.

22. The National Weight Control Registry. The National Weight Control Registry Web site. http://www.nwcr.ws. Accessed June 20, 2014.

23. Food and Nutrition Board, Institute of Medicine. *Dietary Reference Intakes for Energy, Carbohydrate, Fiber, Fat, Fatty Acids, Cholesterol, Protein, and Amino Acids (Macronutrients).* Washington, DC: National Academies Press; 2002. http://www.nap.edu/books/0309085373/html. Accessed June 20, 2014.

24. U.S. Department of Agriculture, U.S. Department of Health and Human Services. *Dietary Guidelines for Americans, 2010.* 7th ed. Washington, DC. U.S. Government Printing Office; 2010. Accessed at http://health.gov/dietaryguidelines/2010.asp, June 20, 2014.

25. Ornish D, Scherwitz LW, Billings JH, et al. Intensive lifestyle changes for the reversal of coronary heart disease. *JAMA.* 1998;280(23):2001–7.

26. Hession M, Rolland C, Kulkarni U, et al. Systematic review of randomized controlled trials of low-carbohydrate vs. low-fat/low-calorie diets in the management of obesity and its comorbidities. *Obes Rev.* 2009;10(1):36–50.

27. Russell WR, Gratz SW, Duncan SH, et al. High-protein, reduced-carbohydrate weight-loss diets promote metabolite profiles likely to be detrimental to colonic health. *Am J Clin Nutr* 2011;93(5):1062–72.

28. Volek JS, Fernandez ML, Feinman RD, et al. Dietary carbohydrate restriction induces a unique metabolic state positively affecting atherogenic dyslipidemia, fatty acid partitioning, and metabolic syndrome. *Prog Lipid Res.* 2008;47:307–18.

29. U.S. Department of Health and Human Services. *2008 Physical Activity Guidelines for Americans.* Washington, DC: U.S. Department of Health and Human Services; 2008. ODPHP Publication No. U0036. Accessed at http://www.health.gov/paguidelines, June 20, 2014.

30. Thompson WG, Cook DA, Clark MM, et al. Treatment of obesity. *Mayo Clin Proc.* 2007;82(1):93–101.

31. U.S. Food and Drug Administration. Clean-up of ineffective ingredients in otc drug products [news release]. November 7, 1990. Accessed at http://pinch.com/skin/docs/FDA-OTC-ingredients-ban. June 20, 2014.

32. U.S. Food and Drug Administration. Phenylpropanolamine (PPA) information page. November 23, 2005. Updated September 3, 2010. Accessed at http://www.fda.gov/drugs/drugsafety/informationbydrugclass/ucm150738.htm, June 20, 2014.

33. U.S. Environmental Protection Agency. Cold, cough, allergy, bronchodilator, and antiasthmatic drug products for over-the-counter human use; partial final rule for combination drug products containing a bronchodilator. U.S. Food and Drug Administration. *Federal Regist.* 2001:66: 49276–8. Accessed at http://www.epa.gov/fedrgstr/EPA-IMPACT/2001/September/Day-27/i24127.htm, June 20, 2014.

34. U.S. Food and Drug Administration. Status of certain additional over-the-counter drug category II and III active ingredients. *Federal Regist.* 2002; 67: 31125–7. Accessed at http://www.fda.gov/OHRMS/DOCKETS/98fr/050902a.htm, June 20, 2014.

35. U.S. Food and Drug Administration. Final rule declaring dietary supplements containing ephedrine alkaloids adulterated because they present an unreasonable risk. *Federal Regist.* 2004;69:6787–854. Accessed at http://www.fda.gov/Food/GuidanceRegulation/GuidanceDocumentsRegulatoryInformation/DietarySupplements/ucm072997.htm, June 20, 2014.

36. U.S. Food and Drug Administration. Chapter 7–Court Decisions [fiscal year 2007]. Accessed at http://www.fda.gov/downloads/ICECI/EnforcementActions/EnforcementStory/EnforcementStoryArchive/UCM090325.pdf, June 20, 2014.

37. U.S. Food and Drug Administration. FDA approves orlistat for over-the-counter use [news release]. February 7, 2008. Accessed at http://www.fda.gov/NewsEvents/Newsroom/PressAnnouncements/2007/ucm108839.htm, June 20, 2014.

38. U.S. Food and Drug Administration Warning: counterfeit Alli [consumer update]. August 9, 2012. Accessed at http://www.fda.gov/ForConsumers/ConsumerUpdates/ucm198557.htm, June 20, 2014.

39. Xenical [prescribing information]. Genentech USA, South San Francisco, CA; January 2012. Accessed at http://www.gene.com/download/pdf/xenical_prescribing.pdf, June 20, 2014.

40. Anderson JW, Schwartz SM, Hauptman J, et al. Low-dose orlistat effects on body weight of mildly to moderately overweight individuals: a 16-week, double-blind, placebo-controlled trial. *Ann Pharmacother.* 2006;40(10):1717–23.

41. Mancini MC, Halpern A. Orlistat in the prevention of diabetes in the obese. *Vasc Health Risk Manag* 2008;4(2):325–36.

42. MacLaughlin HL, Cook SA, Kariyawasam D, et al. Nonrandomized trial of weight loss with orlistat, nutrition education, diet, and exercise in obese patients with CKD: 2-year follow-up. *Am J Kidney Dis.* 2009;55(1):69–76.

43. U.S. Food and Drug Administration. Orlistat (marketed as Alli and Xenical): labeling change. May 26, 2010. Accessed at http://www.fda.gov/Safety/MedWatch/SafetyInformation/SafetyAlertsforHumanMedicalProducts/ucm213448.htm, June 20, 2014.

44. U.S. Food and Drug Administration. Re: docket no. 2006P-0154/CP1 and SUP1. February 7, 2007. Accessed at http://www.fda.gov/ohrms/dockets/dockets/06p0154/06P-0154-pdn0001.pdf, June 20, 2014.

45. Haller CA, Benowitz NF, Jacob P III. Hemodynamic effects of ephedra-free weight-loss supplements in humans. *Am J Med.* 2005;118(9):998–1003.

46. Ulbright CE. *Natural Standard Herb & Supplement Guide: An Evidence-Based Reference.* 1st ed. Maryland Heights, MO: Mosby, Inc.; 2010:799–823.

47. Hasani-Ranjbar S, Nayebi N, Larijani B, et al. A systematic review of the efficacy and safety of herbal medicines used in the treatment of obesity. *World J Gastroenterol.* 2009;15(25):3073–85.

48. Egras AM, Hamilton WR, Lenz TL, Monaghan MS. An evidence-based review of fat modifying supplemental weight loss products. *J Obes.* 2011;2011. Article ID 297315. http://dx.doi.org/10.1155/2011/297315.

49. Dwyer JT, Allison DB, Coates PM. Dietary supplements in weight reduction. *J Am Diet Assoc.* 2005;105(5 suppl 1):S80–6.

50. U.S. Food and Drug Administration. Addressing challenges of economically-motivated adulteration. PowerPoint presentation, May 2009. Accessed at http://www.fda.gov/downloads/NewsEvents/MeetingsConferencesWorkshops/UCM163631.ppt, June 20, 2014.

51. U.S. Food and Drug Administration. Economically motivated adulteration in the dietary supplement market place. PowerPoint presentation, n.d. Accessed at http://www.fda.gov/downloads/NewsEvents/MeetingsConferencesWorkshops/UCM163645.ppt, June 20, 2014.

52. U.S. Food and Drug Administration. Tainted_supplements_CDER. FDA's Medication Health Fraud Page. Accessed at http://www.accessdata.fda.gov/scripts/sda/sdNavigation.cfm?sd=tainted_supplements_cder, June 20, 2014.

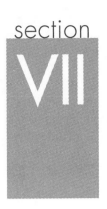
OPHTHALMIC, OTIC, AND ORAL DISORDERS

OPHTHALMIC DISORDERS

Richard G. Fiscella and Michael K. Jensen

The nonprescription ophthalmic market consists of products that treat a wide range of disorders. Little population-based data are available on the epidemiology of these disorders. People with ocular conditions are commonly seen in the primary care provider's office, the emergency department, the eye care provider's office, or the pharmacy. Ocular discomfort associated with dry eye disease may be the most common condition for which nonprescription ophthalmic products can be used. Dry eye disease may affect as many as 5 million people in the United States ages 50 years and older.[1]

Many common conditions that cause ocular discomfort are minor and self-limiting. In some instances, however, relatively minor symptoms may be associated with severe, potentially vision-threatening conditions. Health care providers should be well versed in eye anatomy and physiology (as well as in common ocular conditions) so they can provide the best possible guidance for patients who want help choosing between self-treatment and professional medical care.

Self-treatable ophthalmic disorders occur primarily on the eyelids; however, a few disorders of the eye surface may be responsive to self-treatment. The latter include dry eyes, allergic conjunctivitis, diagnosed corneal edema, presence of loose foreign debris, minor ocular irritation, and the cleaning or lubricating of artificial eyes. *Careful assessment is important,* especially with ongoing symptoms, to rule out more complicated manifestations that may require referral to an eye care specialist.

Role of Eye Anatomy in Ocular Drug Pharmacokinetics

The external location and exposure of the eye make it susceptible to environmental and microbiologic contamination. The eye has many natural defense mechanisms to protect it against contamination, however, and the eyelid is one of its major protective elements (Figure 27–1).

The eyelids are a multilayer tissue covered externally by the skin and internally by a thin, mucocutaneous epithelial layer called the palpebral conjunctiva. The middle portion of the eyelid contains glandular tissue and muscles for lid movement. The glandular tissue found within the eyelid, along with conjunctival goblet cells, secretes the bulk of nonstimulated tears.

The eyelids primarily protect the anterior surface of the eye and spread the tears produced by the glandular tissue over the ocular surface. The lids force the flow of tears toward the nose and into the drainage canals located in the upper and lower eyelids. The drainage canals converge, forming the lacrimal sac between the inner eyelid and nose. The lacrimal sac is drained by a canal opening just below the inferior turbinate of the nasal cavity. A highly vascularized epithelium lines the lacrimal drainage system, and absorption into the systemic circulation along this pathway gives rise to the potential systemic effects of topically administered eye medications.[2]

The tear layer keeps the ocular surface lubricated, provides a mechanism for removing debris that touches the ocular surface, and has potent antimicrobial action provided by specific enzymes and a number of immunoglobulins (including the most prevalent, immunoglobulin A). The tear layer is a complex, multilayer film. The outer lipid layer maintains the eyes' optical properties and reduces evaporation. The middle aqueous layer is largely responsible for the wetting properties of the tear film. The inner mucinous layer allows the outer lipid and middle aqueous layers to maintain constant adhesion across the cornea and conjunctiva. Abnormalities within any one of the tear layers can result in ocular discomfort.

Tears are produced at a rate of 1–2 μL per minute, with a turnover of approximately 16% of the total volume per minute.[3,4] As much as 25% of the total tear volume is lost to evaporation.[3] An ambient tear volume of approximately 7–10 μL is found on the ocular surface at any point in time.[3] During episodes of ocular irritation, reflex tearing is stimulated by the lacrimal gland found underneath the outer portion of the upper eyelid, and tear production increases to greater than 300% of the nonstimulated production rate.[5] Reflex tearing occurs immediately on instillation of a drug into the eye, diluting the drug's concentration. Drug penetration into the eye is reduced because of increased lacrimal drainage and tearing that falls down the cheek. Studies have shown that as much as 90% of an instilled dose of a drug administered to the eye may be lost.[6]

The visible external portion of the eye is composed of the noninnervated sclera and the innervated cornea. The sclera is a tough, collagenous layer that gives the eye rigidity and encases the internal eye structures. The visible sclera is covered by two epithelial layers: the episclera and the bulbar conjunctiva. The bulbar conjunctiva is contiguous with the palpebral conjunctiva at the junction between the eyelid and the ocular surface (the fornix). The episcleral and bulbar conjunctival layers (which contain the vascular and lymphatic systems of the anterior eye

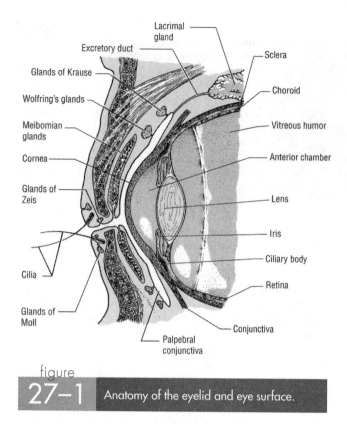

Lacrimal gland
Excretory duct
Glands of Krause
Wolfring's glands
Meibomian glands
Cornea
Glands of Zeis
Cilia
Glands of Moll
Palpebral conjunctiva
Sclera
Choroid
Vitreous humor
Anterior chamber
Lens
Iris
Ciliary body
Retina
Conjunctiva

figure

27–1   Anatomy of the eyelid and eye surface.

surface) are the sources of visible eye redness in ocular irritation or inflammation.

The cornea is an aspherical, vascular tissue that is the principal refractive element of the eye. The cornea is approximately 12 mm wide and 0.5 mm thick and consists of five distinct layers. Of the five corneal layers, the pharmacokinetics of ocularly administered drugs is affected by the outermost epithelium layer, the middle and most abundant stromal layer, and the innermost endothelial layer. The corneal epithelium is lipophilic and facilitates the passage of fat-soluble drugs. However, if a drug is too lipophilic, it may become trapped in the corneal epithelium. The epithelium is often the rate-limiting step in absorption of medication into the anterior chamber. The corneal stroma is hydrophilic and allows the passage of water-soluble drugs.

Damage to the corneal epithelium may often increase drug absorption rates. Comparative studies with intact and compromised epithelium have shown that drug penetration into the aqueous humor may be increased as much as threefold in corneas with compromised epithelium.[7] Corneal epithelium can be compromised by trauma, routine contact lens wear, topical ocular anesthetics, and thermal or ultraviolet (UV) light exposure.

Directly behind the cornea is the anterior chamber, a cavity filled with aqueous humor. The aqueous humor maintains the normal intraocular pressure (IOP) and provides nutritional support for the cornea and crystalline lens. The aqueous humor is produced by the ciliary body and is drained from the anterior chamber through the uveoscleral tract and the trabecular meshwork. The trabecular meshwork, which is located at the junction of the cornea and iris, accounts for approximately 80%–90% of aqueous drainage from the

anterior chamber. The uveoscleral tract (located posterior to the iris and comprising the sclera, ciliary body, and choroid areas) accounts for approximately 10%–20% of aqueous drainage, although this percentage may vary with age and disease state.

During episodes of internal eye inflammation, inflammatory cells may block the drainage system, causing the IOP to rise. Increased IOP is one of the most significant risk factors for primary open-angle glaucoma. Similarly, during episodes of closed-angle glaucoma, the iris physically blocks the trabecular meshwork, which also results in an increase in IOP. Dilating the pupil with mydriatic drugs may precipitate an angle-closure attack. These attacks often occur as the pupil is returning to its normal state several hours after the mydriatic drug has been instilled. Any agent with anticholinergic or dilating effects has the potential to cause angle closure. The most common symptoms are brow ache or headache, often accompanied by nausea and vomiting. These symptoms are severe enough to cause individuals to visit their eye care providers.

The visible, colored portion of the eye, the iris, is located in the anterior segment of the eye, behind the cornea. It functions in much the same way as an aperture on a camera by regulating the amount of light striking the retina. The central opening in the iris is the pupil. The pupillary diameter is controlled by two opposing muscles within the iris: the sphincter and the dilator. The sphincter muscle runs along circular arcs parallel to the pupillary border and causes a miotic (closing) effect through parasympathetic stimulation. The dilator muscles are radial from the pupillary border and cause a mydriatic (opening) effect through sympathetic stimulation. Prostaglandins released by the iris during episodes of inflammation may affect the sphincter muscle, resulting in constriction of the pupil.

The ciliary body is bordered anteriorly by the iris and is continuous posteriorly with the choroid. In addition to producing aqueous humor, the ciliary body participates in focusing the optical mechanism (lens) for near viewing (a process known as accommodation). During episodes of ocular inflammation, the ciliary muscle may go into spasm, resulting in fluctuating vision and pain. Therefore, inhibition of the ciliary muscle (cycloplegia) with anticholinergic agents is a frequent treatment for internal ocular inflammation.

The vitreous cavity, located in the posterior segment of the eye, is the largest portion of the eye and is filled with vitreous humor. Floating spots in the visual field ("floaters") are related to this area. Floaters are deposits of various shapes, sizes, and motility in the vitreous humor; they may be related to degenerative changes in gel that is normally transparent. Problems in this area are not amenable to self-treatment and require professional evaluation because of the possibility of concurrent retinal problems.

The retina is responsible for the initial processing and transmission of light signals. A number of inflammatory conditions of the retina can occur, and most have prominent symptoms. Some, however, have relatively mild symptoms, mimicking common irritative conditions. Trauma, even minor, may cause the retina to separate from its underlying layer (the pigment epithelium), resulting in retinal detachment. The retinal pigment epithelium provides vital "electrical" support to the retina. Macular degeneration, the leading cause of blindness in the United States, is directly related to atrophy in the pigment epithelium. Diabetic retinopathy also is a major cause of vision loss.

Dry Eye Disease

Pathophysiology and Clinical Presentation of Dry Eye

Dry eye disease is among the most common disorders affecting the anterior eye.[1] Most often associated with the aging process (especially with postmenopausal women), dry eye also can be caused by lid defects, corneal defects, loss of lid tissue turgor, Sjögren's syndrome, Bell's palsy, thyroid eye disease, various collagen diseases (e.g., rheumatoid arthritis), and systemic medications. Refractive surgery patients may complain of transient dry eyes for weeks to months after the procedure. This effect is usually mild if it does occur, but it can be more pronounced in some patients. Drugs with anticholinergic properties (e.g., antihistamines and antidepressants), decongestants, diuretics, and beta-blockers are some of the more common pharmacologic causes of dry eye. The condition may be exacerbated by allergens or other environmental conditions (e.g., dry, dusty working situations), or by heating and air conditioning systems that reduce relative humidity, thereby increasing the evaporation of tears.

Dry eye disease is characterized by a white or mildly red eye; patients may complain of a sandy, gritty feeling or a sensation that something is in the eye. Contrary to what the name suggests, dry eye disease often may present with excessive tearing initially. Abnormalities in the tear layer cause less-than-optimal lubrication of the ocular surface, thus producing more inadequate tears and beginning a vicious cycle. Failure to properly diagnose and treat dry eye diseases can result in severe damage to eye tissue, particularly to the corneal surface (see Color Plates, photograph 3). Recent evidence demonstrates that dry eye disease can be linked to a T-cell–mediated inflammatory process, which can respond to immunomodulatory agents (e.g., cyclosporine).[8]

Treatment of Dry Eye Disease

Treatment Goals

The goal in treating dry eye disease is to alleviate and control the dryness of the ocular surface, thereby relieving the symptoms of irritation and preventing possible tissue and corneal damage. Although dry eye disease also has been referred to as "dysfunctional tear syndrome," "keratoconjunctivitis sicca," and "dry eye disease," a recent published report of the International Dry Eye Workshop (DEWS) accepted "dry eye disease" as the most appropriate term.[1,9] The DEWS report, in conjunction with a Delphi panel paper and the recently published preferred practice patterns from the American Academy of Ophthalmology, has introduced a severity scale and an accompanying set of guidelines for treatment of dry eye disease.[9–11]

General Treatment Approach

The primary self-treatment for dry eye disease is the use of ocular lubricants. However, treatment of mild and moderate dry eye disease also includes other pharmacologic and nonpharmacologic recommendations, including education, environmental modifications, eyelid therapy, elimination of offending topical or systemic medications, and use of systemic omega–3 fatty acid supplements (e.g., flax seed oil; Table 27–1). The availability of synthetic chemicals suitable for topical application to the eye has resulted in the development of various solutions (artificial tears) to help alleviate dryness of the ocular surface. Artificial tear products vary by viscosity according to the ingredients used in their preparation. Increasing the viscosity of a product results in a more prolonged ocular contact time and greater resistance to tear dilution. Mild cases of dry eye disease may be treated with less viscous products, whereas more severe cases may require more viscous products. Bland (i.e., nonmedicated) ophthalmic ointment (e.g., petrolatum) is another type of ocular lubricant. Because ointment preparations tend to cause blurred vision, they are typically reserved for use only at bedtime or for severe cases of dry eye. As with ointments, the more viscous the tear drops are, the greater their blurring effect becomes. Vitamin A preparations are also available for treating dry eye disease.

Nonpharmacologic measures (e.g., warm compresses; discontinuing any offending agents; eyelid therapy, consisting of warm compresses and eyelid hygiene) may also increase eye comfort for patients with this disorder. The use of omega-3 oils or flax seed oil in the normal doses recommended by the manufacturer

table

27–1 Treatment Recommendations for Dry Eye Disease by Disease Severity Level

Mild

Education, environmental modifications

Elimination of offending topical or systemic medications

Aqueous enhancement using artificial tear substitutes, gels/ointments

Eyelid therapy (warm compresses and eyelid hygiene)

Treatment of contributing ocular factors such as blepharitis or meibomianitis

Moderate

Same treatments listed for mild disease plus the following treatments:

Anti-inflammatory agents (topical cyclosporine and corticosteroids, systemic omega-3 fatty acid supplements)

Punctal plugs

Spectacle side shields and moisture chambers

Severe

Same treatments listed for mild and moderate disease plus the following treatments:

Systemic cholinergic agonists

Systemic anti-inflammatory agents

Mucolytic agents

Autologous serum tears

Contact lenses

Correction of eyelid abnormalities

Permanent punctal occlusion

Tarsorrhaphy

Source: Adapted from the American Academy of Ophthalmology Preferred Practice Guidelines at www.AAO.org.

is thought to improve lid function, possibly because the products have some anti-inflammatory properties.[9–11]

Eye care providers treat the most severe cases of dry eye disease with punctal plugs, which occlude the lacrimal drainage system to increase the available tear pool. New understanding of the underlying pathophysiology of dry eye disease suggest that patients may benefit from treatment with topical cyclosporine.[8] However, patients with mild dry eye disease may require relief of only ocular surface dryness, whereas patients with more moderate and severe dry eye disease may benefit from a combined approach of immunomodulating agents (e.g., topical cyclosporine in conjunction with ocular surface lubrication); such patients must be referred to an eye care specialist.

Nonpharmacologic Therapy

The primary nondrug measure is avoiding environments that increase evaporation of the tear film. If possible, patients should avoid dry or dusty places. Using humidifiers or repositioning workstations away from heating and air conditioning vents may help alleviate dry eyes. In addition, avoiding prolonged use of computer screens and wearing eye protection (e.g., sunglasses or goggles) in windy, outdoor environments may further help alleviate dry eye problems.

Pharmacologic Therapy

Nonmedicated ointments are commonly used in treating minor ophthalmic disorders, including dry eye. Because ointments can cause blurred vision (resulting in severe vision limitations), combination therapy using artificial tears and nonmedicated ointments is usually recommended. Gels offer some advantage to patients because they disturb vision less compared to ointments and are tolerated better. The effectiveness of retinol solutions for treating dry eye remains speculative.

Artificial Tear Solutions

Although many advances have been made in understanding the mechanisms involved in tear film formation, the role of tears in maintaining a normal conjunctival and corneal surface is still not completely understood. Lubricants that are formulated as artificial tear solutions consist of preservatives, inorganic electrolytes to achieve tonicity and maintain pH, and water-soluble polymeric systems. The lubricating agents in artificial tear products are similar, but buffering agents, preservatives, pH, and other formulation components may vary (Table 27–2). The newer artificial tear substitutes have important properties, including

table 27–2 **Commonly Used Nonprescription Ophthalmic Lubricants**

Trade Name	Primary Ingredients
Artificial Tear Solutions	
Bion Tears[a]	Hydroxypropyl methylcellulose 0.3%; dextran 70, 0.1%
Clear Eyes Contact Lens Relief Drops	Sorbic acid 0.25%; EDTA 0.1%; NaCl; hypromellose; glycerin
Dry Eyes	PVA 1.4%; sodium phosphate; NaCl; BAK 0.01%; EDTA
Eye-Lube-A	Glycerin 0.25%; EDTA; NaCl; BAK
GenTeal Lubricant Eye Drops, Mild and Mild to Moderate	Hydroxypropyl methylcellulose; boric acid; phosphonic acid; NaCl; sodium perborate
HypoTears[b]	PVA 1%; PEG 400; BAK 0.01%
LubriTears	Hydroxypropyl methylcellulose 2906, 0.3%; dextran 70, 0.1%; EDTA; KCl; NaCl; BAK 0.01%
Moisture Eyes[b]	Propylene glycol 1%; glycerin 0.3%; BAK 0.01%
Murine Tears Lubricant	Povidone 0.6%; PVA 0.5%; BAK
Nature's Tears	Hydroxypropyl methylcellulose 2906, 0.4%; KCl; NaCl; sodium phosphate; BAK 0.01%; EDTA
Ocucoat Lubricating[b]	Hydroxypropyl methylcellulose 0.8%; dextran 70, 0.1%; BAK 0.01%
Preservative-Free Moisture Eyes[a]	Propylene glycol 0.95%; boric acid; NaCl; KCl; sodium borate; EDTA
Refresh	PVA 1.4%; povidone 0.6%
Refresh Dry Eye Therapy	Glycerin 1.0%; polysorbate 80, 1.0% (polymer matrix; emulsifying agent; carbomer; castor oil)
Refresh Optive	CMC 0.5%; glycerin 0.9%; Purite[c]; boric acid; calcium chloride; magnesium chloride; KCl; levocarnitine; erythritol
Refresh Optive Sensitive PF	CMC sodium 0.5%; glycerin 0.9%; boric acid, calcium chloride, erythritol, levocarnitine Magnesium chloride, KCL, water (purified), sodium borate, NaCl
Refresh Optive Sensitive PF Advanced	CMC sodium 0.5%, glycerin 1%, polysorbate 80, 0.5%, boric acid, castor oil, erythritol, levocarnitine, carbomer copolymer type A, purified water, Purite; may also contain hydrochloric acid, sodium hydroxide
Refresh Plus[a]	CMC sodium 0.5%
Refresh Tears	CMC sodium 0.5%; Purite[c]

table
27–2 Commonly Used Nonprescription Ophthalmic Lubricants (continued)

Trade Name	Primary Ingredients
Soothe	Restoryl (Drakeol-15 1.0% and Drakeol-35 4.5%); polysorbate 80, 0.4%; octoxynol 40; NaCl; sodium phosphate; EDTA; polyhexamethylene biguanide preservative
Systane	PEG-400, 0.4%; propylene glycol 0.3%; boric acid; calcium chloride; hydroxypropyl guar; magnesium chloride; polyquaternium preservative; KCl; NaCl; zinc chloride; water
Teargen	BAK 0.01%; EDTA; NaCl; PVA
Teargen II	Hydroxypropyl methylcellulose 2910, 4 mg; dextran 70, 0.1%; NaCl; KCl; sodium borate
Tears Naturale	Hydroxypropyl methylcellulose 0.3%; dextran 70, 0.1%; BAK 0.01%
Tears Naturale Forte	Dextran 70, 0.1%; hydroxypropyl methylcellulose 0.3%; glycerin 0.2%; polyquaternium 1, 0.001%; NaCl; KCl; sodium borate
Tears Naturale Free[a]	Hydroxypropyl methylcellulose 0.3%; dextran 70, 0.1%
Tears Naturale II	Hydroxypropyl methylcellulose 0.3%; dextran 70, 0.1%; Polyquad 0.001%
Tears Plus	PVA 1.4%; povidone 0.6%; chlorobutanol 0.5%
Tears Renewed	BAK 0.01%; EDTA; dextran 70, 0.1%; NaCl; hydroxypropyl methylcellulose 2906, 0.3%
Theratears PF[a]	CMC 0.25%
Visine Pure Tears Drops[b]	Glycerin 0.2%; hypromellose 0.2%; PEG 400, 1%
Nonmedicated Ointments	
Artificial Tears PF[a]	White petrolatum; anhydrous liquid lanolin; mineral oil
Dry Eyes	White petrolatum; mineral oil; lanolin
DuraTears Naturale[a]	Petrolatum; mineral oil; lanolin
HypoTears	White petrolatum; light mineral oil
Lacri-Lube N.P.[a]	White petrolatum 57.3%; mineral oil 42.5%; lanolin alcohols
Lacri-Lube S.O.P.	White petrolatum 56.8%; mineral oil 42.5%; lanolin alcohols; chlorobutanol 0.5%
Preservative Free Moisture Eyes PM	White petrolatum 80%; mineral oil 20%
Refresh P.M.[a]	White petrolatum 56.8%; mineral oil 41.5%; lanolin alcohols
Tears Renewed[a]	White petrolatum; light mineral oil
Nonmedicated Gels	
GenTeal Lubricant Eye Gel	Hydroxypropyl methylcellulose 0.3%; sodium perborate 0.028%; carbopol 980; phosphoric acid; sorbitol
Theratears Gel	CMC 1%; KCl; sodium bicarbonate; NaCl; sodium phosphate

Key: BAK = Benzalkonium chloride; CMC = carboxymethylcellulose; EDTA = ethylenediamine tetraacetic acid; KCl = potassium chloride; NaCl = sodium chloride; PEG = polyethylene glycol; PVA = polyvinyl alcohol.

[a] Preservative-free product.

[b] Preservative-free formulation available.

[c] Stabilized oxychloro complex.

their ability to stabilize the tear film, protect the corneal and conjunctival cells, reduce tear evaporation with the combination of lipids, and enhance wound healing and lubrication of the ocular surface.[1]

One class of ophthalmic vehicles or ocular lubricants, in their commonly used ophthalmic formulation concentrations, is the substituted cellulose ethers, which include hydroxypropyl methylcellulose 0.3%–0.8% and carboxymethylcellulose (CMC) 0.5% and 1.0%. These solutions are colorless and vary in viscosity depending on the grade and concentration of the cellulose ether. Polyvinyl alcohol (PVA) 1.4% and povidone 0.6% are two other vehicles commonly used as ocular lubricants.[12–15]

Combining drugs with these vehicles increases the vehicles' viscosity, thereby enhancing the drugs' action. The increased viscosity retards drainage of the active ingredient from the eye, thus increasing the retention time of the active drug and enhancing bioavailability at the external ocular tissues. These effects generally occur without irritation or toxicity to the ocular tissues. Similar to the cellulose ethers, PVA also enhances stability of the tear film without causing ocular irritation or toxicity.

Povidone has surface-active properties similar to those of cellulose ethers. This compound is believed to form a hydrophilic layer on the corneal surface, mimicking natural conjunctival mucin. This mucomimetic property has firmly established the role of povidone as an artificial tear formulation. Because this agent promotes wetting of the ocular surface, mucin- and aqueous-deficient dry eyes appear to benefit from its use.

One example of the most commonly recommended and newer products on the market is Refresh Optive Advanced Lubricant Eye Drops, which contains glycerin (0.9%), polysorbate 80 (0.5%), CMC 0.5%, boric acid, castor oil, erythritol, levocarnitine, and carbomer copolymer type A. This product is reported to be a lipid-based, triple action preparation that helps lubricate and hydrate dry eyes and protects against evaporation of natural tears. Soothe is an artificial tear solution that contains a lipid restorative layer, which provides a barrier to prevent loss of the aqueous component of the tears.

Systane is a lubricant eyedrop that contains a gelling and polymer system. Hydroxypropyl guar binds to the hydrophobic corneal surface, forming a glycocalyx or gel-like environment that stays in contact with the ocular surface for a longer period of time. Systane is said to create an ocular shield, allowing epithelial repair that promotes patient comfort and relief of symptoms. Optive, a combination of CMC and glycerin, is believed to help protect the corneal epithelium through an osmotic protective effect.

Studies have shown that formulations of artificial tear products without preservatives are less likely than those with preservatives to irritate the ocular surface.[10] Providers and patients should be aware, however, that nonpreserved products should be discarded immediately after being opened and used.

Most patients with mild cases of dry eye disease instill drops of artificial tears once or twice per day, typically on arising in the morning and/or before retiring at night (Table 27-3).[11] Recommending drops at least twice per day is a good starting point. The viscosity of the drops and amount used can then be adjusted according to the patient's response. For more severe cases, the dosage can be increased to 3–4 times daily. If the patient's clinical needs and response to therapy indicate more frequent use, these solutions may be given as often as hourly. In many cases, artificial tears may be continued indefinitely, depending on patient response. Preservative-free products or those with less toxic preservatives (e.g., Purite or sodium perborate; see Ophthalmic Preservatives) are preferred in patients with moderate-severe dry eye disease.

Use of ocular lubricants requires balancing the number of drops per day with the viscosity of the recommended solution and the presence of a preservative; as the number of drops per day increases, toxicity from preservatives becomes more likely.[16]

Although PVA is compatible with many commonly used drugs and preservatives, certain compounds (e.g., sodium bicarbonate, sodium borate, the sulfates of sodium, potassium, and zinc) can thicken or gel solutions containing PVA. For example, sodium borate is found in some extraocular irrigating solutions or irrigants and may react with contact lens wetting solutions that contain PVA.[17] Therefore, health care providers must be cautious when recommending solutions containing PVA.

Nonmedicated Ophthalmic Ointments

The primary ingredients in commercial nonprescription ophthalmic ointments (Table 27-2) are white petrolatum 60% (which contains a lubricant and an ointment base), mineral oil 40% (which helps the ointment melt at body temperature), and

table 27-3	**Administration Guidelines for Eyedrops**

1. If you have difficulty determining whether eyedrops have touched your eye surface, refrigerate the solution before instilling it. Do not refrigerate suspensions. Always check the expiration date.
2. Wash hands thoroughly. Wash areas of the face around the eyes. Contact lenses should be removed unless the product is designed specifically for use with contact lenses.
3. Tilt head back. When administering drops to children, have them lie down before placing drops in their eyes.
4. Gently grasp lower outer eyelid below lashes, and pull eyelid away from eye to create a pouch.
5. Place dropper over eye by looking directly at it, as shown in the drawing.

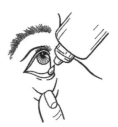

6. Just before applying a single drop, look up.
7. As soon as the drop is applied, release the eyelid slowly. Close eyes gently for 3 minutes by placing your head down as though looking at the floor (using gravity to pull the drop onto the cornea). Minimize blinking or squeezing of the eyelid.
8. Use a finger to put gentle pressure over the opening of the tear duct.
9. Blot excessive solution from around the eye.
10. If multiple medications are indicated, wait at least 5 minutes before instilling the next drop. This pause helps ensure that the first drop is not flushed away by the second and that the second drop is not diluted by the first.
11. If using a suspension, shake well before instilling. If using the suspension with another dosage form, place the suspension drop last, because it has prolonged retention time in the tear film.
12. If both drop and ointment therapy are indicated, instill the drops at least 10 minutes before the ointment so that the ointment does not become a barrier to the drops' penetration of the tear film or cornea.

lanolin (which facilitates incorporation of water-soluble medications and also prevents evaporation).

The principal advantage of nonmedicated (bland) ointments is their enhanced retention time in the eye, which appears to enhance the integrity of the tear film. Therefore, mucin- and aqueous-deficient eyes can benefit from the application of lubricating ointments.

Ointment formulations are usually administered twice daily (Table 27-4). However, depending on the patient's clinical needs and therapeutic response, ointments may be administered as often as every few hours or only occasionally, as needed. Many patients prefer to instill the ointment at bedtime to keep the eyes moist during sleep and improve morning symptoms of dry eye.

Because of the viscosity of the melted ointment base in the tear film, many patients complain of blurred vision when

table
27–4 Administration Guidelines for Eye Ointments

1. Wash hands thoroughly. Wash areas of the face around the eyes.
2. If both drop and ointment therapy are indicated, instill the drops at least 10 minutes before the ointment so that the ointment does not become a barrier to the drops' penetration of the tear film or cornea.
3. Tilt head back.
4. Gently grasp lower outer eyelid below lashes, and pull eyelid away from eye as shown in the drawing.

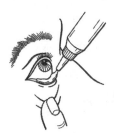

5. Place ointment tube over eye by looking directly at it.
6. With a sweeping motion, place a one-fourth- to one-half-inch strip of ointment inside the lower eyelid by gently squeezing the tube, but avoid touching the tube tip to any tissue surface.
7. Release the eyelid slowly.
8. Close eyes gently for 1–2 minutes.
9. Blot excessive ointment from around the eye.
10. Vision may be blurred temporarily. Avoid activities that require good visual ability until vision clears.

using ointments. This problem can usually be managed by decreasing the amount of ointment instilled or by administering the ointment at bedtime. Providers should routinely counsel patients about the blurred vision associated with eye ointments.

Ointment preparations are generally nonirritating, but preservatives can be toxic to ocular tissues. Some patients develop hypersensitivity reactions, which may prompt them to discontinue therapy. Changing to a single-use, preservative-free formulation (e.g., Duratears Naturale, HypoTears, Lacri-Lube N.P., or Refresh PM) may eliminate symptoms associated with preservative-containing ointments. Preservative-free products are particularly helpful in long-term treatment. As a rule, pharmacists should recommend preservative-free, nonmedicated ointments for the treatment of dry eye to avoid the potential problems associated with preservatives.

Formulation Considerations for Ocular Lubricants and Other Ophthalmic Products

Ocular lubricants and other nonprescription ophthalmic drugs are formulated to reduce the stinging, burning, and other side effects commonly associated with some ophthalmic drugs. These products are comfortable to use because their pH is carefully controlled, and because they use buffers, tonicity adjusters, and preservative systems; therefore, they encourage patients to

adhere to self-treatment. Drug vehicle and preservative systems are among the most important inactive ingredients of these products. Other commonly used vehicles are dextran 70, gelatin, glycerin, hydroxyethylcellulose, methylcellulose, polyethylene glycol, and propylene glycol. Various other ingredients often are included as excipients.

Ophthalmic Preservatives

Preservatives are incorporated into multidose ophthalmic products. These components are intended to destroy or limit the growth of microorganisms inadvertently introduced into the product. Surfactants, one of two distinct groups of preservatives, are usually bactericidal, meaning they disrupt the bacterial plasma membrane. Of the quaternary surfactants, benzalkonium chloride (BAK) and benzethonium chloride are preferred by many manufacturers because of their stability, excellent antimicrobial activity, and long shelf-lives. Unfortunately, these agents can have toxic effects on both the tear film and the corneal epithelium.[18,19] Long-term use of topical products containing BAK can damage conjunctival and corneal epithelial cells. Complications associated with BAK include allergy, fibrosis, dry eye disease, and increased risk of failure of glaucoma surgery.[20] Although only a small percentage of patients with dry eye disease experience BAK toxicity, it may become quite problematic for those exhibiting symptoms. Polyquad, a large-molecular-weight quaternary compound, does not bind to contact lenses and is less toxic than BAK.

Chlorhexidine is useful as an antimicrobial agent in the same range of concentrations as BAK, yet it is used at lower concentrations in commercial ophthalmic formulations. Because it does not alter corneal permeability to the same extent as BAK, chlorhexidine is not as toxic to the eye.

The second distinct group of preservatives includes the metals mercury and iodine, their derivatives, and alcohols. Of the mercurial preservatives, patients who become sensitized to thimerosal develop contact blepharitis or conjunctivitis after several weeks of exposure and must discontinue the use of products that contain it. These products are rapidly disappearing from the marketplace.

Chlorobutanol is less effective than BAK as an antimicrobial preservative and, in fact, tends to disappear from bottles during prolonged storage.[12] However, prolonged use of chlorobutanol does not appear to produce allergic reactions. This preservative is often used in 0.5% concentrations and has both antifungal and antibacterial properties.

Methylparaben and propylparaben, both p-hydroxybenzoic acid derivatives, have a long history of use in some ophthalmic medications (especially in artificial tears and nonmedicated ointments). However, these preservatives are unstable at high pH and can sometimes induce allergic reactions.

Ethylenediamine tetraacetic acid (EDTA) is a chelating agent that preferentially binds and sequesters divalent cations. EDTA assists the action of thimerosal, BAK, and other agents. EDTA can sometimes induce contact allergic reactions.[21]

Sodium perborate, which has been used extensively as a tooth-bleaching agent, has found a new use as an ophthalmic preservative. The first of two so-called "disappearing preservatives," sodium perborate dissociates on contact with the eye to form hydrogen peroxide, which in turn rapidly dissociates to oxygen and water. The amount of hydrogen peroxide formed is so small that it does not produce eye irritation. The second,

Purite (oxychloro complex), also is designed to dissociate on contact with the eye. After exposure to long-wavelength UV light, Purite breaks down quickly to water and sodium chloride. These disappearing preservatives have the advantage of microbial protection while potentially limiting preservative toxicity.

Other less common ophthalmic preservatives include cetylpyridinium chloride, phenylethyl alcohol, sodium propionate, and sorbic acid.

Ophthalmic Excipients

Other useful excipients are antioxidants, wetting agents, buffers, and tonicity adjusters. Antioxidants prevent or delay deterioration of products that are exposed to oxygen. Wetting agents reduce surface tension, allowing the drug solution to spread more easily over the ocular surface. Buffers are added to help maintain a pH range of 6.0–8.0, thereby preventing ocular discomfort on product instillation. Tonicity adjusters allow the medication to be isotonic with the physiologic tear film. Products in the sodium chloride equivalence range of 0.9%–1.2% are considered isotonic; they help reduce ocular irritation and tissue damage. Solutions in the tonicity range of 0.6%–1.8% are usually comfortable when placed on the human eye. Hypertonic solutions used for corneal edema are not well tolerated.

Product Selection Guidelines

In recent years, artificial tear preparations have been introduced in preservative-free formulations and, more recently, in disappearing-preservative formulations. These preparations are beneficial for patients who are sensitive to preservatives such as BAK and thimerosal, those who use drops frequently, and those with compromised corneas. Four solution products (Genteal [Mild to Moderate or Moderate to Severe], Refresh Liquigel, and Refresh Tears) and three lubricant gels (Genteal Lubricant Eye Gel [Mild to Moderate or Moderate to Severe] and Tears Again Gel) are uniquely formulated to allow the preservative to rapidly dissociate into nontoxic components on the ocular surface. True preservative-free artificial tear preparations (e.g., Bion Tears, Celluvisc, HypoTears, and Refresh Plus) are available in a variety of unit-dose dispensers, and some of these products are formulated to provide electrolyte support to the damaged surface epithelium of the eye. Preservative-free formulations not only are more expensive than preserved artificial tear solutions, but also are easily contaminated by the patient during use. Therefore, patients must follow strict hygienic procedures for self-administration and should discard any unused solution immediately after opening and using it.

Clinical results and patient acceptance remain the final criteria for determining a product's efficacy in the treatment of patients with dry eye. Importantly, no single formulation has yet been identified that will universally improve clinical signs and symptoms while maintaining patient comfort and acceptance.[16,17] If symptoms do not improve after use of multiple artificial tear products, the patient should be encouraged to seek professional assessment and care from an eye care provider.

Allergic Conjunctivitis

Pathophysiology and Clinical Presentation of Allergic Conjunctivitis

The list of antigens that can cause ocular allergy is virtually endless, but the most common allergens include pollen, animal dander, and topical eye preparations. Patients with ocular allergy will often report seasonal allergic rhinitis, as well. Allergic conjunctivitis is characterized by a red eye with watery discharge (see Color Plates, photograph 4). The hallmark symptom of ocular allergy is itching. Vision is usually not impaired but may be blurred because of excessive tearing. Contact lenses should not be used until the condition resolves.[22]

Treatment of Allergic Conjunctivitis
Treatment Goals

The goals in treating allergic conjunctivitis are to (1) remove or avoid the allergen, (2) limit or reduce the severity of the allergic reaction, (3) provide symptomatic relief, and (4) protect the ocular surface.

General Treatment Approach

Questioning the patient about exposure to allergens may help identify the offending substance. Removal or avoidance of the responsible allergen is the best treatment, but nonprescription ocular lubricants, ocular decongestants, ocular decongestant/antihistamine preparations, ocular antihistamines/mast cell stabilizers, oral antihistamines, and cold compresses will help relieve symptoms.

Nonpharmacologic Therapy

In addition to removing and/or avoiding exposure to the offending allergen, applying cold compresses to the eyes 3–4 times per day will help reduce redness and itching. Other important measures for avoiding the allergic response include checking the pollen count, keeping doors and windows closed, running air conditioning, using air filters, and so on. If eyes are itchy, cool compresses often help relieve some symptoms.[31]

Pharmacologic Therapy

The first-line treatment of allergic conjunctivitis is to instill artificial tears as needed (see Treatment of Dry Eye). If symptoms persist, the patient should switch to an ophthalmic antihistamine/mast cell stabilizer product. The reclassification of a product from prescription to nonprescription status has been a very favorable improvement for the treatment of allergic conjunctivitis. Ketotifen fumarate 0.025% (Zaditor, Alaway) is very safe and can be used in individuals ages 3 years and older; it is dosed twice daily and is very effective in relieving the signs and symptoms of allergic conjunctivitis. Although a definite time period of treatment has not been well studied, these antihistamine/mast cell stabilizer products have been used for many years in patients, depending on symptoms. An oral antihistamine can be added to the second treatment option, if needed. Medical referral is indicated if symptoms do not resolve.

Nonprescription ophthalmic products designated specifically for treatment of allergic conjunctivitis include decongestants (often in combination with antihistamines) and, more recently, the antihistamine/mast cell stabilizer combination. (See Chapter 11 for discussion of systemic nonprescription antihistamines.)

Ophthalmic Decongestants/ Alpha-Adrenergic Agonists

Four decongestants are available in nonprescription strength for topical application to the eye: phenylephrine, naphazoline, tetrahydrozoline, and oxymetazoline. In nonprescription ophthalmic products, phenylephrine is available in a concentration of 0.12% or lower. Higher concentrations of phenylephrine (2.5% and 10%) are prescription products and are used for pupillary dilation. Naphazoline, tetrahydrozoline, and oxymetazoline are chemically classified as imidazoles. As Table 27–5 shows, these agents are available as solutions in a variety of concentrations.

Phenylephrine acts primarily on alpha-adrenergic receptors of the ophthalmic vasculature to constrict conjunctival vessels, thereby reducing eye redness. The higher-concentration, prescription-only products that contain this agent are generally reserved for the short-term dilation needed for eye examinations. Similar to phenylephrine, the imidazoles have greater

table 27–5	Commonly Used Nonprescription Ophthalmic Products Containing Decongestants, Antihistamines, and/or Astringents
Trade Name	**Primary Ingredients**
Decongestant Eyedrop Products	
All Clear	Naphazoline 0.012%; PEG 300, 0.2%; BAK 0.01%; EDTA
All Clear AR	Naphazoline 0.03%; BAK 0.01%; hydroxypropyl methylcellulose 0.5%; EDTA
Allerest	Naphazoline 0.012%; BAK; EDTA
Clear Eyes	Naphazoline HCl 0.012%; glycerin 0.2%; BAK
Clear Eyes ACR	Naphazoline 0.012%; BAK; EDTA; zinc sulfate 0.25%; glycerin 0.2%
Murine Tears Plus	Tetrahydrozoline HCl 0.05%; povidone 0.6%; PVA 0.5%; BAK
Naphcon	Naphazoline HCl 0.012%; BAK 0.01%
Opti-Clear	Tetrahydrozoline 0.05%; BAK 0.01%; boric acid; EDTA; sodium borate; NaCl
Relief[a]	Phenylephrine; PVA 1.4%; EDTA
Tetrasine Extra	Tetrahydrozoline 0.05%; PEG 400, 1.0%; EDTA; BAK
Visine Advanced Relief	Tetrahydrozoline HCl 0.05%; PEG 400, 1.0%; povidone 1.0%; BAK 0.01%; dextran 70, 1.0%
Visine L.R.	Oxymetazoline HCl 0.025%; BAK 0.01%
Visine Moisturizing	Tetrahydrozoline HCl 0.05%; BAK 0.01%; EDTA; hydroxypropyl methylcellulose 0.5%
Visine Original	Tetrahydrozoline HCl 0.05%; BAK 0.01%
Vision Clear	Tetrahydrozoline 0.05%; BAK 0.01%; boric acid; EDTA; sodium borate; NaCl
Antihistamine/Mast Cell Stabilizer Eyedrop Products	
Zaditor, Alaway	Ketotifen 0.025%; BAK 0.01%; glycerol; sodium hydroxide and/or hydrochloric acid; purified water
Antihistamine/Decongestant Eyedrop Products	
Naphcon A	Pheniramine maleate 0.3%; naphazoline HCl 0.025%; BAK 0.01%
Opcon-A	Pheniramine maleate 0.315%; naphazoline HCl 0.02675%; hydroxypropyl methylcellulose 0.5%; BAK 0.01%
Vasocon A	Antazoline phosphate 0.5%; naphazoline HCl 0.05%; BAK 0.01%
Visine-A	Pheniramine maleate 0.3%; naphazoline HCl 0.025%; BAK 0.01%
Decongestant/Astringent Eyedrop Products	
Clear Eyes ACR	Naphazoline HCl 0.012%; zinc sulfate 0.25%; glycerin 0.2%; BAK
Visine Allergy Relief	Tetrahydrozoline HCl 0.05%; zinc sulfate 0.25%; BAK 0.01%
Zincfrin	Phenylephrine HCl 0.12%; zinc sulfate 0.25%; BAK 0.01%

Key: BAK = Benzalkonium chloride; EDTA = ethylenediamine tetraacetic acid; NaCl = sodium chloride; PEG = polyethylene glycol; PVA = polyvinyl alcohol.

[a] Preservative-free formulation.

table

27-6 Dosage Guidelines for Nonprescription Ophthalmic Decongestants and Antihistamines

Agent	Nonprescription Concentration (%)	Dosage	Duration of Action (hours)	Duration of Use
Decongestant Products				
Phenylephrine	0.12	1–2 drops up to 4 times/day	0.5–1.5	72 hours
Naphazoline	0.1, 0.12, 0.02, 0.03	1–2 drops up to 4 times/day	3–4	72 hours
Oxymetazoline	0.025	1–2 drops every 6 hours	4–6	72 hours
Tetrahydrozoline	0.05	1–2 drops every 4 hours	1–4	72 hours
Antihistamine/Mast Cell Stabilizer				
Ketotifen	0.025	1 drop every 8–12 hours	8–12	>72 hours
Decongestant/Antihistamine Products				
Naphazoline/pheniramine	0.025 (naphazoline) 0.3 (pheniramine)	1–2 drops 3–4 times/day	3–4	72 hours
Naphazoline/antazoline	0.05 (naphazoline) 0.5 (antazoline)	1–2 drops 3–4 times/day		72 hours

alpha- than beta-receptor activity and, therefore, are clinically useful in constricting conjunctival blood vessels. These agents have only minimal effect on the underlying vessels of the episclera and sclera. Vasoconstrictors are effective in constricting conjunctival vessels and in reducing redness, vascular congestion, and eyelid edema, but they do not diminish the allergic response.[23] Table 27–6 lists dosages of ophthalmic decongestants.

When used as directed, ocular decongestants generally do not induce ocular or systemic side effects. However, their availability to and use in children should be monitored carefully. Ingestion of these products can result in coronary emergencies and death. When used excessively or long term, ocular decongestants have the potential to produce rebound conjunctival hyperemia (i.e., rebound conjunctival congestion), allergic conjunctivitis, and allergic blepharitis.[24] Thus, they should not be used for more than 72 hours. Rebound congestion appears to be less likely with topical ocular use of naphazoline or tetrahydrozoline than with oxymetazoline or phenylephrine. Rebound congestion may be experienced within a few days of initiating treatment, although a case was reported within 8 hours of use.[24] Patients with apparent rebound congestion should be referred to an eye care provider for differential diagnosis and management.

Indiscriminate use of decongestants in an irritated eye can induce papillary dilation and may precipitate angle-closure glaucoma in eyes that have narrow anterior chamber angles. Use of these products in angle-closure glaucoma is contraindicated, and providers should counsel patients with angle-closure glaucoma against using these products in treating allergic conjunctivitis.

Some patients may experience epithelial xerosis (abnormal dryness) from prolonged topical instillation of ocular decongestants, which may exacerbate the symptoms of irritation, pain, and dryness associated with allergic conjunctivitis.

Ocular decongestants should be used cautiously by patients with systemic hypertension, arteriosclerosis, other cardiovascular diseases, or diabetes. Adverse cardiovascular events are also possible when these agents are used in patients with hyperthyroidism.[25]

Because of these possible adverse reactions, patients should not use phenylephrine and other ocular decongestants as ocular irrigants. During pregnancy, women should use ocular decongestants sparingly, if at all. Storing solutions at high temperatures may cause ocular reactions and severe mydriatic responses to instillation. If offending ophthalmic signs or symptoms do not resolve within 72 hours, the patient should see an eye care provider.

Ophthalmic Antihistamines and Ophthalmologic Antihistamines/Mast Cell Stabilizers

Two nonprescription antihistamines are available for topical ophthalmic use: pheniramine maleate and antazoline phosphate. Although these antihistamines are effective alone, nonprescription products containing them also contain a decongestant. The two combinations are pheniramine/naphazoline and antazoline/naphazoline (Table 27–5).

Pheniramine and antazoline are in different antihistamine classes, but both act as specific histamine$_1$-receptor antagonists.[26,27] Topical antihistamines are used for rapid relief of symptoms associated with seasonal or atopic conjunctivitis. Using a decongestant with either topical antihistamine has been shown to be more effective than using either agent alone.[28]

Ketotifen fumarate is an ophthalmic antihistamine and mast cell stabilizer. It produces very potent H$_1$-receptor-antagonist activity, thereby preventing acute histamine-mediated allergy symptoms. The mast cell stabilization activity inhibits mast cell degranulation, preventing the release of inflammatory mediators, including histamine. Ketotifen also inhibits eosinophils, thereby inhibiting the release of late-phase mediators. Ketotifen provides relief within minutes, its effects may last up to 12 hours from a single dose, and it does not contain a vasoconstrictor;[23] therefore, it is a very safe product with no concerns for vasoconstrictor overuse.

Table 27–6 provides dosages of the antihistamine combination products. Burning, stinging, and discomfort on instillation are the most common side effects of ophthalmic antihistamines.[29,30]

Ophthalmic antihistamines have anticholinergic properties and may cause pupil dilation. This effect is seen most commonly in people with light-colored irises or compromised corneas (e.g., contact lens wearers).[26] In susceptible patients, pupil dilation can lead to angle-closure glaucoma. Therefore, these drugs are contraindicated in people with a known risk of angle-closure glaucoma.[26] Sensitivity to one of the components is another contraindication.

Product Selection Guidelines

Ketotifen is the safest and most effective product for the treatment of allergic conjunctivitis. It is the greatest improvement in the nonprescription treatment of allergic eye disease in many years. The twice-daily dosing and the safety of this product for children ages 3 years and older make it the primary therapy for patients with signs and symptoms of allergic conjunctivitis.

Although product-to-product comparisons are available for decongestant and antihistamine ophthalmic products, reaching definitive conclusions regarding clinical comparisons of the available nonprescription ocular decongestants is difficult. Naphazoline 0.02%, however, is an excellent choice for nonprescription therapy of mild-moderate conjunctivitis of environmental, viral, or noninfectious origin.

Because rebound congestion appears to be less likely after topical ocular use of naphazoline or tetrahydrozoline, these agents should generally be recommended over phenylephrine or oxymetazoline.

Complementary Therapies

The homeopathic product known as Similasan Eye Drops #2 is indicated for relief from itching and burning caused by allergic reactions. The active homeopathic ingredients are Apis, Euphrasia, and Sabadilla. The efficacy of this formulation has not been established in controlled clinical trials.

Corneal Edema

Pathophysiology and Clinical Presentation of Corneal Edema

Corneal edema may occur from a variety of conditions, including overwear of contact lenses, surgical damage to the cornea, and inherited corneal dystrophies. The edematous area of the cornea is often confined to the epithelium. Because fluid accumulation distorts the optical properties of the cornea, halos or starbursts around lights (with or without reduced vision) are a hallmark symptom of corneal edema. An eye care provider must diagnose this disorder.

Treatment of Corneal Edema
Treatment Goals

The goal in treating corneal edema is to draw fluid from the cornea, thereby relieving the associated symptoms.

General Treatment Approach

Once the initial diagnosis is established, patients can use topical hyperosmotic formulations to treat corneal edema. Of the topical ophthalmic hyperosmotic agents available, only sodium chloride can be obtained without a prescription in both solution and ointment formulations (Table 27–7). Sodium chloride is available as a 2% or 5% solution and as a 5% ointment. First-line treatment is instillation of a 2% solution 4 times per day. If symptoms persist, nighttime use of a 5% hyperosmotic ointment should be added to the regimen.[31] If symptoms do not respond to the augmented treatment, the patient should switch to a 5% hyperosmotic solution and continue nighttime use of the ointment. If symptoms still persist, medical referral is necessary.[31]

Pharmacologic Therapy
Hyperosmotics

Hyperosmotic agents increase the tonicity of the tear film, promoting movement of fluid from the cornea to the more highly osmotic tear film. Normal tear flow mechanisms then eliminate the excessive fluid. Many patients with mild-moderate corneal epithelial edema may experience improved subjective comfort and vision after appropriate use of these medications.

Usually, the patient instills 1 or 2 drops of the solution every 3–4 hours (Table 27–3). The ointment formulation, however, requires less frequent instillation and is usually reserved for use at bedtime to minimize symptoms of blurred vision (Table 27–4). Because vision associated with edematous corneas is often worse upon awakening, several instillations of the solution during the first few waking hours may be helpful.

In general, sodium chloride 5% in ointment form is the most effective in reducing corneal edema and improving vision, but it tends to cause stinging and burning. For that reason, patients often prefer the 2% solution for long-term therapy. Hypertonic saline is nontoxic to the external ocular tissues, and allergic reactions are rare.[31]

The most important contraindication to topical hyperosmotic sodium chloride is its use to clear edematous corneas in patients with traumatized epithelium. The intact corneal epithelium permits only limited permeability to inorganic ions; therefore, an absent or compromised corneal epithelium will result in increased corneal penetration of the hyperosmotic product, reducing its osmotic effect.[31] Patients whose history or physical appearance suggests a damaged corneal epithelium should be referred to an eye care provider immediately. Patients must be directed never to prepare homemade saline solutions for use in the eye because of the risk of infection.

Loose Foreign Substances in the Eye

Pathophysiology and Clinical Presentation of Loose Foreign Substances in the Eye

Despite the protective effect of the eyelids, foreign substances often contact the ocular surface. The immediate response of the eye is watering (tearing). If the substance causes

table
27–7   More Commonly Used Miscellaneous Nonprescription Ophthalmic Products

Trade Name	Primary Ingredients
Hyperosmotics	
AK-NaCl Solution	NaCl 5%; methylparaben 0.023%; propylparaben 0.017%
AK-NaCl Ointment[a]	NaCl 5%; lanolin oil; mineral oil; white petrolatum
Muro 128 Solution 2%	NaCl 2%; hydroxypropyl methylcellulose 2906; methylparaben 0.046%; propylparaben 0.02%; propylene glycol; boric acid
Muro 128 Solution 5%	NaCl 5%; boric acid; hydroxypropyl methylcellulose 2910; propylene glycol; methylparaben 0.023%; propylparaben 0.01%
Muro 128 Ointment[a]	Mineral oil; white petrolatum; lanolin
Irrigant Solutions	
Blinx	NaCl; KCl; sodium phosphate; BAK 0.005%; EDTA 0.02%
Collyrium for Fresh Eyes	Boric acid; sodium borate; BAK
Bausch and Lomb Eye Wash	Sodium borate; boric acid; NaCl; sorbic acid 0.1%; EDTA 0.025%
Eye Stream	Sodium acetate 0.39%; sodium citrate 0.17%; sodium hydroxide and/or hydrochloric acid; BAK
Eye Wash	NaCl; sodium phosphate dibasic; sodium phosphate monobasic; EDTA; preserved with benzalkonium chloride in purified water
Irrigate Eye Wash	NaCl; mono- and dibasic sodium phosphate; EDTA; BAK
Optigene	NaCl; mono- and dibasic sodium phosphate; EDTA; BAK
Visual-Eyes	NaCl; mono- and dibasic sodium phosphate; BAK; EDTA
Prosthesis Lubricant/Cleaner	
Enuclene Solution	Tyloxapol 0.25%; hydroxypropyl methylcellulose 0.85%; BAK 0.02%
SteriLid Eyelid Cleanser	Water; PEG-80; sorbitan laurate; sodium trideceth sulfate

Key: BAK = Benzalkonium chloride; EDTA = ethylenediamine tetraacetic acid; KCl = potassium chloride; NaCl = sodium chloride; PEG = polyethylene glycol.

[a] Preservative-free formulation.

only minor irritation and does not abrade the eye surface, self-treatment is appropriate.[32]

Treatment of Loose Foreign Substances in the Eye
Treatment Goals

The goal in treating loose foreign substances in the eye is to remove the irritant by irrigating the eye. If a known foreign substance is a fragment of wood or metal, it should be treated promptly by an eye care provider because of the potential for penetrating injuries.

General Treatment Approach

If reflex tearing does not remove the foreign substance, the eye may need to be flushed. Lint, dust, and similar materials can usually be removed by rinsing the eye with sterile saline or specific eyewash preparations (irrigants). Outside of a medical setting, treat eyes exposed to loose particles by flushing the eyes with copious amounts of water from a sink faucet or garden hose. If needed, eye ointment can be applied at bedtime.[32]

Pharmacologic Therapy
Ocular Irrigants

An ocular irrigant is used to cleanse ocular tissues while maintaining their moisture; these solutions must be physiologically balanced with respect to pH and osmolality. Because the tissues that the irrigant contacts obtain nutrients elsewhere, the role of irrigants is primarily to clear away unwanted materials or debris from the ocular surface. To reduce risk of contamination, patients should use ocular irrigants only on a short-term basis, and they should be sure that no other ocular pathology is being missed. All ophthalmic irrigating solutions are available without a prescription (Table 27–7).

In the eye care provider's office, irrigating solutions come in handy after certain clinical procedures, and they are often used to wash away mucous or purulent exudates from the eye. They are also administered in the hospital to clean out eyes between changes of ocular dressings.

Ocular irrigants should not be used for open wounds in or near the eyes. Although irrigating solutions may be used to wash out the eyes after contact lens wear, they have no particular value as contact lens wetting, cleansing, or cushioning solutions.

If the patient experiences continuous eye pain, changes in vision, or continued redness or irritation of the eye, or if the ocular condition persists or worsens, evaluation by an eye care provider should be strongly encouraged. Irrigants may be packaged with an eyecup; however, because contamination of the eyecup is possible, it should not be used to rinse the eye.

Minor Eye Irritation

Pathophysiology and Clinical Presentation of Minor Eye Irritation

Nonallergic, minor eye irritation can be caused by a loose foreign substance in the eye; contact lens wear; or exposure of the eye to wind, sun (e.g., snow skiing without protective eye goggles), smog, chemical fumes, or chlorine. Redness of the eye is a common sign of minor irritation. In cases of snow blindness, other burns from UV light, or arc welder's burns, common additional symptoms include pain and the feeling of "sand in the eyes."

Treatment of Minor Eye Irritation

Minor irritation often responds well to artificial tear solutions or nonmedicated ointments (see Treatment of Dry Eye Disease).

Zinc sulfate, a mild astringent, may be recommended for temporary relief of minor ocular irritation. The dosage is 1–2 drops up to 4 times daily.

The homeopathic product known as Similasan Eye Drops #1 is marketed to relieve dryness and redness caused by smog, contact lenses, and other causes. The active homeopathic ingredients are Belladonna, Euphrasia, and Mercurius sublimatus. Controlled clinical trials have not demonstrated the efficacy of this formulation in the treatment of this condition.

Chemical Burn

Pathophysiology and Clinical Presentation of Chemical Burn

Chemical burns may occur from exposure to alkali (e.g., oven cleaners, cement, or lye); acids (e.g., battery acid or vinegar); detergents; and various solvents and irritants (e.g., tear gas or mace). Burns may range from mild to severe, depending on the inciting agent and/or exposure time. Patients complain of pain, irritation, photophobia, and tearing. Signs will vary according to the severity. Less severe signs include superficial punctate keratitis (small pinpoint loss of epithelial cells in the cornea), perilimbal ischemia, chemosis, hyperemia, eyelid edema, hemorrhages, and first- or second-degree burns of the lid and outer skin. More severe signs include corneal edema and opacification, anterior chamber inflammation, increased IOP, and retinal toxicity from scleral penetration. Alkali burns are more penetrating and potentially more damaging to eye tissues than acid burns. Alkali burns often are more resistant

to irrigation and have greater tissue destruction when they penetrate into the deeper (stromal) layers of the cornea. If the burns are more superficial and only several layers of the corneal epithelium have been affected, the cells should be replenished within approximately 24 hours.[32]

Emergent Treatment of Chemical Burn

Emergent treatment includes immediate copious irrigation with sterile saline (Table 27–7) or even tap water, if nothing else is available. Irrigation must be continued until an eye care provider can be seen; if irrigation is stopped prematurely, residual material that may still be under the lid or in the inferior cul-de-sac may cause the pH of the tear film to revert to either acidic or alkaline.[32] Further treatment after irrigation may include the use of cycloplegic agents, topical antibiotics, and analgesics. In more severe cases, if significant inflammation of the anterior chamber or cornea is present, eye care specialists may use topical steroids. Antiglaucoma medications are also used if the IOP is elevated. Follow-up by the eye care provider is required to prevent conjunctival adhesions and corneal complications. Chemical burns are considered ophthalmic emergencies and should be referred to an eye care provider or emergency department immediately.

Artificial Eyes

Besides the obvious aesthetic benefits, clearing dried mucus or fluid secretions from the surfaces of artificial eyes eliminates a potential medium for bacterial growth. A sterile, isotonic buffered solution containing tyloxapol 0.25% and BAK 0.02% is available especially for cleaning and lubricating ophthalmic prostheses. The primary method of preventing bacterial growth is routine hygiene with mild, nonallergenic soap and water.

Tyloxapol is a surfactant that softens solid matter on the prosthesis, and BAK aids tyloxapol in wetting the artificial eye. The solution is used in the same manner as ordinary artificial tears. With the artificial eye in place, 1 or 2 drops of solution should be applied 3 or 4 times daily. In addition, the solution can be used as a cleaner to remove oil or mucous deposits; in this case, the artificial eye is then rubbed between the fingers and rinsed with tap water before reinsertion.

Contact Dermatitis

Pathophysiology and Clinical Presentation of Contact Dermatitis

Contact dermatitis of the eyelid can be a reaction to either an allergen or an irritant. Causes of contact dermatitis include a change in cosmetics or soap, exposure to eye medications, or contact with other foreign substances. The involvement of both eyelids suggests allergy, because both eyes are often exposed. Common symptoms include swelling, scaling, or redness of the eyelid, along with profuse itching. Sunburns of the eyelids and UV burns to the cornea (e.g., recent sun exposure from beach or ski outings without eye protection) should be ruled out.

Treatment of Contact Dermatitis

Questioning the patient about the use of eye medications or new products (e.g., eyeliner or eye shadow) may help identify the offending substance quickly. Discontinuing use of the suspected product is the best treatment. If swelling of the eyelid is marked, nonprescription oral antihistamines (e.g. diphenhydramine) along with cold compresses applied 3–4 times per day will help reduce the inflammation and itching.

Assessment of Ophthalmic Disorders: A Case-Based Approach

For patients who have not seen an eye care provider, the pharmacist or primary care provider must determine whether the ophthalmic disorder is self-treatable or requires medical referral. Great care must be taken when assessing a patient with a new, acute problem. Ocular inflammation and irritation can be caused by many conditions, some of which can be treated safely and effectively with nonprescription ophthalmic products. These products are used primarily to relieve minor symptoms of burning, stinging, itching, and watering. The Food and Drug Administration has suggested that self-treatment may be indicated for tear insufficiency, corneal edema, and external inflammation or irritation.

Cases 27–1 and 27–2 are examples of the assessment of patients with ophthalmic disorders.

---

case 27–1

Relevant Evaluation Criteria	Scenario/Model Outcome
Information Gathering	
1. Gather essential information about the patient's symptoms and medical history, including:	
a. description of symptom(s) (i.e., nature, onset, duration, severity, associated symptoms)	Patient has suffered from allergies over the past couple of weeks this spring. She currently is taking a systemic, nonsedating OTC antihistamine (loratadine 10 mg), but she is still having ocular symptoms. Her ocular irritation and dry eye symptoms are definitely affecting her day-to-day activities. She is willing to do anything to cure the problem.
b. description of any factors that seem to precipitate, exacerbate, and/or relieve the patient's symptom(s)	Symptoms appeared about the same time as last year, at the start of spring. Patient started her loratadine last year and did fine. This year, however, her eyes are itchy, red, and dry, and her eyelids are swollen, even though her systemic complaints seem under control. The dryness and ocular irritation began prior to the allergy season.
c. description of the patient's efforts to relieve the symptoms	The decongestant eyedrops to get the "red out" do not appear to give her any relief from her ocular symptoms.
d. patient's identity	May Wong
e. age, sex, height, and weight	49 years old, female; 5 ft 6 in., 125 lb
f. patient's occupation	Full-time employee; mother of two
g. patient's dietary habits	Normal healthy diet with occasional social drinking; works out on treadmill 4 times weekly.
h. patient's sleep habits	Stays up late and sleeps in as allowed by her schedule.
i. concurrent medical conditions, prescription and nonprescription medications, and dietary supplements	Seasonal allergies (spring and fall): loratadine 10 mg once daily, tetrahydrozoline eyedrops 3–4 times daily in both eyes; glucosamine capsules 2 times daily; aspirin 75 mg daily
j. allergies	Seasonal allergies (spring and fall): loratadine 10 mg once daily, tetrahydrozoline eyedrops 3–4 times daily in both eyes; glucosamine capsules 2 times daily; aspirin 75 mg daily
k. history of other adverse reactions to medications	None
l. other (describe) _____	NA
Assessment and Triage	
2. Differentiate patient's signs/symptoms and correctly identify the patient's primary problem(s).	Patient is experiencing exacerbation of seasonal allergy symptoms. This is the first year she has experienced ocular irritation and dryness; some symptoms have occurred a little earlier than expected.
3. Identify exclusions for self-treatment (Table 27–8 and Figure 27–2).	None

Relevant Evaluation Criteria	**Scenario/Model Outcome**
4. Formulate a comprehensive list of therapeutic alternatives for the primary problem to determine if triage to a health care provider is required, and share this information with the patient or caregiver.	Options include: (1) Refer Mrs. Wong to an eye care provider (optometrist or ophthalmologist). (2) Suggest that Mrs. Wong discontinue her topical decongestant eyedrops and switch to ketotifen topical drops twice daily. (3) Recommend that she continue with her OTC artificial tear solution. (4) Take no action.

Plan

5. Select an optimal therapeutic alternative to address the patient's problem, taking into account patient preferences.	The patient prefers to discontinue her decongestant drops and start the artificial tear product and the new ocular antihistamine:
6. Describe the recommended therapeutic approach to the patient or caregiver.	"Instill 1 drop of the ketotifen eyedrops twice daily in both eyes as described in Table 27–3. Supplement throughout the day with the artificial tear product as much as you desire; however, wait at least 5 minutes after instilling the ketotifen eyedrops."
7. Explain to the patient or caregiver the rationale for selecting the recommended therapeutic approach from the considered therapeutic alternatives.	"You may not need to see an eye care provider if you follow the administration guidelines in Table 27–3."

Patient Education

8. When recommending self-care with nonprescription medications and/or nondrug therapy, convey accurate information to the patient or caregiver:	
a. appropriate dose and frequency of administration	See Table 27–6.
b. maximum number of days the therapy should be employed	See Table 27–6.
c. product administration procedures	See Table 27–3.
d. expected time to onset of relief	See Table 27–6.
e. degree of relief that can be reasonably expected	"Complete symptom control should be possible. Some minor symptoms likely will appear from time to time."
f. most common side effects	"Burning, stinging, and discomfort may occur on instillation of the drops."
g. side effects that warrant medical intervention should they occur	"If the eye pain worsens and the redness continues, see your eye care provider."
h. patient options in the event that condition worsens or persists	"An eye care provider should be consulted if the condition does not improve, or if irritation and pain become intolerable."
i. product storage requirements	"Store under room temperature and away from heat and light. Observe product expiration date."
j. specific nondrug measures	"Remove and/or avoid exposure to the offending allergen (e.g., check pollen count, keep doors and windows closed, run air conditioning, use air filters). In addition, apply cold compresses to the eyes 3–4 times per day to help reduce redness and itching."
Solicit follow-up questions from the patient or caregiver.	(1) "If my eyes still bother me, may I use the drops that I was using previously to get the red out?" (2) "Also, my spouse has tobramycin/dexamethasone eyedrops that he used previously, and they seemed to help him very quickly. May I try his eyedrops?"
Answer the patient's or caregiver's questions.	(1) "No. The get-the-red-out eyedrops actually can cause more ocular redness (rebound) and eye dryness." (2) "The tobramycin/dexamethasone drops (steroid and antibiotic) can cause significant eye complications, such as secondary infection, glaucoma, and cataract."

Evaluation of Patient Outcome

9. Assess patient outcome.	Inform the patient to feel free to contact you if she has any further questions.

Key: NA = Not applicable; NKA = no known allergies; OTC = over-the-counter.

case
27–2

Relevant Evaluation Criteria	Scenario/Model Outcome

Information Gathering

1. Gather essential information about the patient's symptoms and medical history, including:

a. description of symptom(s) (i.e., nature, onset, duration, severity, associated symptoms)

The patient explains that he burned the skin around his eyelids, and his eyes are sore and pretty red. He was working in his bathroom on a clogged sink. He bought a viscous product for clearing drains and poured it in the clogged sink, which contained some water that would not drain. He got the plunger and started plunging the water, and some of the fluid splashed into his face. It burned some of the skin around his eyelids, as well as his eyes. He thought the redness and pain would get better in a few hours, but they seem to be getting worse, especially in the right eye. If he closes his eyes, the pain abates a bit; however, because his symptoms do not seem to be getting any better, he would like assistance choosing a product that might help.

b. description of any factors that seem to precipitate, exacerbate, and/or relieve the patient's symptom(s)

The patient mentions that his eyes hurt when he keeps them open (especially the right one). He also mentions that his vision is sensitive to light and that his eyes feel "gritty" when he leaves them open.

c. description of the patient's efforts to relieve the symptoms

He wears sunglasses to help protect from the glare, but they do not really help the pain or redness. He has taken 2 ibuprofen tablets for the pain, but they are not giving him much relief.

d. patient's identity

Jim Orewell

e. age, sex, height, and weight

35 years old, male, 6 ft 2 in., 195 lb

f. patient's occupation

Accountant

g. patient's dietary habits

Pretty healthy; fishes twice a week; diet low in fatty foods.

h. patient's sleep habits

7 hours a night

i. concurrent medical conditions, prescription and non-prescription medications, and dietary supplements

None; occasional upset stomach relieved by Maalox

j. allergies

None

k. history of other adverse reactions to medications

None

l. other (describe) _____

Patient is an avid runner; runs 4 times per week.

Assessment and Triage

2. Differentiate patient's signs/symptoms and correctly identify the patient's primary problem(s).

3. Identify exclusions for self-treatment.

4. Formulate a comprehensive list of therapeutic alternatives for the primary problem to determine if triage to a health care provider is required, and share this information with the patient or caregiver.

Mr. Orewell has a chemical burn with residual ocular involvement. He needs to be seen immediately by an eye care specialist.

Table 27–8

Options include:

(1) To prevent or reduce scarring of eyelids from chemical burns, he should continue to flush both eyes immediately and for at least 10 minutes.

(2) Patient should use sterile saline or water, if possible. If neither is available, he should flush with tap water.

(3) After flushing eye, he should arrange immediate transportation to an emergency facility.

Plan

5. Select an optimal therapeutic alternative to address the patient's problem, taking into account patient preferences.

Initially, the patient did not want to see an eye doctor; after briefly discussing alkali burns and learning that such burns could continue causing further damage, he said he would go right away.

6. Describe the recommended therapeutic approach to the patient or caregiver.

The patient needs to see an eye doctor right away. In the meantime, he should use an irrigating solution to irrigate his eyes.

7. Explain to the patient or caregiver the rationale for selecting the recommended therapeutic approach from the considered therapeutic alternatives.

"Seeing an eye doctor is the best option. The eye doctor can determine how much damage has been done and if continual treatment is required. The doctor can also recommend a topical treatment for your eyelids."

case

27–2 *continued*

Relevant Evaluation Criteria	Scenario/Model Outcome
Patient Education	
8. When recommending self-care with nonprescription medications and/or nondrug therapy, convey accurate information to the patient or caregiver.	Criterion does not apply in this case.
Solicit follow-up questions from the patient or caregiver.	"Is there anything I should do to prevent this in the future?"
Answer the patient's or caregiver's questions.	"In the future, it is critical to wear protective goggles when working with liquids that may potentially cause chemical burns. Some protection of the skin and face is also suggested to protect from burns."
Evaluation of Patient Outcome	
9. Assess patient outcome.	Contact the patient to find out the results of the eye doctor's examination and treatment.

Table 27–8 describes the major features of disorders that require medical referral. Any self-treated condition that does not resolve within a reasonably short time should be referred to an eye care provider for care.

Patient Counseling for Ophthalmic Disorders

Before counseling a patient, the health care provider should carefully consider the nature and extent of ocular involvement. Patients with acute ocular disease must receive a prompt, definitive diagnosis (including baseline visual acuity) before the provider considers the appropriateness of nonprescription therapy. Some acute conditions (which may or may not involve ocular pain or blurred vision) can be appropriately treated with nonprescription agents, but a recent diagnosis from an eye care provider can give additional reassurance and confidence in recommending such treatment. Although the cost-effectiveness of ophthalmic care can be greatly improved through the use of nonprescription agents, severe visual impairment—including blindness—can be a serious clinical and medicolegal complication if referral for definitive diagnosis and treatment is delayed. After careful consideration of the patient's history, the primary care provider should always counsel patients on the indications

table

27–8 Differentiation of Ophthalmic Disorders That Require Medical Referral

Disorder	Potential Signs/Symptoms	Complications	Treatment Approach
Blunt trauma	Ruptured blood vessels, bleeding into eyelid tissue space, swelling, ocular discomfort, facial drooping	Internal eye bleeding, secondary glaucoma, detached retina, periorbital bone fracture (blow-out fracture)	Medical referral is appropriate.
Foreign particles trapped/embedded in the eye	Reddened eyes, profuse tearing, ocular discomfort	Corneal abrasions/scarring, chronic red eye, intraocular penetration from metal striking metal at high speeds	Medical referral for removal of particles is appropriate.
Ocular abrasions	Partial/total loss of corneal epithelium, blurred vision, profuse tearing, difficulty opening eye	Risk of bacterial/fungal infection with eye exposure to organic material, corneal scarring, anterior chamber rupture	Medical referral is appropriate.
Infections of eyelid/eye surface	Red, thickened lids, scaling	Scarring of lids, dry eye, corneal abrasion or scarring, loss of vision, hordeolum (stye), chalazion (risk of malignancy), and blepharitis (loss of lashes, corneal irritation)	Medical referral is appropriate.

table

27–8 Differentiation of Ophthalmic Disorders That Require Medical Referral (continued)

Disorder	Potential Signs/Symptoms	Complications	Treatment Approach
Eye exposure to chemical splash, solid chemical, or chemical fumes	Reddened eyes, watering, difficulty opening eye	Scarring of eyelids and eye surface, loss of vision	To prevent/reduce scarring of eyelids from chemical burns, flush eye immediately for at least 10 minutes, preferably with sterile saline/water. If neither is available, flush with tap water. After flushing eye, arrange immediate transportation to an emergency facility. No recommendation is noted for chemical neutralization.
Thermal injury to eye (welder's arc)	Reddened eyes, pain, sensitivity to light	Corneal scarring, secondary infection	Medical referral for definitive care (including possible eye patching) is appropriate.
Bacterial conjunctivitis	Reddened eyes with purulent (mucous) discharge, ocular discomfort, eyelids stuck together on awakening	Typically self-limiting in 2 weeks	Medical referral for treatment with topical antibiotics to clear infection more quickly is appropriate; some infections require systemic antibiotic treatment.
Viral conjunctivitis	Reddened eyes with watery discharge, ocular discomfort, hyperemia	Typically self-limiting in 2 or 3 weeks	Medical provider will monitor for corneal involvement. Treatment with topical decongestants to provide comfort is appropriate; cold compresses can be applied.
Chlamydial conjunctivitis	Watery or mucous discharge, ocular discomfort, low-grade fever, possible blurred vision	Scarring	If infection with *Chlamydia* spp. is known or suspected, or if symptoms are too vague to rule out viral or allergic conjunctivitis, medical referral is mandatory.

Source: Reference 32.

for and limitations of self-treatment. The algorithms in Figures 27–2 and 27–3 can assist providers in recommending the appropriate treatment for self-treatable disorders of the eye surface and eyelid, respectively.

Numerous nonprescription ophthalmic products for treating minor ocular irritations are available for self-administration by the patient with minimal or no supervision. These products are also adequate for treating certain clinical conditions diagnosed by primary care providers or eye care providers. First-line therapy should always include counseling on nonpharmacologic treatment. These treatments alone are frequently sufficient to relieve the ocular symptoms or are necessary as an adjunct to the ophthalmic drug therapy. Proper drug instillation technique is critical if the target tissue (the eye) is to receive the maximum benefit from the medication. Ophthalmic solutions and ointments are often used incorrectly. Carefully instructing patients in the proper self-administration procedures can help ensure maximum safety and effectiveness of these agents. Appropriate patient education and counseling must accompany dispensing of any ophthalmic product.

Although drug side effects and interactions are rare with topically applied ophthalmic products, the potential for such effects does exist; therefore, patients should be advised of possible adverse effects, including the clinical signs of drug toxicity or allergy.

The health care provider must actively assist patients in selecting the appropriate product, which will enhance compliance, minimize or avoid side effects, and reduce the attendant costs of therapy. The other major considerations in making therapeutic recommendations include whether the person has

a sensitivity to one of the product constituents, whether the product can be used with contact lenses, and whether the product has the potential to wash out prescription ophthalmic drugs the patient may be using. With the exception of ophthalmic antihistamines and decongestants, little product-to-product comparative research has been done for nonprescription ophthalmic preparations. Therefore, therapy recommendations should be made on the basis of the patient's diagnosis and the products the patient is using. The box Patient Education for Ophthalmic Disorders lists specific information to provide patients.

Evaluation of Patient Outcomes for Ophthalmic Disorders

Patients who self-treat for allergic conjunctivitis, loose foreign substances in the eye, or minor eye irritation should see an eye care provider if symptoms persist after 72 hours of treatment. Dry eye disease is often a chronic disorder, requiring continuous treatment with ophthalmic lubricants. Patients with this disorder should be advised to seek medical care if the symptoms worsen despite diligent self-treatment. Patients with corneal edema should consult an eye care provider if the symptoms persist or worsen despite adherence to the instructions for treating the disorder.

Symptoms of contact dermatitis should resolve quickly once the offending substance is removed. If symptoms persist after 72 hours of antihistamine use, the patient should see an eye care provider.

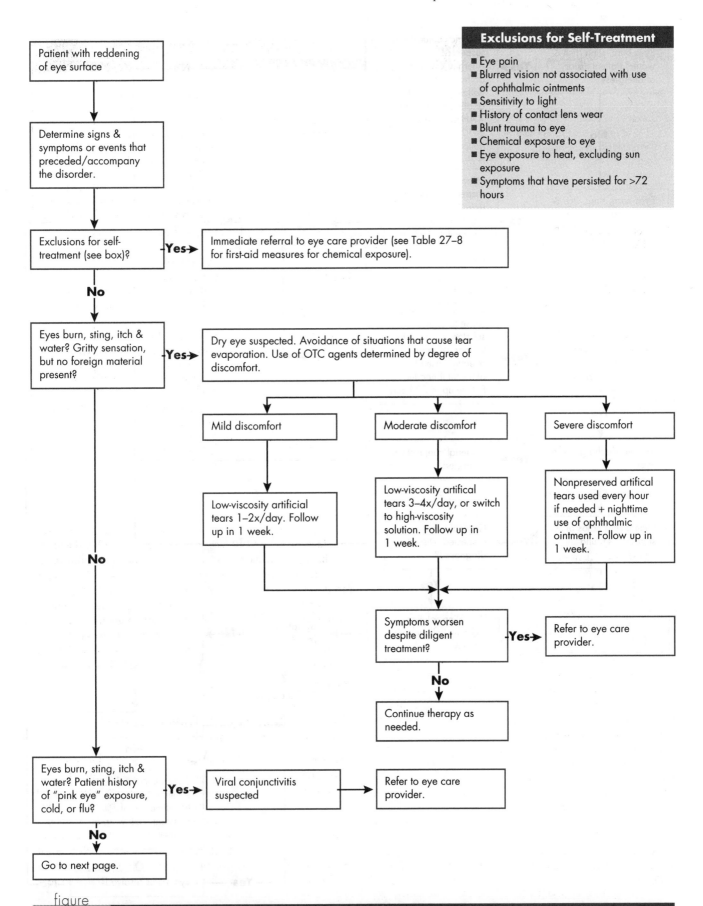

Exclusions for Self-Treatment

- Eye pain
- Blurred vision not associated with use of ophthalmic ointments
- Sensitivity to light
- History of contact lens wear
- Blunt trauma to eye
- Chemical exposure to eye
- Eye exposure to heat, excluding sun exposure
- Symptoms that have persisted for >72 hours

Patient with reddening of eye surface

Determine signs & symptoms or events that preceded/accompany the disorder.

Exclusions for self-treatment (see box)? —Yes→ Immediate referral to eye care provider (see Table 27–8 for first-aid measures for chemical exposure).

No

Eyes burn, sting, itch & water? Gritty sensation, but no foreign material present? —Yes→ Dry eye suspected. Avoidance of situations that cause tear evaporation. Use of OTC agents determined by degree of discomfort.

Mild discomfort

Moderate discomfort

Severe discomfort

Low-viscosity artificial tears 1–2x/day. Follow up in 1 week.

Low-viscosity artifical tears 3–4x/day, or switch to high-viscosity solution. Follow up in 1 week.

Nonpreserved artifical tears used every hour if needed + nighttime use of ophthalmic ointment. Follow up in 1 week.

Symptoms worsen despite diligent treatment? —Yes→ Refer to eye care provider.

No

Continue therapy as needed.

No

Eyes burn, sting, itch & water? Patient history of "pink eye" exposure, cold, or flu? —Yes→ Viral conjunctivitis suspected → Refer to eye care provider.

No

Go to next page.

figure

27–2 Self-care of eye surface disorders. Key: AH = Antihistamine; D/C = discontinue; MCS = mast cell stabilizer; OTC = over-the-counter.

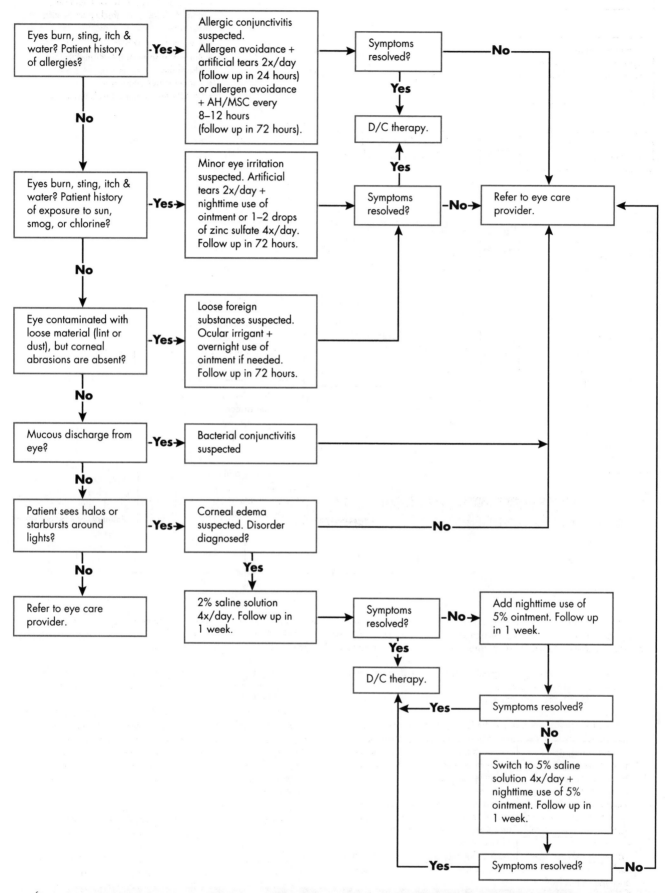

figure
27-2 (continued)

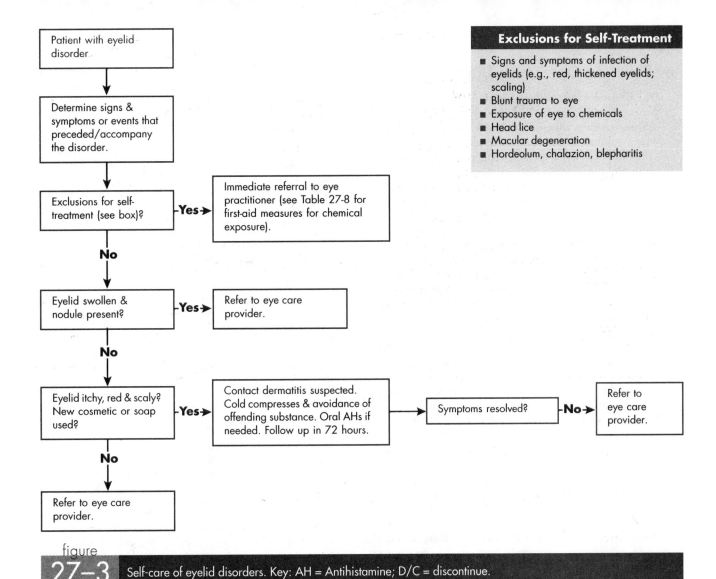

Exclusions for Self-Treatment

- Signs and symptoms of infection of eyelids (e.g., red, thickened eyelids; scaling)
- Blunt trauma to eye
- Exposure of eye to chemicals
- Head lice
- Macular degeneration
- Hordeolum, chalazion, blepharitis

Patient with eyelid disorder

↓

Determine signs & symptoms or events that preceded/accompany the disorder.

↓

Exclusions for self-treatment (see box)? —**Yes**→ Immediate referral to eye practitioner (see Table 27-8 for first-aid measures for chemical exposure).

No ↓

Eyelid swollen & nodule present? —**Yes**→ Refer to eye care provider.

No ↓

Eyelid itchy, red & scaly? New cosmetic or soap used? —**Yes**→ Contact dermatitis suspected. Cold compresses & avoidance of offending substance. Oral AHs if needed. Follow up in 72 hours. → Symptoms resolved? —**No**→ Refer to eye care provider.

No ↓

Refer to eye care provider.

figure

27–3 Self-care of eyelid disorders. Key: AH = Antihistamine; D/C = discontinue.

patient education for
Ophthalmic Disorders

The objectives of self-treatment are to (1) relieve the symptoms of minor ophthalmic disorders using the appropriate nonprescription products or non-drug measures and (2) use nonprescription products as adjunctive treatment of ophthalmic disorders diagnosed by an eye care provider. For most patients, carefully following product instructions and the self-care measures listed here will help ensure good outcomes.

- Remove the causative ocular agent/irritant that predisposes you to your ocular condition or disease.
- If *blunt trauma* to the eye occurs, obtain an eye examination as soon as possible.
- If you have *dry eye disease* and the first ophthalmic lubricants used to treat it are not effective, ask your eye care provider or pharmacist about the following treatment options: increasing the dosage, switching to a product with increased viscosity, and/or switching to a preservative-free product (Table 27-2).
- When treating *allergic conjunctivitis*, do not exceed the recommended dosages of ophthalmic antihistamine/mast cell stabilizer, decongestant, or antihistamine/decongestant products (Tables 27-5 and 27-6). Consult an eye care provider if symptoms persist after 72 hours of treatment.
- Discard or replace eyedrop bottles 30 days after the sterility safety seal is opened. The manufacturer's expiration date does not apply once the seal is broken.
- If *eye exposure to chemicals* occurs, irrigate the eye continuously for 10 minutes with copious amounts of water or eye irrigants (Table 27-7) and seek immediate eye care.

- If *loose foreign substances* such as lint, dust, or pollen enter the eye, flush the substance from the eye using an eye irrigant or water (Table 27-7).
- If a *foreign substance* becomes embedded in the eye or trapped under the eyelid, see an eye care provider. Failure to remove the substance could cause an eye infection or tissue damage.
- Consult an eye care provider before treating *corneal edema*. If hyperosmotic solutions (Table 27-7) are recommended, follow the recommended dosages even though the product may sting. Continual utilization of these products will depend upon the eye care professional's suggestions.
- Note that taking ophthalmic vitamin supplements for macular degeneration along with general multivitamins may result in gastrointestinal upset or vitamin toxicity.
- If *contact dermatitis of the eyelid* occurs, wash the affected areas, identify the cause of the reaction, and try to avoid future contact with the substance. Consult an eye care provider if symptoms persist after 72 hours of use of oral antihistamines.

Key Points for Ophthalmic Disorders

➤ The pharmacist is positioned in the community to treat patients with ophthalmic pathology or to recommend self-management with one or more nonprescription drugs.

➤ Many ophthalmic products are available to manage the symptoms of minor acute or chronic conditions of the eye and eyelid.

➤ By understanding the pathophysiology of certain ocular conditions and knowing how to assess a patient who presents with such conditions, pharmacists should be able to optimize the safe, appropriate, effective, and economical use of nonprescription drugs to manage selected conditions of the eye and eyelid.

➤ Nonprescription ophthalmic products should be used only in cases of minor pain or discomfort. If doubt exists concerning the nature of the problem, the pharmacist should refer the patient for professional care.

➤ Nonprescription ocular medications should not be recommended to patients who have demonstrated an allergy to any of the active ingredients, preservatives, or other excipients in the product.

➤ Patients who are already using a prescription ophthalmic product should use nonprescription products only after consulting with an eye care provider or pharmacist.

➤ Patients with narrow anterior chamber angles or narrow-angle glaucoma should not use topical ocular decongestants because of the risk of angle-closure glaucoma.

➤ Drug administration should be conservative in patients with hyperemic conjunctiva because of the potential for increased systemic drug absorption and the risk of adverse effects.

➤ The lowest concentration and conservative dosage frequencies should be used, especially for ocular decongestants; overuse should be avoided.

➤ Ophthalmic products frequently are used incorrectly; therefore, counseling on appropriate application of products is crucial.

REFERENCES

1. Lemp M. Advances in understanding and managing dry eye disease. *Am J Ophthalmol*. 2008;146(3):350–6.
2. Warwick R, ed. In: *Anatomy of the Eye and Orbit*. 7th ed. Philadelphia, PA: WB Saunders;1975:195–219.
3. Milder B. The lacrimal apparatus. In: Moses RA, Hart WM, eds. *Adler's Physiology of the Eye*. 8th ed. St. Louis, MO: Mosby;1987:15–35.
4. Mishima S, Gasset A, Klyce SO, et al. Determination of tear volume and tear flow. *Invest Ophthalmol*. 1966;5(3):264–76.
5. Jordan A, Baum J. Basic tear flow. Does it exist? *Ophthalmology*. 1980;87(9):920–30.
6. Harris LS, Galin MA. Dose response analysis of pilocarpine-induced ocular hypotension. *Arch Ophthalmol*. 1970;84(5):605–8.
7. Pfister RR, Burstein N. The effects of ophthalmic drugs, vehicles, and preservatives on corneal epithelium: a scanning electron microscope study. *Invest Ophthalmol*. 1976;15(4):246–59.
8. Stern ME, Beurman RW, Fox RI, et al. The pathology of dry eye: the interaction between the ocular surface and lacrimal glands. *Cornea*. 1998;17(6):584–9.
9. Lemp MA, Daudouin C, Baum J, et al. The definition and classification of dry eye disease: report for the Definition and Classification Subcommittee of the International Dry Eye Workshop (2007). *Ocul Surf*. 2007;5(2):75–92;163–78.
10. Behrens A, Doyle JJ, Stern L, et al. Dysfunctional tear syndrome: a Delphi approach to treatment recommendations. *Cornea*. 2006;25(8):900–7.
11. American Academy of Ophthalmology. Dry Eye Syndrome: Preferred Practice Patterns. The American Academy of Ophthalmology, 2011. Accessed at http://www.AAO.org, October 28, 2013.
12. Schilling H, Koch JM, Waubke TN, et al. Treatment of dry eye with vitamin A acid: an impression cytology controlled study. *Fortschr Ophthalmol*. 1989;86(5):530–4.
13. Mullen W, Sheppard W, Leibowitz J. Ophthalmic preservatives and vehicles. *Surv Ophthalmol*. 1973;17(6):469–83.
14. Sabiston DW. The dry eye. *Trans Ophthalmol Soc N Z*. 1969;21:96–100.
15. Linn ML, Jones LT. Rate of lacrimal excretion of ophthalmic vehicles. *Am J Ophthalmol*. 1968;65(91):76–8.
16. Berdy GJ, Abelson MB, Smith LM, et al. Preservative-free artificial tear solutions. *Arch Ophthalmol*. 1992;110(4):528–32.
17. Pensyl CD. Preparations for dry eye and ocular surface disease. In: Bartlett JD, Jaanus SD, eds. *Clinical Ocular Pharmacology*. 5th ed. Boston: Butterworth-Heinemann; 2007:263–78.
18. Fiscella R, Burstein NL. Ophthalmic drug formulations. In: Bartlett JD, Jaanus SD, eds. *Clinical Ocular Pharmacology*. 5th ed. Boston, MA: Butterworth-Heinemann; 2007:17–37.
19. Burstein NL. Preservative cytotoxic threshold for benzalkonium chloride and chlorhexidine digluconate in cat and rabbit corneas. *Invest Ophthalmol Vis Sci*. 1980;19(3):308–13.
20. Debbasch C, Brignole F, Pisella P-J, et al. Quaternary ammoniums and other preservatives' contribution in oxidative stress and apoptosis on Chang conjunctival cells. *Invest Ophthalmol Vis Sci*. 2001;42(3):642–52.
21. Wilson WS, Duncan AJ, Jay JL. Effect of benzalkonium chloride on the stability of the precorneal tear film in rabbit and man. *Br J Ophthalmol*. 1975;59(11):667–9.
22. Mondino BJ, Salamon SM, Zaidman GW. Allergic and toxic reactions in soft contact lens wearers. *Surv Ophthalmol*. 1982;26(6):337–44.
23. Bielory L. Ocular allergy treatment. *Immunol Allergy Clin North Am*. 2008;28(1):189–224.
24. Soparkar CN, Wilhelmus KR, Koch DD, et al. Acute and chronic conjunctivitis due to over-the-counter ophthalmic decongestants. *Arch Ophthalmol*. 1997;115(1):34–8.
25. Portello JK. Mydriatics and mydriolytics. In: Bartlett JD, Jaanus SD, eds. *Clinical Ocular Pharmacology*. 5th ed. Boston, MA: Butterworth-Heinemann;2007:113–23.
26. Adamczyk DT, Jaanus SD. Antiallergy drugs and decongestants. In: Bartlett JD, Jaanus SD, eds. *Clinical Ocular Pharmacology*. 5th ed. Boston, MA: Butterworth-Heinemann;2007:245–61.
27. Krupin T, Silverstein B, Faitt M, et al. The effect of H1-blocking antihistamines on intraocular pressure in rabbits. *Ophthalmology*. 1980; 87(11):1167–72.
28. Abelson MB, Allansmith MR, Freidlaender MH. Effects of topically applied ocular decongestant and antihistamine. *Am J Ophthalmol*. 1980; 90(2):254–7.
29. Petrusewicz J, Kalizan R. Blood platelet adrenoreceptor: aggregatory and antiaggregatory activity of imidazole drugs. *Pharmacology*. 1986;33(5):249–55.
30. Slonim CB, Boone R. The ocular allergic response: a pharmacotherapeutic review. *Formulary*. 2004;39:213–22.
31. Jaanus SD. Antiedema agents. In: Bartlett JD, Jaanus SD, eds. *Clinical Ocular Pharmacology*. 5th ed. Boston: Butterworth-Heinemann;2007:279–81.
32. Khare GD, Symons RCA, Do DV. Common ophthalmic emergencies. *Int J Clin Pract* 2008;62(11):1776–84.

PREVENTION OF CONTACT LENS–RELATED DISORDERS

Aleda M. H. Chen and Tracy R. Frame

Both soft and gas permeable contact lenses are considered Class II medical devices regulated by the Food and Drug Administration (FDA).[1] Similar to legend drugs, contact lenses are available only by prescription in the United States. Contact lenses are made of flexible or rigid plastics that allow the passage of oxygen to the corneal surface. Designed to be easily applied, worn, and removed, with minimal disturbance to ocular physiology, contact lenses are used to correct refractive errors, alter the cosmetic appearance of the wearer, or therapeutically treat diseases of the anterior surface of the eye (i.e., the cornea). Compared with earlier rigid lenses, soft contact lenses have greatly enhanced comfort, and since their introduction in 1971, the contact lens market has significantly expanded. An estimated 125 million people use contact lenses worldwide, including as many as 38 million in the United States. For 2012, the U.S. soft contact lens market was $2.4 billion of the worldwide contact lens market of $7.1 billion.[2] The types of lenses prescribed vary markedly among countries; however, soft lenses dominate 90% of the market, with gas permeable lenses accounting for approximately 20% of prescribed contact lenses in some countries, such as Argentina, Costa Rica, Mexico, Peru, and Venezuela, but only 9% of contact lenses prescribed in the United States.[3] The newest soft lens material, known as silicone hydrogel, continues to dominate the soft lens market, accounting for nearly half of prescribed soft lenses worldwide and 65% in the United States.[2]

As many as 50% of contact lens wearers experience complications; however, this number varies widely by type of lens, wearing schedule, and compliance with care regimens.[4] Contact lenses, even when expertly fit, alter ocular tissues and change the corneal metabolism. The prevention of contact lens–related disorders requires that both patients and health care providers understand the proper fitting, prescribing, and care regimens associated with safe contact lens wear. Failure to do so can greatly increase the chance of corneal infection (ulcers) and other ocular conditions that may result in permanent eye damage and blindness. Preventive measures aimed at improving patient hygiene and appropriate contact lens care, as well as adherence to the recommended replacement frequency, reduce the overall risk of contact lens complications.[5] Fortunately, most complications from contact lens wear are reversible, if attended to promptly. Approximately 25%–33% of patients discontinue wearing their contact lenses periodically or permanently, with lens discomfort

or dryness cited as the most common reason.[6–8] Proper care and fitting of lenses can help eliminate discomfort and encourage patients to continue wearing their lenses.

The fitting and dispensing of contact lenses, traditionally the sole domain of optometrists and ophthalmologists, have undergone dramatic changes in recent years. The Fairness to Contact Lens Consumers Act, passed by Congress in 2003, requires that contact lens prescribers release a copy of the contact lens prescription to patients at the conclusion of the fitting process, whether or not it is requested.[9] This act allows patients to obtain contact lens fitting services from their eye care providers and gives them the freedom to purchase contact lens materials from any legitimate source, including pharmacies.

The availability of contact lenses from nonprofessional sources such as department stores, mail-order services, or the Internet is a significant concern. In these circumstances, after presentation of a valid prescription, contact lenses can be dispensed by any individual, who only has to comply with state and local business statutes that have no stipulations for basic training in eye care or regard for professional or technical licensing in health care. Recent research has shown that individuals who purchase contact lenses from the Internet are less likely to adhere to recommended lens care,[10,11] which is particularly concerning because online sales of glasses and contact lenses are estimated at $350 million for 2012, having grown more than 28% in the past decade.[2]

As this chapter will point out, fitting and dispensing contact lenses involve more than the parameters of the lenses. Patient compliance with care systems, wearing schedules, and replacement schedules must also be considered. Patient education on lens handling and on signs and symptoms of complications are essential parts of the fitting process. Another concern is enforcement of expiration dates for lens prescriptions.

Use of Contact Lenses

Most people can wear one or more types of contact lenses without problems if certain precautions are taken. In a few cases, use of contact lenses is contraindicated.

Indications for Contact Lenses

The primary indication for the use of contact lenses is the correction of refractive errors such as myopia (nearsightedness), hyperopia (farsightedness), astigmatism, and presbyopia. Astigmatism occurs when dissimilar curvatures of the refractive

---

Editor's Note: This chapter is based on the 17th edition chapter of the same title, written by Peter A. Russo, Bruce I. Gaynes, and Janet P. Engle.

surface of the eye result in a blurred image. Gas permeable lenses or toric soft lenses can be used to correct astigmatism.

The benefits of contact lens wear are widely known and include the convenience of freedom from glasses, no obstruction from eyeglass frames, no fogging of lenses caused by sudden temperature changes, improved optics and clarity of vision, wider peripheral field of vision, equal image sizes when refractive disparity exists between eyes, and better function during sporting activities or exercise. Perhaps a significant reason for choosing contact lenses is the perceived improvement in self-image and personal appearance.[12]

The decision to wear contact lenses rather than eyeglasses is sometimes based on therapeutic necessity. For example, in patients with keratoconus (a corneal dystrophy causing a gradual protrusion of the central cornea), satisfactory vision is usually unattainable with ordinary eyeglasses but can be achieved with rigid contact lenses. Another example of therapeutic necessity is the use of soft contact lenses as "bandage" lenses in the case of corneal abrasions. Other, less common, indications for contact lenses include aphakia (absence of the natural lens of the eye), corneal scarring, and disfigured eyes. In these conditions, patients typically see better with contact lenses, and for patients with disfigurement, tinted prosthetic soft contact lenses may improve cosmetic appearance by rendering disfigurement from a variety of conditions virtually unnoticeable.

Contraindications and Warnings for Contact Lenses

Without question, however, there are patients who are poor candidates for contact lens wear and cannot or should not wear contact lenses. Contraindications are often based on lifestyle as well as on medical history. The following are relative contraindications that should be considered on an individual basis before fitting contact lenses:

- Patients who are monocular. The risk of complications such as inflammation or infection that can permanently scar the cornea must be weighed against the need for optimal visual correction. Overnight wear of lenses should absolutely be avoided.
- Patients with active pathology of the lids, cornea, or conjunctiva. Such conditions include blepharitis, corneal infections (e.g., herpes keratitis), or conjunctivitis. Common colds or chronic allergic conditions such as hay fever and asthma also may make contact lens wear extremely uncomfortable or impossible.
- Patients with dry eye (keratitis sicca) unless using bandage soft contact lenses for protection. This area is controversial because some patients with severe dry eye actually benefit from the use of bandage soft contact lenses to protect the ocular surface. Cosmetic lens wearers who have insufficient tear production, a deficiency or excess of mucin, or excessive lipid production, or who need to spend time in excessively dry environments may be unable to use contact lenses successfully. Poor blink rate or incomplete blinking may also contribute to difficulty with lens wear. Postmenopausal women may experience higher rates of dry eye that preclude successful contact lens wear.
- Women who are pregnant or using oral contraceptives. The fluid-retaining properties of estrogen may lead to edema of the cornea, which will alter corneal topography and affect the fit of contact lenses.

- Patients with diabetes. Diabetic patients are advised against continuous-wear contact lenses because of retarded healing processes and reduced corneal sensitivity. This precaution is probably unnecessary for daily wear of lenses unless problems occur.
- Patients who must use eye medications frequently (e.g., treatment of glaucoma). The preservatives in multidose bottles can bind to soft contact lenses and cause toxicity to the corneal epithelium.
- Patients with a vocation or hobby that is not conducive to lens wear (e.g., smoking, chemical environment). Occupational conditions that may prohibit the wearing of contact lenses include exposure to wind, glare, molten metals, irritants, dust and particulate matter, tobacco smoke, chemicals, and chemical fumes. Certain chemical fumes may be particularly hazardous because of the potential concentration of irritants under a rigid lens or inside a soft lens. The lens theoretically prolongs contact of such substances with the cornea and can lead to corneal toxicity.
- Lens wearers who may move from low to high altitude. Moving from a low to a high altitude may cause hypoxia (causing edema of the cornea) or metabolic deficiency, resulting in irritation and corneal abrasions.
- Patients who have shown a pattern of abusing lens wear or multiple episodes of ocular complications.
- Patients who are unable to care for contact lenses appropriately. This group includes young patients who are not properly supervised or older patients who lack the cognitive skills or dexterity to handle contact lenses.

Soft versus Rigid Contact Lenses

There are only two major categories of contact lenses: soft (hydrophilic) and rigid (gas permeable [GP]) lenses. Rigid lenses of non–gas permeable polymethylmethacrylate (PMMA) (often known as "hard" contact lenses) are rarely used owing to their lack of oxygen permeability. Soft and GP lenses are composed of single or multiple plastic monomers; soft lens materials contain water but GP lens materials do not. Soft lenses are popular because of their excellent initial comfort on insertion. Rigid lenses have always provided the best optics and, therefore, superior visual acuity. In the contact lens field, use of the term *hard lenses* during patient counseling is no longer acceptable because it creates a stigma about optimal lens designs for individual needs. Therefore, rigid lenses should simply be referred to as gas permeable lenses. Table 28–1 provides a comparison of PMMA, soft, and GP lenses. Table 28–2 compares the advantages and disadvantages of soft and GP contact lenses with regard to ease of care and handling, potential complications, and other parameters.

Hydrophilic (Soft) Contact Lenses

First introduced in 1971, soft contact lenses have become the lens of choice from the standpoint of health care providers and patients alike. In the United States alone, soft contact lenses represent almost 90% of all contact lens fits.[2] Once limited by poor reproducibility and limited parameter availability, soft contact lenses are now available in any spherical or cylindrical power, and they can correct for presbyopia, myopia or hyperopia, and astigmatism. The primary monomer that soft lenses are manufactured from is 2-hydroxyethyl methacrylate (HEMA). Other monomers used include methacrylic acid (MA) and

table 28–1	Comparison of Contact Lens Characteristics		
	PMMA	**Lens Type Soft**	**Gas Permeable**
Lens Characteristics			
Rigidity	+++	0	+++
Durability	+++	+	++
Oxygen transmission	0	++	+++
Chemical adsorption	0	+++	0
Optical Quality			
Visual acuity	+++	+	+++
Correction of astigmatism	Yes	Toric	Yes
Photophobia	++	+	++
Spectacle blur	+++	0	++
Convenience			
Comfort	+	+++	++
Adaptation period	Weeks	Days	Weeks
Continuous wear	No	Yes	Yes
Intermittent wear	No	Yes	No

Key: PMMA = Polymethylmethylacrylate; + indicates the degree to which the characteristic is present; 0 means the characteristic is not present.

n-vinylpyrrolidone (NVP).[13] The equilibrium point of hydration of polyHEMA soft contact lenses is 38%. As the polymer changes to contain either MA or NVP, the equilibrium water content increases to 60% or more. The hydration characteristic of soft lenses may be adversely influenced by several variables, including temperature, oxidative reactions of lens care solutions, tonicity, and pH.[13]

In 1986, FDA classified soft hydrogel contacts into four categories according to water content and ionic properties (low water non-ionic, high water non-ionic, low water ionic, high water ionic). Soft contact lenses with less than 50 percent water content are considered to be low water. Less reactive surfaces are called non-ionic, and more reactive materials are called ionic.[2] Most eye care providers fit non-ionic soft contact lenses because of the lenses' inherent chemical ability to deter the formation of charged protein and lipid deposits. Ionic lenses have a negative surface charge, which tends to attract more protein deposits compared with non-ionic lenses. Non-ionic lenses are electrically neutral and tend to be less reactive with the tear film, resulting in a more deposit-resistant lens. Originally, soft contact lenses were intended to be cleaned and disinfected daily and replaced on a yearly basis. Compliance was poor because patients opted for convenience over ocular health by not following prescribed daily care regimens, by replacing lenses after years of wear, and by sleeping overnight while wearing lenses, in some cases for weeks at a time. Contact lens complications such as corneal edema, neovascularization, and infiltrates were observed. Oxygen deprivation, or hypoxia, was known to be

a significant factor in many of these complications. The oxygen transmissibility of contact lenses is described by the term Dk/L,[13] where "D" represents gas diffusion, "k" solubility, and "L" the contact lens center thickness in centimeters. A higher Dk/L value allows more oxygen to pass through the lens. As the water content increases, the "k" value and oxygen permeability increase. However, permeability also depends on lens thickness.

Tighter quality control and refinement of manufacturing techniques have led to improved lens reproducibility and to the advent of disposable soft contact lenses. Disposable lenses represent the fastest-growing segment of the soft lens market. A true disposable soft contact lens is worn once and replaced without interval cleaning, implying that it is worn continuously.[2] The advantage of having a clean lens worn on a regular basis appealed to many patients and lessened the incidence of complications from a soiled lens, such as contact lens papillary conjunctivitis. With disposable contact lenses, the traditional yearly replacement schedule has been replaced with soft lenses, which are replaced monthly. However, some patients use soft contact lenses that are replaced biweekly or daily. Silicone hydrogel materials have contributed to the ability to have continuous wear lenses.

Health care providers were hopeful that frequent lens replacement would improve compliance and negate the negative effects of biofilm development on the surface of lenses. Many also believed that silicone hydrogel materials would effectively eliminate inflammatory and infectious complications of contact lens wear, including microbial keratitis, by removing the effects of hypoxia on the corneal epithelium. Although years of clinical use have shown that these materials do, in fact, diminish the hypoxic effect of lens wear, such as redness, limbal neovascularization, and microcystic edema, they have failed to eliminate infectious and inflammatory complications.[14] One study showed identical rates of microbial keratitis for overnight wear of silicone hydrogel materials and use of older HEMA materials.[15] FDA, however, continues to allow two continuous-wear schedules that are lens specific to remain in effect. The first is 6 continuous days and nights of wear, with the lens being discarded on day 7, as implemented during the early days of continuous wear. For some of the most permeable materials, FDA approves 30 nights of continuous wear, followed by replacement of the lens. Patients should be made aware that the continuous wear of contact lenses has clearly been shown to be the greatest risk factor for the most devastating consequences of lens wear, primarily microbial keratitis. Even though lenses are approved for 30 nights of continuous wear, some patients may not be able to tolerate wearing them for this length of time. None of the soft contact lenses on the market, including silicone hydrogel materials, can prevent or protect an individual from inflammatory and infectious complications. This statement emphasizes the importance of patient education and compliance with care regimens, wearing and replacement schedules, and awareness of adverse symptoms to ensure safe contact lens wear.

Even a disposable, continuous-wear lens may be used only on a daily wear basis, and patients should replace lenses at the prescribed interval. When worn on a daily wear basis, these lenses must be cleaned and disinfected regularly. Patients looking to optimize convenience without exposing themselves to the risk of continuous wear should be directed toward daily disposable lenses. Daily disposables have the following advantages: (1) each lens is sterile prior to removal from its package for immediate insertion into the eye; (2) no cleaning regimen

Soft Contact Lenses	GP Contact Lenses
Advantages	
Excellent initial lens comfort	Excellent optics for optimal visual acuity
Rapid adaptation; well suited for intermittent lens wear	Correct nearly all forms of refractive error
Correct nearly all forms of refractive error	Improve vision for conditions with irregular corneas
Ease of fitting	Fit customized to individual patient
Ease of care	Economical
Unlikely to trap foreign material under the lens	Lower incidence of inflammatory/infectious complications
Unlikely to dislodge or fall out; well suited for sporting activities	
Can be tinted for cosmetic or prosthetic purposes (many lenses have light tints to improve visibility when handling)	
Disadvantages	
Not possible to achieve excellent visual acuity for all patients	Longer initial adaptation period
Fluctuations in vision because lens hydration varies with prolonged wear and changes in temperatures and humidity	Capable of trapping foreign material beneath the lens, causing discomfort
Lens fitting not customized to the patient	May dislodge from the eye
More prone to complications, especially from hypoxia	More difficult to fit
Fragility of lenses during handling	Flare around the periphery that may be noticed at night, particularly with large pupils
Lenses susceptible to preservatives in ophthalmic products	
Unable to verify correct eye for each soft lens once packaging is removed or to mark identification (i.e., L or R) on lens surface	

is necessary because the lens is discarded after wear; (3) deposit formation is minimal; and (4) lens-related problems, such as giant papillary conjunctivitis or allergic reactions to lens care solutions, occur less frequently.

Hydrophilic Lens Fitting

Unlike rigid contact lenses, which are typically custom designed, the parameters of the most commonly used soft contact lenses are predetermined by the manufacturer and are proprietary in nature. Often, the lens diameter and base curve are limited to one or two choices at most, providing little flexibility for adjusting fit. In addition, if a lens does not fit correctly or causes some other complication, another lens design must be tried. There are exceptions, and custom soft lenses with a specified diameter, base curve, and power can be ordered.

Hydrophilic Contact Lenses as Therapeutic Devices

Aside from the cosmetic use of contact lenses, hydrophilic lenses have found wide application in the treatment of ocular disease and are being examined for potential use as ocular drug delivery devices. Notably, hydrophilic lenses are employed as an "eye bandage" or bandage lenses to protect the cornea and promote corneal reepithelialization after corneal injury or various corneal surgical procedures. Four soft contact lenses are currently approved by FDA for use therapeutically as bandage

contact lenses in the treatment of corneal abrasions and other ocular surface problems. It is important to counsel patients who are prescribed contact lenses for this purpose to be diligent in cleaning and disinfecting the lenses.[15,16]

Gas Permeable Contact Lenses

Rigid contact lenses preceded soft lenses in the market but were quickly surpassed because of one primary factor: patients have greater initial awareness of rigid lenses on the eye. In terms of optical quality, rigid lenses are far superior to soft lenses. However, patients are willing to sacrifice clarity for comfort. In defense of rigid lenses, initial discomfort can dissipate over several weeks as adaptation occurs and nerve endings on the inner surface of the eyelids become desensitized to the presence of the lens.

The first rigid lenses were conventional hard lenses made of PMMA plastic, which has no oxygen permeability. Despite PMMA being a stable, durable plastic, lenses made with PMMA are rarely used in the United States because of the advantages of GP materials, primarily direct oxygen permeability through the lens. GP lenses are made from monomer components of hydrophobic plastic compounds that allow oxygen to diffuse through the lens.[17] Advantages of GP lenses over soft contact lenses include increased oxygen transmissibility, reduced lipophilicity, and sharper vision. These lenses also have less surface reactivity, thereby decreasing tear film deposits.[17] Other advantages of GP lenses over soft contact lenses include fewer adverse inflammatory or infectious consequences. When properly cared for, GP lenses are durable and can be reused repeatedly for months to years before replacement is necessary, making them more economical than soft lenses. Surface scratches and deposits can be removed with powerful cleaners or in-office polishing machines. The disadvantages of GP lenses include less surface wettability; a negative surface charge, which can attract lysozymes and other positively charged deposits; and greater mass, which can affect lens fit, depending on the type of GP lens.

GP lenses are the lens of choice for dealing with complicated corneal disease such as keratoconus, corneal scarring from disease or trauma, and transplanted corneas or those with high astigmatism. Unlike soft lenses that drape over the surface of the cornea, even if it is irregular, GP lenses create a new refracting surface with a tear layer filling the gap between lens and cornea. GP lenses are available in a wide range of designs, including toric lenses for astigmatism and bifocals for presbyopia. Although far fewer in number, some GP materials are also FDA approved for either 7 or 30 days of continuous wear, depending on the material.

GP Lens Fitting

Most providers who fit contact lenses agree that, compared with soft lenses, fitting GP lenses requires more art and science. Unlike soft lenses, GP lenses are not mass manufactured but rather are custom designed and manufactured on demand, requiring the optometrist to provide the parameters of diameter, base curve, power, and material to order a lens.

Specialty Contact Lenses

Numerous companies manufacture soft contact lenses. The product offerings of many companies overlap to address the most common myopic, hyperopic, and astigmatic refractive errors. Many companies sell prepackaged, mass-produced lenses that consumers can buy in bulk with a prescription. Some offer customized lenses to address unusual needs. Several promote materials that absorb ultraviolet light. Corrective, tinted lenses are available for easier handling and for cosmetic purposes. Translucent tints facilitate handling by increasing the visibility of the lens and enhance eye color. Opaque lenses cover the iris and hide its natural color. These lenses may also be used as a prosthesis to mask corneal scarring. In contrast, all GP lenses are custom made by laboratories that often use proprietary, computer-generated lens designs. These unique designs are aimed at specialty needs such as keratoconus, post–corneal transplant use, scarred corneas, post–refractive surgery use, aphakia, or high astigmatism. Two specialty lenses worth mentioning are lenses for presbyopia and hybrid lenses.

Presbyopia is the loss of accommodation in the aging eye, requiring the addition of plus power (i.e., adjustment for farsightedness) to improve the clarity of vision at a near reading distance. It affects individuals who are near- or farsighted or who have an astigmatism. Presbyopia is not to be confused with cataracts, another common cause of visual loss, which are caused by reduced clarity in the crystalline lens and are usually attributable to long-term oxidation and genetic predisposition. Presbyopes are projected to be the single largest group of contact lens wearers by 2018 at 28%.[18] In glasses, a separate portion of the spectacle lens at the bottom of the lens provides this additional plus power for reading (bifocal glasses). This change

in power is more difficult to accomplish with contact lenses. A common method of correcting presbyopia with contact lenses is monovision, a technique that uses standard lenses, with the dominant eye fit for distance and the other eye fit for near vision. Monovision can be effective, but it can affect depth perception, intermediate vision, and night driving. Today, multifocal contact lenses are being designed to provide binocular vision for patients, which provides a smooth transition from the near, intermediate, and far zones of the lens. The practitioner should discuss the options with the patient to determine what would work best for him or her.[19]

A *hybrid contact lens* is a unique contact lens that combines GP and soft lens materials in the same lens. The overall advantages of this lens are excellent optics through the GP portion of the lens, improved comfort from the soft lens portion, greater oxygen permeability (compared with an earlier version of the lens), and the ability to deal with astigmatism and irregular corneas (e.g., keratoconus and corneal transplant). The disadvantages are expense, difficulty with insertion and removal, longer fitting time, and complications of lens wear. The care of these lenses follows the patterns described for soft contact lenses in later sections.

Formulation Considerations for Lens Care Products

The manufacturing and marketing of contact lenses are regulated by the ophthalmic devices division of FDA.[1] Patients who wear contact lenses should use only lens care products that have been approved by FDA for use with their specific contact lenses.

The basic considerations for a well-formulated contact lens solution include pH, viscosity, isotonicity with tears, stability, sterility, and provisions for maintaining sterility (bactericidal action). The pH range of comfort is not well defined because, although normal tear pH is 7.4, tear pH varies among individuals. It is best to have a weakly buffered solution that can readily adjust to any tear pH, given that highly buffered solutions can cause significant discomfort, even ocular damage, when they are instilled. However, as with therapeutic ophthalmic solutions, the stability of the solution takes precedence over comfort. For that reason, many contact lens solutions are formulated with pH values above or below 7.4. These systems are weakly buffered and are usually well tolerated by the eye. Solutions from different manufacturers should not be mixed because a precipitate may form.[4,20] For instance, a product containing alkaline borate buffers forms a gummy, gel-like precipitate on lenses if mixed with a wetting solution containing polyvinyl alcohol. Furthermore, solutions containing a cationic preservative, such as chlorhexidine, polyquaternium-1, or polyaminopropyl biguanide, should not be mixed with solutions containing an anionic preservative such as sorbic acid; this combination, too, will cause a precipitate to form.

Soft Contact Lens Care

The goals of cleaning a contact lens are to (1) remove debris from the lens surface, (2) prevent the accumulation of proteins from the tear layer on the lens, and (3) disinfect the lens of organisms that can bind to the lens surface and potentially lead to infection. Lens disinfection is a crucial step, although all steps must be completed on a daily basis or after each wearing period to avoid ocular complications.[21] The basic care regimen for soft lenses (Figure 28–1) differs from that for GP lenses.

Since the early days of contact lens use, separate solutions have been available for each step of cleaning, rinsing, disinfecting, storing, and protein removal. These include surfactants for cleaning the lens surface, saline solution for rinsing, disinfecting agents for sterilization, and enzymes for protein removal, in addition to wetting drops for use while lenses are on the eye. To improve convenience and compliance, multipurpose products are available that combine these active ingredients in a biocompatible solution buffered for pH balance for use directly in the eye. Some of these solutions also contain demulcents to increase lubrication and comfort of the eye.

Tables 28–3 and 28–4 provide steps for cleaning soft contact lenses.

Soft Lens Disinfection

The lens care regimen must be primarily built around the use of a disinfecting system. Emphasis must be placed on hand hygiene and adherence to the manufacturer's requirements for each disinfecting system, while stressing the minimum soaking time for disinfection.

Preservatives

The most important point to be made in a discussion of contact lens disinfection regards the preservatives that are used both to keep multiuse solutions sterile and to disinfect the lens. Daily use of the same bottle of any contact lens solution over a long period of time increases the risk of bacterial contamination. The solution must therefore contain a bactericidal agent that is both effective over the long term and nonirritating to the eye with daily use. Despite the presence of preservatives, once opened, any contact lens solution not used within the recommended time frame on the label, typically 1–3 months, must be discarded. Patients should be encouraged to write the date that the bottle is opened on the outside of the bottle.[22]

Edetate disodium and sorbic acid are the most commonly used preservatives in saline, daily cleaners, and wetting drops for

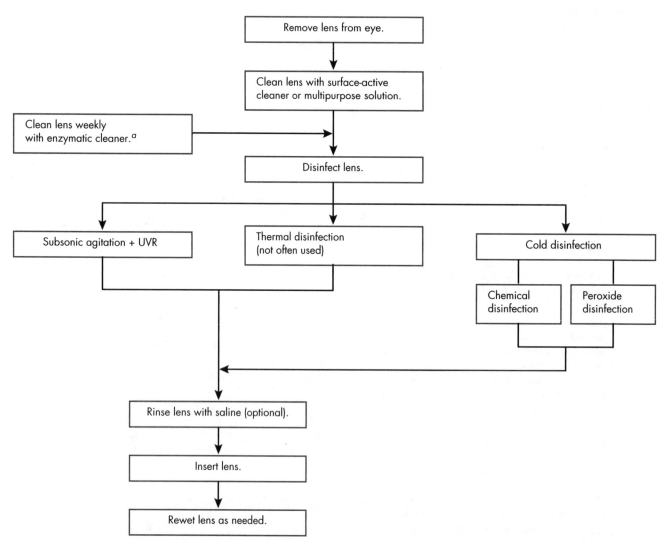

a Step is not necessary for planned replacement or disposable lenses.

figure

28-1   Self-care of soft lenses. Key: UVR, ultraviolet radiation.

table
28–3 General Cleaning Procedures for All Lens Types

- Wash hands with noncosmetic soap and rinse them thoroughly before handling lenses.
- Clean contact lenses only with commercially manufactured products made specifically for that type of lens. Homemade cleansers can scratch the lenses or cause eye irritation or injury.
- Do not mix contact lens care products from different manufacturers unless an eye care provider says the products are compatible.
- When handling lenses over a sink, cover or close the drain to prevent loss of a lens.
- During cleaning, check lenses for scratches, chips, or tears and for the presence of foreign particles, warping, or discoloration. Also, check that lenses are clean and thoroughly rinsed of cleaner. These factors could cause eye discomfort.
- When cleaning a lens, rub it in a back-and-forth, rather than a circular, direction, even if using a no-rub solution.
- Clean the second lens as thoroughly as the first.
- Discard cleansers and other lens care products if the labeled expiration date has passed.

contact lenses; benzalkonium chloride is used less frequently. Polyquaternium and polyhexamethylene biguanide are the preservatives used most commonly as disinfecting agents for soft contact lens solutions; both are recognized as effective antimicrobial agents.[22]

Polyquaternium-1

Polyquaternium-1 (Polyquad) is a quaternary ammonium preservative shown to be effective against certain bacteria, fungi, and yeast. When it was introduced to the market, formulations containing polyquaternium-1 were not compatible with lenses that had high water content because the methacrylic acid component of the lens had the ability to adsorb the preservative at

table
28–4 Specific Cleaning Procedures for Soft Lenses

- Clean regular soft lenses daily with a surface-active cleaner. Clean continuous-wear and disposable soft lenses with a surface-active cleaner after each wearing.
- Wash hands before handling your lenses.
- Place several drops of a cleaning product on the lens; gently rub the lens between the thumb and forefinger or between the fingertip of the forefinger and the palm of the opposite hand for 20–30 seconds, even if using a no-rub product, to ensure protein removal.
- Avoid cutting the lens with a fingernail or scratching the lens surface with grit or dirt on the hands.
- Rinse lenses with a sterile isotonic buffered solution. Never use tap water. It is not isotonic and contains harmful microorganisms.
- Clean lenses at least weekly (or every day if using a daily product) with enzymatic cleaners, either separately from disinfection or as part of the disinfecting process.
- When combining enzymatic cleaning and disinfecting of the lenses as one step, see Table 28–6 for the appropriate combinations of products.
- Discard any enzyme cleaner that is discolored.

toxic levels. However, recent formulations do not seem to have this problem. To date, few toxicity or sensitivity problems have been noted with these formulations.[23]

Polyhexamethylene Biguanide

Polyhexamethylene biguanide, also known as polyaminopropyl biguanide, Dymed, or polyhexanide, is a cationic polymeric biguanide that is effective against certain bacteria and yeast, although its activity against *Acanthamoeba* and fungi is limited. No significant adverse effects of polyaminopropyl biguanide have been reported in lens wearers.

Disinfecting Methods

FDA recommends disinfecting soft contact lenses before each reinsertion.[21,22] Chemical-based disinfection is by far the most popular (Table 28–5). Thermal, or heat, disinfection is no longer a viable method of caring for soft contact lenses. The other alternative is an electronic system, PuriLens, that uses subsonic ultrasound agitation for cleaning and high-intensity ultraviolet light for disinfection. However, one study suggests that additional antimicrobial agents may be needed because some bacteria may survive the disinfection process.[24,25]

table
28–5 Guidelines for Disinfecting Gas Permeable and Soft Lenses

Chemical Disinfection with Hydrogen Peroxide

- Using the cup provided with the hydrogen peroxide product, soak lenses for the length of time specified by the manufacturer. Do not use lens cups or cases that came with other products.
- To disinfect and neutralize in one step, place platinum catalytic disk in lens case and leave the disk there until time to replace it. Add hydrogen peroxide, insert lenses, and leave for at least 6 hours.
- Never place neutralizing solution in a lens case with a catalytic disc. An unwanted chemical reaction may occur, or a gummy residue may form on the disc.
- Before inserting lenses in the eyes, make sure the hydrogen peroxide is completely neutralized by carefully following product instructions.
- Rinse lenses thoroughly with saline before inserting them.

Chemical Preservative Disinfection

- Store lenses for the prescribed period of time (usually a minimum of 4 hours) in a preservative disinfecting solution that is appropriate for the lenses.
- If you experience irritation, rinse lenses thoroughly with saline to remove disinfecting solution.

Combination Enzyme Cleaning and Disinfection

- When combining enzyme cleaning and disinfecting of the lenses as one step, select products compatible with your disinfecting system.
- Add appropriate solution (hydrogen peroxide or chemical disinfecting product) to the storage case of the disinfecting system.
- Add lenses and then add appropriate enzymatic cleaner.
- Follow directions for appropriate disinfecting system listed previously.
- Rinse lenses thoroughly with saline to remove residual enzymes.

In chemical disinfection, lenses are stored for a prescribed period of time (usually 4–6 hours) in a solution containing bactericidal agents that are compatible with soft lens materials. Two basic chemical disinfection methods are available in the United States. The first is based on the original chemical disinfecting solutions, which consisted of antimicrobial preservatives at sufficient concentration in storage solutions composed primarily of saline.[22,26] These original disinfecting solutions contained chlorhexidine and thimerosal, both of which induce sensitivity reactions in many soft lens wearers.[26,27] To avoid this problem, manufacturers are currently marketing solutions with less-sensitizing disinfecting preservatives for soft contact lens care. Some of these preservatives are sorbic acid, polyquaternium-1, polyaminopropyl biguanide, and amidoamine, which are touted as being much less toxic or allergenic than their predecessors. However, some of these agents may also be less effective, especially against fungi and protozoans.[26] The second chemical method uses hydrogen peroxide as the antimicrobial agent. Soft lenses are placed in purified hydrogen peroxide only and disinfected by the liberation of oxygen from peroxide. Household hydrogen peroxide solution should not be used; its pH is too low and it may discolor lenses. After disinfection is completed, the peroxide is neutralized to trace levels by a neutralizing tablet that contains a delayed-release catalase or by the catalytic action of a platinum disc.[28]

One potential disadvantage of hydrogen peroxide disinfection is that patients may mistakenly insert the lens directly from the peroxide solution without neutralization. Patients must be warned not to perform a final rinse with the disinfecting solution prior to inserting their lenses, as they might do with a multipurpose chemical system. Emphasis on the neutralization step is critical. A peroxide-soaked lens placed on the eye will cause a toxic keratitis with symptoms of pain, photophobia, and redness. If this occurs, the patient should immediately remove the lens from the eye and flush the eye copiously with sterile saline solution. If symptoms do not abate, the patient should consult an eye care provider.[28] The catalytic disc used with some systems must be replaced every 3 months. Any sensation of discomfort or burning experienced by the user when inserting contact lenses that have been disinfected with hydrogen peroxide likely means incomplete neutralization and the need to replace the disc. Patients must also be instructed that once disinfection of contact lenses with a hydrogen peroxide system is completed, the remaining liquid is nonpreserved and is not suitable for prolonged storage (maximum of 7 days). Bacterial contamination may occur after that time. Hydrogen peroxide systems are not recommended for patients who wear lenses intermittently; these patients should be advised to switch to a multipurpose solution or to change to daily disposable contact lenses.

Although the catalytic disc systems require only one step, disinfection and neutralization require 6 hours, which decreases the system's flexibility and rules out morning use. Clear Care is the most readily available catalytic disc–based oxidation system. It contains a built-in cleaner and is approved as a "no-rub" product, but it does require a 5-second rinse before disinfection. Clear Care is the only peroxide system approved by FDA for use with silicone hydrogel materials.[29] Unizyme enzymatic cleaner may be added weekly for protein removal. Clear Care can also be used for cleaning, disinfection, and storage of GP lenses, but the lenses require digital rubbing. Oxysept Ultra-Care is a catalase-based system. With this product, the user adds a delayed-release neutralizing tablet at the beginning of the 6-hour disinfecting cycle. Disinfection and neutralization then occur at the appropriate time intervals. This tablet contains catalase and cyanocobalamin; the latter ingredient turns the solution pink, reminding the user that the tablet has been added.[29] The tablet is coated with hydroxypropyl methylcellulose, which helps lubricate the eye if the lens is not rinsed again between disinfection and insertion. A separate daily cleaning step is required. Unizyme enzymatic cleaner may be added weekly for protein removal. Patients using Oxysept UltraCare should know the following:

- This product requires a minimum of 6 hours for complete disinfection of the lenses and neutralization of the peroxide.
- The neutralizing tablet should not be crushed or used if there are cracks in the coating because the tablet will start neutralizing the peroxide before adequate disinfection occurs.
- Pliagel, used for surface-active cleaning, can leave a film on the lenses and lens cup if it is not carefully rinsed off the lenses before peroxide disinfection. This film may result in foaming and overflow of the peroxide–neutralizer solution. If this occurs, lenses should be rinsed more carefully or another surface-active cleaner should be used.
- The user should clean the lens case once a week. Remove lenses from the case if they are not being worn, and then fill the case with fresh Oxysept UltraCare disinfection solution and tighten the cap. Do not add a neutralization tablet. Turn the cup upside down to allow the solution to bathe the upper portion of the cup and cap. Soak the case in this manner until lenses need to be disinfected. Replace the solution for the next disinfection cycle.
- Before lenses are to be inserted in eyes, the case should be turned upside down to ensure full neutralization of all residual disinfecting solution in the case. Then the lenses can be removed from the case and inserted.

Patients also may use Sauflon One-Step (Sauflon), which has a built-in cleaner. Sauflon is considered a no-rub system and contains a rewetting agent. Patients must rinse each side for 5 seconds before disinfection. However, Sauflon is not available in the retail setting and can only be obtained through an eye care professional.[29]

When counseling a patient about the best disinfecting method to use, the primary care provider should consider the patient's compliance, wearing schedule, and convenience. Peroxide-based systems provide excellent disinfection against many organisms and essentially eliminate solution sensitivity issues. They are not well suited, however, for intermittent wear of disposable lenses or for careless patients who may inadvertently instill peroxide in their eye. If the patient has a history of sensitivity reactions to lens solutions or is unsure whether sensitivity exists, it is best to recommend a product containing one of the nonsensitizing preservatives.

Multipurpose Products

Initially manufacturers recommended three separate products for the cleaning, removal of protein, and disinfection of soft contact lenses. However, there has been a trend toward using multipurpose solutions for these functions, and some solutions claim to be effective for all three procedures.

The major problem with a multipurpose solution is that ingredients required in its formulation perform different and somewhat incompatible functions. For example, high concentrations of preservatives are necessary to kill bacteria; however, these same concentrations can cause ocular irritation when placed directly on the eye with a contact lens. If lenses are stored overnight in a cleaning solution containing an anionic surfactant, the detergent may eventually build up on the lens and cause irritation.[30]

Reactions to solutions should always be the differential diagnosis when trying to discern the cause of patient symptoms or findings of surface irritation during an eye examination. Most, if not all, of the chemicals listed as preservatives can cause irritation to the epithelium.[31] If symptoms are related to solution use, possible remedies are to use a final saline rinse prior to lens insertion or to change to another formulation of multipurpose solution that uses a different preservative. Another alternative for patients who are sensitive to chemical-based care systems is the PuriLens system, as discussed earlier.

A common source of confusion among patients is the concept of no-rub multipurpose solutions. The original sequence for cleaning contact lenses was to rub, rinse, and then soak. All of the no-rub products still require thorough rinsing of the lenses first, not just soaking.

Solutions that fail this test can still be approved if they pass the FDA regimen test that requires the manufacturer to recommend the additional steps of rubbing and rinsing in addition to soaking. The point of the requirement is that some mechanical force, either digital rubbing or a steady stream of liquid, is required to debulk the surface of the lens of debris and pathogens.

Patients should be counseled not to "top off" or reuse the contact lens solution in the case, as the solution is less effective once used. Recent research has indicated that when using any multipurpose contact lens solution, the best method of disinfection includes rubbing the contact lens.[32] FDA, American Optometric Association, and American Academy of Ophthalmology all have issued new recommendations that include rubbing each side of the contact lens for 5–10 seconds.[21]

These products are useful for patients with planned replacement lenses, because these lenses are usually discarded before a significant amount of protein or lipid builds up on the lens. Use of these products is usually more of a problem with longer lens replacement schedules.

Cleaning Products

A troublesome aspect of soft lens wear is the accumulation of deposits on the lens. Daily use of separate cleaners and protein removal products, in addition to use of multipurpose solutions, generally is not necessary for disposable lenses that will be discarded after a few weeks of wear. These products should

be recommended if patients have long replacement schedules (>1 month) or demonstrate rapid, heavy formation of deposits on lenses. The nature of deposits varies, but they generally consist of proteins and lipids from lacrimal secretions.

Soft lens cleaning solutions generally contain a nonionic detergent, a wetting agent, a chelating agent, buffers, preservatives, and, in some cases, polymeric cleaning beads. Although the surface-active cleaners are generally quite effective in removing lipid deposits, they remove tenacious protein debris less successfully. Enzymatic cleaners are an additional cleaning aid that can solve this problem. These enzymes hydrolyze polypeptide bonds of protein and dissolve the protein deposits. For the enzyme solution to work properly, however, the lens must be cleaned with a surface-active cleaner first; enzymes are ineffective on debris that covers or is mixed with protein.

Enzymatic cleaners are recommended according to the disinfection system used by the patient. Ultrazyme and Unizyme are used weekly with hydrogen peroxide cleaning systems.[33] These products can be placed in the peroxide solution, thereby cleaning and disinfecting at the same time. For chemical-based systems, OPTI-FREE SupraClens Daily Protein Remover can be added directly to OPTI-FREE multipurpose solutions during the disinfection cycle. SupraClens must be rinsed off before lens insertion. ReNu 1 Step Daily Protein Remover is the companion product for patients using Renu Sensitive Multi-Purpose Solution. If the patient uses another chemical disinfection system, product comparisons are very idiosyncratic unless the patient is allergic to one of the components. Table 28–6 lists characteristics of various enzymatic products. Cleaning with a surface-active cleaner can be done daily or, in the case of continuous-wear lenses, each time they are removed from the eyes. In addition to surfactants, some products contain mild abrasives that aid in the removal of lens deposits. Patients who have difficulty removing deposits from their lenses will benefit from this type of cleaner. These products should be shaken before use. Some patients may have difficulty rinsing these cleaners off their lenses. Care should be taken to ensure that no residue from the cleaning solution remains on the lens prior to insertion. Some surface-active cleaners (e.g., Bausch & Lomb Sensitive Eyes Daily Cleaner) have a lower viscosity and may be easier to rinse off the lens. These products are good choices for patients who have difficulty completely rinsing the cleaner off their lenses.

Products that combine enzymatic cleaning and disinfecting steps tend to increase compliance by decreasing the number of lens care steps that a patient must perform. Of note, in addition

table 28–6	Enzymatic Cleaners		
Trade Name	**Active Ingredient**	**Concurrent Use with Chemical Preservative Disinfection**	**Concurrent Use with Hydrogen Peroxide Disinfection**
OPTI-FREE SupraClens Daily Protein Remover	Liquid pancreatin	Yes, with OPTI-FREE multipurpose solutions	No
ReNu 1-Step Daily Protein Remover	Subtilisin A	Yes, with Renu Sensitive Multi-Purpose Solution	No
Ultrazyme/Unizyme	Subtilisin A	No	Yes

to product patent expirations, which lead to generic formulations, solutions also change in the marketplace according to usage and trends in lens care. Daily cleaners, enzymatic cleaners, and saline solutions are used much less frequently because of the convenience of combination products. Some of the products mentioned in this chapter may be available only through online retailers.

Saline Solutions

A common source of confusion among patients is the use of saline solutions in lieu of disinfecting agents. The hydrophilic soft contact lens must be maintained in a constant state of hydration. Soft lenses in the nonhydrated (dry) state are rigid and extremely brittle, and they should not be handled by the wearer. Furthermore, the hydrated lens must be isotonic with tears, because changes in tonicity can alter the conformation and optical properties of the lens. At one point, isotonic normal saline was the basic solution used for rinsing, thermally disinfecting, and storing soft contact lenses.[27] That regimen is no longer recommended. The health care provider should emphasize that saline used alone lacks disinfecting properties and direct the patient toward a suitable multipurpose or hydrogen peroxide solution.

Saline still has a use as a final rinsing agent prior to insertion, especially for patients who are irritated by the chemicals in multipurpose solutions. Prepared saline is available in either preserved or preservative-free forms. Sorbic acid–preserved products are commonly promoted for sensitive eyes and appear to be acceptable to most wearers. Several preservative-free saline solutions are also available but must be used within 30 days if they are in a multiuse bottle. Patients using nonpreserved saline should be counseled that only aerosolized solutions can be used to rinse lenses just before insertion into the eye. Multipurpose nonpreserved saline (e.g., Unisol 4) should never be used to rinse lenses just before insertion, unless the bottle is new and has not been opened. Once these products have been opened, they should be used only if a disinfection step will be performed before insertion. Patients should avoid using other forms of saline, such as intravenous normal saline or saline squirts. These products are usually too acidic for use with soft contact lenses. Patients should not try to make their own saline solution, as it can become easily contaminated and cause infections.

Rewetting Solutions

Because dryness and discomfort with contact lens wear are common, additional lubricating or wetting drops are often recommended for use while wearing lenses. Exposing lenses to wind and high temperature also causes some dehydration, even with the lens in the eye. These accessory solutions permit lubricating and rewetting and, in some cases, cleaning of the soft lens while on the eye. Patients should be directed toward products specific for use with contact lenses to avoid drops preserved with benzalkonium chloride, as discussed earlier. Preservative-free lubricating drops are also a good alternative. The resulting discomfort is sometimes relieved by 1 or 2 drops of rewetting solution. To minimize contamination, the tip of the applicator bottle should not touch the eye, eyelid, or any other surface.

Generic Solutions

Many generic versions of brand-name solutions are now available. It should be noted, however, that patients who choose to buy generic (e.g., mass merchandiser labeled) multipurpose lens solutions may be purchasing older, potentially obsolete formulas. Mass merchandisers generally purchase older formulations of nationally known brands of multipurpose solutions and then market them under their private label. In addition, the composition of a particular generic formulation can vary because the stores submit bids to manufacturers two to three times per year. Generally, patients should not use generic brands unless they carefully read the label and compare all ingredients with those of the product that was recommended by their eye care or other provider. Manufacturers are not required to use the same name for generic and brand-name ingredients, so comparing formulations may be difficult.[34]

Product Incompatibility

Several incompatibilities may occur during mixing of soft lens products. Most manufacturers test for compatibility within their own product lines; however, compatibility with other manufacturers' products is usually not determined. Generally, chemical disinfecting solutions should not be used interchangeably or concurrently, as discussed earlier.

Product Selection Guidelines

Table 28–7 lists examples of products designed specifically for soft contact lenses.

Insertion and Removal

Table 28–8 provides instructions for inserting and removing soft lenses.

GP Lens Care

The care of GP contact lenses follow the same general guidelines as for soft lenses, but the solutions for GP and soft lenses are not interchangeable. Lens wearers should be advised by their eye care providers about the products and regimens recommended for their particular lenses and advised against substituting other products for those specifically recommended.

Rigid lens care involves the steps of cleaning, disinfecting, soaking, and wetting (Figure 28–2), which should be performed each time the lenses are removed from the eye for optimal lens care. Modern solutions combine these steps in various combinations. Because GP lenses are replaced less frequently, providing more time for deposits to accumulate, separate solutions for daily cleaning and protein removal are still popular. Oxidation systems (hydrogen peroxide) can also be used, but heat disinfection should not be used with GP lenses. Rinsing with tap water is also not recommended because of microorganisms in the water.[35] Tables 28–3, 28–5, 28–6, and 28–9 provide proper cleaning and disinfecting procedures for rigid contact lenses.

Product Selection Guidelines

With the abundance of combination wetting/disinfection solutions now on the market, the appropriate lens care regimen for GP lenses is fairly straightforward. Patients wearing GP lenses should be advised to purchase a surface-active cleaning product, an enzymatic product, and a conditioning or soaking solution,

table 28–7 Selected Products for Soft Lenses

Trade Name	Primary Ingredients
Surface-Active Cleaning Solutions	
Sensitive Eyes Daily Cleaner	Hydroxypropyl methylcellulose; sorbic acid 0.25%; EDTA 0.5%; NaCl; borate buffer; poloxamine
Opti-Clean II Daily Cleaner	Nylon 11; polysorbate 21; hydroxyethyl cellulose; polyquaternium-1; EDTA; boric acid; sodium borate; NaCl
OPTI-FREE Daily Cleaner	Nylon 11; polysorbate 21; hydroxyethyl cellulose; polyquaternium-1 0.001%; EDTA; boric acid; sodium borate; hydrochloric acid and/or sodium hydroxide
Pliagel	Sorbic acid 0.25%; EDTA 0.5%; poloxamer 407; KCl; NaCl
Enzymatic Cleaning Products	
OPTI-FREE SupraClens Daily Protein Remover[a]	Highly purified porcine pancreatin enzymes; PEG; sodium borate
ReNu 1-Step Daily Protein Remover	Subtilisin; glycerin; borate buffers
Ultrazyme Enzymatic Cleaner	Subtilisin A; effervescing agents; buffers
Unizyme Enzymatic Cleaner	Subtilisin A
Hydrogen Peroxide Disinfecting Solutions and Rinsing/Neutralizing Products	
AOSEPT	Disinfecting solution: hydrogen peroxide 3%; NaCl 0.85%; phosphate buffers; phosphoric acid
Clear Care	Hydrogen peroxide 3%; Pluronic
Oxysept UltraCare	Disinfecting solution: hydrogen peroxide 3%; sodium stannate; sodium nitrate; phosphates
Preserved Saline Solutions	
Sensitive Eyes Plus Saline	Sorbic acid 0.1%; NaCl; borate buffer; EDTA
Preservative-Free Saline Products	
Unisol 4	NaCl; sodium borate; boric acid
Rewetting/Lubricating Solutions	
Clerz Plus	Clens 100; Tetronic 1304
Clerz 2	Hydroxyethyl cellulose; sorbic acid 0.1%; EDTA 0.1%; NaCl; KCl; sodium borate
OPTI-FREE Rewetting Drops	Polyquaternium-1 0.001%; citric acid; sodium citrate; NaCl
ReNu Rewetting Drops	Sorbic acid 0.15%; EDTA; borate buffer; poloxamine; NaCl
Multipurpose Solutions	
AQuify	Sorbitol; dexpanthenol; Pluronic F127; tromethamine; polyhexanide; EDTA
Biotrue	Polyaminopropyl biguanide 0.00013%; polyquaternium 0.0001%; hyaluronan; sulfobetaine; poloxamine; boric acid; sodium borate; edetate disodium; NaCl
OPTI-FREE Express or RepleniSH	Polyquaternium-1 0.001%; EDTA; sodium citrate; NaCl; citric acid; myristamidopropyl demethylamine; citrate buffer; C9-ED3A; Tetronic 1304
Renu Fresh	Polyaminopropyl biguanide; EDTA; NaCl; sodium borate; boric acid; poloxamine
Renu Sensitive	Polyaminopropyl biguanide; EDTA; NaCl; sodium borate; boric acid; poloxamine
Complete	Polyhexamethylene biguanide 0.0001%; phosphate buffer; Poloxamer 237; edetate disodium; NaCl; KCl
RevitaLens OcuTech	Alexidine dihydrochloride 0.00016%; polyquaternium-1 0.00030%; boric acid; sodium borate decahydrate; TETRONICa 904; edetate disodium; trisodium citrate dehydrate; NaCl
Naturalens RDS (not for use with silicone hydrogel materials)	Polyhexanide 0.0001%; edetate disodium dehydrate 0.025%; NaCl; bis-tris propane; Pluronic F127; cremophor RH40

Key: EDTA = Ethylenediamine tetraacetic acid; KCl = potassium chloride; NaCl = sodium chloride; PEG = polyethylene glycol.

[a] Preservative-free formulation.

Insertion

- Wash your hands with noncosmetic soap and rinse thoroughly; dry hands with a lint-free towel.
- Remove the lens for the right eye from its storage container.
- Rinse the lens with saline solution to dilute any preservatives left from disinfection (optional).
- Place the lens on the top of a finger, and examine it to be sure it is not inside out. This determination can be made by using the "taco test." Gently fold the lens at the apex (not the edges) between the thumb and forefinger. The edges should look like a taco shell with the edges pointed inward. If the edges roll out, the lens is inverted and must be reversed.
- Examine the lens for cleanliness. If necessary, clean it and rinse again.
- Insert the lens on the right eye using the procedure described for GP lenses (Table 28–11).
- Repeat the process for the left eye.

Removal

- Before removing the lenses, wash hands with a noncosmetic soap; rinse hands thoroughly and dry them with a lint-free towel.
- Using the right middle finger, pull down the lower lid of the right eye. Touch the right index finger to the lens and slide the lens off the cornea, as shown in drawing A.
- Using the index finger and thumb, grasp the lens and remove it (drawing B).
- Repeat the procedure for the left eye.

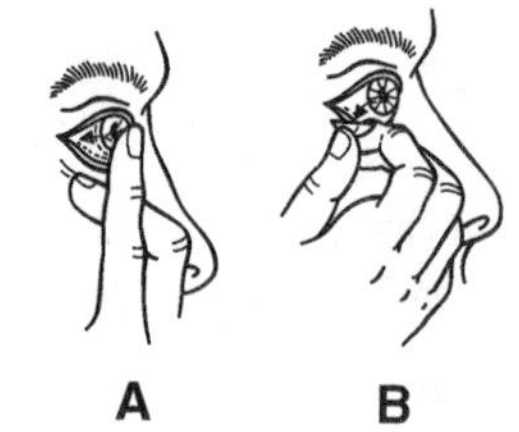

A   B

---

depending on the type of lens worn. A rewetting or reconditioning product should also be recommended. Table 28–10 lists examples of products for GP lenses.

Cleaning Solutions

Normal tears are composed of secretions from many specialized glands lining the lacrimal apparatus, conjunctiva, and lids. Many components are somewhat hydrophobic and tend to adhere to the surface of a rigid lens during normal daily wear.

This residue, primarily proteinaceous debris and lipids, acts as a growth medium for bacteria. If it is not routinely removed by daily cleaning, the residue may harden to form coatings or tenacious deposits that create an irregular surface on the lens. Decreased visual acuity and shorter toleration time are likely consequences of a cloudy lens created by this residue.

Contact lens cleaning solutions typically contain nonionic or amphoteric surfactants that emulsify lipids and aid in solubilizing other debris. Proteins and lipids are soluble in highly alkaline media, but high pH can cause lens decomposition. Weak alkaline solutions may dislodge deposits from the lens in conjunction with the surface tension–lowering properties of the surfactants. Cleaners formulated for tenacious deposits contain silica gel, which acts to mechanically break the adhesive bonds that have formed between the lens and the deposits. Homemade cleaning solutions such as baking soda mixed with

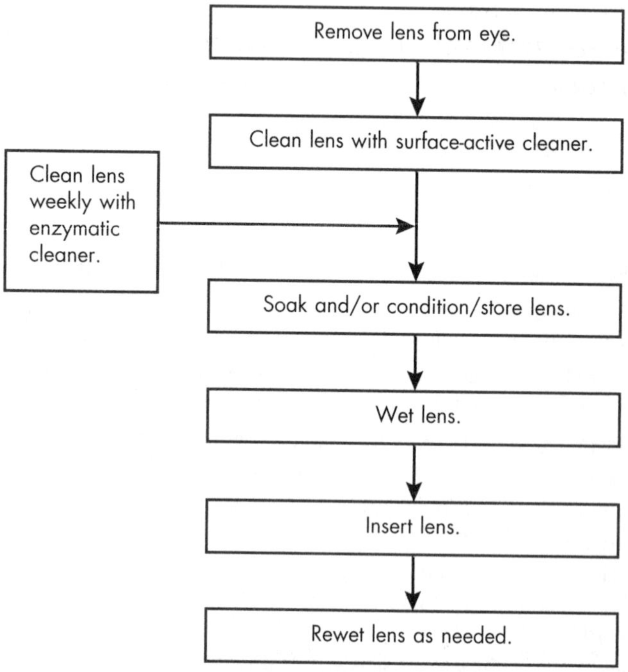

Figure flow diagram:

Remove lens from eye.
↓
Clean lens with surface-active cleaner.   ← Clean lens weekly with enzymatic cleaner.
↓
Soak and/or condition/store lens.
↓
Wet lens.
↓
Insert lens.
↓
Rewet lens as needed.

figure
28–2 Self-care of GP lenses.

- Use the cleansing, soaking, and conditioning products recommended by your eye care provider to clean your lenses.
- If you are unsure of your lens type, ask the eye care provider about proper cleaning procedures.
- Upon removal, apply an appropriate cleaning solution to both surfaces of the lens. Then rub the lens between the forefinger and palm of the opposite hand in a back-and-forth motion to avoid chipping an edge, which may occur if the lens is cleaned between the fingers. Do not apply too much pressure. If debris is still on the lens, soak a cotton swab in the surfactant cleaner, and use the swab to clean the lens.
- Soak and store the lenses in a soaking or conditioning solution recommended by the eye care provider for the specified amount of time. Rewet lenses before inserting them in the eyes.
- Enzymatic cleaning may also be recommended by your eye care provider and is typically performed weekly.

Source: Reference 35.

table

28–10 Selected Products for Gas Permeable Lenses

Trade Name	Primary Ingredients
Cleaning Solutions	
Boston Advance Cleaner[a]	Silica gel; alkyl ether sulfate; ethoxylated alkyl phenol; triquaternary cocoa-based phospholipids
Original Formula Boston Cleaner	Silica gel; alkyl ether sulfate; titanium dioxide; NaCl
Optimum CDS (for cleaning, disinfection, and storage; not for use in the eye)	Lauryl sulfate salt of imidazoline; octylphenoxypolyethoxyethanol; benzyl alcohol 0.3%; disodium edetate 0.5%
Enzymatic Cleaning Products	
Boston One Step Liquid Enzymatic Cleaner	Subtilisin; glycerol
Wetting/Soaking/Disinfecting Solutions	
Boston Advance Comfort Formula Conditioning Solution	Cellulosic viscosifier; polyvinyl alcohol; cationic cellulose derivative polymer; derivatized PEG; chlorhexidine gluconate 0.003%; polyaminopropyl biguanide 0.0005%; EDTA 0.05%
Boston Conditioning Solution	Hydroxyethyl cellulose; polyvinyl alcohol; cationic cellulose derivatives; poloxamer 407; chlorhexidine gluconate 0.006%; EDTA 0.05%
Optimum Wetting/Rewetting	Polyvinyl alcohol; polyvinylpyrrolidone; hydroxyethyl cellulose; NaCl; KCl; sodium carbonate; sodium bisulfite 0.02%; benzyl alcohol 0.1%; disodium edetate 0.1%; sorbic acid 0.05%
Rewetting/Lubricating Solutions	
Boston Rewetting Drops	Hydroxyethyl cellulose; polyvinyl alcohol; cationic cellulose derivatives; poloxamer 407; chlorhexidine gluconate 0.006%; EDTA 0.05%
Multipurpose Solutions	
Boston Simplus	Poloxamine; hydroxyalkylphosphonate; boric acid; sodium borate; NaCl; hydroxypropylmethyl cellulose; Glucam; chlorhexidine gluconate 0.003%; polyaminopropyl biguanide 0.0005%
Naturalens RDS	Polyhexanide 0.0001%; edetate disodium dehydrate 0.025%; NaCl; bis-tris propane; Pluronic F127; cremophor RH40
OPTI-FREE GP	Polyquad (polyquaternium-1) 0.0011%; hydroxypropyl guar; PEG; Tetronic 1304; boric acid; propylene glycol; edetate disodium 0.01%

Key: EDTA = Ethylenediamine tetraacetic acid; KCl = potassium chloride; NaCl = sodium chloride; PEG = polyethylene glycol.

[a] Preservative-free formulation.

distilled water or household cleaning solution should never be used because they may scratch lenses and may not rinse off easily. Use of household cleansers and homemade solutions (including salt tablet solutions) of any kind should be strongly discouraged to prevent lens damage, contamination leading to infection, and ocular irritation.

Soaking Solutions

These solutions are used to store rigid contact lenses after removal and during insertion of the lens in the eye. The solution maintains lenses in a constant state of hydration for maximum comfort and visual acuity, and it aids in removing deposits that accumulate on the lenses during wear. If lenses are allowed to dry out during overnight storage, accumulated deposits are more difficult to remove with normal cleaning.

An ideal soaking solution performs the following functions: (1) converts the hydrophobic lens surface to a hydrophilic surface by means of a uniform film that does not easily wash away; (2) increases comfort by providing cushioning and lubrication between the contacting surfaces; (3) places a viscous coating on the lens to protect it from oil on the fingers during insertion; and (4) stabilizes the lens on the fingertip to ease insertion, particularly for individuals with poor manual dexterity or unsteady hands. Cellulose gum derivatives are often used, but they do not promote uniform wetting of a rigid lens; therefore, polyvinyl alcohol is also often used to decrease surface tension.

Because GP lenses that contain high levels of silicone have decreased surface wettability, conditioning solutions are generally used instead of soaking solutions to aid the formation of a cushioning tear layer. A conditioning solution is essentially a specially formulated wetting solution that enhances wettability of the lens, increases comfort, and disinfects the lens. Saliva should never be used to wet contact lenses because it can lead to infection by many pathogens.

Rewetting Solutions

Rewetting solutions are intended to clean and rewet the contact lens while it is in the eye. These solutions depend on the use of surfactants to loosen deposits; removal is assisted by the natural cleaning action of blinking. Although these products function well to recondition the lens, the cornea benefits more if the lens is actually removed, cleaned, and rewetted. Removing the lens for even a brief time allows the cornea to be resurfaced with a new proteinaceous or mucinaceous layer.

To maintain sterility in rewetting products, preservative levels are carefully selected. Higher levels do not necessarily result in increased effectiveness and may lead to impaired wetting or corneal irritation because of the adsorption of preservatives onto the lens. Most rewetting agents are preserved, multidose products. Patients who use these products frequently should be encouraged to use preservatives such as oxychloro complex or perborates. Patients should be informed that preserved artificial tears and rewetting agents are different; most preserved artificial tears are incompatible with contact lenses.[36]

Enzymatic Solutions

As the silicone content of GP lenses increases, so does the amount of protein adherence. Silicone acrylate lenses have an active surface that promotes the binding of tear constituents. Protein deposits on a lens will decrease the oxygen permeability, and the patient may experience discomfort. If daily cleaning is not sufficient, lenses of this type should be cleaned with an enzymatic product once weekly.[35] Failure to comply with this cleaning step may result in the need for professional polishing or replacement of the lens.

Insertion and Removal

Wearers of GP lenses should be counseled to follow proper insertion and removal procedures (Tables 28–11 and 28–12).

Lens Storage Case

Patient education on the care of all contact lenses must include discussion of the proper care and cleaning of the contact lens storage case as well as the lens material. A dirty lens case can be contaminated with a biofilm that will attract pathogens and increase the risk of infection. The lens case should be cleaned daily. After lens insertion, the case (and lids, if separate) must be emptied, rinsed with the same disinfecting solution, wiped, and air-dried between uses.[37] Tap water should not be used. All solutions should be discarded daily. The case should not be used if cracked and should be replaced periodically, at least every 3 months.[35,37]

Follow-Up Care

Follow-up care is essential for the long-term success of contact lens wear. The minimum recommendation is 1 year between visits in the case of uncomplicated lens wear. These visits allow the prescriber to evaluate the integrity of the lenses worn and the condition of the cornea. Patient education, including the wearing schedule, replacement schedule, and care regimen, should also be reviewed. Regular contact lens follow-up care is an important aspect in the prevention of contact lens complications.

Contact Lens–Related Problems

Both soft and GP contact lenses provide good vision and safe, comfortable wear over years of use, provided they are fitted properly and patients adhere to correct care regimens. Unfortunately, complications of contact lens wear have not been eradicated with advances in material, lens design, and solutions. In general, soft contact lens patients tend to have more complications because there is less tear exchange beneath the lens and because the lenses are worn for longer hours, including overnight. Problems with GP lenses tend to be related to improper fit. Although occasional symptoms of mild redness and discomfort are common with contact lens wear, eye care providers should distinguish more severe symptoms that may cause significant complications, including threats to sight. Whenever a patient presents with signs or symptoms that are believed to be related to contact lens wear, discontinuing lens wear is recommended until the underlying cause is diagnosed and treated. Therefore, every patient should have glasses to wear as a backup to contact lenses.

---

table 28–11   Insertion of Gas Permeable Lenses

- After washing your hands, remove one lens from the lens storage case, rinse it with fresh conditioning/soaking solution, and inspect it for cleanliness and signs of damage (cracks or chips).
- If a wetting or conditioning solution is being used, place a few drops on the lens.
- Place the lens on the top of the index finger, as shown in drawing A.
- Place the middle finger of the same hand on the lower lid and pull it down (drawing B).
- With the other hand, use a finger to lift the upper lid, and then place the lens on the eye (drawing C).
- Release the lids and blink.
- Check vision immediately to see if the lens is in the proper position.
- If vision is blurred, blink three to four times. If vision is still blurred, the lens may be off center, on the wrong eye, or dirty.
  - Instill 1–3 drops of rewetting or reconditioning drops into the eye.
  - If vision is not improved, remove the lens, place several drops of wetting/conditioning solution onto both surfaces, and reinsert lens.
- Repeat all steps with the other lens.

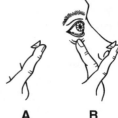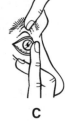

A   B   C

table
28–12   Removal of Gas Permeable Lenses

- Before removing the lens, fill the storage cases with soaking/conditioning solution.
- Remove the top from the cleaning solution.
- Place a hand (or a towel) under the eye.
- Use one of the following methods to remove the lens from the eye.

Two-Finger Method of Removing Lenses

- Place the tip of the forefinger of one hand on the middle of the upper eyelid by the lashes, as shown in drawing A.
- Place the forefinger of the other hand on the center of the lower lid margin (drawing A).
- Push the lids inward and then together, as shown in drawing B. The lens should pop out.
- If the lens becomes decentered onto only the white part of the eye, recenter the lens and try again.

Temporal Pull/Blink Method of Removing Lenses

- Place an index finger on the temporal edge of the lower and upper lids. Initially, widen the eyelids a little (drawing C).
- Stretch the skin outward and slightly upward without allowing the lid to slide over the lens. Blink briskly, as shown in drawing D. The lens will pop out because of the pressure of the eyelids at the top and bottom of the lens. Blinking facilitates removal after the lids have been tightened around the lens.

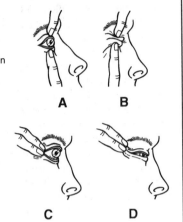

Evaluation of a contact lens–related problem should begin with a thorough history of the problem. During the patient interview, the eye care provider should determine what types of eye problems exist and how long the patient has been experiencing them. Asking the patient whether a history of eye problems exists and what medications are currently being taken will give a general sense of the etiology and urgency of the current eye problem. The answers will also help to determine whether the problem is related to noncompliance with care regimens or to drug–lens interactions. Determining which type of contact lenses a patient is wearing and how long the patient has worn them is crucial in assessing problems that are related to improper lens care or deteriorated lenses. Patients should be asked to describe how they care for their lenses, which lens care products they use, and whether they have recently changed products.

Unfortunately, mild and severe complications of lens wear present with similar symptoms that overlap and vary in degree. For example, mild redness and irritation in both eyes occurring at the end of the day for several weeks or months likely suggest dryness that might resolve with a change in lens material, wearing schedule, or lubricating drops. However, a patient who presents with acute symptoms of marked, sectoral redness in one eye, accompanied by photophobia and pain that started 1 day earlier, suggests a more severe concern, such as a corneal ulcer. The following symptoms are common for lens-related problems:

- *Itching:* Patients are usually not allergic to lens materials, but they may have an allergy to solutions. Itching may also be a sign of allergic conjunctivitis unrelated to lens wear.
- *Blurred vision:* Mild blurring may suggest wrong lens power, lenses switched between eyes, lenses placed on the eye inside out, or debris buildup on the lens. Blurring also accompanies problems with the ocular surface, such as superficial keratitis, corneal abrasion, and corneal edema associated with infiltration or ulceration.
- *Redness:* Redness can occur as a response to numerous insults. The degree of redness typically, but not always, corresponds to the severity of the problem. Mild, diffuse redness can accompany end-of-day dryness, whereas severe redness, especially

sectoral, can indicate a corneal problem. Ocular decongestants reduce mild conjunctival hyperemia associated with prolonged lens wear. However, upon cessation of their use, these topical decongestants can induce a rebound hyperemia, especially if they are used for more than 72 hours. Therefore, routine use of these products should be avoided, and if symptoms persist, the patient should be referred to an eye care provider.

- *Pain:* Pain is a significant finding because it is likely related to the eye's corneal nerve endings. Mild discomfort or irritation is not uncommon among all contact lens wearers. It may be related to the material, lens fit, or a torn or dirty lens. Severe pain or deep aching of the eye can signify corneal abrasions, infiltrates, or ulcers and typically persists even after removal of the lens. These symptoms represent urgent, sight-threatening conditions, and referral to an eye care provider is advised.
- *Fogging:* Misty or smoky vision can be caused by coatings or deposits on lens surfaces or by poor wetting of the lens while on the eye.
- *Photophobia (light sensitivity):* Similar to pain, photophobia suggests complications with the cornea or a symptom of iritis, which should be referred to an eye care provider.
- *Excessive tearing:* Corneal nerves start a feedback loop that promotes tearing; therefore, irritation to the corneal surface, such as a torn or dirty lens, will increase tearing.
- *Flare:* Point sources of light that have a sunburst or streaming quality can be caused by inadequate optic zone size or decentration of a poorly fitting lens.
- *Lens falling out of the eye:* Improper fit is usually the cause; however, even properly fitted rigid lenses may occasionally slide off the cornea or be blinked out of the eye. Soft lenses that dry out on the eye may move excessively and dislocate.
- *Squinting:* This effect is caused by excessive movement of a lens or by a poorly fitted lens. The wearer will squint to center the optical portion of the lens over the pupil. Squinting may also indicate improper lens power.

Symptoms of redness, discomfort, and dryness are the most common complaints and the leading causes of discontinuing lens wear. Even brand new contact lenses disrupt the tear film and alter the environment of the anterior ocular surface. Changes in lens material or solutions, alteration of lens fit, or use of lubricating drops usually improves symptoms.

In contrast, microbial keratitis (corneal ulceration) is the worst complication of contact lens wear. The health care provider should be alert for symptoms of blurred vision, redness, pain, light sensitivity, and watering that often worsen even after discontinuation of lens wear. A white infiltrate visible on the cornea requires urgent referral for evaluation by an eye care provider. Removal of contact lenses and prompt treatment are crucial to improve outcomes.

Overall, distinguishing common lens wear–associated complaints from signs of more severe inflammatory or infectious complications can be difficult. Considerations include whether one or both eyes are involved, the duration of symptoms, the severity of symptoms, and whether symptoms are isolated or found in conjunction with each other. Even experienced health care providers have problems distinguishing inflammatory from infectious complications. Timely referral to an eye care provider is indicated if there is any doubt that symptoms suggest more than lens wear–associated symptoms.

Precautions for Contact Lenses
Adverse Effects of Drugs

Many undesired effects have been reported when a patient who wears contact lenses ingests, applies, or encounters certain drugs (Table 28–13). Wearers of soft hydrophilic contact lenses should be particularly cautious in exposing their lenses to chemicals. These chemicals, many of which penetrate and bind with the lens material, can come from cosmetics, environmental pollutants, and ophthalmic and systemic products. The health care provider must understand these drug-induced problems to counsel patients effectively.

Topical Drugs

In general, patients should be counseled not to place any ophthalmic solution, suspension, gel, or ointment into the eye when contact lenses are in place. A nonprescription ophthalmic product that is not specifically designed for use with contact lenses also should not be used when lenses are in the eye. Soft lenses can absorb chemical compounds from topically administered ophthalmic products.[38] Topical administration of ophthalmic drugs also may have physiologic consequences or may modify pharmacologic responses to drugs. The use of solutions that may be considered benign, such as artificial tears, may reduce tear breakup time and alter the distribution of the mucoid, aqueous, and lipid components of tears, perhaps causing initial discomfort on instillation of the drops.[38] A topical drug administered while soft lenses are in place may have an exaggerated pharmacologic effect. The soft lens may absorb the drug and either release it over time, creating a sustained-release dosage form, or bind it tightly so that none of it is released into the eye. Furthermore, the presence of any kind of contact lens may increase the amount of time the medication is in contact with the eye. Finally, increased drug absorption may occur secondary to a compromised corneal epithelium during contact lens wear.[38] The only exceptions to this rule are products specifically formulated to be used with contact lenses, such as rewetting drops, or those products that an eye care provider has specifically recommended for use with contact lenses.

If a drug solution is instilled into the eye prior to lens insertion, the wearer must not insert a lens until the solution has cleared from the lower eyelid's precorneal (conjunctival) pocket (about 5 minutes). Ideally, when topical ophthalmic ointments, gels, or suspensions are being used, the lenses should not be worn at all.

Airborne Drugs and Particulate Matter

Some drugs that are present in indoor air may damage lenses, so health care providers should be cautious with medications that are administered via inhalation. Similarly, contact lens wearers who have been exposed to a large amount of cigarette smoke have discovered a brown discoloration and nicotine deposits on their lenses.

Systemic Medications

Use of a systemic medication often has far-reaching and unanticipated effects aside from the expected pharmacodynamic actions. Perhaps the most visible manifestation of ocular-related systemic drug toxicity is found among contact lens users who develop ocular discomfort or irritation and contact lens intolerance while using a particular systemic drug. Contact lens patients will often present with complaints of new onset of eye dryness or irritation and intolerance to contact lens wear and request a nonprescription product to provide symptomatic relief. Although such symptoms are similar to other, more common causes, such as contact lens hygiene, health care professionals should consider the pharmacology of specific systemic medications as well as potential relationships between medication initiation and onset of symptoms.[38]

The effects of medications on the eye vary by drug class.[38] As a general rule, compounds with anticholinergic effects can reduce tear volume and induce dry eye, with or without concomitant loss of accommodation and blurry vision.[39] Other classes of drugs, such as hormones (most notably birth control pills), may also alter tear volume and the shape of the corneal surface, resulting in blurring and contact lens intolerance. Some systemic medications are secreted into tears and may interact with (primarily soft) contact lenses. For example, rifampin will stain both lenses and tears orange. Drugs and dietary supplements such as gold salts and garlic are secreted into the tears and may cause ocular irritation. Other drugs may affect tear production, the refractive properties of the eye, the shape of the cornea, or the actual lens (Table 28–13).[40] Some medications may influence the size of the pupil, causing complaints of glare or flare when lenses are in place. Visual performance may be diminished, especially in patients who wear multifocal lenses or GP lenses for which pupil size may determine placement of the reading segment or the optic zone of the lens, respectively.[41]

Use of Cosmetics

Patients who wear contact lenses should choose—and use—cosmetics with care. Individuals should insert lenses before applying makeup and should avoid touching the lens with eyeliner or mascara. Cosmetics, moisturizers, and makeup removers with an aqueous base should be used, because oil-based products may cause blurred vision and irritation if they are deposited on the lens. Water-based products are preferable, and when possible, users should choose makeup that has been specifically

table

28-13   Drug–Contact Lens Interactions

Changes in Tear Film and/or Production

Decreased Tear Volume

Alcohol

Anticholinergic agents

Antihistamines

Beta-blockers

Benzodiazepines

Botulinum toxin type A (Botox)

Conjugated estrogens

Diuretics

Oral contraceptives

Phenothiazines

Serotonin reuptake inhibitors

Sildenafil citrate

Statins

Timolol (topical)

Tricyclic antidepressants

Vardenafil HCl

Increased Tear Volume

Cholinergic agents

Garlic (dietary supplement)

Reserpine

Changes in Lens Color (Primarily Soft Lenses)

Diagnostic dyes (i.e., fluorescein)

Epinephrine (topical)

Fluorescein (topical)

Nicotine

Nitrofurantoin

Phenazopyridine

Phenolphthalein

Phenothiazines

Phenylephrine

Rifampin

Sulfasalazine

Tetracycline

Tetrahydrozoline (topical)

Changes in Tonicity

Pilocarpine (8%)

Sodium sulfacetamide (10%)

Lid/Corneal Edema

Chlorthalidone

Clomiphene

Conjugated estrogens

Oral contraceptives

Primidone

Ocular Inflammation/Irritation

Diclofenac (topical ophthalmic)

Garlic (dietary supplement)

Gold salts

Isotretinoin

Salicylates

Changes in Refractivity (Induction of Myopia)

Acetazolamide

Sulfadiazine

Sulfamethizole

Sulfamethoxazole

Sulfisoxazole

Changes in Pupil Size

Pupillary Dilation

Anticholinergic agents

Antidepressants

Antihistamines

CNS stimulants

Kava

Phenothiazines

Pupillary Miosis

Opiates

Miscellaneous Agents (Effects)

Digoxin (increased glare)

Hypnotics/sedatives/muscle relaxants (decreased blink rate)

Ribavirin (cloudy lenses)

Topical ciprofloxacin/prednisolone acetate (precipitate)

Key: CNS = Central nervous system.

Source: Adapted with permission from Engle JP. Contact lens care. *Am Druggist.* 1990;201:5465. Updated with information from reference 38.

formulated for contact lens wearers. Lens wearers should avoid loose powders (e.g., face, eye) and instead use pressed or cream-based products, if available. Water-resistant mascara (as opposed to waterproof mascara, which requires an oil-based remover) should be applied only to the very tips of the lashes. Eyeliners should never be applied inside the eyelid margin; the liner can clog glands in the eyelid and contaminate the contact lens. Eye makeup should be replaced at least every 3 months.[42]

Aerosol products, in particular, must be used with caution; users should close their eyes when applying the product and step out of the mist before opening their eyes. Nail polish, hand creams, and perfumes should also be applied only after the lenses have been inserted. Men often contaminate their lenses with hair preparations and spray deodorants. Lens wearers should be reminded to take special care to clean their hands thoroughly before handling their lenses. Soaps that contain cold cream or deodorants should be avoided.[42]

Corneal Hypoxia and Edema

An adequate supply of oxygen exists only if the cornea is continuously bathed with oxygenated tears. During blinking, metabolic byproducts from the surface epithelium are flushed from under the contact lenses, and oxygen is brought in as the lenses move toward and away from the cornea. Even when properly fitted, however, both rigid and soft lenses can produce a progressive hypoxia of the cornea while the lenses are in place, especially in individuals who have low blink frequency or incomplete blinks.

Corneal Abrasions

Corneal abrasions are surface defects in the epithelial layer of the cornea. The causes of these abrasions range from poorly fitted lenses or simple overwear to the entrapment of foreign bodies under the lens. The cornea is sensitive to abrasion, so blepharospasm (reflexive lid closure), tearing, and rubbing of

the affected eye occur immediately. However, rubbing the eye can cause more extensive damage while the lens remains in the eye and must be avoided.

Fortunately, the pain associated with corneal abrasion is usually greater than the damage. The epithelium regenerates quickly; most minor epithelial defects generally heal within 12–24 hours. The lens should be left out for 2–7 days. The wearer may then proceed to use a modified break-in schedule suggested by the eye care provider. Corneal abrasions require the attention of an eye care provider.

Exclusions for Self-Care

When lens care is appropriate but the lenses are old or, in the case of hard lenses, chipped or scratched, the patient should see an eye care provider for replacement lenses. Other situations that require referral are suspected vision changes, deep aching of the eyes, last eye examination occurring more than 1 year ago, and a suspected interaction between the lenses and systemic medications. Patients experiencing lens problems that are related to the medical conditions or other factors discussed in Contraindications and Warnings for Contact Lenses should also be referred for further evaluation.

Cases 28–1 and 28–2 illustrate the assessment of patients with contact lens–related problems.

---

case
28–1

Relevant Evaluation Criteria	Scenario/Model Outcome
Information Gathering	
1. Gather essential information about the patient's symptoms and medical history, including:	
a. description of symptom(s) (i.e., nature, onset, duration, severity, associated symptoms)	Patient complains of a "fogginess" in both eyes that is not present when she wears her glasses. She reports that this has been going on for the past 2 days, but it typically occurs toward the end of each month. She wears monthly disposable soft contact lenses and has been wearing the current contact lenses for 3 weeks. She reports changing them on the first of each month and does not sleep in them. The patient's lens care regimen includes soaking the lenses daily by topping off the solution in the case using Biotrue multi-purpose solution, or whatever is on sale when she needs more. She also reports she sometimes forgets to rinse the contact lenses daily.
b. description of any factors that seem to precipitate, exacerbate, and/or relieve the patient's symptom(s)	Patient reports she experiences less itching and redness when she first starts a new pair of contact lenses.
c. description of the patient's efforts to relieve the symptoms	Patient has not tried anything.
d. patient's identity	Emma Smith
e. age, sex, height, and weight	30 years old, female, 5 ft 6 in., 170 lb
f. patient's occupation	Administrative assistant
g. patient's dietary habits	NA
h. patient's sleep habits	Gets about 8 hours of sleep per night.
i. concurrent medical conditions, prescription and nonprescription medications, and dietary supplements	Hypertension; treated with lisinopril
j. allergies	NKA
k. history of other adverse reactions to medications	None
l. other (describe) _____	Nonsmoker, social alcohol use on the weekends

Relevant Evaluation Criteria	Scenario/Model Outcome

Assessment and Triage

2. Differentiate patient's signs/symptoms and correctly identify the patient's primary problem(s).

Discomfort due to poor contact lens hygiene and care

3. Identify exclusions for self-treatment.

None

4. Formulate a comprehensive list of therapeutic alternatives for the primary problem to determine if triage to a health care provider is required, and share this information with the patient or caregiver.

Options include:

(1) Refer the patient to an eye care provider.

(2) Recommend self-treatment.

(3) Take no action.

Plan

5. Select an optimal therapeutic alternative to address the patient's problem, taking into account patient preferences.

Recommend using proper contact lens care and hygiene.

6. Describe the recommended therapeutic approach to the patient or caregiver.

"Your symptoms suggest you are not using an appropriate care regimen for your contacts. Topping off the solution can increase the risk of infection and not rinsing or rubbing your lenses daily can build up proteins on your lens, leading to fogginess. Also, generic solutions may not contain the same ingredients as the brand your eye care provider recommended."

7. Explain to the patient or caregiver the rationale for selecting the recommended therapeutic approach from the considered therapeutic alternatives.

"Fogginess is a common contact lens complaint. Your symptoms are present only when you wear the contact lenses and toward the end of the month when appropriate contact lens care has not been used. This does not cause a concern that requires you to see an eye care provider at this time."

Patient Education

8. When recommending self-care with nonprescription medications and/or nondrug therapy, convey accurate information to the patient or caregiver.

   a. appropriate dose and frequency of administration

"Discard and use new contact lens multipurpose solution daily. Rinse and rub contact lenses to remove proteins daily for at least 20 seconds. Use the recommended contact lens solutions from your eye care provider."

   b. maximum number of days the therapy should be employed

"Use appropriate lens care daily."

   c. product administration procedures

NA

   d. expected time to onset of relief

"Symptoms should resolve within the next day."

   e. degree of relief that can be reasonably expected

"Fogginess should disappear with proper cleaning."

   f. most common side effects

NA

   g. side effects that warrant medical intervention should they occur

"Fogginess that does not go away needs medical attention."

   h. patient options in the event that condition worsens or persists

"See your eye care provider if the fogginess persists even after proper cleaning of the lenses."

   i. product storage requirements

"Solution should be stored at room temperature in a dry place. Contact lens case should be allowed to dry while contact lenses are not in it."

   j. specific nondrug measures

NA

Solicit follow-up questions from the patient or caregiver.

"What if I don't want to have to do this every day?"

Answer the patient's or caregiver's questions.

"You can call your eye care provider and talk to him or her about that. The provider could potentially change you to daily disposable contact lenses."

Evaluation of Patient Outcome

9. Assess patient outcome.

"Please call me and let me know how everything is going and if these suggestions worked for you or if you have any more questions."

Key: NA = Not applicable; NKA = no known allergies.

case
28–2

Relevant Evaluation Criteria	Scenario/Model Outcome

Information Gathering

1. Gather essential information about the patient's symptoms and medical history, including:

   a. description of symptom(s) (i.e., nature, onset, duration, severity, associated symptoms)

   Patient complains of pain and aching in his left eye this morning. He reports he initially woke up with this yesterday morning and thought it would go away when he slept last night, but the pain has become a bit worse, even when he didn't wear his contact lenses all day. He follows all of his eye care provider recommendations for cleaning and use of his GP contact lenses. He reports his last eye exam was over a year and a half ago.

   b. description of any factors that seem to precipitate, exacerbate, and/or relieve the patient's symptom(s)

   Patient reports that not wearing contact lenses helps.

   c. description of the patient's efforts to relieve the symptoms

   The patient has not tried anything to help the situation other than not wearing contact lenses yesterday.

   d. patient's identity

   Ralph Estes

   e. age, sex, height, and weight

   50 years old, male, 6 ft 5 in., 240 lb

   f. patient's occupation

   Engineer

   g. patient's dietary habits

   Patient eats a balanced diet.

   h. patient's sleep habits

   Patient stays up late watching the news but gets about 6 hours of sleep per night.

   i. concurrent medical conditions, prescription and nonprescription medications, and dietary supplements

   Patient has acid reflux and takes Tums as needed.

   j. allergies

   Penicillin

   k. history of other adverse reactions to medications

   None

   l. other (describe) _____

   Patient is nonsmoker and drinks beer at sporting events.

Assessment and Triage

2. Differentiate patient's signs/symptoms and correctly identify the patient's primary problem(s).

   Corneal abrasion, contact lens induced

3. Identify exclusions for self-treatment.

   Possible corneal abrasion caused by overwear, possible poor fit, or a chip or scratch in the lens
   Pain that does not improve with removal of contact lenses

4. Formulate a comprehensive list of therapeutic alternatives for the primary problem to determine if triage to a health care provider is required, and share this information with the patient or caregiver.

   Options include:

   (1) Refer the patient to eye care provider.

   (2) Recommend self-treatment.

   (3) Take no action.

Plan

5. Select an optimal therapeutic alternative to address the patient's problem, taking into account patient preferences.

   Inform patient that he needs to get immediate care from his eye care provider or go to the emergency room to identify the extent of the problem. The patient should not use self-care treatment at this time.

6. Describe the recommended therapeutic approach to the patient or caregiver.

   "Your symptoms suggest that you have injured your eye and you need to go to either your eye care provider or the emergency room immediately."

7. Explain to the patient or caregiver the rationale for selecting the recommended therapeutic approach from the considered therapeutic alternatives.

   "Self-care treatment is not recommended right now, and there are no nonprescription products to treat these problems right now. You need to go to either your eye care provider or the emergency room immediately to prevent any permanent damage, such as vision loss."

case

28–2 *continued*

Relevant Evaluation Criteria	Scenario/Model Outcome
Patient Education	
8. When recommending self-care with nonprescription medications and/or nondrug therapy, convey accurate information to the patient or caregiver.	Criterion does not apply in this case.
Solicit follow-up questions from the patient or caregiver.	"It is a really busy week at work. Do you think I can wait until this evening to contact my eye care provider?"
Answer the patient's or caregiver's questions.	"No. You need to be seen by your eye care provider or an emergency room immediately. You could suffer permanent damage to your eye if it is not treated immediately."
Evaluation of Patient Outcome	
9. Assess patient outcome.	"Please call me and let me know how everything worked out. Also, in the future, feel free to contact me with any questions you may have."

Key: GP = Gas permeable.

Patient Counseling for Prevention of Contact Lens–Related Disorders

Instruction on lens insertion and removal should always be provided at the time lenses are fit. Patients should also be instructed on proper care techniques, with a specific recommendation for a care system. Often the prescriber's advice for a particular product is ignored, and patients select products according to price alone, especially with the availability of generic solutions.

Similar product labels and lack of standardized labeling lead to further confusion. Patients often ask whether it matters which solution they use. The correct answer is that it does matter because solutions can be the cause of contact lens complications. Lens care products are typically formulated for use either with soft or gas permeable lenses and, with a few exceptions, should not be used interchangeably. The box Patient Education for Prevention of Contact Lens–Related Disorders outlines the care regimen for each type of contact lens.

patient education for

Prevention of Contact Lens–Related Disorders

The objective of contact lens care is to prevent lens-related problems such as abrasions or infections of the cornea. For most patients, following the prescribed lens care regimen, product instructions, and self-care measures listed here will help ensure trouble-free use of contact lenses.

General Care Instructions for All Contact Lens Types

- See Table 28–3. Wash hands with noncosmetic soap and rinse them thoroughly before handling or caring for contact lenses.
- Each time contact lenses are removed, clean, rinse, and disinfect them before wearing them again.
- Gently rub both surfaces of the contact lens, rinse thoroughly, and soak lenses overnight in the recommended solution according to the eye care provider's instructions.
- When using contact lens products, use only the products recommended by the prescribing eye care provider.
- Do not change brands or products unless instructed to do so by the eye care provider. (Not all care systems are alike, and some may not be compatible with the contact lenses prescribed.)
- Do not top off a storage solution in the case after the solution has been used.
- Replace soaking/disinfecting solutions in the lens case after each use.
- Store contact lenses in fresh disinfecting solution overnight for the minimum soaking time recommended by the manufacturer to provide adequate disinfection.
- If lenses are worn intermittently, check and replace the solution weekly; consider daily disposable lens wear.

- Discard open bottles of solution if not used within the recommended time frame after being opened. Refer to the package labeling for individual products because the time frame varies from 1–3 months depending on the product. Write the date the solution is first used on the outside of the bottle.
- Store contact lenses in a proper lens case when not in use. Clean the contact lens case daily by rubbing with a disinfecting solution and allowing the case to air-dry.
- Replace the contact lens case every 3 months.
- Saline solution is used only to rinse lenses; saline will not clean or disinfect contact lenses and should not be used as a storage solution.
- Do not use tap water to rinse contact lenses or to clean cases. Never store lenses in tap water.
- Do not place contact lenses in your mouth to clean or lubricate the lens. This practice can result in eye infections.
- To prevent contamination, do not touch dropper tips or the tips of lens care product containers.
- While wearing lenses, use only ophthalmic solutions specifically formulated for contact lens use.
- Avoid swimming, showering, hot tubs, or natural bodies of water while wearing contact lenses unless external eye protection, such as watertight goggles, is used.

patient education for
Prevention of Contact Lens–Related Disorders *(continued)*

- Follow prescribed wearing and replacement schedules.
- Avoid exposing contact lenses to extreme temperatures.
- Avoid wearing oily cosmetics while wearing lenses. Bath oils or soaps with an oil or a cream base may leave a film on the hands, which will be transferred to the lenses. Apply cosmetics after inserting contact lenses.
- To avoid mixing up the lenses, always insert or remove the same lens first. Check hard lenses for a dot in the lens periphery to avoid mixing up the lenses.
- If the lenses are not comfortable after insertion or vision is blurred, check to see if they are on the wrong eyes or are inside out.
- To avoid damaging lenses, either apply aerosol cosmetics and deodorants before lens insertion or keep eyes closed until the air is clear of spray particles.
- Except for prescription continuous-wear lenses, do not wear lenses while sleeping.
- To avoid excessive dryness of the eyes, do not wear lenses while sitting under a hair dryer, overhead fans, or air ducts.
- When lenses are worn outside on windy days, protect the eyes from soot and other particles that may become trapped under the lens and scratch the cornea.
- Use eye protection in industry, sports, or any other occupation or hobby that has the potential for eye damage.
- Do not insert lenses in red or irritated eyes. If the eyes become irritated while lenses are being worn, remove the lenses until the irritation subsides. If irritation or redness does not subside, consult an eye care provider.
- If an eye infection is suspected, see an eye care provider immediately.

Instructions for Soft Lenses

- See Tables 28–3 and 28–4 for guidelines on cleaning and disinfecting soft lenses.

- Handle soft lenses carefully because they are very fragile and can be torn easily.
- Remove these lenses before instilling any ophthalmic preparation not specifically intended for concurrent use with soft contact lenses. Wait at least 20–30 minutes before reinserting the lenses, unless directed otherwise by an eye care provider.
- Do not wear lenses when a topical ophthalmic ointment is being used.
- Do not wear soft contact lenses in the presence of irritating fumes or chemicals.

Instructions for GP Lenses

- See Tables 28–3 and 28–9 for guidelines on cleaning GP lenses.
- Do not use tap water to rinse off cleaner or to rewet lenses. If tap water is used, disinfect lenses before inserting them in the eyes.
- See Table 28–5 for guidelines on using disinfecting systems.

Instructions for Continuous-Wear Lenses (GP or Soft)

- Remove mascara before sleeping because it can flake off during sleep and become trapped underneath the lens.
- If lenses appear to be lost on awakening, check eyes to see whether the lenses were displaced. Soft lenses can fold over on themselves and get lodged underneath the top or bottom eyelid.
- Each morning, check eyes carefully for unusual, persistent redness, discharge, or pain. If redness does not abate within 45 minutes, or if discharge or pain is present, remove the lens and call your eye care provider.
- Check vision after inserting lenses. (Some hazy vision is normal on awakening because of corneal hypoxia, which develops overnight.) Apply a few drops of rewetting solution to improve hydration of the lens and help resolve hypoxia. If the problem is not resolved, remove lenses, clean them, and reinsert. If vision is not improved within an hour, remove lenses and call your eye care prescriber.

Key Points for Prevention of Contact Lens–Related Disorders

➤ Following the prescribed lens care program is the best strategy for avoiding lens wear–related problems.

➤ The health care provider should explain the care regimen for the patient's particular lens type and stress that the patient should use only the products recommended for his or her lenses.

➤ Instructions on avoiding practices or situations that can cause eye irritation or lens damage are also important in educating the patient about successful wearing of contact lenses:

 ➢ Used contact lens solutions should not be "topped off" or reused.

 ➢ Even when using "no-rub" solutions, patients should be counseled to rub and rinse contact lenses to fully remove protein deposits.

➤ The patient should be advised of signs and symptoms that indicate that medical care is needed. Patients should be informed that if eye redness or pain or blurry vision occurs while wearing any form of contact lens, they should immediately remove the lens and see an eye care provider for evaluation prior to reinserting the lens.

REFERENCES

1. U.S. Food and Drug Administration. Device classification. Accessed at http://www.fda.gov/MedicalDevices/DeviceRegulationandGuidance/Overview/ClassifyYourDevice/default.htm#determine, April 30, 2013.
2. Nichols JJ. Annual report: Contact lenses 2012. *Contact Lens Spectr.* January 2013. Accessed at http://www.clspectrum.com/articleviewer.aspx?articleID=107853, April 30, 2013.
3. Morgan PB, Woods CA, Tranoudis IG, et al. International contact lens prescribing in 2012. *Contact Lens Spectr.* January 2013. Accessed at http://www.clspectrum.com/articleviewer.aspx?articleID=107854, April 30, 2013.
4. Forister JFY, Forister EF, Yeung KK, et al. Prevalence of contact lens–related complications: UCLA contact lens study. *Eye Contact Lens.* 2009;35(4):176–80.
5. Yeung KK, Forister JFY, Forister EF, et al. Compliance with soft contact lens replacement schedules and associated contact lens–related ocular complications: UCLA contact lens study. *Optometry.* 2010;81(11):598–607.
6. Richdale K, Sinnott LT, Skadahl E, et al. Frequency of and factors associated with contact lens dissatisfaction and discontinuation. *Cornea.* 2007;26(2):168–74.
7. Young G, Veys J, Pritchard N, et al. A multi-centre study of lapsed contact lens wearers. *Ophthalmic Physiol Opt.* 2002;22(6):516–27.
8. Hickson-Curran S, Chalmers RL, Riley C. Patient attitudes and behaviour regarding hygiene and replacement of soft contact lenses and storage cases. *Cont Lens Anterior Eye.* 2011;34(5):207–15.
9. Federal Trade Commission. FTC issues final rule implementing Fairness to Contact Lens Consumers Act. June 29, 2004. Accessed at http://www.ftc.gov/opa/2004/06/contactlens.htm, April 30, 2013.

10. Fogel J, Zidile C. Contact lenses purchased over the Internet place individuals potentially at risk for harmful eye care practices. *Optometry.* 2008;79(1):23–35.

11. Wu Y, Carnt N, Stapleton F. Contact lens user profile, attitudes, and level of compliance to lens care. *Cont Lens Anterior Eye.* 2010;33(4):183–8.

12. Pesudovs K, Garamendi E, Elliott DB. A quality of life comparison of people wearing spectacles or contact lenses or having undergone refractive surgery. *J Refract Surg.* 2006;22(1):19–27.

13. Jones L. Modern contact lens materials: a clinical performance update. *Contact Lens Spectr.* September 2002:24–35.

14. DeNaeyer GW. Soft lens material choices and selection. *Contact Lens Spectr.* May 2012:38–40.

15. DeNaeyer GW. Therapeutic applications of contact lenses. *Contact Lens Spectr.* May 2010. Accessed at http://www.clspectrum.com/articleviewer. aspx?articleID=104223, April 30, 2013.

16. Gromacki S. The case for bandage soft contact lenses: A primer on the use of these therapeutic lenses to serve and protect the corneas of our patients. *Rev Cornea Contact Lenses.* January 2012. Accessed at http:// www.reviewofcontactlenses.com/content/d/soft_lenses/c/32147, April 30, 2013.

17. Del Pizzo N. Gas permeable (GP) contact lenses. March 2011. Accessed at http://www.allaboutvision.com/contacts/rgps.htm, April 30, 2013.

18. Studebaker J. Soft multifocals: Practice growth opportunity. *Contact Lens Spectr.* June 2009. Accessed at http://www.clspectrum.com/article.aspx? article=103013, April 30, 2013.

19. Morgan PB, Efron N. Contact lens correction of presbyopia. *Cont Lens Anterior Eye.* 2009;32(4):191–2.

20. Mayers M. The dangers of mixing solutions. *Rev Cornea Contact Lenses.* January 2011. Accessed at http://www.reviewofcontactlenses.com/ content/c/26326/, April 30, 2013.

21. U.S. Food and Drug Administration. Ensuring safe use of contact lens solution. Accessed at http://www.fda.gov/forconsumers/consumerupdates/ ucm164197.htm, April 30, 2013.

22. Ward MA. Soft contact lens care products. *Contact Lens Spectr.* July 2003. Accessed at http://www.clspectrum.com/articleviewer.aspx?article id=12384, April 30, 2013.

23. Rolando M, Crider JY, Kahook MY. Ophthalmic preservatives: Focus on polyquarternium-1. *Expert Opin Drug Deliv.* 2011;8(11):1425–38.

24. Hwang TS, Hyon JY, Song JK, et al. Disinfection capacity of PuriLens contact lens cleaning unit against Acanthamoeba. *Eye Contact Lens.* 2004;30(1):42–3.

25. Choate W, Fontana F, Potter J, et al. Evaluation of the PuriLens contact lens care system: An automatic care system incorporating UV disinfection and hydrodynamic shear cleaning. *CLAO J.* 2000;26(3):134–40.

26. Smick KL. The evolution of dual disinfection: where we are today. *Rev Cornea Contact Lenses.* January 2011. Accessed at http://www.reviewof contactlenses.com/content/c/26327/, April 30, 2013.

27. Holden B, Fonn D. The last 25 years of soft lenses. *Contact Lens Spectr.* March 2011. Accessed at http://www.clspectrum.com/articleviewer. aspx?articleID=105287, April 30, 2013.

28. Gromacki SJ. Hydrogen peroxide contact lens disinfection, part 1. *Contact Lens Spectr.* May 2012:23.

29. Gromacki SJ. Hydrogen peroxide contact lens disinfection, part 2. *Contact Lens Spectr.* September 2012. Accessed at http://www.clspectrum.com/ articleviewer.aspx?articleID=107417, April 30, 2013.

30. Lonnen J. Testing care solutions: Need for evolution. *Contact Lens Spectr.* August 2012: 38–42.

31. Bowling EL. Laying the groundwork for successful lens wear. *Contact Lens Spectr.* June 2011. Accessed at http://www.clspectrum.com/ articleviewer.aspx?articleID=105671, April 30, 2013.

32. Zhu H, Bandara MB, Vijay AK, et al. Importance of rub and rinse in use of multipurpose contact lens solution. *Optom Vis Sci.* 2011;88(8):967–72.

33. White P. 2012 contact lenses & solutions summary. July 2012 (supplement). Accessed at http://www.clspectrum.com/content/archive/2012/ july/supplements/class/class-pdf/cls_class.pdf, April 30, 2013.

34. Schacet JL. Taking charge of patients' solution selections. *Rev Cornea Contact Lenses.* January 2012. Accessed at http://www.reviewofcontact lenses.com/content/c/32146/, April 30, 2013.

35. Bennett ES, Heiting G. Caring for gas permeable contact lenses. August 2010. Accessed at http://www.allaboutvision.com/contacts/carergplens. htm, April 30, 2013.

36. Ward MA. Approved GP wetting drops. *Contact Lens Spectr.* January 2011. Accessed at http://www.clspectrum.com/articleviewer.aspx?articleID= 105082, April 30, 2013.

37. Ward MA. GP contact lens care pearls. *Contact Lens Spectr.* October 2012. Accessed at http://www.clspectrum.com/articleviewer.aspx?articleID= 107511, April 30, 2013.

38. Silbert JA. Medications and contact lens wear. *Contact Lens Spectr.* May 2002. Accessed at http://www.clspectrum.com/articleviewer.aspx?article id=12149, April 30, 2013.

39. De Haas EBH. Lacrimal gland response to parasympaticomimetics after parasympathetic denervation. *Arch Ophtalmol.* 1960:64:34–43.

40. Miller D. Systemic medications. *Int Ophthalmol Clin.* 1981;21(2): 177–83.

41. Schornack JA. Drugs and pupillary interaction in contact lens practice. *Contact Lens Spectr.* May 2003;46.

42. Ward MA. Contact lenses and makeup contamination. *Contact Lens Spectr.* February 2013. Accessed at http://www.clspectrum.com/articleviewer. aspx?articleID=107943, April 30, 2013.

OTIC DISORDERS

Judith B. Sommers Hanson

Ear complaints are common and vary from simple complaints of excessive earwax (cerumen) to itching or painful ear infections. Ear disorders affect all ages, with children and geriatric patients being the most prone. Otic disorders account for 1.5% of ambulatory care visits per year.[1] Cerumen impaction can affect up to 10% of children and more than 30% of the elderly nursing home population; it is one of the most common causes of temporary hearing loss in all ages.[2–4] Approximately 12 million patients will visit their primary care physician annually because of cerumen impaction.[5]

Self-treatment with nonprescription medications and complementary therapies should be restricted to external ear disorders, which include disorders of the auricle and the external auditory canal (EAC). Excessive cerumen and water-clogged ears are self-treatable EAC disorders for which the Food and Drug Administration (FDA) has approved nonprescription otic medications. Other self-treatable disorders of the auricle include seborrhea and psoriasis, and allergic and contact dermatitis. Chapters 33 and 34, respectively, provide a detailed discussion of the etiology and treatment of the latter disorders.

Diseases of the head and neck can cause referred pain, which the patient often perceives as pain originating from the ear. The health care provider must attempt to determine the cause of pain prior to recommending self-treatment or medical referral. The assessment of self-treatable otic disorders and discussions for patient counseling and evaluation of patient outcomes are presented later in the chapter. This chapter briefly examines the anatomy and pathophysiology of the ear and associated nonprescription therapies for excessive/impacted cerumen and water-clogged ears.

Pathophysiology of Otic Disorders

The external ear consists of the auricle (also called the pinna), the EAC (Figure 29–1), and the tympanic membrane (eardrum), which separates the external ear from the middle ear.[6] The auricle is composed of a thin layer of highly vascular skin that is tightly bound to cartilage. Adipose, or subcutaneous, tissue, which would insulate blood vessels, is absent except in the lobe. The lobe has fewer blood vessels and is composed primarily of

fatty tissue. The triangular piece of cartilage in front of the ear canal adjacent to the cheek is called the tragus.

The EAC consists of an outer cartilaginous portion, which comprises one-third to one-half of its length, plus an inner body, or osseous, portion.[6] The canal forms a blind cul-de-sac. Children have a shorter, straighter, and flatter EAC than that of adults, whose canal tends to lengthen and form an "S" shape.[7] At the same time, an adult's eustachian tube (part of the inner ear) lengthens downward as it enters the nasal cavity. This shape helps to promote drainage and inhibits aspiration of pharyngeal and nasal contents into the middle ear, which may help to explain why children suffer from more middle ear infections compared with adults.[8]

The skin that covers the auricle is especially susceptible to bleeding when scratched because of the lack of flexibility usually afforded by a subcutaneous layer of fat and the large blood supply to the area.[9] The skin is highly innervated, causing a disproportionate otalgia (ear pain) when inflammation is present. Skin farther into the EAC is thicker, and contains apocrine and exocrine glands as well as hair follicles.[6,7] The skin in the canal is continuous with the outer layer of the tympanic membrane.

Oily secretions from the exocrine glands mix with the milky, fatty fluid from the apocrine glands to form cerumen, which appears on the surface of the skin on the outer half of the EAC. Cerumen lubricates the canal, traps dust and foreign materials, and provides a waxy, waterproof barrier to the entry of pathogens.[7] It also contains various antimicrobial substances, such as lysozymes, and it has an acidic pH, which also aids in inhibition of bacterial and fungal growth.

The canal skin is shed continuously and mixes with cerumen. The debris-laden cerumen slowly migrates outward with jaw movements (such as chewing and talking). This migration serves as a process of self-cleaning.[5] Cerumen may appear dry and flaky or oily and paste-like. Color varies from individual to individual; it can be honey-colored to light gray or tan and may darken on exposure to air.[10]

The natural defenses of the ear canal include the skin layer with its protective coating of cerumen, an acidic pH (<6.5), and hairs that line the outer half of the canal. Together, they protect against injury from foreign material and infection. It is important for the provider to explain the normal role and function of cerumen when educating patients.

Because the EAC forms a blind cul-de-sac, it is especially prone to collecting moisture. Its dark, warm, moist environment is ideal for fungal and bacterial growth. In the preinflammatory stage, moisture, local trauma, or both remove the lipid layer

---

Editor's Note: This chapter is based on the 17th edition chapter of the same title, written by Linda Krypel.

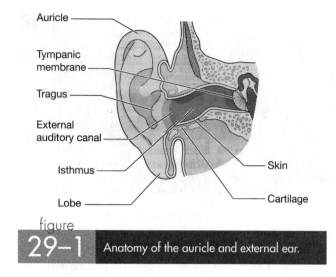

Auricle

Tympanic membrane

Tragus

External auditory canal

Isthmus

Lobe

Skin

Cartilage

figure

29-1 Anatomy of the auricle and external ear.

covering the skin. Local trauma from fingernails, cotton-tipped swabs, or other items inserted into the canal can abrade the skin and allow pathogens to enter. Because a normal, healthy ear canal is impervious to potentially pathogenic organisms, skin integrity generally must be interrupted before an organism can produce an infection. Trauma to the ear from thermal injuries, sports injuries, ear piercing, and poorly fitting or improperly cleaned ear devices or hearing aids can contribute to the breakdown of the EAC's natural defenses.[7] Dermatologic skin disorders, such as contact dermatitis, seborrhea, psoriasis, and malignancies, also compromise these defenses.[6]

Viral illnesses, such as colds and upper respiratory infections, can contribute to the breakdown of natural defenses of the middle and inner ear, especially in children, who are very susceptible to middle ear infections following such illnesses. Because a child's eustachian tube is shorter and angled flatter than that of an adult, it is commonly believed that nasopharyngeal secretions can easily be aspirated and accumulate in the middle ear, leading to proliferation of bacteria.[8] Holding back or trying to stifle a sneeze can force secretions into the middle ear and therefore should be strongly discouraged, even in adults.

Excessive/Impacted Cerumen

Cerumen can be considered an undervalued defense system. Widespread misinformation has often led the public to believe that cerumen production is a pathologic condition and that cerumen must be continually removed. Improper or excessive attempts to remove cerumen can actually damage the EAC.[5]

Pathophysiology of Excessive/ Impacted Cerumen

Individuals who have abnormally narrow or misshapen EACs, excessive hair growth in the canal, overactive ceruminous glands, or who wear hearing aids, earplugs, or sound attenuators often suffer from impacted cerumen caused by the disruption of normal cerumen migration to the outer EAC.[10] Frequent removal and proper cleaning of ear devices may help prevent wax buildup. Older adults often experience impacted cerumen resulting from atrophy of ceruminous glands.[6] This population secretes drier cerumen, which is more difficult to expel from the ear.

Clinical Presentation of Excessive/ Impacted Cerumen

The most common symptoms of impacted cerumen are a sense of fullness or pressure in the ear and a gradual hearing loss, which can lead to a decrease in cognition in the elderly.[5,10] A dull pain is sometimes associated with this disorder, along with vertigo (a sensation of spinning or whirling), tinnitus (ringing, hissing, or buzzing noises in the ear), chronic cough, or mild pain.[3] Hardened cerumen generally does not cling to cotton-tipped applicators, and using them may serve only to remove the protective waxy layer and force the cerumen plug further into the canal. The most important complication of improper cerumen removal results when the delicate skin of the EAC is scratched or damaged, providing an entry point for water and pathogens.[4,7,11] Patients experiencing an abrupt loss of hearing associated with a sharp pain should be referred immediately to their primary care provider because this may indicate a ruptured tympanic membrane. Severe pain should also be referred.

Treatment of Excessive/Impacted Cerumen
Treatment Goals

The goal of treating excessive/impacted cerumen is to soften and remove it using proper methods and safe, effective agents. Proper treatment should eliminate temporary hearing loss and other symptoms.

General Treatment Approach

The initial step in removing impacted cerumen is the use of a safe and effective agent to soften cerumen. Gently irrigating the ear, using an otic bulb syringe filled with warm water, is often recommended after cerumen has been softened. Caution must be used to ensure complete removal of water and to avoid a possible infection attributable to water-clogged ears. Cotton-tipped swabs or other foreign objects should not be used to remove cerumen or water. The algorithm in Figure 29–2 outlines the appropriate self-treatment of excessive/impacted cerumen and lists exclusions for self-treatment.

Nonpharmacologic Therapy

Earwax should be removed only when it has migrated to the outermost portion of the EAC. The only recommended nonpharmacologic method of removing cerumen is to use a wet, wrung-out washcloth draped over a finger. Making this procedure part of daily aural hygiene can prevent impacted cerumen if physiologic abnormalities or physical devices are not the cause of the impaction. This method is not effective once cerumen becomes impacted.

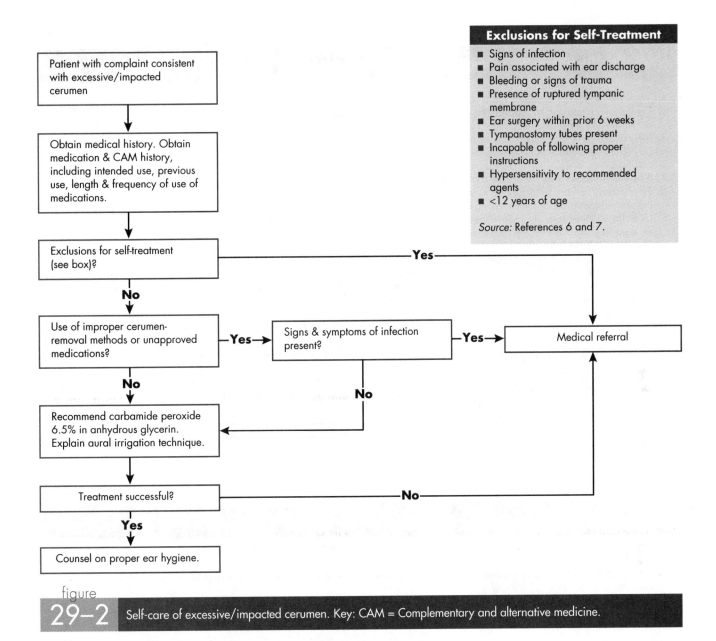

Exclusions for Self-Treatment

- Signs of infection
- Pain associated with ear discharge
- Bleeding or signs of trauma
- Presence of ruptured tympanic membrane
- Ear surgery within prior 6 weeks
- Tympanostomy tubes present
- Incapable of following proper instructions
- Hypersensitivity to recommended agents
- <12 years of age

Source: References 6 and 7.

figure

29–2 Self-care of excessive/impacted cerumen. Key: CAM = Complementary and alternative medicine.

Pharmacologic Therapy

Carbamide peroxide 6.5% in anhydrous glycerin is currently the only FDA-approved nonprescription cerumen-softening agent.[12] Other agents such as mineral oil, olive oil (sweet oil), docusate sodium, glycerin, sodium bicarbonate, and dilute hydrogen peroxide have been used by primary care providers and patients as inexpensive home remedies to soften cerumen. However, no data support these remedies as being more effective than carbamide peroxide in anhydrous glycerin.[3,13]

Carbamide Peroxide

Carbamide peroxide 6.5% in anhydrous glycerin is approved as safe and effective in softening, loosening, and removing excessive earwax in adults and children ages 12 years and older.[12] (See Table 29–1 for proper instillation of eardrops.) Carbamide peroxide is prepared from hydrogen peroxide and urea. When carbamide peroxide is exposed to moisture, nascent oxygen is released slowly and acts as a weak antibacterial. The effervescence that occurs during this process, along with the effect of urea on tissue debridement, helps to mechanically break down and loosen cerumen that has been softened by anhydrous glycerin.[14] Glycerin, which has emollient and humectant properties, is widely used as a solvent and vehicle.[14] It is safe and nonsensitizing when applied to abraded skin.

Any cerumen remaining after treatment may be removed with gentle, warm-water irrigation administered with a rubber otic bulb syringe (Table 29–2). Caution is important in that improper use of an otic syringe can leave excess moisture in the canal or further compress cerumen. Self-use of an oral jet irrigator is not recommended. Either of these actions can also cause otitis externa, perforated tympanic membrane, pain, vertigo, otitis media, and tinnitus.[3,15]

Carbamide peroxide solution is generally considered to be nonirritating and may be used twice daily for up to 4 days. Adverse effects reported after proper use include pain, rash, irritation, tenderness, redness, discharge, or dizziness.[16] If adverse

table
29-1   Guidelines for Administering Eardrops

1. Wash your hands with soap and warm water; then dry them thoroughly.
2. Carefully wash and dry the outside of the ear with a damp washcloth, taking care not to get water in the ear canal. Then dry the ear.
3. Warm eardrops to body temperature by holding the container in the palm of your hand for a few minutes. Do not warm the container in hot water or microwave. Using hot eardrops can cause ear pain, nausea, or dizziness.
4. If the label indicates, gently shake the container to mix contents.
5. Tilt your head (or have the patient tilt his or her head) to the side, as shown in drawing A. Or lie down with the affected ear up, as shown in drawing B. Use gentle restraint, if necessary, for an infant or a young child.
6. Open the container carefully. Position the dropper tip near, but not inside, the ear canal opening. Do not allow the dropper to touch the ear, because it could become contaminated or injure the ear. Eardrop bottles must be kept clean.
7. Pull your ear (or the patient's ear) backward and upward to open the ear canal (drawing A). If the patient is a child younger than 3 years, pull the ear backward and downward (drawing B).
8. Place the proper dose or number of drops into the ear canal. Replace the cap on the container.
9. Gently press the small, flat skin flap (tragus) over the ear canal opening to force out air bubbles and push the drops down the ear canal.
10. Stay (or keep the patient) in the same position for the length of time indicated in the product instructions. If the patient is a child who cannot stay still, the primary care provider may tell you to place a clean piece of cotton gently into the child's ear to prevent the medication from draining out. Use a piece large enough to remove easily, and do not leave it in the ear longer than an hour.
11. Repeat the procedure for the other ear, if needed.
12. Gently wipe excess medication off the outside of the ear, using caution to avoid getting moisture in the ear canal.
13. Wash your hands to remove any medication.

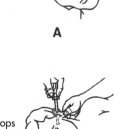
A

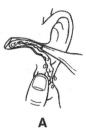
B

Source: *APhA Special Report: Medication Administration Problem Solving in Ambulatory Care.* Washington, DC: American Pharmaceutical Association; 1994:9.

table
29-2   Guidelines for Removing Excessive/Impacted Cerumen

Ceruminolytics

1. Place 5–10 drops of the cerumen-softening solution into the ear canal, and allow it to remain for at least 15 minutes, as described in Table 29–1.
2. Perform this procedure daily for no longer than 4 consecutive days.

Irrigation Technique

The use of ceruminolytics and irrigation together may improve overall removal of impacted cerumen. The ceruminolytic agent is administered first. Then follow the irrigation technique as described below, paying special attention to cautionary instructions.

1. Prepare a warm (not hot) solution of plain water or other solution as directed by your primary care provider. Eight ounces of solution should be sufficient to clean out the ear canal.
2. To catch the returning solution, hold a container under the ear being cleaned. An emesis basin is ideal because it fits the contour of the neck. Tilt the head down slightly on the side where the ear is being cleaned.
3. Gently pull the earlobe down and back to expose the ear canal, as shown in drawing A.
4. Place the open end of the syringe into the ear canal with the tip pointed slightly upward toward the side of the ear canal (drawing A). Do not aim the syringe into the back of the ear canal. Use caution and make sure the syringe does not obstruct the outflow of solution.
5. Squeeze the bulb gently—not forcefully—to introduce the solution into the ear canal and to avoid rupturing the eardrum. (*Note:* Only health professionals trained in aural hygiene should use forced water sprays [e.g., Water Pik] to remove cerumen.)
6. Do not let the returning solution come into contact with the eyes.
7. If pain or dizziness occurs, remove the syringe and do not resume irrigation until a health care provider is consulted.
8. Make sure all water is drained from the ear to avoid predisposing to infection from water-clogged ears.
9. Rinse the syringe thoroughly before and after each use, and let it dry.
10. Store the syringe in a cool, dry place (preferably, in its original container) away from hot surfaces and sharp instruments
11. If cerumen still remains, consult a provider.

A

Source: Adapted with permission from *Ohio Clin.* 1996;14(5):10.

effects develop or symptoms persist after 4 days, the patient should see a primary care provider for evaluation.[17]

Docusate Sodium

Docusate sodium is classified as an emollient and has been topically applied in the ear canal to soften earwax. Evidence for its effectiveness over approved agents is conflicting.[3,13,18,19] Docusate sodium is more expensive, has varying results, and may cause superficial erythema.

Hydrogen Peroxide

Hydrogen peroxide releases nascent oxygen when exposed to moisture and acts as a weak antibacterial.[14] Hydrogen peroxide 3% has been used to flush the ear canal when softening or removing earwax.[3] Because hydrogen peroxide solutions contain water, overuse may predispose the ear to infection from tissue maceration caused by excessive water left in the canal.

Olive Oil (Sweet Oil)

Olive oil is used as an emollient and has been used as a home remedy to soften earwax.[6,17] It has also been used in the ear canal to alleviate itching and pain.[19] Using olive oil to treat ear pain may delay seeking proper treatment.

Product Selection Guidelines

Table 29–3 lists examples of cerumen-softening and other otic products. No nonprescription cerumen-softening agents are approved for patients younger than 12 years. No special consideration is necessary for pregnant, lactating, or geriatric patients.

Complementary Therapies

Although major herbal references do not list herbal remedies for self-treatable otic disorders,[20-22] some folk remedies remain popular in many regions. One of the more interesting—and dangerous—is the use of ear candles to remove cerumen. A hollow candle is burned with one end inserted in the ear canal. The intent is to create negative pressure and draw cerumen from the ear. Studies have shown that this method does not aid in removing cerumen but has caused serious ear injuries and burns to patients.[23] FDA issued an alert warning against the import and sale of these devices in 2007.[24]

A product advertised for ear pain in children contains olive oil, garlic oil, and willow bark; the latter is a form of salicylate.[20,21] Although garlic oil claims to have some antibacterial properties, self-treating ear pain can delay seeking an appropriate diagnosis. Another available herb is chamomilla, which is believed to help with ear inflammation. Although these herbal and homeopathic products are available, no published studies document safety and effectiveness (Table 29–3). (See Chapters 51 and 52 for more information on complementary therapies.)

Water-Clogged Ears

Water-clogged ears is a separate disorder from swimmer's ear (external otitis). FDA has not approved any nonprescription products for preventing or treating external otitis. Manufacturers have argued that removing moisture from water-clogged ears with an approved agent may prevent tissue maceration, a process that can lead to inflammation and infection of the EAC

table 29–3 Selected Products for Otic Disorders[a]

Trade Name	Primary Ingredients
Cerumen-Softening Products	
Auro Ear Drops	Carbamide peroxide 6.5%; anhydrous glycerin
Debrox Earwax Removal Aid Kit	Carbamide peroxide 6.5%; glycerin; packaged with syringe
Ear-Drying Products	
Auro-Dri Drops	Isopropyl alcohol 95%; anhydrous glycerin
Swim Ear Drops	Isopropyl alcohol 95%; anhydrous glycerin
Botanical and Homeopathic Products	
Herbs for Kids Willow/Garlic Ear Oil	Extra virgin olive oil; garlic, calendula; willow bark[b]; usnea; vitamin E oil
Similasan Healthy Relief Homeopathic Ear Drops	Chamomilla HPUS 10X; mercurius solubus HPUS 15X; sulfur HPUS 12X; glycerin
Similasan Ear Wax Relief	Causticum HPUS 12X; Graphites HPUS 15X; Lachesis HPUS 12X; Lycopodium HPUS 12X

Key: HPUS = *Homeopathic Pharmacopoeia of the United States.*
[a] FDA has not approved any product in children < 12 years of age.
[b] Contains salicylate.

(commonly referred to as swimmer's ear). FDA, however, prohibits this extrapolation, and manufacturers may not label their products as preventing swimmer's ear.[25,26]

Pathophysiology of Water-Clogged Ears

Some patients are more prone to retaining water because of the shape of their ear canals or the presence of excessive cerumen. The cerumen can swell, thereby trapping water. Excessive moisture in the ears can result from hot, humid climates, sweating, swimming, bathing, or improper use of aqueous solutions to cleanse the ear. Therefore, simple attempts to remove water by mechanical manipulation may be insufficient. In addition, the use of cotton-tipped applicators has been linked to external otitis.[3,27]

Clinical Presentation of Water-Clogged Ears

A feeling of wetness or fullness in the ear, accompanied by gradual hearing loss, can occur after exposure to any of the etiologic factors. The trapped moisture can compromise the natural defenses of the EAC, causing tissue maceration that, in turn, can lead to itching, pain, inflammation, or infection.[4,7] Severe pain, inflammation, or signs of infection should be referred to a primary care provider.

Treatment of Water-Clogged Ears

Treatment Goals

The goals of treating a water-clogged ear are to dry it using a safe and effective agent and to prevent recurrences in persons who are prone to retaining moisture in the ears.

General Treatment Approach

Before recommending an agent to treat water-clogged ears, the health care provider should determine whether a patient has a ruptured tympanic membrane or has a tympanostomy tube in place. Ear-drying agents are very painful if instilled in either of these situations. Figure 29–2 lists additional exclusions for self-treatment. The algorithm in Figure 29–3 outlines the appropriate treatment of water-clogged ears.

Nonpharmacologic Therapy

Tilting the affected ear downward and gently manipulating the auricle can expel excessive water from the ear. This procedure should be performed after swimming or bathing, or during periods of excessive sweating, especially by persons who are prone to developing this disorder. Using a blow-dryer on a low heat and speed setting around (not directly into) the ear immediately after swimming or bathing may help dry the ear canal. One-time-use water-absorbing earplugs (ClearEars) are available for patients ages 17 years and older. These earplugs will not prevent water from entering the ear during bathing or swimming. When used to dry ears, they should be removed after a maximum

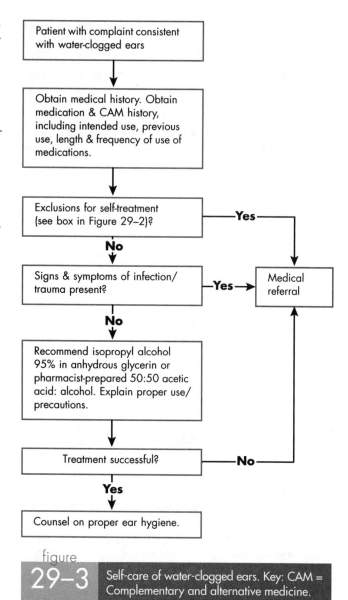

figure
29–3 Self-care of water-clogged ears. Key: CAM = Complementary and alternative medicine.

of 10 minutes and discarded. If these earplugs are accidently ingested, small children or pets can choke as the earplug expands upon contact with the fluid in the throat. No clinical trials of this product have been conducted as of this time.[28] In one study, cotton wool with petrolatum was ranked the most effective for waterproofing ears and the easiest to insert.[29]

Pharmacologic Therapy

FDA has approved only isopropyl alcohol 95% in anhydrous glycerin 5% as a safe and effective "ear-drying aid."[25,26] (See Table 29–3 for examples of products containing these agents.) In addition, a 50:50 mixture of acetic acid 5% (white household vinegar) and isopropyl alcohol 95% has commonly been recommended to help dry water-clogged ears.[4,7]

Ear-drying agents recommended for use in adults and children ages 12 years and older may be used whenever ears are exposed to water. Table 29–1 presents guidelines for administering these agents. Medical referral is necessary if symptoms persist after several days of simultaneous use of ear-drying agents and prevention of exposure of ears to water.

Isopropyl Alcohol in Anhydrous Glycerin

Alcohol is highly miscible with water and acts as a drying agent. In concentrations greater than 70%, alcohol is also an effective skin disinfectant.[14] Glycerin has been used in pharmaceutical preparations for its solvent, emollient, or hygroscopic properties. It is safe but stings when applied to open wounds or abraded skin. Repeated use of alcohol alone can cause overdrying of the canal. The combination of alcohol and glycerin, however, provides a product that reduces moisture in the ear without overdrying.

Acetic Acid

Acetic acid in a 50:50 mixture of acetic acid 5% and isopropyl alcohol 95% has bactericidal and antifungal properties.[14] Species of *Pseudomonas, Candida,* and *Aspergillus* are particularly sensitive to this agent. Care must be taken to advise patients against using cider vinegar instead of white vinegar. Cider vinegar is produced from fruit and contains impurities that could hinder antibacterial activity. A 50:50 mixture of white vinegar 5% and isopropyl alcohol 95% provides an acetic acid 2.5% solution. Concentrations of acetic acid between 2% and 3% may lower the pH of the ear canal below the optimal pH of 6.5–7.5 needed for bacterial growth.[14] The solution is well tolerated and non-sensitizing and does not induce resistant organisms. It may sting or burn slightly, especially if the skin is abraded. The provider should direct the patient in how to properly compound this solution by preparing it from ingredients that are not expired and discarding any remainder after use.

Product Selection Guidelines

Table 29–3 lists examples of ear-drying and other otic products. No nonprescription ear-drying agents are approved for patients younger than 12 years. No special consideration is necessary for pregnant, lactating, or geriatric patients.

Assessment of Otic Disorders: A Case-Based Approach

The most common complaints of ear disorders are otalgia, pruritus (itching), and hearing loss. Evaluating the characteristics of particular symptoms, such as pain and hearing loss, and the specific combination of symptoms is the key to assessing otic disorders. The discussion of common otic symptoms in Cases 29–1 and 29–2

---

case

29–1

Relevant Evaluation Criteria	Scenario/Model Outcome
Information Gathering	

1. Gather essential information about the patient's symptoms and medical history, including:	
a. description of symptom(s) (i.e., nature, onset, duration, severity, associated symptoms)	Two days ago, the patient started to experience a sense of fullness in her left year after her water aerobics class.
b. description of any factors that seem to precipitate, exacerbate, and/or relieve the patient's symptom(s)	She experience hearing loss in her left ear after she tried to dry her ears with a cotton swab after her morning shower. She denies experiencing pain in her ear.
c. description of the patient's efforts to relieve the symptoms	After her water aerobics class, she used isopropyl alcohol 95% in anhydrous glycerin drops to dry the water in her ears.
d. patient's identity	Lillian Keller
e. age, sex, height, and weight	68 years old, female, 5 ft 2 in., 155 lb
f. patient's occupation	Retired; previous occupation was an administrative assistant.
g. patient's dietary habits	Recently began weight-loss program where she purchases 3 meals and 2 snacks per day to limit her caloric intake to 1200–1400 kcal/day.
h. patient's sleep habits	She sleeps 7–8 hours each night.
i. concurrent medical conditions, prescription and nonprescription medications, and dietary supplements	Hypertension: enalapril 10 mg daily; hydrochlorothiazide 25 mg daily; Dyslipidemia: atorvastatin 20 mg daily in the evening; multivitamin; calcium citrate 600 mg and vitamin D 400 IU 2 caplets twice daily; glucosamine 1500 mg with evening meal
j. allergies	NKA
k. history of other adverse reactions to medications	None
l. other (describe) _____	The patient participates in a water aerobics class 5 days a week. Earlier this month the patient began using hearing aids to help improve the overall clarity of her hearing.

Assessment and Triage	

2. Differentiate patient's signs/symptoms and correctly identify the patient's primary problem(s) (Table 29–4).	Lillian is experiencing cerumen impaction that is likely the result of the improper attempt to remove any water from the ear and recently starting to wear hearing aids.

Relevant Evaluation Criteria	Scenario/Model Outcome
3. Identify exclusions for self-treatment (Figure 29–2).	None
4. Formulate a comprehensive list of therapeutic alternatives for the primary problem to determine if triage to a health care provider is required, and share this information with the patient or caregiver.	Options include: (1) Refer Lillian to appropriate health care provider. (2) Recommend nonprescription cerumen-softening agent with proper ear hygiene (Table 29–3). (3) Recommend continuation of nonprescription ear-drying agent (Table 29–3). (4) Recommend self-care until Lillian can see an appropriate health care provider. (5) Take no action.

Plan

5. Select an optimal therapeutic alternative to address the patient's problem, taking into account patient preferences.	The patient would like to try to use a self-care product until she can be seen by her health care provider.
6. Describe the recommended therapeutic approach to the patient or caregiver.	"The cerumen-softening agent carbamide peroxide 6.5% can help soften and aid in the removal of excessive earwax."
7. Explain to the patient or caregiver the rationale for selecting the recommended therapeutic approach from the considered therapeutic alternatives.	"People who wear hearing aids can often experience impacted earwax. Attempting to use cotton swabs to dry the water in your ears added to the cerumen impaction. The cerumen-softening drops with gentle water irrigation can help remove the impacted cerumen."

Patient Education

8. When recommending self-care with nonprescription medications and/or nondrug therapy, convey accurate information to the patient or caregiver.	"You should use proper ear hygiene and avoid placing objects like cotton-tipped swabs in your ears." See the box Patient Education for Self-Treatable Otic Disorders.
a. appropriate dose and frequency of administration	"Place 5–10 drops of the cerumen-softening solution into ear canal, and allow it to remain for at least 15 minutes." "Continue with irrigation technique to assist with cerumen impaction removal."
b. maximum number of days the therapy should be employed	"Do this procedure twice daily for no longer than 4 consecutive days."
c. product administration procedures	See Table 29–1.
d. expected time to onset of relief	"Fullness or pressure sensation relief can often be felt after first treatment. However, it may take additional treatments to fully resolve symptom relief."
e. degree of relief that can be reasonably expected	"Full resolution of symptoms can be expected within 4 days."
f. most common side effects	"The medication may cause bubbling or crackling sound in the ear."
g. side effects that warrant medical intervention should they occur	"You may experience pain, rash, irritation, tenderness, redness, discharge, or dizziness from the medication."
h. patient options in the event that condition worsens or persists	"Stop using the product and see your primary care provider."
i. product storage requirements	"Keep cap on bottle when not in use. Store drops in original carton at room temperature. Rinse syringe thoroughly before and after use, and let dry. Store ear syringe in a cool, dry place and in its original container."
j. specific nondrug measures	See the box Patient Education for Self-Treatable Otic Disorders.
Solicit follow-up questions from the patient or caregiver.	"Will I always have earwax impaction because I started to wear hearing aids?"
Answer the patient's or caregiver's questions.	"Although wearing hearing aids may put you at risk for experiencing cerumen impaction, it does not mean that this will be a continual problem for you. Frequent removal and cleaning of your hearing aids can help prevent earwax buildup. In addition, daily safe ear hygiene techniques will help reduce that risk."

Evaluation of Patient Outcome

9. Assess patient outcome.	Offer to contact the patient in 2 days to evaluate her response.

Key: NKA = No known allergies.

case
29–2

Relevant Evaluation Criteria	Scenario/Model Outcome

Information Gathering

1. Gather essential information about the patient's symptoms and medical history, including:

   a. description of symptom(s) (i.e., nature, onset, duration, severity, associated symptoms)

   Patient reports gradual hearing loss and itchiness over the last 3 days in his right ear and began experiencing intense pain this afternoon in the same ear.

   b. description of any factors that seem to precipitate, exacerbate, and/or relieve the patient's symptom(s)

   The hearing loss began about 2 days after returning home from family vacation at water park. He noticed a small amount of fluid drainage from his ear and felt that excess water was draining from the ear.

   c. description of the patient's efforts to relieve the symptoms

   Patient applied 5–10 drops of water-drying drops (isopropyl alcohol 95% in anhydrous glycerin) in an effort to remove the water that was clogging his ears. The drops provided no relief and caused mild pain when administered.

   d. patient's identity

   David Peterson

   e. age, sex, height, and weight

   43 years old, male, 5 ft 7 in., 145 lb

   f. patient's occupation

   Business analyst

   g. patient's dietary habits

   Eats 3 meals per day, with minimal vegetable intake.

   h. patient's sleep habits

   8 hours nightly

   i. concurrent medical conditions, prescription and nonprescription medications, and dietary supplements

   Allergic rhinitis: fexofenadine 180 mg and pseudoephedrine 240 mg daily; fluticasone propionate 50 mcg nasal spray 2 sprays each nostril daily.
   Sinus headaches: ibuprofen 400 mg twice daily with food as needed

   j. allergies

   NKA

   k. history of other adverse reactions to medications

   None

Assessment and Triage

2. Differentiate patient's signs/symptoms and correctly identify the patient's primary problem(s) (Table 29–4).

   Patient could be suffering from otitis externa rather than excessive water in the ear.

3. Identify exclusions for self-treatment (Figure 29–3).

   Recent onset of intense ear pain

4. Formulate a comprehensive list of therapeutic alternatives for the primary problem to determine if triage to a health care provider is required, and share this information with the patient or caregiver.

   Options include:

   (1) Immediate referral of patient to health care provider for a differential diagnosis.

   (2) Recommend continuation with self-care until patient can see an appropriate health care provider.

   (3) Take no action.

Plan

5. Select an optimal therapeutic alternative to address the patient's problem, taking into account patient preferences.

   Patient should consult a health care provider.

6. Describe the recommended therapeutic approach to the patient or caregiver.

   "You should consult a health care provider for treatment."

7. Explain to the patient or caregiver the rationale for selecting the recommended therapeutic approach from the considered therapeutic alternatives.

   "The best option for you is to discontinue any additional self-treatment and seek immediate care from a health care provider. The recent onset of the pain you are feeling is not due to water in the ears, but rather an ear infection. Nonprescription ear products will not be able to treat this. In your case, you may need prescription ear drops to treat the condition."

case
29–2   *continued*

Relevant Evaluation Criteria	Scenario/Model Outcome
Patient Education	
8. When recommending self-care with nonprescription medications and/or nondrug therapy, convey accurate information to the patient or caregiver.	Criterion does not apply in this case.
Solicit follow-up questions from the patient or caregiver.	"How might I be able to prevent this problem in the future?"
Answer the patient's or caregiver's questions.	"Consider using ear plugs to prevent water from entering your ears when swimming."
Evaluation of Patient Outcome	
9. Assess patient outcome.	Contact patient in 1 day to ensure that he sought medical care.

Key: NKA = No known allergies.

describes the possible causes. Table 29–4 compares the signs and symptoms and other features of common otic disorders, and Table 29–5 describes the common etiologies and treatments for otalgia, otic pruritus, hearing loss, dizziness, and tinnitus.[30-33] A verbal 5-minute hearing loss test is available at the American Academy of Otolaryngology Head and Neck Surgery, Inc., Web site (www.entnet.org/healthinformation/hearing-loss.cfm) and will quickly assess in adults how often and the circumstances when the patient experiences hearing loss.

Patient Counseling for Otic Disorders

Patients who self-treat otic disorders must understand how easily the EAC can be injured. The health care provider should discourage common harmful practices of relieving itching of the ear using cotton swabs, fingernails, or other devices, and instruct patients on the proper methods of removing excessive cerumen and moisture from the ears. Patients who are susceptible to these disorders should be advised to incorporate the proper removal methods as

table
29–4   **Differentiation of Common Otic Disorders**

Disorder	Etiology	Pain	Itching	Loss of Hearing	Discharge	Other Features
Ruptured tympanic membrane	Otitis media or trauma to ear such as sharp blows, diving into water, forceful irrigation of ear	Brief, severe	No	Abrupt	If associated with otitis media	May be associated with otitis media (see subsequent text)
External otitis (swimmer's ear)	Local trauma to EAC caused by excessive moisture or abrasions; subsequent fungal/ bacterial infections	Acute onset, varies from mild to severe, increases with movement of tragus or auricle	Yes	Occasional	Occasionally, clear discharge changing to seropurulent	Swollen ear canal, stuffiness, discharge, swollen lymph nodes, fever, usually occurs in summer or in warm, humid climates
Otitis media	Bacterial infection of middle ear, usually following upper respiratory tract infections	Sharp, steady, frequently unilateral; does not increase with movement of tragus or auricle	No	Is sometimes decreased	Possible exudate through perforated eardrum	Perforated or bulging eardrum, lymph nodes sometimes swollen, fever, dizziness, usually occurs in winter
Foreign object in ear	Insects, insertion of objects by children, hearing aids, sound attenuators	Dull-severe pain with sense of fullness or pressure during chewing	Yes	Yes	Possible exudate from secondary bacterial infection	If obstruction not removed promptly, acute otitis externa and tinnitus may develop

table
29–4 Differentiation of Common Otic Disorders *(continued)*

Disorder	Etiology	Pain	Itching	Loss of Hearing	Discharge	Other Features
Trauma to ear	Burns from curling iron, frostbite, hematomas/ injuries from contact sports or ill-fitting helmets, ear piercing, improper cerumen removal techniques, abrasions of EAC, rapid changes in air pressure	Varies from sharp and steady to brief and severe	Rare	Varies, can be abrupt to seldom	Seldom	Untreated hematomas may cause swelling/ scarring; ear piercing may cause metal sensitivities, keloids, perichondritis, toxic shock syndrome, hepatitis B
Tinnitus	Hearing disorders, blockage of EAC, exposure to high noise levels, acoustic trauma, systemic diseases, drug toxicities (salicylate, quinidine, aminoglycosides, and other antibiotics)	Possible	No	Sometimes	None	Continuous or intermittent alien noises in ear such as ringing, roaring, or humming
Excessive/ impacted cerumen	Overactive ceruminous glands, obstructed migration of cerumen	Rare, dull pain if present	No	Often	None	Sense of fullness or pressure in the ears
Water-clogged ears	Excessive moisture in EAC	None	No	Often	None	Sense of fullness or wetness

Key: EAC = External auditory canal.
Source: References 3, 4, 6, 8, 12, 16, 30, and 33.

table
29–5 Differentiation of Common Otic Disorders

Disorder	Etiology	Treatment
Otalgia	Intrinsic: infection, trauma, foreign objects, perichondritis Extrinsic: dental or jaw problems, nasopharyngeal infections, tumors, cysts, migraine headaches, neuralgias, cervical arthritis	Medical referral unless cause is clearly obvious, self-limiting, and self-treatable; always refer infections; self-care may delay seeking proper treatment
Otic pruritus	Seborrhea, psoriasis, contact dermatitis; infection (external otitis); excessive dryness related to decreased sebum production	See Chapters 33 and 34; medical referral if infection suspected; excessive dryness: 1–2 drops of mineral oil
Hearing loss	Foreign objects or water trapped in EAC; infection, congestion, neoplasms, tympanic membrane perforation, medications, excessive pressure, cerumen, or noise in EAC	Medical referral unless hearing loss is related to excessive water or impacted cerumen
Dizziness	Inner ear lesions, otitis media, rapid change in pressure on the tympanic membrane, migraine headache, ototoxic drugs, postural hypotension, cardiac disease, neoplasms, irrigation of ear canal with very hot or cold water, motion sickness	Medical referral unless related to motion sickness
Tinnitus	See Table 29–4	Check for impacted cerumen; medical referral otherwise
Foreign body	Insects, beads, seeds, small batteries, or other objects	Medical referral; mineral oil can quickly suffocate an insect until removed by a provider; moisture causes seeds to swell, making removal more difficult

Key: EAC = External auditory canal.
Source: References 3, 4, 6–8, 12, and 30–33.

part of their aural hygiene. The provider should explain the proper use and possible adverse effects of all recommended medications. The box Patient Education for Self-Treatable Otic Disorders lists specific information to provide patients.

Evaluation of Patient Outcomes for Otic Disorders

If the symptoms of excessive/impacted cerumen or water–clogged ears persist or worsen after 4 days of proper self-treatment, the patient should consult a primary care provider. The patient should also consult a primary care provider if ear pain or discharge develops during treatment. The provider can follow up by phone in 4 days to determine whether the therapy is successful.

Key Points for Otic Disorders

➤ Limit the self-treatment of otic disorders to minor symptoms such as a sense of fullness, pressure, or wetness in the ears.

➤ Refer for further evaluation patients younger than 12 years, as well as those with signs and symptoms of ear infection, bleeding or signs of trauma, tympanostomy tubes, ruptured tympanic membrane, or ear surgery within the past 6 weeks.

➤ Instruct patients on how to use specific otic products that have been proven safe and effective (Tables 29–1 and 29–2).

➤ Advise patients with self-treatable symptoms to contact a primary care provider if symptoms worsen or do not improve after 4 days.

➤ Advise patients about proper ear hygiene and the importance of cerumen to prevent further problems.

---

patient education for
Self-Treatable Otic Disorders

Excessive/Impacted Cerumen

The objective of self-treatment is to soften and remove excessive or impacted cerumen (earwax) that is already present or to prevent the disorder from recurring in susceptible patients. For most patients, carefully following product instructions and the self-care measures listed here will help ensure optimal therapeutic outcomes.

Nondrug Measures

▪ Use a washcloth draped over a finger to remove earwax from the outer canal.
▪ Do not insert objects in the ear to remove earwax. Such attempts may injure the ear canal or push the wax farther into the canal.
▪ Never use the hollow candle method to remove earwax; it can cause serious ear injury or burns to other areas of the body.

Nonprescription Medications

▪ Cerumen is necessary to lubricate the canal, trap dust and foreign materials, and provide a waxy, waterproof barrier to the entry of pathogens.
▪ Carbamide peroxide and anhydrous glycerin are combined to soften and mechanically break down excessive/impacted cerumen.
▪ See Tables 29–1 and 29–2 for guidelines on using carbamide peroxide to remove excessive or impacted earwax.
▪ Do not let the medication come into contact with the eyes.
▪ Do not use this medication if you have a fever, ear drainage, pain more severe than a dull pain, dizziness, or a ruptured eardrum, or if you had ear surgery within the past 6 weeks.
▪ Do not use this medication to treat inflamed ear tissue, swimmer's ear, or itching of the ear canal.
▪ Prolonged contact between carbamide peroxide solution and skin of the ear canal can cause dermatitis. Discontinue treatment if irritation or a rash appears.
▪ Store product in a cool, dry area and check expiration date before using.

When to Seek Medical Attention

▪ Monitor for changes in your hearing and symptoms of infection such as pain and itching.
▪ If severe pain occurs or your hearing worsens, see a primary care provider immediately. Severe pain may indicate a ruptured eardrum.

Water-Clogged Ears

The objective of self-treatment is to remove water from ears already clogged with water or to prevent the disorder in persons who are susceptible to excessive moisture in the ears. For most patients, carefully following product instructions and the self-care measures listed here will help ensure optimal therapeutic outcomes.

Nondrug Measures

▪ Tilt the affected ear down, and gently manipulate it to help drain water from the ear. Immediately after swimming or bathing, use a blow-dryer on a low heat and speed setting to help dry the ear canal. Do not blow air directly into the ear canal.

Nonprescription Medications

▪ Water can become trapped in the ear, causing a sense of fullness or wetness.
▪ Use a product that reduces moisture content in the ear without overdrying. Isopropyl alcohol 95% in anhydrous glycerin 5% is the only FDA-approved formula.
▪ Do not use the medication if you have a ruptured eardrum or have tympanostomy tubes in place.
▪ Place 5–10 drops of the solution in the ear canal, and allow the solution to remain for 1–2 minutes.
▪ See Table 29–1 for further instructions on instilling the medication.
▪ Do not let the medication come into contact with the eyes.
▪ Discontinue the medication if stinging or burning occurs.
▪ Store product in a cool, dry area and check expiration date before using.

When to Seek Medical Attention

▪ If pain, fever, or discharge develops, see a primary care provider immediately.

Dermatologic Disorders of the Ear

The objective of self-treatment is to relieve the symptoms. For most patients, carefully following product instructions and the self-care measures listed in Chapters 33 and 34 will help ensure optimal therapeutic outcomes.

REFERENCES

1. CDC/National Center of Health Statistics. *National Ambulatory Medical Care Survey: 2010 Summary Tables.* Atlanta, GA: Centers for Disease Control and Prevention; 2010. Accessed at http://www.cdc.gov/nchs/data/ahcd/namcs_summary/2010_namcs_web_tables.pdf, February 15, 2103.

2. Tueh B, Shapiro N, MacLean CH, et al. Screening and management of adult hearing loss in primary care. *JAMA.* 2003;289(15):1976–85.

3. McCarter DF, Courtney AU, Pollart SM. Cerumen impaction. *Am Fam Phys.* 2007;75(10):1523–8.

4. Kesser B. External ear disorders. In: Porter RS, Kaplan JL, eds. *The Merck Manual Online.* Accessed at http://www.merckmanuals.com/professional/ear_nose_and_throat_disorders/external_ear_disorders/external_ear_obstructions.html, April 15, 2013.

5. Roland PS, Smith TL, Schwartz SR, et al. Clinical practice guideline: cerumen impaction. *Otolaryngol Head Neck Surg.* 2008;139(3 suppl 2):S1–21.

6. Beatrice F, Bucolo S, Cavallo R. Earwax, clinical practice. *Acta Otorhinolaryngol Ital.* 2009;29(suppl 1):1–20.

7. Brown K, Banuchi V, Selesnick S. Diseases of the external ear. In: Lalwani AK, ed. *Current Diagnosis and Treatment in Otolaryngology Head and Neck Surgery.* 3rd ed. New York, NY: Lange Medical Books/McGraw Hill; 2012:645–60.

8. National Institute on Deafness and Other Communication Disorders. *Ear Infections in Children.* Rockville, MD: National Institutes of Health; 2010. NIH Publication No. 10-4799. Accessed at http://www.nidcd.nih.gov/staticresources/health/hearing/EarInfectionsFS.pdf, November 20, 2012.

9. Oghalai JS, Brownell WE. Anatomy and physiology of the ear. In: Lalwani AK, ed. *Current Diagnosis and Treatment in Otolaryngology Head and Neck Surgery.* 3rd ed. New York, NY: Lange Medical Books/McGraw Hill; 2012:599–616.

10. Hersh SP. Cerumen: insights and management. *Ann Longterm Care.* 2010;18(7):39–42.

11. Block SL. Otitis externa: providing relief while avoiding complications. *J Fam Prac.* 2005;54(8):669–76.

12. U.S. Food and Drug Administration. Topical otic drug products for over-the-counter human use; final monograph; final rule. *Federal Register.* August 8, 1986;51:28656–61.

13. Burton MJ, Doree CJ. Eardrops for the removal of earwax. *Cochrane Database Syst Rev.* 2009;3:CD004326. doi:10.1002/14651858. CD004326.pub2. Accessed at http://www.thecochranelibrary.com/view/0/index.html.

14. Allen LV, ed. *Remington: The Science and Practice of Pharmacy.* 22nd ed. Philadelphia, PA: Pharmaceutical Press and University of the Sciences, Philadelphia College of Pharmacy; 2013:1081–2, 1631.

15. Folmer RL. Chronic tinnitus resulting from cerumen removal procedures. *Int Tinnitus J.* 2004;10(1):42–6.

16. Eye, ear, nose and throat (EENT) preparations: carbamide peroxide. *AHFS Drug Information.* Bethesda, MD: American Society of Health System Pharmacists; 2007:2807.

17. Carbamide peroxide. Drug Facts and Comparisons. Facts & Comparisons [database online]. St. Louis, MO: Wolters Kluwer Health, Inc; May 2005. Accessed June 29, 2013.

18. Whatley VN, Dodds CL, Paul RI. Randomized clinical trial of docusate, triethanolamine polypeptide, and irrigation in cerumen removal in children. *Arch Pediatr Adolesc Med.* 2003;157:1177–83.

19. Harkin H. Evidence based ear care. *Primary Health Care.* 10;8:25–30. Accessed at http://rcnpublishing.com/doi/abs/10.7748/phc2000.10.10.8.25.c259, April 26, 2013.

20. Olive oil. Drug Facts and Comparisons. Facts & Comparisons [database online]. St. Louis, MO: Wolters Kluwer Health, Inc; May 2005. Accessed June 29, 2013.

21. Willowbark. Drug Facts and Comparisons. Facts & Comparisons [database online]. St. Louis, MO: Wolters Kluwer Health, Inc; May 2005. Accessed June 29, 2013.

22. Office of Dietary Supplements International Bibliographic Information on Dietary Supplements. Accessed at http://ods.od.nih.gov, April 26, 2013.

23. Ernst E. Ear candles: a triumph of ignorance over science. *J Laryngol Otol.* 2004;118(1):1–2.

24. U.S. Food and Drug Administration. Detention without physical examination of ear candles. Important Alert 77-01. June 20, 2013. Accessed at http://www.accessdata.fda.gov/cms_ia/importalert_225.html, May 29, 2014.

25. U.S. Food and Drug Administration. Topical otic drug products for over-the-counter human use; products for drying water-clogged ears; proposed amendment of monograph. *Federal Register.* August 17, 1999;64:44671–74.

26. U.S. Food and Drug Administration. Topical otic drug products for over-the-counter human use; products for drying water-clogged ears; amendment of monograph; lift of partial stay of effective date. *Federal Register.* August 10, 2000;65:48902.

27. Nussinocitch M, Rimon A, Volovitz B, et al. Cotton-tipped applicators as a leading cause of otitis externa. *Int J Pediatr Otohinolaryngol.* 2004;68(4):433–5.

28. ClearEars [package insert]. Cold Springs Harbor, NY: Cirrus Healthcare; 2010.

29. Chisholm EJ, Kuchai R, McPartlin D. An objective evaluation of the waterproofing qualities, ease of insertion and comfort of commonly available earplugs. *Clin Otolaryngol.* 2004;29(2):128–32.

30. Pai S, Parikh, SR. Otitis media. In: Lalwani AK, ed. *Current Diagnosis and Treatment in Otolaryngology Head and Neck Surgery.* 3rd ed. New York, NY: Lange Medical Books/McGraw Hill; 2012:674–81.

31. Dekelboum AM. Diving medicine. In: Lalwani AK, ed. *Current Diagnosis and Treatment in Otolaryngology Head and Neck Surgery.* 3rd ed. New York, NY: Lange Medical Books/McGraw Hill; 2012:739–46.

32. Gates GA, Clark WW. Occupational hearing loss. In: Lalwani AK, ed. *Current Diagnosis and Treatment in Otolaryngology Head and Neck Surgery.* 3rd ed. New York, NY: Lange Medical Books/McGraw Hill; 2012:747–59.

33. Johnson J, Lalwani AK. Vestibular disorders. In: Lalwani AK, ed. *Current Diagnosis and Treatment in Otolaryngology Head and Neck Surgery.* 3rd ed. New York, NY: Lange Medical Books/McGraw Hill; 2012:729–38.

PREVENTION OF HYGIENE-RELATED ORAL DISORDERS

Daniel Forrister

Dental diseases and disorders impact the health and well-being of Americans throughout their lifespan. Dental caries (tooth decay) is the most common childhood condition, being five times more prevalent than asthma and seven times more prevalent than hay fever. Individuals should receive professional care to maintain oral health, yet 50% of the population is in need of dental treatment. Routine dental care is recommended twice per year for children and adults; children should have their first visit to the dentist within 6 months of getting their first tooth or no later than 12 months of age. Fifty percent of children ages 5–9 years have at least one cavity or filling; this number increases to 78% by the time individuals are 17 years of age. Oral health is reflective of overall general health.[1]

Improper oral hygiene is a direct cause of dental caries, periodontal disease (gingivitis and periodontitis), halitosis, and some cases of denture-related discomfort. Nonprescription products for prevention of oral disease are widely available in pharmacies, food stores, and other retail stores; therefore, educating the public about proper use of these products is the key to preventing dental diseases.

The teeth and supporting structures are necessary for normal mastication and articulation, as well as for normal appearance. The primary (deciduous, or baby) dentition first appears at approximately 6 months of age, when the mandibular (lower jaw) central incisors erupt; the process is usually complete with the eruption of the upper second molars at approximately 24 months of age. Each of the upper and lower arches holds 10 deciduous teeth, 20 in all. Generally, the first permanent dentition (adult tooth) appears when the mandibular first molar erupts behind the deciduous second molar at approximately 6 years of age, and the process continues in a regular pattern, usually replacing shedding deciduous teeth. Of the 32 total permanent teeth, 28 are usually present by age 14; third molars (wisdom teeth) may appear between 17 and 21 years of age.

Anatomically, the teeth are viewed grossly as having two parts, the roots and the crown (Figure 30–1). Normally, the roots are below the gingival (gum) line or margin; roots are essential in supporting and attaching the tooth to the surrounding tissues. The crown is above the gingival margin and is responsible for mastication. Each tooth has four major components: enamel, dentin, pulp, and cementum.

Enamel is composed of very hard, crystalline calcium phosphate salts (hydroxyapatite). It is 1.5–2 mm thick at its thickest part and protects the underlying tooth structure. It covers the crown of the tooth, ending around the gum line at the cementoenamel junction. Enamel's hardness enables the crown to withstand the wear of mastication. Dentin, which is softer, lies beneath the enamel and makes up the largest part of the tooth structure. It is transected by microscopic tubules that transport nutrients from the dental pulp. Dentin protects the dental pulp from mechanical, thermal, and chemical irritation. The bone-like cementum is softer than dentin and covers the root of the tooth, extending apically from the cementoenamel junction.

The pulp occupies the pulp chamber and canal. It is continuous with the tissues surrounding the tooth by an opening at the apex of the root (apical foramen). The pulp consists primarily of vascular and neural tissues. The only nerve endings in the pulp are free nerve endings; therefore, any type of stimulus to the pulp is interpreted as pain.

The periodontium comprises the hard and soft tissues that surround the teeth, including the periodontal ligament, the encompassing alveolar bone, and the gingiva. The tooth is suspended hammock-like in bone by the periodontal ligament. The cementum's major function is to attach the tooth to the periodontal ligament by periodontal fibers. The periodontal ligament is connective tissue that attaches the tooth to the surrounding alveolar bone and gingival tissue. The periodontal ligament performs supportive, formative, sensory, and nutritive functions. The alveolar bone forms the sockets of the teeth. The gingiva is the soft tissue surrounding the teeth. Gingiva is categorized as either keratinized attached gingiva or unkeratinized unattached gingiva. Attached gingiva is normally pink, stippled (like an orange peel), and keratinized. It is attached to the cementum by the gingival group of periodontal ligament fibers.

The major salivary glands (parotid, submandibular, and sublingual) are responsible for secreting saliva, an alkaline, slightly viscous, clear secretion that contains enzymes (lysozymes and ptyalin), albumin, epithelial mucin (a mucopolysaccharide), immunoglobulin, leukocytes, and minerals. Normal salivary gland function promotes good oral health in several ways. First, saliva lubricates and facilitates the removal of carbohydrates and microorganisms from the oral cavity. Second, saliva also buffers the decline in pH caused by the acid formed by carbohydrate fermentation. Third, the mineral components of saliva have a protective role in the demineralization and remineralization of tooth enamel.

Editor's Note: This chapter is based on the 17th edition chapter of the same title, written by Amy W. Rudenko.

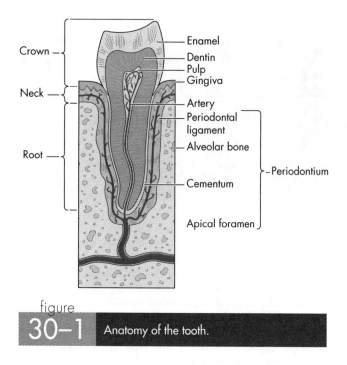

figure

30–1   Anatomy of the tooth.

Caries

The increase in dental caries globally among both children and adults is a great public health concern. Although no consensus exists as to the cause of this increase, health care providers should focus attention on public health strategies that have been successful in reducing caries in the past (e.g., fluoridation of the municipal water supply, topical fluoride treatments, education on proper tooth brushing with a fluoride dentifrice, daily flossing, a proper diet, and regular dental office visits).[2]

Patients with poor oral hygiene are at greatest risk for developing caries. Patients at increased risk for caries include those with orthodontic appliances, xerostomia (dry mouth), and gum tissue recession that exposes root surfaces. Certain medications may cause xerostomia (see Chapter 31); xerostomia is more likely to manifest in patients who have undergone head and neck radiation therapy.

Increased dental caries is also associated with the use of tobacco products, which may be attributable to changes in salivary function, buffering capacity, or composition, including bacterial flora.[3] Because alcohol consumption can cause xerostomia, individuals who consume alcohol may also have a higher risk of caries.

Pathophysiology of Caries

Dental caries is now considered an infectious disease that affects the calcified tissues of the teeth. Certain plaque bacteria generate acid from dietary carbohydrates; the acid demineralizes tooth enamel and dentin, leading to the formation of soft carious lesions (pits or fissures of smooth surface that, if left untreated, will eventually destroy the tooth). Formation of dental caries requires growth and attachment of many cariogenic microorganisms (e.g., *Streptococcus mutans, Lactobacillus casei,* and

Actinomyces viscosus) to exposed tooth surfaces. If oral hygiene is neglected, dental plaque (the biofilm containing these organisms) remains on the tooth surfaces and, in time, attracts more bacteria, thereby promoting decay.

The carious process is characterized by alternating periods of destruction (demineralization) and repair (remineralization). Demineralization is caused by organic acids, (e.g., lactic and formic acids), which are produced (usually anaerobically) by microbial metabolism of low-molecular-weight carbohydrates (sugars) that readily diffuse into plaque. The resulting reduction in pH on the tooth surface causes demineralization of dental enamel. Saliva, which is rich in calcium and phosphate ions, is crucial in remineralizing early carious lesions. The presence of fluoride ions in the mouth also promotes remineralization and slows demineralization, thereby retarding enamel dissolution.

A carious lesion starts slowly on the enamel surface and initially produces no clinical symptoms. Once demineralization progresses through the enamel to the softer dentin, the destruction proceeds much more rapidly, becoming clinically or radiographically evident as a carious lesion. At this point, the patient can become aware of the lesion either by observing it or by experiencing symptoms of sensitivity to stimuli (e.g., heat, cold, or sweet foods) or chewing. If untreated, the carious lesion can damage the dental pulp (with continuous pain as a common symptom) and eventually cause necrosis of vital pulp tissue.

Clinical Presentation of Caries

Plaque is commonly recognized as the source of microbes that cause caries and periodontal disease; therefore, plaque buildup is directly related to the incidence of oral disease. After meals, food residue may be incorporated into plaque by bacterial degradation. Left undisturbed, plaque thickens, and bacteria proliferate. Plaque growth begins in protected cracks and fissures and along the gingival margin. If not removed within 24 hours, dental plaque (especially in areas opposite the salivary glands) begins to calcify by calcium salt precipitation from the saliva, forming calculus, or tartar. This hardened, adherent deposit is removable only by professional dental cleaning.

Calculus is generally considered to be a substrate on which additional plaque can develop and is not considered the primary cause in periodontal disease. However, most periodontists agree that supragingival (above) and subgingival (below the gingival margin) calculus can promote the progression of periodontal disease by accumulating new bacterial plaque in contact with sensitive tissue sites and by interfering with local self-cleaning efforts to remove plaque.

Prevention of Caries
General Approach

The key to preventing caries is controlling dental plaque. Because a combination of diet (carbohydrate substrate), oral bacteria, and host resistance is involved in developing caries, prevention should be aimed at modifying these factors. The frequency of refined carbohydrate intake should be reduced; plaque (which supports cariogenic bacterial growth) should be removed, usually by mechanical means (e.g., brushing and flossing); and host resistance should be increased through appropriate exposure to fluoride ion. Antiplaque products aid in mechanical removal of plaque or retard its buildup. The declining prevalence of dental caries in children in the United States may be attributed to a combination of these interventions (e.g., increased exposure to fluoride in drinking water, dentifrices, and mouth rinses; changed patterns of diet; and overall improved oral hygiene).

Two methods are used to manage plaque: The first is mechanical removal (brushing with a dentifrice and flossing), and the second is chemical management (e.g., using specific products to prevent plaque accumulation or aid its removal). The best way to ensure the health of teeth and gingival tissues is to remove plaque buildup mechanically by brushing at least twice daily and flossing at least once daily. Toothbrushing removes plaque from the lingual (tongue side), buccal (cheek side), and occlusal (biting) surfaces of the teeth. Plaque found on interproximal (between the teeth) surfaces can only be removed efficiently with dental floss and other interdental cleaning aids (e.g., interproximal brush, dental tape, and tapered picks).

Nonpharmacologic Therapy

Dietary Measures

Cariogenic foods and beverages should be avoided in favor of those that are less cariogenic. A food is considered highly cariogenic if it contains more than 15% sugar, clings to the teeth, and remains in the mouth after it is chewed. Conversely, foods are less cariogenic if they have a high water content (e.g., fresh fruit); stimulate the flow of saliva (e.g., carrots and other fibrous foods that require a lot of chewing); or are high in protein (e.g., dairy products). Both the water content of fresh fruit and the resulting flow of saliva tend to wash away the fruit's sugar and neutralize the acid it creates. Milk protein also raises pH and tends to inhibit binding of bacteria.

Oral hygiene products (e.g., mouth rinses and dentifrices) may contain a low concentration of saccharin, which is a potent noncariogenic sugar substitute that appears to present no caries hazard. Other noncariogenic sugar substitutes such as sugar alcohols (sorbitol and xylitol) and aspartame (amino acid methyl ester) are currently used as sweetening agents.

Plaque Removal Devices

Toothbrushes, dental floss, oral irrigating devices, and specialty aids (e.g., interproximal dental brushes) are the primary devices used in facilitating plaque removal.

---

table

30–1   Guidelines for Brushing Teeth

- Brush teeth after each meal or at least twice a day.
- If using toothpaste, apply a small amount of paste to the toothbrush.
- Use a gentle scrubbing motion with the bristle tips at a 45-degree angle against the gum line so that the tips of the brush do the cleaning.
- Do not use excessive force because it may result in bristle damage, cervical abrasion, irritation of delicate gingival tissue, and gingival recession with associated hypersensitivity.
- Brush for at least 2 minutes, cleaning all tooth surfaces systematically.
- Gently brush the upper surface of the tongue to reduce debris, plaque, and bacteria that can cause oral hygiene problems.
- Rinse the mouth, and spit out all the water.

Toothbrushes

The toothbrush is the most universally accepted device available for removing dental plaque and maintaining good oral hygiene.

The proper frequency and method of brushing will vary from patient to patient. Thoroughness of plaque removal without gingival trauma is more important than the method used. Table 30–1 describes the proper method of brushing teeth.

Manual toothbrushes vary in size, shape, texture, and design, with new product designs proliferating rapidly. These toothbrushes have either nylon or natural bristles that are usually rated as soft, medium, or firm.

Powered toothbrushes (which are widely available on the market) are either battery operated or have a rechargeable battery system. The battery-operated devices (e.g., the Arm & Hammer Spinbrush and Colgate 360 Sonic Power Toothbrush) use a rotary and/or vibratory motion and are less expensive, but their effectiveness deteriorates over time as the disposable battery loses power. Rechargeable battery toothbrushes use a rotary and/or vibrating motion (e.g., Oral B) or ultrasonic vibration (e.g., Sonicare and Oral B) to remove plaque. These power brushes tend to be more expensive, but they maintain constant efficiency because of their rechargeability. Powered toothbrushes may benefit certain patients, such as those who are disabled or who have dexterity issues.[1]

Patients can expect best results by using a brush carrying the American Dental Association's (ADA) Seal of Acceptance described in the box The American Dental Association Seal of Acceptance[4] and by following a dental professional's specific

---

the american dental association

Seal of Acceptance

ADA evaluates the safety and efficacy of dental products used by dental professionals and the public through the Council on Scientific Affairs' Seal of Acceptance evaluation program. Manufacturers of dentifrices or mouth rinses with therapeutic potential for gingivitis and supragingival dental plaque control may voluntarily submit data to ADA for evaluation. Product labels and promotional material must also comply with ADA standards.[5]

The ADA Council on Scientific Affairs allows only products that demonstrate a significant effect against gingivitis to make plaque-control or plaque-modification claims. A product that can demonstrate significant plaque reduction but no concomitant significant reduction in gingivitis will not be eligible for acceptance.[10] ADA has approved two statements to be used for products classified under

these guidelines—one for both gingivitis and plaque reduction, and one for gingivitis reduction only:

- [Product name] has been shown to help prevent and reduce [whichever is appropriate] gingivitis [and supragingival plaque accumulation] when used as directed in a conscientiously applied program of oral hygiene and regular professional care. Its effect on periodontitis has not been determined.[10]

Once a product has earned the ADA seal, it may display that seal for 3 years, provided it continues to meet all the requirements.[5] The ADA online home page (www.ada.org) provides searchable access to a current listing of dental consumer products that have been awarded the ADA Seal of Acceptance.

directions for use. The ADA criteria for acceptance are based on safety and efficacy concerns. Research has shown no evidence of a statistically significant difference in the effectiveness between powered and manual toothbrushes. Although electric toothbrushes appear to significantly reduce plaque and gingivitis in both the short- and long-term, the clinical significance of this finding is unknown.[5]

No definite guideline exists as to how often a patient should buy a new toothbrush, although 3 months has been suggested as the average toothbrush life expectancy. Marketing data suggest that consumers, on average, replace their toothbrushes only 1.7 times per year. Two compelling reasons exist for replacing toothbrushes frequently: wear and bacterial accumulation. Different brushing methods cause bristles to wear differently. Worn, bent, or matted bristles do not remove plaque effectively. Therefore, patients should replace toothbrushes at the first sign of bristle wear, rather than after a defined period of use. Ideally, they should rotate among 2 or 3 toothbrushes to allow each to dry completely between uses, thereby decreasing bristle wear and matting. Some brands of toothbrushes have color-impregnated bristles that indicate the need for replacement when the color disappears halfway down the bristles.

Product Selection Guidelines. Dental professionals recommend toothbrushes according to the individual patient's manual dexterity, oral anatomy, and periodontal health. The toothbrush should be of a size and shape to allow the patient to reach every tooth in the mouth. Innovations in head shapes and bristle configurations continue to be introduced in an attempt to improve cleaning contact with tooth and gum line surfaces. Toothbrush firmness is not standardized; toothbrushes designated as soft, medium, or hard may not be comparable across manufacturers. Use of medium- or hard-bristled toothbrushes may result in damage to the tooth enamel and gingival tissue. Softer bristles are more effective at working themselves into crevices and spaces between the teeth, and they are less abrasive on teeth with exposed recession. Many dentists and dental hygienists prefer soft, rounded, multi-tufted, nylon bristle brushes, because nylon bristles are more durable and easier to clean than natural bristles, and because soft, rounded bristle tips are more effective in removing plaque below the gingival margin and on proximal tooth surfaces.

The handle size and shape of a toothbrush should allow the individual to maneuver the brush easily while maintaining a firm grasp. Many modifications (e.g., angle bends or flexible areas in the handle) that may improve contact between the bristles and some less-accessible tooth surfaces have been introduced. Dentists can fabricate customized handles for physically impaired individuals by adding moldable acrylic to the handles.

Children's toothbrushes are smaller than adult toothbrushes and are available in two sizes: baby (for children up to 6 or 7 years of age) and junior (for children 7 years of age to teens). Toothbrush size and shape should be individualized according to the size of the child's mouth. Soft bristles are recommended for children's toothbrushes. Children can usually remove plaque more easily with a brush that has short and narrow bristles.

Dental Floss

Plaque accumulation in the interdental spaces contributes to proximal caries and periodontal pocketing. Interdental plaque removal has been reported to reduce gingival inflammation and prevent periodontal disease and dental caries. Dental flossing is the most widely recommended method of removing dental plaque from proximal tooth surfaces that are not adequately cleaned by toothbrushing alone. By removing plaque and debris interproximally, proper flossing also polishes the tooth surfaces and reduces gingival inflammation. Proper flossing technique requires some finger dexterity and practice. If performed improperly, flossing can injure gingival tissue and cause cervical wear on proximal root surfaces.[1] Table 30–2 describes the proper use of dental floss.

Most floss is a multifilament nylon yarn that is available in waxed or unwaxed form and in varying widths, from thin thread to thick tape. Many brands feature product lines of flosses that are impregnated or coated with additives, such as flavoring, baking soda, and fluoride. In addition, several manufacturers are marketing floss made of materials with superior antishredding properties (e.g., Glide and Oral B Essential). ADA has recognized nearly 30 brands of dental floss and tape as safe and effective.[5]

Product Selection Guidelines. Because no particular product has been proved superior, patient factors (e.g., tightness of tooth contacts, tooth roughness, manual dexterity, and personal preference) should be considered in product selection. Similarly, clinical studies show no difference between various floss types in terms of removing plaque and preventing gingivitis.[6] Evidence does not support concern about waxed floss leaving a residual wax film on tooth surfaces.

Waxed floss may pass interproximally between tight-fitting teeth with less shredding than unwaxed floss. Teflon floss (e.g., Glide), also resists shredding and slips easily between tight teeth. If contacts at the crowns of teeth are too tight to force floss interdentally, floss threaders can be used to pass floss between the teeth and under the replacement teeth (pontics) of fixed bridges. Floss threaders (available in reusable and disposable forms) are usually thin plastic loops or soft plastic, needle-like appliances. Patients who wear braces may find that the use of threaders aids in the flossing process. Electrically powered interdental cleaning devices may be used to remove interproximal debris. However, electrically powered interdental devices or floss threaders should be used cautiously to avoid physical trauma of the gingiva.[7] Floss holders have one or two forks that are rigid enough to keep floss taut and a mounting mechanism that allows quick rethreading of floss. These products are recommended for patients who lack manual dexterity and for caregivers who assist disabled or hospitalized patients.

table 30–2	Guidelines for Using Dental Floss

- Pull out approximately 18 inches of floss, and wrap most of it around the middle finger.
- Wrap the remaining floss around the same finger of the opposite hand. About an inch of floss should be held between the thumbs and forefingers.
- Do not snap the floss between the teeth; instead, use a gentle, sawing motion to guide the floss to the gum line.
- When the gum line is reached, curve the floss into a C-shape against one tooth, and gently slide the floss into the space between the gum and tooth until you feel resistance.
- Hold the floss tightly against the tooth, and gently scrape the side of the tooth with an up and down motion.
- Curve the floss around the adjoining tooth, and repeat the procedure.

Specialty Aids

Cleaning devices that adapt to irregular tooth surfaces better than dental floss are recommended for interproximal cleaning of teeth with large interdental spaces. These large interdental spaces are often characteristic of periodontal disease. The G-U-M Flossbrush is such a device; it features woven dental floss that contains a time-release fluoride system and is molded into a plastic handle for interdental cleaning. The most common aids are tapered triangular wooden toothpicks (Stim-U-Dent), holders for round toothpicks (Perio-Aid), miniature bottle brushes (Proxabrush), rubber stimulator tips, denture brushes, and denture clasp brushes.

Oral Irrigating Devices

Oral irrigators work by directing a high-pressure stream of water through a nozzle to the tooth surfaces. These devices can remove only a minimal amount of plaque from tooth surfaces. Therefore, oral irrigators cannot be viewed as substitutes for a toothbrush, dental floss, or other plaque-removal devices, but they should be considered as adjuncts in maintaining good oral hygiene. These devices are useful for removing loose debris from those areas that cannot be cleaned with a toothbrush (e.g., around orthodontic bands and fixed bridges). Several brands on the market carry the ADA Seal of Acceptance.[5]

Oral irrigators are also valuable as vehicles for administering chemotherapeutic agents that inhibit microbial growth in inaccessible regions of the mouth. Patients with advanced periodontal disease should use these devices only under professional supervision because transient bacteremia may occur after manipulative procedures with the oral irrigator. Oral irrigation devices are also contraindicated in patients who are predisposed to bacterial endocarditis.

Pharmacologic Therapy

Chemical Management of Plaque

Chemical management of plaque and calculus can enhance mechanical removal either by acting directly on the plaque bacteria or by disrupting components of plaque to aid in its removal during routine oral hygiene. The use of chemical agents in plaque control may be particularly appropriate for selected patients who may be unable to brush and floss effectively. Physically or mentally disabled individuals (who may not be able to master the manual techniques necessary to brush and floss effectively) and orthodontia patients (i.e., those with fixed prostheses) may benefit from adding antiplaque agents to their oral hygiene regimen.

Desirable characteristics for antiplaque agents include the following:

- Selective antibacterial activity; interference with the rate of accumulation or metabolism of supragingival plaque
- Substantivity (sustained retention of the agent in the mouth)
- Compatibility with dentifrice ingredients
- Lack of undesirable side effects for the user
- Noninterference with the natural ecology of the normal oral microflora

Use of Fluoride

Fluoride is believed to help prevent dental caries through a combination of effects. When it is incorporated into developing teeth, fluoride systemically reduces the solubility of dental enamel by enhancing the development of a fluoridated hydroxyapatite (which is more resistant to demineralizing acids) at the enamel surface. The topical effect facilitates remineralization of early carious lesions during repeated cycles of demineralization and remineralization. Some evidence exists that fluoride interferes with the bacterial cariogenic process. Fluoride that is chemically bound to organic constituents of plaque may interfere with plaque adherence and may inhibit glycolysis (the process by which sugar is metabolized to produce acid).[1]

Fluoridation of the public water supply is an effective and economically sound public health measure that has played a major role in decreasing the incidence of caries.[8] According to the Centers for Disease Control, nearly 70% of the U.S. population resides in communities in which the public water supply contains either naturally occurring or added fluoride at optimal levels for decay prevention (1 ppm or 1 mg/L). In addition to reducing dental caries in children, fluoridation has benefits that extend through adulthood, resulting in (1) fewer decayed, missing, or filled teeth; (2) greater tooth retention; and (3) a lower incidence of root caries. Systemic fluoride supplementation in children is based on the preventive mechanism of fluoride when incorporated into developing enamel. Current concepts of the action of fluoride relative to its presence in saliva and plaque provide a rationale for its topical application to prevent caries in all age groups. Any decision to supplement fluoride intake must factor in the concentration of fluoride already present in the drinking water.[1] Bottled water does not contain fluoride.

Mouth rinses and gels that contain sodium fluoride are therapeutic topical applications of fluoride for prevention of dental caries (Table 30–3). Fluoride mouth rinsing enables patients to apply fluoride interproximally.

Patients who may benefit from fluoride rinsing include those with orthodontic appliances, those with decreased salivary flow, those at risk for developing root caries, and anyone with difficulty maintaining good oral hygiene. Orthodontic patients are at risk of developing decalcified areas during treatment, and their ability to thoroughly clean interdental spaces may be inhibited.

Because fluoride rinses and gels provide a therapeutic fluoride treatment, package directions should be followed closely to maximize the safe and effective use of these products. Table 30–4 describes the proper method of applying fluoride treatments.[9] When recommending a nonprescription fluoride mouth rinse, the health care provider should stress that parents and caregivers should supervise children younger than 12 years as necessary until they are capable of using the product correctly.

table 30–3 Selected Nonprescription Topical Fluoride Products

Trade Name	Primary Ingredient
ACT Anticavity Fluoride Rinse	Sodium fluoride 0.05%
Gel-Kam Gel	Stannous fluoride 0.4%
Crest Pro-Health For Me Anti-Cavity Fluoride Rinse	Sodium fluoride 0.022%
Phos-Flur Fluoride Rinse	Sodium fluoride 0.044%

- Use topical fluoride treatments no more than once a day.
- Brush teeth with a fluoride dentifrice before using a fluoride treatment.
- If using a fluoride rinse, measure the recommended dose (most commonly 10 mL), and vigorously swish it between the teeth for 1 minute.
- If using a fluoride gel, brush the gel on the teeth. Allow the gel to remain for 1 minute.
- After 1 minute, spit out the fluoride product. Do not swallow it.
- Do not eat or drink for 30 minutes after the treatment.
- Supervise children as necessary until they can use the product without supervision.
- Instruct children younger than 12 years in good rinsing habits to minimize swallowing of the product.
- Consult a dentist or primary care provider before using fluoride products in children younger than 6 years.

Furthermore, children younger than 6 years should use these products only as directed by a dentist or primary care provider.

Dental fluorosis (a mottled appearance of the surface enamel of the tooth) may develop in certain children. Fluorosis develops in children who, during the time of tooth formation, receive optimal fluoride intake from the water supply or from supplements but inadvertently ingest additional fluoride from dentifrices. Although a mild degree of fluorosis is an aesthetic concern, more severe cases can result in pitting and surface defects (see Color Plates, photograph 5).

In response to the aesthetic concerns related to fluorosis, FDA considered issuing comments regarding formulation of a reduced-strength fluoride dentifrice during the anticaries final rule process. FDA determined that, unlike dental caries, mild dental fluorosis does not compromise oral health or tooth function; therefore, the risk of dental caries from inadequate fluoride protection is a greater health hazard than the cosmetic effect of fluorosis.

Dentifrices

Dentifrices (e.g., toothpastes or gels) are used with a toothbrush for cleaning accessible tooth surfaces. Use of a dentifrice enhances removal of dental plaque and stains, resulting in a decreased incidence of dental caries and gum disease, reduced mouth odors, and enhanced personal appearance.

Dentifrices are available as pastes or gels (Table 30–5). The gels and pastes commonly contain an abrasive, a surfactant, a humectant (moistening agent), a binder/thickener, a sweetener, flavoring agents, and one or more therapeutic agents (e.g., fluoride) for anticaries activity.

Dentifrice abrasives are pharmacologically inactive and insoluble compounds; common abrasives include silicates, dicalcium phosphate, alumina trihydrate, calcium pyrophosphate, calcium carbonate, and sodium metaphosphate. Although dentifrices vary in their degree of abrasiveness, factors such as the size and shape of the abrasive particle, individual brushing technique, and individual salivary characteristics affect the abrasive's potential effectiveness.[1] The ideal abrasive would provide maximal cleaning aid while causing minimal damage to tooth surfaces. Unfortunately, because of the variability in patients' brushing

techniques and oral conditions, the ideal dentifrice abrasive does not exist. Low-abrasive dentifrices (including most dentifrice formulations currently marketed in the United States) usually have a low concentration of silica abrasives (10%–25%), whereas high-abrasive dentifrices typically have higher concentrations of the inorganic calcium or aluminum salts previously mentioned (40%–50%). Baking soda, a mild abrasive, is found in a number of dentifrices. Although they are safe to use, toothpastes with baking soda have not been shown to clean teeth better than toothpastes without it.

Fluoride Dentifrices

Fluoride dentifrices are indicated for both preventing and treating carious lesions. All countries that show a reduction in caries use fluoride-containing dentifrices for caries prevention. ADA accepts fluoride-containing toothpaste and fluoride-containing gel dentifrice formulations with compatible abrasives as safe and effective. Concentrations of various fluoride dentifrices are outlined in Table 30–6.

About 10%–20% of patients experience slight (but noticeable) tooth discoloration after using stannous fluoride continuously for 2–3 months. The staining is not permanent and is readily removed at the next professional dental cleaning. Stannous fluoride is for use by adults and children ages 12 years and older.

Tartar-Control Dentifrices

A number of fluoride dentifrices contain anticalculus (tartar control) compounds. Although plaque—not supragingival calculus— is the primary etiologic factor in marginal periodontal disease, reducing calculus formation remains a goal of good oral hygiene. The ingredients that prevent or retard new calculus formation are zinc chloride, zinc citrate, and soluble pyrophosphates (which act to inhibit crystal growth).

ADA regards the inhibition of supragingival calculus as a nontherapeutic use and, therefore, does not evaluate anticalculus claims. However, all advertising claims made for accepted products are reviewed for accuracy. ADA has directed that the following additional statement appear on all package and container labeling for accepted fluoride dentifrice products with calculus-control activity: "[Product name] has been shown to help prevent and reduce [whichever is appropriate] gingivitis and supragingival plaque formation when used as directed in a conscientiously applied program of oral hygiene and regular professional care. Its effect on periodontitis has not been determined."[10]

The use of tartar-control toothpastes has been associated with a type of contact dermatitis in the perioral region. Adding pyrophosphate compounds to these products increases alkalinity and requires increased concentrations of other components for solubilizing (e.g., flavorings and surfactants). The pyrophosphates (either alone or in combination with the higher concentrations of inactive ingredients) are hypothesized to be the cause of irritant contact dermatitis. Patients experiencing such a reaction should be advised to discontinue the tartar-control dentifrice and should switch to a non–tartar-control fluoride product.

Antiplaque/Antigingivitis Dentifrices

Colgate Total contains triclosan, an antibacterial agent and promoter of substantivity that has antigingivitis and antiplaque activity. The product also contains fluoride for caries protection and a copolymer delivery system for the triclosan. This toothpaste is currently accepted by ADA for both antiplaque and

table 30–5 Selected Nonprescription Dentifrices

Trade Name	Primary Ingredients
Fluoride Toothpastes	
Aquafresh Extra Fresh Toothpaste	Calcium carbonate; hydrated silica; sodium monofluorophosphate (fluoride 0.15%)
Colgate Cavity Protection Toothpaste	Dicalcium phosphate dihydrate; sodium monofluorophosphate (fluoride 0.15%)
Crest Cavity Protection Gel	Hydrated silica; sodium fluoride (fluoride 0.15%)
Tartar-Control Toothpastes	
Aquafresh Tartar Protection Whitening Toothpaste	Hydrated silica; sodium fluoride (fluoride 0.15%); tetrapotassium pyrophosphate; tetrasodium pyrophosphate
Colgate Tartar Protection Whitening Toothpaste	Hydrated silica; sodium fluoride (fluoride 0.15%); pentasodium triphosphate; tetrasodium pyrophosphate
Crest Tartar Protection Gel/Toothpaste	Hydrated silica; sodium fluoride (fluoride 0.15%); tetrapotassium pyrophosphate; disodium pyrophosphate; tetrasodium pyrophosphate
Antiplaque/Antigingivitis Toothpastes	
Colgate Total Gum Defense Toothpaste	Hydrated silica; sodium fluoride (fluoride 0.24%); triclosan 0.3%
Crest Pro-Health Clinical Gum Protection Toothpaste	Hydrated silica; stannous fluoride (fluoride 0.16%); sodium hexametaphosphate; trisodium phosphate
Whitening Toothpastes	
Aquafresh Ultimate White Toothpaste	Hydrated silica; sodium fluoride (fluoride 0.15%); titanium dioxide
Colgate Optic White Toothpaste	Sodium monofluorophosphate (fluoride 0.15%); tetrasodium pyrophosphate; hydrogen peroxide
Rembrandt Deeply White Plus Peroxide Whitening Toothpaste	Hydrated silica; urea peroxide; sodium monofluorophosphate
Sodium Lauryl Sulfate-Free Toothpastes	
Biotène Antibacterial Dry Mouth Toothpaste	Lactoperoxidase; glucose oxidase; lysozyme; lactoferrin; sodium monofluorophosphate 0.14%
Sensodyne Iso-Active Toothpaste	Potassium nitrate 5%; sodium fluoride (fluoride 0.15%)
Botanical-Based Toothpastes	
Tom's of Maine Botanically Bright	Peppermint or spearmint; carrageenan; propolis
Jason Powersmile Whitening Toothpaste	Calcium carbonate; carrageenan; bamboo powder; parsley extract; grapefruit seed extract; peppermint; sodium bicarbonate

table 30–6 FDA-Approved Active Ingredients for Anticaries Dentifrices

Ingredient	Concentration (ppm) (dosage form)
Sodium fluoride	850–1150 (paste)
Sodium monofluorophosphate	850–1150 (paste)
Stannous fluoride	850–1150 (paste)

antigingivitis indications.[5,10] Approval was based on clinical data for safety and efficacy. The product is not intended for use in children younger than 6 years.

Whitening/Antistain Dentifrices

Cosmetic dentifrices make no therapeutic claims and are usually chosen by patients because of taste, whitening ability, or antistain properties. Some dentifrices that claim to remove coffee or tobacco stains may contain higher concentrations of abrasives. High-abrasive formulations are not advised for long-term use or for use by patients with exposed root surfaces. Plain baking soda (a water-soluble, mild abrasive) and toothpastes containing baking soda have limited polishing and stain-removal capacity. Other products may contain a pigment (e.g., titanium dioxide) that produces a temporary brightening effect. Rembrandt Whitening

a word about

Tooth-Bleaching Products

The popularity of tooth bleaching has increased in the United States in recent years. Three methods are currently in use: (1) in-office dental bleaching, (2) dental office–supported home bleaching, and (3) nonprescription home bleaching. All three methods use basically the same chemical agents: carbamide peroxide or hydrogen peroxide in various strengths. The in-office method has the advantage of a one-time treatment, but the stronger bleach and the accelerator light are not necessary to obtain the same result with the dental office–supported home-bleaching process. The latter method involves the use of custom trays. With this process, patients can fine-tune the extent of lightening to their own preferences.

The following two nonprescription products (from among many) may aid in lightening teeth:

■ Rembrandt Intense Stain Dissolving Strips contain hydrogen peroxide. The kit contains 56 whitening strips that are applied to upper and lower teeth. Strips dissolve in 5–10 minutes with nothing to remove. The kit is designed for use over a 2-week period.

■ Crest 3D WhiteStrips Vivid provide translucent film strips impregnated with hydrogen peroxide and other ingredients. The strips are peeled away from a protective backing and folded over the six upper or lower front teeth (different strips are provided for upper and lower teeth). The teeth will look as though they are covered with small pieces of transparent food wrap. The strips are applied once a day and left in place for 30 minutes. A kit contains enough strips for 10 days. An Advanced version of the same system is also available over the counter and is used for a longer period of time.

Toothpaste contains a chemical complex of aluminum oxide, a citrate salt, and papain. Whitening dentifrices that contain oxygenating agents rely on a debriding action to remove stained pellicle. Numerous products offer a combination of baking soda and peroxide with fluoride. Whitening dentifrices should not be confused with tooth-bleaching products described in the box A Word about Tooth-Bleaching Products.

Administration Guidelines

Table 30–1 describes the proper method for brushing teeth using a fluoride dentifrice. Children are usually unable to brush by themselves until they are 4 or 5 years of age; to clean their teeth effectively, children may require supervision until 8 or 9 years of age. FDA recommends that parents instruct children ages 6–12 years about good brushing and rinsing habits to minimize swallowing of fluoride. Parents should apply only a pea-sized amount of toothpaste to a child-sized toothbrush and should brush preschoolers' teeth until the children can manage toothbrushing properly without assistance. Children should be taught to rinse thoroughly and expectorate after brushing. Only regular-strength fluoride toothpaste is recommended for use in children 2–6 years of age. Fluoride toothpaste should be used in children younger than 2 years only under the direction of a dentist or primary care provider. Non-fluoridated pediatric toothpastes are advised for young children who may ingest toothpaste instead of rinsing and expectorating.

All fluoride dentifrice products must contain the following warning on the labeling: "Warning: Keep out of the reach of children under 6 years of age. If you accidentally swallow more than used for brushing, seek professional assistance or contact a Poison Control Center immediately."

Product Selection Guidelines

Unless otherwise advised by their dentists, patients (especially those with periodontal disease, significant gum recession, and/or exposed root surfaces) should choose the least abrasive dentifrice that effectively removes stained pellicle. Although dentifrice abrasives do not pose a risk to dental enamel, toothbrushing action and excessive abrasiveness (which may lead to tooth hypersensitivity) can damage the cementum (the softer material of exposed root surfaces) and dentin.

Children younger than 6 years should not use a fluoride dentifrice unless their parents can ensure the children can rinse and expectorate appropriately. Extra-strength fluoride dentifrices may be beneficial to patients who have a greater tendency to develop cavities or who reside in an area with non-fluoridated water.

Flavored gel dentifrices disperse rapidly in the mouth and are popular with children. Manufacturers of gel dentifrices have advertised that children brush longer and more thoroughly because of the gel's consistency, translucence, dispersibility, and flavor. This claim has not been substantiated, but many dentifrices marketed for children are of the gel type. Children's products usually have fruit flavors rather than the breath-freshening minty or cinnamon flavors that adults prefer.

Mouth Rinses

A mouth rinse with plaque- or calculus-control properties is indicated as an adjunct to proper flossing and toothbrushing with fluoride toothpaste. Further research is necessary to determine the efficacy of the antiplaque activity of these products.

Mouth rinse and dentifrice formulations are very similar. As with dentifrices, mouth rinses may be cosmetic or therapeutic (Table 30–7). Both may contain surfactants, humectants, flavor, coloring, water, and therapeutic ingredients.

A mouth rinse approximates a diluted liquid dentifrice that contains alcohol but no abrasive. Alcohol adds bite and freshness, enhances flavor, solubilizes other ingredients, and contributes to the mouth rinse's cleansing action and antibacterial activity. Flavor contributes pleasant taste and breath freshening action. Surfactants are foaming agents that aid in the removal of debris. Other active ingredients may include astringents (alum or zinc chloride), demulcents (sorbitol or glycerin), antibacterial agents (cetylpyridinium chloride or thymol), and fluoride.

Cosmetic mouth rinses freshen the breath and clean some debris from the mouth. Mouth rinses can be classified by appearance, flavor, alcohol content, and active ingredients. In general, mouth rinses are minty or spicy, or medicinal or alcoholic, and contain various ingredients such as (1) glycerin, a topical protectant that tastes sweet and is soothing to oral mucosa; (2) benzoic acid, an antimicrobial agent; or (3) zinc chloride/citrate, an astringent that neutralizes odoriferous sulfur compounds

table 30–7	Selected Nonprescription Mouth Rinses
Trade Name	**Primary Ingredients**
Cosmetic Mouth Rinses	
Biotène	Lactoferrin; lysozyme; lactoperoxidase; aloe vera gel; glucose oxidase
Lavoris	Clove oil; zinc chloride; zinc oxide
Therapeutic Mouth Rinses	
Crest Pro-Health Rinse	Cetylpyridinium chloride 0.07%
Crest Pro-Health Clinical Rinse	Cetylpyridinium chloride 0.1%
Gly-Oxide	Carbamide peroxide 10%
Scope	Cetylpyridinium chloride
Botanical-Based Mouthwashes	
Listerine	Thymol; eucalyptol; methyl salicylate; menthol
Tom's of Maine	Peppermint or spearmint; xylitol; menthol

produced in the oral cavity. The most popular cosmetic mouth rinses are medicinal and mint flavored. Healthy individuals normally have some degree of oral malodor (e.g., morning breath). This malodor results from reduced activity of tongue, cheeks, and salivary flow, which enhances bacterial activity and production of odoriferous sulfur compounds. Therefore, products that are intended to eliminate or suppress mouth odor of local origin in healthy people with healthy mouths are considered by the FDA Advisory Review Panel on Over-the-Counter Oral Health Care Products to be cosmetics, unless they contain antimicrobial or other therapeutic agents. ADA's acceptance program does not evaluate mouth rinses labeled and advertised as only cosmetic agents.

One important consideration is the potential for breath-freshening mouth rinses to disguise or delay treatment of pathologic conditions that may contribute to lingering oral malodor (e.g., periodontal disease, purulent oral infections, and respiratory infections). If marked breath odor persists after proper toothbrushing, the cause should be investigated and not masked with mouth rinse.

Since the 1990s, nonprescription mouth rinses promoted for antiplaque or tartar-control activity have proliferated. Plaque control ingredients include (1) aromatic oils (thymol, eucalyptol, menthol, and methyl salicylate), which are antibacterial and have some local anesthetic activity; and (2) agents with antimicrobial activity (e.g., quaternary ammonium compounds). Listerine, containing the active ingredients thymol, eucalyptol, methyl salicylate, and menthol, was the first mouth rinse to be accepted by ADA as a nonprescription antiplaque/antigingivitis mouth rinse. The phenol oils (active ingredients) control plaque by destroying bacterial cell walls, inhibiting bacterial enzymes, and extracting bacterial lipopolysaccharides. ADA has since added Cool Mint, FreshBurst Listerine, and more than

100 similarly formulated private-label antiseptic mouth rinses to the antiplaque/antigingivitis category of accepted therapeutic products.[5]

Many dental providers have found anecdotally that use of rinses containing phenol oils, methyl salicylate, and alcohol may bring about a sloughing of the oral epithelium, which subsides when the rinse is discontinued. A similar event seems to occur with the use of lozenges or candies containing cinnamon or other common flavoring substances.

Mouth rinses and gels are generally safe when used as directed, but occasional adverse reactions (e.g., burning sensation or irritation) have been reported. Overuse should be discouraged. Consultation with a health professional is indicated if irritation occurs and persists after the patient discontinues use of the product. The detergent sodium lauryl sulfate is present in nearly all toothpastes and has been implicated as a cause of oral mucosal irritations such as aphthous ulcers (canker sores; see Chapter 31).[11] Some dentifrices that do not contain sodium lauryl sulfate are listed in Table 30–5.

Unsupervised use of mouth rinses is contraindicated in patients with mouth irritation or ulceration. These products should be kept out of children's reach. In case of accidental ingestion, the caregiver should seek professional assistance or contact a poison control center.

The alcohol content in mouth rinses ranges from 0% to 27%; the most popular adult mouth rinses contain between 14% and 27%. Ingestion of alcohol-containing products poses a danger for children, who may be attracted by the products' bright colors and pleasant flavors. Toxicity data concerning children's ingestion of alcohol-containing mouth rinses demonstrate that the amount of alcohol in available mouth rinse preparations is sufficient to cause serious illness and injury. Acute alcoholic intoxication and death resulting from high-dose ingestion are possible. For a child weighing 26 pounds, 5–10 ounces of a mouth rinse containing alcohol can be lethal.[1] Responding to concern over the potential danger to children, the Consumer Products Safety Commission issued a final rule that required child-resistant packaging for mouth rinses containing 3 grams or more of absolute alcohol per package—the amount that is present in a small quantity (approximately 2.6 ounces) of a mouth rinse with alcohol 5%: For the purposes of this final rule, the term *mouthwash* includes liquid products that are variously called mouthwashes, mouth rinses, oral antiseptics, gargles, fluoride rinses, antiplaque rinses, and breath fresheners. The rule does not include throat sprays or aerosol breath fresheners. These products should be kept out of children's reach and should not be administered to children younger than 12 years. Labeling includes a warning not to swallow the product but to seek professional assistance or contact a poison control center immediately in case of accidental ingestion.

Special Population Considerations for Plaque Removal

At birth, the 20 primary teeth that will erupt are present but not visible. Oral hygiene must be started early in life. Accordingly, the health care provider should recommend that caregivers remove plaque and milk residue from a baby's mouth after each feeding by wiping the baby's gums with a wet gauze pad. The deciduous teeth will usually start to erupt at about 6 months of age and can decay at any time. "Baby bottle caries" results when an infant is allowed to nurse continuously from a bottle of juice, milk, or sugar water. The prolonged contact of teeth with the cariogenic liquid promotes caries.

When the teeth have erupted, a soft, child-sized toothbrush can be used for cleaning. Parents must do the brushing and should take care to use only a very small amount of fluoride toothpaste or none at all. Children at this age will swallow the toothpaste, which will contribute to overall systemic fluoride ingestion. Therefore, younger children need to be taught the proper brushing technique and should be supervised while brushing.

In patients with fixed orthodontia, very careful attention to oral hygiene to prevent gingivitis and caries is required because of the ease with which plaque accumulates along the orthodontic brackets. Patients with these appliances require a combination of toothbrush types to clean all surfaces effectively. Use of power toothbrushes or oral irrigating devices may help remove plaque and debris around orthodontic bands. Orthodontic patients may want to use a nonprescription fluoride mouth rinse while undergoing treatment.

Patients with removable orthodontic appliances should consult their orthodontist about using a denture cleanser. In addition to brushing orthodontic appliances, some dental providers recommend a denture cleanser to remove plaque, tartar, odor-causing bacteria, and stain that accumulate on orthodontic appliances.

In patients of advanced age who have natural dentition, topical fluoride application in the form of a dentifrice, rinse, or gel is indicated to prevent coronal and root caries. Health care providers should continue to recommend fluoride anticaries products to their older adult patients. When counseling an older patient on oral health care, the provider must consider the patient's medication use. Because this population is more likely to be taking multiple medications, the incidence of drug-induced or disease-related changes in oral physiology is increased.

Assessment of Caries

When asked to recommend plaque-control products, the provider should determine what dental care measures the patient is taking, whether these measures meet recommended oral hygiene standards, and how often the patient sees a dentist. The patient's concern about caries should alert the provider to ask whether the patient has a history of caries or if the patient suspects that a new carious lesion has developed. Refer patients with dental caries symptoms (toothache; tooth sensitivity with chewing; or tooth pain with hot, cold, or sweet foods or beverages) to their dentist for evaluation and treatment.

Patient Counseling for Caries

The provider should tailor all explanations of the purposes of various oral hygiene products and the methods for using them to the patient's level of knowledge. Patients with a history of caries should be encouraged to brush after meals and to consult with a dentist regarding the use of topical fluoride products. If caries recur or are widespread, the patient should be encouraged to visit a dentist for treatment. The provider may recommend products with anticaries agents (e.g., chlorhexidine or xylitol). The provider should explain the precautions for these products as well as the possible adverse effects of some therapeutic

ingredients in other products. Patients should be advised of signs and symptoms that indicate a dental evaluation is necessary. The box Patient Education for Prevention of Caries, Gingivitis, and Halitosis lists specific information to provide patients about plaque-induced oral disorders.

Gingivitis

Periodontal disease (which may result in tooth loss) affects an estimated 47% of U.S. adults ages 30 years and older.[12] Controlling buildup of plaque can prevent or control this common and significant public health problem. All forms of periodontal disease are associated with oral hygiene status, not with age. However, as life spans increase and people retain more teeth later in life, both the number of teeth at risk and the time for development of periodontal disease increase.[1]

Gingivitis, the mildest form of periodontal disease, is common and reversible. Gingivitis may progress to more severe periodontal diseases (e.g., acute necrotizing ulcerative gingivitis and periodontitis, the latter of which can cause significant, irreversible alveolar bone loss).

Gingivitis is inflammation of the gingiva without loss or migration of epithelial attachment to the tooth, but periodontitis occurs when the periodontal ligament attachment and alveolar bone support of the tooth have been compromised or lost. This process involves apical migration of the epithelial attachment. (See Color Plates, photographs 6 and 7.)

Pregnant patients are more susceptible to both dental caries and gingivitis. "Pregnancy gingivitis" is characterized by red, swollen gingival tissue that bleeds easily. Local factors cause this gingivitis, but varying hormone levels may make gingival tissue more sensitive to bacterial dental plaque. These changes in the connective tissues that compose the periodontium appear to be the primary factor leading to pregnancy gingivitis.[1] Pregnancy gingivitis can be prevented or resolved with thorough plaque control. The severity of the inflammatory response and the resulting gingivitis decrease postpartum and return to pre-pregnancy levels after approximately 1 year.

Pathophysiology of Gingivitis

Gingivitis results from the accumulation of supragingival bacterial plaque. If this accumulation is not controlled, the plaque proliferates and invades subgingival spaces. At the same time, specific types of bacteria are associated with plaque at different stages of accumulation; the composition of the bacterial flora changes to a more complex mix of organisms. Although not all gingivitis progresses to periodontitis, the progression from supragingival plaque to gingivitis to periodontitis does occur; therefore, controlling gingivitis is a reasonable approach to limiting periodontitis.[1]

Other possible etiologies include medications such as calcium channel blockers, cyclosporine, and phenytoin. Anticholinergics and antidepressants may cause gingivitis by reducing the flow of saliva. The use of tobacco (both smokeless and smoked) has also been linked to periodontal disease.

Clinical Presentation of Gingivitis

The marginal gingiva (the border of the gingiva surrounding the neck of the tooth) is held firmly to the tooth by a network of collagen fibers. Microorganisms present in the plaque in the gingival sulcus (the space between the gingiva and the tooth) are capable of producing harmful products (e.g., acids, toxins, and enzymes) that damage cellular and intercellular tissue. Early-stage gingivitis symptoms include dilation and proliferation of gingival capillaries, increased flow of gingival fluid, and increased blood flow with resulting erythema of the gingiva. The gingiva may also enlarge, change contour, and appear puffy or swollen as a result of the inflammation (see Color Plates, photograph 6). The inflammatory process of early-stage gingivitis is reversible with effective oral hygiene.

In time and with neglect, some common indications that early-stage gingivitis has become chronic gingivitis include changes in gingival color, size, and shape, as well as changes in the ease with which gingival bleeding occurs. Both the patient and the dental provider can recognize these symptoms. Additionally, the flat knife-edge appearance of healthy gingiva is replaced by a ragged or rounded edge. Progression of these conditions is usually slow and insidious—and often painless.

Left untreated, chronic gingivitis may advance to the inflammatory condition of chronic destructive periodontal disease, or periodontitis (see Color Plates, photograph 7). Bacterial species that predominate in periodontitis but that are not present in healthy periodontium have been found in low proportions in gingivitis. Progression of gingivitis may parallel the increasing proportions of bacterial species implicated in the genesis of periodontitis.

Prevention of Gingivitis

Because prevention of gingivitis and caries depends on calculus prevention and plaque control, the same measures described in Prevention of Caries pertain to gingivitis. The active antigingivitis ingredients in dentifrices, mouth rinses, and other plaque removal and antiplaque products include triclosan, cetylpyridinium chloride, and stabilized stannous fluoride.[13]

Brushing and flossing can cure early gingivitis that arises from irritating food debris and plaque. The most important factors in reversing gingivitis and in preventing and controlling periodontal disease are adequate removal and control of supragingival plaque. Health care providers should immediately refer for dental care any patient who describes bleeding during brushing or shows signs of early gingivitis.

Assessment of Gingivitis: A Case-Based Approach

Before recommending oral hygiene products, the provider should evaluate the patient's oral hygiene regimen. At a minimum, the provider should find out whether the patient has a history of gingivitis, whether signs and symptoms of gingivitis are currently present, and what preventive measures the patient has tried or is using. Checking the patient's medical and medication history will identify asymptomatic patients who are at risk for gingivitis. Refer patients with signs or symptoms

of gingivitis (swollen gums, gums that bleed with brushing or flossing, receding gums, gums that appear darker red than usual) to their dentist for evaluation and treatment.

The provider is quite often alerted to pregnancy gingivitis during counseling on prescription prenatal vitamins. Besides monitoring the pregnant patient's medications for safety, the provider has an opportunity to encourage the patient to have a dental checkup and to stress the importance of careful attention to brushing and flossing to avoid oral health complications.

Patient Counseling for Gingivitis

Because gingivitis is usually not associated with pain, patients are unlikely to seek dental care for this problem alone. More likely, patients will ask for oral hygiene information and product recommendations. The provider may have to suggest oral hygiene methods and alert the patient to the possible adverse effects of certain products. Case 30–1 provides an example of assessment of a patient with gingivitis. The box Patient Education for Prevention of Caries, Gingivitis, and Halitosis lists specific information to provide patients.

The provider should also use this opportunity to warn patients with suspected gingivitis (bleeding, swollen gums) that this disease is a serious problem warranting professional attention. The provider should stress that adherence to an oral hygiene program is vital to preventing gingivitis.

Halitosis

Halitosis (oral malodor, usually known as bad breath) may be a symptom of oral pathology. However, in 90% of cases, poor oral hygiene is the cause.

Pathophysiology of Halitosis

Causes of halitosis may be related to both systemic and oral conditions; however, about 85% of cases are generally related to an oral cause. Oral causes may include dental caries, periodontal disease, oral infections, mucosal ulcerations, tongue coating, and impacted food or debris.[14]

Xerostomia can also cause mouth odor. Medications that have anticholinergic properties often cause xerostomia. Many foods and products such as garlic, tobacco, onions, alcohol, and other substances may contribute to mouth odor, as well.

Most foul breath odors occur because of volatile sulfur compounds (VSCs), which can be produced by breakdown of food debris left in the mouth or by systemic conditions that eliminate VSCs through exhaled air.[15]

Prevention of Halitosis

Prevention of halitosis relies on the removal of plaque and the prevention of calculus formation as described in Prevention of Caries. One of the primary sites for the formation of VSCs

case

30-1

Relevant Evaluation Criteria	Scenario/Model Outcome
Information Gathering	
1. Gather essential information about the patient's symptoms, including:	
a. description of symptom(s) (i.e., nature, onset, duration, severity, associated symptoms)	Patient has been experiencing sore, swollen gums for the past several weeks.
b. description of any factors that seem to precipitate, exacerbate, and/or relieve the patient's symptom(s)	Gum tissue bleeds freely during toothbrushing; bleeding increases with use of dental floss.
c. description of the patient's efforts to relieve the symptoms	Patient has continued brushing teeth twice daily and flossing once daily as normal.
d. patient's identity	Louise Baker
e. age, sex, height, and weight	63 years old, female, 5 ft 3 in., 135 lb
f. patient's occupation	Retired
g. patient's dietary habits	Normal, healthy diet
h. patient's sleep habits	6–8 hours of sleep each night
i. concurrent medical conditions, prescription and non-prescription medications, and dietary supplements	Hypertension: takes lisinopril 10 mg daily and a women's multivitamin daily.
j. allergies	Penicillin
k. history of other adverse reactions to medications	None
l. other (describe) _____	NA
Assessment and Triage	
2. Differentiate patient's signs/symptoms and correctly identify the patient's primary problem(s).	Louise appears to have gingivitis.
3. Identify exclusions for self-treatment.	Bleeding, swollen gums (see the box Patient Education for Prevention of Caries, Gingivitis, and Halitosis)
4. Formulate a comprehensive list of therapeutic alternatives for the primary problem to determine if triage to a medical provider is required, and share this information with the patient or caregiver.	Options include: (1) Refer Louise to a dentist. (2) Recommend appropriate nonprescription products along with education about proper oral care and referral to a dentist. (3) Take no action.
Plan	
5. Select an optimal therapeutic alternative to address the patient's problem, taking into account patient preferences.	Refer patient to a dentist.
6. Describe the recommended therapeutic approach to the patient or caregiver.	"You need to see a dentist because you have signs of gingivitis."
7. Explain to the patient or caregiver the rationale for selecting the recommended therapeutic approach from the considered therapeutic alternatives.	"Although there are steps you can take to improve your oral hygiene, a dentist will need to evaluate your condition and develop a treatment plan. It appears that you are appropriately caring for your teeth and gums, but sometimes changes can occur to your gum tissue. You should get a thorough checkup and cleaning from your dental health provider to ensure that you and your teeth and gums stay healthy."

Relevant Evaluation Criteria	Scenario/Model Outcome
Patient Education	
8. When recommending self-care with nonprescription medications and/or nondrug therapy, convey accurate information to the patient or caregiver.	Criterion does not apply in this case.
Solicit follow-up questions from the patient or caregiver.	"Is there a nonprescription medication that might work?"
Answer the patient's or caregiver's questions.	"Nonprescription medications do not treat gingivitis. They may reduce the symptoms, but ultimately your dental care provider will need to develop a treatment strategy. Once you have been diagnosed, there are nonprescription products you may use as part of your oral care regimen. Gingivitis and periodontal disease, if left untreated, may result in tooth loss and other complications."
Evaluation of Patient Outcome	
9. Assess patient outcome.	Contact Louise in a day or two to ensure she made an appointment and sought medical care.

Key: NA = Not applicable.

is the back of the tongue. Plaque and VSCs in this area of the mouth can seed the tonsillar crypts with malodorous debris. Brushing both the teeth and tongue is helpful, but some dentists have found that the use of a tongue-cleaning device (e.g., a tongue blade) may be the best way to clean the circumvallate papillae area of the tongue. Cleaning this posterior dorsal area not only will remove the fetid VSCs but also will prevent them from spreading to the tonsils.

Zinc salts and chlorine dioxide are most effective in the chemical prevention of oral malodor. The two are combined in 2-part rinses such as Smart-Mouth (Triumph Pharmaceuticals) or as single ingredients in CloSYS (Rowpar Pharmaceuticals). Zinc chloride, citrate, and acetate reduce the receptor binding necessary for VSC production. Chlorine dioxide breaks disulfide bonds and oxidizes the precursors of VSCs. In addition, the zinc salts kill gram-negative bacteria.

Any patient who complains of severe or lingering halitosis without a readily identifiable cause (e.g., smoking) should be advised to see a dentist for a thorough evaluation. Masking foul taste and odor with cosmetic mouth rinses may delay necessary dental or medical assessment and any needed treatment.

Assessment of Halitosis: A Case-Based Approach

When assessing a patient for halitosis, the health care provider should evaluate the patient's dental hygiene. Ideally, the provider should obtain a medication and medical history to determine whether the halitosis might arise from one of the oral pathologies discussed in Pathophysiology of Halitosis (see also Xerostomia in Chapter 31). Refer patients with medical conditions that cause halitosis and patients with halitosis that persists despite proper dental hygiene to their dentist for evaluation and treatment.

Patient Counseling for Halitosis

For patients with mouth odor related to poor dental hygiene, the provider should reinforce proper techniques for maintaining dental hygiene, including brushing and flossing. Providers should also recommend appropriate products and explain their use. The provider should stress to patients whose mouth odor is related to medical conditions that proper oral hygiene is still necessary to prevent tooth and gum problems. The box Patient Education for Prevention of Caries, Gingivitis, and Halitosis lists specific information to provide patients.

Hygiene-Related Denture Problems

Pain along the gingival ridge under a denture prosthesis suggests conditions such as denture stomatitis (an inflammation of the oral tissue in contact with a removable denture), inflammatory papillary hyperplasia, and chronic candidiasis. Denture stomatitis, which results from poor cleaning of dentures, can lead to chronic candidiasis (fungal infection).[16]

Pathophysiology of Hygiene-Related Denture Problems

Dentures accumulate plaque, stain, and calculus by a process very similar to that occurring on natural teeth. The denture plaque mass that is in contact with oral tissues produces predictable toxic results. Poor denture hygiene contributes to fungal and bacterial

Prevention of Caries, Gingivitis, and Halitosis

The primary objective of self-care is the removal of plaque to prevent caries, gingivitis, and halitosis. For most patients, carefully following product instructions and the self-care measures listed here will help ensure good oral hygiene.

Nondrug Measures and Other Considerations

- Avoid cariogenic foods, such as foods that contain more than 15% sugar, that cling to the teeth, and that remain in the mouth after they are chewed.
- Eat low-cariogenic foods, such as foods that have a high water content (e.g., fresh fruit); that stimulate the flow of saliva (e.g., fibrous foods that take longer to chew); or that are high in protein (e.g., dairy products).
- To help prevent mouth odor, maintain proper oral hygiene and limit or avoid foods and products that may cause oral malodor. Also, if you wear dentures, do not wear them while sleeping.
- Note that use of alcohol and tobacco are associated with caries, gingivitis, and halitosis.
- Note that hormonal changes during pregnancy increase the risk of gingivitis.

Plaque Removal
Brushing Teeth

- Mechanically remove plaque buildup by brushing teeth at least twice daily with a fluoride dentifrice. (See Table 30–1 for proper brushing technique.)
- Use a brush with soft nylon bristles.
- Replace the brush when the bristles show signs of wear.
- For children younger than 2 years, clean the teeth with a soft cloth and massage the gums.
- For preschool children, apply a pea-sized amount of toothpaste to a child-sized toothbrush, and brush the child's teeth until the child can brush properly.
- Use only regular-strength fluoride toothpaste for children ages 2–6 years. Consult a dentist before using fluoride toothpastes in children younger than 2 years.
- Teach children how to rinse the mouth and spit out the toothpaste to avoid swallowing fluoride.
- Note that tartar-control toothpastes have been related to a type of contact dermatitis in the perioral region. If you experience itching or irritation of the mouth after brushing, discontinue the tartar-control toothpaste, and switch to a non–tartar-control fluoride toothpaste.
- If you are prone to developing caries or gingivitis, consider using toothpaste classified as having antiplaque/antigingivitis activity. Such toothpastes contain stannous fluoride.
- If you are prone to developing aphthous ulcers, consider using toothpaste that does not contain sodium lauryl sulfate.

Flossing Teeth

- Floss your teeth at least once a day. (See Table 30–2 for proper flossing technique.)
- Use waxed or Teflon-coated floss for teeth with tight contacts.

Using Mouth Rinses and Gels

- To freshen breath, use a mouth rinse that contains zinc chloride and zinc citrate. Zinc chloride and chlorine dioxide are found in Smart-Mouth Tri-Oral 2-part rinse. These ingredients eliminate odoriferous volatile sulfur compounds.
- If you are prone to developing caries or gingivitis, consider using a mouth rinse classified as having antiplaque/antigingivitis activity. Such mouth rinses contain cetylpyridinium chloride or a combination of thymol, eucalyptol, methyl salicylate, and menthol.
- To use plaque-softening mouth rinses (Advanced Formula Plax) effectively, use them before brushing. Vigorously swish 1–2 tablespoons of rinse in the mouth and between the teeth for about 30 seconds, and spit out the rinse. Do not smoke, eat, or drink for 30 minutes following use.
- Note that overuse of mouth rinses containing cetylpyridinium can stain teeth.

Using Topical Fluoride Treatments

- If your drinking water is not fluoridated (including bottled water), or if you are prone to developing caries, consider using topical fluoride treatments. (See Table 30–4 for proper use of these products.)
- Supervise children younger than 12 years until they are capable of using the product correctly.
- Consult a dentist or primary care provider before using these products in children younger than 6 years.

When to Seek Medical Attention

- See a dentist if any of the following occurs:
  - You develop symptoms of a toothache.
  - Your teeth develop a mottled appearance.
  - Your gums bleed, swell, or become red.
  - Mouth odor persists despite regular use of fluoride toothpaste, or the cause of the mouth odor cannot be identified.

---

growth that not only affects the patient aesthetically (unpleasant odors and staining) but also seriously affects the patient's oral health (inflammation and mucosal disease) and ability to wear the dentures successfully.

Chronic atrophic candidiasis (sometimes referred to as denture stomatitis or denture sore mouth) is common in patients with full or partial dentures. This condition may be attributed to infection with *Candida* organisms, which are more prevalent in denture wearers.[1] Symptomatically, the inflamed denture-bearing area may appear granular or erythematous and edematous with soreness or a burning sensation (see Color Plates, photograph 8). Inflammation secondary to *Candida* organisms is generalized to the entire denture-bearing tissue area, whereas inflammation secondary to the trauma of ill-fitting dentures is usually localized to the specific area of the trauma. Failure to remove the denture at bedtime

and clean it regularly worsens this condition. Angular cheilitis (soreness and cracking at corners of the mouth) is commonly associated with chronic atrophic candidiasis, other forms of oral candidiasis, and poor denture fit. The corners of the mouth can often be treated effectively with terbinafine cream. If a staphylococcal organism is also involved, a prescription will be needed.

Prevention of Hygiene-Related Denture Problems

Removing plaque from dentures helps prevent gum infections, staining of dentures, and mouth odor. Specialty brushes and aids are available to remove plaque from hard-to-clean areas (e.g., spaces around a fixed bridge, implant, or orthodontic band) and dentures. Dentures should be cleaned thoroughly at least once daily to remove unsightly stain, debris, and plaque. Abrasive and chemical cleansers formulated specifically for dentures are available (Table 30–8). A combination regimen of brushing dentures with an abrasive cleaner and soaking them in a chemical cleanser is recommended.

Denture cleansers (paste or powder) containing mild abrasives (e.g., calcium carbonate) must be applied properly with specialty brushes adapted to the denture's contour to remove stains, plaque, and calculus. Overly vigorous scrubbing can abrade the denture's acrylic materials and bend the metal clasps. To prevent irritation of oral tissues, the patient should rinse the abrasive cleaner from the denture thoroughly.

The brushing routine can be followed by soaking the denture in an alkaline peroxide cleansing solution to help remove remaining plaque and bacteria. Plaque removal is then enhanced by brushing the denture after it has soaked; instructions for this procedure are included on some products.

The other method of cleaning is to use a soaking solution containing one of the three chemical cleansers: alkaline peroxide, hypochlorite, or dilute acids.

Alkaline peroxide cleaners are the most commonly used chemical denture cleansers. These powders or tablets become alkaline solutions of hydrogen peroxide when dissolved. The ingredients are alkaline detergents and perborates; the latter cause oxygen release for a mechanical cleaning effect. These products are most effective on new plaque and stains when the denture is soaked for 4–8 hours. The alkaline peroxides have few serious disadvantages and do not damage the surface of acrylic resins.

Hypochlorite (bleach) removes stains, dissolves mucin, and is both bactericidal and fungicidal. Denture plaque consists of cells embedded in a matrix that serves as a surface on which calculus may develop. Hypochlorite cleansers act directly on the organic plaque matrix to dissolve its structure, but they cannot dissolve calculus once it has formed. The most serious disadvantage of hypochlorite is that it corrodes metal denture components (e.g., the framework and clasps of removable partial dentures, solder joints, and possibly the pins holding the teeth). The addition of anticorrosive phosphate compounds has greatly reduced this problem, but these products should be used for only 10-minute soaks (to limit exposure) and not more often than once a week.

Acid-containing soaking solutions can also be corrosive to metals, and short soaking times are recommended for these solutions. A sonic or ultrasonic cleaning device, when used with a commercially prepared solution, is easier to use and cleans more effectively than soaking alone. However, some hand brushing may still be required.

All denture-cleansing products should be rinsed off the denture completely before it is inserted into the mouth. If abrasive cleansers come in contact with oral or other mucous membranes, they may cause tissue irritation. Chemical cleansers may cause tissue irritation or possibly severe chemical burns. All denture cleansers should be kept out of children's reach because of the potential for eye or skin irritation and because they are toxic if accidentally ingested. Stains that are resistant to proper denture brushing and soaking in available solutions should be evaluated by a dentist.

Only products that are specifically formulated for denture cleansing should be used. Household cleansers (sometimes used by patients for soaking dentures) are not appropriate and may be ineffective or may damage the denture material. The use of whitening toothpastes (which are formulated for use with natural dentition) should be discouraged because they are too abrasive to be used safely on denture material.

Patients should not soak or clean dentures in hot water or hot soaking solutions, because distortion or warping may occur.

Patients of advanced age or disabled patients may prefer an alkaline peroxide soak solution for daily, overnight cleaning. Unlike alkaline hypochlorite and acid cleansers, alkaline peroxide cleansers do not corrode metal components of dentures.

Assessment of Hygiene-Related Denture Problems

Before recommending any type of oral hygiene product, the health care provider should determine what denture care measures the patient is taking and whether those measures are adequate. At a minimum, the provider should determine whether the patient suffers from denture stomatitis or inflammation secondary to ill-fitting dentures. Patients with denture stomatitis or inflammation secondary to ill-fitting dentures should be referred to their dentist for evaluation and treatment. Case 30–2 illustrates assessment of a patient with a hygiene-related denture problem.

Patient Counseling for Hygiene-Related Denture Problems

Denture wearers may tend to blame the appliances for any oral discomfort rather than their hygiene regimen. The provider should stress that diligent plaque removal from dentures is the key to preventing denture stomatitis. The methods of cleaning dentures, including their advantages and disadvantages, should be explained. The provider should recommend a denture cleanser according to the patient's preferences and reinforce the methods of use. The box Patient Education for Hygiene-Related Denture Problems lists specific information to provide patients.

Key Points for Prevention of Hygiene-Related Oral Disorders

➤ Removing plaque and modifying the diet are the main goals of self-care to prevent caries, gingivitis, and halitosis.

table 30–8	Selected Nonprescription Denture Cleaners
Trade Name	**Primary Ingredients**
Efferdent Plus Tablets	Potassium monopersulfate; sodium bicarbonate; sodium perborate
Polident Dentu-Cream Paste	Dicalcium phosphate dihydrate; calcium carbonate; aluminum silicate
Polident Tablets	Potassium monopersulfate; sodium perborate; sodium carbonate; sodium bicarbonate; citric acid

case
30–2

Relevant Evaluation Criteria	Scenario/Model Outcome
Information Gathering	
1. Gather essential information about the patient's symptoms, including:	
a. description of symptom(s) (i.e., nature, onset, duration, severity, associated symptoms)	The patient feels that he is unable to get his dentures as clean as he would like.
b. description of any factors that seem to precipitate, exacerbate, and/or relieve the patient's symptom(s)	NA
c. description of the patient's efforts to relieve the symptoms	He soaks his dentures in an alkaline peroxide cleanser overnight.
d. patient's identity	Ray Williams
e. age, sex, height, and weight	71 years old, male, 5 ft 9 in., 190 lb
f. patient's occupation	Bank manager
g. patient's dietary habits	Normal healthy diet; enjoys sweet foods.
h. patient's sleep habits	Light sleeper; averages 5–7 hours per night.
i. concurrent medical conditions, prescription and non-prescription medications, and dietary supplements	Seasonal allergic rhinitis (spring and fall): loratadine 10 mg, 1 tablet daily
j. allergies	NKA
k. history of other adverse reactions to medications	Morphine: itching
l. other (describe) _____	NA
Assessment and Triage	
2. Differentiate patient's signs/symptoms and correctly identify the patient's primary problem(s).	Patient seems to have residual plaque on dentures despite daily soaks.
3. Identify exclusions for self-treatment.	None
4. Formulate a comprehensive list of therapeutic alternatives for the primary problem to determine if triage to a medical provider is required, and share this information with the patient or caregiver.	Options include: (1) Refer Ray to a dentist. (2) Recommend appropriate nonprescription products along with education about proper oral care and a referral to a dentist. (3) Take no action.
Plan	
5. Select an optimal therapeutic alternative to address the patient's problem, taking into account patient preferences.	Ray should also be using a denture brush and denture paste daily because soaking only provides superficial cleaning.
6. Describe the recommended therapeutic approach to the patient or caregiver.	"Denture brushes and pastes are specially designed to remove deposits from dentures."
7. Explain to the patient or caregiver the rationale for selecting the recommended therapeutic approach from the considered therapeutic alternatives.	"Effective manual brushing removes more plaque and biofilm from dentures than soaking alone."
Patient Education	
8 When recommending self-care with nonprescription medications and/or nondrug therapy, convey accurate information to the patient or caregiver:	
a. appropriate dose and frequency of administration	"Dentures should be brushed daily."
b. maximum number of days the therapy should be employed	NA
c. product administration procedures	"All surfaces of the denture should be brushed. To avoid breaking the denture, brush it over a folded towel or a sink filled with water. Thoroughly rinse the denture after brushing."
d. degree of relief that can be reasonably expected	"Daily brushing may help remove plaque and stains."

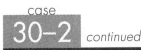

case
30–2 *continued*

Relevant Evaluation Criteria	Scenario/Model Outcome
e. most common side effects	"Only denture paste should be used because dentures are easily scratched by regular toothpastes."
f. side effects that warrant medical intervention should they occur	NA
g. patient options in the event that condition worsens or persists	"A dentist should evaluate stains that are resistant to proper brushing and soaking in available solutions."
h. product storage requirements	NA
i. specific nondrug measures	"Continue regular denture hygiene and maintenance."
Solicit follow-up questions from the patient or caregiver.	"Can I increase the frequency of brushing or use whitening toothpastes to provide additional cleaning?"
Answer the patient's or caregiver's questions.	"No. Brushing too often and using toothpastes other than denture paste may scratch and damage dentures."

Evaluation of Patient Outcome	
9. Assess patient outcome	Ask the patient to call to update you on his response to your recommendations, or follow up with a call in 1 week to evaluate his response.

Key: NA = Not applicable; NKA = no known allergies.

patient education for
Hygiene-Related Denture Problems

The objective of self-care is to prevent bacterial or fungal infections of the mouth by removing plaque from the dentures. For most patients, carefully following product instructions and the self-care measures listed here will help ensure good denture hygiene.

- Thoroughly clean dentures at least once daily to remove unsightly stain, debris, and potentially harmful plaque.
- Preferably, brush dentures with an abrasive cleaner, and then soak them in a chemical cleanser. This combination regimen is more effective in removing plaque and bacteria.
- Apply the abrasive cleaner to the denture, using a brush designed to adapt to the denture's contour.
- Do not scrub the denture surface vigorously; this action can abrade the acrylic materials and bend the metal clasps.
- To prevent irritation of oral tissues, thoroughly rinse the abrasive cleaner from the denture.
- After brushing the dentures, soak them in an alkaline peroxide cleansing solution for 10–20 minutes. Rinse the dentures thoroughly to avoid chemical burns of the mouth.
- If possible, brush the dentures again, and rinse them thoroughly.

- If using an alkaline or sodium hypochlorite cleanser, soak the dentures for only 10 minutes to avoid corrosion of metal denture components.
- Keep all denture cleansers out of children's reach. These agents can cause eye or skin irritation or toxicity if accidentally ingested.
- Do not use household cleansers or whitening toothpastes to clean dentures. These agents may damage denture material.
- Do not soak or clean dentures in hot water or hot soaking solutions. Distortion or warping of the denture may occur.
- Do not sleep while wearing your dentures. Decreased levels of saliva during sleep may contribute to plaque buildup on the denture.

When to Seek Medical Attention

- If your mouth becomes sore or shows sign of infection, see a dentist.

➤ Mechanical removal of plaque by brushing and flossing is essential for good oral health.

➤ Mouth rinses may augment brushing and flossing procedures and may be used to freshen breath and/or as antiplaque/antigingivitis adjuncts.

➤ Topical fluorides may be used in individuals with high caries activity.

➤ Parents must supervise children younger than 12 years as necessary until they can use the products without supervision.

➤ Denture cleaners may be used to remove debris physically and to prevent bacterial and/or fungal infections.

➤ If individuals have specific problems related to the purpose or use of these products, consultation with a dentist should be recommended.

REFERENCES

1. Harris NO, Garcia-Godoy F, Nathe CN. *Primary Preventive Dentistry.* 8th Ed. Upper Saddle River, NJ: Pearson; 2013:3, 40–49, 70–83, 135–44, 148–59, 164–91, 198–217, 223–43, 249–52, 380–1.
2. Bagramian RA, Garcia-Godoy F, Volpe AR. The global increase in dental caries. A pending public health crisis. *Am J Dent.* 2009;22(1):3–8.
3. Warnakulasuriya S. Oral health risks of tobacco use and effects of cessation. *Int Dent J.* 2010;60(1):7–30.
4. Deery C, Heanue M, Deacon S, et al. The effectiveness of manual versus powered toothbrushes for dental health: a systematic review. *J Dent.* 2004;32(3):197–211.
5. Council on Scientific Affairs. *Products of Excellence ADA Seal Program.* Chicago, IL: American Dental Association; 2010.
6. Terzhalmy GT, Bartizek RD, Biesbrock AR. Plaque-removal efficacy of four types of dental floss. *J Periodontol.* 2008;79(2):245–51.

7. Rawal SY, Claman LJ, Kalmar JR, et al. Traumatic lesions of the gingiva: a case series. *J Periodontol.* 2004;75(5):762–9.

8. Bailey W. Populations receiving optimally fluoridated public drinking water – United States, 1992–2006. *MMWR Morb Mortal Wkly Rep.* 2008;57(27):737–41.

9. Gluck GM, Morganstein WM. *Jong's Community Dental Health.* 5th ed. St. Louis, MO: Mosby; 2003:250–9.

10. Council on Scientific Affairs. *Acceptance Program Guidelines: Chemotherapeutic Products for the Control of Gingivitis.* Chicago, IL: American Dental Association; 2008.

11. Moore C, Addy M, Moran J. Toothpaste detergents: a potential source of oral soft tissue damage? *Int J Dent Hyg.* 2008;6(3):193–8.

12. Eke P. Prevalence of periodontitis in adults in the United States: 2009 and 2010. *J Dent Res.* 2012;91(10):914–20.

13. U.S. Food and Drug Administration. Oral health care drug products for over-the-counter human use; antigingivitis/antiplaque drug products; establishment of a monograph. *Federal Register.* 2003;68:32232.

14. Cortelli JR, Barbosa MD, Westphal MA. Halitosis: a review of associated factors and therapeutic approach. *Braz Oral Res.* 2008;22(suppl 1): 44–54.

15. Armstrong B. Halitosis: A review of current literature. *J Dent Hyg.* 2010;84(2):65–74.

16. Gonsalves WC, Chi AC, Neville BW. Common oral lesions: part I. Superficial mucosal lesions. *Am Fam Physician.* 2007;75(4):501–7.

chapter 31

ORAL PAIN AND DISCOMFORT

Nicole Paolini Albanese

Oral pain and discomfort are common ailments that affect people worldwide.[1] Many children experience irritation and soreness during the teething process. In adulthood, oral pain may be associated with sudden exposure of or damage to nerves in a tooth; unexpected cracking or breaking of teeth, fillings, or crowns (caps) may also occur. Similarly, pain in the mucosa of the oral cavity and lips can be generated by injury to the mouth, recurrent aphthous stomatitis (canker sores), or herpes simplex labialis (cold sores). Some adults experience xerostomia (dry mouth) that is significant enough to require treatment with nonprescription medications. Oral pain and discomfort can interfere with daily activities such as drinking, eating, and working; cause mental anxiety and distress; and result in cost to the patient from visits to their health care providers.[2,3] Distinguishing the patient's self-treatable problems from those potentially requiring professional dental or medical care is an important advisory role for oral health care providers.

Tooth Hypersensitivity

Tooth hypersensitivity, or dentin hypersensitivity, is characterized by a short, sharp pain arising from exposed dentin (i.e., mineralized tissue of teeth internal to crown enamel and root cementum) in response to a stimulus (thermal, chemical, or physical) that cannot be ascribed to any other form of dental defect or disease.[4-8] Tooth hypersensitivity affects 15%–20% of the adult population, with peak incidence between the ages of 30 and 39 years.[4]

Pathophysiology of Tooth Hypersensitivity

Two processes are essential for the development of dentin hypersensitivity: (1) dentin must become exposed (lesion localization) through loss of enamel or gingival recession, and (2) the dentin tubules must be open to both the oral cavity and the pulp (lesion initiation).[4-8] The roots of teeth are usually covered by gum tissues (gingiva), but infection (e.g., periodontal disease) or injury (e.g., traumatic brushing) can cause the gums to recede. The cementum covering affected root surfaces may be reduced by further injury (attrition, abrasion, or erosion), eventually exposing the underlying porous dentin. When stimuli such as heat, cold, pressure, or acid touch exposed dentin or reach an open tubule, fluid flow in the dentinal tubule is increased, and the underlying nerves are stimulated, resulting in pain.[4-8]

Enamel, which covers the anatomic crowns of the teeth and is the most mineralized body tissue, is resistant to abrasion by normal toothbrushing, but excessive brushing with an abrasive dentifrice or a medium- or hard-bristled toothbrush can be problematic. The etiology of dental erosion is primarily attributed to the presence of extrinsic or intrinsic acid.[6,7] Extrinsic sources of acid include frequent consumption of acidic medications, foods, or drinks. Persons who regularly consume citrus juices and fruits, carbonated drinks, wines, and ciders may be at risk for tooth hypersensitivity. The most common source of intrinsic acid is regurgitation of gastric contents into the mouth, which occurs with disorders such as gastroesophageal reflux disease or bulimia nervosa.[6,7] Tooth hypersensitivity is more common in individuals with periodontitis or after procedures such as deep scaling, root planing, orthodontic tooth movement, or periodontal (gum) surgery.[4-8] Sensitivity to hot and cold for several weeks after dental therapy is normal. Hypersensitivity can also occur as a result of clenching or grinding teeth and from gumline grooves formed by abrasive or inappropriate toothbrushing technique.[6] Tooth whitening procedures, whether done at home or by a trained clinician, can cause dentin sensitivity. Tooth sensitivity is the most common reason why patients fail to complete or comply with a tooth whitening regimen.[7] Tooth whitening products are discussed in further detail in Chapter 30.

Clinical Presentation of Tooth Hypersensitivity

A patient with tooth hypersensitivity experiences pain from hot or cold and sweet or sour solutions, as well as when hot or cold air touches the teeth. As individual pain thresholds vary, so does the pain experienced from tooth hypersensitivity. Pain varies from mild discomfort to sharp, excruciating pain. Although tooth hypersensitivity is self-treatable, toothache is not; therefore, it is critical to differentiate between these two conditions (Table 31–1). Resolution of pain associated with toothache, fractured dentition, ill-fitting dentures, or suspected infection (abscess) requires professional dental care. Only a dentist can adequately evaluate and treat these conditions; therefore, the patient should see a dentist without delay.

Treatment of Tooth Hypersensitivity
Treatment Goals

The goals of self-treating tooth hypersensitivity are to (1) repair the damaged tooth surface using the appropriate toothpaste and

table

31–1 Differentiation of Tooth Hypersensitivity and Toothache

	Tooth Hypersensitivity	**Toothache**
Etiology	Exposed and open dentin tubules	Bacterial invasion to the pulp
Pathophysiology	Stimuli (heat, cold, pressure, acid) cause fluid in the dentinal tubules to expand and shrink, stimulating pulp nerve fibers and resulting in pain	Inflammatory response to invading bacteria stimulates free nerve endings in the pulp
Causes	Attrition, abrasion, erosion, tooth/restoration fracture, faulty restoration, or gingival recession	Cavitation/decay present in tooth/teeth under existing restoration, tooth/restoration fracture, or trauma to the dentition
Symptoms	A quick, fleeting, sharp, or stabbing pain on stimulation by thermal, chemical, or physical stimuli, which stops after stimuli are no longer present	Pain that remains even in the absence of stimulus; intermittent, short, and sharp pain on stimulation may indicate reversible damage; continuous, dull, and throbbing pain without stimulation usually indicates irreversible damage
Assessment	Hypersensitivity due to attrition, abrasion, or erosion is not serious and is self-treatable; sensitivity due to fracture, faulty restoration, or gingival recession should be referred to a dentist	Requires dental care for resolution

Source: References 4, 6, and 7.

(2) stop abrasive toothbrushing practices. When these goals have been achieved, tooth hypersensitivity may be eliminated.

General Treatment Approach

Pain related to tooth hypersensitivity can be challenging. Acute pain may cause anxiety and the patient may not seek care. Patients will likely not seek treatment by a dentist, but rather will try to self-treat.[5,6] Before recommending self-treatment of tooth pain, the provider should determine if the patient is a self-care candidate. Figure 31–1 outlines the self-treatment of tooth hypersensitivity and lists exclusions for self-care.[5–9]

Nonpharmacologic Therapy

Treatment plans for tooth hypersensitivity should include identification and elimination of predisposing factors, such as extrinsic and intrinsic acid and improper (harsh) toothbrushing technique. Tooth hypersensitivity can be prevented by brushing less vigorously with standard fluoride dentifrice (toothpaste) and a soft-bristled toothbrush. One should avoid brushing teeth within 30–60 minutes of consuming acidic foods or drinks to reduce the effects of acids and abrasions. Dentin permeability can be increased after ingesting acidic foods or beverages.[6] Fluoride is discussed in further detail in Chapter 30.

Pharmacologic Therapy

In general, two pharmacologic mechanisms are designed to treat tooth hypersensitivity. The first involves depolarizing the excited nerves in the tubules and pulp to disrupt the pain stimuli neuronal response.[8] A potassium salt, usually potassium nitrate, diffuses along the dentinal tubules to decrease the excitability of intradental nerves and alter its membrane potential. The potassium nitrate acts on the dentin to block the perception of stimuli that patients with healthy teeth usually do not

experience. The second involves minimizing the flow of fluid by sealing the exposed dentin.[8] A new technology using 8% arginine, an amino acid naturally found in saliva, combined with calcium carbonate works by occluding the exposed dentinal tubules.[8] This treatment prevents the fluid from moving into the tubules, which is the cause of hypersensitivity. Table 31–2 lists selected desensitizing toothpastes and their active ingredients.

Potassium nitrate 5% is the most widely used and generally accepted ingredient used for teeth sensitivity. Most commercially available desensitizing dentifrices are combination products containing potassium nitrate and sodium fluoride, in varying concentrations. Studies have shown these products to be highly efficacious for the treatment of tooth sensitivity.[9,10] The Pro-Argin technology, which combines 8% arginine and calcium carbonate, though highly efficacious,[8,11] is not currently available to consumers for home use.

Guidelines for brushing teeth can be found in the previous chapter (Table 30–1) and can be applied to brushing with desensitizing dentifrices.[9,10] A single application has no effect; for some patients, long-term use (2–4 weeks) may be necessary to relieve the symptoms. The desensitizing dentifrice should be used until the sensitivity subsides or as long as a dentist recommends its use. In about 25% of adults, hypersensitive teeth are a chronic problem and require long-term treatment provided by a dentist.[5,6] If tooth hypersensitivity is not relieved within 14–21 days of using a desensitizing dentifrice, the patient should see a dentist for an in-office method of treatment or an appropriate health care provider for further evaluation.[5,6]

Product Selection Guidelines

Dentifrices containing potassium nitrate 5% are not recommended for children younger than 12 years. Patients with hypersensitive teeth should be cautioned against using high-abrasion toothpastes such as cosmetic pastes that whiten teeth or remove stains.

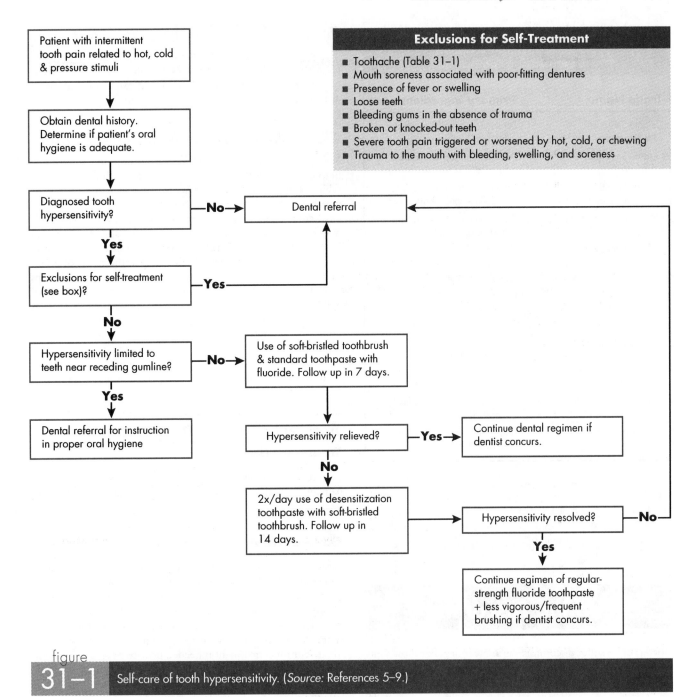

Assessment of Toothache and Tooth Hypersensitivity: A Case-Based Approach

The primary objectives of the assessment are to determine whether the patient has a history of dental problems, whether the patient regularly cares for his or her teeth, and whether the patient receives regular professional dental care. This information will help determine the patient's level of care and risk for a toothache versus tooth hypersensitivity (Table 31–1).

Patient Counseling for Tooth Hypersensitivity

Subsequent to a definite diagnosis of tooth hypersensitivity, patients should be counseled on the proper use of desensitizing toothpastes and safe methods of toothbrushing, as outlined in the box Patient Education for Tooth Hypersensitivity. Patients should use the desensitizing toothpaste for as long as the dentist recommends and then switch to a low-abrasion (nonwhitening) fluoride dentifrice.

Evaluation of Patient Outcomes for Tooth Hypersensitivity

The patient with hypersensitive teeth should use a desensitizing dentifrice for a maximum of 4 weeks. If the pain is resolved, the patient should continue treatment as recommended by a dentist. The patient should be advised to continue the recommended

table

31–2   Selected Nonprescription Desensitizing Toothpastes

Trade Name	Primary Ingredients
Colgate Sensitive Multiprotection	Potassium nitrate 5%; sodium fluoride 0.24%
Colgate Sensitive Pro-Relief Original	Potassium nitrate 5%; sodium fluoride 0.24%
Colgate Sensitive Pro-Relief Enamel Repair	Potassium nitrate 5%; sodium monofluorophosphate 1.14%
Colgate Sensitive Pro-Relief Whitening	Potassium nitrate 5%; sodium fluoride 0.24%
Colgate Total Zx Pro-Shield Plus Sensitivity	Potassium nitrate 0.24%; sodium monofluoride 0.055%; zinc citrate trihydrate 0.096%
Crest Sensitivity: Clinical Sensitivity Relief Extra Whitening	Potassium nitrate 5%; sodium fluoride 0.243%
Crest Sensitivity Whitening Plus Scope	Potassium nitrate 5%; sodium fluoride 0.243%
Sensodyne Maximum Strength with Fluoride	Potassium nitrate 5%; sodium fluoride 0.15%
Sensodyne Pronamel	Potassium nitrate 5%; sodium fluoride 0.15%
Tom's Sensitive	Potassium nitrate 5%; sodium fluoride 0.24%

dental hygiene measures (i.e., brush teeth twice daily and visit the dentist twice a year). If the pain persists or worsens, or if new symptoms develop after 14–21 days, the patient should see a dentist for further evaluation.[5,6,8]

Teething Discomfort

Not all babies suffer discomfort during teething. For those who do, nonprescription products can provide symptomatic relief.

Pathophysiology of Teething Discomfort

Teething is the eruption of the deciduous (primary or baby) teeth through the gingival tissues. Usually, this normal physiologic process is uneventful. However, it can cause pain, sleep disturbances, or irritability in some children.

Clinical Presentation of Teething Discomfort

Mild pain, irritation, reddening, excessive drooling, mouth biting, gum rubbing, low-grade fever, or slight swelling of the gums while teething may precede or accompany sleep disturbances or irritability.[12] Teething is not associated with vomiting, diarrhea, nasal congestion, malaise, fever, or rashes, but these symptoms may be a sign of ear or stomach infection. Bluish, soft, round swellings (called eruption cysts) sometimes form over emerging incisors and molars. Eruption cysts are not the result of infection and will disappear if left alone. In addition, three bumps (called mamelons) may be present on the biting surfaces (incisal edges) of emerging incisors. The mamelons will wear away as the teeth begin to occlude against the opposing dentition. If the underside of the tongue becomes irritated, a dentist may try to smooth the edges of the mamelons to prevent further irritation. Teeth eruption can begin as early as 6 months of age, and for each tooth that erupts, the teething period usually occurs over an 8-day window.[12]

Treatment of Teething Discomfort

Treatment Goals

The goal of self-care of teething discomfort is to relieve gum pain and irritation, thereby reducing the child's irritability and sleep disturbances.[12]

General Treatment Approach

Parents and caregivers should be cautioned to exercise restraint in treating a child's teething discomfort. Eruption cysts are a part of the normal physiologic process and should be left alone to resolve spontaneously. If cut or punctured, the cysts will leave scars that may delay the tooth's eruption. Parents should try all nonpharmacologic measures to determine which ones are helpful. If additional treatment is needed pediatric doses of systemic analgesics can be used.

patient education for
Tooth Hypersensitivity

The objectives of self-treatment of tooth hypersensitivity are to (1) repair the damaged tooth surface using the appropriate toothpaste and (2) stop abrasive toothbrushing practices. For most patients, carefully following product instructions, the dentist's recommendations, and the self-care measures listed here will help ensure optimal therapeutic outcomes.

- If correct brushing techniques with a fluoride toothpaste are ineffective, a desensitizing toothpaste should be used.
- If a desensitizing toothpaste is needed, apply a 1-inch strip of toothpaste to a soft-bristled toothbrush. Brush at least twice daily.
- Note that relief of the sensitivity may take several days to several weeks. The better the patient is at removing bacterial plaque, the quicker the sensitivity will resolve.
- Use the toothpaste for as long as the dentist recommends, and then switch to a low-abrasion (nonwhitening) fluoride dentifrice.

- Note that some cases of hypersensitive teeth require long-term treatment or several repeated treatments.
- Do not use desensitizing toothpastes in children younger than 12 years.
- Do not use high-abrasion toothpastes, such as cosmetic pastes that whiten or remove stains.

When to Seek Medical Attention

- See a dentist if the pain worsens during treatment or if new symptoms develop.

Source: References 5–9.

Nonpharmacologic Therapy

If the baby cooperates, massaging the gum around the erupting tooth may provide relief. Babies may be made more comfortable by giving them a cold teething ring. Teething products made of plastic and filled with fluid should not be subjected to extreme temperatures, like boiling to sanitize or freezing, as this can weaken the plastic and lead to leakage of the fluid.[12] The cold temperature causes local vasoconstriction in addition to the pressure on the gums that the child feels when he or she bit the object. If the child is at an age to tolerate food such as dry toast or teething biscuits, he or she may be given such food to chew. Foods high in sucrose should be avoided.[12]

Pharmacologic Therapy

Pharmacologic management of infant teething discomfort is limited to pediatric doses of systemic analgesics. Topical analgesics that are approved for use in infants carry strict FDA warnings against their use.

Topical Oral Analgesics

Benzocaine is available in concentrations ranging from 5% to 20% are generally not accepted as safe topical anesthetics/analgesics for teething pain. Benzocaine is a drug product classified as Pregnancy Category C.[13]

In the highest concentration approved for nonprescription use (20%), benzocaine is too potent for infants and can even cause death from drug overdose.[12] In April 2011, FDA released a MedWatch safety alert that warned health care providers of the reports linking benzocaine use and methemoglobinemias.[14] Methemoglobinemia is a serious but rare condition whereby the amount of oxygen circulating in the blood is greatly reduced.[12] FDA recommends that benzocaine products not be used on children younger than 2 years, except under the advice and supervision of a health care professional.[12,14] Patients with known hypersensitivity to common local anesthetics should not use a product containing benzocaine. Benzocaine is a known sensitizer (allergen), and its use in these patients can cause a hypersensitivity reaction.

In June 2014, FDA released a Drug Safety Communication that discussed the use of topical agents used for infant and child teething discomfort.[15] The communication warns that prescription oral viscous lidocaine 2% solution should not be used to treat infants and children with teething pain. Further, the agency requires the following *Boxed Warning* be added to these products: "Oral viscous lidocaine solution is not approved to treat teething pain, and use in infants and young children can cause serious harm, including death." In addition, the communication recommends against use of nonprescription topical medications for teething pain, which would include-benzocaine containing products. These products are sold under different brand names, such as Anbesol, Hurricaine, Orajel, Baby Orajel, Orabase, and various store brands. FDA recommends following the American Academy of Pediatrics' recommendations to help lessen teething pain. These modalities are discussed in detail above in the section Nonpharmacologic Therapy.

Systemic Analgesics

Pediatric doses of systemic nonprescription analgesics (e.g., acetaminophen) may be used to relieve teething discomfort.

(See Chapter 5 for discussion of these agents and their recommended dosages.)

Product Selection Guidelines

Topical teething products labeled for the temporary relief of sore gums due to teething in infants and children ages 4 months and older are no longer recommended by FDA as safe and effective.[15] Nonpharmacologic management and systemic analgesics, given at the appropriate pediatric doses, should be used for symptom management.

Assessment of Teething Discomfort: A Case-Based Approach

In most cases, teething discomfort must be assessed on the basis of the parent's description of the child's symptoms. If the child cooperates, visual inspection of the gums may confirm that the child is teething. Nonetheless, the signs and symptoms of teething must be distinguished from those of an infection.

Patient Counseling for Teething Discomfort

Parents should be counseled about both nonpharmacologic and pharmacologic remedies for teething discomfort, as outlined in the box Patient Education for Teething Discomfort. Parents should be urged to contact a primary care provider when uncharacteristic symptoms of teething discomfort are present.

Evaluation of Patient Outcomes for Teething Discomfort

The parent should be asked to call back after 3–5 days of treatment. If neither nonpharmacologic therapy nor nonprescription medications are relieving the symptoms, the parent should be advised to take the baby to a primary care provider, pediatrician, or pediatric dentist. Furthermore, if symptoms uncharacteristic of teething discomfort have developed, the baby should be evaluated by a primary care provider or pediatrician.

Recurrent Aphthous Stomatitis

Recurrent aphthous stomatitis (RAS), also known as canker sore or aphthous ulcer, affects approximately 2.5 billion people worldwide.[16] Prevalence of RAS is influenced by the population, diagnostic criteria, and environmental factors.[17] The onset of RAS appears to peak between the ages of 10 and 19 years.[17] Eighty percent of patients with RAS are considered to have a mild form of the disease. The lesions affect only nonkeratinized mucosa (e.g., labial or buccal) and will spontaneously heal in 10–14 days.[18]

Pathophysiology of Recurrent Aphthous Stomatitis

The cause of RAS is unknown in most patients. Precipitating factors such as local, systemic, immunologic, genetic, allergic, and nutritional have been proposed. Local trauma (e.g., smoking,

Teething Discomfort

The objective of self-treatment of teething discomfort is to relieve gum pain and irritation, thereby reducing the child's irritability and sleep disturbances. For most patients, the parent's or caregiver's careful following of product instructions and the self-care measures listed here will help ensure optimal therapeutic outcomes.

Nondrug Measures

- If possible, massage the gum around the erupting tooth to provide relief.
- Give the baby a cold teething ring or cold wet cloth, or food (e.g., dry toast or teething cookies) to chew.
- The American Dental Association recommends regular dental checkups, which includes a dental visit within 6 months of the child's first tooth but no later than the child's first birthday.

Nonprescription Medications
Topical Analgesics

- Do not use teething preparations containing benzocaine on infants and young children.

- Do not use prescription viscous lidocaine 2% solution on infants and young children.

Systemic Analgesics

- If desired, use pediatric formulations of oral nonprescription analgesics such as acetaminophen to relieve teething discomfort.
- Read the label carefully, and do not exceed recommended doses or frequency of use.

When to Seek Medical Attention

- If the baby is vomiting or has diarrhea, fever, nasal congestion, malaise, pain, or other symptoms not typical of teething discomfort, take the baby to a family physician or pediatrician.

Source: References 12, 14, and 15.

chemical irritation, biting of the inside of cheeks or lips, or injury caused by toothbrushing or braces) has been implicated as a leading cause of lesions.[17,18] Streptococci and Varicella zoster virus have been implicated as microbial causes.[17] Systemic conditions associated with RAS include Behçet's disease, systemic lupus erythematosus, neutrophil dysfunction, inflammatory bowel disease, and human immunodeficiency virus/acquired immunodeficiency syndrome. Nutritional conditions include gluten-sensitive enteropathy and deficiencies of iron; vitamins B_1, B_2, B_6, and B_{12}; and folic acid. A genetic component to the disease is possible, given that 40% of RAS patients have a familial history: children with parents who have RAS have a 90% chance of developing RAS themselves compared with a 20% chance in children whose parents do not have RAS.[17] Additional precipitating or contributing factors may include food allergy (e.g., preservatives) and hormonal changes (e.g., menstrual cycle).[18]

Clinical Presentation of Recurrent Aphthous Stomatitis

RAS appears as an epithelial ulceration on nonkeratinized mucosal surfaces of movable mouth parts, such as the tongue, floor of the mouth, soft palate, or inside lining of the lips and cheeks. Rarely, ulcerations affect keratinized tissue such as the gingiva or the external lips (vermillion). Individual ulcers are usually (1) round or oval, (2) flat or crater-like, and (3) gray to grayish yellow, with an erythematous halo of inflamed tissue surrounding the ulcer (see Color Plates, photograph 9).

RAS occurs in three clinical forms: minor, major, and herpetiform. The RAS form can be distinguished primarily by the number of lesions, the size of the ulcer, and the number of days that the lesion persists. Table 31–3 compares the features of the three forms of RAS and cold sores.[17,21–23] Some patients may experience a pricking or burning sensation (prodrome) about 2–48 hours before the lesion actually appears.[17] The lesions can be very painful, with the pain increasing with eating and drinking, and may inhibit normal eating, drinking, swallowing, talking, and routine oral hygiene. Usually, fever or

lymphadenopathy does not accompany RAS; however, such symptoms may arise if a secondary bacterial infection is present.

Treatment of Recurrent Aphthous Stomatitis

RAS cannot be cured; however, nonprescription medications can provide symptomatic relief.

Treatment Goals

The primary objective of self-treatment of RAS is to relieve pain and irritation so the lesions can heal, and the patient can eat, drink, and perform routine oral hygiene. The secondary objective is to prevent complications, such as secondary infection.[19]

General Treatment Approach

If possible, the lesions should be inspected to determine whether their appearance and location are characteristic of RAS. If possible, factors that may have led to development of the ulcer should be identified, and precipitating or contributing factors should be removed. For example, if trauma is suspected, perhaps a gentler toothbrush and gentler brushing technique could be suggested. It is also helpful to determine whether the patient has a history of RAS. If the treatments used are appropriate and have been successful for the patient, they should be continued. Figure 31–2 outlines the self-treatment of RAS and lists exclusions for self-care.[13,17–20]

Nonpharmacologic Therapy

If a nutritional deficiency (e.g., iron, folate, or vitamins) is diagnosed as a contributing factor, the patient should increase consumption of foods high in these nutrients or take nutritional supplements. For patients in whom a food allergy is thought to be a contributing factor, elimination of the offending agent from the diet may help to improve or resolve RAS.

table
31–3   **Differentiation of RAS and HSL**

	RAS (canker sores)			HSL (cold sores)
	Minor	**Major**	**Herpetiform**	
Manifestation	Oval, flat ulcer; erythematous tissue around ulcer	Oval, ragged, gray/yellow ulcers; crater form	Small, oval ulcers in crops, similar to minor RAS	Red, fluid-filled vesicles; lesions may coalesce; crusted when mature
Location	All areas except gingiva, hard palate, vermilion (border of the oral mucosa and external skin)	Any intraoral area, but prefers lips, soft palate and throat	Any intraoral area	Junction of oral mucosa and skin of lip and nose
Incidence	13%–26%	1.5%–3%	0.5%–1%	20%–30%
Incidence among RAS sufferers	80%	10%	5%–10%	NA
Number of lesions	1–5	Several (1–10)	10–100 (in crops)	Several
Size of lesion	<0.5 cm	>0.5 cm	<0.5 cm	1–3 mm
Duration (days)	10–14	≥6 weeks	7–10	10–14
Pain	None-moderate	None-moderate	Moderate-severe	None-moderate
Scarring	None	Common	None	Rare
Comments	Immunologic defect	Immunologic defect	Immunologic defect	Induced by HSV-1

Key: HSL = Herpes simplex labialis; HSV-1 = herpes simplex virus-1; NA = not applicable; RAS = recurrent aphthous stomatitis.
Source: References 17 and 21–23.

Because stress may play a role in the development of RAS, relaxation and stress removal may be useful and have shown reductions in ulcer frequency.[17] The box Patient Education for Recurrent Aphthous Stomatitis lists additional non-pharmacologic therapy.

Pharmacologic Therapy

Several types of nonprescription medications (oral debriding and wound-cleansing agents, topical oral anesthetics, topical oral protectants, oral rinses, and systemic analgesics) provide symptomatic relief of RAS, but they do not prevent its recurrence. Table 31–4 lists a variety of the commercially available products for oral pain and discomfort and their pregnancy category rating, if known.

Oral Debriding and Wound-Cleansing Agents

Oral debriding agents and wound cleansers may be used to (1) aid in the removal of debris or phlegm, mucus, or other secretions associated with a sore mouth; (2) cleanse minor wounds or minor gum inflammation; and (3) cleanse recurrent aphthous ulcers. Products that release nascent oxygen can be used as debriding and cleansing agents to provide temporary relief of RAS discomfort. Hydrogen peroxide and carbamide peroxide release oxygen immediately on contact with tissue enzymes (catalase and peroxidase), but tissue and bacterial exposure to the oxygen is very brief.[20,24]

For direct application, a few drops of carbamide peroxide (10%–15%) or hydrogen peroxide (1.5%) are applied to the affected area and allowed to remain in place for 1 minute. As a rinse, carbamide peroxide drops are placed on the tongue, mixed with saliva, and swished in the mouth for 1 minute. An aqueous solution of hydrogen peroxide 3% should be mixed with an equal amount of water before rinsing the mouth. Some products (e.g., Peroxyl Rinse) are a solution of hydrogen peroxide 1.5% and should be used without dilution. Prolonged rinsing with oxidizing products can lead to soft-tissue irritation, transient tooth sensitivity from decalcification of enamel, cellular changes, and overgrowth of undesirable organisms that will possibly lead to a black, hairy tongue.[20]

Topical Oral Anesthetics

Topical oral anesthetic/analgesic products, including benzocaine 5%–20%, benzyl alcohol 0.05%–0.1%, butacaine sulfate 0.05%–0.1%, dyclonine 0.05%–0.1%, hexylresorcinol 0.05%–0.1%, and salicylic alcohol 1%–6%, are generally recognized for temporary relief of pain associated with RAS.[17] To reduce the incidence of RAS, patients should also avoid the use of dentifrices containing sodium lauryl sulfate.[17,18]

Topical Oral Protectants

Oral mucosal protectants are pharmacologically inert substances that coat and protect the ulcerated area. Coating the ulcer with a topical oral protectant can be effective in protecting ulcerations, decreasing friction, and giving temporary symptomatic relief. These products create a barrier by using a paste, an adhering film, or a dissolvable patch to cover the lesion. Some products are available in combination with an oral anesthetic. Products

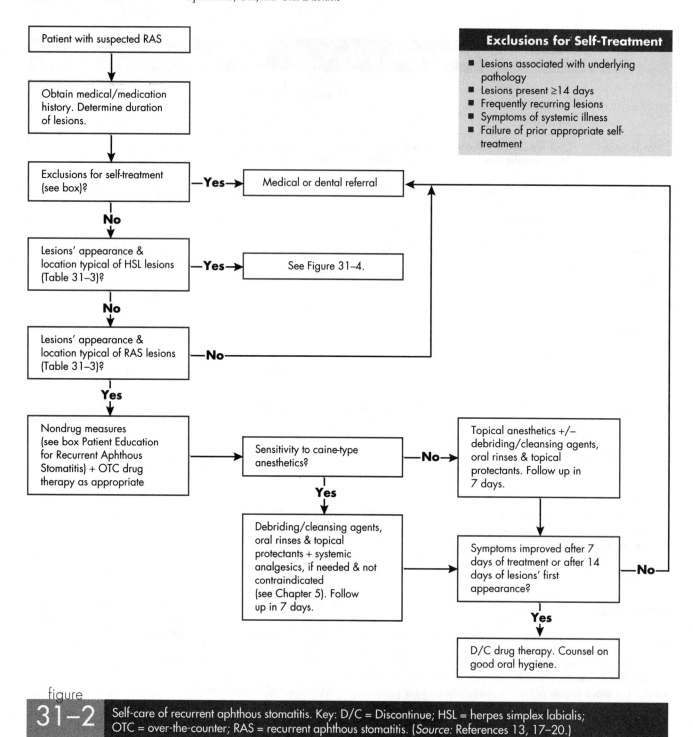

Exclusions for Self-Treatment

- Lesions associated with underlying pathology
- Lesions present ≥14 days
- Frequently recurring lesions
- Symptoms of systemic illness
- Failure of prior appropriate self-treatment

figure
31–2 Self-care of recurrent aphthous stomatitis. Key: D/C = Discontinue; HSL = herpes simplex labialis; OTC = over-the-counter; RAS = recurrent aphthous stomatitis. (*Source:* References 13, 17–20.)

available as a patch or dissolving disc must be placed against the sore for 10–20 seconds. Once the disc adheres to the lesion, the barrier is formed and the disc will stay in place until dissolved, about 8–12 hours.[25]

Oral Rinses

Rinsing the mouth with an antiseptic rinse will hasten the healing of the lesions. Saline rinses (1–3 teaspoons of salt in 4–8 ounces of warm tap water) may soothe ulcers and can be used before topical application of a medication. Similarly, a paste

of baking soda applied to the lesions for a few minutes may soothe irritation.

Systemic Analgesics

Systemic nonprescription analgesics (e.g., aspirin, nonsteroidal anti-inflammatory drugs, and acetaminophen) give additional relief of mouth discomfort. (See Chapter 5 for discussion of these agents and their recommended dosages.) Aspirin should not be retained in the mouth before swallowing, nor placed in the area of the oral lesions. The acid can

Recurrent Aphthous Stomatitis

The primary objective of self-treatment of RAS is to relieve pain and irritation so the lesions can heal and so the patient can eat, drink, and perform routine oral hygiene. The secondary objective is to prevent complications, such as secondary infection. For most patients, carefully following product instructions and the self-care measures listed here will help ensure optimal therapeutic outcomes.

Nondrug Measures

- If a deficiency of iron, folate, or vitamin B_{12} is diagnosed as a contributing factor, increase consumption of foods high in these nutrients, or take nutritional supplements.
- Avoid spicy or acidic foods until the lesions heal.
- Avoid sharp foods that may cause increased trauma to the lesion.
- If desired, apply ice directly to the lesions in 10-minute increments but not longer than 20 minutes in a given hour.
- Do not use heat. If an infection is present, heat may spread the infection.

Nonprescription Medications

- If longer-lasting relief is desired, nonprescription medications such as debriding and cleansing agents, topical oral anesthetics, topical oral protectants, oral rinses, and systemic analgesics can be used.

Oral Debriding and Wound Cleansing Agents

- Use a product containing one of the following ingredients: carbamide peroxide 10%–15% or hydrogen peroxide 1.5%. Apply after meals up to 4 times daily.
- Do not use these medications longer than 7 days. Chronic use can cause tissue irritation, decalcification of enamel, and black hairy tongue.
- Do not swallow these medications.

Topical Oral Anesthetics

- Use products containing one of the following medications: benzocaine 5%–20%, benzyl alcohol 0.05%–0.1%, butacaine sulfate 0.05%–0.1%, dyclonine 0.05%–0.1%, hexylresorcinol 0.05%–0.1%, or salicylic alcohol 1%–6%.

- Do not use benzocaine if you have a history of hypersensitivity to other benzocaine-containing products.

Topical Oral Protectants

- Use topical oral protectants or denture adhesives to coat and protect the lesions. These agents will also provide temporary relief of discomfort.
- Apply these products as needed.

Oral Rinses

- Rinse the mouth with Original Listerine Antiseptic to hasten healing of the lesions.
- Rinse the mouth with a saline solution to soothe discomfort or to prepare the lesion for application of a topical medication. For saline solution, add 1–3 teaspoons of salt to 4–8 ounces of warm tap water.

Systemic Analgesics

- Oral analgesics (e.g., aspirin, NSAID, or acetaminophen) can be used for additional relief of mouth discomfort.
- Do not hold aspirin in the mouth or place it on oral lesions. The acid can cause a chemical burn and tissue damage.

When to Seek Medical Attention

- See a primary care provider if any of the following occur:
  - Symptoms do not improve after 7 days of treatment with oral debriding or wound-cleansing agents.
  - The lesions do not heal in 14 days.
  - Symptoms worsen during self-treatment.
  - Symptoms of systemic infection, such as fever, rash, or swelling, develop.

Source: References 13, 17–20, 24, and Camphor and phenol. Clinical Pharmacology, 2012. Tampa, FL: Elsevier/Gold Standard. Accessed at http://www.clinicalpharmacology.com, August 14, 2013.

table
31–4 Selected Nonprescription Medications for RAS and HSL

Trade Name	Primary Ingredients	Pregnancy Category
Oral Debriding and Wound-Cleansing Agents[a]		
Cankaid Liquid Oral Antiseptic	Carbamide peroxide 10%	ID
Gly-Oxide Antiseptic Oral Cleanser	Carbamide peroxide 10%	ID
Orajel Antiseptic Rinse for Mouth Sores	Hydrogen peroxide 1.5%	C
Colgate Peroxyl Mouth Sore Rinse	Hydrogen peroxide 1.5%	C
Topical Oral Anesthetics		
Anbesol Regular Strength Gel/Liquid	Benzocaine 10%	C
Zilactin-B Gel	Benzocaine 10%	C
Anbesol Maximum Strength Gel	Benzocaine 20%	C
Kank-A Liquid	Benzocaine 20%	C
Orabase Paste	Benzocaine 20%	C
Benzodent	Benzocaine 20%	C

table
31–4   **Selected Nonprescription Medications for RAS and HSL** *(continued)*

Trade Name	Primary Ingredients	Pregnancy Category
Orajel Mouth Sore Gel	Benzocaine 20%; benzalkonium chloride 0.02%; zinc chloride 0.1%	C
Campho-Phenique Gel/Liquid	Camphor 10.8%; phenol 4.7%	ID
Blistex Lip Medex Ointment	Camphor 1%; menthol 1%; phenol 0.54%; petrolatum 59.14%	ID
Carmex Lip Balm Ointment	Menthol 0.7%; camphor 1.7%; phenol 0.4%	ID
Herpicin-L Lip Balm	Dimethicone 1%; meradimate 5%; octinoxate 7.5%; octisalate 5%; oxybenzone 5%	ID
Topical Oral Protectants[a]		
Canker Cover	Menthol 2.5 mg	ID
Oral Rinses		
Original Listerine Antiseptic	Eucalyptol 0.092%; menthol 0.042%; methyl salicylate 0.060%; thymol 0.064%	ID
Topical Treatments[b]		
Abreva	Docosanol 10%	ID

Key: HSL = Herpes simplex labialis; ID = insufficient data to determine pregnancy category; RAS = recurrent aphthous stomatitis.

[a] Use limited to RAS.

[b] Use limited to HSL.

Source: References 13, 20, 24, and Docosanol. Lexi-Drugs Online. Hudson, OH: Lexi-Comp. Accessed at http://www.crlonline.com, August 14, 2013; Menthol. Lexi-Drugs Online. Hudson, OH: Lexi-Comp. Accessed at http://www.crlonline.com, August 11, 2013; and Camphor and phenol. Clinical Pharmacology, 2012. Tampa, FL: Elsevier/Gold Standard. Accessed at http://www.clinicalpharmacology.com, August 14, 2013.

cause a chemical burn with subsequent tissue damage (see Color Plates, photograph 10).

Product Selection Guidelines

Patients with known hypersensitivity to common local anesthetics should not use a product containing a local anesthetic. Benzocaine is a known sensitizer (allergen), and its use in these patients can cause a hypersensitivity reaction. Patients with known sensitivity to aspirin should avoid salicylic acid. Various dosage forms exist (e.g., liquid, gel, rinse, and dissolvable patch); however, drug delivery is a major concern because topical applications can be easily washed away by saliva. Gels are the preferred drug delivery application because they are easy to apply and are not easily washed away.[17–19] A topical anesthetic will provide short-term relief of the pain and discomfort associated with RAS, and the oral debriding agents will help to keep the ulcer clean. Using both of these agents should help alleviate immediate discomfort and heal the ulcer quickly.

Assessment of Recurrent Aphthous Stomatitis: A Case-Based Approach

Controlling the pain and preventing infection are the primary concerns when RAS is suspected. If possible, factors that may have precipitated or contributed to the development of the ulcer should be identified and then removed. The patient should be asked about previous self-treatments and their effectiveness.

If the treatments used are appropriate and have been successful for the patient, they should be continued.

Case 31–1 provides an example of the assessment of a patient with RAS.

Patient Counseling for Recurrent Aphthous Stomatitis

All nonpharmacologic and pharmacologic measures for treating RAS, as outlined in the box Patient Education for Recurrent Aphthous Stomatitis, should be explained to the patient. The patient should also be cautioned about using ineffective or harmful therapies. Possible adverse effects, contraindications, and precautions should then be explained for all nonprescription agents. In addition, patients must be alerted to the conditions that warrant dental or medical evaluation.

Evaluation of Patient Outcomes for Recurrent Aphthous Stomatitis

Minor RAS lesions are typically self-limiting and resolve within 14 days. Oral debriding and wound-cleansing agents are labeled for use for up to 7 days. If the symptoms have improved, the patient should discontinue treatment but continue other dental hygienic measures (e.g., twice-daily toothbrushing). Symptoms that are unimproved or that have worsened during treatment require medical evaluation.

case
31–1

Relevant Evaluation Criteria	Scenario/Model Outcome

Information Gathering

1. Gather essential information about the patient's symptoms and medical history, including:

   a. description of symptom(s) (i.e., nature, onset, duration, severity, associated symptoms)

      Patient noticed a burning/prickling sensation about a day ago. When she looks in her mouth she notices an oval shaped lesion that looks bumpy and is grayish in color.

   b. description of any factors that seem to precipitate, exacerbate, and/or relieve the patient's symptom(s)

      Patient was recently diagnosed with a gluten sensitivity.

   c. description of the patient's efforts to relieve the symptoms

      Patient has not tried anything yet.

   d. patient's identity

      Rebecca Sithgib

   e. age, sex, height, and weight

      32 years old, female, 5 ft 9 in., 155 lb

   f. patient's occupation

      High school German teacher

   g. patient's dietary habits

      Excellent eater, although she admits to having a "sweet tooth."

   h. patient's sleep habits

      6–8 hours nightly

   i. concurrent medical conditions, prescription and non-prescription medications, and dietary supplements

      Multivitamin × 2 years; Nuvaring × 2 months

   j. allergies

      NKDA

   k. history of other adverse reactions to medications

      None

   l. other (describe) _____

      NA

Assessment and Triage

2. Differentiate patient's signs/symptoms and correctly identify the patient's primary problem(s) (Table 31–3).

      Given the location and appearance of the lesion it is highly likely that the patient has RAS. She is at high risk for developing RAS given that she has gluten sensitivity and fluctuation in hormone levels that is associated with recent insertion of a Nuvaring.

3. Identify exclusions for self-treatment (Figure 31–2).

      None

4. Formulate a comprehensive list of therapeutic alternatives for the primary problem to determine if triage to a health care provider is required, and share this information with the patient or caregiver.

      Options include:

      (1) Refer Rebecca to an appropriate health care provider.

      (2) Recommend an OTC product to treat RAS.

      (3) Recommend other self-care options until Rebecca can see an appropriate provider.

      (4) Take no action.

Plan

5. Select an optimal therapeutic alternative to address the patient's problem, taking into account patient preferences.

      An oral debriding and wound-cleansing agent, e.g., hydrogen peroxide 1.5% (Peroxyl), and a topical anesthetic, e.g., benzocaine 20% (Anbesol) would be appropriate initial options. (Table 31–4 lists other options.)

6. Describe the recommended therapeutic approach to the patient or caregiver.

      "A topical anesthetic will provide short-term relief of the pain and discomfort. An oral debriding and wound-cleansing agent will help to keep the ulcer clean to aid in healing."

7. Explain to the patient or caregiver the rationale for selecting the recommended therapeutic approach from the considered therapeutic alternatives.

      "Using both of these agents should help to ease your discomfort as well as heal the ulcer quickly. If you are not experiencing pain or discomfort the topical anesthetic does not need to be used."

Patient Education

8. When recommending self-care with nonprescription medications and/or nondrug therapy, convey accurate information to the patient or caregiver:

   a. appropriate dose and frequency of administration

      "The debriding and cleansing mouth rinse can be used up to 4 times a day (after meals)."

   b. maximum number of days the therapy should be employed

      "Do not use the product for more than 7 days."

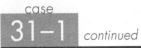

case

31-1   *continued*

Relevant Evaluation Criteria	Scenario/Model Outcome
c. product administration procedures	See the box Patient Education for RAS.
d. expected time to onset of relief	See the box Patient Education for RAS.
e. degree of relief that can be reasonably expected	"The discomfort should dissipate within 7 days and the ulcer should begin improving. It should be completely resolved within 14 days from the day it started."
f. most common side effects	See the box Patient Education for RAS.
g. side effects that warrant medical intervention should they occur	See the box Patient Education for RAS.
h. patient options in the event that condition worsens or persists	See the box Patient Education for RAS.
i. product storage requirements	"Store in a cool, dry place out of children's reach."
j. specific nondrug measures	See the box Patient Education for RAS.
Solicit follow-up questions from the patient or caregiver.	"Should I maintain my normal oral hygiene routine?"
Answer the patient's or caregiver's questions.	"Yes. Continue to brush and floss twice a day, and use a toothpaste that contains fluoride."
Evaluation of Patient Outcome	
9. Assess patient outcome.	Ask the patient to call to update you on her response to your recommendations; or you could call her in a week to evaluate response.

Key: NKDA = No known drug allergies; NA = not applicable; OTC = over-the-counter; RAS = recurrent aphthous stomatitis.

Minor Oral Mucosal Injury or Irritation

Pathophysiology of Minor Oral Mucosal Injury or Irritation

Minor wounds or inflammation resulting from minor dental procedures; accidental injury (e.g., biting of the cheek or abrasion from sharp, crisp foods); or other irritations of the mouth, gums, or palate may be treated with various nonprescription medications.

Treatment of Minor Oral Mucosal Injury or Irritation

Treatment of mouth injury (traumatic laceration or ulcer) and irritation is similar to that for RAS. Mouth injury and irritation differ from RAS with regard to etiology and certain treatment considerations.

Treatment Goals

The goals of treating minor mucosal injury and irritation are to (1) control discomfort and pain, (2) aid healing with the appropriate use of nonpharmacologic and pharmacologic measures, and (3) prevent secondary bacterial infection.

General Treatment Approach

Treatment should focus first on relieving discomfort. Application of ice can relieve discomfort. Local anesthetics, oral analgesics, and saline rinses are safe and effective. Once the discomfort has resolved, patients should focus on healing the affected area. Homemade sodium bicarbonate rinses and oral debriding and wound–cleansing agents can help achieve this objective. Finally, concomitant use of oral protectants can relieve discomfort and aid healing by protecting the area from further irritation. Figure 31–3 outlines this approach and lists exclusions for self-care.[21-23]

Nonpharmacologic Therapy

When tissues of the lips, cheeks, or palate are bruised, direct application of ice may reduce the swelling. Ice should be applied in 10-minute increments but not longer than 20 minutes in a given hour. Longer application times may cause local tissue damage. Sodium bicarbonate solutions (1/2–1 teaspoon of household baking soda in 4 ounces of water) can act as an oral debriding agent and wound cleanser.[23] The solution is swished in the mouth over the affected area for at least 1 minute and then expectorated. Sodium bicarbonate's mucolytic action is related to its alkalinity. Saline rinses (1–3 teaspoons of salt in 4–8 ounces of warm tap water) can cleanse and soothe the affected area.

Pharmacologic Therapy

As with RAS, topical analgesics/anesthetics, oral protectants, and oral debriding and wound–cleansing agents are the mainstay of pharmacologic therapy. The Pharmacologic Therapy section

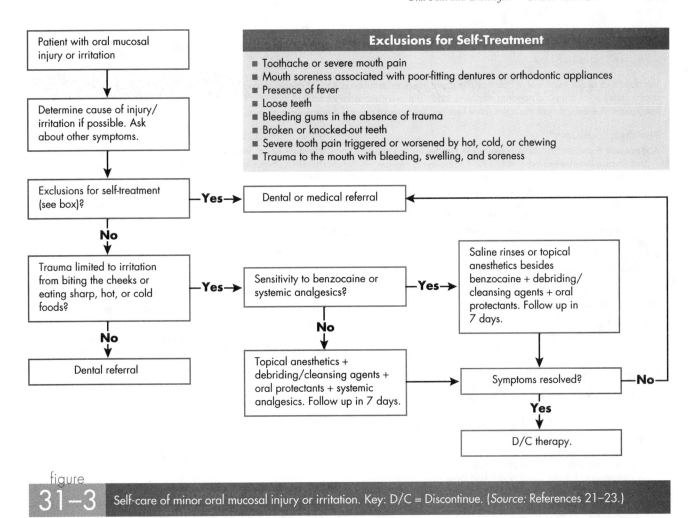

Exclusions for Self-Treatment

- Toothache or severe mouth pain
- Mouth soreness associated with poor-fitting dentures or orthodontic appliances
- Presence of fever
- Loose teeth
- Bleeding gums in the absence of trauma
- Broken or knocked-out teeth
- Severe tooth pain triggered or worsened by hot, cold, or chewing
- Trauma to the mouth with bleeding, swelling, and soreness

figure
31–3   Self-care of minor oral mucosal injury or irritation. Key: D/C = Discontinue. (*Source:* References 21–23.)

for treatment of RAS discusses these agents in further detail. In addition to these agents, astringents may be used. Astringents cause tissues to contract or arrest secretions by causing proteins to coagulate on a cell surface.[26] Dentists may suggest that their patients use oxidizing mouth rinses or topically applied steroids (which are available only by prescription) as an adjunctive treatment of specific conditions or as a postoperative aid to cleaning the affected area, relieving discomfort, and assisting the healing process.

Assessment of Minor Oral Mucosal Injury or Irritation: A Case-Based Approach

The cause and nature of the injury or irritation are the primary considerations in patient assessment. If the disorder is self-treatable, the patient should be asked whether the injury or irritation has occurred previously, how it was treated, and whether the patient has known contraindications to the nonprescription medications used to treat the disorder.

Patient Counseling for Minor Oral Mucosal Injury or Irritation

Once the problem is determined to be minor irritation or injury of the mouth, the patient should be counseled on (1) the

steps in the treatment regimen, (2) the purpose of each agent, and (3) the length of time the products can be used safely. Signs and symptoms that indicate infection should also be explained. (See the box Patient Education for Minor Oral Mucosal Injury or Irritation.)

Evaluation of Patient Outcomes for Minor Oral Mucosal Injury or Irritation

Minor injury or irritation should resolve within 7 days of treatment and within 10 days of the initial insult or injury.[26] If the symptoms are resolved, no further treatment is necessary. If symptoms persist or worsen, or swelling, rash, or fever develops, the patient should be evaluated by a primary care provider.

Herpes Simplex Labialis

Herpes simplex labialis (HSL), also known as cold sores or fever blisters, is a disorder caused by a virus of the family Herpesviridae. Herpes simplex virus 1 (HSV-1) is primarily associated with oral and labial lesions, whereas herpes simplex virus 2 (HSV-2) usually produces genital sores. However, preference of a specific HSV type for an anatomic site is changing, in part

patient education for
Minor Oral Mucosal Injury or Irritation

The objectives of self-treatment of minor oral mucosal injury or irritation are to (1) control discomfort and pain, (2) aid healing with the appropriate use of drug and nondrug measures, and (3) prevent secondary bacterial infection. For most patients, carefully following product instructions and the self-care measures listed here will help ensure optimal therapeutic outcomes.

Nondrug Measures

- Rinse with a sodium bicarbonate solution to remove injured tissue and cleanse the affected area. Add 1/2–1 teaspoon of sodium bicarbonate to 4 ounces of water. Swish the solution in the mouth over the affected area for at least 1 minute, then spit out the solution. This can be done up to four times a day.
- Use saline rinses to cleanse and soothe the affected area. Add 1–3 teaspoons of salt to 4–8 ounces of warm tap water. This can be done up to 4 times a day.
- For bruised lips or cheeks, apply ice in 10-minute increments to reduce swelling. Do not apply ice longer than 20 minutes in a given hour.

Nonprescription Medications

- If longer-lasting relief is desired, use the following types of non-prescription medications: debriding and cleansing agents, topical oral anesthetics, topical oral protectants, and systemic analgesics.

Debriding and Cleansing Agents

- Use a product containing one of the following ingredients: carbamide peroxide 10%–15%, hydrogen peroxide 1.5%, or perborates.
- Do not use these medications longer than 7 days. Chronic use can cause tissue irritation, decalcification of enamel, and black hairy tongue.
- Do not swallow these medications.
- These products should be used after meals (3–4 times a day), and the patient should avoid eating or drinking for at least 30 minutes after application. Swish the liquid around the mouth for 10–15 minutes (or as long as the patient can; no longer than 15 minutes).

Topical Oral Anesthetics

- Use a product containing one of the following medications: benzocaine 5%–20%, benzyl alcohol 0.05%–0.1%, butacaine sulfate 0.05%–0.1%, dyclonine 0.05%–0.1%, hexylresorcinol 0.05%–0.1%, or salicylic alcohol 1%–6%.
- Do not use benzocaine if you have a history of hypersensitivity to other benzocaine-containing products.
- Avoid potentially inflammatory products containing substantial amounts of menthol, phenol, or camphor. These agents may cause tissue irritation and damage or systemic toxicity.
- These products should be used after meals (3–4 times a day), and the patient should avoid eating or drinking for at least 30 minutes after application.

Topical Oral Protectants

- Use topical oral protectants or denture adhesives to coat and protect the lesions.
- These products should be used after meals (3–4 times a day), and the patient should avoid eating or drinking for at least 30 minutes after application.

Systemic Analgesics

- If desired, take an oral analgesic (e.g., aspirin, NSAID, or acetaminophen) for additional relief of mouth discomfort.
- Do not hold aspirin in the mouth or place it on oral lesions. The acid can cause a chemical burn and tissue damage.

When to Seek Medical Attention

- See a primary care provider if any of the following occur:
  - Symptoms persist after 7 days of treatment.
  - Symptoms worsen during self-treatment.
  - Symptoms of systemic infection such as fever, redness, or swelling develop.

Source: References 21, 23, 24, and Camphor and phenol. Clinical Pharmacology, 2012. Tampa, FL: Elsevier/Gold Standard. Accessed at http://www.clinicalpharmacology.com, August 14, 2013.

because of varying sexual practices.[23] Any of the human herpes viruses (e.g., cytomegalovirus and Epstein–Barr virus), not just HSV-1 and 2, can cause oral lesions. Anyone who comes in contact with the herpes virus can potentially become infected. After the primary infection, HSV can be latent and reactivate at a later date as the more commonly known herpes labialis or "cold sore."[21]

Pathophysiology of Herpes Simplex Labialis

HSV is contagious and believed to be transmitted by direct contact. Fluid from herpes vesicles contains live virus and may transmit the virus from patient to patient. Because the virus remains viable on surfaces for several hours, contaminated objects may also be a source of infection. Transmission commonly occurs through kissing or sharing utensils or drinks.[21] HSV enters the host through a break in the skin or intact mucous membranes. Once the virus has infected a host, it remains in a latent state in the trigeminal ganglia. The virus can be reactivated upon exposure to a trigger, such as ultraviolet radiation, stress, fatigue, cold, and windburn. Other possible triggers include fever, injury, menstruation, dental work, infectious diseases, and factors that depress the immune system (e.g., chemotherapy or radiation therapy).[21] Although the virus can go through periods of dormancy and reactivation, the person is infected for life. Upon reactivation, the lesions often arise repeatedly in the same location.

Clinical Presentation of Herpes Simplex Labialis

HSL is so named because it commonly occurs on the lip or on areas bordering the lips; the usual site is at the junction of mucous membrane and skin of the lips or nose. However, these lesions may also occur intraorally (primarily involving keratinized mucosa such as the hard palate or gingiva). The lesions are recurrent, painful, and cosmetically objectionable. HSL lesions are often preceded by a prodrome in which the patient notices burning, itching, tingling, or numbness in the area of the forthcoming lesion. Other symptoms include pain, fever, bleeding, swollen lymph nodes, and malaise.

The lesion first becomes visible as small, red papules of fluid-containing vesicles 1–3 mm in diameter. Often, many lesions coalesce to form a larger area of involvement. An erythematous, inflamed border around the fluid-filled vesicles may be present. A mature lesion often has a crust over the top of many coalesced, burst vesicles; its base is erythematous (see Color Plates, photograph 11). Pustules or pus present under the crust of a herpes virus lesion may indicate a secondary bacterial infection; prompt evaluation and treatment with an appropriate antibiotic, if indicated, are appropriate. Table 31–3 further describes the clinical presentation of HSL and compares its features with those of RAS.

A related disease, acute (primary) herpetic gingivostomatitis, is seen mainly in children but can occur in adults, especially those who are immunocompromised. Although the oral lesions of this disease can develop anywhere on the oral mucosal surface, they commonly occur on the lips, areas bordering the lips, or the gums. Herpetic gingivostomatitis is distinguished from RAS gingivostomatitis by infected gums that are very red and covered by a pseudomembrane or that are studded with ulcerations. Other symptoms of herpetic gingivostomatitis may include submandibular lymphadenitis, swallowing difficulties, and halitosis. Referral to a health care professional would be warranted if this is suspected.

The appearance of HSL and RAS should be easy to distinguish from oral candidiasis, which develops as part of yeast infections. In the mouth, candidiasis is often referred to as thrush and is characterized by white plaques with a milk curd appearance. These plaques, which are attached to the oral mucosa, can usually be detached easily, displaying erythematous, bleeding, sore areas beneath (see Color Plates, photograph 8).

Treatment of Herpes Simplex Labialis

Although the etiologies of HSL and RAS differ, global treatment of these disorders is similar. The patient should be instructed to avoid circumstances that induce more lesions (e.g., stress), keep the lesions free of counterirritants, and keep existing lesions as clean as possible, thereby avoiding secondary infections. Table 31–4 lists common classes of nonprescription medications used to treat RAS and HSL. (*Note:* Of the products listed in Table 31–4, oral debriding and wound-cleansing agents and oral mucosal protectants are not used to treat HSL.)

Treatment Goals

The objectives of self-treatment of herpes simplex labialis (cold sores) are to (1) relieve pain and irritation while the sores are healing, (2) prevent secondary infection, and (3) prevent spread of the lesions.

General Treatment Approach

The lesions should be inspected to determine whether their appearance and location are characteristic of HSL. If possible, factors that may have led to development of lesions should be identified; then precipitating or contributing factors should be removed. For example, if trauma is suspected, perhaps a gentler toothbrush and gentler brushing technique could be suggested. It is also helpful to determine whether the patient has a history of HSL. The patient's medical history should be obtained to determine whether an underlying pathology predisposes the patient to recurrent HSL or could complicate treatment. The patient should be asked about previous self-treatments and their effectiveness. If the treatments used are appropriate and have been successful for the patient, they should be continued. Treatment should focus on

cleansing the affected area, protecting the lesions from infection, and relieving the discomfort of burning, itching, and pain. Figure 31–4 outlines the self-treatment of HSL and lists exclusions for self-care.[21,22,27–29]

Nonpharmacologic Therapy

Lesions should be kept clean by gently washing with mild soap solutions. Handwashing is important in preventing lesion contamination and minimizing autoinoculation of herpes virus. The lesion should be kept moist to prevent drying and fissuring. Cracking of the lesions may render them more susceptible to secondary bacterial infection, may delay healing, and usually increases discomfort. Factors that delay healing (e.g., stress, local trauma, wind, excessive sun exposure, and fatigue) should be avoided. Patients who identify sun exposure as a precipitating event should be advised to routinely use a lip and face sunscreen product. (See Chapter 38 for more detail about sunscreens and sun protection factor [SPF] requirements.)

Pharmacologic Therapy

Topical skin protectants help to protect the lesions from infection, relieve dryness, and keep the lesions soft. These products should be used after meals (3–4 times a day), and the patient should avoid eating or drinking for at least 30 minutes after application.[22]

Externally applied analgesics/anesthetics, in bland, emollient vehicles, also relieve the discomfort of burning, itching, and pain, but they do not reduce the duration of symptoms. Ingredients that are generally used include benzocaine 5%–20%, dibucaine 0.25%–1%, dyclonine hydrochloride 0.5%–1%, benzyl alcohol 10%–33%, camphor 1%–20%, and menthol 0.1%–1%. Menthol in concentrations greater than 1% can stimulate cutaneous sensory receptors and produce a counterirritant effect and therefore are contraindicated.[30]

Docosanol 10% (Abreva) is the only FDA-approved nonprescription product proven to reduce the duration and severity of symptoms. The agent inhibits direct fusion between the herpes virus and the human cell plasma membrane, thereby preventing viral replication.[28] Docosanol should be applied at the first sign of an outbreak (prodromal stage), 5 times a day until the lesion is healed, but for no more than 10 days. Treatment with docosanol reduces the median time to healing by approximately 1 day (18 hours) compared with placebo. Docosanol-treated patients also note a significant reduction in the duration of symptoms, including pain and/or burning, itching, or tingling, compared with placebo (20% reduction in the median time to complete cessation of these symptoms).[28] Systemic therapy should always be considered superior to topical therapy. If evidence of secondary bacterial infection (e.g., failure of crusting to occur or persistence of erythematous border) is seen, topical application of a thin layer of triple-antibiotic ointment 3–4 times daily is recommended. (See Chapter 40 for more information about these agents.) Systemic nonprescription analgesics may provide additional pain relief.

Studies suggest that patients suffering from sideropenia, a condition resulting from a deficiency of iron in the body, and who have recurrent HSL may experience fewer episodes following treatment with iron replacement therapy.[26]

HSL is not considered a steroid-responsive dermatosis; therefore, the use of topical steroids is contraindicated. Products

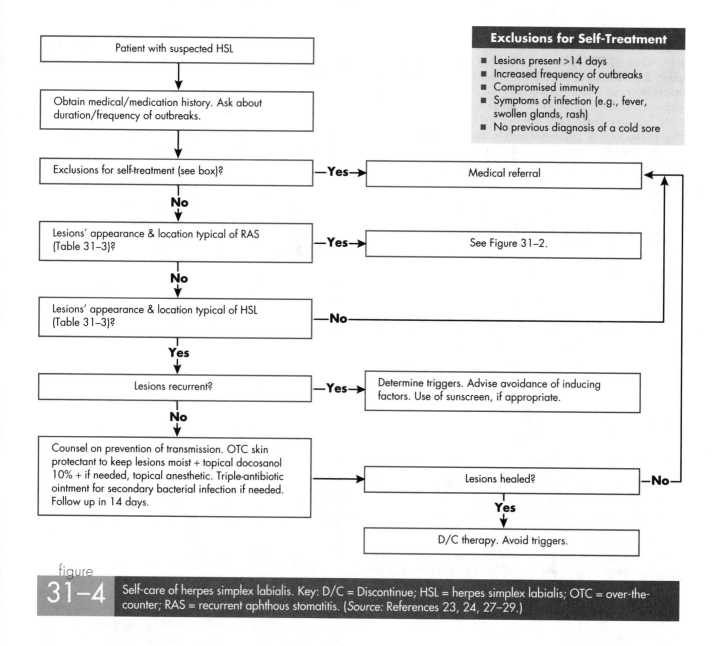

Exclusions for Self-Treatment

- Lesions present >14 days
- Increased frequency of outbreaks
- Compromised immunity
- Symptoms of infection (e.g., fever, swollen glands, rash)
- No previous diagnosis of a cold sore

figure

31–4   Self-care of herpes simplex labialis. Key: D/C = Discontinue; HSL = herpes simplex labialis; OTC = over-the-counter; RAS = recurrent aphthous stomatitis. (*Source:* References 23, 24, 27–29.)

that are highly astringent should also be avoided. Tannic acid and zinc sulfate should be avoided because their frequent application to the lip and oral cavity could cause oral mucosal absorption and toxicity.[31,32]

Complementary Therapies

The essential oil of *Melaleuca alternifolia,* or tea tree oil, has activity against HSV in vitro. Studies have shown that, compared with placebo, the healing time is reduced with use of tea tree oil and is similar to that of topical acyclovir 5%.[33] Lysine has preventive effects and has been shown to decrease the frequency of outbreaks when taken daily.[27,34] Extract of the leaves of *Melissa officinalis,* or lemon balm, have also been used in patients with HSL. Studies comparing lemon balm with placebo have shown a reduction in symptoms, shortened healing time, prevention of infection spread, and patient preference for lemon balm.[34]

Assessment of Herpes Simplex Labialis: A Case-Based Approach

Although many of the same nonprescription medications are indicated for RAS and HSL, the disorders still need to be differentiated. Because herpes simplex lesions are contagious, additional measures are necessary to prevent transmission of the virus. The patient's medical history should be obtained to determine whether an underlying pathology predisposes the patient to recurrent HSL or could complicate treatment.

Case 31–2 provides an example of the assessment of a patient with HSL.

Patient Counseling for Herpes Simplex Labialis

Patient counseling should stress that HSL lesions are contagious and should explain appropriate measures to prevent transmission of the virus, as outlined in the box Patient Education for Herpes

case

31–2

Relevant Evaluation Criteria	Scenario/Model Outcome

Information Gathering

1. Gather essential information about the patient's symptoms and medical history, including:

   a. description of symptom(s) (i.e., nature, onset, duration, severity, associated symptoms)

   Patient is complaining of a burning, itching, tingling feeling on the top of his lip, which he has had for almost 3 weeks. He reports that he has had about 6 cold sores over the past 4 months.

   b. description of any factors that seem to precipitate, exacerbate, and/or relieve the patient's symptom(s)

   Patient reports that he is under a lot of stress as he has been studying for his law school admission tests for the past 4 months.

   c. description of the patient's efforts to relieve the symptoms

   He has tried to put ice on it to relieve the burning and itching, which works until the ice melts. He has also used Carmex and Blistex, which did help with the pain and discomfort.

   d. patient's identity

   William Thanyou

   e. age, sex, height, and weight

   22 years old, male, 6 ft 1 in., 180 lb

   f. patient's occupation

   Student

   g. patient's dietary habits

   Eats a lot of fast food, pasta, and pizza.

   h. patient's sleep habits

   Roughly 6 hours nightly

   i. concurrent medical conditions, prescription and non-prescription medications, and dietary supplements

   Seasonal allergies for which he takes loratadine. Exercise-induced asthma for which he uses albuterol before exertion.

   j. allergies

   NKDA

   k. history of other adverse reactions to medications

   None

   l. other (describe) _____

   NA

Assessment and Triage

2. Differentiate patient's signs/symptoms and correctly identify the patient's primary problem(s) (Table 31–3).

   Patient's signs and symptoms seem to be consistent with recurrent HSL or "cold sore." He seems to be in the prodrome stage, in which a lesion has yet to appear.

3. Identify exclusions for self-treatment (Figure 31–4).

   Increased frequency of breakouts, and lesions present for >14 days.

4. Formulate a comprehensive list of therapeutic alternatives for the primary problem to determine if triage to a health care provider is required, and share this information with the patient or caregiver.

   Options include:

   (1) Refer William to an appropriate health care provider.

   (2) Recommend an OTC product to treat the HSL outbreak.

   (3) Recommend self-care until William can see an appropriate provider.

   (4) Take no action.

Plan

5. Select an optimal therapeutic alternative to address the patient's problem, taking into account patient preferences.

   William is not a self-care candidate because he meets two exclusion criteria.

6. Describe the recommended therapeutic approach to the patient or caregiver

   William should consult an appropriate health care provider for treatment.

7. Explain to the patient or caregiver the rationale for selecting the recommended therapeutic approach from the considered therapeutic alternatives.

   "Seeing a health care provider is best because you have had these symptoms for 3 weeks and you have had frequent episodes over the past 4 months."

Patient Education

8. When recommending self-care with nonprescription medications and/or nondrug therapy, convey accurate information to the patient or caregiver.

   Criterion does not apply in this case.

Relevant Evaluation Criteria	Scenario/Model Outcome
Solicit follow-up questions from the patient or caregiver.	"Is there something I can use to help with the pain and discomfort until I can see my physician tomorrow?"
Answer the patient's or caregiver's questions.	"Any product containing benzocaine 20% would provide acute relief (Table 31–4)."
Evaluation of Patient Outcome	
9. Assess patient outcome.	Contact the patient in a day or two to ensure that he made an appointment and sought medical care.

Key: HSL = Herpes simplex labialis; NA = not applicable; NKDA = no known drug allergies.

Simplex Labialis. Patients should be advised that the disorder is self-limiting, and that pharmacologic therapy can keep the lesions moist and supple, decrease the itching and pain, protect the lesions from secondary bacterial infection, and help reduce the duration of active infection. The action of each recommended product, its proper use, and possible adverse effects should also be explained.

Evaluation of Patient Outcomes for Herpes Simplex Labialis

In immunocompetent patients, HSL is typically mild and self-limiting, resolving within 10–14 days.[21,22,28] If the symptoms have resolved, no further treatment is necessary. However, if the condition worsens (pain and itching persist, redness increases, or signs of secondary infection are apparent), the patient should see his or her primary care provider.

Xerostomia

Xerostomia, commonly referred to as dry mouth, is a syndrome in which salivary flow is limited or completely arrested. A person with normal salivary flow reportedly produces up to 1.5 liters of saliva every 24 hours. Between 10%–50% of the population is said to be afflicted with persistent dry mouth.[35]

Pathophysiology of Xerostomia

Patients with certain disease states, including Sjögren syndrome (an autoimmune condition in which the salivary glands become partly or completely dysfunctional and patients typically present with dry mouth and/or dry eyes), diabetes mellitus, depression, and Crohn's disease, are prone to xerostomia. Radiation therapy of the head and neck can cause atrophy of the salivary glands. After this treatment, the vast majority of patients have

patient education for

Herpes Simplex Labialis

The objectives of self-treatment of herpes simplex labialis (cold sores) are to (1) relieve pain and irritation while the sores are healing, (2) prevent secondary infection, and (3) prevent spread of the lesions. For most patients, carefully following product instructions and the self-care measures listed here will help ensure optimal therapeutic outcomes.

Nondrug Measures

- Keep labial or extraoral lesions clean by gently washing them with mild soap solutions.
- Wash hands frequently to prevent contaminating the lesions and to avoid spreading the virus.
- Avoid factors believed to delay healing such as stress, injury to the lesions, wind, excessive sun exposure, and fatigue.
- If outbreaks are related to sun exposure, use a lip and face sunscreen, with appropriate SPF protection, routinely. Refer to Chapter 38, Sun-Induced Skin Disorders, for further discussion related to SPF.

Nonprescription Medications

- Use topical anesthetics such as benzocaine or dibucaine to relieve burning, itching, and pain. Do not use benzocaine if you have a history of hypersensitivity to other benzocaine-containing products.
- If using products containing camphor and menthol, make sure the concentration of camphor does not exceed 3% and the concentration of menthol does not exceed 1%.
- Do not apply hydrocortisone to the lesions.

- If evidence of secondary bacterial infection is seen, apply a thin layer of triple-antibiotic ointment 3–4 times daily.
- Apply topical agent docosanol 10% (Abreva) to limit the burning, tingling, and itching sensations. Docosanol 10% can also speed up the healing process, thus reducing the duration of the symptoms.
- If desired, take an oral nonprescription analgesic (e.g., aspirin, NSAID, or acetaminophen) for additional pain relief.
- Do not hold aspirin in the mouth or place it on oral lesions. The acid can cause a chemical burn and tissue damage.
- These products should be used after meals (3–4 times a day), and the patient should avoid eating or drinking for at least 30 minutes after application.

When to Seek Medical Attention

See a primary care provider if any of the following occurs:
- The lesions do not heal in 14 days.
- The self-treatment measures do not relieve discomfort.
- Symptoms of systemic illness such as fever, malaise, rash, or swollen lymph glands occur.
- Symptoms change or worsen.

Source: References 21, 23, 27, 29, and 34.

compromised salivary function for the rest of their lives. Medications that have anticholinergic activity or cause depletion of salivary flow volume (e.g., antihistamines, decongestants, antihypertensives, diuretics, antidepressants, antipsychotics, and sedatives) can cause xerostomia.[36] Older patients who are more likely to be taking multiple medications for chronic diseases may be more greatly affected. However, if xerostomia is drug induced and the medication can be discontinued, the condition may be reversed in some cases.[37] Nonpharmacologic causes of xerostomia include use of alcohol, tobacco, caffeine, or hot spicy food; salivary gland stones (sialolithiasis); and mouth breathing.

Clinical Presentation of Xerostomia

Xerostomia can result in difficulty talking and swallowing, stomatitis, burning tongue, and halitosis. Unmoistened food cannot be tasted; therefore, xerostomia can cause loss of appetite and eventual decline in nutritional status.[35,36] Patients' teeth can become hypersensitive, which can be related to a decrease in salivary flow and the lack of buffering capacity that saliva provides.[36] Xerostomia can also result in a higher-than-normal incidence of cervical caries (decay around the root surfaces of teeth) despite excellent oral hygiene. This result can occur because saliva is responsible for washing away food and debris from the teeth, and if saliva is absent and cannot do this, tooth decay can result.[36] Depending on the status of a patient's dentition, this disorder can increase the incidence of caries, gingivitis, and more severe periodontal disease, or reduce denture-wearing

time. Furthermore, reduced flow of saliva can disturb the balance of microflora in the oral cavity and predispose it to candidiasis.

Treatment of Xerostomia

Dry mouth should never be discounted as inconsequential. Failure to treat it can result in serious complications for some patients.

Treatment Goals

The objectives of self-treatment of xerostomia (dry mouth) are to (1) relieve the discomfort of dry mouth, (2) reduce the risk of dental decay, and (3) prevent and treat infections and periodontal disease.

General Treatment Approach

The patient should stop using substances that dry the mouth or erode tooth enamel. If possible, medications that are known to cause xerostomia should be discontinued. To reduce the risk of caries, the patient must maintain good oral hygiene. In mild cases, using sugarless sweets and chewing gums or sucking on ice chips can help to stimulate residual salivary flow.

Commercial artificial saliva products can be used as needed to relieve soft-tissue discomfort. Figure 31–5 outlines the self-treatment of xerostomia and lists exclusions for self-care.[35–38]

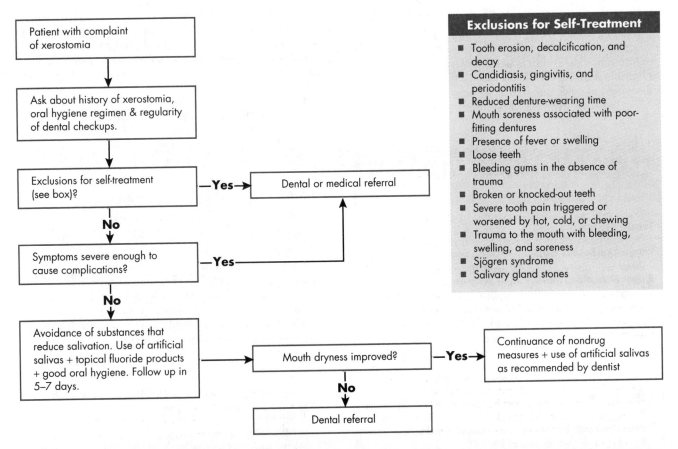

figure
31–5 Self-care of xerostomia. (*Source:* References 35–38.)

Nonpharmacologic Therapy

The patient should avoid substances that reduce salivation, including tobacco (smoked and smokeless), caffeine, hot spicy foods, and alcohol (including mouth rinses). Medication schedules should be modified in consultation with the treating health care provider to coincide with periods of natural stimulation. For example, patients could take medications that cause dry mouth 1 hour prior to meals, because eating naturally stimulates an increase in salivary flow. Consequently, the duration of dry mouth would be reduced.

To prevent tooth decay, the xerostomic patient should limit intake of sugary (e.g., candy), starchy (e.g., cookies, potato chips), and acidic foods (e.g., orange juice) that may have been tolerated before but now pose significant danger to the patient's oral health.[38] Sugar promotes the bacterial production of acid, which causes tooth decay. Acidic foods may also decrease the pH of saliva, resulting in caries and tooth erosion. Chewing gum sweetened with sugar alcohols (e.g., xylitol), however, may be beneficial. Chewing gum increases salivary flow, and xylitol has not been shown to be cariogenic.[35,36] Increasing water intake, especially if it is fluoridated, would also benefit the patient. Using a humidifier at home can help to add moisture in the air, which may provide some level of relief.[38] Finally, the use of very soft-bristle toothbrushes will help prevent decay by minimizing tissue abrasion.

Pharmacologic Therapy

Artificial saliva products are the primary agents for relieving the discomfort of dry mouth. They are designed to mimic natural saliva both chemically and physically. However, they do not contain the many naturally occurring protective components that are present in innate saliva. Because these products do not stimulate natural salivary gland production, they must be considered replacement therapy, not a cure for xerostomia. However, such products can be used on an as-needed basis in patients with little or no saliva flow. Table 31–5 lists selected nonprescription saliva substitutes and other xerostomia products.

table

31–5 Selected Nonprescription Saliva Substitutes and Other Xerostomia Products

Trade Name	Primary Ingredients
Biotene Oral Balance Gel/Liquid Biotene Moisturizing Mouth Spray	Glucose oxidase 10,000 units; lactoferrin 16 mg; Lacto-peroxidase 15,000 units; lysozyme 16 mg; sodium monofluorophosphate 0.14% (w/v fluoride ion)
Entertainer's Secret Spray	Sodium carboxymethylcellulose; dibasic sodium phosphate; potassium chloride; parabens; aloe vera gel; glycerin
Biotene Dry Mouth Gum	Sorbitol; gum base; xylitol; maltitol syrup
Biotene Dry Mouth Toothpaste	Sodium monofluorophospate 0.14%

Key: w/v = Weight per volume.

Product Selection Guidelines

The majority of artificial saliva products are available as sprays and gels; however, gums and toothpastes are also available. Proper use of a gel involves placing approximately a 1/2-inch length of gel onto the tongue and spreading it thoroughly in the mouth. These products can be used at any time; a minimum suggested use is after meals and before going to bed. Products that contain preservatives, such as methyl- or propylparaben, may cause hypersensitivity reactions in certain patients. Patients on low-sodium diets should avoid artificial salivas that contain sodium.

Assessment of Xerostomia: A Case-Based Approach

The patient should be asked about his or her history of xerostomia, oral hygiene practices, and regularity of dental visits. The patient's symptoms should be evaluated to determine whether the symptoms have progressed to the point that complications are likely. A review of the patient's medical and medication history can identify medical conditions and/or medications known to reduce salivation. Furthermore, the reviewer should determine whether lifestyle or other practices could be contributing to the condition. Asking the patient whether he or she has concurrent dry eyes or joint symptoms will assess the risk for Sjögren's syndrome. Similarly, the patient should be questioned as to whether any salivary gland pain or swelling occurs with meals to assess the risk for salivary gland stones.

Patient Counseling for Xerostomia

It is generally necessary for xerostomic patients to have professional dental management of their condition in addition to the self-care methods discussed previously and outlined in the box Patient Education for Xerostomia. Patients should be encouraged to practice good oral hygiene measures and to see their dentist regularly. In addition, patients should be given appropriate information about nonpharmacologic and pharmacologic measures they can use to keep the oral cavity moist and to treat dry mouth to minimize their increased risk for tooth decay associated with xerostomia. Finally, patients must be alerted to signs and symptoms that indicate complications from dry mouth.

Evaluation of Patient Outcomes for Xerostomia

The patient with xerostomia should return for evaluation after 5–7 days of self-treatment. If the mouth dryness is improved, the patient should continue using artificial saliva and fluoride products as recommended by a health care provider. The patient should also be advised to continue the nonpharmacologic measures. If the dryness becomes worse or symptoms of complications develop, the patient should return to a dental health care provider for further evaluation.

Key Points for Oral Pain and Discomfort

➤ Tooth hypersensitivity and teething are not serious and are self-treatable problems.
➤ Self-treatment of toothache should be limited to the temporary relief of pain, because professional treatment is required for complete resolution of pain.

patient education for
Xerostomia

The objectives of self-treatment of xerostomia (dry mouth) are to (1) relieve the discomfort of dry mouth, (2) reduce the risk of dental decay, and (3) prevent and treat infections and periodontal disease. For most patients, carefully following product instructions and the self-care measures listed here will help ensure optimal therapeutic outcomes.

Nondrug Measures

- To prevent reduced levels of saliva, avoid use of cigarettes and smokeless tobacco.
- Do not drink or use products that contain alcohol (including mouth rinses) or medications that cause depletion of salivary flow.
- Avoid food or drinks that contain caffeine.
- Avoid hot spicy foods.
- To prevent tooth decay, limit consumption of sugary (e.g., candy), starchy (e.g., cookies, potato chips), and acidic foods (e.g., orange juice). Do not suck on hard candy or lozenges sweetened with sugar.
- If desired, chew gum sweetened with sugar alcohols, such as xylitol, to help increase flow of saliva.
- If possible, take medications 1 hour before meals so that the natural saliva flow caused by food can counteract any mouth dryness.

- To help prevent tooth decay, use a very soft toothbrush to reduce abrasion of the teeth.
- Drink water.
- Use a humidifier at home to help "moisten" the air.

Nonprescription Medications

- Use artificial saliva products that contain fluoride to relieve the discomfort of dry mouth and prevent tooth decay.
- If you are on a low-sodium diet, avoid artificial salivas that contain sodium.
- Brush and floss your teeth at least twice daily using a regular toothpaste with fluoride, and see your dentist regularly.

When to Seek Medical Attention

- If your symptoms do not improve or if they worsen, see a dentist.

Source: References 35–38.

➤ RAS is amenable to self-treatment of the relief of pain and irritation so the lesions can heal, thereby allowing the patient to eat, drink, and perform routine oral hygiene while preventing further complications.

➤ Minor oral mucosal injury or irritation may be self-treated by controlling discomfort and pain, by using drug and nondrug measures appropriately to aid healing, and by preventing secondary bacterial infection.

➤ The goals of self-treatment of HSL (cold sores) are to relieve pain and irritation while the sores are healing, prevent secondary infection, and prevent spread of the lesions to other areas of the body and other individuals.

➤ Self-treatment of xerostomia (dry mouth) can relieve discomfort from dry mouth, thereby reducing the risk of dental decay as well as preventing and, at times, treating infections.

➤ If conditions worsen or persist after self-treatment and nondrug measures, medical referral for further treatment is imperative.

REFERENCES

1. Petersen PE, Bourgeois D, Ogawa H, et al. The global burden of oral diseases and risks to oral health. *Bull World Health Organ.* 2005;83(9):661–9.
2. Benjamin RM. *Oral Health: The Silent Epidemic.* Rockville, MD: U.S. Department of Health and Human Services, Office of the Surgeon General; 2010. Public Health Reports; No 125:158–9.
3. U.S. Department of Health and Human Services. *Oral Health in America: A Report of the Surgeon General.* Rockville, MD: U.S. Department of Health and Human Services, National Institute of Dental and Craniofacial Research; 2000.
4. Cummins D. Dentin hypersensitivity: from diagnosis to a breakthrough therapy for everyday sensitivity relief. *J Clinical Dent.* 2009;20(spec iss):1–9.
5. Cummins D. Advances in the clinical management of dentin hypersensitivity: a review of recent evidence for the efficacy of dentifrices in providing instant and lasting relief. *J Clinical Dent.* 2011;22:100–7.
6. Jones JA. Dentin hypersensitivity: etiology, risk factors, and prevention strategies. *Dent Today.* 2011;30(11):108, 110, 112–3.
7. Pashley DH, Haywood VB, Collins MA, et al. Dentin hypersensitivity: consensus-based recommendations for the diagnosis and management of dentin hypersensitivity. *Inside Dentistry.* 2008;4(9):1–16.
8. Li Y. Innovations for combating dentin hypersensitivity: current state of the art. *Compend Contin Educ Dent.* 2012;33(spec no 2):10–6.
9. Rosing CK, Fiorini T, Liberman DN, et al. Dentine hypersensitivity: analysis of self-care products. *Braz Oral Res.* 2009;23(suppl 1):56–63.
10. Poulsen S, Errboe M, Lescay-Mevil Y, et al. Potassium containing toothpastes for dentine hypersensitivity. *Cochrane Database Syst Rev.* 2012;4: CD001476. doi:10.1002/14651858.CD001476.pub2. Accessed at http://www.thecochranelibrary.com/view/0/index.html.
11. Schiff T, Delgado E, Zhang YP, et al. Clinical evaluation of the efficacy of an in-office desensitizing paste containing 8% arginine and calcium carbonate in providing instant and lasting relief of dentin hypersensitivity. *Am J Dent.* 2009;22(spec no A):8a–15a.
12. Markman L. Teething: facts and fiction. *Pediatr Rev.* 2009;30(8):e59–64.
13. Benzocaine. Lexi-Drugs Online. Hudson, OH: Lexi-Comp. Accessed at http://www.crlonline.com, August 11, 2013.
14. U.S. Food and Drug Administration. MedWatch safety alert. Benzocaine topical products: sprays, gels and liquids—risk of methemoglobinemia. April 7, 2011. Accessed at http://www.fda.gov/safety/medwatch/safetyinformation/safetyalertsforhumanmedicalproducts/ucm250264.htm, April 19, 2013.
15. U.S. Food and Drug Administration. Drug Safety Communications. FDA recommends not using lidocaine to treat teething pain and requires new *Boxed Warning.* June 24, 2014. Accessed at http://www.fda.gov/downloads/Drugs/DrugSafety/UCM402241.pdf, July 13, 2014.
16. Lalla RV, Choquette LE, Feinn RS, et al. Multivitamin therapy for recurrent aphthous stomatitis: a randomized, double-masked, placebo-controlled trial. *J Am Dent Assoc.* 2012;143(4):370–6.
17. Chavan M, Jain H, Diwan N, et al. Recurrent aphthous stomatitis: a review. *J Oral Pathol Med.* 2012;41(8):577–83.
18. Scully C. Clinical practice. Aphthous ulceration. *N Engl J Med.* 2006; 355(2):165–72.
19. Messadi DV, Younai F. Aphthous ulcers. *Dermatol Ther.* 2010;23(3):281–90.
20. Carbamide peroxide. Lexi-Drugs Online. Hudson, OH: Lexi-Comp. Accessed at http://www.crlonline.com, August 11, 2013.
21. Gonsalves WC, Chi AC, Neville BW. Common oral lesions: part I. Superficial mucosal lesions. *Am Fam Physician.* 2007;75(4):501–7.
22. Munoz-Corcuera M, Esparza-Gomez G, Gonzalez-Moles MA, et al. Oral ulcers: clinical aspects. A tool for dermatologists. Part I. Acute ulcers. *Clin Exp Dermatol.* 2009;34(3):289–94.
23. Klein RS. Treatment of herpes simplex virus type 1 infection in immunocompetent patients. UpToDate; 2012. Accessed at http://www.uptodate.com, August 11, 2013.
24. Hydrogen peroxide. Clinical Pharmacology, 2012. Tampa, FL: Elsevier/Gold Standard. Accessed at http://www.clinicalpharmacology.com, August 14, 2013.

25. Shemer A, Amichai B, Trau H, et al. Efficacy of a mucoadhesive patch compared with an oral solution for treatment of aphthous stomatitis. *DrugsRD.* 2008;9(1):29–35.

26. Burgess JA, van der Ven PF, Martin M, et al. Review of over-the-counter treatments for aphthous ulceration and results from use of a dissolving oral patch containing glycyrrhiza complex herbal extract. *J Contemp Dent Pract.* 2008;9(3):88–98.

27. Elish D, Singh F, Weinberg JM. Therapeutic options for herpes labialis: experimental and natural therapies. *Cutis.* 2005;76(1):38–40.

28. McCarthy JP, Browning WD, Teerlink C, et al. Treatment of herpes labialis: comparison of two OTC drugs and untreated controls. *J Esthet Restor Dent.* 2012;24(2):103–9.

29. Docosanol. Lexi-Drugs Online. Hudson, OH: Lexi-Comp. Accessed at http://www.crlonline.com, August 14, 2013.

30. Menthol. Lexi-Drugs Online. Hudson, OH: Lexi-Comp. Accessed at http://www.crlonline.com, August 11, 2013.

31. Tannic acid. Natural Standard Database. Somerville, MA: Natural Standard. Accessed at http://www.naturalstandard.com, August 14, 2013.

32. Zinc sulfate. Lexi-Drugs Online. Hudson, OH: Lexi-Comp. Accessed at http://www.crlonline.com, August 14, 2013.

33. Carson CF, Ashton L, Dry L, et al. Melaleuca alternifolia (tea tree) oil gel (6%) for the treatment of recurrent herpes labialis. *J Antimicrob Chemoth.* 2001;48(3):450–1.

34. Gaby AR. Natural remedies for herpes simplex. *Altern Med Rev.* 2006; 11(2):93–101.

35. Furness S, Worthington HV, Bryan G, et al. Interventions for the management of dry mouth: topical therapies. *Cochrane Database Syst Rev.* 2011(12):CD008934. doi:10.1002/14651858. CD008934. pub2. Accessed at http://www.thecochranelibrary.com/view/0/index. html.

36. Rayman S, Dincer E, Almas K. Xerostomia. Diagnosis and management in dental practice. *NY State Dent J.* 2010;76(2):24–7.

37. Gonsalves WC, Wrightson AS, Henry RG. Common oral conditions in older persons. *Am Fam Physician.* 2008;78(7):845–52.

38. Singh M, Tonk RS. Xerostomia: etiology, diagnosis, and management. *Dent Today.* 2012;31(10):80, 82–3.

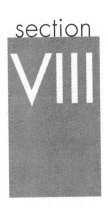
DERMATOLOGIC DISORDERS

ATOPIC DERMATITIS AND DRY SKIN

Kimberley W. Benner

An estimated 5% of the U.S. population suffers from a chronic skin, hair, or nail disorder, and many other Americans experience acute or seasonal disorders.[1] In the United States alone, millions are estimated to suffer from some type of eczematous condition, with atopic dermatitis (AD) specifically reported as a worldwide problem. Furthermore, most patients with this condition are believed either to be undertreated or to use primarily nonprescription medications.[2] Therefore, it is essential for health care providers to be able to recognize and differentiate common skin disorders, suggest appropriate treatment, and know when to refer patients to a primary care provider or dermatologist.

Dermatitis is a nonspecific term describing numerous dermatologic disorders that are generally characterized by erythema and inflammation. The terms *eczema* and *dermatitis* are used interchangeably to describe a group of inflammatory skin disorders of unknown etiology. AD (or atopic eczema) is a form of eczema, which is a general term meaning "to boil over" in Greek; it describes inflammatory skin conditions that are typically erythematous, edematous, papular, and crusty.[3] Many types of eczema exist, including allergic or irritant contact dermatitis, AD, drug-related eczematous dermatitis, eczematous insect bite reaction, and photo-eczematous eruption.[4] Dry skin is a common complaint in many dermatoses, particularly AD. This chapter focuses on AD and dry skin. Although dry skin is often not severe, it may be associated with decreased quality of life for patients with mild-moderate dryness because of the accompanying pruritus and, in some cases, infection, pain, and inflammation that may occur. Many patients are affected by dry skin, and its incidence increases with age.[5]

Role of Skin in Drug Absorption

The skin is involved in numerous physical and biochemical processes. Skin thickness is variable but averages about 1–2 mm. The thickest skin is on the palms and soles, and the thinnest skin is on the genitalia. Thinner skin areas are more permeable, allowing substances to be absorbed more easily than through thicker skin. Although skin is exposed to a variety of chemical and environmental insults, it demonstrates remarkable resiliency and recuperative ability.[6]

Human skin has three functionally distinct regions: epidermis, dermis, and hypodermis (Figure 32–1). The epidermis, the outermost thin layer of the skin, regulates the water content of the skin and controls drug transport into the lower layers and systemic circulation. The middle layer, the dermis, is 40 times thicker than the epidermis and contains nerve endings, vasculature, and hair follicles. The hypodermis primarily provides nourishment and cushioning for the upper two layers.

The most important function of skin and its appendages (hair and nails) is to protect the body from external harmful agents such as pathogenic organisms and chemicals. The skin's ability to do this depends on age, immunologic status, underlying disease states of the individual, medications, and preservation of an intact stratum corneum. Skin is also important in hydroregulation, controlling moisture loss from the body and moisture penetration into the body. If the stratum corneum becomes dehydrated, it loses elasticity and its permeation characteristics are altered. As individuals age, their skin becomes more fragile, requiring a longer recovery time after injury.[5,7]

A drug applied topically must be released from its vehicle if it is to exert an effect at the desired site of activity (skin surface, epidermis, or dermis). Release occurs at the area of contact between the skin surface and the applied layer of product. The physical–chemical relationship between the drug and the vehicle determines the rate and amount of drug released. Considerations such as the drug's solubility in the vehicle, its diffusion coefficient in the vehicle, and its partition coefficient into the sebum and stratum corneum are significant to its efficacy.[8] The major mechanism of drug absorption is passive diffusion through the stratum corneum, followed by transport through the deeper epidermal regions and then the dermis. Drug movement into and through the skin is enhanced or inhibited to varying degrees depending on the physical–chemical properties of a drug, the sebum, and the location of the skin. The stratum corneum provides the greatest resistance and is often a rate-limiting barrier to percutaneous absorption. The hydration status of the stratum corneum can affect drug diffusion. Occlusion increases hydration of the stratum corneum, which enhances the transfer of most drugs.[8] Wounds, burns, chafed areas, and dermatitis can alter the integrity of the stratum corneum and can result in artificial shunts of the percutaneous absorption process. Inflammation can also enhance percutaneous absorption of topically applied medications, which may result in higher systemic drug levels. Therefore, caution should be used in applying topical medication to compromised skin, particularly if large surface areas are involved.

Topical medications are used to treat many common skin disorders in infants and children. Treatment of any unknown

Editor's Note: This chapter is based on the 17th edition chapter of the same title, written by Steven A. Scott.

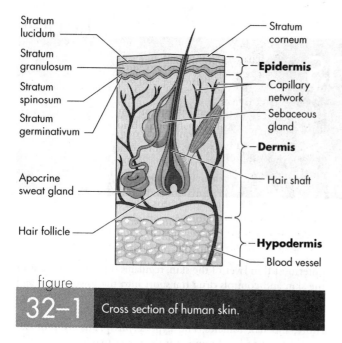

32-1 Cross section of human skin.

32-1 Diagnostic Criteria for Atopic Dermatitis

A pruritic skin disorder, plus three or more of the following criteria:
- Onset at younger than 2 years
- History of skin crease involvement (including cheeks in children younger than 10 years)
- History of generally dry skin
- Personal history of other atopic disease, that is, asthma (or history of any atopic disease in first-degree relative in children younger than 4 years)
- Visible flexural dermatitis (or dermatitis of cheeks/forehead and other outer limbs in children younger than 4 years)

Source: References 21 and 22.

skin disorder in infants younger than 1 year should be initiated only after seeking the advice of a primary care provider. Infants have a reduced capability to biotransform drugs absorbed by the cutaneous route because they have immature hepatic enzyme systems. In addition, because the ratio of surface area to body weight in a neonate is approximately two to three times that of an adult, the proportion of drug absorbed per kilogram of body weight is greater in a newborn.[9]

Atopic Dermatitis

AD is a common, pervasive inflammatory condition of the epidermis and dermis that is characterized by episodic flares and periods of remission. AD is estimated to effect from 10% to 20% of children and many of these individuals have symptoms into adulthood.[10,11] Sixty percent of patients are diagnosed within the first year of life while another 30% manifests before the age of 5 years.[12,13] In adults the prevalence is estimated at 1%–3% with the overall lifetime prevalence reported at 7%.[10] Prevalence worldwide is increasing, possibly because of air pollution, industrialization, urbanization, dietary modifications, and higher socioeconomic class.[11,14] The atopic triad is asthma, allergic rhinitis, and atopic dermatitis. Asthma and allergic rhinitis can occur in up to 80% of patients with AD, either in childhood or as individuals age.[15] This phenomenon has been referred to as the "atopic march."[12] Eighty percent of AD is classified as mild and can be safely treated with nonprescription products.[16] In addition, many patients with AD do not seek medical care and therefore are likely to look for advice regarding self-care of this disorder.[17]

Pathophysiology of Atopic Dermatitis

AD has a genetic basis, but its expression is modified by a broad spectrum of exogenous manifestations.[17] Atopic skin is inflamed with an expression of cytokines and chemokines; inflammatory cytokines such as interleukin-4 and 13 and tumor necrosis factor are produced.[11,12] A protein in the epidermal differentiation complex, filaggrin (FLG), is related to the development of AD. Even one mutation in FLG increases one's risk of AD, and 35 mutations are known to exist in the FLG gene.[3] The filaggrin mutation can lead to the deficient skin barrier characteristic of AD.[18] This mutation leads to irritation in atopic skin caused by increased penetration of allergens, a decrease in skin barrier proteins, higher peptidase activity, and lack of protease inhibitors.[19] In addition, because of a decreased concentration of lipid and ceramides, atopic skin has a decreased ability to retain moisture.[20] Seventy percent of AD cases have an atopic family history; if one parent is atopic, the rate of similar symptoms in their children is approximately 50%, whereas if both parents are atopic, this risk rises to 79%.[3]

AD is diagnosed according to clinical criteria (Table 32–1).[21,22] No established confirmatory laboratory tests exist, although many patients have shown an elevated immunoglobulin (Ig) E level and peripheral blood eosinophilia. This elevated IgE level typically does not appear early on, and in some children may never occur.[23] The SCORAD (SCORing Atopic Dermatitis) Index was developed to create a consensus on assessment methods for AD and measures the severity of the AD. The index grades or rates the following items: erythema, edema, papulation (formation of papules), excoriations (abrasion of the epidermis by trauma), lichenification (increased epidermal markings), oozing/crusting, and dryness. The index also uses a visual analogue scale to rate daily pruritus and sleepiness. A SCORAD index of less than 25 is considered mild, 25–50 moderate, and greater than 50 severe.[24]

Clinical Presentation of Atopic Dermatitis

Although AD is often first manifested in infancy, it is rarely present at birth. If it does develop early in life, it typically occurs within the first year, often beginning at 2–3 months of age. Infantile or childhood AD initially appears as erythema and scaling of the infant's cheeks, which may progress to affect the face, neck, forehead, and extremities (see Color Plates, photographs 12A, B, and C). Crusts and pustules can form from the effects of scratching and rubbing. Remission usually occurs by the end of the second year with xerosis (dry skin) often continuing into adulthood.[25] In older patients, AD presents quite differently when compared with children and may be less severe.[11,25] Plaques appear erythematous, scaly, exudative, or lichenified. Areas affected include antecubital and popliteal fossae, neck, forehead, eyes and hands.[25] The cause in adults is often environmental, attributed to chemicals or skin trauma.[19] Pruritus, the hallmark symptom of AD, causes morbidity and is sometimes referred to as the "itch that rashes." Patients with AD react more readily and more persistently to pruritic-inducing stimuli. Scratching and lichenification can produce a vicious cycle and lead to excoriation.[3,19] It is important to note that patients can present atypically, and any undiagnosed skin lesions that do not improve over time or that get worse with self-treatment should be evaluated by a physician.

AD has three clinical forms. Acute AD, characterized by intensely pruritic, erythematous papules or vesicles over erythematous skin, is often associated with excoriation and serous exudate. Subacute AD is characterized by erythematous, excoriated papules and plaques that can be scaly. Chronic AD is characterized by thickened plaques of skin and accentuated skin markings.[26] In chronic AD, all three stages of skin reactions frequently coexist in the patient.

Secondary or associated cutaneous infections, especially bacterial, can be common, difficult to prevent, and typically aggravate AD. More than 90% of the skin lesions in patients with AD (in contrast to 5% of unaffected individuals) harbor *Staphylococcus aureus (S. aureus)*.[12,17] Although *S. aureus* is the most common cause of infection, streptococci may also be found alone or in association with *S. aureus*. Infections present as yellowish crusting of the eczematous lesions.

Patients with AD may also develop infections with viruses, such as herpes simplex or *Molluscum contagiosum*.[12,26] Although true infection of the skin is more common in children with AD, colonization is higher in adult patients.[11] Patients should be counseled to seek medical attention promptly when signs of bacterial or viral skin infection, such as pustules (circumscribed, elevated lesions, 1 cm in diameter containing pus), vesicles (especially exudate or pus-filled), and crusting (dried exudate), are noticed.[17]

Treatment of Atopic Dermatitis
Treatment Goals

The goals of self-treatment of AD are to (1) stop the itch–scratch cycle, (2) maintain skin hydration, (3) avoid or minimize factors that trigger or aggravate the disorder, and (4) prevent secondary infections.

General Treatment Approach

To prevent unrealistic expectations, health care providers should stress to patients that AD cannot be cured but that most patients' symptoms can be managed satisfactorily. The disorder should be explained as being multifactorial, and just as there is no cure, there is no single cause. Often no explanation can be found for a particular flare-up of the disorder, and many factors can contribute simultaneously.

Enhancing hydration in atopic skin can be achieved through nonpharmacologic measures and through the use of emollients and moisturizers. Hydrocortisone relieves itching and inflammation, and cool water compresses relieve weeping vesicles. An effective preventive measure is to minimize exposure to factors known to trigger AD. The algorithm in Figure 32–2 outlines the self-treatment of this disorder and lists exclusions for self-treatment.[12,13,26]

Nonpharmacologic Therapy

The variability in severity and age of onset requires tailoring treatment to a patient's needs and preferences, bearing in mind the patient's age, gender, and social conditions, along with the site(s) and severity of the lesions. Successful treatment of AD includes (1) skin hydration; (2) the identification and elimination of triggers; and (3) the use of topical therapy and possibly systemic therapy for refractory cases.

Education on trigger avoidance and hydration of the skin are of utmost importance in the prevention as well as treatment of AD. Common triggers that patients should avoid are listed in Table 32–2.[12,18,27] Compared with nonaffected individuals, skin in a patient with AD may be more susceptible to irritants. Therefore, additional preventive measures and lifestyle changes can be made in patients with AD. One suggestion is to use cotton sheets washed in gentle detergents with a second rinse cycle. Laundering and thoroughly rinsing new clothing with unscented laundry detergent is recommended, as is avoiding fabric softeners. If used, liquid fabric softeners are preferred over dryer sheets. Bathing can be helpful in AD sufferers; bathing can hydrate the stratum corneum, remove allergens and irritants, cleanse and debride crusts, and enhance the effects of moisturizers and topical steroids.[13,28] However, baths should be kept to a minimum (3–5 minutes and every other day), and bath water should be tepid; putting colloidal oatmeal in the water can be considered. Common bar soaps are often too drying and irritating for some AD patients.[29] Because of this, mild nonsoap cleansers (e.g., Cetaphil) are often recommended. After bathing, skin should be patted dry or air dried, followed by application of moisturizers to help to seal in the water. Patients should be reminded to use sunscreens outside; however, zinc and titanium should be avoided as they can aggravate some lesions.

Although allergens such as plant or animal proteins from food, pollens, or pets can aggravate AD, the role of food allergies in exacerbating AD is unclear. In about one-third of children, food allergies may exacerbate moderate-severe AD.[30] These allergies often include egg, milk, peanut, soy, and wheat. The more severe the AD and younger the patient, the more likely food is the triggering allergen. Although many children who have AD caused by food allergies can outgrow the allergy (and the AD as well), children who present with food allergies and AD should be evaluated by a physician.[16,31] Restricting offending foods, especially in children, creates overwhelming compliance problems. Moreover, although dietary restriction may produce some improvement in the disorder initially, complete resolution is unlikely to occur. Therefore, reserving dietary management for patients who have severe symptoms and are unresponsive to other treatments is probably best.[12] Patients with AD are often intolerant of sudden and extreme changes in temperature and humidity. High temperature may enhance perspiration, leading to increased itching. Low humidity, often found in heated buildings during the winter, dries the skin and increases itching. Use of humidifiers in dry environments can provide some benefit.

Because the pruritus is often bothersome for many patients, keeping the fingernails short, smooth, and clean is important to avoid introduction of bacteria via microfissures; patients can consider the use of cotton gloves at night to prevent constant scratching of the itchy skin. Excessive scratching can result in open sores that may need to be treated with a topical antibiotic. Use of bacitracin/polymyxin B ointment (Polysporin) may be preferred to bacitracin/polymyxin B/neomycin ointment, given that some patients may be sensitized to neomycin.[32]

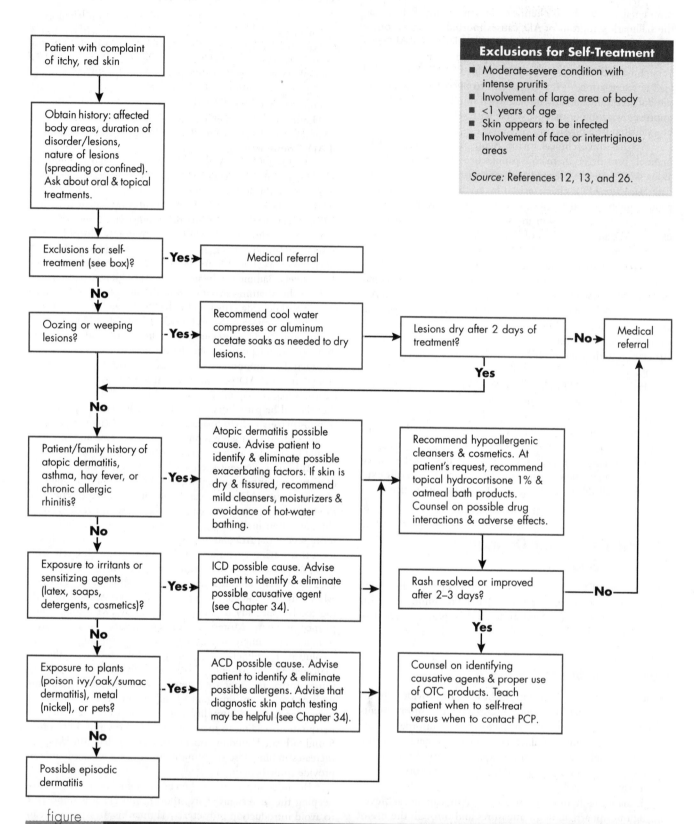

Exclusions for Self-Treatment
- Moderate-severe condition with intense pruritis
- Involvement of large area of body
- <1 years of age
- Skin appears to be infected
- Involvement of face or intertriginous areas

Source: References 12, 13, and 26.

figure

32–2 Self-care of dermatitis. Key: ACD = Allergic contact dermatitis; ICD = irritant contact dermatitis; OTC = over-the-counter; PCP = primary care provider.

table	
32–2	**Triggers Associated with Atopic Dermatitis**

Food allergens (e.g., egg, milk, peanut, soy, wheat, nuts)

Aeroallergens (e.g., dust mites, cat dander, molds, grass, ragweed, pollen)

Stress

Air pollutants (tobacco smoke or traffic exhaust)

Cosmetics/fragrances/astringents

Exposure to temperature extremes (heat/cold)

Electric blankets

Excessive hand or skin washing

Use of irritating soaps, detergents, and scrubs

Tight-fitting or irritating clothes (wool or synthetics)

Dyes and preservatives

Source: References 12, 18, and 27.

Because maintaining skin hydration and patency is important, the use of emollients should be included. Emollients are considered standard of care and often referred to as "steroid sparing."[13,33] Studies have shown their use improves skin response rate in AD.[13,34] Moisturization with emollients at least twice daily is recommended for preventive and maintenance therapy to keep skin soft and pliable. Use of creams or ointments is recommended over lotions to keep the skin soft and hydrated. Oil-in-water preparations (creams and lotions) are often more cosmetically acceptable, but they need to be applied more frequently than ointments because their ability to maintain moisture in the skin is often more short-lived. If applied correctly, creams and lotions should have a good emollient effect and not produce dryness.

Other preventive measures, such as breast-feeding and delaying introduction of solid food, remain controversial. Few studies have looked at these interventions and their role in the prevention of AD; guidelines state that no definite evidence indicates that breast-feeding and solid food introduction will significantly affect AD.[13] Although more recent literature suggests that exclusive breast-feeding can decrease the incidence of AD, no convincing evidence exists that delaying solid foods will help.[12,35]

Pharmacologic Therapy

Hydrocortisone in an oil-in-water base is the primary nonprescription pharmacologic agent used to treat AD. This agent is classified as a low-potency corticosteroid and is primarily used to decrease inflammation and relieve itching. This corticosteroid is safe to use short term on virtually any area of the body (including the face, neck, axillae, and groin) and safe to use in children older than 2 years.[13,26] When used properly, hydrocortisone 0.5% and 1% products are associated with a very low risk of local and systemic adverse effects compared with high-potency topical corticosteroid products. Hydrocortisone cream is often the preferred product for most patients with AD because of patient preference for a less greasy preparation.[28] Ointment formulations, while often greasy, are preferred on areas of thick skin or if a patient's skin is dry, lichenified, or scaly.[26,36,37]

These products are usually applied 1–2 times daily during AD flare-ups, usually before application of any moisturizers.[8,12,36] Ointments should be avoided if the AD lesions are weeping, and all hydrocortisone products should be avoided if the skin is open or cracked.[38] Refractory cases of AD should be referred to a physician but can further be treated with higher-potency topical corticosteroids; topical calcineurin inhibitors, such as tacrolimus or pimecrolimus; or systemic immunomodulators (e.g., cyclosporine, azathioprine, or methotrexate)[28,39]; however, these agents require a prescription and thus are not covered in detail in this chapter.

Because of the risk of infections, as previously mentioned, preventing and managing infections is important in an AD patient. Topical mupirocin may be initially effective, but the patient will need referral to a physician and require a short course of an oral antistaphylococcal antibiotic, such as cephalexin or penicillin. The benefits of topical or oral antibiotics in improving AD lesions remain under debate.

Guidelines state the use of systemic and topical antibiotics may reduce skin colonization[13] whereas more recent information suggests topical antibiotics are not effective and should not be used long term.[18,28] The use of antiseptics, while of limited benefit, can also be considered, but can be associated with a drying effect. Data on the use of chlorhexidine, triclocarban, and fusidic acid are conflicting, and thus the guidelines do not specifically recommend their use.[13]

Complementary Therapies

Few complementary therapies exist to manage atopic dermatitis. The use of probiotics, such as lactobacillus, *may* delay the presentation of AD, although more studies are needed to determine the exact dose, duration, and safety of the use of probiotics.[13,40] The use of phototherapy in patients with AD may be beneficial.[13] Coal tar has also shown benefit in other dermatologic conditions and likewise can be useful in refractory AD, particularly in combination with phototherapy.[3] Safety of the coal tar and phototherapy combination therapy in children, however, has not been established.[41] The use of certain Chinese herbal mixtures has shown benefit in AD,[3] but recent guidelines state insufficient evidence to support their use.[39] Other botanicals used in skin disorders are mentioned in Chapter 51. Although time consuming for patients and caregivers, the use of "wet wraps" (applying a steroid or emollient to affected lesions, then wrapping the lesions in a wet then dry layer, and retaining the wraps for an overnight period) can increase skin hydration and help decrease scratching.[12] A growing body of literature and evidence is available on the use and efficacy of wet wraps.[42,43]

Dry Skin

Xerosis, or dry skin, is the result of decreased water content of the skin with resultant abnormal loss of cells from the stratum corneum. Environmental dry skin is often associated with long, hot showers or not consuming enough water. The prevention and care of dry skin may become a major focus for health care providers as the population of older adults continues to increase. Among those caring for these older adults, a heightened awareness exists that prophylactic dry skin care can reduce morbidity by minimizing the risk of skin breakdown and, therefore, can ultimately reduce the cost of dermatologic health care.[5]

Dry skin is a common problem and affects more than 50% of older adults. It is also the most common cause of pruritus.[44] Dry skin is a frequent cause of pruritus in cooler climates during the winter season (i.e., "winter itch"). Individuals who live or work in arid, windy, or cold environments also have an increased risk for dry skin.

Pathophysiology of Dry Skin

Dry skin can result from various etiologies. It can be caused by disruption of keratinization and desquamation.[44] Dry skin may also occur secondary to prolonged detergent use, malnutrition, or physical damage to the stratum corneum. Furthermore, dry skin may signal a systemic disorder such as hypothyroidism or dehydration. Dry skin is related to decreased water retention in the stratum corneum—not to a lack of natural skin oils. Dry air allows the outer skin layer to lose moisture, become less flexible, and crack when flexed, leading to an increased rate of moisture loss. Exposure of skin to high wind velocity will result in moisture loss.

With advancing age, the epidermis changes because of abnormal maturation or adhesion of the keratinocytes, resulting in a superficial, irregular layer of corneocytes. This disorder may be described as a thinning of the entire epidermis, which produces a roughened skin surface. The skin's hygroscopic substances also decrease in quantity with advancing age. Hormonal changes that accompany aging result in lowered sebum output. Older patients also typically have inadequate water intake, which contributes to this disorder.[5,45]

Clinical Presentation of Dry Skin

Dry skin is characterized by one or more of the following signs and symptoms: roughness, scaling, loss of flexibility, fissures, inflammation, and pruritus. Common clinical findings include fine platelike scaling, particularly on the arms and legs, that may be associated with a "cracked" appearance (eczema craquelé) or fish-scaling (ichthyosis) appearance of the skin.[44]

Treatment of Dry Skin
Treatment Goals

The goals of self-treatment of dry skin are to (1) restore skin hydration, (2) restore the skin's barrier function, and (3) educate the patient about prevention and treatment of this chronic disorder.

General Treatment Approach

Treatment involves recognizing the problem as well as modifying the environment (humidity) and bathing habits to maintain skin hydration. Nonprescription products such as bath oils, emollients and moisturizers containing humectants, keratolytic agents, or both, aid in restoring and maintaining barrier function. If needed, topical hydrocortisone can be used to reduce pruritus and erythema.[46]

---

table
32–3   **Dry Skin Therapy**

- Take tub baths with addition of bath oil 2–3 times per week for brief periods (3–5 minutes). Take sponge baths on other days.
- Bathe in tepid water, not more than 3°F above body temperature.
- Within 3 minutes of getting out of the tub, pat the body dry, leaving beads of moisture, and generously apply body lotion to trap the moisture.
- Apply the body lotion at least 3 more times during the day to the whole body (preferably) or at least the most affected areas.
- Additional measures include:
  - Use corticosteroid ointments rather than creams if indicated for short-term use.
  - Keep room humidity high.

Nonpharmacologic Therapy

The most important aspects of care are the proper use of emollients and modifications to bathing practices. Products such as oilated oatmeal or bath oil added near the end of the bath may be used to enhance skin hydration. The patient should apply oil-based emollients immediately after bathing while the skin is damp and should reapply them frequently. The room humidity should be increased with a portable cool-mist humidifier, or a humidification unit can be added to the home heating system. The patient should be encouraged to stay well hydrated by drinking ample water daily unless contraindicated by any medical disorders. Table 32–3 reviews nonpharmacologic therapy of dry skin.

Pharmacologic Therapy

Dry skin is more prone to itching, inflammation, and development of secondary infections. Most moisturizers are mixtures of oils and water, but more severe cases of dry skin may require a product containing a humectant (e.g., glycerin, urea, lactic acid) to enhance hydration. Other agents that can be added to these emollients or moisturizers include alpha hydroxy acids and lipid moisturizers such as phospholipids and ceramides.[44]

Dry skin responds minimally to topical corticosteroid therapy, although short-term (≤7 days) use of topical corticosteroids may reduce symptoms of erythema and pruritus.[44] If resolution does not occur within 1 week, a primary care provider should be consulted because other options may be required to improve the dry skin.

Treatment of Atopic Dermatitis and Dry Skin

Nonprescription products for dermatitis and dry skin that restore skin hydration include bath products and emollients, which can contain hydrating, keratolytic, and keratin-softening agents. Often these products are combined in commonly available nonprescription products (Table 32–4). Many ingredients are available for use on AD lesions or dry skin; these products are reviewed below. These products can be recommended according to patient preference and therapeutic response.

table

32–4 Selected Nonprescription Dry Skin Products

Trade Name	Primary Ingredients
Petrolatum-Containing Products	
Absorbase Ointment[a]	Petrolatum; mineral oil; ceresin wax; wool wax alcohol; potassium sorbate
AmLactin Cream/Lotion	Ammonium lactate 12%
Aquaphor Ointment	Petrolatum 41%; water
Cetaphil Gentle Cleansing Bar[a]	Sodium cocoyl isethionate; stearic acid; sodium tallousate; PEG-20; petrolatum
Eucerin Cream[a]	Petrolatum; mineral oil; mineral wax; wool wax alcohol
Jergens Advanced Therapy Ultra Healing Lotion	Petrolatum; mineral oil; dimethicone; cetearyl alcohol; cetyl alcohol; glycerin; allantoin
Moisturel Cream/Lotion[a]	Petrolatum; dimethicone; cetyl alcohol; glycerin
Vaseline Dermatology Formula Lotion	White petrolatum 5%; mineral oil 4%; dimethicone 1%; glyceryl stearate; cetyl alcohol; glycerin
Colloidal Products	
Aveeno Daily Moisturizing Lotion[a]	Dimethicone 1.25%; cetyl alcohol; oat kernel flour; glycerin
Aveeno Moisturizing Bath Treatment Formula[a]	Mineral oil; colloidal oatmeal 43%
Aveeno Moisturizing Cream/Lotion[a]	Petrolatum; dimethicone; isopropyl palmitate; cetyl alcohol; colloidal oatmeal 1%; glycerin
Aveeno Skin Relief Moisturizing Lotion[a]	Dimethicone 1.25%; menthol 0.1%; oat kernel flour
Aveeno Soothing Bath Treatment Formula[a]	Colloidal oatmeal 100%
Neosporin Eczema Essentials[a]	Colloidal oatmeal; ceramide; mineral oil
Urea-Containing Products	
Carmol 10 Lotion	Urea 10%
Carmol 20 Cream	Urea 20%
Lac-Hydrin Five Lotion	Urea 5%
Counterirritants	
Sarna Anti-Itch Lotion	Camphor 0.5%; menthol 0.5%; carbomer 940; cetyl alcohol; DMDM hydantoin; glyceryl stearate; petrolatum
Miscellaneous Emollients	
Cetaphil Gentle Skin Cleanser Liquid[a]	Cetyl alcohol; stearyl alcohol; PEG
Gold Bond Ultimate Healing Lotion	Glycerin; petrolatum; cetyl alcohol; aloe; cetearyl alcohol; propylene glycol; glyceryl stearate
Keri Original Formula Therapeutic Dry Skin Lotion	Mineral oil; lanolin oil; glyceryl stearate; propylene glycol
Lubriderm Advanced Therapy Lotion	Cetyl alcohol; glycerin; mineral oil; PEG-40; emulsifying wax; vitamin E
Lubriderm Daily Moisturizing Lotion	Mineral oil; petrolatum; sorbitol; lanolin; lanolin alcohol; triethanolamine
Neutrogena Body Oil	Isopropyl myristate; sesame oil
Neutrogena Soap	TEA-stearate; triethanolamine; glycerin
Nivea Body Lotion	Mineral oil; glycerin isopropyl palmitate; vitamin E; lanolin alcohol
Purpose Gentle Cleansing Bar	Sodium tallowate; sodium cocoate; glycerin; BHT

Key: BHT = Butylhydroxytoluene; DMDM = dimethylol dimethyl; PEG = polyethylene glycol; TEA = triethanolamine.
[a] Fragrance-free formulation.

Bath Products

Bath Oils

Bath oils generally consist of a mineral or vegetable oil plus a surfactant. Mineral oil products are absorbed better than vegetable oil products. Some commercially available bath oil products are combined with colloidal oatmeal in an attempt to provide better relief of itching. Because these commercial products can be expensive, some providers recommend preparing these products at home by processing instant (unflavored) oatmeal in a blender and placing in the bath water. Bath oils are minimally effective in improving a dry skin disorder because they are greatly diluted in water.

When applied as wet compresses, bath oils (1 teaspoon in one-fourth cup of warm water) help lubricate dry skin and may allow a decrease in the frequency of full-body bathing. Bath oils make the tub and floor slippery, creating a safety hazard, especially for older adults or children.

Cleansers

Typical bath soaps generally contain salts of long-chain fatty acids (commonly oleic, palmitic, or stearic acid) and alkali metals (e.g., sodium or potassium). Combined with water, these products act as surfactants that remove many substances from the skin, including the lipids that normally keep the skin soft and pliable. Providers often recommend special soaps, such as those including glycerin, that contain extra oils to minimize the drying effect of washing. However, these soaps usually lather and clean poorly. Glycerin soaps, which are transparent and more water soluble, have a higher oil content than standard soaps because of the addition of castor oil. They are closer to a neutral pH and are regarded as less drying than traditional soaps, which are alkaline. Although little objective proof exists to prove their superiority, glycerin soaps are advertised for, and well accepted by, people with skin disorders. Mild cleansers such as Cetaphil or pHisoDerm can be recommended if soap is to be avoided. Many products for dry skin are oil free and consist primarily of surfactants. Although these products claim to have a low potential for irritation, clear evidence of enhanced benefit over soaps is lacking.

Emollients and Moisturizers

Emollients function by filling the space between the desquamating skin scales with oil droplets, but their effect is only temporary. Other products include lubricants (i.e., products that increase skin slip in dry skin), moisturizers (i.e., products that impart moisture to the skin, thereby increasing skin flexibility), and repairing or replenishing products (i.e., those intended to reverse the appearance of aging skin). Most moisturizers consist of water (60%–80%), which functions as a diluent and evaporates, leaving behind the active agents; lipids (essential fatty acids) to augment the skin barrier; emulsifiers, which keep water and lipids in one continuous phase; humectants, which help skin retain water; preservatives; fragrance (or may be fragrance free); and color (dyes). Specialty additives, such as vitamins (vitamins A, C, D, and B complex), which have no known clinical effect, and natural moisturizing factors (e.g., lactate, urea, ammonia, uric acid, and glucosamine) can also be added and are reported to regulate the moisture content of the stratum corneum. A newer lipid additive, ceramide, is being added to some emollient agents for added skin barrier protection.[28] Facial moisturizers are either oil-in-water emulsions or water-in-oil emulsions. The differences between moisturizer products are due to the addition of fragrances, exotic oils, vitamins, protein or amino acid products, and other minor moisturizing aids. The selection of an appropriate facial moisturizer depends on skin type. Products for those with an oily complexion are oil free or contain small amounts of light oils (mineral oil) with silicone derivatives and talc, clay, starch, or synthetic polymers (oil control). Products for individuals with normal skin contain predominantly water, mineral oil, and propylene glycol, with very small amounts of petrolatum or lanolin. These products leave an oilier residue on the face than oil-free formulations. Dry skin products contain water, mineral oil, propylene glycol, and larger amounts of petrolatum or lanolin.

Body moisturizers come in lotions, creams, ointments, and butters. Creams, ointments, and butters are more difficult to spread, especially in hairy areas. Butters are stiffer moisturizing formulations sold in jars and often contain shea butter, which is extracted from the nut of the African shea tree. Patients with tree nut allergies appear to be able to use these products without fear of an allergic reaction. Hand moisturizers are much heavier than body or facial emollients. The simplest and most economical hand ointment is petroleum jelly. Although it is greasy, which may lead to poor compliance, petroleum jelly is effective when applied at bedtime and covered with wraps or clothing. Because sebum and skin surface lipids contain a relatively high concentration of fatty acid glycerides, vegetable and animal oils derived from avocado, cucumber, mink, peanut, safflower, sesame, turtle, and shark liver are included in dry skin products, presumably because of their unsaturated fatty acid content. Although use of these oils contributes to skin flexibility and lubricity, their occlusive effect is less than that of white petrolatum. Use of these products should be avoided in individuals with an allergy to any component.

Emollients, both occlusive and moisturizing, are used to prevent or relieve the signs and symptoms of dry skin. These products act primarily by leaving an oily film on the skin surface through which moisture cannot readily escape. Cosmetically, emollients make the skin feel soft and smooth by helping reestablish the integrity of the stratum corneum. Lipid components make the scales on the skin translucent and flatten them against the underlying skin. This flattening eliminates air between the scales and the skin surface, which is partly responsible for a white, scaly appearance.[47]

Frequency of application depends on the severity of the dry skin disorder and the hydration efficiency of the occlusive agent. Generally, moisturizers must be applied 3–4 times daily to achieve maximum benefit. For dry hands, the patient may need to apply the occlusive agent after each hand washing, as well as at numerous other times during the day.

Emollient products are available as petrolatum-containing ointments that are typically greasy and generally lack consumer appeal because of their texture, difficulty of spreading and removing, and staining properties. To avoid a greasy feel, patients should gently warm the product in the hands, apply a very thin layer, and massage it gently, but thoroughly, into the skin. If an ointment is needed for maximal penetration in an area of thick skin, such as the soles of the feet, a sock could be worn to minimize the mess. Ointments are inappropriate for oozing AD because they do not allow the lesions to dry and ultimately heal. In addition, ointments may be too occlusive in very warm weather, making creams a better choice.[28]

Lotions and creams are either water-in-oil or oil-in-water emulsions. As the lipid content of the moisturizer increases, the occlusive effect increases. In most cases, patients prefer the less effective oil-in-water emulsions for their cosmetic acceptability. These agents help alleviate the pruritus associated with dry skin by virtue of their cooling effect as water evaporates from the skin surface. Lotions may be preferred when dryness is not as severe or in warm weather, when the occlusive properties of ointments is an issue.[28] Lanolin, a natural product derived from sheep wool, is found in many nonprescription moisturizing products. Patients rarely develop an allergic reaction to this substance, presumably because its wool wax fraction is recognized as antigenic. Patients with a previous history of allergic reactions to lanolin should generally avoid lanolin-containing products.[27] Petrolatum should not be applied over puncture wounds, infections, or lacerations because its high-occlusive property may lead to maceration and further inflammation. Application of petrolatum to intertriginous areas (e.g., armpits, groin, and perianal region), mucous membranes, and acne-prone areas should be minimized; only a preparation with a low concentration of petrolatum is tolerated in these areas.

Humectants

Humectants or hydrating agents are hygroscopic materials that are often added to emollient bases. Commonly used hydrating agents are glycerin, propylene glycol, urea, and phospholipids. Humectants draw water into the stratum corneum to hydrate the skin. Humectants are distinct from emollients, which serve to retain water already present.

Because of glycerin's hygroscopic properties, high concentrations may actually increase water loss by drawing water from the skin rather than from the atmosphere. At lower concentrations (i.e., 5%), humectants such as glycerin help decrease water loss by keeping water in close contact with skin and accelerating moisture diffusion from the dermis to the epidermis. In addition, glycerin lubricates the skin surface. Propylene glycol is a viscous, colorless, odorless solvent with hygroscopic properties. It is less viscous than glycerin and is included in many skin care formulations for its humectant action. Urea is mildly keratolytic and increases water uptake in the stratum corneum, giving it a high water-binding capacity. Urea has a direct effect on stratum corneum elasticity because of its ability to bind to skin protein.[44] Concentrations of 10% have been used on simple dry skin; 20%–30% formulations have been used to treat more resistant dry skin disorders. Lotion and cream formulations containing urea may be better at helping to remove scales and crusts, whereas urea in emollient ointments may be better at rehydrating the skin. However, urea preparations can cause stinging, burning, and irritation, particularly on broken skin.[48]

Alpha Hydroxy Acids

Alpha hydroxy acids include ammonium lactate and lactic acid. These acids can increase the hydration of human skin and, at low concentrations, may act as a modulator of epidermal keratinization rather than as a keratolytic agent. Lactic acid may be added to urea preparations in creams and lotions for both its stabilizing and its hydrating effects.[44]

Allantoin

Allantoin and allantoin complexes soften keratin by disrupting its structure. A product of purine metabolism, allantoin is

considered a relatively safe skin protectant for adults, children, and infants when applied in concentrations of 0.5%–2.0%.[24] However, it is less effective than urea.[48]

Topical Hydrocortisone

Hydrocortisone (0.5% or 1%) is currently the only corticosteroid available without a prescription for the topical treatment of dermatitis. Although its exact mechanism is unknown, hydrocortisone most likely suppresses cytokines associated with the development of inflammation and itching, which is associated with various dermatoses. Food and Drug Administration monograph indications for use of hydrocortisone include temporary relief of itching associated with minor skin irritations, inflammation, and rashes caused by dermatitis, seborrheic dermatitis, insect bites, poison ivy/oak/sumac dermatitis, soaps, detergents, cosmetics, and jewelry.[49] Concentrations of 0.5% or 1% are considered appropriate for treating localized dermatitis. Many commercially available nonprescription hydrocortisone products now also contain aloe. The inclusion of aloe may serve as a potential irritant to some patients with dermatitis; thus, products with aloe should be avoided in this population. (See Chapter 40 for more information on aloe.)

Hydrocortisone should be applied sparingly to the affected area 1–2 times a day. For mild dry skin, a cream is acceptable; however, an ointment formulation generally provides the best results for chronic, nonoozing dermatoses.

Maximizing the application of moisturizers (lotions, creams, ointments) to dry, itchy skin disorders may lessen the frequency that medicated products, such as hydrocortisone, have to be applied.[26,38]

Hydrocortisone should not be applied to infected skin; it may mask the symptoms of dermatologic infections and allow the infection to progress. Topical hydrocortisone rarely produces systemic complications because its systemic absorption is relatively minimal (approximately 1%). Therefore, the risk of adrenal suppression, growth suppression, osteoporosis, and other metabolic complications is slight when low-potency hydrocortisone is used on a short-term basis or rotated with other agents.[28] Certain local adverse effects such as skin atrophy rarely occur with nonprescription concentrations; they are more common with the more potent prescription products.[28,36] Because response to topical hydrocortisone may decrease with continued use owing to tachyphylaxis, intermittent courses of therapy are advised when possible. This can include use of hydrocortisone daily during periods of flare-ups with once weekly dosing, or no hydrocortisone at all, during remission phases, with continued maintenance strategies (i.e., emollient use).[27,39]

Antipruritics

The pruritus associated with dermatitis may be mediated through several mechanisms, which may explain how local anesthetics, antihistamines, and hydrocortisone (discussed previously) are useful as antipruritics. Cooling the area through application of a soothing, bland lotion, such as Lubriderm, may reduce the extent of the pruritus, but this effect is only transitory.

The itching sensation is mediated by the same nerve fibers that carry pain impulses. Local anesthetics block conduction along axonal membranes, thereby relieving itching as well as pain. However, because local anesthetics may cause systemic side effects, they should not be used on large areas of the body or over long periods of time, particularly if the skin is raw or blistered. Nonprescription topical anesthetics that appear to be safe and effective are pramoxine, lidocaine, and benzocaine. Topical anesthetics may be applied to affected areas 3 or 4 times daily, but caution should be used because these agents may have a sensitizing effect in some patients. Guidelines do not recommend routine use of these local anesthetics.[18] Counterirritants such as camphor and menthol, in concentrations of 0.5%–1%, are available in or can also be added to lotions and creams and can serve as an inexpensive antipruritic.[48]

Itching may also be mediated by various endogenous substances, including histamine. Therefore, topical antihistamines (e.g., diphenhydramine) are effective in alleviating this symptom, as well as exerting a topical anesthetic effect. Although topical antihistamines may provide some short-term relief of itching, their use is not recommended, and furthermore, may be associated with sensitization.[13,18,31] Local anesthesia may be the more important mechanism of action, given that the cause of itching in many disorders (e.g., atopic dermatitis) is most likely caused by cytokine release and may not be related to histamine release at all.

Oral antihistamines have traditionally been used to treat the itching of dermatologic disorders. Some researchers claim that the antipruritic effect is a result of the sedative side effect; others claim the efficacy is caused by antihistaminic activity, although with a delayed onset of several days. Oral antihistamines are not recommended for the routine treatment for pruritus in AD because of the lack of demonstrated efficacy and the hypothesis that the pruritus in AD is often not histamine related.[13,18,20] However, an oral antihistamine may help with sleep in the patient who has been staying up all night scratching, and if concurrent depression is a problem, an antidepressant with anticholinergic properties may further help with itching. In either case, sedation may be a problem as may the anticholinergic side effects in patients with disorders such as benign prostatic hypertrophy or closed-angle glaucoma.[38]

Product Selection Guidelines

When deciding which product to recommend for dermatitis or dry skin, the provider must evaluate the active ingredients and the vehicle. Primary active ingredients contained in nonprescription skin products are water and oil. However, a variety of secondary ingredients is added to enhance product elegance and stability, and many of these ingredients, such as preservatives, have the potential to produce contact dermatitis through either an irritant or a sensitizing effect.[38]

The type of vehicle (e.g., ointment, cream, lotion, gel, solution, or aerosol) may significantly affect treatment of dermatitis and should be selected based on patient preference and location of lesions. If a drying effect is desired, the provider may recommend solutions, gels, and occasionally creams. However, components may quickly diffuse into the underlying tissue and possibly cause irritation. If lubrication is needed, creams and lotions are preferable. Notably, creams may be less potent than ointments and contain preservatives previously mentioned as potential irritants. Lotions (and gels) are not as greasy, and both dry quickly. Lotions can be useful in hairy areas, as can foams and mousses. If the lesion is dry, thick, or fissured, an ointment is the vehicle of choice. However, use of ointments in intertriginous areas (e.g., groin, axillae) should be avoided because of the potential for maceration.[37] Also, in the acute phase of AD, the occlusive effects of an ointment may cause further irritation.

Assessment of Atopic Dermatitis and Dry Skin: A Case-Based Approach

For most forms of dermatitis, the initial signs and symptoms are similar. A diagnosis of AD is often made after excluding other dermatologic disorders such as contact dermatitis (see Chapter 34) or scaly dermatoses (see Chapter 33). Because AD is primarily a disease of the young, patient age is important in assessment. The provider should determine whether the patient (or the patient's family) has a history of atopic disorders. Inquiries should be made regarding onset and duration of the eruption, anatomic location, and distribution of the lesions.

When recommending the use of an appropriate nonprescription product or making a medical referral, the provider must consider the cosmetic, psychological, and work- or recreation-related aspects of a dermatologic disorder in addition to the underlying pathology. If the dermatologic disorder has a significant psychological component and it has not responded to first-line nonprescription treatments, the patient may benefit from referral to a provider who can assist the patient with alternative remedies such as behavioral modification and stress-reducing therapies.

Dry skin is typically visible, with roughness and scaling. Questions about bathing habits, the soaps and detergents used, medications recently started, and other medical disorders that may predispose a patient's skin to excessive dryness should be asked. Patients should note that changes in climate, such as winter air and air from heating sources that dry the skin, can affect their skin.

Care is warranted when making recommendations for the treatment of pruritic skin disorders in special populations. A wide variety of disorders can be associated with pruritus during pregnancy.[50] Although recommending the use of emollients for dry, pruritic skin is generally safe, pregnant patients should be instructed to contact their obstetrician for a more thorough investigation of the skin disorder if the symptoms do not respond adequately in 2–3 days. Although emollients are generally safe to use on dry skin of infants and children, a provider should be consulted prior to recommending the use of any topical medication, such as hydrocortisone, for a prolonged period of time (>7 days).[5] In addition, lower-potency corticosteroids (such as hydrocortisone) are preferred in children, and the use of occlusion (with diapers or tight clothing) should be avoided since this can increase absorption.[36] Older patients are especially prone to dry skin and dermatologic disorders associated with reduced peripheral circulation. Dry skin in these patients will likely respond better to the routine application of moisturizing creams and ointments rather than lotions. In addition, care should be used when recommending sedating antihistamines for pruritus because these patients are more likely to experience cognitive and anticholinergic side effects associated with these agents. Similarly, bath products that may result in a slippery bathtub should be used with caution in older patients, given their propensity for falls and subsequent complications.

Cases 32–1 and 32–2 are examples of the assessment of patients with AD or dry skin, respectively.

Patient Counseling for Atopic Dermatitis and Dry Skin

Patients with AD should be counseled on achieving control of their disease, the chronic nature of the condition, exacerbating factors, and appropriate treatment options.

case

32–1

Relevant Evaluation Criteria	Scenario/Model Outcome

Information Gathering

1. Gather essential information about the patient's symptoms and medical history, including:

   a. description of symptom(s) (i.e., nature, onset, duration, severity, associated symptoms)

   Patient presents with persistent itching on the wrist and elbow areas, which has intensified during the past 3–4 months. The skin is dry and thickened, and within the past week yellowish exudates and crusting have been present in both areas.

   b. description of any factors that seem to precipitate, exacerbate, and/or relieve the patient's symptom(s)

   She states that symptoms seem to have worsened after moving to a new house. The itching is much worse and has resulted in frequent scratching.

   c. description of the patient's efforts to relieve the symptoms

   She has tried hydrocortisone 1% cream applied twice daily but it has not helped to date.

   d. patient's identity

   Cathy Smith

   e. age, sex, height, and weight

   28 years old, female, 5 ft, 4 in., 135 lb

   f. patient's occupation

   Salesperson

   g. patient's dietary habits

   Normal diet

   h. patient's sleep habits

   6–7 hours per night

   i. concurrent medical conditions, prescription and nonprescription medications, and dietary supplements

   Allergic rhinitis: loratadine 10 mg once daily

   j. allergies

   House dust

   k. history of other adverse reactions to medications

   None

   l. other (describe) _____

   Cathy was diagnosed with atopic dermatitis at 12 years of age. It has been controlled fairly well with topical corticosteroids used on an as-needed basis.

Assessment and Triage

2. Differentiate patient's signs/symptoms and correctly identify the patient's primary problem(s).

   Patient has lesions associated with atopic dermatitis that vary with time and are likely to worsen with continued irritation from scratching.

3. Identify exclusions for self-treatment. (Figure 32–2).

   The recent development of yellow exudates may indicate a secondary infection; thus, any form of self-treatment should be avoided. Further evaluation should take place prior to using any pharmacologic agent on a chronic basis.

4. Formulate a comprehensive list of therapeutic alternatives for the primary problem to determine if triage to a health care provider is required, and share this information with the patient or caregiver.

   Options include:

   (1) Refer Cathy to a primary care provider or dermatologist for a differential diagnosis.

   (2) Recommend an appropriate nonprescription product.

   (3) Recommend an appropriate nonprescription product until Cathy can be seen by a health care provider or dermatologist.

   (4) Take no action.

Plan

5. Select an optimal therapeutic alternative to address the patient's problem, taking into account patient preferences.

   A topical emollient cream or lotion should be applied 3–4 times daily to the lesions, using clean hands. Cathy should try to keep the lesions and surrounding skin as clean as possible. In addition, she should be seen by her primary care provider or a dermatologist. Hydrocortisone should be avoided because it could delay the healing of a skin infection. She should continue to take her loratadine for her allergic rhinitis that may also minimize the skin itch.

6. Describe the recommended therapeutic approach to the patient or caregiver.

   "Until you can see your primary care provider or a dermatologist, you may apply a topical emollient cream or lotion 3–4 times daily to the lesions. You may have a skin infection, so you should stop using the hydrocortisone because it could delay the healing of the infection. Continue to take the loratadine; it may help to minimize the itching."

7. Explain to the patient or caregiver the rationale for selecting the recommended therapeutic approach from the considered therapeutic alternatives.

   "Because of the likelihood of a skin infection, it is important to be sure what the lesions are prior to recommending any long term treatment with any pharmacologic agent, such as hydrocortisone."

case
32–1 *continued*

Relevant Evaluation Criteria	Scenario/Model Outcome
Patient Education	

8. When recommending self-care with nonprescription medications and/or nondrug therapy, convey accurate information to the patient or caregiver.

"Try not to scratch the lesions; wearing cotton gloves at night may help with this." See the box Patient Education for Atopic Dermatitis and Dry Skin for additional information that can be discussed with the primary care provider or a dermatologist.

Solicit follow-up questions from the patient or caregiver.

"Is there a nonprescription medication that might help?"

Answer the patient's or caregiver's questions.

"Use of a nonprescription topical antibiotic ointment may not be adequate therapy to eradicate the skin infection. Nonprescription medications are not appropriate to recommend without a definite diagnosis from a health care provider or dermatologist."

Evaluation of Patient Outcome	

9. Assess patient outcome.

Contact the patient in a day or two to ensure that she made an appointment and sought further medical care.

case
32–2

Relevant Evaluation Criteria	Scenario/Model Outcome
Information Gathering	

1. Gather essential information about the patient's symptoms and medical history, including:

   a. description of symptom(s) (i.e., nature, onset, duration, severity, associated symptoms)

   The patient presents with pruritic, scaly skin on both forearms and lower legs. He claims the soles of his feet and palms of his hands are very rough, with some fissures. Significant flaking is observed, especially in the morning.

   b. description of any factors that seem to precipitate, exacerbate, and/or relieve the patient's symptom(s)

   He states the symptoms are more bothersome in the winter months and have worsened as he has aged.

   c. description of the patient's efforts to relieve the symptoms

   He has tried a store-brand lotion on most mornings with minimal improvement.

   d. patient's identity

   Ellis Taylor

   e. age, sex, height, and weight

   79 years old, male, 5 ft 7 in., 230 lb

   f. patient's occupation

   Retired engineer

   g. patient's dietary habits

   MNT diet for patients with diabetes

   h. patient's sleep habits

   7–9 hours of sleep per night

   i. concurrent medical conditions, prescription and nonprescription medications, and dietary supplements

   Hypertension: lisinopril 20 mg once daily; prophylaxis for CVD: ASA 81 mg once daily; type 2 DM: metformin 500 mg twice daily

   j. allergies

   None

   k. history of other adverse reactions to medications

   None

   l. other (describe) _____

   Ellis bathes 5–6 times per week in a tub for 30 minutes at a time. He lives in Madison, Wisconsin. He keeps the temperature in his home at 75 degrees and says that he uses a humidifier in his bedroom during the winter months.

Assessment and Triage	

2. Differentiate patient's signs/symptoms and correctly identify the patient's primary problem(s).

Ellis has dry skin that is most likely caused by environmental factors in combination with his advancing age.

3. Identify exclusions for self-treatment (Figure 32–2).

None

case
32-2 *continued*

Relevant Evaluation Criteria	Scenario/Model Outcome
4. Formulate a comprehensive list of therapeutic alternatives for the primary problem to determine if triage to a health care provider is required, and share this information with the patient or caregiver.	Options include: (1) Refer Ellis to a health care provider or dermatologist. (2) Recommend appropriate nonprescription product(s) and nondrug measures. (3) Recommend appropriate self-care until Ellis can see an appropriate provider. (4) Take no action.

Plan

5. Select an optimal therapeutic alternative to address the patient's problem, taking into account patient preferences.	A nonprescription emollient will be appropriate for this patient. Applying white petrolatum at bedtime on his arms, legs, and feet and then covering them with sleeves or stockings, as appropriate, will provide the fastest results. Once the disorder improves, a moisturizing cream can be used 2–3 times daily in place of the petrolatum. Hand lotion should be used 4–5 times daily. If intense itching is troublesome, hydrocortisone 1% cream or ointment may be applied to the affected area 2–4 times daily in addition to the emollients.(Table 32–3 provides other information on dry skin therapy.)
6. Describe the recommended therapeutic approach to the patient or caregiver.	See Table 32–3 and the box Patient Education for Atopic Dermatitis and Dry Skin.
7. Explain to the patient or caregiver the rationale for selecting the recommended therapeutic approach from the considered therapeutic alternatives.	"Your skin condition can be managed but not cured with nonprescription topical therapy plus changes to your bathing habits."

Patient Education

8. When recommending self-care with nonprescription medications and/or nondrug therapy, convey accurate information to the patient or caregiver:	
a. appropriate dose and frequency of administration	See the box Patient Education for Atopic Dermatitis and Dry Skin.
b. maximum number of days the therapy should be employed	"It is likely the emollient will need to be used chronically. Avoid daily prolonged use (>7 days) of topical hydrocortisone, if possible." (See the box Patient Education for Atopic Dermatitis and Dry Skin.)
c. product administration procedures	See the box Patient Education for Atopic Dermatitis and Dry Skin.
d. expected time to onset of relief	See the box Patient Education for Atopic Dermatitis and Dry Skin.
e. degree of relief that can be reasonably expected	See the box Patient Education for Atopic Dermatitis and Dry Skin.
f. most common side effects	See the box Patient Education for Atopic Dermatitis and Dry Skin.
g. side effects that warrant medical intervention should they occur	See the box Patient Education for Atopic Dermatitis and Dry Skin.
h. patient options in the event that condition worsens or persists	See the box Patient Education for Atopic Dermatitis and Dry Skin.
i. product storage requirements	See the box Patient Education for Atopic Dermatitis and Dry Skin.
j. specific nondrug measures	See the box Patient Education for Atopic Dermatitis and Dry Skin.
Solicit follow-up questions from the patient or caregiver.	"Can I just use my Jergen's Lotion rather than using the Vaseline on my feet and legs?"
Answer the patient's or caregiver's questions.	"Ointments such as Vaseline hold moisture in the skin better than creams or lotions do. Although you may be able to use only your lotion after your disorder improves, you would have to apply it 4–5 times daily to achieve the same results that Vaseline will provide."

Evaluation of Patient Outcome

9. Assess patient outcome.	Ask the patient to call you to report how he responds to the recommended therapy, or call the patient in a week to evaluate his response.

Key: ASA = Acetyl salicylic acid; CVD = cardiovascular disease; DM = diabetes mellitus; MNT = medical nutrition therapy.

patient education for

patient education for
Atopic Dermatitis and Dry Skin

The primary objectives of self-treating atopic dermatitis are to (1) stop the itch–scratch cycle, (2) maintain skin hydration, (3) avoid or minimize factors that trigger or aggravate the disorder, and (4) prevent secondary infections. The primary objective in self-treating dry skin—restoring skin moisture and the skin's barrier function—can also help relieve the discomfort of atopic dermatitis. For most patients, carefully following product instructions and the self-care measures listed here will help ensure optimal therapeutic outcomes. Understanding that patience is required is key with a treatment plan for AD because some therapeutic measures can be time-consuming to implement and often a delay occurs in time to maximal benefit.

Atopic Dermatitis
Nondrug Measures

- Avoid factors that trigger allergic reactions. Do not wear tight clothing. Remain in areas that have a moderate temperature and low humidity.
- Bathe or shower every other day, if possible. Take short (3–5 minutes) showers or baths, using warm (tepid) water and a nonsoap cleanser.
- If possible, substitute sponge baths (with tepid water) for full-body bathing.
- Pat dry after bath or shower.
- To dry weeping lesions, apply cool tap water compresses for 5–20 minutes, 4–6 times daily.
- To prevent injury to the affected area caused by scratching, keep your fingernails short, smooth, and clean. At night, wear cotton gloves or socks on your hands to lessen scratching.

Nonprescription Medications

- To decrease itching, bathe in tepid water that contains colloidal oatmeal, or add bath oil to the water near the end of the bath.
- Gently wash the affected areas with a nonsoap cleanser before applying any emollient or medication. Gently pat skin dry, and apply an emollient within 3 minutes after washing while skin is still damp.
- Wash hands before and after applying any medication.
- Apply a thin layer of medication over the affected areas.
- Apply hydrocortisone 1–2 times daily to dry lesions to relieve itching. Do not use this medication longer than 7 days.
- With proper use of medications and nondrug measures, noticeable improvement can be observed in 24–48 hours.
- Although completely eliminating the rash and itch is possible, the lesions likely could get worse, especially during the winter and summer months.

When to Seek Medical Attention

- Thinning of the skin while using hydrocortisone should be reported to a primary care provider.

- If the atopic dermatitis does not improve or worsens after 2–3 days of treatment, consult a primary care provider.

Dry Skin
Nondrug Measures

- Avoid excessive bathing; take brief (3- to 5-minute) full-body baths 2–3 times per week, using bath oil and warm (tepid) water.
- If possible, take sponge baths on other days using warm water to maintain skin hydration.
- Pat dry after bathing or showering.
- Drink plenty of water daily.
- Moisturizer should be generously applied 3–4 times daily and continued as long as dry skin persists.
- Moisturizers should be applied within 3 minutes after bathing, plus an additional 3 times per day.
- Although getting rid of the dry skin completely may be difficult, initial improvement should be seen within 24 hours.
- Avoid caffeine, spices, and alcohol because they can contribute to dehydration.
- Keep the room humidity higher than normal to minimize evaporation from the skin.

Nonprescription Medications

- Add products such as oilated oatmeal or bath oil near the end of your bath to improve skin hydration. Colloidal oatmeal products, if used on a regular basis, may clog plumbing pipes and can leave the tub slick.
- Apply an oil-based emollient immediately after bathing while your skin is damp. Reapply the emollient frequently.
- For more severe cases of dry skin, use a product that contains urea or lactic acid.
- Apply nonprescription topical hydrocortisone ointment to reduce inflammation and itching. Do not use this medication longer than 7 days.

When to Seek Medical Attention

- If skin dryness worsens after 7 days of treatment, consult a health care provider.

Patients with dry skin should be informed that they have more control over mild-moderate forms of this disorder than over most other types of dermatologic disorders. The provider should also explain factors that cause dry skin and the appropriate measures for restoring barrier function. The box Patient Education for Atopic Dermatitis and Dry Skin lists specific information to provide patients.

Evaluation of Patient Outcomes for Atopic Dermatitis and Dry Skin

A patient with dry skin should be reevaluated in 7 days after initiation of therapy. Visual assessment is the best method of determining treatment response. Therefore, a scheduled visit is the preferred follow-up method. If the symptoms have not improved or have worsened (continued or additional itching, redness, scaling, lesions, or tissue breakdown), medical referral is appropriate.

Key Points for Atopic Dermatitis and Dry Skin

➤ Most patients with mild-moderate AD or dry skin are candidates for self-treatment with a combination of non-prescription and nonpharmacologic therapies.

➤ Refer patients with yellow, crusting, eczematous AD lesions and all children younger than 1 year of age with AD to a primary care provider or dermatologist for evaluation and treatment.

➤ Question patients presenting with dry or eczematous skin lesions about exposure to soaps, detergents, fragrances, chemicals, irritants, changes in temperature, allergens, and other triggers; then provide information about avoiding such triggers.

➤ Counsel patients with dry skin disorders to take brief baths, use tepid water, pat dry, and apply moisturizers within 3 minutes of completing the bath or shower.

➤ Advise patients to use mild skin cleansers and to apply copious quantities of moisturizers 3–4 times daily.

➤ Educate the patient with chronic dry skin disorders about the importance of stopping the itch–scratch cycle and maintaining adequate hydration.

➤ Advise patients to use ointment-based products, whenever possible, to maximize the hydrating properties of the product. Cream-based products can be recommended for patients who will not comply with use of ointments.

➤ Instruct patients how to properly apply topical emollients, anti-inflammatory agents, and antipruritic agents, using the smallest amount possible and thoroughly rubbing in.

➤ Advise patients with self-treatable symptoms to contact their primary care provider if symptoms worsen or do not improve within 7 days.

REFERENCES

1. Weller R, Hunter JAA, Savin J, et al. *Clinical Dermatology*. 4th ed. Hoboken, NJ: Wiley-Blackwell; 2008:1–14.
2. Hanifin JM, Reed ML. A population-based survey of eczema prevalence in the United States. *Dermatitis*. 2007;18(2):82–91.
3. Atopic dermatitis, eczema, and noninfectious immunodeficiency disorders. In: James WD, Berger TG, Elston DM, eds. *Andrews' Diseases of the Skin: Clinical Dermatology*. 11th ed. London: Saunders Elsevier; 2011:62–70.
4. Weinberg MA. Diagnosis and treatment of acute inflammatory dermatoses. *US Pharm*. April 2009;34(4):HS-1–6.
5. House AA. Issues in geriatric dermatology. In: Olsen CG, Tindall WN, Clasen ME, eds. *Geriatric Pharmacotherapy: A Guide for the Helping Professional*. Washington, DC: American Pharmacists Association; 2007:137–61.
6. Micali G, Lacarrubba F, Bongu A, et al. The skin barrier. In: Freinkel R, Woodely D, eds. *The Biology of the Skin*. New York, NY: Parthenon; 2001:227.
7. Law RM, Law DTS. Dermatologic drug reactions and common skin conditions. In: DiPiro JT, Talbert RL, Yee GC, et al., eds. *Pharmacotherapy: A Pathophysiologic Approach*. 8th ed. New York, NY: McGraw-Hill; 2011: 1661–72.
8. Burkhart C, Morrell D, Goldsmith L. Dermatological pharmacology. In: Brunton L, ed. *Goodman and Gilman's the Pharmacological Basis of Therapeutics*. 12th ed. New York, NY: McGraw-Hill; 2011:1803–32.
9. Buck ML. Pediatric pharmacotherapy. In: Alldredge BK, Corelli RL, Ernst ME, et al., eds. *Applied Therapeutics: The Clinical Use of Drugs*. 10th ed. Philadelphia, PA: Lippincott Williams and Wilkins; 2013:2265–76.
10. National Institute of Arthritis and Musculoskeletal and Skin Diseases. Handout on health: atopic dermatitis. August 2011. Accessed at http://www.niams.nih.gov/health_info/Atopic_Dermatitis/#b, October 21, 2013.
11. Eichenfield LR, Ellis CN, Mancini AJ, et al. Atopic dermatitis: epidemiology and pathogenesis update. *Semin Cutan Med Surg*. 2012;31(3 suppl): S3–5.
12. Krakowski AC, Eichenfield LF, Dohil MA. Management of atopic dermatitis in the pediatric population. *Pediatrics*. 2008;122(4):812–24.
13. Hanifin JM, Cooper KD, Ho VC, et al. Guidelines for the care of atopic dermatitis. *J Am Acad Dermatol*. 2004;50(3):391–404.
14. Deckers IAG, McLean S, Linssen S, et al. Investigating international time trends in the incidence and prevalence of atopic eczema 1990–2010: a systematic review of epidemiological studies. *PLoS One*. 2012;7(7):e39803.
15. Bieber T, Cork M, Reitamo S. Atopic dermatitis: a candidate for disease-modifying strategy. *Allergy*. 2012;67(8):969–75.
16. Sabin BR, Peters N, Peters AT. Atopic dermatitis. *Allergy Asthma Proc*. 2012;33(suppl 1):S67–9.
17. Thompson J, Avery M, Honeywell M, et al. Atopic dermatitis: a review of clinical management. *US Pharm*. 2006;31:89–96.
18. Ring J, Alomar A, Bieber T, et al. Guidelines for treatment of atopic eczema (atopic dermatitis) part I. *J Eur Acad Dermatol Venereol*. 2012;26(8): 1045–60.
19. Law RM, Kwa PG. Atopic dermatitis. In: DiPiro JT, Talbert RL, Yee GC, et al., eds. *Pharmacotherapy: A Pathophysiologic Approach*. 8th ed. New York, NY: McGraw-Hill; 2011:1707–16.
20. Condren M, Miller JL. Pediatric dermatology. In: Benevades S, Nahata MC. *Pediatric Pharmacotherapy*. Lenexa, KS: American College of Clinical Pharmacy; 2013:92–107.
21. Akdis CA, Akdis M, Bieber T, et al. Diagnosis and treatment of atopic dermatitis in children and adults: European Academy of Allergology and Clinical Immunology/American Academy of Allergy, Asthma and Immunology/PRACTALL Consensus Report. *J Allergy Clin Immunol*. 2006;118:152–69.
22. Brenninkmeijer EEA, Schram ME, Leeflang MMG, et al. Diagnostic criteria for atopic dermatitis: a systematic review. *Br J Dermatol*. 2008;158(4): 754–65.
23. Beiber T. Mechanisms of disease: Atopic dermatitis. *N Engl J Med*. 2008; 358(14):1483–94.
24. Oranje AP, Glazenburg EJ, Wolkerstorfer A, et al. Practical issues on interpretation of scoring atopic dermatitis: the SCORAD index, objective SCORAD and three-item severity score. *Br J Dermatol*. 2007; 157(4):645–8.
25. Ellis CN, Mancini AJ, Paller AS, et al. Understanding and managing atopic dermatitis in adult patients. *Semin Cutan Med Surg*. 2012;31(3 suppl): S18–22.
26. Berke R, Singh A, Guralnick M. Atopic dermatitis: an overview. *Am Fam Physician*. 2012;86 (1):35–42.
27. Jaffe R. Atopic dermatitis. *Prim Care*. 2000;27(2):503–13.
28. Paller AS, Simpson EL, Eichenfield LF, et al. Treatment strategies for atopic dermatitis: optimizing the available therapeutic options. *Semin Cutan Med Surg*. 2012;31(3 suppl):S10–7.
29. White MI, McElwan-Jenkinson D, Lloyd DH. The effect of washing on the thickness of the stratum corneum in normal and atopic individuals. *Br J Dermatol*. 1987;116(4):525–30.
30. Lieberman JA, Sicherer SH. The diagnosis of food allergy. *Am J Rhinol Allergy*. 2010;24(6):439–43.
31. Boguniewicz M, Schmid-Grendelmeier P, Leung DYM. Atopic dermatitis. *J Allergy Clin Immunol*. 2006;118(1):40–3.
32. Menezes de Padua CA, Schnuch A, Lessmann H, et al. Contact allergy to neomycin sulfate: results of a multifactorial analysis. *Pharmacoepidemiol Drug Saf*. 2005;14(10):725–33.
33. Grimalt R, Menegeaud V, Cambazard F. Study Investigators' Group. The steroid-sparing effect of an emollient therapy in infants with atopic dermatitis: a randomized controlled study. *Dermatology*. 2007; 214(1):61–7.
34. Hanifin JM, Hebert AA, Mays SR, et al. Effects of a low-potency corticosteroid lotion plus a moisturizing regimen in the treatment of atopic dermatitis. *Arch Dermatol*. 2001;137:1110–2.
35. Greer FR, Sicherer SH, Burks AW, and the Committee on Nutrition and Section on Allergy and Immunology. Effects of early nutritional interventions on the development of atopic disease in infants and children: the role of maternal dietary restriction, breastfeeding, timing of introduction of complementary foods, and hydrolyzed formulas. *Pediatrics*. 2008; 121:183–91.
36. Lee NP, Arriola ER. Topical corticosteroids: back to basics. *West J Med*. 1999;171(5–6):351–3.
37. Ference JD, Last AR. Choosing topical corticosteroids. *Am Fam Physician*. 2009;79(2):135–40.
38. Buys LM. Treatment options for atopic dermatitis. *Am Fam Physician*. 2007;75(4):523–8.

39. Ring J, Alomar A, Bieber T, et al. Guidelines for treatment of atopic eczema (atopic dermatitis) part II. *J Eur Acad Dermatol Venereol.* 2012; 26(9):1176–93.

40. Wickens K Black PN, Stanley TV, et al. A differential effect of two probiotics in the prevention of eczema and atopy: a double-blind, randomized, placebo-controlled trial. *J Allergy Clin Immunol.* 2008;122(4):788–94.

41. Pughdal KV, Schwartz RA. Topical tar: Back to the future. *J Am Acad Dermatol.* 2009;61(2):294–302.

42. Devillers AC, Oranje AP. Wet-wraps treatment in children with atopic dermatitis: a practical guide. *Pediatr Dermatol.* 2012;29(1):24–7.

43. Song T. The efficacy of wet wrap treatment in children with atopic dermatitis. *J Allergy Clin Immunol.* 2012;127:AB36.

44. Zagaria MAE. Xerosis: treating clinically dry skin. *US Pharm.* 2006;31: 28–32.

45. Hutchison LC. Biomedical principles of aging. In: Hutchison LC, Sleeper RB, eds. *Fundamentals of Geriatric Pharmacotherapy.* Bethesda, MD: American Society of Health-System Pharmacists; 2010:53–69.

46. Habif TP. Eczema and hand dermatitis. In: Habif TP, ed. *Clinical Dermatology.* 5th ed. St. Louis, MO: Mosby Elsevier; 2009:100–10.

47. Lazar AP, Lazar P. Dry skin, water, and lubrication. *Dermatol Clin.* 1991; 9(1):45–51.

48. Knutson K, Pershing LK. Topical drugs. In: Hendrickson R, Beringer P, Der Marderosian AH, et al., eds. *Remington: The Science and Practice of Pharmacy.* 21st ed. Philadelphia, PA: Lippincott Williams & Wilkins; 2005: 1277–93.

49. U.S. Food and Drug Administration. Hydrocortisone monograph. Accessed at http://www.fda.gov/Drugs/default.htm, April 29, 2013.

50. Moses S. Pruritus. *Am Fam Physician.* 2003;68(6):1135–42.

SCALY DERMATOSES

Richard N. Herrier

Dandruff, seborrheic dermatitis, and psoriasis are chronic scaly dermatoses. These disorders involve the uppermost layer of skin, the epidermis. They all have scales as a primary manifestation. Dandruff or seborrhea is a less inflammatory form of seborrheic dermatitis with relatively fine scaling confined to the scalp. Seborrheic dermatitis, which involves the scalp, face, and chest (usually the sternum), has significant inflammation. Psoriasis is a highly inflammatory skin condition with raised plaques and adherent thick scales that can have profound physical, psychological, and economic consequences.[1]

Nonprescription products are appropriate treatment for most cases of dandruff and seborrheic dermatitis. Mild psoriasis may be responsive to nonprescription treatment, but the initial diagnosis of psoriasis and the management of acute flares require the attention of a dermatologist.

Dandruff

Dandruff is a chronic, mildly inflammatory scalp disorder that results in excessive scaling of the scalp. It is a substantial cosmetic concern and is associated with social stigma. Previously thought to be a separate entity, this disorder represents the less inflammatory end of the seborrheic dermatitis spectrum. Authorities disagree as to whether inadequate shampooing exacerbates dandruff; however, they agree that a consistent washing routine is important in managing the condition.[1,2]

Dandruff occurs in approximately 1%–3% of the population. Dandruff is uncommon in children and generally appears at puberty, reaches a peak in early adulthood, levels off in middle age, and is less prominent after 75 years of age.[1] Dandruff shows no gender preference, and bald spots are typically dandruff free. Dandruff is less severe during the summer.[1,2] The specific cause of accelerated cell growth seen in dandruff is unclear, but the *Malassezia* species of yeasts is generally agreed to be responsible for the accelerated cell turnover and inflammation seen in both dandruff and seborrheic dermatitis.[3]

Pathophysiology of Dandruff

Dandruff is a hyperproliferative epidermal disorder, characterized by an accelerated epidermal cell turnover (twice that of normal scalp) and an irregular keratin breakup pattern, resulting in the shedding of large, nonadherent white scales.[1] With dandruff, crevices occur deep in the stratum corneum, resulting in cracking, which generates relatively large scales.[1] If the large scales are broken down to smaller units, the dandruff becomes less visible. The accelerated cell turnover rate is thought to be caused by the irritant inflammatory effects of fatty acids and cytokines produced by *Malassezia* species.[2]

Clinical Presentation of Dandruff

Dandruff is diffuse rather than patchy and is minimally inflammatory. Scaling, the only visible manifestation of dandruff, is the result of an increased rate of cell turnover on the scalp and the sloughing of large white or gray scales. Although not universal in all patients, pruritus is common. The crown of the head is often a prime location for formation of dandruff flakes.

Treatment of Dandruff
Treatment Goals

The goals of self-treating dandruff are to (1) reduce the epidermal turnover rate of the scalp skin by reducing the number of *Malassezia* species in the scalp, (2) minimize the cosmetic embarrassment of visible scaling, and (3) minimize itch.

General Treatment Approach

Washing the hair and scalp with a general-purpose nonmedicated shampoo every other day or daily is often sufficient to control mild-moderate dandruff. If it is not, the health care provider may recommend nonprescription medicated antidandruff products.

Contact time is the key to effectiveness when using medicated shampoos containing pyrithione zinc or selenium sulfide that suppress the replication of *Malassezia* species.[4,5] The patient should massage the medicated shampoo into the scalp and leave on the hair for 3–5 minutes before rinsing. Repeated rinsing (2–3 times) after the desired contact time is suggested with medicated shampoos containing selenium sulfide to ensure

Editor's Note: This chapter is based on the 17th edition chapter of the same title, written by Steven A. Scott.

that a residue is not left on the hair, which may result in its discoloration. Medicated shampoos should be used daily for 1 week, then used 2–3 times weekly for 2–3 weeks and thereafter once weekly or every other week to control the condition. Scalp scrubbers are useful in all patients to help ensure adequate contact of the medicated shampoo with the scalp, especially in patients with longer hair.

An agent that reduces *Malassezia* counts on the scalp (e.g., pyrithione zinc or selenium sulfide) is generally recommended initially. Alternatively, nonprescription ketoconazole shampoo, an antifungal shampoo that also has anti-*Malassezia* activity, can be used. Shampoos containing a cytostatic agent such as coal tar are usually reserved for second-line therapy because they may discolor light hair as well as clothing and jewelry and are of limited efficacy. These agents reduce scaling by decreasing the epidermal turnover rate. A keratolytic shampoo containing salicylic acid or sulfur may also be used but requires far longer treatment periods and is of limited efficacy (see Treatment of Scaly Dermatoses). If dandruff proves resistant to these agents after 4–8 weeks of appropriate use, the patient should be referred to a primary care provider for treatment with products containing a higher concentration of selenium sulfide or ketoconazole.[1]

Seborrheic Dermatitis

Seborrheic dermatitis is a subacute or chronic inflammatory disorder that occurs predominantly in the areas of greatest sebaceous gland activity (e.g., scalp, face, and chest).[3–5] Seborrheic dermatitis is a common chronic, red, scaly, itchy rash typically seen within the first 3 months of life and around the fourth to the seventh decade of life. Seborrheic dermatitis is common in infants and affects 2%–5% of adults (more commonly men). Seborrheic dermatitis is typically more severe in winter and may be aggravated by emotional stress.

Pathophysiology of Seborrheic Dermatitis

Seborrheic dermatitis is more inflammatory than dandruff and is marked by accelerated epidermal proliferation in areas with dense distribution of sebaceous glands, which is caused by elevated levels of *Malassezia*.[3] Whereas normal epidermal cell turnover is 25–30 days, it is 9–10 days for seborrheic dermatitis compared with 13–15 days for dandruff.[1] The characteristic accelerated cell turnover and enhanced sebaceous gland activity give rise to prominent yellow, greasy scales displayed in the condition.

Clinical Presentation of Seborrheic Dermatitis

Seborrheic dermatitis occurs in the scalp, eyebrows, glabella, eyelid margins (blepharitis), cheeks, paranasal areas, nasolabial folds, beard area, presternal area, central back, retroauricular (behind the ear) creases, and in and about the external ear canal. The disorder typically presents as dull, yellowish, oily, scaly areas on red skin that are fairly well demarcated. Pruritus is common.[1]

The infantile form, which occurs in the first months of life as greasy scales and scale crusts on a bright erythematous base, affects the scalp (cradle cap), retroauricular creases, lateral neck, and intertriginous folds. Cradle cap usually clears without treatment by age 8–12 months as the hormones passed from the mother to the child before birth gradually disappear. The disease rarely presents again until puberty.

The most common form in adults is characterized by yellow, greasy scales on the scalp that often extend to the middle third of the face with subsequent eyebrow involvement (see Color Plates, photograph 13). For some unknown reason, seborrheic dermatitis is frequently seen in patients with Parkinson's disease. Typically, seborrheic dermatitis on the scalp is manifested by greasy, scaling patches or plaques, exudation, and thick crusting. On the face, flaky scales or yellowish scaling patches on red, itchy skin are seen in the eyebrows and glabella. Red scaling, fissures, and swelling may be present in the ear canals, around the auditory meatus, in the postauricular region, or under the earlobe. V-shaped areas of the chest and back and, much less frequently, intertriginous areas such as the side of the neck, axillae, submammary region, umbilicus, and genitocrural folds may also be involved. In adults, the disease lasts for years to decades, with periods of improvement in warmer seasons and periods of exacerbation in the colder months.

Treatment of Seborrheic Dermatitis
Treatment Goals

The goals of self-treatment of seborrheic dermatitis are to (1) reduce inflammation and the epidermal turnover rate of the scalp skin by reducing the level of *Malassezia* species, (2) minimize or eliminate visible erythema and scaling, and (3) minimize itch.

General Treatment Approach

The treatment of seborrheic dermatitis is similar to that of dandruff but is often more aggressive because of the inflammatory nature of the disease. Patients should be informed about the chronic nature of the disease, and they need to understand that therapy works by controlling the disease rather than by curing it. Therapy is directed toward loosening and removal of scales and crusts, inhibiting yeast colonization, controlling secondary infection, and reducing erythema and itching. When a medicated shampoo containing pyrithione zinc, selenium sulfide, or ketoconazole is used for treatment, patients should work the shampoo into the scalp and then leave the lather on the hair and affected areas for 3–5 minutes. Initially, the shampoo should be used daily for the first week or two, then 2–3 times per week for the next 4 weeks. When the condition is controlled, the shampoo is applied once a week to prevent relapse. Commercially available products containing salicylic acid and sulfur are of limited effectiveness because they are slow acting, producing therapeutic effects in months rather than days.

In infants, seborrheic dermatitis is usually self-limited and treated primarily by gently massaging the scalp with baby oil, followed by the use of a nonmedicated shampoo to remove scales.[1] For cases that do not respond to this treatment, the patient should be referred to a pediatrician. In adults, regardless of the location of any skin lesions, shampooing is the foundation of treatment, since once the disorder is controlled, at least weekly use of shampoos containing pyrithione zinc, selenium sulfide, or ketoconazole prevents relapses. If the odor of a medicated shampoo is objectionable, it can be followed by a more cosmetically acceptable shampoo or conditioner. A regular non-medicated shampoo or liquid dishwashing soap (e.g., Dawn) can be used to soften and remove crusts or scales.[5] Seborrheic dermatitis can also be treated by applying the shampoo containing pyrithione zinc or selenium sulfide to the affected areas of the skin at the same time the shampoo is massaged into the scalp and hair, washing it off 5 minutes later when the shampoo is rinsed out of the hair. Topical corticosteroids are not useful in treating dandruff; however, these agents are needed more frequently to treat the greater levels of inflammation in seborrheic dermatitis. These products may be used to manage seborrheic dermatitis whenever erythema persists after therapy with medicated shampoos. Hydrocortisone ointment should be applied no more than twice daily, because of the reservoir effect of the stratum corneum that slowly releases the corticosteroid over time. Treat until symptoms subside for up to 7 consecutive days. Use of nonprescription hydrocortisone should not exceed 7 consecutive days. If the condition worsens or symptoms persist longer than 7 days, a primary care provider should be consulted. A more potent topical corticosteroid may be indicated.[5]

Psoriasis

Psoriasis is a chronic inflammatory disease estimated to afflict 1%–3% of Americans.[7,8] Lesions are often localized, but they may become generalized over much of the body surface. Remissions and exacerbations are unpredictable. Approximately 30% of people with psoriasis find that lesions may clear spontaneously.[7,8] Unrelenting generalized psoriasis may cause enough psychological distress to adversely affect the patient's quality of life. Treatment of moderate-severe psoriasis can produce a significant physical and economic burden.[8]

The incidence of psoriasis is distributed almost equally among men and women. Psoriasis is seen in all races and geographic regions, but the incidence is lower among people living in countries close to the equator and among people of African American, Native American, and Asian descent.[6–8]

The cause of psoriasis is unknown. However, exacerbations of psoriasis can be triggered by the following:

- Environmental factors such as physical, ultraviolet, and chemical injury.
- Various infections (streptococcal infection but also acute viral infections and human immunodeficiency virus infections).
- Prescription drug use (e.g., beta-blockers, lithium, antimalarials, indomethacin, and quinidine) and withdrawal of systemic corticosteroids.
- Psychological stress.
- Endocrine/hormonal changes.
- Obesity.
- Use of alcohol and tobacco.

Pathophysiology of Psoriasis

Accelerated epidermal proliferation leading to excessive scaling on raised plaques is one hallmark symptom of psoriasis. Epidermal cell turnover rate is approximately 4 days in a psoriatic plaque. The duration of psoriasis is variable, and lesions may last a lifetime or disappear quickly. When lesions disappear, they may leave the skin either hypopigmented or hyperpigmented. The disease course is marked by spontaneous exacerbations and remissions, and it tends to be chronic and relapsing.[8]

Clinical Presentation of Psoriasis

Regardless of the clinical form, psoriasis is usually symmetrical. Plaque psoriasis is the most common form, occurring in more than 90% of patients. Lesions start as small papules that grow and unite to form plaques. These lesions are well-circumscribed, sharply demarcated, light pink to bright red or maroon plaques, with overlying opaque, thick, adherent, white scales that can be pulled off in layers (see Color Plates, photographs 14A, B, and C). When the scale is lifted from the base of the plaque, punctate bleeding points sometimes occur at the sites of scale removal (Auspitz sign). The most common locations are the extensor surfaces of the elbow and knees, the lumbar region of the back, the scalp, the posterior auricular area, the external auditory canal, and the glans penis.

Treatment of Psoriasis
Treatment Goals

The goals of self-treatment of psoriasis are to (1) control or eliminate the signs and symptoms (inflammation, scaling, and itching) and (2) prevent or minimize the likelihood of flare-ups.

General Treatment Approach

The Food and Drug Administration (FDA) recommends that only very mild cases of psoriasis be self-treated (up to a few isolated lesions no larger than a quarter). Larger areas of involvement, involvement of the face, or the presence of joint pain dictate that the patient be treated by a dermatologist with more effective prescription medications. Individuals with moderate-severe cases, involving more than 5% of body surface area, should be treated by a dermatologist.[7,9] Cases not responding to emollients and nonprescription strengths of hydrocortisone or cases in children younger than 2 years should also be referred to a dermatologist.

Numerous nondrug measures can be used by patients in the treatment of psoriasis. Although these treatments can help symptoms and enhance the local effectiveness of nonprescription products, these measures alone are unlikely to control the signs and symptoms of the disorder. Patients should avoid physical, chemical, or ultraviolet (UV) trauma to the skin because of the Koebner phenomenon where lesions develop at the site of skin trauma. Scale removal is an important treatment modality because scales facilitate the continuation of psoriatic plaques and interfere with the penetration of topical agents. Patients with psoriasis should be encouraged to bathe with lubricating bath products (see Chapter 32) 2–3 times per week using tepid water. Loose scales can be removed by gently rubbing with a soft cloth. Emollients (e.g., Lubriderm Lotion or Nivea Cream) should be applied to the lesions within minutes of bathing. Pruritic dry skin is common in psoriasis, and emollients and lubricating bath products often provide some relief for these symptoms. Daily lubrication of the skin after a bath or shower is an essential part of therapy. Emollients moisturize, lubricate, and soothe dry and flaky skin, as well as reduce fissure formation within plaques and help maintain flexibility of the surrounding skin. To be effective, they need to be applied liberally with gentle rubbing, up to 4 times daily.

Hydrocortisone ointment 1% is the nonprescription treatment of choice for individual acute lesions. Acute localized flares, characterized by bright red lesions, call for soothing local therapy with emollients and hydrocortisone ointment. Many patients respond well to simple measures, whereas others have a form of disease that requires more aggressive treatments.[8]

For patients who are not candidates for nonprescription treatment, the selection of therapy must be individualized based on the site, severity, duration, previous treatment, and age of the patient. Treatment may be topical, systemic, or a combination of both. Factors in determining appropriate therapy include body surface area affected by psoriasis, age, cost, and ability of the patient to comply with the regimen. In most cases, psoriasis will not be controlled by nonprescription treatment, and referral to a dermatologist will be necessary. Prescription topical agents such as calcipotriol, tazarotene, and more potent corticosteroids are effective. For moderate-severe or recalcitrant psoriasis, more aggressive treatment is necessary. Treatment options available in many dermatologists' offices include phototherapy with narrow-band UVB radiation and a combination of methoxsalen (a chemical photosensitizing psoralen) and UVA radiation. Other treatment options include systemic agents, such as oral retinoids (acitretin), methotrexate, cyclosporine, and the newer biologics (adalimumab, etanercept, infliximab, and ustekinumab).[7]

Psoriasis cannot be cured, and remissions do occur. During flare-ups, however, signs and symptoms can usually be controlled adequately with appropriate patient education and treatment. The patient should be reassured that, in most cases, control is possible. This reassurance increases compliance with burdensome and prolonged treatment regimens. In addition, if the patient can be helped to gain some understanding and acceptance of the condition, that knowledge may reduce the patient's emotional stress and psychogenic exacerbations. Prevention of flare-ups should be emphasized. Flare-ups can be prevented by minimizing identified precipitating factors, such as emotional stress, skin irritation, and physical trauma.

Treatment of Scaly Dermatoses

A variety of products, often in the form of a medicated shampoo, with varying mechanisms of action, is used to treat scaly dermatoses. In addition, hydrocortisone is used to control the inflammation associated with seborrheic dermatitis and psoriasis. Table 33–1 summarizes the concentrations and indications of currently approved agents,[6,10] and the algorithm in Figure 33–1 outlines self-treatment with these agents.

Patients should shampoo with a nonmedicated, nonresidue shampoo to remove scalp and hair dirt, oil, and scales before using a medicated shampoo. Many shampoos leave a residue on the hair shaft and scalp that may aggravate scaly dermatoses of the scalp. Nonresidue shampoos (e.g., Johnson's and Johnson's Baby Shampoo) do not interfere with these scalp conditions; rather they leave the scalp clean and receptive to optimal effects from medicated shampoos. A nonresidue shampoo application and rinse may be followed by a medicated shampoo, left on the scalp for up to 5 minutes. The patient can use this treatment daily, if needed, until symptoms are relieved and then 2–3 times weekly.[5]

table

33–1 Concentrations of Approved Nonprescription Ingredients for Products Used to Treat Scaly Dermatoses

Ingredient	Concentration (%)		
	Dandruff	Seborrheic Dermatitis	Psoriasis
Coal tar	0.5–5	0.5–5	0.5–5
Hydrocortisone		0.5–1	0.5–1
Ketoconazole	1	1	1
Pyrithione zinc (brief exposure)	0.3–2	0.95–2	2
Pyrithione zinc (residual)	0.1–0.25	0.1–0.25	0.25
Salicylic acid	1.8–3	1.8–3	1.8–3
Selenium sulfide	1	1	1
Sulfur	2–5	2–5	

Source: References 6 and 10.

Anti-Malassezia Agents

Pyrithione Zinc

Pyrithione zinc's mechanism of action is its anti-*Malassezia* activity, which reduces the yeast count in the scalp and skin. Product effectiveness is influenced by several factors. Pyrithione zinc binds strongly to both hair and the external skin layers of the scalp, and the extent of binding correlates with clinical performance.

For pyrithione zinc products intended to be applied and washed off within minutes (brief exposure), FDA recommends concentrations of 0.3%–2.0% for treating dandruff and 0.95%–2.0% for treating seborrheic dermatitis. Shampoos and soaps are currently available in 1% and 2% concentrations. Pyrithione zinc shampoo is well tolerated when used as directed and is not associated with any major adverse effects. Contact with the eyes should be avoided to prevent stinging.

Selenium Sulfide

Selenium sulfide and pyrithione zinc have a similar mechanism of action.[3] Like pyrithione zinc, selenium sulfide is more effective with longer contact time and therefore should be applied in a similar manner.[4,5] Selenium sulfide in prescription strength must be rinsed from the hair thoroughly or discoloration may result, especially in blond, gray, or dyed hair. Frequent use may leave a residual odor and an oily scalp.

Selenium sulfide is approved in a 1% concentration in nonprescription products to treat dandruff and seborrheic dermatitis. A 2.5% lotion formulation is available by prescription for use in resistant cases and other topical fungal infections. The risk of irritation of the mucous membranes and scalp from selenium sulfide is minimal, and no adverse effects are associated with routine use of the 1% shampoo. Contact with the eyelids should be avoided because of the potential for eye irritation.

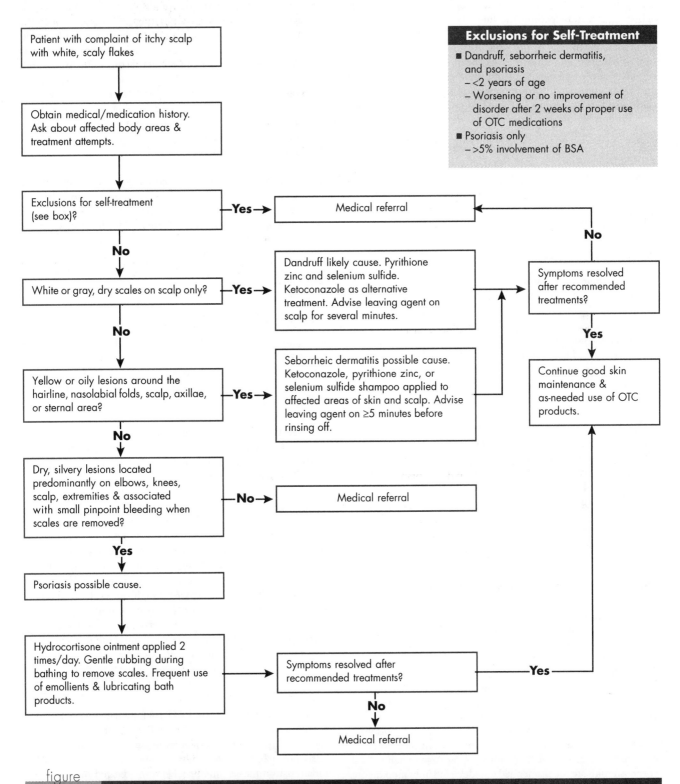

Exclusions for Self-Treatment

- Dandruff, seborrheic dermatitis, and psoriasis
  - <2 years of age
  - Worsening or no improvement of disorder after 2 weeks of proper use of OTC medications
- Psoriasis only
  - >5% involvement of BSA

Patient with complaint of itchy scalp with white, scaly flakes

Obtain medical/medication history. Ask about affected body areas & treatment attempts.

Exclusions for self-treatment (see box)? —**Yes**→ Medical referral

No

White or gray, dry scales on scalp only? —**Yes**→ Dandruff likely cause. Pyrithione zinc and selenium sulfide. Ketoconazole as alternative treatment. Advise leaving agent on scalp for several minutes.

No

Yellow or oily lesions around the hairline, nasolabial folds, scalp, axillae, or sternal area? —**Yes**→ Seborrheic dermatitis possible cause. Ketoconazole, pyrithione zinc, or selenium sulfide shampoo applied to affected areas of skin and scalp. Advise leaving agent on ≥5 minutes before rinsing off.

No

Dry, silvery lesions located predominantly on elbows, knees, scalp, extremities & associated with small pinpoint bleeding when scales are removed? —**No**→ Medical referral

Yes

Psoriasis possible cause.

Hydrocortisone ointment applied 2 times/day. Gentle rubbing during bathing to remove scales. Frequent use of emollients & lubricating bath products. → Symptoms resolved after recommended treatments? —**Yes**→

No

Medical referral

Symptoms resolved after recommended treatments? —**No**→ Medical referral

Yes

Continue good skin maintenance & as-needed use of OTC products.

figure

33–1 Self-care of scaly dermatoses. Key: BSA = Body surface area; OTC = over-the-counter.

Ketoconazole

Ketoconazole, a synthetic azole antifungal agent, is available as a nonprescription shampoo formulation. Ketoconazole 1% is active against most pathogenic fungi but is indicated specifically for *Malassezia*. Therefore, it is used to treat dandruff and seborrheic dermatitis of the scalp. Although the fungal etiology of dandruff and seborrhea has been debated, the efficacy of newer antifungal agents against these conditions has caused an FDA review panel for nonprescription products to endorse these agents for treatment of these two common skin disorders.

Patients should use ketoconazole shampoo twice a week for 4 weeks, with at least 3 days between each treatment. Once the condition is controlled, the shampoo can be applied once weekly to prevent relapse. Adverse effects associated with 1% ketoconazole shampoo are minimal, but hair loss, skin irritation, abnormal hair texture, and dry skin have been reported. Patients should be advised to avoid contact of ketoconazole shampoo with the eyes because irritation may occur.

Cytostatic Agents

Although their mechanism of action is not completely understood, topical cytostatic agents are known to decrease the rate of epidermal cell replication. This action increases the time required for epidermal cell turnover, which in turn allows the possibility of normalizing epidermal differentiation, resulting in a slow decline in visible scales. However, these products have limited efficacy and multiple other issues that make them poor alternatives to anti-*Malassezia* products.

Coal Tar

Coal tar products have long been popular for treating dandruff, seborrheic dermatitis, and psoriasis. Many nonprescription products are available but are of limited usefulness because of their potentially unacceptable cosmetic properties and limited clinical efficacy.

For many years, the therapeutic response to coal tar products was believed to be caused solely by its phototoxicity. Now it is believed that the beneficial effect of coal tar lies primarily in its ability to cross-link with DNA and arrest excessive skin cell proliferation.

Coal tar is available in concentrations of 0.5%–5% as creams, ointments, pastes, lotions, bath oils, shampoos, soaps, and gels for self-treatment of dermatologic disorders. This variety of dosage forms is partly a result of an attempt to develop a cosmetically acceptable product, one that masks the odor, color, and staining properties of crude coal tar that most patients find esthetically unappealing.

Side effects are associated with the use of coal tar, including folliculitis (particularly of the axilla and groin); stains to the skin and hair (particularly blond, gray, and dyed hair); photosensitization; and irritant contact dermatitis.[2] Rarely, the disorder may worsen on exposure to coal tar products. This situation is of particular concern in the acute phase of psoriasis, when topical corticosteroids are recommended to reduce inflammation before coal tar preparations are used.

Coal tar products may be applied to the body, arms, and legs, preferably at bedtime. Because coal tar stains most materials, the patient should use bed linen and clothing for which staining would not present a problem. Overnight application is followed by a bath in the morning to remove residual coal tar and loosen psoriatic scales. Patients using coal tar preparations should avoid sun exposure for 24 hours after application.

Keratolytic Agents

The keratolytic agents salicylic acid and sulfur can be used in dandruff and seborrheic dermatitis products to loosen and lyse keratin aggregates, thereby facilitating their removal from the scalp in smaller particles. These agents act by dissolving the "cement" that holds epidermal cells together. Vehicle composition, contact time, and concentration are important factors in the success of a keratolytic agent. Keratolytic concentrations in nonprescription scalp products (Table 33–2) are not sufficient to impair the normal skin barrier, but they do affect the abnormal, incompletely keratinized stratum corneum. These products have very limited efficacy and are very slow acting, taking weeks to months to see any visible improvement.

Keratolytic agents may produce several adverse effects, and patients should be counseled accordingly. These agents have a primary, concentration-dependent irritant effect, particularly on mucous membranes and the conjunctiva of the eye. They also have the potential of acting on hair and skin keratin; therefore, extended use may alter hair appearance. The directions and precautions for the use of keratolytic shampoos are similar to those for shampoos containing other therapeutic agents, with the exception that prolonged use is usually necessary to obtain a therapeutic response.

Salicylic Acid

Salicylic acid decreases skin pH, which causes increased hydration of keratin and therefore facilitates its loosening and removal. Topical salicylic acid is useful for psoriasis when thick scales are present. However, application over extensive areas should be avoided because of the potential for percutaneous absorption.

Salicylic acid has been approved in concentrations of 1.8%–3% for the self-treatment of dandruff, seborrheic dermatitis, and psoriasis. At these concentrations, the keratolytic effect typically takes 7–10 days.

Sulfur

Sulfur is believed to cause increased sloughing of cells and to reduce corneocyte counts. Sulfur has been approved in concentrations of 2%–5% for the self-treatment of dandruff only. Although it is approved as a single-entity active ingredient, sulfur is often combined with salicylic acid. Although not an FDA-approved indication, this combination has been commonly used for the self-treatment of seborrheic dermatitis.[9] The use of nonprescription topical preparations containing sulfur has not been associated with any significant adverse effects.

Topical Hydrocortisone

Topical hydrocortisone 0.5% and 1% is available without a prescription and is FDA approved for inflammatory skin conditions such as allergic contact dermatitis, insect bites, eczema, and psoriasis. It may be useful for seborrheic dermatitis accompanied by inflammation that is unresponsive to medicated shampoos and is the non-prescription treatment of choice for mild psoriasis.[3–6]

Nonprescription hydrocortisone products can play a role in managing mild psoriasis. Topical corticosteroids have several effects (e.g., anti-inflammatory, vasoconstrictive, and immunosuppressive) on cellular activity, which can result in decreased redness and itching. Hydrocortisone ointment is the most potent and effective dosage form. The activity of the ointment can be enhanced in psoriasis by waiting 30 minutes after its application

Trade Name	Primary Ingredients
Anti-Malassezia Products	
Denorex Everyday Shampoo	Pyrithione zinc 2%
DHS Zinc Shampoo	Pyrithione zinc 2%
Head & Shoulders Dandruff Shampoo	Pyrithione zinc 1%
Head & Shoulders Intensive Treatment Shampoo	Selenium sulfide 1%
Nizoral AD Shampoo	Ketoconazole 1%
Sebulon Shampoo	Pyrithione zinc 2%
Selsun Blue Medicated Treatment Shampoo	Selenium sulfide 1%
Zincon Shampoo	Pyrithione zinc 1%
ZNP Cleansing Bar	Pyrithione zinc 2%
Cytostatic Products	
Balnetar Bath Oil	Coal tar 2.5% in mineral oil
DHS Tar Shampoo	Coal tar 0.5%
DHS Tar Gel Shampoo	Coal tar 0.5%
Neutrogena T/Derm Body Oil	Tar 5% (equivalent to coal tar 1.2%)
Neutrogena T/Gel Extra Strength Therapeutic Shampoo	Tar 4% (equivalent to coal tar 1%)
Neutrogena T/Gel Shampoo	Tar 2% (equivalent to coal tar 0.5%)
Pentrax Shampoo	Coal tar extract 5%
Keratolytics	
MG217 Medicated Tar-Free Shampoo	Salicylic acid 3%; sulfur 5%
Neutrogena Healthy Scalp Anti-Dandruff Shampoo	Salicylic acid 1.8%
Sebucare Lotion	Salicylic acid 1.8%
Sebulex Conditioning Shampoo with Protein	Salicylic acid 2%; sulfur 2%
Sulfoam Medicated Antidandruff Shampoo	Sulfur 2%
Sulray Cleansing Bar	Sulfur 5%
Sulray Dandruff Shampoo	Sulfur 2%
X-Seb Shampoo	Salicylic acid 4%
Combination Products	
Neutrogena T/Sal Maximum Strength Therapeutic Shampoo	Salicylic acid 3%; coal tar extract 2%
P&S Plus Gel	Coal tar solution 8%; salicylic acid 2%
Scalpicin Maximum Strength Foam/Solution	Salicylic acid 3%; menthol
Sebutone Shampoo	Coal tar 0.5%; sulfur 2%; salicylic acid 2%
X-Seb Plus Shampoo	Pyrithione zinc 1%; salicylic acid 2%
X-Seb T Shampoo	Coal tar solution 10%; salicylic acid 4%
X-Seb T Plus Shampoo	Coal tar solution 10%; salicylic acid 3%; menthol 1%

and then covering the area of the psoriatic plaque with a greasy emollient such as petrolatum, which acts as an occlusive dressing.

Adverse effects associated with the use of topical corticosteroids include local atrophy after prolonged use, as well as the aggravation of certain cutaneous infections. The possibility of systemic sequelae exists and is enhanced by the use of the more potent compounds, use of occlusive dressings, or application to large areas of the body.

Assessment of Scaly Dermatoses: A Case-Based Approach

Differentiation of the scaly dermatoses involves several factors. The appearance of the scales in the early stages of a disorder is not always definitive. In these cases, the presence and nature of other symptoms or the location of the dermatitis provides additional important clues to its assessment. Factors that precipitate

table
33-3 Distinguishing Features of Scaly Dermatoses

	Dandruff	Seborrheic Dermatitis	Psoriasis
Location	Scalp	Adults and children: head and trunk	Scalp, elbows, knees, trunk, lower extremities
Exacerbating factors	Generally a stable condition, exacerbated by dry climate	Exacerbated by many external factors, notably Parkinson's disease	Exacerbated by irritation, stress, climate, medications, infection, endocrine factors
Appearance	Thin, white, or grayish flakes; even distribution on scalp	Macules, patches, and thin plaques of discrete yellow, oily scales on red skin	Discrete symmetrical, red plaques with sharp border; silvery white scale; small bleeding points when scale is removed; difficult to distinguish from seborrhea in early stages or in intertriginous zones
Inflammation	Absent	Present	Present
Epidermal hyperplasia	Absent	Present	Present
Epidermal kinetics	Turnover rate 2 times faster than normal	Turnover rate about 3 times faster than normal	Turnover rate about 5–6 times faster than normal
Percentage of incompletely keratinized cells	Rarely exceeds 5% of total corneocyte count	Commonly makes up 15%–25% of corneocyte count	Commonly makes up 40%–60% of corneocyte count

Source: References 1 and 2.

or exacerbate the disorder are also helpful in defining the disorder. Table 33–3 describes the distinguishing features of these three dermatoses. Cases 33–1 and 33–2 illustrate the assessment of patients with scaly dermatoses.

Patient Counseling for Scaly Dermatoses

Patients need to know that scaly dermatoses are rarely cured by pharmacotherapy; rather, nonprescription agents help control the signs and symptoms of the disorders. Patients should also

be advised that fluctuation in severity of seborrheic dermatitis and psoriasis may be related to emotional, physical, or environmental factors.

Explanations of the proper use of antifungal, cytostatic, and keratolytic agents should include information about the length of time to leave the agent on the affected area. Possible side effects with recommended agents should also be explained. Finally, patients should be advised of signs and symptoms that indicate medical attention is needed. The box Patient Education for Dandruff and Seborrheic Dermatitis and the box Patient Education for Psoriasis list specific information to provide patients.

case
33-1

Relevant Evaluation Criteria	Scenario/Model Outcome
Information Gathering	

1. Gather essential information about the patient's symptoms, including:

a. description of symptom(s) (i.e., nature, onset, duration, severity, associated symptoms)	Patient complains of yellow, oily scales along his hairline and around his nose. Some minor erythema is also present in these areas.
b. description of any factors that seem to precipitate, exacerbate, and/or relieve the patient's symptom(s)	The condition has grown worse since the onset of cold weather.
c. description of the patient's efforts to relieve the symptoms	Washing the face twice daily with hand soap has not proven beneficial.
d. patient's identity	Robert Plant
e. age, sex, height, and weight	57 years old, male, 5 ft 9 in., 185 lb
f. patient's occupation	Sales manager
g. patient's dietary habits	Normal healthy diet
h. patient's sleep habits	6–7 hours per night
i. concurrent medical conditions, prescription and nonprescription medications, and dietary supplements	Depression: sertraline 50 mg daily; hypertension: hydrochlorothiazide 25 mg daily

case
33–1 *continued*

Relevant Evaluation Criteria	Scenario/Model Outcome
j. allergies	NKA
k. history of other adverse reactions to medications	None
l. other (describe) _____	NA

Assessment and Triage

2. Differentiate patient's signs/symptoms and correctly identify the patient's primary problem(s) (Table 33–3).

Robert appears to have seborrheic dermatitis on his face. His scalp should be examined closely for involvement as well.

3. Identify exclusions for self-treatment (Figure 33–1).

None

4. Formulate a comprehensive list of therapeutic alternatives for the primary problem to determine if triage to a medical provider is required, and share this information with the patient or caregiver.

Options include:

(1) Recommend self-care with an appropriate OTC product and non-drug measures.

(2) Recommend self-care with an appropriate OTC product and non-drug measures until a PCP or dermatologist can be consulted.

(3) Refer Robert to a PCP or dermatologist.

(4) Take no action.

Plan

5. Select an optimal therapeutic alternative to address the patient's problem, taking into account patient preferences.

OTC treatment with pyrithione zinc shampoo can be used initially. Ketoconazole or selenium sulfide shampoo is a good alternative agent to recommend if the patient prefers to use an alternative product. Hydrocortisone 1% ointment can be added to red areas if 1 week of treatment with medicated shampoo does not resolve redness.

6. Describe the recommended therapeutic approach to the patient or caregiver.

"For the first week, shampoo the hair with the medicated shampoo and apply it to the affected areas of the face daily. Leave on for 5 minutes, then rinse off. For the next 4 weeks, repeat the above procedure only 2–3 times per week. Regardless of the location of the lesions, the hair needs to be shampooed to prevent relapse. Once the condition is controlled, the hair should be shampooed at least once a week to prevent relapse."

7. Explain to the patient or caregiver the rationale for selecting the recommended therapeutic approach from the considered therapeutic alternatives.

"You may use the pyrithione zinc, selenium sulfide, or ketoconazole shampoo according to personal preference and cost."

Patient Education

8. When recommending self-care with nonprescription medications and/or nondrug therapy, convey accurate information to the patient or caregiver:

See the box Patient Education for Dandruff and Seborrheic Dermatitis.

Solicit follow-up questions from the patient or caregiver.

"What should I use on my hair on the days I do not use the medicated shampoo?"

Answer the patient's or caregiver's questions.

"Any type of nonmedicated shampoo is fine to use. One that does not leave a residue is preferred. Once your condition is controlled, daily use of a shampoo is not necessary unless your scalp is especially oily."

Evaluation of Patient Outcome

9. Assess patient outcome.

Contact the patient in a week to assess his progress in resolving his seborrheic dermatitis.

Key: NA = Not applicable; NKA = no known allergies; OTC = over-the-counter; PCP = primary care provider.

case

33-2

Relevant Evaluation Criteria	Scenario/Model Outcome

Information Gathering

1. Gather essential information about the patient's symptoms, including:

    a. description of symptom(s) (i.e., nature, onset, duration, severity, associated symptoms)

      The patient has had shiny scales bilaterally on her elbows for greater than 6 months. Some minor bleeding occurs when the scales are removed. She now complains of the development of lesions on both of her knees.

    b. description of any factors that seem to precipitate, exacerbate, and/or relieve the patient's symptom(s)

      The lesions appeared to worsen after her recent divorce from her husband.

    c. description of the patient's efforts to relieve the symptoms

      Use of hydrocortisone 1% cream once daily has been marginally effective. Use of lotion on the lesions is soothing.

    d. patient's identity

      Elaine Abel

    e. age, sex, height, and weight

      43 years old, female, 5 ft 6 in., 195 lb

    f. patient's occupation

      Factory line worker

    g. patient's dietary habits

      Normal diet

    h. patient's sleep habits

      Averages 6–8 hours per night.

    i. concurrent medical conditions, prescription and nonprescription medications, and dietary supplements

      Diabetes mellitus × 2 years: fairly well controlled with metformin 500 mg twice daily; hypothyroidism × 15 years: well controlled with levothyroxine 100 mcg once daily; allergic rhinitis × 20+ years: controlled with loratadine 10 mg once daily

    j. allergies

      Penicillin: rash

    k. history of other adverse reactions to medications

      None

    l. other (describe) _____

      Elaine showers once or twice daily.

Assessment and Triage

2. Differentiate patient's signs/symptoms and correctly identify the patient's primary problem(s) (Table 33–3).

    Elaine possibly has a flare of psoriasis. The type of lesions and bilateral appearance support this assessment.

3. Identify exclusions for self-treatment (Figure 33–1).

    The worsening symptoms and appearance of the lesions on the patient's knees indicate a worsening condition that requires more than self-care.

4. Formulate a comprehensive list of therapeutic alternatives for the primary problem to determine if triage to a medical provider is required, and share this information with the patient or caregiver.

    Options include:

    (1) Refer Elaine to a dermatologist for a differential diagnosis.

    (2) Recommend an OTC product (hydrocortisone ointment 1% and emollient therapy) to use until the physician appointment.

    (3) Take no action.

Plan

5. Select an optimal therapeutic alternative to address the patient's problem, taking into account patient preferences.

    Refer the patient to a dermatologist for a differential diagnosis and treatment.

6. Describe the recommended therapeutic approach to the patient or caregiver.

    "Contact your dermatologist to accurately diagnose your condition. Until the time of your appointment, you could switch to applying hydrocortisone ointment 1% to the affected areas 2 times daily. Wait 30 minutes and then liberally apply an emollient."

7. Explain to the patient or caregiver the rationale for selecting the recommended therapeutic approach from the considered therapeutic alternatives.

    "You need to see a dermatologist because OTC therapy won't be as effective as prescription medications for disease as extensive as yours."

case

33-2 *continued*

Relevant Evaluation Criteria	Scenario/Model Outcome
Patient Education	
8. When recommending self-care with nonprescription medications and/or nondrug therapy, convey accurate information to the patient or caregiver.	See the box Patient Education for Psoriasis for nondrug measures to treat psoriasis.
Solicit follow-up questions from the patient or caregiver.	"I saw on the Internet that treatment with coal tar products is an option for psoriasis. Should I use one of these products?"
Answer the patient's or caregiver's questions.	"Although coal tar products have been used for a long time, topical corticosteroid therapy is now considered the first-line topical therapy for most patients. The smell and mess associated with using coal tar products are major drawbacks, plus they have limited efficacy."
Evaluation of Patient Outcomes	
9. Assess patient outcome.	Call patient in 2 days to make sure she was able to get an appointment with the dermatologist.

Key: OTC = Over-the-counter.

patient education for

Dandruff and Seborrheic Dermatitis

The primary objective of self-treating dandruff and seborrheic dermatitis is to reduce the turnover rate of skin cells, which is responsible for the scaly lesions. Controlling inflammation and itching of the affected areas is another treatment objective. Although these disorders are chronic and incurable, carefully following product instructions and the self-care measures can help ensure optimal therapeutic outcomes for many patients.

General Measures

- Shampoo the hair with the medicated shampoo 3–7 times a week initially, leaving the shampoo on the hair for 5 minutes. Work the shampoo into the scalp and simultaneously apply the shampoo to the affected area of the face. Rinse the scalp and face thoroughly after 5 minutes. Use a scalp scrubber to ensure penetration to the scalp. Repeat this procedure.
- Use the shampoo for a minimum of 2 weeks to determine effectiveness; after 4 weeks of use, apply the shampoo once a week to control the condition.
- If used, apply a thin layer of the hydrocortisone cream no more than 2 times daily. Wash the affected areas before use.
- With use of medication and proper nondrug therapy, noticeable improvement could be observed within 7–14 days. Complete control of the condition is possible with weekly use of the medicated shampoo. It is likely that exacerbations may occasionally appear, especially during the winter months.
- Stinging or burning may occur if medicated shampoo enters the eyes.

Dandruff

- Use a medicated shampoo containing pyrithione zinc or selenium sulfide. If these agents are ineffective, refer to a physician or dermatologist.
- Coal tar can stain light hair and cause folliculitis (inflammation of hair follicles), dermatitis, and photosensitization (sensitivity of the skin to sunlight).

- Shampoo the hair with the medicated shampoo, and leave it on the hair for 3–5 minutes. Rinse the hair thoroughly and repeat. Rinse hair thoroughly after use of the medicated shampoo.

Seborrheic dermatitis

- Use a medicated shampoo containing ketoconazole, pyrithione zinc, or selenium sulfide. Shampoo the hair and scalp, and apply shampoo directly to any lesions on the face and hairline. More aggressive doses of the anti-*Malassezia* shampoos are used for seborrheic dermatitis than for dandruff. Daily use for seborrheic dermatitis is appropriate for the first week; after that reduce use to 2–3 times a week. Regardless of the location of the lesions, the hair needs to be shampooed. The scalp always has the highest concentration of *Malassezia* yeast and is the source of the yeast that causes skin lesions on the face. Washing the hair at least weekly with anti-*Malassezia* shampoos is absolutely essential to preventing relapse, even if lesions were only on the face.
- If redness persists after therapy with medicated shampoos, apply hydrocortisone ointment 2 times a day until symptoms subside, and then apply the ointment intermittently to control acute exacerbations. Do not use this agent longer than 7 days. Prolonged use can cause rebound flare-ups when the hydrocortisone is discontinued.

When to Seek Medical Attention

- Consult a primary care provider or dermatologist if the condition does not improve or if it worsens after 1–2 weeks of treatment with nonprescription medications.

patient education for
Psoriasis

The primary objective of self-treating psoriasis is to reduce the turnover rate of skin cells, which is responsible for the scaly lesions. Controlling inflammation and itching of the affected areas and hydrating the skin are other treatment objectives. Although psoriasis is chronic and incurable, carefully following product instructions and self-care measures can help ensure optimal therapeutic outcomes for many patients.

- For itchy, dry skin, use emollients and lubricating bath products (see Chapter 32). Remove scales by gently rubbing them with a soft cloth after the bath. Do not rub vigorously.
- For psoriasis involving more than one or two coin-sized lesions, refer to a dermatologist.
- Prevent flare-ups by minimizing factors such as emotional stress, skin irritation, and physical trauma that you know will exacerbate the disorder.

When to Seek Medical Attention

- If you have psoriasis lesions plus joint pain, see a dermatologist for treatment.
- If hydrocortisone ointment and emollients are not effective, or if the area affected is more than a few less-than-quarter-size lesions, see a dermatologist for treatment with prescription products.
- Consult a dermatologist if the condition does not improve or if it worsens after 2 weeks of treatment with nonprescription medications.

Evaluation of Patient Outcomes for Scaly Dermatoses

Follow-up on the patient's progress should occur after 1 week of self-treatment. If the symptoms have worsened after this period, the patient should consult a primary care provider. If the disorder has not worsened, the provider should ask the patient to return after a second week of treatment. If the symptoms persist or have worsened after this period, the patient should consult a primary care provider.

Key Points for Scaly Dermatoses

- ➤ Mild-moderate scaly dermatoses can often be effectively managed with topical nonprescription products.
- ➤ Product selection should be based on an evaluation of the patient's history and prior response to treatment, as well as a careful evaluation of the risks and benefits of using the nonprescription products.
- ➤ The provider should be sure to educate patients about the proper application of topical therapy, which greatly impacts the efficacy of therapy.

REFERENCES

1. James WD, Berger TG, Elston DM. *Andrews' Diseases of the Skin: Clinical Dermatology.* 11th ed. Philadelphia, PA: Saunders Elsevier; 2011.
2. Schwartz RA, Janusz CA, Janniger CK. Seborrheic dermatitis: an overview. *Am Fam Physician.* 2006;74(1):125–30.
3. Hay RJ. *Malassezia,* dandruff and seborrheic dermatitis: an overview. *Brit J Derm.* 2011:165(suppl 2):2–8.
4. Shin H, Kwon OS, Won CH, et al. Clinical efficacies of topical agents for the treatment of seborrheic dermatitis of the scalp: a comparative study. *J Dermatol.* 2009;36(3):131–7.
5. Stefanaki I, Katsambas A. Therapeutic update on seborrheic dermatitis. *Skin Therapy Lett.* 2010;15(5):1–4.
6. Wolff K, Goldsmith LA, Katz SI, et al., eds. *Fitzpatrick's Dermatology in General Medicine.* 7th ed. New York, NY: McGraw-Hill; 2008.
7. Herrier, RN. Advances in the treatment of moderate to severe psoriasis. *Am J Health Syst Pharm.* 2011;68(9):795–806.
8. Luba KM, Stulberg DL. Chronic plaque psoriasis. *Am Fam Physician.* 2006;73(4):636–44.
9. Menter A, Gottlieb A, Feldman S, et al. Guidelines of care for the management of psoriasis and psoriatic arthritis. *J Am Acad Dermatol.* 2008;58(5):826–50.
10. U.S. Food and Drug Administration. Final rule: dandruff, seborrheic dermatitis and psoriasis drug products for over-the-counter human use. *Federal Register.* December 4, 1991;56:63554–69.

CONTACT DERMATITIS

Kimberly S. Plake and Patricia L. Darbishire

Contact dermatitis is a condition characterized by inflammation, redness, itching, burning, stinging, and vesicle and pustule formation on dermal areas exposed to irritant or antigenic agents.[1,2] The two primary types of contact dermatitis, classified by etiology and presentation, are discussed separately in this chapter. Irritant contact dermatitis (ICD) is an inflammatory reaction of the skin caused by exposure to an irritant. Allergic contact dermatitis (ACD) is an immunologic reaction of the skin caused by exposure to an antigen.[2]

Irritant Contact Dermatitis

The majority of ICD cases are related to occupation, particularly jobs that involve work with water or exposure to irritant substances. ICD occurs frequently in the home; however, the only available statistics are those associated with employment. According to the U.S. Bureau of Labor Statistics (BLS), work-related skin disorders comprised 16.0% of total workplace injuries in 2011. Individuals employed in forestry, agriculture, and fishing industries have the greatest incidence of ICD, at 9.2 per 10,000 workers in each of these sectors. Workers in manufacturing, education, and health services sectors follow, with incidence of 4.6 per 10,000 workers in each of the sectors.[3]

The BLS annual survey of occupational illnesses reveals that occupational dermatitis in private industry accounts for approximately 57.1% of all occupational skin diseases, with 41.2% of the cases of contact dermatitis identified as ACD, 26.1% as ICD, and 32.7% as unspecified or other types of dermatitis.[4] The actual number of cases is estimated to be 10–50 times greater than the reported number because of changes in industry procedure, underreporting of incidents, and limitations in data collection for the BLS survey.[5] The estimated cost for managing contact dermatitis is $1 billion annually, which includes treatment and workdays lost.[6]

Pathophysiology of Irritant Contact Dermatitis

ICD is common in individuals who work in environments such as personal service (e.g., hair stylists) and health care. Substances associated with ICD are listed in Table 34–1. Individuals who must wash their hands frequently, handle food, or have repeated contact with other irritants are at increased risk.[7-9] Most instances of ICD occur on exposed skin surfaces, especially the face and dorsal surfaces of the hands and forearms. ICD may appear after a single exposure to an irritant or after multiple exposures to the same agent. Mechanisms responsible for causing ICD include disruption of the skin barrier, changes in the cells of the epidermis, and release of proinflammatory cytokines.[7] The substance or irritant may directly damage the epidermal cells by being directly absorbed through the cell membrane and destroying cell systems. Another mechanism may be through the release of cytokines as a result of chemical exposure.[7,10]

Several factors may affect the magnitude of the skin response. The presence of existing skin conditions, such as atopic dermatitis, can result in a more profound dermatitis because of the increased or enhanced permeability of the dermis. The quantity and concentration of substance exposure also affect the severity of the response. Chemical irritants, acids, and alkalis are likely to produce immediate and severe inflammatory reactions. Mild irritants, such as detergents, soaps, and solvents, often require repeated exposures before the dermatitis appears. Occlusive clothing and diapers can prolong skin contact with the irritant, allowing greater skin penetrability of the irritant and leading to a more severe reaction. In addition, environmental factors, such as warmer ambient temperature and higher humidity, may contribute to more severe ICD.

Clinical Presentation of Irritant Contact Dermatitis

Following exposure to an irritant, the skin becomes inflamed, swells, and turns erythematous. Symptoms often are delayed and generally do not occur immediately after exposure. ICD presents primarily as dry or macerated, painful, cracked, and inflamed skin. Itching, stinging, and burning commonly occur with the rash. The inflammatory reaction varies, ranging from these initial symptoms to ulcer formation and localized necrosis. Within days, the dermatitis may crust. If the patient avoids further contact with the irritant, the dermatitis generally resolves in several days. In patients chronically exposed to an irritant, the affected areas of skin will remain inflamed, may develop fissures and scales, and may become hyper- or hypopigmented.[10,11] Some patients who are chronically exposed to irritants recover

table 34–1 Selected Common Substances Associated with Irritant Contact Dermatitis

- Acids, strong (e.g., hydrochloric, nitric, sulfuric, hydrofluoric)
- Alkalis, strong (e.g., sodium, potassium, calcium hydroxides)
- Detergents, soaps, and hand sanitizers
- Epoxy resins
- Ethylene oxide
- Fiberglass
- Flour
- Oils (e.g., cutting, lubricating)
- Oxidants, plasticizers, and activators in athletic shoes
- Oxidizing agents
- Reducing agents
- Solvents
- Urine/feces
- Water
- Wood dust and products

Source: Adapted from references 8 and 9.

completely, whereas others improve but continue to have recurrences. In some patients who are chronically exposed to an irritant, necrosis, inflammation, and crusting comparable to or worse than the original insult may be observed.[12] Chronic forms of ICD can present with lichenification, or leathery thickening of the skin.

Treatment of Irritant Contact Dermatitis

Treatment Goals

The goals in self-treating ICD are to (1) remove the offending agent and prevent future exposure to the irritant; (2) relieve the inflammation, dermal tenderness, and irritation; and (3) educate the patient on self-management to prevent or treat recurrences.

General Treatment Approach

The primary treatment advice is avoidance of further irritant exposure, institution of preventive measures, and patient education.

Nonpharmacologic Therapy

Regardless of the severity, the area of initial exposure to the irritant should be washed with copious amounts of tepid water and cleansed with a mild or hypoallergenic soap, such as Cetaphil or Dove.[7] Immediately washing exposed areas will reduce contact time with the irritant and, if a dermal response occurs, help in localizing symptoms.

Preventive Measures

Educating the patient in techniques to reduce risk of exposure is fundamental. Using protective clothing, gloves, or other equipment, and limiting the time skin areas are occluded through frequent changes in coverings will aid in reducing irritant exposure. Emollients, moisturizers, and barrier creams, especially those with dimethicone, are recommended in the treatment and prevention of ICD because they assist in repairing the epidermal barrier.[7]

Pharmacologic Therapy

Liberal application of emollients to the affected area will help restore moisture to the stratum corneum and serve as a protectant from further exposure to the effects of a wet working environment. Colloidal oatmeal baths may help in relieving itching.[7] Topical corticosteroids have questionable efficacy in the treatment of ICD and are generally not considered optimal therapy.[7,13] The use of topical caine-type anesthetics should be avoided because of their ability to cause ACD.

Allergic Contact Dermatitis

Three thousand chemicals have been cited as causes of ACD.[14] Poison ivy, oak, or sumac (*Toxicodendron* genus) is a common cause of ACD in the United States. Metal allergy, most often precipitated by nickel, is also a common cause. Approximately 19% of patients patch-tested for allergies are allergic to nickel.[15] Dermatitis caused by nickel is generally localized to areas at point of contact, such as where jewelry is worn on the ears or around the neckline or other areas that may touch jewelry with nickel.[14] Products containing latex commonly cause allergic reactions in health care workers, and latex found in waistbands and socks can cause ACD. Fragrances, cosmetics, and skin care products can also cause ACD.[14] Table 34–2 lists selected allergenic substances.[5,13–16]

Pathophysiology of Allergic Contact Dermatitis

ACD is an inflammatory dermal reaction related to exposure to an allergen that activates sensitized T cells, which migrate to the site of contact and release inflammatory mediators. ACD ordinarily does not appear on first contact. Several steps must occur before the dermatitis is manifested. An initial exposure to the antigen must take place to sensitize the immune system. This process is known as the induction phase. With the immune system now sensitized, the next contact with the antigen induces a type IV delayed hypersensitivity reaction, which is a cell-mediated (antigen-sensitized T cell) immune reaction that can take 24 hours to 21 days to develop. This reaction results in the dermatitis and symptoms associated with ACD.[17–19] In people previously sensitized, the rash and related symptoms typically appear within 24–48 hours after exposure.[20]

Urushiol-Induced ACD

In the United States, four species of *Toxicodendron* plants, which belong to the family Anacardiaceae, are primarily responsible for dermatoses associated with exposure to plants (Table 34–3).[20–23] Many of these plants were previously considered to belong to the genus *Rhus,* but *Toxicodendron* is now the accepted genus for this group of antigenic plants and is used throughout this chapter. The change in genus and the difficulty in classifying these plants are the result of variability in plant morphology.

As much as 80% of the U.S. population is estimated to be sensitive to urushiol, the oleoresin in plants of the genus *Toxicodendron.*

table 34-2 Selected Common Allergens Associated with Allergic Contact Dermatitis

Allergen	Sources of Allergen
Balsam of Peru	Cough syrups, flavors
Benzocaine	The caine-type anesthetics have crossover allergy to other caine-type local anesthetics, topical medications (for skin, eye, ear), other oral medications
Chromium salts	Potassium dichromate electroplating, cement, leather-tanning agents, detergents, dyes
Cobalt chloride	Cement, metal plating, pigments in paints
Colophony (rosin)	Rosin cake for string instrument bows, sport rosin bags, cosmetics, adhesives
Epoxy resins	Constituents prior to mixing and hardening
Formaldehyde	Germicides, plastics, clothing, glue, adhesives
Fragrances	Cosmetics, household products, eugenol, cinnamic acid, geraniol, oak moss absolute
Lanolin	Lotions, moisturizers, cosmetics, soaps
Latex	Gloves, syringes, vial closures, elastic waistbands, socks, condoms
Nickel sulfate	In jewelry, blue jean studs, utensils, pigments, coins, tools, many metal alloys encountered daily
Neomycin sulfate	Medications, antibiotic ointments, other aminoglycosides
Plants	*Toxicodendron* species (poison ivy, oak, sumac), primrose (*Primula obonica*), tulips, others
Rubber (carba mix)	Added ingredients, accelerators, activators, other processing chemicals
Thimerosal	Preservative in many medications, injectables, cosmetics

Source: References 13, 15, and 16.

table 34-3 *Toxicodendron* Plants Indigenous to North America

Plant	Other Common Names	Common Geographic Location
Poison ivy (*Toxicodendron radicans*)	Poison vine, mark weed, three-leaved ivy, poor man's liquid amber	Exists throughout North America, ranging throughout the United States (central plains, Midwest, south central, southeastern, lower Mississippi Valley regions); Canada (Ontario, Nova Scotia); and Mexico
Poison oak, Eastern (*Toxicodendron toxicarium*)		Exists widely in the southeastern United States
Poison oak, Western (*Toxicodendron diversilobum*)		Exists throughout the Pacific Coast
Poison sumac (*Toxicodendron vernix*)	Poison elder, poison ash	Exists from Quebec to Florida, primarily in the eastern third of the U.S. coast

Source: Adapted from references 20–23.

Urushiol, an antigen, enters the skin within 10 minutes, starting the sensitivity process. Poison ivy/oak/sumac dermatitis has been reported in patients as young as 3 years of age. Sensitivity to urushiol increases into adulthood, with adult sensitization patterns occurring after 10 years of age.[24] However, sensitivity seems to be reduced in elderly individuals.[11,22]

If patients have sensitivity to any one *Toxicodendron* species, they are usually allergic to all members of the genus. These species are most easily identified as having three leaves emanating from a central stem, with the middle leaflet appearing at the terminal end of the stem. The plants flower in the spring and produce small, waxy, white, five-petaled flowers. In the late fall, the leaves turn brilliant red or orange, and the plants develop berries that are greenish white, pale yellow, or tan. A saying taught to children to help identify the plant and avoid exposure to urushiol is "Leaves of three; let it be!" In general, this statement is true, but other members of the genus differ in the number of leaflets attached to the central stalk and in the berry and leaf morphology.[20,22]

Urushiol is quite sensitive to oxidation by ambient air. It changes in appearance from clear fluid to a black inky lacquer that becomes tarry and may harden on the damaged portion of the plant in a matter of minutes. The release of urushiol from the plant can occur only through damage to the plant itself, either through direct damage by an individual who bruises the plant or by damage from natural causes (e.g., wind, rain, insects, or animals). The antigenic urushiol is contained and carried only within resin canals of the plant.[20,22]

Urushiol is not a volatile substance, but it has been implicated in dermatitis when the plant is burned because smoke emanating from burned plants contains the antigen. Urushiol carried by smoke particulates is capable of affecting body surface areas ordinarily viewed as protected, such as the lungs. This source of exposure is a primary occupational hazard in persons who fight forest fires.[20,22] Unwashed contaminated hands and fingers may also transfer urushiol to other body surfaces and to other individuals. Dermatitis can occur on all skin surfaces, including the eyes, lips, underarms, buttocks, anus, and genitalia.

Poison Ivy

The most common *Toxicodendron* plant found throughout the United States is poison ivy (*Toxicodendron radicans* and *Toxicodendron rydbergii*). Poison ivy is quite common throughout the central and northeastern United States and Canada. It has been described as a climbing shrub or hairy vine that commonly grows up poles, trees, and building walls (see Color Plates, photograph 15A). It also grows along roads, hiking trails, streams, dry rocky canyons, and embankment slopes. *T. radicans* is composed of nine subspecies that can exist as a shrub or a climbing vine, whereas *T. rydbergii* is a dwarf shrub that has large, broad, spoon-shaped leaves with a hairy underside. *T. rydbergii* is the principal variety of poison ivy growing in the northern United States and southern Canada. *T. radicans* grows across much of the United States as a climbing vine with aerial rootlets.[20,22–23]

Poison Oak

Poison oak has two species indigenous to the United States: *Toxicodendron diversilobum,* which inhabits the West Coast, and *Toxicodendron toxicarium,* which inhabits the East Coast. Both species possess leaves similar to those of oak trees, with most plants having an unlobed leaf edge and commonly displaying 3 leaflets per stem. The leaves and berries can be covered with fine hairs (see Color Plates, photograph 15B). The plant ordinarily exists as a nonclimbing shrub but is capable of climbing as high as 131 feet (40 meters). Western poison oak (*T. diversilobum*) differs by usually possessing between 3 and 11 leaflets per stem; its leaves are quite similar to California live oak. Poison oak grows along streams, in thickets, on wooded slopes, and in dry woodlands. As a rule, poison oak grows well at altitudes below 4000–5000 feet.[20,22,23]

Poison Sumac

Poison sumac (*Toxicodendron vernix*) grows in remote areas of the eastern third of the United States in peat bogs and swampy areas. It appears as a shrub or small tree, attains a height of roughly 9.8 feet (3 meters), and may somewhat resemble elder or ash trees, hence its other names, "poison elder" and "poison ash." Its leaves are odd numbered and pinnate and may be almost 16 inches (40 cm) long, with 7–13 leaflets. The edges of the leaves are smooth and come to a tip.[20,22,23] (See Color Plates, photograph 15C.)

Clinical Presentation of Allergic Contact Dermatitis

General Presentation

ACD can be distinguished from ICD by the distribution and presentation of the rash. Both ICD and ACD can occur anywhere on the body where there is exposure to an irritant, but ICD is usually limited to the hands and forearms as a result of occupational exposure. The rash in ACD is limited to the area of antigen contact and the area immediately surrounding the antigen contact. For example, reactions to latex gloves involve only the hands or areas covered by the glove. Sensitivity to latex in undergarments occurs in areas touched by the latex, such as the waist (by waistbands) or calves (from men's socks). Urushiol-induced ACD, however, can be linear or occur over a broader area because urushiol is transferred from hands or inanimate objects, such as clothing, to other parts of the body. ACD usually presents with papules, small vesicles, and sometimes large bullae over inflamed, swollen skin. Significant itching is a prominent feature of ACD. Chronic forms of ACD can present with lichenification.

Presentation of Urushiol-Induced Dermatitis

Presentation of this condition is highly variable and depends on the sensitivity of the patient and extent of exposure. The dermal reaction to urushiol is an intense itching of the exposed skin surfaces, followed by erythema. As the dermatitis progresses, vesicles or bullae form depending on an individual's sensitivity. The vesicles or bullae may break open, releasing their fluid (see Color Plates, photograph 16A). Papules and plaques may develop in addition to or instead of vesicles and bullae. Vesicular

fluid does not contain any antigenic material and cannot cause further transfer of the dermatitis. Streaks of vesicles that correspond to the points of urushiol contact from the damaged plant suggest poison ivy or oak exposure (see Color Plates, photograph 16C). Oozing and weeping of the vesicular fluid continues to occur for several days and cannot cause further spread of the dermatitis. In the last stage of the dermatitis, the affected area develops crusts and begins to dry (see Color Plates, photograph 16B).

Severity of Poison Ivy/Oak/Sumac Dermatitis

Mild dermatitis is characteristically seen as linear streaks. Clinically, the dermatitis is localized on unprotected areas of the body exposed to the urushiol oil. Itching may be minimal. Signs of moderate dermatitis include the appearance of erythema, bullae, papules, vesicles, and inflammation of the exposed skin, in addition to pruritus. Severe dermatitis is distinguished by extensive involvement and edema of the extremities and/or face. Marked swelling of the eyelids without associated swelling of other parts of the face may occur[23] and is caused by rubbing the eyelids with urushiol-contaminated fingers and hands. Often the eyelids are swollen closed. Extreme itching, irritation, and formation of numerous vesicles and bullae may also be present. Furthermore, daily activities may be hampered. Dermatitis or edema affecting large areas of the face, eyes, or genitalia requires immediate medical referral for systemic therapy.

Complications of Poison Ivy/ Oak/Sumac Dermatitis

Patients may continue to scratch for several days after exposure and excoriate the surface dermal layer, leading to open lesions and the potential for secondary wound infections. Common microbes found in infected poison ivy dermatitis include *Staphylococcus aureus,* group A *Streptococcus,* and *Escherichia coli.*[25] In addition to these microbes, other organisms may be identified, depending on where the infection originated on the skin.

Treatment of Allergic Contact Dermatitis

Treatment Goals

The goals of self-treating ACD are to (1) remove and avoid further contact with the offending agent, (2) treat the inflammation, (3) relieve itching and excessive scratching that may lead to open lesions and potential secondary skin infections, and (4) relieve the accumulation of debris that arises from oozing, crusting, and scaling of the vesicle fluids.

Treated or untreated dermatitis will naturally resolve in approximately 10–21 days as a result of the patient's own immune system. Topical nonprescription products may be used for symptomatic relief. Patients will seek advice on treatment because of the intensity of itching and discomfort associated with a mild localized rash, or because of the widespread nature of the dermatitis and the magnitude of symptoms.

General Treatment Approach

Removing the known antigen from the skin as soon as possible may reduce the chance of and severity of the immune response (e.g., not wearing jewelry, switching to underwear and socks without latex, not wearing a leather watch band, washing urushiol-contaminated clothes, or showering or washing the affected area with mild soap and tepid water).

Customarily, the first several days after the initial appearance of ACD are usually the most uncomfortable for the patient. Treatment for the allergic reaction depends on the severity of the symptoms from the antigenic reaction (Figure 34–1). Hydrocortisone 1% cream may be applied to localized patches of rash that have intense pruritus and erythema. Hydrocortisone reduces the inflammation, helps relieve the itching, and as a cream, allows weeping lesions to dry. The patient also may use astringent compresses and baths to dry oozing vesicles.

Other potential options for areas of nonweeping lesions include products containing calamine, as well as colloidal oatmeal products. Calamine assists in the drying of poison ivy lesions. Application of products containing calamine leaves a visible pink film, which may not be esthetically pleasing for some patients. Colloidal oatmeal relieves the itching associated with rash. Care needs to be taken with the use of colloidal oatmeal because it makes the bathtub extremely slippery.

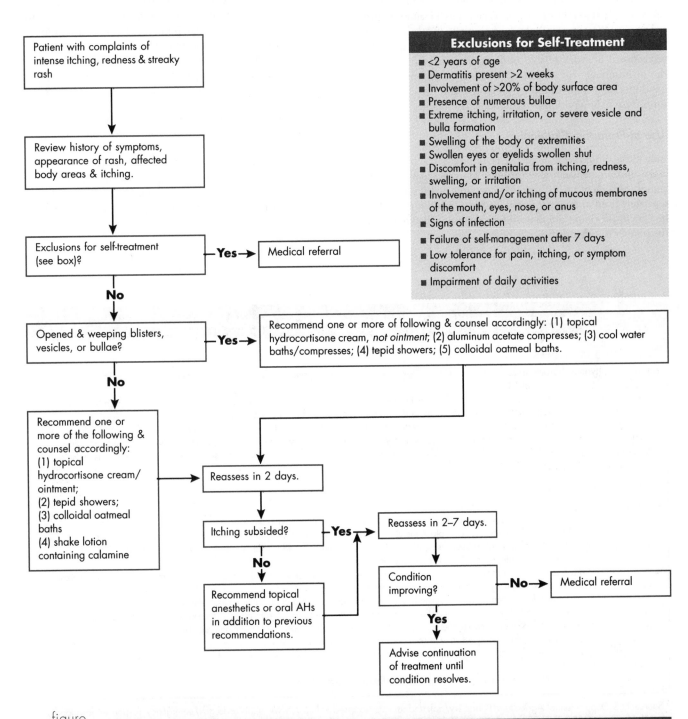

figure
34—1 Self-care of allergic contact dermatitis. Key: AH = Antihistamine.

Medical referral for definitive care is appropriate for children younger than 2 years and for patients with involvement of the eyes, eyelids, and genitals or with extensive involvement of more than 20% of the skin surface. Referral is also appropriate when signs of infection or numerous large bullae are present or when self-treatment for 7 days fails to resolve the rash.

Nonpharmacologic Therapy
Prevention of Urushiol-Induced ACD

Individuals at risk should familiarize themselves with descriptions and photographs of *Toxicodendron* plants. Health care providers can educate patients presenting with ACD by giving them descriptions and photographs of the plants. Patients involved in recreational or work-related outdoor activities should survey the surrounding vegetation to determine the potential risk of exposure. Table 34–4 describes preventive and protective measures for avoiding poison ivy/oak/sumac dermatitis.

Use of Protective Clothing

Individuals should wear protective clothing that can be removed and washed immediately after exposure. They should use ordinary laundry detergent to wash clothes contaminated with urushiol separately from noncontaminated clothing. In addition, washing bed linens after exposure to urushiol is recommended to prevent the transfer to other parts of the body.

Use of Barrier Products

IvyBlock lotion is the only barrier product approved by the Food and Drug Administration (FDA) to provide protection against exposure to poison ivy/oak/sumac. This product's active ingredient is an organoclay known as quaternium-18 bentonite (bentoquatam).[26,27] The product contains 5% bentoquatam in a lotion containing alcohol. Bentoquatam is a nonsensitizing and nonirritating organoclay that appears to possess little antigenicity or toxicity when applied topically. The mechanism by which this ingredient works is not known, but it is believed to physically block urushiol from being absorbed into the skin. It is effective in protecting patients from exposure to the urushiol common to all *Toxicodendron* plants, through both direct contact and airborne particles in smoke from burned plants.

IvyBlock lotion claims to protect when it is topically applied at least 15 minutes before exposure to *Toxicodendron*. The lotion should be shaken vigorously before generously applying it to clean dry skin. It should leave a smooth wet film of lotion where it is applied. One may determine skin coverage by looking for the faint white coating that appears when the lotion has dried. It should be reapplied once every 4 hours or as needed after the initial application to maintain effective protection. After the period of exposure has ended, the patient may remove the lotion by washing with soap and water.[27] This product is flammable and should not be used around the eyes or applied to an existing poison ivy rash. In addition, its use is not recommended in children younger than 6 years.

table
34–4 Preventive and Protective Measures for Poison Ivy/Oak/Sumac Dermatitis

Preventive Measures
- Learn the physical characteristics and usual habitat of *Toxicodendron* plants. Survey the area when outdoors to assess potential risk for exposure to *Toxicodendron* plants.
- Eradicate *Toxicodendron* plants near your residence either by mechanically removing the plant and its roots or by applying an herbicide recommended by the state farm bureau or the USDA extension services. Do not burn the leaves of plants.
- Apply bentoquatam on exposed areas of the body to reduce the risk of contamination before visiting an outdoor site with high likelihood of contact with poison ivy/oak/sumac. Repeat application every 4 hours until your potential exposure has ended. This application should be followed by flushing the area with water to remove bentoquatam and any urushiol deposited on the skin surface. Bentoquatam is flammable, so avoid use near open flames.

Protective Measures
- Wear protective clothing to cover exposed areas.
- Cover your nose and mouth with a protective mask when removing or eradicating *Toxicodendron* plants.
- Remove all clothing worn during exposure, and place the clothing directly into a washing machine, separately from other clothes.
- Wash the suspected areas of exposure as soon as possible with soap and water or with other suggested removal products.
- If thorough washing is not possible, rinse with water as soon as possible.
- At the earliest convenience, take a shower instead of a bath, using soap and water. Avoid tub baths right after exposure because oleoresin may remain in the tub and potentially affect other unexposed areas.
- Clip fingernails and meticulously clean under fingernails to avoid transferring trapped urushiol to clean skin surfaces.
- Using ordinary detergent and hot water, wash all clothing exposed to urushiol separately from other clothes in a washing machine. If clothes are dry cleaned to remove urushiol, warn cleaning personnel of the possible contamination. Put contaminated clothing in a plastic bag for transport.
- As soon as possible after use, thoroughly wash with soap and water—or with water alone—any shoes, gloves, jackets, or other protective garments; sports equipment; garden and work tools; and equipment that is capable of carrying urushiol. Wear vinyl gloves for washing contaminated objects.
- Cleanse the fur of pets after known or suspected exposures to *Toxicodendron* plants.

Source: U.S. Department of Agriculture. Poison ivy/oak and sumac. Accessed at http://www.aphis.usda.gov/emergency_response/downloads/health/Appendix%203-6-C%20Poison%20Ivy,%20Oak%20and%20Sumac.pdf, August 2, 2015; U.S. Department of Agriculture. Outsmarting poison ivy and its relatives. Accessed at http://www.fs.fed.us/t-d/pubs/htmlpubs/htm07672313/, August 2, 2014; and Centers for Disease Control and Prevention. Poisonous plants. Accessed at http://www.cdc.gov/niosh/topics/plants/, August 2, 2014.

Eradication of Toxicodendron *Plants*

The eradication of *Toxicodendron* plants has been suggested in situations in which extremely sensitive individuals are affected by close proximity to the plant and its oleoresin. Two methods of eradication have been recommended: either mechanically removing (hand grubbing plants and the root system using protective equipment, such as gloves and long sleeves and pants) or applying an appropriate herbicide. When considering the use of herbicides, patients should contact the U.S. Department of Agriculture's Extension Service, review information on the Web site (www.nifa.usda.gov/Extension/index.html), or contact the appropriate state or county agency to determine the recommended herbicide and prescribed methods of application to *Toxicodendron* species indigenous to the area.

Patients presenting with *Toxicodendron* ACD in midwinter or during off-season periods may have recently used urushiol-contaminated objects. Urushiol is inactivated by exposure to wet environmental conditions but remains active within dead and dried parts of plants and on inanimate objects for long periods of time. An object is easily contaminated with the oleoresin. It is not unusual for objects to become contaminated in one growing season; the contaminating urushiol retains its antigenicity throughout the winter and causes rashes with each use of the object in succeeding seasons. Implicated sources of nonseasonal poison ivy rash and recurrent seasonal rashes include urushiol-contaminated shoes, boots, clothing, garden and work tools, golf clubs, baseball bats, fishing rods, other recreational equipment, and the fur of domestic pets.[20]

Removal of Antigen at Time of Exposure

If preventive measures were not taken, individuals exposed to urushiol can reduce its contact with skin and transfer to other body areas by immediately washing exposed areas with mild soap and water. Urushiol is water-insoluble; however, immediate washing may avoid or reduce the severity of the rash. Once urushiol has entered the skin and attached to tissue proteins, it can no longer be removed. Washing done within 10 minutes of contact with urushiol has been shown to be the most effective.[28] Even up to 30 minutes postexposure, washing may remove oleoresin that remains on the skin's surface and has not entered the dermal layers. There is a misconception that a rash from urushiol spreads. The appearance of spreading is attributed to the transfer of urushiol by the hands; to additional exposure to urushiol-contaminated objects, clothing, or linens; or to the intensity of the exposure to urushiol.

Washing while in the field is difficult, but using large volumes of water will assist in rinsing away much of the surface irritant and oleoresin. Historically, many home remedies included vigorous scrubbing of contaminated skin surfaces with a harsh soap or household bleach. Other cleansers and organic solvents have been used to rinse urushiol from skin surfaces, including isopropyl alcohol and hand sanitizers; however, these are not generally recommended to remove the antigen. Instead, the current recommendation is to use a mild face soap and water to wash all body areas believed to have been exposed to urushiol. Good handwashing, including meticulous cleansing under or clipping of the fingernails, is necessary to avoid contaminating additional skin surfaces.

Zanfel is marketed as a nonprescription wash to prevent or relieve the rash associated with urushiol. Two small studies suggest that Zanfel reduces the redness and blistering after urushiol exposure.[29–31] With application, Zanfel can immediately relieve pain and itching and is especially useful for spot treatments to areas that continue to itch. Anecdotally, it also has been used to clean equipment such as garden tools that are exposed to urushiol. To use Zanfel, one should wet the affected area, measure 1½ inches of the product into one palm, wet both hands and rub the product into a paste, rub both hands on the affected area (up to 3 minutes) until there is no sign of itching, and rinse the affected area thoroughly.[32] If itching returns after several hours, the product may be used again. Compared with other products, Zanfel is considered expensive, making cost a consideration when selecting this product.

Tecnu Outdoor Skin Cleanser was originally developed as an agent to wash away radioactive matter from the skin surface of exposed individuals. This product is recommended for use after exposure to urushiol and should be rubbed into the affected area as soon after exposure as possible. Label directions indicate that it can be used up to 8 hours after exposure, with the objective of limiting exposure to other areas. The patient should cleanse the contaminated area for a minimum of 2 minutes. No water is required for the initial cleansing application. The cleanser may be wiped away with a cloth or rinsed with cool water. The manufacturer recommends using the product before eating, smoking, or using the bathroom in an effort to minimize transfer of urushiol to uncontaminated skin.

A study that compared untreated urushiol exposures and exposures cleaned with Tecnu, Dial Ultra dishwashing soap, and Goop grease remover found that all three provided good protection against poison ivy rash when used to cleanse skin exposed to urushiol.[29,33] The difference in protective ability among the products was not significant, so cost can be a consideration in selecting a product.

Relief of Itching

For the symptoms of ACD, the primary nondrug measure is to take cold or tepid soapless showers to temporarily relieve the pruritus. A tepid shower is approximately 90°F (32.2°C) or cooler. Hot showers, those with temperatures of 105°F (40.5°C), may cause scalding or thermal skin injuries (second-degree burns) and may intensify the pruritus. Patients can shower using hypoallergenic soap to maintain cleanliness. They should never use harsh soaps or vigorously scrub affected areas. Along with applying topical treatment, all patients should trim their fingernails to reduce the risk of secondary bacterial skin infections from scratching.

Pharmacologic Therapy
Itching

Topical ointments and creams containing anesthetics (e.g., benzocaine), antihistamines (e.g., diphenhydramine), or antibiotics (e.g., neomycin) should not be used. These agents are known sensitizers and can cause a drug-induced ACD superimposed on the existing ACD.[20,22] Although topical antihistamines are not indicated, nonprescription, first-generation oral antihistamines can be used to assist with itching and offer sedation at night. If sedation is a concern, nonsedating antihistamines can be used. If itching is not alleviated by nonprescription oral antihistamines, patients should be referred to a primary care provider (PCP) for further care.

Weeping

Astringents retard weeping, oozing, discharge, or bleeding from dermatitis when applied to unhealthy serous skin or mucous membranes. They decrease edema, exudation, and inflammation by reducing cell membrane permeability and by hardening the intercellular cement of the capillary epithelium. When applied as a wet dressing or compress, astringents cool and dry the skin through evaporation. They cause vasoconstriction and reduce blood flow in inflamed tissue. They also cleanse the skin of exudates, crust, and debris. Because astringents generally have low cell penetrability, their activity is limited to the cell surface and interstitial spaces. The protein precipitate that forms may serve as a protective coat, allowing new tissues to grow underneath.[34]

Aluminum acetate solution USP, or Burow's solution, contains approximately 5% aluminum acetate. The drying ability of aluminum acetate solution probably involves complexing of the astringent agent with proteins, thereby altering the proteins' ability to swell and hold water. The solution must be diluted 1:40 with water before use. A 1:40 dilution of Burow's solution may be prepared from prepackaged tablets or powder by adding 1 tablet or package to 1 pint of cool tap water.[14] The patient may soak the affected area 15–30 minutes 2–4 times daily. Alternatively, the patient may loosely apply a compress of washcloths, cheesecloth, or small towels; the compress is prepared by soaking the materials in the solution and then gently wringing them so that they are wet but not dripping. The dressings should be rewetted and applied every few minutes for 20–30 minutes, 4–6 times daily. Any remaining solution should be discarded and a fresh solution prepared for each application. Burow's solution is useful in softening and removing crusting, and it also has a mild antipruritic effect. Less expensive alternatives to aluminum acetate include isotonic saline solution (1 teaspoon of salt in 2 cups of water), tap water, diluted white vinegar (one-fourth cup per 1 pint of water), and unchlorinated water.

Hydrocortisone 1% cream will reduce weeping by treating the immune-mediated inflammation. Ointments should not be applied to open lesions because removal from the skin is more difficult. Ointments may also trap bacteria beneath the oleaginous film, leading to secondary infections.

Inflammation

Hydrocortisone is the most effective form of topical therapy for treating symptoms of mild-moderate ACD that does not involve edema and extensive areas of the skin. Hydrocortisone is a low-potency corticosteroid capable of vasoconstriction, thereby reducing inflammation and relieving pruritus associated with ACD. It is available topically with nonprescription strengths of 0.5% and 1%. It has been approved for use in eczema, psoriasis, insect bites, seborrheic dermatitis, and allergic contact dermatitis, including poison ivy/oak/sumac. An FDA advisory panel and dermatologists believe that hydrocortisone is safe to apply to all parts of the body except the eyes and eyelids. Although systemic absorption is nominal when used on intact skin, use of topical hydrocortisone over large surface areas, prolonged use, use with an occlusive dressing, or use when skin integrity is compromised can lead to systemic absorption. Hydrocortisone cream can be applied as frequently as two to four times per day.[35]

Generally, topical hydrocortisone is well tolerated, with limited adverse reactions. When adverse reactions occur, they typically include burning and irritation. No dressing or bandages should be applied when hydrocortisone is used as a self-care treatment. Topical hydrocortisone should not be used on children younger than 2 years, except on a PCP's advice. Hydrocortisone should not be used if the dermatitis persists longer than 7 days, or if symptoms clear and then reappear in a few days, unless patients have consulted with a PCP.

When greater than 20% of the body is affected, systemic therapy is recommended and patients should be referred to a PCP.[24]

Product Selection Guidelines
Special Populations

Treatment of contact dermatitis in pediatric patients is similar to the approach in adults. Nondrug therapies and pharmacologic therapies such as emollients, barrier creams, and topical corticosteroids can be used in pediatric patients as described for adults (refer to product label instructions). Use of pharmacologic products in pediatric patients younger than 2 years is discouraged without the advice of a PCP.

Topical preparations are generally considered safe for use during pregnancy, as long as they are not used for long periods of time or over extensive areas of the body. Hydrocortisone is considered a Pregnancy Category C product, but the risk is considered limited with low-potency (nonprescription) formulations.[36,37] Other topical preparations (e.g., calamine, colloidal oatmeal, and aluminum acetate) have an "undetermined" pregnancy category. The same precautions described for self-treatment in adults apply to pregnant women. For other treatments, pregnant patients should be referred for medical evaluation.

In geriatric patients, first-generation antihistamines (e.g., diphenhydramine) should be avoided because of sedation and other anticholinergic effects. In addition, itching is of concern in geriatric patients because scratching increases the risk for skin tears and accompanying infections.

Patient Factors and Preferences

Nonprescription medications for ACD are available in numerous dosage forms. The choice of dosage form depends on several factors, including the severity of the dermatitis and the presence of vesicles (dry or weeping). Ointments hold moisture within the skin and act as a reservoir for the active ingredient, keeping it on the affected site. They are also effective for use on dry or cracked skin.[13] However, ointments tend to hold in the heat of inflamed skin and may intensify itching in the early stages of treatment of urushiol-induced rash. Ointments should not be applied to open lesions because their removal from the skin is more difficult, and they may trap bacteria beneath the oleaginous film, leading to secondary infections. As a result, ointments are not recommended in plant-based ACD and where weeping lesions are present.

Applying a cream base allows vesicle fluid to flow freely from the blisters and does not trap bacteria because the medication is quickly absorbed into the skin. Because a cream is an oil-in-water emulsion, it tends to be drying and is best for open weeping lesions. In addition, creams are more cosmetically appealing and feel more pleasant to patients.[13] Gels offer ease of application and a rapid absorption of active ingredients into the skin. Some gels may contain alcohol or similar organic solvents that may cause irritation or burning when applied to open lesions.

Spray products provide the easiest form of drug application. They allow even distribution to larger areas and are convenient to use. Another advantage of a spray product is that it does not

table

34–5 Selected Products for Poison Ivy/Oak/Sumac Dermatitis

Aveeno Soothing Bath Treatment	Colloidal oatmeal 100%
Burow's Solution	Aluminum acetate 5%
Calamine Lotion	Calamine 8%
Cortaid	Hydrocortisone 1% or 0.5%
Domeboro Astringent Solution Powder Packets	Aluminum sulfate 1347 mg; calcium acetate 952 mg

require touching the area of dermatitis, which may curtail additional scratching. However, aerosol sprays may contain propellants that cause additional inflammation and/or alcohol that causes excessive drying and irritation. Table 34–5 lists selected products that contain primarily colloidal oatmeal, pharmacologic treatments, or bentoquatam. (See Chapter 36 for products that contain local anesthetics, hydrocortisone, or topical antihistamines.)

Assessment of Contact Dermatitis: A Case-Based Approach

Circumstances surrounding the occurrence of the dermatitis can help determine the type of dermatitis (Table 34–6). The factors that help to distinguish ICD from ACD include (1) history of irritant or allergen exposure, (2) history of known sensitivity on previous exposure, (3) time from exposure (at home, work, or recreation) to appearance of rash, (4) distribution and appearance of the lesions, (5) severity of symptoms, and (6) improvement of

the dermatitis with avoidance of irritants.[2,4] Much of the information distinguishing between ICD and ACD is obtained by taking the patient's history; the distribution and appearance of lesions will be the only factor directly observable at the time of the patient visit. Determining the type and success of previous treatments of similar rashes will aid in selecting the appropriate nonprescription medications.

Cases 34–1 and 34–2 illustrate the assessment of patients with contact dermatitis.

Patient Counseling for Contact Dermatitis

Counseling of a patient who presents with possible ICD or ACD, but who cannot identify contact with irritant chemicals, allergens, or *Toxicodendron* plants, should begin with a review of chemicals or allergens likely to cause dermatitis. Then preventive and protective measures, as well as nonprescription pharmacologic treatment options, should be explained. Counseling for nonprescription agents should include their purpose and appropriate use, their possible adverse effects, expected time to experience relief, and signs and symptoms that indicate the need for medical referral for further evaluation. The box Patient Education for Contact Dermatitis lists specific information to provide patients.

Evaluation of Patient Outcomes for Contact Dermatitis

Follow-up on the patient's progress should occur after 5–7 days of treatment; that is, the patient should be encouraged to call for additional advice if the itching has not subsided significantly

table

34–6 Differentiation of Irritant and Allergic Contact Dermatitis

Symptom or Characteristic	Irritant Contact Dermatitis	Allergic Contact Dermatitis
Itching	Yes, later	Yes, early
Stinging, burning	Early	Late or not at all
Erythema	Yes	Yes
Vesicles, bullae	Rarely or no	Yes
Papules	Rarely or no	Yes
Dermal edema	Yes	Yes
Time to reaction (rash) after exposure	Minutes to hours	Days, slower reaction
Appearance of symptoms in relation to exposures	Initial or repetitive exposures	Delayed
Causative substances	Water, urine, flour, detergents, hand sanitizers, soap, alkalis, acids, solvents, salts, surfactants, oxidizers	*Toxicodendron* plants, fragrances, nickel, latex, benzocaine, neomycin, leather
Substance concentration at exposure	Important	Less important
Mechanism of reaction	Direct tissue damage	Immunologic reaction
Common location	Hands, wrist, forearms, diaper area	Anywhere on body that comes in contact with antigen
Presentation	No clear margins	Clear margins based on contact of offending substance

Source: Adapted from references 13, 14, and 23.

case
34–1

Relevant Evaluation Criteria	Scenario/Model Outcome

Information Gathering

1. Gather essential information about the patient's symptoms and medical history, including:

   a. description of symptom(s) (i.e., nature, onset, duration, severity, associated symptoms)

   Patient has irritated hands and wishes to treat the condition. He works full-time as a nurse. He noticed that his hands were becoming more irritated over the past month. Patient's hands appear dry and cracked. He complains of itching and redness. No vesicles, bullae, open lesions, or signs of infection are present. Irritation is confined to the hands.

   b. description of any factors that seem to precipitate, exacerbate, and/or relieve the patient's symptom(s)

   Symptoms worsened as the weather got colder and as he started working more shifts. Dryness and itching progressively increased over the last month.

   c. description of the patient's efforts to relieve the symptoms

   He has not tried any treatments.

   d. patient's identity

   John Darby

   e. age, sex, height, and weight

   54 years old, male, 6 ft 3 in., 210 lb

   f. patient's occupation

   Surgical nurse

   g. patient's dietary habits

   Normal diet with frequent use of alcohol

   h. patient's sleep habits

   Averages 8 hours per night.

   i. concurrent medical conditions, prescription and nonprescription medications, and dietary supplements

   Ibuprofen 600 mg by mouth every 6 hours as needed for arthritis

   j. allergies

   Codeine

   k. history of other adverse reactions to medications

   None

   l. other (describe) _____

   NA

Assessment and Triage

2. Differentiate patient's signs/symptoms and correctly identify the patient's primary problem(s).

   John is suffering from irritant contact dermatitis. The likely sources are the continuous use of hand sanitizers and gloves, as well as constant handwashing.

3. Identify exclusions for self-treatment (Figure 34–1).

   None

4. Formulate a comprehensive list of therapeutic alternatives for the primary problem to determine if triage to a medical provider is required, and share this information with the patient or caregiver.

   Options include:

   (1) Refer John to the appropriate health care provider.

   (2) Recommend self-care with a nonprescription product and/or nondrug measures.

   (3) Recommend self-care until John can be seen by an appropriate health care provider.

   (4) Take no action.

Plan

5. Select an optimal therapeutic alternative to address the patient's problem, taking into account patient preferences.

   John should take protective measures when at work to prevent irritant exposure to liquids. He should use a mild cleanser, such as Cetaphil. He should apply hand lotion frequently. He can consider wearing gloves if they are not a source of irritation.

6. Describe the recommended therapeutic approach to the patient or caregiver.

   "Completely dry your hands after washing with a mild cleanser such as Cetaphil; then use a hypoallergenic hand lotion. Apply moisturizer at night and cover with cotton gloves overnight."

7. Explain to the patient or caregiver the rationale for selecting the recommended therapeutic approach from the considered therapeutic alternatives.

   "Drying your hands will cleanse them of irritants. The hypoallergenic hand lotion will relieve dryness. The addition of cotton gloves will increase the moisture retained in your skin."

Relevant Evaluation Criteria	Scenario/Model Outcome
Patient Education	

8. When recommending self-care with nonprescription medications and/or nondrug therapy, convey accurate information to the patient or caregiver:

a. appropriate dose and frequency of administration	See the box Patient Education for Contact Dermatitis.
b. maximum number of days the therapy should be employed	See the box Patient Education for Contact Dermatitis.
c. product administration procedures	See the box Patient Education for Contact Dermatitis.
d. expected time to onset of relief	See the box Patient Education for Contact Dermatitis.
e. degree of relief that can be reasonably expected	"Complete symptomatic relief is likely."
f. most common side effects	See the box Patient Education for Contact Dermatitis.
g. side effects that warrant medical intervention should they occur	See the box Patient Education for Contact Dermatitis.
h. patient options in the event that condition worsens or persists	"You should consult a primary care provider if the condition does not improve or if irritation is intolerable."
i. product storage requirements	See the box Patient Education for Contact Dermatitis.
j. specific nondrug measures	See the box Patient Education for Contact Dermatitis.
Solicit follow-up questions from the patient or caregiver.	"When should the irritation get better?"
Answer the patient's or caregiver's questions.	"You should see a difference in 1 week. If you do not see improvement, contact your primary care provider."

Evaluation of Patient Outcome	
9. Assess patient outcome.	Ask the patient to contact you and report how he responded to the recommended therapy, or call him in a week to evaluate his treatment outcome.

Key: NA = Not applicable.

Relevant Evaluation Criteria	Scenario/Model Outcome
Information Gathering	

1. Gather essential information about the patient's symptoms and medical history, including:

a. description of symptom(s) (i.e., nature, onset, duration, severity, associated symptoms)	Patient complains of redness, swelling, and mild itching on her ears. Symptoms have worsened over the past 2 weeks.
b. description of any factors that seem to precipitate, exacerbate, and/or relieve the patient's symptom(s)	She notices some relief at night.
c. description of the patient's efforts to relieve the symptoms	Patient reports that no treatment has been used.
d. patient's identity	Anna Jones
e. age, sex, height, and weight	21 years old, female, 5 ft 8 in., 130 lb
f. patient's occupation	College student
g. patient's dietary habits	Normal diet with junk food
h. patient's sleep habits	5 hours a night
i. concurrent medical conditions, prescription and nonprescription medications, and dietary supplements	Yasmin, 1 tablet by mouth daily Albuterol inhaler, 1–2 puffs as needed prior to exercising
j. allergies	Nickel
k. history of other adverse reactions to medications	NA
l. other (describe) _____	NA

case
34-2 *continued*

Relevant Evaluation Criteria	Scenario/Model Outcome

Assessment and Triage

2. Differentiate patient's signs/symptoms and correctly identify the patient's primary problem(s).

Anna is suffering from an allergic reaction to a new pair of earrings. Her symptomatology (e.g., redness, swelling, and mild itching), has worsened over time as a result of continued daily exposure.

3. Identify exclusions for self-treatment (Figure 34–1).

None

4. Formulate a comprehensive list of therapeutic alternatives for the primary problem to determine if triage to a medical provider is required, and share this information with the patient or caregiver.

Options include:

(1) Refer Anna to the appropriate health care provider.

(2) Recommend self-care with a nonprescription product and/or nondrug measures.

(3) Recommend self-care until Anna can see an appropriate health care provider.

(4) Take no action.

Plan

5. Select an optimal therapeutic alternative to address the patient's problem, taking into account patient preferences.

Anna should begin self-care using hydrocortisone 1% cream.

6. Describe the recommended therapeutic approach to the patient or caregiver.

"Discontinue wearing the earrings and avoid all nickel-containing jewelry. Apply a small amount of hydrocortisone on your earlobe two times a day until symptoms resolve. The rash should resolve in 7–10 days. Contact your primary care provider if the rash worsens or persists."

7. Explain to the patient or caregiver the rationale for selecting the recommended therapeutic approach from the considered therapeutic alternatives.

"Allergic contact dermatitis can be effectively treated using hydrocortisone cream."

Patient Education

8. When recommending self-care with nonprescription medications and/or nondrug therapy, convey accurate information to the patient or caregiver.

   a. appropriate dose and frequency of administration

See the box Patient Education for Contact Dermatitis.

   b. maximum number of days the therapy should be employed

See the box Patient Education for Contact Dermatitis.

   c. product administration procedures

See the box Patient Education for Contact Dermatitis.

   d. expected time to onset of relief

See the box Patient Education for Contact Dermatitis.

   e. degree of relief that can be reasonably expected

"Complete symptomatic relief is likely."

   f. most common side effects

See the box Patient Education for Contact Dermatitis.

   g. side effects that warrant medical intervention should they occur

See the box Patient Education for Contact Dermatitis.

   h. patient options in the event that condition worsens or persists

"A primary care provider should be consulted if the condition does not improve or if irritation is intolerable."

   i. product storage requirements

See the box Patient Education for Contact Dermatitis.

   j. specific nondrug measures

See the box Patient Education for Contact Dermatitis.

Solicit follow-up questions from the patient or caregiver.

"Can I wear any jewelry?"

Answer the patient's or caregiver's questions.

"Yes, you can wear earrings once the rash is resolved, as long as they do not contain nickel. Because you are allergic to nickel in earrings, you may experience the same type of rash from other jewelry or clothing items containing nickel."

Evaluation of Patient Outcome

9. Assess patient outcome.

Ask the patient to contact you and report if the recommended therapy resolved the rash, or call the patient in a week to evaluate her response to the therapy.

Key: NA = Not applicable.

Irritant Contact Dermatitis

The goals in self-treating ICD are to (1) remove the offending agent and prevent future exposure to the irritant; (2) relieve the inflammation, dermal tenderness, and irritation; and (3) educate the patient on self-management to prevent and treat recurrences. For most patients, carefully following product instructions and the self-care measures listed here will help ensure optimal therapeutic outcomes.

Nondrug Measures

■ Avoid or limit contact with common skin irritants, such as detergents, soaps, and solvents.
■ Change clothing, diapers (if applicable), and gloves used for cleaning more frequently.
■ Wash the affected area gently to remove the skin irritant.

Nonprescription Medications

■ To help soothe the affected area, apply compresses of cool tap water or aluminum acetate for 20 minutes, 4–6 times daily.
■ Use emollients liberally to restore moisture to skin.
■ If itching keeps you awake at night, take a sedating oral antihistamine, such as diphenhydramine or doxylamine, and follow the label instructions. These medications can cause drowsiness that might extend to the next morning.
■ Store nonprescription medications in a cool, dry place out of children's reach.
■ Rash and itching should improve within 5–7 days. If either rash or itching worsens, consult your primary care provider.
■ Using nonprescription medications longer than 7 days for dermatitis without consulting a physician is not recommended.

Allergic Contact Dermatitis

The goals of self-treating ACD are to (1) remove and/or avoid further contact with the offending agent, (2) treat the inflammation, (3) relieve itching and excessive scratching that may lead to open lesions and potential secondary skin infections, and (4) relieve the accumulation of debris that arises from oozing, crusting, and scaling of the vesicle fluids. For most patients, carefully following product instructions and the self-care measures listed here will help ensure optimal therapeutic outcomes.

Nondrug Measures

■ Use the measures outlined in Table 34–4 to prevent poison ivy/oak/sumac dermatitis.
■ Take tepid, soapless showers to relieve itching.
■ When cleansing the affected areas, do not use harsh cleansers or scrub vigorously.
■ To avoid potential allergic reactions, use hypoallergenic cosmetics and soapless cleansers.

Nonprescription Medications

■ Use clean white cloths to apply cool water compresses; apply for 20–30 minutes as often as needed or desired. Use a fresh solution with each new application.
■ If desired, to reduce inflammation and the itching and redness, apply topical hydrocortisone cream *only* as follows:
  – Apply a small amount to affected areas up to 2–4 times a day.
  – Avoid applying the cream around the eyes or eyelids.
■ To avoid infection, do not apply ointments to open lesions.
■ Apply aluminum acetate (Burow's solution) compresses to areas with vesicles, bullae, and/or weeping lesions as follows:
  – Mix a prepackaged tablet or packet of aluminum acetate with a pint of cool tap water, wet a cloth with the solution, and apply the compress to rash areas.
  – Apply compresses for 30 minutes at least 4 times a day or as needed.
  – Prepare fresh Burow's solution for each application.
■ Use colloidal oatmeal baths or soaks to soothe and cleanse areas of the rash and to reduce itching:
  – Sprinkle a 30 gram packet or a cup full of milled oatmeal into fast-running bath water, and mix the water to avoid lumping of the oatmeal.
  – Soak for 15–20 minutes in the oatmeal bath at least twice a day.
  – Pat skin dry rather than wiping it.
  – Be careful; oatmeal baths can leave the tub quite slippery.
■ Store nonprescription medications in a cool, dry place out of children's reach.
■ Using nonprescription medications for dermatitis longer than 7 days without consulting a physician is not recommended.

When to Seek Medical Attention

■ Contact a primary care provider for the following situations:
  – The rash does not begin to improve in 7 days.
  – Symptoms become worse.
  – The rash spreads.
  – The rash covers large areas of the face or causes swelling of the eyelids.
  – The rash involves the genitals.

---

within 5–7 days. If, at follow-up, the rash has significantly increased in size, affects the eyes or genitals, or covers extensive areas of the face, the patient must be referred to his or her PCP. Overall, complete remission of the dermatitis may take up to 3 weeks. However, the patient should see slow but steady reduction in itching, weeping, and dermatitis after 5–7 days of therapy.

Key Points for Contact Dermatitis

➤ The leading cause of ICD is constant unprotected exposure to wet environments that may contain irritant substances such as detergents and cleaning solutions.

➤ ACD is produced through sensitization to an antigenic substance.

➤ Many substances are antigenic. Common antigens include fragrances, metals, medications, plants, and chemicals. Urushiol from poison ivy/oak/sumac is one of the most common allergens.

➤ Patients who are sensitive to irritants, allergens, or urushiol should take precautions to eliminate exposure by avoiding these agents, limiting exposure time, and wearing protective clothing and equipment.

➤ In the case of poison ivy, avoiding geographic areas with endemic *Toxicodendron* plants is helpful. Patients should be advised to wear clothing (e.g., gloves, long sleeves, and long pants) that limits exposure of the skin to the environment.

In addition, to reduce the risk of dermatitis, patients sensitive to urushiol may liberally apply bentoquatam barrier lotion every 4 hours until the exposure period is over.

➤ Once exposed to an irritant or antigen, the patient should bathe with mild soap and water or use large volumes of cool water immediately after exposure to reduce the risk of dermatitis.

➤ ACD may begin as localized streaks or patches of highly pruritic rash that with time may become more numerous or coalesce into larger plaques on exposed dermal areas. The rash may affect the eyelids or face and, in some cases, areas ordinarily considered to be protected.

➤ Patients should be referred for further evaluation if there is involvement of the face, genitalia, or anus; considerable edema anywhere on the body (including eyelids); or extensive lesions covering a large portion of the body.

➤ Treatment of localized, pruritic rash consists of a topical application of hydrocortisone cream, compresses, or baths. Weeping vesicles or bullae may be treated with aluminum acetate compresses as an astringent with soothing and drying properties.

➤ Irritant and allergic contact dermatitis will resolve in approximately 10–21 days with or without topical therapy. Nonprescription medications primarily relieve symptoms.

REFERENCES

1. Cohen DE, Heidary N. Treatment of irritant and allergic contact dermatitis. *Dermatol Ther.* 2004;17(4):334–40.

2. Wolff K, Johnson RA, Suurmond D. Contact dermatitis. In: *Color Atlas and Synopsis of Clinical Dermatology.* 5th ed. New York, NY: McGraw-Hill; 2005:18–32.

3. Bureau of Labor Statistics. Incidence rates of nonfatal occupational illness, by industry and category of illness, 2011. Accessed at http://www.bls.gov/iif/oshwc/osh/os/ostb3186.pdf, May 23, 2013.

4. Bureau of Labor Statistics. Number of nonfatal occupational injuries and illnesses involving days away from work by nature of injury or illness, gender, and length of service with employer, private industry, 2010. Accessed at http://www.bls.gov/iif/oshwc/osh/case/ostb2871.pdf, May 23, 2013.

5. Cashman MW, Reutemann PA, Erhlich A. Contact dermatitis in the United States: epidemiology, economic impact, and workplace prevention. *Dermatol Clin.* 2012;30(1):87–98.

6. National Institute for Occupational Safety and Health (NIOSH). Developing dermal policy based on laboratory and field studies: a new National Institute for Occupational Safety and Health (NIOSH) research program in response to the National Occupational Research Agenda (NORA). Accessed at http://www.cdc.gov/niosh/docs/2000-142/pdfs/2000-142.pdf, May 23, 2013.

7. Hogan DJ. Contact dermatitis, irritant. Accessed at http://emedicine.medscape.com/article/1049353-overview, May 23, 2013.

8. Lushniak BD. Occupational skin diseases. Occupational and environmental medicine. *Prim Care.* 2000;27:895–915.

9. Koch P. Occupational contact dermatitis, recognition and management. *Am J Dermatol.* 2001;2:353–65.

10. Slodownik D, Lee A, Nixon R. Irritant contact dermatitis: a review. *Australas J Dermatol.* 2008;49:1–11.

11. Honari G, Talor JS, Sood A. Occupational skin diseases due to irritants and allergens. In: Goldsmith LA, Katz SI, Gilchrest BA, et al., eds. *Fitzpatrick's Dermatology in General Medicine.* 8th ed. New York, NY: McGraw-Hill; 2012.

12. Aajjachareonpong P, Cahill J, Keegel T, et al. Persistent post-occupational dermatitis. *Contact Dermat.* 2004;51:278–81.

13. Crowe MA. Pediatric contact dermatitis. Accessed at http://emedicine.medscape.com/article/911711-clinical, May 23, 2013.

14. Hogan DJ. Allergic contact dermatitis. Accessed at http://emedicine.medscape.com/article/1049216-overview, May 23, 2013.

15. Zug KA, Warshae EM, Fowler JF, et al. Patch test results of the North American Contact Dermatitis Group 2005–2006. *Dermatitis.* 2009;20(3):149–60.

16. Scheman A, Jacob S, Zirwas M, et al. Contact allergy: alternatives for the 2007 North American Contact Dermatitis Group (NACDG) standard screening tray. *Disease-a-Month.* 2008;54(1–2):7–156.

17. Funk JO, Maibach HI. Horizons in pharmacologic intervention in allergic contact dermatitis. *J Am Acad Derm.* 1994;31(6):999–1014.

18. Gayer KD, Burnett JW. Toxicodendron dermatitis. *Cutis.* 1988;42(2):99–100.

19. Epstein WL. Plant-induced dermatitis. *Ann Emerg Med.* 1987;16(9):950–5.

20. Gladman AC. Toxicodendron dermatitis: poison ivy, oak, and sumac. *Wilderness Environ Med.* 2006;17(2):120–8.

21. Botanical Dermatology Database. Anacardiaceae. Accessed at http://www.botanical-dermatology-database.info/BotDermFolder/ANAC-1.html, May 23, 2013.

22. Allen PLJ. Leaves of three, let them be: if it were only that easy. *Dermatol Nurs.* 2006;18(3):236–42.

23. Reitschel RL, Fowler JF, eds. *Fisher's Contact Dermatitis: Allergic Sensitization to Plants.* 6th ed. Lewiston, NY: BD Decker; 2008:405–53.

24. Beltrani VS, Bernstein IL, Cohen DE, et al. Contact dermatitis: a practice parameter. *Ann Allergy Asthma Immunol.* 2006;97:S1–38.

25. Brook I. Secondary bacterial infections complicating skin lesions. *J Med Microbiol.* 2002;51(10):808–12.

26. Marks JG Jr, Fowler JG Jr, Sheretz EF, et al. Prevention of poison ivy and poison oak allergic contact dermatitis by quaternium-18 bentonite. *J Am Acad Dermatol.* 1995;33(2 pt 1):212–6.

27. IvyBlock Lotion [package insert]. Plymouth, MA: EnviroDerm Pharmaceuticals; 1998.

28. Fisher AA. Poison ivy/oak dermatitis, part 1: prevention soap and water, topical barriers, and hyposensitization. *Cutis.* 1996;57(6):384–6.

29. Boelman DJ. Treating poison ivy, oak, and sumac. *Am J Nurs.* 2010;210(6):49–52.

30. Davila A, Lucas J, Laurora M, et al. A new topical agent, Zanfel, ameliorates urushiol-induced toxicodendron allergic contact dermatitis. *Ann Emerg Med.* 2003;42(suppl):601.

31. Stankewicz H, Cancel G, Eberhardt M, et al. Effective topical treatment and post-exposure prophylaxis of poison ivy: objective confirmation. Seattle: American College of Emergency Physicians; 2007. Abstract 81.

32. Zanfel [package insert]. Peoria, IL: Zanfel Laboratories; 2013. Accessed at http://www.zanfel.com/help/productfaq.html.

33. Epstein WL. Topical prevention of poison ivy/oak dermatitis. *Arch Dermatol.* 1989;125(4):499–501.

34. Knutson K, Pershing LK. Topical drugs. In: Hendrickson R, Beringer P, Der Marderosian AH, et al., eds. *Remington: The Science and Practice of Pharmacy.* 21st ed. Philadelphia, PA: Lippincott, Williams & Wilkins; 2005:1277–93.

35. U.S. Food and Drug Administration. Hydrocortisone [monograph]. Accessed at http://www.fda.gov/Drugs/default.htm, May 20, 2014.

36. Conover EA. Herbal agents and over-the-counter medications in pregnancy. *Best Pract & Res Clin Endo and Metab.* 2003;17(2):237–51.

37. Chi CC, Mayon-White RT, Wojnarowska FT. Safety of topical corticosteroids in pregnancy: a population-based cohort study. *J Invest Derm.* 2011;131(4):884–91.

DIAPER DERMATITIS AND PRICKLY HEAT

Nicholas E. Hagemeier

Irritant contact diaper dermatitis, commonly referred to as diaper rash, is an acute inflammation of the skin occurring in the region of the perineum, buttocks, lower abdomen, and inner thighs. Despite the common perception that diaper dermatitis is a condition occurring in infancy, it can and does occur in any population in which incontinence presents.[1] Given the prevalence of diaper dermatitis in the infant population, this chapter focuses primarily on infant diaper dermatitis. Information presented in this chapter may be generalized to the adult population. Readers are referred to Chapter 49 for specific information regarding treatment of adult incontinence.

Prickly heat, also known as miliaria, miliaria rubra, or heat rash, is a transient inflammation of the skin that appears as a very fine, pinpoint, and usually red raised rash. It can appear on any part of the body that has sweat glands (e.g., groin, chest, and axillae). In most circumstances, neither diaper dermatitis nor prickly heat causes serious illness. These conditions typically produce discomfort, irritation, and itching. They may lead to fussiness, agitation, and irritability, especially in the infant population. Diaper dermatitis and prickly heat can also be devoid of any discomfort.

Diaper Dermatitis

Both irritant contact and allergic contact diaper dermatitis can present in the diaper area.[2] This chapter focuses primarily on irritant contact diaper dermatitis, given the prevalence of this form. For ease of reading, irritant contact diaper dermatitis is referred to simply as diaper dermatitis or diaper rash throughout the chapter. Allergic contact dermatitis is also discussed briefly.

Diaper dermatitis is the most common dermatologic disorder of infancy, resulting in more than 1 million provider office visits per year.[3] The majority of diaper dermatitis cases appear in infants 2 years of age and younger.[3,4] Diaper dermatitis can present as early as 7 days after birth.[4] Given the common nature of diaper dermatitis, the actual incidence of the condition is likely underreported. Literature has suggested a prevalence rate of 4%–35% in the first 2 years of life.[3] However, a majority of children experience diaper dermatitis at least once by the time they are out of diapers. The steady decline in the number of cases of diaper rash in infants since the 1970s is attributed to the increased use of disposable diapers. The decline was accelerated

in the 1980s and 1990s with improvements in diaper technology and the rise of superabsorbent core materials and breathable diaper coverings.[5–7]

Pathophysiology of Diaper Dermatitis

Diaper dermatitis can be caused by multiple factors. Occlusion, moisture, microbes, gastrointestinal tract proteolytic enzymes and bile salts, a shift from the normal acidic skin pH (pH 4.0–5.5) to a more alkaline pH, mechanical chafing, and friction can cause skin compromise and in additive or synergistic ways present as diaper dermatitis.[1,4,8–15]

The skin of the infant perineal region is about one-half to one-third the thickness of adult skin. Because the perineal region is typically occluded by a diaper, this area tends to hold moisture and wetness, predisposing it to irritation and infection.[16] Frequent urination and defecation, combined with infrequent changing of the diaper, contributes to increased skin moisture. The typical infant begins to urinate within 24 hours after birth. Urination occurs in infants up to 20 times a day until they are approximately 2 months old; thereafter, the frequency decreases to about 8 times a day until age 8 months. Defecation occurs from 3–6 times a day up to about age 8 months. As the infant's autonomic and muscular control develops, defecation gradually declines to 1–3 times a day. In the first months of life, infants commonly need in excess of 6 diaper changes per day. Skin left in contact with wetness for long periods becomes waterlogged or hyperhydrated, which plugs sweat glands, increases susceptibility to abrasion and frictional harm, and diminishes the barrier function of the stratum corneum in the diaper area. Diminished barrier capabilities in turn make the skin more susceptible to irritation, absorption of chemicals, and opportunistic microbes.

Urine and fecal bacteria can contribute to skin breakdown. Urea-splitting bacteria from the colon are believed to convert urine contents into ammonia. Ammonia raises the pH of the skin, making it more susceptible to damage or infection. This etiologic factor has been lessened by the use of absorbent disposable diapers, which minimize mixing of urine and feces in the diaper area.[5,17] Mechanical irritation can also lead to epidermal breakdown, allowing other irritants (e.g., fecal bacteria) to harm the skin. Tight-fitting, stiff, or rough diapers and the use of occlusive plastic or rubberized covers or pants over cloth diapers can contribute to occlusion and mechanical friction of the skin.

Medications and foods that affect the motility or microbial flora of the gastrointestinal tract, or that hinder autonomic control of urination and defecation may contribute to diaper dermatitis. Foods high in hexitols, sorbitol, sucrose, and fructose may induce diarrhea and predispose to diaper rash. Dairy products can also induce diarrhea, especially in the presence of lactose intolerance. Variations in infant feeding preferences can also influence prevalence of diaper dermatitis. Breast-fed infants have decreased incidences of diaper rash compared with bottle-fed infants.[18] The feces of breast-fed infants are less copious, less alkaline, and less caustic to the skin. Transitions in the type of food consumed (e.g., from breast milk to solid foods) can also contribute to diaper rash.

Some products (e.g., antioxidants, detergent or soap residues, household cleaning products, lotions, sunscreens, insect repellents), plant materials (e.g., ragweed and thistle), and diaper product ingredients can produce an allergic contact dermatitis that resembles diaper dermatitis.[19] Although many of these agents commonly are not purposefully used in the diaper region, they may have an unexpected effect on skin under a diaper should they be placed in the diaper region through accident or ignorance. Chemicals used to launder reusable cloth diapers, for example, can contribute to diaper rash and skin irritation if the diapers are not adequately washed and rinsed. Harsh chemicals used to clean and sanitize the diapers may leave chemical residues that exacerbate diaper dermatitis. Allergic contact dermatitis in the diaper region routinely presents only where contact with the allergen has occurred, often sparing the inguinal skin folds. Allergic contact dermatitis should be considered when standards of care do not lead to healing in the diaper area (see Chapter 34 for a discussion of allergic contact dermatitis).[2]

Clinical Presentation of Diaper Dermatitis

Diaper dermatitis usually presents as red to bright red (erythematous), sometimes shiny, wet-looking patches and lesions on the skin (see Color Plates, photograph 17). Lesions may appear dusky maroon or purplish on darker skin. Generally, diaper dermatitis occurs on the skin spaces covered by the diaper, but severe cases can spread outside the diaper area. If an infant, for example, lies primarily on his or her abdomen, the rash may appear more anterior to the perineum. In the same manner, if the infant lies primarily on his or her back, the rash may appear more posterior to the perineum.

A disconcerting feature of diaper rash is that it can perceivably present in a matter of hours, yet it can often take days to completely resolve. Most likely, the process of skin breakdown is not pronounced or visible initially, yet the skin breakdown quickly transitions from unobservable to observable. The entire process from normal to noticeably erythematous skin takes longer than the time between normal diaper changes.

Although uncommon, severe diaper dermatitis can progress to maceration, papule formation, the presence of vesicles or bullae, oozing, erosion of the skin, or ulceration. Diaper rash can also predispose infants to secondary infections and genital damage. As skin pH changes, it can foster the growth of opportunistic infections that can be bacterial (e.g., *streptococci* or *staphylococci*), fungal (e.g., yeasts), and viral (e.g., herpes simplex) in nature. If infection is a concern, visual inspection of the diaper area is beneficial for proper diagnosis. *Candida* infections, for example, can present in the diaper area secondary to diaper dermatitis. The presentation

of a *Candida* infection is distinct from that of uncomplicated diaper dermatitis. The typical *Candida* superinfection presents as papular or pustular lesions around the margins of the diaper dermatitis. Pustules can also present outside the primary diaper dermatitis area (satellite lesions). Additionally, *Candida* infections in the diaper area often present in the skin folds or creases, whereas the skin folds can serve to protect areas from diaper dermatitis. Untreated or infected diaper dermatitis can progress to skin ulceration, infections of the penis or vulva, and urinary tract infections. Such developments require medical referral.

Diaper rash can also be a manifestation of other diseases, such as Kawasaki's syndrome, granuloma gluteale infantum, cytomegalovirus infection, and nutritional deficiencies. Infants born to immunocompromised mothers (e.g., those with HIV; genital herpes; other chronic, congenital, or sexually transmitted infections) should be considered at increased risk for unusual manifestations of diaper rash or diaper rash–like presentations. Primary infections of the skin can resemble diaper rash and be misdiagnosed. Inguinal swelling, fever, chills, tachycardia, blisters, vesicles, and irregular borders bounded by bumps or vesicles are indicators of infections that require medical referral.[4,20] Diaper rash can exist concurrently with other skin conditions such as psoriasis and seborrhea.[10] Skin conditions that can occur on other parts of the body can exist in the diaper region and may be misdiagnosed as diaper dermatitis.

Treatment of Diaper Dermatitis
Treatment Goals

The goals of diaper dermatitis treatment are to (1) relieve the symptoms, (2) rid the patient of the rash, (3) discourage infection, and (4) prevent recurrences.

General Treatment Approach

The general treatment approach for diaper rash is the use of nonpharmacologic therapy or a combination of pharmacologic and nonpharmacologic therapy as outlined in Figure 35–1.

The best treatment for diaper dermatitis is prevention. The ideal, yet often impractical, preventive therapy would be to change the diaper immediately after the individual defecates or urinates. Self-treatment will often involve increased vigilance in keeping the infant dry and use of skin protectants in the diaper area. Self-treatment should be limited to diaper dermatitis that is uncomplicated (e.g., absence of comorbid conditions or symptoms) and mild-moderate (e.g., absence of oozing or blood at lesion sites, or lesions present <7 days) in presentation. Figure 35–1 presents a thorough list of characteristics of complicated and severe diaper dermatitis. Medical referral should occur when diaper dermatitis manifests one or more of the exclusions listed.

Nonpharmacologic Therapy

Nonpharmacologic therapy plays an integral role in the treatment of diaper dermatitis. The goals of nonpharmacologic therapy are to (1) reduce occlusion, (2) reduce contact time of urine and feces with skin, (3) reduce mechanical irritation and trauma to the inguinal and perineal skin, (4) protect the skin from further irritation, (5) encourage healing, and (6) discourage the onset of secondary infection.

Person with reddened, maroon, or purplish skin under diaper area. Affected skin may also be shiny or wet looking.

↓

Obtain medical history. Determine longevity & extent of dermatitis. Ask about other symptoms, including behavioral changes. Ask about attempts to treat the dermatitis.

↓

Exclusions for self-treatment (see box)? —**Yes**→ Medical referral

No

↓

Recommend OTC protectants up to 7 days. If warranted, recommend more frequent diaper changes & better diaper hygiene.

↓

Lesions healed after 7 days of treatment? —**Yes**→ Advise parent that prophylactic use is safe if such use is desired.

No

↓

Medical referral

Exclusions for Self-Treatment of Diaper Dermatitis and Prickly Heat

- Lesions present >7 days
- Lesions have not improved in 7 days despite appropriate care
- Therapy complicated by secondary infection (viral, bacterial, or fungal)
- Lesions part of or caused by another disease state
- Presence of *diaper dermatitis* outside diaper region
- *Diaper dermatitis* possibly associated with urinary tract infection (painful urination) or disfigurement of penis or vulva
- Presence of broken skin (ulceration, blistering, or peeling of skin) due to disease progression or patient action (e.g., scratching)
- Onion-skin–like appearance or bulla formation in affected area
- Oozing, blood, vesicles, or pus at lesion sites
- Chronic or frequently recurrent lesions
- Presence of constitutional symptoms (e.g., fever, diarrhea, nausea, vomiting, swollen inguinal lymph nodes, rapid pulse, or rash or skin lesions on other parts of body)
- Significant behavioral changes in patient (e.g., lethargy, incessant crying) associated with the rash
- Comorbid conditions (e.g., HIV, organ transplantation, immune suppressive therapy, a history of dermal hepatic infections)

Source: References 4, 10, 20, and 28.

figure

35–1   Self-care of diaper dermatitis. Key: HIV = Human immunodeficiency virus; OTC = over-the-counter.

Treatment of uncomplicated diaper dermatitis should be initiated with nonpharmacologic therapy. Increasing the frequency of diaper changes to a minimum of six per day is advisable. Increased vigilance in combination with increased frequency of diaper changes will often alleviate mild symptoms.

Should wiping be needed, gentle rubbing or patting with a bland, soft cloth or wipe is appropriate. Most commercially available baby wipes are now low in abrasives and chemically bland for use on diaper rash. Sensitive–skin baby wipe products are readily available to consumers. Used with finesse and gentle wiping,

infant wipes are as mild as or milder than washcloths.[21] Few baby wipes still contain alcohol, perfumes, soap, or other ingredients that can cause contact dermatitis or actually burn or sting the infant. Products that list such ingredients on the label should be avoided. Importantly, the unsoiled part of a diaper should not be used to clean or wipe the infant because it may harbor bacteria.

During each diaper change, careful flushing of the skin with plain water followed by gentle nonfriction drying is encouraged. One nonpharmacologic treatment modality is to let the infant's diaper area air dry prior to rediapering; however, the risk exists that the infant may have more urine or bowel contents to evacuate while air drying. Regardless of the technique used, thorough drying before rediapering is essential to good diaper-changing procedures.

As the technology of disposable diapers has improved, the disposable diaper has become a critical component of non-pharmacologic therapy for diaper rash.[5,7] Some disposable diapers have absorptive materials that pull moisture away from direct contact with the skin to reduce skin hyperhydration and mixing of urine with feces. Some disposable diapers have a protectant (e.g., petrolatum) already in the diaper. Research has indicated that use of disposable diapers compared with cloth diapers decreases the incidence of severe diaper dermatitis.[6,22,23] If cloth diapers are used, diapers should be laundered with a mild detergent and extra rinse cycles employed if sanitizing agents are used in the laundering process.

Pharmacologic Therapy

The goals of pharmacologic therapy are to (1) protect the skin from further contact with urine and feces, (2) soothe any discomfort caused by the lesions, (3) encourage healing, and (4) discourage the onset of secondary infection.

Skin Protectants

Protectants are the only products considered safe and effective for use in diaper dermatitis without medical referral. The Food and Drug Administration (FDA) has approved 17 ingredients, all skin protectants, for treatment of diaper dermatitis (Table 35–1).[24] Two or more of the approved ingredients are

commonly combined in commercial products for treating diaper dermatitis. Importantly, some products contain an approved ingredient in combination with other ingredients that are unsafe or of dubious value for treating diaper rash. The other ingredients may be unsuitable or even toxic when applied to skin compromised by diaper dermatitis. Therefore, a general rule of thumb is to suggest the simplest possible products that contain FDA-approved ingredients. By law, products that contain antimicrobials, topical analgesics, and antifungals cannot claim they are for treatment of diaper dermatitis. Ingredients routinely included in skin-protectant formulations but not approved for treatment of diaper dermatitis are provided in Table 35–2.

Of the 17 skin protectants listed in Table 35–1, a select few are commonly incorporated into trade-name skin-protectant products. Useful comparative studies of the skin protectants are lacking. Zinc oxide is one of the most commonly employed semisolid skin protectants in products that treat diaper dermatitis. A major drawback of many zinc oxide ointment preparations and other hydrophobic diaper dermatitis preparations is the necessity of soap to remove the product from the skin. However, the hydrophobic nature of the preparations is beneficial in forming a protective barrier for the compromised skin. Some zinc oxide preparations are formulated to be more washable and creamlike and therefore easier to apply and remove. However, one must weigh the ease of use with the ability of the preparation to adequately protect the skin.

Petrolatum and white petrolatum are commonly used oleaginous ingredients that serve as excellent skin protectants. These products are ubiquitous ointment bases. Petrolatum may be listed as an active or inactive ingredient in skin protectant formulations. Lanolin is a bacteriostatic product obtained from a fatty substance found in wool and is also commonly used in skin-protectant products. It can be used alone or in combination with other skin protectants. Lanolin is a common contact sensitizer, and although approved for use in diaper dermatitis, risk should be noted if applied in the diaper area where the skin is inflamed and more likely vulnerable to contact allergens.

Calamine is a mixture of zinc and ferrous oxides. It has absorptive, antiseptic, and antipruritic properties and is available in numerous dosage forms. Mineral oil coats the skin with a water-impenetrable film that must be washed off with each diaper change to avoid buildup in pores and subsequent folliculitis. Mineral oil is often used in small quantities in skin protectant

table
35–1   FDA-Approved Skin Protectants to Treat Diaper Rash

Agent	Concentration (%)
Allantoin	0.5–2
Calamine	1–25
Cocoa butter	50–100
Cod liver oil (in combination)	5.0–13.56
Colloidal oatmeal	≤0.007
Dimethicone	1–30
Glycerin	20–45
Hard fat	50–100
Kaolin	4–20
Lanolin	12.5–50
Mineral oil	50–100
Petrolatum	30–100
Topical cornstarch	10–98
White petrolatum	30–100
Zinc acetate	0.1–2
Zinc carbonate	0.2–2
Zinc oxide	1–25

Source: Reference 24.

table
35–2   Selected Nonmonograph Ingredients in Diaper Dermatitis Products

Aloe	Lavender
Beeswax	Peruvian balsam
Calendula	Sodium bicarbonate
Castor oil	Sweet clover
Chamomile	Tea tree oil
Comfrey	Vitamin A
Flower extract	Vitamin D
Goldenseal	Vitamin E
Jojoba	

products. It is often listed as an inactive ingredient in formulations despite FDA approval for use as an active ingredient. Dimethicone is a silicone-based oil that repels water and soothes and counteracts inflammation. It is used in combination with other skin protectants such as petrolatum.

Topical cornstarch and talc are used almost exclusively as loose powders. Topical cornstarch is an absorbent material, whereas talc functions as a lubricant. Both products carry warnings against inhalation of the powder because of a history of injury and fatality from improper use around infants. The warning states, "Keep powder away from child's face to avoid inhalation, which can cause breathing problems."[24] Powders should be carefully applied with as little aerosolization as possible. Concerns about inhalation of powders have caused some health care providers to suggest pouring the powder into the hands away from the infant and gently rubbing it onto the perineal area, whereas others recommend avoiding any use of powders around infants. Talc specifically should not be applied to broken or oozing skin; it can cake on the edges of wounds and precipitate infection or retard healing.

Overall, skin protectants serve as physical barriers between the skin and external irritants. Protectants also serve as lubricants in areas in which skin-to-skin or skin-to-diaper friction could aggravate diaper rash or predispose the area to diaper rash. Protectants absorb moisture or prevent moisture from coming into direct contact with skin. Protective effects of these products allow the body's normal healing processes to work. Because skin protectants are remarkably safe, their use as either treatment or prophylaxis is acceptable. Research suggests that applying a skin protectant regularly with each diaper change is one element of preventing diaper dermatitis.[12]

When diaper dermatitis is present and pharmacologic therapy is indicated, the provider should inform caregivers about their choices between semisolid and powdered protectants. Caregivers may be more comfortable with a semisolid product if they are anxious about the inhalation warning on powders, or when hands-on application is not painful or uncomfortable to the child. Fortunately, the products in this category are relatively inexpensive, and socioeconomic status tends not to be a major issue in treating diaper dermatitis. Table 35–3 lists selected widely available trade-name products and their active ingredients.

Skin-protectant dosing and application are straightforward. The protectant is applied liberally to the skin in the diaper area. Special attention should be paid to completely cover erythematous areas with the protectant if diaper dermatitis is already present. Overapplication (overdosage) of approved skin protectants is not a concern. Underapplication, however, can reduce the protective effectiveness of the product. The protectant should be reapplied as needed and with every diaper change. Diaper rash that does not necessitate medical referral commonly improves dramatically within 24 hours of initiating pharmacologic and nonpharmacologic treatment.

Contraindicated Agents

Topical nonprescription antibiotic and antifungal agents are not appropriate to use in the self-treatment of diaper dermatitis. If an infection is suspected, medical referral is advised. Topical analgesics are not recommended because they can alter sensory perception in a population that often cannot communicate perceptual changes. These agents may also excoriate macerated skin, cause pain, retard healing, and further complicate diaper dermatitis.

table 35–3	Selected Nonmonograph Ingredients in Diaper Dermatitis Products
Trade Name	**Primary Ingredients (and selected additional ingredients)**
A + D Original Ointment	Petrolatum 53.4%; lanolin 15.5%
A + D Zinc Oxide Ointment	Zinc oxide 10%; dimethicone 1%
Aquaphor Healing Ointment	Petrolatum 41% (lanolin; mineral oil)
Balmex Diaper Rash Cream	Zinc oxide 11.3% (dimethicone, mineral oil)
Boudreaux's Butt Paste	Zinc oxide 16% (castor oil; mineral oil; Peruvian balsam[a]; petrolatum)
Caldesene Baby Cornstarch Powder with Zinc Oxide	Talc 81%[a]; zinc oxide 15%
Desitin Maximum Strength Original Paste	Zinc oxide 40% (cod liver oil; lanolin; petrolatum; talc[a])
Flanders Buttocks Ointment	White petrolatum 66.2%; zinc oxide 13.4% (beeswax; castor oil[a]; mineral oil; Peruvian balsam[a])
Lansinoh Diaper Rash Ointment	Dimethicone 5%; lanolin 15.5%; zinc oxide 5.5% (chamomile[a]; corn starch; jojoba[a]; petrolatum)
Triple Paste Medicated Ointment	Zinc oxide 12.8% (corn starch; lanolin; white petrolatum)
Vitacilina Bebe Diaper Rash Ointment	Petrolatum 34.6%; zinc oxide 30%; allantoin 1% (corn starch; mineral oil; vitamin A[a]; vitamin D[a])

[a] Nonmonograph ingredients.

Hydrocortisone is indicated for minor skin irritation, but it should not be used in diaper dermatitis without supervision by a medical provider, especially in infants. Hydrocortisone can increase the risk of secondary infection via immune response suppression. Additionally, the diaper area is a significant portion of the infant's body surface area. Hydrocortisone absorption into the skin is enhanced under occlusive conditions. When applied to macerated skin or a large surface area, absorption of hydrocortisone may lead to serum levels that interfere with the infant's pituitary–adrenal axis. Nonprescription hydrocortisone is labeled not to be used in patients younger than 2 years. (See Chapter 34 for additional information on the use of hydrocortisone.)

Product Selection Guidelines

Whereas no particular product among the approved products possesses evidence-based advantages, personal preferences for particular product characteristics will likely determine which product caregivers use to treat diaper dermatitis. As previously mentioned, some commonly used products contain nonapproved (i.e., nonmonograph) ingredients. These products may be used for formulation purposes, or they may be unregulated nutraceuticals listed as inactive or active ingredients. Unapproved ingredients could also be included in preparations to support marketing claims. For example, camphor may be present to provide a "medicated" fragrance; aloe may be present to appeal to the public perception that aloe is a wound-healing agent; or vitamins may be present to convey "natural" characteristics. To make the claim to treat diaper dermatitis, the product must, however, meet the FDA-published guidelines for active ingredients. Although the products used in diaper dermatitis generally have a wide margin of safety, they should not be recommended indiscriminately.

Complementary Therapies

Complementary therapies are not recommended for use in newborns and infants because evidence is lacking regarding their safety and effectiveness in these populations. The amount and effect of systemic absorption are unknown. Appropriateness of product strength is often unknown. Although some of these

agents have been used without incident in adults, no credible data exist on their safety or efficacy in infants.

Assessment of Diaper Dermatitis: A Case-Based Approach

When a caregiver or patient consults a health care provider about a suspected diaper rash, the provider should evaluate the presentation of the diaper rash itself and determine the extent to which factors conducive to exacerbation of diaper dermatitis are present. The provider should visually inspect the diaper dermatitis if appropriate. If inappropriate, the provider should use open-ended questioning techniques to gain a description of the dermatitis. Case 35–1 illustrates assessment of patients with diaper dermatitis. If the dermatitis is deemed to be uncomplicated diaper dermatitis warranting self-care, nonpharmacologic and

case

35-1

Relevant Evaluation Criteria	Scenario/Model Outcome
Information Gathering	
1. Gather essential information about the patient's symptoms and medical history, including:	
a. description of symptom(s) (i.e., nature, onset, duration, severity, associated symptoms)	Mr. Charles indicates that his 8-month-old daughter is quite irritable and has a rash on her "bottom." He indicates that the rash presented this morning out of nowhere. He describes his daughter's groin area as very red, shiny, and sensitive to touch. His daughter cries as if in pain during diaper changes when the diaper area is cleaned with a baby wipe. Mr. Charles indicates that his daughter has had this type of rash before but never so badly that it made her cry. Previous occurrences have resolved without the need to seek medical advice.
b. description of any factors that seem to precipitate, exacerbate, and/or relieve the patient's symptom(s)	None noted.
c. description of the patient's efforts to relieve the symptoms	Mr. Charles has been using a moisturizer cream on the diaper area since this morning, but he cannot remember the name of it. He bought some sensitive-skin baby wipes to see if that would cause less pain when cleaning his daughter's diaper area.
d. patient's identity	Neva Charles
e. patient's age, sex, height, and weight	8 months old, female, 26 in., 18 lb
f. patient's occupation	NA
g. patient's dietary habits	Breast-fed 5 times daily; eats baby cereal and baby food; also eats soft table food.
h. patient's sleep habits	Normal for age
i. concurrent medical conditions, prescription and non-prescription medications, and dietary supplements	None
j. allergies	NKA
k. history of other adverse reactions to medications	None noted.
l. other (describe) _____	NA
Assessment and Triage	
2. Differentiate the patient's signs/symptoms and correctly identify the patient's primary problem(s).	Symptoms suggest mild-moderate diaper rash in the inguinal area. The quick presentation of the rash and the painfulness and irritability support this diagnosis.
3. Identify exclusions for self-treatment (Figure 35–1).	None noted.

COLOR PLATES

COLOR ILLUSTRATION CONTRIBUTORS

Allergan, Inc.

Lawrence R. Ash

Umberto Benelli (eyeatlas.com)

Jean A. Borger

Richard C. Childers

Stanley Cullen

emedicine.com, Inc.

Jeffery A. Goad

Alfred C. Griffin (deceased)

Harold L. Hammond

Hollister Incorporated

Christopher Huerter

Thomas C. Orihel

Joan Lerner Selekof

R. Gary Sibbald

George Yatskievych

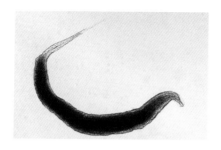

1A

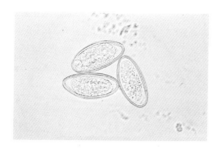

1B

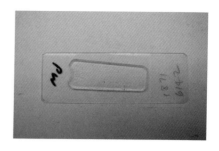

1C

1A, B, and C Pinworm infection, the most common worm infestation in the United States, is caused by ingestion of pinworm eggs from fecally contaminated hands, food, clothing, or bedding. **A,** The adult pinworm is a small (1-cm long), white, thread-like worm with a pin-shaped, pointed tail. **B,** The mature female stores approximately 11,000 eggs in her body, which she deposits in the perianal region of the host, usually at night. Reinfection occurs when the hatched larvae return to the large intestine or when eggs are transferred from the anus to the mouth and swallowed. **C,** Commercial pinworm detection kits use a sticky paddle, instead of tape, to affix the adult pinworm to a slide, which is then examined microscopically (see Chapter 18). (Photographs 1A and B courtesy of Lawrence R. Ash, PhD, and Thomas C. Orihel, PhD, © 1997, *Atlas of Human Parasitology.* 4th ed. Chicago: ASCP Press; 1997. Photograph 1C courtesy of Jeffery A. Goad, PharmD, University of Southern California, School of Pharmacy, Los Angeles, © 2003.)

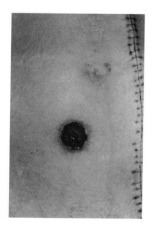

2A

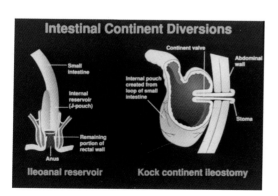

2B

2A–B There are three major types of ostomies: ileostomy, colostomy, or urinary diversion. **A,** In an ileostomy, a portion of the ileum is brought through the abdominal wall. **B,** The two most common types of continent ileostomies are the ileoanal reservoir and the Kock continent ileostomy. The ileoanal reservoir is created by stripping diseased mucosa from the rectum, creating an internal pouch from the ileum, and pulling the distal end of the pouch through the rectum and attaching it. In the Kock continent ileostomy, an internal pouch is created from the ileum and an intussusception of the bowel is used to create a "nipple."

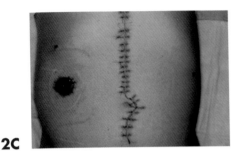

2C

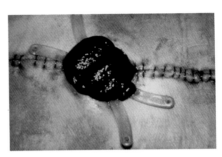

2D

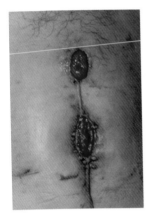

2E

2C–F Colostomies are located on the ascending, transverse, or descending/sigmoid colon. **C,** Ascending colostomies are uncommon. The ascending colon is retained, but the rest of the large bowel is removed or bypassed. The stoma is usually on the right side of the abdomen. The transverse colon is the site of most temporary colostomies. A loop of the transverse colon is lifted through the abdominal incision, and a rod or bridge is placed under the loop to give it support. **D,** Loop colostomies have one large opening, but two tracts. The proximal tract discharges fecal material; the distal tract secretes small amounts of mucus. **E,** In a double-barrel transverse colostomy, the bowel is completely divided by bringing both the proximal end and the distal end through the abdominal wall and suturing them to the skin. **F,** Descending and sigmoid colostomies are fairly common and generally are on the left side of the abdomen.

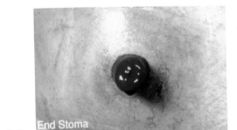

End Stoma

2F

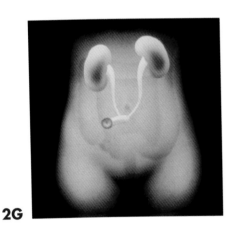

2G

2G–I Urinary diversion surgery diverts the urinary stream through an opening in the abdominal wall. **G,** In the ileal conduit, the most common type of urinary diversion, ileal and colon conduits are created after removal of the bladder by implanting the ureters into an isolated loop of bowel, the distal end of which is brought to the surface of the abdomen. **H,** Mucous shreds will be present if the bowel is used to create the diversion. **I,** In a ureterostomy, one or both ureters are detached from the bladder and brought to the outside of the abdominal wall, where a stoma is created. This procedure is used less frequently because the ureters tend to narrow unless they have been dilated permanently by previous disease (see Chapter 21). (Copyrighted photographs 2B, D, and G courtesy of Hollister Incorporated, Libertyville, Illinois. Copyrighted photographs 2A, C, E, F, H, and I courtesy of Joan Lerner Selekof, BSN, CWOCN, University of Maryland Medical Center, Baltimore, Maryland.)

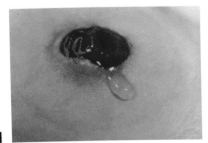

2H

2I

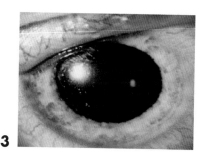

3 **Severe dry eye** can result from failure to properly diagnose and treat dry eye diseases. Severe damage to eye tissue, particularly the corneal surface, can occur (see Chapter 27). (Photograph courtesy of Allergan, Inc., Irvine, California.)

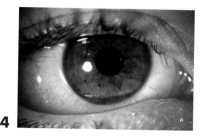

4 **Allergic conjunctivitis** is characterized by itchy, red eyes with a watery discharge. Vision is usually not impaired, but it may be blurred because of excessive tearing (see Chapter 27).

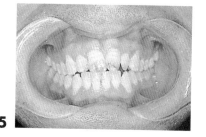

5 **Dental fluorosis (mottled enamel)** occurs during the time of tooth formation and is caused by the long-term ingestion of drinking water containing fluoride at concentrations greater than 1 ppm. Discoloration of the teeth varies, depending on the level of fluoride in the water, and ranges from white flecks or spots to brownish stains, small pits, or deep irregular pits that are dark brown in color (see Chapter 30).

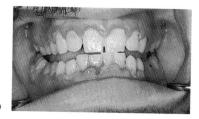

6 **Chronic gingivitis,** an asymptomatic inflammation of the gingivae (gums) at the necks of the teeth, is an early stage of periodontitis and is usually caused by poor oral hygiene. The gingivae are erythematous (red) and may have areas that appear swollen and glossy. In addition, mild hemorrhage may occur during toothbrushing (see Chapter 30).

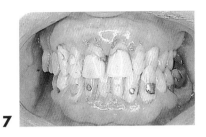

7 Chronic periodontitis (pyorrhea), an inflammation of the tissues surrounding the teeth, including the gingivae, periodontal ligaments, alveolar bone, and the cementum (bony material covering the root of a tooth), is caused by plaque accumulation resulting from poor oral hygiene. The gingivae may be erythematous and swollen, and may recede from the necks of the teeth. The condition is not painful and usually is accompanied by halitosis, loosening of the teeth, and mild hemorrhage during toothbrushing (see Chapter 30).

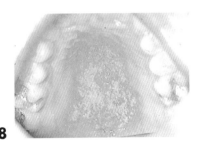

8 Candidiasis (candidosis, moniliasis, thrush), an infection caused by overgrowth of *Candida albicans,* tends to occur in people with debilitating or chronic systemic disease or those on long-term antibiotic therapy. Candidiasis commonly presents as a whitish-gray to yellowish, soft, slightly elevated pseudomembrane-like plaque on the oral mucosa; the plaque is often described as having a milk curd appearance. If the membrane is stripped away, a raw bleeding surface remains. A dull, burning pain is often present (see Chapters 30 and 31).

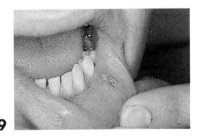

9 Recurrent aphthous ulcers (canker sores) are recurrent, painful, single, or multiple ulcerations of bacterial origin. The central ulceration is sharply demarcated, often has a gray to grayish-yellow surface of necrotic debris, and is surrounded by an erythematous margin (see Chapter 31).

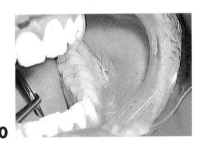

10 Aspirin burn results from the topical use of aspirin to relieve toothache. An aspirin tablet is placed against the tooth, where it is held in place by pressure from the buccal (cheek) mucosa. The mucosa becomes necrotic and is characterized by a white slough that rubs away, revealing a painful ulceration (see Chapter 31).

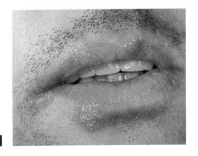

11 Herpes simplex lesions of the mouth and the eye usually start as a small cluster of vesicles (tiny blisters) that subsequently heal over with a serosanguineous (blood-tinged) crust. Local stinging, burning, and pain often herald the onset of lesions. Eye involvement should always be referred to an ophthalmologist (see Chapter 31).

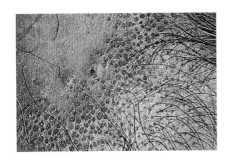

22

22 Comedonic acne (noninflammatory) occurs when follicles become plugged with sebum, forming a comedone on the surface. The black color is caused by oxidation of lipid and melanin, not dirt as is commonly believed (see Chapter 37).

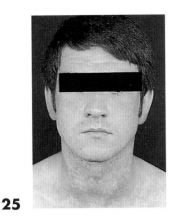

23

23 Pustular acne (inflammatory) presents as inflamed papules that are formed when superficial hair follicles become plugged and rupture at a deeper level. Superficial inflammation results in pustules; deep lesions cause large cysts to form with possible resultant scarring (see Chapter 37).

24

24 Sunburn presents as an erythema that occurs after excessive sun exposure; severe burns can result in large blister formation. Proper sunscreen application can provide photoprotection for susceptible patients (see Chapters 38 and 40).

25

25 Drug-induced photosensitivity is a reaction that occurs on sun-exposed surfaces of the head, neck, and dorsum (back) of the hands. The erythema does not occur on photoprotected areas, such as under the nose and chin, behind the ears, and between the fingers (see Chapters 38 and 40).

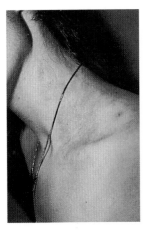

26

26 Cosmetic-induced photosensitivity can be caused by ingredients in certain topical colognes and perfumes. This reaction produces a local erythema that leaves characteristic postinflammatory pigmentation (see Chapters 38 and 40).

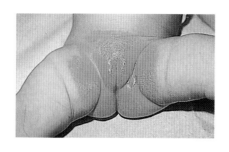

17   **Diaper dermatitis** presents as erythema of the groin (crease area around the genitals) and is common in infants. The case shown here was caused by a contact allergen. Contact irritants, such as urine and feces, and secondary bacterial and yeast infections may also cause problems in this area (see Chapter 35). (Photograph reprinted with permission from emedicine.com, Inc., © 2003.)

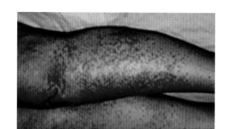

18   **Miliaria rubra (heat rash)** is an obstruction of sweat glands. Superficial involvement results in only tiny vesicles (blisters) appearing on the skin surface (miliaria crystallina). When deeper inflammation is present, the surrounding erythema is characteristic of miliaria rubra (see Chapter 35). (Photograph reprinted with permission from emedicine.com, Inc., © 2003.)

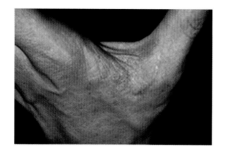

19   **Scabies** is caused by a small mite that burrows under the superficial skin layers. Small linear blisters that cause intense itching can be seen between the finger webs, on the inner wrists, in the axilla, around the areola (nipple) of the breast, and on the genitalia (see Chapter 36). (Photograph reprinted with permission from emedicine.com, Inc., © 2003.)

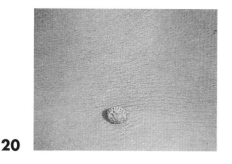

20   **Ticks** can attach to human skin and burrow into superficial skin layers. With careful examination, the back of the organism is usually visible on the skin surface. Ticks are vectors of several systemic diseases (see Chapter 36).

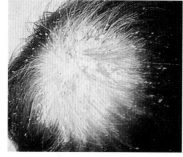

21A   **21B**

21A and B   **Pediculosis humanus capitis** is a louse infestation of the scalp. **A,** Examination of the scalp hair in this infestation shows tiny nits (eggs) attached to the hair shaft. **B,** The organism shown is only occasionally seen (see Chapter 36).

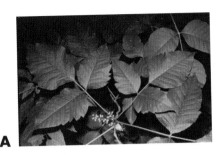

15A

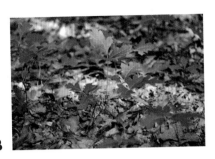

15B

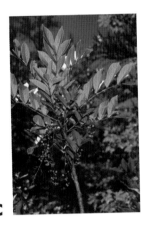

15C

15A, B, and C   Poison ivy, oak, and sumac account for the majority of plant-induced allergic contact dermatitis. **A,** In the United States, poison ivy is the most common of the three plants. It usually grows as a scrambling shrub or a climbing hairy vine that often grows up poles, trees, and building walls. Its leaves are usually large, broad, and spoon-shaped. **B,** Two species of poison oak are indigenous to the United States; both possess leaves with unlobed edges that look similar to those of oak trees. Eastern poison oak (*Toxicodendron toxicarium*) commonly displays three leaflets, whereas Western poison oak (*Toxicodendron diversilobum*) has between 3 and 11 leaflets per stem. Poison oak usually grows as a shrub capable of reaching heights of 131 feet (40 meters). **C,** Poison sumac (*Toxicodendron vernix*) grows in remote areas of the eastern one third of the United States in peat bogs and swampy areas. It grows as a shrub or small tree and attains a height of about 9.8 feet (3 meters). Its pinnate leaves have smooth edges that come to a tip and may be almost 16 inches (40 cm) in length. The leaves are odd numbered, ranging between 7 and 13 leaflets (see Chapter 34). (Photographs courtesy of George Yatskievych, PhD, Missouri Botanical Garden, St. Louis, © 2000.)

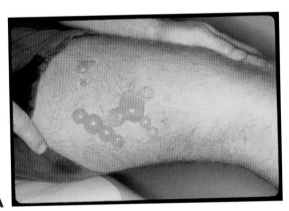

16A

16A, B, and C   Poison ivy dermatitis is often associated with **(A)** fluid-filled vesicles (blisters) or bullae, depending on a person's sensitivity. **B,** Oozing and weeping of the vesicular fluid occur for several days, until the affected area develops crusts and begins to dry. **C,** Streaks of vesicles that correspond to the points of urushiol contact from the damaged plant are highly suggestive of poison ivy exposure. Similar reactions can also be caused by poison oak and poison sumac (see Chapter 34). (Photographs courtesy of Christopher Huerter, MD, Creighton University Medical Center, Omaha, Nebraska, © 2002.)

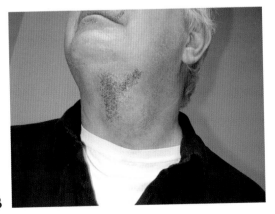

16B

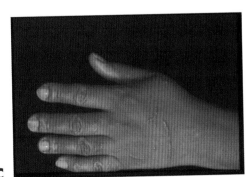

16C

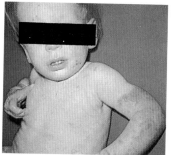

12A

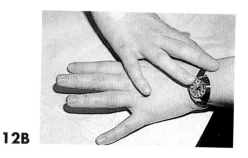

12B

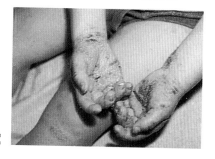

12C

12A, B, and C   Atopic dermatitis (eczema) is an inflammatory condition that occurs **(A)** on the extensor surface of the elbows and knees during the first year of life and then **(B)** involves predominantly the flexors. **C,** The hands, feet, and face are often involved as well. The dermatitis is characterized by erythema, scale, increased skin surface markings, and crusting; secondary infection is common (see Chapter 32).

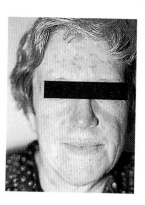

13

13   Seborrheic dermatitis is a red scaling condition of the scalp, midface, and upper midchest of adults. This dermatitis is marked by characteristic greasy, yellowish scaling and is associated with erythema (see Chapter 33).

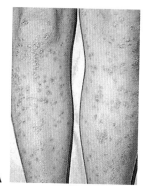

14A

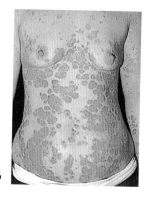

14B

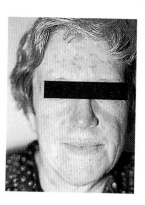

14C

14A, B, and C   Psoriasis is a scaling condition in which erythematous plaques (red raised areas) are covered by a thick adherent scale. The borders of the lesions are well developed and vary from guttate (very small drop-shaped plaques) to much larger plaques: **(A)** guttate, **(B)** medium-size plaques, **(C)** large plaques (see Chapter 33).

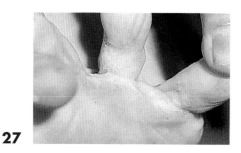

27

27 Tinea pedis infection of the toes characteristically starts between the fourth and fifth web space and spreads proximally. Scaling can progress to maceration with resultant small fissures (see Chapter 41).

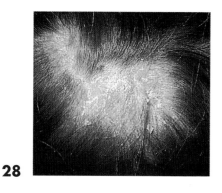

28

28 Tinea capitis, a fungal infection of the scalp, is marked by scale on the scalp with local breaking or loss of hair; erythema (redness) is usually not observed (see Chapter 41).

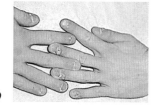

29

29 Common warts are viral-induced lesions that present as localized rough accumulations of keratin (hyperkeratosis) containing many tiny furrows. If the wart's surface is pared, small bleeding points can be seen (see Chapter 42).

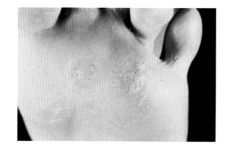

30

30 Plantar warts, caused by a viral infection, are often found on the plantar surface of the foot and present with hard, localized accumulations of keratin. The punctate bleeding points seen when the lesions are pared distinguish plantar warts from calluses (see Chapter 42). (Photograph reprinted with permission from emedicine.com, Inc., © 2003.)

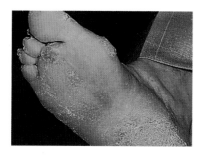

31

31 Calluses are thickened scales that often form on joints and weight-bearing areas. A callus on the plantar surface of the foot is shown here (see Chapter 43).

case
35-1 *continued*

Relevant Evaluation Criteria	Scenario/Model Outcome
4. Formulate a comprehensive list of therapeutic alternatives for the primary problem to determine if triage to a medical provider is required, and share this information with the patient or caregiver.	Options include: (1) Refer Neva immediately to her pediatrician or other PCP. (2) Recommend self-care until an appropriate PCP can be consulted. (3) Recommend self-care with nonprescription pharmacologic product. (4) Recommend self-care with nonpharmacologic methods. (5) Recommend both nonpharmacologic treatment and nonprescription pharmacologic treatment. (6) Take no action.

Plan

5. Select an optimal therapeutic alternative to address the patient's problem, taking into account patient preferences.	Recommend that Mr. Charles use both nonprescription and nonpharmacologic modalities to treat Neva's diaper rash. Specifically recommend increased diaper changes, air drying in between diaper changes, and liberal application of Desitin Maximum Strength Original Paste with every diaper change as needed. Desitin can also be used to prevent diaper rash and can therefore be applied after Neva's current diaper rash heals.
6. Describe the recommended therapeutic approach to the patient or caregiver.	"A zinc oxide–based skin protectant such as Desitin should protect the skin and thereby allow it to heal. Nonpharmacologic therapy is just as important because it will promote healing and meet goals of treatment."
7. Explain to the patient or caregiver the rationale for selecting the recommended therapeutic approach from the considered therapeutic alternatives.	"Neva meets none of the exclusion criteria that would indicate medical referral is preferred. Mild-to-moderate diaper dermatitis can be effectively managed with nonpharmacologic and nonprescription pharmacologic therapy."

Patient Education

8. When recommending self-care with nonprescription medications and/or nondrug therapy, convey accurate information to the patient or caregiver.	See Nondrug Measures in the box Patient Education for Diaper Dermatitis.
a. appropriate dose and frequency of administration	"Apply Desitin paste liberally with every diaper change and as needed."
b. maximum number of days the therapy should be employed	"Desitin can be applied to treat and prevent diaper rash. There is no maximum length of therapy with this medication."
c. product administration procedures	"Wash hands and clean diaper region with a soft cloth or baby wipe. Allow the area to dry thoroughly. Thereafter, apply Desitin to the diaper region liberally. A glove may be worn if preferable. Overapplication presents no danger to Neva. Change diapers every 3–4 hours as a minimum."
d. expected time to onset of relief	"Neva's diaper rash will likely be noticeably improved by tomorrow."
e. degree of relief that can be reasonably expected	"You can expect the rash to be less tender tomorrow. Application of the skin protectant will likely soothe the pain associated with the rash."
f. most common side effects	"No side effects are associated with this product."
g. side effects that warrant medical intervention should they occur	NA
h. patient options in the event the condition worsens or persists	See the box Patient Education for Diaper Dermatitis and Figure 35–1.
i. product storage requirements	"Store away from children."
j. specific nondrug measures	See the box Patient Education for Diaper Dermatitis.
Solicit follow-up questions from the patient or caregiver.	"Should I use the creamy Desitin or the original Desitin paste?"
Answer the patient's or caregiver's questions.	"Whereas both products will help Neva's condition, I suggest the original paste because it is thicker, creates a better barrier, and may allow Neva's diaper area to heal more quickly."

Evaluation of Patient Outcome

9. Assess patient outcome.	Call Mr. Charles in 2 days to evaluate Neva's response to the suggested treatment regimen.

Key: N/A = Not applicable; NKA = no known allergies; PCP = primary care provider.

pharmacologic suggestions can be made by the provider. From a nonpharmacologic perspective, the caregiver should be asked what type of diaper is being used and how frequently diapers are changed. Drawing on that response, the provider must consider whether increasing the frequency of diaper changes and other nonpharmacologic measures are likely sufficient to heal the diaper dermatitis or whether pharmacologic treatment is warranted. Given minimal risk associated with pharmacologic treatment options, said options are often appropriate to suggest to the caregiver.

Patient Counseling for Diaper Dermatitis

The health care provider should review with the caregiver proper cleaning of the diaper area. Additionally, the provider should advise the caregiver to avoid occlusion of the area, when feasible, and to avoid prolonged contact of urine or feces with the infant's skin. The provider should explain the proper methods of applying nonprescription skin protectants and should describe to the caregiver signs and symptoms that indicate the dermatitis has worsened and warrants medical attention. The box Patient Education for Diaper Dermatitis lists specific information to provide caregivers.

Evaluation of Patient Outcomes for Diaper Dermatitis

Treatment of diaper dermatitis should be relatively short. If 7 days of treatment have elapsed and the condition is not healed, medical referral should occur. At the conclusion of therapy, the

skin should return to its pre–diaper dermatitis condition. If diaper dermatitis presents routinely or presents in a severe manner, prophylactic use of skin protectants is suggested, given the safety of preparations presented in Table 35–1.

Prickly Heat

Prickly heat, sometimes referred to as heat rash or miliaria, can occur at any age in anyone who has active sweat glands. The condition affects up to 40% of infants.[25] It is likely significantly underreported, given that it is less troublesome than diaper dermatitis and clears up very rapidly if left alone or if its cause is removed. Prickly heat often presents in hot working conditions and with activities in which sweating occurs (e.g., manual labor, exercise, or athletics).[26,27]

Pathophysiology of Prickly Heat

Prickly heat results from blocked or clogged sweat glands.[28] (See Chapter 37 for a review of the anatomy of the sweat gland.) The inability of sweat to escape the pores causes dilation and rupture of epidermal sweat pores, causing an acute inflammation of the dermis that may manifest as stinging, burning, or itching.

Prickly heat can arise from normal skin with little or no anatomic prodrome. The condition is most often associated with very hot, humid weather or can occur during illnesses that cause significant or profuse sweating. It also results from the inability of the skin to "breathe" because of excessive clothing,

---

patient education for
Diaper Dermatitis

The goals of diaper rash treatment are to (1) relieve the symptoms, (2) rid the patient of the rash, (3) discourage infection, and (4) prevent recurrences.

For most patients, carefully following product instructions and the self-care measures listed here will help ensure optimal therapeutic outcomes.

Nondrug Measures
- Change diapers frequently, at least six times a day, to prevent exposure of the infant's skin to moisture and feces.
- Do not use rubber or plastic pants over cloth diapers. Tightly covering the skin encourages skin breakdown.
- During every diaper change, use plain water to clean the diaper area. Gently dry area or allow it to air dry.
- Do not wipe the infant with any part of the diaper. Even areas that appear clean may be contaminated with fecal bacteria.
- Avoid starched or very stiff diapers.
- Avoid commercial baby wipes that contain alcohol, perfumes, and soap, which may burn or sting the skin.
- If feasible, allow the infant to go without a diaper, even for short instances, in an effort to dry the rash.

Nonprescription Medications
- To treat diaper rash, use a product containing one or more of the skin protectants listed in Table 35–1. The product can be used even after the rash clears to prevent recurrences.
- Do not use products that contain ingredients listed in Table 35–1 if they are combined with benzocaine or an antibacterial such as

benzethonium chloride. Benzocaine can cause an allergic reaction; antibacterials are not suitable for use on diaper rash.
- Do not use hydrocortisone.
- Do not use topical (external) analgesics such as phenol, menthol, methyl salicylate, or capsaicin to treat diaper rash. These medications are inappropriate for use on infant skin and may cause harm.
- Powders for children or infants should be gently poured into the hands and then rubbed onto the skin, using a sufficient amount to cover the affected area. Do not vigorously shake powders near infants. Avoid infant inhalation of powders.
- Apply cream or ointment liberally, by hand or with a disposable or washable spatula, to cover the affected area.
- If using mineral oil, wash it off at every diaper change to avoid clogging skin pores.
- Throw away products that are discolored or whose expiration dates have passed. (The health care provider should point out expiration dates on the products.)

When to Seek Medical Attention
- Consult a primary care provider if any of the exclusions in Figure 35–1 apply.

very tight clothing, or clothing that is occlusive, such as leather, polyester, or athletic protective or safety garments and devices.

Clinical Presentation of Prickly Heat

The pinpoint-size lesions that are the hallmark of prickly heat are raised and red or maroon, forming erythematous papules (see Color Plates, photograph 18). The lesions may appear in small numbers clustered together or spread over the occluded area on a pink to red field (miliaria rubra). Common sites for prickly heat dermatitis include the axillae, chest, upper back, back of the neck, abdomen, and inguinal area. The lesions often trace the pattern of the occlusion and, in uncomplicated cases, do not extend beyond the occluded area. If lesions are not resolved in a reasonable length of time (approximately 3–10 days), they can evolve into the same kinds of complications seen in diaper dermatitis (e.g., infection, pustule formation, or generalized dermatitis). Complications are extremely rare.

Treatment of Prickly Heat
Treatment Goals

The primary goal in the treatment of prickly heat is removal of the causative agent or agents. Lesions associated with prickly heat usually resolve without pharmacologic treatment if the cause is removed. A secondary goal in the treatment of prickly heat is alleviation of symptoms associated with the condition.

General Treatment Approach

The nonpharmacologic treatment goals for prickly heat include (1) eliminating occlusion of skin, (2) protecting skin from further irritation, (3) promoting healing of skin, and (4) discouraging onset of secondary infection.

Pharmacologic therapy and nonpharmacologic therapy have the same goals. Pharmacologic products help (1) keep skin dry, (2) promote healing, (3) soothe any discomfort caused by lesion(s), and (4) discourage onset of secondary infection. The algorithm in Figure 35–2 outlines the self-treatment of prickly heat.

Nonpharmacologic Therapy

Nondrug therapy for prickly heat consists of taking measures to decrease sweating and increase air flow to the affected area. If the sweating is caused by a fever, the use of internal antipyretics, if not contraindicated, is appropriate. Wearing loose, light-colored, and lightweight clothing is palliative in prickly heat and is also good prevention in that it allows airflow to the skin. Health care providers should warn patients not to apply oleaginous substances to prickly heat lesions because these substances plug pores that need to be patent.

Pharmacologic Therapy

Nonprescription treatment of prickly heat should be limited to mild-moderate, uncomplicated cases. Affected areas should not be occluded during therapy. Overall, this disorder can be ameliorated in less time and with less total drug exposure than diaper dermatitis.

Emollients, Skin Protectants, and Antipruritics

The choice of a drug product should be limited to one product that relieves burning and itching but does not block skin exposure to the air. Water-washable antipruritic products as well as bland emollients and protectants that soothe the skin and maintain skin moisture and texture can be used to treat the symptoms of prickly heat while the condition resolves. Colloidal oatmeal bath products and lotions have been employed for their antipruritic and soothing properties. Powders should be used only prophylactically to absorb moisture and keep skin dry, rather than as treatment of active prickly heat. (See Table 35–4 for selected trade-name products and Chapter 32 for a discussion of skin emollients.)

Other Pharmacologic Agents

As with diaper dermatitis, hydrocortisone is contraindicated in infants. In adults, hydrocortisone may be useful if the body surface area involved is 10% or less. (See Figure 40–4 for information on calculating body surface area.) Because prickly heat rapidly clears without drug therapy, the only actual use for hydrocortisone when treating prickly heat is to relieve itching. Topical antihistamines and local anesthetics (see Chapter 36) carry the risk of sensitization, but they can be employed as antipruritic agents.

Product Selection Guidelines

When treating prickly heat, the skin needs to dry and dissipate moisture. Therefore, only water-washable, cream-based products should be applied to prickly heat to relieve symptoms. For moisture absorption and prevention of wetness, powders are a reasonable choice. However, prolonged use or overuse of powders can lead to clogged pores and can actually precipitate prickly heat. When applied to the chest or neck, cornstarch or talc powder should be placed in the hand and applied manually to the skin with light friction. Any product that has an ingredient (e.g., phenols or boric acid) that could be toxic if absorbed through thin, compromised skin should not be recommended for use on infants. Bathing children and infants with prickly heat in colloidal oatmeal or lukewarm water may be recommended as a first option.

Assessment of Prickly Heat: A Case-Based Approach

Patient assessment for prickly heat involves identifying the site(s) of the lesions and potential causes of the exacerbation. If the patient is an infant, the health care provider should gather information regarding potential environmental characteristics (e.g., sleeping conditions or presence/absence of air conditioning) that could be exacerbating the condition.

Case 35–2 provides an example assessment of a patient with prickly heat.

Patient Counseling for Prickly Heat

The health care provider should stress to the patient that prickly heat is usually easily treated by removing factors that clog skin pores, while also explaining appropriate nonpharmacologic and

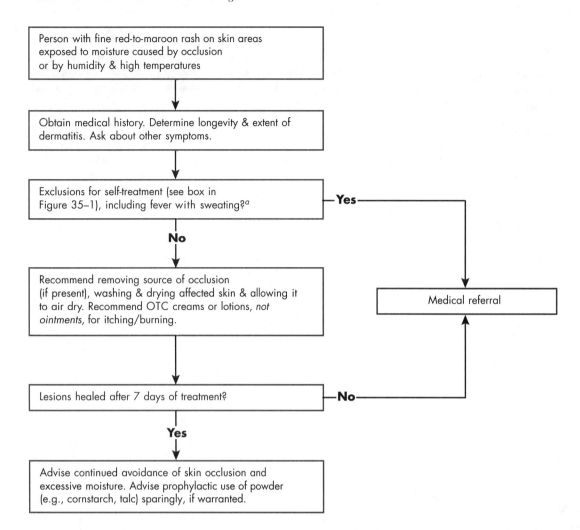

Person with fine red-to-maroon rash on skin areas exposed to moisture caused by occlusion or by humidity & high temperatures

↓

Obtain medical history. Determine longevity & extent of dermatitis. Ask about other symptoms.

↓

Exclusions for self-treatment (see box in Figure 35-1), including fever with sweating?*a* —— **Yes** ——→ Medical referral

↓ **No**

Recommend removing source of occlusion (if present), washing & drying affected skin & allowing it to air dry. Recommend OTC creams or lotions, *not ointments,* for itching/burning.

↓

Lesions healed after 7 days of treatment? —— **No** ——→ Medical referral

↓ **Yes**

Advise continued avoidance of skin occlusion and excessive moisture. Advise prophylactic use of powder (e.g., cornstarch, talc) sparingly, if warranted.

a High fever without sweating, high pulse rate, possible increased respiration, or hot, flushed dry skin (patient seems to be "burning up") may indicate hyperpyrexia ("heatstroke" or "sunstroke"). Refer the patient immediately to a PCP and/or transport patient to an emergency facility. Slow or weak pulse; lethargy; cold, pale, clammy skin; absence of fever; or disorientation may indicate heat exhaustion. Move patient to a cool environment, and have the patient recline and take regular sips of water or slightly salty liquids or electrolyte solutions every few minutes.

figure

35-2 Self-Care of prickly heat. Key: OTC = Over-the-counter; PCP = primary care provider.

table

35-4 **Selected Nonprescription Products for Prickly Heat**

Trade Name	Primary Ingredients
Aveeno Daily Moisturizing Lotion	Colloidal oatmeal
Extra Strength Benadryl Itch Stopping Cream	Diphenhydramine HCl 2%; zinc acetate 0.1%
Cortizone-10 Maximum Strength Anti-Itch Cream	Hydrocortisone 1%
Eucerin Skin Calming Itch Relief Treatment	Menthol
Lubriderm Daily Moisture Lotion	Water; glycerin; mineral oil

pharmacologic measures for healing or alleviating symptoms of prickly heat. The provider should explain that excessive use of skin protectants can exacerbate the disorder. The box Patient Education for Prickly Heat lists specific information to provide patients.

Evaluation of Patient Outcomes for Prickly Heat

Treatment of prickly heat should be relatively short. Considerable improvement is commonly noted in as little as 24 hours after nonpharmacologic and pharmacologic treatment initiation. If the condition is not completely resolved or has worsened after 7 days of treatment, the patient should be referred

Relevant Evaluation Criteria	Scenario/Model Outcome
Information Gathering	
1. Gather essential information about the patient's symptoms and medical history, including:	
a. description of symptom(s) (i.e., nature, onset, duration, severity, associated symptoms)	Patient states he has "some sort of itchy rash" on several parts of his body, including his back and thighs. He has had the rash for about 3 days. He states that the rash is not painful.
b. description of any factors that seem to precipitate, exacerbate, and/or relieve the patient's symptom(s)	Patient has had previous rashes that look identical to this rash. He tends to get the rash more often in the summer when he's working construction, but he sometimes has it in the winter months as well.
c. description of the patent's efforts to relieve the symptoms	Patient tries to prevent rash through good personal hygiene techniques (e.g., taking showers more frequently) and applying a thick cream to problem areas to keep them moist; however, these measures do not always keep him from getting the rash.
d. patient's identity	C. A. Robison
e. age, sex, height, and weight	38 years old, male, 5 ft 11 in., 180 lb
f. patient's occupation	Construction worker
g. patient's dietary habits	Normal diet; minimal vegetables; 8 cups of coffee per day
h. patient's sleep habits	Averages 7 hours of sleep nightly.
i. concurrent medical conditions, prescription and non-prescription medications, and dietary supplements	None noted.
j. allergies	Allergy to tramadol (hives)
k. history of other adverse reactions to medications	NA
l. other (describe) _____	C. A. is a very fit individual who, in addition to his job, coaches a local high school cross-country team. He often joins his students on runs.
Assessment and Triage	
2. Differentiate patient's signs/symptoms and correctly identify the patient's primary problem(s).	Prickly heat secondary to sweating and possibly occlusive clothing
3. Identify exclusions for self-treatment (see Figure 35–1).	None
4. Formulate a comprehensive list of therapeutic alternatives for the primary problem to determine if triage to a medical provider is required, and share this information with the patient or caregiver.	Options include: (1) Refer C. A. to a dermatologist or his PCP. (2) Recommend self-care until an appropriate PCP can be consulted. (3) Recommend self-care with nonprescription product(s). (4) Recommend self-care with nonpharmacologic methods. (5) Recommend both nonprescription self-care products and non-pharmacologic treatment. (6) Take no action.
Plan	
5. Select an optimal therapeutic alternative to address the patient's problem, taking into account patient preferences.	Application of nonprescription hydrocortisone product would likely minimize itching associated with C. A.'s prickly heat while his condition heals. Because of the relatively large surface area (thighs and back) where the prickly heat presents, a thin layer of hydrocortisone should be applied 3–4 times per day (see Chapter 34). A powder to keep the affected areas dry could also be used judiciously. Patient education about the cause of prickly heat is important in prevention of future occurrences.
6. Describe the recommended therapeutic approach to the patient or caregiver.	"I suggest discontinuation of the 'thick cream' because such a product can exacerbate prickly heat. A topical antihistamine will help with the itching associated with your prickly heat. It will not heal the prickly heat, but you should notice that the prickly heat heals itself in as little as 24 hours. It's important to take appropriate steps to minimize occlusion in the affected areas and to keep those areas clean and dry."

case
35-2 *continued*

Relevant Evaluation Criteria	Scenario/Model Outcome
7. Explain to the patient or caregiver the rationale for selecting the recommended therapeutic approach from the considered therapeutic alternatives.	See outcome discussion in #6.

Patient Education

8. When recommending self-care with nonprescription medications and/or nondrug therapy, convey accurate information to the patient or caregiver:

a. appropriate dose and frequency of administration	"Extra Strength Benadryl Itch Stopping Cream: Apply to affected area(s) not more than 4 times daily as needed. Johnson's Baby Powder: Apply 1 time daily after showering. Do not inhale powder."
b. maximum number of days the therapy should be employed	"Both can be applied as needed; however, topical antihistamines should not be applied for more than 7 consecutive days."
c. product administration procedures	See the box Patient Education for Prickly Heat.
d. expected time to onset of relief	"Twenty-four hours or less if nonpharmacologic measures are employed as directed."
e. degree of relief that can be reasonably expected	"Itching should be minimized. Skin should return to pre–prickly heat condition."
f. most common side effects	"The cream has no common side effects. The powder can clog pores if used in excess."
g. side effects that warrant medical intervention should they occur	NA
h. patient options in the event that condition worsens or persists	"If condition persists after 7 days of treatment, see your primary care provider to rule out other conditions."
i. product storage requirements	"Keep product out of reach of children."
j. specific nondrug measures	See Nondrug Measures in the box Patient Education for Prickly Heat.
Solicit follow-up questions from the patient or caregiver.	"I sometimes shower multiple times per day. Should I apply the powder after every shower?"
Answer the patient's or caregiver's questions.	"Applying too much powder can actually make you more likely to get prickly heat because the powder can clog the pores through which your sweat is excreted. I suggest applying the powder after the shower that will get you through the part of your day when you are most likely to sweat."

Evaluation of Patient Outcome

9. Assess patient outcome.	Call Mr. Robison in 2 days to evaluate his response to the suggested treatment regimen.

Key: NA = Not applicable; PCP = primary care provider.

for further evaluation. Monitoring of treatment success involves simple observation of lesions. At the end of therapy, skin should return to its precondition state.

Key Points for Diaper Dermatitis and Prickly Heat

Diaper Dermatitis

➤ Diaper dermatitis is exacerbated by moisture and occlusion.
➤ Increasing the frequency of diaper changes (i.e., decreasing contact time between skin and excrement) plays a major role in the nonpharmacologic treatment of diaper dermatitis.

➤ Pharmacologic treatment should be limited to products containing FDA-approved ingredients indicated for the treatment of diaper dermatitis (Table 35–1); exotic additives and complementary therapies should be avoided.
➤ Apply hydrophobic skin protectants liberally to diaper dermatitis areas; overapplication should not be a concern.
➤ Do not use hydrocortisone in the self-treatment of diaper dermatitis.
➤ The majority of diaper rash cases will resolve when occlusion and wetness are adequately suppressed.
➤ Cases of diaper dermatitis that are still present after 7 days of treatment should be referred for further evaluation.

patient education for
Prickly Heat

The objectives of self-treatment are to (1) relieve the discomfort of prickly heat and (2) eliminate its cause. For most patients, following product instructions and the self-care measures listed here will help ensure optimal therapeutic outcomes.

Nondrug Measures

- To prevent clogging skin pores, avoid excessive sweating by resting, cooling off, or going to a cool environment.
- Wear loose, light-colored, porous, and lightweight clothing to allow airflow to the skin.
- Shower, bathe, or change clothes immediately after heavy sweating, and wear loose-fitting clothes when such activity is anticipated. Remember to drink plenty of fluids and allow the body to cool down after any strenuous activity.

Nonprescription Medications

- Unless a primary care provider advises otherwise, use systemic analgesics (e.g., aspirin, acetaminophen, or ibuprofen) to reduce a fever and the sweating it can cause. (See Chapter 5 for dosing information.)
- Do not apply oily substances to prickly heat lesions because they clog skin pores.
- Use powdered skin protectants to absorb moisture and help prevent wetness (Table 35–3). Place cornstarch or talc powder in the hand, and apply to the skin with light friction. Note that prolonged

use or overuse of powders can lead to clogged pores and can precipitate prickly heat.

- Do not use hydrocortisone on infants. However, it may be used to relieve itching in adult cases of prickly heat if no more than 10% of the body surface area is involved.
- Water-washable emollients applied in a thin film twice a day can help the skin return to normal (see Chapter 32).
- If redness, burning, itching, peeling, or swelling develops after a product is applied, rinse any remaining product off the skin and avoid further use.
- For older children and adults, consider using oral antihistamines for relief of itching.
- To soothe discomfort in adults or infants, wash the affected skin with bland soap or soak the skin in a colloidal oatmeal solution.
- The condition should show observable improvement in 24 hours.

When to Seek Medical Attention

- If the condition persists after 7 days of treatment, consult a primary care provider.

Prickly Heat

➤ Prickly heat is exacerbated by moisture and occlusion.

➤ The majority of prickly heat cases will resolve when occlusion and wetness are adequately suppressed.

➤ Cases of prickly heat that persist after 7 days of treatment should be referred for further evaluation.

➤ Pharmacologic treatment of prickly heat should be targeted at providing relief from itching or burning.

➤ Products containing emollients or anti-itch ingredients in water-washable dosage forms are favored in the treatment of prickly heat. Powders may be used to help dry the skin, but they must be used judiciously to prevent clogged pores.

REFERENCES

1. Foureur N, Vanzo B, Meaume S, et al. Prospective aetiological study of diaper dermatitis in the elderly. *Br J Dermatol.* 2006;155(5):941–6.
2. Ravanfar P, Wallace JS, Pace NC. Diaper dermatitis: a review and update. *Curr Opin Pediatr.* 2012;24(4):472–9.
3. Ward DB, Fleischer Jr AB, Feldman SR, et al. Characterization of diaper dermatitis in the United States. *Arch Pediatr Adolesc Med.* 2000; 154(9):943–6.
4. Nield LS, Kamat D. Prevention, diagnosis, and management of diaper dermatitis. *Clin Pediatr (Phila).* 2007;46(6):480–6.
5. Erasala GN, Romain C, Merlay I. Diaper area and disposable diapers. *Curr Probl Dermatol.* 2011;40:83–9.
6. Akin F, Spraker M, Aly R, et al. Effects of breathable disposable diapers: reduced prevalence of Candida and common diaper dermatitis. *Pediatr Dermatol.* 2001;18(4):282–90.
7. Odio M, Friedlander SF. Diaper dermatitis and advances in diaper technology. *Curr Opin Pediatr.* 2000;12(4):342–6.
8. Shin HT. Diaper dermatitis that does not quit. *Dermatol Therapy.* 2005;18(2):124–35.
9. Adam R. Skin care of the diaper area. *Pediatr Dermatol.* 2008;25(4):427–33.
10. Scheinfeld N. Diaper dermatitis: a review and brief survey of eruptions of the diaper area. *Am J Clin Dermatol.* 2005;6(5):273–81.
11. Borkowski S. Diaper rash care and management. *Pediatr Nurs.* 2004; 30(6):467–70.
12. Atherton DJ. A review of the pathophysiology, prevention and treatment of irritant diaper dermatitis. *Curr Med Res Opin.* 2004;20(5):645–9.
13. Adalat S, Wall D, Goodyear H. Diaper dermatitis—frequency and contributory factors in hospital attending children. *Pediatr Dermatol.* 2007; 24(5):483–8.
14. Berg RW. Etiologic factors in diaper dermatitis: a model for development of improved diapers. *Pediatrician.* 1986;14(suppl 1):27–33.
15. Stamatas GN, Zerweck C, Grove G, et al. Documentation of impaired epidermal barrier in mild and moderate diaper dermatitis in vovi using noninvasive methods. *Pediatr Dermatol.* 2011;28(2):99–107.
16. Wolf R, Wolf D, Tuzun B, et al. Diaper dermatitis. *Clin Dermatol.* 2000; 18(6):657–60.
17. Beguin AM, Malaquin-Pavan E, Guihaire C, et al. Improving diaper design to address incontinence associated dermatitis. *BMC Geriatr.* 2010; 10(86):1–10.
18. Benjamin L. Clinical correlates with diaper dermatitis. *Pediatrician.* 1987; 14(suppl 1):21–6.
19. Smith WJ, Jacob SE. The role of allergic contact dermatitis in diaper dermatitis. *Pediatr Dermatol.* 2009;26(3):369–70.
20. Gupta AK, Skinner AR. Management of diaper dermatitis. *Int J Dermatol.* 2004;43(11):830–4.
21. Odio M, Streicher-Scott J, Hansen RC. Disposable baby wipes: efficacy and skin mildness. *Dermatol Nurs.* 2001;13(2):107–13.
22. Liu N, Wang X, Odio M. Frequency and severity of diaper dermatitis with use of traditional Chinese cloth diapers: observations in 3- to 9-month-old children. *Pediatr Dermatol.* 2011;28(4):380–6.
23. Lavender T, Furber C, Campbell M, et al. Effect on skin hydration of using baby wipes to clean the napkin area of newborn babies: assessor-blinded randomised controlled equivalence trial. *BMC Pediatr.* 2012; 12(59):1–9.
24. U.S. Skin protectant drug products for over-the-counter human use: final monograph. *Federal Register.* June 4, 2003;68(107):33362–81.
25. Feng E, Janniger CK. Miliaria. *Cutis.* 1995;55(4):213–6.
26. Howe AS, Boden BP. Heat-related illness in athletes. *Am J Sports Med.* 2007;35(8):1384–95.
27. Schwerha JJ. Heat-related illnesses: opportunities for prevention. *J Occup Environ Med.* 2010;52(8):844–5.
28. Zaidi Z, Lanigan SW. Diseases of the sebaceous, sweat, and apocrine glands. In: *Dermatology in Clinical Practice.* 1st ed. London: Springer; 2010: 337–57.

INSECT BITES AND STINGS AND PEDICULOSIS

Wayne Buff and Patricia H. Fabel

Insect bites and stings are common, and anyone who spends time outdoors is at risk. These injuries usually cause only a local reaction, but they can produce a mild allergic reaction or life-threatening anaphylaxis in patients who are sensitive. About 0.5% of the population may show signs of systemic allergic reactions to insect stings, and simultaneous multiple insect stings of 500 or more may cause death from toxicity. In the United States, more people die of insect stings than of bites from all poisonous animals combined. The exact number of people who experience systemic allergic reactions to insect bites is unknown.

Despite the potentially fatal consequences, encounters with biting and stinging insects are typically brief. Pediculosis (lice infestation) and scabies, by contrast, are parasitic infections, and the arachnids remain on the host until eradicated. Approximately 10–12 million people in the United States are affected by pediculosis each year, most of them children ages 3–12 years.

This chapter covers the stings of insects only but discusses the bites of both insects and arachnids (e.g., ticks, mites, spiders, and lice). The term *insect* is used to cover general statements about these invertebrates.

Insect Bites

Pathophysiology and Clinical Presentation of Insect Bites

Bites from insects (e.g., mosquitoes, fleas, and bedbugs) and from arachnids (e.g., ticks and chiggers) are nonvenomous. Each insect has distinctive biting organs and salivary secretions that contribute to the characteristic signs and symptoms for each type of bite.

Mosquitoes

Mosquitoes are found in abundance worldwide, particularly in humid, warm climates. After landing on the skin, mosquitoes inject an anticoagulant saliva into the victim, which causes the characteristic welt and itching.

Malaria and West Nile virus are serious systemic infections that are transmitted by mosquitoes. In 2012, West Nile virus human infection was reported in 48 states in the United States.[1]

Although most infected patients do not experience symptoms,[2] about 20% of infected patients experience flu-like symptoms with fever and fatigue. Symptoms can progress to muscle weakness, encephalitis, or meningitis. Controlling mosquito populations is particularly important in preventing the spread of this disease.[3]

Fleas

Fleas are tiny bloodsucking insects that can be found worldwide but breed best in a humid climate. Humans are often bitten after moving into a vacant flea-infested habitat or when living with infested pets. Fleabites are usually multiple and grouped and, in humans, occur primarily on legs and ankles. Each lesion is characterized by an erythematous region around the puncture and intense itching. In addition to being annoying, fleas can transmit diseases such as bubonic plague and endemic typhus.

Sarcoptes scabiei

Scabies, commonly called "the itch," is a contagious parasitic skin infection caused by *Sarcoptes scabiei,* a very small and rarely seen arachnid mite. The mites burrow up to 1 cm into the stratum corneum, and the females deposit eggs in their "tunnels." Common infestation sites are interdigital spaces of fingers, flexor surfaces of the wrists, external male genitalia, buttocks, and anterior axillary folds (see Color Plates, photograph 19). Scabies infection is characterized by inflammation and intense itching. Mites are transmitted from an infected individual to others through physical contact. A scabies infection requires prescription therapy rather than nonprescription treatment.

Bedbugs

Bedbugs usually hide and deposit their eggs in crevices of walls, floors, picture frames, bedding, folds of linens, corners of suitcases, and furniture during the day; they bite their victims at night. The increased mobility of society worldwide has heightened concern for an increased incidence of bedbug infestations in the United States in places frequented by travelers, such as hotels.[4] Bedbug bites typically appear along exposed areas of skin, such as the head, neck, and arms. Bites occur in clusters of twos and threes and usually in a straight line. The reaction to a bedbug bite can range from irritation at the site to a small dermal hemorrhage, depending on the sensitivity of the individual.[5]

Ticks

Ticks feed on the blood of humans and animals. During feeding, the tick's mouthparts are introduced into the skin, enabling it to hold firmly (see Color Plates, photograph 20). If the tick is removed but the mouthparts are left behind, intense itching and nodules requiring surgical excision may develop. If left attached, the tick becomes fully engorged with blood and remains for up to 10 days before dropping off. Ticks should be removed intact with fine tweezers within 36 hours. Tick removal by heating methods, such as a match or hot nail, or by painting substances onto the tick, such as nail polish or petrolatum, is not recommended because these methods can irritate the tick, causing it to secrete more saliva or even regurgitate gut contents, thereby increasing the likelihood of transmission of a tick-borne illness.[6]

The local reaction to tick bites consists of itching papules that disappear within 1 week. Certain species of ticks, however, can transmit systemic diseases such as Rocky Mountain spotted fever and Lyme disease. Rocky Mountain spotted fever, transmitted by wood ticks or dog ticks, is characterized by severe headache, rash, high fever, and extreme exhaustion.[7] Lyme disease is caused by a spirochete found in deer ticks that is transmitted into the victim after the tick is attached for 36 hours.[7] In 2009, Lyme disease was reported in 46 states in the United States, including the District of Columbia, with the highest number of cases in the northeast and upper Midwest.[8] Most acute stages of Lyme disease are heralded by skin rash and flu-like symptoms. The rash appears first as a papule at the bite site and may become an enlarged circle with a clear center called a "bull's-eye." Tender urticarial lesions appear 3–32 days after the bite and disappear spontaneously within 3–4 weeks. If left untreated, complications such as neurologic symptoms, cardiac disturbances, musculoskeletal symptoms, and arthritis may occur. Early diagnosis and prompt treatment by a health care provider are essential to prevent development of these serious manifestations.

Chiggers

Chiggers, or red bugs, live in shrubbery, trees, and grass. After attaching to the skin, the larvae secrete a digestive fluid that causes cellular disintegration of the affected area, a red papule, and intense itching. This fluid also causes the skin to harden and form a tiny tube in which the chigger lies and continues to feed until engorged. It then drops off and changes into an adult.

Spiders

Although all species of spiders are poisonous, most are unable to penetrate the skin because their fangs are too short or too fragile. The black widow, brown recluse, and hobo spiders are three major exceptions. Deaths from spider bites are rare, but symptoms can be serious. Reaction to black widow bites includes delayed intense pain, stiffness and joint pain, abdominal disturbances, fever, chills, and dyspnea. Brown recluse bites can cause these symptoms as well as a spreading ulcerated wound at the bite site. Hobo spider bites typically present with a moderate-severe, slow-healing wound.[9] If a spider bite is suspected but cannot be confirmed, the wound area should be monitored for these symptoms.

Complications of Insect Bites

Secondary bacterial infection of insect bites can occur if skin of the affected area is abraded from scratching. Skin infections such as impetigo may be a complication of insect bites; these infections may appear as yellow crusting, purulent drainage, and/or significant redness and swelling of the skin around the bite.

Treatment of Insect Bites

Specific nonprescription external analgesics are labeled for use in treating minor insect bites.

Treatment Goals

The goals of self-treating insect bites are to relieve symptoms and prevent secondary bacterial infections.

General Treatment Approach

Application of an ice pack wrapped in a washcloth may provide sufficient relief of the pain and irritation of bites from mosquitoes, chiggers, bedbugs, or fleas; apply the ice pack to the affected area for up to 10 minutes with at least 10 minutes between applications. If this treatment does not work, applying an external analgesic to the site should relieve symptoms. Patients should be advised to avoid scratching the bite. Prevention of future insect bites is also important.

Self-treatment of insect bites with a nonprescription product is appropriate if the reaction is confined to the site and the patient is older than 2 years. No effective nonprescription product is available to treat scabies. Patients with bites from ticks and spiders require medical referral because of possible systemic effects. Figure 36–1 outlines treatment of insect bites and lists exclusions for self-treatment.

Nonpharmacologic Therapy

Nondrug measures include the two methods of preventing insect bites: avoiding insects and using repellents. Specific measures are discussed in the box Patient Education for Insect Bites.

Avoidance of Insects

Recommendations for avoiding insects are included in the box Patient Education for Insect Bites.

Use of Insect Repellents

Insect repellents are useful in preventing bites from insects such as mosquitoes, fleas, and ticks, but these products are not effective in repelling stinging insects. Selection of an insect repellent should be based on product ingredients, concentration, and the anticipated type and length of exposure. Most commercial products contain n,n-diethyl-m-toluamide, commonly called DEET; concentrations ranging from 7%–100% are available. Other ingredients that may be combined with DEET include ethylbutylacetylaminopropionate (IR3535) and dimethyl phthalate (Table 36–1).

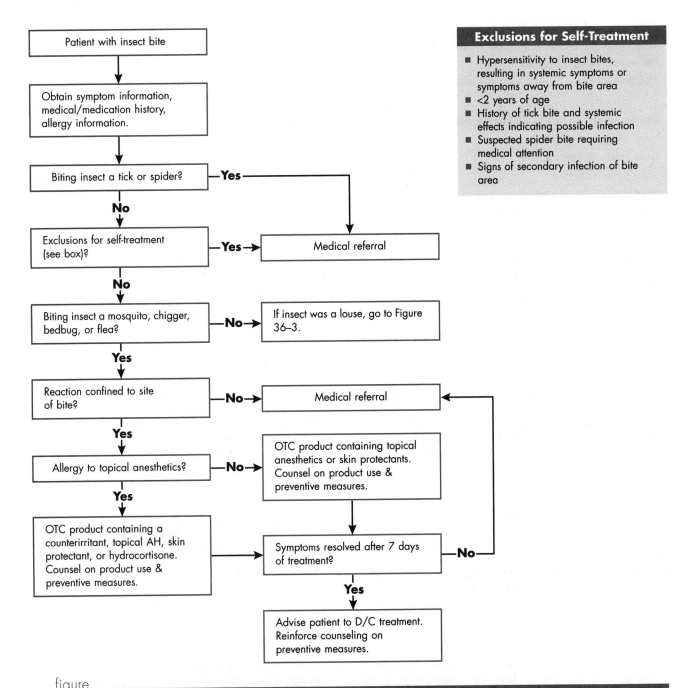

Exclusions for Self-Treatment

- Hypersensitivity to insect bites, resulting in systemic symptoms or symptoms away from bite area
- <2 years of age
- History of tick bite and systemic effects indicating possible infection
- Suspected spider bite requiring medical attention
- Signs of secondary infection of bite area

figure

36–1 Self-care of insect bites. Key: AH = Antihistamine; D/C = discontinue; OTC = over-the-counter.

table

table 36–1 Selected Nonprescription Insect Repellents

Trade Name	Primary Ingredients
Cutter Skinsations Pump	DEET 7%; aloe vera; vitamin E
Cutter Advanced Sport Insect Repellent	Picaridin 15%
Deep Woods Off! For Sportsmen Insect Repellent I Pump Spray	DEET 100%
Off! Insect Repellent II Aerosol	DEET 15%
Off! Skintastic Family Formula Pump or Aerosol	DEET 7%
Off! Light and Fresh Towelettes	DEET 5.6%; aloe vera
Skin-So-Soft Bug Guard Plus IR3535 Insect Repellent Spray	IR3535 7.5%
Repel Lemon Eucalyptus Lotion	Lemon eucalyptus oil
Repel Sportsman Formula Aerosol	DEET 29%
Repel Sun and Bug Lotion	DEET 20%; ethyl hexyl-p-methoxy-cinnamate 7.5%; oxybenzone 5%
Fite Bite Permethrin Clothing Spray	Permethrin 0.5%

Key: DEET = N,N-Diethyl-m-toluamide.

N,N-Diethyl-m-Toluamide

The best all-purpose repellent is n,n-diethyl-m-toluamide, or DEET.

Repellents protect the skin against insect bites. The exact mechanism of action is not fully known, but DEET, like other repellents, does not kill insects. The volatile repellent, when applied to skin or clothing, releases vapors that tend to discourage the approach of insects.

Repellents, available in sprays, solutions, creams, wipes, and other forms, are applied as needed to skin or clothing according to package directions, which usually is no more frequently than every 4–8 hours. Concentrations below 30% are preferable for children, but use of DEET insect repellents on children younger than 2 months should be discouraged.[10] Products with DEET concentrations ranging from 10%–40% provide adequate effect and sufficient protection for adults in routine situations. Products containing 50%–100% DEET generally are promoted for adults with high exposure to insects for long periods and when high heat and humidity may decrease adherence of the product; higher concentrations of DEET may be associated with higher incidence of skin reactions.[11] Table 36–2 provides a summary from the Environmental Protection Agency regarding the application and safe use of DEET products.[12,13]

Skin irritation is the most frequent DEET-related problem, with occlusion of the application area possibly contributing to skin rashes or eruptions.[13] Central nervous system reactions, including seizures, ataxia, hypotension, encephalopathy, and angioedema, have been reported in association with improper use or ingestion.[14–16] These products are considered safe if used appropriately, even in women who are pregnant or breast-feeding.[15,16] Table 36–2 lists warnings and precautions for use of DEET.

Other Insect Repellents

Alternative products include citronella, lemon eucalyptus oil, soybean oil, cedar oil, lavender oil, tea tree oil, garlic, thiamin, and scented moisturizers in mineral oil (e.g., Skin-So-Soft). These products generally have been found to be less effective than DEET as repellents against mosquitoes, particularly with regard to length of action. Picaridin, an alternative to DEET, is being promoted as having less odor and being less irritating to skin.[14] Insect repellents containing permethrin 0.5% are designed for use only on clothing and camping equipment.

Pharmacologic Therapy

External analgesics such as local anesthetics, topical antihistamines, hydrocortisone, and some counterirritants are

table 36–2 EPA Guidelines for Safe Use of DEET

- Read and follow all directions and precautions on the product label.
- Do not apply over cuts, wounds, or irritated skin.
- Do not apply to hands or near eyes and mouth of young children.
- Do not allow young children to apply this product.
- Use just enough repellent to cover exposed skin and/or clothing.
- Apply the sunscreen first, followed by the repellent, when sunscreen needs to be used in conjunction with a repellent.
- Do not use under clothing.
- Avoid overapplication of this product.
- After returning indoors, wash treated skin with soap and water.
- Wash treated clothing before wearing it again.
- Use of this product may cause skin reactions in rare cases.
- Do not spray in enclosed areas.
- To apply to face, spray on hands first, and then rub on face.
- Do not spray directly onto face.

Key: DEET = N,N-Diethyl-m-toluamide; EPA = Environmental Protection Agency.
Source: References 12 and 13.

approved for treating pain and itching associated with insect bites. These agents are not approved for use in children younger than 2 years.

Topical skin protectant agents may be used to reduce inflammation and promote healing. First-aid antiseptics and antibiotics can help prevent secondary infections (see Chapter 40).

Systemic antihistamines often are used in treating itching related to insect bites, but this use is not a label indication. Chapter 11 discusses systemic antihistamines in detail.

Local Anesthetics

Local anesthetics such as benzocaine, pramoxine, benzyl alcohol, lidocaine, dibucaine, and phenol are approved in topical preparations for relief of itching and irritation caused by insect bites.

Local anesthetics cause a reversible blockade of conduction of nerve impulses at the site of application, thereby producing loss of sensation. Phenol exerts topical anesthetic action by depressing cutaneous sensory receptors.

Topical preparations containing local anesthetics are applied in the form of creams, ointments, aerosols, or lotions. These products are generally applied to the bite area up to 3–4 times daily for no longer than 7 days.

Local anesthetics are relatively nontoxic when applied topically as directed, and systemic absorption does not typically occur with these topical products. However, allergic contact dermatitis may occur. Pramoxine and benzyl alcohol do not commonly cause adverse effects and exhibit less cross-sensitivity compared with other local anesthetics. Dibucaine, a common allergen, may cause systemic toxicity if excessive absorption occurs. Convulsions, myocardial depression, and death have been reported from systemic absorption.[17] Phenol solutions of greater than 2% are irritating and may cause sloughing and necrosis of skin, but the concentration of phenol in nonprescription products ranges from 0.5%–1.5%. Nonprescription products containing phenol should not be applied to extensive areas of the body, especially under compresses or bandages, because of the risk of skin damage and systemic absorption.[17] Products containing phenol should be avoided in pregnant patients and children.

Topical Antihistamines

Diphenhydramine hydrochloride in concentrations of 0.5%–2% is the agent used in most products that contain a topical antihistamine.

Topical antihistamines exert an anesthetic effect by depressing cutaneous receptors and are approved for temporary relief of pain and itching related to minor insect bites.[18] Products are available in several topical dosage forms; they are generally applied to the bite area up to 3–4 times daily for no longer than 7 days.

Although absorption occurs through skin, topical antihistamines generally are not absorbed in sufficient quantities to cause systemic side effects, even when applied to damaged skin. Systemic absorption is of more concern when these products are used over large body areas, especially in young children. Topical antihistamines can cause photosensitivity and hypersensitivity reactions; continued use of these agents for 3–4 weeks increases the possibility of contact dermatitis.

Counterirritants

Low concentrations of the counterirritants camphor and menthol are used in some topical analgesic products. Chapter 7 discusses these agents in more detail. These products generally are applied to the bite area 3–4 times daily for up to 7 days.

Camphor

At concentrations of 0.1%–3%, camphor depresses cutaneous receptors, thereby relieving itching and irritation by exerting an anesthetic effect. However, camphor-containing products can be very dangerous if ingested. Patients should be warned to keep these products out of children's reach.

Menthol

In concentrations of less than 1%, menthol depresses cutaneous receptors and exerts an analgesic effect. Menthol is considered a safe and effective antipruritic when applied to the affected area in concentrations of 0.1%–1%.

Hydrocortisone

Hydrocortisone 1% topical preparations are indicated for temporary relief of minor insect bites.

A wide variety of topical hydrocortisone dosage forms are available and should be applied as directed to the bite area 3 or 4 times daily for up to 7 days. Chapter 34 provides more information about topical hydrocortisone.

Skin Protectants

Medications such as zinc oxide, calamine, and titanium dioxide are applied to insect bites mainly in the form of lotions, ointments, and creams. These agents act as protectants and tend to reduce inflammation and irritation. Zinc oxide works as a mild astringent with weak antiseptic properties.[18] Zinc oxide and calamine also absorb fluids from weeping lesions.

The Food and Drug Administration (FDA) considers nonprescription drugs containing zinc oxide and calamine to be safe and effective in concentrations of 1%–25%. Although its mechanism of action is similar to that of zinc oxide, titanium dioxide's safety and effectiveness have not been determined by FDA. These preparations should be applied to the affected area as needed. They have minimal adverse effects and are recommended for adults, children, and infants.

Product Selection Guidelines

Sensitization, specifically contact dermatitis, can occur with local anesthetics. If these agents are preferred, pramoxine and benzyl alcohol have a low incidence of adverse effects. Dibucaine and phenol have the most potential for adverse effects, especially if systemic absorption occurs from improper application.

Adverse effects and systemic absorption generally are not a concern with short-term use of the topical antihistamine diphenhydramine hydrochloride. However, its prolonged use can cause allergic or photoallergic contact dermatitis. Similarly, short-term use of hydrocortisone usually does not cause adverse effects or clinically significant systemic absorption. Patients with scabies, bacterial infections, or fungal infections should

Trade Name	Primary Ingredients
Local Anesthetics	
Itch-X Gel/Pump Spray	Pramoxine HCl 1%; benzyl alcohol 10%
Lanacane Aerosol Spray	Benzocaine 20%
Nupercainal Ointment	Dibucaine 1%
Solarcaine Medicated First Aid Aerosol Spray	Benzocaine 20%; triclosan 0.13%
Unguentine Maximum Strength Cream	Benzocaine 5%; resorcinol 2%
Topical Antihistamines	
Di-Delamine Gel/Spray	Diphenhydramine HCl 1%; tripelennamine 0.5%; benzalkonium chloride 0.15%; menthol
Maximum Strength Benadryl Cream/Spray	Diphenhydramine HCl 2%
Counterirritants	
Blue Star Ointment	Camphor 1.2%
Sarna Lotion	Camphor 0.5%; menthol 0.5%
Corticosteroids	
Cortaid with Aloe Cream/Ointment	Hydrocortisone 0.5%; aloe vera
Cortaid Intensive Therapy Cooling Spray	Hydrocortisone 1%
Cortizone-5 Cream	Hydrocortisone 0.5%
Maximum Strength Cortaid Cream/Ointment	Hydrocortisone 1%
Combination Products	
Aveeno Anti-Itch Cream/Lotion	Pramoxine HCl 1%; calamine 3%; camphor 0.3%
Benadryl Itch Stopping Gel Extra Strength	Diphenhydramine HCl 2%; zinc acetate 1%; camphor
Caladryl Clear Lotion	Diphenhydramine HCl 1%; zinc oxide 2%; camphor
Campho-Phenique Gel	Camphor 11%; phenol 5%; eucalyptus oil
Chigarid	Camphor 2.8%; phenol 2%; eucalyptus oil 0.5% in collodion
Medi-Quik Spray	Lidocaine 2%; benzalkonium chloride 0.2%; camphor
Sting-Kill Swabs	Benzocaine 19%; menthol 0.9%

not use hydrocortisone without medical supervision because it can worsen or mask these disorders. Camphor-containing products can be very dangerous if ingested, making them an inappropriate choice for use in children. Patients must understand that topical antipruritics and anesthetics should not be used for longer than 7 days.

The patient's preference of dosage forms should also guide product recommendations. Table 36–3 lists selected trade-name products in various dosage forms.

Assessment of Insect Bites: A Case-Based Approach

The type of insect that inflicted the patient's injury should be determined first. Patients with suspected spider or tick bites require a medical referral because of the risk of complications. For other insect bites, the seriousness of the reaction should be

evaluated before a nonprescription product or nondrug measure is recommended. If a nonallergic reaction is present, the appropriate external analgesic for symptomatic relief should be recommended. Recommending a skin protectant to reduce irritation and inflammation or to prevent secondary bacterial infection is appropriate.

Patient Counseling for Insect Bites

Counseling for insect bites includes an explanation of how to treat the injury and how to prevent recurrences. Nondrug measures and proper use of recommended nonprescription products should be explained. The explanation should include potential adverse effects of these agents, plus signs and symptoms that indicate the injury needs medical attention. Appropriate use of insect repellents to prevent further bites should also be discussed. The box Patient Education for Insect Bites lists specific information to provide patients.

Insect Bites

The objectives of self-treatment for insect bites are to (1) relieve swelling, pain, and itching; (2) prevent scratching that may lead to secondary bacterial infection; (3) monitor for infections transmitted by ticks; and (4) prevent future insect bites. For most patients, carefully following product instructions and the self-care measures listed here will help ensure optimal therapeutic outcomes.

Nondrug Measures

- Apply ice pack promptly to bite area to reduce swelling, itching, and pain.
- Avoid scratching affected area; keep fingernails trimmed.
- Remove ticks with tweezers by grasping the tick's head and gently pulling; the head should be removed. Keep the removed tick in a sealed container for future identification in case of systemic symptoms. After removal of the tick, clean the area with rubbing alcohol to disinfect the skin.
- Do not wear rough, irritating clothing over bite area.

Preventive Measures

- To prevent exposure, cover skin as much as possible with clothing and socks and cuff clothing around ankles, wrists, and neck.
- Avoid swamps, dense woods, and dense brush that harbor mosquitoes, ticks, and chiggers.
- Keep pets free of pests.
- Remove standing water from around the home to reduce breeding areas for mosquitoes.
- Limit the amount of time spent outside at dawn and dusk.
- Use barriers such as window screens and netting.
- Apply insect repellent according to package recommendations to repel biting insects (see Table 36–2); these repellents do not deter stinging insects.
- To prevent transmission of scabies, avoid close, physical contact with infected individuals.

Nonprescription Medications
Topical Analgesics

- Use an external analgesic to relieve pain and itching of insect bites. Choice of medications includes local anesthetics, topical antihistamines, counterirritants, and hydrocortisone.

- These products can be applied to the bite area 3–4 times daily. Do not use on children younger than 2 years. Do not use longer than 7 days.
- Note that local anesthetics can cause sensitization. If these agents are preferred, pramoxine and benzyl alcohol are less likely to cause adverse effects.
- Do not use dibucaine in large quantities, particularly over raw surfaces or blistered areas. Such use could cause myocardial depression, convulsions, or death.
- Do not apply phenol to extensive areas of the body or under compresses and bandages. Such application increases the possibility of skin damage or systemic absorption.
- Do not use topical diphenhydramine longer than the recommended 7 days. Prolonged use can cause hypersensitivity reactions or systemic effects.
- Do not use hydrocortisone on scabies, bacterial infections, or fungal infections without a medical recommendation. Hydrocortisone can mask or worsen these disorders.
- Do not allow children to ingest camphor-containing products. Camphor is toxic when ingested.

Skin Protectants

- If needed to reduce irritation or inflammation, or if bacterial infection is a concern, use a skin protectant such as zinc oxide or calamine.
- Apply protectant to affected area as needed up to 4 times daily.
- Protectants can be applied to skin of children younger than 2 years.
- Some insect bite products contain external analgesics and skin protectants.

When to Seek Medical Attention

- Seek medical attention if the condition worsens during treatment or if symptoms persist after 7 days of topical treatment.

Evaluation of Patient Outcomes for Insect Bites

Follow-up should occur after 7 days of self-treatment. The patient should be advised to seek medical attention if symptoms such as redness, itching, and localized swelling worsen during treatment, or if the patient develops secondary infection, fever, joint pain, or lymph node enlargement. Medical attention is also necessary if symptoms persist after 7 days of treatment.

Insect Stings

Pathophysiology and Clinical Presentation of Insect Stings

Venomous insects such as bees, wasps, hornets, yellow jackets, and fire ants belong to the order Hymenoptera. They attack their victims to defend themselves or to kill other insects.

The injected venom contains allergenic proteins and pharmacologically active molecules. Because venom contents vary within the Hymenoptera order, venom is discussed in general terms.

Most people will complain of pain, itching, and irritation at the site following an insect sting, but they will have no systemic symptoms. Individuals who are allergic to insect stings may experience hives, itching, swelling, and burning sensations of the skin. Although anaphylaxis is rare, those with severe allergies may experience a fall in blood pressure, light-headedness, chest tightness, dyspnea, and even loss of consciousness.

Wild Honeybees, Wasps, Hornets, and Yellow Jackets

Wild honeybees are most commonly found in the western and midwestern United States; they usually nest in hollow tree trunks. Because the honeybee stinger is barbed, it remains embedded in the skin, even after the bee pulls away or is brushed off, and continues to inject venom. Paper wasps, hornets, and yellow jackets are found more commonly in the southern, central, and southwestern United States. Paper wasps tend to nest in high places, under eaves of houses or on branches of high trees, whereas hornets prefer to nest in hollow spaces, especially hollow trees. Yellow jackets, considered the most common stinging culprits, usually nest in low places, such as burrows in the ground, cracks in sidewalks, or small shrubs. The stinging mechanism of wasps, hornets, and yellow jackets resembles that of the honeybee, except their stingers are not barbed. Their stingers can be withdrawn easily after venom is injected, enabling them to sting repeatedly.

Fire Ants

Fire ants, imported from South America early in the 20th century, are now found in the southern and western United States, live in underground colonies, and form large raised mounds. Some ants only bite, whereas others bite and sting simultaneously; however, the bite is believed to cause the reactions. Fire ant bites cause intense itching, burning, vesiculation, tissue necrosis, and anaphylactic reactions in hypersensitive persons.

Treatment of Insect Stings

Although labeling of nonprescription products for insect-related injuries mentions only "insect bites" as an indication, it is generally accepted that FDA had intended the term to also cover insect stings.

Treatment Goals

The goal of self-treating insect stings is to relieve the itching and pain of cutaneous nonallergic reactions. Allergic reactions require medical referral.

General Treatment Approach

Removal of the stinger and application of an ice pack in 10-minute intervals are the first steps in treating insect stings. Application of a local anesthetic, skin protectant, antiseptic, or counterirritant to the sting site is appropriate if the reaction is confined to the site and if no exclusions for self-treatment apply. Figure 36–2 lists exclusions for self-treatment and outlines the treatment of insect stings.

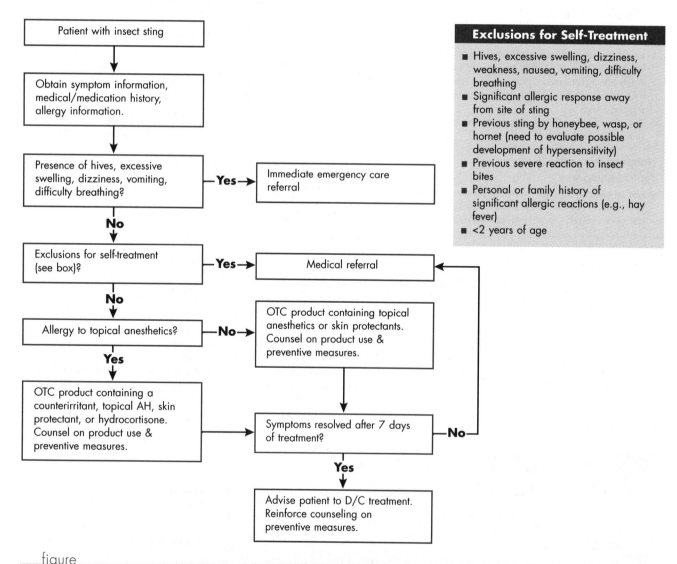

Exclusions for Self-Treatment

- Hives, excessive swelling, dizziness, weakness, nausea, vomiting, difficulty breathing
- Significant allergic response away from site of sting
- Previous sting by honeybee, wasp, or hornet (need to evaluate possible development of hypersensitivity)
- Previous severe reaction to insect bites
- Personal or family history of significant allergic reactions (e.g., hay fever)
- <2 years of age

figure
36–2 Self-care of insect stings. Key: AH = Antihistamine; D/C = discontinue; OTC = over-the-counter.

Avoiding future insect stings can prevent an individual from developing allergic reactions to stings. If symptoms of an allergic reaction develop, emergency treatment should be administered, and the patient should seek medical attention. Patients with severe allergic reactions should be advised to wear a bracelet or carry a card identifying the nature of the allergy. They should also contact their primary care provider about carrying an injectable form of epinephrine.

Nonpharmacologic Therapy

Prompt application of cold packs to the sting site in 10-minute intervals helps slow absorption and reduce itching, swelling, and pain. Removal of the honeybee's stinger and venom sac, which are usually left in the skin, is important. The patient should remove the stinger before all venom is injected; approximately 2–3 minutes are needed to empty all contents from the honeybee's venom sac. The patient should not use tweezers or squeeze the sac because rubbing, scratching, or grasping it releases more venom. Scraping away the stinger with a fingernail or the edge of a credit card minimizes the venom flow. After the stinger is removed, an antiseptic, such as hydrogen peroxide or alcohol, should be applied.

Measures to avoid attracting stinging insects are included in the Patient Education for Insect Stings box.

Pharmacologic Therapy

The section Treatment of Insect Bites discusses the following external analgesics approved for treatment of insect bites and, by inference, insect stings: local anesthetics, topical antihistamines, counterirritants, hydrocortisone, and skin protectants.

Product labels for systemic antihistamines do not include treatment of itching associated with insect stings as an indication, even though these products are often used for this purpose.

Complementary Therapies

Meat tenderizer has been used on insect stings to "break down" proteins in venom. Ammonia and baking soda have been used to "neutralize" venom in insect bites. These products may affect itching. Most reports of their success are anecdotal, however, and currently their effectiveness has not been determined.

Assessment of Insect Stings

The critical determination in assessing a patient with an insect sting is whether the patient is allergic to the venom. Patients experiencing allergic reactions should be referred immediately for emergency medical attention.

Patient Counseling for Insect Stings

The health care provider should advise the patient that local reactions to insect stings usually are transient, but that severe reactions to insect stings can occur if sensitization to the insect venom develops with repeated exposure. The symptoms of allergic reactions should be explained. Patients who have a known hypersensitivity to insect stings should have epinephrine injection available at all times for emergency self-treatment.

For nonallergic reactions to stings, the provider should recommend one or more topical medications to manage immediate symptoms. The patient should be advised about adverse effects and any contraindications. The box Patient Education for Insect Stings lists specific information that should be provided.

---

patient education for
Insect Stings

The objectives of self-treatment for insect stings are to (1) relieve the swelling, pain, and itching of insect stings; (2) monitor any reaction to the sting to determine whether an allergic reaction is developing; and (3) prevent future insect stings. For most patients, carefully following product instructions and the self-care measures listed here will help ensure optimal therapeutic outcomes.

Nondrug Measures

- For honeybee stings, removing the honeybee stinger immediately is important. Scraping the stinger away with the edge of a credit card is effective. Try not to squeeze or rub the stinger; these actions will actually release more venom.
- Apply an ice pack or a cold compress promptly to the sting site to help slow absorption of the venom. This action will reduce itching, swelling, and pain.
- Avoid scratching the affected area; keep fingernails trimmed. Gloves or mittens may be used on small children during sleep to avoid unconscious scratching.
- To avoid attracting stinging insects, avoid wearing perfume, scented lotions, and brightly colored clothes; control odors in picnic and garbage areas; change children's clothing if it becomes contaminated with summer foods such as fruits; wear shoes when outdoors; and destroy nests of stinging insects near homes.
- If you are hypersensitive to stings, wear a bracelet or carry a card showing the nature of the allergy.

Nonprescription Medications

- For nonallergic stings, apply a topical nonprescription external analgesic such as a local anesthetic, topical antihistamine, counterirritant, or hydrocortisone to the affected site to relieve pain and itching. A skin protectant can also be recommended to prevent irritation and inflammation as well as prevent secondary bacterial infection.
- These products can be applied 3–4 times daily for up to 7 days.

When to Seek Medical Attention

- If you have experienced previous severe reactions to insect stings, seek emergency medical care immediately. If a primary care provider has prescribed epinephrine or an oral antihistamine and you have it on your person, administer it according to the primary care provider's instructions.
- Seek medical attention if you develop symptoms of an allergic reaction, such as hives, excessive swelling, dizziness, vomiting, or difficulty breathing.
- Seek medical attention if the pain and itching worsen during treatment or if they do not improve after 7 days of topical treatment.

Evaluation of Patient Outcomes for Insect Stings

Follow-up for nonallergic reactions to insect stings should occur within 7 days. The patient should be advised to seek medical attention if symptoms of pain, itching, and localized swelling worsen during the treatment period or persist after 7 days of treatment. Symptoms of secondary infection or fever also warrant medical attention. Follow-up for patients who have allergic reactions should occur the same day, if possible.

Case 36–1 illustrates assessment of a patient who has an insect sting.

case 36-1

Relevant Evaluation Criteria	Scenario/Model Outcome
Information Gathering	
1. Gather essential information about the patient's symptoms and medical history, including:	
a. description of symptom(s) (i.e., nature, onset, duration, severity, associated symptoms)	A mother comes into the pharmacy concerned after her son has just been "bitten" by something in their back yard. Her 9-year-old son had been playing all morning and suddenly ran into the house frantic and complaining of pain on his left forearm. The father had previously noticed many burrows in the backyard with what appeared to be wasps near the burrows. The son is now stating that the site has begun to itch and pain is subsiding upon coming to the pharmacy.
b. description of any factors that seem to precipitate, exacerbate, and/or relieve the patient's symptom(s)	Mother states that she used ice on the affected area with some relief.
c. description of the patient's efforts to relieve the symptoms	The mother is aware of wasp nests in the backyard and warned her son to stay away from the burrows. In an attempt to reduce swelling and relieve pain, the mother used ice on the affected area.
d. patient's identity	Timmy Smith
e. age, sex, height, and weight	9 years old, male, 48 in., 65 lb
f. patient's occupation	4th-grade student
g. patient's dietary habits	Timmy appears to be well nourished, and proper diet is confirmed by the mother.
h. patient's sleep habits	Timmy regularly gets 8–9 hours of sleep per night.
i. concurrent medical conditions, prescription and non-prescription medications, and dietary supplements	Multivitamin, chewable
j. allergies	None
k. history of other adverse reactions to medications	None
l. other (describe) _____	NA
Assessment and Triage	
2. Differentiate patient's signs/symptoms and correctly identify the patient's primary problem(s).	Patient's "bite" appears to be an insect sting, and the suspected cause is a wasp. Suspicion confirmed by multiple wasp nests in the backyard where the patient was playing prior to complaining about the sting. Patient's affected site also confirms the suspected sting with mild pain, redness, and now itching. No stinger appears to be present at affected area.
3. Identify exclusions for self-treatment (Figure 36–1).	None
4. Formulate a comprehensive list of therapeutic alternatives for the primary problem to determine if triage to a medical provider is required, and share this information with the patient or caregiver.	Options include: (1) Removal of stinger and application of an ice pack in 10-minute intervals are the first step. (2) Application of local anesthetic, topical antihistamine, counterirritant, antiseptic, or hydrocortisone including the following: a. anesthetic: Lanacane Aerosol Spray (benzocaine 20%) b. antihistamine: Maximum Strength Benadryl Cream/Spray (diphenhydramine 2%) c. counterirritant: Blue Star Ointment (camphor 1.2%) d. antiseptic: hydrogen peroxide of alcohol e. hydrocortisone: Cortizone-5 Cream (hydrocortisone 0.5%)

case
36–1 *continued*

Relevant Evaluation Criteria	Scenario/Model Outcome
	(3) Refer Timmy to his PCP.
	(4) Recommend self-care until the PCP can be consulted.
	(5) Take no action.

Plan

5. Select an optimal therapeutic alternative to address the patient's problem, taking into account patient preferences.	Because the affected area is confined to the sting site, no stinger is present, and the patient is older than 2 years, he is eligible for self-treatment. Now that the pain has subsided and the patient's chief complaint is itching at the sting site, relieving the itching is the most important therapeutic factor.
6. Describe the recommended therapeutic approach to the patient or caregiver.	"You should begin application of a topical antihistamine to Timmy's affected area: – Apply a thin layer to affected area 3–4 times a day. – Ice may also be continued in 10-minute intervals to help alleviate discomfort. – If symptoms persist after 7 days of treatment, alert the child's PCP."
7. Explain to the patient or caregiver the rationale for selecting the recommended therapeutic approach from the considered therapeutic alternatives.	"Because Timmy's pain is subsiding and itching is the chief complaint, topical antihistamines and ice are preferred over other therapies to relieve these symptoms."

Patient Education

8. When recommending self-care with nonprescription medications and/or nondrug therapy, convey accurate information to the patient or caregiver.	
a. appropriate dose and frequency of administration	"Apply a thin layer of Maximum Strength Benadryl Cream to the affected area 3–4 times a day."
b. maximum number of days the therapy should be employed	"Apply no longer than 7 days."
c. product administration procedures	"Apply to affected areas per package insert directions."
d. expected time to onset of relief	"Product should take effect quickly."
e. degree of relief that can be reasonably expected	"Symptoms should be largely depressed, but total relief may not be achieved until the bite has completely healed in a few days."
f. most common side effects	"Photosensitivity and rash are the most common side effects."
g. side effects that warrant medical intervention should they occur	"If rash or skin irritation worsens after discontinuation, seek medical attention for the child."
h. patient options in the event that condition worsens or persists	"If signs of infection from the bite occur, seek medical attention for the child."
i. product storage requirements	"Product may be stored at room temperature."
j. specific nondrug measures	"Keep people away from wasp burrows; contact professional pesticide company for eradication of wasp nests."
Solicit follow-up questions from the patient or caregiver.	"What if my son develops an allergic reaction to the insect sting?"
Answer the patient's or caregiver's questions.	"If symptoms of an allergic reaction develop, emergency treatment should be administered, and you should seek immediate medical attention for your son. Patients with severe allergic reactions might be advised to carry a bracelet or card identifying the allergy and to carry an injectable form of epinephrine. Your son's primary care provider can prescribe the injectable epinephrine if it is needed."

Evaluation of Patient Outcome

9. Assess patient outcome.	Ask the mother to call to update you on her son's response to your recommendations, or you could call her in a week to evaluate his response.

Key: NA = Not applicable; PCP = primary care provider.

Pediculosis

Pathophysiology and Clinical Presentation of Pediculosis

Lice are irritating pests, and lice infestations in the United States are common. Three types of lice that infest humans are head lice (*Pediculus humanus capitis*), body lice (*Pediculus humanus corporis*), and pubic lice (*Phthirus pubis*).

Head Lice

Head lice are the most common cause of lice infestation, and outbreaks of lice infestation are common in places such as schools and day care centers. Infestations are spread through close personal contact or sharing personal items such as caps, hairbrushes, and combs. Outbreaks usually peak after the opening of schools each year, between August and November. All socioeconomic groups are affected. Head lice create problematic infestations, but they generally do not contribute to the spread of other diseases in the United States.[19]

Head lice usually infest the head and live on the scalp (see Color Plates, photographs 21A and B). A lice egg or nit is about 1 mm in diameter and is typically found within 4 mm of the scalp. Once hatched, the louse must begin feeding within 24 hours or it dies. The nymph, or newly hatched, immature louse, resembles an adult and matures within 8–9 days. Without treatment, this cycle may repeat every 3 weeks.[19] The bite of a louse causes an immediate wheal to develop around the bite, with a local papule appearing within 24 hours. Itching and subsequent scratching may result in secondary infection. Adult lice, which are about the size of a sesame seed, are often difficult to locate because they move, but nits and nit casings generally can be spotted at the base of hair shafts when hair is parted for physical inspection. Hair inspections should focus on the crown of the head, near ears, and at the base of the neck. The grayish nits blend in well with the hair, but nit casings (hatched nits) are a lighter color and are more easily located. Nits and nit casings may be differentiated from dandruff, dirt, and so forth because of their firm attachment to the hair shaft. The presence of black powdery specks, lice feces, is also evidence of an infestation.

Body Lice

Body lice (or "cooties") live, hide, and lay their eggs in clothing, particularly in the seams and folds of underclothes. They periodically attack body areas for blood feedings and can transmit infections such as typhus and trench fever.[20] Body lice infestations generally occur in individuals who do not shower or change clothing frequently, such as the homeless.[20]

Pubic Lice

Pubic lice or "crabs," referring to their crab-like appearance, are generally transmitted through high-risk sexual contact, but they may also spread by way of toilet seats, shared undergarments, or bedding. The lice usually are found in the pubic area but may infest armpits, eyelashes, mustaches, beards, and eyebrows.[21]

Treatment of Pediculosis

Nonprescription pediculicide agents, appropriate hair combing for nit removal, and home vacuuming and cleaning of personal items are primary treatments for lice infestation.[19]

Treatment Goals

The goal of treating pediculosis is to rid the infested patient of lice by killing adult and nymph lice and by removing nits from the patient's hair.

General Treatment Approach

A pediculicide is applied to the infested body area for the designated amount of time to rid the patient of lice. The hair is then combed with a lice or nit comb to remove nits from the hair shaft; combing will also remove dead lice. Once rid of lice, patients should be instructed on how to avoid future infestations. Figure 36–3 outlines treatment of lice infestations and lists exclusions for self-treatment.

Nonpharmacologic Therapy

Because none of the pediculicides kills 100% of lice eggs, careful visual inspection of the hair for nits and combing with a nit comb, such as the LiceMeister comb, to remove nits are helpful in treating and controlling head lice.[19] Direct physical contact with an infested individual should be avoided, and articles such as combs, brushes, towels, caps, and hats should not be shared. Clothing and bedding should be washed in hot water and dried in a clothes dryer to kill lice and their nits; an alternative to washing would be to seal contaminated items in a plastic bag for 2 weeks. Hairbrushes and combs should be washed in very hot water. Carpets, rugs, and furniture should be vacuumed thoroughly and regularly.[19] Use of insecticidal sprays on these items is not generally recommended because lice usually survive for less than 48 hours when not in contact with a host.[19] Given the increasing resistance to pediculicides, some patients are choosing to use nondrug therapy exclusively; these nondrug methods, specifically combing and vacuuming, can be effective, but they are labor intensive and tedious.[22] Complete head shaving has also been used as a lice treatment, but the social stigma involved makes this a questionable option. Body lice are controlled by appropriate body hygiene and frequent changing and appropriate laundering of clothing and bed linens.[21]

Pharmacologic Therapy

Two nonprescription pediculicide agents are available for treating pediculosis: permethrins and synergized pyrethrins. Patients should be warned about overusing these agents because of an apparent increasing trend of lice resistance to pediculicides, including the nonprescription products; the resistance may be caused by overuse, improper use, or insufficient contact time.[19,23,24]

Synergized Pyrethrins

Pyrethrins are synergized by addition of piperonyl butoxide, a petroleum derivative. Pyrethrins are approved for treating head and pubic lice.

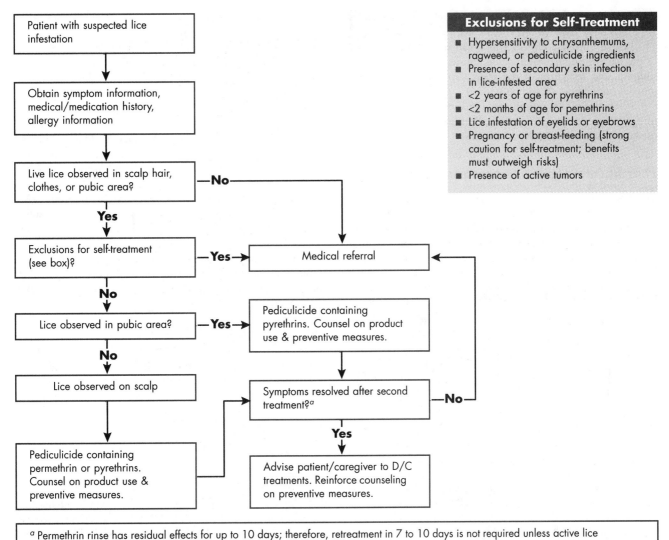

Exclusions for Self-Treatment

- Hypersensitivity to chrysanthemums, ragweed, or pediculicide ingredients
- Presence of secondary skin infection in lice-infested area
- <2 years of age for pyrethrins
- <2 months of age for pemethrins
- Lice infestation of eyelids or eyebrows
- Pregnancy or breast-feeding (strong caution for self-treatment; benefits must outweigh risks)
- Presence of active tumors

a Permethrin rinse has residual effects for up to 10 days; therefore, retreatment in 7 to 10 days is not required unless active lice are detected.

figure

36–3 Self-care of pediculosis. Key: D/C = Discontinue.

Pyrethrins block nerve impulse transmission, causing the insect's paralysis and death. Addition of piperonyl butoxide to pyrethrins synergizes their insecticidal effect through inhibition of pyrethrin breakdown, increasing insecticide levels within the louse.[19,25] Excessive contact time or occlusion of the scalp after product application may increase skin absorption of topical pyrethrins.

Pyrethrins, in concentrations ranging from 0.17%–0.33%, generally are used in combination with 2%–4% piperonyl butoxide. This combination is considered an effective pediculicide when applied topically as shampoos, foams, solutions, or gels. The medication is applied to the affected area for 10 minutes, and then the treated area is rinsed or shampooed as recommended. Combing with a lice comb should follow treatment. The treatment is repeated in 7–10 days to kill any remaining nits that have since hatched. The drug should not be applied more than twice in 24 hours.

When applied according to directions, pyrethrins have a low order of toxicity. Most adverse reactions are cutaneous and include irritation, erythema, itching, and swelling.[19,26] Contact with eyes and mucous membranes should be avoided.

Individuals allergic to pyrethrins or chrysanthemums should not use this agent; ragweed-sensitive individuals risk cross-sensitivity.

Permethrin

Permethrin, a synthetic pyrethroid, is available as a nonprescription cream rinse for treating head lice. Permethrin acts on the nerve cell membrane of lice. It disrupts the sodium channel, delaying repolarization and causing paralysis and death of the parasite.

When permethrin is applied, an estimated less than 2% is absorbed, after which the agent is metabolized.

Nonprescription permethrin is indicated for treating head lice only.

The 1% cream rinse is applied in sufficient quantities to cover or saturate washed hair and scalp. It is left on the hair for 10 minutes before rinsing; the hair is then combed with a lice comb. The rinse has residual effects for up to 10 days; therefore, retreatment in 7–10 days is not required unless active lice are detected.

Primary adverse effects, which can occur in up to 10% of the patient population, include transient pruritus, burning, stinging, and irritation of the scalp. Contact with eyes and mucous membranes should be avoided.

Permethrin is contraindicated in patients who are sensitive to pyrethrins or chrysanthemums. Permethrin should not be used on infants younger than 2 months.

Pharmacotherapeutic Comparison

When treatment involves a single application of a pediculicide, permethrin is more effective than the pyrethrin and piperonyl butoxide combination. However, no significant difference exists in effectiveness of these agents when treatment consists of two applications.[23]

Product Selection Guidelines

Preparations that contain pyrethrins may be used on children ages 2 years and older, but they should be used in pregnancy and lactation only if prescribed by a health care provider.

Pyrethrins may be recommended for treating pubic lice. For treatment of head lice, pyrethrins or permethrin may be selected on the basis of preferred dosage form, desire for single application, or patient allergies and sensitivities. Table 36–4 lists selected trade-name products containing these agents.

Complementary Therapies

Lice enzyme shampoos, which claim to break down the lice exoskeleton, are being promoted as an alternative to traditional pediculicides. A product containing 10% tea tree oil and 1% lavender oil applied weekly for 3 weeks was more effective at eradicating lice than a pyrethrin/piperonyl butoxide product applied twice (1 week apart).[27] Tea tree oil must be used with caution because of potential significant allergic reactions and possible liver toxicity.[28] Other oil-based products such as petroleum jelly and mayonnaise are also being used on the basis of the theory that they impair lice respiration; however, these products are not very effective and most likely only slow the movement of lice.[19,26] Dangerous alternative treatments such as gasoline and kerosene should always be avoided because of their flammability and potential for toxicity.[19,22]

Emerging Therapies

A new potential treatment under study is a class of products called DSP (Dry-on, Suffocation-based Pediculicide) lotions. The first DSP product to be tested, the Nuvo method, also marketed as Cetaphil cleanser, is a nontoxic lotion that "shrink wraps" lice. It is applied to hair and dried with a hairdryer to form a shrink-wrap film over hair and lice. The lotion covers breathing holes, suffocating the louse. A growing body of evidence suggests suffocation products may be more effective than pyrethrins/piperonyl butoxide.[27]

Dimethicone 4% lotion has also been shown to cure pediculosis while causing less irritation than traditional therapy. Furthermore, dimethicone works by coating the lice and irreversibly immobilizing them within 5 minutes of application.[29]

The LouseBuster is a machine that applies heat to the hair and scalp, dehydrating and killing lice and nits. Preliminary evidence suggests this procedure kills more than 90% of nits.[30] Unfortunately, it is expensive and requires a certified technician to operate the machine.

Assessment of Pediculosis: A Case-Based Approach

In many cases of pediculosis, visual inspection of the scalp will verify the presence or absence of head lice or nits. Similarly, presence of body lice can be determined by identifying adult lice and nits in seams of clothing. If a patient does not want such an inspection or if lice have not been confirmed by another health care provider, a pediculicide should not be recommended. When the disorder is confirmed, the appropriate pediculicide should be recommended.

Case 36–2 illustrates assessment of a patient who has a head lice infestation.

Patient Counseling for Pediculosis

Control of pediculosis requires both pharmacologic and non-pharmacologic intervention. The health care provider should reassure parents of children with head lice that the condition is not the result of poor hygiene. Patients with confirmed head or pubic lice infestations should be counseled on which product is best for the situation and how to use the product properly; preventive measures should also be discussed. Additional information regarding patient counseling for pediculosis can be found in the box Patient Education for Pediculosis.

Evaluation of Patient Outcomes for Pediculosis

Follow-up of lice infestations should occur within 10 days. If signs of lice infestation persist after a second application of a pediculicide, the patient should be advised to seek medical

table 36–4	Selected Nonprescription Pediculicides
Trade Name	**Primary Ingredients**
A-200 Lice Killing Shampoo	Pyrethrins 0.33%; piperonyl butoxide 3%
RID Lice Killing Shampoo, Maximum Strength	Pyrethrins 0.33%; piperonyl butoxide 4%
RID Mousse Foam, Maximum Strength	Pyrethrins 0.33%; piperonyl butoxide 4%
Nix Cream Rinse Lice Treatment	Permethrin 1%
Pronto Lice Killing Shampoo	Pyrethrins 0.33%; piperonyl butoxide 4%

case

36–2

Relevant Evaluation Criteria	Scenario/Model Outcome
Information Gathering	

1. Gather essential information about the patient's symptoms and medical history, including:

   a. description of symptom(s) (i.e., nature, onset, duration, severity, associated symptoms)

   > A frantic woman comes into the pharmacy asking about OTC options for head lice. She says that her 7-year-old daughter has just returned from summer camp complaining of an "itchy" scalp that started a day or so ago. Her daughter admits to sharing another girl's cap the day before leaving camp and denies any itching previously while away at camp. Upon further inspection, the woman noticed small red bumps clustered throughout the scalp and on the base of the neck. She also noticed tiny light colored "dandruff looking things" attached firmly to the hair shaft. She reports her daughter's complaints are severe itching and mild pain on scalp.

   b. description of any factors that seem to precipitate, exacerbate, and/or relieve the patient's symptom(s)

   > The woman explains that she has just picked up her daughter from camp when she noticed her daughter scratching her head aggressively. The mother noted that the skin had been broken in multiple locations on the scalp because of scratching; also the skin appears red and swollen in certain areas of the scalp. She inspected her daughter's scalp once they returned home and was not able to comment on any precipitating or exacerbating symptoms.

   c. description of the patient's efforts to relieve the symptoms

   > The woman has taken all of her daughter's clothes out of her suitcase and placed them in a large plastic bag to be washed when she goes home.

   d. patient's identity

   > Caroline Davis

   e. age, sex, height, and weight

   > 7 years old, female, 45 in., 52 lb

   f. patient's occupation

   > Second-grade student

   g. patient's dietary habits

   > Mother says that Caroline usually eats a well-balanced diet.

   h. patient's sleep habits

   > Caroline usually sleeps about 9 hours per night.

   i. concurrent medical conditions, prescription and nonprescription medications, and dietary supplements

   > None

   j. allergies

   > Chrysanthemums (rash), amoxicillin (rash)

   k. history of other adverse reactions to medications

   > None

   l. other (describe) _____

   > NA

| **Assessment and Triage** | |

2. Differentiate patient's signs/symptoms and correctly identify the patient's primary problem(s).

   > Patient has observable nit casings and small red papules throughout the scalp and base of the neck. Patient has recently returned from summer camp and reports sharing headwear with another child, a common occurrence associated with head lice infestation.

3. Identify exclusions for self-treatment (Figure 36–3).

   > Patient presents with broken skin caused by aggressive scratching. Signs of secondary infection appear to be present. Also, patient has documented an allergy to chrysanthemums, which would prohibit treatment with OTC synergized pyrethrins and permethrins.

4. Formulate a comprehensive list of therapeutic alternatives for the primary problem to determine if triage to a medical provider is required, and share this information with the patient or caregiver.

   > Options include:
   >
   > (1) Purchase nit comb for nit observation and removal.
   >
   > (2) Prior to nit comb use, recommend OTC pediculicide:
   >
   >   a. A-200 Lice Killing Shampoo
   >
   >   b. RID Lice Killing Shampoo, Maximum Strength
   >
   >   c. RID Mousse Foam, Maximum Strength
   >
   >   d. Pronto Lice Killing Shampoo
   >
   >   e. OTC permethrin products should be avoided because of chrysanthemum allergy
   >
   > (3) Recommend immediate medical attention.
   >
   > (4) Take no action.

case

36-2 *continued*

Relevant Evaluation Criteria	Scenario/Model Outcome
Plan	
5. Select an optimal therapeutic alternative to address the patient's problem, taking into account patient preferences.	The patient should seek medical attention because of suspected secondary infection from lice bites and scratching. Also, because of documented chrysanthemum allergy, OTC pyrethrins and permethrins cannot be used.
6. Describe the recommended therapeutic approach to the patient or caregiver.	"Your scalp shows redness, swelling, and broken skin from scratching. These are an indication of secondary infection and could possibly require antibiotic treatment."
7. Explain to the patient or caregiver the rationale for selecting the recommended therapeutic approach from the considered therapeutic alternatives.	"A suspected secondary infection and a significant allergy have been documented. You should be seen by a PCP to confirm the infection; self-treatment is not appropriate at this time."
Patient Education	
8. When recommending self-care with nonprescription medications and/or nondrug therapy, convey accurate information to the patient or caregiver.	Criterion does not apply in this case.
Solicit follow-up questions from the patient or caregiver	"How do I avoid future contraction and spread of pediculosis?"
Answer the patient's or caregiver's questions.	"Direct physical contact with an infected individual should be avoided. Personal articles of the infected individual such as combs, brushes, towels, caps, and hats should not be shared. An infected person's clothing and bedding should be washed in hot water and dried in a clothes dryer to kill lice and nits. Once prescribed, use a pediculicide as directed. If lice are still present, this process may be repeated in 7–10 days. Do not overuse the pediculicide because overuse increases the resistance of lice to treatment."
Evaluation of Patient Outcome	
9. Assess patient outcome.	Contact the patient in a day or two to ensure that she made an appointment and sought medical care.

Key: NA = Not applicable; OTC = over-the-counter; PCP = primary care provider.

attention. Overuse of these products should be discouraged and nonpharmacologic control measures emphasized.[22]

Key Points for Insect Bites and Stings and Pediculosis

➤ Insect stings and bites cause local irritation, inflammation, swelling, and itching; a cold pack may be applied to reduce local symptoms.
➤ For relief of the itching and pain resulting from insect bites, topical nonprescription preparations that contain local anesthetics, antihistamines, hydrocortisone, or counterirritants can be used in patients ages 2 years and older.
➤ In hypersensitive people, anaphylactic reactions may pose serious emergency problems; these patients require immediate medical attention.

➤ Suspected spider bites should be referred; nonprescription treatments are not appropriate. If possible, the spider should be sealed in a container for identification.
➤ A tick should be removed by grasping it near the head with tweezers and gently pulling to cause the tick to release from the skin. The patient should be monitored for systemic effects such as Lyme disease and Rocky Mountain spotted fever.
➤ Appropriate use of insect repellents containing DEET will help prevent insect bites from mosquitoes, ticks, and chiggers.
➤ Exposure to mosquito bites warrants monitoring the patient for symptoms of West Nile virus.
➤ Nondrug measures are an important component in treatment of lice infestation.
➤ Available nonprescription pediculicides contain either synergized pyrethrins or permethrin.
➤ Pediculicides are designed for initial treatment and retreatment in 7–10 days; hair should be combed with a nit comb after treatment. Overuse should be avoided because resistance to pediculicides is a growing problem and affects the products' effectiveness.

patient education for
Pediculosis

The objectives for self-treatment of pediculosis are to (1) rid the body of lice and nits and (2) implement measures to prevent future infestations. For most patients, carefully following product instructions and the self-care measures listed here will help ensure optimal therapeutic outcomes.

Nondrug Measures

- Wash hairbrushes, combs, and toys of infested patients in water at a temperature of 130°F (39.4°C) or higher for 10 minutes.[17]
- Use water at a temperature of 130°F (39.4°C) or higher to wash the clothes, bedding, and towels of infested patients. Dry the items on the hottest dryer setting that the fabric permits.[17]
- Objects or clothing that cannot be washed should be sealed in plastic bags for the length of the louse's life cycle (2 weeks) so that it is unable to feed on a host.
- Avoid close physical contact with an infested patient; do not share articles such as combs, brushes, towels, caps, and hats.
- Vacuum living areas thoroughly and regularly during treatment period.
- Visually inspect the hair and scalp before, during, and after treatment for evidence of lice or nits:
  - Use a nit comb diligently to remove nits.
  - Comb the hair in segments. (Individual hairs can be trimmed if nit removal proves difficult.)

Nonprescription Medications

- Treatment of other family members should be determined on the basis of presence of lice or nits and the family members' level of contact with the infested individual; unnecessary treatment should be avoided.
- Application steps for a pyrethrin shampoo include the following:
  - Apply sufficient quantity to wet the dry hair and scalp. (Foams should also be applied to dry hair.)
  - Allow the treatment to remain for 10 minutes.

- Work the shampoo into a lather and then rinse thoroughly. (Remove foams with shampoo or soap and water.)
  - Use a nit comb to remove dead lice and eggs as described previously.
- Application steps for a permethrin cream rinse include the following:
  - Shampoo with regular shampoo, rinse, and towel dry hair.
  - Apply sufficient cream rinse to wet hair and scalp.
  - Allow the treatment to remain for 10 minutes; then rinse and towel dry.
  - Use a nit comb as described previously.
- Avoid contact of the pediculicide with eyes and mucous membranes.
- The pediculicide can cause temporary irritation, erythema, itching, swelling, and numbness of the scalp; itching should be relieved in a few days.
- For pyrethrin products, repeat entire process in 7–10 days; permethrin products can be used again in 7–10 days if lice or nits are detected. Because of treatment resistance, proper use of these products is required and overuse must be avoided.
- If desired, contact the National Pediculosis Association at www.headlice.org or 1-781-449-6487 for information about treatment of lice infestations.

When to Seek Medical Attention

- Significant skin irritation or excessive exposure of eyes or mucous membranes to pediculicides warrants medical intervention.
- Seek medical attention if symptoms of lice infestation persist after the second treatment.

REFERENCES

1. Centers for Disease Control and Prevention. Division of Vector-Borne Diseases West Nile Virus. 2012 West Nile virus update: December 11. Updated April 9, 2013. Accessed at http://www.cdc.gov/ncidod/dvbid/westnile/index.htm, April 15, 2013.
2. Centers for Disease Control and Prevention. West Nile virus: what you need to know. CDC Fact Sheet. Updated September 12, 2012. Accessed at http://www.cdc.gov/ncidod/dvbid/westnile/wnv_factsheet.htm, April 15, 2013.
3. Carson PJ, Konewko P, Wold KS, et al. Long-term clinical and neuropsychological outcomes of West Nile Virus infection. *Clin Infect Dis.* 2006;43(6):723–30.
4. Kolb A, Needham GR, Neyman KM, et al. Bedbugs. *Dermatol Ther.* 2009;22(4):347–52.
5. Silverman A, Qu L, Low J, et al. Assessment of hepatitis B virus DNA and hepatitis C virus RNA in the common bedbug and kissing bug. *Am J Gastroenterol.* 2001;96(7):2194–8.
6. Centers for Disease Control and Prevention. Tick removal. Updated July 26, 2012. Accessed at http://www.cdc.gov/ticks/removing_a_tick.html, April 20, 2013.
7. Bratton RL, Corey GR. Tick-borne disease. *Am Fam Physician.* 2005; 71(12):2323–30.
8. Centers for Disease Control and Prevention. Lime disease statistics. Updated September 10, 2012. Accessed at http://www.cdc.gov/lyme/stats/index.html, April 20, 2013.
9. Centers for Disease Control and Prevention. NIOSH workplace safety and health topics. venomous spiders. Updated February 24, 2012. Accessed at http://www.cdc.gov/niosh/topics/spiders/, April 20, 2013.
10. Civen R, Villacorte F, Robles DT, et al. West Nile virus infection in the pediatric population. *Pediatr Infect Dis J.* 2006;25(1):75–8.
11. Fradin M, Day J. Comparative efficacy of insect repellents against mosquito bites. *N Engl J Med.* 2002;347(1):13–8.
12. Centers for Disease Control and Prevention. West Nile virus. Questions and answers. Insect repellent use and safety. Updated August 27, 2012. Accessed at http://www.cdc.gov/ncidod/dvbid/westnile/qa/insect_repellent.htm, April 20, 2013.
13. U.S. Environmental Protection Agency. Insect repellents: DEET. Accessed at http://www2.epa.gov/insect-repellents/deet, September 15, 2014.
14. Katz TM, Miller JH, Hebert AA. Insect repellents: historical perspectives and new developments. *J Am Acad Dermatol.* 2008;58(5):865–71.
15. Koren G, Matsui D, Bailey B. DEET-based insect repellants: safety implications for children and pregnant and lactating women. *CMAJ.* 2003;169(3):209–11.
16. Sudakin D, Trevathan W. DEET: a review and update of safety and risk in the general population. *J Toxicol.* 2003;42(6):831–9.
17. Dibucaine. Lexi-Drugs Online™ [database online]. Hudson, OH: Lexi-Comp, Inc. Accessed at http://www.crlonline.com, April 20, 2013.
18. Zinc oxide. Lexi-Drugs Online™ [database online]. Hudson, OH: Lexi-Comp, Inc. Accessed at http://www.crlonline.com, April 20, 2013.
19. Frankowski BL, Bocchini JA, Council on School Health, et al. Head lice. *Pediatrics.* 2010;126(2):392–403.
20. Raoult D, Roux V. The body louse as a vector of reemerging human diseases. *Clin Infect Dis.* 1999;29(4):888–911.
21. Leone PA. Scabies and pediculosis pubis: an update of treatment regimens and general review. *Clin Infect Dis.* 2007;44(suppl 3):S153–9.

22. Pray S. Pediculicide resistance in head lice: a survey. *Hosp Pharm.* 2003;38:241–6.

23. Meinking T, Serrano L, Hard B, et al. Comparative in vitro pediculicidal efficacy of treatments in a resistant head lice population in the United States. *Arch Dermatol.* 2002;138(2):220–4.

24. Meinking T, Entzel P, Villar M, et al. Comparative efficacy of treatments for pediculosis capititis infestations. *Arch Dermatol.* 2001;137(3): 287–91.

25. Burkhart C. Relationship of treatment-resistant head lice to the safety and efficacy of pediculicides. *Mayo Clin Proc.* 2004;79(5):661–6.

26. Pearlman D. Nuvo lotion and the future of head-lice treatment. *Pediatrics.* 2005;115(5):14523.

27. Barker SC, Altman PH. A randomized assessor blind, parallel group comparative efficacy trial of three products for the treatment of head lice in children—melaleuca oil and lavender oil, pyrethrins and piperonyl butoxide, and a suffocation product. *BMC Dermatol.* 2010;10:1–7.

28. HeadLice.org. Alternative treatments: what the NPA Is saying about mayonnaise, vaseline, and tea tree oil. Accessed at http://www.headlice.org/faq/treatments/alternatives.htm, April 20, 2013.

29. Burgess I, Brown C, Lee P. Treatment of head louse infestation with 4% dimeticone lotion: randomized controlled equivalence trial. *Br Med J.* 2005:330(7505);1423–5.

30. Goates BM, Atkin JS, Wilding KG, et al. An effective nonchemical treatment for head lice: a lot of hot air. *Pediatrics.* 2006;118(5):1962–70.

ACNE

Karla T. Foster and Cynthia W. Coffey

Acne vulgaris (AV) is a common inflammatory skin disease of the pilosebaceous glands resulting in lesions most commonly found on the face, but also located on the neck, chest, upper back, and shoulders. More than 81%–95% of adolescent boys and 79%–82% of adolescent girls are affected.[1] Traditionally known as a disease affecting adolescents, AV incidence has been rising in adults, particularly in women older than 25 years.[2] The cause of this increase is unknown. Acne is reportedly more prevalent in male patients before 16 years of age. However, it is more prevalent in female patients after 23 years of age.[3] Although the peak prevalence of acne is during the adolescent years, the mean age for treatment of acne is 24 years, with roughly 10% of visits occurring between 35 and 44 years of age.[3] An estimated 45 million people are affected by AV in the United States.[1]

Many adolescents will achieve spontaneous remission of their acne, whereas some patients will experience acne into adulthood (3% of adult men and 12% of adult women) and may already have scarring by 18 years of age.[2,4] Although patients may tend to overestimate the severity of their acne, health care providers tend to underestimate the impact of the disease on patients. The effect of acne on patients should not be overlooked: Whether or not physical scarring exists, the potential for psychological scarring exists. Associations have been shown between acne and lower self-esteem and a negative impact on quality of life similar to that in patients with asthma or epilepsy.[5] In 2001, health care expenditures for acne were reported at over $1 billion.[1] The direct costs related to acne are $2.2 billion annually, and the indirect costs are $620 million annually in the United States.[6,7]

A wide variety of nonprescription treatment options are available for AV. Prescription anti-acne product sales have been declining over recent years, whereas nonprescription counter sales have steadily increased.[1] Sales of prescription anti-acne products were estimated at $3.3 million in 2006 and $3.6 million in 2011.[8] The nonprescription market is estimated to be more than two to four times the size of the prescription market. One nonprescription medication, Proactiv, was projected to generate over $800 billion in revenue in 2010.[1] Although most nonprescription acne medications are not marketed to the extent of Proactiv, their market share continues to grow. Health care providers can help patients make informed choices about their selection of acne products. This interaction also represents an opportunity for providers to introduce a new group of consumers to the value of pharmaceutical care.

Pathophysiology of Acne

Acne is the result of several pathologic processes that occur within the pilosebaceous unit located in the dermis, or middle layer of the skin (Figure 37–1A). These units, consisting of a hair follicle and associated sebaceous glands, are connected to the skin surface by a duct (infundibulum) lined with epithelial cells through which the hair shaft passes. The sebaceous glands produce sebum. Sebum normally functions to protect the skin from light and retain moisture. It possesses an antibacterial property that is both pro- and anti-inflammatory and is involved in the wound-healing process.[9] Further insight into the molecular function of the sebaceous glands has helped to further explain the role of these glands in skin function. The sebaceous gland also acts as an endocrine organ and responds to changes in androgens and hormones similar to the action of the hypothalamus–pituitary–adrenal axis. Corticotrophin-releasing hormone (CRH) influences the sebaceous glands' endocrine function.[10] CRH is the primary hormone involved in neuroendocrine and behavioral responses to stress. In acne-prone skin, CRH is found throughout the sebaceous glands and has been associated with the immune and inflammatory processes that lead to stress-induced acne.[9]

The formation of acne is multifactorial. In addition to the intricate pathophysiology, genetics and gender play an important role. Ebede et al. describe one study of 200 patients with postadolescent acne and found that 50% of patients reported at least one first-degree family relative with acne. The mean prevalence in adolescents ranges from 70%–80%. The prevalence of acne is significantly higher among women than among men in all age groups.[11]

The pathologic factors involved in the development of acne are (1) androgenic hormonal triggers, (2) excessive sebum production, (3) alteration in the keratinization process, (4) proliferation of *Propionibacterium acnes,* and (5) resulting inflammatory responses.[4,10]

The rise in androgenic hormones coincides with the start of puberty and the appearance of acne. The conversion of testosterone to dihydrotestosterone stimulates an increase in the size and metabolic activity of sebaceous glands. The excessive sebum serves as a breeding ground for *P. acnes* as the comedo develops.

Increases in androgen levels are also partly responsible for abnormal follicular desquamation within the infundibulum. Some evidence exists in the role of sebum lipid abnormalities, such as deficiencies of linoleic acid and excesses of free fatty acids, in hyperkeratinization. Linoleic acid is an essential fatty

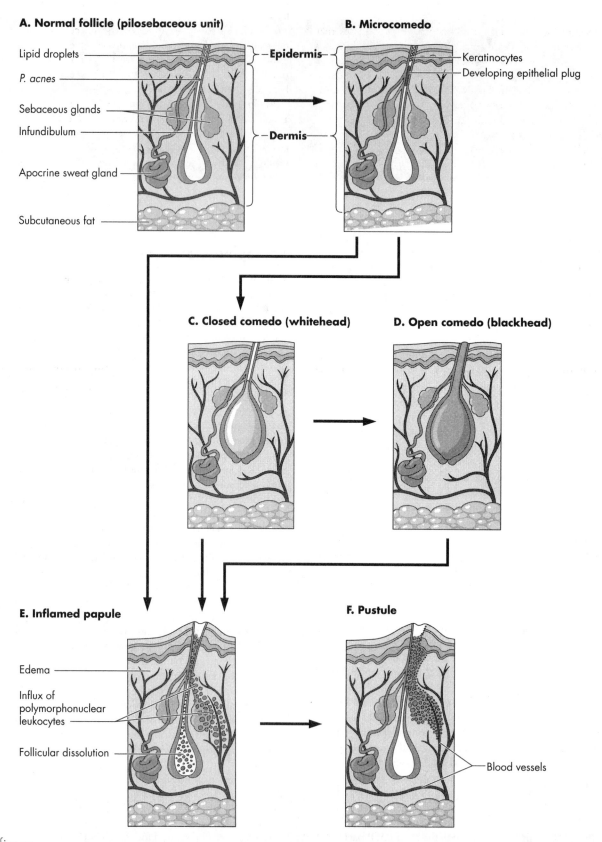

A. Normal follicle (pilosebaceous unit)

Lipid droplets

P. acnes

Sebaceous glands

Infundibulum

Apocrine sweat gland

Subcutaneous fat

Epidermis

Dermis

B. Microcomedo

Keratinocytes

Developing epithelial plug

C. Closed comedo (whitehead)

D. Open comedo (blackhead)

E. Inflamed papule

Edema

Influx of polymorphonuclear leukocytes

Follicular dissolution

F. Pustule

Blood vessels

figure

37–1   Pathogenesis of acne. Key: *P. acnes = Propionibacterium acnes. (Source:* Adapted with permission from Fulton JE, Bradley S. *Cutis.* 1976:7:560.)

acid that cannot be synthesized in vivo, only obtained through diet. Low levels of linoleic acid have been cited in patients with acne.[9] Sebum includes several matrix metalloproteinases that have a prominent role in inflammatory matrix remodeling and proliferative skin disorders.[10] Evidence also exists that follicular keratinocytes release interleukin-1, which may stimulate comedones formation. Regardless of the cause, hyperproliferation of these keratinocytes results in cell cohesion and formation of a plug that blocks the follicular orifice. This plug distends the follicle to form a micro comedo, the initial pathologic lesion of acne (Figure 37–1B). As more cells and sebum accumulate, the micro comedo enlarges and becomes visible as a closed comedo, or whitehead, that is, a small, pale nodule just beneath the skin surface (Figure 37–1C). If the contents of the plug cause distension of the pore's orifice, the plug will protrude from the pore, causing an open comedo or blackhead. The lesion is named a blackhead because of the presence of melanin and oxidation of lipids upon exposure to air. Comedones are the precursors of other acne lesions.[4]

Behind the plug, the buildup of sebum is an ideal habitat for proliferation of *P. acnes*. This bacterium breaks down sebum into highly irritating free fatty acids through production of lipases; *P. acnes* is also responsible for the production of pro-inflammatory mediators that induce pro-inflammatory cytokines.[4] As a result of the irritation and inflammation, localized tissue destruction occurs. Toll-like receptors (TLR) are mammalian proteins that have emerged as a vital regulator of host responses to infection.[10,12] Research shows that cytokine induction by *P. acnes* occurs through TLR-2, which stimulates inflammatory lesions. In acne, TLR-2 invokes a significant inflammatory response as well as cellular apoptosis and tissue injury.[13] Redness and inflammation in and around the follicular canal constitute a papule (Figure 37–1E). A pustule (Figure 37–1F; see also Color Plates, photograph 23) possesses the same qualities as a papule but has visible purulence in the center of the lesion. Nodules result from disruption of the

follicular wall and release of its contents into the surrounding dermis.[14]

Several factors contribute to the exacerbation of existing acne and cause periodic flare-ups of acne in some patients (Table 37–1).[6,10,15] Recent information about the molecular function of the sebaceous glands has helped explain the role of these glands in skin function.[16]

Diet as a cause of acne flare-ups has been speculated on and dismissed in the past. However, recent research does show a link between diet and acne.[10,12,17] Several epidemiologic studies have correlated acne with the Western diet.[18] In a 2002 study with 1300 patients from two non-Westernized societies who had their skin examined by a general practitioner trained in diagnosing acne, no cases of acne were found. Researchers concluded that this finding must be related to the societies' diet. Several studies comparing the diets of Western civilizations to non-Westernized cultures have made similar correlations. The non-Westernized civilization had low-glycemic-load diets. These diets do not include refined cereals, chips, cookies, and bread.[19] Foods with a high-glycemic load elevate plasma concentrations of insulin, which regulates insulin-like growth factor-1 (IGF-1) and IGF-binding protein, promotes unregulated tissue growth, and enhances androgen synthesis. Hormones, such as androgens and IGF-1, act on sebaceous glands and keratinocytes. Dietary milk also causes a rise in IGF-1 through a high rise in blood glucose and serum insulin levels.[20] Newer research discusses the role of diet and medication in controlling acne.[12] Melnik discusses the role of mammalian target of rapamycin complex 1 (mTORC1) as a nutrient-derived signal involved in the exacerbation of acne through diet. The mTORC1 signal is activated in the presence of foods with a high glycemic load, high fat intake, high dairy intake, and high meat consumption. These foods are characteristic of foods found in the Western diet.[21] The mTORC1 kinase integrates signals of cellular energy, growth factors (insulin, IGF-1), and protein-derived signals, predominantly leucine, which is

table
37–1   Exacerbating Factors in Acne

Factor	Description of Factor
Acne mechanica	Local irritation or friction from occlusive clothing, headbands, helmets, or other friction-producing devices Excessive contact between face and hands, such as resting the chin or cheek on the hand
Excoriated acne	A form of acne caused by constant picking, squeezing, or scratching at the skin. This causes the acne to look worse
Acne cosmetic	Noninflammatory comedones on the face, chin, and cheek caused by occlusion of the pilosebaceous unit by oil-based cosmetics, moisturizers, pomades, or other health and beauty products
Chloracne	An acneiform eruption caused by exposure to chlorine compounds
Occupational acne	Exposure to dirt, vaporized cooking oils, or certain industrial chemicals, such as coal tar and petroleum derivatives
Drug-induced acne	Anabolic steroids, corticosteroids, isoniazid, lithium, phenytoin
Stress and emotional extremes	May induce expression of neuroendocrine modulators and release of CRH, which play a role in centrally and topically induced stress of the sebaceous glands and possibly progression of acne[6]
High-humidity environments and prolonged sweating	Hydration-induced decrease in size of pilosebaceous duct orifice and prevention of loosening of comedone
Hormonal alterations	Increased androgen levels induced by medical conditions, pregnancy, or medications

Key: CRH = Corticotrophin-releasing hormone.
Source: References 6, 10, and 15.

provided in high amounts by milk proteins and meat with resultant increases in androgen and sebum production, respectively, which further perpetuates the pathogenesis of acne.[21] Melnik goes on to explain that the role of diet in acne pathogenesis is still controversial. However, the discovery of nutrient signaling pathways, like mTORC1, help explain the link between diet and acne exacerbation.

Clinical Presentation of Acne

Acne lesions can generally be classified as noninflammatory or inflammatory. Noninflammatory lesions consist of either open or closed comedones. These lesions are often the first to manifest in the early stages of puberty and often appear initially on the forehead. With the progression of puberty and with age, especially in women, lesions tend to appear on areas of the body below the neck, such as the chest and back. Women in their 30s and 40s not uncommonly have acne that is concentrated on the chin and along the jaw line. Inflammatory lesions are further characterized as papules, pustules, or nodules. On presentation to a provider, the patient may exhibit one or more types of lesions. Acne severity is defined by the number and type of acne lesions. The Food and Drug Administration (FDA) has called on industry to develop a global grading acne system for accessing overall acne severity. FDA noted that a number of acne grading systems exist with small differences between them or inadequately defined grades of severity. Table 37–2 describes the recommended comprehensive acne grading scale.[22]

table 37–2	Assessment of Acne Severity
Grade of Acne	**Description**
0	Clear skin with no inflammatory or non-inflammatory lesions
1	Almost clear; rare noninflammatory lesions with no more than one small inflammatory lesion
2	Mild severity; greater than Grade 1; some noninflammatory lesions with no more than a few inflammatory lesions (papules/pustules only, no nodular lesions)
3	Moderate severity; greater than Grade 2; up to many noninflammatory lesions and may have some inflammatory lesions, but no more than one small nodular lesion
4	Severe; greater than Grade 3; up to many noninflammatory and inflammatory lesions, but no more than a few nodular lesions

Source: Reference 22.

Note: The Case Report Forms for acne studies can allow for reporting by investigators of lesions worsening beyond grade 4 with treatment. It is recommended that enrollment of acne vulgaris patients not include patients with nodulocystic acne. Patients who worsen beyond grade 4 are to be described in the safety evaluation.

If acne lesions persist beyond the mid-20s or develop in the mid-20s or later, the symptoms may signal rosacea, rather than acne vulgaris. A differential diagnosis is necessary because the treatment of rosacea, although similar to that for acne, has unique elements.

Complications associated with acne include scarring and negative psychosocial impact. An acute complication of acne is postinflammatory erythema or hyperpigmentation.[4]

Treatment of Acne

In most cases, acne is self-limiting and can be controlled to varying degrees. Adherence to therapeutic regimens will reduce symptoms and minimize scarring. Because acne persists for long periods, treatment must be long term, continuous, and consistent.

Treatment Goals

Patients and providers should identify any exacerbating factors of acne (Table 37–1). It is also imperative that patients and providers classify the acne (Table 37–2) to allow selection of the most appropriate therapeutic options.[23–25] Once the classification has been determined, treatment should be initiated and adherence to medication therapy should be encouraged.[10]

General Treatment Approach

Zaenglein and Thiboutot recommend that one or more acne treatments, either topical or topical and systemic, be combined to target a greater number of pathogenic factors.[26] The treatment of acne depends on the severity of the disease (Table 37–2). Patients with mild-moderate acne may self-treat with nonprescription topical products. Topical antimicrobial products are just as efficacious as oral antimicrobial agents in patients with moderate acne.[27] Oral antibiotics should be reserved for more severe cases of acne. Patients under the care of a provider should be instructed to avoid use of nonprescription products unless the provider recommends their use. Combining some nonprescription products with prescription acne drugs may decrease a patient's ability to tolerate prescribed topical drugs.

Nonpharmacologic Therapy

Patients with acne should eliminate exacerbating factors of acne (Table 37–1). This measure should promote understanding and prevention of the disease as well as adherence to therapy. Patients seeking self-care options should cleanse the skin with a mild soap or nonsoap cleanser twice daily. The use of abrasive products and excessive cleansing may worsen the acne. Self-care options should also include staying well hydrated. Dehydration may increase the inflammatory chemicals in the cell and may cause dysfunction in the natural desquamation process of the stratum corneum. Decker and Graber explain that the normal skin has a pH of 5.3–5.9. Washing the face with harsh soaps that can increase the pH by at least 2.0 units can cause skin dryness and create an environment for growth of *P. acnes*.[1] Patients should also consider dietary changes by eliminating or cutting back on high-glycemic-load foods to determine whether the acne improves or remains the same.[12]

Physical Treatments

Physical treatments have increased in popularity (Table 37–3).[1,28] A wide range of self-applied, acrylate glue–based material strips can aid in the extraction of impacted comedones. These products are a better alternative to picking the acne, which can result in scarring.[29] Professional comedo extraction is a useful adjunct to the overall acne regimen and often results in immediate improvement; the risks include tissue damage or scarring if these procedures are not done correctly. In addition, FDA has approved several light-based therapies for the treatment of acne. These treatments target reduction of *P. acnes* and disruption of sebaceous gland function. *P. acnes* produce porphyrin compounds during normal metabolism. Porphyrins absorb visible light at a variety of wavelengths, which excites the porphyrin compound, causing oxygen and free radicals. The oxygen radicals are thought to destroy *P. acnes* by damaging lipids in the cell wall of the organism.[10] For now, light therapy is considered a device to be used in conjunction with traditional pharmacologic therapy for acne.[17] More well-designed trials that include light therapy as a standard of treatment are needed.[10,17]

Pharmacologic Therapy

Topical therapy is the standard of care in acne treatment.[30] Health care providers should be familiar with the several nonprescription products available for treatment of acne.

Benzoyl Peroxide

Many are familiar with benzoyl peroxide (BP), the most common topical antibiotic acne product available both with and without a prescription. BP has keratolytic, comedolytic, and antibacterial properties against skin *P. acnes*. BP kills bacteria by introducing oxygen into the environment, thereby killing *P. acnes*, which can thrive only in an oxygen-free environment.

BP has been the mainstay of treatment for type I acne since the 1930s.[1] In March 2010, FDA issued a final rule for topical acne drug products that included BP as a generally recognized as safe and effective (Category I) active ingredient in nonprescription topical acne product. BP had been classified as Category III since 1995 because of concern about benzoyl's weak mutagenic effect in vitro and BP's tumor promotion potential. FDA concluded that BP in concentrations of 2.5%–10% should be switched from class III to class I based on animal studies that suggest BP is not carcinogenic or photocarcinogenic.[31]

BP has the ability to prevent or eliminate the development of treatment resistance by *P. acnes*, which has increased with the use of conventional antibiotics (macrolides and tetracyclines) over the last three decades.[16,30] Resistant strains have been found in 50% of acne patients who had close contact with a resistant organism.[16] *Close contact* is defined as those individuals living in the same household with family members with acne. The use of BP in combination with antibiotics has been recommended to minimize *P. acnes* resistance.[16] BP is often used in combination with other oral or topical antibiotics. In a recent literature review, BP was more effective than topical antibiotics such as clindamycin and erythromycin. In addition, BP in combination with either of these antibiotics was more effective and better tolerated than either of the antibiotics alone.[16]

Nonprescription formulations of BP are available in concentrations of 2.5%–10%. Higher strengths of BP have the same antibacterial effects as the lower strengths.[1] Higher strengths may cause more skin irritation.[17] All new users of nonprescription acne products should test the product by applying it sparingly to one or two small affected areas over the first 3 days. If discomfort does not occur, the product should be used according to label directions.[31] Avoidance of contact with clothes or hair is advised because this product may cause bleaching. In addition, avoidance of excessive sun exposure and use of a sunscreen product are recommended. Minor improvement may occur with daily application of BP; the number of applications can be increased or decreased until a mild peeling occurs. Some patients may experience only mild erythema and scaling during the first few days, which usually subside within 1 or 2 weeks. Allergic contact dermatitis reactions, characterized by a sudden onset of erythema and vesiculation, are considered rare and occur in a minority of the population (1 in 500).[1] A 2014 FDA Drug Safety Communication reported rare but serious allergic reactions to BP and salicylic acid that ranged from symptoms of local irritation to local and systemic hypersensitivity, including anaphylaxis.[32] FDA has not determined if the products active ingredients, inactive ingredients, or both are responsible for these reactions. Use of BP products should be discontinued when

table 37–3	Description of Physical Treatments
Implement	**Treatment**
Scrubs	Abrasion opens closed comedones and prevents their progression. However, the abrasive nature of this action could damage the integrity of the skin.
Cleansing cloth	Cloths are less abrasive than scrubs while providing conditioning and exfoliation of the skin.
Cosmetic adhesive pads	Pads were developed to remove adherent corneocytes, dirt, oil, or loosen open comedones from the skin.
Brushes	Oscillating motion of the brush is used to deeply cleanse the skin while removing makeup. The impact of this treatment has not been clinically evaluated.
Heating devices	Heating devices are marketed to directly treat AV by contacting the lesion. The device is thought to treat acne through heat and phototherapy.
Light therapy	Use of limited-spectrum wavelength, such as blue light (peak at 415 nm) and mixed blue and red light (peak at 415 and 660 nm) has been found to be effective in reducing acne lesions after 4–12 weeks.

Source: References 1 and 28.

an allergic reaction such as itching or hives occurs. Medical attention should be sought for hypersensitivity reactions such as throat tightness; difficulty breathing; feeling faint; or swelling of the eyes, face, lips, or tongue. The box Patient Education for Acne lists other precautions for use of BP.

Other FDA–approved topical anti–acne ingredients include hydroxy acids in various strengths, sulfur 3%–10% (in single-ingredient products), and a combination of sulfur 3%–8% with either resorcinol 2% or resorcinol monoacetate 3%.[33,34]

Hydroxy Acids

Keratolytic agents such as alpha hydroxy acids (AHAs) and beta hydroxy acids (BHAs) are also common nonprescription acne

---

patient education for
Acne

The goal of self-treatment is to control mild acne, thereby preventing more serious forms from developing. Acne usually goes away without treatment. Symptoms can usually be managed with diligent and long-term treatment. The best approaches to controlling acne are using cleansers and medications to keep the pores open and avoiding situations that worsen acne. For most patients, carefully following product instructions and the self-care measures listed here will help ensure optimal therapeutic outcomes.

Disease Information

- Acne is the result of several pathologic processes that occur within the pilosebaceous unit located in the dermis, or middle layer of the skin.
- Acne can be controlled by using certain medications, but it cannot be cured.

Nondrug and Preventive Measures

- Cleanse skin thoroughly but gently twice daily to produce a mild drying effect that loosens comedones. Use a mild, oil-free cleanser and warm water.
- To prevent or minimize acne flare-ups, avoid or reduce exposure to environmental factors such as dirt, dust, petroleum products, cooking oils, or chemical irritants.
- To prevent friction or irritation that may cause acne flare-ups, do not wear tight-fitting clothes, headbands, or helmets; avoid resting the chin on the hand.
- To minimize acne related to cosmetic use, do not use oil-based cosmetics and shampoos.
- To prevent excessive hydration of the skin, which can cause flare-ups, avoid areas of high humidity. In addition, do not wear tight-fitting clothes that restrict air movement.
- Avoid stressful situations when possible and practice stress-management techniques. Stress can worsen existing acne.
- Do not pick or squeeze pimples, which can further irritate skin and possibly lead to worsening of acne and scarring.
- Note that sexual activity plays no role in the occurrence or worsening of acne, although the onset of sexual activity and occurrence of acne may be simultaneous or take place within the same time span.

Nonprescription Medications

- Most common available nonprescription products contain BP, salicylic acid, or sulfur, and they come in a variety of formulations (e.g., cleansers, creams, gels, and astringents).
- BP is the most effective and widely used nonprescription medication for treating acne.

Benzoyl Peroxide

- BP inhibits the growth of *Propionibacterium acnes,* the bacteria involved in acne development; it also helps unclog pores by causing a mild peeling effect.
- Do not use BP if you have very sensitive skin or are sensitive to BP.
- When using this product, avoid unnecessary sun exposure and use a sunscreen.
- Avoid contact of BP with eyes, lips, mouth, and nose, as well as cuts, scrapes, and other abrasions, to avoid possible excessive irritation.
- Avoid contact of BP with hair and dyed fabrics, which may be bleached by this product.

- Skin irritation, characterized by redness, burning, itching, peeling, or possibly swelling, may occur with the recommended treatment regimen. Irritation may be reduced by using the product less frequently or in a lower concentration.
- Note that use of other acne medications with this product may cause excessive dryness and peeling. Do this only as directed by a health care provider.
- After the initial 1–2 weeks of treatment, applications can be increased up to 2–3 times per day over a period of 2–3 days, as tolerated.
- Slight improvement may be noticed in as little as a few days, but maximum effectiveness may take up to 4–6 weeks of continued use.
- If treatment is tolerated, but the problem persists, the strength may be increased to 5% after 1 week and to 10% after 2 weeks, if necessary.
- Continue the treatment regimen even after lesions have cleared to prevent the formation of new ones.

Salicylic Acid

- Salicylic acid helps unclog pores by causing slight peeling.
- This medication is less effective than BP.
- Salicylic acid can be used once or twice daily as a cleanser or as a topical gel.
- Gel formulations should be applied to only the affected area.
- If excessive peeling occurs, limit use to once daily or every other day.
- Salicylic acid may cause sun sensitivity, so use a sunscreen (see the previous section Benzoyl Peroxide).
- Maximum effectiveness and duration of use are similar to those of BP.
- Lack of response after 6 weeks is an indication of need for medical referral.

Sulfur

- Sulfur is believed to work by inhibiting the growth of *P. acnes.*
- This medication can be applied 1–3 times daily, but its use is limited by its chalky yellow color and characteristic unpleasant odor.
- Use of sulfur is mostly adjunctive; it is not as effective as BP.
- Do not use in patients with allergy to sulfa drugs.

When to Seek Medical Attention

- If severe skin irritation or sensitivity develops, stop use of BP and sunscreen, and see a health care provider.
- If improvement has not occurred after 6 weeks of treatment with BP, seek medical evaluation.
- If you experience tightness in the throat; breathing problems; feeling faint; or swelling of the eyes, face, tongue, or lips with use of either BP or salicylic acid, seek emergency medical attention.

products. Hydroxy acids are considered less potent and are often used when patients cannot tolerate other topical acne products.[30] Some hydroxy acids have comedolytic properties and are moderately effective in the treatment of acne.[16]

AHAs are natural exfoliating acids that occur in sugar cane, milk products, and fruits; the most common AHAs are glycolic, lactic, and citric acids, respectively.[1] AHAs are not able to penetrate the pilosebaceous unit to cause a comedolytic effect. AHAs are available in several nonprescription formulations in concentrations of 4%–10% or through dermatologists at higher concentrations. In a study comparing BP with AHAs, BP demonstrated a superior effect at 8 weeks. However, once acne is controlled, a light chemical peel with AHAs may be useful to help correct scarring and hyperpigmentation.[16]

Polyhydroxyl acids are a new category of AHA that has fewer side effects such as irritation and stinging. They are marketed for patients with more clinical sensitivity. They are also said to have moisturizing and humectant properties.[1] Lactobionic acid has been said to inhibit the breakdown of matrix metalloproteinase enzymes that occurs because of sun exposure. This reduces the appearance of photoaging on the skin.[1]

Salicylic acid, often described as a BHA, is a comedolytic agent available in various nonprescription acne products in concentrations of 0.5%–2%.[1,17] The comedolytic effect is concentration dependent. Higher concentrations are used for prescriptions and chemical peels.[1] Salicylic acid provides a milder, less-effective alternative to prescription agents such as topical retinoids.[17] In cleansing preparations, salicylic acid is considered adjunctive treatment. This agent is a phytohormone and is chemically similar to the active component of aspirin. Salicylic acid is lipid soluble and able to penetrate the pilosebaceous unit to produce a comedolytic effect.[17] Salicylic acid products also offer protection from the sun by inhibiting ultraviolet radiation B (UVB)-induced formation of sunburn cells that occurs after the cell has been exposed to UVB rays that cause an irreversible damage the cell's DNA and by increasing the removal of UVB-induced dimers (premutagenic lesions) in living skin equivalents.[17] However, patients using these products should continue to wear a broad-spectrum sunscreen to protect skin from further skin damage. BHA products are contraindicated in diabetic patients or patients with poor blood circulation. Use of these products should be limited to the affected area. Use of the products over a large area for prolonged periods could result in toxicity. Signs of salicylate toxicity include nausea, vomiting, dizziness, loss of hearing, tinnitus, lethargy, hyperpnea, diarrhea, psychic disturbances, toxic inner ear damage,

hypoglycemia, and hypersensitivity.[17] In 2014, FDA warned of potentially life-threatening hypersensitivity reactions for nonprescription acne products containing salicylic acid or BP (see section Benzoyl Peroxide).[32]

Sulfur

Sulfur, precipitated or colloidal, is included in acne products as a keratolytic and antibacterial in concentrations of 3%–10%.[1,34] It is generally accepted as effective in promoting the resolution of existing comedones but, on continued use, may have a comedogenic effect. Alternative forms of sulfur such as sodium thiosulfate, zinc sulfate, and zinc sulfide are not recognized as safe and effective.

Side effects with these products are rare but include the noticeable odor and dry skin, depending on the formulation used.[17] Sulfur is usually combined with other topical nonprescription agents such as resorcinol.[1]

Sulfur/Resorcinol

Combinations of sulfur 3%–8% with resorcinol 2% or resorcinol monoacetate 3%, which enhances the effect of sulfur, are available in nonprescription acne products.[17,34] The products function primarily as keratolytics, fostering cell turnover and desquamation. Resorcinol is not effective when used as a monotherapy. However, it is believed to have antibacterial, antifungal, and keratolytic effects when used with other anti-acne products such as sulfur.[1] Resorcinol produces a reversible, dark brown scale on some darker-skinned individuals.[17]

Pharmacotherapeutic Comparison

Table 37–4 provides a comparison of the therapeutic properties of the major acne products.[1,24,34,35]

Product Selection Guidelines

Skin cleansers and topical acne products are available in a variety of vehicles and strengths. Medicated cleansing products (bars and liquids) are not of much value; they leave little active ingredient residue on the skin. Generally, gels are the most effective formulations because they are astringents and remain on the skin the longest. Gels and solutions have a drying effect that may sometimes cause contact dermatitis. However, these dosage forms are not greasy and may be more beneficial in patients with oily

table
37–4   Comparison of Nonprescription Topical Acne Agents

	Benzoyl Peroxide	Hydroxy Acids	Sulfur	Resorcinol
Bactericidal	Yes	No	No	Yes (also has antifungal properties)
Keratolytic	Yes	Yes	Yes	Yes
Comedolytic	Yes	Yes (BHAs)	Yes	No
Concentration	2.5%–10%	0.5%–2%	3%–10%	2% 3%–8% (in combination with sulfur)

Key: BHA = Beta hydroxy acid.
Source: References 1, 24, 34, and 35.

skin. Creams and lotions are generally less irritating to the skin compared with gels and solutions. Lotions and creams with a low fat content are intended to counteract drying (astringent effect) and peeling (keratolytic effect).[36] They are acceptable alternatives to the more-effective gels and are recommended for dry or sensitive skin and for use during dry winter weather. Ointment vehicles are not used because they are occlusive and tend to worsen acne. Patients should start with the lowest strength available and gradually increase the concentration to minimize the irritating effects of the product. Table 37–5 lists selected nonprescription trade-name acne products in these and other formulations.

Many patients will use nonprescription medications in combination with prescription products to manage acne. Product selection is important for the successful treatment and management of acne. It is important that patients seek medical referral for proper diagnosis and grading of acne. For example, women who experience acne related to hormonal imbalance may benefit more from correction of the imbalance with hormone therapy such as oral contraceptives, whereas a peripubertal teenager or young adult may benefit more from consultation on avoidance of comedogenic products and adherence with nonprescription products such as BP.[29]

Special Populations

Pregnant patients may have problems with acne because of hormonal imbalances. In most cases, if pregnancy occurs during treatment with any acne medication, the medication should be discontinued and the obstetrician should be advised of current or previous product use because of the potential for teratogenic effects. Topical BP, sulfur, and hydroxy acids are all Pregnancy Category C.[1,37]

Acne occurs in all age groups, including the pediatric population. This population comprises neonates, infants, and young children. Most infantile and neonatal acne is self-limiting; however, differential diagnoses by appropriate health care providers, which may include a pediatric endocrinologist, are needed for treatment recommendations. The first detailed evidenced-based clinical guidelines by the American Acne and Rosacea Society were endorsed by the American Academy of Pediatrics and published in May 2013.[38]

Complementary Medicine, Vitamins, and Vitamin Analogues

Tea tree oil is widely known for its antibacterial and antifungal properties. *Staphylococcus aureus,* a common pathogen found on the skin, is sensitive to tea tree oil. Tea tree oil also has anti-inflammatory properties.[1] Terpen-4-ol, the active ingredient in tea tree oil, has been postulated to suppress production of inflammatory mediators and inflammation.[1]

Oral zinc may be considered an alternative to tetracyclines.[16,17] Zinc is bacteriostatic against *P. acnes,* inhibits chemotaxis, and has shown effectiveness against severe acne. One study found that zinc was 17% less effective than minocycline but that zinc could be used as an alternative to tetracycline therapy, especially in the summer, because it does not cause phototoxicity. However, zinc's adverse effects of nausea, vomiting, and diarrhea have made it a less attractive therapy. Poor patient compliance as a result of these side effects has limited its use.

table 37–5	**Selected Nonprescription Acne Products**	
Benzoyl Peroxide Products		
Proactiv Repairing Treatment		Benzoyl peroxide 2.5%
ZAPZYT Maximum Strength 10% Benzoyl Peroxide Acne Treatment Gel		Benzoyl peroxide 10%
PanOxyl Acne Foaming Wash 10% Benzoyl Peroxide		Benzoyl peroxide 10%
Salicylic Acid Products		
Neutrogena Oil-Free Acne Stress Control Salicylic Acid Acne Treatment, Power-Foam Wash		Salicylic acid 0.5%
Olay Total Effects Blemish Control Salicylic Acid Acne Cleanser		Salicylic acid 2%
NeoStrata Bionic Face Cream		Gluconolactone 8%; lactobionic acid 4%
Alpha Hydroxy Acid Products		
Alpha Hydrox AHA Souffle 12% Glycolic AHA		Glycolic acid
Gly Derm Lotion Lite		Glycolic acid
Alpha/Beta Hydroxy Acid Products		
M.D. Forte Skin Rejuvenation Hydra-Masque		Glycolic acid; salicylic acid
Polyhydroxy Acid Product		
NeoStrata Bionic Face Cream		Gluconolactone 8%; lactobionic acid 4%
Sulfur Product		
De La Cruz Sulfur Ointment 10% Acne Medication Ointment		Sulfur 10%
Sulfur/Resorcinol Product		
Clearasil Stayclear Acne Treatment Cream, Sulfur Resorcinol Medication		Resorcinol 2%; sulfur 8%
Physical Treatments		
Olay Pro-X Advanced Cleansing System, Brush		Acne brush
Garnier Skin Care Clean+ Refreshing Remover Cleansing Towelettes, cleansing cloth		Cleansing cloth
Zeno Heat Treat Blemish Prevention Kit		Heat therapy
Bioré Deep Cleansing Pore Strips		Comedone extraction strip
Proactiv Clearzone Acne Clearing Device		Light therapy

Vitamin A is naturally occurring and is a retinol. Vitamin A is transformed into several metabolites. One metabolite, retinoic acid, is used in cosmetics to help eliminate wrinkles and fine lines. Theoretically, retinol should also work against acne. However, few studies exist to validate this claim. Oral vitamin A or retinol may be beneficial in acne in doses up to 300,000 units daily for women and 500,000 daily for men. Common adverse effects include xerosis and chelitis. Nicotinamide is used both orally and topically for AV. Nicotinamide is an active form of niacin and has been postulated to have several roles in the treatment of acne. It is an anti-inflammatory that improves the texture of photoaged skin and decreases sebum production.[39] Data on nicotinamide's role in acne are still limited, and more research needs to be facilitated to assess the role of nicotinamide in acne.

Assessment of Acne: A Case-Based Approach

Patient assessment begins with asking questions to define the condition. Physical assessment, which involves observing the affected area and questioning the patient further, is the next step in evaluating the disorder. This evaluation helps determine whether the condition is acne vulgaris or another dermatologic condition with similar signs and symptoms. Physical assessment also determines whether the severity of the condition precludes self-treatment (Figure 37–2). Before self-care is

recommended, an assessment of current medication use (prescription and nonprescription) is necessary to reveal prescribed treatments for the disorder or use of medications known to cause acne (Table 37–1).

Cases 37–1 and 37–2 are examples of assessment of patients presenting with acne.

Patient Counseling for Acne

The success of the treatment regimen depends largely on the patient. Therefore, it is crucial that the provider educate the patient on the causes of acne, correct any misconceptions, and clearly explain the rationale for treatment. Patient buy-in will facilitate adherence and increase the likelihood of a successful outcome. The provider must also evaluate the patient's maturity and willingness to comply with a skin care program that involves a continued daily regimen of washing affected areas and applying medication. Reassurance and emotional support are

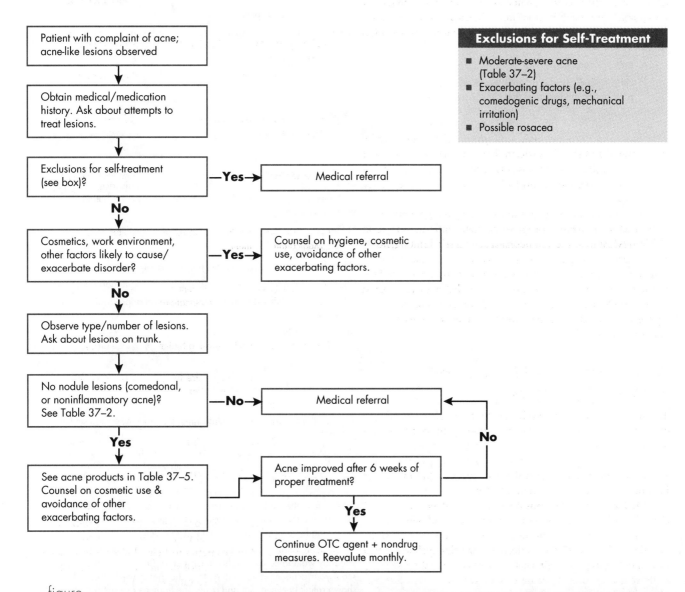

figure 37–2 Self-care of acne. Key: OTC = Over-the-counter.

case
37–1

Relevant Evaluation Criteria	Scenario/Model Outcome

Information Gathering

1. Gather essential information about the patient's symptoms and medical history, including:

   a. description of symptom(s) (i.e., nature, onset, duration, severity, associated symptoms)

   Patient has come into the pharmacy complaining of breakouts on the forehead over the last 3 weeks. He describes them as small bumps on his forehead.

   b. description of any factors that seem to precipitate, exacerbate, and/or relieve the patient's symptom(s)

   He complains that this started once it got warm outside. He started baseball season and needs to wear his uniform and hat. He noticed the acne about 3 weeks ago, and he cannot seem to get a handle on his breakouts.

   c. description of the patient's efforts to relieve the symptoms

   He says that he is now washing his face with soap and water about 4 or 5 times a day to keep it clean, but the acne seems worse.

   d. patient's identity

   Dylan McGhee

   e. age, sex, height, and weight

   16 years old, male, 6 ft 1 in., 185 lb

   f. patient's occupation

   Student and baseball player

   g. patient's dietary habits

   Eats healthy for dinner. Usually eats whatever he has time to eat for breakfast and lunch.

   h. patient's sleep habits

   Stays up late studying.

   i. concurrent medical conditions, prescription and non-prescription medications, and dietary supplements

   NA

   j. allergies

   NKDA

Assessment and Triage

2. Differentiate patient's signs/symptoms and correctly identify the patient's primary problem(s).

   Exacerbation of acne could be caused by patient's baseball cap that is worn during baseball season. Patient also washes his face very often and uses a soap that could be very drying, hence contributing to his worsening acne.

3. Identify exclusions for self-treatment (Figure 37–2).

   None

4. Formulate a comprehensive list of therapeutic alternatives for the primary problem to determine if triage to a medical provider is required, and share this information with the patient or caregiver.

   Options include:

   (1) Refer Dylan to an appropriate health care provider.

   (2) Recommend self-care with an OTC product and nondrug measures.

   (3) Recommend self-care until Dylan can see an appropriate health care provider.

   (4) Take no action.

Plan

5. Select an optimal therapeutic alternative to address the patient's problem, taking into account patient preferences.

   Recommend self-care options to Dylan.

6. Describe the recommended therapeutic approach to the patient or caregiver.

   "Try a self-care option that includes nondrug measures and an OTC product."

7. Explain to the patient or caregiver the rationale for selecting the recommended therapeutic approach from the considered therapeutic alternatives.

   "Your acne could be caused by the baseball cap. The cap may occlude your skin and cause your pores to clog with sweat and oil. Try removing your cap or wearing a looser cap during games. You should remove your cap when you are not in the sun. You could also try benzoyl peroxide 2.5% to treat the existing acne and prevent new acne. I also recommend that you wash your face twice a day with a mild cleanser. Soap may be too drying for your skin and could make your acne worse."

   "In addition, although your diet is typical of young adults your age, you may want to consider a healthier diet for breakfast and lunch to see if your acne improves with dietary changes as well. Research has shown a link between diet and acne. The findings are still controversial, but some patients may find that changing their diet helps improve their acne symptoms."

case
37-1 *continued*

Relevant Evaluation Criteria	Scenario/Model Outcome
Patient Education	

8. When recommending self-care with nonprescription medications and/or nondrug therapy, convey accurate information to the patient or caregiver:

a. appropriate dose and frequency of administration	See the box Patient Education for Acne.
b. maximum number of days the therapy should be employed	See the box Patient Education for Acne.
c. product administration procedures	See the box Patient Education for Acne.
d. expected time to onset of relief	See the box Patient Education for Acne.
e. degree of relief that can be reasonably expected	"Slight improvement may be noticed in as little as a few days, but maximum effectiveness may take up to 6 weeks of continued use."
f. most common side effects	See the box Patient Education for Acne.
g. side effects that warrant medical intervention should they occur	"If severe irritation or sensitivity develops, stop use of BP and sunscreen, and see a health care provider."
h. patient options in the event that condition worsens or persists	"If your acne worsens, see a health care provider."
i. product storage requirements	See the box Patient Education for Acne.
j. specific nondrug measures	See the box Patient Education for Acne.
Solicit follow-up questions from the patient or caregiver.	"Can I use the higher strength of benzoyl peroxide to get rid of the acne faster?"
Answer the patient's or caregiver's questions.	"Studies have shown that lower strengths of benzoyl peroxide are just as effective as higher strengths. You should start with the lowest strength first to avoid irritation of your skin."

Relevant Evaluation Criteria	Scenario/Model Outcome
Evaluation of Patient Outcome	
9. Assess patient outcome.	Contact the patient in 3 weeks to see if he has noticed any improvement in his acne symptoms. Ask him to call in 6 weeks to discuss whether his acne symptoms are controlled.

Key: BP = Benzoyl peroxide; NA = not applicable; NKDA = no known drug allergies; OTC = over-the-counter.

case
37-2

Relevant Evaluation Criteria	Scenario/Model Outcome
Information Gathering	

1. Gather essential information about the patient's symptoms and medical history, including:

a. description of symptom(s) (i.e., nature, onset, duration, severity, associated symptoms)	Patient has come into the pharmacy for advice on recurrent facial acne.
b. description of any factors that seem to precipitate, exacerbate, and/or relieve the patient's symptom(s)	She always had occasional acne that coincided with her menstrual cycle. However, now that she is pregnant, her acne seems out of control.
c. description of the patient's efforts to relieve the symptoms	She has not really tried anything yet.
d. patient's identity	Daphne Turner
e. age, sex, height, and weight	28 years old, female, 5 ft 5 in., 145 lb
f. patient's occupation	Teacher
g. patient's dietary habits	Normal healthy diet with a recent occasional increase in cravings for ice cream
h. patient's sleep habits	Sleeps well. Her bedtime is 10:30 pm.

case
37–2 continued

Relevant Evaluation Criteria	Scenario/Model Outcome
i. concurrent medical conditions, prescription and non-prescription medications, and dietary supplements	Prenatal vitamin once a day
j. allergies	Penicillin
k. history of other adverse reactions to medications	None
l. other (describe) _____	NA

Assessment and Triage

2. Differentiate patient's signs/symptoms and correctly identify the patient's primary problem(s).	Patient's acne may have flared because of pregnancy and fluctuation in hormones.
3. Identify exclusions for self-treatment (Figure 37–2).	Pregnancy
4. Formulate a comprehensive list of therapeutic alternatives for the primary problem to determine if triage to a medical provider is required, and share this information with the patient or caregiver.	Options include: (1) Refer Daphne to an appropriate health care provider. (2) Recommend self-care with an OTC product and nondrug measures. (3) Recommend self-care. (4) Take no action.

Plan

5. Select an optimal therapeutic alternative to address the patient's problem, taking into account patient preferences.	Refer Daphne to an appropriate health care provider.
6. Describe the recommended therapeutic approach to the patient or caregiver.	"Most over-the-counter and prescription drugs for acne may not be safe for you to use during pregnancy."
7. Explain to the patient or caregiver the rationale for selecting the recommended therapeutic approach from the considered therapeutic alternatives.	"You should talk to your health care provider for recommendations on how to treat your acne. Most over-the-counter drugs used for acne are a Pregnancy Category C drug. You will need to talk with a health care provider to determine which drugs may be safe for you during pregnancy."

Patient Education

8. When recommending self-care with nonprescription medications and/or nondrug therapy, convey accurate information to the patient or caregiver:	Criterion does not apply in this case.
Solicit follow-up questions from the patient or caregiver.	"Can I use some of the acne towelettes on my skin?"
Answer the patient's or caregiver's questions.	"You should still consult your health care provider because some of the towelettes have medication on them that could be absorbed by your skin."

Evaluation of Patient Outcome

9. Assess patient outcome.	Contact the patient in 3 days to see whether she was able to set up an appointment with her health care provider.

Key: NA = Not applicable; OTC = over-the-counter.

often necessary to reduce patient concern because acne cannot be cured—only controlled. The box Patient Education for Acne lists specific information to provide patients.

The Internet lists supplemental information about acne in lay language, including discussions of acne, nonprescription drugs used to treat it, and treatment expectations. Selected sites that appear to provide accurate information are listed in Table 37–6. If not copyrighted, these materials can be printed and given to the patient during the consultation. If the material is copyrighted, the provider should instead give the patient the Web site address.

table
37–6 Selected Web Sites for Acne Information

Organizations	Web Site
Acne.com	www.acne.com
Acne.org	www.acne.org
Food and Drug Administration	www.fda.gov

Evaluation of Patient Outcomes for Acne

Although the patient may expect complete resolution of the acne, an improvement in the disorder, as defined by a decrease in both the number and severity of lesions, is a more realistic expectation for effective self-treatment. The provider should determine whether patients whose acne shows no improvement after 6 weeks of self-treatment or 6 months with diet change are following the recommended regimen. If they have been adherent, medical referral is appropriate. Patients who have not diligently followed the regimen should be encouraged to do so. The provider should again explain the expected results and the rigor with which treatment must be pursued. If some improvement is evident, the provider may suggest monthly follow-up to check for improvement in the condition and potential adjustment of the maintenance regimen.

Key Points for Acne

➤ Acne cannot be cured, but it may be controlled enough to improve cosmetic appearance and prevent development of severe acne with resultant scarring.

➤ Adherence to any regimen to treat acne is a crucial factor in achieving a successful outcome.

➤ Minimizing environmental and physical factors that exacerbate acne can help limit the extent of the condition.

➤ Pharmacologic and nonpharmacologic therapies should be tailored to the patient.

➤ According to current guidelines, medical referral is the preferred initial step before implementing nonprescription therapy.

➤ Some people have chronic acne into adulthood and must care for their skin for a long time before improvement will occur.

➤ If given proper counseling, including empathy and reassurance, patients with acne may understand that the condition may not exist forever.

REFERENCES

1. Decker A, Graber EM. Over-the-counter acne treatments. *J Clin Aesthetic Dermatol*. 2012;5(5):32–40.
2. Purdy S, de Berker D. Acne vulgaris. *Clin Evid* (Online). 2011 Jan 5;2011.
3. Collier CN, Harper JC, Cafardi JA, et al. The prevalence of acne in adults 20 years and older. *J Am Acad Dermatol*. 2008;58(1):56–9.
4. Yan AC. Current concepts in acne management. *Adolesc Med Clin*. 2006; 17(3):613–37; abstract x–xi.
5. Keri J, Shiman M. An update on the management of acne vulgaris. *Clin Cosmet Investig Dermatol CCID*. 2009;2:105–10.
6. Bickers DR, Lim HW, Margolis D. The burden of skin diseases: 2004 a joint project of the American Academy of Dermatology Association and the Society for Investigative Dermatology. *J Am Acad Dermatol*. 2006;55(3):490–500. Accessed at http://www.lewin.com/~/media/lewin/site_sections/publications/april2005skindisease, October 29, 2013.
7. Bhambri S, Del Rosso JQ, Bhambri A. Pathogenesis of acne vulgaris: recent advances. *J Drugs Dermatol JDD*. 2009;8(7):615–8.
8. Consumer Healthcare Products Association OTC sales by category. Accessed at http://www.chpa.org/OTCsCategory.aspx, October 31, 2013.
9. Makrantonaki E, Ganceviciene R, Zouboulis C. An update on the role of the sebaceous gland in the pathogenesis of acne. *Dermatoendocrinol*. 2011;3(1):41–9.
10. Thiboutot D, Gollnick H, Bettoli V, et al. New insights into the management of acne: an update from the Global Alliance to Improve Outcomes in Acne group. *J Am Acad Dermatol*. 2009;60(5 suppl):S1–50.
11. Ebede TL, Arch EL, Berson D. Hormonal treatment of acne in women. *J Clin Aesthet Dermatol*. 2009;2(12):16–22.
12. Kurokawa I, Danby FW, Ju Q, et al. New developments in our understanding of acne pathogenesis and treatment. *Exp Dermatol*. 2009;18(10): 821–32.
13. Hari A, Flach TL, Shi Y, et al. Toll-like receptors: role in dermatological disease. *Mediat Inflamm*. 2010.2010:437246. doi: 10.1155/2010/437246. Epub 2010 Aug 22.
14. Farrar MD, Ingham E. Acne: inflammation. *Clin Dermatol*. 2004;22(5): 380–4.
15. Kraft J, Freiman A. Management of acne. *CMAJ*. 2011;183(7):E430–5.
16. Gollnick H, Cunliffe W, Berson D, et al. Management of acne: a report from a Global Alliance to Improve Outcomes in Acne. *J Am Acad Dermatol*. 2003;49(1 suppl):S1–37.
17. Bowe WP, Shalita AR. Effective over-the-counter acne treatments. *Semin Cutan Med Surg*. 2008;27(3):170–6.
18. Degitz K, Ochsendorf F. Pharmacotherapy of acne. *Expert Opin Pharmacother*. 2008;9(6):955–71.
19. Bowe WP, Joshi SS, Shalita AR. Diet and acne. *J Am Acad Dermatol*. 2010;63(1):124–41.
20. Lolis MS, Bowe WP, Shalita AR. Acne and systemic disease. *Med Clin North Am*. 2009;93(6):1161–81.
21. Melnik B. Dietary intervention in acne. *Dermatoendocrinol*. 2012; 4(1):20–32.
22. U.S. Food and Drug Administration. Guidance for Industry. Acne Vulgaris: Developing Drugs for Treatment. September 2005. Accessed at http://www.fda.gov/ohrms/dockets/98fr/2005d-0340-gdl0001.pdf, August 2, 2014.
23. Federman DG, Kirsner RS. Acne vulgaris: pathogenesis and therapeutic approach. *Am J Manag Care*. 2000;6(1):78–87; quiz 88–9.
24. Baldwin HE. The interaction between acne vulgaris and the psyche. *Cutis Cutan Med Pr*. 2002;70(2):133–9.
25. Van de Kerkhof PCM, Kleinpenning MM, de Jong EMGJ, et al. Current and future treatment options for acne. *J Dermatol Treat*. 2006;17(4): 198–204.
26. Zaenglein AL, Thiboutot DM. Expert committee recommendations for acne management. *Pediatrics*. 2006;118(3):1188–99.
27. Sagransky M, Yentzer BA, Feldman SR. Benzoyl peroxide: a review of its current use in the treatment of acne vulgaris. *Expert Opin Pharmacother*. 2009;10(15):2555–62.
28. Rathi SK. Acne vulgaris treatment: the current scenario. *Indian J Dermatol*. 2011;56(1):7–13.
29. Brown SK, Shalita AR. Acne vulgaris. *Lancet*. 1998;351(9119):1871–6.
30. Strauss JS, Krowchuk DP, Leyden JJ, et al. Guidelines of care for acne vulgaris management. *J Am Acad Dermatol*. 2007;56(4):651–63.
31. U.S. Food and Drug Administration. Classification of benzoyl peroxide as safe and effective and revision of labeling to Drug Facts format; topical acne drug products for over-the-counter human use. Final rule. *Federal Register*. March 4, 2010;75(42):9767–77. Accessed at http://www.gpo.gov/fdsys/pkg/FR-2010-03-04/html/2010-4424.htm, July 19, 2014.
32. U.S. Food and Drug Administration. Drug Safety Communications. FDA warns of rare but serious hypersensitivity reactions with certain over-the-counter topical acne products. Accessed at http://www.fda.gov/downloads/Drugs/DrugSafety/UCM402663.pdf, August 7, 2014.
33. Baxi S. OTC products for the treatment of acne. US Pharm. 2007; 32(7):13–7. Accessed at http://www.uspharmacist.com/content/t/dermatology,acne/c/10277/, April 3, 2013.
34. U.S. Food and Drug Administration. Microbial drug products for over-the-counter human use; subpart D-topical acne drug products. CFR: Code of Federal Regulations Title 21, Part 333. Accessed at http://edocket.access.gpo.gov/cfr_2006/aprqtr/pdf/21cfr333.110.pdf, April 3, 2013.
35. Goodman G. Managing acne vulgaris effectively. *Aust Fam Physician*. 2006;35(9):705–9.
36. Zouboulis CC, Böhm M. Neuroendocrine regulation of sebocytes—a pathogenetic link between stress and acne. *Exp Dermatol*. 2004; 13(suppl 4):31–5.
37. Whitney KM, Ditre CM. Management strategies for acne vulgaris. *Clin Cosmet Investig Dermatol*. 2011;4:41–53.
38. Eichenfield LF, Krakowski AC, Piggott C. Evidence-based recommendations for the diagnosis and treatment of pediatric acne. *Pediatrics*. 2013;131(suppl 3):S163–86.
39. Ebanks JP, Wickett RR, Boissy RE. Mechanisms regulating skin pigmentation: the rise and fall of complexion coloration. *Int J Mol Sci*. 2009;10(9):4066–87.

PREVENTION OF SUN-INDUCED SKIN DISORDERS

Kimberly M. Crosby and Katherine S. O'Neal

Current research has demonstrated that exposure to ultraviolet radiation (UVR) is cumulative and can produce serious, long-term problems. The most common skin problem caused by excessive UVR exposure is sunburn. However, other conditions either are directly caused or exacerbated by exposure to UVR, including premature aging, skin cancers, cataracts, and photodermatoses.

Long-term UVR exposure and damage can result in histopathologic changes in the skin, resulting in premature aging of the skin or photoaging. These changes may result in wrinkling of the skin, discolorations, and other signs of skin damage. Chapter 39 provides an in-depth discussion of photoaging and its treatment.[1–5]

Photodermatoses can be defined as a heterogenous group of skin disorders that are induced or exacerbated (photoaggravated) by radiation of varying wavelengths. More than 20 disorders are classified as photodermatoses (Table 38–1). The common factor in the development of a photodermatosis is the onset or exacerbation of signs and symptoms after exposure to UVR. In addition to the idiopathic photodermatoses, UVR can precipitate or exacerbate many photoaggravated dermatologic conditions, including herpes simplex labialis (cold sores), systemic lupus erythematosus (SLE) and associated skin lesions, and melasma, which may affect pregnant women and women taking oral contraceptives.[1–3]

The most serious skin disorder caused by UVR is skin cancer. Cumulative exposure from childhood to adulthood, even without serious sunburn, may predispose a person to develop precancerous and cancerous skin conditions. Epidemiologic studies conducted since the 1950s demonstrate a strong relationship between chronic, excessive, and unprotected sun exposure and human skin cancer. Nonmelanoma skin cancers are the most common type of cancer malignancy in the United States. In the United States in 2006, an estimated 2 million people were treated for basal and squamous cell carcinomas (nonmelanoma skin cancers, NMSC). An estimated 76,250 people were diagnosed with malignant melanoma in 2012. Although skin cancers are a significant cause of morbidity and mortality associated with UVR exposure, most NMSCs can be cured, and melanoma is highly treatable if detected early.[3–5]

Avoiding excessive exposure to UVR through the use of sunscreens and other sun protection measures will reduce the incidence of the sun-induced skin disorders: sunburn, premature aging of the skin, photodermatoses, skin cancer, and other long-term dermatologic effects. Education about the safe and effective use of sunscreen and suntan products is a public health need. To perform this function, health care providers should be aware of the hazards of UVR and the criteria for selecting and properly using sunscreen products. Providers are encouraged to become involved in educational efforts to help minimize the morbidity and mortality associated with UVR exposure.[4,5]

Pathophysiology of Sun-Induced Skin Disorders

Ultraviolet Radiation

The UV spectrum is divided into three major bands: ultraviolet C (UVC), ultraviolet B (UVB), and ultraviolet A (UVA); all three cause or exacerbate sun-induced skin disorders. Because most UVC radiation (wavelength between 200 and 290 nm) is screened out by the ozone layer of the upper atmosphere, little of it reaches Earth; however, UVC is emitted by some artificial sources of UVR. Most of the UVC that strikes the skin is absorbed by the dead cell layer of the stratum corneum.

UVB (wavelength between 290 and 320 nm) is the most active UVR wavelength for producing erythema, which is why it is called sunburn radiation. The intensity of UVB radiation reaching the Earth is the highest from 10:00 am to 4:00 pm.

UVB is considered the primary inducer of skin cancer; however, its carcinogenic effects are believed to be augmented by UVA. UVB is also primarily responsible for wrinkling, epidermal hyperplasia, elastosis, and collagen damage. The only true therapeutic effect of UVB exposure is vitamin D_3 synthesis in the skin.[5–8] The amount of UVB needed for vitamin D production is dependent on both patient and environmental factors (e.g., location, altitude, cloud cover, time of year, skin pigmentation, and age). However, with the wide availability of vitamin D supplementation in foods and the availability of vitamin D supplements, the need for UVB exposure to increase vitamin D production is not necessary. The American Academy of Dermatology position statement on vitamin D states that UV radiation exposure should not be used as a source of vitamin D because of the risks associated with UV radiation.[7–9]

Previously, only UVB was believed to produce premature aging effects on the skin and increase skin cancer risk; however, evidence now exists that UVA radiation (wavelength between 320 and 400 nm) is involved in suppression of the immune system and damage to DNA, which result in premature photoaging and skin cancers.[5,6] In addition, UVA can produce photosensitivity reactions in patients who have ingested or applied photosensitizing agents. Although approximately 20 times more UVA than

table 38-1 Common Photodermatoses

Idiopathic Disorders

Actinic prurigo	Polymorphous light eruption
Chronic actinic dermatitis	Solar urticaria
Hydroa vacciniforme	

Photoaggravated Dermatoses

Atopic dermatitis	Pellagra
Chronic actinic dermatitis	Pemphigus
Cutaneous T-cell lymphoma	Porphyrias
Dermatomyositis	Psoriasis
Disseminated superficial actinic porokeratosis	Reticular erythematous mucinosis
	Rosacea
Drug-induced photosensitivity	Systemic lupus erythematosus
Erythema multiforme	Transient acantholytic dermatosis
Herpes simplex labialis	
Lichen planus actinicus	

Source: References 1 and 2.

UVB reaches Earth at noon (30 times more in winter), erythemogenic activity is relatively weak in the UVA band.[10]

The Food and Drug Administration (FDA) sets standards for sunlamp products and UV lamps. However, these regulations do not include any specified limits on the amount of UVA and UVB emitted from tanning devices. The only requirement is that the ratio of UVB to UVA must not exceed 0.05 (5%). Most tanning beds or devices use UVR sources that emit more than 96% UVA and less than 4% UVB, a different mix of UVR than that obtained from natural sunlight. Tanning bed use has been associated with an increased risk of skin cancers.[6,11–13] Health care providers should advise parents and patients about the long-term hazards related to tanning devices; in addition, providers should explain that tanning devices currently provide no accepted health benefits.

Many factors contribute to the amount of UVR exposure received. Contrary to popular opinion, cloud cover filters very little UVR; 70%–90% of UVR will penetrate clouds, depending on the clouds' density. However, clouds tend to filter out the infrared radiation that contributes to the sensation of heat, creating a false sense of security against a burn.[14] White or light-colored surfaces (e.g., snow or sand) reflect the UVR that strikes them.[15] Also, the irradiance of UVB increases by 4% for every 1000-foot increase in altitude. These factors all contribute to the overall radiation received, and severe sunburn may result even if the person is sitting in the shade or if there is cloud cover.[16,17] Water reflects no more than 5% of UVR, allowing the remaining 95% to penetrate and burn the swimmer. Therefore, time in the water, even if the swimmer is completely submerged, should be considered part of the total time spent in the sun. Dry clothes reflect almost all UVR; however, if light passes through dry clothing when held up to the sun, UVR will also penetrate the clothing. Tightly woven material offers the greatest protection.[15,17] Wet clothes allow transmission of approximately 50% of UVR.

Although UVB does not penetrate window glass, UVA does. Most automobile windshields are made from laminated glass that filters most of the UVA. However, side windows are not made from laminated glass; therefore, a significant amount of UVA may pass through to persons in the vehicle. Therefore, patients sensitive to UVA (e.g., those with photodermatoses or those taking photosensitizing drugs) should use appropriate sunscreens even when driving with the windows closed.[18]

The Environmental Protection Agency has developed a UV index that uses a scale to rate the amount of skin-damaging UV radiation that reaches the earth's surface at any instance in time (Table 38–2). As the rating increases, the risk of exposure increases. When a UV index is given in the United States, it typically is given for noon; however, the UV index changes throughout the day. Factors that influence the UV index are time of day (UVR exposure is greater at midday than in the early morning or late afternoon); ozone (limited amounts of ozone increase the amount of UVR exposure); altitude (higher altitudes receive greater UVR exposure); season (spring and summer have greater UVR exposure); surface (reflective surfaces increase UVR exposure); latitude (UVR exposure increases closer to the equator); and land cover (less tree cover increases UVR exposure).[19]

Sunburn and Suntan

The degree to which a person will develop a sunburn or a tan depends on several factors, including type and amount of radiation received, thickness of the epidermis and stratum corneum, skin pigmentation, skin hydration, and distribution and concentration of peripheral blood vessels. Most UVR that strikes the skin is absorbed by the epidermis.

A sunburn involves a number of mediators, including histamine, lysosomal enzymes, kinins, and at least one prostaglandin. These mediators produce peripheral vasodilatation as the UVR penetrates the epidermis; then an inflammatory reaction involving a lymphocytic infiltrate develops. Swelling of the endothelium and leakage of red blood cells from capillaries will also occur. Although the exact mechanism is not fully understood, UVB radiation is believed to produce erythema by first causing damage to cellular DNA. The intensity of the UVB-induced erythema peaks at 12–24 hours after exposure.[14]

A tan is produced when UVR stimulates the melanocytes in the skin layers to generate more melanin, and when UVR oxidizes the melanin already in the epidermis. Both processes serve as protective mechanisms to diffuse and absorb additional UVR. However, tanning does not protect an individual from developing skin cancer, photodermatoses, premature photoaging,

table 38-2 Global Solar UV Index

Rating Number	Interpretation of UVR Exposure Risk
1–2	Low
3–5	Moderate
6–7	High
8–10	Very high
11+	Extreme

Key: UV = Ultraviolet; UVR = ultraviolet radiation.
Source: Reference 19.

or other UVR-related negative health risks. Tanning also does not protect against future sunburns. Although UVA and UVB both contribute to the tanning process, they induce pigmentation by different mechanisms. UVA produces a tan by inducing an immediate pigment darkening, resulting from photooxidation of existing melanin and redistribution of melanocytes. The pigment darkening begins to be visible rapidly after exposure and may last for 2 hours after UVR exposure. UVB acts by stimulating melanocyte activity and increasing the number of melanocytes in the skin. This delayed tanning of the skin becomes visible 3–4 days after exposure to UVR and will last from 10 to 30 days depending on skin type and amount of UVR exposure.[14]

Photodermatoses

Photodermatoses can be classified into 4 main categories: immunologically-mediated reactions; drug- or chemical-induced photosensitivity; defective DNA disorders; and photoaggravated disorders. The exact pathologic mechanism for the development of these abnormal reactions to UVR is unknown. UVB most often is responsible for the reactions; however, UVA and some visible light may also cause photodermatoses.

Photosensitivity encompasses two types of conditions: photoallergy and phototoxicity. Drug photoallergy (a relatively uncommon immunologic response) involves an increased, chemically induced reactivity of the skin to UVR and/or visible light. UVR (primarily UVA) triggers an antigenic reaction in the skin. This reaction, which is not dose related, usually is seen after at least one prior exposure to the involved chemical agent or drug.

Like photoallergy, phototoxicity is an increased, chemically induced reactivity of the skin to UVR and/or visible light. However, phototoxicity is not immunologic. It is often seen on first exposure to a chemical agent or drug, is dose related, and usually exhibits no drug cross-sensitivity. Some drugs associated with phototoxicity are listed in Table 38–3. This type of reaction is not limited to drugs but is also associated with plants, cosmetics, and soaps.[2]

table 38–3	Selected Medications (by Drug Category) Associated with Photosensitivity Reactions

Anticancer Drugs
Dacarbazine
Daunorubicin
Fluorouracil
Methotrexate
Vinblastine

Anticonvulsants
Carbamazepine
Gabapentin
Lamotrigine
Phenytoin

Antidepressants
Bupropion
Selective serotonin reuptake inhibitors
Trazodone
Venlafaxine

Antihistamines
Cetirizine
Diphenhydramine

Antihypertensives
Angiotensin-converting enzyme inhibitors
Calcium channel blockers
Hydralazine
Labetalol
Methyldopa
Minoxidil
Sotalol

Anti-Infectives
Azithromycin
Ceftazidime
Dapsone
Gentamicin
Griseofulvin
Itraconazole
Ketoconazole
Metronidazole
Pyrazinamide
Quinolones
Ritonavir
Saquinavir
Sulfonamides
Tetracyclines
Trimethoprim
Trovafloxacin
Zalcitabine

Antimalarials
Chloroquine
Quinine

Antipsychotics/Phenothiazines
Haloperidol
Olanzapine
Ziprasidone

Coal Tar and Derivatives
DHS Tar Gel Shampoo
Ionil T Plus Shampoo
Neutrogena T/Derm Body Oil
Neutrogena T/Gel Extra Strength

Diuretics
Acetazolamide
Amiloride
Furosemide
Metolazone
Triamterene
Thiazide diuretics

Nonsteroidal Anti-Inflammatory Drugs
Celecoxib
Ibuprofen
Indomethacin
Methoxsalen
Naproxen
Psoralen
Trioxsalen

Sunscreens
Aminobenzoic acid
Aminobenzoic acid derivatives
Benzophenones
Cinnamates
Homosalate
Menthyl anthranilate
Oxybenzone

Miscellaneous
Amiodarone (antiarrhythmic)
Benzoyl peroxide
Gold salts (antiarthritic)
Isotretinoin (antiacne)
Quinidine sulfate (antiarrhythmic)
Retinoids
Statins

Source: Reference 1 and Stein KR, Scheinfeld NS. Drug-induced photoallergic and phototoxic reactions. *Expert Opin Drug Saf.* 2007;6(4):431–43.

Skin Cancer

The majority of NMSCs occur on the most exposed areas of the body (the face, head, neck, and backs of the hands). The two most common types of NMSC are basal cell carcinoma (BCC) and squamous cell carcinoma (SCC). BCC is often an aggressive, invasive disorder of the epidermis and dermis that can cause serious damage to the skin and underlying tissue. However, it rarely metastasizes. SCC is found in epithelial keratinocytes and grows very slowly.

The pathophysiology of melanoma differs from that of the NMSCs. Although most melanomas come from normal skin, about 30% arise from existing nevi (moles). Some of the risk factors for skin cancer include a family or personal history of melanoma; sun sensitivity (e.g., difficulty tanning or burning easily); large numbers of atypical nevi; a previous history of SCC or BCC; tanning bed use; and a history of excessive sun exposure and sunburns. Regardless of risk factors, skin cancer may develop in all individuals with increased exposure to UVR.[5] A growing amount of evidence supports the supposition that sun exposure plays a role in the development of all types of skin cancers.[20]

Clinical Presentation of Sun-Induced Skin Disorders

Sunburn

Sunburn is, in fact, a burn. It most often is seen as a superficial burn with a reaction that ranges from mild erythema to tenderness, pain, and edema (see Color Plates, photograph 24). Severe reactions to excessive UVR exposure can sometimes produce burns that range in severity from superficial partial-thickness to full-thickness with the development of vesicles (blisters) or bullae (many large blisters), as well as fever, chills, weakness, and shock. Shock caused by heat prostration or hyperpyrexia can lead to death. (See Chapter 40 for treatment of sunburn.)

Drug Photosensitivity

Drug photoallergy presents similar to allergic contact dermatitis (e.g., poison ivy) and is characterized by pruritus with erythematous papules, vesicles, bullae, and/or urticaria (see Color Plates, photograph 25). Phototoxicity is most likely to appear as exaggerated sunburn with pruritis,[1] but urticaria may also occur (see Color Plates, photograph 26).

Photodermatoses

Each photodermatosis has a unique morphology. Polymorphous light eruption alone can have multiple morphologic presentations of pruritus with papules, vesicles, plaques, and/or urticaria.

Premature Aging

This condition is characterized by wrinkling and yellowing of the skin. Conclusive evidence reveals that prolonged exposure to UVR results in elastosis (degeneration of the skin due to a breakdown of the skin's elastic fibers). Pronounced drying, thickening, and wrinkling of the skin also may result. Other physical changes include cracking, telangiectasia (spider vessels), solar keratoses (growths), and ecchymoses (subcutaneous hemorrhagic lesions).[2,5,14] (See Chapter 39 for measures for reversing photoaging.)

Skin Cancer

BCC is a translucent nodule with a smooth surface. It is usually firm to the touch and may be ulcerated or crusted. It is generally found as an isolated lesion on the nose or other parts of the face, although multiple lesions are sometimes found. SCC, on the other hand, is a slow-growing, isolated papule or plaque on sun-exposed areas of the body.

Self-examination for melanoma uses four factors (A-B-C-D) for evaluation: Asymmetric shape; Border irregularity or poorly defined border; Color variation within the same mole or a change in color; and Diameter larger than 6 mm. A mole with these characteristics and any new growth or change in appearance of the skin (including the lips) should be evaluated by a dermatologist.[17]

Prevention of Sun-Induced Skin Disorders

The short-term goals in preventing sun-induced skin disorders are relatively simple: avoid or minimize sunburn, photosensitivity reactions, and UVR-induced or -exacerbated photodermatoses. The expected long-term outcomes are prevention of skin cancer and avoidance of premature aging of the skin.

UVR-induced skin disorders can be prevented by minimizing exposure to UVR and by using sunscreen agents. The sunscreen product selected and the degree of protection will vary, depending on the patient's intended use for the product and the conditions under which the product will be used (Figure 38-1).

The greater the risk a patient has of developing a UVR-induced skin disorder, the greater the need to avoid sun exposure. However, most people do not spend warm, sunny afternoons sitting inside, nor do they go to the beach or pool wearing lots of clothing. Providers can assist the patient in striking a balance between completely avoiding sun exposure, wearing protective clothing, and using sunscreen products. If, however, the patient suffers from a UVR-induced skin disorder (e.g., SLE), few options are available. With regard to preventing sunburn, the patient's natural skin type will be the primary factor in determining the sun protection factor (SPF) of the sunscreen product to be used. The lighter the natural skin color (and the more *quickly* a burn develops), the higher the SPF required for the sunscreen product to prevent sunburn.

Avoidance of Sun Exposure

Although unrealistic, complete avoidance of UVR is often the best approach for patients who have the physical characteristics or history listed in Table 38-4. For people who refuse to stay indoors or who must be outdoors for extended periods, wearing protective clothing (e.g., a hat with a 4-inch brim, long pants, and a long-sleeved shirt) should be recommended. In situations in which the patient is unwilling or unable to avoid the sun or to wear protective clothing, the next best choice is to use a sunscreen product.[21]

Measures of UVR Protection

SPF

Purchasers of sunscreens are usually familiar with SPF, which is one parameter for determining a sunscreen's effectiveness for UV protection. Another parameter, minimal erythema dose (MED), is used to calculate a sunscreen's SPF. The MED

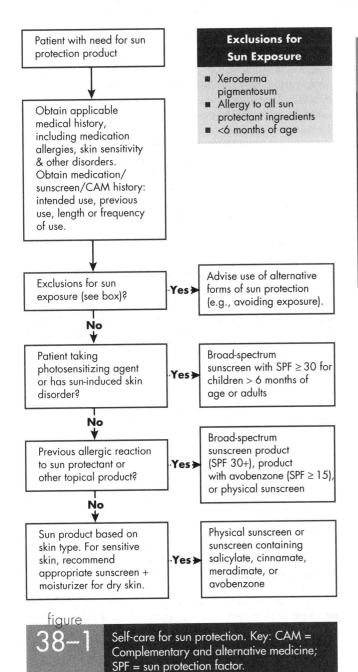

Patient with need for sun protection product

↓

Obtain applicable medical history, including medication allergies, skin sensitivity & other disorders. Obtain medication/sunscreen/CAM history: intended use, previous use, length or frequency of use.

↓

Exclusions for sun exposure (see box)? —**Yes**→ Advise use of alternative forms of sun protection (e.g., avoiding exposure).

↓ **No**

Patient taking photosensitizing agent or has sun-induced skin disorder? —**Yes**→ Broad-spectrum sunscreen with SPF ≥ 30 for children > 6 months of age or adults

↓ **No**

Previous allergic reaction to sun protectant or other topical product? —**Yes**→ Broad-spectrum sunscreen product (SPF 30+), product with avobenzone (SPF ≥ 15), or physical sunscreen

↓ **No**

Sun product based on skin type. For sensitive skin, recommend appropriate sunscreen + moisturizer for dry skin. —**Yes**→ Physical sunscreen or sunscreen containing salicylate, cinnamate, meradimate, or avobenzone

figure 38-1 Self-care for sun protection. Key: CAM = Complementary and alternative medicine; SPF = sun protection factor.

table 38-4 **Patient Risk Factors for the Development of UVR-Induced Problems**

- Fair skin that always burns and never tans
- A history of one or more serious or blistering sunburns
- Blonde or red hair
- Blue, green, or gray eyes
- A history of freckling
- A previous growth on the skin or lips caused by UV exposure
- The existence of a UV-induced disorder
- A family history of melanoma
- Current use of an immunosuppressive drug
- Current use of a photosensitizing drug
- Excessive lifetime exposure to UVR, including tanning beds and booths
- History of an autoimmune disease

Key: UV = Ultraviolet light; UVR = ultraviolet radiation.
Source: Reference 17.

rating of 10. The higher the SPF, the more effective the agent is in preventing sunburn. If 60 minutes of sun exposure normally is required for someone to experience two MEDs (a bright erythematous sunburn), a sunscreen with an SPF of 6 will allow that person to stay in the sun 6 times longer (or 6 hours) before receiving the same degree of sunburn (assuming the sunscreen is reapplied at the recommended intervals). The SPF is product specific, because it is calculated on the basis of the final formulation of the product and cannot be determined on the basis of the active ingredient alone.[18,19] A product with an SPF of 15 blocks 93% of UVB. Raising the SPF to 30 increases UVB protection to only 96.7%, and an SPF of 40 blocks 97.5%.[19] A hypothetical SPF of 70 would increase UVB protection to only 98.6%.[21,22]

Measures of UVA Protection

With concern growing about the long-term adverse effects of UVA, the utility of the SPF value in measuring photoprotection from UVA has been questioned. FDA has concluded that both UVA and UVB radiation protection can be assessed effectively by the SPF test in combination with a new broad-spectrum in vitro test. Products that pass the new test will offer higher protection against both UVA and UVB, and they will be labeled as broad-spectrum sunscreens.[23]

Use of Sunscreens

On June 17, 2011, FDA announced new requirements for nonprescription sunscreens. These changes are outlined in four regulatory documents: a final rule, a proposed rule, an advanced notice of proposed rulemaking, and a draft guidance for industry.[23–27] These regulations became effective in June 2012.

The final rule mandates that all sunscreens labeled as broad spectrum must pass FDA's new, standardized broad-spectrum procedure that measures a product's UVA protection relative to its UVB protection. This procedure is in addition to the standardized sun protection factor test mandated previously. Only broad-spectrum sunscreens with an SPF value of 15 or higher will be able to claim to reduce the risk of skin cancer and early

is defined as the "minimum UVR dose that produces clearly marginated erythema in the irradiated site, given as a single exposure."[20,21] It is a dose of radiation, not a grade of erythema. Generally, two MEDs will produce a bright erythema; four MEDs, a painful sunburn; and eight MEDs, a blistering burn. However, because of variations in thickness of the stratum corneum, different parts of the body may respond differently to the same MED. Furthermore, the MED for heavily pigmented blacks is estimated to be 33 times higher than that for lightly pigmented whites.

The important measure for sunscreens is the SPF, which is derived by dividing the MED on protected skin by the MED on unprotected skin. For example, if a person requires 25 mJ/cm² of UVB radiation to experience 1 MED on unprotected skin and requires 250 mJ/cm² of radiation to produce 1 MED after applying a given sunscreen, the product would be given an SPF

skin aging if they are used as directed along with other skin protection measures. Broad-spectrum sunscreens with an SPF value between 2 and 14 and products that protect against only UVB (not broad spectrum) can claim only to help prevent sunburn. Products that are not broad spectrum must carry a label warning: "Skin Cancer/Skin Aging Alert: Spending time in the sun increases your risk of skin cancer and early skin aging. This product has been shown only to help prevent sunburn, not skin cancer or early skin aging."[23]

A sunscreen's efficacy is also related to its substantivity—that is, its ability to remain effective during prolonged exercising, sweating, and swimming. This property can be a function of the active sunscreen, the vehicle, or both. Generally speaking, products with cream-based (water-in-oil) vehicles appear more resistant to removal by water than those with alcohol bases. The final rule prohibits "waterproof," "sweatproof," and "sunblock" claims, because these terms overstate product effectiveness. Further, water-resistance claims on the front label must indicate whether the sunscreen remains effective for either 40 or 80 minutes while swimming or sweating. These times are based on the standard testing procedure. Products that are not water resistant must instruct consumers to wear a water-resistant product while swimming or sweating. Finally, all sunscreen products must include standard "Drug Facts" labeling on the back or side of the container.[23]

The final rule limited the maximum SPF value on sunscreen levels to "50+." This rule is based on the lack of sufficient evidence that products with SPF values higher than 50 provide more protection than products with SPF values of 50.[24,25]

The application dosage forms eligible for review and inclusion in the final monograph are oils, lotions, creams, gels, butters, pastes, ointments, sticks, and sprays. Other application dosage forms (e.g., towelettes and wipes) are not considered in the final monograph.[26–28]

The draft guidance for industry is an enforcement guide for manufacturers of sunscreens. It provides information to help manufacturers understand how to label and test their products in light of the new final rule, proposed rule, and advance notice of proposed rulemaking.[27]

Types of Sunscreens

According to the therapeutic definitions, topical sunscreens can be divided into two major subgroups: chemical sunscreens and physical sunscreens. Chemical sunscreens work by absorbing and thus blocking the transmission of UVR to the epidermis. An active ingredient absorbs at least 85% of the radiation in the UV range at wavelengths from 290 to 320 nm, but the agent may or may not allow transmission of radiation to the skin at wavelengths longer than 320 nm. Physical sunscreens are generally opaque and act by reflecting and scattering UVR, rather than by absorbing it. An opaque sunscreen active ingredient reflects or scatters all light in the UV and visible ranges at wavelengths from 290 to 777 nm. The sunscreen thereby minimizes suntan and sunburn.

The final monograph (FM) for sunscreens includes 15 chemical agents and 2 physical agents as safe and effective for use as sunscreens. Table 38–5 lists these agents, their UVR absorbance range, and their maximum concentrations. Because the SPF is product-specific and does not depend on the sunscreen's active agent alone, the FM has eliminated a required minimum strength for sunscreens that contain a single active ingredient.[28–30]

Aminobenzoic Acid and Derivatives

Aminobenzoic acid (formerly para-aminobenzoic acid [PABA]), once was the most widely used sunscreen agent; however, it has been replaced by other agents, because it is a major sensitizer. Because of the continuing confusion about the name of this common sunscreen agent, the FM requires that product labels list it as "aminobenzoic acid"; in addition, each time this name appears on product labeling, it must be followed by "(PABA)" so patients know which chemical entity they are using.

Aminobenzoic acid is an effective UVB sunscreen, especially when formulated in a hydroalcoholic base (maximum of 50%–60% alcohol). The SPF of such formulations increases proportionally as the concentration of aminobenzoic acid increases from 2% to 5%. One advantage of this agent is its ability to penetrate into the horny layer of the skin and provide lasting protection. Its substantivity on sweating skin is significant but is reduced on skin that is immersed in water. The only recommended derivative of aminobenzoic acid is padimate O.

The disadvantages of alcoholic solutions of aminobenzoic acid include contact dermatitis, photosensitivity, stinging and drying of the skin, and yellow staining of clothes on exposure to the sun. Products containing padimate O will not cause staining of the clothing, which may offer an advantage over aminobenzoic acid–containing products. Patients who have experienced a photosensitivity reaction to a sunscreen product containing aminobenzoic acid or any of its derivatives should avoid using these products.[10,21,22,30]

Anthranilates

The anthranilates are ortho-aminobenzoic acid derivatives. Meradimate, the menthyl ester of anthranilic acid, is a weak UV sunscreen with maximal absorbance in the UVA range. It is usually found in combination with other sunscreen agents to provide broader UV coverage.[10,21,22,30,31]

Benzophenones

The benzophenone group comprises three agents: dioxybenzone, oxybenzone (benzophenone-3), and sulisobenzone (benzophenone-4). As a group, these agents are primarily UVB absorbers, with maximum absorbance between 282 and 290 nm. However, their absorbance extends well into the UVA range (up to 350 nm with oxybenzone, and up to 380 nm with dioxybenzone). Because of the possibility of allergic reactions to aminobenzoic acid and its derivatives and their broad spectrum of action, many sunscreen products now contain benzophenones in their formulations. Oxybenzone, also found in some cosmetic formulations, is a significant sensitizing agent among sunscreens. As the use of these agents has increased, reports of sensitivity to the benzophenones have also increased.[10,21,22,30]

Cinnamates

Cinnamates include cinoxate, octinoxate, and octocrylene. As shown in Table 38–5, cinoxate and octinoxate have similar absorbance ranges and maximum absorbances. Octocrylene, however, has an absorbance range of 250–360 nm, well into the UVA range. Octocrylene is currently found in more commercial sunscreen preparations than it was in the past, possibly reflecting its broader spectrum of absorbance. It is also an effective photostabilizer. Octocrylene can decrease the rate that other sunscreens

table

38–5 Sunscreens Considered Safe and Effective

Sunscreen Agent	UV Spectrum Activity	Maximum Range (nm)	Approved Maximum Concentration (%)
ABA and Derivatives			
Aminobenzoic acid (PABA)	UVB	288.5	15
Padimate O	UVB	310	8
Anthranilates			
Meradimate	UVA II	340[a]	5
Benzophenones			
Dioxybenzone	UVB, UVA II	282[b]	3
Oxybenzone	UVB, UVA II	290[c]	6
Sulisobenzone	UVB, UVA II	285[d]	10
Cinnamates			
Cinoxate	UVB	310	3
Octocrylene	UVB, UVA II	303	10
Octinoxate	UVB	308–310	7.5
Dibenzoylmethane Derivatives			
Avobenzone[e]	UVA I	360	3
Salicylates			
Homosalate	UVB	306	15
Octisalate	UVB	305	5
Trolamine salicylate	UVB	298	12
Miscellaneous			
Ensulizole	UVB	302	4
Ecamsule (terephthalylidene dicamphor sulfonic acid)	UVB, UBA	345	2
Titanium dioxide[f]	290–770	—	25
Zinc oxide[f]	290–770	—	24

Key: ABA = Aminobenzoic acid; UVA = ultraviolet A; UVB = ultraviolet B.
[a] Values are achieved when used in combination with other sunscreen agents.
[b] Second peak occurs at 217 nm.
[c] Second peak occurs at 329 nm.
[d] Second peak occurs at 324 nm.
[e] Agent is currently marketed through a new drug application.
[f] Agent scatters (rather than absorbs) radiation in the 290–770 nm range.
Source: References 10, 21, 22, 24, and 30–32.

degrade when they are exposed to sun. It is often combined with other sunscreens to improve their stability.[29]

Unfortunately, cinnamates do not adhere well to the skin and must rely on the vehicle in a given formulation for their substantivity.[10,21,22,30,31]

Dibenzoylmethane Derivatives

Avobenzone (butyl methoxydibenzoylmethane, originally known as Parsol 1789) is the first of a new class of sunscreen agents effective throughout the entire UVA range (320–400 nm;

full spectrum). It has maximum absorbance at approximately 360 nm. Although avobenzone absorbs UVR throughout the UVA spectrum, its absorption capacity falls off sharply at 370 nm. Therefore, reactions from photosensitive drugs and chemicals that are highly reactive in the 370–400 nm range could still occur. Avobenzone, however, offers the best protection in the UVA range compared with the other chemical sunscreens on the market. It is commonly included in sunscreen products to increase UVA coverage. Avobenzone is easily degraded by exposure to sunlight; it is found in newer sunscreen products combined with octocrylene, salicylates, methylbenzylidene camphor, and micronized zinc oxide and/or titanium dioxide to enhance stability of the product and to extend the product's spectrum of coverage through the UVA and UVB spectrum.[10,21,22,30]

Salicylates

Salicylic acid derivatives are weak sunscreens and must be used in high concentrations. They do not adhere well to the skin and are easily removed by perspiration or swimming.[10,30,31]

Other Chemical Sunscreens

Ensulizole does not fit into any of the above classes. It is a pure UVB sunscreen with an absorbance range of 290–320 nm. Ecamsule (terephthalylidene dicamphor sulfonic acid) is a new molecule that FDA approved in 2006. It is a water-resistant broad-spectrum sunscreen. Ecamsule is often combined with octocrylene to increase its stability to light.[10,31]

Physical Sunscreens

Physical sunscreens (zinc oxide and titanium dioxide) are considered broad-spectrum UV protectants. They are used most often on small and prominently exposed areas by patients who cannot limit or control their exposure to the sun (e.g., lifeguards). Earlier formulations of these agents were opaque and had an undesirable sticky or gritty sensation. Current formulations contain micro- or nano-sized particles of the agent. These formulations are transparent, which improves their cosmetic appeal. Because titanium dioxide increases the effective SPF of a product and extends the spectrum of protection well into the UVA range, the number of commercial products containing this agent has increased. The FM allows zinc oxide to be used alone or in combination with any of the other sunscreen agents except avobenzone; the exception results from a lack of data on effectiveness.[10,21,22,30]

Combination Products

FDA has not recommended limits on the number of sunscreen agents that may be used together. However, each sunscreen agent must contribute to the efficacy of a product and must not be included merely for marketing promotion purposes. Therefore, the FM requires that each active ingredient contribute a minimum SPF of not less than 2; in addition, the finished product must have a minimum SPF of not less than the number of sunscreen active ingredients used in the combination multiplied by 2.[22]

Dosage and Administration Guidelines

The two major causes of poor sun protection with sunscreen use are application of inadequate amounts and infrequent reapplication. Although many sunscreen products that prevent burning of the lips (or nose) are available, the lips are often neglected. Products for the lips differ in ingredients and in the UVA and UVB spectrum, but they carry most of the same labeling used on sunscreen lotions (including the SPF). The SPF of these products is usually at least 15. Studies have shown that lip protection not only helps prevent drying and burning of the lips, but that it also helps prevent the development of cold sores or fever blisters triggered by the herpes simplex virus in patients who are susceptible to recurrent outbreaks.

For maximum effectiveness, sunscreens must be applied liberally to all exposed areas of the body and reapplied at least as often as the label recommends. FDA–approved labeling recommends that sunscreens be applied 15–30 minutes before UV exposure and at least every 2 hours thereafter. Reapplication after every episode of swimming, towel drying, or excessive sweating is also recommended.[33]

The FDA standard for application of sunscreens is 2 mg/cm^2 of body surface area. This standard means that, for sufficient protection, the average adult in a bathing suit should apply nine portions of sunscreen of approximately one-half teaspoon each, or approximately 4 and one-half teaspoons (22.5 mL) total. The sunscreen should be distributed as follows:

- Face and neck: one-half teaspoon.
- Arms and shoulders: one-half teaspoon to each side of body.
- Torso: one-half teaspoon each to front and back.
- Legs and tops of feet: 1 teaspoon to each side of body.

Because of the cost of sunscreen products and the need to apply them often and in sufficient amounts, people may use far less sunscreen than is necessary to provide adequate protection. Exposure to UVR should be within the limits of the SPF value of the sunscreen for the individual using the sunscreen. A higher SPF may be needed for longer or more intense exposure to UVR. The final rule requires that the sunscreen label recommend the following with regard to sunscreen application: Regardless of the water resistance of the product, it should be applied 15 minutes before sun exposure. Non–water-resistant products should be reapplied at least every 2 hours. Water-resistant products should be reapplied every 2 hours, after 40 or 80 minutes of swimming or sweating (as designated on the label), and immediately after towel drying.[23]

Safety Considerations

The development of a rash, vesicles (blisters), hives, or exaggerated sunburn after use of the sunscreen product is most likely a sign of either a photosensitivity or allergic reaction.[1–3] Product labels must state the following: "Stop use if skin rash occurs."[22] The patient should be referred for medical evaluation of the situation. The degree of the reaction will determine what type of medical intervention (if any) is necessary.

If a patient has experienced a prior reaction to a sunscreen product, the product's name and ingredients should be identified, if possible. This action may be difficult, because product formulations change frequently. Photosensitivity and contact dermatitis are more likely to occur with aminobenzoic acid and its derivatives, although the benzophenones, cinnamates, homosalate, avobenzone, and meradimate have also been reported to produce both conditions. In a French study of contact dermatitis, 15.4% of patients were found to have an allergy to sunscreens, with almost one-half attributed to oxybenzone.[34] Although no evidence exists of significant effects from eye contact, FDA requires the label warning "Keep out of eyes."

Additional Product Considerations
Sunscreens in Cosmetic Products

The FM addresses a gray area that has allowed the proliferation of cosmetics claiming to offer sun protection. It stipulates that sunscreen products will be classified as drugs rather than cosmetics, because consumers expect that sunscreens will protect them from some of the sun's damaging effects. However, cosmetics that contain sunscreen agents will be classified as cosmetics as long as no therapeutic claims are made and the sunscreen is intended for a nontherapeutic, nonphysiologic purpose. If the cosmetic makes a claim for use as a sunscreen product, it will have to include the appropriate labeling. Under the directions for use, the optional statement "for sunscreen use" may be added.[22,23]

Product Selection Guidelines

Two primary factors will determine the best product for a given patient: the intended use of the product and specific patient characteristics. The decision of which sunscreen product to use must be based on the information obtained from both categories.

Intended Use

Some patients may want to use sunscreens to prevent sunburn or the photoaging effects of UVR or to protect themselves from skin cancer. Others may need protection from sun exposure because they are taking photosensitive drugs or they suffer from a photodermatosis.

The higher the SPF of the sunscreen product, the greater the protection it provides against sunburn and tanning. Studies have shown that sunscreens can protect against the long-term hazards of skin cancer.[10,21] Considerable research is currently being conducted on all aspects of UVR and its effects. However, experts are debating whether low-SPF products protect individuals from UV skin damage or allow them to receive dangerously high levels of UVR over extended periods of time. Because of the known hazards associated with UVR, FDA and other organizations such as the American Academy of Dermatology recommend the use of sunscreen products of at least SPF 15. Generally, if a product is to be used to prevent skin cancer, reduce the chances of a photosensitivity reaction, or reduce the risk of triggering a skin disorder induced or aggravated by UVR, a broad-spectrum SPF value of 15 or higher is recommended.

Patient Factors

For patients not concerned with photosensitivity, photodermatoses, or prevention of skin cancer, product selection is much simpler. The following factors can serve as a guide in selecting products with the appropriate properties for a patient's particular situation.

The most important factors in product selection are the individual's natural skin type and tanning history. An SPF product of 30+ should be used by people who burn easily and tan minimally at best. If the individual plans to swim, participate in vigorous activity (e.g., sand volleyball), or work outdoors, the sunscreen product must be able to adhere to the skin more substantially than if the individual just lies on the beach. The expected duration of the physical activity can also help to determine which sunscreen to use. Water-resistant products are usually effective for at least 40 or 80 minutes when used during the above activities.[23]

At least one-third of the current commercial products are labeled "noncomedogenic," "fragrance-free," and "hypoallergenic." Noncomedogenic products do not plug the pores and, therefore,

do not exacerbate acne. This property is especially important for teenagers, who usually spend more time outdoors than other age groups and generally would prefer not to use comedogenic sunscreens. Many patients are sensitive to various ingredients (e.g., fragrances, emulsifiers, and preservatives). These patients should try to choose fragrance-free formulations or those that are hypoallergenic. In a randomized, placebo-controlled study of adverse reactions to sunscreens, 16% of subjects developed a local reaction to the topically applied product.[35] Of these subjects, 53% agreed to patch testing and photopatch testing. None of this subset showed an allergic sensitivity to the sunscreen agents. Instead, all the reactions were found to be caused by formulation ingredients, such as fragrances and preservatives. This finding reinforces the belief that most sensitivity may be caused by ingredients other than sunscreens. Although it may not be possible to figure out which specific ingredient a patient is sensitive to, patients who have a history of sensitivity to certain types of ingredients would do well to use a fragrance-free, hypoallergenic product.

Some patients have normally dry skin; sunbathing can further exacerbate this problem. These patients should avoid ethyl and isopropyl alcohols, which are included in a number of commercial sunscreen products and can further dry the skin.

Use in Special Populations

Absorptive characteristics of human skin in children younger than 6 months differ from those of adult skin. The metabolic and excretory systems of infants are not fully developed to handle any sunscreen agent absorbed through the skin. Therefore, only patients older than 6 months are considered to have skin with adult characteristics. FDA requires that sunscreen products be labeled with the statement "children under 6 months of age: ask a doctor." Caregivers should be extremely wary regarding sun exposure in children, especially infants. Although the evidence is not yet conclusive, researchers and providers agree that use of an SPF-15 product starting after 6 months of age and continuing throughout one's lifetime can reduce the incidence of long-term skin damage due to UVR. A product with an SPF of 30+ may result in even higher reductions in sunburn, premature skin aging, skin cancer, and other skin problems. No special consideration is needed for the use of sunscreen-containing products in the elderly or in pregnant or lactating women.[23–28,36]

Assessment of Sun-Induced Skin Disorders: A Case-Based Approach

The approach to UVR-induced skin disorders differs from that used in most self-care situations. These disorders are addressed from a preventive, rather than a treatment, standpoint.

Consequently, assessment of the patient should focus on the *intended use* of the product. Clinical providers' interventions with patients occur in two primary situations. The first situation occurs when a patient requests a recommendation for a sunscreen product to prevent a burn and/or to allow development of a tan. The second situation is initiated by the provider when a patient is placed on a drug that can produce a photosensitivity reaction. In this second scenario, no real patient assessment is needed, because prevention of exposure to UVR is the standard approach.

Cases 38–1 and 38–2 illustrate the assessment of patients with sun-induced skin disorders.

case
38–1

Relevant Evaluation Criteria	Scenario/Model Outcome

Information Gathering

1. Gather essential information about the patient's symptoms and medical history, including:

   a. description of symptom(s) (i.e., nature, onset, duration, severity, associated symptoms)

   The patient would like help picking out a sunscreen to take with her on vacation to the Bahamas. She is concerned that she could get a bad sunburn because she will be out in the sun for several hours most days. She has light skin and usually burns before she tans. She typically uses a product with an SPF of 12. She has a history of multiple sunburns (ranging from mild to severe) on her face and exposed areas.

   b. description of any factors that seem to precipitate, exacerbate, and/or relieve the patient's symptom(s)

   Staying completely out of the sun has been the only thing she has found that keeps her from getting burned, but she doesn't want to have to spend this vacation indoors.

   c. description of the patient's efforts to relieve the symptoms

   She has tried using sunscreens with an SPF of 25 in the past. She applied them while she was outside in the sun, and usually only one time.

   d. patient's identity

   Cecelia Jones

   e. age, sex, height, and weight

   30 years old, female, 5 ft 2 in., 130 lb

   f. patient's occupation

   Paralegal

   g. patient's dietary habits

   Tries to eat a well-balanced diet.

   h. patient's sleep habits

   Typically gets 6–8 hours of sleep per night.

   i. concurrent medical conditions, prescription and non-prescription medications, and dietary supplements

   Allergic rhinitis: loratadine 10 mg daily; contraception: Yasmin 1 tablet by mouth daily

   j. allergies

   NKA

   k. history of other adverse reactions to medications

   None

   l. other (describe) _____

   NA

Assessment and Triage

2. Differentiate patient's signs/symptoms and correctly identify the patient's primary problem(s).

   The patient desires a sunscreen product that will allow her to spend time in the sun while on vacation.

3. Identify exclusions for sun exposure (Figure 38–1).

   None

4. Formulate a comprehensive list of therapeutic alternatives for the primary problem to determine if triage to a health care provider is required, and share this information with the patient or caregiver.

   Options include:

   (1) Use an OTC sunscreen product regularly while in the sun.

   (2) Avoid sun exposure by staying in the shade or indoors.

   (3) Take no action.

Plan

5. Select an optimal therapeutic alternative to address the patient's problem, taking into account patient preferences.

   Regularly using a sunscreen product while outdoors will allow the patient to enjoy the outdoor activities she would like to do on vacation.

6. Describe the recommended therapeutic approach to the patient or caregiver.

   "Use a sunscreen product of SPF 15 or greater that provides both UVA and UVB coverage. A product that is water resistant will be a better choice if you plan to be in the water during the day. Apply the product liberally to all sun-exposed areas of the body."

7. Explain to the patient or caregiver the rationale for selecting the recommended therapeutic approach from the considered therapeutic alternatives.

   "Correct use of a sunscreen product will allow you to enjoy time outdoors without getting a sunburn. With past burns, you may not have applied an appropriate amount of sunscreen or the right type: a broad spectrum sunscreen that provides both UVA and UVB coverage."

Relevant Evaluation Criteria	Scenario/Model Outcome
Patient Education	
8. When recommending self-care with nonprescription medications and/or nondrug therapy, convey accurate information to the patient or caregiver.	Apply the sunscreen product every day 15–30 minutes prior to going out into the sun. Reapply non–water resistant sunscreen at least every 2 hours and every 40 or 80 minutes as directed on the product label if sweating or in the water. You will need to apply the sunscreen as follows:
	■ Face and neck: one-half teaspoon.
	■ Arms and shoulders: one-half teaspoon to each side of body.
	■ Torso: one-half teaspoon each to front and back.
	■ Legs and tops of feet: 1 teaspoon to each side of body.
Solicit follow-up questions from the patient or caregiver.	"What sunscreen should I choose? Is there a specific one I should get?"
Answer the patient's or caregiver's questions.	"There are many sunscreens that are effective. The most important thing to look for is a broad-spectrum sunscreen that blocks both UVA and UVB. Also, you should use a water-resistant product if you will be in the water or sweating."
Evaluation of Patient Outcome	
9. Assess patient outcome.	NA

Key: NA = Not applicable; NKA = no known allergies; OTC = over-the-counter; SPF = sun protection factor; UVA = ultraviolet A; UVB = ultraviolet B.

Relevant Evaluation Criteria	Scenario/Model Outcome
Information Gathering	
1. Gather essential information about the patient's symptoms and medical history, including:	
a. description of symptom(s) (i.e., nature, onset, duration, severity, associated symptoms)	The patient has a history of psoriasis, and she has noticed that her condition and medication for the psoriasis make her more sensitive to the sun. Any sunburn will exacerbate her psoriasis. She would like something to help her worsening psoriasis symptoms. She noticed a worsening of her psoriasis when in the sun for too long this weekend, and she got a sunburn. Her psoriasis symptoms have gotten much worse since the sun exposure.
b. description of any factors that seem to precipitate, exacerbate, and/or relieve the patient's symptom(s)	Sun exacerbates her psoriasis symptoms. So far, nothing has helped relieve her exacerbation.
c. description of the patient's efforts to relieve the symptoms	She used sunscreen prior to being in the sun, but she failed to reapply it throughout the day.
d. patient's identity	Sarah-Anne Smith
e. age, sex, height, and weight	25 years old, female, 5 ft 8 in., 145 lb
f. patient's occupation	Teacher
g. patient's dietary habits	She eats at home for most meals and tries to eat a healthy diet. Occasionally (1–2 meals per week) she eats out or picks up fast food.
h. patient's sleep habits	She gets between 7–8 hours of sleep a night.
i. concurrent medical conditions, prescription and nonprescription medications, and dietary supplements	Psoriasis: topical triamcinolone 0.5% cream applied 3 times daily.
j. allergies	Penicillins
k. history of other adverse reactions to medications	None

case
38–2 *continued*

Relevant Evaluation Criteria	Scenario/Model Outcome
Assessment and Triage	
2. Differentiate patient's signs/symptoms and correctly identify the patient's primary problem(s).	Patient with history of psoriasis that is exacerbated by sunburns or excessive sun exposure.
3. Identify exclusions for sun exposure (Figure 38–1).	None
4. Formulate a comprehensive list of therapeutic alternatives for the primary problem to determine if triage to a health care provider is required, and share this information with the patient or caregiver.	Options include: (1) Avoidance of additional sun exposure until her psoriasis symptoms improve. (2) Use of a sunscreen product in future sun exposures. (3) Referral to her dermatologist.
Plan	
5. Select an optimal therapeutic alternative to address the patient's problem, taking into account patient preferences.	Because the patient has had a worsening of her psoriasis secondary to sun exposure, she should follow up with her dermatologist to assess her symptoms. In the future, she should use sunscreen regularly when exposed to the sun.
6. Describe the recommended therapeutic approach to the patient or caregiver.	"You should see your dermatologist for treatment of your worsening psoriasis symptoms. In the future, apply a sunscreen at least 15 minutes prior to sun exposure, and reapply it every 2 hours during sun exposure for non–water-resistant products. Also, you should consider wearing a long-sleeved shirt and a hat with a 4-inch brim prior to sun exposure, and you should avoid sunburns."
7. Explain to the patient or caregiver the rationale for selecting the recommended therapeutic approach from the considered therapeutic alternatives.	"Psoriasis is commonly aggravated by sun exposure."
Patient Education	
8. When recommending self-care with nonprescription medications and/or nondrug therapy, convey accurate information to the patient or caregiver.	Criterion does not apply in this case.
Solicit follow-up questions from the patient or caregiver.	"Is there any sunscreen that only needs to be used once a day?"
Answer the patient's or caregiver's questions.	"No. All sunscreens, even water-resistant ones, must be reapplied."
Evaluation of Patient Outcome	
9. Assess patient outcome.	NA

Key: NA = Not applicable.

Patient Counseling for Sun-Induced Skin Disorders

Health care providers can provide a great service by counseling patients about the suntanning process and about properly selecting and using sunscreens. One study reported that among the participants, 13% of children and 9% of adults had experienced a sunburn during the previous week; in addition, the study found a relationship between sunburn and a parental attitude that tanning is healthy.[29]

One simple way to find out whether a patient is using a sunscreen properly is to ask how long the current bottle has lasted. When applied properly, according to the suggested dosing guidelines and in accordance with the appropriate substantivity of the product, a sunbather could easily use about 1 ounce every 80–90 minutes. This use would amount to several ounces a day and several bottles per week. Incredibly, many frequent sunbathers use only one bottle in an entire season. This diminished usage demonstrates the importance of individuals' receiving adequate counseling to get the protection they desire. The box Patient Education for Protection from Sun Exposure lists specific information to provide patients.

Patients should also be advised to wear sunglasses to protect their eyes from sun-induced damage. The box A Word about Sun-Induced Ocular Damage describes the categories of available sunglasses and their UVR filtration properties.[31]

patient education for
Protection from Sun Exposure

The objectives of self-treatment depend on a patient's specific goal or health status. Protection from sun exposure can prevent sunburn or tanning, photosensitivity reactions in susceptible persons, or exacerbation of sun-induced photodermatoses. The primary long-term benefits are to prevent skin cancer and premature aging of the skin. For most patients, carefully following product instructions and the self-care measures listed here will help ensure optimal therapeutic outcomes.

Avoiding/Minimizing Sun Exposure

- Avoid exposure to the sun and other sources of ultraviolet radiation (UVR), such as tanning beds/booths and sunlamps.
- The sun's rays are the most direct and damaging between 10:00 am and 4:00 pm. Avoid sun exposure as much as possible during this time of day.
- Sunburn can occur on a cloudy or overcast day; 70%–90% of UVR penetrates clouds.
- Wear protective clothing (e.g., long pants, a long-sleeved shirt, and a hat with a brim). Tightly woven fabrics that do not allow light to pass through will provide the most protection.
- Use a beach umbrella or other protection to reduce UVR.
- Water and wet clothing allow significant transmission of UVR. Even if the body is completely submerged, consider time in the water as part of the total time spent in the sun.

Use of Sunscreens

- An SPF of 15 or greater provides the greatest protection against sunburn and other UVB-induced skin problems.
- A broad-spectrum sunscreen product (e.g., avobenzone used in combination with padimate O and/or octocrylene, meradimate, titanium dioxide, or one of the benzophenones) provides optimal protection against UVA and UVB sun exposure. This type of sunscreen is especially recommended if you have a sun-induced disorder, if you are taking photosensitizing drugs, or if you just want to reduce sun exposure as much as possible to prevent long-term effects.
- Apply first dose 15 minutes before exposure.

- Apply approximately 1 ounce of sunscreen over the exposed areas of the body, avoiding contact with the eyes. The sunscreen should be distributed as follows: 1/2 teaspoon to the face and neck area, 1/2 teaspoon to the arms and shoulders, 1/2 teaspoon to the front and back each, and 1 teaspoon to each side on the leg and top of the foot.
- Use the most substantive sunscreen available; water-resistant sunscreens are recommended if you will be in water or perspiring excessively.
- Reapply the sunscreen according to the label instructions, usually every 40 minutes or 80 minutes (as directed on the label) for water-resistant sunscreens while swimming or sweating or after towel drying. Apply every 2 hours for non–water-resistant products or for water-resistant products if you are not swimming or sweating.
- Always check the expiration date on the sunscreen product. Sunscreens can lose their effectiveness.
- Higher altitudes and lower latitudes increase the amount of UVR to which an individual is exposed. Take proper precautions (e.g., use a sunscreen with a high SPF) to protect skin from UVR.
- Snow and sand reflect UVR. Take proper precautions to protect exposed skin (e.g., wear sunglasses and use high SPF sunscreens).
- Keep sunscreen out of direct sun, which can reduce its potency.
- Continue to use a sunscreen as long you are taking a photosensitizing drug or exhibiting signs and symptoms of photodermatitis.
- Avoid sunscreens containing aminobenzoic acid derivatives, benzophenones, cinnamates, or meradimate if you have had a prior allergic reaction to a sunscreen product.
- Stop using the sunscreen if redness, itching, rash, or exaggerated sunburn occurs.

Key: SPF = Sun protection factor; UVA = ultraviolet A; UVB = ultraviolet B.

Evaluation of Patient Outcomes for Sun-Induced Skin Disorders

The short-term outcomes for sunscreen use are readily apparent. Twenty-four hours after use, there will be no obvious sunburn, photosensitivity reaction, or eruption of photodermatosis. This success indicates that the appropriate sunscreen agents and/or SPF were used. However, the long-term effects of UVR (e.g., skin cancer or premature aging of the skin) may take up to 20–30 years to become evident.

Key Points for Sun-Induced Skin Disorders

➤ UVR (UVA and UVB) triggers a variety of photodermatoses and causes sunburn, photosensitivity, skin cancer, premature aging of the skin, cataracts, and a variety of other medical problems.
➤ There is no safe form of UVR exposure. Tanning and use of tanning beds can result in negative health effects.
➤ The effects of UVR are cumulative over one's lifetime.

a word about
Sun-Induced Ocular Damage

Recent studies have demonstrated a relationship between both UVA and UVB in cataract formation. UVR has been shown to cause temporary injuries such as photokeratitis (a painful type of snow blindness associated with highly reflective surfaces). Another concern involves an increase in the incidence of uveal (iris plus ciliary body) melanoma. These concerns are even more serious because of the erroneous belief that all sunglasses screen out UVR. In response, the Sunglass Association of America, working with FDA, has developed a voluntary labeling program. Abbreviated information concerning sunglasses' UVR-screening properties is directly attached to each pair, and brochures describing the appropriate use of each type of lens are available at outlets selling the sunglasses.[37]

According to its UVR filtration properties, each pair of sunglasses is placed in one of the following three categories:

1. Cosmetic sunglasses block at least 70% UVB and 20% UVA. They are recommended for activities in nonharsh sunlight (e.g., shopping).
2. General-purpose sunglasses block at least 95% UVB and 60% UVA. With shades that range from medium to dark, they are recommended for most activities in sunny environments (e.g., boating, driving, flying, or hiking).
3. Special-purpose sunglasses block at least 99% UVB and 60% UVA. They are recommended for activities in very bright environments (e.g., ski slopes and tropical beaches).[37]

Key: FDA = Food and Drug Administration; UVA = ultraviolet A; UVB = ultraviolet B; UVR = ultraviolet radiation.

➤ The best protection against UVR is avoidance. The next best approach is to wear a hat, long sleeves, pants, and UV-protective sunglasses.

➤ Maximum protection is provided by using a broad-spectrum sunscreen of SPF 15+.

➤ Because broad-spectrum sunscreens provide added UVA protection, they are the best sunscreen for preventing long-term effects, regardless of the patient's history.

Providers need to appreciate sunscreen products as therapeutic agents rather than cosmetics. Unfortunately, most patients have the latter view. This perception makes good patient counseling even more important. Reinforcing the need for proper selection of the appropriate sunscreen product and correct use of these products are key to educating the public and reducing the risks of UVR exposure.

REFERENCES

1. Bylaite M, Grigaitiene J, Lapinskaite GS. Photodermatoses: classification, evaluation and management. *Br J Dermatol.* 2009;161(suppl 3):61–8.

2. Vandergriff TW, Bergstresser PR. Abnormal responses to ultraviolet radiation: idiopathic, probably immunologic, and photoexacerbated. In: Goldsmith LA, Katz SI, Gilchrest BA, et al., eds. *Fitzpatrick's Dermatology in General Medicine.* 8th ed. New York: McGraw-Hill; 2012:Chap 91. Accessed at http://www.accessmedicine.com/content.aspx?aID=56051339, April 23, 2013.

3. Lim HW. Abnormal responses to ultraviolet radiation: photosensitivity induced by exogenous agents. In: Goldsmith LA, Katz SI, Gilchrest BA, et al., eds. *Fitzpatrick's Dermatology in General Medicine.* 8th ed. New York: McGraw-Hill; 2012:Chap 92. http://www.accessmedicine.com/content.aspx?aID=56051779. Accessed April 23, 2013.

4. American Cancer Society. *Cancer Facts & Figures 2012.* Atlanta, GA: American Cancer Society, Inc.; 2012.

5. Gonzaga ER. Role of UV light in photodamage, skin aging, and skin cancer. *Am J Clin Dermatol.* 2009;10(suppl 1):19–24.

6. El Ghissassi F, Baan R, Straif K, et al. A review of human carcinogens—Part D: radiation. *Lancet Oncol.* 2009;10(8):294–304.

7. Reichrath J. Skin cancer prevention and UV-protection: how to avoid vitamin D-deficiency? *Br J Dermatol.* 2009;161(suppl 3):54–60.

8. Diehl JW, Chiu MW. Effects of ambient sunlight and photoprotection on vitamin D status. *Dermatol Ther.* 2010;23(1):48–60.

9. American Academy of Dermatology. Position statement on Vitamin D. January 19, 2011. Accessed at http://www.aad.org/forms/policies/uploads/ps/ps-vitamin%20d%20postition%20statement.pdf, September 15, 2014.

10. Palm MD, O'Donoghue MN. Update on photoprotection. *Dermatol Ther.* 2007;20(5):360–76.

11. O'Riordan DL, Field AE, Geller AC, et al. Frequent tanning bed use, weight concerns, and other health risk behaviors in adolescent females (United States). *Cancer Causes Control.* 2006;17(5):679–86.

12. International Agency for Research on Cancer Working Group on Artificial Ultraviolet (UV) Light And Skin Cancer. The association of use of sunbeds with cutaneous malignant melanoma and other skin cancers: a systematic review. *Int J Cancer.* 2007;120(5):1116–22.

13. U.S. Food and Drug Administration. Sunlamp products and ultraviolet lamps intended for use in sunlamp products. 21 CFR 1040. *Federal Register.* 1992;20:519–22.

14. Young AR, Walker SL. Acute and chronic effects of ultraviolet radiation on the skin. In: Wolff K, Goldsmith LA, Katz SI, et al., eds. *Fitzpatrick's Dermatology in General Medicine.* 7th ed. New York: McGraw-Hill; 2007:Chap 89. Access Medicine Online Electronic Medical Library. Available to subscribers at http://www.accessmedicine.com.

15. U.S. Environmental Protection Agency. *The Burning Facts.* Washington, DC: U.S. Environmental Protection Agency; September 2006. Publication No. EPA430-F-060-013.

16. Averbach H. Geographic variation in incidence of skin cancer in the United States. *Public Health Rep.* 1961;76:345–8.

17. American Cancer Society. Skin cancer prevention and early detection. July 6, 2010. Accessed at http://www.cancer.org/cancer/cancercauses/

sunanduvexposure/skincancerpreventionandearlydetection/skin-cancer-prevention-and-early-detection-intro, June 24, 2011.

18. Tuchinda C, Srivannaboon S, Lim HW. Photoprotection by window glass, automobile glass, and sunglasses. *J Am Acad Dermatol.* 2006;54(5):845–54.

19. U.S. Environmental Protection Agency. *A Guide to the UV Index.* Washington, DC: U.S. Environmental Protection Agency; May 2004. Publication No. EPA30-F-04-020. Accessed at http://www.epa.gov/sunwise/publications.html, June 24, 2011.

20. Brash DE, Heffernan T, Nghiem P. Carcinogenesis: ultraviolet radiation. In: Wolff K, Goldsmith LA, Katz SI, eds. *Fitzpatrick's Dermatology in General Medicine.* 7th ed. New York: McGraw-Hill; 2008:Chap 112. Access Medicine Online Electronic Medical Library. Available to subscribers at http://www.accessmedicine.com. Accessed July 14, 2011.

21. Kullavanijaya P, Lim HW. Photoprotection. *J Am Acad Dermatol.* 2005;52(6):937–58.

22. U.S. Food and Drug Administration. Over-the-counter human drugs; labeling requirements; delay of implementation date. Final rule: delay of implementation date of certain provisions. *Federal Register.* 2004;69:53801–04.

23. U.S. Food and Drug Administration. Labeling and effectiveness testing; sunscreen drug products for over-the-counter human use. Final rule. *Federal Register.* 2011;76(117):35620–65. Accessed at http://www.regulations.gov/#!documentDetail;D=FDA-1978-N-0018-0698, June 24, 2011.

24. U.S. Food and Drug Administration. Revised effectiveness determination; sunscreen drug products for over-the-counter human use. *Federal Register.* 2011;76(117):35672–8. Accessed at http://www.regulations.gov/#!documentDetail;D=FDA-1978-N-0018-0699, June 24, 2011.

25. U.S. Food and Drug Administration. SPF labeling and testing requirements and drug facts labeling for over-the-counter sunscreen drug products; agency information collection activities; proposed collection. *Federal Register.* 2011;76(117):35678–81. Accessed at http://www.regulations.gov/#!documentDetail;D=FDA-2011-N-0449-0001. Accessed June 24, 2011.

26. U.S. Food and Drug Administration. Sunscreen drug products for over-the-counter human use; request for data and information regarding dosage forms; advanced notice of proposed rulemaking; request for data and information. *Federal Register.* 2011;76(117):35669–72. Accessed at http://www.regulations.gov/#!documentDetail;D=FDA-1978-N-0018-0697, June 24, 2011.

27. U.S. Food and Drug Administration. Guidance for Industry. Enforcement Policy—OTC Sunscreen Drug Products Marketed Without an Approved Application. Draft Guidance. June 2011. Accessed at http://www.fda.gov/downloads/Drugs/GuidanceComplianceRegulatoryInformation/Guidances/UCM259001.pdf, June 24, 2011.

28. U.S. Food and Drug Administration. Sunscreen drug products for over-the-counter human use. Final monograph. *Federal Register.* 1999;64:27666–93.

29. Wang SQ, Balagula Y, Osterwalder U. Photoprotection: a review of the current and future technologies. *Dermatol Ther.* 2010;23(1):31–47.

30. Tuchinda C, Lim HW, Osterwalder U, et al. Novel emerging sunscreen technologies. *Dermatol Clin.* 2006;24(1):105–17.

31. U.S. Food and Drug Administration. Sunscreen drug products for over-the-counter human use. Final monograph; technical amendment. *Federal Register.* 2002;67:41821–3.

32. Burnett ME, Hu JY, Wang SQ. Sunscreens: Obtaining adequate photoprotection. *Dermatologic Therapy.* 2012;25(3):244–51

33. Centers for Disease Control and Prevention. Sunburn and sun protective behaviors among adults aged 18–29 years—United States, 2000–2010. *Morb Mortal Wkly Rep MMWR* 2012;61(18):318–30.

34. Journe F, Marguery MC, Rakotondrazafy J, et al. Sunscreen sensitization: a 5-year study. *Acta Derm Venereol.* 1999;79(3):211–3.

35. Foley P, Nixon R, Marks R, et al. The frequency of reactions to sunscreens: results of a longitudinal population-based study on the regular use of sunscreens in Australia. *Br J Dermatol.* 1993;128(5):512–8.

36. U.S. Food and Drug Administration. Should you put sunscreen on infants? Not usually. Update for consumers. June 25, 2013. Accessed at http://www.fda.gov/forconsumers/consumerupdates/ucm309136.htm, October 31, 2013.

37. Sunglass Association of America. *SAA UV Labeling Program.* Norwalk, CT: Sunglass Association of America; 1997.

SKIN HYPERPIGMENTATION AND PHOTOAGING

Katherine S. O'Neal and Kimberly M. Crosby

Photoaging of the skin is directly related to exposure to ultraviolet radiation (UVR). Skin hyperpigmentation may result from serious or benign medical conditions. This chapter focuses on the treatment of hyperpigmentation and photoaging once they have occurred. Nonprescription products used to minimize sun exposure are discussed in Chapter 38.

Hydroquinone, a skin-bleaching agent, can be used for self-treatment of hyperpigmentation. However, this may soon change if the Food and Drug Administration (FDA) rules to remove this product from the market. Alpha hydroxy acids (AHAs), promoted as nonprescription treatments for photoaging, are used to treat both disorders.

Skin Hyperpigmentation

Hyperpigmentation, manifested as an area of skin darker than the surrounding skin, is usually a benign phenomenon. Hyperpigmentation may be perceived by the patient as a disfigurement, especially when the altered pigmentation occurs on the face and neck and is in noticeable contrast to the surrounding normal skin color. Although products used to treat hyperpigmentation serve a cosmetic function, it is important to emphasize that they are drugs with potential toxicity and side effects. Pigment disorders may also present with both hypo- and hyperpigmented skin or skin that may appear mottled.

Pathophysiology of Skin Hyperpigmentation

Systemic as well as localized skin diseases may cause pigment cells to become overactive (resulting in skin darkening) or underactive (resulting in skin lightening). Endocrine imbalances caused by Addison's disease, Cushing's disease, or hyperthyroidism and conditions such as pregnancy are capable of altering skin pigmentation. Metabolic alterations affecting the liver, as well as certain nutritional deficiencies, can be associated with diffuse melanosis. Inflammatory dermatoses (e.g., contact dermatitis from poison ivy or acne lesions) or physical trauma to the skin (e.g., thermal burn) may cause prolonged postinflammatory hyperpigmentation. In addition, certain drugs (Table 39–1) have an affinity

for melanin and may cause hyperpigmentation. Skin hyperpigmentation resulting from these conditions may occur as a result of increased melanin, increased melanocytes, or deposits of other darkening chemicals in the skin.[1–3] Melanocytes (pigment cells) produce melanosomes, pigment granules that contain the protein melanin, a brown-black pigment. These cells can be viewed as tiny one-celled glands with long projections used to pass pigment particles into the keratinocytes, from which the particles migrate upward to the skin surface. The human epidermis has about 800–1000 melanocytes per square millimeter. The melanocyte density is the same in all races. However, the proportion and distribution of these cells throughout the epidermis differ. The melanocyte is believed to provide protection from UVR. Dark skin usually has more active melanocytes compared with light skin, which explains why UVR-induced skin cancers of all types are less common in dark skin than in light skin.[4–6]

Three types of hyperpigmentation may be self-treated with topical nonprescription agents: ephelides, solar lentigines, and melasma.[7] Ephelides, or freckles, are spots of uneven skin pigmentation that first appear in childhood, are exacerbated by the sun, and tend to fade with reduced sun exposure. Melasma (also called chloasma), a condition in which macular hyperpigmentation appears, usually on the face or neck, is often associated with pregnancy ("the mask of pregnancy") or the use of oral contraceptives, as well as with sun exposure. Solar or "senile" lentigines (age spots or liver spots) appear on exposed skin surfaces, particularly in fair-skinned people, and are induced by UVR.

Clinical Presentation of Skin Hyperpigmentation

Depending on the etiology of hyperpigmentation, patients can present with varying signs and symptoms. Most notably, patients complain of persistent macular discoloration on the face or other sun-exposed areas. Discoloration typically consists of a more intense brown coloration than that of surrounding normal skin and may range from dark to faint in appearance. Clinical evidence of hyperpigmentation and photoaging, as well as response to treatment, is not easily quantifiable by standard light photography or by routine clinical evaluation. Fluorescence photography is used to detect subtle but significant decreases in diffuse and mottled hyperpigmentation after topical treatment, which helps to clinically evaluate and effectively assess the efficacy of topical products.[8]

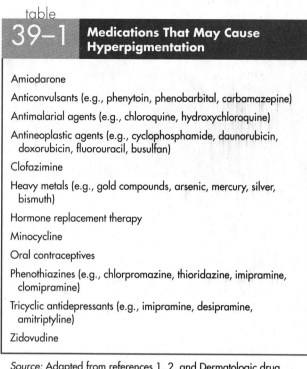

table

39–1 Medications That May Cause Hyperpigmentation

Amiodarone

Anticonvulsants (e.g., phenytoin, phenobarbital, carbamazepine)

Antimalarial agents (e.g., chloroquine, hydroxychloroquine)

Antineoplastic agents (e.g., cyclophosphamide, daunorubicin, doxorubicin, fluorouracil, busulfan)

Clofazimine

Heavy metals (e.g., gold compounds, arsenic, mercury, silver, bismuth)

Hormone replacement therapy

Minocycline

Oral contraceptives

Phenothiazines (e.g., chlorpromazine, thioridazine, imipramine, clomipramine)

Tricyclic antidepressants (e.g., imipramine, desipramine, amitriptyline)

Zidovudine

Source: Adapted from references 1, 2, and Dermatologic drug reactions and common skin conditions. In: Dipiro JT, Talbert RL, Yee GC, et al., eds. *Pharmacotherapy: A Pathophysiologic Approach.* 8th ed. New York, NY: McGraw-Hill Professional; 2011:1661–72.

Treatment of Skin Hyperpigmentation

Treatment Goals

The goal of treating skin hyperpigmentation is to diminish the degree of pigmentation of affected areas so the skin tone of these areas is consistent with surrounding normal skin.

General Treatment Approach

The approaches to treat hyperpigmentation have expanded significantly within the past 10 years. The treatment generally falls into two categories: stopping the skin cells from overproducing melanin (the cells responsible for giving the skin its pigment) and physically removing the top few layers of the skin's surface through chemical or mechanical exfoliation. Although good results can be achieved using either approach, the best results are accomplished through a combination of the two.

Exfoliation used to treat hyperpigmentation involves physically buffing away surface-layer skin (microdermabrasion) and applying chemical agents (e.g., AHAs). Although microdermabrasion is a routine procedure in salons, the recommendation is to seek an experienced practitioner. Because of the risk of microdermabrasion tearing the skin, chemical peeling is a better option for sensitive skin. Abrading skin may also cause irradiation and burning.

Skin-bleaching agents diminish hyperpigmentation by inhibiting melanin production within skin.[9] As discussed in the section Treatment of Photoaging, the combination of hydroquinone with an antioxidant and exfoliant is considered efficacious, giving patients acceptable outcomes with minimal adverse effects.[3,9–11]

To prevent negation of the effects of treatment, patients must avoid even minimal exposure to UVR, and they must use sunscreen agents and protective clothing on an ongoing

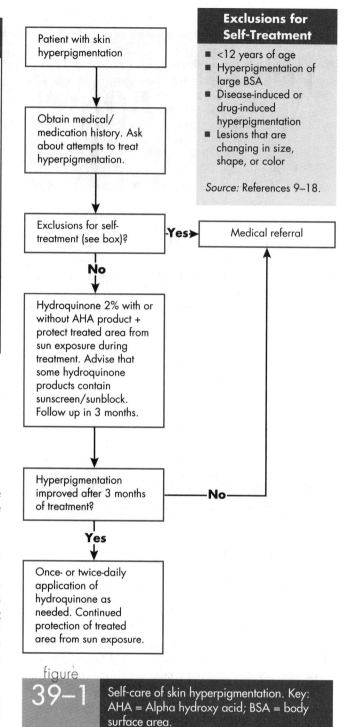

figure

39–1 Self-care of skin hyperpigmentation. Key: AHA = Alpha hydroxy acid; BSA = body surface area.

basis, even after discontinuing the bleaching agent. The algorithm in Figure 39–1 outlines the self-treatment of skin hyperpigmentation.[9–18]

Pharmacologic Therapy

Management of hyperpigmentation as directed by a primary care provider may include topical prescription agents composed of ingredients known to cause lightening of the skin, such as tretinoin (retinoic acid), azelaic acid, hydroquinone, and corticosteroid, and may include laser therapy. Combination products or laser therapy may sometimes be effective for postinflammatory hyperpigmentation that is resistant to nonprescription treatment.[12]

A number of nonprescription agents have been used in skin-bleaching preparations. These agents have included hydroquinone 2%, ascorbic acid, *N*-acetyl glucosamine, glycolic acid, vitamin C, licorice extract, niacinamide, and kojic acid. Newer products are being formulated with synthetic oligopeptide, rucinol, tranexamic acid, deoxyarbutin, dioic acid, and aloesin.[3,13] However, only preparations containing hydroquinone were submitted to the FDA Advisory Review Panel on Over-the-Counter Miscellaneous External Drug Products, and products containing this agent remain the most effective nonprescription skin-bleaching products available. Table 39–2 lists selected trade-name products.

Hypopigmentation treatment options are often limited. Treating hypopigmentation may involve the use of topical products, light or laser treatment, or surgical skin grafting. Nonprescription skin-staining products such as Dy-O-Derm or Chromelin Complexion Blender, which contain dihydroxyacetone (the active ingredient in self-tanning products and treatment for vitiligo), may be used to adjust color in lightened skin areas to approximate natural darker tones in mixed hypo- and hyperpigmented disorders.[14] Once the desired skin color is attained, applications may be decreased from daily to every fourth to seventh day to maintain the desired outcome. These products have a higher

concentration of dihydroxyacetone compared with self-tanning products and are not intended for widespread application over the body.

Hydroquinone

Hydroquinone (*p*-dihydroxybenzene) in concentrations of 1.5%–2% is currently available for nonprescription use for the treatment of skin hyperpigmentation.[7] It is considered to be the mainstay and gold standard of hyperpigmentation therapy.[3,10,13] However, the safety of bleaching creams that contain hydroquinone continues to be reviewed in the literature.[14–15] In 2006, FDA proposed withdrawing the tentative final monograph approving skin-bleaching creams to replace it with a final rule stating that all drug products (including hydroquinone) used for skin lightening in nonprescription products are no longer generally recognized as safe and effective owing to the potential increased risk of cancer and ochronosis. If this final monograph is published, hydroquinone products will be removed from the nonprescription marketplace. In December 2009, a nomination was approved for additional studies to be conducted by the National Toxicology Program (NTP) to determine if the use of hydroquinone poses a risk to humans.[17] At the time this book went to press, the NTP review process was still ongoing.[17] In the interim, FDA believes that hydroquinone should remain available as a nonprescription OTC drug product.

Hydroquinone and its derivatives act by reducing conversion of tyrosine to dopa and, subsequently, to melanin by inhibiting the enzyme tyrosinase. Other possible mechanisms of action include destruction of the melanocyte or melanosomes.[9–10] The 2% concentration is safer and produces results equivalent to those of higher concentrations.[15] Exfoliants such as topical glycolic acid (an AHA) or topical tretinoin are sometimes combined with hydroquinone to increase efficacy compared with hydroquinone monotherapy.[18]

Hydroquinone 2% should be rubbed gently but thoroughly into affected areas twice daily. The agent should be applied to clean skin before application of moisturizers or other skin care products. It should not be applied to damaged skin or near the eyes. If no improvement is seen within 2 months, its use should be discontinued and a primary care provider should be consulted.[9,19] Once the desired benefit is achieved, hydroquinone can be applied as often as needed in a once- or twice-daily regimen to maintain lightening of the skin. Because of the lack of safety data, hydroquinone is not recommended for children younger than 12 years. Contraindications to the use of hydroquinone include hypersensitivity to the product. Although not directly contraindicated, it should be used during pregnancy only if absolutely needed.[19]

Adverse effects, such as tingling or burning on application, are mild with low concentrations of topical hydroquinone.[11] Patients may want to apply the agent to a small test area and check for signs of irritation after 24 hours. Higher concentrations frequently irritate the skin and, if used for prolonged periods, may cause side effects, including epidermal thickening, ochronosis, and colloid milium.[11,19]

The effectiveness of hydroquinone varies among patients. Results are best on lighter skin and lighter lesions. In dark skin, the response to hydroquinone depends on the amount of pigment present. Although treatment may not lead to complete disappearance of hypermelanosis, the results are often satisfactory enough to reduce self-consciousness. A disadvantage of

table 39–2	Selected Nonprescription Skin Bleaching/Fading Products
Trade Name	**Primary Ingredients**
Clinicians Complex 6% Skin Bleaching Cream	Hydroquinone 2%; kojic acid 2%
La Roche-Posay Mela-D Skin Lightening Daily Lotion	Hydroquinone 2%
Topix HQS-2 Skin Lightening Cream	Hydroquinone 2%; benzophenone 1.5%
DDF Fade Gel 4	Hydroquinone 2%; kojic acid; azelaic acid; salicylic acid
Glymed Plus Derma Pigment Bleaching Fluid	Hydroquinone 2%
SkinCeuticals Pigment Regulator	Kojic acid 2%; emblica extract 2%; glycolic acid
Murad Age Spot and Pigment Lightening Gel	Hydroquinone 2%; glycolic acid
Exuviance Brighten Up Kit	Hydroquinone 2%; glycolic acid; PHA/kojic acid complex
Alpha Hydrox Spot Light Skin Lightener	Hydroquinone 2%; glycolic acid 10%; vitamin E
Lumixyl	Synthetic oligopeptide 0.1%
Philosophy Miracle Worker Dark Spot Corrector	Niacinamide
Shiseido White Lucent Intensive Spot Targeting Serum	Tranexamic acid
Noreva IKLEN Depigmenting Serum	Rucinol

Key: PHA = Polyhydroxy acids.

treatment with hydroquinone is that it tends to overshoot the intended degree of lightening and may produce treated areas that are lighter than the surrounding normal skin color. Therefore, the patient must carefully observe the degree of lightening as the treatment progresses and must subsequently decrease applications when sufficient lightening has occurred.

A decrease in skin color usually becomes noticeable in about 4 weeks; however, the time of onset varies from 3 weeks to 2 months. The reduced pigmentation lasts for 2–6 months but can be reversed by exposing skin to UVR. Although sunscreens may help to prevent repigmentation, even visible light may cause some darkening. Therefore, a sunscreen containing opaque ingredients, such as zinc oxide or titanium dioxide, is preferable for sun protection.[2] Some nonprescription hydroquinone products are formulated to include a sunscreen.

In some cases, lesions become slightly darker before fading. A transient inflammatory reaction may develop after the first few weeks of treatment. Inflammation makes subsequent lightening more likely, although inflammation can occur without subsequent depigmentation. Mild inflammation is not an indication to stop therapy except when the reaction increases in intensity, at which point a patch test for allergy to hydroquinone can be done. Most reactions, however, are irritant rather than allergic in nature. Topical hydrocortisone may be used temporarily to alleviate the inflammatory reaction. A few cases of reversible brown discoloration of nails after application of hydroquinone have been reported.[20]

Alternative Agents

Synthetic Oligopeptide

A clinical trial demonstrated that synthetic oligopeptide 0.01% produced improvement in hyperpigmentation. The oligopeptide's mechanism of action, inhibiting tyrosinase, is similar to that of hydroquinone. The study found that the product was well tolerated and less toxic than hydroquinone. This agent is currently available only in the nonprescription product Lumixyl. It has not been approved by FDA as a skin-bleaching product. A pea-size amount should be applied twice daily, with results expected in 8–16 weeks.[21–23]

Kojic Acid

Kojic acid, a product derived from certain species of fungus (e.g., *Acetobacter*, *Aspergillus*, and *Penicillium*), can be found in cosmetic products promoted for the treatment of hyperpigmentation. This product is usually found in combination with AHAs, with or without hydroquinone. It is dosed and applied according to the product type (e.g., cream, soap, lotion, and drops). Kojic acid works by inhibiting the production of tyrosinase. Adverse effects associated with this product include contact dermatitis and erythema. One study comparing the combination of kojic acid and glycolic acid with that of hydroquinone and glycolic acid demonstrated similar results between the two therapies.[3,10–12]

Rucinol

Rucinol is a resorcinol derivative that has a unique mechanism of action that inhibits both tyrosinase and tyrosinase-related protein-1 (TRP-1), which is an enzyme used in melanin synthesis.[10,13] Several studies have demonstrated that rucinol serum

or cream, applied twice daily, improved pigmentation within 8–12 weeks and was tolerated well.[10,13,23]

Tranexamic Acid

Tranexamic acid (trans-4-aminomethylcyclohexanecarboxylic acid) is an agent that has been available for many years but is receiving more attention as a result of the hydroquinone controversy. It works by inhibiting plasmin.[9,13,24] Plasmin indirectly leads to decreased tyrosinase activity in melanocytes. Although some studies have shown no benefit, a few have shown improvement within 12 weeks of beginning use.[24] Studies have evaluated topical, intravenous, and oral dosage forms. The most common side effects of the topical form were irritation to the applied area. Currently, tranexamic acid can be found as an adjunct ingredient in some nonprescription serums.

Mandelic Acid

Mandelic acid is one type of AHA and is derived from almonds. It is used in the treatment of several skin conditions, including hyperpigmentation. When combined with salicylic acid and administered as a peel, it has fewer side effects than a glycolic peel and has demonstrated better efficacy.[25]

Niacinamide

Niacinamide is a form of vitamin B_3. Although most pharmacologic treatments of hyperpigmentation disrupt tyrosinase activity, niacinamide instead works by preventing the transfer of melanin to keratinocytes. Another form of vitamin B_3, niacin, has been shown to significantly decrease hyperpigmentation and is associated with only mild side effects.[26–27]

Product Selection Guidelines

Product selection should be based on a suitable dosage form (e.g., cream, lotion, or gel) for the patient's skin type (dry, normal, or oily) and anatomic site (face or neck). For example, an emollient cream-based product may be more suitable for dry skin, whereas a gel-based preparation may be preferable for an oily skin type.

Assessment of Skin Hyperpigmentation: A Case-Based Approach

Assessment should involve evaluating the affected areas to determine whether they are characteristic of freckles, melasma, or lentigines. The patient's medication history and health status are important factors in pinpointing possible causes of the hyperpigmentation.

Case 39–1 is an example of the assessment of a patient with skin hyperpigmentation.

Patient Counseling for Skin Hyperpigmentation

The types of hyperpigmentation that are self-treatable should be explained to the patient, and the importance of avoiding sun exposure during and after treatment should be stressed. The

case
39–1

Relevant Evaluation Criteria	Scenario/Model Outcome

Information Gathering

1. Gather essential information about the patient's symptoms and medical history, including:

    a. description of symptom(s) (i.e., nature, onset, duration, severity, associated symptoms)

       The patient has been experiencing darkening areas of skin on her forehead, which first appeared 6 months ago.

    b. description of any factors that seem to precipitate, exacerbate, and/or relieve the patient's symptom(s)

       Patient says that she has been on an oral contraceptive for 2 years. The skin areas appear darker when the patient spends more time in sunlight.

    c. description of the patient's efforts to relieve the symptoms

       The patient has tried topical moisturizing lotions and hydroquinone 2% per the pharmacist's recommendation 3 months ago, but she has seen little improvement. Patient inquires about trying Lumixyl next.

    d. patient's identity

       Judy Blume

    e. age, sex, height, and weight

       20 years old, female, 5 ft 6 in., 160 lb

    f. patient's occupation

       Full-time college student

    g. patient's dietary habits

       Diet is well balanced. She drinks wine and beer occasionally.

    h. patient's sleep habits

       She averages 5 hours per night during the week and 10 hours on the weekend.

    i. concurrent medical conditions, prescription and nonprescription medications, and dietary supplements

       Birth control: Yaz 1 tablet every day; headaches or menstrual cramps: ibuprofen 200 mg as needed; polycystic ovaries: Glucophage XR 500 mg daily

    j. allergies

       None

    k. history of other adverse reactions to medications

       None

    l. other (describe) _____

       NA

Assessment and Triage

2. Differentiate patient's signs/symptoms and correctly identify the patient's primary problem(s).

    The patient has hyperpigmentation on her forehead, which appeared 6 months ago. Patient started taking an oral contraceptive agent 2 years ago, which may have contributed to the hyperpigmentation. The areas turn darker when exposed to sunlight, but they have not really changed since they appeared.

3. Identify exclusions for self-treatment (Figure 39–1).

    The patient has tried OTC products, including hydroquinone, unsuccessfully for 3 months.

4. Formulate a comprehensive list of therapeutic alternatives for the primary problem to determine if triage to a medical provider is required, and share this information with the patient or caregiver.

    Options include:

    (1) Refer Judy to a health care provider or dermatologist for further evaluation.

    (2) Discontinue oral contraceptive.

    (3) Take no action.

Plan

5. Select an optimal therapeutic alternative to address the patient's problem, taking into account patient preferences.

    Patient should be referred to a health care provider or dermatologist because the OTC treatment has been unsuccessful.

6. Describe the recommended therapeutic approach to the patient or caregiver.

    "Because you have tried self-treatment unsuccessfully for 3 months, you should see a health care provider or dermatologist for further evaluation."

7. Explain to the patient or caregiver the rationale for selecting the recommended therapeutic approach from the considered therapeutic alternatives.

    "Continuing treatment with the current product or trying another OTC option will most likely not provide any benefit. A health care provider or dermatologist can evaluate your condition and suggest other treatments."

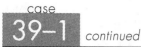

case

39-1 *continued*

Relevant Evaluation Criteria	Scenario/Model Outcome
Patient Education	
8. When recommending self-care with nonprescription medications and/or nondrug therapy, convey accurate information to the patient or caregiver.	Criterion does not apply in this case.
Solicit follow-up questions from the patient or caregiver.	"A friend told me about Lumixyl. Can't I try it first?"
Answer the patient's or caregiver's questions.	"Lumixyl is not FDA approved yet. Hydroquinone is currently the best OTC product available, and because you tried it for 3 months with no improvement, I would recommend that you be seen for further evaluation."
Evaluation of Patient Outcomes	
9. Assess patient outcome.	Contact the patient in a couple of days to ensure that she made an appointment for further evaluation.

Key: FDA = Food and Drug Administration; NA = not applicable; OTC = over-the-counter.

product instructions should be reviewed with the patient to ensure a successful therapeutic outcome. The box Patient Education for Skin Hyperpigmentation lists specific information to provide patients.

Evaluation of Patient Outcomes for Skin Hyperpigmentation

Follow-up on the patient's progress should occur after 3 months of therapy. Follow-up can be achieved through a telephone call or a scheduled visit. If the pigmented area shows no improvement, the patient should consult a primary care provider or a

dermatologist. If the desired outcome has been achieved, the patient should continue applying the agent once or twice daily to maintain lightening of the skin.

Photoaging

Photoaging, also referred to as premature aging or dermatoheliosis, is the pattern of characteristic skin changes associated with sun exposure. Most fair-skinned Americans will have some signs of photodamaged skin by 50 years of age. A variety of therapies

patient education for

Skin Hyperpigmentation

The objective of self-treatment with skin-bleaching products is to diminish the degree of pigmentation in affected areas. For most patients, carefully following product instructions and the self-care measures listed here will help ensure optimal therapeutic outcomes.

Hydroquinone

- Use hydroquinone to lighten only limited areas of hyperpigmented skin that show brownish discoloration.
- Do not use these products on nevi (moles) or reddish or bluish areas, such as port wine discoloration.
- Time to initial response averages 6–8 weeks, but it may take up to 3 months to see noticeable results.
- Test for possible irritant reactions to the product by applying it to a small test area and by checking the area for redness, itching, or swelling after 24 hours.
- Do not apply the product near the eyes or to damaged skin.
- Apply a thin layer of the product to clean, dry skin in the affected area only. Rub product into the skin gently but thoroughly.
- If moisturizers or other topical agents are being used at the same time, apply the hydroquinone first.

- When you are outdoors for even a short time, apply an opaque sunblock or broad-spectrum sunscreen (see Chapter 38) to the affected area after applying the hydroquinone, unless the product already contains a sunscreen in the formulation.
- Once the desired lightening of skin is reached, apply the hydroquinone once or twice daily to prevent hyperpigmentation from recurring. Continue to protect the treated area from sun exposure.

When to Seek Medical Attention

- Consult a primary care provider if:
  - No improvement is seen after 3 months of using hydroquinone.
  - Skin pigmentation becomes darker during treatment with hydroquinone.

are available to treat photodamaged skin; these therapies range from use of topical products and cosmetics to more invasive procedures such as face-lifts, botulinum toxin A injections, and laser resurfacing. Although some products are available by prescription only, many others are nonprescription, with AHAs being widely used to combat photoaged skin.[28]

Pathophysiology of Photoaging

Aging skin results from a combination of intrinsic and extrinsic factors. Clinical and histologic changes that occur intrinsically include genetically controlled skin and muscle changes, expression lines, sleep lines, and hormonal changes. The second component, extrinsic aging, relates to environmental influences such as UVR, smoking, wind, and chemical exposure.[29–31] Medications known to induce photosensitivity can contribute to photoaging by making the skin sensitive to UVR (see Chapter 38).

Prematurely aged facial skin, with creases and wrinkles, dry texture, and blotchy hyperpigmentation, is largely attributed to cumulative UVR, or photoaging. Exposure to ultraviolet B (UVB) (290–320 nm) is primarily responsible for photoaging, although the longer ultraviolet A (UVA) wavelengths (320–400 nm) also contribute to damage. The amount of UVA present in sunlight is 10 times that of UVB, which allows greater amounts of skin exposure. UVA can penetrate into the deeper dermal layer and can work synergistically with UVB to cause photodamage and skin cancers.

Microscopically, sun-damaged skin shows dysplasia (abnormal tissue development), atypical keratinocytes, and occasional cell necrosis. Irregularity of epidermal cell alignment is also common. Loss of collagen and elastin is seen deeper in the dermal layer.[29–31]

Clinical Presentation of Photoaging

Clinical signs of photoaging include changes in color, surface texture, and functional capacity (Table 39–3). Photoaged skin may have a sallow yellow color with discoloration and may

show telangiectasias (visible distended capillaries). Textural changes include loss of smoothness, loss of subcutaneous tissue around the mouth, and epidermal thinning around the lips. As sebaceous glands hypertrophy, the skin begins to show coarse texture with increased pore size. In addition, fine vellus hairs can develop into unwanted terminal hairs. Other manifestations of photoaged skin may include development of precancerous (actinic keratosis) and cancerous (basal cell, squamous cell, and melanoma) tumor development.[28–31] Cosmetically, patients may notice freckling, discolorations, or "crow's feet" (small parallel lines around the eyes). Postmenopausal skin is susceptible to reduced estrogen receptor stimulation of dermal metabolism and undergoes significant changes in collagen and moisture content. These changes lead to signs of skin aging, as evidenced by diminished elasticity and wrinkles.[32]

Treatment of Photoaging
Treatment Goals

The first goal is to prevent or minimize the likelihood of skin photoaging by using appropriate sun protection, including sunscreens.[33] The goals of treating photoaging are to (1) reverse cumulative skin damage with prescription and nonprescription products and (2) maintain the skin and protect it from further extrinsic damage by making lifestyle changes and, most important, protecting the skin from further and prolonged sun exposure.

General Treatment Approach

The first step in preventing and treating photoaged skin is for the patient to commit to daily sun protection. Broad-spectrum sunscreens (UVA and UVB coverage) with a sun protection factor (SPF) of 15 or greater can minimize further photodamage during UVR exposure[29] (see Chapter 38).

Proper cleansing of the skin removes bacteria, dirt, desquamated keratinocytes, cosmetics, sebum, and perspiration. However, excessive use of soap leads to xerosis, eczematous dermatitis, and other skin conditions.[34]

Pharmacologic Therapy

Within the vast array of available nonprescription products for skin care, the division of categories is blurred. Cosmetics and moisturizers are not pharmaceuticals, whereas antiperspirants and sunscreens are considered nonprescription pharmaceuticals. Although "cosmeceuticals" are an undefined category of products recognized by providers and dermatologists, no final regulatory guidance is currently available for these products from FDA. Many cosmeceutical ingredients, such as AHAs, function as active pharmaceuticals that are known to have a sustained effect on the skin.[35]

Various topical products are being used to treat aging skin. These products include coenzyme Q10, *N*-furfuryladenine (Kinerase), AHAs, and beta hydroxy acids (BHAs). Of the vitamins, only A, C, B$_3$, and E have the most evidence supporting their use in treatment and/or prevention of photoaging.[36]

Alpha and Beta Hydroxy Acids

Current labeling on AHA cosmetic products includes recommendations for melasma, acne, solar lentigines, and fine wrinkling of photoaging.[10] The AHAs are used in various concentrations

table **39–3**	**Glogau Classification of Photoaging**
Type I (Mild)	No wrinkles, early photoaging, mild pigment changes 20–30 years of age
Type II (Moderate)	Wrinkles in motion, early-to-moderate photoaging, keratoses palpable 30–40 years of age
Type III (Advanced)	Wrinkles at rest, advanced photoaging, obvious dyschromia and keratoses ≥50 years of age
Type IV (Severe)	Only wrinkles, severe photoaging, yellow-gray skin ≥60 years of age

Source: Glogau RG. Aesthetic and anatomic analysis of the aging skin. *Semin Cutan Med Surg.* 1996;15(3):134–8.

and in a wide array of available products. Most AHAs are sold as cosmeceuticals; however, some are sold as cosmetics, and yet others are sold as pharmaceuticals through a primary care provider. These products range in concentration from 2% to 20% (as nonpeeling AHAs). As peeling agents (as used by estheticians or dermatologists), they come in concentrations greater than 20%.

Of the available nonprescription products, AHAs currently play a major role in reliably reversing and cosmetically improving aging skin.[10,37] Many types of AHAs are available, with the most common being lactic and glycolic acids (Table 39–4). The Cosmetic Ingredient Review Expert Panel, the cosmetic industry's self-regulatory body, concluded that use of AHAs in cosmetic products is safe if (1) concentrations are less than or equal to 10%, (2) the final pH is greater than or equal to 3.5, and (3) the product is formulated with a sunscreen or includes directions to use a sunscreen.[38]

Of the BHAs, salicylic acid is used widely, even as a chemical peel.[39–40] Compared with AHA products, BHAs are more lipophilic and demonstrate keratolytic effects. Products containing BHAs as the active ingredients may be beneficial to acne-prone skin.

Polyhydroxy acids are the new generation of AHAs that appear to have results similar to those of the alpha and beta hydroxy products, but with less irritation.[33]

Used appropriately, AHA products act as exfoliants by causing detachment of keratinocytes, resulting in a smoother, nonscaly skin surface with eventual normalization of keratinization. The effect of the AHA product depends on the concentration and pH.[33] The lower the pH, the more effective the product, and the higher the AHA concentration, the more deeply it affects the stratum corneum. By improving skin elasticity, AHAs have been shown to make skin more flexible and less vulnerable to cracking and flaking. Long-term use has led to an increase in skin collagen and elastin.[33,37] Regular application of AHAs results in smoother skin texture, lessening of fine lines, and normalization of pigmentation.[37]

Guidelines for treatment with AHAs include identification of patient factors such as medications, prior procedures, and medical history, all of which may affect treatment outcome and realistic patient expectations.[41] Care should be taken to apply AHAs to completely dry skin, with an estimated wait time of 10–15 minutes after cleansing the face. It is also prudent to begin application gradually, starting every other night for approximately 1 week and then increasing as tolerated to a maximum of twice-daily application. AHA products may make the skin more sensitive to sun exposure. Patients should be advised to use daily sunscreen or sunblock with an SPF of 15 or greater during use of AHAs and after their discontinuation.[29]

Common adverse effects of AHA and BHA products include mild, transient stinging, burning, pruritus, skin lightening, and dryness. BHA products may be less irritating. Many of these effects can be ameliorated if products are used with caution and proper counseling. Patients should also note that other topically applied products, both medications and cosmetics, may contain active ingredients capable of exacerbating irritation (e.g., AHA, BHA, and hydroquinone).

Retinol and Retinaldehyde

Retinol has been incorporated into many skin care products. It is very unstable and, with light exposure, easily degrades to biologically inactive forms.[33] Retinol is transformed into retinaldehyde and then into retinoic acid with a two-step enzymatic process involving dehydrogenase in human keratinocytes. Topical retinaldehyde not only is well tolerated by human skin but has also been shown to have several effects identical to that of tretinoin.

Ascorbic Acid (Vitamin C)

Ascorbic acid (vitamin C) is a plentiful antioxidant in the skin.[33] It neutralizes reactive oxygen species caused by UV irradiation and functions as a scavenger of free radicals. Ascorbic acid could be used topically for the prevention and correction of human skin aging. Several studies with human volunteers have appeared in the literature in the past few years that suggest some anti-aging potential after topical ascorbic acid application. It is also reported that ascorbic acid has at least some photoprotective properties.

Idebenone

Ubiquinone (ubidecarenone; coenzyme Q10) is a lipophilic antioxidant that is synthesized by all mammalian cells and is critical for the protection of mitochondrial membranes.[33] Idebenone is a synthetic derivative of ubiquinone that is more soluble and has potent antioxidant properties. It has been suggested that by quenching free radicals in the epidermis, it has a beneficial effect on preventing and/or reversing photoaging. These products are

table **39–4**	**Selected Nonprescription Products for Photoaged Skin**
Trade Name	**Active Ingredients**
Alpha Hydroxy Acid Products	
DermaQuest Skin Therapy	Glycolic acid 5%; azelaic acid 2.5%; salicylic acid 2%
Dr. Michelle Copeland AHA Face Cream	Glycolic acid 10%
M.D. Forte Facial Cleanser III	Glycolic acid 20%
Alpha Hydrox AHA Enhanced Anti-Wrinkle Crème	Glycolic acid 10%
Aqua Glycolic Hand and Body Lotion	Glycolic acid 14%
Peter Thomas Roth Glycolic Acid Hydrating Gel	Glycolic acid 10%
DDF Glycolic Exfoliating Oil Control Gel	Glycolic acid 10%
Reviva Labs Glycolic Acid Cream Exfoliation and Cell Renewal	Glycolic acid 10%
Alpha Hydrox AHA Souffle	Glycolic acid 12%
Peter Thomas Roth Glycolic Acid Moisturizer	Glycolic acid 10%
Beta Hydroxy Acid Products	
Paula's Choice Exfoliating 2% BHA Lotion	Salicylic acid 2%
Peter Thomas Roth Beta Hydroxy 2% Acne Wash	Salicylic acid 2%

often found in cosmetic creams and lotions promoted as anti-aging and/or antioxidant products.

Product Selection Guidelines

Skin type should determine the product type chosen. Creams are appropriate for drier skin types, lotions are best for combination or normal skin, and gels or solutions are useful for oilier skin. Use of products with higher concentrations and a lower pH may produce faster results. However, the patient should be warned that these products may also cause greater skin irritation.

There are limited data on the safety of AHAs in special populations, such as pregnant or lactating women and pediatric and geriatric populations. AHA products appear to be safe when used topically in adults.[42]

Assessment of Photoaging: A Case-Based Approach

If visual inspection of the patient's skin indicates photoaging, the patient should be questioned about his or her history of UVR (sunlight as well as artificial light) exposure. Knowing whether the patient's current occupational or recreational habits require excessive exposure is useful not only in determining the cause of the skin disorder but also in developing a treatment plan. It is important to assess for a history of diseases or medications that may predispose the patient to premature photodamage or photosensitivity. The patient's health status, lifestyle practices, and daily skin maintenance regimen are other pertinent assessment criteria.[28]

Case 39–2 is an example of assessment of a patient with photoaging.

case

39–2

Relevant Evaluation Criteria	Scenario/Model Outcome
Information Gathering	
1. Gather essential information about the patient's symptoms and medical history, including:	
a. description of symptom(s) (i.e., nature, onset, duration, severity, associated symptoms)	Patient complains of observable photoaging on her skin, which includes increased pore size, wrinkles, dry skin, and dark skin pigmentation.
b. description of any factors that seem to precipitate, exacerbate, and/or relieve the patient's symptom(s)	These skin changes have been occurring over the past several years and are progressively becoming more noticeable.
c. description of the patient's efforts to relieve the symptoms	She uses daily moisturizer but wants to "clean up her face" with something stronger.
d. patient's identity	Dora Norris
e. age, sex, height, and weight	50 years old, female, 5 ft 4 in., 145 lb
f. patient's occupation	Executive assistant
g. patient's dietary habits	Patient eats fast food often while running errands for her boss. She denies drinking alcohol.
h. patient's sleep habits	Normal sleep schedule; she averages 7 hours per night.
i. concurrent medical conditions, prescription and non-prescription medications, and dietary supplements	Asthma: Advair 250/50 mcg 1 puff twice daily, Ventolin HFA as needed; osteoporosis prevention: calcium 600 mg + vitamin D 400 international units
j. allergies	None
k. history of other adverse reactions to medications	None
l. other (describe) _____	NA
Assessment and Triage	
2. Differentiate patient's signs/symptoms and correctly identify the patient's primary problem(s).	The patient has increased pore size, wrinkles, dry skin, and hyperpigmented areas on her face caused by photoaging.
3. Identify exclusions for self-treatment.	The patient has no exclusions for self-treatment.
4. Formulate a comprehensive list of therapeutic alternatives for the primary problem to determine if triage to a medical provider is required, and share this information with the patient or caregiver.	Options include: (1) Refer Dora to a health care provider or dermatologist for further evaluation. (2) Recommend a 2-month trial of an OTC AHA product and use of daily sunscreen. (3) Take no action.

case
39-2 *continued*

Relevant Evaluation Criteria	Scenario/Model Outcome

Plan

5. Select an optimal therapeutic alternative to address the patient's problem, taking into account patient preferences.

The patient would like to try an OTC product.

6. Describe the recommended therapeutic approach to the patient or caregiver.

"Apply chosen AHA product, such as Thomas Roth Glycolic Acid Hydrating Gel, to clean, dry face. Wait about 10 minutes after cleansing face to apply. Start out applying every other night for 1 week, and increase as tolerated to a maximum of twice daily."

7. Explain to the patient or caregiver the rationale for selecting the recommended therapeutic approach from the considered therapeutic alternatives.

"Seeing a dermatologist may not be necessary with proper use of this product. Wrinkles will not be completely removed because they are part of the natural aging process."

Patient Education

8. When recommending self-care with nonprescription medications and/or nondrug therapy, convey accurate information to the patient or caregiver:

   a. appropriate dose and frequency of administration

   "AHA product should be applied to a clean, dry face. Wait 10–15 minutes after drying face before applying product. Start out gradually with 1 application every other day, and increase to a maximum of twice daily as tolerated."

   b. maximum number of days the therapy should be employed

   "Improvement may be seen in as little as 4 weeks but may take as long as 2 months."

   c. product administration procedures

   "The product should be applied after cleansing the face."

   d. expected time to onset of relief

   "Improvement is usually seen in 1 month."

   e. degree of relief that can be reasonably expected

   "Fine lines may be reduced, pore size may decrease, and dryness should be improved. All signs of wrinkles, however, may not completely disappear."

   f. most common side effects

   "Mild irritation may occur. In addition, the areas being treated may appear to be lighter than surrounding skin."

   g. side effects that warrant medical intervention should they occur

   "If the treated areas of skin become severely irritated or darken significantly, you should see your health care provider or a dermatologist."

   h. patient options in the event that condition worsens or persists

   "If no improvement is seen within 2 months, you should see your health care provider or a dermatologist."

   i. product storage requirements

   "When not in use, the product should be stored at normal room temperature and tightly closed."

   j. specific nondrug measures

   "This product may make the skin more sensitive to sun exposure. A sunscreen with an SPF of at least 15 should be applied daily while using this product and for up to a week afterward."

   Solicit follow-up questions from the patient or caregiver.

   (1) "May I use this product more than twice a day?"

   (2) "Should I always wear sunscreen or only when I am using this product?"

   Answer the patient's or caregiver's questions.

   (1) "No. This product should be used a maximum of twice daily."

   (2) "This product will increase the overall sensitivity of your skin to the sun. In addition because you are in the car often during your work-day, it is advisable to use a daily moisturizer or foundation with an SPF of at least 15."

Evaluation of Patient Outcome

9. Assess patient outcome.

Ask the patient to call you to update you on her response to your recommendation; or you could call her in a month to evaluate response.

Key: AHA = Alpha hydroxy acid; NA, = not applicable; OTC = over-the-counter; SPF = sun protection factor.

The objectives of self-treatment are to (1) reverse skin damage by using available nonprescription products and (2) protect the skin from further damage by making lifestyle changes and protecting skin from sun exposure. For most patients, carefully following product instructions and the self-care measures listed here will help ensure optimal therapeutic outcomes.

Alpha Hydroxy Acids

- Protect the skin from sun exposure by covering it with clothing. FDA recommends advising patients to wear long-sleeved clothing and hats with brims of at least 4 inches. Patients should also use a sunblock or sunscreen product with an SPF of 15 or greater during use of alpha hydroxy acids (AHAs) and regularly in the future to prevent further damage.
- To prevent dry skin, cleanse the skin with a mild soap or a soap-free liquid cleanser. Do not cleanse skin more often than twice daily. Apply a pea-sized amount of an AHA product to clean, dry skin.
- To minimize transient mild tingling and stinging, wait 10–15 minutes after cleansing the face to apply an AHA product.
- Excessive skin dryness or irritation warrants decreased application.

- Note that AHA products contain an active ingredient and that the use of other products, including cosmetics, could result in skin irritation, including mild stinging, burning, or erythema.
- Do not apply the product too close to the eyes or mucous membranes.
- Begin applying this product once at bedtime every other day for approximately 1 week. Gradually increase application to twice a day.
- Use a daily moisturizer with sunscreen after applying the AHA product to minimize dry skin and maintain the antiphotoaging effect.
- Store this product in a cool dry place out of children's reach.
- Discontinue the AHA product if severe irritation, such as redness or excessive dryness, or a rash occurs.

Patient Counseling for Photoaging

Patients should be advised that premature wrinkling, creases, dry texture, and blotchy hyperpigmentation are not inevitable.[30] The provider should be proactive in identifying and recommending products that are appropriate for a specific patient. The box Patient Education for Photoaging lists specific information to provide patients.

Evaluation of Patient Outcomes for Photoaging

Patients treated with nonprescription products for photoaging should set a reasonable goal. Obviously, these preparations cannot "erase wrinkles." The provider should monitor the progress of the treatment and be sensitive to issues that may require medical referral.

Key Points for Skin Hyperpigmentation and Photoaging

- ➤ Photoaging and hyperpigmentation are cosmetically unacceptable skin conditions. Patients who have reasonable expectations should be able to achieve even skin tone and to minimize appearance and occurrence of fine wrinkling with the use of nonprescription products.
- ➤ Hydroquinone is the only FDA-approved nonprescription skin-bleaching product. Patients should apply a 2% concentration to skin up to twice daily, as tolerated.
- ➤ Patients younger than 12 years, those with large areas of hyperpigmentation or disease- or drug-induced hyperpigmentation, or those with lesions that have changed in size, shape, or color should consult their primary care provider.
- ➤ Patients should be referred to a primary care provider if no improvement occurs within 3 months or if skin darkens during treatment of hyperpigmentation.

- ➤ Patients should avoid applying hydroquinone-containing products near the eye area or on damaged skin areas.
- ➤ Patients using AHAs to reduce photoaging should be advised to apply AHAs up to twice daily to dry skin. Patients who do not see a desired improvement in skin appearance in 2 months or who experience excessive irritation or drying of the skin should contact their primary care provider.
- ➤ Patients who use products to prevent photoaging or hyperpigmentation should be instructed to protect their skin from daily sun exposure by using a sunscreen with SPF 15 or greater to maintain results.

REFERENCES

1. Nicolaidou E, Antoniou C, Katsambas A. Origin, clinical presentation and diagnosis of facial hypermelanoses. *Dermatol Clin.* 2007;25(3):321–6.
2. Plensdorf S, Martinez J. Common pigmentation disorders. *Am Fam Physician.* 2009;79(2):109–16.
3. Callender VD, St. Surin-Lord S, Davis EC, et al. Postinflammatory hyperpigmentation. *Am J Clin Dermatol.* 2011;12(2):87–99.
4. Park H, Yaar M, Lee J, et al. Biology of melanocytes. In: Goldsmith LA, Katz SI, Gilchrest BA, eds. *Fitzpatrick's Dermatology in General Medicine.* 8th ed. New York: McGraw-Hill; 2012. Access Medicine Online Electronic Medical Library. Accessed at http://www.accessmedicine.com, April 24, 2013.
5. Parvez S, Kang M, Chung H, et al. Survey and mechanism of skin depigmenting and lightening agents. *Phytother Res.* 2006;20(11):921–34.
6. Fisher JM, Fisher DE. From suntan to skin cancers: molecular pathways and prevention strategies. *Targ Oncol.* 2008;3:41–4.
7. U.S. Food and Drug Administration. Skin bleaching drug products for over-the-counter human use; proposed rule. *Federal Register.* 2006;71:51146–55.
8. Rigopoulos D, Gregoriou S, Katsambas A. Hyperpigmentation and melasma. *J Cosmet Dermatol.* 2007;6(3):195–202.
9. Sheth VM, Pandya AG. Melasma: a comprehensive update: part II. *J Am Acad Dermatol.* 2011;65(4):699–714.
10. Arefiev KL, Hantash BM. Advances in the treatment of melasma: a review of the recent literature. *Dermatol Surg.* 2012;38(7 pt 1):971–84.
11. Gupta AK, Gover MD, Nouri K, et al. The treatment of melasma: a review of clinical trials. *J Am Acad Dermatol.* 2006;55(6):1048–65.
12. Davis E, Callender V. Postinflammatory hyperpigmentation: a review of the epidemiology, clinical features, and treatment options in skin of color. *J Clin Aesthetic Dermatol.* 2010;3(7):20–31.

13. Konda S, Geria AN, Halder RM. New horizons in treating disorders of hyperpigmentation in skin of color. *Semin Cutan Med Surg.* 2012;31(2):133–9.

14. Rajatanavin N, Suwanachote S, Kulkollakarn S. Dihydroxyacetone: a safe camouflaging option in vitiligo. *Int J Dermatol.* 2008;47(4):402–6.

15. Nordlund JJ, Grimes PE, Ortonne JP. The safety of hydroquinone. *J Eur Acad Dermatol Venereol.* 2006;20(7):781–7.

16. Draelos Z. Skin lightening preparations and the hydroquinone controversy. *Dermatol Ther.* 2007;20(5):308–13.

17. U.S. Food and Drug Administration. Hydroquinone studies under the National Toxicology Program (NTP). Accessed at http://www.fda.gov/AboutFDA/CentersOffices/OfficeofMedicalProductsandTobacco/CDER/ucm203112.htm, April 24, 2013.

18. Azzam OA, Leheta TM, Nagui NA, et al. Different therapeutic modalities for treatment of melasma. *J Cosmet Dermatol.* 2009;8(4):275–81.

19. McEvoy GK, ed. Hydroquinone. In: *AHFS Drug Information 2007.* Bethesda, MD: American Society of Health-System Pharmacists; 2007:3551–2.

20. Ladizinski B, Mistry N, Kundu RV. Widespread use of toxic skin lightening compounds: medical and psychosocial aspects. *Dermatol Clin.* 2011; 29(1):111–23.

21. Hantash BM, Jimenez F. A split-face, double-blind, randomized and placebo-controlled pilot evaluation of a novel oligopeptide for the treatment of recalcitrant melasma. *J Drugs Dermatol.* 2009;8(8):732–5.

22. Ubeid AA, Zhao L, Wang Y, et al. Short-sequence oligopeptides with inhibitory activity against mushroom and human tyrosinase. *J Invest Dermatol.* 2009;129:2242–9.

23. Woolery-Lloyd H, Kammer JN. Treatment of hyperpigmentation. *Semin Cutan Med Surg.* 2011;30(3):171–5.

24. Tse TW, Hui E. Tranexamic acid: an important adjuvant in the treatment of melasma. *J Cosmet Dermatol.* 2012;12(1):57–66.

25. Garg VK, Sinha S, Sarkar R. Glycolic acid peels versus salicyclic-mandelic acid peels in active acne vulgaris and post-acne scarring and hyperpigmentation: a comparative study. *Dermatol Surg.* 2008;35(1):59–65.

26. Hakozaki T, Minwalla L, Zhuang J, et al. The effect of niacinamide on reducing cutaneous pigmentation and suppression of melanosome transfer. *Br J Dermatol.* 2002;147(1):20–31.

27. Navarrete-Solis J, Castandeo-Cazares JP, Torres-Alvarez B, et al. A double-blind, randomized clinical trial of niacinamide 4% versus hydroquinone 4% in the treatment of melasma. *Dermatol Res Pract.* 2011;2011:379173. doi: 10.1155/2011/379173. Epub 2011 Jul 21.

28. Drake L, Dinehart S, Farmer E, et al. Guidelines of care for photoaging/photodamage. *J Am Acad Dermatol.* 1996;35(3 pt 1):462–4.

29. Rabe JH, Mamelak AJ, McElgunn PJ, et al. Photoaging: mechanisms and repair. *J Am Acad Dermatol.* 2006;55(1):1–19.

30. Yarr M, Gilchrest B. Aging of skin. In: Goldsmith LA, Katz SI, Gilchrest BA, eds. *Fitzpatrick's Dermatology in General Medicine.* 8th ed. New York, NY: McGraw-Hill; 2012. Access Medicine Online Electronic Medical Library. Accessed at http://www.accessmedicine.com, April 24, 2013.

31. Yaar M, Gilchrest BA. Photoaging: mechanism, prevention and therapy. *Br J Dermatol.* 2007;157(5):874–87.

32. Archer DF. Postmenopausal skin and estrogen. *Gynecol Endocrinol.* 2012;28(suppl 2):2–6.

33. Antoniou C, Kosmadaki MG, Stratigos AJ, et al. Photoaging: prevention and topical treatments. *Am J Clin Dermatol.* 2010;11(2):95–102.

34. Baumann L. Cosmetics and skin care in dermatology. In: Goldsmith LA, Katz S, Gilchrest BA, eds. *Fitzpatrick's Dermatology in General Medicine.* 8th ed. New York, NY: McGraw-Hill; 2012. Access Medicine Online Electronic Medical Library. Accessed at http://www.accessmedicine.com, April 24, 2013.

35. Newburger AE. Cosmeceuticals: myths and misconceptions. *Clin Dermatol.* 2009;27(5):446–52.

36. Zussman J, Ahdout J, Kim J. Vitamins and photoaging: do scientific data support their use? *J Am Acad Dermatol.* 2010;63(3):507–25.

37. Huang CK, Miller TA. The truth about over-the-counter topical anti-aging products: a comprehensive review. *Aesthetic Surg J.* 2007;27(4):402–12.

38. U.S. Food and Drug Administration. Guidance for industry. Labeling for topically applied cosmetic products containing alpha hydroxy acids as ingredients. January 2005. Accessed at http://www.fda.gov/Cosmetics/GuidanceRegulation/GuidanceDocuments/ucm090816.htm, April 24, 2013.

39. Fabbrocini G, De Padova MP, Tosti A. Chemical peels: what's new and what isn't new but still works well. *Facial Plast Surg.* 2009;25(5):329–36.

40. Kessler E, Flanagan K, Chia C, et al. Comparison of α- and β-hydroxy acid chemical peels in the treatment of mild to moderately severe facial acne vulgaris. *Dermatol Surg.* 2008;34(1):45–51.

41. Landau M. Chemical peels. *Clin Dermatol.* 2008;26(2):200–8.

42. Cosmetic ingredient review. Final report on the safety assessment of glycolic acid, ammonium, calcium, potassium, and sodium glycolates, methyl, ethyl, propyl, and butyl glycolates, and lactic acid, ammonium, calcium, potassium, sodium, and TEA-lactates, methyl, ethyl, isopropyl, and butyl lactates, and lauryl, myristyl, and ceryl lactates. *Int J Toxicol.* 1998;17(suppl 1):1–242.

MINOR BURNS, SUNBURN, AND WOUNDS

Daphne B. Bernard

Pharmacists often provide guidance to consumers needing treatment for minor burns and wounds. A quick assessment helps to identify appropriate products and procedures to manage cuts, burns, and scrapes and to speed the healing process. Burn and wound care management can be quite resource intensive, with much of the cost related to fees for emergency department visits and the expense of the medications and supplies used for wound healing. Thousands of people seek medical treatment for skin injuries each year. For example, approximately 450,000 patients per year are estimated to receive burn injuries that require medical treatment.[1] Because patients commonly use self-care in burn and wound management, a thorough knowledge of skin injuries and how they heal is essential. Although the skin is well adapted to heal minor burns and wounds over time, use of the proper dressing and appropriate use of antiseptics and antibiotics will facilitate healing, minimize scar formation, and prevent secondary bacterial skin infections. All health care providers must perform an accurate assessment of the injury to determine whether self-care or referral for further evaluation is appropriate.

Pathophysiology of Minor Burns, Sunburn, and Wounds

Skin injuries are described according to the cause and depth of damage. Acute wounds include burns, abrasions, punctures, and lacerations. These wounds are typically caused by trauma, and with proper care, tend to heal within 1 month in healthy adults. On the other hand, any wound that does not heal properly through the normal stages of wound healing is considered a chronic wound and requires triage with more intense medical care. Chronic wounds will not be discussed in this chapter.

Burns are wounds caused by thermal, electrical, chemical, or ultraviolet radiation (UVR) exposure.

Thermal burns result from skin contact with flames, scalding liquids, or hot objects (e.g., irons, oven broiler elements, hot pans, curling irons, or radiators) or from the inhalation of smoke or hot vapors. Figure 40–1 shows a cross-section of the anatomy of the skin and the depths of injury caused by thermal burns. (See Chapter 32 for further discussion of skin anatomy and physiology.)

Chemical burns occur secondary to exposure to corrosive or reactive chemicals that cause tissue damage, ulceration and sloughing. The necrotic tissue often acts as a reservoir allowing continued absorption of the chemical. This may result in

prolonged cutaneous damage and tissue injury.[2] If not adherent to the skin, clothing that has been exposed to chemicals should be removed to prevent continued burn insult to the affected skin. The provider should refer all patients with chemical burns to the emergency department for evaluation.

Sunburn is caused by too much exposure to ultraviolet A (UVA) and ultraviolet B (UVB) light produced from natural sunlight and by commercial tanning beds and tanning lamps. (see Color Plates, photograph 24).[3] (See Chapter 38 for a discussion of UVR bands.) Photosensitive reactions (phototoxicity and photoallergy) are related to the coadministration of drugs and chemicals but are often mistaken as sunburn (see Color Plates, photographs 25 and 26). The clinical presentation of phototoxicity includes erythema that resembles sunburn, which desquamates (peels) within several days.[4]

Abrasions usually result from a rubbing or friction injury to the epidermal portion of the skin and extend to the uppermost portion of the dermis. *Punctures* usually result from a sharp object that has pierced the epidermis and may reach into the dermis or deeper tissues. *Lacerations* result from sharp objects cutting through the various layers of the skin.[5]

Self-treatment of acute wounds such as abrasions, lacerations, punctures, and burn wounds that do not extend beyond the dermis is generally deemed appropriate.

Understanding the physiology of wound healing is just as important as understanding the pathology of the wound itself. Skin integrity depends on a delicate balance between structure and function. When a burn or wound disturbs this balance, prompt restoration is required to ensure body homeostasis and proper wound healing. Wound healing begins immediately after injury and consists of three overlapping phases: inflammatory, proliferative, and maturation (remodeling).[6]

The *inflammatory phase* is the body's immediate response to injury. This phase, which lasts approximately 3–4 days, is responsible for preparing the wound for subsequent tissue development and consists of two primary parts: hemostasis and inflammation. Hemostasis is initiated by the release of thromboplastin from injured cells to form a clot to stop bleeding and allow healing to proceed. Later in the inflammatory phase, debris and bacteria are removed from the wound bed. Collagen is formed to stimulate wound healing, and epithelial cells migrate to cover the wound bed and provide the initial (one-cell-thick) layer of new skin that will cover the wound.[6]

In the next phase of healing, the *proliferative phase,* the wound is filled with new connective tissue and covered with new epithelium. This phase starts on about day 3 and continues

Depth of Burn   **Level**

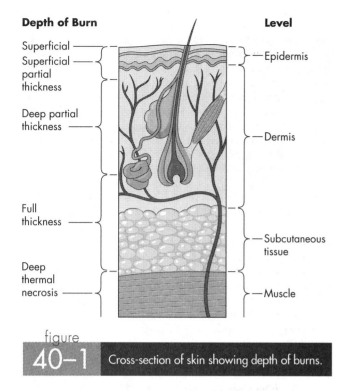

figure
40-1
Cross-section of skin showing depth of burns.

for about 3 weeks. It involves the formation of granulation tissue, which is a collection of new connective tissue (fibroblasts and newly synthesized collagen), new capillaries, and inflammatory cells.[6]

The final phase of healing is known as the *maturation* or *remodeling phase*. This is the longest phase, beginning at about week 3, when the wound is completely closed by connective tissue and resurfaced by epithelial cells. It involves a continual process of collagen synthesis and breakdown, replacing earlier, weak collagen with high-tensile-strength collagen; this process peaks approximately 60 days after the injury occurred.[6]

Several local and systemic factors can affect how efficiently and to what extent a wound will heal. Local factors include tissue perfusion and oxygenation, infection, and wound characteristics. The most important systemic factors that can affect the healing process are poor vascularization, bacterial contamination, inadequate nutrition, coexisting medical conditions, and medications.

Poor vascularization delays wound healing. The resulting poor oxygenation leads to impaired leukocyte activity, decreased production of collagen, decreased epithelialization, and reduced resistance to infection. Common disorders that may cause decreased perfusion include diabetes, severe anemia, hypotension, peripheral vascular disease, and congestive heart failure.[7]

Wound infection occurs when there is deposition and multiplication of organisms in tissue with an associated host reaction. Some wound infections are caused by fungi and protozoa, but most minor wound infections are caused by bacteria, especially *Streptococcus pyogenes, Enterococcus faecalis,* and *Staphylococcus aureus.* When the number of bacteria is excessive, wounds can become infected. Localized infection in the wound delays collagen synthesis and epithelialization, prolongs the inflammatory phase, and causes additional tissue destruction.[8]

Adequate nutrition provides the building blocks for wound repair. Protein, carbohydrates, vitamins, and trace elements are needed for collagen production and cellular energy.[9] Vitamin supplements are commonly used to manage wound healing. Vitamin C has many roles in wound healing, and a deficiency

in this vitamin has multiple effects on tissue repair. Vitamin C deficiencies result in impaired healing and have been linked to decreased collagen synthesis and fibroblast proliferation, decreased angiogenesis, and increased capillary fragility. Also, vitamin C deficiency leads to an impaired immune response and increased susceptibility to wound infection. Vitamin E also has anti-inflammatory properties and has been suggested to have a role in decreasing excess scar formation in chronic wounds. Animal experiments have indicated that vitamin E supplementation is beneficial to wound healing and topical vitamin E has been widely promoted as an antiscarring agent.[10]

It is commonly recognized that, in healthy older adults, the effect of aging causes a temporal delay in wound healing but not an actual impairment in terms of the quality of healing.[11] Patients who are obese have problems with poor perfusion (adipose tissue lacks blood flow) and tend to have delayed wound healing.[12]

Poorly controlled diabetes is usually associated with reduced collagen synthesis, impaired wound contraction, delayed epidermal migration, and reduced polymorphonuclear leukocyte chemotaxis and phagocytosis. Strict professional attention should be given to wounds in patients with diabetes because of these inherent difficulties.[13]

Some medications have the capacity to affect wound healing, such as those that interfere with clot formation or platelet function or with inflammatory responses and cell proliferation. Glucocorticosteroids inhibit wound repair through global anti-inflammatory effects and suppression of cellular wound responses, including fibroblast proliferation and collagen synthesis. Systemic steroids cause wounds to heal with incomplete granulation tissue and reduced wound contraction. In addition, chemotherapeutic drugs delay cell migration into the wound, decrease early wound matrix formation, lower collagen production, impair proliferation of fibroblasts, and inhibit contraction of wounds[12] Patients who are taking these medications should be carefully followed by a wound care specialist to ensure that proper healing occurs.

Local features that may impair wound closure include poor oxygenation resulting from inadequate perfusion, with chronic hypoxia and inflammation largely secondary to infection; the presence of necrotic tissue, eschar (i.e., scab), or foreign bodies (e.g., glass and dirt); inadequate moisture; and infection.[14] Providers who are aware of and can recognize problems associated with these local factors can provide more effective wound care management instructions to ensure faster wound healing.

Clinical Presentation of Minor Burns, Sunburn, and Wounds

The clinical presentation of burns, sunburn, and wounds is largely determined by the depth of skin damage. For simplification, this depth classification (Figure 40–2) has been divided into four descriptive stages.

Stage I skin injuries (i.e., minor sunburn and superficial burn) involve only the epidermis, with no loss of any skin layers, and consist primarily of reddened, nonblanching unbroken, nonblistering skin. Minor sunburn causes a superficial burn injury characterized by erythema and slight dermal edema that results from an increase in blood flow to the affected skin. The increased blood flow begins approximately 4 hours after exposure, peaking between 12 and 24 hours after exposure. Other superficial burns usually result from a brief exposure to low heat, causing a painful area of erythema similar to sunburn but without significant damage to epithelial cells. Avoidance of additional injury and symptomatic relief of pain and fever are

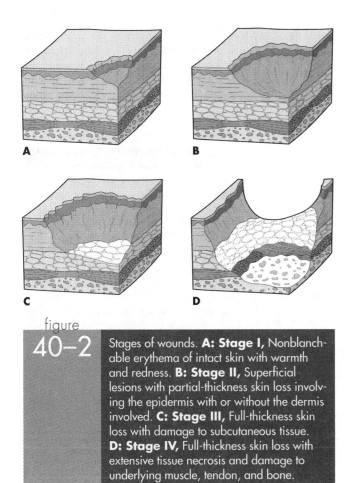

figure

40–2   Stages of wounds. **A: Stage I,** Nonblanchable erythema of intact skin with warmth and redness. **B: Stage II,** Superficial lesions with partial-thickness skin loss involving the epidermis with or without the dermis involved. **C: Stage III,** Full-thickness skin loss with damage to subcutaneous tissue. **D: Stage IV,** Full-thickness skin loss with extensive tissue necrosis and damage to underlying muscle, tendon, and bone.

usually the only treatment required. The majority of superficial burns can be managed through self-care or ambulatory care centers and will heal within 3–6 days.[15]

Stage II skin injuries (i.e., severe sunburn, abrasions, superficial lacerations and punctures, superficial partial-thickness burns, and deep partial-thickness burns) include blistering or partial-thickness skin loss that involves all the epidermis and part of the dermis. Because the injury involves a break in the skin, drainage from the wound area may occur, in addition to pain, edema, and erythema. Severe sunburns fall into this category and result in blisters that will desquamate or "peel" over a period of several days. There is a slight chance of bacterial infection because of the loss of the outer skin barrier (see Color Plates, photograph 24). Pain, edema, and skin tenderness accompany erythema. Systemic symptoms such as vomiting, low-grade fever, chills, weakness, and shock may be seen in patients in whom a large portion of the skin surface has been affected. After exfoliation and for several weeks thereafter, the skin will be more susceptible than normal to sunburn.[15] In addition to sun exposure, stage II burns result from higher levels of heat or longer exposures than in superficial burns. Damage to the epidermis and dermis layers produces painful blistering and can be superficial partial-thickness or deep partial-thickness burns. These burns often occur from a splash or spill of hot liquid, brief contact with a hot object, flash ignition, chemical contact, and exposure to a flame. Stage II burns are painful and sensitive to temperature and air. In addition, blanching occurs, indicating loss of blood vessels to the area. The burn's appearance may be a patchy white-to-red area, and large blisters may be present. Pain may be more intense than in superficial burns because of the irritation to nerve endings, although some areas may lack sensation. Wound resurfacing can occur because of surviving nests

of epithelial cells that line the hair follicles and sweat glands. In this case, healing may be slow and scarring is likely to occur.

Stage II burns are prone to infection because of the loss of barrier function and vasculature. Infection will worsen the severity of a burn injury or its depth, or both. If the damage does not involve the deeper proliferating area of the epidermis (e.g., superficial partial-thickness burns), rapid regeneration of a normal epidermis usually results within 2–3 weeks, with minimal or no scarring. If more of the dermis is involved (e.g., deep partial-thickness burns), the wound will take longer to heal (up to 6 weeks) and may cause thick scar formation (hypertrophic scarring or cheloid), as well as contractures of the skin and underlying tissues that can affect use of the involved areas.

Small stage II burns on 1%–2% of body surface area (BSA) can usually be managed through self-care. However, superficial partial-thickness burns that occur on a child or a patient with multiple medical problems or that cover more than 10% of BSA require hospitalization with fluid restoration. All stage II burns that fail to heal within 2–3 weeks or those that exhibit pain, redness, exudate formation, fever, odor, or malaise that persists days or weeks after the initial injury should be referred for medical evaluation. Finally, patients with deep partial-thickness burns should be examined in a hospital's emergency department. These burn injuries can convert to full-thickness injuries if not properly and promptly managed.[15]

Stage III skin injury (i.e., full-thickness burns and deep lacerations and punctures) includes full-thickness skin loss with damage to the entire epidermis, dermis, and dermal appendages and may involve subcutaneous tissue. Heat exposure that is more extensive than deep partial-thickness burns will cause death of the full thickness of skin in the affected area, resulting in a dry, leathery area that is painless and insensate. Deep punctures and lacerations can be quite painful. Deep lacerations bleed profusely, and underlying tissue layers may be visible in the wound bed. The body attempts to heal these wounds by sloughing off the dead layer and contracting the wound. Hospitalization is normally required for treatment of full-thickness burns.[15] Patients suffering from deep lacerations or punctures should seek emergency care as soon as possible.

Stage IV skin injury is an extension of *Stage III* stage III but also involves the subcutaneous tissue and underlying muscle, tendon, and bone.[5] Understanding these stages helps in selecting appropriate dressings for proper wound closure.

Figures 40–1 and 40–2 illustrate the depth and associated stages of skin injury.

Treatment of Minor Burns, Sunburn, and Wounds
Treatment Goals

The goals in treating acute, minor skin injury are to relieve symptoms, to promote healing by protecting the burn or wound from infection and further trauma, and to minimize scarring. Treatment should include a stepwise approach that involves cleansing the damaged area, selectively using antiseptics and antibiotics, and closing or covering with an appropriate dressing.

General Treatment Approach

The extent and depth of stage I and II burns should be assessed for self-treatment, both initially and again in 24–48 hours. The inflammatory response to a burn injury evolves over the first 24–48 hours; therefore, the initial appearance of the injury often leads to an underestimation of its actual severity. If the patient has none of the exclusions for self-treatment listed in Figure 40–3, the provider should treat the patient (or guide the patient's treatment) using the treatment approach outlined in the algorithm. If the burned area is 2% of BSA or larger and consists of superficial partial-thickness or greater injury, medical

attention is needed. Figure 40–4 illustrates the rule-of-nine method for estimating the percentage of BSA. Stage III and IV skin injury (e.g., animal or human bites, puncture wounds, and severe burns) require immediate medical evaluation. Specifically, these injuries require primary care provider consultation to assess the need for systemic or topical prescription antibiotics

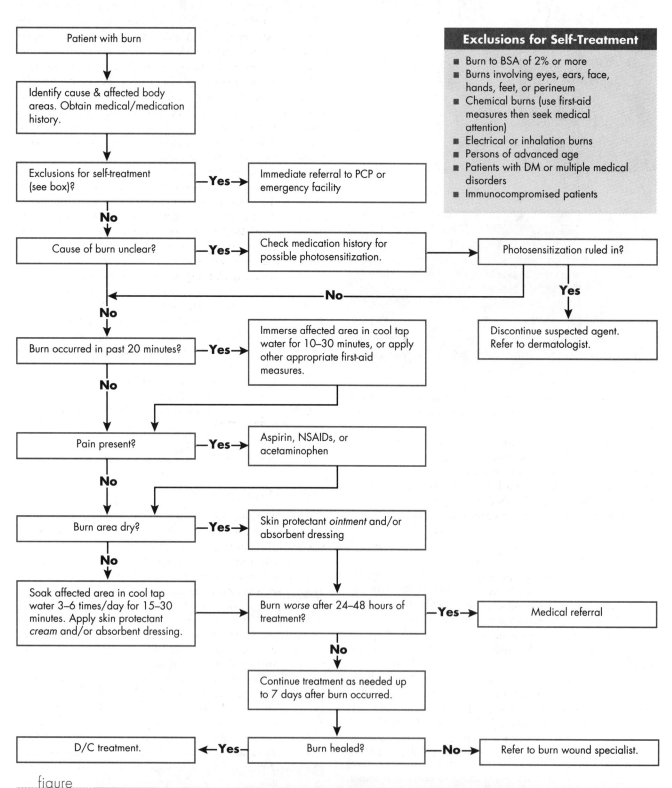

figure
40–3 Self-care of minor burns and sunburn. Key: BSA = Body surface area; D/C = discontinue; DM = diabetes mellitus; NSAID = nonsteroidal anti-inflammatory drug; PCP = primary care provider.

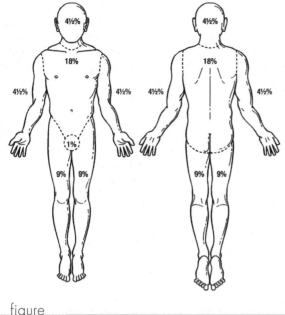

figure

40–4 Rule-of-nine method for quickly establishing the percentage of adult body surface burned. (*Source:* Adapted with permission from *The Guide to Fluid Therapy.* Deerfield, IL: Baxter Laboratories; 1969:111.)

and a tetanus booster to prevent infection from the tetanus toxin occasionally found in dust, soil, and animal waste.

Uncontaminated acute skin injuries at stages I and II (Figure 40–2), such as minor cuts, scrapes, and burns, require only basic supportive measures, including irrigation with saline or water for removal of debris from the damaged area and use of a wound dressing to keep the area moist and to prevent entry of bacteria into the affected area. Topical nonprescription antibiotic and antiseptic preparations can also be useful in preventing secondary infection, especially when debris or other foreign particulate matter that increases the risk of infection is present. Figure 40–5 outlines the triage and treatment of acute skin injuries.

Nonpharmacologic Therapy

Nonpharmacologic therapy used in the treatment of stage I and II skin injuries primarily involves first-aid measures to relieve pain, prevent contamination, and promote healing. The approach involves steps to remove exposure to the offending agent, stop bleeding and weeping from exudates, cool a burn, provide pain relief, decrease infection risk, and protect the area from further trauma.

Wound irrigation is often necessary to clean the wound surface by removing dirt and debris. Normal saline or water is sufficient for irrigation; however, mechanical removal of debris with clean gauze is sometimes appropriate. Minor abrasions and lacerations should be cleansed with water or sterile saline to remove any debris. They should then be covered with an appropriate wound dressing.

The patient or provider should inspect puncture wounds to ensure that no foreign bodies are retained and update tetanus prophylaxis, if necessary. If no debris is present, the wound should then be cleansed with either water or sterile saline. The wounds should be left open and soaked with soapy water for 30 minutes, at least 4 times a day initially, to allow for proper healing.[11] The wound should then be covered with an appropriate wound dressing.

Specific first-aid measures for the care of burns are described in Figure 40–3. Reducing further trauma to the site of skin injury caused by burns is done by immediately removing the source of heat and actively cooling the burn wound with cool tap water (lavage, soaks, compress or immersion). Continuous cooling for the first 10 minutes dissipates heat, reduces pain, delays onset and minimizes the extent of burn edema by decreasing the histamine release from the skin mast cells. Cooling beyond 10 minutes may provide pain relief to the patient. It is best to avoid the application of ice or ice-cold water because this may cause numbness and intense vasoconstriction, resulting in further tissue damage. Chemical burns should be irrigated with copious amounts of water to reduce the size and extent of the injury.[16]

A nonadherent, hypoallergenic dressing may be applied to the wound to protect the damaged area and speed wound healing (Table 40–1). Minor skin injuries usually heal without additional treatment. Patients should be advised not to pull at loose skin or peel off burned skin because viable skin may be removed in the process, thereby delaying healing.

In the case of chemical burns, the patient should immediately remove any clothing on or near the affected area. The affected area should then be washed with tap water for at least 15 minutes or longer until the offending agent has been removed. This treatment, however, should not delay transport to a hospital emergency department.

If the eye is involved, the eyelid should be pulled back and the eye irrigated with tap water for at least 15–30 minutes. The irrigation fluid should flow from the nasal side of the eye to the outside corner to prevent washing the contaminant into the other eye. The area poison control center should be contacted immediately at 800-222-1222 for treatment recommendations. Referral for further evaluation is frequently encouraged for eye injuries, and medical attention should be sought as soon as possible.

Wound Dressing

Traditional wound management involves leaving the wound open to air or covering it with a nonocclusive textile dressing (gauze). However, this type of management leads to eschar (i.e., scab) formation, which impedes reepithelialization of wounds and creates unwanted scars (Figure 40–6A). Wound dehydration with delayed healing and increased risk of bacterial entry into the wound may also occur. Removal of gauze dressings often tears away not only the eschar but also the new tissue under the eschar. These cumulative problems have led primary care providers and nurses to develop new treatment strategies that are based on creating a moist wound environment (Figure 40–6B). Providing a moist wound environment reduces the loss of protein, electrolytes, and fluid from the wound to help to minimize pain and infection.[17] Providers should still recommend the use of gauze and gauze-type adhesive dressings under certain circumstances; for example, gauze pads may be used with more advanced semiocclusive dressings such as foams for better exudate absorption. Gauze dressings also assist with the removal of eschar and necrotic tissue when wound debridement is necessary. In addition, gauze-type adhesive bandages may be used for stage I skin injuries for which the possible removal of excess granulation tissue is not a concern.

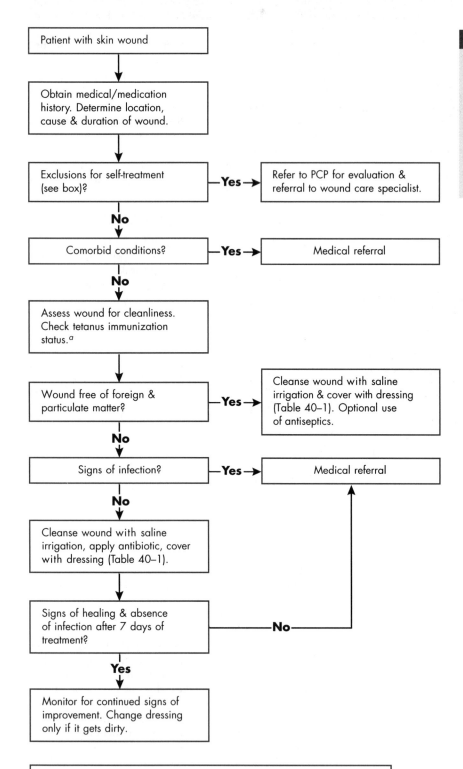

table

40–1 Options in Wound Dressing

Description (Trade Name)[a]	Uses/Indications	Advantages	Disadvantages
Gauze Dressings			
Nonocclusive fiber dressing with loose, open weave (Bulky Bandage, Conform, Kerlix Rolls and Sponges, Kling)	Stages II–IV Minimal to heavy exuding wounds/topicals Debridement Wound rehydration May use with semiocclusive dressings	Readily available in many sizes Deep wound packing May use with infected wounds/topicals Nonocclusive Conformable	Wound bed may desiccate if dressing is dry Nonselective debridement May cause bleeding/pain on removal Need secondary dressing Frequent dressing changes
Nonadherent (Gauze-Type) Dressings			
Nonadherent, porous dressings lightly coated (Adaptic, Nexcare Pads, Release, Telfa, Vaseline Gauze)	Skin donor sites Stage II, shallow stage III Staple/suture lines Abrasions Lacerations Punctures May use with semiocclusive dressings	Readily available Less adherent than plain gauze Lightly coated dressings allow exudate to flow through	Need secondary dressing May cause bleeding/pain on removal Some impregnated dressings may delay healing May require frequent dressing changes Some may cause exudate pooling
Foams			
Semipermeable, nonwoven, absorptive, inert polyurethane foam dressings (Allevyn, EPIGARD, Epi-Lock, Hydrasorb, Lyofoam; Figure 40–6C)	Stage II, shallow stage III Minimal-to-moderate drainage First- and second-degree burns Contraindicated in third-degree burns	Most are nonadhesive Some can be used with infected wounds/topicals Thermal insulation Reduce pain Nonocclusive Moist environment Conformable Less frequent dressing changes Trauma-free removal Absorbent	Most require secondary dressing May require cutting May cause wound desiccation May be difficult to determine wound contact surface
Alginates			
Hydrophilic, nonwoven dressings composed of calcium-sodium (percentages vary) alginate fibers. Alginates are processed from brown seaweed into pad or twisted fiber form. Exudate transforms fibers to gel at wound interface (AlgiDERM, Algosteril, Band-Aid Brand Quick Stop Adhesive Bandages, Kaltostat, Sorbsan)	Light-to-heavy exuding wounds Stages II, III, IV Skin donor sites	Absorptive Reduce pain Nonocclusive Moist environment Conformable Easy, trauma-free removal Can use on infected wounds Accelerate healing time Less frequent dressing changes Potential to aid in control of minor bleeding	Require secondary dressing Characteristic odor May need wound irrigation May desiccate May promote hypergranulation
Carbon-Impregnated (Odor-Control) Dressings			
Dressings with an outer layer of carbon for odor control (Carboflex, Lyofoam C)	Malodorous wounds	Control odor	Require appropriate seal or odor may escape Carbon is inactivated when it becomes wet
Composite/Island Dressings			
Nonadherent, absorptive center barrier with adhesive at perimeter (Allevyn Island, Lyofoam A, Nu-Derm, Viasorb)	Stages II, III Moderate-to-heavy exuding wounds	Nonadherent over wound Semiocclusive Autolysis Suture/staple lines Protective and reduce pain No secondary dressing required Impermeable to fluids/bacteria	May cause periwound trauma on removal

table

40–1   Options in Wound Dressing *(continued)*

Description (Trade Name)[a]	Uses/Indications	Advantages	Disadvantages
Hydrocolloids			
Wafer dressings composed of hydrophilic particles in an adhesive form covered by a water-resistant film or foam (Band-Aid Brand Advanced Healing Strips, Comfeel Plus, Cutinova, DuoDERM CGF Dressing, Exuderm, Tega-sorb, ULTEC; Figure 40–6D)	Stages I, II, shallow stage III Clean, granular wounds Autolysis Minimal-to-moderate exuding wounds Can use with absorption products and alginates	Occlusive Manage exudate by particle swelling Autolysis Long wear time Self-adherent Impermeable to fluids/bacteria Conformable Protective Thermal insulation Reduce pain Moist environment	For uninfected wounds only May cause periwound trauma on removal Difficult wound assessment Characteristic odor Impermeable to gases Some may leave residue on skin or in wound
Transparent Adhesive Films			
Semiocclusive, translucent dressings with partial or continuous adhesive composed of polyurethane or copolyester thin film (BIOCLUSIVE, Blisterfilm, CarraFilm, OpSite, Suresite, Tegaderm; Figure 40–6E)	Stages I, II, shallow stage III Clean granular wounds Minimally exuding wounds Autolysis Can use with absorption products and alginates Can be used in conjunction with some enzymatic debriders	Semiocclusive Gas permeable Easy inspection Autolysis Protective Impermeable to fluids/bacteria Comfortable Self-adherent Reduce pain Moist environment Shear resistant	For uninfected wounds only Not absorptive May cause periwound trauma on removal With continuous adhesive, may reinjure wound on removal With large amounts of exudate, maceration may occur
Hydrogels/Gels			
Nonadherent, nonocclusive dressings with high moisture content that come in the form of sheets and gels (Aquasite, Bioflex RX 1267P, Elasto-Gel, FlexiGel, New Skin Burn Relief Dressings, 2nd Skin Hydrogel Moist Gel Pads, Vigilon; Figure 40–6F)	Stages II, III, some approved for stage IV Granular or necrotic wound beds Autolysis Some used on partial- and full-thickness burns Punctures	Nonadherent Most are nonocclusive Trauma-free removal Varying absorption capabilities Conformable Some can be used in conjunction with topicals Thermal insulation Reduce pain Moist environment	Most require secondary dressings May macerate periwound skin Some products may dehydrate Slow-to-minimal absorption rate in most Most require frequent/daily dressing change
Antimicrobial			
Dressings that contain an antimicrobial agent to reduce bacterial contamination (Acticoat, Actisorb Silver 200, Avance, Aquacel, Iodoflex)	Stages II, III, and IV All locally infected wounds	Nonadherent Absorbent Reduce infection	Use caution in patients with thyroid disease because of increased iodine absorption Skin allergy

[a] The trade names listed for each type of wound dressing are given as examples of available products; however, these products do not constitute an all-inclusive list of available wound-dressing products.

Source: Adapted with permission from an unpublished document prepared by McIntosh A, Raher E. Silver Cross Hospital, Joliet, IL; 1991.

Selection Criteria for Wound Dressings

Choosing the right dressing depends on proper assessment of skin injury and of characteristics of the wound bed. Healing requires the appropriate type and amount of moisture in the wound bed to enhance healing. The role of a wound dressing is to provide the right environment to enhance and promote wound healing. A moist healing environment stimulates cell proliferation and encourages epithelial cells to migrate. Moisture-retentive dressings also act as a barrier against bacteria and absorb excess wound fluid, creating opportune conditions for healing. Today's wound dressings can also help decrease or eliminate pain, reduce the need for dressing changes, and provide autolytic debridement. Used appropriately, they are also cost-effective.[18]

Understanding the potential use and function of specific wound dressings should guide the provider in proper product selection. Also, wound dressing requirements may change with each healing phase. In terms of promoting moist wound healing,

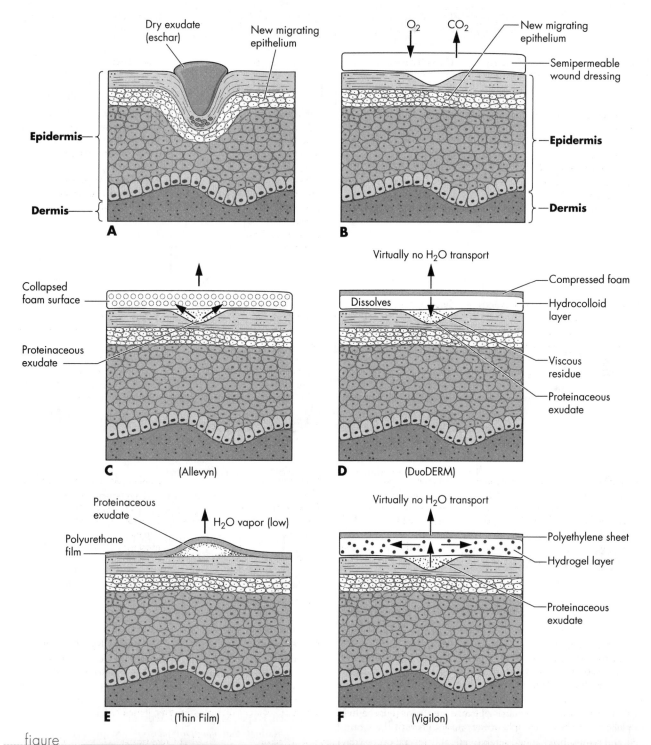

figure 40–6 Mechanisms by which semipermeable wound dressings create a moist environment for wound healing. **A,** Regenerating epidermal cells are forced to "tunnel" below the dry wound eschar to attain wound closure. This tunneling delays wound closure. **B,** Semipermeable wound dressings prevent formation of eschar by maintaining optimal moisture level at the wound bed. Unhindered by the presence of a dry eschar, migrating epithelial cells are able to migrate and close the wound. **C,** Mechanism of action of a hydrophilic polyurethane foam dressing (Epi-Lock). **D,** Mechanisms of action of a hydrocolloid wound dressing (DuoDERM). **E,** Mechanism of water vapor transmission in thin films. **F,** Mechanism of action of a hydrogel wound dressing (Vigilon). (*Source:* Adapted with permission from Syzcher M, Lee SJ. Modern wound dressings: a systemic approach to wounds. *J Biomater Appl.* 1992;7:142–213.)

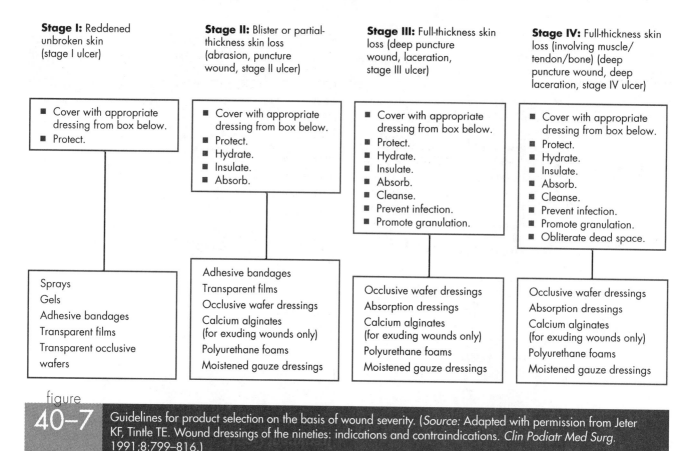

Stage I: Reddened unbroken skin (stage I ulcer)

- Cover with appropriate dressing from box below.
- Protect.

Stage II: Blister or partial-thickness skin loss (abrasion, puncture wound, stage II ulcer)

- Cover with appropriate dressing from box below.
- Protect.
- Hydrate.
- Insulate.
- Absorb.

Stage III: Full-thickness skin loss (deep puncture wound, laceration, stage III ulcer)

- Cover with appropriate dressing from box below.
- Protect.
- Hydrate.
- Insulate.
- Absorb.
- Cleanse.
- Prevent infection.
- Promote granulation.

Stage IV: Full-thickness skin loss (involving muscle/tendon/bone) (deep puncture wound, deep laceration, stage IV ulcer)

- Cover with appropriate dressing from box below.
- Protect.
- Hydrate.
- Insulate.
- Absorb.
- Cleanse.
- Prevent infection.
- Promote granulation.
- Obliterate dead space.

Sprays
Gels
Adhesive bandages
Transparent films
Transparent occlusive wafers

Adhesive bandages
Transparent films
Occlusive wafer dressings
Calcium alginates (for exuding wounds only)
Polyurethane foams
Moistened gauze dressings

Occlusive wafer dressings
Absorption dressings
Calcium alginates (for exuding wounds only)
Polyurethane foams
Moistened gauze dressings

Occlusive wafer dressings
Absorption dressings
Calcium alginates (for exuding wounds only)
Polyurethane foams
Moistened gauze dressings

figure 40–7 Guidelines for product selection on the basis of wound severity. (*Source:* Adapted with permission from Jeter KF, Tintle TE. Wound dressings of the nineties: indications and contraindications. *Clin Podiatr Med Surg.* 1991;8:799–816.)

the wound dressing may be used to absorb excess moisture, maintain optimal moisture, or provide moisture where it is lacking. Table 40–1 and Figure 40–7 describe the major categories of available wound care products and give an overview of their indications, advantages, and disadvantages.[18,19]

Types of Wound Dressings

Gauze

Gauze is available in a variety of forms and is generally used to care for minor burns and wounds that are draining or those requiring debridement. It is available in woven and nonwoven forms and can be impregnated with nonadherent products such as petrolatum as well as with antiseptics and antimicrobials. Some advantages of gauze are that it is readily available in many sizes and forms, it is affordable, and it can be combined with other topical products. Disadvantages of gauze are that it must be held in place by a second agent, its fibers may adhere to the wound bed, and it must be changed often (preferably several times a day) to prevent the wound from drying out. In addition, gauze alone is not recommended for moist wound treatment. Examples of gauze products include Kerlix, Kling, and Conform.[18]

Antimicrobial

Antimicrobial dressings contain products like silver and iodine and are often used in the management of wounds that are colonized or infected. As exudates from the wound bed are slowly absorbed, silver and iodine are gradually released to decrease the bacterial load within the wound bed. Examples include Acticoat, Actisorb, and Iodoflex.[20]

Specialty Wound Dressings

Often the practitioner must maintain a delicate balance of moisture and wound healing.[18] Specialty dressings are available that absorb excess moisture (e.g., foams, alginates), maintain moisture (e.g., hydrocolloid and transparent film dressings), or provide moisture where it is lacking (e.g., hydrogels).

Dressings that absorb moisture are beneficial early in the inflammatory phase of healing. The wound tissue may be overly moist as a result of the accumulation of fluid evaporated by exposed damaged tissue and from blood and serous drainage. A wound that is "too wet" may result in maceration of the tissue.[21] A wound that exudes moderate-to-high levels of drainage requires an absorbent dressing (e.g., foam, alginates, carbon-impregnated, and composite dressings). These dressings offer the benefit of requiring fewer dressing changes compared with nonabsorbent dressings, enabling undisturbed wound healing. Examples include Kaltostat, Repel, Mepilex, and Actisorb.

Dressings that maintain moisture are preferred as healing moves to the proliferative phase, with the formation of new connective tissue. Dressings that maintain natural moisture, such as hydrocolloid and transparent film dressings, are preferred in this phase.[18,19] Examples include Exuderm and Suresite.

Dressings that provide moisture are preferred when a dry wound that is covered with dead tissue needs to be rehydrated before optimal healing can occur. Providing moisture will soften and remove the dead tissue while promoting autolytic debridement, which facilitates the migration of newly formed epithelial tissue to the wound bed. A wound dressing must contain water to effectively add moisture to a wound and promote healing. Hydrogel dressings can consist of 80%–99% water on a nonadherent, cross-linked polymer, and they have varying absorptive properties.[19,22,23] Examples include AquaSite and FlexiGel.

Adhesive Bandages

Most superficial wounds (minor abrasions and lacerations) may simply require the application of adhesive gauze-type bandages such as regular Band-Aid brand bandages. Recognition of the importance of the moist wound-healing method has led to the development and marketing of more moisture retaining hydrocolloid-based bandages that promote wound healing (e.g., Band-Aid Brand Advanced Healing Strips and New Skin). Alternatives to conventional bandages are cyanoacrylate tissue adhesives, also known as liquid adhesive bandages (e.g., Liquiderm), which are used for small cuts and abrasions. These bandages are preferred for either cosmetic purposes (i.e., when a wound is located on the face) or when a more flexible dressing product is needed (i.e., when a wound is located on the finger or elbow). Adhesive bandages are often preferred by patients because they are waterproof, require no needles for wound closure, and have antimicrobial properties against gram-positive organisms.[24]

Surgical Tape

As the name implies, surgical tape is primarily used to hold in place bandages that cover a wound or surgical incision. The tape should be chosen on the basis of its adhesive properties, but it should be easy to remove. To minimize skin irritation, paper and cloth tapes should not contain latex and should be hypoallergenic. The most adherent, and potentially irritating, tape is clear surgical tape. Thus, it should be reserved for wounds that do not require frequent dressing changes (e.g., to secure IVs or surgical drains). Examples include Blenderm, Medipore, and Micropore.

Pharmacologic Therapy

Various products are useful in treating minor burns, sunburn, and wounds. Some agents cleanse the area and/or relieve pain, swelling, and/or inflammation. Others either protect the damaged area from infection or otherwise aid in healing the skin.

Systemic Analgesics

An initial step in treating the patient with a minor skin injury is to recommend short-term administration of a systemic analgesic, preferably one with anti-inflammatory activity, such as the NSAIDs (e.g., aspirin, naproxen, or ibuprofen). As prostaglandin inhibitors, NSAIDs may decrease erythema and edema in the injured area. NSAIDs may be especially beneficial in the patient with mild sunburn, especially in the first 24 hours after overexposure to UVR. Their use has been shown to decrease inflammation caused by exposure to UVR. However, this effect has been found to last only about 24 hours,[25] possibly because the initial inflammation of sunburn is mediated by prostaglandins, whereas the later inflammation is associated primarily with leukocytes. For patients who cannot tolerate NSAIDs, acetaminophen can provide pain relief, although it is a weak prostaglandin inhibitor and is not an anti-inflammatory agent. (See Chapter 5 for discussion of dosages and safety considerations for systemic analgesics.)

table 40–2	Skin-Protectant Ingredients Used in Treatment of Minor Burns and Sunburn

Ingredient	Proposed Concentrations (%)
Allantoin	0.5–2
Cocoa butter	50–100
Petrolatum	30–100
Shark liver oil	3
White petrolatum	30–100

Source: U.S. Food and Drug Administration. Skin protectant drug products for over-the-counter human use. Final rule. *Federal Register.* 2003;68:33377.

Skin Protectants

The Food and Drug Administration (FDA) has recognized the skin protectants in Table 40–2 as safe and effective for the temporary protection of minor burns and abrasions.

Skin protectants benefit patients with minor skin injuries by making the damaged area less painful. They protect the area from mechanical irritation caused by friction and rubbing, and they prevent drying of the stratum corneum. Products that prevent dryness and provide lubrication should be selected. Generally, the patient may apply a skin protectant as often as needed. If the skin injury has not improved in 7 days or if it worsens during or after treatment, the patient should seek medical attention promptly.

Topical Anesthetics

The pain of minor burns, wounds, and sunburn can be attenuated by the judicious use of topical anesthetics. Agents proposed as safe and effective in providing temporary relief of pain specifically associated with minor burns are listed in Table 40–3.

Topical anesthetics relieve pain by inhibiting the transmission of pain signals from pain receptors. Relief is short lived, lasting only 15–45 minutes.[26]

Benzocaine (0.5%–20%) and lidocaine (2%–5%) are the two anesthetics most often used in nonprescription drug preparations. Dibucaine (0.25%–1%), tetracaine (0.5%–2%), butamben (1%), and pramoxine (0.5%–1%) are also found in external anesthetic preparations. The higher concentrations of the topical anesthetics are appropriate for skin injuries in which the skin is intact. Lower concentrations are preferred when the skin surface is not intact because drug absorption is enhanced. These agents should be applied only to small areas of no more than 1%–2% of BSA to avoid systemic toxicity.[26,27]

Topical anesthetics should be applied no more than 3 or 4 times daily. Because their duration of action is short, continuous pain relief cannot be obtained with these agents. Increasing the number of applications increases the risk of a hypersensitivity reaction and, more important, the chance for systemic toxicity.

Benzocaine produces a hypersensitivity reaction in about 1% of patients, a higher incidence than that seen with lidocaine. In contrast, benzocaine is essentially free of systemic toxicity, whereas the systemic absorption of lidocaine can lead to a number of side

table

40–3   Nonprescription Topical Analgesic Ingredients for Treatment of Minor Burns and Sunburn

Agent	FDA-Approved Concentrations (%)
Amine and Caine-Type Local Anesthetics	
Benzocaine	5–20
Butamben picrate	1
Dibucaine	0.25–1
Dibucaine hydrochloride	0.25–1
Dimethisoquin hydrochloride	0.3–0.5
Dyclonine hydrochloride	0.5–1
Lidocaine	0.5–4
Lidocaine hydrochloride	0.5–4
Pramoxine hydrochloride	0.5–1
Tetracaine	1–2
Tetracaine hydrochloride	1–2
Antihistamines	
Diphenhydramine hydrochloride	1–2
Tripelennamine hydrochloride	0.5–2

Source: Federal Register. 1983;48:6820–33.

effects. However, systemic toxicities caused by lidocaine are rare if the product is used on intact skin, on localized areas, and for short periods.[26]

First-Aid Antiseptics

Antiseptics are chemical substances designed for application to intact skin up to the edges of a damaged skin area for disinfection purposes. When effective antisepsis is combined with proper skin injury care technique, including gentle handling of tissue, the infection rate is low. Ideally, antiseptics should exert a sustained effect against all microorganisms, without causing tissue damage. However, even therapeutic concentrations of antiseptics can harm tissue. For example, alcohol-containing preparations should not be used within the wound bed because they dehydrate the area and also cause pain and cell damage. Therefore, antiseptics should be used to disinfect only intact skin surrounding the wound after the removal of all organic matter.

Antiseptic active ingredients recognized as safe and effective for use include hydrogen peroxide topical solution USP, ethyl alcohol (48%–95%), isopropyl alcohol (50%–91.3%), iodine topical solution USP, iodine tincture USP, povidone/iodine complex (5%–10%), and camphorated phenol (Tables 40–4 and 40–5).[27]

Hydrogen Peroxide

Hydrogen peroxide 3% topical solution USP is a widely used antiseptic. Enzymatic release of oxygen occurs when the hydrogen peroxide comes in contact with the skin, causing an effervescent, mechanical cleansing action. Hydrogen peroxide should

table

40–4   Nonprescription First-Aid Antiseptic Ingredients

Antiseptic Agents	Concentration (%)
Ethyl alcohol	48–95
Isopropyl alcohol	50.0–91.3
Hydrogen peroxide topical solution	USP
Iodine tincture	USP
Iodine topical solution	USP
Phenol	0.5–1.5
Povidone/iodine complex	5–10
Quaternary ammonium compound	0.13

Source: Federal Register. 1994;59:31435–6.

be used where released gas can escape; therefore, it should not be used in abscesses, nor should bandages be applied before the compound dries. Because of the limited bactericidal effect and the risk of tissue toxicity, hydrogen peroxide has little benefit over soapy water for antisepsis.

Ethyl Alcohol

Alcohol has good bactericidal activity in 20%–70% concentrations. Caution must be used, however, when applying it to the intact skin surrounding the injured area, given that inadvertent, direct application of alcohol to the wound bed can cause tissue irritation. Ethyl alcohol may be used 1–3 times daily, and the wound may be covered with a sterile bandage only after the washed area has dried.[27]

table

40–5   Selected Nonprescription Wound Irrigant and Antiseptic Products

Trade Name	Primary Ingredients
Wound Irrigants	
Wound Wash Saline Aerosol	
Saline Wound Flush	Sodium chloride 0.9%
Antiseptics	
Betadine Skin Cleanser Liquid	Povidone/iodine 7.5%
Campho-Phenique Gel/Liquid	Camphor 10.8%; phenol 4.7%
Hibiclens	Chlorhexidine gluconate 4%
Neosporin Wound Cleanser	Benzalkonium chloride 0.013%

Source: Wolters Kluwer Health Inc. Genitourinary irrigants. Drug Facts and Comparisons. eFacts. Accessed at http://online.factsandcomparisons.com/MonoDisp.aspx?monoid=fandc-hcp11913&book=DFC&fromtop=true&search=676999%7c5&isStemmed=True&asbooks=, July 28, 2014; and Wolters Kluwer Health, Inc. Antiseptics and germicides. Drug Facts and Comparisons eFacts. Accessed at http://online.factsandcomparisons.com/MonoDisp.aspx?monoid=fandc-hcp10207&book=DFC, July 28, 2014.

Isopropyl Alcohol

Compared with ethyl alcohol, isopropyl alcohol 70% aqueous solution has somewhat stronger bactericidal activity and lower surface tension. Isopropyl alcohol is generally used for its cleansing and antiseptic effects on intact skin. It should not be used to clean open wound beds because of possible cytotoxic effects and higher reported infection rates. Isopropyl alcohol also has a greater potential for drying the skin (astringent action) because its lipid solvent effects are stronger than those of ethyl alcohol. Similar to ethyl alcohol, isopropyl alcohol is flammable and must be kept away from a flame.[27]

Iodine

An iodine solution USP of iodine 2% and sodium iodide 2.5% is used as an antiseptic for superficial skin injuries. An iodine tincture USP of iodine 2%, sodium iodide 2.5%, and alcohol (approximately 50%) is less preferable than the aqueous solution because the tincture is irritating to the tissue. Strong iodine solution (Lugol's solution) must not be used as an antiseptic. In general, bandaging should be discouraged after iodine application to avoid tissue irritation. Iodine solutions stain skin, may be irritating to tissue, and may cause allergic sensitization in some people. Iodine products are recommended if patients have chlorhexidine allergy.[28]

Povidone/Iodine

Povidone/iodine is a water-soluble complex of iodine with povidone. It contains 9%–12% available iodine, which accounts for its rapid bactericidal activity. Povidone/iodine is nonirritating to skin and mucous membranes. However, when used as a wound irrigant, povidone/iodine is absorbed systemically; the extent of iodine absorption is related to the concentration used and the frequency of application. The final serum level also depends on the patient's intrinsic renal function. When severe burns and large wounds are treated with povidone/iodine, iodine absorption through the skin and mucous membranes can result in excess systemic iodine concentrations, possibly causing transient thyroid dysfunction, clinical hyperthyroidism, and thyroid hyperplasia.[28]

Camphorated Phenol

Oily solutions of phenol and camphor are often used as nonprescription first-aid antiseptics. These products contain relatively high concentrations of phenol (4%) and must be used with caution. If oleaginous phenolic solutions are applied to moist areas, the phenol is partitioned out of the vehicle into water, resulting in caustic concentrations of phenol on the skin. These damaging effects can be avoided by applying these products only to dry, intact skin. Wounds treated with camphorated phenol should not be bandaged because the moisture would result in tissue damage.[29]

First-Aid Antibiotics

Nonprescription first-aid antibiotics available in the United States consist of the active ingredients bacitracin, neomycin, and polymyxin B sulfate (Table 40–6).[30] These topical agents help prevent infection in minor cuts, wounds, scrapes, and burns. They are especially beneficial if the wound contains debris or foreign matter. Topical and, in some cases, oral antibiotics are indicated in contaminated wounds that have a moderately high

table **40–6**	**Selected Nonprescription Antibiotic Products**
Trade Name	**Primary Ingredients**
Betadine First Aid Antibiotics + Moisturizer Ointment	Polymyxin B sulfate 10,000 U/g; bacitracin zinc 500 U/g
Q-tips Treat & Go	Cotton swabs containing bacitracin 500 U/g
Gold Bond First Aid Antibiotic Ointment	Bacitracin zinc 500 U/g; polymyxin B sulfate 10,000 U/g; neomycin base 3.5 mg/g; pramoxine HCL 10 mg
Neosporin Ointment	Polymyxin B sulfate 5000 U/g; bacitracin zinc 400 U/g; neomycin base 3.5 mg/g
Neosporin Plus Pain Relief Ointment	Bacitracin zinc 500 U/g; polymyxin B sulfate 10,000 U/g; neomycin base 3.5 mg/g; pramoxine HCL 10 mg
Neosporin Plus Pain Relief Cream	Polymyxin B sulfate 10,000 U/g; neomycin base 3.5 mg/g; pramoxine HCl 10 mg
Polysporin Ointment/Powder	Polymyxin B sulfate 10,000 U/g; bacitracin zinc 500 U/g

Source: Wolters Kluwer Health, Inc. Antiinfectives-topical. Antibiotic agents. Drug Facts and Comparisons eFacts. Accessed at http://online.factsandcomparisons.com/MonoDisp.aspx?monoid=fandc-hcp10163&book=DFC, July 28, 2014.

risk of infection. However, clean wounds free of contamination have a low infection rate and do not warrant the use of prophylactic antibiotics. If questions arise concerning the degree of contamination and the need for oral antibiotics, the patient should seek medical attention.

Topical antibiotic preparations should be applied to the wound bed after cleansing and before applying a sterile dressing. Special caution should be taken when applying these preparations to large areas of denuded skin, however, because the potential for systemic toxicity can increase. Prolonged use of these agents may result in the development of resistant bacteria and secondary fungal infection. If significant signs of improvement are not seen within 7 days, the patient should seek medical attention.

Bacitracin

Bacitracin is a polypeptide bactericidal antibiotic that inhibits cell wall synthesis in several gram-positive organisms. The development of resistance in previously sensitive organisms is rare. Minimal absorption occurs with topical administration. The frequency of allergic contact dermatitis (erythema, infiltration of macrophages, papules, edematous, or vesicular reaction) is approximately 2%. Topical nonprescription preparations usually contain 400–500 U/g of ointment and are applied 1–3 times a day.[30]

Neomycin

Neomycin is an aminoglycoside antibiotic; it exerts its bactericidal activity by irreversibly binding to the 30S ribosomal subunit to inhibit protein synthesis in gram-negative organisms and some species of *Staphylococcus*. Neomycin has been demonstrated to decrease the severity of clinical infection 48 hours after treatment in tape-stripped wounds. Resistant organisms may develop. Neomycin applied topically produces a relatively high rate of hypersensitivity; reactions occur in 3.5%–6% of patients. Although neomycin is not absorbed when applied to intact skin, application to large areas of denuded skin may cause systemic toxicity (ototoxicity and nephrotoxicity). It is most frequently used in combination with polymyxin and bacitracin in a concentration of 3.5 mg/g to prevent the development of neomycin-resistant organisms. Applications are made 1–3 times a day. [30]

Polymyxin B Sulfate

Polymyxin B sulfate is a polypeptide antibiotic that is effective against several gram-negative organisms because it alters the bacterial cell wall permeability. Topical preparations may be compounded in either a solution or ointment base, and numerous prepackaged antibiotic combinations containing polymyxin B are available. Applications are usually made 1–3 times a day. [30]

Product Selection Guidelines

If a topical anesthetic is to be used, the provider should recommend the most appropriate product formulation. These products are available as ointments, creams, solutions (lotions), and sprays (aerosols).

Ointments are oleaginous-based preparations. They provide a protective film to impede the evaporation of water from the wound area, which helps keep the skin from drying. However, if the skin is broken, an ointment may not be appropriate because of its impermeability. The presence of excessive moisture trapped beneath the ointment may promote bacterial growth or maceration of the skin, thereby delaying healing. Ointments are more appropriate for minor burns and wounds in which the skin is intact. Creams are emulsions that allow some fluid to pass through the film and are best for broken skin. Generally, it is easier to apply and remove creams than ointments. To prevent contamination of the preparation, the patient should not apply ointments and creams directly from the container onto the burn or wound. A preferred technique is to apply the topical product to a clean or gloved hand or gauze and then apply it directly to the injury site.

Lotions spread easily and are easier to apply when the burn or wound area is large. However, lotions that produce a powdery cover should not be used on a wound bed because they tend to dry the area, are difficult (and possibly painful) to remove, and provide a medium for bacterial growth under the caked particles.

Generally, aerosol and pump sprays are more costly than other topical dosage forms. Sprays offer the advantage of precluding the need to physically touch the injured area, so there is less pain associated with applying the medication. Proper application requires holding the container approximately 6 inches from the wound and spraying for 1–3 seconds. This method decreases the chances of chilling the area. However, sprays are not usually protective in that the aerosol is typically water or alcohol based and will evaporate. In addition, alcohol-based sprays can irritate and dehydrate the wound bed.

Table 40–7 lists selected trade-name topical products appropriate for treating minor burns, sunburn, and wounds.

table

40–7 Selected Nonprescription Topical Products for Minor Burns, Sunburn, and Wounds

Trade Name	Primary Ingredients
Skin Protectants	
A + D Original Ointment	Petrolatum 80.5%; lanolin 15.5%; cod liver oil (contains vitamins A and D)
Zinc oxide, Desitin Ointments	Zinc oxide 20% or 25%; white petrolatum
Local Anesthetics	
Americaine Aerosol	Benzocaine 20% ointment
ELA-Max 4%	Lidocaine 4%
Dermoplast Pain-Relieving Spray	Benzocaine 20%; menthol 0.5%
Dibucaine Topical Ointment	Dibucaine 1%
Itch-X Spray/Gel	Pramoxine HCl 1%; benzyl alcohol 10%
Solarcaine Aloe Extra Burn Relief Gel/Spray	Lidocaine 0.5%
Xylocaine Ointment	Lidocaine 2.5%
Local Anesthetics/Antiseptics	
Bactine First Aid Antiseptic Spray	Lidocaine HCl 2.5%; benzalkonium chloride 0.13%
Dermoplast Antibacterial Spray	Benzocaine 20%; benzethonium chloride 0.2%
Lanacane Maximum Strength Anti-Itch Cream	Benzocaine 20%; benzethonium chloride 0.1%
Bicozene	Benzocaine 6%; resorcinol 2%

Source: Wolters Kluwer Health, Inc. Protectants. Drug Facts and Comparisons eFacts. Accessed at http://online.factsandcompari sons.com/MonoDisp.aspx?monoid=fandc-hcp14800&book=DFC, July 28, 2014, and Wolters Kluwer Health, Inc. Ester local anesthetics. Drug Facts and Comparisons eFacts. Accessed at http://online. factsandcomparisons.com/MonoDisp.aspx?monoID=fandc-hcp10282, July 28, 2014.

Normal saline is the preferred choice for effective wound irrigation. The issue of which is the best antiseptic solution to use remains unresolved. When choosing an antiseptic product, one must consider tissue toxicity and costs of the different ingredients.

A topical antibiotic applied 1–3 times a day to a contaminated wound is effective in eradicating bacteria and producing faster wound healing when the agent is combined with appropriate cleansing of the wound and the use of proper dressings.

Complementary Therapies

Natural products such as honey, *Calendula officinalis, Aloe vera, Garcinia morella,* and *Datura metol* are said to have healing properties. [31,32] (See Chapter 51 for a more in-depth review of natural products for skin.)

Aloe vera gel is obtained from the mucilaginous center of the leaf of the aloe vera plant. It has been used for many centuries and is the major ingredient in various commercial skin and wound-care products. The aloe vera gel contains vitamins A, B, C, and E; enzymes; polysaccharides; amino acids; sugars; and minerals. In the management of acute and chronic wounds, several reports of studies using aloe vera have demonstrated variable results. [31]

Calendula officinalis has been widely used in homeopathic medicine for the treatment of many diseases. It is thought to promote wound healing by its reported anti-inflammatory and antibacterial properties. Results of one study indicate the effectiveness of *C. officinalis* extract for enhancing the antioxidant defense mechanism, thereby decreasing burn injury in a group of rats exposed to burn injury. [32]

The use of honey in wound management dates back many centuries. Honey consists of approximately 40% fructose, 30% glucose, 5% sucrose, and 20% water. It also contains several amino acids, antioxidants, vitamins, minerals, glucose oxidase (which produces hydrogen peroxide), and gluconic acid. Honey is highly viscous and delivers a moist wound healing environment. Also, because of the hyperosmolarity of honey, it is able to absorb the exudates from the wound and enable the wound to heal in a moist environment. Honey also has antibacterial, anti-inflammatory, and antifungal properties. [33]

One prospective randomized trial of honey versus silver sulfadiazine (SSD) for superficial burns demonstrated that honey dressings showed greater efficacy over SSD cream for treating superficial and partial-thickness burns; however, honey dressings are not advocated by burn centers. [34]

Assessment of Minor Burns, Sunburn, and Wounds: A Case-Based Approach

The assessment approach for burns differs slightly from the approach for wounds. When a patient presents with a burn, the severity of the burn should be immediately assessed by determining the depth of the injury and the percentage of BSA involved. The percentage of the adult body that has been burned can be estimated by the rule-of-nine method (Figure 40–4). The total BSA is divided into 11 areas, each accounting for 9% or a multiple of 9. An easy way to estimate the percentage of burned BSA is to use the back of the hand as 1% of BSA. The rule of nine is reliable for adults but inaccurate for children and patients with small body surfaces.

Case 40–1 is an example of the assessment of a patient with a minor burn.

case 40–1

Relevant Evaluation Criteria	Scenario/Model Outcome
Information Gathering	
1. Gather essential information about the patient's symptoms and medical history, including:	
a. description of symptom(s) (i.e., nature, onset, duration, severity, associated symptoms)	The patient describes intense pain and a dark pink burn on her right arm. She says that she accidentally touched the oven door when reaching in to retrieve a baked dish 2 days ago. The lesion is approximately 1 inch by 3 inches with nonraised edges.
b. description of any factors that seem to precipitate, exacerbate, and/or relieve the patient's symptom(s)	The patient says that the pain is worse when she moves her right arm and when she showers.
c. description of the patient's efforts to relieve the symptoms	The patient has not tried anything other than keeping the area dry to "help it heal faster."
d. patient's identity	Gena Davies
e. age, sex, height, and weight	42 years old, female, 5 ft 5 in., 160 lb
f. patient's occupation	Bus driver
g. patient's dietary habits	Eats a regular diet filled with meats and potatoes.
h. patient's sleep habits	At least 7 hours nightly
i. concurrent medical conditions, prescription and non-prescription medications, and dietary supplements	Hyperlipidemia: pravastatin 20 mg daily; hypothyroidism: levothyroxine 125 mcg daily
j. allergies	Aspirin
k. history of other adverse reactions to medications	None
l. other (describe) _____	The patient uses her arms a lot when driving the bus route 5 days a week. She also likes to do garden work regularly.
Assessment and Triage	
2. Differentiate patient's signs/symptoms and correctly identify the patient's primary problem(s).	Gena is suffering from a first-degree superficial thermal burn secondary to coming into contact with a hot oven.
3. Identify exclusions for self-treatment (Figure 40–3).	None

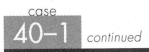

Relevant Evaluation Criteria	Scenario/Model Outcome
4. Formulate a comprehensive list of therapeutic alternatives for the primary problem to determine if triage to a health care provider is required, and share this information with the patient or caregiver.	Options include: (1) Refer Gena to an appropriate health care provider. (2) Recommend self-care with a nonprescription skin protectant and nondrug measures. (3) Recommend self-care until Gena can see an appropriate provider. (4) Take no action.

Plan

5. Select an optimal therapeutic alternative to address the patient's problem, taking into account patient preferences.	Gena should use a nonprescription skin protectant or topical analgesic along with nondrug measures to treat her problem.
6. Describe the recommended therapeutic approach to the patient or caregiver.	"Cleanse the area with water and a mild soap. Apply a skin protectant ointment such as cocoa butter or petrolatum to the burn area several times a day to reduce pain, keep the wound area moist, and protect the wound from mechanical irritation. Cover the burn with a transparent film dressing to provide additional protection."
7. Explain to the patient or caregiver the rationale for selecting the recommended therapeutic approach from the considered therapeutic alternatives.	"Minor burns can be properly managed with nonprescription skin protectants and nondrug measures as long as there are no exclusions for self-treatment, as in your case."

Patient Education

8. When recommending self-care with nonprescription medications and/or nondrug therapy, convey accurate information to the patient or caregiver:	
a. appropriate dose and frequency of administration	See the box Patient Education for Minor Burns and Sunburn.
b. maximum number of days the therapy should be employed	See the box Patient Education for Minor Burns and Sunburn.
c. product administration procedures	See the box Patient Education for Minor Burns and Sunburn.
d. expected time to onset of relief	"You should experience relief in about 7 days."
e. degree of relief that can be reasonably expected	"The burn can be healed by using a skin protectant and recommended nondrug measures properly."
f. most common side effects	See the box Patient Education for Minor Burns and Sunburn.
g. side effects that warrant medical intervention should they occur	See the box Patient Education for Minor Burns and Sunburn.
h. patient options in the event that condition worsens or persists	See the box Patient Education for Minor Burns and Sunburn.
i. product storage requirements	"Store in a cool, dry place out of children's reach."
j. specific nondrug measures	See the box Patient Education for Minor Burns and Sunburn.
Solicit follow-up questions from the patient or caregiver.	"Will the burn heal faster if I 'dry it out'?"
Answer the patient's or caregiver's questions.	"Drying the burn area leads to scab formation, which can delay wound healing and possibly lead to unwanted scarring. Providing a moist wound environment is ideal to aid in healing."

Evaluation of Patient Outcome

9. Assess patient outcome.	"If you provide me with your phone number, I will give you a call in 7–10 days to see how your wound is healing."

When a patient presents with a minor wound, the type, depth, location, and degree of contamination should be assessed. Visual inspection of the affected area usually provides an accurate evaluation of these factors. The wound should also be assessed for signs of infection, including whether drainage of yellow or greenish fluid (pus) is present or whether the skin around the wound has become increasingly erythematous, swollen, and painful. Because noninfectious processes such as drug-induced eruptions could be involved, the patient's health status and current medication use should also be determined. Antimicrobial agents should generally be recommended when secondary infection is present or might occur.

Case 40–2 is an example of the assessment of a patient with a minor wound.

case

40–2

Relevant Evaluation Criteria	Scenario/Model Outcome

Information Gathering

1. Gather essential information about the patient's symptoms and medical history, including:

   a. description of symptom(s) (i.e., nature, onset, duration, severity, associated symptoms)

   The patient approaches the pharmacy counter asking for "something for a swollen tongue that hurts really bad." Upon questioning, she says she had her tongue pierced four days ago, and it's been hurting and swollen ever since. She grimaces and slowly opens her mouth to reveal a tongue with a swollen dark yellow-brownish center that has a red tear in the middle.

   b. description of any factors that seem to precipitate, exacerbate, and/or relieve the patient's symptom(s)

   She says the pain that now extends to her jaws and neck keeps her from eating and drinking. Nothing has relieved the discomfort at this point other than keeping her mouth closed as much as possible. The pain is getting worse.

   c. description of the patient's efforts to relieve the symptoms

   The patient has tried liquid Tylenol with little relief.

   d. patient's identity

   Kim Summers

   e. age, sex, height, and weight

   27 years old, female, 5 ft 5 in., 160 lb

   f. patient's occupation

   Hair stylist

   g. patient's dietary habits

   Vegetarian

   h. patient's sleep habits

   6–8 hours a night

   i. concurrent medical conditions, prescription and non-prescription medications, and dietary supplements

   Norethindrone and ethinyl estradiol 777, 1 per day

   j. allergies

   NKA

   k. history of other adverse reactions to medications

   None

   l. other (describe) _____

   None

Assessment and Triage

2. Differentiate patient's signs/symptoms and correctly identify the patient's primary problem(s).

   Patient is suffering from inflammation and pain from a possible wound infection.

3. Identify exclusions for self-treatment (Figure 40–5).

   Involvement of mucous membrane

4. Formulate a comprehensive list of therapeutic alternatives for the primary problem to determine if triage to a health care provider is required, and share this information with the patient or caregiver.

   Options include:

   (1) Refer patient to an appropriate health care provider.

   (2) Recommend self-care with a nonprescription analgesic and nondrug measures.

   (3) Recommend self-care until patient can see an appropriate health care provider.

   (4) Take no action.

Plan

5. Select an optimal therapeutic alternative to address the patient's problem, taking into account patient preferences.

   Patient should consult a health care provider.

6. Describe the recommended therapeutic approach to the patient or caregiver.

   "You should consult a health care provider for treatment because self-treatment is not recommended."

7. Explain to the patient or caregiver the rationale for selecting the recommended therapeutic approach from the considered therapeutic alternatives.

   "Seeing a health care provider is best because your problem is severe and debilitating. You may also have a bacterial infection that requires a prescription antibiotic. Finally, you are at high risk for serious foot problems because you have diabetes."

case

40–2 continued

Relevant Evaluation Criteria	Scenario/Model Outcome
Patient Education	
8. When recommending self-care with nonprescription medications and/or nondrug therapy, convey accurate information to the patient or caregiver.	Criterion does not apply in this case.
Solicit follow-up questions from the patient or caregiver.	"Is there anything I can put on my tongue to help stop the pain?"
Answer the patient's or caregiver's questions.	"Yes. There is a viscous lidocaine solution that your prescriber may recommend."
Evaluation of Patient Outcome	
9. Assess patient outcome.	Contact the patient in a day or two to ensure that she made an appointment and sought medical care.

Key: NKA = No known allergies.

Patient Counseling for Minor Burns, Sunburn, and Wounds

Once a burn is assessed as self-treatable, the patient's immediate concern, relieving the pain and swelling, should be addressed. Some patients may not realize the potential complications of even minor burns; therefore, advice on how to protect the injury is vital in preventing possible infection and minimizing scarring.

After a 24- to 48-hour follow-up evaluation of the burn, either continuation of self-treatment or referral for further evaluation should be recommended. If self-treatment continues, the patient needs to know how long healing of the burn will take, as well as the signs and symptoms that indicate worsening of the injury. Burned skin is more susceptible to sunburn for several

weeks after initial injury, so avoiding sun exposure and using sunscreen agents during this period are recommended. The box Patient Education for Minor Burns and Sunburn lists specific advice for successful treatment of these injuries.

When assessing a wound, the provider should remember that minor cuts and abrasions may be self-treated, whereas chronic and more severe acute wounds or those that appear infected should first be evaluated by a primary care provider (Figure 40–5). Irrigation with soapy water or normal saline is generally recommended if a wound is dirty. Patients should be instructed to change the dressing only when it is dirty or not intact. The provider should ensure that the patient understands the basic steps in wound care, especially the selection of appropriate wound dressings. An explanation of basic skin physiology and the wound-healing process will enhance patient

patient education for

Minor Burns and Sunburn

The objectives of self-treatment are to (1) relieve the pain and swelling, (2) protect the burned area from further physical injury, and (3) avoid infection and scarring of the burned area. For most patients, carefully following product instructions and the self-care measures listed here will help ensure optimal therapeutic outcomes.

Nondrug Measures

- Treat superficial burns with no blistering as follows:
  - Immerse the affected area in cool tap water for 10–30 minutes.
  - Cleanse the area with water and a mild soap.
  - Apply a nonadherent dressing or skin protectant to the burn.
- For small burns with minor blistering, follow the first two steps above, but use a hydrocolloid dressing to protect the burn.
- If possible, avoid rupturing blisters.
- For sunburns, avoid further sun exposure and follow the previous procedures according to whether blistering is present.

Nonprescription Medications

- For superficial burns (including sunburn) with unbroken skin, treat the affected area with thin applications of skin protectants or topical anesthetics using a tissue to reduce the risk of infection from the fingertips.

- If the skin is broken, use topical antibiotics to prevent infection.
- If nutritional status is poor, take supplements for vitamins A, B, and C.
- Do not apply camphor, menthol, or ichthammol to the burn.
- For temporary relief of pain, take aspirin, acetaminophen, ibuprofen, or naproxen (see Chapter 5 for dosage guidelines and safety considerations).

When to Seek Medical Attention

- If a skin rash, weight gain, swelling, or blood in the stool occurs while taking pain relievers, report these side effects to a primary care provider.
- Report immediately to a primary care provider any redness, pain, or swelling that extends beyond the boundaries of the original injury.
- If the burn seems to worsen or is not healed significantly in 7 days, see a primary care provider for further treatment.

Acute Wounds

The objective of self-treatment is to promote healing by protecting the wound from infection or further trauma. For most patients, carefully following product instructions and the self-care measures listed here will help ensure optimal therapeutic outcomes.

- Position the wound above the level of the heart to slow bleeding and relieve throbbing pain.
- If the wound is dirty, irrigate it with tepid tap water or normal saline solution, which is not toxic to cells. Use antiseptic solutions selectively and cautiously. Any inflammation should subside within 12–24 hours.
- When cleansing with soapy water, wash hands, apply mild liquid soap (e.g., Dove soap) to a wet cotton ball, and gently wash the wound area; rinse the wound under running warm water and gently pat the area dry.
- Cover the wound with a dressing that will keep the wound site moist. Make sure the dressing is the appropriate size and contour for the affected body part.
- Continue using a wound dressing until the wound bed has firmly closed and signs of inflammation in surrounding tissue have subsided. This process usually takes 2–3 weeks. Failure to keep the wound covered may delay healing.

- Avoid disrupting the dressing unnecessarily; change it only if it is dirty or is not intact. Most dressings should be changed every 3–5 days. Frequent changes may remove resurfacing layers of epithelium and slow the healing process. Change dressing if excessive fluid is released.
- Use a mild analgesic to control pain.
- All wound dressings should be kept in their original packaging and stored away from moisture.
- Observe the wound for signs of infection. Redness, swelling, and exudate are a normal part of healing; foul odor is not.

When to Seek Medical Attention

- Consult a primary care provider if infection is suspected or the wound does not show signs of healing after 7 days of self-treatment.

---

compliance. The box Patient Education for Acute Wounds lists specific information to provide patients. The patient should be referred for further treatment if the wound does not show signs of healing after 7 days of self-treatment.

Evaluation of Patient Outcomes for Minor Burns, Sunburn, and Wounds

Burn should be reassessed after 24–48 hours because the full extent of skin damage may not be initially apparent. If the burn has progressed or worsened, the patient should be referred to an appropriate health care provider for further evaluation.

Minor wounds should exhibit decreased redness during healing. Signs that indicate the need for further evaluation include cellulitis or tissue infection, such as increasing redness, pain, and swelling that extend beyond the boundaries of the original wound, and contact dermatitis from topical treatment.

The patient's progress should be checked after 7 days to assess the healing process; therefore, a scheduled visit to see the provider is preferable. If the wound shows no signs of healing or has worsened (i.e., foul odor, worsened inflammation), the patient should be referred for more aggressive therapy.

Key Points for Minor Burns, Sunburn, and Wounds

➤ Minor burns and sunburn can often be treated with self-care. However, deeper burn injuries or burns affecting more than 1%–2% of BSA require medical attention.
➤ Burn injuries may increase in severity over the first 24–48 hours, so reassessment is always necessary.
➤ Patient complaints usually focus on pain. Skin protectants and dressings should be recommended, and aspirin or NSAIDs are often helpful if not contraindicated. The type of dressing or skin protectant used depends on whether the wound is dry or weeping. Blisters should not be ruptured.

Topical hydrocortisone or anesthetics may provide additional relief in some patients but should be used sparingly on broken skin. Counterirritants such as camphor, menthol, and ichthammol should be avoided.

➤ Vitamins, whether systemic or topical, are generally of no value unless the patient is malnourished.
➤ Photosensitization reactions can often be assessed by reviewing the patient's history and must be distinguished from ordinary sunburns.
➤ Self-treatment of minor acute wounds is appropriate.
➤ First-aid antibiotics are used to prevent infection.
➤ Moist wound healing is now considered the standard of care.
➤ Proper selection of first-aid products, including appropriate wound dressing, is essential.

REFERENCES

1. American Burn Association. Burn incidence and treatment in the United States: 2011 fact sheet. Accessed at http://www.ameriburn.org/resources_factsheet.php, June 27, 2011.
2. Rice RH, Mauro TM. Chapter 19. Toxic responses of the skin. In: Rice RH, Mauro TM, eds. *Casarett & Doull's Essentials of Toxicology.* 2nd ed. New York: McGraw-Hill; 2010. Accessed at http://www.accesspharmacy.com/content.aspx?aID=6484631, June 8, 2013.
3. Marneros AG, Bickers DR. Chapter 56. Photosensitivity and other reactions to light. In: Fauci AS, Kasper DL, Jameson JL, et al., eds. *Harrison's Principles of Internal Medicine.* 18th ed. New York: McGraw-Hill; 2012. Accessed at http://www.accesspharmacy.com/content.aspx?aID=9098703, June 8, 2013.
4. Bickers DR. Photosensitivity and other reactions to light. In: Fauci AS, ed. *Harrison's Principles of Internal Medicine.* 16th ed. New York, NY: McGraw Hill Inc.; 2005:324–39.
5. Internal Medicine and Pediatric Clinic of New Albany. Skin wounds (lacerations, punctures, and abrasions). 2007. Accessed at http://www.impcna.com/intranet/Nelson%20Pediatric/Emergency/SkinWounds%5B1%5D.pdf, September 18, 2014.
6. Hanson D, Langemo D, Thompson P, et al. Understanding wound fluid and the phases of healing. *Adv Skin Wound Care.* 2005;18(7);360–2.
7. Guo S, Dipietro LA. Factors affecting wound healing. *J Dent Res.* 2010;89(3):219–29.
8. Wound infection. *Nurs Times.* 2005;101(8):32. Accessed at http://www.nursingtimes.net/wound-infection/203984.article, June 8, 2013.

9. Demling RH. Nutrition, anabolism, and the wound healing process: an overview. *Eplasty.* 2009;9:e9-65–94.

10. Arnold M, Barbul A. Nutrition and wound healing. *Plast Reconstr Surg.* 2006;117(7 suppl):42S–58S.

11. Keylock KT, Vieira VJ, Wallig MA, et al. Exercise accelerates cutaneous wound healing and decreases wound inflammation in aged mice. *Am J Physiol Regul Integr Comp Physiol.* 2008;294(1):R179–84.

12. Franz MG, Steed DL, Robson MC. Optimizing healing of the acute wound by minimizing complications. *Curr Probl Surg.* 2007;44(11):691–763.

13. Velander P, Theopod C, Hirsch T, et al. Impaired wound healing in an acute diabetic pig model and the effects of hyperglycemia. *Wound Repair Regen.* 2008;16(2):288–93.

14. Menke NB, Ward KR, Witten TM, et al. Impaired wound healing. *Clin Dermatol.* 2007;25(1):19–25.

15. Alsbjorn B, Gilbert P, Hartmann B, et al. Guidelines for the management of partial-thickness burns in a general hospital or community setting—recommendations of a European working party. *Burns.* 2007; 33(2):155–60.

16. Shrivastava P, Goel A. Pre-hospital care in burn injury. *Indian J Plast Surg.* 2010;43(suppl):S15–22.

17. Sarabahi S. Recent advances in topical wound care. *Indian J Plast Surg.* 2012;45(2):379–87.

18. Baranoski S. Choosing a wound dressing, part 1. *Nursing.* 2008;38 (1):60–1.

19. Baranoski S. Choosing a wound dressing, part 2. *Nursing.* 2008; 38(2):14–5.

20. Jones V, Grey J, Harding K. ABC of wound healing: wound dressing. *BMJ.* 2006;332(7554):777–80.

21. Thompson G, Stephen-Hayes J. An overview of wound healing and exudates management. *Br J Community Nurs.* 2007;12(12):S22, S24–6, S28–30.

22. Lee K and Mooney DJ. Alginate: properties and biomedical implications. *Prog Polym Sci.* 2012;37(1):106–26.

23. Okan D, Woo K, Ayello E. The role of moisture balance in wound healing. *Adv Skin Wound Care.* 2007;20(1):39–53.

24. Laccourreye O, Cauchois R, El Sharkawy L, et al. Octylcyanoacrylate (Dermabond) for skin closure at the time of head and neck surgery: a longitudinal prospective study. *Ann Chir.* 2005;130(10):624–30.

25. Young AR, Walker SL. Acute and chronic effects of ultraviolet radiation on the skin. In: Wolff K, Goldsmith LA, Katz SI, et al., eds. *Fitzpatrick's Dermatology in General Medicine.* 7th ed. New York, NY: McGraw-Hill, Inc.; 2007.

26. McEvoy GK, Miller J, eds. Antipruritics and local anesthetics. In: *AHFS Drug Information.* Bethesda, MD: American Society of Health-System Pharmacists; 2007:2844–5.

27. Wolters Kluwer Health, Inc. Antiseptics and germicides. Drug Facts and Comparisons eFacts. Accessed at http://online.factsandcomparisons.com/MonoDisp.aspx?monoid=fandc-hcp10207&book=DFC, July 28, 2014.

28. Eloot S, Dhondt A, Hoste E, et al. How to remove accumulated iodine in burn-injured patients. *Nephrol Dial Transplant.* 2010;25(5):1614–20.

29. Wolters Kluwer Health, Inc. Topical combinations: Miscellaneous. Drug Facts and Comparisons eFacts. Accessed at http://online.factsandcomparisons.com/MonoDisp.aspx?monoID=fandc-hcp12094&quick=243282%7c5&search=243282%7c5&isstemmed=True&NDCmapping=-1&fromTop=true#firstMatch, July 28, 2014.

30. Robertson DB, Maibach HI. Chapter 61. Dermatologic pharmacology. In: Katzung BG, Masters SB, Trevor AJ, eds. *Basic & Clinical Pharmacology.* 12th ed. New York: McGraw-Hill; 2012. Accessed at http://www.accesspharmacy.com/content.aspx?aID=55832444, June 9, 2013.

31. Khorasani G, Hosseinimehr SH, Azadbakht M, et al. Aloe vs silver sulfadiazine creams for second degree burns: a randomized controlled study. *Surg Today.* 2009;39(7):587–91.

32. Chandran O, Kuttan R. Effect of *Calendula officinalis* flower extract on acute phase proteins, antioxidant defense mechanism and granuloma formation during thermal burns. *J Clin Biochem Nutr.* 2008;43(2):58–64.

33. Bittmann S, Luchter E, Thiel M, et al. Does honey have a role in paediatric wound management? *Br J Nurs.* 2010;19(15):19–24.

34. Malik KI, Malik MA, Aslam A. Honey compared with silver sulphadiazine in the treatment of superficial partial-thickness burns. *Int Wound J.* 2010;7(5):413–17.

chapter

FUNGAL SKIN INFECTIONS

41

Gail D. Newton

Fungal skin infections, or dermatomycoses, are among the most common cutaneous disorders.[1] Dermatomycoses are often referred to as ringworm because their characteristic lesions are ring shaped with clear centers and red, scaly borders. However, these lesions can vary from the ring form and may present as single or multiple lesions that range from mild scaling to deep granulomas (inflamed, nodular lesions).

Fungal infections are usually superficial and can involve the hair, nails, and skin. The term *tinea* refers exclusively to dermatophyte infections. Most often, tinea infections are named according to the area of the body that is affected (e.g., scalp [tinea capitis], groin [tinea cruris], body [tinea corporis], feet [tinea pedis], and nails [tinea unguium]). These infections are generally caused by three genera of fungi. Species of *Candida* and other yeasts may also be involved[2]; however, currently available nonprescription antifungals are not indicated for self-management of cutaneous infections secondary to yeasts.[3]

Although many pathogenic fungi exist, the overall prevalence of actual superficial fungal infections is remarkably low. An estimated 10%–20% of the U.S. population suffer from a tinea infection at any one time.[4,5] Many degrees of susceptibility, from instantaneous "takes" by a single spore to severe trauma with massive exposure, produce a clinical infection. Trauma to the skin, especially trauma that produces blisters (e.g., from wearing ill-fitting footwear), appears to be significantly more important than simple exposure to the offending pathogens to the occurrence of human fungal infections.[5] Other predisposing factors for the development of tinea infections include diabetes mellitus and other diseases associated with immune system depression, use of immunosuppressive drugs, impaired circulation, poor nutrition and hygiene, occlusion of the skin, and warm, humid climates.[5,6]

The most prevalent cutaneous fungal infection in humans is tinea pedis (dermatophytosis of the foot, or athlete's foot). Tinea pedis afflicts approximately 26.5 million people in the United States every year; 7 of every 10 sufferers are male. Approximately 45% will suffer with tinea pedis episodically for more than 10 years. When exposure to infectious environments is equal, the incidence of tinea pedis infections in women approaches that in men.[4,5,7,8] Tinea pedis is rare among blacks but common in whites, particularly whites who live in urban tropical areas.[9] An estimated 70% of people will be afflicted with tinea pedis in their lifetime. Although tinea pedis may occur at all ages, it is more common in adults, presumably because of their increased opportunities for exposure to pathogens.[5]

The risk for development of tinea pedis is greater in individuals who use public pools or bathing facilities than in the general population. However, tinea pedis may be acquired in the home if one or more members of the household are already infected. High-impact sports that cause chronic trauma to the feet (e.g., long-distance running) also predispose athletes to tinea pedis.[10–12] The trauma affords infecting fungi the opportunity to invade the outer layers of the skin. In addition, wearing socks and shoes exacerbates the problem by impeding the dispersion of heat and the evaporation of moisture, both of which facilitate fungal growth. In contrast, individuals who most often use footwear that allows the feet to remain cool and dry (e.g., sandals) are less likely to develop tinea pedis.

Tinea unguium (ringworm of the nails or onychomycosis) causes about half of all nail disorders and is sometimes associated with tinea pedis. The estimated prevalence of tinea unguium is between 2% and 8% percent, depending on the population.[13] The Food and Drug Administration (FDA) has not approved self-treatment of onychomycosis with topical nonprescription antifungals. Rather, the affected nail must be treated with systemic drug therapy (e.g., terbinafine or itraconazole) or removed surgically to rid the area of the offending fungus.

The next two most common infections are tinea corporis and tinea cruris. Tinea corporis, also called ringworm of the body, is most common in prepubescent individuals. It is frequently transmitted among children in day care centers and among child participants in contact sports, such as wrestling. However, it is also more common in adults and children who live in hot, humid climates. Individuals who are under stress or overweight are also at increased risk to develop tinea corporis.[14,15]

Tinea cruris, or jock itch, is most common during warm weather, but it can occur at any time of the year if the skin in the groin area stays warm and moist for long periods. For example, sweating or prolonged contact with wet clothing provides an ideal environment for the growth of fungi. Tinea cruris occurs more often in men than in women and rarely affects children. Close indirect or direct physical contact between infected males and noninfected females does not mitigate the higher prevalence of tinea cruris in males. For example, females who live in the same household with infected males do not develop infections at the same rate as noninfected males in the same household.[5]

Although its true incidence is unknown, tinea capitis, or ringworm of the scalp, occurs most often in children because they are more likely to have contact with infected individuals and because they are less attentive than adults to personal hygiene. Compared with black males and white children, black female children are infected more often, possibly because of the hair care products and practices (e.g., occlusive hair dressings and tight braiding) that are unique to this population.[5,14]

Tinea capitis can be spread by direct contact with an infected person, but it is often spread by contact with infected fomites (e.g., using infected combs, hats, toys, or telephones; wearing infected clothing; using infected towels; or sleeping on infected linens). In some instances, tinea capitis is spread through contact with other infected individuals or with infected cats or dogs.[16] As with onychomycosis, tinea capitis cannot be managed with topical nonprescription antifungals.

Pathophysiology of Fungal Skin Infections

Tinea infections are caused by three genera of pathogenic fungi: *Trichophyton, Microsporum,* and *Epidermophyton.* Tinea pedis and tinea cruris are caused by species of *Epidermophyton* and *Trichophyton.* Species of *Trichophyton* and *Microsporum* cause ringworm of the scalp. *Trichophyton* species also cause ringworm of the nails or onychomycosis. All species of the three genera can cause tinea corporis.[5] Fungal transmission can occur through contact with infected people, animals, soil, or fomites. Dermatophytes are classified according to their habitat: anthropophilic (humans), zoophilic (animals), and geophilic (soil). Most tinea infections are caused by person-to-person contact with individuals infected with anthropophilic dermatophytes.[14]

In addition to specific fungi, other environmental factors such as climate and social customs contribute to dermatophytosis development. Footwear is a key variable, as illustrated by the incidence of tinea pedis in any population that wears occlusive footwear, especially in the summer and in tropical or subtropical climates. Nonporous shoe material increases temperature and hydration of the skin, which interferes with the barrier function of the stratum corneum. Similarly, sweating or wearing wet clothing for long periods of time can predispose individuals to the development of tinea corporis and tinea cruris.

Chronic health problems and medications that weaken or suppress the immune system can also increase the risk for development of tinea infections. For example, patients with diabetes or human immunodeficiency virus and elderly persons taking medications such as glucocorticoids should be instructed to monitor themselves for signs and symptoms of tinea infections. They should also be instructed about the importance of proper hygiene and diet for the prevention of tinea infections and other health problems.

After a dermatophyte is inoculated into the skin under suitable conditions, a tinea infection progresses through several stages. The stages include periods of incubation and then enlargement, followed by a refractory period and a stage of involution. During the incubation period, the dermatophyte grows in the stratum corneum, sometimes with minimal signs of infection. After the incubation period and once the infection is established, two factors appear to play a role in determining the size and duration of the lesions: the growth rate of the organism and the epidermal turnover rate.[17] The fungal growth rate must equal or exceed the epidermal turnover rate, or the organism will be quickly shed.

Dermatophytid infestations remain within the stratum corneum. Resistance to the spread of infection seems to involve both immunologic and nonimmunologic mechanisms. For example, the presence of a serum inhibitory factor (SIF) appears to limit the growth of dermatophytes beyond the stratum corneum. SIF is not an antibody but a dialyzable, heat-labile component of fresh

sera. It appears that SIF chelates the iron that dermatophytes need for continued growth.[17] Once in the stratum corneum, dermatophytes produce keratinases and other proteolytic enzymes that cause allergic reactions when they reach living epidermis.[5]

The major immunologic defense against fungal skin infections is the type IV delayed-hypersensitivity response. The refractory period precedes complete development of this cell-mediated immunity. The fungal growth rate typically exceeds epidermal turnover, and inflammation and pruritus are at their peak. After development of an adequate immune response, symptoms of superficial fungal infections diminish, and the infection may clear spontaneously during the involution period. Patients with chronic infections typically present with much less inflammation. This presentation may be caused by a suppressed hypersensitivity response, which in turn reduces the inflammatory response.[2]

Clinical Presentation of Fungal Skin Infections

The clinical spectrum of tinea infections ranges from mild itching and scaling to a severe, exudative inflammatory process characterized by denudation, fissuring, crusting, and/or discoloration of the affected skin. Individuals experiencing their first tinea infection and patients with infections secondary to zoophilic fungi tend to present with greater inflammation.[14] Table 41–1 summarizes key differences between fungal skin infections, contact dermatitis, and bacterial skin infections to distinguish the underlying cause of a patient's symptoms from other conditions that may have a similar clinical presentation.

Tinea Pedis

Clinically, tinea pedis has four accepted variants; two or more of these types may overlap. The most common is the chronic intertriginous type,[5] characterized by fissuring, scaling, or maceration in the interdigital spaces; malodor; pruritus; and/or a stinging sensation on the feet (see Color Plates, photograph 27). Typically, the infection involves the lateral toe webs, usually between either the fourth and fifth or the third and fourth toes. From these sites, the infection may spread to the sole or instep of the foot but rarely to the dorsum. Warmth and humidity aggravate this condition; consequently, hyperhidrosis (excessive sweating) becomes an underlying problem and must be treated along with the dermatophyte infestation.[5]

Normal resident aerobic diphtheroids may become involved in the tinea pedis process. After initial invasion of the stratum corneum by dermatophytes, enough moisture may accumulate to trigger a bacterial overgrowth. Increased moisture and temperature then lead to the release of metabolic products that diffuse easily through the underlying horny layer already damaged by fungal invasion. In more severe cases, gram-negative organisms intrude and may exacerbate the condition, causing skin maceration, white hyperkeratosis, or erosions with increased patient symptomatology.[5]

The second variant of tinea pedis foot is known as the chronic papulosquamous pattern.[5] It is usually found on both feet and is characterized by mild inflammation and diffuse, moccasin-like scaling on the soles of the feet. Tinea unguium of one or more toenails may also be present and may continue to fuel the infection. The toenails must first be cured with oral drug therapy, such as itraconazole, ketoconazole, or terbinafine,

table

41–1 Differentiation of Fungal Skin Infections and Skin Disorders with Similar Presentation

Criterion	Fungal Skin Infections	Contact Dermatitis	Bacterial Skin Infection
Location	On areas of the body where excess moisture accumulates, such as the feet, groin area, scalp, and under the arms	Any area of the body exposed to the allergen/irritant; hands, face, legs, ears, eyes, and anogenital area involved most often	Anywhere on the body
Signs	Presents either as soggy malodorous, thickened skin; acute vesicular rash; or fine scaling of affected area with varying degrees of inflammation; cracks and fissures may also be present	Presents as a variety of lesions: raised wheals, fluid-filled vesicles, or both	Presents as a variety of lesions from macules to pustules to ulcers with redness surrounding the lesion; lesions are often warmer than surrounding, unaffected skin
Symptoms	Itching and pain	Itching and pain	Irritation and pain
Quantity/severity	Usually localized to one region of the body but can spread	Affects all areas of exposed skin but does not spread	Usually localized to one region of the body but can spread
Timing	Variable onset	Variable onset from immediately after exposure to 3 weeks after contact	Variable onset
Cause	Superficial fungal infection	Exposure to skin irritants or allergens	Superficial bacterial infection
Modifying factors	Treated with nonprescription astringents, antifungals, and nondrug measures to keep the area clean and dry	Treated with topical antipruritics, skin protectants, astringents, and nondrug measures to avoid reexposure	Treated with prescription antibiotics

or they must be removed surgically to rid the area of the offending fungus.

The third variant of tinea pedis is the vesicular type, usually caused by *Trichophyton mentagrophytes* var. *interdigitale.*[5] Small vesicles or vesicopustules are observed near the instep and on the mid-anterior plantar surface. Skin scaling is seen on these areas as well as on the toe webs. This variant is symptomatic in the summer and is clinically quiescent during the cooler months.

The acute ulcerative type is the fourth variant of tinea pedis. It is often associated with macerated, denuded, weeping ulcerations on the sole of the foot. Typically, white hyperkeratosis and a pungent odor are present. This type of infection, which is complicated by an overgrowth of opportunistic, gram-negative bacteria such as *Proteus* and *Pseudomonas,* has been called a "dermatophytosis complex," and it may produce an extremely painful, erosive, purulent interspace that can impede the patient's ability to walk.[5]

Tinea Unguium

Nails affected by tinea unguium gradually lose their normal shiny luster and become opaque. If left untreated, the nails become thick, rough, yellow, opaque, and friable. The nail may separate from the nail bed if the infection progresses secondarily to subungual hyperkeratosis. Ultimately, the nail may be lost altogether. Subungual debris also provides an excellent medium for the growth of opportunistic bacteria and other microorganisms, which can lead to further infectious complications.[5]

Tinea Corporis

Tinea corporis may have a diverse clinical presentation. Most often, the lesions, which involve glabrous (smooth and bare) skin, begin as small, circular, erythematous, scaly areas. The lesions spread peripherally, and the borders may contain vesicles or pustules. Infected individuals may also complain of pruritus.[18]

Tinea corporis can occur on any part of the body. However, the location of the infection can provide clues to the type of infecting dermatophyte. For example, zoophilic dermatophytes often infect areas of exposed skin such as the neck, face, and arms. In contrast, infections secondary to anthropophilic dermatophytes often occur in occluded areas or in areas of trauma.[5]

Tinea Cruris

Tinea cruris is more common in males and occurs on the medial and upper parts of the thighs and the pubic area. The lesions have well-demarcated margins that are elevated slightly and are more erythematous than the central area; small vesicles may be seen, especially at the margins. Acute lesions are bright red, and chronic cases tend to have more of a hyperpigmented appearance; fine scaling is usually present. This condition is generally bilateral with significant pruritus; however, the lesions usually spare the penis and scrotum. This characteristic can help to distinguish tinea cruris from candidiasis, which also causes lesions in these areas.[19] Pain may also be present during periods of sweating or when the skin becomes macerated or infected by a secondary microorganism.[4,5]

Tinea Capitis

Clinically, tinea capitis may present as one of four variant patterns, depending on the causative dermatophyte. In noninflammatory tinea capitis, lesions begin as small papules surrounding individual hair shafts. Subsequently, the lesions spread centrifugally to involve all hairs in their path. Although there is some scaling of the scalp, little inflammation is present (see Color Plates, photograph 28). Hairs in the lesions are a dull gray color and usually break off above the scalp level.[5]

The inflammatory type of tinea capitis produces a spectrum of inflammation, ranging from pustules to kerion formation.

Kerions are weeping lesions whose exudate forms thick crusts on the scalp.[8] In addition to fever and pain, individuals with this type of tinea capitis may experience a higher degree of pruritus. Regional lymph nodes may also be enlarged.[5]

The black dot variety of tinea capitis was named for the appearance of infected areas of the scalp. The location of arthrospores on the hair shaft causes hairs to break off at the level of the scalp, leaving black dots on the scalp surface. Hair loss, inflammation, and scaling with this type of tinea capitis range from minimal to extensive. Therefore, this variant is especially challenging to diagnose.[5,20,21]

The favus variant of tinea capitis typically presents as patchy areas of hair loss and scutula (yellowish crusts and scales). Ultimately, these lesions can coalesce to involve a major portion of the scalp. If left untreated, this condition can lead to secondary bacterial infections, scalp atrophy, scarring, and permanent hair loss.[5]

Treatment of Fungal Skin Infections

Treatment Goals

The goals of treating fungal skin infections are to (1) provide symptomatic relief, (2) eradicate existing infection, and (3) prevent future infections.

General Treatment Approach

In many instances, patients can effectively self-treat tinea pedis, tinea corporis, and tinea cruris with nonprescription topical antifungals and nonpharmacologic measures. However, individuals with tinea unguium or tinea capitis should be referred to a primary care provider for treatment.

Patients who want to improve the appearance of the nail during prescription treatment of tinea unguium can use Fungal Nail Revitalizer to reduce nail discoloration and to smooth out the thick, rough nail. This product contains calcium carbonate (a strong alkali) and urea (a protein denaturant) to debride nail tissue. The patient should apply the cream over the entire surface of the infected nail, scrub this area for at least 1 minute with the provided nailbrush, and then wash and dry the nail completely. For optimum results, this procedure should be performed daily for 3 weeks. Patients should be advised that this product will improve only the appearance of the nails and that it will not treat the tinea infection.

Before recommending therapy, the provider must be reasonably sure that the lesions are consistent with a tinea infection. Their appearance should conform to the descriptions provided in Clinical Presentation of Fungal Skin Infections, and photographs 27 and 28 of tinea lesions (see Color Plates) should be consulted for comparison. Furthermore, the lesions should not resemble any other skin conditions covered in this text. When in doubt about the true cause of a condition, the patient should be advised to consult a primary care provider or dermatologist. Figure 41–1 outlines the appropriate self-treatment options for fungal skin infections.

A number of topical antifungals are available in a variety of dosage forms for self-treatment of fungal skin infections. The selection of a particular product depends on the type of infection and on individual patient characteristics and preferences. For example, in acute, inflammatory tinea pedis, characterized by reddened, oozing, and vesicular eruptions, the inflammation

must be counteracted with solutions of astringent aluminum salts before antifungal therapy can be instituted.

A critical determinant of the outcome of therapy is the patient's ability to adhere to the recommended therapy for the appropriate length of time. Adherence may be difficult because these conditions may take between 2 and 4 weeks to resolve. Patients may be tempted to terminate therapy when their symptoms subside but before the infection has been eradicated. Another determinant of therapeutic outcome relates to the patient's adherence to the nonpharmacologic measures intended to complement the effects of nonprescription antifungals and to prevent future infections. These measures include keeping the skin clean and dry, avoiding the sharing of personal articles, and avoiding contact with infected fomites or persons who have a fungal infection.

Nonpharmacologic Therapy

The box Patient Education for Fungal Skin Infections located at the end of the chapter describes nonpharmacologic measures intended to complement the effects of nonprescription antifungals and to prevent future infections. The patient should follow these measures during and after treatment of the infection.

Pharmacologic Therapy

An antifungal ingredient must have at least one well-designed clinical trial that demonstrates its effectiveness in treating tinea infections before FDA will classify it as a monograph antifungal.[22] Butenafine hydrochloride, clioquinol, clotrimazole, haloprogin, miconazole nitrate, terbinafine hydrochloride, tolnaftate, and various undecylenates are considered safe and effective for nonprescription use in the treatment of fungal skin infections.[3] These agents are labeled for treatment of athlete's foot, jock itch, and body ringworm. The recommended treatment period is a minimum of 1–4 weeks.

Clotrimazole and Miconazole Nitrate

Topical clotrimazole and miconazole nitrate are imidazole derivatives that demonstrate fungistatic/fungicidal activity (depending on concentration) against *Trichophyton mentagrophytes, Trichophyton rubrum, Epidermophyton floccosum,* and *Candida albicans.*

These agents act by inhibiting the biosynthesis of ergosterol and other sterols and by damaging the fungal cell wall membrane, thereby altering its permeability and resulting in the loss of essential intracellular elements. These drugs have also been shown to inhibit the oxidative and peroxidative enzyme activity that results in intracellular buildup of toxic concentrations of hydrogen peroxide; this toxicity may then contribute to the degradation of subcellular organelles and to cellular necrosis. In *C. albicans* infections, these drugs have been shown to inhibit the transformation of blastospores into the invasive mycelial form that causes infection.

FDA classifies clotrimazole 1% and miconazole nitrate 2% as safe and effective for topical nonprescription use in treating tinea pedis, tinea cruris, and tinea corporis. Clotrimazole and miconazole nitrate are applied once in the morning and once in the evening. For athlete's foot and ringworm, these drugs should be applied twice daily for 4 weeks; for jock itch they should be applied twice daily for 2 weeks.

Rare cases of mild skin irritation, burning, and stinging have occurred with use of nonprescription topical antifungals.

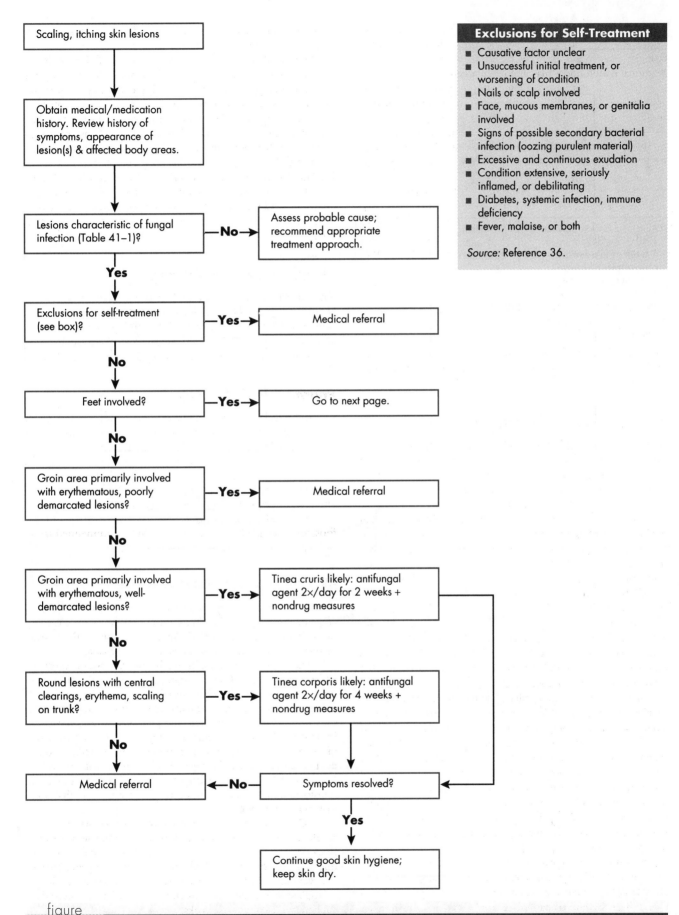

figure

41–1   Self-care of fungal skin infections.

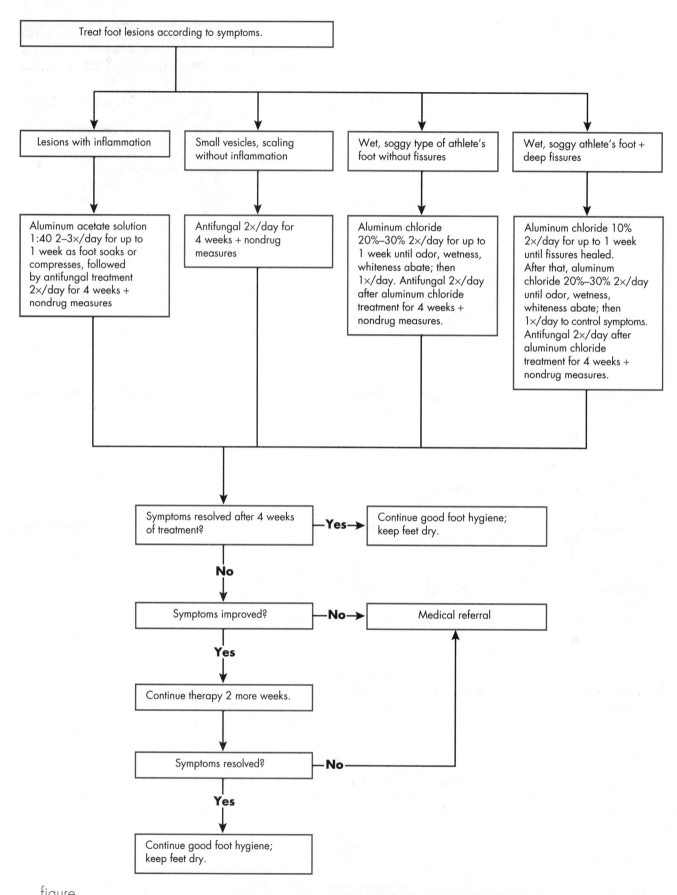

figure
41–1   (continued)

No drug–drug interactions have been reported with topical use of clotrimazole and miconazole nitrate for up to 4 weeks.[3]

Terbinafine Hydrochloride

Topical terbinafine hydrochloride 1% was reclassified as a nonprescription medication in 1999.

This antifungal agent inhibits squalene epoxidase, a key enzyme in fungi sterol biosynthesis. This action results in a deficiency in ergosterol and a corresponding accumulation of squalene within the fungal cell, causing fungal cell death.

Terbinafine hydrochloride is indicated for interdigital tinea pedis, tinea cruris, and tinea corporis caused by *E. floccosum, T. mentagrophytes,* and *T. rubrum.* Similar to miconazole and clotrimazole, terbinafine hydrochloride should be applied sparingly to the affected area twice daily.

In clinical trials, this drug demonstrated that it could cure tinea pedis with 1 week of treatment. However, complete resolution of symptoms may require up to 4 weeks of treatment. For athlete's foot between the toes, patients should apply terbinafine twice a day for 1 week. For athlete's foot on the bottom or sides of the foot, it should be applied twice a day for 2 weeks. For jock itch and ringworm, patients should apply terbinafine once a day for 1 week or as directed by a primary care provider.

Clinical trials to date have demonstrated a low incidence of side effects for terbinafine hydrochloride. These side effects include irritation (1%), burning (0.8%), and itching/dryness (0.2%).[23,24] No drug–drug interactions have been reported with topical use of this agent.

Butenafine Hydrochloride

Topical butenafine hydrochloride 1% was reclassified as a nonprescription medication in 2001. Like terbinafine, this antifungal agent is a squalene epoxidase inhibitor. This action results in a deficiency in ergosterol, a corresponding accumulation of squalene within the fungal cell, and eventually cell death.

Butenafine hydrochloride is indicated as a cure for tinea pedis between the toes, tinea cruris, and tinea corporis caused by *E. floccosum, T. mentagrophytes,* and *T. rubrum.* Similar to other nonprescription topical antifungals, butenafine hydrochloride also relieves the itching, burning, cracking, and scaling that can accompany these conditions. This agent's effectiveness on infection of the bottom or sides of the foot is unknown.

Patients suffering from tinea pedis should be advised to apply a thin film to affected skin between and around toes twice daily for 1 week, once a day for 4 weeks, or as directed by a primary care provider. Patients with tinea cruris or tinea corporis should apply a thin film to the affected area once daily for 2 weeks or as directed by a primary care provider.

Effective treatment rates of butenafine for interdigital tinea pedis with 1-week and 4-week application durations are reported to be approximately 38% and 74%, respectively. In clinical trials, Lotrimin Ultra kept users free of tinea pedis for up to 3 months.[25] To date, clinical trials demonstrate a low incidence of side effects for this agent. Further, no drug–drug interactions have been reported with its topical use.

Tolnaftate

Topical tolnaftate has demonstrated clinical efficacy since its commercial introduction in the United States in 1965. In addition, it was the standard against which the efficacy of other topical antifungals was compared for many years.

Although tolnaftate's exact mechanism of action has not been reported, it is believed that tolnaftate distorts the hyphae and stunts the mycelial growth of the fungi species. Tolnaftate is the only nonprescription drug approved for both preventing and treating tinea infections.[3] It acts on fungi that are typically responsible for tinea infections, including *T. mentagrophytes, T. rubrum,* and *E. floccosum.*

Tolnaftate is valuable primarily in the dry, scaly lesions. Relapse of superficial fungal infections has occurred after tolnaftate therapy has been discontinued. Relapse may be caused by inadequate duration of treatment, patient nonadherence with the medication, or use of tolnaftate when an oral antifungal should have been used.

As a cream, tolnaftate is formulated in a polyethylene glycol 400/propylene glycol vehicle. The 1% solution is formulated in polyethylene glycol 400 and may be more effective than the cream. The solution solidifies when exposed to cold but liquefies with no loss in potency if allowed to warm. These vehicles are particularly advantageous in superficial antifungal therapy because they are nonocclusive, nontoxic, nonsensitizing, water miscible, anhydrous, easy to apply, and efficient in delivering the drug to the affected area.

The topical powder formulation of tolnaftate uses cornstarch/talc as the vehicle. The two agents combined absorb excess moisture in the affected area that allows fungus to thrive. The topical aerosol formulation of tolnaftate includes talc, alcohol, and the propellant vehicle.

Tolnaftate (1% solution, cream, gel, powder, spray powder, or spray liquid) is applied sparingly twice daily. Effective therapy usually takes 2–4 weeks, although some individuals (patients with lesions between the toes or on pressure areas of the foot) may require treatment lasting 4–6 weeks. Tolnaftate is well tolerated when applied to intact or broken skin, although it usually stings slightly when applied. Delayed hypersensitivity reactions to tolnaftate are extremely rare. No drug–drug interactions have been reported with topical use of tolnaftate.

Clioquinol/Haloprogin/Undecylenic Acid

Although FDA has approved clioquinol 3%, haloprogin 1%, and undecylenic acid and undecylenate salts for nonprescription use, no commercially available nonprescription topical antifungals currently contain these agents.

Salts of Aluminum

Because aluminum salts do not have any direct antifungal activity, these drugs were not included in the FDA final monograph for topical antifungal drug products. Rather, they are approved for the relief of inflammatory conditions of the skin, such as tinea pedis. However, their effectiveness as astringents and their possible use in treating tinea pedis merit their inclusion in this chapter. Historically, aluminum acetate has been the foremost astringent used for both the acute, inflammatory type and the wet, soggy type of tinea pedis. Aluminum chloride is also used to treat the wet, soggy type of infection.

Aluminum salts do not cure athlete's foot entirely but are useful when combined with other topical antifungal drugs. Application of aluminum salts merely shifts the disease process back to the simple dry type of athlete's foot, which can then be controlled with other agents, such as tolnaftate or an imidazole.

The action and efficacy of aluminum salts appear to be two pronged. First, these compounds act as astringents. Their drying ability probably involves complexing of the astringent agent with proteins, thereby altering the proteins' ability to swell and hold water. Astringents decrease edema, exudation, and inflammation by reducing cell membrane permeability and by hardening the intercellular cement of the capillary epithelium. Second, aluminum salts in concentrations greater than 20% possess antibacterial activity, which may help to prevent the development of secondary bacterial infections. Aluminum chloride solution (20%) may exhibit that activity in two ways: by directly killing bacteria and by drying the interspaces. Solutions of 20% aluminum acetate and 20% aluminum chloride demonstrate equal in vitro antibacterial efficacy.

Aluminum acetate for use in tinea pedis is generally diluted with about 10–40 parts of water. Depending on the situation, the whole foot may be immersed in the solution for 20 minutes up to 3 times a day (every 6–8 hours), or the solution may be applied to the affected area in the form of a wet dressing.

For patient convenience, aluminum acetate solution (Burow's solution) or modified Burow's solution (which includes dextrin, polyethylene glycol and sodium bicarbonate as inactive ingredients) is available for immediate use in solution or in forms to be dissolved in water (powder packets, powder, and effervescent tablets) (see Chapter 34).

Aqueous solutions of 20%–30% aluminum chloride have been the most beneficial for the wet, soggy type of athlete's foot.[7] Twice-daily applications are generally used until the signs and symptoms (odor, wetness, and whiteness) abate. After that, once-daily applications may control the symptoms. In hot, humid weather, the original condition may return within 7–10 days after the application is stopped.

Because aluminum salts penetrate the skin poorly, their toxicity is low. However, a few cases of irritation have been reported in patients with deep fissures. Therefore, the use of concentrated aluminum salt solutions on severely eroded or deeply fissured skin is contraindicated. In this case, the salts must be diluted to a lower concentration (10% aluminum chloride) for initial treatment.

Solutions of aluminum acetate or aluminum chloride have the potential for misuse (e.g., accidental childhood poisoning by ingestion of the solutions or the solid tablets), so precautions must be taken to prevent this misuse. Products containing these ingredients are intended for external use only and should not be applied near the eyes. Prolonged or continuous use of aluminum acetate solution may produce tissue necrosis. In the acute inflammatory stage of tinea pedis, this solution should be used less than 1 week. The provider should instruct the patient to discontinue its use if inflammatory lesions appear or worsen.

Pharmacotherapeutic Comparison

All the topical antifungals approved for treating cutaneous fungal infections have demonstrated effectiveness. The allure of butenafine hydrochloride and terbinafine hydrochloride is their ability to cure athlete's foot in some patients after 1 week. However, a close analysis of the data demonstrates that the number of patients achieving complete resolution of the problem is low, and that the effectiveness of these agents parallels that of other antifungals previously approved for nonprescription use (e.g., clotrimazole and miconazole nitrate).[26]

Controlled studies have demonstrated the efficacy of clotrimazole and miconazole nitrate for tinea pedis and other kinds of fungal infections (see Chapter 8). Both agents would be expected to demonstrate efficacy comparable to that of tolnaftate for tinea infections. If patient factors (e.g., nonadherence or improper foot hygiene) can be ruled out as a cause of treatment failure, both can be suggested as alternative treatment modalities.

Product Selection Guidelines

Cutaneous antifungals are available as ointments, creams, powders, and aerosols (Table 41–2). Creams or solutions are the most efficient and effective dosage forms for delivery of the active ingredient to the epidermis. Sprays and powders are less effective because often they are not rubbed into the skin. They are probably more useful as adjuncts to a cream or a solution or as prophylactic agents in preventing new or recurrent infections.

Patient adherence is influenced by product selection. Therefore, the provider should recommend a drug and dosage form that are likely to cause the least interference with daily habits and activities, without sacrificing efficacy. For example, elderly patients may require a preparation that is easy to use. Obese patients, in whom excessive sweating may contribute to the disease, should sprinkle talcum powder on the feet and in the shoes as adjunctive therapy to keep the feet dry. Under certain circumstances, the provider may need to instruct the caregiver instead of the patient in the proper use of foot products.

Before recommending a nonprescription product, the provider should review the patient's medical history. For example, patients with diabetes should have their blood glucose levels under control because increased glucose in perspiration may promote fungal growth. Patients with allergic dermatitides often have a history of asthma, hay fever, or atopic dermatitis; therefore, they are extremely sensitive to many oral and topical agents. Acquiring a good medical history may aid in distinguishing a tinea infection from atopic dermatitis and may avoid the recommendation of a product that might cause further skin irritation.

In addition, product line extensions that carry the same brand name do not necessarily have the same active ingredient(s). For example, the cream and solution formulations of Lotrimin AF contain clotrimazole 1%, whereas the topical spray and powder formulations contain miconazole nitrate 2%. Indeed, Lotrimin Ultra, the newest line extension, contains butenafine hydrochloride. It is economically prudent for the manufacturer to create a line extension with a different active ingredient for an already-approved brand name. Filing New Drug Applications (NDAs) for new brand names of antifungal products with different active ingredients would be prohibitively expensive. Similarly, Desenex spray liquid and spray powder formulations contain miconazole nitrate 2%, whereas these products formerly contained undecylenic acid and zinc undecylenate in a 25% concentration. In addition, Desenex Max Antifungal Cream now contains terbinafine 1%.

Complementary Therapies

Bitter orange, tea tree oil, and garlic have been used with some success in the management of fungal skin infections, with few or no side effects. None of the studies that examined these

table

41-2 Selected Nonprescription Topical Antifungal Products

Trade Name	Active Ingredient	Directions for Use
Cruex Antifungal Spray Powder	Miconazole 2%	Spray a thin layer over affected area twice daily for 2 weeks.
Desenex Antifungal Liquid Spray	Miconazole 2%	Spray a thin layer over affected area twice daily for 4 weeks.
Lamisil AT Antifungal Gel,	Terbinafine HCl 1%	For athlete's foot between the toes, apply once a day for 1 week. For jock itch and ringworm, apply once a day (morning or night) for 1 week.
Lamisil AT Cream	Terbinafine HCl 1%	For athlete's foot between the toes, apply twice a day (morning and night) for 1 week. For athlete's foot on the bottom or sides of the foot, apply twice a day (morning and night) for 2 weeks. For jock itch and ringworm, apply once a day (morning or night) for 1 week.
Lotrimin AF Clotrimazole Cream	Clotrimazole 1%	For athlete's foot and ringworm, use twice daily for 4 weeks. For jock itch, use daily for 2 weeks.
Lotrimin AF Antifungal Jock Itch Powder Aerosol Spray	Miconazole nitrate 2%	For athlete's foot and ringworm, use twice daily for 4 weeks. For jock itch, use twice daily for 2 weeks.
Lotrimin Ultra Antifungal Cream	Butenafine 1%	For athlete's foot between the toes, apply to affected skin between and around the toes twice a day for 1 week (morning and night), or once a day for 4 weeks. For jock itch and ringworm, apply once a day to affected skin for 2 weeks.
Micatin Antifungal Cream	Miconazole nitrate 2%	For athlete's foot and ringworm, use twice daily for 4 weeks. For jock itch, use twice daily for 2 weeks.
Tinactin Athlete's Foot Cream	Tolnaftate 1%	For athlete's foot and ringworm, use daily for 4 weeks. For jock itch, use daily for 2 weeks.
Tinactin Powder Spray	Tolnaftate 1%	For athlete's foot and ringworm, spray twice daily for 4 weeks. For prevention, spray 1–2 times daily.

ingredients included more than 60 patients, but the results suggest that further investigation of each complementary therapy is warranted.

Bitter orange has the least evidence of safety and efficacy. However, in one controlled trial, topical application of oil of bitter orange 3 times daily demonstrated benefit in most patients with tinea corporis, tinea cruris, or tinea pedis in 1–4 weeks. The only reported side effect was mild, local irritation.[27]

Investigations into the efficacy of tea tree oil for tinea pedis have yielded mixed results. In one study that compared tolnaftate 1% cream with tea tree oil 10% cream, both agents were equally effective in relieving the scaling, inflammation, itching, and burning, but neither agent was more effective than placebo in achieving mycologic cure.[28] Results of two other studies suggest that tea tree oil 25% and 50% appear to result in both symptomatic and mycologic cure of tinea pedis. However, the mycologic cure rates were inferior to those for butenafine and clotrimazole.[29,30]

Research relative to the efficacy of topical garlic for the management of tinea infections has been positive. For example, application of a garlic gel containing 0.6% ajoene (i.e., a constituent of garlic believed to have antifungal activity) was demonstrated to be as effective as terbinafine 1% cream in a study of subjects with either tinea corporis or cruris.[31] In another study, the use of ajoene 0.4% as a cream resulted in clinical and mycologic cure of all research subjects after 2 weeks of use.[32] In the most recent study, researchers reported evidence that ajoene 1% cream produces a higher mycologic cure rate than that of ajoene 0.6% and terbinafine 1% creams.[33] (For an in-depth discussion of garlic, see Chapter 51.)

Assessment of Fungal Skin Infections: A Case-Based Approach

Fungal skin infections must be differentiated from bacterial skin infections and noninfectious dermatitis. If possible, the provider should examine the affected area to determine whether the disorder's manifestation is typical of a fungal infection (Table 41–1).[34] The only true determinant of a fungal infection is a clinical laboratory evaluation of tissue scrapings from the affected area.

The provider should question the patient thoroughly regarding the condition and its characteristics to determine symptoms, extent of disease, previous patient adherence with medications, and any compounding disorders (e.g., diabetes or obesity) that might render the patient susceptible. Patients with diabetes, for example, may present with a mixed dermatophytid and monilial infection. In general, it is appropriate to inspect the affected area if privacy and sanitary conditions allow. Inspection is especially appropriate for patients with diabetes.

Cases 41–1 and 41–2 are examples of the assessment of patients with a fungal skin infection.

case

41-1

Relevant Evaluation Criteria	Scenario/Model Outcome
Information Gathering	
1. Gather essential information about the patient's symptoms and medical history, including:	
a. description of symptom(s) (i.e., nature, onset, duration, severity, associated symptoms)	The patient presents to the pharmacy with redness in the shape of eyeglasses on her nose and around both eyes. Scaling and weeping vesicles on both eyelids extend into both eyebrows. The patient has an open sore on the bridge of her nose that she admits she caused by scratching the area. She also complains of intense itching. Her symptoms began about a month ago, right after she started to swim competitively at school.
b. description of any factors that seem to precipitate, exacerbate, and/or relieve the patient's symptom(s)	She says that the itching is worse after she removes her swim goggles.
c. description of the patient's efforts to relieve the symptoms	She has tried hydrocortisone ointment with no relief.
d. patient's identity	Sara Lansbury
e. age, sex, height, and weight	21 years old, female, 5 ft 6 in, 128 lb
f. patient's occupation	College student
g. patient's dietary habits	Patient is a vegetarian.
h. patient's sleep habits	Number of hours that patient sleeps each night varies.
i. concurrent medical conditions, prescription and non-prescription medications, and dietary supplements	Seasonal allergies: Claritin D in the spring and fall
j. allergies	Ragweed and maple trees
k. history of other adverse reactions to medications	None
l. other (describe) _____	Patient has a history of ringworm during swim season.
Assessment and Triage	
2. Differentiate patient's signs/symptoms and correctly identify the patient's primary problem(s) (Table 41–1).	Patient is suffering from inflammation, weeping, denudation, and intense itching on her face, secondary to ringworm.
3. Identify exclusions for self-treatment (Figure 41–1).[36]	Severe symptoms, eye involvement, eyebrow involvement
4. Formulate a comprehensive list of therapeutic alternatives for the primary problem to determine if triage to a medical provider is required, and share this information with the patient or caregiver.	Options include: (1) Refer patient to an appropriate health care provider. (2) Recommend self-care with a nonprescription antifungal and nondrug measures. (3) Recommend self-care until patient can see an appropriate health care provider. (4) Take no action.
Plan	
5. Select an optimal therapeutic alternative to address the patient's problem, taking into account patient preferences.	Patient should consult a health care provider.
6. Describe the recommended therapeutic approach to the patient or caregiver.	"You should consult a health care provider for treatment."
7. Explain to the patient or caregiver the rationale for selecting the recommended therapeutic approach from the considered therapeutic alternatives.	"This option is best because your problem is severe and is affecting skin near your eyes. You will need oral medication that is available only by prescription to treat your condition."

case
41-1 *continued*

Relevant Evaluation Criteria	Scenario/Model Outcome
Patient Education	
8. When recommending self-care with nonprescription medications and/or nondrug therapy, convey accurate information to the patient or caregiver.	Criterion does not apply in this case.
Solicit follow-up questions from the patient or caregiver.	"One of my teammates said that I should suffocate the ringworms by applying clear nail polish on the itchy spots. Does this really work?"
Answer the patient's or caregiver's questions.	"Ringworm is not actually caused by worms. It is caused by a fungus that lives in the superficial skin layers. Nail polish will have no effect on your symptoms. It can, however, cause severe irritation if you get it in your eyes."
Evaluation of Patient Outcome	
9. Assess patient outcome.	Contact the patient in a day or two to ensure that she made an appointment and sought medical care.

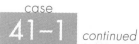

case
41-2

Relevant Evaluation Criteria	Scenario/Model Outcome
Information Gathering	
1. Gather essential information about the patient's symptoms and medical history, including:	
a. description of symptom(s) (i.e., nature, onset, duration, severity, associated symptoms)	The patient describes intense itching and a red, scaly rash on and between the third, fourth, and fifth toes of each foot. He says that the symptoms began a week ago, soon after he began his summer job at a lawn maintenance service.
b. description of any factors that seem to precipitate, exacerbate, and/or relieve the patient's symptom(s)	The patient says that the itching is worse after he gets home from work in the evening.
c. description of the patient's efforts to relieve the symptoms	The patient has not tried anything other than scratching the affected area when the itching becomes unbearable.
d. patient's identity	Robert Grees
e. age, sex, height, and weight	17 years old, male, 5 ft 11 in., 175 lb
f. patient's occupation	Lawn maintenance worker
g. patient's dietary habits	Eats fast food for breakfast and lunch.
h. patient's sleep habits	6–7 hours nightly
i. concurrent medical conditions, prescription and non-prescription medications, and dietary supplements	None
j. allergies	None
k. history of other adverse reactions to medications	None
l. other (describe) _____	NA
Assessment And Triage	
2. Differentiate patient's signs/symptoms and correctly identify the patient's primary problem(s) (Table 41-1).	Robert is suffering from a scaling red rash and itching secondary to athlete's foot. He likely contracted this problem from mowing lawns.
3. Identify exclusions for self-treatment (Figure 41-1).[36]	None

case
41-2 *continued*

Relevant Evaluation Criteria	Scenario/Model Outcome
4. Formulate a comprehensive list of therapeutic alternatives for the primary problem to determine if triage to a medical provider is required, and share this information with the patient or caregiver.	Options include: (1) Refer Robert to an appropriate health care provider. (2) Recommend self-care with a nonprescription antifungal and nondrug measures. (3) Recommend self-care until Robert can see an appropriate provider. (4) Take no action.

Plan

5. Select an optimal therapeutic alternative to address the patient's problem, taking into account patient preferences.	Robert should use a nonprescription antifungal and nondrug measures to treat his problem.
6. Describe the recommended therapeutic approach to the patient or caregiver.	"Regular use of any of the commercially available nonprescription antifungals in any dosage form except a spray or powder should alleviate the problem. However, for the medication to be optimally effective, you will have to take several measures to keep the affected area clean and dry."
7. Explain to the patient or caregiver the rationale for selecting the recommended therapeutic approach from the considered therapeutic alternatives.	"Athlete's foot can be effectively managed with nonprescription antifungals and nondrug measures (keeping the area clean and dry) as long as there is no evidence of secondary infection or preexisting medical conditions that would preclude self-treatment, as in your case. Sprays and powders are less effective because they often are not rubbed into the skin."

Patient Education

8. When recommending self-care with nonprescription medications and/or nondrug therapy, convey accurate information to the patient or caregiver:	
a. appropriate dose and frequency of administration	See the box Patient Education for Fungal Skin Infections.
b. maximum number of days the therapy should be employed	See the box Patient Education for Fungal Skin Infections.
c. product administration procedures	See the box Patient Education for Fungal Skin Infections.
d. expected time to onset of relief	"Itching may be relieved somewhat within a few days, but eradication of the causative microorganism may take up to 4 weeks."
e. degree of relief that can be reasonably expected	"Athlete's foot can be cured if you use the antifungal and nondrug measures properly."
f. most common side effects	See the box Patient Education for Fungal Skin Infections.
g. side effects that warrant medical intervention should they occur	See the box Patient Education for Fungal Skin Infections.
h. patient options in the event that condition worsens or persists	See the box Patient Education for Fungal Skin Infections.
i. product storage requirements	"Store in a cool, dry place out of children's reach."
j. specific nondrug measures	See the box Patient Education for Fungal Skin Infections.
Solicit follow-up questions from the patient or caregiver.	"Why do I have this? I am not an athlete."
Answer the patient's or caregiver's questions.	"Your feet are sweating more than usual now because you are working outside. As a result, the skin on your feet remains damp until you remove your shoes and socks after work. Moisture helps the fungus that causes ringworm to thrive."

Evaluation of Patient Outcome

9. Assess patient outcome.	Ask the patient to call to update you on his response to your recommendations. Or you could call him in a week to evaluate the outcome.

Key: NA = Not applicable.

The most common complaint of patients with a cutaneous fungal infection is pruritus. However, if fissures are present, particularly between the toes, painful burning and stinging may also occur. If the area is abraded, denuded, or inflamed, weeping or oozing may be present in addition to pain. Some patients may merely remark on the bothersome scaling of dry skin, particularly if the infection involves the soles of the feet. In other instances, small vesicular lesions may combine to form a larger bullous eruption marked by pain and irritation, or the only symptoms may be brittleness and discoloration of a hypertrophied nail.

The provider should seek to distinguish a tinea infection from diseases with similar symptoms, such as bacterial infection, irritant contact dermatitis, allergic contact dermatitis, and atopic dermatitis. For this reason, the manifestation of these disorders is briefly discussed here. In children, peridigital dermatitis or atopic dermatitis is more common than tinea pedis. Shoe dermatitis is perhaps the most common form of allergic contact dermatitis from clothing. Therefore, the provider should inquire about the type of footwear worn by the patient and about recent footwear changes. Since 1950, the increased use of rubber and adhesives in footwear has paralleled the increase in reports of shoe dermatitis in the dermatologic and podiatric literature. Contact allergy to accelerators (the chemical compounds used to speed the processing of rubber used in sponge-rubber insoles for tennis shoes) has also been reported.[35] In addition to accelerators, antioxidants have been implicated as major chemical allergens, and various phenolic resins used in adhesives are also troublesome. The patient is usually unaware that his or her footwear may be causing the problem.

Hyperhidrosis of interdigital spaces and of the sole of the foot is common, as is infection of the toe webs by gram-negative bacteria. In hyperhidrosis, tender vesicles cover the sole of the foot and toes, and these areas may be quite painful. The skin generally turns white, erodes, and becomes macerated. This condition is accompanied by a foul foot odor. A soggy wetness of the toe webs and the immediately adjacent skin characterizes infection by gram-negative bacteria; the affected tissue is damp and softened. The last toe web (adjacent to the little toe) is the most common area of primary or initial involvement because it is deeper and extends more proximally than the web between the other toes. Furthermore, abundant exocrine sweat glands, a semiocclusive anatomic setting, and the added occlusion provided by footwear enhance development of the disease at this site. The provider must be careful not to confuse this condition with soft corns, which also appear between the fourth and fifth toes.

Patient Counseling for Fungal Skin Infections

The proper application technique for topical antifungals and required duration of therapy should be described to the patient to prevent over- or undermedication. The patient should be told to apply the medication regularly throughout a complete course of therapy. Information that will help to control or eradicate the infection and that will minimize the likelihood of recurrent infections may also be provided. This information should address proper care of the infected skin site, appropriate laundry techniques and products, minimal use of occlusive clothing, and avoidance of habits or behavior that may lead to recurring infections. The patient should also be told which conditions indicate the need to consult a primary care provider (e.g., the development of a secondary bacterial infection). The box Patient Education for Fungal Skin Infections lists specific information to provide patients.

---

patient education for
Fungal Skin Infections

The objectives of self-treatment are to (1) relieve itching, burning, and other discomfort; (2) inhibit the growth of fungi and cure the disorder; and (3) prevent recurrent infections. For most patients, carefully following product instructions and the self-care measures listed here will help ensure optimal therapeutic outcomes.

Nondrug Measures

- To prevent spreading the infection to other parts of the body, either use a separate towel to dry the affected area or dry the affected area last.
- Do not share towels, clothing, or other personal articles with household members, especially when an infection is present.
- Launder contaminated towels and clothing in hot water, and dry them on a hot dryer setting to prevent spreading the infection.
- Cleanse skin daily with soap and water, and thoroughly pat dry to remove oils and other substances that promote growth of fungi.
- If possible, do not wear clothing or shoes that cause the skin to stay wet. Wool and synthetic fabrics prevent optimal air circulation.
- If needed, allow shoes to dry thoroughly before wearing them again. Dust shoes with medicated or nonmedicated foot powder to help keep them dry.
- If needed, place odor-controlling insoles in casual or athletic shoes. These insoles also provide some support and cushioning for the feet. Change insoles routinely every 3–4 months or more often if their condition warrants. Take care that the shoe fit is not compromised by the insoles.
- As with all topical medications, discontinue the use of an antifungal if irritation, sensitization, or worsening of the skin condition occurs.

- Avoid contact with people who have fungal infections. Wear protective footwear (e.g., rubber or wooden sandals) in areas of family or public use, such as home bathrooms or community showers.

Nonprescription Medications

- Ask a health care provider for assistance in picking the appropriate antifungal agent and dosage form for your infection.
- Available agents include butenafine, clotrimazole, miconazole nitrate, terbinafine, and tolnaftate.
- It usually takes 2–4 weeks to cure tinea infections. Some cases may require 4–6 weeks of treatment.
- Apply the antifungal to the clean, dry affected area as directed (in the morning or evening if once daily, or both times if twice daily). Massage the medication into the area. Note that creams and solutions are easier to work into the skin; therefore, they are probably more effective treatment forms.
- Avoid getting the product in your eyes.
- Wash hands thoroughly with soap and water before and after applying the product.
- Topical antifungals themselves may cause itching, redness, and irritation.
- Tolnaftate may sting slightly upon application.

- When the medication is to be applied to pressure areas of the foot, where the horny skin layer is thicker, apply a keratolytic agent (e.g., Whitfield's ointment) to the affected area first to help the antifungal penetrate the skin.
- If oozing lesions are present, apply aluminum acetate solution (1:40) to the area before applying the antifungal:
  - Soak the area in an aluminum acetate solution for 20 minutes up to 3 times a day (every 6–8 hours), or apply the solution to the affected area in the form of a wet dressing.
  - Note that aluminum acetate solution (Burow's solution) or modified Burow's solution is available for immediate use as a solution or as forms to be dissolved in water (powder packets, powder, and effervescent tablets).
  - Avoid getting the product in your eyes.

- To avoid skin damage, use the solution for no more than 1 week. Discontinue use of the solution if inflammatory lesions appear or worsen.
- For the wet, soggy type of athlete's foot, apply to or soak foot in aluminum acetate solution (1:40) before applying the antifungal:
  - Soak feet with aluminum acetate solution (1:40) twice daily until the odor, wetness, and whiteness are gone. After that, soak once daily to control the symptoms.
  - If deep fissures are present in the skin, use a more dilute solution of aluminum acetate for initial treatment.

When to Seek Medical Attention

- Discontinue use of the product and contact a primary care provider if itching or swelling occurs, or if the infection worsens.
- Consult a primary care provider if the infection worsens or persists beyond the recommended length of therapy.

Evaluation of Patient Outcomes for Fungal Skin Infections

In general, the patient should begin to see some relief of the itching, scaling, and/or inflammation within 1 week. If the disorder shows improvement within this time frame, continuing treatment for 1–3 weeks (depending on the type of tinea infection and medication being used) should be recommended. If the disorder has not improved or has worsened, referring the patient to a primary care provider for more aggressive therapy is appropriate. Recurrent skin infections may be a sign of undiagnosed diabetes, immunodeficiency, or another organic problem that requires medical evaluation.

Key Points for Fungal Skin Infections

➤ Tinea corporis, tinea cruris, and tinea pedis can be treated with nonprescription drugs. Clotrimazole, miconazole nitrate, terbinafine hydrochloride, butenafine hydrochloride, tolnaftate, and undecylenic acid and its derivatives are efficacious for this purpose.

➤ The effectiveness of topical antifungals will be limited unless the patient eliminates other predisposing factors to tinea infections.

➤ These drugs are effective in all their delivery vehicles, but the powder forms should be reserved only for extremely mild conditions or as adjunctive therapy.

➤ Because solutions and creams can spread beyond the affected area, they should be used sparingly.

➤ When recommended for suspected or actual dermatophytosis, these topical antifungals should be used twice daily (morning and night). Treatment should be continued for 2–4 weeks, depending on the symptoms. After that time, the patient and/or provider should evaluate the effectiveness of the therapy.

➤ To minimize nonadherence, the provider should advise patients that alleviation of symptoms will not occur overnight. Patients should also be cautioned that frequent recurrence of any of these problems is an indication that they should consult a primary care provider.

➤ Immunocompromised patients and those with diabetes or circulatory problems should be treated by a primary care provider.

REFERENCES

1. Hay RJ, Roberts SOB, MacKenzie DWR. In: Campion RH, Burton JL, Ebling FJG, eds. *Textbook of Dermatology.* 6th ed. Oxford, UK: Blackwell Scientific Publications; 1999:1127–216.
2. Freeberg IM, Eisen AZ, Wolff K, et al., eds. *Dermatology in General Medicine.* 5th ed. New York, NY: McGraw-Hill; 1999.
3. *Federal Register.* 1993;58:49890–9.
4. Drake LA, Dinehart SM, Farmer ER, et al. Guidelines for care of superficial mycotic infections of the skin: tinea corporis, tinea cruris, tinea faciei, tinea manuum and tinea pedis. *J Am Acad Dermatol.* 1996;34(2 pt 1):282–6.
5. Fitzpatrick TB, Eisen AZ, Wolf K, et al., eds. *Dermatology in General Medicine.* 7th ed. New York, NY: McGraw-Hill; 2007.
6. Lesher J, Levine N, Treadwill P. Fungal skin infections. *Patient Care.* 1994;28:16–44.
7. Shrum JP, Millikan LE, Bataineh O. Superficial fungal infections in the tropics. *Dermatol Clin.* 1994;12(4):687–93.
8. Bergus GR, Johnson JS. Superficial tinea infections. *Am Fam Physician.* 1993;48(2):259.
9. Evans EG. Tinea pedis: clinical experience and efficacy of short treatment. *Dermatology.* 1997;194(suppl 1):3–6.
10. Aly R. Ecology and epidemiology of dermatophyte infections. *J Am Acad Dermatol.* 1994;31(3 pt 2):S21.
11. Auger P, Marquis G, Joly J, et al. Epidemiology of tinea pedis in marathon runners: prevalence of occult athlete's foot. *Mycoses.* 1993;36(1–2):35–43.
12. Griffin LY. Common sports injuries of the foot and ankle seen in children and adolescents. *Orthop Clin North Am.* 1994;25(1):83–93.
13. Szepietowski JC, Reich A, Carlowska E, et al. Factors influencing coexistence of toenail onychomycosis with tinea pedis and other dermatomycoses. *Arch Dermatol.* 2006;142(10):1279–84.
14. What causes athlete's foot? *Mayo Clin Women's Healthsource.* 2009;13(12):8.
15. Odom R. Pathophysiology of dermatophyte infections. *J Am Acad Dermatol.* 1993;28(5 pt 1):S2–7.
16. Pray SW. *Nonprescription Product Therapeutics.* 2nd ed. Philadelphia, PA: Lippincott Williams & Wilkins; 2006:591.
17. Dahl MV. Dermatophytosis and the immune response. *J Am Acad Dermatol.* 1994;31(3 pt 2):S34–41.
18. Pray, SW. Recognizing and eradicating tinea pedis (athlete's foot). *US Pharm.* 2010;35(8):10–5.
19. Weinstein A, Berman B. Topical treatment of common superficial tinea infections. *Am Fam Physician.* 2002;65(10):2095–102.
20. Elewski BE, Silverman RA. Clinical pearl: diagnostic procedures for tinea capitis. *J Am Acad Dermatol.* 1996;34(3):498–9.

21. Drake LA, Dinehart SM, Farmer ER, et al. Guidelines for care of superficial mycotic infections of the skin: tinea capitis and tinea barbae. *J Am Acad Dermatol*. 1996;34(2 pt 1):290.

22. *Federal Register*. 1982;47:12480–566.

23. Savin RC. Treatment of chronic tinea pedis (athlete's foot type) with topical terbinafine. *J Am Acad Dermatol*. 1990;23(4 pt 2):786–9.

24. Savin RC, Zaias N. Treatment of chronic moccasin-type tinea pedis with terbinafine: a double-blind, placebo-controlled trial. *J Am Acad Dermatol*. 1990;23(4 pt 2):804–7.

25. Center for Drug Evaluation and Research. Approval package for: application number: 020663, trade name: MENTAX CREAM 1%, generic name: butenafine HCl cream; sponsor: Penederm, Inc.; approval date: December 31, 1996. Accessed at http://www.accessdata.fda.gov/drugsatfda_docs/label/2001/20524s5lbl.pdf, May 13, 2013.

26. Gupta AK, Einarson TR, Summerbell RC, et al. An overview of topical antifungal therapy in dermatomycoses: a North American perspective. *Drugs*. 1998;55(5);645–74.

27. Ramadan W, Ibrahim S, Sonbol F. Oil of bitter orange: new topical antifungal agent. *Int J Dermatol*. 1996;35(6):448–9.

28. Tong MM, Altman PM, Barneston RS. Tea tree oil in the treatment of tinea pedis. *Australas J Dermatol*. 1992;33(3):145–9.

29. Buck, DS, Nidor DM, Addino JD. Comparison of two topical preparations for the treatment of onychomycosis: Melaleuca alternifolia (tea tree) oil and clotrimazole. *J Fam Pract*. 1994:38(6):601–5.

30. Syed TA, Qureshi ZA, Ali SM, et al. Treatment of toenail onychomycosis with 2% butenafine and 5% Melaleuca alternifolia (tea tree) oil in cream. *Trop Med Int Health*. 1999:4(4):284–7.

31. Ledezma E, Lopez JC, Marin P, et al. Ajoene in the topical short term treatment of tinea cruris and tinea corporis in humans. Randomized comparative study with terbinafine. *Arzneimittelforschung*. 1999: 49(6):554–7.

32. Ledezma E, DeSousa L, Jorquera A, et al. Efficacy of ajoene, an organosulphur derived from garlic, in the short-term efficacy of tinea pedis. *Mycoses*. 1996:39(9–10);393–5.

33. Ledezma E, Marcano K, Jorquera A, et al. Efficacy of ajoene in the treatment of tinea pedis: a double-blind comparative study with terbinafine. *J Am Acad Dermatol*. 2000;43(5 pt 1):829–32.

34. Bruinsma W, ed. *A Guide to Drug Eruptions*. 6th ed. Amsterdam, The Netherlands: Free University Press; 1995.

35. Jung JH, McLaughlin JL, Stannard J, et al. Isolation, via activity-directed fractionation, of mercaptobenzothiazole and dibenzothiazyl disulfide as 2 allergens responsible for tennis shoe dermatitis. *Contact Dermat*. 1988;19:254–9.

36. U.S. Food and Drug Administration. Topical anti-microbial drug products for over-the-counter-human use. CFR: Code of Federal Regulations. Title 21, Part 333, Section 333.150. Accessed at http://www.gpo.gov/fdsys/pkg/CFR-2001-title21-vol5/xml/CFR-2001-title21-vol5-part333.xml, May 14, 3013.

WARTS

Donna M. Adkins

W arts, or verrucae, are a common skin disorder caused by human papillomaviruses (HPVs).[1–12] Approximately 7%–10% of the general population has warts. This percentage does not include nongenital warts.[1] Approximately 70% of warts are common warts.[2–4] Warts occur more frequently in children and adolescents than in infants and adults, with the peak incidence among 12- to 16-year-olds.[1,2,5] Warts are a benign condition and often go away without treatment. Approximately 23% of warts regress within 2 months, 30% within 3 months, and 65%–78% within 2 years.[1,6,11] This chapter discusses treatments for common and plantar warts that are found on areas of the body and are amenable to self-treatment.

High-quality, consistent data on warts are limited. Several risk factors exist for the development of warts, such as having previous or existing warts; having a depressed immune system; going barefoot, especially on wet surfaces; using swimming pools and public showers; working in a meat handling occupation; and biting one's fingernails.[1–3,5]

HPV infection occurs via person-to-person contact, auto-inoculation, or fomites found on contaminated surfaces.[1,3,7] When minor skin abrasions are present, HPV may enter the epidermal layer and infect the basal keratinocytes.[1] HPV infection is limited to the epidermal tissues and does not spread systemically.[11] Although different types of HPV are not found exclusively in specific areas of the body, different types do preferentially infect nonkeratinized mucous membranes rather than keratinized stratified squamous epithelium.[1] The incubation period may be long (i.e., 8 months).[2] The manifestation of warts may depend on the immune response of the infected individual. How quickly warts are cleared is influenced by factors such as viral type, patient immune status, and the extent and duration of time the warts have been present.[1]

Pathophysiology of Warts

HPVs are double-stranded DNA viruses.[1–6,8] More than 150 related viruses and more than 200 subgroups have been identified through DNA sequencing.[2] Warts may affect skin and mucous membranes anywhere on the body.[9] Specific HPV types cause warts in specific areas of the body.[4] HPV-2, HPV-4,

HPV-27, and HPV-57 are the most common cause of warts on the hands. HPV-1 is the most common cause of warts on the feet.[7,12]

Clinical Presentation

The appearance, size, shape, and response to treatment of individual warts vary by HPV type and the specific location of the warts on the body.[1,3,9] Table 42–1 describes the categories of warts.

Common warts are skin-colored or brown, hyperkeratotic, dome-shaped papules with a rough cauliflower-like appearance; they frequently occur on the hands.[1,2] Common warts are often painless.[2] Plantar warts are skin-colored callous-like lesions that occur on the feet.[2] Because of their deeply penetrating sloping sides and central depressions, plantar warts may be painful, especially if they occur in a weight-bearing location.[1] When tightly clustered, multiple plantar warts may appear as one large wart. In this presentation, the warts are called a mosaic wart.[1,2]

Plantar warts can be confused with corns or calluses.[1] If there is any question about whether the lesion is a wart, the patient should be referred to a medical provider for evaluation and treatment. To distinguish plantar warts from calluses, the provide may remove the outer keratinous layer of the lesion. When the surface layer is removed, the warts exhibit pinpoint bleeding, which resembles small black seeds. The bleeding is from thrombosed capillaries in the warts.[1]

Plantar warts can also be confused with malignant growths.[6] The latter are usually very painful and discolored, and they bleed and grow quickly.[7] Patients with lesions displaying these characteristics should be referred for medical evaluation and treatment.

Treatment of Warts

No single regimen is universally effective in the treatment of warts.[1,4,9] Although several treatment options are available for relief of symptoms associated with warts and for their removal, none cure the HPV infection.[1,4,9] Limited high-quality evidence exists for the efficacy of most wart treatments, and a placebo effect cannot be ruled out.[1,4,7]

Because many warts will resolve without treatment, one treatment option is a wait-and-see approach. However, many patients seek treatment because of the pain, cosmetic appearance,

Editor's Note: This chapter is based on the 17th edition chapter of the same title, written by Nicholas G. Popovich and Gail D. Newton.

table

42–1   Types of Nongenital Warts

Type	Common Location	Commonly Occurs in	Characteristics
Common (verruca vulgaris)	Hands	Children and adolescents	Skin colored or brown, dome-shaped, hyperkeratotic papules with a rough surface
Flat (verruca plana)	Face	Children	Smooth, flat topped, yellow-brown papules; common in children but rare in adults
Plantar (verruca vulgaris)	Feet	Adolescents and young adults	Skin-colored, flat, callous-like papules on the feet
Mosaic	Feet	Adolescents and young adults	Multiple, closely grouped plantar warts
Periungual	Nails	Persons who bite their nails	Thickened, fissured, cauliflower-like skin around the nail plate
Filiform	Face		Rapidly growing, thread-like projections

Source: References 1, 2, 5, and 9.

and social stigma associated with warts or because of concern about transmitting warts to others. The decision to treat a wart is based on the patient's desire for treatment; the presence of pain or bleeding, disabling/disfiguring lesions, or large or multiple lesions; the desire to prevent transmission of the warts; and the presence of an immunocompromising condition.[4,8] Warts often recur after treatment. Some warts, especially recurrent or recalcitrant warts, will require a combination of treatments.[1]

Treatment Goals

The goals for the treatment of warts are to (1) eliminate signs and symptoms associated with the warts, (2) remove the wart without scarring, (3) prevent recurrence of the warts, and (4) prevent spread of HPV through autoinoculation of one's self or transmission to others.[8]

General Treatment Approach

Determining the optimal treatment for a patient with warts depends on a number of factors, including the patient's age; the type, number, size, location, and duration of the lesions; the patient's immune status; the cost of therapy; access to therapies; side effects; and treatment preference.[1,4]

Although approximately 70% of warts will resolve after 2 years, even without treatment, only 46% of affected individuals will remain wart free.[6] Warts are less likely to resolve spontaneously in adults, immunocompromised patients, and patients with persistent warts.[1] A wait-and-see approach allows the continued spread of warts through autoinoculation and transmission to others.[4,6,7] Patient education regarding the cause of warts and ways to prevent their transmission to others is a key part of the treatment plan for any patient with warts.

Figure 42–1 outlines the treatment of warts and lists exclusions for self-treatment. A medical provider should evaluate patients with multiple warts, warts in any area other than the hands and feet, large warts, and/or painful warts to determine whether the warts may be caused by a more serious condition. Patients with poor circulation or decreased sensitivity (e.g., patients with diabetes mellitus or peripheral vascular disease) should not self-treat warts because of the potential for injury.

Nonpharmacologic Therapy

Nonpharmacologic therapies focus mainly on preventing the spread of the HPV virus. To prevent spreading warts through autoinoculation, patients should be instructed to avoid cutting, shaving or picking at warts; to wash hands before and after treating or touching warts; to keep feet clean and dry; to use a designated towel to dry warts; and to avoid using the designated towel to dry other body areas. To prevent transmission of the virus to others, patients should be instructed to avoid sharing towels, razors, socks, shoes, and so; to keep the wart covered; and to not walk barefoot, especially in bathrooms or in public places.

Pharmacologic Therapy
Salicylic acid

Salicyclic acid is a keratolytic agent available in three different formulations for use in self-treatment of common and plantar warts: salicylic acid 12%–40% in a plaster vehicle, salicylic acid 17% in a collodion vehicle, and salicylic acid 15% in a karaya gum glycol plaster vehicle.[2,13] Table 42–2 lists selected products that contain salicyclic acid products. Salicylic acid concentrations of 17% or less are generally used for common warts, and higher concentrations (i.e., 40%) are used for plantar warts.[9]

Salicyclic acid slowly destroys the virus-infected cells. It may also induce an immune response secondary to mild irritation.[1,3–5,9] The Food and Drug Administration (FDA) recommends that use of salicylic acid for self-treatment of warts be restricted to common and plantar warts.[13] Self-treatment is not recommended for other types of warts because of the difficulty in accurately recognizing and treating warts without medical oversight. A medical provider should evaluate patients with painful plantar warts and lesions that are not easily recognizable as common or plantar warts.

The advantages of topical nonprescription products that contain salicylic acid include low cost, ease of access, few adverse effects if used as directed, and a reasonable effectiveness.[1,3,5] Compared with placebo, salicyclic acid is more effective in treating warts at all locations but may be more effective for warts on the hands than those on the feet.[5] Disadvantages include the need for consistent, frequent application; the potential for damage to healthy skin surrounding the wart; and the duration of treatment

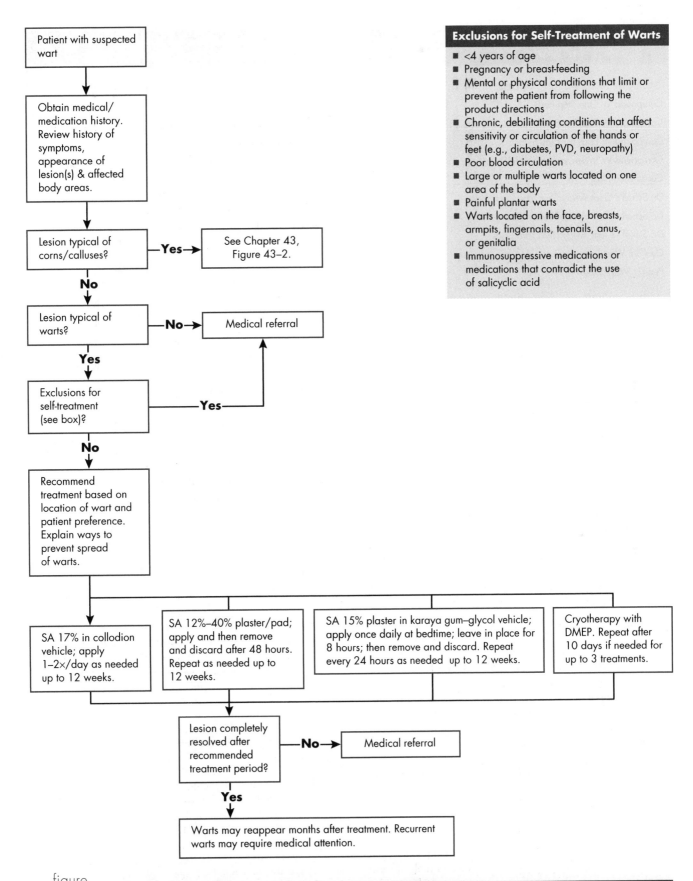

Exclusions for Self-Treatment of Warts

- <4 years of age
- Pregnancy or breast-feeding
- Mental or physical conditions that limit or prevent the patient from following the product directions
- Chronic, debilitating conditions that affect sensitivity or circulation of the hands or feet (e.g., diabetes, PVD, neuropathy)
- Poor blood circulation
- Large or multiple warts located on one area of the body
- Painful plantar warts
- Warts located on the face, breasts, armpits, fingernails, toenails, anus, or genitalia
- Immunosuppressive medications or medications that contradict the use of salicyclic acid

Patient with suspected wart

Obtain medical/medication history. Review history of symptoms, appearance of lesion(s) & affected body areas.

Lesion typical of corns/calluses? — **Yes**→ See Chapter 43, Figure 43–2.

No

Lesion typical of warts? — **No**→ Medical referral

Yes

Exclusions for self-treatment (see box)? — **Yes**→

No

Recommend treatment based on location of wart and patient preference. Explain ways to prevent spread of warts.

SA 17% in collodion vehicle; apply 1–2×/day as needed up to 12 weeks.

SA 12%–40% plaster/pad; apply and then remove and discard after 48 hours. Repeat as needed up to 12 weeks.

SA 15% plaster in karaya gum–glycol vehicle; apply once daily at bedtime; leave in place for 8 hours; then remove and discard. Repeat every 24 hours as needed up to 12 weeks.

Cryotherapy with DMEP. Repeat after 10 days if needed for up to 3 treatments.

Lesion completely resolved after recommended treatment period? — **No**→ Medical referral

Yes

Warts may reappear months after treatment. Recurrent warts may require medical attention.

figure

42–1 Self-care of warts. Key: DMEP = Dimethyl ether and propane; PVD = peripheral vascular disease; SA = salicylic acid.

table

42–2 Selected Self-Care Products for Warts

Salicylic Acid 40% Products

Compound W One Step Pads

Compound W Pads for Feet

Compound W Pads for Kids

Compound W Waterproof Invisible Strips

Curad Mediplast Pads

Dr. Scholl's Clear Away One Step Clear Strips

Dr. Scholl's Clear Away Plantar Discs

Dr. Scholl's Clear Away Ultra Thin Discs

DuoFilm Wart Remover Patch for Kids

PediFix Wart Stick

Salicylic Acid 17% Products

Compound W Fast Acting Gel

Compound W Fast Acting Liquid

Dr. Scholl's Clear Away Fast Acting Liquid

DuoFilm Wart Remover Liquid

Salicylic Acid 15% Products

Trans-Ver-Sal 12 MM Adult Patch

Trans-Ver-Sal 20 MM Adult Patch

Cryotherapy Products (dimethyl ether; propane)

Dr. Scholl's Freeze Away Wart Remover

Kids Wartner Wart Removal System

Wartner Plantar Wart Removal System

Wartner Wart Removal System

Cryotherapy Products (dimethyl ether; propane; isobutene)

Compound W Freeze Off Wart Removal System

table

42–3 Guidelines for Treating Warts with Selected Salicylic Acid Products

Salicyclic Acid 40% Plasters/Pads/Strips[14]

- Wash the affected area.
- May soak the affected area for 5 minutes in warm water.
- Dry the affected area thoroughly.
- Apply disc of appropriate size to wart and cover with pad. Or trim a plaster to fit the wart, apply plaster, and cover with an occlusive tape.
- Remove plasters/pads/strips after 48 hours.
- Repeat procedure every 48 hours as needed until the wart is removed. These products may be used for up to 12 weeks.

Salicyclic Acid 17% Liquid in Collodion Vehicle[15]

- Wash the affected area.
- May soak the affected area for 5 minutes in warm water.
- Dry the affected area thoroughly.
- Apply one drop at a time to cover the wart. Protect adjacent healthy skin from coming into contact with the drug.
- Let solution dry completely.
- Cover wart with self-adhesive cover-up discs or an occlusive tape.
- Repeat procedure 1–2 times a day until the wart is removed. This product may be used for up to 12 weeks.

Salicyclic Acid 15% Patch in Karaya Gum Vehicle[16]

- Wash the affected area.
- Dry the affected area thoroughly.
- Use a file to gently remove the keratinous surface.
- Trim patch to fit wart.
- Apply a drop of warm water to the wart.
- Apply patch at bedtime and allow patch to remain on wart for at least 8 hours.
- Cover patch with occlusive tape.
- Remove patch after at least 8 hours.
- Repeat daily until the wart is removed. This product may be used up to 12 weeks.

needed to see a therapeutic response.[1,3,5,9] Side effects include skin irritation and the potential for systemic toxicity.[1,3,9]

In most instances, warts will begin to improve within a couple of weeks of treatment with salicylic acid. Self-treatment of common and plantar warts should not continue past 12 weeks. A medical provider should evaluate patients who have warts that do not completely resolve after 12 weeks.

Table 42–3 provides guidelines for using salicylic acid products.[14–16]

Cryotherapy

Health care providers have used cryotherapy with liquid nitrogen and other agents for many years to treat warts in their offices.[6] Cryotherapy destroys the wart by freezing the wart tissue.[6,9] Liquid nitrogen can freeze tissue to temperatures around $-196°C$.[3,7] As temperatures fall to -5 to$-15°C$, extracellular ice crystals form.[6] At $-40°C$ and below, intracellular ice crystals form.[6] As tissue freezes, microthrombi form, leading to ischemic necrosis and destruction of the HPV-infected keratinocytes.[6] The freezing also causes local inflammation that may clear the wart through a cell-mediated response.[1,4]

FDA has approved a mixture of dimethyl ether and propane for the self-treatment of common and plantar warts. Compared with liquid nitrogen used in physician's offices, nonprescription products containing dimethyl ether reach only temperatures around $-70°C$.[1,3]

Nonprescription cryotherapy products have similar, but product-specific, directions for preparing the applicator. Table 42–4 provides guidelines for using cryotherapy products and illustrates the procedural differences between two selected nonprescription cryotherapy products.[17–19] The cryotherapy is applied directly to the wart. Patients must follow the directions carefully to avoid

table

42–4 **Guidelines for Treating Warts with Selected Cryotherapy Products**

General Guidelines

- Wash hands before and after use.
- Soak the wart in warm water for 5 minutes; then use a file or pumice stone to remove the keratinous surface.
- Do not hold the canister close to your face, body, or clothing.
- Discard the foam applicator after a single use.
- Repeat after 14 days, if needed.
- Do not use product if:
  - You cannot follow the instructions exactly as written.
  - You are not sure if the condition is a wart.
  - The wart is on children younger than 4 years.
  - You are pregnant or breast-feeding.
  - You have diabetes or poor circulation.
  - The wart is on thin, sensitive, or irritated skin such as the face, breasts, genitals, or arm pits.

Compound W Freeze Off[17,18]

- Keep the protective cap on the canister. Hold the Compound W Freeze Off applicator by the plastic stick. Attach the applicator to the canister by firmly inserting the applicator stick into the opening.
- Place the canister on a sturdy surface.
- Remove the protective cap from the canister. Keeping the can upright, press the dispensing valve all the way down for 3–5 seconds to saturate the applicator. Release your finger from the dispensing valve when droplets start to fall from the applicator tip.
- Turn the canister so that the applicator is pointing straight down and wait 15 seconds.
- Position the wart so that it faces upward.
- While keeping the applicator pointing straight down, lightly place the tip of the applicator on the center of the wart. Do not press the valve while the applicator is in contact with the skin. The applicator should be applied to the skin for no more than 40 seconds. Do not dab applicator onto the wart.
- Replace the protective cap after use.
- This product may be used for up to 3 treatments.

Wartner Wart Removal System[17,19]

- Holding the end of the foam applicator between the thumb and index finger, squeeze until a small opening appears.
- Slide the opening of the foam applicator over the stick of the holder until the stick is no longer visible. You will find the holder in the bag containing the foam applicators.
- Insert the holder with the applicator in the opening on the top of the cap so that the foam applicator is no longer visible.
- Place the aerosol spray can on a sturdy surface.
- Holding the can firmly at the bottom, press down the valve for 2–3 seconds.
- Leave the foam applicator on the holder and wait 20 seconds.
- Lightly place the tip of the foam applicator to the wart.
  - Apply 20 seconds for common warts.
  - Apply 40 seconds for plantar warts.
- This product may be used for up to four treatments.

damaging the healthy skin surrounding the wart. A blister will form under the wart and, after about 10 days, the wart will fall off. Applicators must not be used more than once to avoid reinfecting the tissue or spreading the virus to others.

With regard to evaluating the effectiveness of cryotherapy in the treatment of both common and plantar warts, cryotherapy is no more effective than salicyclic acid or placebo.[3,5,9] One study found that cryotherapy may be more effective than salicyclic acid for warts on the hands but not on the feet.[20]

The use of two freeze–thaw cycles during a treatment may improve the clearance of plantar warts, but this approach has not been shown to improve clearance of common warts on the hands.[1,3,11] Aggressive cryotherapy treatments are more effective (52%) than gentle treatments (31%) but have an increased incidence of adverse effects.[1,3,5,9] Treating the wart every 2–3 weeks with cryotherapy yields the best results.[5,11]

The advantages of nonprescription cryotherapy products include their easy access and lower cost, compared with the liquid nitrogen used in the physician's office, and one treatment may be sufficient to clear the wart. Disadvantages of cryotherapy include pain and the potential for damage to healthy skin surrounding the wart, and self-treatments may not be as effective as the liquid nitrogen used in the physician's office. Potential adverse effects include blistering, scarring, hypo- or hyperpigmentation, and tendon damage or nerve damage with aggressive therapy.[1,3 9]

In most instances, warts will resolve after one treatment with cryotherapy. Self-treatment of common and plantar warts may be repeated every 2–3 weeks. Treatments should not continue beyond 3 months or a maximum of four treatments. If this regimen does not completely resolve the wart, the patient should be referred to a medical provider for evaluation and treatment.

Other Pharmacologic Therapies

Numerous prescription products, laser treatments, immunotherapies, and combinations of treatments are used to treat warts. Discussion of prescription products and procedures is outside the scope of this chapter. Limited or inconsistent data exist for the effectiveness of using products other than salicyclic acid and cryotherapy for self-treatment of common and plantar warts.

Complementary Therapies
Folklore

Some of the numerous folk remedies for warts include the following: "Rub dry toast on a wart then bury it at night by the full moon and by the next full moon it will be gone," and, as described in the Foxfire 40th Anniversary Book, "Take a knife, and on the wart make a cross over the top. It works with the sap of the trees."[21] Folk remedies such as these are often based on anecdotal successes and highlight the probability that many warts resolve spontaneously without treatment.[1]

Vitamin A

Retinoids such as vitamin A regulate epithelial cell differentiation and keratin expression. Vitamin A may interfere with HPV replication. One case report of a 30-year-old woman found vitamin A to be effective in clearing recalcitrant warts. The woman's warts had been present for a 9-year period despite various treatments. The treatment required 6 months to clear the largest wart. The report noted that untreated warts on the opposite hand cleared without application of vitamin A, which may illustrate either a placebo effect or an unknown mechanism of action.[12]

Dietary Zinc

Deficiencies of zinc lead to decreased immunity.[1,10] Dietary zinc is postulated to improve immune response and inhibit HPV replication.[10] One placebo-controlled trial evaluated 10 mg/kg/day of zinc to treat recalcitrant warts. Complete clearance was reported in 87% of the treatment group versus no clearance in the placebo group.[1,10]

Garlic (*Allium sativum*)

Garlic is thought to inhibit cellular proliferation of virus-infected cells.[1,22] One placebo-controlled trial reported that application of chloroform extracts of garlic resulted in complete resolution of warts for all 23 patients after 1–2 weeks, with no recurrence after 3–4 months.[1,22]

Essential Oils

Essential oils contain a combination of oils with antiviral properties. One case report[23] of a woman with ovarian cancer found essential oils to be effective in clearing recalcitrant warts. Essential oils were applied directly on the wart; then a salicylic acid plaster (40%) followed by an adhesive bandage was used to cover the wart. The woman's warts cleared after 17 days of treatment with essential oils and salicylic acid and did not return. It is difficult to determine whether the essential oils contributed to the effectiveness of the salicylic acid.

Occlusion with Duct Tape

Duct tape has become a popular, inexpensive treatment for warts.[1] The mechanism by which duct tape clears warts is still unclear, but local irritation may cause stimulation of the patient's immune response.[5]

One randomized controlled study[24] compared duct tape occlusion with cryotherapy for the treatment of common warts. In one treatment group, liquid nitrogen was applied to warts every 2–3 weeks, for a maximum of six treatments or until the warts resolved. In the other treatment group, duct tape was applied to the wart, left in place for 6 days, removed in the evening of the sixth day, and replaced with a new piece of duct tape the next morning; this procedure was repeated for up to 2 months or until the wart resolved. The treated warts were completely resolved in 84.6% of the patients in the duct tape group and 60% of the patients in the cryotherapy group.[1,5]

Another randomized controlled trial[25] yielded conflicting results. This trial compared occlusion of warts with either duct tape or moleskin. In each group the wart was shaved and the pad applied for 1 week. The wart was then debrided with an emery board, and the pad was reapplied for an additional week. This procedure was repeated for up to 2 months or until the wart resolved. Six months later, patients were asked if the wart had recurred. The treatment groups demonstrated no difference in resolution or recurrence of the warts.[5,25]

More evidence on the effectiveness of therapy with duct tape is needed. Duct tape may have a place in therapy for small children with warts or in combination with other treatments.[1]

Assessment of Warts: A Case Based Approach

When a patient presents with a wart-like lesion, the provider should gather information from multiple sources to determine whether the lesion is suitable for self-treatment and whether available treatments are appropriate for that individual. Before a treatment plan is recommended, the provider should inspect the wart to accurately identify the lesion as a wart and to determine whether self-treatment is appropriate. The provider should question the patient about medication use and the existence of medical conditions that would preclude self-treatment. The patient should also be asked about previous attempts to treat the lesion and whether those attempts were successful. Patient preferences for type of treatment may be used to help guide product selection. Table 42–5 compares characteristics of warts, corns, calluses, and malignant growths. Cases 42–1 and 42–2 illustrate the assessment of patients with warts.

table
42–5   Differentiation of Warts and Skin Disorders with Similar Presentation

Criterion	Warts	Corns	Calluses	Malignant Growth
Location	Any area of skin susceptible to the virus	Over bony prominences in the feet	Weight-bearing areas of the feet	Any area of the skin
Signs	Rough cauliflower-like appearance; plantar warts disrupt normal skin ridges	Raised, sharply demarcated, hyperkeratotic lesions with a central core	Raised, yellowish thickening of the skin; broad based with diffuse borders; normal pattern of skin ridges	Bleeding; swelling; red, discolored, or multicolored and swollen
Symptoms	Usually not painful but pain may occur if the wart is located in areas undergoing repeated pressure (i.e., soles of the feet)	Pain	Pain	Pain
Quantity/severity	Varies; may grow to approximately 1 inch in diameter	Varies; a few millimeters to 1 cm	Varies; a few millimeters to several centimeters	Varies; grows rapidly
Timing	Incubation period may be several months in length; may progressively enlarge	Variable onset; may progressively enlarge	Variable onset; may progressively enlarge	Variable onset; grows rapidly
Cause	HPV infection of the epidermal layer	Friction	Friction, walking barefoot, structural foot problems	Mutations related to damaged DNA cause skin cells to grow unchecked
Modifying factors	Prevention of spread; treatment with salicylic acid or cryotherapy	Alleviation of causative factors	Alleviation of causative factors	Surgical removal; prescription medications

case
42–1

Relevant Evaluation Criteria	Scenario/Model Outcome

Information Gathering

1. Gather essential information about the patient's symptoms and medical history, including:

    a. description of symptom(s) (i.e., nature, onset, duration, severity, associated symptoms)

> A female high school student, accompanied by her mother, tells you she has a rough spot on the bottom of her great right toe and asks if you can suggest anything to help her get rid of the lesion. When she first noticed the lesion 6 weeks ago, it was smaller than a pea but has gradually enlarged over the last several weeks. She says it is not painful, but she is concerned about how it looks and that it is getting larger. There is no inflammation, bleeding, significant discoloration, or discharge from the lesion.

    b. description of any factors that seem to precipitate, exacerbate, and/or relieve the patient's symptom(s)

> She plays high school basketball and has gym class 3 times a week. After gym and the games, she showers barefoot in the communal showers.

    c. description of the patient's efforts to relieve the symptoms

> She has not tried to treat the lesion.

    d. patient's identity

> Marri Nelson

    e. age, sex, height, and weight

> 16 years old, female, 5 ft 4 in., 125 lb

    f. patient's occupation

> High school student

    g. patient's dietary habits

> She follows no particular diet. Her food choices are usually healthy. She sometimes skips breakfast.

    h. patient's sleep habits

> 7–8 hours a night

    i. concurrent medical condition, prescription and non-prescription medications, and dietary supplements

> No medical conditions; medication(s): generic multivitamin daily, vitamin D 400 IU daily

    j. allergies

> None

    k. history of other adverse reactions to medications

> None

    l. other (describe) _____

> She lives at home and shares a bathroom with her two siblings. She is not pregnant or sexually active.

Relevant Evaluation Criteria	Scenario/Model Outcome

Assessment and Triage

2. Differentiate patient's signs/symptoms and correctly identify the patient's primary problem(s).

Marri most likely has a plantar wart.

3. Identify exclusions for self-treatment (Figure 42–1).

None

4. Formulate a comprehensive list of therapeutic alternatives for the primary problem to determine if triage to a medical provider is required, and share this information with the patient or caregiver.

Options include:

(1) Recommend self-care with a nonprescription wart removal product and nondrug measures.

(2) Recommend self-care until Marri can consult a medical provider for evaluation and treatment.

(3) Refer Marri for medical evaluation and treatment

(4) Take no action.

Plan

5. Select an optimal therapeutic alternative to address the patient's problem, taking into account patient preferences.

Because Marri is concerned about the wart's cosmetic appearance and the possibility that it will continue to enlarge, and because there is significant possibility of transmitting the virus to others, pharmacologic treatment of the wart should be considered. Because the wart is a single, small, nonpainful lesion confined to one area, and the patient has no identifiable exclusions for self-treatment, she can be treated with a nonprescription wart removal product. She can prevent transmitting the wart to others by wearing shoes or covering the wart, especially when showering at the gym or when using her bathroom.

6. Describe the recommended therapeutic approach to the patient or caregiver.

See Figure 42–1 and the box Patient Education for Warts.
"Salicylic acid in a pad or strip would be a good choice in this situation. Salicylic acid pads/strip products have to be applied every 48 hours. The pad should be covered with occlusive tape. Salicyclic acid therapy might take up to 12 weeks for the wart to resolve."

7. Explain to the patient or caregiver the rationale for selecting the recommended therapeutic approach from the considered therapeutic alternatives.

"Salicylic acid in a strip/pad form is an appropriate recommendation for you because salicylic acid is effective for this type of wart, easy to use, and less painful than some other treatment options. Cryotherapy is another self-care option for the treatment of warts. However, cryotherapy is more painful than salicyclic acid, and small warts may be adequately treated with salicylic acid."

"Your wart is not severe enough to warrant a referral to a health care provider at this time. Self-treatment is more cost-effective and should provide acceptable results in resolving your wart."

Patient Education

8. When recommending self-care with nonprescription medications and/or nondrug therapy, convey accurate information to the patient or caregiver.

"Table 42–4 and the box Patient Education for Warts provide information on removing warts safely. Also, be sure to read and follow the directions that come with the product."

"The wart may be soaked in warm water for 5 minutes to soften the outer surface. The pad/strip should be applied directly over the wart. Remove the pad/strip every 48 hours and replace it with a new one. Treatment with salicylic acid may be continued for up to 12 weeks."
"If there is any irritation to the healthy tissue surrounding the wart, wash the area immediately with soap and water."

Solicit follow-up questions from patient or caregiver.

(1) "Is there anything I can do to prevent the spread of the wart?"

(2) "What should I do if the wart is not gone after 12 weeks?"

(3) "Should I cover the wart?"

Answer patient or caregiver's questions.

(1) "See the box patient Education for Warts for preventive measures."

(2) "If after 12 weeks of treatment, the wart is still present, you should consult a health care provider."

(3) "Yes. Covering the wart helps prevent spreading warts to others."

Evaluation of Patient Outcome

9. Assess patient outcome.

Follow up in 4–6 weeks to assess the patient's progress in clearing the wart with the recommended therapy.

case

42–2

Relevant Evaluation Criteria	Scenario/Model Outcome

Information Gathering

1. Gather essential information about the patient's symptoms and medical history, including:

a. description of symptom(s) (i.e., nature, onset, duration, severity, associated symptoms)

A middle-aged male asks for something to get rid of a callus-like lesion on the bottom of his foot. When he first noticed the lesion 3 months ago, it was about the size of a dime but has enlarged to the size of a quarter. The lesion is on the ball of the foot and appears to be multiple lesions fused together. He complains of discomfort when walking. There is no inflammation, bleeding, significant discoloration, or discharge from the growth.

b. description of any factors that seem to precipitate, exacerbate, and/or relieve the patient's symptom(s)

None

c. description of the patient's efforts to relieve the symptoms

He has soaked his feet and applied lotions regularly in an attempt to soften the lesion. He attempts to shave the lesion regularly.

d. patient's identity

Lee Williams

e. age, sex, height, and weight

45 years old, male, 5 ft 11 in., 200 lb

f. patient's occupation

High school gym teacher and football coach

g. patient's dietary habits

He attempts to follow a healthy diet but frequently indulges in concentrated sweets.

h. patient's sleep habits

6–7 hours a night

i. concurrent medical condition, prescription and nonprescription medications, and dietary supplements

Hypertension: lisinopril 10 mg daily; type 2 diabetes: metformin 1000 mg twice daily, Lantus 40 units at bedtime, and gabapentin 100 mg 3 times daily

j. allergies

None

k. history of other adverse reactions to medications

None

l. other (describe) _____

He walks 3–5 days a week.

Assessment and Triage

2. Differentiate patient's signs/symptoms and correctly identify the patient's primary problem(s).

Lee most likely has multiple plantar warts.

3. Identify exclusions for self-treatment (Figure 42–1).

Diabetes; neuropathy; multiple, large, painful warts

4. Formulate a comprehensive list of therapeutic alternatives for the primary problem to determine if triage to a medical provider is required, and share this information with the patient or caregiver.

Options include:

(1) Recommend self-care with a nonprescription wart removal product and nondrug measures.

(2) Recommend self-care until Lee can consult a medical provider for evaluation and treatment.

(3) Refer Lee for medical evaluation and treatment.

(4) Take no action.

Plan

5. Select an optimal therapeutic alternative to address the patient's problem, taking into account patient preferences.

Lee should be referred to a health care provider for evaluation and treatment because the multiple warts seem to have coalesced into what appears to be one large wart, and because he has decreased sensation secondary to diabetic neuropathy.

6. Describe the recommended therapeutic approach to the patient or caregiver.

"You should consult a health care provider to evaluate and treat the wart."

7. Explain to the patient or caregiver the rationale for selecting the recommended therapeutic approach from the considered therapeutic alternatives.

"Self-treatment is not recommended because multiple warts have coalesced to form one large wart, and because you have decreased feeling in your feet, making it possible for you to injure your feet with the nonprescription wart removal products."

case

42–2 *continued*

Relevant Evaluation Criteria	Scenario/Model Outcome
Patient Education	
8. When recommending self-care with nonprescription medications and/or nondrug therapy, convey accurate information to the patient or caregiver.	Criterion does not apply in this case.
Solicit follow-up questions from patient or caregiver.	(1) "Is there anything I can do to keep from getting this again?"
	(2) "Will these spread to other people or other areas of my body?"
Answer patient or caregiver's questions.	(1) "It is common for warts to recur even after treatment. The box Patient Education for Warts lists things you can do to reduce the risk of reinfection."
	(2) "Warts are spread through person-to-person contact or by contact with contaminated surfaces such as towels or exercise equipment. The box Patient Education for Warts provides information on how to prevent spreading warts to other areas of your body or to other persons."
Evaluation of Patient Outcome	
9. Assess patient outcome.	The patient should follow-up with the health care provider as directed.

Patient Counseling for Warts

Patients must understand that warts are caused by the HPV virus and are contagious. Providers should discuss with patients measures to prevent the spread of warts to other parts of the body or to other individuals. Providers should also point out the differences between available products, including their indications, contraindications, warnings, and precautions. The box Patient Education for Warts lists specific information for patients who are using either salicylic acid products or cryotherapy products. If warts persist despite self-treatment, patients should be referred to a medical provider for evaluation and treatment.

Evaluation of Patient Outcomes for Warts

Salicyclic acid may require up to 12 weeks of daily treatment to completely resolve the wart. Patients should see some improvement in 1–2 weeks. A follow-up should be scheduled at 4–6 weeks to evaluate the wart. If the wart does not appear to be resolved, the patient should be encouraged to continue treatment. If the wart has not cleared after 12 weeks, prescription therapies may be warranted. The patient should be referred to a health care provider for further evaluation and treatment.

Cryotherapy may be repeated after 10 days for up to three treatments. If the wart is not cleared after three treatments, the patient should see a health care provider.

patient education for

Warts

When treating warts, the goals are to (1) eliminate signs and symptoms associated with the warts, (2) remove the wart without causing scars, (3) prevent the wart from recurring, and (4) prevent spreading of warts to self or others. To ensure the best possible treatment outcomes, patients must follow product instructions carefully and must consistently use measures to prevent the spread of warts.

Nondrug Measures
- To decrease the chances of getting warts, avoid nail-biting; do not go barefoot; do not cut, shave, or pick at warts; wash hands before and after treating or touching warts; keep feet clean and dry; use one specific towel to dry warts; and do not use the same towel to dry other areas of the body.
- To avoid spreading warts to others, do not share towels, razors, socks, shoes, etc.; keep the wart covered; and do not walk barefoot, especially in bathrooms or in public places.

Nonprescription Medications
- Select only nonprescription salicylic acid products approved for self-treatment of warts. Follow the instructions on the label closely.
- Make sure to use these products only on common or plantar warts. Do not use on moles, birthmarks, warts with hairs growing from them, irritated or inflamed skin, or infected skin.

- If you are not 100% certain that the condition is a wart, consult a health care provider before using these products.
- Do not use these products to treat warts on the face, mucous membranes, armpits, breasts, genitals, or around fingernails.
- Do not use these products on children who are younger than 4 years, women who are pregnant or breast-feeding, or patients who have diabetes or poor circulation.
- Keep these products away from the eyes. If they come into contact with the eyes, seek medical help immediately.
- Do not apply these products to healthy skin. If they come into contact with healthy skin, wash the area with soap and water immediately.
- Some of these products are flammable or contain collodions that are poisonous if ingested. Keep away from heat and out of children's reach.

- Improvement should be seen within a week or two of beginning treatment. The wart should completely clear within 6–12 weeks. Self-treatment should not continue longer than 12 weeks.
- Warts may recur after treatment.

Nonprescription Cryotherapy

- Follow the instructions on the label closely.
- Use these products only on common or plantar warts. Do not use on moles, birthmarks, warts with hairs growing from them, irritated or inflamed skin, or infected skin.
- If you are not 100% certain that the condition is a wart, consult a health care provider before using these products.
- Do not use these products to treat warts on the face, mucous membranes, armpits, breasts, genitals, or around fingernails.

- Do not use these products on children who are younger than 4 years, women who are pregnant or breast-feeding, or patients who have diabetes or poor circulation.
- You will feel an aching, stinging sensation when the product is applied.
- A blister will form and the wart should fall off after about 10 days.
- If the wart does not completely clear after the first treatment, the procedure may be repeated in 10–14 days. The product should not be used more than 3 times.

When to Seek Medical Attention

- Stop using the products and consult a medical provider if severe irritation or pain occurs immediately after application.
- If the wart has not cleared after 12 weeks of treatment, consult a health care provider.

Key Points for Warts

➤ Because many warts will resolve without treatment, a wait-and-see approach may be an appropriate treatment option in some patients. However, this approach allows the continued transmission of the highly contagious HPV virus.

➤ Patients with diabetes, poor circulation, or immunodeficiencies should not self-treat with salicyclic acid or cryotherapy without first consulting a health care provider.

➤ The nonprescription drug of choice for common and plantar warts is salicyclic acid.

➤ Plantar warts should be treated with higher concentrations of salicyclic acid (≤40%). Warts on the hands or areas with thinner epidermis should be treated with lower concentrations of salicyclic acid (<17%)

➤ DMEP products are available for home cryotherapy treatments, but cryotherapy is no more effective than salicylic acid.

➤ The directions for use of nonprescription salicyclic acid and cryotherapy products should be followed to prevent injury to healthy tissue surrounding the wart.

➤ Patients who experience adverse effects from nonprescription wart removal products or have warts that recur frequently should be evaluated by a health care provider.

REFERENCES

1. Lipke MM. An armamentarium of wart treatments. *Clin Med Res.* 2006;4(4):273–93.
2. Pray WS, Pray GE, Pray M. Removing warts with nonprescription treatments. *US Pharm.* 2011;36(8):15–23.
3. Mulhem E, Pinelis S. Treatment of non-genital cutaneous warts. *Am Fam Phys.* 2011;84(3):288–93.
4. Micali G, Dall'Oglio F, Nasca MR, et. al. Management of cutaneous warts. *Am J Clin Dermatol.* 2004;5(5):311–7
5. Kwok CS, Gibbs S, Bennett C, et al. Topical treatments for cutaneous warts. *Cochrane Database Syst Rev.* 2012;9:CD001781. doi: 10.1002/14651858.CD004976.pub3. Accessed at http://www.thecochranelibrary.com/view/0/index.html.
6. Nguyen NV, Burkhart CG. Cryotherapy treatment of warts: dimethyl ether and propane versus liquid nitrogen—case report and review of the literature. *J Drugs Dermatol.* 2011;10(10):1174–6.
7. Watkins P. Identifying and treating plantar warts. *Nurs Stand.* 2006;20(42):50–4.

8. Drake LA, Celley RI, Cornelison R. Guidelines of care: guidelines of care for warts: human papillomavirus. *J Am Acad Dermatol.* 1995;32:98–103.
9. Dall'Oglio F, D'Amico V, Nasca MR, et al. Treatment of cutaneous warts: an evidence-based review. *Am J Clin Dermatol.* 2012;13(2):72–96.
10. Al-Gurairi FT, Al-Waiz M, Sharquie KE. Oral zinc sulphate in the treatment of recalcitrant viral warts: randomized placebo controlled clinical trial. *Br J Dermatol.* 2002;146:423–31.
11. Kuykendall-IVY TD, Johnson SM. Evidence based review of management of non-genital cutaneous warts. *Cutis.* 2003;71:213–22.
12. Gaston A, Garry R. Topical vitamin A treatment of recalcitrant common warts. *Virol J.* 2012;9:21.
13. *Federal Register.* 1990;55:33246–56.
14. Compound W [product information]. Compound W (Prestige Brands) Web site. Accessed at http://compoundw.com/products/wart-remover-pads, April 1, 2013.
15. Compound W [product information]. Compound W (Prestige Brands) Web site. Accessed at http://www.compoundw.com/products/wart-remover-liquid, April 1, 2013.
16. Trans-Ver-Sal (Dermal Patch) [package insert]. Accessed at http://home.intekom.com/pharm/allergan/transver.html, April 1, 2013.
17. Newton GD, Pray WS, Popovich NG. New OTC drugs and devices 2003: a selective review. *J Am Pharm Assoc.* 2004;44:211–25.
18. Compound W Freeze Off [patient instruction leaflet]. Compound W (Prestige Brands) Web site. Accessed at https://compoundw-prod-uploads.s3.amazonaws.com/cms_page_media/27/compoundw.com_en_products_freeze-off-wart-removal-english.pdf, September 15, 2014.
19. Wartner Wart and Veruca Remover Instruction Leaflet. Wartner Web site. Accessed at http://wartner.eu/wp-content/uploads/Wartner-Corporate-Leaflet-Unilingual.pdf, April 2, 2013.
20. Bruggink SC, Gussekloo J, Berger MY, et al. Cryotherapy with liquid nitrogen versus topical salicylic acid application for cutaneous warts in primary care: randomized controlled trial. *CMAJ.* 2010;182(15):1624–30.
21. Cheek A, Nix LH, eds. *The Foxfire 40th Anniversary Book: Faith, Family, and the Land.* New York, NY: Anchor; 2006.
22. Dehghani F, Merat A, Panjehshahin MR, et al. Healing effect of garlic extract on warts and corns. *Int J Dermatol.* 2005;44:612–5.
23. Forbes MA, Schmidt MM. Use of essential oils to clear plantar warts. *Nurse Pract.* 2006;31(3):53–7.
24. Christakis DA, Lehmann HP. Is duct tape occlusion therapy as effective as cryotherapy for the treatment of the common wart? *Arch Pediatr Adolesc Med.* 2002;156:975–7.
25. Wenner R, Askari SK, Cham PM, et al. Duct tape for the treatment of common warts in adults: a double-blind randomized controlled trial. *Arch Dermatol.* 2007;143:309–13.

MINOR FOOT DISORDERS

chapter 43

Cynthia W. Coffey and Karla T. Foster

Often neglected, overlooked, and unprotected, the feet contain nearly one quarter of all the bones in the body. The foot is intricately designed to absorb shock from pressure and assist in movement. On average, a person walks 115,000 miles in a lifetime, which is equivalent to circling the world nearly four times. Seventy-five percent of all Americans will develop foot-related disorders.[1] Individuals who exercise regularly are at risk for foot disorders. Without adequate precautions, particular problems and injuries, particularly those involving the feet, can arise.[1] Among the most common foot disorders are ingrown toenails, bunions, and corns and calluses. Therefore appropriate education and training for the prevention and treatment of minor foot disorders are important.[1,2]

In some instances, self-care of foot disorders is inappropriate. Children with a congenital malformation, a deformity, or a specific disease that affects the foot (e.g., juvenile arthritis) need medical care by an orthopedic surgeon or a podiatrist. Adolescents may experience rapid growth, and growth plates in their feet may subsequently become stressed and irritated. Athletic activity at this age can also contribute to secondary conditions, especially if activity-associated injuries to the feet are not properly treated. Osteoarthritis, for example, can develop secondary to a foot injury. Patients may also encounter foot problems related to aging (e.g., arthritis) and disease (e.g., peripheral vascular disease). In particular, diabetes and arthritis can cause secondary foot problems. Therefore, patients should check their feet regularly for foot disorders. Common foot disorders could result in more serious injuries in patients with comorbid disorders (e.g., diabetes) and may be indicative of other serious underlying conditions.[3] In some instances, foot disorders or inappropriate foot care practices may be life threatening to patients with diabetes, severe arthritis, and impaired circulation (see the box A Word about Chronic Diseases and Foot Disorders).[3–7] For most patients, however, such problems cause nominal measures of discomfort and impaired mobility.

Pathophysiology of the Foot

At birth, an infant's foot has 33 joints, 19 muscles, 107 ligaments, and cartilage that will develop into 26 bones. The feet continue to develop and mature until ages 14–16 years for females and ages 15–21 years for males. Women and men will generally begin to notice changes in their feet in their 40s and 50s, respectively.[8] After years of bearing the body's weight, feet tend to broaden and flatten, thus stretching ligaments and causing bones to shift positions. These changes subject feet to stress, which is compounded by prolonged standing. An estimated 40% of the U.S. population spends about 75% of their workday on their feet, increasing the potential for painful foot conditions.[1,2]

Corns and Calluses

Although corns and calluses are common foot disorders, they should not be ignored. They may indicate a biomechanical problem and lead to serious complications in predisposed patients.

Pathophysiology of Corns and Calluses

Under normal conditions, the cells in the skin's basal cell layer (stratum basale) undergo mitotic division at a rate equal to the continual surface cellular desquamation, leading to complete replacement of the epidermis in approximately 1 month. During corn or callus development, however, friction and pressure increase mitotic activity of the basal cell layer, leading to the migration of maturing cells through the prickle cell (stratum spinosum) and granular (stratum granulosum) skin layers (see Chapter 32, Figure 32–1). As more cells reach the outer skin surface, they produce a thicker horny layer (stratum corneum). This process is a natural protective mechanism of the skin surface and may signal biomechanical problems resulting in abnormal weight distribution on the foot. When friction or pressure is relieved, mitotic activity returns to normal, causing remission and disappearance of the lesion.[8–11]

Clinical Presentation of Corns and Calluses

Corns and calluses are similar in that both produce a marked hyperkeratosis of the stratum corneum, but they have marked differences.

Corns

A corn (clavus) is a small, raised, sharply demarcated, hyperkeratotic lesion with a central core; the lesion is caused by pressure from underlying bony prominences or joints (Figure 43–1).

a word about

Chronic Diseases and Foot Disorders

Some chronic diseases predispose certain patients to foot complications. Patients who have diabetes often have poor circulation and diminished limb sensitivity, which make them especially vulnerable to infectious foot problems. Other susceptible patients include those with peripheral vascular disease or arthritis. The health care provider can identify these patients by asking about daily medication use or reviewing the patient's drug profile. Typical drug use patterns for high-risk patients include insulin; oral antidiabetic drugs (e.g., glipizide, glyburide, metformin, acarbose, and nateglinide); drugs for circulation disorders (e.g., clopidogrel, cyclandelate, isoxsuprine, papaverine, and pentoxifylline); drugs for neuropathic pain (e.g., gabapentin and duloxetine); and drugs for arthritic disorders (e.g., aspirin and other NSAIDs).

If not properly supervised in patients with impaired circulation, self-treatment with nonprescription products may induce more inflammation, ulceration, or even gangrene, particularly in cases of vascular insufficiency in the foot. Patients with diabetes and those with peripheral circulatory impairments are particularly susceptible to gangrene. In addition, simple lesions may mask more serious abscesses or ulcerations. If left medically unattended, these lesions may lead to conditions such as osteomyelitis, which may require hospitalization and aggressive intravenous antibiotic therapy.

Diabetes Mellitus[3-6]

Patients who have poorly controlled diabetes are at greater risk for lower extremity complications, which result in increased health care costs, decreased quality of life, and increased morbidity. Two major causes of foot ulcerations are peripheral neuropathy, which results in loss of injury perception and subsequently excessive plantar pressure, which contributes to decreased mobility and foot deformities. Patients with diabetes also contribute to foot complications by poor foot hygiene such as extreme hot water soaks, inappropriate footwear, and lack of daily foot self-examinations. Patients with diabetes need to be educated on proper foot care, such as trimming toenails appropriately, not applying creams/lotions between the toes, keeping socks clean and dry, performing foot examinations at home, and having foot examinations at the health care provider's office. (See Chapter 45 for further discussion of diabetes management.)

Peripheral Vascular Disease[4,6]

Patients with peripheral vascular disease often have poor circulation of the feet and legs. Because of decreased blood flow and low oxygen perfusion, skin ulcerations and decreased wound healing may be problematic in these patients. They may complain of persistent and unusual feelings of cold, numbness, tingling, burning, or fatigue. Other symptoms may include discolored skin, dry skin, absence of hair on the feet or legs, or a cramping or tightness in the leg muscles.

The provider should palpate for pedal pulses. The most discriminating questions that a provider can ask this type of patient are (1) Do you experience aching in your calves when you walk? (2) Do you have to hang your feet over the edge of the bed during sleep to relieve the soreness in your calves? A yes response to either question warrants referral to a primary care provider or podiatrist.

Localized redness or unilateral coldness may indicate a possible blockage (a clot) of circulation to the foot. Sometimes the involved foot or lower leg will appear physically larger than the other, may be red or waxy in appearance, may have no hair growth on the toes, and will exhibit thickened nails. If the medication history of the patient with suspected circulatory problems does not indicate the use of medications intended to relieve such symptoms, the patient should be referred immediately for further evaluation.

A daily footbath is a simple measure to assist patients with peripheral vascular disease. After the foot is patted dry, an emollient foot cream can be applied to aid the skin in retaining moisture and pliability. The footbath will also soften brittle toenails for clipping and filing. The feet should be kept warm and moderately exercised every day.

Arthritis[6]

Osteoarthritis is a noninflammatory, degenerative joint disease that occurs primarily in older people. Degeneration of the articular cartilage and changes in the bone result in a loss of resilience and a decrease in the skeleton's shock-absorption capability. This condition, however, is also experienced by individuals in their late teens and early 20s as a secondary complication of a previous athletic injury. This condition might be evidenced by the development of hallux limitus or rigidus of the big toe (e.g., a painful flexion or extension of the big toe related to stiffness and spur formation in the metatarsophalangeal joint or a stiff toe, respectively). Subsequently, these patients have a lot of difficulty with their shoes not fitting properly. They may also develop an osteoarthritic condition in the ankle joint. Referral for further evaluation is appropriate. Most patients with rheumatoid arthritis eventually have foot involvement. The major forefoot deformities in these patients are painful metatarsal heads, hallux valgus, and clawfoot. Corrective surgical procedures are often indicated to reduce pain and improve function and mobility. Little evidence exists that conventional nonsurgical therapy (e.g., orthopedic shoes, metatarsal inserts, conventional arch supports, and metatarsal bars) is effective for these deformities.

Proper palliative foot care is especially important for arthritic patients. They should wear properly fitted shoes, pad their shoes with insoles to protect their feet from the shock of hard surfaces, and undergo regular podiatric or medical examinations. (See Chapter 7 for use of topical or systemic nonprescription analgesics for osteoarthritis.)

The central core of the corn differentiates it from a wart (see Chapter 42, Table 42–5).

Misidentification of warts and corns is common. Differentiation can be made by shaving the central core. A corn has a hard center, whereas a wart will bleed because of the multiple capillary loops in its center.[9] Corns are yellowish gray and well circumscribed, with diameters of 1 cm or less. The base of the corn is on the skin surface; its apex points inward and presses on the nerve endings in the dermis, causing pain.[7,12]

Polished, shiny, dry hard corns (heloma durum) are the most prevalent and usually occur on the bulb of the great toe, the dorsum of the fourth or fifth toe, or tips of the middle toes. Soft corns (heloma molle) are whitish thickenings of the skin and

may be extremely painful. Accumulated perspiration macerates the epidermis, giving this corn a soft appearance. Soft corns may occur between any adjacent toes but are most frequently found between the fourth and fifth toe.[8,9]

Pressure from inappropriate, tight-fitting shoes is the most frequent cause of pain from corns. As narrow-toed or high-heeled shoes crowd toes into a narrow toe box, the most lateral toe, the fifth, sustains the most pressure and friction and is the usual site of a corn. The resulting pain may be severe and sharp (when downward pressure is applied) or dull and discomforting. Consumer research approximates that 82% of women ages 35–54 years suffer moderate-severe pain from corns and that 35% are consequently limited or restricted in their activities.[7,10,12]

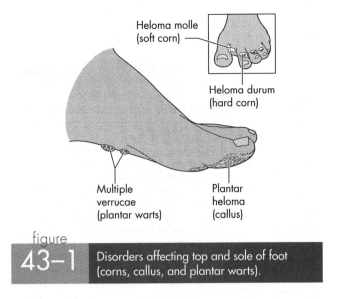

Heloma molle
(soft corn)

Heloma durum
(hard corn)

Multiple
verrucae
(plantar warts)

Plantar
heloma
(callus)

figure

43–1

Disorders affecting top and sole of foot
(corns, callus, and plantar warts).

Calluses

A callus has a broad base, with relatively even thickening of skin, and is generally found on the bottom of the foot in areas such as the heel, ball of the foot, toes, and sides of the foot (Figure 43–1). A callus has indefinite borders and ranges from a few millimeters to several centimeters in diameter. The indefinite borders help health care providers differentiate calluses from corns, which have well-circumscribed margins. A callus is usually raised and yellow, and it has a normal pattern of skin ridges on its surface. Calluses form on joints and weight-bearing areas of the hands and feet[7,9,10,12] (see Color Plates, photograph 31).

Friction (caused by loose-fitting shoes or tight-fitting hosiery), walking barefoot, and structural biomechanical problems contribute to the development of calluses. Structural problems include improper weight distribution, pressure, and development of bunions with age. Calluses can be symptomatic and protective.

Discrete-nucleated and diffuse-shearing calluses are most commonly found on the feet. The discrete-nucleated callus is smaller and has a localized translucent center; this type of callus is painful with applied pressure because of its central keratin plug. The diffuse-shearing callus covers a larger surface area and does not have a central core; therefore, this callus is not associated with pain.[9,10,12]

Treatment of Corns and Calluses

Treatment Goals

The goals of self-treatment are to (1) provide symptomatic relief, (2) remove corns and calluses, and (3) prevent their recurrence by correcting underlying causes.

General Treatment Approach

Although effective nonprescription products are available for removing corns and calluses, ultimate success depends on eliminating the causes. The algorithm in Figure 43–2 outlines self-treatment of corns and calluses and lists exclusions for self-treatment.

Nonpharmacologic Therapy

Daily soaking of the affected skin area (for at least 5 minutes in warm, not hot, water) throughout the treatment period aids in softening dead tissue for removal. After normal washing of the foot, dead tissue should be removed gently, rather than forcibly, to avoid further damage. A callus file or pumice stone effectively accomplishes this purpose. Power-operated foot files may be too aggressive. Sharp knives or razor blades should not be used because these instruments may lacerate the skin, which could allow bacteria to enter the wound and result in localized infection.[9,11]

Cushioning pads are another option. Circular foam cushioning pads may aid in relieving painful pressure from inflamed tissue. Some podiatrists recommend that patients change the pads every day. Many providers, however, are concerned that the pad adhesive may degrade the skin, leading to infection. Disadvantages associated with older pads have been overcome with polymer gel pads (e.g., Bunion Guard, available from the Mayo Clinic), which provide a protective cushion without leaving a sticky residue. Another advantage of gel pads is that the smooth outer surface does not cause snags and runs in socks and hosiery.[9,13] Silicone toe sleeves impregnated with mineral oil (i.e., Pedifix Visco-Gel Toe Protector) are another option for toes affected by corns. The mineral oil is slowly released to soften the skin. The sleeves also protect and cushion the corn area. A foam spacer or lamb's wool may be used to provide relief in areas with soft corns. Placement of a metatarsal pad may help relieve pain and pressure from a diffuse-shearing callus.[8,14]

Eliminating the pressure and friction that induce corns and calluses entails using well-fitting, nonbinding footwear that evenly distributes body weight[14] (Table 43–1). For anatomic foot deformities, orthopedic corrections must be made. These measures relieve pressure and friction, which allow normal mitosis of the basal cell layer to resume. The stratum corneum will normalize after topical keratolytics are applied and total desquamation of the hyperkeratotic tissue occurs. Orthotics (i.e., arch supports) may be needed to help compensate for deformities by redistributing the mechanical forces. Ultimately, surgical correction of toe deformities and resection of the underlying bone may be necessary.

Pharmacologic Therapy
Salicylic Acid

Salicylic acid, the oldest of the keratolytic agents, is formulated in varying strengths (0.5%–40%). For the treatment of corns and calluses, the approved concentration ranges are 6%–17% in hydrisalic gel, 12%–40% in a plaster vehicle, and 12%–27.5% in a collodion-like vehicle.[15–17]

Salicylic acid is believed to act on hyperplastic keratin, without affecting viable epidermis. Product application will cause the area to swell, soften, macerate, and then desquamate the affected epithelium. The Food and Drug Administration (FDA) has stated that presoaking the affected area produced no significant positive effects before application of salicylic acid. In its final rule, FDA proposed allowing manufacturers of these products to use the following statement as an optional direction to the consumer: "May soak corn/callus (or wart) in warm water for 5 minutes to assist in removal."[15–17]

The FDA advisory review panel evaluated more than 20 agents for the treatment of corns and calluses. Of these agents,

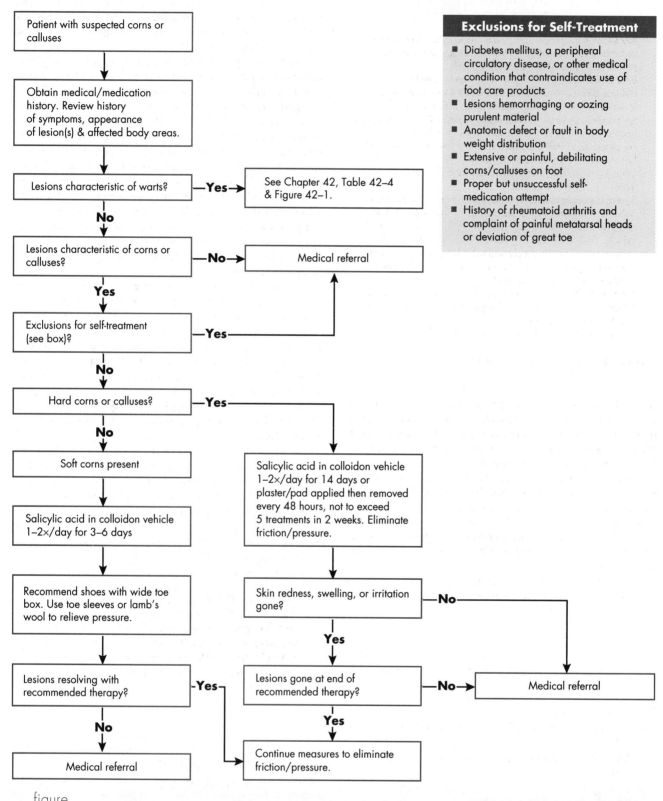

figure

43–2 Self-care of corns and calluses.

table

43–1 Selection of Properly Fitted Footwear

- Buy shoes in the proper size (width and length). To obtain an accurate measurement, ask a trained salesperson to measure your feet. Recheck shoe size every 2 years.
- Base shoe length on the longest toe of your longest foot. The distance between the tip of the shoe and the longest toe is approximately one-half inch. In an athletic shoe, 1 inch is needed.
- For proper arch length, choose a shoe in which the first metatarsal head of the foot fits the metatarsal break of the shoe.
- For proper shoe width, choose a shoe that feels comfortable at the first metatarsal joint (i.e., toes do not feel cramped in the toe box).
- Once the shoe size is determined, choose a shoe shaped to match the shape of your foot.
- If you have abnormalities of the toes (e.g., hammer toes) or use orthotics or padding in your shoes, select a shoe with a toe box of adequate depth (vertical height) to prevent friction of the tops of the toes. A wide toe box will help relieve pressure between toes.
- Make sure the heel fits snugly and helps hold the foot straight.
- If you are physically active, make sure the shoe's midsole provides adequate cushioning and support.
- Try on both shoes at the time of purchase, preferably wearing a pair of socks or stockings of the type that will usually be worn with the new pair of shoes.
- If your feet tend to swell, select shoes at the end of the day.

Source: References 1, 8, 10, 14, and 23.

only salicylic acid in a plaster, pad, disk, gel, or collodion vehicle dosage form is approved as safe and effective for nonprescription marketing for the removal of corns and calluses (Table 43–2). FDA recognized that the term *plaster* includes disks and pads because these dosage forms are similar.[16,17]

Salicylic acid is usually applied to a corn, callus, or common wart in a collodion or collodion-like vehicle. These vehicles contain pyroxylin and various combinations of volatile solvents (e.g., ether, acetone, or alcohol) or a plasticizer, which is usually castor oil. Pyroxylin is a nitrocellulose derivative that remains on the skin as a water-repellent film after the volatile solvents have evaporated.[15–17]

The advantages of collodions and liquid dosage forms are that they form an adherent flexible or rigid film and prevent

table

43–2 Selected Corn and Callus Products

Trade Name	Primary Ingredients
Curad Mediplast Corn, Callus & Wart Remover	Salicylic acid 40%
Dr. Scholl's Corn/Callus Remover Liquid	Salicylic acid 12.6%
Hydrisalic Gel	Salicylic acid 6%
Dr. Scholl's Cushlin Gel Corn/Callus Remover Disk	Salicylic acid 40%
Freezone One Step Corn/Callus Remover Pads	Salicylic acid 40%

Source: Reference 15.

moisture evaporation. These qualities aid penetration of the active ingredient into the affected tissue and result in sustained local action of the drug. The delivery systems are largely water insoluble, as are most of their active ingredients, such as salicylic acid. They are also less prone than other aqueous solutions to run onto surrounding skin.[15–17]

A disadvantage of collodions is that they are extremely flammable and volatile. Some patients may inhale and abuse these vehicles. Another disadvantage is the occlusion of normal water transport through the skin, which allows systemic absorption of some drugs (e.g., salicylic acid). Percutaneous absorption may be problematic with prolonged use on large surface areas of children and patients with renal or hepatic impairment because salicylic acid is largely metabolized in the liver and excreted in the urine. Although occlusive vehicles can enhance the percutaneous absorption of salicylic acid, it is highly unlikely that salicylate toxicity will result during corn, callus, or wart therapy at recommended dosages. However, if symptoms of possible salicylism (nausea, vomiting, dizziness, hearing loss, tinnitus, lethargy, hyperpnea, diarrhea, or psychiatric disturbances) occur, use of these products should be discontinued immediately.[15–17]

Salicylic acid may also be delivered to the skin through the use of a plaster, disk, or pad. This delivery system provides direct and prolonged contact of the drug with the affected area, resulting in quicker resolution of the condition. Salicylic acid plaster is a uniform solid or semisolid adhesive mixture of salicylic acid in a suitable base that is spread on appropriate backing material (e.g., felt, moleskin, cotton, or plastic). The usual concentration of salicylic acid in the base is 40%; these dosage forms may be applied directly to the corn or callus.[9,15–17] Table 43–3 provides instructions for applying salicylic acid products.

Caution should be used while applying topical salicylic acid because misapplication may lead to inflammation or ulcer formation (see the box A Word about Chronic Diseases and Foot Disorders). These products may be hazardous in pregnancy and should not be used in patients who are breast-feeding because of systemic absorption and the potential for Reye's syndrome. Salicylic acid may be used in pediatric patients older than 2 years at concentrations of 1.8%–6%. FDA requires the following warning on salicylic acid product labels:

> Do not use this product on irritated skin, any area that is infected or reddened, moles, birthmarks, warts with hair growing from them, genital warts, warts on the face, or warts on the mucous membranes, such as inside the mouth, nose, anus, genitals, or lips. Do not use if you are diabetic, or if you have poor blood circulation.[15–17]

Assessment of Corns and Calluses: A Case-Based Approach

A private area where patients can be comfortable removing their shoe(s) allows direct inspection of the feet and enables accurate assessment of the nature and extent of the problem and its underlying cause. The patient should be asked about any self-care attempts and their outcome. The patient's health status and current medication regimen should also be assessed. Lifestyle factors

table

43–3 Guidelines for Treating Corns and Calluses with Salicylic Acid Products

- ▓ Wash and dry the affected area thoroughly before applying any product.
- ▓ May soak the affected foot in warm water for 5 minutes. Then remove the macerated, soft white skin of the corn or callus by scrubbing gently with a rough towel, pumice stone, or callus file. Do not debride the healthy skin.

Salicylic Acid 12%–17.6% in Collodion-Like Vehicle

- ▓ Apply product no more than twice daily. Morning and evening are usually the most convenient times.
- ▓ Do not let adjacent areas of normal healthy skin come in contact with the drug. If this happens, immediately wash off the solution with soap and water.
  - – Petroleum jelly applied to the healthy skin will serve as protection if delivery of the medication to the intended treatment area might be unsuccessful.
- ▓ Apply 1 drop at a time directly to the corn or callus until the affected area is well covered. Do not overuse the product.
- ▓ Allow the drops to dry and harden so the solution does not run.
- ▓ The solution is applied once or twice daily for up to 14 days.
- ▓ After use, cap the container tightly to prevent evaporation and to prevent the active ingredients from assuming a greater concentration.
- ▓ Store the product in an amber or light-resistant container away from direct sunlight or heat.

Salicylic Acid 12%–40% Plasters/Pads

- ▓ If using plaster, trim the plaster to follow the contours of the corn or callus. Apply the plaster to the affected skin, and cover it with adhesive occlusive tape.
- ▓ If using medicated disks with pads, apply the appropriately sized disk directly on the affected area, and then cover the disk with the pad.
- ▓ Remove the plaster/pad and occlusive tape within 48 hours.
- ▓ After removing the softened skin, reapply the plaster every 48 hours as needed to remove the corn/callus but not longer than 14 days.
  - – Seek medical attention if redness or irritation of the skin occurs or if corn or callus is not removed after 14 days of treatment.

Source: References 8 and 15–17.

(e.g., occupation, daily exercise, and footwear); underlying pathology (e.g., circulatory or neurologic disorders); the possibility of an aggravating event; and the walking/working surface must also be evaluated. This information should be recorded and regularly updated in the patient's medication profile.

Case 43–1 illustrates the assessment of a patient with corns.

Patient Counseling for Corns and Calluses

Remission of corns and calluses can take several days to several months. Patients suffering from corns and calluses should understand that effective treatment and maintenance depend on eliminating predisposing factors that contributed to the foot

case

43–1

Relevant Evaluation Criteria	Scenario/Model Outcome
Information Gathering	
1. Gather essential information about the patient's symptoms and medical history, including:	
a. description of symptom(s) (i.e., nature, onset, duration, severity, associated symptoms)	The patient describes thick, yellowish patches of rough skin on her heels and on her fourth and fifth toes.
b. description of any factors that seem to precipitate, exacerbate, and/or relieve the patient's symptom(s)	The patient says she does not have any pain, but she is irritated because her feet snag her hosiery and socks. She feels her feet look horrible when she is barefoot or wearing sandals.
c. description of the patient's efforts to relieve the symptoms	The patient has not tried anything other than applying lotion to her feet after showering.
d. patient's identity	Erin Mathers
e. age, sex, height, and weight	37 years old, female, 5 ft 7 in, 148 lb
f. patient's occupation	Florist
g. patient's dietary habits	Fruit, toast, or yogurt for breakfast; too busy for lunch; eats on the run a lot for dinner because of her child's ball schedule.
h. patient's sleep habits	4–7 hours nightly
i. concurrent medical conditions, prescription and non-prescription medications, and dietary supplements	Allergies: cetirizine 10 mg nightly and mometasone nasal 2 sprays each nostril daily

case

43–1 *continued*

Relevant Evaluation Criteria	Scenario/Model Outcome
j. allergies	Seasonal allergies
k. history of other adverse reactions to medications	None
l. other (describe) _____	None

Assessment and Triage

2. Differentiate patient's signs/symptoms and correctly identify the patient's primary problem(s).	Erin has developed diffuse shearing calluses (Figure 43–1).
3. Identify exclusions for self-treatment (Figure 43–2).	None
4. Formulate a comprehensive list of therapeutic alternatives for the primary problem to determine if triage to a health care provider is required, and share this information with the patient or caregiver.	Options include: (1) Refer Erin to an appropriate health care provider. (2) Recommend self-care with a nonprescription callus remover and nondrug measures. (3) Recommend self-care until Erin can see an appropriate provider. (4) Take no action.

Plan

5. Select an optimal therapeutic alternative to address the patient's problem, taking into account patient preferences.	Erin should use a nonprescription callus remover, callus cushioning pads, and nondrug measures to treat her condition.
6. Describe the recommended therapeutic approach to the patient or caregiver.	"Daily foot soaks, pumice stone or foot file may be used to reduce roughness of your calluses. Completely dry the feet before applying the callus remover. Applying cushioning pads will help to reduce pressure point areas on your feet, allowing the calluses to improve. You should also consider selection of appropriate shoes as outlined in Table 43–1."
7. Explain to the patient or caregiver the rationale for selecting the recommended therapeutic approach from the considered therapeutic alternatives.	"Calluses can be removed by nonprescription products and the use of foot files. However, it is important to assess the cause of the callus formation and correct the cause with appropriate footwear."

Patient Education

8. When recommending self-care with nonprescription medications and/or nondrug therapy, convey accurate information to the patient or caregiver.	See Table 43–3 for instructions for applying salicylic acid products. Also see the box Patient Education for Corn and Calluses. Erin should see a response to treatment recommendations within 14 days.
Solicit follow-up questions from the patient or caregiver.	(1) "Would it be better to go without shoes as often as possible, rather than wearing my dress shoes?" (2) "Can I speed up the process by cutting the callus down with a razor blade before applying the nonprescription medication?"
Answer the patient's or caregiver's questions.	(1) "Selecting a shoe that fits appropriately will prevent rubbing of the foot or a too snug fit, which will eliminate the cause of a callus and protect against callus formation." (2) "It is best to soak the feet and use foot files to pare down the callus. Do not cut on your feet because of the risk of injury and infection."

Evaluation of Patient Outcome

9. Assess patient outcome.	Ask Erin to call in 14 days to update you on the response to your treatment recommendations. Or you could call her into the pharmacy to evaluate the response.

The objectives of self-treatment are to (1) provide symptomatic relief, (2) remove corns or calluses, and (3) prevent their recurrence by correcting underlying causes. For most patients, carefully following product instructions and the self-care measures listed here will help ensure optimal therapeutic outcomes.

Nondrug Measures

- To avoid spreading the infection to another body site, clean the instruments used to remove dead skin after each use.
- Do not use sharp knives or razor blades to remove dead skin from corns and calluses. These instruments may cause bacterial infections.
- If you have trouble applying the product only to the affected area, apply petroleum jelly to healthy skin surrounding the treatment area before applying the corn and callus remover.
- For temporary relief of painful pressure in the area under a corn or callus, cover the affected area with a pad.
- Consult a health care provider if the symptoms described come back.

Preventive Measures

- To eliminate the pressure and friction that cause corns and calluses, wear well-fitting shoes that evenly distribute body weight (Table 43–1).
- Consult a podiatrist about foot deformity corrections.

Nonprescription Medications

- To remove corns and calluses, use a salicylic acid product labeled for use on these types of lesions (Table 43–2).
- Do not use this product on irritated, infected, or reddened skin.
- Do not use this product if you are diabetic or have poor blood circulation.
- Salicylic acid is poisonous. Do not allow it to come in contact with the mouth, and keep it out of children's reach.
- Note that the medication sloughs off skin and may leave an unsightly pinkish tinge to the skin.

When to Seek Medical Attention

- Stop treatment and consult a health care provider if swelling, reddening, or irritation of the skin occurs, or if pain occurs immediately with product application.

problem. It is important to discuss the need for wearing footwear of adequate width and length. Pads and cushions also help to reduce the pressure and shearing associated with corn and callus development.

The patient or caregiver should be counseled on how to use nonprescription medications that remove corns and calluses. Because many products contain corrosive materials, they must be applied to only the corn or callus. Patients should be alerted that products containing collodions are poisonous when ingested and that these products, as well as all other medications, should be stored out of children's reach. The box Patient Education for Corns and Calluses lists specific information to provide patients.

Evaluation of Patient Outcomes for Corns and Calluses

The progress of patients with hard corns or calluses should be checked after 14 days of treatment. The affected area should be visually inspected to determine whether the corns or calluses have decreased in size or resolved. The methods used to eliminate the corns or calluses should also be evaluated. If these conditions are still present, the patient should seek further medical evaluation.

Bunions

Nearly half of Americans have bunions. Women are 10 times more likely than men to develop bunions because of improperly fitting shoes with narrow toe boxes or too-high heels. Often, several family members suffer from this disorder. Obesity can

also lead to a higher prevalence of bunion formation. However, despite a positive family history, aggravating circumstances (e.g., wearing tight shoes) must also be present for a bunion to actually develop.[14,18,19]

Pathophysiology of Bunions

The hallux, or great toe, and the inner side of the foot provide the elasticity and mobility needed to walk or run. Prolonged pressure over the prominent, angulated metatarsophalangeal joint of the great toe from external shoe irritation may result in painful inflammation, swelling, and exostosis over the involved bony joint structure (Figure 43–3). This process may result in bunion formation, as shown in Figure 43–4.

Bunions can be caused by various conditions. Pressure on the metatarsal head of the great toe may result from the manner in which a person sits, walks, or stands. In women, pressure from high-heeled shoes and too-narrow or too-shallow toe boxes forces the side of the toe inward and can aggravate the condition. Friction on the toes from bone malformations (wide heads or lateral bending) is also a major factor in bunion production, as are biomechanical defects. Vigorous exercise such as running or jumping can cause or exacerbate existing bunions. Bunions can increase the severity of a hallux valgus deformity, a deviation of the great toe, toward the lateral side of the foot.[14,16,18]

Clinical Presentation of Bunions

Bunions are usually asymptomatic but may become quite painful, swollen, red, and tender. The bunion itself is usually covered by an extensive keratinous overgrowth. The bunion may have a fluid-filled sack called bursitis. Patients may experience increased pain or decreased movement of the great toe.[18–20]

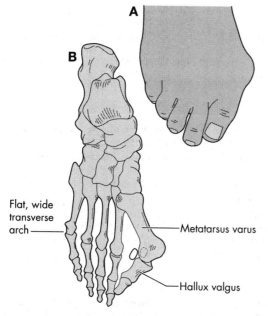

figure
43-3

Two views of hallux valgus. **A,** Gross representation of hallux valgus. **B,** Bone structure of hallux valgus.

Labels on figure: Flat, wide transverse arch; Metatarsus varus; Hallux valgus

Treatment of Bunions

Corrective steps to alleviate bunions often depend on the degree of discomfort. In some cases, corrective surgery is necessary.

Treatment Goals

The self-treatment goals are to (1) decrease irritation of the affected area and (2) prevent worsening of the condition by correcting the cause.

General Treatment Approach

Bunions are not amenable to topical drug therapy, and the chronic use of oral nonprescription analgesics is not suggested. Management of the bunion should address the cause (e.g., tight-fitting or high-heeled shoes, excessive pronation of the foot, or a previous injury). Therefore, self-treatment includes avoiding high-heeled

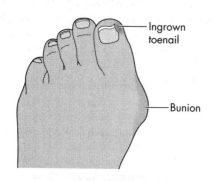

figure
43-4

Bunion and ingrown toenail.

Labels on figure: Ingrown toenail; Bunion

shoes; using protective padding (e.g., bunion pads or toe separators); and taking oral anti-inflammatory drugs on a short-term basis, if needed. Self-treatment relieves only the swelling caused by shoe friction; therefore, well-fitted shoes with a wide toe box should be worn at all times to prevent subsequent flares of inflammation. If shoe adjustments fail to alleviate pain, medical referral is indicated. Physical therapy may be beneficial to provide relief from pain and inflammation. Orthotics may help control irregularities of the foot movement.[18] Self-treatment of bunions and exclusion criteria are outlined in Figure 43–5.

Nonpharmacologic Therapy
Selection of Footwear

Table 43–1 provides guidelines for selecting properly fitted footwear.

Bunion Pads/Cushions

Topical nonprescription padding (e.g., moleskin) can be helpful and may be all that is necessary to decrease the irritation and inflammation from footwear. Before the protective pad is applied, the foot should be bathed and thoroughly dried. The pad is then cut into a shape that conforms to the bunion. If the intention is to relieve the pressure from the center of the bunion area, the pad should be cut to surround the bunion. Precut pads are available for immediate patient use. To minimize the risk of skin maceration and ulceration, the patient should avoid constant skin contact with adhesive-backed pads, unless their use is recommended by a podiatrist or health care provider.[13,21–22]

For patients who are allergic to adhesives, a nonmedicated, nonadhesive gel bunion cushion (i.e., Bunion Guard) can be used for up to 3 months. Toe separators (i.e., Bunion Relievers) may also be used in conjunction with pads to align crooked toes and relieve irritation between toes.[13]

Larger footwear may be necessary to compensate for the space taken up by the pad; in fact, failure to increase shoe size appropriately may cause pressure in other areas. In addition, protective pads should not be used on bunions when the skin is broken or blistered. Abraded skin should receive palliative treatment before pads are applied. If symptoms persist, these patients should consult a podiatrist or orthopedist.

Assessment of Bunions: A Case-Based Approach

Measures discussed in Assessment of Corns and Calluses: A Case-Based Approach also apply to bunions. Specific information to obtain from patients includes the bunion's location, duration, and possible association with specific footwear, as well as the degree of discomfort it causes. Asking about methods used to relieve symptoms (e.g., shoes, cushioning pads, or NSAIDs) is also important.

Patient Counseling for Bunions

It should be stressed to patients that effective, long-term treatment of bunions is to remove the source of irritation. Patients who do not achieve permanent relief by changing footwear

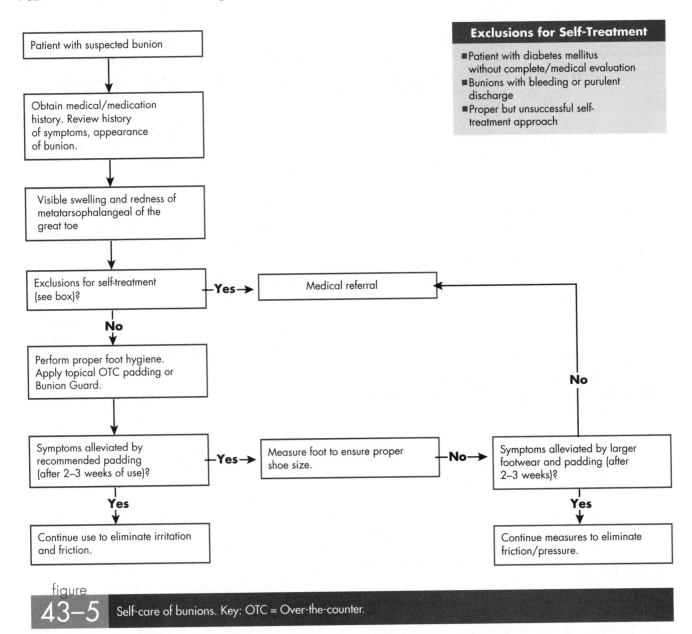

Exclusions for Self-Treatment

- Patient with diabetes mellitus without complete/medical evaluation
- Bunions with bleeding or purulent discharge
- Proper but unsuccessful self-treatment approach

figure

43–5   Self-care of bunions. Key: OTC = Over-the-counter.

should consult a podiatrist or orthopedist to determine whether anatomic defects are causing bunions. The proper short-term use of bunion pads and cushions should be explained to patients who want to use them. In addition, nondrug measures such as applying ice to relieve pain and inflammation can be recommended.[13,21,22] The box Patient Education for Bunions lists specific information to provide patients.

Evaluation of Patient Outcomes for Bunions

Bunions that are not caused by biomechanical defects of the foot may take a few weeks to resolve, depending on the severity of the irritation. Follow-up should occur after 2–3 weeks to determine whether wearing new shoes and using bunion cushions or pads have eliminated the discomfort. If the patient is still experiencing discomfort, medical referral is appropriate.[21,22]

Tired, Aching Feet and Other Painful Disorders

With every step taken (8000–10,000 steps each day), gravity-induced pressure of up to twice the body's weight bears down on each foot, releasing powerful shocks of energy that the foot's natural padding must struggle to absorb.[1,20,23] In an unpadded shoe, the shock as the foot strikes the ground is absorbed throughout the foot, ankle, leg, and back. This shock can fatigue muscles, resulting in tired, aching feet and/or back pain.[20,23,24]

An estimated two-thirds of Americans suffer from tired, aching feet (the most common foot problem). In addition, 2 million adults are estimated to suffer from heel pain. People simply do not realize the daily abuse their feet must endure.[25]

Pathophysiology of Tired, Aching Feet and Other Painful Foot Disorders

Aching feet can be caused by increased frequency of standing and/or walking (especially on hard surfaces), age-related erosion of the fat padding on the bottom of the foot, circulatory or neurologic disorders, and poor-fitting/inappropriate footwear.[20,23,25]

Because the cause of heel pain is difficult to determine, treatment can often be prolonged and expensive. The three common types of heel pain are heel spurs (i.e., bony growths on the underside of the heel bone),[20,24] plantar fasciitis (strain on the connective tissue that attaches the arch to the front of the heel),[26] and Sever's disease (calcaneal apophysitis).[12,27]

Heel spurs are the result of strained foot muscles and the wearing away of the fat tissue surrounding the heel bone. Incorrect walking or running technique, excessive running, poor-fitting shoes, obesity, and aging are common contributors to this condition.[9,18]

Plantar fasciitis is caused by high arches, flat feet, repetitive stress during athletic activity, pronated feet, or prolonged standing. This disorder can be determined by the patient's description of the pain and its occurrence.[16,18,19,24,26]

Sever's disease is heel pain seen in children that is precipitated by running, jumping, and excessive walking. It predominately occurs in males between ages 8 and 15 years and usually resolves once the bone has completed growth or activity is lessened.[27]

Clinical Presentation of Tired, Aching Feet, and Other Painful Foot Disorders

Individuals who suffer from tired, aching feet most often describe either general foot pain or heel pain. Calcium deposits may form on the calcaneous bone (heel spurs) from constant foot stress. Heel spurs are detected via X-ray; they cause pain of increasing intensity after prolonged periods of rest. Plantar fasciitis usually presents with pain from the first moment the person gets out of bed in the morning or stands up after sitting; the pain results from tissue contraction. The sensation on the bottom of the heel is quite painful, and the patient may complain of a burning sensation.[12,14,16,18,26] Sever's disease presents with no swelling, skin changes, erythema, or visible abnormalities. The squeeze test aids in the diagnosis of Sever's disease: pressure is applied at the point of attachment of the calcaneal apophysis to the main body of the os calcis to determine if the patient experiences pain.[27]

Treatment of Tired, Aching Feet and Other Painful Foot Disorders
Treatment Goals

The primary goal in self-treating tired, aching feet, and other painful foot disorders is to provide additional support and shock absorbance for the feet in order to reduce foot pain and fatigue. Stretching muscles to prevent limitations on daily activities is also desired.

General Treatment Approach

The first measure to avoid tired, aching feet is to use well-fitted footwear that has sufficient padding and cushioning (Table 43–1). Wearing sport-specific shoes with good arch support (e.g., running shoes) is an excellent measure for preventing heel pain. Individuals should purchase shoes carefully to ensure a proper fit.[14,18]

Individuals who are physically active or stand for prolonged periods during the day may need to take additional measures, such as replacing worn shoes or heel pads, using a night splint, strapping or taping the arch, decreasing the amount of weight-bearing activity, and, if necessary, entering a weight-reduction program.[24] Oral nonprescription anti-inflammatory agents and topical anti-inflammatory treatments such as ice applications (Table 43–4) are also appropriate. Magnesium sulfate baths (Epsom salts) have historically been used for soothing tired aching muscles, sprains, and bruising, but no scientific evidence supports these claims. When self-treatment fails, patients should be referred to an appropriate health care provider for evaluation of possible bony malalignments and possible orthotic therapy. Figure 43–6 outlines self-treatment of tired, aching feet and other painful foot disorders.

table 43-4   Guidelines for Applying Cold Compresses

Ice Bag Method

- Fill the ice bag with crushed or shaved ice to one-half to two-thirds of its capacity, if possible. These forms of ice will ensure greater contact with the injured body part.
- If needed, break ice into walnut-sized pieces with no jagged edges. An overfilled bag will be difficult to apply because it will not rest on the contour of the body area.
- After filling the bag, squeeze out trapped air. Then dry the outside of the bag and check for leaks.
- Bind the injured body part with a wet elastic wrap, and then apply the ice bag. The wet wrap aids transfer of cold to the injured area.
- If the ankle is being treated, keep it in a dorsiflexed position (foot toward the nose) when it is wrapped in the elastic bandage.
- Apply the ice bag to the specific body part.
- To avoid tissue damage, apply the ice bag for 10 minutes and then remove it for 10 minutes. If the bag is not cloth covered, wrap the injured area or the ice bag in a thin towel to prevent tissue damage.
- Follow this procedure 3–4 times a day.
- For most injuries, continue the cryotherapy until swelling decreases or for a maximum of 12–24 hours. Application of ice may be necessary for up to 48–72 hours, depending on the severity of the injury. (For example, the maximum swelling of ankle injuries may occur up to 48 hours after the injury.)
- Before storing the ice bag, drain it and allow it to air dry. If possible, turn it inside out for more efficient drying. Cap the bag and store it in a cool, dry place.

Cold Wraps

- To activate a single-use cold pack, squeeze the middle of the pack to burst the bubble. This action initiates an endothermic reaction of ammonium nitrate, water, and special additives.
- For a reusable cold wrap (cold pack or gel pack), store it in the freezer for 2 hours. Do not put the cloth cover in the freezer.
- Remove the cold wrap from the freezer, insert it in the cloth cover, and apply it to the injured body part.
- If the cold wrap is uncomfortable, remove it for 1–2 minutes and then reapply it.
- Alternate application of the cold wrap (10 minutes on; 10 minutes off) 3–4 times a day for 24–48 hours.
- After use, store the cold wrap in the freezer.
- Although some gel packs are nontoxic, keep all cold wraps out of children's reach.

Source: References 25 and 39

Nonpharmacologic Therapy

Shoe Inserts, Partial Insoles, and Heel Cups/Cushions

Full-shoe inserts, which can provide cushioning and absorb shock, are available in various sizes and thicknesses to accommodate most individuals. These inserts help decrease the incidence of lower back pain associated with the impact from walking. The patient must select an insert that conforms to the type of shoe worn.[8,9]

Partial insoles are preferred when a patient needs cushioning or support in a certain portion of the shoe. For example, metatarsal arch supports, which fit into the ball-of-foot region of a woman's shoe, help lift the arch behind the toes to alleviate pain associated with the spreading of the foot, a condition that occurs with increasing age. There are inserts specifically designed to fit in high heels (e.g., Dr. Scholl's for Her High Heel Insoles). Finally, the arch support insert is intended to cushion and support painful longitudinal arches.[9,14]

A heel cup or heel cushion may be indicated, depending on the location and extent of the pain. For example, a heel cushion might be appropriate when the pain is confined to the bottom of the heel. A heel cushion supports the entire heel as it elevates the sensitive area to prevent further irritation. Alternatively, when the pain is widespread and diffuse, a heel cup might be more appropriate. Heel cups help relieve the pain caused by the breakdown of the heel's natural padding or by intense athletic activity.

Caution should be used when selecting shoe inserts. If an insole affects the patient's gait, the patient should be referred to a podiatrist or pedorthist; the latter specializes in the designing, manufacturing, modifying, and fitting of footwear and orthotics. Insoles should be used only to cushion the foot, not to correct malformation, which requires a specialist's attention.

Compression Stockings

Compression stockings are also an option to enhance support for individuals who spend many hours on their feet. Compression stockings may be purchased without a prescription in compressions ranging from 15 to 40 mm Hg. These stockings will decrease inflammation by improving circulation, thereby reducing fatigue of the feet, legs, and back.[28,29]

Assessment of Tired, Aching Feet and Other Painful Disorders

Treatment of tired, aching feet requires evaluation of lifestyle factors (e.g., occupation, daily exercise, and footwear); the possibility of underlying pathology (e.g., circulatory or neurologic disorders); the possibility of an aggravating event; and the walking/working surface. If underlying pathology is suspected, the patient should be referred to a primary care provider or podiatrist for initial evaluation.

Patient Counseling for Tired, Aching Feet and Other Painful Foot Disorders

The provider can play an integral role in counseling patients on preventing and treating foot disorders caused by friction and excessive impact. The cornerstone of preventing these disorders is selecting the appropriate footwear. If the disorder persists after a change in footwear, the provider can help patients select in-shoe supports and advise them of other measures to reduce the impact of weight-bearing activities. The box Patient Education for Tired, Aching Feet and Other Painful Foot Disorders lists specific information to provide patients.

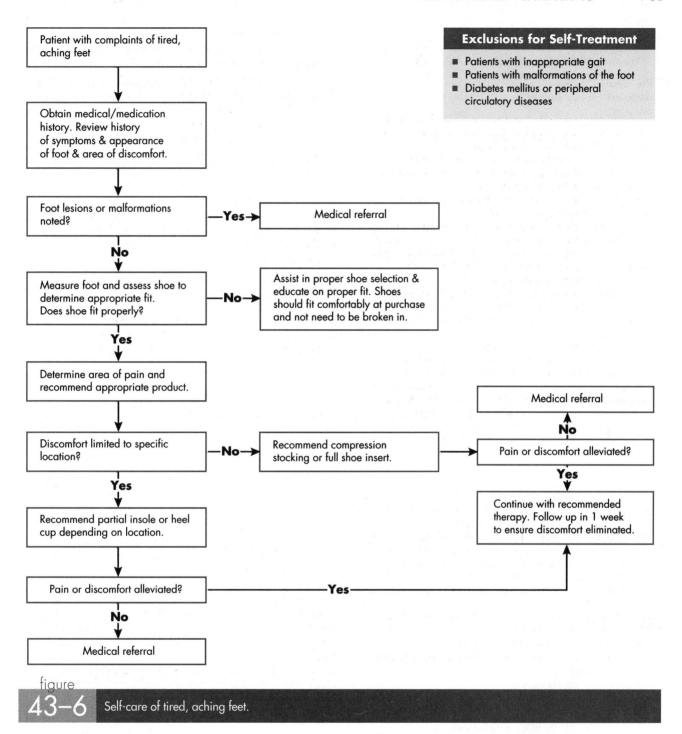

Patient with complaints of tired, aching feet

↓

Obtain medical/medication history. Review history of symptoms & appearance of foot & area of discomfort.

↓

Foot lesions or malformations noted? —**Yes**→ Medical referral

No ↓

Measure foot and assess shoe to determine appropriate fit. Does shoe fit properly? —**No**→ Assist in proper shoe selection & educate on proper fit. Shoes should fit comfortably at purchase and not need to be broken in.

Yes ↓

Determine area of pain and recommend appropriate product.

↓

Discomfort limited to specific location? —**No**→ Recommend compression stocking or full shoe insert. → Pain or discomfort alleviated? —**No**→ Medical referral

Yes ↓ (Discomfort limited to specific location)

Recommend partial insole or heel cup depending on location.

↓

Pain or discomfort alleviated? —**Yes**→ Continue with recommended therapy. Follow up in 1 week to ensure discomfort eliminated.

No ↓

Medical referral

Pain or discomfort alleviated? **Yes** ↓ Continue with recommended therapy. Follow up in 1 week to ensure discomfort eliminated.

figure 43-6 Self-care of tired, aching feet.

Evaluation of Patient Outcomes for Tired, Aching Feet and Other Painful Foot Disorders

Resolution of pain in the soles or heels of the feet depends on whether the patient has exclusions for self-treatment and how long the foot problem has persisted. Follow-up should occur after 1 week to determine whether the use of new shoes and/or in-shoe supports has eliminated the discomfort. If the symptoms persist, the patient should consult a podiatrist for evaluation.

Exercise-Induced Foot Injuries

Providers should be aware of possible exercise-induced foot injuries, particularly those caused by running, jogging, or other high-impact physical activities (Figure 43–7). Often, individuals fail to take certain precautions and dive head first into a strenuous exercise program. To minimize potential injuries and dangers, individuals who are typically sedentary, are older than 35 years, have hypertension, or have a history of heart disease or diabetes should seek medical evaluation before beginning a strenuous exercise program. Patients with potential orthopedic problems may benefit from walking instead of performing strenuous forms of exercise.[30]

Treatment of Exercise-Induced Foot Injuries

Treatment Goals

The goals in self-treating exercise-induced foot problems are to (1) relieve any pain, (2) prevent secondary bacterial infection if

the skin is broken, and (3) institute measures to prevent further injury.

General Treatment Approach

Measures to prevent exercise-induced injuries entail using suitable footwear that fits properly (Table 43–1); running on the proper surface; using correct posture (i.e., running erect); and stretching muscles before exercising. Most running injuries can be successfully treated with measures such as shoe modifications, shoe inserts, and in-shoe supports, as discussed in the section Treatment of Tired, Aching Feet and Other Painful Foot Disorders.

If an injury to the leg or foot occurs, activity must usually be interrupted to allow the injured leg or foot to rest. Relative rest (i.e., avoiding activities that produce the symptoms) is often indicated. Alternative exercise such as swimming, rowing, and/or bicycling (stationary or outdoor) should be encouraged.

If the injury warrants it, the patient can be instructed on selecting and using nonprescription accessories (e.g., cryotherapy, a compression ice wrap, ice bags, compression bandages, arch supports, and heel cushions) that will alleviate injuries or problems. Systemic analgesics can also relieve the pain and inflammation of minor foot injuries (see Chapter 5).

Nonpharmacologic Therapy

Table 43–5 provides specific recommendations for self-treatment of the discussed exercise-induced foot injuries.[28–39]

Athletic Footwear

Appropriate footwear can be a powerful tool for manipulating human movement and can greatly influence the healing of injured tissues, both positively and negatively. The importance of appropriate footwear has been reported by Cheung and Ng.[37] Their study demonstrated that the type of footwear chosen by recreational runners is important to prevent injury. Consequently, inappropriate or worn-out shoes can result in

figure
43–7
Selected foot and leg injuries associated with excessive impact shock.

table
43–5 Differentiation and Management of Exercise-Induced Foot Injuries

Type of Injury	Common Causes	Pathophysiology	Signs/Symptoms	Recommendations
Shin splints	Overzealous workout; inappropriate stretching; running/walking on sloped or hard surfaces; wearing ill-fitting footwear; overstriding	Excessive pronation weakens/strains posterior tibialis; anterior tibial muscle stretches away from periosteum that lines shinbone	Pain in medial lower third of shin, or below knee and above ankle; pain worsens with exercise; cramping, burning, and tightness on anterior lateral section of shin	PRICE or RICE therapy; acetaminophen or ibuprofen; shoe orthotic; medical referral
Stress fracture	Running on hard, rigid surfaces; rapid increase in physical activity; jumping; estrogen deficiency; nutritional deficiencies; obesity; ill-fitting footwear	Outer cortex of long bones of leg or foot cracks from alternation in tensile forces sent by ligaments, tendons, and muscles	Deep pain in lower leg; tender to the touch; swelling; pain worsens with exercise	Medical referral; complete rest; NSAID therapy
Achilles tendonitis	Running on hills or in sand; ill-fitting footwear; excessive pronation; arthritis	Inflammation of Achilles tendon; rupture of tendon	Posterior heel pain; tenderness; swelling	Medical referral
Blisters	Repetitive movement; ill-fitting footwear; tight hosiery	Continual friction on small surface of foot separates stratum corneum and stratum lucidum skin layers, causing space between layers to fill with fluid	Accumulation of fluid beneath stratum corneum; may be painful	Do not remove blister; protect with topical bandage; medical referral for drainage, if needed
Ankle sprains	Ankle rotating outside acceptable range	Lateral ligament damage	Pain; bruising; tenderness; difficulty walking	PRICE or RICE therapy; compression bandage
Intermetatarsal neuritis	Small toe box space	Inflammation of nerves from compression of or entanglement between metatarsal heads and digital bases	Pain and numbness between toes	Proper footwear
Toenail loss	Long, thick toenails in small toe box space; friction and pressure from running in "stop and go" sports, such as tennis	Fluid beneath nail plate pushes toenail from nail bed	Dark discoloration from blood underneath nail plate; pain at toe; nail loss	Referral to podiatrist or PCP

Key: NSAID = Nonsteroidal anti-inflammatory drug; PCP = primary care provider; PRICE = protection, rest, ice, compression, elevation; RICE = rest, ice, compression, elevation.
Source: References 28–39.

foot injuries and pain. Athletic shoes should be replaced after 200–400 miles of use, as detailed by Meadows.[38]

Compression Bandages

Typically, a compression bandage (e.g., Ace Bandages) is used for an ankle or knee sprain. If a compression bandage is to be used, the width of the bandage depends on the injury site. For example, a foot or an ankle requires a 2- to 3-inch bandage.[39] Table 43–6 describes the proper method of applying this type of bandage.

Cryotherapy

Applying cold compresses to an injury such as a muscle sprain anesthetizes the area and decreases the pain and inflammation. Ice bags or cold wraps are useful for cold application in 10-minute increments. Table 43–4 describes the proper method of cold application to injuries.

Contrast Bath Soaks

For acute injury, cold application is beneficial during the first 48 hours to decrease ensuing inflammation. After the acute injury, some podiatrists advocate the use of alternating applications of cold therapy and warm therapy for chronic, nagging pain. Specifically, the cold therapy is intended to decrease inflammation. The warm therapy attempts to bring increased blood flow to the affected area and effect smooth muscle relaxation.

Assessment of Exercise-Induced Foot Injuries

The provider may be called on to play a triage role in treating an exercise-induced injury to the foot (Figure 43–8). Identifying the location of the pain will help determine the type and extent of the injury. Asking about the nature and duration of the pain will help in determining whether the injury is self-treatable.

table
43–6 Application Guidelines for Compression Bandages

- Choose the appropriate size of bandage for the injured body part. If you are unsure of the size, purchase a product designed for the appropriate body part.
- Recommended elastic bandage widths according to coverage area:
  - 2 inches: foot, wrist, ankle
  - 3 inches: elbow, knee, ankle
  - 4 inches: knee, lower leg, shoulder
  - 6 inches: shoulder, upper leg, chest
- Unwind about 12–18 inches of bandage at a time, and allow the bandage to relax.
- If ice is also being applied to the injured area, soak the bandage in water to aid the transfer of cold (Table 43–4).
- Wrap the injured area by overlapping the previous layer of bandage by about one-third to one-half of its width.
- Tightly wrap the point most distal from the injury. For example, if the ankle is injured, begin wrapping just above the toes.
- Decrease the tightness of the bandage as you continue to wrap. (Follow package directions on how far to extend the bandage past the injury.) If the bandage feels tight or uncomfortable or if circulation is impaired, remove the compression bandage and rewrap it. Cold or swollen toes and fingers indicate that the bandage is too tight.
- After using the bandage, wash it in lukewarm, soapy water; do not scrub it. Rinse the bandage thoroughly, and allow it to air-dry on a flat surface. Roll up the bandage to prevent wrinkles, and store it in a cool, dry place. Do not iron the bandage to remove wrinkles.

Source: Reference 39.

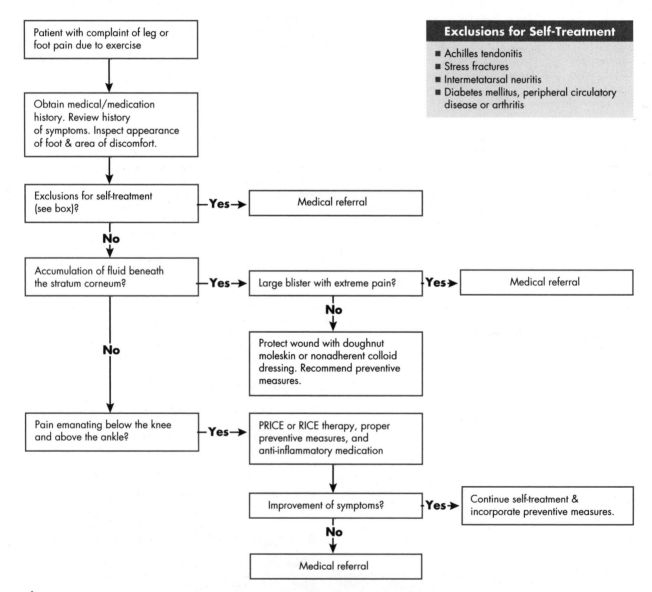

figure

43–8 Self-care of exercise-induced injuries. Key: PRICE = Protection, rest, ice, compression, and elevation; RICE = rest, ice, compression, and elevation.

Patient Counseling for Exercise-Induced Foot Injuries

Rest and appropriate preventive measures for the patient's particular injury should be explained. When rest alone does not relieve foot discomfort, the proper use of oral nonprescription analgesics, compression bandages, and cryotherapy should be recommended. The correct procedure for wrapping a bandage, which is also described on the package, should be reviewed with the patient. If inappropriate use of a compression bandage is a concern, simply elevating the body part and applying an ice pack should be recommended. If warranted by the severity of the injury, medical referral should be recommended. The box Patient Education for Exercise-Induced Injuries lists specific information to provide patients.

Evaluation of Patient Outcomes for Exercise-Induced Injuries

Follow-up of patients who have shin splints or ankle sprains should occur 7 days after the use of compression bandages, cryotherapy, or other anti-inflammatory therapy to determine symptom resolution. If symptoms of swelling and/or pain persist, medical referral is appropriate. Patients with blisters on the feet or under the toenail should also be reevaluated after 7 days of the recommended therapy. If signs of infection are present or the toenail has separated from the nail bed, medical referral is appropriate.

Ingrown Toenails

The most frequent cause of ingrown toenails, or onychocryptosis, is incorrect trimming of the nails. The correct method is to cut the nail straight across, without tapering the corners. Wearing pointed-toe or tight shoes or too-tight hosiery has also been implicated. Other causes are hyperhidrosis, trauma, obesity, and excessive pressure on the toes. Direct pressure on a toe can force the lateral or medial edge of the nail into the soft tissue. The embedded nail may then continue to grow, resulting in swelling and inflammation of the nail fold.[8,10,38,40]

Bedridden patients may develop ingrown toenails if tight bedcovers press the soft skin tissue against the nails. Nail curling, which can be hereditary or secondary to incorrect nail trimming, onychomycosis, or a systemic, metabolic disease, can also result in ingrown toenails.

---

patient education for
Exercise-Induced Injuries

The objectives of self-treatment are to (1) rest the injured foot or limb to allow healing, (2) relieve discomfort, and (3) take measures to prevent further injury. For most patients, carefully following product instructions and the self-care measures listed here will help ensure optimal therapeutic outcomes.

General Measures

- When a leg or foot injury occurs, rest the injured limb. If desired, perform other types of exercise that do not put a great deal of force on the feet, such as swimming or bicycling (stationary or outdoor).
- Take the following actions to prevent exercise-induced injuries:
  - Stretch muscles before exercising.
  - Choose sport-specific shoes with good arch support for athletic activities.
  - Run or walk on a relatively smooth, level, and resilient surface.
  - Keep the back straight when running.

Shin Splints

- Rest the feet and apply an ice bag or a cold wrap to the painful area (Table 43–4).
- If desired, take aspirin or NSAIDs to relieve pain and reduce tissue inflammation.
- Do not use analgesics to suppress pain or to increase your endurance during a workout.

When to Seek Medical Attention

- Seek medical attention if the discomfort becomes a cramping, burning tightness that repeatedly occurs at the same distance or time during a run.

Blisters

- To prevent blisters during running, wear moisture-wicking socks (i.e., wool or acrylic). If desired, wear two pairs of socks with ordinary talcum powder sprinkled between them. Using an acrylic sock next to the foot will assist in drawing moisture from the foot.

- Apply compound tincture of benzoin or a flexible collodion product (e.g., New Skin) to the blister before exercise to decrease pain and accelerate healing by promoting reepithelialization.
- Apply an antiperspirant that contains aluminum chloride 20% to decrease incidence of blisters.
- If blisters break, apply a first-aid antibiotic to the broken skin to prevent secondary bacterial infection.
- Cover blistered area with moleskin to protect the surface.

Ankle Sprains

- Although maximum swelling will not occur for 48 hours, begin treatment as soon as possible.
- Stay off the injured foot, wrap a compression bandage around the ankle, apply ice, and elevate the ankle. (Tables 43–4 and 43–6 provide guidelines on applying ice and compression bandages.)

When to Seek Medical Attention

- Seek medical attention if swelling persists more than 72 hours.

Toenail Blisters/Loss

- To prevent blisters under the toenail, keep toenails trimmed and run in properly fitted shoes.
- Should a blister develop, do not disturb or puncture the blister roof.

When to Seek Medical Attention

- If the toenail separates from the skin or is lost, consult a primary care provider or podiatrist for proper treatment.

Pathophysiology of Ingrown Toenails

An ingrown toenail occurs when the nail curves and embeds into the flesh at the corner(s) of a toe, causing pain (Figure 43–4). Puncturing of the skin that is accompanied by soft tissue hypertrophy and subsequent invasion by opportunistic resident foot bacteria can cause a superficial infection. Swelling, inflammation, and ulceration are secondary complications that can arise from an ingrown toenail.[38]

Treatment of Ingrown Toenails

Treatment Goals

The goals of self-treating ingrown toenails are to (1) relieve pressure on the toenails, (2) relieve pain, and (3) prevent recurrence of the disorder.

General Treatment Approach

Patient education is the best means of preventing the development of ingrown toenails. In the early stages of development, therapy is directed at providing adequate room for the nail to resume its normal position adjacent to soft tissue. This therapy is accomplished by relieving the external source of pressure. Warm water soaks for 10–20 minutes several times a day until resolution will help soften the area. Topical antiseptics prescribed by a primary care provider can be applied to prevent possible opportunistic infections. Insertion of small cotton wisps or dental floss under the impinged nail edge has a 79% rate of symptomatic improvement. No evidence is linked to secondary infection from the cotton wisps or dental floss.[40] Medical referral is necessary if the condition is recurrent or gives rise to an oozing discharge, pain, or severe inflammation. Sometimes surgery is warranted; with subsequent systemic antibiotic therapy, the toe may take up to 3–4 weeks to heal. The most common surgical procedure is removal of the lateral edge of the nail followed by chemical matricectomy using phenolization. This process destroys the exposed nail-forming matrix.[38,40] Figure 43–9 outlines self-treatment options for ingrown toenails.[37]

Pharmacologic Therapy
Sodium Sulfide Gel

Dr. Scholl's Ingrown Toenail Pain Reliever contains sodium sulfide 1%. The gel is applied topically, and a retainer ring is

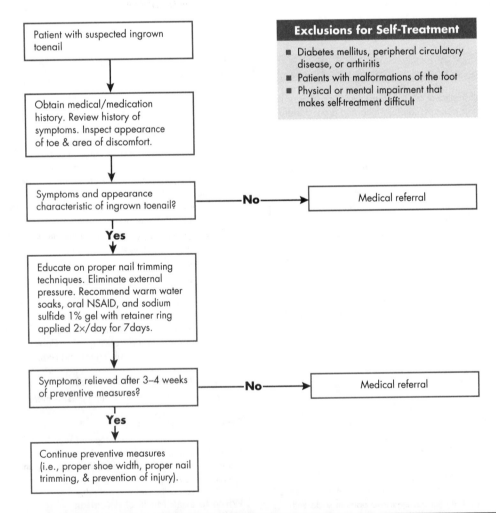

Exclusions for Self-Treatment

- Diabetes mellitus, peripheral circulatory disease, or arthiritis
- Patients with malformations of the foot
- Physical or mental impairment that makes self-treatment difficult

Patient with suspected ingrown toenail

↓

Obtain medical/medication history. Review history of symptoms. Inspect appearance of toe & area of discomfort.

↓

Symptoms and appearance characteristic of ingrown toenail? —**No**→ Medical referral

↓ **Yes**

Educate on proper nail trimming techniques. Eliminate external pressure. Recommend warm water soaks, oral NSAID, and sodium sulfide 1% gel with retainer ring applied 2×/day for 7days.

↓

Symptoms relieved after 3–4 weeks of preventive measures? —**No**→ Medical referral

↓ **Yes**

Continue preventive measures (i.e., proper shoe width, proper nail trimming, & prevention of injury).

figure
43–9   Self-care of ingrown toenails. Key: NSAID = Nonsteroidal anti-inflammatory drug.

then placed around the affected area to help maintain the product at the site of action. The mechanism of action of sodium sulfide 1% is relief of pain by softening the nail or by hardening the nail bed. It may be applied twice daily for up to 7 days for relief of the discomfort of ingrown toenails.[41–43] Providers must be aware of misleading trade-name products marketed for ingrown toenails. Products such as Outgro Pain-Relieving Formula contain benzocaine 20% to relieve pain associated with ingrown toenails, but this agent does not treat the underlying problem.[43–45]

Patients with ingrown toenails often fail to realize that oral medications to alleviate pain and inflammation may help their condition. Provided no contraindications exist for their use by a particular patient, oral aspirin, ibuprofen, or naproxen may be recommended; all are proven analgesics with anti-inflammatory activity (see Chapter 5).

Assessment of Ingrown Toenail

The provider can play a vital role in recommending measures for relieving acute pain from ingrown toenails and in preventing their recurrence. For relief of ingrown toenail, initial recommendations include warm bath soaks to soften the skin and oral anti-inflammatory therapy for temporary pain relief. If the toenail or nail bed is infected, immediate referral is warranted.

Patient Counseling for Ingrown Toenails

The box Patient Education for Ingrown Toenails lists specific information to provide patients.

Evaluation of Patient Outcomes for Ingrown Toenails

Patient evaluations should be made after 3–4 weeks to determine whether pressure relief and preventive measures have been successful. Medical referral is appropriate if the condition shows no improvement or worsens or if there is a discharge from the site of irritation.

Hyperhidrosis

Hyperhidrosis, or excessive sweating, comprises two types: primary focal hyperhidrosis and secondary hyperhidrosis. The incidence of hyperhidrosis is 2.8% of the U.S. population; it occurs equally in men and women.[46,47] It is most prevalent in people ages 25–64 years.[46] Hyperhidrosis is a complicated process that involves sympathetic and parasympathetic pathways.[46]

Primary focal hyperhidrosis is defined as visible, excessive sweating that has lasted 6 months without cause and that has two or more of the following characteristics: bilateral and symmetrical presentation, one or more episodes a week, hindrance of social activities, family history of the disorder, and absence of sweating during sleep.[44] This disorder seems to begin during childhood. Symptoms of hyperhidrosis usually improve with age. Family history is positive in 30%–50% of patients.[47] Hyperhidrosis can be embarrassing to affected individuals and may affect their daily activities, lifestyle, and social interactions. Although psychological morbidity is prevalent in most patients experiencing hyperhidrosis, few people seek medical attention for the disorder.

Secondary hyperhidrosis can have a focal or generalized presentation that affects the entire body. Secondary hyperhidrosis is usually caused by a variety of medical conditions. Examples include endocrine disorders (e.g., hyperthyroidism or diabetes mellitus); pregnancy; neurologic disorders; malignant disorders; cardiovascular disorders; respiratory failure; licit and illicit drug use; and alcohol abuse.[47] This discussion will focus on primary focal hyperhidrosis because nonprescription medications are available to treat it.

Pathophysiology of Hyperhidrosis

Primary focal hyperhidrosis occurs mainly in the palms, plantar surfaces, and axillae. The more than 4 million sweat glands in the body are classified as either eccrine or apocrine, with eccrine glands making up 75% of the total. Eccrine glands primarily produce colorless, odorless sweat and are located all over the body. They are more concentrated in the soles of the feet, forehead, and palms. The apocrine glands are scented sweat glands

---

patient education for
Ingrown Toenails

The ultimate goals for self-treatment of ingrown toenails are to relieve the pain and pressure associated with the condition and to prevent recurrence.

- Ensure that shoes fit properly to eliminate pressure on the toenails (Table 43–1).
- Prevent recurrence of ingrown toenails by cutting toenails straight across, rather than at an angle.
- Decrease pain and swelling of the ingrown toenail by taking a nonsteroidal anti-inflammatory medication such as ibuprofen or naproxen.

- Relieve impingement of the nail by soaking your feet in warm water to soften the nail and the skin around it.
- Place cotton wisps or dental floss under the edge of the ingrown nail for almost immediate pain relief.

located in the axillae and genital areas. The pathophysiology of hyperhidrosis is not fully understood, but it may be caused by dysfunction of the autonomic nervous system. It seems that once sweating begins, a vicious cycle predominates, and evaporative cooling of the skin increases a reflex sympathetic outflow, which actually increases sweating.[47]

Clinical Presentation of Hyperhidrosis

The most common sign of hyperhidrosis is profuse sweating.[47] Excessive sweating is considered to be any amount of sweat that interferes with daily life and activities. Laboratory diagnosis is not necessary. The starch–iodine test has been used to identify the primary area of sweating. Starch is applied to the area previously covered by an iodine solution. The starch/iodine solution turns a dark blue color wherever excessive sweating is present. This test helps direct treatment to the affected areas and allows providers to note improvement in treated areas as a subsequent decrease in the focal area.[46,48]

No physical complications are associated with focal hyperhidrosis. Some patients may experience odor problems from sweaty feet or underarms. Psychological complications may result from the embarrassment of hyperhidrosis. More than 35% of patients report they have altered their lifestyle by decreasing leisure activity time because of hyperhidrosis. Simple social interactions such as shaking hands, holding hands, and hugging may be difficult.

Treatment of Hyperhidrosis
Treatment Goals

The main goal of treatment is to eliminate profuse sweating in a cost-effective, minimally invasive method. Several types of treatments are available.

General Treatment Approach

Patients should consider convenience, ease of administration, side effects, and cost in choosing the best self-treatment. Figure 43–10 outlines this process.

Nonpharmacologic Therapy

One of the primary concerns of this disorder is its psychosocial implications. Psychotherapy has been beneficial in a small number of cases.[49] Few noninvasive methods to treat hyperhidrosis are available because the disease involves mainly the autonomic nervous system. Several surgical and nonsurgical treatments are available. Iontophoresis is used as a second-line therapy for hyperhidrosis.[46–48] This treatment, which involves the passage of a direct electrical current onto the skin, is safe and effective for plantar hyperhidrosis. Its mechanism of action may be related to induction of hyperkeratosis of the sweat pores, which obstructs sweat flow and secretion.[46–50]

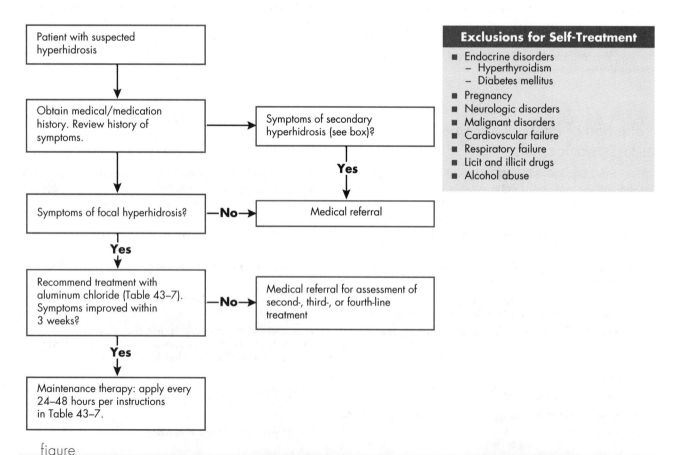

figure
43–10 Self-care of hyperhidrosis.

Pharmacologic Therapy

Several pharmacologic treatments are available for hyperhidrosis. Aluminum chloride is recommended as first-line treatment in hyperhidrosis because it is inexpensive and relatively easy to administer.[46][47,50] The same treatments used in axillary hyperhidrosis are used for treatment of plantar hyperhidrosis. The most common nonprescription treatments are topical aluminum salts. Aluminum salts indicated for treatment of excessive perspiration are commonly found in nonprescription antiperspirants. Their mechanism of action is related to mechanical obstruction of the eccrine gland duct or atrophy of eccrine secretory ducts.[46] Aluminum chloride solutions are available in concentrations of 20%–25%. The nonprescription antiperspirant Certain Dri contains 12% aluminum chloride and is available as a roll-on antiperspirant. Drysol is a common prescription drug used to treat hyperhidrosis; it contains aluminum chloride hexahydrate 20% topical solution in absolute anhydrous ethyl alcohol.

Frequent applications, every 24–48 hours, of products that contain aluminum chloride are needed; improvement may be seen as early as 3 weeks. Patients should apply the product sparingly at bedtime and wash it off after 6–8 hours. To prevent stinging and burning, patients should not apply the product after bathing or shaving, or to broken, irritated skin.[46-48] The short duration of action and frequency of repeated applications make these products inconvenient for patients. The side effects associated with use of aluminum chloride solution include localized burning, stinging, and irritation. Hydrocortisone can be applied if irritation occurs. These agents may be used on the hands, axillae, or feet. Products containing aluminum chloride should not be used on children and patients with reduced renal function. Also, patients who are pregnant or lactating should not use these products because their safety for use in these patients has not been studied.

Botulinum toxin A (Botox), a neurotoxin produced by clostridium botulinum, is a third-line treatment that is available by prescription and administered by a health care provider. It inhibits the release of acetylcholine, which causes excessive perspiring, from sympathetic nerves.[46] Botulinum toxin A is indicated for axillary hyperhidrosis and has shown great promise in treating the disorder.

Some patients with hyperhidrosis who do not want to consider surgery or prescription medications have found that insoles such as Summer Soles and other foot inserts help keep the feet comfortable. They prevent the slipping and sliding in shoes that sometimes occur when the feet are wet. These products, which are made of a wool and rayon blend that absorbs sweat, are available online and in some shoe stores. Some patients may add talcum powder to their shoes or apply it to their feet. However, this measure does not stop or slow the physiologic sweating that occurs with hyperhidrosis. The water and powder combination can also result in a glue-like substance.

Assessment of Hyperhidrosis: A Case-Based Approach

For proper assessment of hyperhidrosis, the patient's medical history and medication history related to this disorder are needed. Most often, patients with hyperhidrosis have had symptoms since childhood. A comfortable screening area may allow observation of the bilateral excessive sweating. The health care provider should also discuss treatment options and determine the patient's comfort level with the treatment standards and the expense and invasiveness of the therapies.

Case 43–2 illustrates the assessment of a patient with hyperhidrosis.

---

case
43–2

Relevant Evaluation Criteria	Scenario/Model Outcome
Information Gathering	
1. Gather essential information about the patient's symptoms and medical history, including:	
a. description of symptom(s) (i.e., nature, onset, duration, severity, associated symptoms)	Patient presents with perfuse sweating of her feet that makes wearing shoes uncomfortable.
b. description of any factors that seem to precipitate, exacerbate, and/or relieve the patient's symptom(s)	Warm weather or situations that make her nervous make her symptoms worse.
c. description of the patient's efforts to relieve the symptoms	The patient has tried rubbing aluminum chloride hexahydrate solution (Drysol) on her feet every other night. She also uses Summer Soles in her shoes during the summer so that she can wear sandals without her feet slipping.
d. patient's identity	Connie Smith
e. age, sex, height, and weight	35 years old, female, 5 ft 6 in, 145 lb
f. patient's occupation	Nurse
g. patient's dietary habits	Vegetarian; eats three meals and two snacks a day.
h. patient's sleep habits	Averages 5–6 hours per night.
i. concurrent medical conditions, prescription and nonprescription medications, and dietary supplements	Known diagnosis of plantar and palmer hyperhidrosis. Takes 1 One A Day vitamin daily with her breakfast.

case

43-2 *continued*

Relevant Evaluation Criteria	Scenario/Model Outcome
j. allergies	NKDA
k. history of other adverse reactions to medications	None
l. other (describe) _____	Connie says that she is tired of this situation and would like advice on what she should do about her sweaty feet.

Assessment and Triage

2. Differentiate patient's signs/symptoms and correctly identify the patient's primary problem(s).	The patient is experiencing plantar hyperhidrosis.
3. Identify exclusions for self-treatment (Figure 43–10).	None
4. Formulate a comprehensive list of therapeutic alternatives for the primary problem to determine if triage to a health care provider is required, and share this information with the patient or caregiver.	Options include: (1) Recommend OTC products for focal hyperhidrosis. (2) Refer patient for plantar hyperhidrosis. (3) Take no action.

Plan

5. Select an optimal therapeutic alternative to address the patient's problem, taking into account patient preferences.	Patient should consult a health care provider because the response to treatment of her hyperhidrosis with topical preparations and nonpharmacologic measures has been inadequate. Options such as Botox therapy or surgical treatment may be warranted.
6. Describe the recommended therapeutic approach to the patient or caregiver.	"You should consult a health care provider about your hyperhidrosis."
7. Explain to the patient or caregiver the rationale for selecting the recommended therapeutic approach from the considered therapeutic alternatives.	"This option is best because you have tried nonprescription products without success. Second-line therapy is iontophoresis. You will need to consult your health care provider for details about iontophoresis or other possible options."

Patient Education

8. When recommending self-care with nonprescription medications and/or nondrug therapy, convey accurate information to the patient or caregiver.	Criterion does not apply in this case.
Solicit follow-up questions from the patient or caregiver.	"Is this a common problem in women?"
Answer the patient's or caregiver's questions.	"Hyperhidrosis occurs in 2.8% of the population; it occurs equally in men and women."

Evaluation of Patient Outcome

9. Assess patient outcome.	Contact Connie in a day or two to ensure that she made an appointment and sought medical care.

Key: NDKA = No known allergies; OTC = over-the-patient education for counter.

Patient Counseling for Hyperhidrosis

The box Patient Education for Hyperhidrosis provides specific information for patients.

Evaluation of Patient Outcomes for Hyperhidrosis

Patients and health care providers should discuss the expectations of the treatment modalities used for hyperhidrosis. In addition, patients may need to incorporate a routine to allow continued compliance with treatments that require consistent reapplications. The patients' quality of life should be discussed to determine whether the treatments are effective in improving daily activities.

Key Points for Minor Foot Disorders

➤ The nonprescription drug of choice to treat corns and calluses is salicylic acid in a collodion-like vehicle or plaster form.

➤ Predisposing factors responsible for corns and calluses must be corrected.

➤ Patients should also be cautioned that frequent recurrence of any of these foot disorders is an indication to consult a podiatrist or health care provider.

➤ Patients with diabetes, circulatory problems, and/or arthritis should be counseled to avoid self-medicating with any topical or oral nonprescription drug without first checking with their health care provider.

➤ Nonprescription products are powerful drugs and may exacerbate certain conditions; the provider must monitor patient progress carefully and be attuned to patient comments that might indicate the occurrence of drug-related problems.

➤ Providers should be prepared to educate and assist patients who develop exercise-induced injuries.

➤ Most exercise-induced injuries can be treated with shoe modifications, in-shoe supports, modified training methods, ice applications, and stretching exercises.

➤ Maintaining good foot hygiene is an important component of overall health care.

➤ Talking with patients about proper foot hygiene is an important aspect of caring for the patient as a whole.[50]

➤ Aluminum salts are commonly used in nonprescription products used to treat focal hyperhidrosis, which occurs in the palms, plantar surfaces, and axillae.

REFERENCES

1. Georgia Podiatric Medical Association. Foot facts. Accessed at http://www.gapma.com/Foot-Facts, March 15, 2013.

2. Khan M. Podiatric management in epidermolysis bullosa. *Dermatol Clin.* 2010;28(2):325–33.

3. Singh N, Armstrong DG, Lipsky BA. Preventing foot ulcers in patients with diabetes. *JAMA.* 2005;293(2):217–28.

4. Stolt M, Suhonen R, Puukka P, et al. Foot health and self-care activities of older people in home care. *J Clin Nurs.* 2012;21(21–22):3082–95.

5. Smith RG. Common foot disorders in patients with diabetes. *Drug Top.* 2005;149(9):57–66.

6. Schroeder SM, Blume P. Foot infections. Accessed at http://www.emedicine.com/orthoped/topic601.htm, April 1, 2013.

7. Corns and calluses—baby your feet. *Mayo Clin Health Lett.* 2008;26(4):7. Accessed at http://healthletter.mayoclinic.com/health/pdf/88/200804.PDF, September 15, 2014.

8. Auerbach. *Wilderness Medicine.* 6th ed. Maryland Heights, MO: Mosby; 2011:Chap 29.

9. Lyman TP, Vlahovac TC. Foot care from A to Z. *Dermatol Nurs.* 2010;22(5):2–7.

10. Menz HB, Morris ME. Footwear characteristics and foot problems in older people. *Gerontology.* 2005;51(5):346–51.

11. All Children's Hospital, John Hopkins Medicine. Blisters, calluses, and corns. Accessed at http://www.allkids.org/body.cfm?id=1905&category=20169&ref=84428, July 31, 2014.

12. DeLee D. *Orthopaedic Sports Medicine.* 3rd ed. Philadelphia, PA: Saunders; 2010:Chap 25.

13. Mayo Clinic Store: Healthy Living. 2013–2014 Medical Supplies Catalog. Accessed at http://www.mayoclinic.org/mcitems/mc1200-mc1299/mc1234-20.pdf, April 28, 2013.

14. How your feet work—and three steps for keeping them healthy. *Harvard Health Lett.* 2009;34(10):3–5.

15. Salicylic acid topical. Facts and Comparisons eAnswers [subscription database]. Accessed at http://online.factsandcomparisons.com, July 9, 2011.

16. U.S. Food and Drug Administration. Wart remover drug products for over-the-counter human use. Final monograph. *Federal Register.* 1990;55(358):33258–62.

17. U.S. Food and Drug Administration. Wart remover drug products for over-the-counter human use. Correction. *Federal Register.* 1990;55:33246–56.

18. Ioli JP. What to do about bunions. *Harvard Women's Health Watch.* 2011;18(10):4–6.

19. Stern MJ. Family Footcare, PC. Bunions. Accessed at http://www.familyfootcare.org/Bunion%20Article.htm, July 31, 2014.

20. California Podiatric Medical Association. Top 10 foot problems. Accessed at https://www.podiatrists.org/visitors/foothealth/other/common, July 31, 2014.

21. Mayo Clinic. Bunions: lifestyle and home remedies. Accessed at http://www.mayoclinic.com/health/bunions/DS00309, April 28, 2013.

22. Mayo Clinic. Metatarsalgia: causes. Accessed at http://www.mayoclinic.org/diseases-conditions/metatarsalgia/basics/causes/con-20022369, September 15, 2014.

23. Cushing M. *You Can Cope with Peripheral Neuropathy: 365 Tips for Living A Better Life.* New York, NY: Demos Medical Publishing; 2009:Chap 2.

24. Kennedy JG, Knowles B, Dolan M, et al. Foot and ankle injuries in the adolescent runner. *Curr Opin Pediatr.* 2005;17(1):34–42.

25. The New York Times Health. Foot pain in-depth report. Accessed at http://www.nytimes.com/health/guides/symptoms/foot-pain/print.html?module=Search&mabReward=relbias%3Ar, July 31, 2014.

26. Adams SB, Theodore GH. Extracorporeal shock wave therapy for treatment of plantar fasciitis. *Orthopaed J Harvard Med School Online.* Accessed at http://orthojournalhms.org/volume5/manuscripts/ms13.htm, April 1, 2013.

27. Weineer D, Morscher M, Dicintio M. Calcaneal apophysitis: simple diagnosis, simpler treatment. *J Fam Practice.* 2007;56(5):352–5.

28. Bope ET, Kellerman RD. *Conn's Current Therapy.* 1st ed. Philadelphia, PA: Saunders; 2013.

29. Flore R, Gerardino L, Santoliquido A, et al. Reduction of oxidative stress by compression stockings in standing workers. *Occup Med* (Oxford). 2007;57:337–41.

30. McDermott AY, Mernitz H. Exercise and older patients: prescribing guidelines. *Am Fam Physician.* 2006;74:437–44.

31. McKeon P, Mattacola C. Interventions for the prevention of first time and recurrent ankle sprains. *Clin Sports Med.* 2008;27:371–82.

32. Badlissi et al. Foot musculoskeletal disorders, pain, and foot-related functional limitation in older persons. *JAGS.* 2005; 53:1029–33.

33. Habif TP. *Clinical Dermatology: A Color Guide to Diagnosis and Therapy.* 5th ed. Maryland Heights, MO: Mosby; 2010: Chap 25.

34. Rout R, Tedd H, Lloyd R, et al. Morton's neuroma: diagnostic accuracy, effect on treatment time and costs of direct referral to ultrasound by primary care physicians. *Qual Prim Care.* 2009;17(4):277–82.

35. Franson J. Intermetatarsal compression neuritis. *J Clin Podiatr Med Surg.* 2006;23(3):569–78.

36. Mailler-Savage EA, Adams BB. Skin manifestations of running. *J Am Acad Dermatol.* 2006;55(2):290–301.

37. Cheung RT, Ng G. Influence of different footwear on force of landing during running. *Phys Ther.* 2008;88(5):620–8. 2008 Feb 14 [Epub ahead of print].

38. Meadows M. Taking care of your feet. *FDA Consum.* 2006;40(2);16–24.

39. Nicola TL. Rehabilitation of running injuries. *Clin Sports Med.* 2012; 31(2):351–72.

40. Heidelbaugh JJ, Lee H. Management of the ingrown toenail. *Am Fam Physician.* 2009;79(4):303–8.

41. U.S. Food and Drug Administration. Ingrown toenail relief drug products for over-the-counter human use. Final rule. *Federal Register.* 2003; 68(88):24347–9.

42. Sodium sulfide gel. MedFacts Patient Information. Baltimore, MD: Wolters Kluwer Health, Inc.; 2010.

43. U.S. Food and Drug Administration. Ingrown toenail relief drug products for over-the-counter human use. Final rule. *Federal Register.* 1993; 58(88):47602–6.

44. U.S. Food and Drug Administration. Ingrown toenail relief drug products for over-the-counter human use. Tentative final monograph. *Federal Register.* 1982;47:39120–5.

45. Benzocaine. Lexi-Drugs Online™ [subscription database]. Hudson, Ohio: Lexi-Comp, Inc.; 2010. Accessed at http://online.lexicomp, April 30, 2013.

46. Haider A, Solish N. Focal hyperhidrosis: diagnosis and management. *CMAJ.* 2005;172(1):69–75.

47. Haider A, Solish N. Hyperhidrosis: an approach to diagnosis and management. *Dermatol Nurs.* 2004;16(6):515–23.

48. Heit J. Hyperhidrosis. Medline Plus Medical Encyclopedia. Accessed at http://www.nlm.nih.gov/medlineplus/ency/article/007259.htm, April 30, 2013.

49. Connolly M, de Berker D. Management of primary hyperhidrosis: a summary of the different treatment modalities. *Am J Clin Dermatol.* 2003;4(10):681–97.

50. Thomas I, Brown J, Vafaie J. Palmoplantar hyperhidrosis: a therapeutic challenge. *Am Fam Physician.* 2004;69(5):1117–20.

chapter

HAIR LOSS

44

Tricia M. Berry

Significant numbers of men and women experience hair loss, with up to 50% of men and women affected at some point in their life.[1] Hair loss has many potential contributing factors (Table 44–1).[1–9] Regardless of the cause, hair loss can have a significant psychological and social impact. Individuals affected by hair loss often experience low self-esteem; personal, social, and work-related challenges; and psychiatric disorders, such as depression and anxiety.[10] The economic impact is also substantial, with patients spending approximately $3.5 billion each year on products and procedures to treat hair loss.[11]

Hair loss is broadly categorized as nonscarring or scarring alopecia. Forms of nonscarring alopecia include androgenetic alopecia (AGA, or pattern hereditary hair loss); alopecia areata (rapid onset, patchy hair loss); anagen effluvium (rapid shedding of growing hairs); telogen effluvium (rapid shedding of resting hairs); cosmetic hair damage; and trichotillomania (a compulsive pulling out of one's hair). Types of hair loss secondary to medication use, acute or chronic illness, or dietary changes typically are also nonscarring. Table 44–2 provides information on common types of nonscarring alopecia.[1,3,7,12–14] Scarring alopecia may be related to conditions such as discoid lupus erythematosus, syphilis, sarcoidosis, tinea capitis, or lichen planus.

AGA is the most common form of hair loss and the only type of alopecia to be approved by the Food and Drug Administration (FDA) for nonprescription therapy. AGA is characterized by progressive, patterned hair loss from the scalp. Caucasian men are more likely than men of other ethnicities to experience baldness and more extensive hair loss.[12] By age 30, about 30% of white men have AGA, with the incidence increasing to 50% by age 50 and 80% by age 70.[12] Although the prevalence of hair loss in women is lower, it is still significant, with approximately 40%–50% of women developing female pattern hair loss (FPHL) by age 70.[1,3]

Pathophysiology of Hair Loss

Hair follicle activity is cyclic (Figure 44-1). A variety of triggers can alter the hair follicle cycle, resulting in hair loss. In AGA, the hair follicle undergoes a stepwise miniaturization and change in growth dynamics. With each successive cycle, the anagen phase becomes shorter and the telogen phase becomes longer. Consequently over time, the anagen-to-telogen ratio decreases from 12:1 to 5:1. Because telogen hairs are more loosely anchored

to follicles, their presence in increased numbers eventually manifests as increased shedding. In addition, the catagen phase lengthens, reducing the number of hairs. As telogen hairs are shed, they are gradually replaced by vellus-like (short and fine) hairs or by anagen hairs that are too short to reach the surface.

Hair follicles and their sebaceous glands produce enzymes that convert weak androgens to estrogens, testosterone, and dihydrotestosterone (DHT) (Figure 44-2). These enzymes are believed to maintain androgen balance in the follicle, thereby regulating the hair cycle. Testosterone and DHT stimulate production of growth factors and proteases, affect vascularization of the follicle and the composition of basement membrane proteins, and alter the amounts of cofactors required for follicle metabolism.

DHT is believed to be a primary repressor of hair growth. It binds five times more readily than testosterone to androgen receptors. Increased 5-alpha-reductase–mediated conversion of testosterone to DHT in the balding areas of women with AGA also supports the contention that DHT is important in this process. Women with this disease rarely lose all their hair, not only because they have less 5-alpha-reductase but also because they have more aromatase that converts testosterone into estradiol.[15] In addition, women are more likely to have follicles with fewer localized androgen receptors and, therefore, are more likely to retain actively growing hair.[16]

Chemotherapeutic agents (e.g., antimitotic drugs) are identified as a potential cause of anagen effluvium. They cause narrowing of the hair shaft, which may fracture the hair or stop hair growth. Current nonprescription drug therapies are not FDA approved for the treatment of alopecia caused by anagen effluvium.

Hair care products and hair-grooming methods associated with scarring or burns on the scalp may result in scarring alopecia. Traction alopecia is seen primarily in individuals who braid their hair tightly every day. Braiding traumatizes the hair follicles, causing hairs to loosen and break. Patients who use oily moisturizers to make hair more manageable and to stop the scalp from flaking may develop folliculitis and hair loss. Hot combs used to straighten hair may cause scalp inflammation and result in scarring alopecia.[14]

Scaly dermatoses, such as psoriasis and seborrheic dermatitis, may also lead to scarring alopecia. Nonprescription agents marketed for the treatment of psoriasis and seborrheic dermatitis are not effective in treating alopecia. Chapter 33 provides additional information on the self-care of scaly dermatoses.

table

44-1 Causes of Hair Loss

General Causes	Specific Examples
Hormonal changes	Menopause Pregnancy Post-partum Hyperandrogenic conditions (e.g., polycystic ovary syndrome)
Physiologic stress	Surgery Trauma Fever, infections Hemorrhage
Chronic illnesses	Eating disorders (e.g., anorexia, bulimia) Endocrine disorders (e.g., hypo/hyperthyroidism, hypopituitarism, diabetes mellitus, growth hormone deficiency, hyperprolactinemia) Autoimmune diseases (e.g., rheumatoid arthritis, lupus) Hepatic or renal failure Infections (e.g., HIV, syphilis)
Medications	Beta-blockers (e.g., propranolol, metoprolol) ACE-inhibitors (e.g., enalopril, captopril) Allopurinol Anticonvulsants (e.g., phenytoin, carbamazepine, valproate) Anticoagulants (e.g., warfarin, heparin) Antidepressants (e.g., SSRIs, tricyclic antidepressants) Androgenic action (e.g., oral contraceptives, danazol, testosterone, anabolic steroids) Cholesterol-lowering drugs (e.g., clofibrate, gemfibrozil) Chemotherapeutic agents
Dietary changes or deficiencies	Rapid weight loss Strict vegetarian diet Protein restriction/deficiency Zinc, biotin, or iron deficiencies
Local trauma	Tinea capitis Hair care practices Compulsive hair pulling (trichotillomania)
Genetics	HLA genes, such as HLA-DRB1*0401 and DQB1*0301, in alopecia areata[7] Polymorphisms in the androgen-receptor gene in AGA[8,9] Chromosome 3q26 and 20p11 in AGA[9]

Key: ACE = Angiotensin-converting enzyme; AGA = androgenetic alopecia; HIV = human immunodeficiency virus; SSRI = selective serotonin reuptake inhibitor.

Source: References 1–9.

Untreated or improperly treated tinea capitis may lead to hair loss. This disease must be treated with systemic antifungals; hair regrowth occurs after eradication of the dermatophyte.

Psychological stress may potentiate several types of hair loss, although the literature on this subject is conflicting. Trichotillomania, a compulsive psychiatric disorder most common in children, involves an individual repetitively pulling or plucking hairs, leading to patchy hair loss.

Clinical Presentation of Hair Loss

The scalp of a patient with AGA shows no signs of inflammation or scarring. Hair loss is gradual; in contrast to other alopecias, the number of hairs that come out during brushing or shampooing does not suddenly increase. Typically, male pattern hair loss (MPHL) is insidious in onset and usually does not start until after puberty. Progression fluctuates considerably, with 3–6 months of accelerated loss followed by 6–18 months of no loss. Most men take 15–25 years to lose their hair. The loss begins with a recession of the frontal hairline and continues with thinning at the vertex until only a fringe of hair at the occipital and temporal margins remains. The pattern and extent of MPHL are often characterized with the Norwood Scale; images are viewable at the referenced Web site.[17]

In women with alopecia, hair loss is typically more diffuse. FPHL manifests as gradual hair thinning over the crown and mid-frontal portion of the scalp. Several scales (e.g., Ludwig, Sinclair, and Savin) have been used to classify the extent of FPHL.[4,18] The Ludwig and Savin scales use similar images for degrees of hair loss; these images can be viewed at the referenced Web site.[18] In contrast, the Sinclair Scale uses 5 ratings for severity of hair loss.[4] These scales are helpful in visualizing the typical progression of hair loss in male and FPHL, but they may have limited clinical utility when making assessments and recommendations within a community setting.

FPHL is often classified as AGA; genetic components along with hormonal factors contribute to the hair loss.[3,8,19] Women with AGA may present with symptoms of hyperandrogenism (an excess of androgen), such as significant acne, hirsutism (hairiness in other parts of the body), menstrual irregularities, and infertility. It is conceivable that a patient with FPHL may be using a hair regrowth treatment agent on the scalp while using an anti-hirsute agent (e.g., topical eflornithine or oral spironolactone [off label]) to remove excess hair on the face. Androgen excess may indicate serious metabolic disturbances, such as cardiovascular disease, diabetes mellitus, polycystic ovarian syndrome, and endometrial cancer.[19] Women with multiple symptoms should be referred for medical evaluation and treatment.[1,8,19]

Alopecia areata has three stages: sudden loss of hair in patches, enlargement of the patches, and regrowth. The cycle may take months, sometimes years, and can occur in any hair-bearing area. Up to 5% of patients lose all their scalp hair (alopecia totalis), and 1% of patients lose all their body and scalp hair (alopecia universalis). Hair loss may accompany or be preceded by nail pitting or other nail abnormalities, itching, tingling, burning, or other painful sensations in the patch of hair loss.

Telogen effluvium (also known as diffuse alopecia) can be acute (lasting <6 months) or chronic (lasting >6 months). The precipitating factor usually precedes shedding by 1–6 months, but identifying a specific causal event is often difficult, if not impossible. This point is especially important to note with medication use because hair loss will often occur one to several months after the patient has begun a particular drug therapy. Health care providers should assess the start date of all medications as a part of the clinical workup of patients with telogen effluvium. This type of hair loss is usually reversible.[1]

Hair loss may be assessed by using a variety of tests (e.g., biopsy of the scalp, daily hair loss count, and hair–pull test).[2,20] A hair–pull test is done by holding 40–60 hairs between the thumb and forefinger and firmly (but not forcefully) pulling the hairs away from the scalp. A positive test, noted when more than 10% of the hairs come out, suggests specific types of alopecia

table
44–2 Characteristics of Common Types of Nonscarring Alopecia

Type of Hair Loss	Etiology	Epidemiology	Clinical Presentation
Androgenetic alopecia/ pattern hereditary hair loss	Hormonal, hereditary	Female: 40%–50% by age 70 years[1,3] Male: 80% by age 70 years[12] Affects white men more often than men of other ethnicities[12]	Gradual onset with progression of patterned hair loss Female: Central portion of scalp, sparing frontal hairline; wide midline part on the crown with progression to diffuse thinning over crown Male: Top rear of the head (vertex), frontal hairline, and occipital regions
Alopecia areata	Autoimmune	2% of U.S. population; affects men and women of all races equally; most cases (70%) occur in children and young adults[7]	Abrupt onset (may wax and wane with relapses); usually patchy but can be generalized; can occur in any hair-bearing area: axillary, pubic, and other body hair often not affected, but eyebrows and eyelashes can be lost and sometimes are only sites affected[14]
Anagen effluvium	Chemotherapy, radiation, heavy metal poisoning	Data not available	Abrupt loss of 80%–90% of body hair
Telogen effluvium	Metabolic or hormonal disturbances, stress; severe illness or injury; medications[1]	Exact prevalence unknown; can occur in either gender at any age, but not common in childhood[3,13]	Generalized, abrupt onset (often with trigger factor); rapid hair thinning without bare patches
Cosmetic hair damage	Hair care practices (e.g., braiding, permanents, bleaching)	Any age; associated with specific social, cultural, and cosmetic practices[1]	Gradual or abrupt loss on any area of the scalp depending on cause; broken hairs with blunt rather than tapered tips
Trichotillomania	Psychiatric compulsive disorder	More common in children but may persist into adulthood[1]	Twisted and broken-off hairs are visible in patchy areas across the scalp[1]
Tinea capitis[a]	*Trichophyton tonsurans*	Any age; common in childhood[1]	Any area of the scalp; usually round patch(es) of hair loss

[a] May also be considered scarring alopecia.

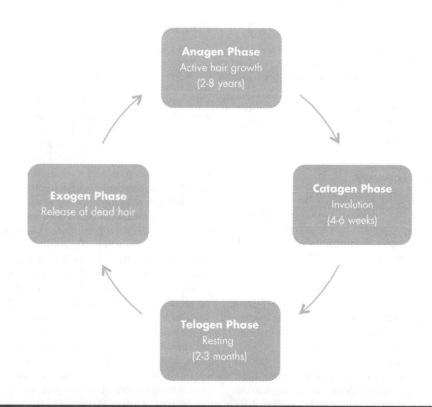

figure
44–1 Hair follicle cycle.

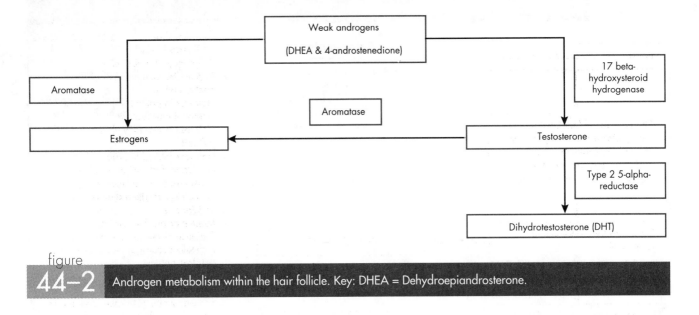

44–2

Androgen metabolism within the hair follicle. Key: DHEA = Dehydroepiandrosterone.

(e.g., effluvium or alopecia areata).[2,13] All patients presenting with hair loss that is not considered androgenetic should be referred to a primary care provider for complete medical evaluation.

Treatment of Hair Loss

Treatment Goals

The goal in self-treating hair loss is to achieve an appearance the patient considers acceptable.

General Treatment Approach

Treatment goals for hair loss can be accomplished through the following nonprescription measures: (1) nonpharmacologic therapy such as cosmetic camouflage and/or (2) the use of topical minoxidil to stimulate hair growth, if applicable. With the exception of AGA, all other types of hair loss should be referred to a health care provider to determine the cause and proper treatment. The algorithm in Figure 44–3 outlines the self-treatment of hair loss and lists specific exclusions for self-treatment.

Nonpharmacologic Therapy

Hair loss that is dramatic and extensive can be emotionally distressing. Camouflaging thinning hair with wigs and hair weaves may help relieve the distress of hair loss. Technological advances have made production of custom wigs that match the wearer's original hair a standard practice. These advances have tremendously improved the psychological impact of hair loss. Approaches to treating less severe hair loss include hair sprays, gels, colorants, permanents, and scalp camouflaging products (e.g., topical hair fibers, powder cakes, scalp lotions, scalp sprays, and hair crayons); these products can create an illusion of fullness without decreasing hair loss.[21]

Scalp massage, frequent shampooing, and electrical stimulation have been proposed as treatments for hair loss; however, these remedies are considered ineffective.[22] Although its efficacy remains unknown, low-level light therapy is a safe therapy marketed for hair growth.[23]

Both acute and chronic telogen effluvium should be referred to a health care provider for further evaluation. Acute telogen effluvium usually resolves spontaneously, and treatment is limited to comforting and reassuring the patient. Chronic telogen effluvium is slower to resolve, but the patient will still need comfort and reassurance. If a patient's hair loss is caused by poor diet or iron deficiency, the patient may benefit from consulting a dietitian. In deficiency states, increasing protein intake or taking iron supplements may be simple solutions to reversing hair loss.

Surgical transplantation of terminal hair follicles from another anatomic site is an alternative nonpharmacologic approach to hair loss. This method may be useful in frontal and vertex hair loss.

Pharmacologic Therapy

Minoxidil

Minoxidil, the only FDA-approved self-treatment option for AGA, is available as a 2% and 5% hydroalcoholic solution and a 5% solvent-free foam. Minoxidil can be applied by various methods (Table 44–3), depending on the applicator (spray, dropper, and rub-on assembly).[24] Treatment is indicated for baldness at the crown of the head in men and for hair thinning at the fronto-parietal area in women.[25] The 2% and 5% products are approved for use in both men and women. When used orally to control hypertension, minoxidil is a potassium channel opener and vaso-dilator. When used topically for hair loss, the drug appears to act by increasing cutaneous blood flow directly to hair follicles, which increase in size after treatment.[26] Minoxidil also promotes and maintains vascularization of hair follicles in alopecia.[26,27] Minoxidil, which has been shown to directly stimulate follicular hypertrophy and prolong the anagen phase,[26] may transform resting (telogen phase) hair follicles into active (anagen phase) hair follicles.[24] After up to 12 months of therapy, a subset of these same patients also revealed a reduction in the percentage of telogen hairs.

For men undergoing hair transplantation whose hair follicles may be viable but not functioning optimally in the area to be transplanted, topical minoxidil can increase hair density, speed regrowth in transplanted follicles, and complement the surgical outcome by minimizing the likelihood of progression of hair loss.[28]

After initiation of minoxidil treatment, an increase in hair loss may occur within the first few weeks of product usage.[29]

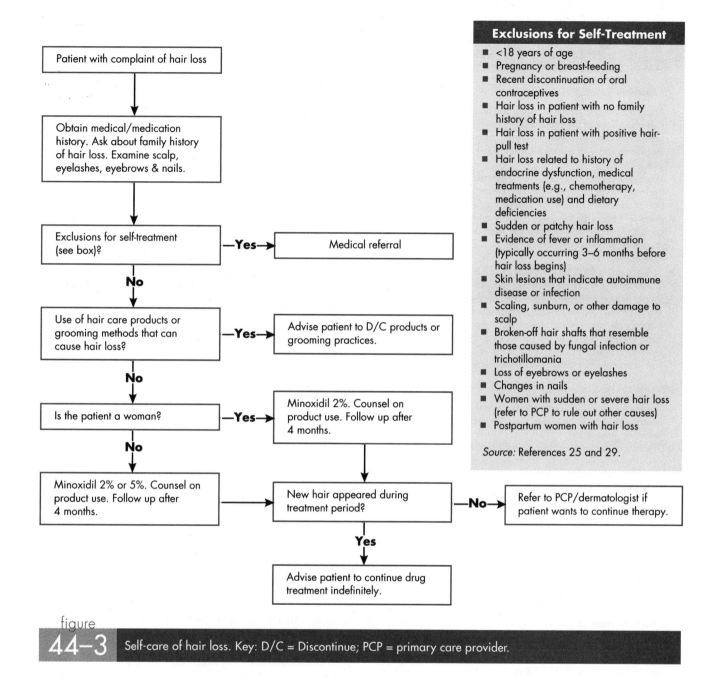

Exclusions for Self-Treatment

- <18 years of age
- Pregnancy or breast-feeding
- Recent discontinuation of oral contraceptives
- Hair loss in patient with no family history of hair loss
- Hair loss in patient with positive hair-pull test
- Hair loss related to history of endocrine dysfunction, medical treatments (e.g., chemotherapy, medication use) and dietary deficiencies
- Sudden or patchy hair loss
- Evidence of fever or inflammation (typically occurring 3–6 months before hair loss begins)
- Skin lesions that indicate autoimmune disease or infection
- Scaling, sunburn, or other damage to scalp
- Broken-off hair shafts that resemble those caused by fungal infection or trichotillomania
- Loss of eyebrows or eyelashes
- Changes in nails
- Women with sudden or severe hair loss (refer to PCP to rule out other causes)
- Postpartum women with hair loss

Source: References 25 and 29.

figure 44–3 Self-care of hair loss. Key: D/C = Discontinue; PCP = primary care provider.

Several months may elapse before hair growth is apparent. If increased hair density fails to appear after 4 months of using minoxidil, the patient should consider ending treatment and discussing other options with a health care provider. For many patients, increased hair density is minimal and treatment response is difficult to assess. Once the drug is discontinued, hair density returns to pretreatment levels in a matter of months; therefore, the patient must continue to use the product indefinitely to maintain new growth.[25]

Several studies have evaluated the effectiveness and safety of minoxidil 2% and 5% preparations. In a 48-week study, men using 5% minoxidil had an earlier response and greater hair regrowth (45% more hair regrowth) than did men using 2% minoxidil.[30] Increased frequency in itching and local irritation was also noted in the 5% minoxidil treatment group compared with the 2% minoxidil group.[30] A randomized, double-blind, placebo-controlled trial compared the efficacy and safety of 5% topical minoxidil with 2%

topical minoxidil and placebo in the treatment of FPHL.[31] Both 5% and 2% minoxidil were superior to placebo, and the 5% topical minoxidil group showed statistically significant benefits over the 2% topical minoxidil group.[31] The incidence of itching, local irritation, and hypertrichosis in the group receiving 5% minoxidil was greater than that of the 2% minoxidil and placebo groups; however, both concentrations were considered well tolerated with no evidence of systemic side effects.[31] In a randomized, single-blind trial studying 113 women with androgenetic alopecia, once-daily 5% minoxidil foam was found to be as effective as twice-daily 2% minoxidil solution; the 5% concentration was also associated with several aesthetic and practical advantages.[32]

Primary care providers may consider treating male patients who have failed nonprescription minoxidil with finasteride 1 mg tablets daily. Finasteride is the only currently FDA-approved prescription product for treatment of alopecia in male patients. Finasteride has been studied in female patients; however, the

table
44-3 Administration Guidelines for Nonprescription Minoxidil

Minoxidil Solution

- Apply minoxidil to clean, dry scalp and hair.
- Rub about 1 mL of the product into the affected area of the scalp twice daily (morning and night). Some products have a measuring cap with a 1 mL fill line. Do not apply more often than twice daily.
- Wash and dry hands after applying the medication. If it gets into the eyes, mouth, or nose, rinse these areas thoroughly.
- Do not double the dose if you miss an application.
- Allow 2–4 hours for the drug to penetrate the scalp. Do not participate in any activity that might wash away or dilute the drug (e.g., bathing or swimming without a cap) for 2–4 hours after application.
- At night, apply the drug 2–4 hours before bedtime; if minoxidil is not fully dry, it can stain clothing and bed linen.
- Do not dry the scalp with a hair dryer after applying the drug. This action will reduce the drug's effectiveness.
- If applicable, apply hair grooming and styling products (e.g., sprays, mousses, or gels) or coloring agents, permanents, or relaxing agents after the minoxidil has dried. These products usually do not affect the efficacy of topical minoxidil.

Minoxidil Foam

- The foam may melt on contact with warm skin. Therefore, wash hands in cold water before applying. Dry hands thoroughly before applying foam.
- Within the thinning hair area, part the hair into one or more rows to maximize contact of the foam with the scalp. The hair should be completely dry before application.
- Holding the can upside down, apply one-half of a capful of the foam to the fingertips. The 5% product for men should be applied twice daily, in the morning and at night. The 5% product for women should be applied once daily.
- Using the fingertips, spread the foam over the thinning scalp area, and then massage gently into the scalp. Wash hands thoroughly after application.
- Allow the product to dry completely before lying down or applying grooming, styling, or coloring products.

Source: References 25 and 29.

results have shown the drug to be no better than placebo in women.[23] Topical minoxidil solution 2% has also been investigated in combination with oral finasteride 1 mg in male patients. The outcomes of this study indicate a higher percentage of responders with the combination treatment than with either agent alone. It is inferred that efficacy may be enhanced by the two-drug regimen, which acts on multiple AGA etiologies.[33]

The most common side effect associated with minoxidil—local itching, irritation, and dryness or scaling at the site of application—may be related to the hydroalcoholic/propylene glycol vehicle. A 5% minoxidil topical formulation in a propylene glycol-free foam vehicle is available to reduce the risk of local side effects.

The most common side effect of long-term use is transient hypertrichosis (excessive hair growth), usually on the forehead and cheeks. Occasionally, patients may notice hypertrichosis on the chest, back, forearms, and ear rims, which could indicate that the product has been applied excessively.[34] Rare side effects include acne at the site of application, increased hair loss, inflammation (soreness) of the hair roots, reddened skin,

swelling of the face, and allergic dermatitis.[25,29] No differences in side effects or other problems were demonstrated in a limited number of older patients (≤65 years of age).

Minoxidil is absorbed through the skin in relatively low concentrations; documented systemic side effects are rare. In the unlikely event of an accidental ingestion, the patient should seek emergency medical attention. Symptoms may include the following[29]:

- Low blood pressure (dizziness, confusion, fainting, and lightheadedness)
- Blurred vision or other changes in vision
- Headache or chest pain
- Irregular heart rate
- Swollen hands or feet
- Flushing of the skin
- Numbness or tingling of the face, hands, or feet

Although minoxidil-induced hemodynamic changes have not been detected in most controlled clinical studies, patients with cardiovascular disorders may have an increased risk of cardiotoxicity.[35]

The use of topical minoxidil is not associated with any known drug interactions. However, the concurrent use of guanethidine could potentiate orthostatic hypotension, and the concurrent use of oral minoxidil could increase its systemic levels and enhance its effects. Topical application of corticosteroids, petrolatum, or retinoids (e.g., Retin-A) to the scalp in combination with minoxidil may increase absorption of minoxidil and the risk of side effects. In addition, minoxidil should not be used for 24 hours before or after application of a permanent, hair color, or hair relaxant.[25, 29]

Patients who are allergic to minoxidil or to any component of the preparation should avoid this medication, as should patients with scalp damage from psoriasis, severe sunburn, or abrasions, which may increase minoxidil absorption.

Topical minoxidil has a Pregnancy Category C rating; its effect on nursing babies is not known. Therefore, pregnant and lactating women should be advised to consult a primary care provider before using minoxidil.

The solution formulation is alcohol based and will burn or irritate eyes, mucous membranes, and abraded skin. When spraying either formulation of the product, the patient should avoid inhalation. If the product gets into the eyes, mouth, or nose, the patient should thoroughly rinse these areas. Patients should wash and dry their hands after using the product. These precautions are also intended to prevent the systemic entry of minoxidil by alternative routes. Products containing minoxidil should not be used on any other part of the body.[29]

Researchers have found little evidence of a potential effect of minoxidil on systemic endocrine functions.[36] Measurement of plasma testosterone and excretion of urinary hydroxysteroids and ketosteroids in hypertensive patients who had been treated with oral minoxidil did not reveal any effects. Moreover, although serum cortisol, testosterone, and thyroid indexes are apparently unchanged by topical minoxidil, modification of follicular testosterone metabolism does occur.[37]

Safety and efficacy of the product in children younger than 18 years have not been established, so the use of minoxidil in this population is contraindicated.

Product Selection Guidelines

Either the 2% or 5% formulations can be recommended for use by women; however, men are usually advised to use the 5%

table 44–4 — Selected Nonprescription Hair Regrowth Products

Trade Name	Primary Ingredient
Minoxidil Topical Solution (various manufacturers)	Minoxidil 2%
Minoxidil Topical Solution 5% for Men (various manufacturers)	Minoxidil 5%
Rogaine Extra Strength Topical Solution for Men (Johnson & Johnson Healthcare)	Minoxidil 5%
Rogaine Men's Topical Solution (Johnson & Johnson Healthcare)	Minoxidil 2%
Rogaine Men's Topical Foam (Johnson & Johnson Healthcare)	Minoxidil 5%
Rogaine Women's Topical Solution (Johnson & Johnson Healthcare)	Minoxidil 2%

Source: Reference 25.

concentration. One study demonstrated a lower incidence of contact dermatitis with foam products, which do not contain propylene glycol, than with topical solutions.[3,23] Accordingly, the foam formulation *may* be more desirable in patients with a history of sensitive skin or dermatitis. Patient preference for method of application is a critical factor in product selection. Patients with impaired vision or physical dexterity may find the rub-on method of application preferable to using sprays or droppers. Table 44–4 lists examples of commercially available products.

Complementary Therapies

In the past, FDA advisory panels have proposed removing from the market a number of ingredients that were known to be safe for external use but lacked scientific data to support their purported efficacy in preventing hair loss or promoting hair growth.[38] The false claims generally are no longer made, but many of these ingredients are still available today in nonprescription lotions and shampoos. In addition, oral and topical dietary supplements marketed to improve the structure and function of hair growth have become more popular. Ingredients included in shampoos, topical solutions, and dietary supplements for hair loss include amino acids, aminobenzoic acid, B vitamins, jojoba oil, lanolin, maidenhair fern (*Adiantum capillis-verneris*), polysorbates 20 and 660, royal jelly (white secretion of *Apis melliferis* worker bees), tetracaine hydrochloride, urea, and wheat germ oil.[14,22,37,39] Saw palmetto demonstrated increased hair growth in 6 of 10 men with AGA in one randomized, double-blind, placebo-controlled study.[23]

Assessment of Hair Loss: A Case-Based Approach

Before treatment for hair loss, the provider should first identify any possible underlying medical cause. To assess alopecia areata or telogen effluvium, the provider can direct the patient to perform a gentle hair-pull test. The patient should be referred to a dermatologist if a pull-test is positive. However, the test may be falsely negative if the patient's hair has been recently combed, brushed, or shampooed.[6] If pathology-induced and active hair loss is ruled out, the provider should determine whether the balding fits the criteria for AGA.

Cases 44–1 and 44–2 illustrate the assessment of patients with hair loss.

case 44–1

Relevant Evaluation Criteria	Scenario/Model Outcome
Information Gathering	
1. Gather essential information about the patient's symptoms and medical history, including:	
a. description of symptom(s) (i.e., nature, onset, duration, severity, associated symptoms)	Patient has had gradual hair loss at the temples and a recently a little thinning at the vertex; no signs of inflammation or scarring on scalp.
b. description of any factors that seem to precipitate, exacerbate, and/or relieve the patient's symptom(s)	None
c. description of the patient's efforts to relieve the symptoms	Has changed shampoos several times with no noticeable change/improvement in hair loss
d. patient's identity	Michael Jones
e. age, sex, height, and weight	42 years old, male, 5 ft 10 in., 170 lb
f. patient's occupation	Accountant
g. patient's dietary habits	Skips breakfast, eats out for lunch during the week; eats with family in the evening.
h. patient's sleep habits	Sleeps ~6 hours nightly.
i. concurrent medical conditions, prescription and nonprescription medications, and dietary supplements	Patient in good health; takes no prescribed medications; has taken 2 fish oil capsules daily for several years to "improve cholesterol."
j. allergies	Penicillin (skin rash)

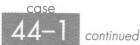

case
44–1 *continued*

Relevant Evaluation Criteria	Scenario/Model Outcome
k. history of other adverse reactions to medications	None
l. other (describe) _____	Father and maternal uncles suffer from male pattern baldness. Michael prefers to use a topical treatment because he is concerned about the side effects of systemic therapy.

Assessment and Triage

2. Differentiate patient's signs/symptoms and correctly identify the patient's primary problem(s).	The patient has androgenetic alopecia, as evidenced by gradual hair loss at temple and vertex. He has no signs of inflammation or scarring on scalp. Eyebrows and eyelashes are normal.
3. Identify exclusions for self-treatment (Figure 44–3).	None
4. Formulate a comprehensive list of therapeutic alternatives for the primary problem to determine if triage to a medical provider is required, and share this information with the patient or caregiver.	Options include:
	(1) Recommend self-care using OTC minoxidil topical treatment and/or camouflage measures.
	(2) Refer Michael to a PCP for treatment.
	(3) Recommend self-care until a PCP can be consulted.
	(4) Take no action.

Plan

5. Select an optimal therapeutic alternative to address the patient's problem, taking into account patient preferences.	Topical minoxidil 2% or 5% solution or foam
6. Describe the recommended therapeutic approach to the patient or caregiver.	"Apply approximately 1 milliliter of minoxidil 5% topical foam twice daily to a clean, dry scalp."
7. Explain to the patient or caregiver the rationale for selecting the recommended therapeutic approach from the considered therapeutic alternatives.	"The most effective nonsystemic therapy is topical minoxidil 5%. A solution or foam is available. The foam formulation may cause less irritation."

Patient Education

8. When recommending self-care with nonprescription medications and/or nondrug therapy, convey accurate information to the patient or caregiver:	
a. appropriate dose and frequency of administration	See Table 44–3.
b. maximum number of days the therapy should be employed	See the box Patient Education for Hair Loss.
c. product administration procedures	See Table 44–3.
d. expected time to onset of relief	See the box Patient Education for Hair Loss.
e. degree of relief that can be reasonably expected	"Progressive hair loss will be slowed."
f. most common side effects	See the box Patient Education for Hair Loss.
g. side effects that warrant medical intervention should they occur	See the box Patient Education for Hair Loss.
h. patient options in the event that condition worsens or persists	See the box Patient Education for Hair Loss.
i. product storage requirements	See the box Patient Education for Hair Loss.
j. specific nondrug measures	"Minimize exposure to agents that may trigger hair loss."
Solicit follow-up questions from the patient or caregiver.	"How can I tell if I am responding to the treatment?"
Answer the patient's or caregiver's questions.	"Hair density will increase if the treated area involves early thinning. Look for fine, short hairs as a first response."

Evaluation of Patient Outcome

9. Assess patient outcome.	You can ask the patient to call you right away with significant concerns of side effects (skin irritation, redness) and to monitor and report any hair regrowth in 1–4 months.

Key: OTC = Over-the-counter; PCP = primary care provider.

case

44–2

Relevant Evaluation Criteria	Scenario/Model Outcome

Information Gathering

1. Gather essential information about the patient's symptoms and medical history, including:

a. description of symptom(s) (i.e., nature, onset, duration, severity, associated symptoms)

Patient has noticed a sudden increase in hair loss in the shower and in her hair brush, resulting in noticeable thinning over the past few weeks. No signs of inflammation or scarring on scalp are present. No bare patches are noted but hair pull-test is positive.

b. description of any factors that seem to precipitate, exacerbate, and/or relieve the patient's symptom(s)

None

c. description of the patient's efforts to relieve the symptoms

Patient has not tried anything for the hair loss.

d. patient's identity

Katherine James

e. age, sex, height, and weight

41 years old, female, 5 ft 4 in., 165 lb

f. patient's occupation

High school science teacher

g. patient's dietary habits

Started Weight Watchers to improve health and lose weight.

h. patient's sleep habits

Sleeps ~7–8 hours a night.

i. concurrent medical conditions, prescription and non-prescription medications, and dietary supplements

DVT 3 months ago after a significant car accident: warfarin 8 mg daily × 3 months

j. allergies

None

k. history of other adverse reactions to medications

None

l. other (describe) _____

"It seems like everything has been falling apart since my car accident 3 months ago. There is no history of hair loss among family members."

Assessment and Triage

2. Differentiate patient's signs/symptoms and correctly identify the patient's primary problem(s).

The patient likely has telogen effluvium, as evidenced by the positive hair-pull test and rather sudden onset of hair loss. She has no signs of inflammation or scarring on the scalp. Eyebrows and eyelashes are normal, with no bare patches noted. Several possible causes include medications and possible stress/injury associated with the car accident.

3. Identify exclusions for self-treatment (Figure 44–3).

Hair loss with positive hair-pull test, hair loss related to medications

4. Formulate a comprehensive list of therapeutic alternatives for the primary problem to determine if triage to a medical provider is required, and share this information with the patient or caregiver.

Options include:

(1) Refer Katherine to a PCP for evaluation and treatment.

(2) Recommend self-care until a PCP can be consulted.

(3) Take no action.

Plan

5. Select an optimal therapeutic alternative to address the patient's problem, taking into account patient preferences.

Refer Katherine to PCP for evaluation and treatment.

6. Describe the recommended therapeutic approach to the patient or caregiver.

"Minimize or eliminate exposure to triggers for hair loss. For example, reduce stress and discontinue warfarin when the recommended duration of treatment is fulfilled."

7. Explain to the patient or caregiver the rationale for selecting the recommended therapeutic approach from the considered therapeutic alternatives.

If possible causes of hair loss can be identified and eliminated or minimized, hair loss will stop or lessen and hair will regrow.

Relevant Evaluation Criteria	Scenario/Model Outcome
Patient Education	
8. When recommending self-care with nonprescription medications and/or nondrug therapy, convey accurate information to the patient or caregiver.	See the box Patient Education for Hair Loss for specific nondrug measures.
Solicit follow-up questions from the patient or caregiver.	"Will my hair grow back if my medications are adjusted?"
Answer the patient's or caregiver's questions.	"You will also need to minimize new triggers for hair loss. Hair density will gradually increase as the causes of your hair loss are removed. Look for fine, short hairs as a first response."
Evaluation of Patient Outcome	
9. Assess patient outcome.	Ask the patient to report to you the outcome of the PCP evaluation and recommendations.

Key: DVT = Deep venous thrombosis; PCP = primary care provider.

Patient Counseling for Hair Loss

Patients should be advised that most treatment regimens for hair loss do not alter its progression, especially if the hair loss has gone on for a prolonged period of time. Patients who want to use nonprescription minoxidil should be informed that the longer the hair thinning or loss has continued, the less likely it is that treatment will elicit a regrowth response. If the patient still wants to use minoxidil, the provider should review product instructions with the patient, making sure that the patient understands the possible adverse effects and the signs and symptoms that indicate the need for medical attention. In addition, the patient should be counseled that if hair regrowth is achieved, long-term continuation of minoxidil will be necessary to maintain the regrowth. If the patient is concerned about long-term continuation of treatment regimens to maintain the effect or is not achieving desired endpoints with minoxidil, cosmetic products, camouflaging options, and hair transplants/surgical interventions may be acceptable alternatives. The box Patient Education for Hair Loss lists specific information to provide patients.

patient education for
Hair Loss

The goal in self-treating hair loss is to achieve an appearance the patient considers acceptable. This objective can be accomplished through nonprescription means by recommending (1) cosmetic camouflage and/or (2) the use of topical minoxidil to stimulate hair growth, when appropriate. To ensure optimal therapeutic outcomes, it is essential that patients carefully follow product packaging information and consider the following measures.

Nondrug Measures
- If desired, use wigs to cover severe hair loss until hair is regrown.
- For less severe hair loss, use hair sprays, gels, colorants, permanents, or hair-building products in moderation to create the illusion of full hair. These cosmetics will not affect the rate of hair loss.
- Avoid the use of oily hair products that can cause folliculitis.
- Avoid hairstyles that pull on the hair, such as tight braids.
- Avoid heat from hair dryers and curling/flat irons because their use can make the hair more brittle.

Nonprescription Medications
- Note that use of minoxidil must be continuous and indefinite to maintain regrowth. It may take up to 4 months to see any results. If treatment is interrupted, regrowth will typically be lost within 4 months or less, and progression of hair loss will begin again.
- Minoxidil is not recommended in patients who are pregnant, breast-feeding, or planning to become pregnant while using this product. Consult a primary care provider before you use this product.
- See Table 44-3 for instructions on how to use this product.

- Do not apply the product more often than directed. More frequent applications will not achieve better regrowth or a faster response but may increase side effects.
- Do not apply the product to damaged or inflamed areas of the scalp, including areas with active scalp psoriasis or eczema lesions and open scalp wounds of any kind.
- Note that local itching or irritation at the site of application may occur. More rarely, allergic contact dermatitis or transient hypertrichosis (unwanted facial hair growth) may occur.
- Keep product container in a cool, dry place, but do not put it in the refrigerator.
- Keep the product out of children's reach. Ingestion of minoxidil is potentially hazardous, and a poison control center should be contacted immediately.
- The solution is flammable. Keep away from fire or flame.
- Do not use on infants or children ages 18 years or younger.
- Do not use if you have heart disease except under the supervision of a primary care provider.
- If hair fails to appear within the time specified on the product (generally 4–6 months) despite consistent use of the product, consider stopping the treatment and seeing your primary care provider for further evaluation.

Source: References 25 and 29.

Evaluation of Patient Outcomes for Hair Loss

Patients should use minoxidil for the minimum recommended period. If new hair growth does not occur after using minoxidil 2% or 5% for 4 months, the patient should consider ending treatment. If new hair does appear within the recommended period, the patient should be advised to continue the drug treatment indefinitely.

Key Points for Hair Loss

➤ Minoxidil is not effective for everyone.

➤ Positive treatment results may take several weeks to be noticed. Hair loss will recur if therapy is stopped.

➤ Adherence is critically important for pharmacologic treatment.

➤ Offering cosmetic solutions may also be helpful.

➤ Patients, particularly women, are seeking treatment not only for hair loss but also for lost self-esteem resulting from the association of hair loss with illness and advanced age.

➤ Providers should dispense medication with a dose of emotional support and should describe the limitations of the existing treatment.

REFERENCES

1. Mounsey AL, Reed SW. Diagnosing and treating hair loss. *Am Fam Physician*. 2009;80(4):356–62, 373–4.

2. Harrison S, Bergfield W. Diffuse hair loss: its triggers and management. *Cleve Clin J Med*. 2009;76(6):361–7.

3. Shapiro J. Hair loss in women. *N Eng J Med*. 2007;357(16);1620–30.

4. Dinh QQ, Sinclair R. Female pattern hair loss: current treatment concepts. *Clin Inter Aging*. 2007;2(2):189–99.

5. Shinkai K, Roujeau J, Stern RS, et al. Cutaneous drug reactions. In: Longo DL, Fauci AS, Kasper DL, et al., eds. *Harrison's Principles of Internal Medicine*. 18th ed. New York: McGraw-Hill; 2012: Chap 55. Accessed at http://accesspharmacy.mhmedical.com/content.aspx?bookid=331&Sectionid=40726780, February 22, 2014.

6. American Hair Loss Association. Drug induced hair loss. Accessed at http://www.americanhairloss.org/drug_induced_hair_loss/, February 22, 2014.

7. Alzolibani AA. Epidemiologic and genetic characteristics of alopecia areata (part 1). *Acta Dermatoven APA*. 2011;20(4):191–8.

8. Mesinkovska NA, Bergfeld WF. Hair: What is new in diagnosis and management? Female pattern hair loss update: diagnosis and treatment. *Dermatol Clin*. 2013;31(1):119–27.

9. Rathnayake D, Sinclair R. Male androgenetic alopecia. *Expert Opin Pharamcother*. 2010;11(8):1295–304.

10. Hunt N, McHale S. The psychological impact of alopecia. *BMJ*. 2005; 331(7522):951–3.

11. Hume AL. Viviscal: an answer for hair loss in women? *Pharmacy Today*. 2013;9:22.

12. Stough D, Stenn K, Haber R, et al. Psychological effect, pathophysiology, and management of androgenetic alopecia in men. *Mayo Clin Proc*. 2005;80(10):1316–22.

13. Shapiro J, Wiseman M, Lui H. Practical management of hair loss. *Can Fam Physician*. 2000;46:1469–77.

14. Dawber R, Van Neste D, eds. Hair loss/hair dysplasia. *Hair and Scalp Disorders: Common Presenting Signs, Differential Diagnosis and Treatment*. 2nd ed. London, UK: Martin Dunitz; 2004:51–154.

15. Sawaya ME, Price VH. Different levels of 5 alpha-reductase type I and II, aromatase, and androgen receptor in hair follicles of women and men with androgenetic alopecia. *J Invest Dermatol*. 1997;109(3):296–300.

16. Randall VA, Hibberts NA, Thornton MJ, et al. The hair follicle: a paradoxical androgen target organ. *Horm Res*. 2000;54(5–6):243–50.

17. American Hair Loss Association. The Norwood Scale. Accessed at http://www.americanhairloss.org/men_hair_loss/the_norwood_scale.asp, June 16, 2013.

18. American Hair Loss Association. Degree of hair loss. Accessed at http://www.americanhairloss.org/women_hair_loss/degree_of_hair_loss.asp, June 16, 2013.

19. van Zuuren EJ, Fedorowicz Z, Carter B, et al. Interventions for female pattern hair loss. *Cochrane Database System Rev*. 2012;5:CD007628. doi: 10.1002/14651858.CD007628.pub3. Accessed at http://www.thecochranelibrary.com/view/0/index.html.

20. Sinclair R, Patel M, Dawson TL, et al. Hair loss in women: medical and cosmetic approaches to increase scalp hair fullness. *Br J Derm*. 2011;165(supp 3):12–8.

21. Donovan JC, Shapiro RL, Shapiro P, et al. A review of scalp camouflaging agents and prostheses for individuals with hair loss. *Dermatol Online J*. 2012;18(8):1.

22. Ross E, Shapiro J. Management of hair loss. *Dermatol Clin*. 2005: 23;227–43.

23. Rogers NE, Avram MR. Medical treatments for treatment of male and female pattern hair loss. *J Am Acad Dermatol*. 2008;59(4):547–66.

24. Tosti A, Duque-Estrada B. Treatment strategies for alopecia. *Expert Opin Pharmacother*. 2009;10(6):1017–26.

25. Minoxidil topical. Facts and Comparisons eAnswers. Accessed at http://online.factsandcomparisons.com, June 15, 2013.

26. Otomo S. Hair growth effect of minoxidil. *Nippon Yakurigaku Zasshi*. 2002;119(3):167–74.

27. Lachgar S, Charveron M, Gall Y, et al. Minoxidil upregulates the expression of vascular endothelial growth factor in human hair dermal papilla cells. *Br J Dermatol*. 1998;138(3):407–11.

28. Avram MR, Cole JP, Gandelman M, et al. The potential role of minoxidil in the hair transplantation setting. *Dermatol Surg*. 2002;28(10):894–900.

29. McNeill-PPC, Inc. Rogaine. Accessed at http://www.rogaine.com, June 15, 2013.

30. Olsen EA, Dunlap FE, Funicella T, et al. A randomized clinical trial of 5% topical minoxidil versus 2% topical minoxidil and placebo in the treatment of androgenetic alopecia in men. *J Am Acad Dermatol*. 2002;47(3):377–85.

31. Lucky AW, Piacquadio DJ, Ditre CM, et al. A randomized, placebo-controlled trial of 5% and 2% topical minoxidil solutions in the treatment of female pattern hair loss. *J Am Acad Dermatol*. 2004;50(4):541–53.

32. Blume-Peytavi U, Hillmann K, Dietz E, et al. A randomized, single-blind trials of 5% minoxidil foam once daily versus 2% minoxidil solution twice daily in the treatment of androgenetic alopecia in women. *J Am Acad Dermatol*. 2011;65(6):1126–34.

33. Khandpur S, Suman M, Reddy BS. Comparative efficacy of various treatment regimens for androgenetic alopecia in men. *J Dermatol*. 2002;29(8):489–98.

34. Peluso AM, Misciali C, Vincenzi C, et al. Diffuse hypertrichosis during treatment with 5% topical minoxidil. *Br J Dermatol*. 1997;136(1):118–20.

35. Satoh H, Morikaw S, Fujiwara C, et al. A case of acute myocardial infarction associated with topical use of minoxidil (RiUP) for treatment of baldness. *Jpn Heart J*. 2000;41(4):519–23.

36. Nguyen KH, Marks JG Jr. Pseudoacromegaly induced by the long-term use of minoxidil. *J Am Acad Dermatol*. 2003;48(6):962–5.

37. Sato T, Tadokoro T, Sonoda T, et al. Minoxidil increases 17 beta-hydroxysteroid dehydrogenase and 5 alpha-reductase activity of cultured human dermal papilla cells from balding scalp. *J Dermatol Sci*. 1999;19:123–5.

38. Hanover L. Hair replacement. *FDA Consum*. 1997;31:7–10.

39. Maidenhair fern and royal jelly monographs. In: Fetrow CW, Avila JR, eds. *Professional's Handbook of Complementary & Alternative Medicines*. Philadelphia, PA: Lippincott Williams & Wilkins; 2004:530, 718.

OTHER MEDICAL DISORDERS

chapter

SELF-CARE COMPONENTS OF SELECTED CHRONIC DISORDERS

45

Timothy R. Ulbrich and Daniel L. Krinsky

Chronic diseases affect approximately one in two adult Americans (133 million) and account for 7 of 10 deaths in the United States each year.[1] These diseases put a significant burden on the U.S. health care system, including both direct and indirect costs. Chronic diseases most often have a gradual onset, have no cure, change over time, and require significant interventions, including pharmacologic and nonpharmacologic management.

Self-care management of chronic disease requires an educated and involved patient.[2] Although active engagement is vital, it can be difficult, considering the physical, emotional, and psychological toll chronic diseases may impart. Other comorbid conditions, persistent symptoms, daily medication use, poor communication among patients and health care providers, subpar family support, financial stressors, and the need to interpret and treat symptoms may contribute to less than ideal patient involvement in self-care activities. Therefore, cooperative identification and management of these barriers by providers and patients are essential to achieve the common goal of optimal condition management.

Modifiable risk factors such as tobacco use, lack of exercise, poor nutrition, and excessive alcohol use may contribute to worsening or causing chronic diseases. Therefore, behavioral changes such as tobacco cessation, moderation of alcohol use, improvement in nutrition, and participation in more physical activity may prevent and lessen the suffering associated with chronic diseases. Determining the patient's readiness to change a behavior, providing proper education on the benefits to making lifestyle changes, and setting realistic goals may help improve the success of a plan to eliminate some or all of the modifiable risk factors.

The day-to-day monitoring and adjustments by the patient are central to achieve optimal outcomes. This model of self-care engagement requires the patient to think outside the traditional role of depending only on the provider to achieve optimal care. For this shift to happen, providers must empower patients to actively engage in self-care. Patients who voice their goals of therapy and regularly participate in their care may better adhere to their regimen, thereby increasing the likelihood of achieving set goals. Providers can assist patients by cultivating a relationship that will allow them to assess the patient's capability for self-care, identify gaps in the patient's knowledge, teach patients proper self-care strategies, and monitor self-care measures.

This chapter explores commonly encountered chronic medical conditions that involve extensive self-care, including diabetes mellitus, asthma, osteoporosis, heart failure, hypertension, and dyslipidemia.

Diabetes Mellitus

As defined by the American Diabetes Association (ADA), diabetes mellitus is a group of metabolic diseases characterized by hyperglycemia resulting from defects in insulin secretion, insulin action, or both.[3] Although several types of diabetes are recognized, types 1 (5%–10% of patients) and 2 (90%–95% of patients) account for the majority of cases.

More than 25.8 million people in the United States, or 8.3% of the population, have diabetes.[4] Of these, 7 million individuals are undiagnosed cases. Another 79 million Americans older than 20 years are estimated to have prediabetes. In 2007, the total annual combined direct and indirect costs attributed to diabetes were estimated to be $174 billion.[4] Because most health care expenditures are related to treatment of long-term diabetes complications, focus should be on prevention, early diagnosis, and aggressive metabolic control.

Pathophysiology of Diabetes Mellitus

Working in conjunction with counterregulatory hormones (e.g., glucagon, epinephrine, norepinephrine, growth hormone, and cortisol), endogenous insulin maintains normal blood glucose (BG) concentrations between 60 and 100 mg/dL. A defect in insulin action or secretion, or a combination of the two, results in hyperglycemia categorized as type 1, type 2, or prediabetes. Type 1 diabetes is often caused by autoimmune-mediated pancreatic beta-cell destruction that leads to absolute insulin deficiency. Type 2 diabetes is caused by insulin resistance, impaired insulin secretion, and increased hepatic glucose production. Prediabetes precedes type 2 diabetes and is diagnosed by an impaired fasting glucose level, oral glucose tolerance test, or A1C (glycosylated hemoglobin) test that is elevated but not to the extent of that of a patient with type 2 diabetes.

Clinical Presentation of Diabetes Mellitus

Type 1 diabetes is typically characterized by individuals who present with a younger age of onset (usually <30 years), are thin in physique, and may or may not have a family history of diabetes. In contrast, type 2 diabetes is characterized by individuals who present with an older age of onset (usually >40 years), are overweight, obese, or both, and have a family history of diabetes.

For individuals with new-onset diabetes mellitus, as plasma glucose concentrations rise to exceed the normal renal threshold of 180 mg/dL, glycosuria produces an osmotic diuresis and potential dehydration resulting in polyuria (frequent urination), especially at night (nocturia). Dehydration can progress to significant hypovolemia (decrease in volume of circulating blood), electrolyte loss, and cellular dehydration, causing dry mouth and polydipsia (increased thirst). A lack of insulin production or presence of insulin resistance prevents cells from using circulating plasma glucose, and the nervous system signals polyphagia (hunger accompanied by increased appetite). The onset of clinical symptoms is usually more rapid and pronounced for patients with type 1 diabetes and often follows a stressful event. For patients with type 2 diabetes, symptoms of long-term diabetes complications may appear before elevated plasma glucose is detected.

Chronic hyperglycemia is associated with the development and progression of complications affecting major organs and physiologic systems. Complications of diabetes are categorized as microvascular and macrovascular. Achieving reductions in A1C, a marker for longer-term glycemic control, lowers the overall risk of developing microvascular complications.

Microvascular complications affect the eyes (retinopathy), nervous system (neuropathy), and kidneys (nephropathy). Among adults ages 20–74 years in the United States, diabetes is the leading cause of new-onset blindness.[4] More than 60% of patients with diabetes have mild-moderate damage to their nervous system. Severe peripheral neuropathy is a main contributor to lower-extremity amputations. Although peripheral neuropathy is one example, patients can experience other disorders (e.g., gastroparesis and erectile dysfunction) as a result of nerve damage. Finally, diabetes is the leading cause of kidney failure in the United States.[4]

Macrovascular complications include atherosclerosis, contributing to peripheral vascular disease (PVD), cardiovascular disease (CVD), and stroke. Heart disease is the leading cause of diabetes-related deaths,[4] and compared with people without diabetes, those with diabetes have two to four times the risk of heart attack and stroke.

In addition to micro- and macrovascular complications, patients with diabetes may have abnormalities in immune function that increase their rates of morbidity and mortality from infection.

Poorly controlled diabetes is a risk factor for the development of oral and dental complications, including gingivitis, periodontitis, dental caries, oral mucosal diseases, oral infections, salivary dysfunction, and taste disturbances. Maintaining glucose control and good dental hygiene, having regular checkups with a dentist, and smoking cessation can decrease the risk of developing oral and dental complications.

Treatment of Diabetes Mellitus

Patients can reduce their risk of developing or decrease the progression of diabetes complications by instituting self-care and other preventive measures. Providers should educate patients about the role of self-care and other preventive measures and encourage their use (Table 45–1). The provider should review lifestyle modifications with the patient and stress their importance

in controlling the disorder. However, medical referral for further evaluation is needed if the assessment process reveals any of the following:

- No formal diagnosis of diabetes
- Uncontrolled diabetes (signified by symptoms or blood glucose readings that identify hypo- or hyperglycemia)
- Concurrent condition (e.g., acute illness) or medication (e.g., steroids) that may be affecting the patient's blood glucose and that has not been evaluated by the provider
- No visit (or missed visit) to a primary care provider in the last year
- History of hypo- or hyperglycemia severe enough to warrant medical attention
- Nonadherence to any provider-recommended prescription medications, nonprescription medications, or self-care measures
- Pregnancy
- Perception that prescription medications are ineffective
- Unknown status of other comorbid conditions (e.g., dyslipidemia)
- Use of dietary supplements without provider's knowledge or without achieving set goals

In addition to self-care measures, patients with diabetes should receive medical care from an interprofessional team with expertise in diabetes.[3] Effective diabetes management is patient centered, taking into account factors such as the patient's health beliefs, attitudes, preferences, practices, health literacy, daily routines, and socioeconomic situation that may affect his or her self-care abilities. Collaborative diabetes management therefore includes patients, their families, and caregivers as central members of the team.

Because heart disease is the leading cause of diabetes-related deaths, proper management and prevention of disease-related risk factors such as hypertension and dyslipidemia are essential. Patients with hypertension and/or dyslipidemia in conjunction with diabetes are treated to more stringent goals than those without diabetes.

Treatment Goals

Glycemic control is the cornerstone of diabetes management. It includes preventing hypoglycemic and hyperglycemic occurrences. Treatment goals should be individualized, taking into account patient-specific factors, such as age (e.g., children, adolescents, and the elderly), pregnancy status, and comorbid conditions. Table 45–2 summarizes the ADA recommendations for nonpregnant adults with diabetes. The diabetes guidelines issued by the American Association of Clinical Endocrinologists have stricter goals than the ADA guidelines.

General Treatment Approach

A diabetes care plan should include the following eight steps:

1. Assessment of the patient's knowledge (e.g., of disease state and goals of therapy), current care regimen, comorbid conditions, and any factors (e.g., cultural, health literacy, and socioeconomic) that may affect the patient's care.
2. Meal planning and healthy eating instructions.
3. Physical activity recommendations.
4. Self-monitoring of BG and, when appropriate, ketone concentrations.

Self-Monitoring of Blood Glucose

- Determine patient's frequency of BG testing (e.g., fasting, preprandial, postprandial, or bedtime) and target BG goals.
- Discuss signs and symptoms of low BG episodes, and have patient test when symptoms arise and record the date, time, and BG value for evaluation.
- Educate patient on proper management of hypoglycemic episodes.

Medical Nutrition Therapy

- Tailor nutrition and physical activity to individual patient characteristics, such as timing of meals, glycemic control, and comorbid conditions.
- Educate patient on ways to maintain a healthy weight.
- Refer patient to a dietitian if necessary.

Tobacco Use

- Assess the patient's willingness to quit.
- Recommend tobacco cessation (see Chapter 47).

Eye Care

- Recommend an annual eye examination after an initial dilated and comprehensive eye exam. Less frequent examinations (e.g., every 2–3 years) may be an option after having one or more normal examinations.
- Review any topical eye preparations for potential contraindication.
- Recommend medical attention if vision changes or eye irritation occurs.

Dental Care

- Recommend professional teeth cleaning and oral health evaluation by a dentist twice each year.
- Recommend that teeth be brushed and flossed twice daily.
- Recommend a dental consult at the first sign of any gum abnormalities (e.g., bleeding).
- Have patient review dental care products with a dentist before use.

Skin Care

- Recommend daily bathing with mild soap and drying skin thoroughly.
- Recommend that skin be inspected daily—head to toe—for signs of potential infection.
- Instruct patient to cleanse minor cuts and scratches promptly with soap and water.
- Instruct patient to avoid topical drying agents (e.g., alcohol, except for use when sterilizing for insulin injection) or salicylic acid–containing products.

Foot Care

- Perform annual foot examination.
  - Have patient remove shoes at each visit with the primary care provider for visual inspection.
  - Evaluate for any changes in foot appearance or tactile sensation.
  - Advise patients identified at high risk of ulcers (e.g., neuropathy) to see a podiatrist regularly.
- Teach patient to clean and inspect feet daily for any changes (e.g., corn, callus, open wound, or fungal infection).
- Instruct patient that nails should be trimmed carefully, preferably straight across, and filed with an emery board to the contour of the toe.
- Instruct patient to avoid walking barefoot.
- Recommend use of soft cotton, synthetic blend, or wool socks to absorb moisture.
- Recommend that patient wear properly fitting, comfortable shoes and use caution when "breaking in" new shoes.
- Recommend that patient inspect shoes for foreign objects before inserting feet.
- Recommend that patient (1) use moisturizing lotion sparingly for the tops and bottoms of dry feet, (2) allow feet to completely dry before wearing shoes to prevent excess moisture, and (3) avoid use of moisturizers between the toes.

Medication Adherence: Information for Patients

- Discuss each medication's indication.
- Advise patient to take medications as prescribed. Patient should not discontinue medications without consulting provider.
- If indicated, advise patient to take low-dose aspirin daily to prevent heart attack and stroke.
- Advise patient to avoid taking any nonprescription medications, herbal products, or supplements without first discussing them with a provider.
- Advise patient to consult with a health care provider about strategies to help keep track of medications and daily doses.
- Confirm that all immunizations are up to date.

Sick Day Management

- Establish a sick day plan for insulin use during an acute illness.
- Recommend testing of BG and urine ketones (especially with type 1 diabetes) frequently during acute illness. During a period of illness, blood glucose levels may be elevated and patients may have an altered caloric intake.
- Advise patient to maintain ample hydration with noncaloric liquids.

Key: BG = Blood glucose.

table
45–2   ADA Treatment Goals for Nonpregnant Adults with Diabetes

Glycemic Control	
Hemoglobin A1C	<7.0%[a,b]
Fasting plasma glucose	70–130 mg/dL (3.9–7.2 mmol/L)
Peak postprandial plasma glucose[c]	<180 mg/dL (<10.0 mmol/L)
Body mass index	<25.0 kg/m²
Blood pressure	<140/80 mm Hg
Immunizations	Influenza vaccination annually Pneumococcal vaccination All others should be up to date (e.g., tetanus, hepatitis A and B, and zoster)

Key: ADA = American Diabetes Association; A1C = glycosylated hemoglobin.

[a] Reference to a normal range for patients without diabetes of 4.0%–6.0% using a Diabetes Control and Complications Trial–Based Assay.

[b] Lower (e.g., <6.5%) or higher (e.g., <8%) A1C goals may be considered in individual patients.

[c] Postprandial plasma glucose measured 1–2 hours from the start of the meal.

5. Safe and effective use of medication therapy.
6. Patient self-management education.
7. Assessment of adherence to self-monitoring of blood glucose (SMBG), medical nutrition therapy (MNT), and other non-pharmacologic and pharmacologic therapy.
8. Follow-up care to alter or adjust the plan as needed to achieve metabolic goals, which could be accomplished by sending written or verbal documentation directly to the provider or instructing the patient to talk with the provider and review the diabetes care plan during follow-up visits. Depending on the patient comfort level and relationship with the provider, the latter option may allow the patient to be empowered and active in his or her treatment regimen.

Nonpharmacologic Therapy
Medical Nutrition Therapy

Coupled with regular physical activity, MNT is an essential nonpharmacologic component of diabetes care. Rather than focusing on the need to "diet" or "lose weight," the term "nutrition" is used to emphasize the importance of eating for a healthy lifestyle and achieving and maintaining metabolic goals.

The concepts of MNT are similar for patients with types 1 and 2 diabetes, but treatment goals differ. For patients with type 1 diabetes, the goals are to integrate insulin regimens with usual habits of eating and physical activity, and to ensure normal growth and development during childhood and adolescence. Because obesity and a sedentary lifestyle are key issues in type 2 diabetes, the main objectives are healthy eating habits (including caloric and fat restriction), moderate weight loss, and increased physical activity to achieve optimal metabolic goals.

Current guidelines for meal planning entail an individualized approach and should involve the patient in the decision-making process, taking into account personal and cultural preferences.[5] If necessary, a referral should be made to a dietitian or certified diabetes educator. Clinical studies have reported significant benefits of MNT, including 0.25%–2.9% reductions in A1C at 3–6 months, 15–25 mg/dL reductions in low-density lipoprotein cholesterol, and improved blood pressure.[3]

Macronutrients

In general, the optimal mix of macronutrients (i.e., carbohydrate, protein, and fat) is individualized. A meal plan high in fresh fruits and vegetables and moderate in starches is recommended. High-fiber starches (e.g., legumes, whole-grain breads, and fiber-rich cereals with a goal of 14 grams fiber per 1000 kcal per day, or 25–38 grams fiber per day) are preferred over low-fiber starches (e.g., mashed potatoes, pasta, and rice).

Not all carbohydrates affect plasma glucose concentrations equally. Elevated glucose concentrations are determined by both the quality (e.g., glycemic index) and the total quantity of carbohydrates (e.g., glycemic load [GL]) consumed. Glycemic index is a system that ranks carbohydrates on a scale of 0%–100% based on their potential to raise plasma glucose concentrations immediately after they are consumed. Diets with low-glycemic-index foods (e.g., some fresh fruits and vegetables, beans, oatmeal, and whole-grain pasta) may improve glucose and lipid concentrations in people with diabetes. Not all fruits and vegetables have a low glycemic index and therefore should be considered on an individual basis. GL is the total glycemic response to a food or meal and is based on the grams of carbohydrates consumed. GL is calculated by multiplying the glycemic index percentage by the total grams of carbohydrates per serving. ADA states that the use of glycemic index or GL may be beneficial for glycemic control.[3]

With regard to fat, the main goal for people with diabetes is to reduce CVD risk factors. Less than 10% of the total daily caloric intake should come from saturated fats, with mono-unsaturated oils (e.g., olive oil) favored; consumption of trans fats should be minimized. A daily cholesterol intake of less than 300 mg/day and two or more servings of fish per week are recommended.

Lifestyle changes, moderate daily physical activity, and portion-size control for carbohydrates, protein, and fats are the critical factors in controlling obesity in patients with diabetes. Sodium intake should be limited (<2300 mg/day), especially when hypertension is present.[5] All health professionals should encourage patients to keep a meal plan and physical activity log to track the effects of food, physical activity, and medication on BG. In addition, patients should learn how to interpret these data and to identify patterns to make a cause-and-effect relation for glycemic control.

Use of Sweeteners and Sugar-Free Products

Both nutritive (caloric) and nonnutritive (noncaloric) sweetening agents are available and are good alternatives to using table sugar. Consuming large amounts of sugar alcohols (e.g., sorbitol, mannitol, xylitol, maltitol, lactitol, erythritol, isomalt, and hydrogenated starch hydrolysates) may cause diarrhea, resulting from the laxative effects of polyols.

Currently the Food and Drug Administration (FDA) has approved six nonnutritive sweeteners, including saccharin

(Sweet'N Low), sucralose (Splenda), acesulfame potassium (Sweet One, Sunett), aspartame (Equal, NutraSweet), neotame, and stevia (Truvía). Aspartame contains phenylalanine in a high enough concentration that it should be avoided in patients with phenylketonuria.

Sugar-free products such as cough and cold medications are preferred for patients with diabetes to avoid unnecessary elevations in BG. While using sugar-containing products, patients should monitor their BG closely. Occasional use of a sugar-containing product at the recommended dose is unlikely to cause significant BG elevations. However, several doses of a medication in an uncontrolled type 1 diabetic patient who is ill may exacerbate or precipitate diabetic ketoacidosis (DKA). (See the section Ketones.)

Use of Alcohol

Patients with diabetes should be educated that alcohol (1) is considered a fat (7 cal/g) in the meal plan and (2) increases insulin response. Acute alcohol consumption can cause and prolong hypoglycemia, especially if consumed on an empty stomach.

Adult patients choosing to drink alcohol should be advised as follows:[5]

- Limit daily intake to no more than two alcoholic beverages for men and one for women.
- One drink is considered 12 ounces of beer, 5 ounces of wine, or 1.5 ounces of distilled spirits (hard alcohol). Each contains 15 grams of alcohol.
- Calories from alcoholic beverages and sugar-containing mixes must be included as an addition to the regular meal plan.
- To reduce hypoglycemia risk, consume alcohol with food.
- Refrain from drinking if you are pregnant, overweight, or have other medical problems such as pancreatitis, advanced neuropathy, hypertriglyceridemia, or alcohol abuse.

Physical Activity

Patients with diabetes benefit from an active lifestyle. Regular physical activity can improve glycemic control (increases insulin sensitivity), facilitate weight loss (reduces body fat and increases muscle mass), reduce cardiovascular risk factors (reduces low-density lipoprotein cholesterol and triglycerides; increases high-density lipoprotein cholesterol with weight loss; improves blood pressure), and improve self-esteem.[6] Regular physical activity can even prevent the onset of type 2 diabetes.[7]

Before increasing physical activity, patients should undergo medical evaluation to screen for any underlying diabetes-related complications that may limit certain activities. The patient's lifestyle, preferences, metabolic goals, complications, and limitations should be considered to create an individualized fitness program. The current ADA recommendation for adults with diabetes is a minimum of 150 minutes per week of moderate-intensity aerobic physical activity. Moderate intensity is defined as reaching 50%–70% of the maximum heart rate or working hard enough to increase heart rate and break a sweat while being able to maintain a conversation. The 150 minutes per week should be divided over at least 3 days of the week with a gap of no more than 2 days in a row without exercise. An additional 2 days per week of resistance training should be recommended for patients with type 2 diabetes. Patients of advanced age should start slowly (5–10 minutes a day) and increase the amount of time gradually

as tolerated. Patients are encouraged to use the large muscle groups and participate in aerobic activities (e.g., walking, swimming, and biking). Some modifications of physical activity are needed for patients with certain diabetes-related complications. For example, patients with moderate or worsening retinopathy should avoid activities that elevate blood pressure or are strenuous (e.g., heavy competitive sports and power weightlifting). Patients who have neuropathy with loss of protective sensation should avoid repetitive sports such as prolonged walking or jogging, although low-impact alternatives may be recommended by their provider with close follow-up.[3]

Effects of physical activity on BG vary in type 1 diabetes. In general, patients who use insulin may need to consume extra carbohydrates or adjust insulin to account for the potential hypoglycemic effects of physical activity. Patients with type 1 diabetes may be at risk of hypoglycemia up to 8–15 hours after prolonged physical activity. Table 45–3 provides guidelines for patients who perform physical activity. Patients should be reminded to include their physical activity in their daily log.

Use of Tobacco Products

Tobacco use is associated with an increased risk of mortality, macrovascular complications, and early microvascular complications. Therefore, providers should encourage cessation of all tobacco products (see Chapter 47).

table 45–3	**Education for Patients with Diabetes Who Conscientiously Perform Physical Activity**

- Wear properly fitted shoes and a diabetes identification bracelet.
- Perform SMBG before and after physical activity. SMBG testing during physical activity may be necessary for prolonged physical activity.
- Perform a 5- to 10-minute, low-intensity, aerobic (e.g., walking or bicycling) warm-up (to prepare the muscles and heart) and cooldown (to bring heart rate down).
- Adjust insulin or carbohydrate intake if needed because physical activity may cause hypoglycemia if medication doses and/or carbohydrate intake is not adjusted accordingly. Before physical activity, if glucose concentration is normal or low (e.g., <100 mg/dL), consume a 10- to 15-gram carbohydrate snack (e.g., one small apple, 6-ounce cup of yogurt, or four to six whole-grain crackers), and add an additional snack if needed after the activity.
- To avoid increased absorption of regular or rapid-acting insulin (and possible hypoglycemia) from physical activity, inject insulin into the abdomen or do physical activities 30 minutes to 1 hour after insulin administration.
- Avoid physical activity if glucose concentration is greater than 250 mg/dL in the presence of ketosis (particularly in patients with type 1 diabetes). Use caution if BG concentrations are greater than 300 mg/dL without ketosis.
- Late-onset hypoglycemia can occur 8–15 hours after the physical activity, especially in patients with type 1 diabetes. If a patient performs physical activities during the day, recommend an increase in carbohydrate intake and performing SMBG during the night to detect nocturnal hypoglycemia.

Key: BG = Blood glucose; SMBG = self-monitoring of blood glucose.
Source: References 3 and 6.

Monitoring of Glycemic Control

With knowledge of their glycemic status, patients may be better able to self-manage their diabetes. Glycemic testing methods can be divided into two main categories: day-to-day glycemic measures (e.g., BG, blood ketones, and urine ketones) and chronic glycemic control measures (e.g., A1C and glycated serum proteins). Home testing products for urine protein are also available.

Self-Monitoring of Blood Glucose

Over the past decade, SMBG has become the standard for day-to-day assessment of glycemic control. SMBG provides patients with immediate feedback. Patients can recognize glucose patterns to track whether daily goals are being met, to prevent or detect hypoglycemia, and to evaluate glycemic response to foods, physical activity, or medication changes. Providers use SMBG data to help patients make changes to their diabetes care plan.

For most patients who have type 1 diabetes or who are using multiple insulin injections a day or pump therapy, self-monitoring should occur at a minimum for the following: prior to meals and snacks, periodic postprandially, at bedtime, prior to exercise, when low BG is expected, after treating low BG until returning to normoglycemic, and before critical tasks such as driving or operating machinery. This may be 6–8 times per day or more. For patients who are not on insulin therapy or are on a single insulin injection, self-monitoring may be useful as a guide to the success of therapy, and whether to monitor or not should be decided collaboratively by the patient and provider. The decision to test and the frequency of testing should be patient specific and should include factors such as the impact on quality of life and cost.

More frequent monitoring may be necessary for patients prone to hypoglycemia and during illness, or for dose changes in insulin or other diabetes medication, physical activity, diet changes, or travel. The patient must be trained in SMBG technique, instructed on appropriate timing for testing, and given specific guidelines for therapy alterations.[3]

Several factors play a role in SMBG product selection, including costs of necessary supplies and special considerations for individual patients (e.g., manual dexterity and visual acuity). Although SMBG offers many benefits, some drawbacks include out-of-pocket expense and time required for testing, possible invasive finger or skin punctures, motivation, and health literacy (e.g., cognition) required to perform SMBG and to learn to interpret test results.

BG Monitoring with Glucose Monitors

A glucose monitor used in conjunction with reagent strips measures the specific BG concentration. All monitors are calibrated and will generally analyze the BG concentration according to programmed data. All monitors provide a digital display of the BG concentration, although the display size may vary. Most have memories for later recall of recent BG concentrations. If meters have a capacity to download information, it may be saved, printed, and copied into the electronic medical record. Patients who are blind or visually impaired may benefit from monitors with audio features.

Many factors are used to select a monitor for an individual patient, first of which is generally the cost of the meter and test strips, which may be driven by the patient's insurance coverage where applicable. Additional factors may include the monitor size, size of display, blood sample size, capabilities for alternate site testing, timing devices, calibration, accuracy, ease of use, effect of temperature on accuracy, memory or data management and download features, battery types, need for cleaning, accessories required, audio capabilities, and price. A comprehensive list and description of blood glucose monitors is published annually in the ADA *Diabetes Forecast*. The 2013 guide can be found free online at www.diabetesforecast.org/2013/jan/blood-glucose-meters-2013.html.

Even when BG monitors are used properly, calibrated frequently, and interpreted correctly, accuracy can vary by up to 20%. Most glucose monitors report plasma glucose concentrations (similar to laboratory-reported results), but a few report capillary (whole blood) glucose concentrations. Because BG concentrations in plasma are approximately 11% higher than those in whole blood, patients should know which results their monitors yield to determine their glycemic goals.[8] Therefore, education about the type of meter being used (capillary versus plasma) is essential if patients will be making treatment decisions (e.g., adjusting an insulin dose) based on the reading obtained. Plasma monitors should be recommended when possible to avoid any confusion in differences between laboratory- and meter-reported values.

Many BG monitors allow blood sampling at alternate sites from the fleshy part of the palm, forearm, upper arm, thigh, and calf. Blood flow to the finger is faster than that to the forearm. Therefore, when glucose concentrations are rapidly fluctuating (e.g., after meals, during hypoglycemia, or with increased physical activity), alternate site testing should be avoided because a finger stick will reflect the change in BG before the alternate sites will.[9]

Tips for improving accuracy of SMBG via finger stick can be found in Table 45–4. For patients who intend to use alternate sites, providers should spend sufficient time reviewing the technique and assessing the patient's understanding of alternate site testing.

Proper education in the methods for self-monitoring, the differences between individual monitors, the importance of timing and frequency, and the interpretation and application of test results will encourage patients to perform SMBG consistently.[9] Return demonstration by the patient is necessary to ensure the patient's understanding of the procedure and to correct any errors as they are observed. Patients should be encouraged to maintain accurate records of SMBG and to return with their logbook, which should also contain records of medication use (e.g., name, dose, and time taken), diet changes, activities, and body weight. In addition, computerized data management systems that come with some monitors can be used at home or in the health care provider's workplace. The programs include software for downloading monitor information, modules for personal digital assistants, electronic logbooks, and Web-based programs to help patients track SMBG trends.

Lancets and Blood Sampling Equipment

Most BG testing requires the use of lancets and lancet devices. Several lancing devices are available and are provided with BG monitors. These devices allow a finger stick with less associated pain, because most have an auto-retractable needle and the amount of skin penetration can be adjusted in some products. Lancing devices should not be shared because they can harbor blood-borne pathogens and promote infection. Obtaining an adequate blood sample is essential for test accuracy. Providers should instruct patients on proper techniques for improving accuracy (Table 45–4).

table

45-4

Tips for Improving Accuracy of Finger Stick Technique

Using Test Strips

- Properly store test strips at room temperature in the original vial or container.
- Avoid exposing test strips to changes in temperature, humidity, and light.
- Check expiration date on test strips.
- Code monitor for the batch of test strips (if applicable).
- Use control solutions to verify test strips are working properly.

Using Glucose Monitor

- Follow manufacturer's directions for calibrating monitor and using control solutions.

Obtaining an Adequate Blood Sample

- Gather all necessary supplies (e.g., monitor, test strips, lancet, lancet device, and tissue).
- Vigorously clean hands with warm soapy water to increase blood circulation.
- Allow hands to dry completely to avoid diluting the blood sample.
- If alcohol must be used to clean hands, wait 1 minute to ensure alcohol has completely evaporated.
- Dry hands thoroughly.
- Hang hand below heart for 30–60 seconds to increase blood flow to fingers.
- Using the other hand, apply pressure on the finger from the base to the finger pad.
- If possible, rotate the fingertip for each self-monitored BG test.

Lancing the Finger

- Use a lancet device with an adjustable puncture depth, and adjust as needed to ensure adequate blood drop.
- Point fingers to the ground and lance the side of the fingertip.
- Avoid lancing finger pads because the presence of more nerves in these areas may cause pain.
- If lancing the index finger or thumb causes pain, avoid these areas as well.

Applying the Drop of Blood

- Ensure adequate size of blood drop is applied to test strip.
- If necessary, apply light pressure on the finger from the base to the finger pad to increase size of blood drop.
- Quickly place drop of blood on test strip. Method varies with monitor type. Refer to monitor instructions for proper technique.

Continuous Glucose Monitoring

An alternative method of monitoring glucose control is using a continuous glucose monitoring (CGM) system. A CGM device contains a sensor that is inserted into the subcutaneous tissue and then records glucose concentrations at a regular interval (e.g., every 1 or 5 minutes). The sensor stays in place for several days up to a week, depending on the device, before being replaced. Although not intended for day-to-day glucose monitoring, CGM offers the advantage of detecting glucose fluctuations, excursions, and trends throughout the day (e.g., unrecognized nocturnal or daytime hypoglycemia, or 3- to 4-hour postprandial hyperglycemia) that go unnoticed if only A1C and SMBG values are used as guides for treatment. Results from CGM allow better pattern management, particularly for insulin users. Challenges with CGM include insurance coverage and the need for

a motivated patient who will wear the device and then obtain and record SMBG readings.

Testing for Ketones, Microalbumin, and Protein

Ketones

The development of self-monitoring of blood ketone levels has revolutionized the process of detecting or predicting ketoacidosis. When the body does not have sufficient insulin, BG concentrations rise and the body's cells become energy deprived. During these times of low carbohydrate availability, the liver breaks down fat to produce ketone bodies (acetoacetate, 3-beta-hydroxybutyrate, and acetone). A sufficient blood concentration of ketones can result in diabetic ketoacidosis, a potentially fatal condition. Because ketones in the blood overflow into the urine, urinary ketone concentrations can be tested. The basis for the urinary ketone testing is that sodium nitroprusside alkali turns lavender in the presence of acetoacetate. These tests require comparing the color change to a reference chart. Several urine ketone testing products are available (e.g., Ketostix Reagent Strips, KetoCare Ketone Test Strips, and DiaScreen 1K).

In addition to testing BG, certain monitors (e.g., Precision Xtra) are capable of using test strips designed to detect 3-beta-hydroxybutyrate concentrations in the blood. This type of meter may eliminate the need for two different testing devices. Unlike urine ketone tests, blood ketone tests provide a real-time picture. Because ketone bodies will be detected in the blood first, blood tests allow earlier detection and treatment of ketoacidosis. Another advantage of blood ketone testing over urine ketone and tablet testing is the lack of false positives in the presence of vitamin C or during exposure to ambient air.

It is important to note that DKA, which occurs most often in type 1 diabetic patients, differs from hyperglycemic hyperosmolar nonketotic syndrome (HHNS), which is more common in elderly patients with type 2 diabetes. The primary cause of DKA is insulin deficiency, whereas the primary cause of HHNS is prolonged hyperglycemia paired with dehydration. DKA can present with a lower BG (e.g., >240 mg/dL) compared with HHNS (e.g., >600 mg/dL). In addition, DKA is classified by the presence of ketones at elevated BG levels, whereas in HHNS usually few or no ketones are produced. Ketone urine or blood monitoring should be recommended any time a condition exists that may lead to poor glycemic control (e.g., illness) for patients who are prone to elevated ketones. Patients should be counseled on the proper methods of testing for ketones in the urine and blood.

Microalbumin and Protein

Detection of microalbuminuria (trace protein in the urine) is an early sign of kidney damage. ADA recommends annual screening to measure urine albumin in patients with type 1 diabetes start 5 years after diagnosis and for all patients with type 2 diabetes.[3]

A nonprescription test for microalbumin is available (Kidney Screen At Home), but the urine specimen is mailed to a laboratory for analysis and reporting. Large protein particles in the urine can be determined by using an array of products (e.g., Albustix and Chemstrip). When testing at home, patients should note that, in addition to kidney damage secondary to diabetes, other factors may cause microalbuminuria, such as uncontrolled blood pressure, intense exercise, heart failure, or a recent urinary tract infection. The presence of microalbumin and protein in the urine should be reported to the primary care provider.

Self-Monitoring of Glycosylated Hemoglobin

Compared with SMBG, A1C and glycated protein testing provide useful information about a patient's glycemic control over a longer period. Traditionally, these tests were performed in a laboratory setting from venipuncture samples. New technology allows home or clinic testing with smaller blood samples.

Plasma glucose binds to red blood cells. A1C is formed at a rate directly proportional to the BG concentration over the previous 120 days (lifespan of the average erythrocyte). Because A1C concentrations correlate with the weighted mean plasma glucose values over the preceding 2–3 months, A1C may be used to assess overall glycemic control in patients with diabetes. Patients may find it easier to understand their glycemic control if they use an estimated average glucose (eAG). The eAG is calculated by using the formula eAG = 28.7 × (A1C − 46.7). For example, A1C values of 7% and 10% are equivalent to eAG values of 154 mg/dL and 240 mg/dL, respectively. Providers can refer patients to a useful online eAG calculator (professional. diabetes.org/glucosecalculator.aspx).

In general, ADA recommends testing A1C twice yearly in patients who are stable and meeting their glycemic goals, and every 3 months for patients who are not at goal or whose therapy has changed.[3] The exact testing frequency should be based on clinical judgment. The normal nondiabetic A1C range is 4%–6%. According to ADA guidelines, the goal for most people with diabetes is less than 7%. Several nonprescription A1C kits are available (e.g., A1CNow, AccuBase A1c Test Kit, A1c At Home, and BIOSAFE Hemoglobin A1c Test Kit). (See Chapter 48 for further discussion of home A1C tests.)

Identification Tags

Persons with diabetes should consider wearing a visible identification bracelet, necklace, or tag that indicates the person has diabetes and takes medication. Specifically, patients requiring insulin therapy should be strongly encouraged to wear an identification tag in the case of an emergency secondary to hypoglycemia. Patients should also be encouraged to carry an identification card (e.g., in a wallet) that includes their name, address, and telephone number; the amount and type of medication used; and the name and telephone number of the patient's primary care provider. This information may be lifesaving in the event of hypoglycemia or ketoacidosis that requires emergency services or hospitalization.

Travel Supplies and Preparations

Patients with diabetes who are planning to travel should pack enough diabetes supplies for the entire trip, plus at least 1 additional week's supply (or double what they anticipate needing). Patients should be advised to carry their supplies with them, not in checked luggage. The following is a travel checklist:

- A written note from patient's provider indicating the need for diabetes supplies (especially syringes and needles)
- Extra vials of insulin, as applicable
- Extra supply of syringes and needles because access may be limited (patients should refrain from prefilling syringes for a trip because of potential for leakage and the potential for compromised stability)
- Extra insulin pump supplies

- Extra supply of all oral medications in their original prescription bottles
- Extra SMBG supplies (e.g., glucose monitor, test strips, control solutions, lancets and devices, and batteries if needed)
- Written prescriptions for medications, including insulin and diabetes supplies (e.g., syringes and test strips), in case of an emergency
- A summary of the patient's current medication regimen and emergency contact information
- Identification cards and a diabetes identification bracelet or tag
- Snacks and glucose tablets (and glucagon kit for insulin users) as preparation for schedule changes or prevention of hypoglycemia (see the section Hypoglycemia)
- If traveling abroad, the names of English-speaking primary care providers in each city and some cards with several key phrases in the language of the country being visited (e.g., "I have diabetes" and "Please get me a doctor") to access care

Travelers should monitor their caloric intake carefully and allow time for physical activity. Because most airlines currently provide limited or no meal options onboard, patients should plan accordingly to bring their food. Patients should wear comfortable well-fitting shoes if they intend to walk more than usual during the trip. They should also anticipate changes in activity level because of extra walking and potentially erratic meals. Insulin users should be educated that time zone changes of 2 or more hours usually require insulin dose adjustments. They can work with their providers on specific adjustments to their basal and/or mealtime insulin doses. More frequent SMBG may be necessary.

Pharmacologic Therapy

Pharmacologic treatment options for patients with type 1 diabetes include insulin therapy delivered by injection or insulin pump. Because they are unable to produce insulin, patients with type 1 diabetes must inject themselves with insulin each day. Insulin therapy should be tailored to balance the effects of diet and physical activity.

Patients with prediabetes may be able to normalize their BG concentrations with diet, physical activity, and weight loss alone. However, some may benefit from the addition of pharmacotherapy. Patients with type 2 diabetes require MNT and physical activity combined with pharmacologic intervention.

Insulin

Insulin is the primary medication used to treat type 1 diabetes. Insulin is also commonly used in the treatment of type 2 diabetes. Although primary care providers prescribe insulin therapy, other health care providers, especially pharmacists, are often consulted by both primary care providers and patients about insulin and issues related to its use (e.g., initiation, adjustments, monitoring, injection technique, etc.). Thus, health care providers should be knowledgeable about insulin products and their use.

Insulin stimulates uptake and storage of glucose as glycogen (in muscles and the liver) and synthesis of fatty acids and triglycerides. In addition, insulin decreases hepatic glucose output, lipolysis, and ketone production. Finally, insulin enhances amino acid incorporation into proteins.

Human insulin is available without a prescription, whereas insulin analogues and oral agents require a prescription. In the United States, insulin is commercially available in concentrations of 100 units/mL (designated as U-100) and 500 units/mL (designated as U-500). The goal of insulin therapy in patients with type 1 diabetes is to mimic physiologic pancreatic insulin secretion to maintain normal plasma glucose concentrations. Physiologic insulin therapy provides basal and bolus (mealtime) needs. Doses are adjusted according to BG response, glycemic goals, and other patient-specific variables (e.g., BG concentrations, growth, diet, activity, and ketosis). Dosing regimens are also tailored to patients' lifestyle and routine (e.g., number of daily meals and snacks, sleep, and work schedules). Insulin doses are adjusted based on patient response to therapy as evidenced by trends in A1C and fasting, preprandial and postprandial plasma glucose concentrations, and incidence of hypoglycemia and hyperglycemia. Patients can learn to manage and adjust their daily insulin requirements on the basis of BG concentrations, diet, and activity levels.

Insulin therapy in patients with type 2 diabetes is mainly determined by the amount of glycemic control and duration of disease. Patients with type 2 diabetes whose BG is not controlled with noninsulin BG-lowering agents may require insulin therapy to achieve glycemic goals. In some cases, patients with newly diagnosed type 2 diabetes with severe hyperglycemia may require insulin therapy alone or in combination with other medications to reduce A1C values and BG concentrations.

The most common side effect of insulin therapy is hypoglycemia. Many other factors (e.g., a decrease or inconsistency in mealtime carbohydrate content, physical activity, alcohol intake, and medications) can contribute to hypoglycemic episodes. For this reason, when adjusting insulin therapy, providers should carefully assess the relationship of insulin dose and timing with patient BG trends, including hypoglycemic or hyperglycemic episodes. Patients with comorbid conditions, such as gastroparesis or reduced renal function, may be at increased risk of hypoglycemia. Insulin doses should be adjusted accordingly.

Weight gain is another common side effect. It is usually caused by increased efficiency of glucose and fat storage resulting from insulin therapy. Hypoglycemic episodes, which stimulate appetite, also contribute to weight gain because patients consume additional calories to correct the low BG.

Some patients experience local reactions on insulin injection, such as pain, redness, bruising, burning, stinging, or irritation. Using a new syringe or pen needle with each injection may help minimize or alleviate pain associated with injections. Reminding patients to inject insulin at room temperature minimizes pain associated with cold insulin injections. Proper insulin injection technique minimizes redness, swelling, and bruising. Good hygiene along with proper use and storage of syringes and other delivery devices minimizes the risk of infection.

Hyperglycemia

Hyperglycemia can occur if an insulin dose is missed or if the dose is insufficient to meet metabolic needs or carbohydrates that are consumed. Hyperglycemic symptoms—frequent urination, dehydration, thirst, increased appetite—usually occur at BG concentrations greater than 180 mg/dL. If ketosis develops, the patient's breath may have a fruity odor. Untreated hyperglycemia requires immediate medical attention because it could progress to DKA or HHNS, followed by coma and death.

Morning hyperglycemia may result from an asymptomatic nocturnal hypoglycemia (Somogyi effect) in patients who are otherwise well controlled on intensive insulin regimens. In response to hypoglycemia, the body secretes epinephrine, which induces hepatic glucose production and results in morning hyperglycemia. Another reaction that can present with a similar morning hyperglycemia is termed the "dawn phenomenon."[10] As part of the circadian rhythm, hormones such as growth hormone, cortisol, and epinephrine are released during the night. In response, the plasma glucose concentration rises in the early morning hours, and insulin is released from the functioning pancreas. In people with diabetes, the insulin release may not occur, resulting in morning hyperglycemia. Thus, a Somogyi effect is caused by too much insulin, whereas the dawn phenomenon is caused by too little insulin. Patients with morning hyperglycemia should monitor their plasma glucose concentration between 2 am and 3 am to determine whether it is low (Somogyi effect), normal, or high (dawn phenomenon). They should record the results along with any changes in their diet and physical activities, and seek assistance in interpreting the results and adjusting therapy accordingly.

Hypoglycemia

Several factors can contribute to hypoglycemia, including insufficient caloric intake (e.g., skipping or delaying meals, and/or vomiting), inaccurate insulin dose (e.g., too high, frequent adjustments, inadequate preparation, and/or irregular timing), concomitant use of hypoglycemic drugs, drug interactions, very tight glycemic control, and physical activity. Although a BG concentration of less than 70 mg/dL indicates hypoglycemia, some patients experience symptoms at higher glucose concentrations. Early warning symptoms may be both autonomic (e.g., trembling, shaking, sweating, palpitations, and/or tachycardia) and neuroglycopenic (e.g., slow thinking, difficulty concentrating, slurred speech, lack of coordination, and/or dizziness). Some patients may be hypoglycemic without experiencing any symptoms, a serious condition called hypoglycemia unawareness.

Mild-moderate hypoglycemic symptoms usually are rapidly relieved by ingestion of glucose. As a preventive measure, people with diabetes should always carry a source of fast-acting carbohydrate (Table 45–5). At the onset of hypoglycemic symptoms, patients should check their plasma glucose value if a BG monitor is available. If a patient is experiencing hypoglycemia symptoms, it is safer to initiate treatment with carbohydrates even if the plasma glucose value is not known. If a patient is able to test and determine that the blood sugar is low, he or she should follow

table 45–5 **Selected Fast-Acting Carbohydrates for Treating Hypoglycemia (15 grams)**

Source	Quantity
Milk (low-fat or nonfat)	8 ounces (1 cup)
Fruit juice (e.g., apple, orange)	4 ounces (1/2 cup)
Soft drink (nondiet)	4 ounces (1/2 cup)
Sugar	1 tablespoon or 3 cubes
Raisins	2 tablespoons
Hard candies (e.g., peppermint, butterscotch, Skittles, Life Savers, jelly beans)	3 pieces of hard candy, such as peppermint or butterscotch, or 5–6 pieces of Skittles, Life Savers, or jelly beans

Glucose Tablets

Various products on the market with different amounts of glucose per tablet and flavors available

Glucose Gels

Various products on the market with different amounts of glucose per tablet and flavors available

the "rule of 15." According to the "rule of 15," the patient should consume 15–20 grams of carbohydrates once hypoglycemia is determined. If symptoms persist or BG concentrations are still below 70 mg/dL after 15 minutes, an additional 15 grams of carbohydrates should be consumed.[3] Patients who take alpha-glucosidase inhibitors (acarbose or miglitol) should use oral glucose during an episode of hypoglycemia since the medication will inhibit the breakdown of more complex sugars (e.g., sucrose from table sugar or fructose from juices).

Once hypoglycemia is treated, if mealtime is not within 1 hour, a small snack containing a carbohydrate plus protein (e.g., crackers and peanut butter, piece of fruit and cheese, or a small protein-containing sandwich) should be consumed to prevent further hypoglycemia. BG should be monitored frequently to prevent recurrent hypoglycemia.

Severe hypoglycemia, which may result in unconsciousness, coma, seizures, and inability to swallow, should be treated with glucagon.[3] All patients using insulin should have a glucagon emergency kit, particularly those with type 1 diabetes. Available by prescription, these kits contain a 1 mg ampule of glucagon, a syringe of diluent, and administration directions. Glucagon is indicated when an individual becomes unconscious because of hypoglycemia. For this reason, family members, other patient caregivers, and co-workers should be taught to mix and administer glucagon by subcutaneous or intramuscular injection. The usual dose is 1 mg for adults and children weighing 20 kg or more, and 0.5 mg for children weighing 20 kg or less. Glucagon may cause vomiting, lasting up to 24 hours. Unconscious individuals should therefore be turned on their side before glucagon is administered, to prevent choking. Glucagon usually works within 5–10 minutes, but the effects are short lived. If no response is seen after 5–10 minutes, a second injection may be given. If this is ineffective, the caregiver should call 911 immediately. Once an individual is conscious and can swallow, the caregiver should give a carbohydrate liquid (e.g., juice, milk, or nondiet soft drink) followed by a carbohydrate snack (small sandwich or crackers with peanut butter). For the next 24 hours, regular SMBG and adequate food intake are necessary to replenish hepatic glycogen stores. The primary care provider should be informed of the episode.

Insulin Administration, Contamination, and Storage

Unless age (e.g., the very young) or physical or mental impairments preclude self-injection, a patient should be trained on (1) how to prepare his or her dose for subcutaneous injection, (2) the location of acceptable self-injection sites, and (3) proper subcutaneous injection technique. Table 45–6 describes the steps for preparing an insulin dose using a syringe and insulin vial or a prefilled insulin-delivery device.

Injection Sites, Routes, and Absorption Rates.
Insulin injection site may influence insulin absorption. Acceptable subcutaneous injection sites include the abdomen, upper arms (deltoid region), thighs (anterior and lateral aspects), and buttocks (Figure 45–1). If a patient chooses the upper arms or buttocks, self-injection may be difficult and assistance may be required.

Different anatomic sites differ in their rates of absorption. The abdomen is considered the preferred site for subcutaneous injection of insulin by most experts because insulin absorption is more predictable. Patients should avoid the area within 2 inches around the navel. Rotation of injection sites within an anatomic area helps prevent lipohypertrophy or lipoatrophy. Proper subcutaneous injection technique for use of nonprescription

---

table 45–6 **Guidelines for Preparing a Dose of Insulin Using a Vial and Syringe**

- Wash hands with soap and warm water.
- Check the insulin label on the vial to verify the type of insulin to be injected.
- Visually inspect the insulin vial for signs of contamination or degradation (e.g., white clumps or color changes).
- Remove the cap and wipe the top of the vial with an alcohol swab or cotton ball dipped in alcohol.
- Remove the protective coverings over the plunger and needle of the syringe.
- Taking care not to touch the needle, draw up air equal to the insulin dose to be administered into the syringe.
- Inject the air into the insulin vial.
- With the syringe still inserted, invert the vial and withdraw the insulin dose.
- Be sure to keep the hub of the needle below the surface of the insulin to prevent creating air bubbles within the syringe.
- If bubbles are present, inject the insulin back into the vial and pull the dose back into the syringe.
- Remove the syringe from the vial and self-inject dose, using proper injection technique (Table 45–7).

---

insulin syringes is depicted in Figure 45–2 and described step by step in Table 45–7. Injection technique may need to be altered for certain patients (e.g., 45-degree injection angle for infants and extremely thin individuals with minimal subcutaneous fat). Nonprescription insulin syringes differ in size (e.g., 6 mm, 8 mm, and 12.7 mm) compared to the prescription pen needles that are shorter in length (e.g., 4 mm, 5 mm, 8 mm, and 12.7 mm). Where possible, the shortest length should be used to ensure the injection is provided in the subcutaneous area and not in the muscle. Pinching the skin provides a firm injection surface and lifts the fat off the muscle to avoid intramuscular or intravenous injection. Properly injected insulin should leave only a needle puncture dot; bruising generally should not occur. Patients should be instructed to inject and leave the needle in place for 5–10 seconds to prevent the leakage of insulin.

Injection pain can be reduced by injecting insulin at room temperature, ensuring air bubbles are not present in the syringe, and penetrating the skin quickly in one motion. Patients who routinely experience soreness, pain, bruising, welts, or redness should have their injection technique evaluated by a health care provider. In patients complaining of pain, bruising, or redness, the provider should ensure that the patient is not reusing needles.

Subcutaneous absorption rates can be highly variable within and across patients. Patients should be educated about the influence of factors such as physical activity, massage, temperature, and smoking on insulin absorption. Performing physical activity or massaging the injection area can increase absorption rates. Heat from hot weather, a hot bath or shower, or a sauna can increase peripheral blood flow, which can increase absorption rates. Cold has the opposite effect. A smoker may require a higher amount of insulin than a nonsmoker because of a decrease in insulin absorption and an increase in insulin resistance secondary to smoking. Therefore, upon cessation of smoking, patients should monitor their BG more closely to determine if a reduction of the insulin dose is warranted.

Storage of Insulin.
Insulin preparations must be stored carefully to maintain stability and maximum potency. Patients

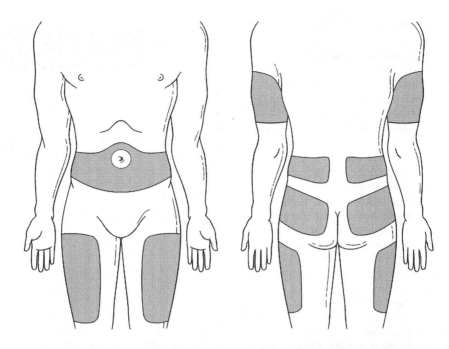

figure
45–1
Body map of subcutaneous insulin injection sites.

should inspect their insulin for visible changes in appearance before each injection. Because patients should inspect for visible changes in their insulin, including the presence of particulates, it is important to note that regular insulin is a clear suspension, whereas NPH insulin is a cloudy suspension. Color changes may be associated with protein denaturation and should be interpreted as evidence of potency loss.

Unopened insulin vials and cartridges may be stored in the refrigerator (36°F–46°F [2°C–8°C]) until the expiration date listed on the product. Insulin should never be frozen. The refrigerator door is usually a good storage location to ensure that insulin does not become frozen. The stability of unopened and in-use insulin vials or cartridges stored at room temperature varies depending on the product. Providers should contact individual manufacturers with specific questions about the stability of individual insulin products and devices under different storage or exposure conditions.

Patients who transport insulin regularly (e.g., to and from school or work, or while running errands) should be reminded to insulate insulin from heat, direct sunlight, and excess agitation. Patients should never store insulin in the car. Insulin should be carried in an insulated pack (e.g., cold pack) by patients when traveling by bus, train, or air to ensure proper storage conditions.

Product Selection Guidelines

Insulin Delivery Devices and Injection Aids. Providers should ensure that patients purchase the right type of supplies to facilitate insulin administration. Insulin available in vials must be administered with syringes. Durable (reusable)

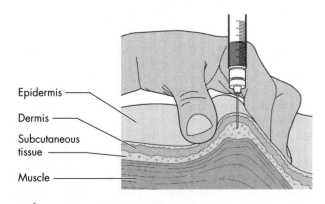

Epidermis
Dermis
Subcutaneous tissue
Muscle

figure
45–2
Correct method of subcutaneous insulin injection.

table
45–7
Subcutaneous Self-Injection Technique of OTC Insulin Syringes

- Determine the appropriate size of the needle (e.g., 6 mm, 8 mm, 12.7 mm). A shorter length needle is preferred where possible to allow for a subcutaneous injection with minimal risk of entering the muscle.
- Prepare insulin dose for administration (Table 45–6).
- Pinch the area to be injected. This is especially important when using longer OTC needles compared to the shorter prescription pen needles (e.g., 4 mm).
- Insert the needle at a 90-degree angle to the skin in the center of the pinched area (a 45-degree angle for insertion may be used in small children and very thin adults).
- Release the pinch.
- Press down on the syringe or device plunger to inject insulin.
- Hold the syringe or device in the area for 5–10 seconds to ensure full delivery of insulin. This step is particularly important for insulin pen devices.
- Remove the syringe or device.

Key: OTC = Over-the-counter.

and disposable insulin pens and other delivery devices provide added convenience and ease of use, especially in patients with impaired vision or dexterity. A resource guide with information on selected insulin syringes, other delivery aids, and related products currently available in the United States is published annually in an issue of ADA's *Diabetes Forecast* (available free online at www.diabetesforecast.org/landing-pages/lp-consumer-guide.html). Insulin pumps are an alternative delivery device available for use in selected patients.

Insulin syringes are plastic, disposable syringes that come with very fine, well-lubricated needles. Insulin syringes are designed for U-100 insulin and are marked in insulin units. Marker increments may differ among syringes; this should be pointed out to patients. Depending on the manufacturer, insulin syringes are available in 0.3, 0.5, and 1 mL capacities, which hold 30, 50, and 100 units, respectively. Patients should be reminded to purchase syringes closely matched to their individual insulin dose(s). For example, a patient taking 38 units of regular insulin should use a 0.5 mL syringe to draw up insulin to the 38-unit mark. Because U-500 insulin syringes are not available, patients initiated on U-500 insulin should have the dose expressed as a volume, and a tuberculin syringe marked in volume should be supplied to a patient. If tuberculin syringes are not readily available or covered by insurance, the patient will need to know how much U-500 insulin to pull up in the U-100 syringe. If the prescriber did not provide the conversion value, the pharmacist dispensing the insulin should do so and ensure that the patient understands proper use of the U-500 insulin to avoid a potential error.

Today's needles have virtually no "dead space" or air space at the needle's hub to reduce a potential source of dosing error. Several needle lengths, including 1/2, 3/8, and 5/16 inch, are available. Needles also come in a variety of gauges (e.g., 28–31). The higher the gauge, the finer is the needle, which lessens injection site pain. Silicone coating eases insertion, also reducing pain.

For patients who would rather not use a sharps container, a device such as the BD Safe-Clip Device (www.bd.com/us/diabetes/page.aspx?cat=7002&id=7416) lets users clip off the needle into a device that stores hundreds of needles until disposal is necessary. A selected list of related products and services is published in the *Diabetes Forecast* Consumer Guide (www.diabetesforecast.org/landing-pages/lp-consumer-guide.html). Patients should consult with their local jurisdiction about sharps disposal or call the Coalition for Safe Community Needle Disposal at 800-643-1643 for instructions for proper needle disposal.

Several types of insulin injection aids and devices are available for patients who have an aversion to or difficulty with self-injection. Such products include syringe magnifiers, needle guides and vial stabilizers, syringe insertion aids, insulin pens, and jet injectors. Syringe magnifiers enlarge the marks on a syringe barrel, making them easier to see for visually impaired patients. Patients should be reminded that, depending on the manufacturer, magnifiers work only with specific syringe brands. Needle guides and vial stabilizers are available to help patients with limited dexterity safely insert syringes into vials and draw up accurate insulin doses. Insertion aids and jet injectors may be useful for patients with needle or self-injection phobias.

Special Populations. Children and adolescents with diabetes differ from their adult counterparts in many ways. These differences include insulin sensitivity related to growth and puberty, neurologic vulnerability to hypoglycemia, and the ability to provide self-care.[3] Diabetes care and education for children and adolescents should therefore be delivered by health care providers experienced in the unique physiologic, developmental,

emotional, and psychosocial aspects and challenges faced by this population and their families.

Women with diabetes who are trying to conceive should receive special preconception care to ensure the health and safety of themselves and the developing fetus. Diabetes can increase the risk of complications during pregnancy, including fetal malformations. Women with diabetes need to be educated about the importance of family planning and good glycemic control before conception and throughout pregnancy. Insulin is used for glycemic control during pregnancy, and dosing may need to be adjusted to ensure good glycemic control throughout pregnancy.[3]

Older individuals with diabetes have higher rates of co-existing comorbid conditions, disability, and early death than do older individuals without diabetes.[3] Individuals who are physically, functionally, and cognitively intact with a normal life expectancy should have the same goals of therapy and self-care as their younger counterparts. However, special considerations for self-care measures and medication therapy, including insulin, may be relevant for certain individuals. In older patients whose physical, functional, or cognitive abilities are impaired or diminished, or those who have significantly reduced life expectancies, less aggressive metabolic goals should be considered. Their abilities for self-care management should also be assessed. Depending on their individual situations, these patients may be less likely to benefit from reducing the risk of microvascular and macrovascular complications and more likely to have serious adverse events from hypoglycemic episodes. For example, patients who are at a significant risk for falls may be treated less aggressively to avoid impaired consciousness caused by hypoglycemia. Glycemic goals, however, must be tempered to avoid potential consequences of uncontrolled hyperglycemia, such as dehydration, poor wound healing, and hyperglycemic hyperosmolar coma.

Chronic conditions can also affect glycemic control in patients with diabetes. Patients with significantly decreased renal function may have decreased insulin clearance and should be closely monitored for hypoglycemic episodes. Patients undergoing hemodialysis may have fluctuating BG concentrations and should be closely monitored. Certain medications, such as beta-adrenergic blockers, corticosteroids, diuretics, niacin, hormonal contraceptives, protease inhibitors, and atypical antipsychotics, can alter BG concentrations. Beta-blockers can mask symptoms associated with hypoglycemia, such as tachycardia and tremor, so patients should be counseled about how to recognize hypoglycemia. Patients taking hypoglycemic agents or insulin in combination with medications known to raise or lower BG or medications that can alter their physiologic response to hypoglycemia should be instructed to perform SMBG regularly and to carefully monitor for other symptoms of hypoglycemia.

Aspirin Therapy

Rheologic changes contribute to diabetes-related PVD and CVD, and platelets in patients with diabetes are hypersensitive to platelet aggregates. People with type 2 diabetes and CVD overproduce thromboxane, a potent vasoconstrictor and platelet aggregate. Low-dose aspirin therapy (75–162 mg/day) should be recommended for secondary prevention in patients with diabetes and a history of CVD, and for primary prevention for patients with type 1 or type 2 diabetes not at an increased risk for bleeding with a 10-year cardiovascular risk score greater than 10%. This includes most men older than 50 years and women older than 60 years who have one or more additional risk factors for CVD (e.g., family history, hypertension, smoking, etc.). Recommending low-dose aspirin therapy for patients with diabetes who have a 10-year risk score of 5%–10% depends on the provider's clinical judgment. Finally, low-dose aspirin therapy for patients with diabetes who have a 10-year risk score of less than 5% is not recommended. This would include most men younger than 50 years and women younger than 60 years who do not have additional risk factors for CVD.[3]

Immunizations

Individuals with diabetes who are 6 months of age and older should receive an annual influenza vaccine. The pneumococcal vaccine should also be given to all patients with diabetes who are 2 years of age and older. A one-time pneumococcal revaccination is recommended for patients older than 64 years who were previously immunized more than 5 years earlier when they were younger than 65 years. The hepatitis B vaccine should be administered to unvaccinated adults (ages 19–59 years) with diabetes, and consideration should be given for administration to those who are unvaccinated over the age of 60.[3] Patients should also be able to show current immunization status for other vaccinations, such as tetanus-diphtheria, hepatitis A, and hepatitis B.

Complementary Therapies

People with diabetes are 1.6 times more likely to use some form of complementary and alternative medicine, including herbal products or dietary supplements, than are people without diabetes.[11] (For an in-depth discussion of natural products as they may relate to patients with diabetes, see Chapter 51.)

Electronic Management Resources for Patients with Diabetes

Advances in technology make diabetes disease management and monitoring much easier. From BG monitors customized for iPhones, mobile applications, and Web sites that allow tracking progress, a vast array of tools is available to make patients' lives easier. Directing patients to free online tools is a great way to keep them actively involved in managing their diabetes.

Many online management Web sites allow patients to track daily blood sugar values and other labs, insulin usage, medication, food consumption, and activity. Data are stored on a secure Web site in a quick, easy-to-read format. Three of the more comprehensive online management tools, discussed below, are ADA's 24/7, My Diabetes Home, and SugarStats.com.

Diabetes 24/7 (247.diabetes.org) allows patients to quickly and easily input and share all valuable health care information with their health care team. ADA has integrated its online management system with Microsoft's HealthVault. The benefit of being linked with HealthVault is that the patient can securely import data from physicians' offices, the hospital laboratory, or the local pharmacy and share that information with anyone he or she chooses. Diabetes 24/7 allows users to monitor their disease by tracking the following: BG, A1C, blood pressure, cholesterol, daily activity levels, weight, and medications. Users can print reports for their caregivers with the most up-to-date information and bring this to their visits. Target goals and times can also be programmed, allowing patients to set and meet individualized goals. Using this system allows patients to quickly and accurately assess response to treatment, and depending on the degree to which they are empowered to make changes, adjust their regimen for better results. Overall, Diabetes 24/7 is extremely functional and easy to use.

The My Diabetes Home (mydiabeteshome.com) Web site provides a "fun, motivational and personalized dashboard" with quick access to tools and resources. This system allows its users to record, track, and monitor medications and certain laboratory information such as BG, blood pressure, weight, cholesterol, and A1C values. Once data are input, comprehensive myVisits reports can be generated, printed, and shared with the patient's health care providers. For more visually oriented patients, custom graphs are available, which provide a great illustration of patient health over time. This site also provides access to a team of health care professionals, including an endocrinologist, registered dieticians, pharmacists, and certified diabetes educators who can provide additional information and suggestions. The site also provides links to money-saving opportunities such as coupons, patient assistance programs, and other cost-saving opportunities that can be used at local pharmacies. Last, My Diabetes Home offers a unique feature called myArticles. Experts have researched the best articles available, and all the information is tailored to fit each patient's specific needs on topics such as fitness tips, blood sugar management ideas, recipe options, and nutrition plans.

A third online management resource is SugarStats.com. This site also has links for inputting data (via multiple devices including smartphones) such as medications, blood sugar and A1C readings, foods, and exercise. Information can be shared with providers electronically, or charts, reports, and graphs can be printed.

Assessment of Diabetes Mellitus: A Case-Based Approach

If a patient describes classic symptoms of diabetes, the health care provider should ask whether a primary care provider has made this diagnosis. If not, screening for diabetes is appropriate. For asymptomatic individuals, ADA recommends that a laboratory-based glucose test be considered to detect type 2 diabetes or prediabetes in individuals who are overweight or obese and have one or more risk factors (e.g., family history, physical in-activity, hypertension, etc.). If normal, patients should be retested every 3 years.[3] Patients with risk factors for diabetes should be considered for testing more frequently and at an earlier age (see Pathophysiology of Diabetes Mellitus). Screening can start with the diabetes risk calculator developed by ADA (www.diabetes.org/diabetes-basics/prevention/diabetes-risk-test/). Individuals with a high risk of prediabetes or diabetes can then be tested for capillary BG (finger stick). High-risk patients identified during screening should be referred to a primary care provider for follow-up.

When working with a patient with newly diagnosed diabetes, the provider should determine all medications and supplements the patient takes, any known drug allergies, any concurrent diseases or infections, and relevant social history (e.g., tobacco use, alcohol use, and insurance coverage). Providers should sensitively assess the patient's beliefs, attitudes, and knowledge about the disease and the effect of diabetes care on the patient's lifestyle. These assessments allow development of a culturally sensitive diabetes education and care plan centered on the patient's expectations and needs. Providers should be prepared to negotiate treatment and adherence strategies, provide information, and answer the patient's questions about diabetes and related conditions. Case 45–1 illustrates assessment of patients with type 2 diabetes mellitus.

Relevant Evaluation Criteria	Scenario/Model Outcome

Information Gathering

1. Gather essential information about the patient's symptoms and medical history, including:

a. description of symptom(s) (i.e., nature, onset, duration, severity, associated symptoms)

The patient presents to the pharmacy with a refill for metformin 500 mg (twice daily) for diabetes. She complains of feeling shaky, lightheaded, and dizzy. These symptoms have worsened over the last 2 hours.

b. description of any factors that seem to precipitate, exacerbate, and/or relieve the patient's symptom(s)

When asked about recent blood glucose readings, the patient notes she has a meter at home but does not typically check on a regular basis. Last time she checked was 1 week ago in the morning before breakfast and it was 98. She notices that she feels more of these symptoms since also starting glipizide XL 10 mg once daily a few days ago. When you check today in the pharmacy, the reading is 52 mg/dL.

c. description of the patient's efforts to relieve the symptoms

Sitting down helps some but not very much.

d. patient's identity

Sandra Dippel

e. age, sex, height, and weight

77 years old, female, 5 ft 2 in., 105 lb

f. patient's occupation

Retired (former elementary school teacher)

g. patient's dietary habits

Consumes approximately 1600 calories per day and classifies her diet as "pretty normal" where she rarely eats out and tries to cook for herself at home.

h. patient's sleep habits

6 hours (12 am to approximately 6 am)

i. concurrent medical conditions, prescription and non-prescription medications, and dietary supplements

Diabetes (type 2): metformin 500 mg twice daily, glipizide XL 10 mg every morning; dyslipidemia: simvastatin 20 mg at bedtime

j. allergies

NKA

k. history of other adverse reactions to medications

NA

l. other (describe) _____

None

Assessment and Triage

2. Differentiate patient's signs/symptoms and correctly identify the patient's primary problem(s).

The patient has type 2 diabetes and is presenting with symptoms of hypoglycemia since recently starting a new medication (glipizide XL 10 mg). According to the patient's age, weight, and blood glucose level that was at goal when self-checking approximately 1 week ago before starting the glipizide, the dose is likely too high and needs to be adjusted. She has other comorbidities (dyslipidemia) that highlight the need for appropriate blood glucose control. Her age, weight, and gender may put her at risk for a fracture from a fall secondary to her symptoms of low blood sugar.

3. Identify exclusions for self-treatment.

Sandra has hypoglycemia signified by her reading at the pharmacy today and symptoms since initiating a new medication. Also, the status of her comorbidity of dyslipidemia is unknown.

4. Formulate a comprehensive list of therapeutic alternatives for the primary problem to determine if triage to a health care provider is required, and share this information with the patient or caregiver.

Options include:

(1) Refer Sandra to receive immediate medical treatment.

(2) Treat the low blood glucose in the pharmacy, and then recommend follow-up as soon as possible with her PCP.

(3) Provide Sandra with instructions to self-treat her low blood sugar on her own, and then encourage a follow-up appointment as soon as possible with her PCP.

Plan

5. Select an optimal therapeutic alternative to address the patient's problem, taking into account patient preferences.

Recommend treating the low blood glucose in the pharmacy and then referring for appropriate follow-up with the PCP as soon as possible.

Acute plan: Take 15 grams of carbohydrates (e.g. glucose tablets, small glass of a soft drink or juice). Have the patient wait in the pharmacy in an observable place for approximately 15 minutes. At that point, recheck the blood glucose level, and if it is still below 70 mg/dL, have her take an additional 15 grams of carbohydrates. Continue this process until the blood glucose is >70 mg/dL. At that time, if a meal is not planned within the hour, the patient should consume a small snack containing a carbohydrate plus a protein

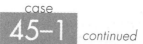

case

45–1 *continued*

Relevant Evaluation Criteria	Scenario/Model Outcome
	(e.g., crackers and peanut butter). If her blood glucose level is not improving (and/or continues to drop) despite treatment, the pharmacist should call 911. **Once resolved:** In addition, refer the patient to her PCP for a follow-up. Because Sandra is at risk for hypoglycemia, suggest initiation of self-monitoring of blood glucose. According to ADA guidelines, the evidence for self-testing for patients not on multiple-dose insulin therapy is mixed. However, in this case, self-testing for a period of time until seeing the PCP may be warranted because of the episode of hypoglycemia. Therefore, until Sandra can see her PCP, recommend that she monitor and record her blood glucose level once daily, alternating testing between fasting and 2 hours after the biggest meal of the day. These values can be shared with the PCP. Counsel her on proper use of the blood glucose meter, as well as management and identification of the signs and symptoms of hypoglycemia. At the conclusion of the session, Sandra should demonstrate her understanding of how to test her blood glucose. Stress to Sandra that it is not ideal to use another patient's blood glucose meter and supplies.
6. Describe the recommended therapeutic approach to the patient or caregiver.	"You are currently experiencing low blood sugar that needs to be treated. I would like you to consume these carbohydrates and sit here in the waiting area so I can observe you over the next 15 minutes. After 15 minutes, I will recheck your blood sugar to see if it is above 70 mg/dL and to determine how you are feeling. If your blood sugar is not above 70 in 15 minutes, I will have you take another dose of carbohydrates. We will repeat that process until your sugar is above 70 mg/dL." "Now that your blood sugar is at the recommended level, you should follow up with your primary care provider. In the meantime, I recommend that you test your blood sugar once daily (alternating between first thing in the morning before you eat breakfast and 2 hours after your biggest meal of the day). Please record your blood sugar values to share with your PCP during the follow-up visit."
7. Explain to the patient or caregiver the rationale for selecting the recommended therapeutic approach from the considered therapeutic alternatives.	"You need to see a primary care provider because of the symptoms you are having and the other conditions you have that may increase your risk for further problems. It is important for your provider to know of these symptoms so that proper adjustments can be made to your medication therapy to achieve the desired goals. In the meantime, it is important that you check your blood sugar regularly. This will help you identify trends in your daily values, and your provider will have more information about your blood sugar levels at your visit."

Patient Education

8. When recommending self-care with nonprescription medications and/or nondrug therapy, convey accurate information to the patient or caregiver.	Criterion does not apply in this case.
Solicit follow-up questions from the patient or caregiver.	"Is there anything I can do to prevent this from happening again?"
Answer the patient's or caregiver's questions.	"Yes, it is important that you follow up with your primary care provider as soon as possible to determine the best medications for you that will help control your blood sugar but will not cause it to go too low. In the meantime, I am going to call your PCP to let him or her know what happened and to determine the appropriate immediate steps that need to be taken, such as potentially stopping the glipizide XL medication and checking your blood sugar."

Evaluation of Patient Outcome

9. Assess patient outcome.	Contact the patient in a day to ensure she made a follow-up appointment with her PCP, to determine how she is feeling, and to assess her understanding of using a blood glucose monitor.

Key: ADA = American Diabetes Association; NA = not applicable; NKA = no known allergy; PCP = primary care provider.

For overweight patients with type 2 diabetes, providers should also discuss weight loss (see Chapter 26). Education should focus on the link between overweight or obesity and type 2 diabetes, as well as the importance of weight loss in helping control the disease. The overall health benefits of weight reduction should also be discussed. Learning that weight loss and consistent physical activity may obviate the need for medications may motivate an individual to lose weight.

Patient Counseling for Diabetes Mellitus

Adhering to healthy eating, regular physical activity, and medication regimens is often a challenge for individuals with diabetes. Providers can assist patients to overcome barriers to adhering to their diabetes therapies while also providing encouragement and counseling on meal planning and physical activity. Each patient encounter is an opportunity for the provider to evaluate and educate patients. A good way to start a conversation and help identify patient knowledge and commitment to self-care is asking simple questions such as the following: "What are your blood glucose readings running these days?" "What was your last A1C value?" If insulin was prescribed, the provider should explain the various diabetes care products, teach the patient how to use the selected products, and review the symptoms and treatment of hyper- and hypoglycemia. Patients should be encouraged to return for reevaluation of injection technique, self-monitoring of their BG, and adherence to a prescribed self-care routine. Moreover, providers should be familiar with new medications and devices, as well as keep abreast of current practice guidelines for the care of people with diabetes. The box Patient Education for Diabetes Mellitus lists specific information to provide patients.

patient education for
Diabetes Mellitus

The primary objective of diabetes self-care is to achieve and maintain metabolic control. Secondary benefits of meeting metabolic goals are to (1) prevent or reverse diabetes complications, (2) maintain normal daily activities with maximum lifestyle flexibility, (3) avoid weight gain by following a proper nutrition and physical activity plan, (4) avoid infection, and (5) achieve a sense of well-being. For most patients, carefully following product instructions (including instructions on the proper use of insulin) and the self-care measures listed here will help ensure optimal therapeutic outcomes.

Nondrug Measures

- Recognize that having diabetes requires lifestyle and behavioral changes.
- Consult with your primary care provider, dietitian, nurse, or pharmacist to develop a nutrition plan and physical activity program that suits your lifestyle.
- Learn how to read food labels.
- Involve your entire family in your healthy lifestyle changes.
- Knowledge is power. Know your glucose and other diabetes-related goals (Table 45–2). Learn about your disease and the ways you can take control of your diabetes.
- Where indicated check your BG (blood glucose) regularly and know what makes your glucose concentrations go up and down (e.g., foods, activity, medications, and/or stress).
- Use a logbook to document BG results, diet, physical activity, insulin, or other medication administration changes, and bring it with you to every health care visit.
- To avoid being overwhelmed, set realistic, achievable goals. Make one or two specific changes at a time and recognize your accomplishments.
- If you have a diabetes complication, consult a diabetes specialist. Practice the preventive measures listed in Table 45–1.
- When performing physical activities conscientiously, follow the guidelines in Table 45–3.
- Where indicated monitor your BG several times each day (e.g., before meals, 2 hours after meals, or at bedtime). If a BG reading is greater than 240 mg/dL, check urine ketones. If your values indicate a problem, see your primary care provider for adjustments to your therapy.
- If you use tobacco products, it is strongly advised you quit. A tobacco cessation program, which includes counseling and smoking cessation medications, is highly recommended (see Chapter 47).
- See your primary care provider if you have cuts or bruises that are not healing.

Nonprescription and Prescription Medications

- Follow your prescribed medication regimen, including insulin, carefully.
- Inject your insulin at the proper sites, and rotate your injection sites (Figure 45–1).
- Follow the guidelines in Tables 45–6 and 45–7 for preparing and injecting insulin doses.
- Know the signs and symptoms related to low or high BG concentrations as well as appropriate monitoring and management strategies.
- Discuss with your primary care provider taking a low dose of aspirin daily to prevent heart attack and stroke.
- Take your medications as directed by your provider. Do not stop taking any of your medications unless you first discuss it with your provider.
- Do not start taking any nonprescription medications or complementary therapies without first discussing them with your pharmacist or primary care provider. Consult your pharmacist for safe nonprescription medication options to treat self-limiting conditions such as allergies, cough, or upset stomach.
- Read the labels of nonprescription medications to identify sugar and alcohol content. Avoid medications that contain sugar or alcohol.
- Certain cold medications, such as pseudoephedrine, may raise BG concentrations and blood pressure levels. Talk to your provider or pharmacist before selecting any allergy, cough, or cold preparations.
- Talk to your pharmacist about strategies to help you remember to take your medications.

When to Seek Medical Attention

- If you use insulin and experience symptoms of hypoglycemia (e.g., sweating, hunger, rapid heartbeat, and/or confusion), hyperglycemia (e.g., frequent urination, dehydration, thirst, and/or increased appetite), or ketoacidosis (e.g., BG greater than 240 mg/dL plus urine ketones and flulike symptoms, confusion, and/or stupor), contact your primary care provider.

Evaluation of Patient Outcomes for Diabetes Mellitus

ADA recommends specific therapeutic goals for people with diabetes (Table 45–2). If the patient is not achieving these outcomes, adherence to the care plan should be assessed. Nonadherent patients should be reevaluated and, if necessary, reeducated about the need for and benefits of the care plan. If nonadherence is not the problem, medical referral is appropriate. In addition, weight management should be closely monitored in patients with type 2 diabetes.

Key Points for Diabetes Mellitus

➤ Early detection; extensive patient education; and early, aggressive glycemic control through MNT, physical activity, and pharmacologic therapy can prevent the development and progression of the long-term complications, morbidity, and mortality associated with diabetes.

➤ Familiarity with the most current standards for diabetes screening and management is imperative to reducing and eliminating health disparities associated with diabetes risk, outcomes, morbidity, and mortality, and to improving care for all patients with diabetes.

➤ Patients should be educated about diabetes, the role of BG control in the prevention of long-term complications, self-care strategies (including SMBG and MNT), and pharmacologic therapy.

➤ Providers should be familiar with and assist patients in selecting BG monitors and related supplies.

➤ Patients using insulin therapy should be educated about insulin and related supplies, proper injection site and technique, insulin storage, and potential adverse events and their management.

➤ Providers and patients should negotiate adherence strategies tailored to patient-specific factors such as, but not limited to, food and activity preferences; sleep, mealtime, and work schedules; insurance status; and income.

➤ Patients with diabetes should be educated about the safety and efficacy of nonprescription medications for self-care of limited acute conditions and about complementary and alternative medicines.

Asthma

Asthma remains one of the most common chronic health conditions in the United States. The most recent statistics describing asthma prevalence suggest that almost 26 million people in the United States had this condition in 2010. This includes approximately 7 million children younger than 18 years and almost 19 million adults. Of patients diagnosed with asthma, just over half have had at least one asthmatic attack on an annual basis (55.8% in 2001, 51.9% in 2009). Hospital outpatient department visits per 100 persons with asthma have ranged from a low of 4.8 (2006, 2009) to a high

of 7.6 (2003), with a slight downward trend from 2008 to 2009. Emergency department visits per 100 persons with asthma ranged from 7 (2006) to 9.5 (2002) with the rate holding steady for the last 2 years of the survey (2008 and 2009; 8.2 and 8.4, respectively). For all the preceding parameters, those in the age group of 4 years and younger had the highest incidence. The overall death rate has decreased from 2.1 per 10,000 persons with asthma in 2003 to 1.4 in 2009. Asthma more negatively affects some subsets of the population. Data for 2009 for hospital outpatient department visits for blacks were twice the rate for whites, while the rate for the Hispanic or Latino population was similar to whites. The rate of physician office visits for blacks and Hispanics/Latinos was 50% more than for whites and blacks, and Hispanic/Latinos had at least twice the rate of emergency department visits compared with whites. Blacks with asthma were twice as likely to die compared with whites or Hispanics and Latinos.[12] In addition to the factors mentioned above, the following groups tend to have a higher incidence of asthma: children (boys in particular), adult women, Puerto Ricans, residents in the northeast corridor of the United States, those living in poverty, and people exposed to certain chemicals in the workplace.[13]

Pathophysiology of Asthma

The exact etiology of asthma is unknown.[14] Potential causes or risks for developing asthma include positive family history, concurrent atopy (increased production of immunoglobulin E, or IgE, after allergen exposure), smoking or exposure to secondhand smoke, higher body mass index, and severe viral respiratory infections during the first 3 years of life. Once asthma develops, various stimuli (often called "triggers"; Table 45–8) can precipitate asthma symptoms. Not all patients with asthma have the same triggers, and the response of an individual to a particular trigger can change over time.

Although bronchoconstriction may be responsible for some acute asthma symptoms, inflammation is largely responsible for severe and persistent asthma symptoms.[15] Once exposed to a trigger, an immediate or early asthmatic response occurs within minutes. The mechanism of this response includes degranulation of mast cells to release histamine and leukotrienes, which causes bronchoconstriction. As the airways narrow, the peak expiratory flow (PEF) decreases and may result in wheezing, chest tightness, cough, and shortness of breath.

A significant number of patients with asthma also have reflux, yet the specific relationship between gastroesophageal reflux disease (GERD) and asthma or worsening asthma is still not completely clear.[16] Initial studies demonstrated that proton pump inhibitor therapy may improve symptoms and pulmonary function in some patients with GERD and asthma,[17] but some newer data show proton pump inhibitors offer little to no benefit.[18]

Although some asthma patients insist that certain foods make them wheeze or experience shortness of breath, confirmed asthmatic reactions to food are uncommon.[19] Even when the trigger is known, prospective identification and avoidance of foods containing these compounds can be challenging. Questionnaires to help identify these triggers are available (see Nonpharmacologic Therapy and Table 45–9).

table 45-8	**Examples of Asthma Triggers**	
Environmental	**Drugs or Chemicals**	**Conditions or Events**
Animals (e.g., cats, dogs, rodents)	Aspirin	Allergic rhinitis
Cockroaches	Beta-adrenergic blockers	Emotional stress, excitement
Cold air	Food or drug preservatives (e.g., metabisulfite)	Exercise
House dust mites	Household cleaning agents	GERD
Indoor irritants (e.g., wood-burning stoves)	NSAIDs	Menstruation, pregnancy
Outdoor air pollution (e.g., vehicle emissions, sulfur dioxide, ozone, nitrogen oxides)	Occupational exposure to dust, chemicals, irritants	Panic attacks
Indoor or outdoor molds and fungi	Perfumes	Viral respiratory infections
Pollen (e.g., grass, weeds, trees)		
Tobacco smoke		
Food allergies (such as seafood, shellfish)		

Key: GERD = Gastroesophageal reflux disease; NSAID = nonsteroidal anti-inflammatory drug.

table 45-9	**Example of a Trigger Screen Tool**[a]

Thinking about how you have felt in the past month, please answer the following questions:

- Do you ever have problems with wheezing or catching your breath when exposed to cold air?
- Do you wheeze when dusting, vacuuming, or using cleaning solvents in the home?
- Do you wheeze, cough, or sneeze, or become short of breath when around household pets such as cats or dogs?
- Do you have problems breathing when exposed to high levels of stress or excitement?
- Have you ever noticed wheezing or worsening shortness of breath before or during your menstrual period?
- Have you ever had a reaction such as shortness of breath, or swollen throat, lips, or tongue after you took medications such as aspirin or ibuprofen?
- Do you have breathing problems after eating shellfish, peanuts, or any other foods?
- Do you have breathing problems when exposed to latex (e.g., rubber gloves or balloons)?
- Does it take you a long time to get over a viral cold?
- Do you have chronic heartburn?
- Do you have problems breathing at work yet are fine during holidays or weekends spent at home?
- Does anyone else at work appear to have similar symptoms?
- Do you typically have a runny nose and watery eyes and experience repetitive sneezing during outdoor activities?
- Are these symptoms worse during:
  Early spring?
  Late spring?
  Late summer to fall?
  Summer and fall?
- Do you experience shortness of breath during or after exercise?

If you answered yes to any of the above questions, please show this questionnaire to your primary care provider.

[a] See Chapter 11 for more information on allergies and their triggers.

Clinical Presentation of Asthma

Key features of asthma are recurrent bouts of wheezing, shortness of breath, chest tightness, and cough, especially at night and in the early morning hours. Asthma symptoms vary in duration, severity, and frequency. Exacerbation severity is assessed based on symptom severity. Patients with asthma need to monitor for worsening control and try to identify the onset of acute asthma exacerbations. A drop in PEF can be the first sign of an impending exacerbation and may precede the onset of significant symptoms.

Other conditions may present with asthma-like symptoms (Table 45–10). In assessing someone who presents with shortness of breath, inquiring about a prior diagnosis of asthma, tobacco use, and onset and duration of symptoms is important. If the individual does not have a prior diagnosis of asthma or if the symptoms are different or more severe than usual, a medical referral is necessary for further evaluation (Table 45–11). Symptoms usually respond to medications; however, severe asthma exacerbations may require emergent care and systemic corticosteroids. Even patients with mild asthma can develop life-threatening exacerbations.

Treatment of Asthma

Ideally, most treatment for asthma should be in the ambulatory setting and should focus on preventing symptoms rather than treating asthma exacerbations. Patients with asthma need to know how to take their medications, monitor for worsening symptoms, manage environmental triggers, and recognize when to seek medical care. Developing an optimal, comprehensive, and individualized asthma care plan requires a partnership between individuals with asthma and their primary care providers. Therefore, self-*care* is a critical part of management. However, isolated self-*treatment* of asthma-like symptoms is potentially dangerous because other serious conditions, such as heart failure, can cause similar symptoms. In addition, mild

table

45–10 Comparison of Selected Conditions That May Present with Respiratory Symptoms

	Asthma	COPD	Respiratory Infection	Heart Failure
Signs	Decreased PEF Increased heart rate Increased respiratory rate	Progressive decline in PEF and FEV$_1$ Polycythemia Signs of right heart failure Pulmonary hypertension Decreased oxygen saturation Pursed lip breathing Increased heart rate Increased respiratory rate	Increased heart rate Increased respiratory rate Fever Increased white blood cell count	Ejection fraction <40% Lower-extremity edema, S$_3$ heart sound Positive hepatojugular reflex Jugular venous distension
Symptoms	Wheezing Cough Chest tightness	Progressive dyspnea on exertion Productive cough Wheezing	Productive cough Nasal congestion Rhinorrhea	Dyspnea on exertion Orthopnea
Onset	Often occurs in childhood, but can develop in adults	Usually the fourth or fifth decade of life Progressive; symptoms develop over years	Any age Symptoms acute, sudden	Older adults
Etiology	Often atopy	Most commonly tobacco smoking	Viruses Bacteria	Hypertension Coronary artery disease
Exacerbating factors	Trigger exposure	Continued smoking		Heavy salt intake Myocardial infarction Nonadherence with medications

Key: COPD = Chronic obstructive pulmonary disease; FEV$_1$ = forced expiratory volume at 1 second; PEF = peak expiratory flow.

table

45–11 Comparison of Indications for Self-Treatment with Nonprescription Medications versus Medical Care for Asthma

Self-treatment *may* be appropriate when:

- The current symptoms are mild, intermittent (less than twice weekly), and of short duration (e.g., <24 hours) OR
- A prior diagnosis of intermittent asthma has been made by a primary care provider AND
- The individual knows the warning symptoms indicating the need for urgent medical care AND
- The individual does not have any other serious concurrent diseases that might impair oxygenation or breathing (e.g., COPD, coronary artery disease) AND
- The individual is 5 years of age or older and not pregnant AND
- The current asthma symptoms are consistent with previous symptoms AND
- The nonprescription medications are for short-term (<24 hours) treatment of mild symptoms until the individual can be seen by a primary care provider

Referral for medical care *should* be made when:

- The symptoms are of moderate severity (e.g., affect activities or sleep) or are more frequent than twice weekly OR
- The symptoms have lasted more than 24 hours OR
- The symptoms do not respond to nonprescription asthma medications within 24 hours OR
- The symptoms differ in quality or severity from those in previous episodes OR
- Signs or symptoms of a respiratory or sinus infection are also present (e.g., fever or purulent nasal discharge) OR
- The individual does not have a previous diagnosis of asthma OR
- The individual has a concurrent condition with symptoms (e.g., cough, wheeze, or shortness of breath) that may be similar to asthma (e.g., heart failure, chronic obstructive pulmonary disease, or vocal cord dysfunction) OR
- The individual has a history of asthma episodes severe enough to require systemic corticosteroids or urgent medical care OR
- The individual is taking (or nonadherent to) other prescription long-term controller medications for asthma OR
- The individual does not have an asthma care provider or has not seen the asthma care provider in the last year OR
- The individual is pregnant or a child younger than 5 years of age OR
- The individual perceives that the prescription medications are not effective

Key: COPD = Chronic obstructive pulmonary disease.

asthma symptoms may escalate into serious exacerbations if inadequately treated.

Treatment Goals

Optimal asthma management and therapy imply that *all* goals are met, which include the following:

- Achieving and maintaining control of symptoms; one tool to assess symptom control is the Asthma Control Test, a series of five questions patients with asthma should answer prior to each visit to a health care provider and take to each visit to help with therapy assessment and response.[20]
- Having normal activity levels
- Infrequently using an inhaled short-acting beta$_2$-agonist (less than twice per week)
- Maintaining pulmonary function as close to normal as possible (PEF $\geq$ 80% of personal best)
- Preventing recurrent exacerbations and the need for urgent care visits
- Providing optimal pharmacologic therapy with minimal or no adverse effects
- Meeting the patient's and his or her family's expectations of asthma care[21]

Even relatively mild-moderate asthma symptoms can significantly impair quality of life. Because most symptoms are readily responsive to medications, the patient needs to understand that frequent symptoms (even mild ones) can and should be prevented. Patients with asthma also need to be confident that they can successfully prevent escalation of symptoms into significant asthma exacerbations. Most patients realize that severe symptoms requiring the need for urgent medical care represent uncontrolled asthma. All these issues should be addressed in a self-management asthma action plan.

General Treatment Approach

Asthma medications are categorized into two groups. Quick-relief medications are used as needed to treat symptoms. Long-term control medications are used daily to prevent symptoms. Inhaled medications have fewer adverse reactions compared with systemic medications. However, the effectiveness of inhaled medications is severely limited when poor device technique decreases drug delivery to the lungs. A detailed discussion of the therapeutic options and rationale for the treatment of asthma in adults and children can be found in the guidelines from the National Asthma Education Prevention Program[21] and the Global Initiative for Asthma.[14]

A comprehensive, individualized *asthma self-care plan* includes when to use long-term control medications and quick-relief medications, how to use asthma devices to optimally deliver medications, how to avoid and minimize effects of asthma triggers, how to prevent the escalation of asthma symptoms into exacerbations, and how to recognize warning signs that require emergent medical treatment. Specific recommendations are provided for when to use quick-relief medications (e.g., prior to exposure to known triggers) and how much to use (e.g., "x" number of puffs every "y" hours). Figure 45–3 is an example of a symptom-based asthma self-care plan. Some self-care plans include recommendations based on the patient's personal best PEF.

Another issue to consider related to asthma treatment is the cost of care. For some individuals, physician office and prescription co-payments are much less than the cost for self-care options. However, for others with little or no insurance, the only options would be nonprescription products and emergency care, with little or no emphasis on preventive care. Determining the significance of health care costs early in the patient assessment process is recommended.

Nonpharmacologic Therapy

Because exposure to triggers can lead to worsening asthma symptoms and because each patient's asthma triggers are different, a comprehensive, individualized trigger management plan should be developed. Once triggers are identified, suggestions are incorporated into the self-care plan to minimize exposure to triggers at home, work, or school. Specific triggers that occur frequently and require further attention include allergy symptoms, exposure to medications that may exacerbate asthma symptoms, and exposure to tobacco smoke.

Proper management of allergy symptoms may improve upper-airway hyperreactivity and asthma symptoms. Labels on first-generation antihistamines (e.g., diphenhydramine) caution persons with asthma against using these agents because of concern that the anticholinergic properties may thicken mucus and decrease mucociliary clearance. These effects are generally minor and are outweighed by the benefits of treating allergic rhinitis in asthma patients. The second-generation antihistamines (e.g., loratadine, cetirizine, and fexofenadine) have little to no anticholinergic properties and do not carry this labeling precaution.

Because certain medications can worsen symptoms, patients with asthma should be cautious about the use of aspirin and nonprescription nonsteroidal anti-inflammatory drugs (NSAIDs) used to treat fever, pain, or inflammation. These medications pose an increased risk of aspirin sensitivity (see Chapters 5 and 6). Symptoms of aspirin sensitivity can be severe and life-threatening and may include itchy or watery eyes, itchy rashes, rashes around the mouth, nasal congestion, hives, worsening asthma, cough or wheezing, and anaphylaxis.[22] Significant potential for cross-sensitivity exists with NSAIDs such as ibuprofen and naproxen. Someone with aspirin sensitivity can usually tolerate acetaminophen. Patients sensitive to aspirin should be cautioned to check the labels of analgesic and antipyretic medications before use to see if they contain NSAIDs. Aspirin-sensitive patients should also be cautioned to avoid other agents that contain salicylates such as oil of wintergreen and bismuth subsalicylate.

Finally, patients with asthma and their family members should be urged not to smoke because tobacco smoke may trigger an asthma exacerbation. Mothers who smoke during pregnancy increase their children's risk of acquiring asthma.[23] Children exposed to secondhand tobacco smoke are more likely to develop asthma and have poorer asthma control. Providers should educate all patients who use tobacco products about options for cessation (see Chapter 47). The commercially available forms of nicotine replacement therapy may be effective as part of a comprehensive tobacco cessation plan. However, the prescription nicotine nasal spray and inhaler are not recommended for people with asthma because nicotine could irritate the airways and trigger an exacerbation.

Pharmacologic Therapy

Few nonprescription medications are available to manage asthma (Table 45–12).[24–27] Patients who are started on a metered-dose inhaler (MDI) should receive counseling for proper technique

ASTHMA ACTION PLAN

St.Louis Regional *Asthma Consortium*
Sponsored by the American Lung Association of Eastern Missouri

Name: _____

Provider: _____

Date: _____

Phone for doctor or clinic: _____

After office hours call: _____

GREEN ZONE

- Breathing is good
- No cough or wheeze
- Can work and play

YOU'RE OK! TAKE ALL OF THESE MEDICATIONS EVERY DAY!

Medicine	How much to take	When to take it
_____	_____	_____
_____	_____	_____
_____	_____	_____

20 minutes before physical activity, use this medicine: _____

YELLOW ZONE

- You are feeling sick or it's harder to breathe

CAUTION! TAKE 2 PUFFS (OR 1 NEBULIZER TREATMENT) OF YOUR QUICK RELIEVER MEDICINE NOW: _____
YOU MAY REPEAT THIS EVERY 20 MINUTES FOR 2 MORE TIMES.
IF YOU ARE NO BETTER CALL YOUR DOCTOR
IMMEDIATELY AT _____ !

| Cough | Wheeze | Tight chest | Wake up at night |

Medicine	How much to take	When to take it
_____	_____	_____
_____	_____	_____

RED ZONE

- Medicine is not helping
- Breathing is hard and fast
- Nose opens wide
- Can't walk or talk well
- Ribs show

DANGER!
TAKE 4 MORE PUFFS (OR 1 NEBULIZER TREATMENT) OF YOUR QUICK RELIEVER MEDICINE NOW.
CALL 9-1-1 OR GO DIRECTLY TO THE NEAREST HOSPITAL!

Medicine	How much to take	When to take it
_____	_____	_____
_____	_____	_____

---

figure 45-3 Sample asthma self-care plan. (*Source:* Reprinted with the permission of the St. Louis Regional Asthma Consortium.)

table
45–12 | Medications Included in Nonprescription Products for the Treatment of Asthma

Drug	Mechanism	Dosage and Administration		Safety Considerations
Racepinephrine (e.g., Asthmanefrin) nebulizer solution	Bronchodilator	Adults and children 4 years and older 2.25% racepinephrine HCl. For use in an atomizer (EZ Breathe Atomizer). Add contents of one vial (0.5 mL) of solution to atomizer. Adults and children ≥ 4 years of age: 1–3 inhalations. Do not use more than every 3 hours and not more than 12 inhalations in 24 hours.		Relative contraindications include pregnancy, hyperthyroidism, hypertension, heart disease, use of other medications (prescription, nonprescription, or herbal therapy). Do not use this product if it is brown in color or cloudy.
Ephedrine/guaifenesin combination products	Bronchodilator + expectorant	Bronkaid Dual Action Formula	Ephedrine 25 mg Guaifenesin 400 mg	1 tablet every 4 hours as needed; do not exceed 6 tablets per day. Do not use in children < 12 years old.	Ephedrine side effects include palpitations, tachycardia, arrhythmias, seizures, hypokalemia, angina, hyperglycemia, hypotension, and hypertension.
		Primatene Tablets	Ephedrine 12.5 mg Guaifenesin 200 mg	1–2 tablets every 4 hours as needed; do not exceed 12 tablets per day. Do not use in children < 12 years old.	Guaifenesin: Case reports have linked nephrolithiasis to guaifenesin alone and in combination with ephedrine.
		Dynafed Asthma Relief Tablets	Ephedrine 25 mg Guaifenesin 200 mg	1/2–1 tablet every 4 hours as needed; do not exceed 6 tablets per day.	
		Mini Two Way Action Asthma Relief Tablets	Ephedrine 25 mg Guaifenesin 200 mg	1/2–1 tablet every 4 hours as needed; do not exceed 6 tablets per day.	

Source: References 24–27.

Closed Mouth Technique

- Step 1
  — Remove dust cap from inhaler.
  — Attach inhaler to spacer/holding chamber if you have one.
  — Shake the inhaler well, as shown in drawing A.

A

- Step 2
  — Blow out all the air in your lungs (see drawing B).

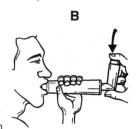

B

- Step 3
  — Seal lips tightly around the mouthpiece.
  — Press down on the inhaler to release medicine as you breathe in slowly until your lungs are full.
  — If using a spacer/holding chamber press down on the inhaler and then wait 5 seconds before breathing in (see drawing C).

C

- Step 4
  — Hold your breath for 10 seconds to allow medicine to reach deeply into your lungs (see drawing D).

 10, 9, 8, …

D

- Step 5
  — Blow out the air in your lungs (see drawing E).

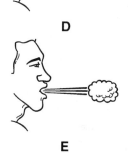

E

Open Mouth Technique

- Step 1
  — Take off the cap.
  — Shake the inhaler (see drawing F).

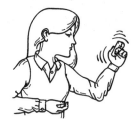

F

- Step 2
  — Stand up and tilt head back a little (see drawing G).

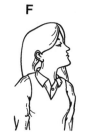

G

- Step 3
  — Place your hand between your mouth and the inhaler. This will help measure how far away the inhaler should be from your mouth (see drawing H).

- Step 4
  — Take a cleansing breath, in and out.

H

- Step 5
  — Open your mouth wide.
  — Start to breathe in slowly.
  — Push down on the medicine and continue to breathe in (see drawing I).

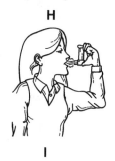

- Step 6
  — Hold your breath.
  — Count to 10 and then breathe out.

I

- Step 7
  — If asthma care plan instructs you to use 2 puffs, wait 15–30 seconds and repeat steps 1–6.

figure

45–4 Guidelines for using a metered-dose inhaler.

(Figure 45–4). Nonprescription medications are generally indicated only for mild infrequent symptoms. Patients who have more frequent or serious symptoms should be referred to a primary care provider so a long-term controller medication can be prescribed. Figure 45–5 lists additional exclusions for self-care. All patients with asthma should be followed closely by a primary care provider.

The pharmacist should review with the patient the lifestyle modifications listed in the Nonpharmacologic Therapy section. The importance of these measures in controlling asthma-related symptoms and complications should be discussed.

Bronchodilators

Two nonselective beta-agonists, epinephrine and ephedrine, are available without a prescription (Table 45–12). Sales of

ephedrine fall under the Combat Methamphetamine Epidemic Act of 2005 and therefore have purchase restrictions, such as quantity limits, placement where customers do not have direct access, and required proof of identification. Because nonselective beta-agonists also act on alpha-receptors, they can constrict blood vessels and increase blood pressure, potentially causing arrhythmias, nervousness, and palpitations. Generally, nonprescription beta-agonists have a shorter duration of action requiring more frequent administration, and they have a greater potential for side effects and abuse compared with prescription beta-agonist medications. Asthmanefrin, introduced fall 2012, is a racemic epinephrine solution for inhalation available over the counter. Primatene Mist was removed from the market in 2011 because of concerns about chlorofluorocarbons and the environment. According to the package labeling, Asthmanefrin is indicated "for temporary relief of shortness of breath,

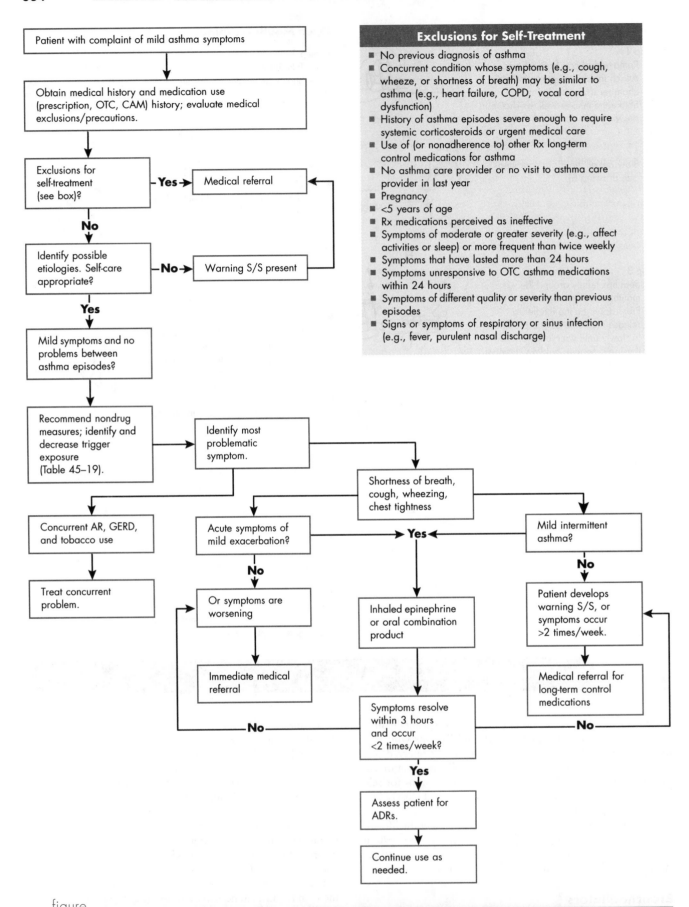

Exclusions for Self-Treatment

- No previous diagnosis of asthma
- Concurrent condition whose symptoms (e.g., cough, wheeze, or shortness of breath) may be similar to asthma (e.g., heart failure, COPD, vocal cord dysfunction)
- History of asthma episodes severe enough to require systemic corticosteroids or urgent medical care
- Use of (or nonadherence to) other Rx long-term control medications for asthma
- No asthma care provider or no visit to asthma care provider in last year
- Pregnancy
- <5 years of age
- Rx medications perceived as ineffective
- Symptoms of moderate or greater severity (e.g., affect activities or sleep) or more frequent than twice weekly
- Symptoms that have lasted more than 24 hours
- Symptoms unresponsive to OTC asthma medications within 24 hours
- Symptoms of different quality or severity than previous episodes
- Signs or symptoms of respiratory or sinus infection (e.g., fever, purulent nasal discharge)

figure 45–5 Self-care of asthma. Key: ADR = Adverse drug reaction; AR = allergic rhinitis; CAM = complementary and alternative medicine; COPD = chronic obstructive pulmonary disease; GERD = gastroesophageal reflux disease; OTC = over-the-counter; Rx = prescription; S/S = signs and symptoms.

tightness of chest, and wheezing due to bronchial asthma." Dosing recommendations are provided for individuals 4 years of age and older, with 1–3 inhalations every 3 hours up to a maximum of 12 inhalations in 24 hours. The medication is available as a 2.25% solution in 0.5 mL, 5 vials in foil pouches. The manufacturer, Nephron Pharmaceuticals Corporation, offers two packages: a starter kit that includes the EZ Breathe Atomizer and 10 vials of medication, and the refill package that includes 30 vials of medication.[27] In September 2013, FDA warned Nephron Pharmaceuticals Corporation that aerosolized Asthmanefrin is an unapproved new drug and that the claim as an alternative to Primatene Mist CFC Inhaler is false or misleading.[28] On September 30, 2013, FDA warned patients and health care professionals about safety concerns with Asthmanefrin.[29] Adverse events reported to FDA in the past year include chest pain, nausea and vomiting, increased blood pressure, increased heart rate, and hemoptysis.

Combination Bronchodilator Products

Compared with inhaled medications, nonprescription oral products (Table 45–12) have a greater potential for side effects because of their systemic absorption. An expectorant, guaifenesin, is often included in combination products, but its efficacy in asthma has not been shown (see Chapter 12). Guaifenesin has no bronchodilatory effects but is marketed to assist with loosening phlegm and thinning bronchial secretions (to increase cough productivity), although efficacy has not been established.

Influenza Vaccine

All patients with asthma who are 6 months of age and older should receive an influenza vaccination yearly.[21] In addition to the traditional influenza vaccine, FDA approved two new versions of influenza vaccines at the end of 2012/early 2013. One product, Flublok, indicated for patients ages 18–49, is manufactured using an insect virus expression system in combination with recombinant DNA technology. The second product, Flucelvax, indicated for patients ages 18 years and older, is manufactured using the familiar cell culture technology; however, animal cells are used rather than the traditional fertilized chicken egg model. Both manufacturing processes allow quick production cycles in case of a pandemic.[30,31]

The live intranasal influenza vaccine, FluMist, is not recommended for patients with a history of asthma or reactive airways disease and should not be administered to children younger than 5 years with recurrent wheezing because of the risk of wheezing after vaccination.[32]

Pneumococcal Polysaccharide Vaccine, Polyvalent (PPSV23)

The Advisory Committee on Immunization Practices recommends pneumonia vaccination for all patients with asthma between ages 19 to 64 years. A second pneumococcal dose is recommended for those 65 years and older, and for those who received their first dose when they were younger than 65 and 5 or more years have expired since the first dose.[33]

Product Selection Guidelines

Special Population Considerations

Persons of Advanced Age. Older patients with asthma should be strongly cautioned against self-treating with nonprescription asthma medications because of the risk of cardiovascular adverse effects with these products. Elderly persons with a new-onset breathing problem should be referred to their primary care provider to rule out other causes of shortness of breath that mimic asthma, such as congestive heart failure, pneumonia, and chronic obstructive pulmonary disease (COPD) (Table 45–10). Dexterity issues (e.g., secondary to arthritis) may make using asthma devices correctly difficult for elderly people.

Pregnant Patients. Pregnant women with asthma should be urged not to use nonprescription asthma medications without the knowledge of their primary care provider. Poorly controlled asthma can worsen outcomes of the pregnancy. Ephedrine and epinephrine are both Pregnancy Category C drugs that stimulate alpha- and beta-adrenergic receptors.[34] Inhaled prescription bronchodilators (e.g., albuterol)[35] are preferred, because localized delivery and selective beta2-adrenergic activity limit fetal drug exposure.

Pediatric Patients. Children with wheezing or a chronic cough but without a diagnosis of asthma should be referred to rule out other causes. Providers caring for school-age children should know local laws that may allow children to carry and administer asthma medications at school. Children should be encouraged to carry their quick-relief medications so they can promptly respond to asthma symptoms and minimize asthma exacerbations when away from home. Written permission from the parents and provider may be required. The school nurse should also have a copy of the child's asthma self-care plan, enabling the nurse to respond appropriately to acute asthma exacerbations that develop at school. Student athletes should check with school administrators before self-administering nonprescription asthma medications. The National Collegiate Athletic Association does not permit the use of ephedrine,[36] and Olympic athletes are not permitted to use stimulants.

Patient Preferences

Inhaled delivery systems are generally preferred to minimize systemic absorption and side effects such as increased heart rate, anxiety, and tremor. Administering medication by MDI is usually less expensive than using a nebulizer and does not require special equipment.

Complementary Therapies

Although not well studied, complementary and alternative medicine (CAM) therapy use among asthma patients is relatively common. The 2006–08 Asthma Call-back Survey solicited information from parents of 5435 children with asthma to determine CAM use. Almost 27% used some form of CAM, including herbal products, vitamins, and breathing techniques (the most popular). Children with financial issues to more traditional therapies and those with poorly controlled asthma were most likely to use CAM.[37] Data from an Asthma Call-back Survey, part of the 2006 Behavioral Risk Factor Surveillance System, analyzed CAM use in adults. Findings suggested approximately 40% of adults stated they used some form of CAM, including vitamins, herbs, homeopathy, aromatherapy, and nonsystemic interventions such as breathing techniques, acupuncture, acupressure, yoga, and reflexology. Those more likely to use CAM were female, were nonwhite, had lower annual incomes, had an emergency room visit for asthma care, and had more disability days related to their asthma.[38]

For an in-depth discussion of natural products as it may relate to patients with asthma, see Chapter 51.

Assessment of Asthma: A Case-Based Approach

To correctly assess whether a patient's breathing problems meet criteria for self-treatment (Table 45–11), the provider needs to gather information from the patient regarding signs, symptoms, and duration of the problem. Other disease states with signs and symptoms similar to asthma should be ruled out (Table 45–10). The provider should also inquire about the patient's current use of prescription and nonprescription medications, CAM therapies, and dietary habits before recommending a nonprescription agent for asthma.

Patient Counseling for Asthma

Educating patients with asthma is extremely important. Even people with mild asthma can have exacerbations; therefore, all patients with asthma must know how to self-monitor and recognize asthma symptoms, and what action to take if they have symptoms that do not respond to quick-relief medications. Health care providers should assess each patient's readiness to learn about asthma, assist the patient in identifying individualized goals, and identify and correct any misconceptions about asthma or medications. Concerns or fears about asthma or asthma medications should be elicited and addressed.

Peak Flow Meters

The airflow and the relative diameter of the larger airways can be assessed by the forced expiratory volume at 1 second (FEV_1) and the PEF. FEV_1 measures the amount of air expired in the first second as the subject forcefully exhales from a maximum inspiration. The PEF is the maximum flow at the outset of forced expiration. PEF meters are handheld devices, available by prescription or over the counter.[39] These meters are relatively inexpensive and portable, which makes PEF monitoring suitable for home assessment of asthma. Guidelines for use are included in Figure 45–6. Home monitoring of PEF is recommended for patients who have moderate-severe persistent asthma, a history of a severe exacerbation, an unexplained response to environmental or occupational exposures, and for those who may not correctly perceive airflow obstruction and worsening symptoms.[21]

Predicted values for PEF and FEV_1 are determined in part by the individual's age, gender, and height. A value greater than 80% of the predicted value is considered within normal limits. However, significant individual variation exists based on body type and ethnic background. Therefore, "personal best" PEF is recommended for use in asthma self-care plans.[21] The personal best PEF is the highest value achieved by the patient over

- **Step 1**
  — Get your peak flow meter, a pencil, and your asthma care plan ready.

- **Step 2**
  — Some peak flow meters have a mouthpiece.
  — Put the mouthpiece on the meter, as shown in drawing A.

A

- **Step 3**
  — Move the indicator to the bottom of the numbered scale to set the meter to zero. See drawing B.

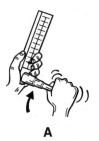

B

- **Step 4**
  — Stand up.
  — Keep the meter upright so the numbers run up and down.
  — Do not cover the hole in the back of the meter or the numbers in the front with your fingers. (See finger positions in drawing C.)
  — Take a deep breath, filling your lungs completely.

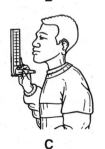

C

- **Step 5**
  — Place the mouthpiece in your mouth and close your lips tightly around it, as shown in drawing D.
  — Do not put your tongue inside the hole or your teeth on the mouthpiece.
  — Blow out as hard and as fast as you can in a single blow.

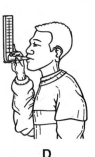

D

- **Step 6**
  — Find your number on the scale.
  — The button will go up and stay at the number you blew (see drawing E).

- **Step 7**
  — Repeat steps 1–6 two more times.
  — Record the best of the three blows in your asthma diary.
  — Check your asthma care plan for further instructions regarding the number you blew (the red, yellow, and green zones).

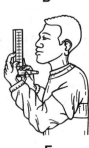

E

figure
45–6 Guidelines for using peak expiratory flow meters.

a 2-week period of monitoring when the patient is well. To determine the PEF, patients check their PEF twice daily, once in the morning and again in the late afternoon or early evening hours, 15–20 minutes after using the quick-relief inhaler.[21] For routine home monitoring, patients check their PEF daily in the morning when they first wake up and before taking their asthma medication.

Many patients with moderate-severe persistent asthma should monitor PEF daily as part of their asthma self-care plan. The green, yellow, and red zone method discussed in the section Asthma Self-Care Plans is often used. The green zone is a PEF reading of at least 80% of the predicted or personal best value, the yellow zone is 50%–79%, and the red zone is less than 50%. Readings are recorded in a diary that is brought to each primary care visit. A decrease in the PEF may precede symptoms of a significant asthma exacerbation; this is why having a self-care plan is critical.

Valved Holding Chambers and Spacers

One of the challenges of using inhaled medications is ensuring optimal delivery of the active drug to the desired site of action, in this case the lungs. Technique with traditional press-and-breathe MDIs is often less than ideal, resulting in medication being sprayed in the mouth, back of the throat, and even the nose. To better ensure drug delivery to the lungs, patients are encouraged to use a valved holding chamber (VHC) with their inhaler. This chamber attaches to the inhaler and allows the user to actuate the inhaler, placing a dose of medicine in the chamber that is then inhaled into the lungs. The VHC has a valve that keeps the medication in the chamber until the patient inhales it through the mouthpiece (which is different from a spacer that only creates additional space between the inhaler and the patient's mouth). Holding chambers also come with different sized masks that fit over a patient's mouth and nose; these are very useful for younger patients. Anyone using an MDI should use a VHC to help ensure optimal medication delivery to the lungs.

Asthma Self-Care Plans

Patients who have moderate-severe persistent asthma or a history of a severe exacerbation should have an asthma self-care plan (Figure 45–3), which provides guidance for symptom treatment and when to seek immediate medical attention. Self-care plans are developed with a health care provider and encourage communication and partnership between individuals and their providers. The self-care plan should be concise and easily understandable and empower patients to take charge of their asthma.

Self-care plans allow patients to make decisions regarding when to seek medical care. Typically, self-care plans are divided into several sections based on the PEF zones. Green-zone plans focus on what to do when the patient feels well and has normal lung function. Green-zone directions encourage adherence with long-term controller medications. Yellow-zone directions provide guidance when PEF readings are in the 50%–80% range of one's personal best, or when symptoms begin or persist. The red-zone section details management of an episode that is severe (e.g., when PEF is <50% of one's personal best) or does not improve with initial treatment. Copies of self-care plans should be given to school nurses, teachers, and day care personnel to ensure prompt treatment of asthma episodes that occur when children are away from the home.

Nonadherence to Prescription Asthma Medications

Adherence rates with asthma medications are inconsistent and dependent on the type of medication and method of determination.[40] Inhalers are the mainstay of therapy, but some people may feel they are somewhat bulky to carry. Nonadherence to long-term control medications is a significant problem, often because the benefits are not immediate. Adherence can usually be improved if the person (1) accepts the diagnosis of asthma, (2) believes that asthma may be dangerous or is a problem, (3) believes that he or she is at risk for more serious breathing or health problems, (4) believes that the treatment is safe, (5) feels in control, and (6) feels that communication with the primary care provider is good. Therefore, education regarding asthma and asthma medications can improve adherence with medications and self-care plans.

The box Patient Education for Asthma offers specific information to provide patients.

Evaluation of Patient Outcomes for Asthma

Acute asthma symptoms should respond to inhaled bronchodilators quickly (within 1 hour). Medical attention should be sought if symptoms worsen or keep returning for longer than 24–48 hours, or if PEF readings remain in the yellow zone for 2 or more days. If any symptoms of severe asthma exacerbations or imminent respiratory arrest develop, immediate medical attention should be sought.

Patients with persistent asthma should be scheduled for follow-up appointments at least every 6 months with their health care provider to assess the adequacy of their self-care plan and achievement of their goals (Table 45–13). Patients with asthma-like symptoms who are not candidates for self-care should be referred to their health care providers (Table 45–11).

Key Points for Asthma

➤ Candidates for self-care of asthma are few. Medical referral is appropriate for those with persistent asthma or those with concurrent diseases but no prior diagnosis of asthma (Table 45–11).

➤ Nonprescription medications should be used for mild, infrequent symptoms or exacerbations lasting less than 2 days.

➤ All patients with asthma need to know warning signs and symptoms of severe asthma exacerbations and need to recognize when to seek urgent care.

➤ Education regarding asthma, appropriate medication use, and self-monitoring is a crucial part of asthma self-care.

➤ Self-care plans should be developed in a partnership between patients, family members where appropriate, and their health care providers. All patients with moderate-to-severe persistent asthma should have a written self-care plan.

➤ Environmental and trigger control can help reduce symptoms of asthma.

➤ Certain concomitant conditions (e.g., GERD, allergic rhinitis, and tobacco use) can worsen asthma symptoms and should be treated individually.

The objectives of self-treatment are to (1) identify candidates for self-care (Table 45–11), (2) prevent acute asthma exacerbations with quick-relief medications, and (3) have tools available to manage acute exacerbations (Figure 45–3). Asthma is an inflammatory disorder characterized by periods of stable lung function coupled with acute exacerbations. Symptoms of an acute exacerbation include wheezing, chest tightness, shortness of breath, and cough. For most patients, carefully following product instructions and the self-care measures listed here will help ensure optimal therapeutic outcomes.

Nondrug Measures

- Identify and control environmental triggers (Table 45–8).
- Stop smoking cigarettes.
- Control concomitant disease states (e.g., GERD, allergic rhinitis, and tobacco use).

Nonprescription Medications

- See Table 45–12 for examples of available medications.
- Two types of nonprescription asthma medications are available: inhaled and oral.
  - Inhaled medications contain epinephrine or racepinephrine.
  - Possible adverse drug effects of inhaled medications include nervousness and rapid heartbeat.
  - Oral medications include ephedrine and guaifenesin.
  - Possible adverse drug effects of oral medications include nervousness, tremor, sleeplessness, nausea, and loss of appetite.
- Precautions and contraindications for inhaled and oral asthma medications include the following:
  - Do not use unless a diagnosis of asthma has been made.
  - Do not take with monoamine oxidase inhibitors.
  - Use only under the supervision of a health care professional if you have heart disease, high blood pressure, thyroid disease,

diabetes, or difficulty with urination because of enlargement of the prostate gland.
  - Do not use if you have been hospitalized for asthma or if you are taking a prescription medication for asthma.
- Monitoring parameters include relief of symptoms and occurrence of adverse effects:
  - If acute symptoms do not improve or become worse within 20 minutes of use of nonprescription bronchodilator medications, seek immediate medical attention.
  - Monitor continuously for adverse effects such as palpitations, angina, anxiety, nervousness, tremor, agitation, dizziness, insomnia, and restlessness. Discontinue use and notify provider if experiencing unwanted adverse effects.
- See Figure 45–3 for safe administration of medication.
- See Table 45–12 for recommended daily dose.
- Store epinephrine inhalers at room temperature (68°F–77°F). Do not store near open flame or heat above 120°F.
- Store combination oral products in a cool, dry place. Do not take products after expiration date on packaging.

When to Seek Medical Attention

- Seek a medical referral if symptoms occur or nonprescription bronchodilator is used more than twice a week.

Key: GERD = Gastroesophageal reflux disease.

table
45–13   Asthma Therapeutic Goals and Monitoring Parameters

Therapeutic Goal	Monitoring Parameter
Control of symptoms	Symptom frequency: 1–2 times per week; symptoms resolve within several minutes after bronchodilator
Normal pulmonary function	Peak expiratory flow rate: >80% of personal best PEF *consistently* every day
Normal activity levels	Few missed school or work days; able to perform desired activities (e.g., play, activities of daily living, etc.)
Prevention of recurrent episodes of asthma (minimize the need for urgent care visits)	No hospitalizations or emergency department visits: goal is none; have regular follow-ups for asthma
Prevention of adverse effects	No increased heart rate, insomnia, palpitations, nervousness, anxiety
Meeting expectations of asthma care	Achievement of patient's goals (e.g., able to perform desired activities): participates in care, is comfortable asking questions, is confident in dealing with symptoms and triggers

Key: PEF = Peak expiratory flow.

Osteoporosis and Osteopenia

Osteoporosis is a silent disease affecting more than 9 million Americans, with 48 million affected by low bone mass. An estimated 54 million adults older than 50 years have osteoporosis or osteopenia; that number is expected to grow to 64 million by 2020.[41] The majority (80%) of osteoporosis cases affect women. Costs to the U.S. health care system for osteoporosis-related fractures were approximately $19 billion dollars in 2005; costs in 2025 are expected to rise to $25 billion.[42] Fractures may result in physical symptoms such as pain or disability, as well as psychological symptoms such as depression and decreased feeling of self-worth because of limited mobility. The importance of appropriate screening, prevention, and treatment is apparent, considering the impact of fractures on morbidity and mortality in the elderly.

Osteopenia is defined by the World Health Organization as a bone density between 1.0 and 2.5 standard deviations below the mean for young normal adults (T-score between −1.0 and −2.5). In contrast, *osteoporosis* is defined as a bone density 2.5 or more standard deviations below the young normal mean (T-score at or below −2.5). In addition, patients who have had a previous fracture are classified to have "severe" or "established" osteoporosis.[42]

Pathophysiology of Osteoporosis and Osteopenia

Osteoporosis and osteopenia are a result of progressive bone loss after peak mass is achieved between 18 and 25 years of age. Bone is made of collagen and minerals. The balance of these substances for flexibility and strength is essential to maintain bone function and decrease risk of a fracture. An imbalance of bone remodeling (removing older bone while building new bone) can result in bone loss and subsequent risk for fractures. This imbalance most often occurs with increasing age and the onset of menopause.[42]

Clinical Presentation of Osteoporosis and Osteopenia

Patients with osteopenia or osteoporosis typically are asymptomatic unless they present secondary to a complication from the disease (e.g., fracture). In addition, patients with degrading bone loss may attribute their pain to other sources (e.g., arthritis) of pain and not associate it with osteopenia or osteoporosis. Other signs and symptoms or complications that patients may or may not be aware of are decreased immobility, shortened stature, and pain.

Treatment of Osteoporosis and Osteopenia
Treatment Goals

The primary goals are to prevent osteopenia and osteoporosis from developing or progressing and to prevent morbidity and mortality associated with complications secondary to osteopenia and osteoporosis (e.g., fractures). Other goals of therapy include prevention of hospital visits, improved quality of life through improved mobility, prevention or management of pain, and participation in activities of daily living.[42]

General Treatment Approach

The provider should review lifestyle modifications with the patient and stress their importance in controlling the disorder. However, medical referral for further evaluation is needed if the assessment process reveals any of the following:

- No formal diagnosis (or identified risk factors) of osteoporosis or osteopenia
- Concurrent use of a medication (e.g., steroids) that may affect bone density or strength and that has not been evaluated by the primary care provider
- No visit (or missed visit) to a provider in the last year
- Nonadherence to provider-recommended prescription medications, nonprescription medications, or self-care measures
- Inability to assess the dietary intake of calcium and vitamin D
- Perception that prescription medications are ineffective
- Signs of bone loss (pain, immobility, shortened stature) that have not been evaluated by the provider
- Use of dietary supplements without the provider's knowledge or without achieving set goals

Besides increasing age and onset of menopause, other factors put an individual at risk for bone loss (Table 45–14). Current recommendations are that all postmenopausal women and men 50 years of age and older should be assessed for osteoporosis risk factors to determine the need for bone mineral density (BMD) testing. According to the National Osteoporosis Foundation, women older than 65 years and men older than 70 years should receive BMD testing (hip or spine acceptable locations).[42] Providers must play a role in encouraging appropriate screening and prevention measures given the tendency of

table
45–14 Selected Risk Factors Associated with Osteoporosis

Dietary	Medications	Other Factors
Decreased calcium intake	Aluminum (antacids)	Age
Increased caffeine intake	Anticonvulsants	Gender
Increased sodium intake	Aromatase inhibitors	Decreased physical activity or limited mobility
Increased vitamin A intake	Barbiturates	Increased alcohol intake (>3 drinks per day)
Vitamin D insufficiency	Glucocorticoids	Smoking
		Low body mass index
		Previous fracture
		Onset of menopause

Note: This list does not include all factors that may contribute to osteoporosis and/or related factors (e.g., genetics, endocrine disorders, etc.). For an inclusive list, see reference 42.

individuals at risk to avoid screenings for a silent disease such as osteoporosis. Although screening tools are available for providers to use in the community setting, a thorough evaluation of the accuracy of the tool should be completed.

Besides factors that contribute to weakening of bone structure, providers should also focus on factors that may lead to falls, such as lack of assistive devices, loose floor items that may lead to tripping, poor lighting, dehydration, medications that cause drowsiness or sedation, and poor balance. An assessment of the patient's home and close collaboration with a caregiver may prevent a fall and the resulting fracture.[42]

Recommendations for individuals to reduce the risk of osteopenia and osteoporosis and ultimately a fracture are listed in Table 45–15.

Nonpharmacologic Therapy

Self-care measures for the prevention and management of osteoporosis include adherence to medications (prescription and nonprescription), completion of weight-bearing (e.g., walking, jogging, or dancing) and muscle-strengthening exercises (e.g., weight and resistance training) where appropriate, following a diet that allows adequate intake of vitamins and minerals while maintaining a healthy body weight, and avoiding detrimental behaviors such as smoking and excessive consumption of alcohol.[42]

Pharmacologic Therapy

Assessment of dietary intake of calcium and vitamin D should be completed prior to making a recommendation for additional supplemental use. A thorough discussion of the evidence regarding the use of calcium and vitamin D, the recommended intake, types, and formulations of calcium and vitamin D can be found in Chapter 22.

Assessment of Osteoporosis and Osteopenia: A Case-Based Approach

Case 45–2 provides an example of how to assess a patient with risk factors for osteoporosis or osteopenia.

Patient Counseling for Osteoporosis and Osteopenia

Patient counseling for self-care of osteopenia and osteoporosis should be complementary to assessment, treatment, or monitoring by the patient's primary care provider. Counseling should focus on engaging the patient in appropriate self-care measures outlined in Table 45–15. The patient should be educated on the impact of untreated osteoporosis and osteopenia as well as the importance and efficacy of pharmacologic and nonpharmacologic measures. The box Patient Education for Osteoporosis lists specific information to provide patients.

Evaluation of Patient Outcomes for Osteoporosis and Osteopenia

Evaluation of outcomes associated with osteopenia and osteoporosis should be completed by the patient's provider. Self-care measures should complement rather than replace the provider recommendation(s).

table 45–15	General Recommendations to Prevent Osteoporosis and Osteopenia
Prevention/Treatment Parameter	**Recommendation**
Calcium intake	See Table 22-4 for specific recommended calcium intakes based on age and gender
Vitamin D intake	See Table 22-3 for specific recommended vitamin D intakes based on age and gender
Exercise	Regular weight-bearing and muscle-strengthening exercises (after evaluation by a primary care provider)
Tobacco use	Cessation[a]
Alcohol intake	No more than moderate use of alcohol (≥3 drinks per day may be harmful to bone health)
Bone mineral density testing	▪ Assessment of need for BMD (based on risk factors) for postmenopausal women and men ages 50–69 years ▪ BMD recommended for women 65 years and older, and men 70 years and older

[a] All patients with osteoporosis who are using tobacco products should be advised to quit. Please refer to Chapter 47 for a more in-depth description of smoking cessation.

Key: BMD= Bone mineral density.

Source: Adapted from reference 42.

Heart Failure

Heart failure (also known as congestive heart failure or chronic heart failure) is a condition characterized by the heart's inability to pump enough blood (and subsequently oxygen) to fulfill the body's requirements. Affecting approximately 5.1 million people in the United States over the age of 20, heart failure will cost the U.S. health care system approximately $32 billion in 2013.[43] More prevalent in the aging populations, heart failure leads to poor quality of life and early mortality. Heart failure is classified by the American College of Cardiology Foundation and the American Heart Association (AHA) as Stages A–D and by the New York Heart Association as Classes I–IV. An increase in stage or class indicates an increase in disease severity.[44,45]

case
45–2

Relevant Evaluation Criteria	Scenario/Model Outcome

Information Gathering

1. Gather essential information about the patient's symptoms and medical history, including:

   a. description of symptom(s) (i.e., nature, onset, duration, severity, associated symptoms)

          Patient presents to the pharmacy with questions about using a calcium supplement.

   b. description of any factors that seem to precipitate, exacerbate, and/or relieve the patient's symptom(s)

          She asks if she should be taking calcium every day for her "bones." She is concerned because she doesn't feel she has any problems with her bones.

   c. description of the patient's efforts to relieve the symptoms

          NA

   d. patient's identity

          Mildred Phillips

   e. patient's age, sex, height, and weight

          71 years old, female, 5 ft 5 in., 111 lb

   f. patient's occupation

          Retired from 45 years as an elementary school teacher; still likes to work around the house with her husband

   g. patient's dietary habits

          Relatively normal diet with limited meat and vegetable consumption, but she does attempt to have at least 3 helpings of fruit/day.

   h. patient's sleep habits

          8–9 hours per night

   i. concurrent medical conditions, prescription and non-prescription medications, and dietary supplements

          Hypertension: metoprolol succinate 50 mg by mouth every morning; osteoarthritis of the knee: acetaminophen 325 mg every 4–6 hours

   j. allergies

          NKA

   k. history of other adverse reactions to medications

          None

   l. other (describe) _____

          Has smoked one pack per day for the last 40 years. Occasional alcohol use (less than 1 glass of wine/week).

Assessment and Triage

2. Differentiate the patient's signs/symptoms and correctly identify the patient's primary problem(s).

          The patient has several risk factors (age, smoking history, likely post-menopausal, gender, low body mass index) that would indicate she is at risk for osteoporosis or osteopenia. An assessment of the patient's dietary consumption of calcium and vitamin D should be completed.

3. Identify exclusions for self-treatment.

          See exclusions for self-treatment in the Osteoporosis and Osteopenia section, subsection General Treatment Approach. Mildred has no formal diagnosis of osteoporosis or osteopenia but does have several risk factors that warrant initiation of calcium/vitamin D therapy.

4. Formulate a comprehensive list of therapeutic alternatives for the primary problem to determine if triage to a medical provider is required, and share this information with the patient or caregiver.

          Options include:

          (1) Refer Mildred to her PCP.

          (2) Recommend OTC calcium and vitamin D supplementation after assessing her dietary consumption.

          (3) Recommend that OTC calcium and vitamin D supplementation be initiated until Mildred can see her PCP.

          (4) Take no action.

Plan

5. Select an optimal therapeutic alternative to address the patient's problem, taking into account patient preferences.

          The patient prefers starting OTC calcium and vitamin D supplementation until she can be evaluated by her PCP.

6. Describe the recommended therapeutic approach to the patient or caregiver.

          "Because you are not consuming enough calcium and vitamin D in your diet, you should increase your dietary intake of calcium and start taking calcium and vitamin D supplementation. In addition, you should stop smoking, perform weight-bearing exercises, and see your primary care provider to obtain a referral for a bone mineral density scan."

case
45–2 *continued*

Relevant Evaluation Criteria	Scenario/Model Outcome
7. Explain to the patient or caregiver the rationale for selecting the recommended therapeutic approach from the considered therapeutic alternatives.	"Calcium and vitamin D are essential to help build bone growth and to prevent complications associated with bone loss, such as fractures. In addition, a referral to your primary care provider is necessary to assess whether a bone scan should be completed. A bone scan will measure the density (or thickness) of your bones to determine how much bone loss has taken place. The results of the scan will allow the provider to determine whether to continue the plan as is or whether to add a prescription medication. Finally, with the more recent data suggesting possible increased risk of cardiovascular complications in patients using calcium supplements, versus receiving calcium in the diet, you should discuss this issue with your provider."

Patient Education

8. When recommending self-care with nonprescription medications and/or nondrug therapy, convey accurate information to the patient or caregiver:	
a. appropriate dose and frequency of administration	See Chapter 22 for a discussion of the types, dosages, and formulations of calcium and vitamin D. The dose should be divided to twice daily to allow adequate absorption.
b. maximum number of days the therapy should be employed	"You should take the supplement(s) until the provider visit, which should be scheduled as soon as possible."
c. product administration procedures	"Take the supplement by mouth. The absorption of some medications may be affected by calcium, so please talk to a primary care provider before starting any new medications."
d. expected time to onset of relief	NA
e. degree of relief that can be reasonably expected	NA
f. most common side effects	"Upset stomach and headache may occur."
g. side effects that warrant medical intervention should they occur	"If you have continued constipation while taking these supplements, see your primary care provider."
h. patient options in the event that condition worsens or persists	"If you experience signs of bone loss, specifically pain, shortened stature, or fractures, see your primary care provider immediately." [Because the patient does not have any symptoms, it is unlikely that the patient will know if the condition is worsening unless she experiences the signs just described.]
i. product storage requirements	NA
j. specific nondrug measures	"Getting a referral for a bone mineral density scan is important. The scan will let you know how much, if any, bone loss has occurred. In the meantime, you can minimize bone loss if you stop smoking and start performing weight-bearing exercises."
Solicit follow-up questions from the patient or caregiver.	(1) "Will the calcium and vitamin D affect any of my other medications?" (2) "What are common dietary sources of calcium?"
Answer the patient's or caregiver's questions.	(1) "In general, the absorption of some medications may be affected by calcium, so please talk to a primary care provider before starting any new medications. With regard to your current regimen (metoprolol), take the calcium and vitamin D 1–3 hours after your metoprolol." (2) "Common dietary sources of calcium include dairy foods (milk, yogurt, cheese), green leafy vegetables (spinach, broccoli, kale), beans/peas, and fish (salmon, sardines)."

Evaluation of Patient Outcome

9. Assess patient outcome.	Contact the patient in a week or two to ensure that she made a follow-up appointment with her PCP, to determine how she is tolerating the supplement, and to assess her status with regard to tobacco cessation.

Key: NA = Not applicable; NKA = no known allergies; OTC = over-the-counter; PCP = primary care provider.

Pathophysiology of Heart Failure

Defined as the ineffectiveness of the heart to pump enough blood to meet the metabolic needs of the body, heart failure is often the result of an acute event that damages the myocardium (i.e., myocardial infarction) or long-term damage that is secondary to a cardiovascular condition (e.g., hypertension).[45] Although these are common causes, heart failure can result from any condition that compromises the ability of the myocardium to contract (systolic dysfunction) or relax (diastolic dysfunction). To compensate for the inability to pump sufficient blood, the body relies on secondary mechanisms such as increased contractility through sympathetic nervous system stimulation and initiation of the renin–angiotensin–aldosterone system. These compensatory mechanisms ultimately lead to vasoconstriction, hypertrophy and remodeling of the ventricles, and sodium and water retention. Although these mechanisms are designed to be short term, they often persist and lead to exacerbation of heart failure.

Clinical Presentation of Heart Failure

Patients with heart failure most often present with dyspnea and fatigue. These, in addition to the compensatory mechanisms, can lead to the retention of fluids and subsequently pulmonary congestion and/or peripheral edema. Because patients present at different stages of the disease and may have various comorbidities, the symptoms can vary significantly. Other common signs and symptoms or complications include exercise intolerance, orthopnea, cough, fatigue, and cool extremities.

Treatment of Heart Failure
Treatment Goals

General treatment goals for heart failure include (1) improving quality of life, (2) reducing or relieving symptoms, (3) prolonging survival, and (4) reducing exacerbations that would lead to hospitalizations and/or discomfort to the patient. Because heart failure is not reversible, it is also prudent to treat the underlying

cause if applicable (e.g., diabetes, hypertension, etc.) to prevent or slow the progression of the disease.

General Treatment Approach

The approach for treatment of heart failure should focus on accurate staging of the disease, identifying and treating any risk factors (e.g., smoking) or comorbid conditions (e.g., hypertension), and using pharmacologic and nonpharmacologic treatment options. In 2009, the American College of Cardiology and AHA issued an update for the diagnosis and management of chronic heart failure in adults.[44] The pharmacist should review lifestyle modifications with the patient and stress their importance in controlling the disorder. However, medical referral for further evaluation is needed if the assessment process reveals any of the following:

- No formal diagnosis of heart failure
- Another comorbid condition (e.g., asthma or COPD) that may make it difficult to distinguish heart failure–related symptoms (e.g., difficulty breathing)
- No visit to a primary care provider in the last year
- Nonadherence to provider-recommended prescription medications, nonprescription medications, or self-care measures
- Perception that prescription medications are ineffective
- Use of dietary supplements without provider's knowledge or without achieving set goals

Nonpharmacologic Therapy

Patients should always be assessed, monitored, and treated by a primary care provider; treatment should not be solely self-managed. Self-care for patients with heart failure may be especially challenging in light of other comorbid conditions (e.g., hypertension, diabetes, etc.) that result in complex medical regimens, dietary restrictions, required monitoring, the burden of decision-making, and/or feeling ill.[46] For example, a patient with heart failure and diabetes may be burdened with monitoring both conditions, adhering to dietary modifications for sodium and carbohydrate intake, and having to make several decisions based on findings throughout the day.

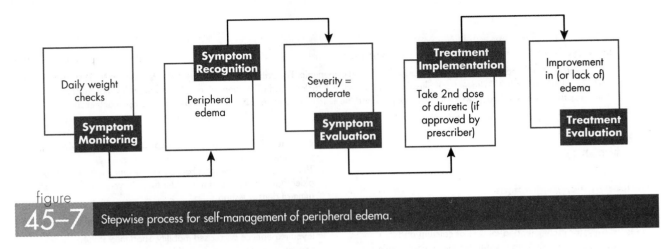

figure
45-7   Stepwise process for self-management of peripheral edema.

Although the data are inconsistent and limited in terms of effectiveness of self-management interventions on clinical markers (e.g., mortality and readmissions),[47,48] self-care measures for patients with heart failure are recommended by AHA.[46] Patients should be educated and ultimately should be responsible for recognizing and evaluating symptoms, determining the need for treatment, implementing treatment (if approved by provider), and evaluating that change. Figure 45–7 highlights an example of how a patient with heart failure can participate in appropriate self-care.[46]

Consideration should be given to screening patients with heart failure to assess for any medications that may be exacerbating symptom control. NSAIDs should be avoided where possible because of sodium retention, peripheral vasoconstriction, and potential to decrease the effectiveness of diuretics and angiotensin-converting enzyme inhibitors.[44] In addition, products such as stimulant laxatives and nonprescription products containing diuretics may lead to dehydration and electrolyte imbalances. Patients may be self-treating symptoms with nonprescription diuretics (e.g., caffeine, pamabrom, and pyrilamine), and should consult their prescriber to avoid potential harm. These diuretics may alter electrolyte levels and are typically contained in products marketed to women with premenstrual symptoms. In addition, sympathomimetics such as pseudoephedrine may lead to an increase in blood pressure, heart rate, and systemic vascular resistance and should be avoided. Caution should also be given to products that are high in sodium or potassium, or other medications that may alter electrolyte levels, such as nonprescription supplements (e.g., potassium).

Table 45–16 provides a summary of nonpharmacologic recommendations for patients with heart failure. Although the data are limited and inconsistent regarding sodium intake in patients with heart failure, the AHA consensus statement recommends a maximum daily dose of 2.3 grams. Patients should be educated on foods that are typically higher in sodium, such as processed meats, canned products, frozen dinners, and cheeses. Fluid restriction is important for several apparent reasons in patients with heart failure and should be an education point to patients, considering the generally held concept that more water is better.[46]

In terms of body weight, the conventional thought is less is better. However, patients with heart failure may be the exception. Although the data are not conclusive, patients with a higher weight show lower mortality and hospitalization rates than those with a normal body mass index (BMI). Because cachexia in chronic diseases such as heart failure often predicts a worse prognosis, the current recommendation is to endorse weight loss for patients with a BMI of 40 or higher to achieve a BMI less than 40. However, patients who have a BMI of 30 or higher are not currently recommended to lose weight, but rather to focus on signs of weight loss, muscle wasting, and a loss of appetite. Finally, in an effort to decrease inflammation and improve the delivery of oxygen, routine exercise should be recommended and tailored on the basis of the severity of the patient's symptoms.[46]

Pharmacologic Therapy

Currently, no nonprescription pharmacologic agents are recommended for the treatment of heart failure. However, providers

table
45-16   **Nonpharmacologic Recommendations for Patients with Heart Failure**

Nonpharmacologic Category	Recommendation
Sodium consumption	Maximum of 2.3 g/day
Fluid intake	<2 L/day[a]
Tobacco use	Cessation or prevention of use[b]
Weight loss	Encouraged only if BMI ≥ 40
Exercise	Recommended (tailored by the provider on the basis of symptom control)
Immunizations	Influenza yearly (inactivated); pneumococcal (maximum of 2 doses in a lifetime)[c]

[a] Patients with mild-moderate heart failure symptoms may not benefit from fluid restriction.

[b] All patients with heart failure who are using tobacco products should be advised to quit. See Chapter 47 for a more in-depth description of smoking cessation.

[c] Specific immunizations listed in the Centers for Disease Control and Prevention Adult Immunization Schedule. Consideration should also be given to routine tetanus vaccinations and other vaccines where appropriate (i.e., high-risk situations).

Source: Adapted from reference 46.

and patients should share responsibility in ensuring that vaccine records are up to date. Where applicable, adults with heart failure should be up to date on tetanus; diphtheria and pertussis; varicella; zoster; and measles, mumps, and rubella. In addition, patients with heart failure should receive an annual influenza vaccine and the pneumococcal vaccine (maximum of 2 doses in a lifetime).

Complementary Therapies

The use of nonprescription medications[49] and CAM[49,50] by patients with heart failure is significant, leading to potential harm if not evaluated appropriately. Patients with heart failure are specifically at risk for adverse effects because symptom control is often achieved with specific adjustments of prescription medications and monitoring of nonpharmacologic factors such as salt and fluid intake. Although very few herbal supplements are used for heart failure specifically, providers should assess all herbal medications being used for other comorbid conditions. (See Chapter 51 for a more in-depth discussion of herbal supplements related to cardiovascular health.)

Patient Counseling for Heart Failure

Patient counseling for self-care of heart failure should be complementary to the assessment, treatment, and monitoring being delivered by a provider. Counseling should focus on engaging the patient in appropriate nonpharmacologic measures (Table 45–16) and stressing the importance of these measures.

Effective complementary therapies for heart failure control are limited. However, patients may be using these therapies for other comorbid conditions (e.g., diabetes, hypertension, etc.). Patients should be asked about use of these products and, if applicable, warned of possible effects on control of heart failure symptoms.

The patient should be educated on common signs and symptoms of heart failure and the impact that comorbid disease states can have on symptom control and progression. The box Patient Education for Heart Failure lists specific information to provide patients.

Evaluation of Patient Outcomes for Heart Failure

Evaluation of outcomes associated with heart failure should be completed by the patient's provider. Self-care measures should complement rather than replace the provider's recommendations.

Hypertension

High blood pressure (hypertension) contributes to heart disease and stroke, the first and fourth leading causes of death in the United States, respectively. Affecting approximately one in three adult Americans,[51] hypertension cost the U.S. health care

---

patient education for
Heart Failure

The objectives of self-treatment measures for heart failure are to (1) prevent exacerbation of symptoms, (2) prevent progression of the disease, and (3) improve overall quality of life. For most patients, carefully following their primary care provider's treatment plan and the self-care measures listed here will help ensure optimal therapeutic outcomes.

Nondrug Measures
- Patients can play a role in managing heart failure by:
  - Monitoring fluid, salt, and alcohol intake. Foods that typically have high sodium content include processed meats, canned products, frozen dinners, and cheeses.
  - Stopping the use of tobacco (if applicable).
  - Maintaining an appropriate weight.
  - Participating in a planned and monitored exercise regimen.
- See Table 45–16 for specific recommendations.

Nonprescription Medications
- Currently, no nonprescription medications are recommended for the treatment of heart failure. Follow carefully your primary care provider's instructions for prescription medications.
- The following nonprescription medications can worsen heart failure and should be avoided:
  - Ibuprofen and naproxen can cause sodium retention and peripheral vasoconstriction and possibly can decrease the effectiveness of prescribed diuretics and angiotensin-converting enzyme inhibitors.
  - Stimulant laxatives may lead to dehydration and electrolyte imbalances.
  - Nonprescription products containing diuretics (e.g., caffeine, pamabrom, and pyrilamine) may also lead to dehydration and

electrolyte imbalances. These diuretics are typically contained in products marketed to treat premenstrual symptoms.
  - Do not use nonprescription diuretics to self-treat symptoms of heart failure unless the use is approved by your primary care provider.
  - Products that are high in sodium or potassium, or other medications that may alter electrolyte levels, such as nonprescription potassium supplements, can also cause electrolyte imbalances.
  - Pseudoephedrine, which is used to treat nasal congestion, may lead to an increase in blood pressure and/or heart rate.
- Keep up to date on vaccinations for tetanus, varicella, zoster (if >50 years), and measles, mumps, and rubella.
- Make sure you receive an influenza vaccine every year.
- Recommendations for the pneumonia vaccine are to take the first dose between the ages of 19–64 years. A second dose is recommended for those 65 years and older. Make sure the two doses are administered 5 years apart.

When to Seek Medical Attention
- If you experience excessive fluid retention, weight gain (from fluid retention), shortness of breath, fatigue or weakness, rapid or irregular heartbeat and/or persistent cough or wheezing, please consult with your primary care provider or seek immediate care.

system approximately $51 billion in direct and indirect costs in 2009.[43] Lifetime prevalence of hypertension is high, with 90% of people who are normotensive at age 55 and older becoming hypertensive.[52] Persistent hypertension may lead to the development of coronary artery disease, stroke, and renal failure. In light of the effects that hypertension can have on cardiovascular and kidney health and its effect in patients with other comorbid conditions (e.g., diabetes), appropriate management and self-care of hypertension are essential.

Pathophysiology of Hypertension

Blood pressure is a result of the resistance of the blood vessels from the force of blood contracted from the heart. Arterial blood pressure is recorded as millimeters of mercury (mm Hg) and reported as systolic blood pressure (during cardiac contraction) and diastolic blood pressure (after contraction when the heart chambers are filling). In the majority of individuals, hypertension has an unknown etiology (essential or primary hypertension). Although the condition cannot be cured, it can be treated with various pharmacologic and nonpharmacologic measures. In patients with a known cause of hypertension (secondary hypertension), the cause may be removed if possible (e.g., excessive sodium use), or the hypertension may be treated if the cause cannot be removed (e.g., necessary therapy for chronic asthma with a steroid). The most common causes of secondary hypertension are renal dysfunction and medications that increase blood pressure.[53]

The exact mechanism leading to essential hypertension is unknown, but several theories include factors that affect the renin–angiotensin–aldosterone system, a defect in neuronal regulation, a defect in sodium excretion, a deficiency of vasodilation substances (e.g., prostacyclin and bradykinin), or an excess of vasoconstriction substances (e.g., angiotensin II). It is hypothesized that a combination of these factors, rather than a single factor alone, is likely.[53]

Clinical Presentation of Hypertension

Patients with hypertension traditionally present asymptomatic and appear otherwise healthy unless they have subsequent cardiovascular risk factors such as diabetes, obesity, and tobacco use. In addition, the patient may or may not have previous signs of complications such as target organ damage secondary to hypertension. Examples of complications secondary to hypertension include stroke, retinopathy, myocardial infarction, chronic kidney disease, or peripheral artery disease. Therefore, proper screening of blood pressure values is essential for early recognition of a condition that can have silent symptoms with detrimental long-term effects.

Treatment of Hypertension
Treatment Goals

The primary goal of treatment of hypertension is to reduce morbidity and mortality. Numerous pharmacologic options are available and usually are necessary for patients to achieve desired

blood pressure goals. The pharmacist should review lifestyle modifications with the patient and stress their importance in controlling the disorder. However, medical referral is needed if the assessment process reveals any of the following:

- No formal diagnosis of hypertension
- No visit to a primary care provider in the last year
- Concurrent medication (e.g., stimulants) that may affect the patient's blood pressure and has not been evaluated by the prescriber
- Nonadherence to provider-recommended prescription medications, nonprescription medications, or self-care measures
- Perception that prescription medications are ineffective
- Use of dietary supplements without the provider's knowledge or without achieving set goals

General Treatment Approach

Hypertension is classified as normal, prehypertension, stage 1 hypertension, or stage 2 hypertension. The classification of hypertension determines pharmacologic and nonpharmacologic measures necessary to achieve the desired goals. In light of the correlation between risk factors and the additional risk from hypertension, the focus should be on managing and addressing these factors early and often. (See Table 45–17 for risk factors for hypertension.)

Nonpharmacologic Therapy

Appropriate self-care measures include self-monitoring of blood pressure, reducing body weight, adopting the dietary approach to stopping hypertension (DASH diet), increasing physical activity, abstaining from smoking, and moderating the amount of alcohol use.[52] Key components of the DASH diet[54] are provided in Table 45–18. Additional information about smoking cessation can be found in Chapter 47. The correlation between several of these risk factors and a corresponding reduction in systolic blood pressure is outlined in Table 45–19.

Home blood pressure monitoring may have a small effect in improving blood pressure and adherence in patients with

table 45–17	Selected Risk Factors for Developing or Worsening Hypertension
Medications	**Other Factors**
Amphetamines	Increased caffeine intake
Decongestants	Increased sodium intake
Erythropoietin	Increased alcohol intake
Estrogen derivatives	Advanced age
Nicotine	Females who are postmenopausal
Nonsteroidal anti-inflammatory drugs	Decreased physical activity
Steroids	Tobacco smoke
Venlafaxine (Effexor, Effexor XR)	

table 45–18 Key Components of the Dietary Approach to Stopping Hypertension (DASH) Diet

Food Group	Recommendation
Fat-free or low-fat milk products	2–3 servings per day
Fruits	4–5 servings per day
Grains	6–8 servings per day
Lean meats, poultry, fish	6 or fewer servings per day
Nuts, seeds, and legumes	4–5 servings per week
Vegetables	4–5 servings per day
Sodium	Start with 2300 mg/day and then decrease to 1500 mg/day.
Potassium	A potassium-rich diet (from fruits and vegetables rather than supplements) may help reduce blood pressure.

Source: Adapted from references 52 and 54.

Note: Based on a 2000 calorie per day diet.

table 45–19 Effect of Managing Risk Factors on Systolic Blood Pressure

Lifestyle Modification	Recommendation	Approximate Reduction in Systolic Blood Pressure
Adopt DASH eating plan.	Follow a diet rich in fruits, vegetables, and low-fat dairy products. Reduce intake of saturated and total fat.	8–14 mm Hg
Reduce weight.	Achieve a body mass index of 18.5–24.9	5–20 mm Hg
Increase physical activity.	Participate in regular aerobic exercise (≥30 minutes/day) for most days of the week.	4–9 mm Hg
Reduce intake of dietary sodium.	Reduce sodium intake to ≤2.4 grams of sodium or 6 grams of sodium chloride.	2–8 mm Hg
Consume alcohol in moderation.	≤2 drinks for men per day ≤1 drink for women per day	2–4 mm Hg

Key: DASH = Dietary approach to stopping hypertension.

Source: Adapted from reference 52.

hypertension.[55,56] Steps to obtaining an accurate blood pressure reading are listed in Table 45–20.[57] Specific patients who may benefit from home monitoring include patients with white coat hypertension (elevated blood pressure in a clinical setting but not in other settings); patients with periodic hypotensive episodes; and patients using pharmacologic or nonpharmacologic measures who are monitoring the progress in disease control. Home blood pressure monitoring should complement rather than replace provider monitoring. Therefore, patients who are self-monitoring should be encouraged to keep a record or logbook of their home readings and bring them to provider visits to help identify patterns or trends in blood pressure over time. Limitations of home monitoring should be considered, such as using devices that are not validated or that have not been calibrated according to manufacturer-recommended frequency,

dexterity needed for measuring, cost of devices, and potential for patients to make changes in therapy based on readings without consulting the prescriber. (See Chapter 48 for additional information on home blood pressure monitors.).

Patients should be advised that some nonprescription preparations, including decongestants with sympathomimetic activity (e.g., phenylephrine and pseudoephedrine),

table 45–20 Steps to Obtaining an Accurate Blood Pressure Measurement

1. The patient should be seated quietly for a minimum of 5 minutes with feet flat on the floor and the arm supported at heart level.
2. Caffeine and nicotine consumption should be avoided for 30 minutes prior to a reading.
3. An appropriate size cuff should be used for the measurement.
4. The palpatory method should be used to estimate the systolic blood pressure. While palpating the radial pulse, inflate the cuff at a steady rate until the pulse can no longer be felt. Then, further inflate the cuff by about 20 mm Hg. Slowly release the valve on the inflating bulb and allow the pressure to drop by about 5 mm Hg per second. The point at which the palpation of the radial pulse reappears is the systolic blood pressure.
5. Place the bell of the stethoscope over the brachial artery.
6. Inflate the cuff to approximately 30 mm Hg above the estimated systolic blood pressure (completed in step 4).
7. Deflate the cuff slowly at a rate of 2–3 mm Hg per second. The first audible Korotkoff sound is the systolic blood pressure. The last audible sound is the diastolic blood pressure.
8. Deflate the cuff completely.
9. Record the measurement to the nearest 2 mm Hg.
10. Two measurements should be taken and the average should be recorded. Wait 1–2 minutes between measurements.

Source: Adapted from reference 57.

may increase blood pressure. At higher doses (210–240 mg), pseudoephedrine has been shown to increase blood pressure and heart rate, which are undesirable in a patient with hypertension. In addition, central nervous system stimulation and risk of stroke (in patients with hypertension) may occur with pseudoephedrine use.[58] Although the doses that caused ill effects are relatively high compared with normal dosing, pseudoephedrine should be avoided if possible in patients with hypertension. A further review of decongestants can be found in Chapter 11.

Complementary Therapies

An in-depth discussion of natural products that are widely used for hypertension and/or overall cardiovascular health can be found in Chapter 51.

Patient Counseling for Hypertension

Patient counseling for self-care of hypertension should be complementary to the assessment, treatment, and monitoring being delivered by a provider. Counseling should focus on engaging the patient in the appropriate nonpharmacologic measures outlined in Tables 45–18 and 45–19. Natural products for the management of hypertension are available. A further discussion of those agents can be found in Chapter 51. The patient should be educated on the impact of uncontrolled hypertension and the importance and efficacy of nondrug measures. The box Patient Education for Hypertension lists specific information to provide patients.

Evaluation of Patient Outcomes for Hypertension

Evaluation of outcomes associated with hypertension should be completed by the patient's primary care provider. Self-care measures should complement but not replace the provider's recommendation(s).

Dyslipidemia

Coronary heart disease (CHD) is the leading cause of death in the United States, contributing to over 600,000 deaths in 2008. Hypercholesterolemia, elevated low-density lipoproteins (LDLs), and decreased high-density lipoproteins (HDLs) are directly linked to CHD and cerebrovascular accidents. Approximately 43% of individuals older than 20 years in the United States have total cholesterol (TC) levels of 200 mg/dL or higher, 31% have LDL levels of 130 mg/dL or higher, and 22% have HDL levels less than 40 mg/dL.[43] Genetic and environmental factors leading to high TC, high LDL, and low HDL make appropriate pharmacologic and nonpharmacologic treatment essential.

Pathophysiology of Dyslipidemia

Lipids in the body (cholesterol, triglycerides, and phospholipids) are transported by proteins, known as lipoproteins. The major classes of lipoproteins include LDLs, HDLs, and very low-density lipoproteins (VLDLs). VLDLs are carried in blood circulation as triglycerides (TGs). Although lipids are essential for cell membrane formation, hormone synthesis, and a source of free fatty acids, elevated levels of lipoproteins may result in coronary, cerebrovascular, or peripheral vascular disease. Dyslipidemia is defined by some combination of elevated TC, LDL, and TG levels and/or low HDL levels. Atherosclerosis of the blood vessels leading to the myocardium is the most significant consequence of dyslipidemia. The risk factor of dyslipidemia is additive to other factors for CHD, such as smoking, hypertension, and diabetes. Prevention is key, considering that a previous myocardial infarction or a diagnosis of CHD increases the risk of a myocardial infarction significantly.

Clinical Presentation of Dyslipidemia

Similar to hypertension, patients with dyslipidemia traditionally present asymptomatic and appear otherwise healthy unless they have subsequent cardiovascular risk factors or complications

---

patient education for
Hypertension

The objectives of self-treatment are to prevent progression of the disease and prevent morbidity and mortality. For most patients, carefully following their primary care provider's treatment plan and the self-care measures listed here will help ensure optimal therapeutic outcomes.

Nondrug Measures
- Manage risk factors for elevated systolic blood pressure by:
  - Adopting the DASH diet (Table 45–19):
    - Reducing excessive body weight
    - Participating in physical activity
    - Minimizing dietary sodium intake
  - Moderating alcohol consumption
  - Stopping use of tobacco (if applicable)
  - Self-monitoring blood pressure

Nonprescription Medications
- Currently, no nonprescription medications are recommended for the treatment of hypertension. Follow carefully your health care provider's instructions for prescription medications.

When to Seek Medical Attention
- If you measure an abnormal elevated blood pressure reading or experience a headache, visual abnormalities or loss of vision, chest pain, or confusion, consult your primary care provider or seek immediate medical care.

consistent with metabolic syndrome, or they present acutely with chest pain, palpitations, sweating, anxiety, or similar symptoms that may signify angina or myocardial infarction. Diagnosis of dyslipidemia is most often completed by laboratory tests of some combination of TC, LDL, TGs, and HDL. (See Chapter 48 for more information on nonprescription cholesterol tests.)

Treatment of Dyslipidemia
Treatment Goals

The primary goal of therapy is to prevent first-time (primary prevention) or recurrent (secondary prevention) cardiovascular events associated with atherosclerosis, such as myocardial infarctions, angina, heart failure, stroke, and/or peripheral artery disease. After baseline cholesterol levels are obtained, pharmacologic and/or nonpharmacologic agents may or may not be warranted. Patient-specific risk factors (e.g., age, family history, smoking, hypertension, and HDL level) are used to determine the risk category and ultimately the goal LDL. The 10-year risks (of myocardial infarction or death) are calculated based on the Framingham risk scores, which are calculated using age, gender, HDL, TC, blood pressure, and smoking status.[59]

The pharmacist should review lifestyle modifications with the patient and stress their importance in controlling the disorder. However, medical referral for further evaluation is needed if the assessment process reveals any of the following:

- No formal diagnosis of dyslipidemia
- No visit (or missed visit) to a primary care provider in the last year
- Nonadherence to any provider-recommended prescription medications, nonprescription medications, or self-care measures
- Unknown status of other comorbid conditions (e.g., hypertension)
- Perception that prescription medications are ineffective
- Use of dietary supplements without provider's knowledge or without achieving set goals

General Treatment Approach

Patients with an elevated fasting lipid panel may be initiated on nonpharmacologic and pharmacologic treatment regimens depending on the goals of therapy. Individuals 20 years of age and older should have a fasting evaluation of TC, LDL, HDL, and TGs at least every 5 years. If an atypical result is obtained, the patient should be classified accordingly, and further evaluation (family history, secondary causes, risk factors [Table 45–21]), and/or treatment should be initiated. Comorbidity of diabetes, which is defined as a CHD risk equivalent, means that a patient with diabetes and no known CHD has the same level of risk as someone with known CHD but without diabetes. Patients with diabetes are therefore treated to a more-aggressive LDL goal. In terms of treating LDL, certain risk factors may modify the treatment goal.[59] These include the following:

- Age (men ≥ 45 years; women ≥ 55 years or premature menopause without estrogen replacement therapy)
- Family history of premature CHD
- Cigarette smoking
- Hypertension (≥140/90 mm Hg or on medications for hypertension)
- Low HDL cholesterol (defined as <40 mg/dL)

table
45–21 Selected Factors Contributing to Dyslipidemia

Conditions	Medications
Obesity	Beta-blockers
Diabetes mellitus	Estrogens/progestins
Hypothyroidism	Glucocorticoids
Obstructive liver disease	Isotretinoin
Systemic lupus erythematous	Protease inhibitors
	Thiazide diuretics

Note: This list does not include every condition/medication that may cause dyslipidemia.

A family history of premature CHD is defined as a myocardial infarction or sudden death before 55 years of age for male relatives and 65 years for female relatives. The term *relatives* as used here refers to a father, mother, or other first-degree male or female relative.[59]

Nonpharmacologic Therapy

Nonpharmacologic treatment options, including therapeutic lifestyle changes (TLC), should be the forefront of the management of dyslipidemia. Dietary counseling or referral to a dietitian for education on intake of fat, saturated fats, and TC may be beneficial for preventing the progression of atherosclerosis. TLC focuses on reducing the intake of saturated fats and cholesterol, increasing the intake of plant stanols/sterols and fiber, reducing weight, and increasing the amount of physical activity (Table 45–22). This regimen may prevent or delay the need for drug therapy if implemented early and aggressively. Unless patients are at very high risk of developing CHD (e.g., have severe hypercholesterolemia, a CHD risk equivalent, strong family history), a minimum of a 3-month trial of TLC should be used before initiation of drug therapy.[59,60]

The following dietary considerations should be given for patients with dyslipidemia to reduce cardiovascular risk[59,60]:

- Consuming 20–30 grams of dietary fiber per day, of which 5–10 grams minimum should be soluble fiber

table
45–22 Key Components of the TLC Diet

Category	Recommendation
Saturated fat	<7% of total daily calories
Fat	25%–35% of total daily calories
Dietary cholesterol	<200 mg/day
Sodium	≤2400 mg/day

Key: TLC = Therapeutic lifestyle changes.
Source: Adapted from reference 59.

The objective of self-treatment is to prevent progression of the disease and prevent morbidity and mortality. For most patients, carefully following their health care provider's treatment plan and the self-care measures listed here will help ensure optimal therapeutic outcomes.

Nondrug Measures

■ Self-management of dyslipidemia includes implementing the therapeutic lifestyle changes diet as outlined in Table 45–23.

Nonprescription Medications

■ Currently, no nonprescription medications are recommended for the treatment of dyslipidemia. Follow carefully your primary care provider's instructions for any prescription medications.

When to Seek Medical Attention

■ If you experience any signs or symptoms such as chest pain, shortness of breath, cold sweats, nausea/vomiting, and/or upper body aches/pains, seek immediate medical care. These may be signs or symptoms of a heart attack that is secondary to high cholesterol, among other factors.

■ Substituting nonhydrogenated unsaturated fats for saturated and trans fats
■ Increasing the amount of omega-3 fatty acids consumed from marine and plant sources
■ Increasing the amount of fruits and vegetables with a low glycemic index (measure of the effect of carbohydrates on BG, reported as a percentage)
■ Substituting whole grains for simple carbohydrates

Fiber intake, although recommended, is often lower than desired. The two types of fiber include insoluble and soluble, defined by their ability to dissolve in water or gastrointestinal fluids. Soluble fiber is preferred in aiding the lowering of cholesterol and can be found in dietary sources such as oat bran, barley, nuts, seeds, beans, lentils, peas, and some fruits and vegetables. A more in-depth discussion of fiber can be found in Chapter 23.

Although the majority of Americans do not participate in regular moderate physical activity, the benefits have been well documented in terms of weight control, blood pressure control, improved insulin resistance, dyslipidemia management, and a decrease in cardiovascular events among patients with cardiovascular disease.[60] In terms of dyslipidemia, regular moderate physical activity can have improvements on all components, including LDL, HDL, and TGs. The amount and level of change depend on the level at baseline as well as the duration and intensity of exercise. The current AHA recommendation for most healthy individuals is 30 minutes of moderate aerobic exercise at least 5 days per week or 25 minutes of vigorous aerobic exercise 3 days a week. Moderate intensity is defined as working hard enough to increase heart rate and break a sweat while being able to maintain a conversation. This time may be accumulated in smaller sessions (e.g., 10–15 minutes). Higher intensity and durations may be needed for patients who are trying to achieve more weight loss versus weight maintenance.[61] In addition to aerobic exercise, individuals should participate in moderate to high intensity muscle-strengthening exercises for a minimum of 2 days per week. Patients who are at higher risk for cardiovascular events or who are concerned about how to start an exercise regimen should contact their primary care provider.

Complementary Therapies

For an in-depth discussion of natural products as it may relate to patients with dyslipidemia, see Chapter 51. Further discussion on niacin can be found in Chapter 22.

Patient Counseling for Dyslipidemia

Patient counseling for self-care of dyslipidemia should be complementary to the assessment, treatment, and monitoring being delivered by a provider. Counseling should focus on engaging the patient in the appropriate nonpharmacologic measures outlined in Table 45–22.

Natural products for the management of hyperlipidemia are available and widely used. A further discussion of these agents can be found in Chapter 51. The patient should be educated on the impact of uncontrolled hyperlipidemia. The box Patient Education for Dyslipidemia lists specific information to provide patients.

Evaluation of Patient Outcomes for Dyslipidemia

Evaluation of outcomes associated with hyperlipidemia should be completed by the patient's provider. Self-care measures should complement but not replace the provider's treatment plan.

REFERENCES

1. Centers for Disease Control and Prevention. Chronic diseases and health promotion. Updated on August 13, 2012. Accessed at http://www.cdc.gov/chronicdisease/overview/index.htm, April 11, 2013.
2. McWilliam CL. Patients, persons or partners? Involving those with chronic disease in their care. *Chronic Illn.* 2009;5:277–92.
3. American Diabetes Association. Standards of medical care in diabetes—2013. *Diabetes Care.* 2013;36(suppl 1):S11–66.
4. Centers for Disease Control and Prevention. *National Diabetes Facts Sheet: National Estimates and General Information on Diabetes and Prediabetes in the United States, 2011.* Atlanta, GA: U.S. Department of Health and Human Services, Centers for Disease Control and Prevention; 2011.
5. Evert AB, Boucher JL, Cypress M, et al. Nutrition therapy recommendations for the management of adults with diabetes. *Diabetes Care.* 2013;36(11):3821–42.
6. Mullooly CA. Physical activity. In: Mensing C, ed. *The Art and Science of Diabetes Self-Management Education.* 1st ed. Chicago, IL: American Association of Diabetes Educators; 2006:297–330.
7. Colberg SR, Sigal RJ, Fernhall B, et al. Exercise and type 2 diabetes: the American College of Sports Medicine and the American Diabetes Association: joint position statement. *Diabetes Care.* 2010;33(12):e147–67.
8. Sacks DB, Arnold M, Bakris GL, et al. Guidelines and recommendations for laboratory analysis in the diagnosis and management of diabetes mellitus. *Diabetes Care.* 2011;34(6):e61–99.

9. Austin MM, Haas L, Johnson T, et al. Self-monitoring of blood glucose: benefits and utilization. *Diabetes Educ.* 2006;32:836–47.

10. Kroon LA, Assemi M, Carlisle BA. Diabetes mellitus. In: Koda-Kimble MA, Young LY, Kradjan WA, et al., eds. *Applied Therapeutics.* 9th ed. Baltimore, MD: Lippincott Williams & Wilkins; 2009:Chap 50.

11. Egede LE, Ye X, Zheng D, et al. The prevalence and pattern of complementary and alternative medicine use in individuals with diabetes. *Diabetes Care.* 2002;25:324–9.

12. Mooman JE, Atkinson LJ, Bailey CM, et al. *National Surveillance of Asthma: United States, 2001–2010.* National Center for Health Statistics. Vital Health Stat 3(35). 2012. Accessed at http://www.cdc.gov/nchs/data/series/sr_03/sr03_035.pdf, May 5, 2013.

13. Healthy People 2020. Topics and Objectives: Respiratory diseases, Overview. U.S. Department of Health and Human Services. 2010. Accessed at http://www.healthypeople.gov, May 5, 2013.

14. Global Initiative for Asthma. *Global Strategy for Asthma Management and Prevention,* 2009 (updated). Accessed at http://www.ginasthma.org, April 26, 2013.

15. Bousquet J, Jeffery PK, Busse WW, et al. Asthma: from bronchoconstriction to airways inflammation and remodeling. *Am J Respir Crit Care Med.* 2000;161(5):1721–45.

16. Parsons JP, Mastronarde JG. Gastroesophageal reflux disease and asthma. *Curr Opin Pulm Med.* 2010;16(1):60–63.

17. McCallister JW, Parsons JP, Mastronarde JG. The relationship between gastroesophageal reflux and asthma: an update. *Ther Adv Respir Dis.* 2011;5(2):143–50.

18. Chan WW, Chiou E, Obstein KL, et al. The efficacy of proton pump inhibitors for the treatment of asthma in adults: a meta-analysis. *Arch Intern Med.* 2011;171(7):620–29.

19. James JM. Respiratory manifestations of food allergy. *Pediatrics.* 2003; 111(6 pt 3):1625–30.

20. Asthma Control Test. Accessed at http://www.asthma.com/resources/asthma-control-test.html?cc=p1113c00145:e1:d1:w1:p20&pid=333640&google=e_&rotation=10970&banner=81018&kw=333640, October 21, 2013.

21. National Heart, Lung, and Blood Institute, National Asthma Education and Prevention Program. *Expert Panel Report 3: Guidelines for the Diagnosis and Management of Asthma: Full Report 2007.* Bethesda, MD: U.S. Department of Health and Human Services, National Institutes of Health; August 28, 2007. NIH Publication No. 07-4051. Accessed at http://www.nhlbi.nih.gov/guidelines/asthma/asthgdln.pdf, April 26, 2013.

22. Stevenson DD. Aspirin sensitivity and desensitization for asthma and sinusitis. *Curr Allergy Asthma Rep.* 2009;9(2):155–63.

23. Metsios GS, Flouris AD, Koutedakis Y. Passive smoking, asthma and allergy in children. *Inflamm Allergy Drug Targets.* 2009;8(5):348–52.

24. Bronkaid® product information. Accessed at http://www.bronkaid.com/en/product-information/index.php, August 28, 2014.

25. Wyeth Consumer Heathcare. Primatene® Tablets [consumer information]. Wyeth Consumer Healthcare. Accessed at http://www.primatenetablets.com/productsprimatene_tablets, April 26, 2013.

26. Epinephrine monograph. Lexi-Drugs Online™ [subscription database]. Hudson, OH: Lexi-Comp. Accessed at http://online.lexi.com/crlsql/servlet/crlonline, April 27, 2013.

27. Nephron Pharmaceuticals Corporation. Asthmanefrin [product information]. Accessed at http://www.asthmanefrin.com. April 22, 2013.

28. U.S. Food and Drug Administration. Warning Letter to Nephron Pharmaceuticals Corp., FLA-13-30, September 24, 2013. Accessed at http://www.fda.gov/ICECI/EnforcementActions/WarningLetters/2013/ucm370008.htm, October 7, 2013.

29. U.S. Food and Drug Administration. Safety concerns with Asthmanefrin and the EZ Breathe atomizer. Accessed at http://www.fda.gov/Drugs/DrugSafety/ucm370483.htm?source=govdelivery&utm_medium=email&utm_source=govdelivery, October 2, 2013.

30. Flublok [product information]. Protein Sciences Corporation, Meriden, CT. Accessed at http://www.flublok.com, February 22, 2013.

31. Flucelvax [product information]. Novartis, Cambridge, MA. Accessed at http://www.flucelvax.com, February 22, 2013.

32. Influenza virus vaccine live/attenuated monograph. Lexi-Drugs Online™ [subscription database]. Hudson, OH: Lexi-Comp. Accessed at http://online.lexi.com/crlsql/servlet/crlonline, May 3, 2013.

33. Centers for Disease Control and Prevention. Updated immunization schedule for adults 19 years of age and older. *MMWR Morb Mortal Wkly Rep.* 2013;62(1):9–19. Accessed at http://www.cdc.gov/mmwr/preview/mmwrhtml/su6201a3.htm, April 22, 2013.

34. Briggs GG, Freeman RK, Yaffe SJ. Epinephrine and ephedrine. In: *Drugs in Pregnancy and Lactation.* 9th ed. Philadelphia, PA: Lippincott Williams & Wilkins; 2011:495–7.

35. American College of Gynecology. ACOG practice bulletin no. 90: asthma in pregnancy. *Obstet Gynecol.* 2008;111(2 pt 1):457–64.

36. National Collegiate Athletic Association. 2013–14 NCAA Banned Drugs. Updated November 15, 2013. Health and Safety Policy. Accessed at http://www.ncaa.org/health-and-safety/policy/2013-14-ncaa-banned-drugs, August 15, 2014.

37. Shen J, Oraka E. Complementary and alternative medicine (CAM) use among children with current asthma. *Prev Med.* 2012;54(1):27–31.

38. Marino LA, Shen J. Characteristics of complementary and alternative medicine use among adults with current asthma, 2006. *J Asthma.* 2010;47(5):521–5.

39. U.S. Food and Drug Administration, Division of Cardiovascular, Respiratory, and Neurological Devices. Guidance Document. Guidance for labeling peak flow meters for over the counter sale. Rockville, MD: Food and Drug Administration; June 8, 1993. Accessed at http://www.fda.gov/downloads/MedicalDevices/DeviceRegulationandGuidance/GuidanceDocuments/UCM081354.pdf, April 25, 2013.

40. Lim KG, Rank MA, Li JT, et al. How well does patient self-report predict asthma medication possession? Implications for medication reconciliation and adherence assessment. *J Asthma.* 2010;47(8):878–82.

41. National Osteoporosis Foundation. NOF releases new data detailing prevalence of osteoporosis. April 18, 2013. Accessed at http://www.nof.org/news/2948, August 15, 2014.

42. National Osteoporosis Foundation. *Clinician's Guide to Prevention and Treatment of Osteoporosis.* Washington, DC: National Osteoporosis Foundation; 2010. Accessed at http://nof.org/hcp/resources/913, September 15, 2014.

43. Go AS, Mozaffarian D, Roger VL, et al. Heart disease and stroke statistics—2013 update: A report from the American Heart Association Statistics Committee and Stroke Statistics Subcommittee. *Circulation.* 2013;127(1):e6–245.

44. Jessup M, Abraham WT, Casey DE, et al. 2009 Focused update: ACCF/AHA guidelines for the diagnosis and management of heart failure in adults: a report of the American College of Cardiology Foundation/American Heart Association Task Force on Practice Guidelines developed in collaboration with the International Society for Heart and Lung Transplantation. *J Am Coll Cardiol.* 2009;53:1343–82.

45. Uddin N, Patterson JH. Current guidelines for treatment of heart failure: 2006 update. *Pharmacotherapy.* 2007;27(4 pt 2):12S–7S.

46. Riegel B, Moser DK, Anker SD, et al. State of the science: promoting self-care in persons with heart failure; a scientific statement from the American Heart Association. *Circulation.* 2009;120(12):1141–63.

47. Ditewig JB, Blok H, Havers J. Effectiveness of self-management interventions on mortality, hospital readmissions, chronic heart failure hospitalization rate and quality of life in patients with chronic heart failure: a systematic review. *Patient Educ Couns.* 2010;78:297–315.

48. Powell LH, Calvin JE, Richardson D, et al. Self-management counseling in patients with heart failure: the heart failure adherence and retention randomized behavioral trial. *JAMA.* 2010;304(12):1331–8.

49. Pharand C, Ackman ML, Jackevicius CA, et al. Use of OTC and herbal products in patients with cardiovascular disease. *Ann Pharmacother.* 2003; 37(6):899–904.

50. Zick SM, Blume A, Aaronson KD. The prevalence and pattern of complementary and alternative supplement use in individuals with chronic heart failure. *J Card Failure.* 2005;11(8):586–9.

51. National Center for Health Statistics. *Health, United States, 2011.* Hyattsville, MD: National Center for Health Statistics; 2011. Accessed at http://www.cdc.gov/nchs/data/hus/hus11.pdf, April 11, 2013.

52. Chobanian AV, Bakris GL, Black HR, et al., and the National High Blood Pressure Education Program Coordinating Committee. Seventh report of the Joint National Committee on Prevention, Detection, Evaluation, and Treatment of High Blood Pressure. JNC 7-complete version. *Hypertension*. 2003;42:1206–52.

53. Saseen JJ, Maclaughlin EJ. Hypertension (pathophysiology and clinical presentation). In: DiPiro JT, Talbert RL, Yee GC, et al., eds. *Pharmacotherapy: A Pathophysiologic Approach*. 7th ed. New York, NY: McGraw-Hill Professional; 2008:140–46.

54. National Heart, Lung, and Blood Institute. *Your Guide to Lowering Your Blood Pressure with DASH*. Bethesda, MD: National Institutes of Health; 1998 (revised April 2006). NIH Publication No. 06-4082. Accessed at http://www.nhlbi.nih.gov/health/resources/heart/hbp-dash-index.htm, September 15, 2014.

55. Bray EP, Holder R, Mant J, et al. Does self-monitoring reduce blood pressure? Meta-analysis with meta-regression of randomized controlled trials. *Ann Med*. 2010;42(5):371–86.

56. Hein AW, Verberk WJ, Kroon AA, et al. Effect of self-measurement of blood pressure on adherence to treatment in patients with mild-to-moderate hypertension. *J Hypertens*. 2010;28(3):622–7.

57. Pickering TG, Hall JE, Appel LG, et al. Recommendations for blood pressure measurement in humans and experimental animals: part 1: blood pressure measurement in humans: a statement for professionals from the Subcommittee of Professional and Public Education of the American Heart Association Council on High Blood Pressure Research. *Circulation*. 2005;111:697–716.

58. Cantu C, Arauz A, Murilla-Bonilla LM, et al. Stroke associated with sympathomimetics contained in over-the-counter cough and cold drugs. *Stroke*. 2003;34(7):1667–73.

59. Expert Panel on Detection, Evaluation and Treatment of High Blood Cholesterol in Adults. Executive summary of the third report of the National Cholesterol Education Program (NCEP) Expert Panel on Detection, Evaluation and Treatment of High Blood Cholesterol in Adults (Adult Treatment Panel III). *JAMA*. 2001;285:2486–97.

60. Houston MC, Fazio S, Chilton FH, et al. Nonpharmacologic treatment of dyslipidemia. *Prog Cardiovasc Dis*. 2009;52(2):61–94.

61. Haskell WL, Min Lee I, Pate RR, et al. Physical activity and public health: updated recommendation for adults from the American College of Sports Medicine and the American Heart Association. *Circulation*. 2007;116(9):1081–93.

chapter 46

INSOMNIA, DROWSINESS, AND FATIGUE

Sarah T. Melton and Cynthia K. Kirkwood

Insomnia

Insomnia is one of the most common patient complaints, ranking third behind headache and the common cold. Insomnia is a symptom with diverse etiologies, and it can progress to a disorder.[1] Insomnia occurs when a person has trouble falling or staying asleep, wakes up too early and cannot return to sleep, or does not feel refreshed after sleeping. Patients with other sleep disorders, such as sleep apnea, narcolepsy, and restless legs syndrome, also seek nonprescription sleep aids. Because of potentially significant adverse clinical effects, patients with these disorders preferably should see a sleep specialist.

Although the average adult requires 8 or more hours of sleep nightly, the typical American gets 6.7 hours.[2] An estimated 64% of the U.S. population experiences sleep problems at least a few nights a week with 7% of adults reporting the use of alcohol, 7% a nonprescription sleep aid, and 8% a prescription hypnotic to manage their insomnia.[2] Patients with insomnia are significantly more likely to report being unable to work efficiently, exercise, eat healthfully, and engage in leisure activities because they are too sleepy.[2]

Total annual cost estimates for insomnia in the United States range from $30 billion to $107.5 billion, depending on the prevalence rates assumed.[3] Compared with patients without insomnia, this disorder is associated with a significant economic burden for younger (ages 18–64) and older (ages ≥ 65) patients in terms of the average and indirect costs.[4] More than half of adults older than 65 report at least one sleep complaint, with 3%–21% of men and 7%–29% of women reporting the use hypnotics.[5] Five percent of older adults reported using nonprescription medications every night or a few nights a week.[6] This group also has an increased incidence of sleep apnea and restless legs syndrome. Significant morbidity is associated with obstructive sleep apnea, including increased mortality from cardiovascular death.[7] As a result, complaints of insomnia in older patients should be carefully evaluated.

Despite these data, only a small percentage of patients with a sleep disorder actually tell their medical provider.[1] The combination of frequent misuse of hypnotics and availability of nonprescription agents makes insomnia a disorder of significant concern.

Pathophysiology of Insomnia

Physiologically, sleep can be categorized into different stages by using the sleeping electroencephalogram (EEG) in conjunction with electro-oculography and electromyography. Stage 1 sleep is a transitional stage, occurring as the patient falls asleep; the EEG resembles the waking state more than sleep. Stage 2 sleep constitutes about 50% of sleep time and is light sleep. Stages 3 and 4, collectively known as deep sleep or delta sleep, are characterized by the patterns of delta waves, or slow-frequency waves, on the EEG. Rapid eye movement (REM) sleep is neither light nor deep, and the EEG manifests an increase in high-frequency waves. REM sleep is characterized by physiologic activity compared with other sleep stages; skeletal muscle movement is inhibited. The eyes move rapidly from side to side, while blood pressure, heart rate, temperature, respiration, and metabolism are increased.[7,8]

Upon falling asleep, an individual progresses through four stages. The first REM period, usually 5–7 minutes in length, starts in about 70–90 minutes. The time from falling asleep to the first REM period is referred to as REM latency. The sleep cycle then repeats about every 70–120 minutes, with each progressive REM period becoming longer and the time spent in deep sleep becoming shorter. Prolonged suppression of REM sleep can result in psychological and behavioral changes.[7,8]

Sleep physiology changes with increasing age. Among older adults, the total duration of sleep is shorter, the number of nocturnal awakenings increases, and less time is spent in stage 4 and REM sleep. Sleep latency usually remains normal with increasing age. Despite these changes, older adults cannot be assumed to require less sleep.[7]

Insomnia can be classified as transient, short term, or chronic according to the duration of sleep disturbance. Transient insomnia is often self-limiting, lasting less than 1 week. Short-term insomnia usually lasts from 1–3 weeks.[3] Chronic, or long-term, insomnia persists for more than 3 weeks to years and is often the result of medical problems, psychiatric disorders, or substance abuse.[1,3]

Insomnia can also be classified on the basis of an identifiable cause. Primary insomnia is the term used to describe patients who have sleep difficulty for at least 1 month, that affects psychosocial functioning, and that is not caused by another sleep disorder, general medical disorder, psychiatric disorder, or medication (or secondary insomnia).[9] All underlying causes of insomnia must be identified and managed to relieve the sleep disturbance.[1,3,9]

Difficulty falling asleep is often associated with acute life stresses or medical illness, anxiety, and poor sleep habits. The severity of stressful situations can affect the length of insomnia. Travel, hospitalization, or anticipation of an important or stressful event can cause transient insomnia. If more severe stressors, such as the death of a loved one, recovery from surgery, or divorce, are present, transient insomnia can become short-term insomnia. Unless managed appropriately, short-term insomnia can progress to chronic insomnia.

Shift workers often complain of sleep disturbances, excessive sleepiness, or both. Sleep problems occur more frequently in individuals who must rotate shifts. Some nighttime workers adjust to their change in sleep schedule, whereas others never do. Some individuals are extremely sensitive to the stimulant effects of caffeine and nicotine. Drinking caffeinated beverages in the late afternoon or evening hours can cause insomnia. Late-night exercise and late-evening meals as well as environmental distractions, such as noise, lighting, uncomfortable temperatures, or new surroundings, can also interfere with sleep.[7,8]

Several medical disorders, in addition to psychiatric disorders, are associated with chronic insomnia (Table 46–1). Chronic insomnia is a key complaint of patients experiencing pain syndromes. Chronic insomnia can also be secondary to use of medications or other substances, sleep–wake schedule disorders, or primary sleep disorders.[9] Early morning awakening is often associated with depression. Nonprescription hypnotics are generally not helpful in patients with chronic insomnia, and medical referral is indicated.

Medications, including both prescription and nonprescription drugs, can produce either insomnia or withdrawal insomnia (Table 46–2).[1,7,8] Antidepressants, antihypertensive agents, and sympathomimetic amines (e.g., pseudoephedrine, phenylephrine) are commonly associated with causing insomnia. Alcohol can cause insomnia after acute use and as a withdrawal effect after chronic use.

table 46–2 Drugs That Can Exacerbate Insomnia

Drugs That Can Cause Insomnia	Drugs That Can Produce Withdrawal Insomnia
Alcohol	Alcohol
Anabolic steroids	Amphetamines
Antidepressants (e.g., bupropion, fluoxetine, venlafaxine)	Antihistamines (first generation)
Anticonvulsants (e.g., felbamate)	Barbiturate
Antihypertensives (e.g., clonidine)	Benzodiazepines
Antineoplastics	Illicit drugs (e.g., cocaine, marijuana, phencyclidine)
Amphetamines	Monoamine oxidase inhibitors
Anorexiants (e.g., phentermine)	Opiates
Beta-adrenergic agonists (e.g., albuterol)	Tricyclic antidepressants
Beta-blockers (especially propranolol)	
Caffeine	
Corticosteroids	
Decongestants (e.g., pseudoephedrine, phenylephrine)	
Diuretics (at bedtime)	
Levodopa	
Nicotine	
Oral contraceptives	
Thyroid preparations	

Source: References 1, 7, and 8.

table 46–1 Medical Disorders Associated with Insomnia

General Medical Disorders	Psychiatric Disorders
Allergies	Anxiety disorders
Arthritis	Depression
Benign prostatic hyperplasia	**Sleep Disorders**
Chronic pain syndromes	Psychophysiologic insomnia
Diabetes mellitus	Restless legs syndrome
Gastroesophageal reflux disease	Shift-work sleep disorder
Heart failure	Sleep apnea
Peptic ulcer disease	**Other Conditions**
Respiratory Disorders	Menopause
Asthma	Pregnancy
Chronic obstructive pulmonary disease	

Source: References 1, 3, 5, and 7.

Clinical Presentation of Insomnia

Patients with insomnia may have varying complaints, such as difficulty falling asleep, frequent awakening, early morning awakening and inability to fall back to sleep, disturbed quality of sleep with unusual or troublesome dreams, or just poor sleep in general. Their actual duration of sleep, as determined by sleep laboratory studies, may or may not differ from that of individuals who report normal sleep. However, these patients usually report that they need more than 30 minutes to fall asleep and/or that their duration of sleep is less than 6–7 hours nightly. Patients who complain of insomnia characterized by frequent nighttime awakenings or early morning awakenings with difficulty going back to sleep or those with symptoms of 4 weeks or longer should be referred to their health care provider for further evaluation.

Sleep-deprived individuals are highly symptomatic, and their quality of life is negatively affected. Some impairment in daytime functioning is necessary for a diagnosis of insomnia, and most untreated patients with insomnia report symptoms of fatigue, drowsiness, anxiety, irritability, depression, decreased concentration, and memory impairment. If untreated, insomnia is associated with an increase in accidents as well as a rise in morbidity and mortality rates from general medical and psychiatric disorders, such as cardiovascular disease, pain syndromes, depression, anxiety, and substance abuse.[1]

Treatment of Insomnia

Treatment Goals

Treatment goals are to improve the patient's presenting symptoms, quality of life, and functioning.

General Treatment Approach

For patients with transient or short-term insomnia but no underlying medical or psychiatric conditions that cause insomnia, reestablishing the normal sleep cycle with good sleep hygiene practices, with or without a nonprescription sleep aid, should help normalize sleep patterns. The algorithm in Figure 46–1 outlines the assessment and self-treatment of transient and short-term insomnia, and it lists exclusions for self-treatment.

Nonpharmacologic Therapy

The sleep hygiene measures in Table 46–3 are recommended for all patients with insomnia.[10] In many patients with sleep disturbances, these measures should be tried before starting drug therapy. Patients should be encouraged to try one or two measures at a time.

Pharmacologic Therapy

When the Food and Drug Administration (FDA) issued its final monograph on nonprescription sleep aids in 1989, diphenhydramine (HCl and citrate salts) was the only sleep aid deemed to be safe and effective for self-administration.[11]

Antihistamines

Diphenhydramine and doxylamine are members of the ethanolamine group of antihistamines. Ethanolamines affect sleep through their affinity for blocking histamine$_1$ and muscarinic receptors.[12] Although the safety and efficacy of doxylamine have not been fully established, FDA has allowed the drug to remain on the market.[13] Few studies supporting the efficacy of doxylamine as a hypnotic are available.[1,13]

Both diphenhydramine and doxylamine are well absorbed from the gastrointestinal tract with similar times to maximum plasma concentrations (1–4 hours and 2–3 hours, respectively). The elimination half-life of diphenhydramine is 2.4–9.3 hours, whereas that of doxylamine is 10 hours.[11,13] Diphenhydramine is metabolized in the liver through two successive N-demethylations, and its apparent half-life can be prolonged in patients with hepatic cirrhosis.[11] Studies have shown a positive relationship between diphenhydramine plasma concentrations and drowsiness and cognitive impairment. Maximum sedation with diphenhydramine occurs between 3 and 6 hours after a dose.[11]

The primary indication for diphenhydramine in insomnia is the symptomatic management of transient and short-term sleep difficulty, particularly in individuals who complain of occasional problems falling asleep. The efficacy of diphenhydramine in patients with chronic insomnia is poor.[1] Tolerance to the sedative

effect of diphenhydramine was reported to develop quickly, within days of repeated use in healthy volunteers.[14]

Although the usual diphenhydramine dosage is 50 mg nightly, some individuals benefit from a 25 mg dosage. Intermittent use for 3 days with an "off" night to assess sleep quality without medication may reduce tolerance to the hypnotic effect. Diphenhydramine should be used for no more than 7–10 consecutive nights because insomnia may be a symptom of an undiagnosed medical or psychiatric illness that requires further evaluation.[11]

Additive sedation or anticholinergic effects occur when diphenhydramine is used in combination with other medications that have these properties.[12] Diphenhydramine, an inhibitor of the hepatic enzyme CYP2D6, causes more than a twofold decrease in the clearance of metoprolol, especially in women.[15] In patients on multiple medications, particularly older patients, diphenhydramine may reduce the clearance of drugs metabolized by CYP2D6, such as venlafaxine, codeine, or propranolol. These potential interactions should be carefully monitored.

Anticholinergic toxicity can result from excessive antihistamine dosages. Other factors, including drug interactions, intentional overdosage, or individual sensitivity, can also lead to toxicity.[12,16] Central nervous system (CNS) anticholinergic toxicity is one of the primary presenting features of antihistamine excess. Patients exhibiting excessive anticholinergic effects can be anxious, excited, delirious, hallucinating, or stuporous. In more severe cases, coma or seizures may occur. Other physical signs of anticholinergic toxicity include dilated pupils, flushed skin, hot and dry mucous membranes, and elevated body temperature. Tachycardia and moderate QTc prolongation on the electrocardiogram are common. In severe cases, rhabdomyolysis, dysrhythmias, cardiovascular collapse, and death can occur.[11,12,16] In the case of diphenhydramine overdose, patients should be referred for emergency treatment, which includes gastric lavage and activated charcoal via gastric tube, and further symptomatic treatment.

The primary adverse effects of diphenhydramine and doxylamine are anticholinergic.[11,13] Dry mouth and throat, constipation, blurred vision, urinary retention, and tinnitus commonly occur. Older patients, patients with comorbid general medical disorders, and patients taking multiple medications are particularly susceptible to developing adverse effects.

Diphenhydramine is contraindicated in several situations. Older men with prostatic hyperplasia and difficulty urinating should not use diphenhydramine because urinary retention can occur. Because anticholinergic agents can increase intraocular pressure, angle-closure glaucoma is another contraindication. Patients with cardiovascular disease, such as angina or arrhythmias, may be particularly susceptible to the anticholinergic adverse effects and should not use these agents.[12] Anticholinergic agents decrease cognition and increase confusion in patients with dementia; diphenhydramine should be avoided in these patients.

Patients should be cautioned to avoid performing tasks that require their full attention or coordination, such as driving, cooking, or operating machinery, until their response is known. They should be discouraged from drinking alcoholic beverages while taking diphenhydramine. Some patients can develop excitation from diphenhydramine and other highly anticholinergic antihistamines.[12] This paradoxical effect occurs more often in children, older patients, and patients with organic mental

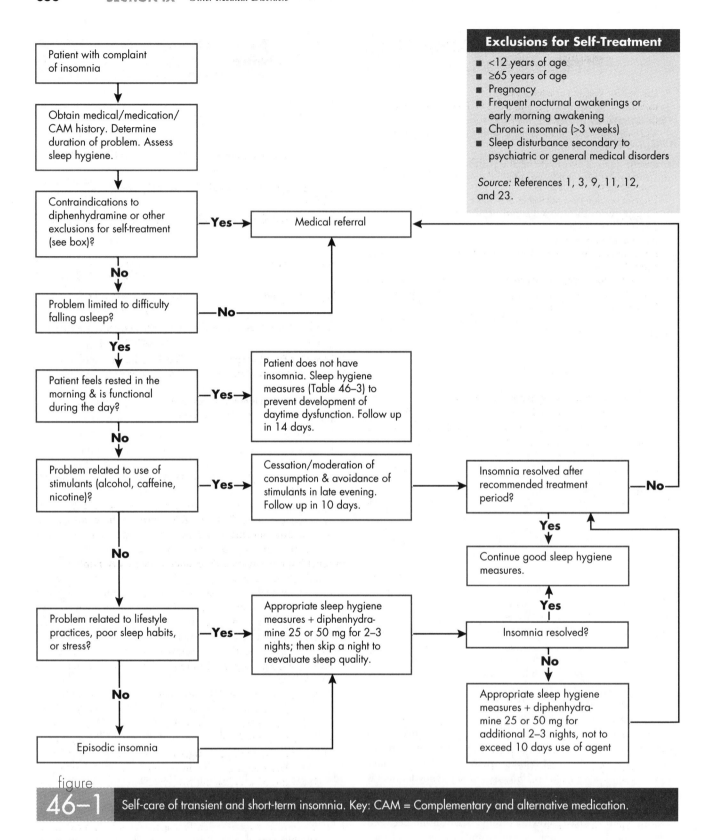

Exclusions for Self-Treatment

- <12 years of age
- ≥65 years of age
- Pregnancy
- Frequent nocturnal awakenings or early morning awakening
- Chronic insomnia (>3 weeks)
- Sleep disturbance secondary to psychiatric or general medical disorders

Source: References 1, 3, 9, 11, 12, and 23.

figure

46-1   Self-care of transient and short-term insomnia. Key: CAM = Complementary and alternative medication.

disorders. Symptoms include nervousness, restlessness, agitation, tremors, insomnia, delirium, and, in rare cases, seizures.

Combination products containing diphenhydramine and acetaminophen, ibuprofen, or aspirin are available,[12] although no published studies establish whether these products are of additive benefit in inducing sleep in patients who complain of insomnia caused by pain.

Several case reports have been published of diphenhydramine abuse in patients taking antipsychotic medications.[17] Animal studies indicate that selected antagonists of the histamine₁ receptors enhance dopamine release in the mesolimbic areas similar to that produced by cocaine.[18] Health care providers should carefully assess for abuse in individuals making repeated purchases for diphenhydramine, especially in patients being treated for psychosis.[17]

<table>
<thead>
<tr><th colspan="2">table
46–3   **Principles of Good Sleep Hygiene**</th></tr>
</thead>
</table>

- Use bed for sleeping or intimacy only.
- Establish a regular sleep pattern. Go to bed and arise at about the same time daily, even on the weekends.
- Make the bedroom comfortable for sleeping. Avoid temperature extremes, noise, and light.
- Engage in relaxing activities before bedtime.
- Avoid using electronic devices (particularly videos, television, and tablets) around bedtime.
- Exercise regularly but not within 2–4 hours of bedtime.
- If hungry, eat a light snack, but avoid eating meals within 2 hours before bedtime.
- Avoid daytime napping.
- Avoid using caffeine, alcohol, or nicotine for at least 4–6 hours before bedtime.
- If unable to fall asleep, do not continue to try to sleep; rather, get out of bed and perform a relaxing activity until you feel tired.
- Do not watch the clock at night.

Source: References 7–10.

Ethanol

Use of alcohol to induce sleep is common in patients with chronic insomnia and is associated with hazardous drinking behavior.[19] Ethanol, in both low and high quantities, initially improves sleep in people who do not abuse alcohol, but sleep disturbances occur in the second half of the night at high doses. Tolerance quickly develops after the initial beneficial effects, often leading to the use of higher doses. Individuals with heavy or continuous alcohol use usually experience restless sleep, often awaken within 2–4 hours, and have reduced total sleep duration. People who chronically drink alcohol usually have a marked disorganization of the sleep cycle. A worsening of sleep or rebound insomnia can occur when alcohol use ceases.[20]

Alcohol is present in some nonprescription combination cold products, such as NyQuil Liquid, which contains 10% alcohol by volume. Products of this type are marketed to induce sleep. Data are limited, however, regarding the efficacy and safety of these products as hypnotics. The multiple ingredients in these products increase the risk of adverse effects and interactions with other drugs.

Pharmacotherapeutic Comparisons

Most clinical trials indicate that diphenhydramine is effective in decreasing time to fall asleep (sleep latency) and in improving the reported quality of sleep for individuals with occasional insomnia.[11] Compared with placebo, diphenhydramine improved sleep efficiency for 2 weeks in patients with mild insomnia.[21] In general, diphenhydramine is not as effective as benzodiazepine hypnotics and should not be recommended for a chronic sleep disturbance.[1]

Product Selection Guidelines

Because the value of doxylamine as a hypnotic is not well established, only diphenhydramine should be recommended to patients for such use. Nonprescription diphenhydramine is available as capsules, gelcaps, tablets, chewable tablets, solutions, and elixirs (Table 46–4), allowing different patient preferences.[12]

<table>
<thead>
<tr><th colspan="2">table
46–4   **Selected Nonprescription Sleep Aid Products**</th></tr>
<tr><th>Trade Name</th><th>Primary Ingredients</th></tr>
</thead>
<tbody>
<tr><td colspan="2">**Single-Entity Antihistamine Products**</td></tr>
<tr><td>Unisom SleepGels Maximum Strength Capsules, liquid filled</td><td>Diphenhydramine HCl 50 mg</td></tr>
<tr><td>Sominex Nighttime Sleep Aid Tablets</td><td>Diphenhydramine HCl 25 mg</td></tr>
<tr><td>ZzzQuil Liquid Sleep-Aid Liquid</td><td>Diphenhydramine HCL 50 mg</td></tr>
<tr><td colspan="2">**Antihistamine/Analgesic Combination Products**</td></tr>
<tr><td>Advil PM Caplets</td><td>Diphenhydramine citrate 38 mg; ibuprofen 200 mg</td></tr>
<tr><td>Bayer PM Caplets</td><td>Diphenhydramine citrate 38 mg; aspirin 500 mg</td></tr>
<tr><td>Excedrin PM Geltabs/Caplets/Tablets</td><td>Diphenhydramine citrate 38 mg; acetaminophen 500 mg</td></tr>
<tr><td>Tylenol PM Extra Strength Geltabs/Gelcaps/Caplets</td><td>Diphenhydramine HCl 25 mg; acetaminophen 500 mg</td></tr>
</tbody>
</table>

Note: Information is not all inclusive. Products may have changed formulations since time of publication.

Special Populations

The safety of antihistamines during pregnancy has not been established.[12] Therefore, the benefit–risk ratio of using these drugs to manage insomnia during pregnancy should be carefully evaluated. In April 2013, FDA approved the combination of doxylamine succinate and pyridoxine HCl for treatment of pregnant women experiencing nausea and vomiting. This product has been given a Pregnancy Category A. Diphenhydramine is classified as Pregnancy Category B based on safety studies conducted in animals. Most epidemiologic studies have not demonstrated increased risk of teratogenicity with the use of diphenhydramine during the first trimester, but one trial reported cleft palate alone and with other fetal abnormalities.[11] Nevertheless, rather than recommending a nonprescription product, pregnant women should be referred for further medical evaluation.

An increased risk of CNS adverse effects can occur in breast-fed neonates after maternal intake of a sedating antihistamine. The intermittent use of low doses of diphenhydramine by the mother after the last daytime feeding would lessen potential drug effects in the infant. Use of large dosages for sustained periods of time may inhibit lactation and cause drowsiness in breast-fed infants.[22] Continued use of sedating antihistamines for insomnia are not recommended for use in nursing mothers.[11-13]

Children and adolescents may present with insomnia because of a circadian rhythm disorder. Teenagers should be asked about their use of nonprescription remedies and intake of caffeine, nicotine, or alcohol. Behavioral interventions and good sleep hygiene are first-line treatment for insomnia in children and adolescents. Diphenhydramine and doxylamine are not indicated to treat insomnia in children younger than 12 years. Diphenhydramine may cause paradoxical excitation in younger children and is not recommended to induce sleep in infants.[11] Anticholinergic toxicity is common in children, and the symptoms may be more severe. Diphenhydramine toxicity was reported in children using the topical application over large areas of their bodies, as well as in those using both the topical and oral preparations.[11] FDA requires a warning statement advising consumers not to use oral nonprescription diphenhydramine products with any other product containing diphenhydramine, including topical agents.[11]

Treatment of insomnia in older adults consists of behavioral therapy and pharmacotherapy with approved agents. The Beers criteria recommend avoiding the use of anticholinergic drugs in older adults.[23] Diphenhydramine has caused cognitive impairment and falls in older patients.[1,24] Therefore, nonprescription antihistamines should not be recommended to treat insomnia in this age group, and the patients should be referred to their health care provider for further evaluation.

Complementary Therapies

Complementary therapies such as melatonin, valerian, and kava are commonly used for insomnia (see chapter 51). In a representative sample of the U.S. population, 5.2% used melatonin and 5.9% used valerian.[25] The decision to use natural products for insomnia was made in consultation with a health care provider less than 50% of the time.[25]

A report on the safety and effectiveness of melatonin found that, for most sleep disorders, its benefits are limited.[26] Melatonin may be effective in short-term treatment of delayed sleep phase syndrome (i.e., a sleep pattern characterized by a delayed onset of sleep by 2 or more hours from normal, resulting in a later bedtime and wake time).[26] Evidence of its efficacy is conflicting and limited.

Valerian (*Valeriana officinalis*) has limited benefit in insomnia compared with placebo.[27] Clinical trials have used 400–900 mg of the valerian root extract. Continuous nightly use for several days or weeks is required for effect, so valerian is not useful for acute insomnia. Patients using large dosages of valerian over several years can experience severe benzodiazepine–like withdrawal symptoms and cardiac complications.[27] Valerian should be slowly tapered after extended use.

Kava (*Piper methysticum*) has been used in insomnia and has been associated with severe hepatotoxicity.[28] Therefore, kava should not be recommended as a sleep aid.

The American Academy of Sleep Medicine recommends that dietary supplements not be used to treat insomnia or any other sleep problem, unless approved by a health care provider, because of the risk of adverse effects and drug interactions.[29] (See Chapter 51.)

Complementary therapies such as acupuncture, tai chi, and light therapy may be useful in the treatment of insomnia.[1,28] However, these treatments have not been adequately evaluated.

Assessment of Insomnia: A Case-Based Approach

In assessing whether to recommend a nonprescription sleep aid, the provider should determine whether use of such products is appropriate, what nondrug interventions should be recommended, and whether referral to another health care provider is indicated. Identifying acute causes of insomnia, poor sleep hygiene practices, or underlying medical disorders can assist the provider in making a recommendation.

Case 46–1 illustrates the assessment of a patient with insomnia.

Patient Counseling for Insomnia

Patients with sleep disorders should be encouraged to practice good sleep hygiene measures. For some patients, these measures alone will resolve insomnia. If use of a nonprescription sleep aid is appropriate, the dosage guidelines and recommended duration of therapy should be reviewed with the patient. Potential adverse effects, drug interactions, and any precautions or warnings should be carefully explained. In addition, patient education should include the signs and symptoms that indicate the need for further visits to the provider. Taking more than one product (i.e., prescription, nonprescription, and dietary supplements) concomitantly to treat insomnia should be discouraged; this approach increases the risk of adverse effects. The box Patient Education for Insomnia lists specific information to provide patients.

Evaluation of Patient Outcomes for Insomnia

Successful outcomes include decreased time to fall asleep, improved sleep quality, and decreased daytime fatigue and drowsiness. The patient should be advised to seek medical evaluation if sleep has not improved in 10 days.[12]

Key Points for Insomnia

➤ Refer patients with chronic insomnia or sleep disturbance caused by an underlying disorder for medical evaluation.
➤ Advise patients with self-treatable symptoms that if symptoms worsen or do not improve after 10 days, they should contact their health care provider.
➤ Counsel patients with insomnia on nondrug measures such as good sleep hygiene (Table 46–3).
➤ Refer children younger than 12 years, pregnant women, and adults older than 65 years with insomnia to their health care provider.
➤ Advise patients about the different dosage forms of sleep aids so they can select a product that is best suited for them.
➤ Advise patients that diphenhydramine is the only antihistamine recommended as a sleep aid for occasional insomnia.
➤ Counsel patients that nonprescription sleep aids can cause next-day sedation.
➤ Counsel patients on the adverse effects of diphenhydramine and other sleep aids, particularly drowsiness and the additive CNS depressant effects of alcohol and other sedating drugs.
➤ Advise patients not to take other oral medications that contain diphenhydramine with a nonprescription sleep aid that also contains diphenhydramine.
➤ Advise patients not to apply topical products that also contain diphenhydramine.
➤ Advise patients to discuss the potential risks and benefits of complementary therapies with their health care provider before selecting an agent.

Relevant Evaluation Criteria	Scenario/Model Outcome

Information Gathering

1. Gather essential information about the patient's symptoms and medical history, including:

a. description of symptom(s) (i.e., nature, onset, duration, severity, associated symptoms)

Patient complains of difficulty sleeping for the past 2 weeks. He feels tired and irritable during the day and an overwhelming need for a nap midday.

b. description of any factors that seem to precipitate, exacerbate, and/or relieve the patient's symptom(s)

Difficulty falling asleep began after the patient was laid off from his job as a computer programmer. Previously, he typically slept well.

c. description of the patient's efforts to relieve the symptoms

He tries to stay up until he is sleepy at night. He states that he lies in bed and begins worrying when he cannot fall asleep. He watches the alarm clock, knowing that he has to get up in a few hours to continue a job search. When he can't fall asleep, he usually turns on the television or plays games on his computer.

d. patient's identity

Mitchell Gibbs

e. age, sex, height, and weight

26 years old, male, 5 ft 11 in., 190 lb

f. patient's occupation

Computer programmer; currently unemployed

g. patient's dietary habits

Patient usually eats fast food at least once daily. He drinks 3–4 cups of coffee in the morning, 2–3 Diet Coke sodas through the day, and a 5-hour ENERGY Extra Strength in the afternoon when he feels tired.

h. patient's sleep habits

Stays up late working on his computer or watching television. Often sleeps in on the weekends until noon to "make up for lost sleep." He takes an hour-long nap in the afternoon 2–3 times weekly.

i. concurrent medical conditions, prescription and non-prescription medications, and dietary supplements

Allergic rhinitis: Allegra D 24-hour allergy and congestion (fexofenadine 180 mg and 240 mg pseudoephedrine) daily; nasal saline prn

j. allergies

Penicillin: throat swelling

k. history of other adverse reactions to medications

None

l. other (describe) _____

Drinks two to three beers every night to help him go to sleep. Denies use of tobacco.

Assessment and Triage

2. Differentiate patient's signs/symptoms and correctly identify the patient's primary problem(s).

Poor sleep, likely secondary to the stress of loss of job and poor sleep hygiene. Possible use of alcohol on a daily basis, use of a decongestant, and excessive caffeine are disrupting sleep.

3. Identify exclusions for self-treatment (Figure 46–1).

None

4. Formulate a comprehensive list of therapeutic alternatives for the primary problem to determine if triage to a health care provider is required, and share this information with the patient or caregiver.

Options include:

(1) Refer Mitchell to his health care provider.

(2) Recommend diphenhydramine until Mitchell can make an appointment with his health care provider.

(3) Recommend diphenhydramine and good sleep hygiene, including limiting daily alcohol and caffeine use and engaging in regular physical activity.

(4) Take no action.

Plan

5. Select an optimal therapeutic alternative to address the patient's problem, taking into account patient preferences.

Diphenhydramine 50 mg tablets and good sleep hygiene measures, as well as limited alcohol and caffeine consumption.

6. Describe the recommended therapeutic approach to the patient or caregiver.

"Take 1 diphenhydramine 50 mg tablet ½–1 hour before your antici-pated bedtime every night for 3 nights. Skip 1 night and evaluate your ability to sleep. If not improved, continue diphenhydramine for 3 more nights, and reevaluate ability to sleep without it. If symptoms persist for 10 days, seek medical evaluation."

"Follow measures for positive sleep hygiene (Table 46–3). Limit alcohol consumption to 1–2 beers or less, consumed no later than 2 hours before bedtime. Limit overall intake of caffeine, and at a minimum, avoid caffeine 6 hours before bedtime."

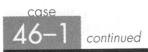

Relevant Evaluation Criteria	**Scenario/Model Outcome**
7. Explain to the patient or caregiver the rationale for selecting the recommended therapeutic approach from the considered therapeutic alternatives.	"A consistent sleep pattern will help resolve your insomnia. Seeing your health care provider may not be necessary if you take the diphenhydramine and follow good sleep hygiene measures. Poor sleep practices are a common cause of insomnia. If these practices are continued, they can create a chronic sleep disturbance. A medicine such as diphenhydramine can facilitate falling asleep, but it must be combined with measures of good sleep hygiene."
	"Alcohol in more than modest quantities can disrupt sleep and make insomnia worse. Therefore, alcohol consumption should be limited and avoided before bedtime. In addition, caffeine is a stimulant that promotes wakefulness. Caffeine intake should be limited and not occur within 6 hours of bedtime. Reduce intake of sodas and stop the 5-hour ENERGY Extra Strength drinks. The Diet Coke contains 47 mg of caffeine in each 12-ounce drink. The 5-hour ENERGY Extra Strength contains 242 mg of caffeine, which is equivalent to 2.5 cups of coffee. All dietary (e.g., coffee, sodas, and energy drinks) and hidden sources of caffeine (e.g., chocolate) should be identified."
	"The pseudoephedrine in the Allegra-D 24-hour tablets may also contribute to insomnia. You may take Allegra 24-hour tablets without the decongestant for your allergies."

Patient Education

8. When recommending self-care with nonprescription medications and/or nondrug therapy, convey accurate information to the patient or caregiver.	"Take diphenhydramine 50 mg nightly for 3 nights; then reevaluate sleep for 1 night without the medication. Do not exceed this nightly dose. Always use sleep aids in combination with good sleep hygiene measures (Table 46–3). Do not take sleep aids nightly longer than 10 days without seeing your health care provider."
	"Avoid drinking alcohol with the diphenhydramine because of the risk of increased sedation and negative effects of alcohol on sleep patterns."
	"Adverse effects may include sedation, next-morning hangover, and anticholinergic effects (e.g., dry mouth, urinary retention, blurry vision, and constipation)."
Solicit follow-up questions from the patient or caregiver.	(1) "May I repeat the dose of diphenhydramine if I do not fall asleep within 2 hours?"
	(2) "May I take diphenhydramine with my Allegra-D allergy medication?"
Answer the patient's or caregiver's questions.	(1) "No. Repeating the dose increases the risk of side effects and will likely not improve sleep."
	(2) "You should continue the saline nasal spray while using the diphenhydramine. Do not take the Allegra-D on the days you take diphenhydramine because both are antihistamines."

Evaluation of Patient Outcome

9. Assess patient outcome.	Contact the patient in 2–3 days to assess efficacy of diphenhydramine and improved sleep hygiene measures. Remind the patient that if the insomnia continues for longer than 10 days he should make an appointment for evaluation with his health care provider.

Drowsiness and Fatigue

Drowsiness or fatigue may be acute in onset or chronic and can increase the risk of workplace or transport–related accidents, as well as adversely impact productivity, mood, and overall health.[30,31] Evidence indicates an increased incidence of sleep-related crashes in young drivers who report an average of less than 6 hours of sleep per night.[32]

Caffeine is the most frequently used CNS stimulant in the world. An estimated 90% of adults report routine caffeine intake, an average of 227 mg daily (1.3 mg/kg), through ingestion of coffee, tea, and soft drinks. Youths consume less caffeine than adults daily; caffeine consumption averaged 69.5 mg (0.55 mg/kg) in those ages 12–17 years and 21 mg (0.4 mg/kg)

patient education for
Insomnia

The objectives of self-treatment are to (1) improve the duration and quality of sleep, (2) reduce fatigue and drowsiness during the day, (3) improve daytime functioning, and (4) minimize adverse effects of treatment. Carefully following product instructions and the self-care measures listed here will help ensure optimal therapeutic outcomes for most patients.

Disease Information

- Insomnia is difficulty getting enough sleep or trouble sleeping without interruption. Insomnia may be described as difficulty falling asleep, waking up too early, or waking up periodically during the night. Insomnia can cause fatigue and drowsiness during the day. Insomnia is *chronic* when it happens almost nightly for at least 1 month. Insomnia can be caused by medical or psychiatric conditions, mental stress or excitement, or certain daytime and bedtime habits. If prescribed a medication that can exacerbate insomnia, talk with your health care provider about taking the medication in the morning (e.g., corticosteroids).

Nondrug Measures

- See Table 46–3 for nondrug measures to prevent insomnia.
- Using principles of good sleep hygiene can help improve bad sleep habits and enhance quality sleep.
- If insomnia worsens or continues beyond 2 weeks, seek medical attention.

Nonprescription Medications

- Do not drive or operate machinery after taking sleep aids, including melatonin and valerian.
- Diphenhydramine is not expected to harm an unborn baby. Tell your doctor if you are pregnant or plan to become pregnant during treatment.

- Diphenhydramine may pass into breast milk and may harm a nursing baby. Antihistamines may also slow breast milk production. Do not use this medicine without medical advice if you are breast-feeding a baby.

Diphenhydramine

- Establish a regular bedtime and take diphenhydramine 30–60 minutes before you want to go to sleep. Do not take more than 50 mg of diphenhydramine each night.
- After 2–3 nights of improved sleep, skip taking the medication for one night to see if the insomnia is relieved.
- Do not take the medication longer than 10 days. Longer use will cause tolerance to the medication's sleep-inducing effects but not necessarily to its side effects, and you may have an underlying disorder that is causing insomnia.
- Note that diphenhydramine can cause morning grogginess or excessive sedation, dry mouth, blurred vision, constipation, and difficulty urinating (particularly in older men).
- Do not take diphenhydramine with alcohol; alcohol can increase the effects of the medication on the central nervous system. Alcohol also disrupts the sleep cycle.
- Do not take diphenhydramine with prescription sleep aids to improve sleep further.
- Consult your health care provider before taking diphenhydramine with other medications.

---

in those ages 2–11 years.[33] Energy drinks are popular with adolescents and young adults. Table 46–5 lists the caffeine content of common beverages. Caffeine is in many nonprescription, prescription, and dietary supplements. Total daily caffeine intake leads to adverse effects, withdrawal reactions, or, rarely, drug interactions.

Pathophysiology of Drowsiness and Fatigue

Daytime drowsiness and fatigue are most often caused by inadequate sleep, both insufficient duration and quality of sleep. The degree of sleepiness is determined by two factors that regulate sleep and wakefulness: (1) a homeostatic process involving an increase in sleepiness as time since the most recent period of sleep increases and (2) a circadian process by which the master biologic clock in the suprachiasmatic nucleus varies alertness over the course of the 24-hour day.[34] Other possible contributing factors include the use of CNS depressants, such as antihistamines, antipsychotics, anticonvulsants, and opioids. Dopamine agonists, antibiotics, and antihypertensive agents may also increase the risk of drowsiness. Increased susceptibility to the sedating effects of these agents can be particularly troublesome in older patients. Other etiologies include depression, cancer, anemia, hypothyroidism, and chronic pain, overexertion, or imbalances in diet and exercise.[30,31]

table
46–5 Caffeine Content in Common Beverages

Coffees, Teas, and Soft Drinks	Ounces	Caffeine Content (mg)
Coffee	8	108
Coffee, decaffeinated	8	6
Starbucks coffee, tall	12	260
Starbucks coffee, grande	16	330
Espresso	2	100
Instant coffee	8	57
Brewed tea, U.S. brands	8	40
Snapple Iced Tea	8	21
Mountain Dew	12	54
Diet Coke	12	46.5
Coca-Cola	12	34.5
Dr. Pepper	12	41

Note: The listed caffeine content for the brewed coffees and teas may vary according to brewing methods.

Clinical Presentation of Drowsiness and Fatigue

The subjective experience of sleepiness includes yawning, eye rubbing, tendency to fall asleep, and decreased ability to focus and concentrate. Self-reported measures of sleepiness include the Stanford Sleepiness Scale and the Epworth Sleepiness Scale.[35]

Treatment of Drowsiness and Fatigue

Treatment Goals

The goal in treating daytime drowsiness and fatigue is to identify and eliminate the underlying cause to improve mental alertness and productivity. The algorithm in Figure 46–2 outlines the approach to self-treatment.

General Treatment Approach

Many consumers use dietary sources of caffeine to self-treat occasional symptoms of fatigue and drowsiness. Nonprescription caffeine-containing products may also be used. Caffeine as a supplement, or in dietary form, is not a substitute for adequate sleep. Before recommending any caffeine-containing nonprescription product, the health care provider should rule out any drug-induced cause of daytime drowsiness and fatigue. If symptoms are chronic, especially with 7–8 hours of sleep, referral is indicated.

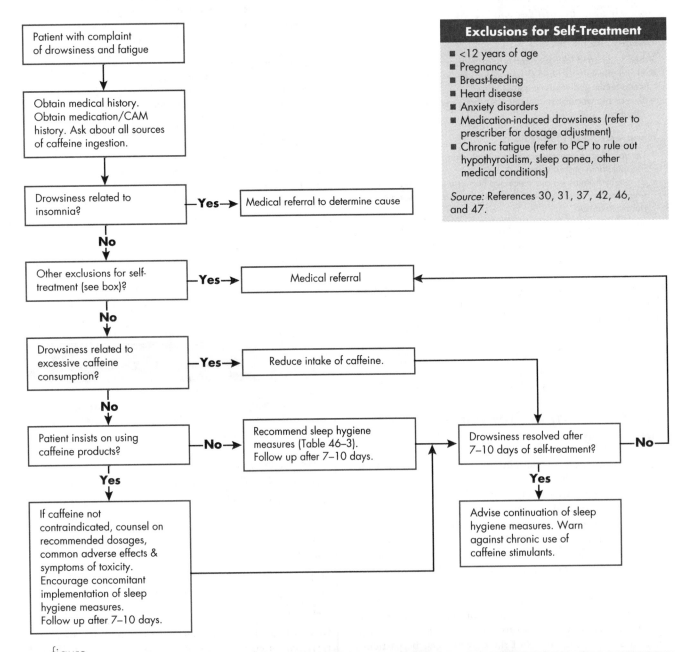

Exclusions for Self-Treatment

- <12 years of age
- Pregnancy
- Breast-feeding
- Heart disease
- Anxiety disorders
- Medication-induced drowsiness (refer to prescriber for dosage adjustment)
- Chronic fatigue (refer to PCP to rule out hypothyroidism, sleep apnea, other medical conditions)

Source: References 30, 31, 37, 42, 46, and 47.

figure
46–2   Self-care of drowsiness and fatigue. Key: CAM = Complementary and alternative medication; PCP = primary care provider.

Nonpharmacologic Therapy

Good sleep hygiene principles should be emphasized (Table 46–3).

Pharmacologic Therapy

Caffeine is a nonselective adenosine antagonist at the A_1 and A_{2A} receptors. Adenosine acts centrally to promote sleep. Secondary effects on other neurotransmitters such as dopamine and acetylcholine may also increase alertness.[36]

Low-to-moderate caffeine doses increase arousal, decrease fatigue, and elevate mood; higher doses are associated with anxiety, nausea, jitteriness, and nervousness.[37] Caffeine possesses weak bronchodilatory action and stimulates the sympathetic nervous system. Moderate caffeine doses (250 mg) can cause a transient increase in heart rate and blood pressure.[38]

Caffeine is completely absorbed, reaching a peak concentration within 30–75 minutes. It is rapidly and widely distributed with an almost immediate effect on alertness. Caffeine is metabolized in the liver by the CYP1A2 isoenzyme; the primary demethylated metabolite is paraxanthine, which predominantly exerts a sympathomimetic effect. Other active metabolites are theobromine and theophylline. Paraxanthine can accumulate with higher dosages and reduce the clearance of caffeine. The elimination half-life is 3–6 hours.[38]

Caffeine is the only FDA-approved nonprescription stimulant, and Table 46–6 lists selected trade-name caffeine-containing products. The labeled dosages of approved nonprescription supplements for adults and children 12 years of age and older is 100–200 mg every 3–4 hours as needed. Caffeine is marketed for occasional use to help restore mental alertness or wakefulness.[39]

Rapid tolerance to the effects of caffeine on the respiratory and cardiovascular systems is common. Habitual caffeine drinkers who routinely consume as little as 1–2 cups of coffee and abruptly discontinue caffeine may experience mild signs and symptoms of withdrawal. Symptoms include headache, fatigue, decreased concentration, and irritability, starting within 12–24 hours after cessation and persisting for 1–5 days.[40]

An exaggerated pharmacologic effect can occur when nonprescription caffeine is combined with dietary sources, or with prescription or nonprescription medications that contain caffeine (Table 46–6). Caffeine may increase the absorption of aspirin or reduce the clearance of theophylline to cause additive sympathetic effects such as an increased heart rate.

The CYP1A2 isoenzyme can be induced or inhibited by other drugs. The routine use of high dosages of caffeine (400 mg/day) could theoretically saturate the binding sites and increase the risk of interactions with drugs that share this metabolic pathway, such as clozapine. Cigarette smoking increases the clearance of caffeine by 56%.[41] When quitting smoking, individuals should be counseled to reduce their caffeine intake by half.[42] Conversely, hormonal contraceptives and ciprofloxacin can inhibit the CYP1A2 isoenzyme. The clinical significance of these interactions is unknown, but at-risk patients should be cautioned to moderate their use of caffeine. They should also be monitored for signs of such interactions. Genetic polymorphisms at CYP1A2 and adenosine receptors may also influence response to caffeine.[37]

Patients on monamine oxidase inhibitors or with existing coronary heart disease, uncontrolled hypertension, or preexisting arrhythmias should be counseled to avoid nonprescription caffeine-containing preparations and to moderate their intake of dietary caffeine. The consumption of coffee increases blood pressure. An increase in systolic blood pressure by 2 mm Hg occurred after acute administration of caffeinated coffee for 1–12 weeks.[43] A small increase in blood pressure was demonstrated in healthy individuals and patients with hypertension after chronic consumption of caffeine (4.2 mm Hg systolic; 2.4 mm Hg diastolic).[43]

When taken before sleep, caffeine delays sleep onset, reduces deep sleep, and increases nocturnal awakenings. After sleep deprivation, caffeine improved psychomotor performance, maintained alertness, and reduced fatigue.[40] In driving simulation tests, caffeine 200 mg was compared with placebo on driving performance and sleepiness during early morning hours.[44] After "restricted sleep," caffeine reduced early morning sleepiness for 2 hours; after "no sleep," caffeine delayed sleep by only 30 minutes. Patients should be counseled that caffeine cannot compensate for an inadequate amount of sleep.

The use of caffeinated coffee to counter the effects of excessive alcohol ingestion is a common practice. In a randomized, double-blind study, the effect of caffeine (200 and 400 mg) versus placebo on driving performance was measured in a driving simulator in alcohol-impaired adults.[45] Both doses of caffeine were effective in counteracting "brake latency" but did not counteract other driving impairments caused by the alcohol. In 2010, FDA banned production of caffeinated alcoholic beverages secondary to safety concerns.[46]

Patients should be cautioned about excessive consumption of caffeine in weight-loss supplements and energy sports drinks. Natural caffeine, other methylxanthines, and caffeine-containing herbs, such as guarana, green tea, yerba mate, and cola nut, are common ingredients in products that are marketed to young consumers for energy or weight loss, but the caffeine content is often not listed on the label.[46] Table 46–7 lists the amount of caffeine that is contained in both selected weight-loss dietary supplements and sports energy drinks.

table **46–6**	**Selected Caffeine-Containing Products**
Trade Name	**Caffeine Content (mg)**
Nonprescription Caffeine-Only Products	
NoDoz Maximum Strength	200
Vivarin	200
Nonprescription Combination Products	
Anacin Tablets	32
Excedrin Migraine Caplets	65
Midol Complete Caplets	60
Prescription Combination Products	
Cafergot	100
Fioricet	40
Fiorinal	40

Note: Information is not all inclusive. Products may have changed formulations or caffeine content since time of publication.

table 46–7	Caffeine Content in Selected Dietary Supplements and Energy Drinks	
Trade Name	**Caffeine Content per Serving (mg)**	
Dietary Supplements		
Dexatrim Max Daytime Appetite Control	200	
Metabofit Blend	264[a]	
Energy Drinks[b]		
Monster Energy	80[c]	
Red Bull	80[d]	
Rockstar Juiced	80[e]	

Note: Information is not all inclusive. Products may have changed formulations or caffeine content since time of publication.

[a] Total amount of methylxanthines from natural sources.

[b] Caffeine content based on serving size sold.

[c] Also contains 1000 mg taurine, 200 mg Panax ginseng, and guarana seed extract.

[d] Also contains 1000 mg taurine.

[e] Also contains 1000 mg taurine, 25 mg Panax ginseng, and 25 mg guarana seed extract.

Product Selection Guidelines

Special Populations

Nonprescription oral caffeine tablets do not have an FDA Pregnancy Category.[47] Caffeine freely crosses the placenta.[47] The American College of Obstetricians and Gynecologists has concluded that moderate caffeine consumption (≤200 mg/day) does not contribute to miscarriages or preterm births.[48] Total daily caffeine intake should be limited to less than 200 mg during pregnancy. The American Academy of Pediatrics considers usual dietary amounts of caffeine compatible with breast-feeding.[48] Infants unable to metabolize caffeine or those who receive large quantities of caffeine through breast milk may have symptoms of nervousness, increased heart rate, sleeplessness, poor feeding, and irritability. Nursing women should consume caffeine only in small-to-moderate amounts, preferably after breast-feeding to minimize effects on the infant.

Children are more susceptible to the cardiovascular and CNS adverse effects of caffeine because of their lower body weight. In one study of adolescents (ages 12–17 years), dosages of 50 mg, 100 mg, and 200 mg of caffeine per day significantly increased diastolic blood pressure.[49] Nonprescription caffeine products are not indicated in children younger than 12 years.

The elimination half-life of caffeine is prolonged in older adults, increasing their susceptibility to an exaggerated pharmacologic effect and interference with sleep.[42] Older adults should avoid consuming caffeine in the diet or as an ingredient in a medication after dinner.

Complementary Therapies

Ginseng is frequently used to boost physical and mental energy and a sense of well-being. A review of randomized controlled trials reveals contradictory scientific evidence to support these claims (see Chapter 51). Caffeine-containing dietary supplements that patients may be using include cola nut, guarana, and yerba mate. Ingredients purported to counteract fatigue that are often found in sports energy drinks include taurine and guarana, although the amounts are unlikely to produce either therapeutic or adverse effects.

Assessment of Drowsiness and Fatigue: A Case-Based Approach

When assessing a patient with a complaint of daytime drowsiness, the provider should determine the cause of the patient's fatigue. Evaluating the patient's medical or psychiatric problems, current medication use, dietary caffeine consumption, sleep patterns, and lifestyle will help in determining the underlying cause. Given the lack of data supporting the efficacy of caffeine, and the adverse effects associated with recommended and excessive dosages, health care providers should recommend improved sleep hygiene and lifestyle modifications or medical referral before recommending the use of a caffeine-containing product.

Case 46–2 provides an example of the assessment of a patient with drowsiness and fatigue.

Patient Counseling for Drowsiness and Fatigue

Counseling on the treatment of drowsiness and fatigue should focus on practicing good sleep hygiene and eliminating factors that may interfere with normal sleep. If a caffeine product is indicated, the health care provider should review dosage guidelines with the patient and emphasize the potential adverse effects and drug interactions. The patient should be counseled on symptoms of excessive caffeine ingestion, such as irritability, tremor, rapid pulse, dizziness, or heart palpitations. Regular users of caffeine should also be counseled on withdrawal symptoms such as headache and anxiety, which can occur if caffeine from any source is stopped abruptly. The box Patient Education for Drowsiness and Fatigue lists information to provide patients.

Evaluation of Patient Outcomes for Drowsiness and Fatigue

Successful outcomes include daytime alertness, increased productivity, and peak performance with respect to psychomotor tasks and cognitive function, including attention and concentration. An individual should seek medical evaluation if, after 7–10 days, drowsiness and fatigue persist despite the limited use of caffeine and the establishment of good sleep hygiene.

Key Points for Drowsiness and Fatigue

➤ Advise patients that caffeine appears to be safe and effective in low-to-moderate doses in the diet, as well as for occasional use as a nonprescription supplement during completion of tasks of short duration when enhanced alertness is desired.

case

46–2

Relevant Evaluation Criteria	Scenario/Model Outcome

Information Gathering

1. Gather essential information about the patient's symptoms and medical history, including:

a. description of symptom(s) (i.e., nature, onset, duration, severity, associated symptoms)

Patient requests help in choosing a product to help her stay awake. She is extremely tired and wants to be more alert during the day. She has become increasingly fatigued with decreased concentration. Her husband has complained that she is "too moody" and wants her to pull herself together, especially regarding housework and cooking. She falls asleep easily but wakes earlier than usual.

b. description of any factors that seem to precipitate, exacerbate, and/or relieve the patient's symptom(s)

Patient retired 4 years ago and volunteers at her church and a local food bank and belongs to a weekly book club. Over the past month, she either had no energy to volunteer or left early to return home to take a nap. She describes her mood as "low" and lacks the ability to concentrate on reading a book, let alone attend the book club.

c. description of the patient's efforts to relieve the symptoms

The patient recently increased coffee intake from 1 regular cup daily to 2–3 cups spread out over the day.

d. patient's identity

Brenda Loving

e. age, sex, height, and weight

69 years old, female, 5 ft 2 in., 118 lb

f. patient's occupation

Retired mathematics teacher

g. patient's dietary habits

Vegetarian and adheres to a no-added-salt diet. Usually drinks 1 cup of coffee daily but has increased consumption over the past 2 weeks.

h. patient's sleep habits

Falls asleep around 9 pm nightly and has early morning awakening with trouble getting back to sleep. Has trouble getting out of bed in the morning because her arms and legs feel heavy.

i. concurrent medical conditions, prescription and non-prescription medications, and dietary supplements

Atrial fibrillation: diltiazem extended-release 180 mg daily; atenolol 25 mg daily; aspirin 81 mg daily; urinary incontinence: tolterodine 2 mg twice daily; hot flashes: black cohosh 40 mg daily

j. allergies

Sulfa drugs: rash

k. history of other adverse reactions to medications

Codeine caused severe nausea.

l. other (describe) _____

NA

Assessment and Triage

2. Differentiate patient's signs/symptoms and correctly identify the patient's primary problem(s).

Daytime fatigue

3. Identify exclusions for self-treatment (Figure 46–2).

OTC stimulants should not be used in patients with heart disease.

4. Formulate a comprehensive list of therapeutic alternatives for the primary problem to determine if triage to a health care provider is required, and share this information with the patient or caregiver.

Options include:

(1) Refer Brenda to her health care provider.

(2) Recommend an OTC stimulant until Brenda can make an appointment to see her health care provider.

(3) Recommend good sleep hygiene and an OTC stimulant to prevent fatigue.

(4) Take no action.

Plan

5. Select an optimal therapeutic alternative to address the patient's problem, taking into account patient preferences.

The patient should be referred to her health care provider for evaluation for depression. Patient findings that suggest depression are daytime fatigue, loss of interest in usual activities, decreased concentration, a "low mood," and waking up early in the morning with a heavy feeling in her extremities. Sleep hygiene education (Table 46–3) should be offered. Stimulants should not be recommended because a psychiatric condition is the cause of the fatigue and caffeine can prolong the half-life of aspirin.

6. Describe the recommended therapeutic approach to the patient or caregiver.

"You should make an appointment to see your health care provider."

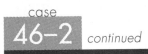

Relevant Evaluation Criteria	Scenario/Model Outcome
7. Explain to the patient or caregiver the rationale for selecting the recommended therapeutic approach from the considered therapeutic alternatives.	"Because this problem of fatigue may be caused by depression, you should make an appointment with your health care provider for a physical examination. Stimulant medication is not indicated at this time because your provider will have to decide the best method of treatment. Even before you see your health care provider, you should reduce your intake of coffee and begin sleep hygiene measures."

Patient Education

8. When recommending self-care with nonprescription medications and/or nondrug therapy, convey accurate information to the patient or caregiver.	Criterion does not apply in this case.
Solicit follow-up questions from the patient or caregiver.	"Can I still drink one cup of coffee a day?"
Answer the patient's or caregiver's questions.	"Yes. Continue with your previous routine."

Evaluation of Patient Outcome

9. Assess patient outcome.	Contact the patient in 1–2 days to ensure that she made an appointment and sought medical care.

Key: NA = Not applicable; OTC = over-the-counter.

➤ Instruct patients that caffeine is most effective when taken intermittently at dosages of 100 or 200 mg every 3–4 hours as needed.

➤ Pregnant or nursing women, children younger than 12 years, patients with heart disease, and patients with anxiety disorders should avoid caffeine.

➤ Health care providers should be aware of the prescription and nonprescription medications and diet supplements that contain caffeine, as well as the patient's dietary consumption of caffeine.

➤ Adverse effects of caffeine are more likely to occur in occasional users and patients of advanced age.

➤ Advise patients taking higher daily dosages of caffeine that drug interactions can occur with some medications.

➤ Counsel patients that dietary supplements should not be used to increase energy or decrease fatigue.

patient education for
Drowsiness and Fatigue

The objective of self-treatment is to maintain wakefulness. For most patients, improved sleep hygiene will help ensure optimal therapeutic outcomes. If the patient insists on taking a caffeine-containing product, carefully following product instructions and the self-care measures listed here will help ensure optimal therapeutic outcomes for most patients.

Disease Information
■ Symptoms of drowsiness and fatigue often include yawning, a tendency to fall asleep, and decreased ability to focus and concentrate.

Nondrug Measures
■ Practice principles of good sleep hygiene (Table 46–3.)
■ If drowsiness or fatigue persists or recurs, consult your health care provider.

Nonprescription Medications
■ Do not exceed the recommended dose of 200 mg every 3–4 hours. Note that higher doses of caffeine may cause side effects and that chronic use may result in tolerance as well as withdrawal symptoms upon abrupt discontinuation.
■ Do not use caffeine tablets in combination with coffee or other caffeinated products, including dietary supplements.

■ Do not use if pregnant or breast-feeding.
■ Do not use in children younger than 12 years.
■ If you are taking clozapine, hormonal contraceptives, or ciprofloxacin, consult your health care provider before using caffeine-containing products.
■ If you have a history of peptic ulcer disease, psychiatric disorders, symptomatic heart disease, or uncontrolled hypertension, consult your health care provider before using caffeine products.

When to Seek Medical Attention
■ Seek medical attention immediately if the following symptoms of caffeine toxicity occur at the same time:
  – Increases in heart rate and blood pressure
  – Headache
  – Symptoms of anxiety and insomnia
  – Increase in hand tremor

REFERENCES

1. National Institutes of Health. NIH State-of-the-Science Conference Statement on Manifestations and Management of Chronic Insomnia in Adults. *NIH Consen Sci State.* 2005;22(2):1–30. Accessed at http://consensus.nih.gov/2005/insomniastatement.pdf, July 17, 2013.

2. National Sleep Foundation. 2009 Sleep in America Poll. Accessed at http://www.sleepfoundation.org/article/sleep-america-polls/2009-health-and-safety, October 30, 2013.

3. Rosekind MR, Gregory KB. Insomnia risks and costs: health, safety, and quality of life. *Am J Manag Care.* 2010;16(8):617–26.

4. Ozminkowski RJ, Wang S, Walsh JK. The direct and indirect costs of untreated insomnia in adults in the United States. *Sleep.* 2007;30(3):263–73.

5. Tariq SH, Pulisetty S. Pharmacotherapy for insomnia. *Clin Geriatr Med.* 2008;24:93–105.

6. National Sleep Foundation. 2002 Sleep in America Poll. Accessed at http://www.sleepfoundation.org/article/sleep-america-polls/2002-adult-sleep-habits, July 17, 2013.

7. Bloom HG, Ahmed I, Alessi CA, et al. Evidence-based recommendations for the assessment and management of sleep disorders in older persons. *J Am Geriatr Soc.* 2009;57(5):761–89.

8. Morin AK, Jarvis CI, Lynch AM. Therapeutic options for sleep maintenance and sleep-onset insomnia. *Pharmacotherapy.* 2007;27(1):89–110.

9. Kraus SS, Rabin LA. Sleep America: managing the crisis of adult chronic insomnia and associated conditions. *J Affect Disord.* 2012;138(3):192–212.

10. Harsora P, Kessmann J. Nonpharmacologic management of chronic insomnia. *Am Fam Physician.* 2009;79(2):125–30.

11. Diphenhydramine. In: McEvoy GK, Snow EK, eds. *AHFS Drug Information 2013.* Bethesda, MD: American Society of Health-System Pharmacists. STAT!Ref Online Electronic Medical Library.

12. Antihistamine drugs. In: McEvoy GK, Snow EK, eds. *AHFS Drug Information 2013.* Bethesda, MD: American Society of Health-System Pharmacists. STAT!Ref Online Electronic Medical Library.

13. Doxylamine. In: McEvoy GK, Snow EK, eds. *AHFS Drug Information 2013.* Bethesda, MD: American Society of Health-System Pharmacists. STAT!Ref Online Electronic Medical Library.

14. Roth J, Roehrs T. Efficacy and safety of sleep-promoting agents. *Med Sleep Clin.* 2008;3:175–87.

15. Sharma A, Pibarot P, Pilote S, et al. Toward optimal treatment in women: the effect of sex on metoprolol-diphenhydramine interaction. *J Clin Pharmacol.* 2010;50(2):214–25.

16. Church MK, Maurer M, Simons FER, et al. Risk of first-generation H₁-antihistamines: a GA²LEN position paper. *Allergy.* 2010;65(4):459–66.

17. Thomas A, Nallur DG, Jones N, et al. Diphenhydramine abuse and detoxification: a brief review and report. *J Psychopharmacol.* 2009;23(1):101–5.

18. Tanda G, Kopajtic TA, Katz JL. Cocaine-like neurochemical effects of antihistaminic medications. *J Neurochem.* 2008;106(1):147–57.

19. Vinson DC, Manning BK, Galligher JM, et al. Alcohol and sleep problems in primary care patients: a report from the AAFP National Research Network. *Ann Fam Med.* 2010;8(6):484–92.

20. Roth T. Does effective management of sleep disorders reduce substance dependence? *Drugs.* 2009;69(suppl 2):65–75.

21. Morin CM, Koetter U, Bastien C, et al. Valerian-hops combination and diphenhydramine for treating insomnia. *Sleep.* 2005;28(11):1465–71.

22. Diphenhydramine. U.S. National Library of Medicine, Toxicology Data Network, LactMed database. Accessed at http://toxnet.nlm.nih.gov, July 17, 2013.

23. The American Geriatrics Society. American Geriatrics Society updated Beers Criteria for potentially inappropriate medication use in older adults. *J Am Geriatr Soc.* 2012;60(4):616–31.

24. Basu R, Dodge H, Stoehr GP, et al. Sedative-hypnotic use of diphenhydramine in a rural, older adult, community-based cohort: effects on cognition. *Am J Geriatr Psychiatry.* 2003;11(2):205–13.

25. Bliwise DL, Ansari FP. Insomnia associated with valerian and melatonin usage in the 2002 National Health Interview Survey. *Sleep.* 2007;30(7):881–4.

26. Buscemi N, Vandermeer B, Pandya R, et al. *Melatonin for Treatment of Sleep Disorders. Summary. Evidence Report/Technology Assessment No. 108.* Rockville, MD: Agency for Healthcare Research and Quality; November 2004. AHRQ Publication No. 05-E002-1.

27. Taibi DM, Landis CA, Petry H, et al. A systematic review of valerian as a sleep aid: safe but not effective. *Sleep Med Rev.* 2007;11(3):209–30.

28. National Center for Complementary and Alternative Medicine. Accessed at http://nccam.nih.gov/, July 17, 2013.

29. American Academy of Sleep Medicine (AASM). AASM Position Statement: Treating Insomnia with Herbal Supplements. Accessed at http://www.aasmnet.org/Articles.aspx?id=254, October 15, 2013.

30. Rosenthal TC, Majeroni BA, Pretorius R, et al. Fatigue: an overview. *Am Fam Physician.* 2008;78(10):1173–9.

31. Schwartz JRL, Roth T, Hirshkowitz M, et al. Recognition and management of excessive sleepiness in the primary care setting. *Prim Care Companion J Clin Psychiatry.* 2009;11(5):197–204.

32. Martiniuk AL, Senserrick T, Lo S, et al. Sleep-deprived young drivers and the risk for crash: the DRIVE Prospective Cohort Study. *JAMA Pediatr.* 2013;167(7):647–55.

33. Frary CD, Johnson RK, Wang MQ. Food sources and intakes of caffeine in the diets of persons in the United States. *J Am Diet Assoc.* 2005;105(1):110–3.

34. Silver R, LeSauter J. Circadian and homeostatic factors in arousal. *Ann NY Acad Sci.* 2008;1129:263–74.

35. Task Force for the Handbook of Psychiatric Measures. *Handbook of Psychiatric Measures.* Washington, DC: American Psychiatric Association; 2000:682–5.

36. Ferré S. An update on the mechanisms of the psychostimulant effects of caffeine. *J Neurochem.* 2008;105(4):1067–79.

37. Yang A, Palmer AA, de Wit H. Genetics of caffeine consumption and responses to caffeine. *Psychopharmacol.* 2010;211(3):245–57.

38. Roehrs T, Roth T. Caffeine: sleep and daytime sleepiness. *Sleep Med Rev.* 2008;12(2):153–62.

39. U.S. Food and Drug Administration. Stimulant drug products for over-the-counter human use. CFR: Code of Federal Regulations. Title 21, Part 340, Section 340.50. Revised April 1, 2010. Accessed at http://www.accessdata.fda.gov/scripts/cdrh/cfdocs/cfcfr/cfrsearch.cfm, July 4, 2013.

40. Snel J, Lorist MM. Effects of caffeine on sleep and cognition. In: Van Dongen HPA, Kerkhof GA, eds. *Progress in Brain Research.* Volume 190. London: Elsevier; 2011;105–17.

41. Drug Interactions with Smoking. Rx For Change. Accessed at http://smokingcessationleadership.ucsf.edu/Downloads/DRUG_INTERACTIONS_SMOKING.pdf, August 6, 2014.

42. Kroon LA. Drug interactions with smoking. *Am J Health-System Pharmacy.* 2007;64(18):1917–21.

43. Higdon JV, Frei B. Coffee and health: a review of recent human research. *Crit Rev Food Sci Nutr.* 2006;46(2):101–23.

44. Reyner LA, Horne JA. Early morning driver sleepiness: effectiveness of 200 mg caffeine. *Psychophysiology.* 2000;37(2):251–6.

45. Liguori A, Robinson JH. Caffeine antagonism of alcohol-induced driving impairment. *Drug Alcohol Depend.* 2001;63(2):123–9.

46. U.S. Food and Drug Administration. Update on Caffeinated Alcoholic Beverages. FDA Announces Progress on Removal of Certain Caffeinated Alcoholic Beverages from the Market. November 24, 2010. Accessed at http://www.fda.gov/NewsEvals/PublicHealthFocus/UCM234900.htm, July 4, 2013.

47. Caffeine. Clinical Pharmacology. Elsevier Gold Standard. Accessed at www.clinicalpharmacology.com, October 11, 2013.

48. American College of Obstetricians and Gynecologists Committee on Obstetric Care. Moderate caffeine consumption during pregnancy. *Obstet Gynecol.* 2010;116(2 pt 1):467–8.

49. Temple JL, Dewey AM, Briatico LN. Effects of acute caffeine administration on adolescents. *Exp Clin Psychopharmacol.* 2010;18(6):510–20.

TOBACCO CESSATION

Beth A. Martin and Maria C. Wopat

In 1982, the U.S. Surgeon General C. Everett Koop stated that cigarette smoking was the "chief, single, avoidable cause of death in our society and the most important public health issue of our time."[1] This statement remains true over 3 decades later. In the United States, cigarette smoking is the leading known cause of preventable death,[2] responsible for an estimated 443,595 deaths each year.[3] In addition to lives lost, the economic impact of smoking is enormous, costing society approximately $193 billion annually for smoking-attributable health expenditures and lost productivity.[3]

The negative effects of smoking are both well established and well publicized, yet an estimated 42.1 million adult Americans (18.1% overall in 2012; 20.5% of males and 15.8% of females) smoked either every day (77.8%) or some days (22.2%).[4] The prevalence of smoking varies by sociodemographic factors, including gender, race/ethnicity, education level, age, and socioeconomic status. The prevalence of smoking in the United States was highest among non-Hispanic American Indians/Alaska Natives (21.8%) and lowest among non-Hispanic Asians (10.7%). Smoking is more common among people ages 25–44 years (21.6%) and people of lower educational levels and those living below the federal poverty level (27.9%).[4] The median prevalence of smoking varies by state, with Utah exhibiting the lowest prevalence at 11.8% and Kentucky exhibiting the highest at 29.0%.[5] Smoking incidence differs in patients with various medical conditions, with the greatest prevalence among patients with mental illness. This population consumed about 30.9% of all cigarettes sold in the United States during 2009–2011.[6]

Despite tobacco control efforts at the state and national levels, tobacco use is a prevailing public health issue of great importance, and only Utah has met the *Healthy People 2020* target goal of a 12% or lower prevalence of smoking.[7] Globally, nearly 6 million deaths attributable to tobacco occur annually; unless tobacco control efforts are able to reverse this trend, the number of annual deaths is likely to exceed 8 million by 2030.[8]

Pathophysiology of Tobacco Use and Dependence

In 1988, the U.S. Surgeon General released a landmark report that concluded that tobacco products are effective nicotine delivery systems capable of inducing and sustaining chemical dependence.[9]

The primary criteria used to categorize nicotine as an addictive substance included its (1) psychoactive effects, (2) use in a highly controlled or compulsive manner, and (3) reinforcement of behavioral patterns of tobacco use. The underlying pharmacologic and behavioral processes associated with tobacco dependence are considered to be similar to those that determine addiction to drugs such as heroin and cocaine.[9]

As with other addictive substances (e.g., opiates, cocaine, and amphetamines), nicotine stimulates the mesolimbic dopaminergic system in the midbrain, inducing pleasant or rewarding effects that promote continued use.[10] This effect is also known as the dopamine reward pathway. Nicotine binds to the $alpha_4beta_2$ nicotinic cholinergic receptors in the ventral tegmental area of the brain, triggering the release of dopamine in the nucleus accumbens. Psychosocial, behavioral, genetic, and environmental factors also play an important role in establishing and maintaining dependence.[10,11] For example, smoking commonly is associated with specific activities such as driving, talking on the telephone, eating, drinking coffee or alcohol, and being around others who smoke. Over time, the habitual use of cigarettes under these circumstances can lead to the development of smoking routines that can be difficult to break. Indeed, specific environmental situations can become powerful conditioned stimuli or cues associated with smoking and are capable of triggering "automatic" smoking patterns.[10]

Tobacco use dramatically increases one's odds of dependence, disease, disability, and death. Cigarettes are carefully engineered and heavily marketed products. For example, although the design of cigarettes and other tobacco products has evolved over the past five decades (e.g., filtered, menthol, low-tar, "light" cigarettes; e-cigarettes; dissolvable tobacco), overall disease risk has not been reduced among smokers.[11] The tobacco industry spends nearly $18.50 to market its products for every $1 that states spend on tobacco control.[12] Cigarettes are the *only* marketed consumable product that, when used persistently, will kill half or more of its users.[13]

Cigarette smoke, which is classified by the Environmental Protection Agency (EPA) as a Class A carcinogen (i.e., a carcinogen with no safe level of exposure for humans), is a complex mixture of thousands of compounds—including nitrogen, carbon monoxide, ammonia, hydrogen cyanide, benzene, and nicotine—in gaseous and particulate phases. The particulate fraction, excluding the nicotine and water components, is collectively referred to as tar. Numerous carcinogens, including polycyclic aromatic hydrocarbons (PAHs) and nitrosamines, have been identified in the tar fraction of tobacco smoke.[11,14]

Editor's Note: This chapter is based on the 17th edition chapter of the title "Smoking Cessation," written by Karen Suchanek Hudmon, Lisa A. Kroon, and Robin L. Corelli.

Nicotine, the addictive component of tobacco, is distilled from burning tobacco and carried in tar droplets to the small airways of the lung, where it is absorbed rapidly into the arterial circulation and distributed throughout the body. Nicotine readily penetrates the central nervous system and is estimated to reach the brain within seconds after inhalation.[15] Nicotine binds to receptors in the brain and other organs, inducing a variety of predominantly stimulatory effects on the cardiovascular, endocrine, nervous, and metabolic systems.[10,16] Pharmacodynamic effects associated with nicotine administration include arousal and increases in the heart rate and blood pressure. In the brain, smoking leads to the activation of nicotinic cholinergic receptors and release of numerous neurotransmitters, which induce a range of effects such as pleasure (dopamine), arousal (acetylcholine and norepinephrine), cognitive enhancement (acetylcholine), appetite suppression (dopamine, norepinephrine, and serotonin), learning and memory enhancement (glutamate), mood modulation (serotonin), and reduction of anxiety and tension (beta-endorphin and gamma-aminobutyric acid).[10,11,15]

Clinical Presentation of Tobacco Use and Dependence

Most chronic tobacco users develop tolerance to the effects of nicotine, and abrupt cessation precipitates symptoms of nicotine withdrawal.[10] The symptoms and their severity vary from person to person but generally include irritability, frustration, anger, anxiety, depression, difficulty concentrating, impatience, insomnia, and restlessness.[17,18] Other symptoms that patients might report include cravings, impaired performance, constipation, cough, dizziness, and increased dreaming. Typically, the physiologic nicotine withdrawal symptoms manifest within the first 1–2 days, peak within the first week, and gradually dissipate over 2–4 weeks.[18] Increased appetite and weight gain may persist for 6 or more months after quitting.[17]

According to reports issued by the U.S. Surgeon General in 2004[2] and 2010,[11] smoking adversely affects nearly every organ system in the body and plays a causal role in the development of numerous diseases, including many cancers (Table 47–1). Furthermore, smoking cigarettes with lower machine-measured

table
47–1   Health Consequences of Smoking

Cancer

Acute myeloid leukemia

Bladder

Cervical

Esophageal

Gastric

Kidney

Laryngeal

Lung

Oral cavity and pharyngeal

Pancreatic

Cardiovascular Diseases

Abdominal aortic aneurysm

Coronary heart disease (e.g., angina pectoris, ischemic heart disease, myocardial infarction)

Cerebrovascular disease (e.g., transient ischemic attacks, stroke)

Peripheral arterial disease

Pulmonary Diseases

Acute respiratory illnesses
  Upper respiratory tract (e.g., rhinitis, sinusitis, laryngitis, pharyngitis)
  Lower respiratory tract (e.g., bronchitis, pneumonia)

Chronic respiratory illnesses
  Chronic obstructive pulmonary disease
  Respiratory symptoms
  Poor asthma control
  Reduced lung function

Reproductive Effects

Reduced fertility in women

Pregnancy and pregnancy outcomes
  Preterm, premature rupture of membranes
  Placenta previa
  Placental abruption
  Preterm delivery
  Low infant birth weight

Infant mortality
  Sudden infant death syndrome (SIDS)

Other Effects

Cataract

Osteoporosis (reduced bone density in postmenopausal women, with increased risk of hip fracture)

Periodontitis

Peptic ulcer disease (in patients infected with *Helicobacter pylori*)

Surgical outcomes
  Poor wound healing
  Respiratory complications

Source: References 2 and 11.

yields of tar and nicotine provides no clear benefit to health. Involuntary exposure to secondhand smoke, which includes the smoke emanating from a cigarette and that exhaled by the smoker, is associated with adverse health effects in nonsmokers, including cardiovascular disease, respiratory disease, and lung cancer.[19] Even low levels of exposure, such as secondhand smoke exposure, lead to rapid increases in endothelial dysfunction and inflammation, which lead to acute cardiovascular events and thrombosis.[11] In children, secondhand smoke exposure can increase the risk of ear infections, precipitate more frequent and severe asthma attacks, worsen respiratory symptoms (e.g., coughing, sneezing, shortness of breath), increase the risk of respiratory infections, and increase the risk for sudden infant death syndrome (SIDS).[19] There is no risk-free level of exposure to tobacco smoke.[11,20]

Tobacco smoke interacts with medications through pharmacokinetic or pharmacodynamic mechanisms that can lead to reduced therapeutic efficacy or, less commonly, increased toxicity. Most of the pharmacokinetic interactions are the result of induction of hepatic cytochrome P450 (CYP) enzymes (primarily the CYP1A2 isoenzyme) by PAHs present in tobacco smoke.[21] Induction of the CYP1A2 isoenzyme can increase the hepatic metabolism of certain drugs (Table 47–2), potentially

resulting in a reduced therapeutic response or a need for higher dosages in smokers; conversely, the dosages of some drugs might need to be reduced in patients who quit smoking.[21] Similarly, the clearance of caffeine is significantly increased (by 56%) in smokers. Following cessation, ex-smokers who drink caffeinated beverages should be advised to decrease their usual caffeine intake to avoid higher levels of caffeine, which may induce symptoms similar to nicotine withdrawal.

A significant pharmacodynamic drug interaction occurs with tobacco smoke and combination hormonal contraceptives (pills, patch, and ring). Data indicate that cigarette smoking substantially increases the risk of serious adverse cardiovascular events (e.g., stroke, myocardial infarction, and thromboembolism) in women using oral contraceptives.[22–26] This risk is markedly increased in women ages 35 years or older who smoke 15 or more cigarettes per day.[22] Accordingly, most experts consider use of hormonal contraceptives to be a contraindication in smokers; therefore, an alternative form of contraception should be used.[23,26] Additional interactions, with their corresponding underlying mechanisms, are provided in Table 47–2.[21,27] During the course of routine patient care, it is important to assess for potential drug and smoking interactions and to make appropriate adjustments to the medication regimen.

table 47–2	**Drug Interactions with Tobacco Smoke**
Drug/Class (Trade Name)	**Mechanism of Interaction and Effects**
Pharmacokinetic Interactions	
Alprazolam (Xanax)	Conflicting data on significance, but possible decreased plasma concentrations (up to 50%); decreased half-life (35%).
Bendamustine (Treanda)ᵃ	Metabolized by CYP1A2. Manufacturer recommends using with caution in smokers owing to likely decreased bendamustine concentrations, with increased concentrations of its two active metabolites.
Caffeineᵃ	Increased metabolism (induction of CYP1A2); increased clearance (56%). Caffeine levels are likely increased after cessation.
Chlorpromazine (Thorazine)	Decreased area under the curve (AUC) (36%) and serum concentrations (24%). Decreased sedation and hypotension possible in smokers; smokers may require increased dosages.
Clopidogrel (Plavix)ᵃ	Increased metabolism (induction of CYP1A2) of clopidogrel to its active metabolite. Clopidogrel's effects are enhanced in smokers (≥10 cigarettes/day): significant increased platelet inhibition, decreased platelet aggregation. Although improved clinical outcomes have been shown, may also increase risk of bleeding.
Clozapine (Clozaril)ᵃ	Increased metabolism (induction of CYP1A2); decreased plasma concentrations (18%). Increased levels may occur upon cessation; closely monitor drug levels and reduce dose as required to avoid toxicity.
Erlotinib (Tarceva)ᵃ	Increased clearance (24%); decreased trough serum concentrations (twofold).
Flecainide (Tambocor)	Increased clearance (61%); decreased trough serum concentrations (25%). Smokers may need increased dosages.
Fluvoxamine (Luvox)ᵃ	Increased metabolism (induction of CYP1A2); increased clearance (24%); decreased AUC (31%); decreased plasma concentrations (32%). Dosage modifications are not routinely recommended, but smokers may need increased dosages.
Haloperidol (Haldol)	Increased clearance (44%); decreased serum concentrations (70%).
Heparin	Mechanism unknown but increased clearance and decreased half-life are observed. Smoking has prothrombotic effects. Smokers may need increased dosages owing to pharmacokinetic (PK) and pharmacodynamic (PD) interactions.

table
47–2 **Drug Interactions with Tobacco Smoke** *(continued)*

Drug/Class (Trade Name)	Mechanism of Interaction and Effects
Insulin, subcutaneous	Possible decreased insulin absorption secondary to peripheral vasoconstriction; smoking may cause release of endogenous substances that cause insulin resistance. PK and PD interactions are likely not clinically significant; smokers may need increased dosages and should monitor blood sugar closely.
Irinotecan (Camptosar)[a]	Increased clearance (18%); decreased serum concentrations of active metabolite, SN-38 (~40%; via induction of glucuronidation); decreased systemic exposure resulting in lower hematologic toxicity; may reduce efficacy. Smokers may need increased dosages.
Mexiletine (Mexitil)	Increased clearance (25%; via oxidation and glucuronidation); decreased half-life (36%).
Olanzapine (Zyprexa)[a]	Increased metabolism (induction of CYP1A2); increased clearance (98%). Dosage modifications are not routinely recommended, but smokers may need increased dosages.
Propranolol (Inderal)	Increased clearance (77%; via side-chain oxidation and glucuronidation).
Ropinirole (Requip)[a]	Decreased maximum concentration (30%) and AUC (38%) in study with patients with restless legs syndrome. Smokers may need increased dosages.
Tacrine (Cognex)[a]	Increased metabolism (induction of CYP1A2); decreased half-life (50%); serum concentrations threefold lower. Smokers may need increased dosages.
(Theo Dur, etc.)[a]	Levels should be monitored if smoking is initiated, discontinued, or changed. Maintenance doses are considerably higher in smokers. Increased clearance with secondhand smoke exposure.
Theophylline	Increased metabolism (induction of CYP1A2); increased clearance (58%–100%); decreased half-life (63%).
Tizanidine (Zanaflex)	Decreased AUC (30%-40%) and decreased half-life (10%) observed in male smokers.
Tricyclic antidepressants (e.g., imipramine, nortriptyline)	Possible interaction with tricyclic antidepressants in the direction of decreased blood levels, but the clinical significance is not established.
Warfarin	Increased metabolism (induction of CYP1A2) of R-enantiomer; however, S-enantiomer is more potent, and the effect on the international normalized ratio (INR) is inconclusive. Consider monitoring INR more closely upon smoking cessation.

Pharmacodynamic Interactions

Benzodiazepines (diazepam, chlordiazepoxide)	Decreased sedation and drowsiness, possibly caused by nicotine stimulation of central nervous system.
Beta-blockers	Less effective antihypertensive and heart rate control effects, possibly caused by nicotine-mediated sympathetic activation. Smokers may need increased dosages.
Corticosteroids, inhaled[a]	Smokers with asthma may have less of a response to inhaled corticosteroids.
Hormonal contraceptives[a]	Increased risk of cardiovascular adverse effects (e.g., stroke, myocardial infarction, thromboembolism) in women who smoke and use oral contraceptives. Ortho Evra patch users shown to have twofold increased risk of venous thromboembolism compared with oral contraceptive users, likely owing to increased estrogen exposure (60% higher levels). Increased risk with age and with heavy smoking (≥15 cigarettes per day) that is quite marked in women ≥35 years old.
Opioids (propoxyphene, pentazocine)	Decreased analgesic effect; smoking may increase the metabolism of propoxyphene (15%–20%) and pentazocine (40%). Mechanism is unknown. Smokers may need increased opioid dosages for pain relief.

Key: PD = Pharmacodynamic; PK = pharmacokinetic.

Note: Many interactions between tobacco smoke and medications have been identified. In most cases, the tobacco smoke—not the nicotine—causes these drug interactions. Tobacco smoke interacts with medications through PK and PD mechanisms. PK interactions affect the absorption, distribution, metabolism, or elimination of other drugs, potentially causing an altered pharmacologic response. The majority of PK interactions with smoking are the result of induction of hepatic cytochrome P450 enzymes (primarily CYP1A2). PD interactions alter the expected response or actions of other drugs. The amount of tobacco smoking necessary to have an effect has not been established, and the assumption is that any smoker is susceptible to the same degree of interaction. Those exposed regularly to secondhand smoke may also be at risk.

[a] Clinically significant interaction.

Source: Reproduced with permission from Rx for Change: Clinician-Assisted Tobacco Cessation program. The Regents of the University of California. Copyright © 1999–2015.

TIME ELAPSED

20 minutes after quitting: Blood pressure drops to a level close to that before the last cigarette. Temperature of hands and feet increases to normal.

8 hours after quitting: Blood levels of carbon monoxide drop to normal.

24 hours after quitting: Chance of having a heart attack decreases.

2 weeks to 3 months after quitting: Circulation improves, and lung function improves by up to 30%.

1 to 9 months after quitting: Coughing, sinus congestion, fatigue, and shortness of breath decrease, and cilia regain normal function in the lungs, increasing the ability to handle mucus, clear the lungs, and reduce infection.

1 year after quitting: Excessive risk of coronary heart disease is half that of a smoker's.

5 years after quitting: Risk of stroke is reduced to that of a nonsmoker 5 to 15 years after quitting.

10 years after quitting: Lung cancer death rate is about half that of continuing smokers. Risk of cancer of the mouth, throat, esophagus, bladder, kidney, and pancreas also are lower than that of continuing smokers.

15 years after quitting: Risk of coronary heart disease is similar to that of a nonsmoker.

figure

47–1 Health benefits of smoking cessation. (*Source:* Reference 28.)

Benefits of Tobacco Cessation

The 1990 Surgeon General's Report on the health benefits of smoking cessation outlined the numerous and substantial health benefits realized when patients quit smoking.[28] Some health benefits are incurred shortly after quitting (e.g., within 2 weeks to 3 months), and others are incurred over time (Figure 47–1). On average, cigarette smokers die approximately 10 years earlier than nonsmokers; among those who continue smoking, at least half will eventually die of a tobacco-related disease. Quitting at ages 30, 40, 50, and 60 years results in a gain of 10, 9, 6, and 3 years of life, respectively.[13] Thus, although it is important to educate tobacco users that it is never too late to quit and achieve many of the associated health benefits, there are significant benefits to quitting earlier in life.

Smoking Cessation Treatment

Treatment Goals

Tobacco dependence is a chronic disease characterized by multiple failed attempts to quit before long-term cessation is achieved. Because tobacco use is a complex, addictive behavior, helping patients quit and preventing relapse are best achieved by combining appropriate pharmacotherapy with counseling.[29] For any patient who uses tobacco, the primary goal is complete, long-term abstinence from all nicotine-containing products.

General Treatment Approach

Most smokers use no cessation treatments for their quit attempts, also known as quitting "cold turkey,"[30] and approximately 95%

of all attempts to quit using this method end in relapse.[29] Yet decades of research clearly show that patients who receive assistance have increased odds of quitting. In 2008, the U.S. Public Health Service published an updated clinical practice guideline for treating tobacco use and dependence,[29] which presents evidence-based recommendations and effective strategies for health care providers who provide tobacco cessation counseling. Although even brief advice from a provider is associated with increased odds of quitting,[29,31] more intensive counseling (longer and more frequent counseling sessions, or greater overall contact time) and use of pharmacotherapy (excluding patients who should not self-treat with medications, as listed in Figure 47–2) result in increased quit rates. Two particularly effective types of counseling are practical counseling (behavior change counseling, including problem-solving and skills training) and social support delivered as part of treatment.[29]

Patients who receive a tobacco cessation intervention from a provider (nonphysician or physician) are 1.7 and 2.2 times as likely to quit (and remain tobacco free at >5 months after cessation), respectively, than are patients who do not receive an intervention from a provider.[29] Self-help materials are only slightly better than no provider intervention. Although the length of an intervention increases effectiveness, even minimal interventions (<3 minutes) increase cessation rates.[29] In a meta-analysis of 46 studies, four or more intervention sessions were found to approximately double cessation rates.[29]

Although the use of pharmacotherapy substantially increases patients' chances of quitting, the addition of counseling further increases cessation rates (1.4 times as likely to quit).[29] Similarly, adding pharmacotherapy to counseling increases cessation rates. Therefore, cessation interventions should consist of pharmacotherapy (one or a combination of medications) and counseling, when medications are not contraindicated (see Special Populations).[29] Figure 47–2 outlines a self-treatment approach for tobacco cessation.

Nonpharmacologic Therapy

Helping Patients Quit: The 5 A's Approach (Comprehensive Counseling)

As delineated in the Clinical Practice Guideline for Treating Tobacco Use and Dependence,[29] the five key components of comprehensive counseling for tobacco cessation are (1) asking patients whether they use tobacco, (2) advising tobacco users to quit, (3) assessing patients' readiness to quit, (4) assisting patients with quitting, and (5) arranging follow-up care. These steps are referred to as the "5 A's."[29]

Ask about Tobacco Use

A key first step in the cessation process, and in all patient interactions, is asking about tobacco use. Because tobacco use is the primary known preventable cause of mortality in the United States, and because tobacco smoke interacts with multiple medications, screening for tobacco use is crucial and should be a routine component of care. The following question can be used to identify all types of tobacco use, even for infrequent users: "Do you ever smoke or use any type of tobacco?" In clinic or hospital settings, tobacco use status should be considered a vital sign and collected routinely, along with blood pressure, pulse, weight, temperature, and respiratory rate.[29] In community pharmacies, tobacco use status should be assessed, documented

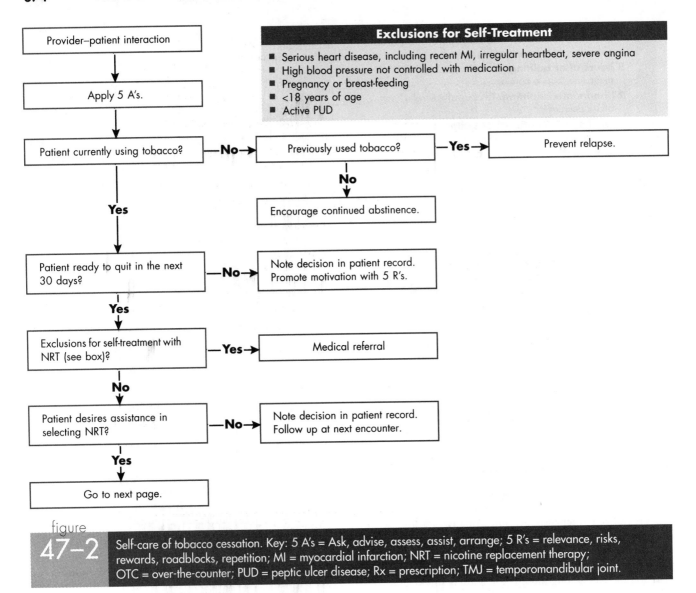

Exclusions for Self-Treatment

- Serious heart disease, including recent MI, irregular heartbeat, severe angina
- High blood pressure not controlled with medication
- Pregnancy or breast-feeding
- <18 years of age
- Active PUD

figure
47–2   Self-care of tobacco cessation. Key: 5 A's = Ask, advise, assess, assist, arrange; 5 R's = relevance, risks, rewards, roadblocks, repetition; MI = myocardial infarction; NRT = nicotine replacement therapy; OTC = over-the-counter; PUD = peptic ulcer disease; Rx = prescription; TMJ = temporomandibular joint.

in the patient profile, and reassessed periodically. Asking about exposure to secondhand smoke should also be considered.

Advise to Quit

All tobacco users should be advised to quit. The advice should be clear, strong, and personalized, yet be delivered with sensitivity and in a tone of voice that communicates concern for the patient and a willingness to assist the patient with quitting when he or she is ready. When possible, primary care providers should individualize the message by linking their advice to the patient's health status, current medication regimen, personal reasons for wanting to quit, or the effect of tobacco on others. An example of this approach would be "Ms. Bettis, I see that you now are on two different inhalers for your emphysema. Quitting smoking is the single most important treatment for your emphysema and can improve how well your inhalers work. I strongly encourage you to quit, and I would like to help you."

Assess Readiness to Quit

Because many patients will not be ready to quit when they are first approached, it is important for providers to gauge each

patient's readiness to quit before recommending a treatment regimen. Patients should be categorized as (1) not ready to quit in the next month; (2) ready to quit in the next month; (3) a recent quitter, having quit in the past 6 months; or (4) a former user, having quit more than 6 months ago.[29] This classification defines the provider's next course of action, which is to provide counseling that is tailored to the patient's readiness to quit. The following approach is an example for a current smoker: "Mr. Crosby, what are your thoughts about quitting? Is this something that you might consider doing in the next month?" Counseling a patient who is ready to quit in the next month should differ from counseling a patient who is not considering quitting in the near future.

Assist with Quitting

Important elements of the assisting component of treatment include (1) helping patients to make the decision to quit and (2) setting a quit date. Providers should be empathetic and acknowledge that quitting is a challenge for most patients. As such, the goal is to help maximize each patient's chances of success by designing an individualized treatment plan.

All patients attempting to quit should be encouraged to use pharmacotherapy combined with counseling. This combination

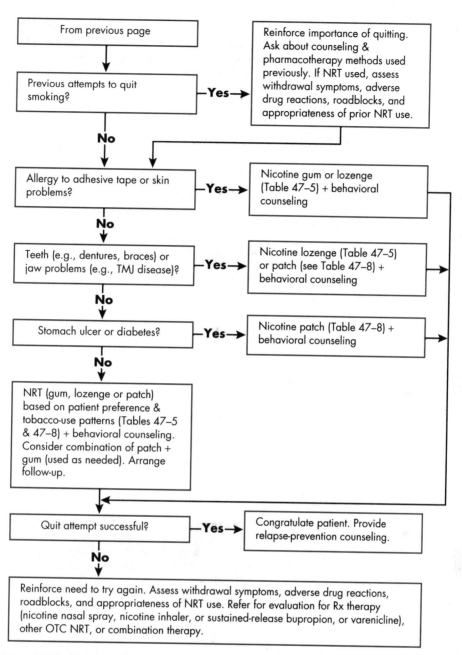

figure
47–2 (continued)

will yield higher quit rates than either approach alone, except for special circumstances or specific populations for which there is inadequate evidence of the combined method's effectiveness (pregnant women, smokeless tobacco users, individuals smoking fewer than 10 cigarettes per day, and adolescents).[29] Counseling interventions, which focus on promoting behavior change and enhancing adherence with medication regimens, include individualized counseling (e.g., in person or by telephone), a group cessation program, an Internet-based program, or a combination of these approaches.

Arrange Follow-Up Counseling

Because a patient's ability to quit increases substantially when multiple counseling interactions are provided, arranging follow-up counseling is an important, yet typically neglected, element of treatment for tobacco dependence. Follow-up contact should occur soon after the quit date, preferably during the first week. Follow-up does not have to be done in person and could be performed by telephone or e-mail. A second follow-up contact is recommended within the first month after quitting.[29] Additional follow-up contacts should occur periodically to monitor patient progress (including adherence with pharmacotherapy) and to provide ongoing support. Quit rates at 5 or more months after cessation are associated with the total number of person-to-person contacts (both individual and group): 12.4% for 0–1 contact, 16.3% for 2–3 contacts, 20.9% for 4–8 contacts, and 24.7% for more than 8 contacts.[29] A dose-response relationship has also been seen for length of contact.[29]

Counseling Interventions for Quitting

When counseling a patient, a provider's goal is to facilitate the process of change by helping to ready patients for their permanent cessation. It is important that providers convey the view of quitting as a learning process that might take months or even years to achieve, rather than a now-or-never event.

Counseling Patients Who Are Not Ready to Quit

When counseling patients who are not ready to quit, an important first step is to encourage the patient to start thinking about quitting and to consider making a commitment to quit sometime in the foreseeable future. Sometimes patients who are not ready truly do not understand the need to quit. In general, most smokers will recognize the need to quit but are not yet ready to make the commitment to quit. Many patients will have tried to quit multiple times and relapsed; thus, they might feel too discouraged to try again.

Strategies for working with patients who are not ready to quit include increasing patient awareness of the available treatment options, having patients identify their reasons for smoking and for wanting to quit, and identifying barriers to quitting. Providers also can engage patients in thinking about quitting by raising awareness of specific drug interactions between medications and tobacco smoke (Table 47–2) and how tobacco use can induce or exacerbate medical conditions (e.g., chronic obstructive pulmonary disease and coronary heart disease). Providers should also discuss the importance of preventive health, such as the recommendation for all adult smokers, ages 19–64, to receive the pneumococcal vaccine to aid in the prevention of invasive pneumococcal disease.[32]

Although it may be useful to provide patients with information about the medications available for quitting, it is not appropriate to recommend a treatment regimen until a patient is ready to quit in the near future (e.g., within the next month). A treatment goal at this stage should be to promote motivation to quit. Providers can encourage patients to seriously consider quitting by asking the following series of three questions:

1. "Do you ever plan to quit?"
   If the patient responds "no," the provider should inquire, "What would have to change for you to decide to quit?" If the patient indicates that nothing would change his or her opinion about quitting, then the provider should offer to assist if or when the patient changes his or her mind. If the patient responds "yes," the provider should continue to question 2.
2. "How would it benefit you to quit now, instead of later?"
   Quitting generally becomes more difficult the longer a patient smokes. Most patients will agree that there is never an ideal time to quit, and that postponing quitting has more negative effects than positive.
3. "What would have to change for you to decide to quit sooner?"
   This question probes patients' perceptions about quitting and can reveal specific barriers to quitting that can be discussed and addressed.

Motivation can also be enhanced by applying the "5 R's: relevance, risks, rewards, roadblocks, and repetition."[29]

Relevance

The intervention begins by encouraging patients to think about why quitting is important to them. Because information has a greater effect if it takes on a personal meaning, counseling should be framed to relate to the patient's risk of disease or exacerbation of disease, other health concerns, family or social situation (e.g., having children with asthma), age, and other patient factors such as prior experience with quitting.

Risks

This intervention entails asking patients to identify negative health consequences of smoking, such as acute risks (e.g., shortness of breath, exacerbation of asthma, pregnancy complications, or infertility); long-term risks (e.g., cancer and cardiac and pulmonary disease); and environmental risks (e.g., effects of secondhand smoke on others, including children and pets). The risks also include patients demonstrating unhealthy behaviors around children and adolescents such as smoking near them.

Rewards

Patients can be asked to identify specific benefits of quitting, such as improved health, enhanced physical performance, acuity of taste and smell, reduced expenditures for tobacco, less time wasted or work missed, reduced health risks to others (e.g., fetus, children, or housemates), and reduced aging of the skin.

Roadblocks

This step entails helping patients identify significant barriers to quitting and helping them develop coping skills to address or circumvent each barrier. Common barriers include nicotine withdrawal symptoms, fear of failure, a need for social support while quitting, depression, concern about weight gain, and a sense of deprivation or loss.

Repetition

The provider continues to work with patients who are either not motivated to quit or who have been unsuccessful in quitting. Discussing circumstances in which smoking occurs will help identify triggers for relapse and should be viewed as part of the learning process. It is also beneficial to repeat the intervention steps whenever possible.

Counseling Patients Who Are Ready to Quit

The goal for patients who are ready to quit in the next month is to achieve cessation by providing an individualized treatment plan that addresses the key issues listed in Table 47–3. The first step is to discuss the patient's tobacco use history by inquiring about levels of smoking (cigarettes/day), number of years smoked, methods used previously for quitting (if any), and reasons for previous failed quit attempts. Providers should understand fully the patient's preferences for the different pharmacotherapies for quitting and work with patients in selecting the quitting methods (e.g., medications or behavioral counseling programs). It is important to recognize that pharmacotherapy might not be desirable or affordable for all patients. However, providers should educate patients that medications, when taken correctly, can substantially increase the likelihood of quitting successfully,[29] and that the costs of continuing smoking far outweigh the costs of the medications.

Ideally, patients will select a quit date that is within the next 2 weeks, allowing ample time to prepare themselves and their environment before the actual quit date. This preparation includes removing all tobacco products and ashtrays from the home, car, and workplace. Patients should be advised to discuss

table

47–3   Key Topics for Individualized Tobacco Cessation Plans

Topic	Description

Assess tobacco use history	▨ Current use:
	  – Type(s) and amount of tobacco used
	▨ Past use:
	  – Duration of smoking
	  – Recent changes in levels of use
	▨ Past quit attempts:
	  – Number of attempts, date of most recent attempt, duration of abstinence
	  – Previous methods: What did or did not work? Why or why not?
	  – Prior experience with cessation pharmacotherapy: agent used, adequacy of dose, adherence, duration of treatment
	  – Reasons for relapse
	▨ Reasons or motivation for wanting to quit (or stay quit)
	▨ Confidence in ability to quit (or stay quit)
	▨ Triggers for smoking
	▨ Routines and situations associated with smoking
	▨ Stress-related smoking
	▨ Social support for quitting
	▨ Concerns about weight gain
	▨ Concerns about withdrawal symptoms

Facilitate the quitting process	▨ Discuss methods for quitting: pros and cons of the different methods ▨ Set a quit date, ideally within the next 2 weeks ▨ Discuss coping strategies ▨ Discuss withdrawal symptoms ▨ Discuss concept of a slip (occasional smoking) versus full relapse ▨ Provide medication counseling: adherence and proper use ▨ Offer to assist throughout the quit attempt

Arrange and provide follow-up counseling	▨ Monitor the patient's progress throughout the quit attempt
	▨ Evaluate the current quit attempt
	  – Status of attempt
	  – Slips (occasional smoking) and relapses
	  – Medication use:
	    ▢ Adherence with regimen
	    ▢ Plans for discontinuation
	  – Address temptations and triggers; discuss relapse prevention strategies
	  – Provide encouragement throughout the quit attempt
	▨ Follow-up contacts (face-to-face, by telephone, or by e-mail): first contact during first week after quitting, second contact within the first month, additional contacts scheduled as needed

Source: Reproduced with permission from Rx for Change: Clinician-Assisted Tobacco Cessation program. The Regents of the University of California. Copyright © 1999–2015.

their desire to quit with their family, friends, and coworkers and to request their support and assistance. Having patients think about when and why they smoke can help them anticipate situations that might trigger a desire to smoke and contribute to relapse. Additional counseling strategies to address with patients during a quit attempt are listed in Table 47–4. Patients should be counseled on proper medication use (including administration), side effects, and adherence, and it is crucial to emphasize the importance of receiving behavioral counseling throughout the quit attempt. Additionally, patients should be advised to adhere to the entire course of pharmacotherapy, even though most withdrawal symptoms subside within 2–4 weeks.[18]

Counseling Patients Who Recently Quit

Patients who recently quit will face frequent, difficult challenges in countering withdrawal symptoms and cravings or temptations to use tobacco. An important step is to help them identify situations that might trigger relapse and to suggest appropriate coping strategies. Because smoking is a habitual behavior, patients should be advised to alter daily routines that were previously associated with tobacco use. These changes help to disassociate the behaviors from the tobacco.

Many people who quit using tobacco will experience cravings for years and even decades after quitting. Thus, relapse prevention counseling should be part of every follow-up contact with patients who have recently or ever quit smoking. Patients who slip and smoke a cigarette (or use any form of tobacco) or experience a full relapse back to habitual smoking should be encouraged to think through the scenario in which smoking first recurred and identify the trigger for relapse. Identifying triggers will provide valuable information for future quit attempts.

Counseling Patients Who Are Former Smokers

The strategies to be applied for former tobacco users are similar but typically less intensive than those to be applied

table
47–4   Cognitive and Behavioral Strategies for Smoking Cessation

Cognitive strategies focus on retraining of the way a patient thinks. Often, patients mentally deliberate on the fact that they are thinking about a cigarette, and this leads to relapse. Patients must recognize that thinking about a cigarette does not mean they need to have one.

Review of the commitment to quit, with focus on the downside of tobacco	Remind oneself that cravings and temptations are temporary and will pass. Announce, either silently or aloud, "I want to be a nonsmoker," and the temptation will pass.
Distractive thinking	Practice deliberate, immediate refocusing of thinking when cued by thoughts about tobacco use.
Positive self-talks, pep talks	Say "I can do this," and remember difficult situations in which tobacco use was avoided with success.
Relaxation through imagery	Mentally focus on a scene, place, or situation that is peaceful, relaxing, and positive.
Mental rehearsal, visualization	Prepare for situations that might arise by envisioning how best to handle them. For example, envision what would happen if offered a cigarette by a friend, mentally craft and rehearse a response, and perhaps even practice it by saying it aloud.

Behavioral strategies involve specific actions to reduce the risk of relapse. For maximal effectiveness, patient-specific triggers for smoking should first be identified; then these behavioral strategies should be considered before quitting. Below are some strategies for responding to several common cues or triggers for relapse.

Stress	Anticipate upcoming challenges at work, at school, or in personal life. Develop a substitute plan for smoking during times of stress (e.g., practice deep breathing, take a break or leave the situation, call a supportive friend or family member, perform self-massage, or use nicotine replacement therapy).
Alcohol	Drinking alcohol can lead to relapse. Consider limiting or abstaining from alcohol during the early stages of quitting.
Other smokers	Quitting is more difficult when other smokers are around. This is especially difficult if there is another smoker in the household. During the early stages of quitting, limit prolonged contact with individuals who are smoking. Ask coworkers, friends, and housemates not to smoke in your presence.
Oral gratification needs	Have nontobacco oral substitutes (e.g., gum, sugarless candy, straws, toothpicks, lip balm, toothbrush, nicotine replacement therapy, and bottled water) readily available.
Automatic smoking routines	Anticipate routines that are associated with tobacco use and develop an alternative plan. Examples: ■ Smoking with morning coffee: Change morning routine; drink tea instead of coffee; take shower before drinking coffee; take a brisk walk shortly after awakening. ■ Smoking while driving: Remove all tobacco from car; have car interior detailed; listen to an audiobook or talk radio; use oral substitute. ■ Smoking while on the phone: Stand while talking; limit call duration; change phone location; keep hands occupied by doodling or sketching. ■ Smoking after meals: Get up and immediately do dishes or take a brisk walk after eating; call a supportive friend.
Postcessation weight gain	Most tobacco users gain weight after quitting. Most quitters will gain less than 10 pounds, but a broad range of weight gain is reported, with up to 10% of quitters gaining as much as 30 pounds.[29] In general, attempting to modify multiple behaviors at one time is not recommended. If weight gain is a barrier to quitting, engage in regular physical activity and adhere to a healthy diet (as opposed to strict dieting). Carefully plan and prepare meals; increase fruit, vegetable, and water intake to create a feeling of fullness; and chew sugarless gum or eat sugarless candy. Consider use of pharmacotherapy shown to delay weight gain (e.g., 4 mg nicotine gum, 4 mg nicotine lozenge, or bupropion).
Cravings for tobacco	Cravings for tobacco are temporary and usually pass within 5–10 minutes. Handle cravings by using distractive thinking, taking a break, changing activities or tasks, taking deep breaths, or performing self-massage.

Source: Reproduced with permission from Rx for Change: Clinician-Assisted Tobacco Cessation program. The Regents of the University of California. Copyright © 1999–2015.

for recent quitters. The goal for former tobacco users is to remain tobacco free for life. Providers should evaluate their patient's resolve for staying tobacco free and ongoing coping strategies; that is, has the patient had any strong temptations to use tobacco or has there been any occasional use of tobacco products? Also, it is important to ensure that patients are appropriately terminating or tapering pharmacotherapy products. Patients who have been tobacco free should be congratulated for their success. For patients who have intermittently used tobacco, situations in which tobacco use occurred should be reviewed, and additional coping strategies should be discussed.

Helping Patients Quit: The Ask-Advise-Refer Approach (Brief Intervention)

Providers should familiarize themselves with local resources for tobacco cessation, including group programs and telephone quit lines. When time or lack of expertise limits the ability to provide comprehensive cessation counseling, providers are encouraged to apply an abbreviated 5 A's model, whereby they *ask* about tobacco use, *advise* tobacco users to quit, and *refer* patients to other resources, including local services and group counseling programs, for additional assistance. Telephone-based counseling is available throughout the United States. These services provide low-cost interventions that can reach patients who might otherwise have limited access to medical treatment because of geographic location or lack of financial resources. In clinical trials, telephone counseling services for which at least some of the contacts are initiated by the quit line counselor were shown to be effective in promoting abstinence.[29] Combining medication with quit line counseling significantly improves abstinence rates compared with medication alone.[29] The national telephone number for the toll-free tobacco quit line is 1-800-Quit-Now.

Pharmacologic Therapy

Although in some situations pharmacotherapy should be used with caution or only under the supervision of a primary care provider (see Special Populations), most patients who are attempting to quit should be advised to incorporate pharmacotherapy in their treatment plan. Currently, seven first-line agents are approved by the Food and Drug Administration (FDA) for smoking cessation[29]: five formulations of nicotine replacement therapy (NRT), sustained-release bupropion, and varenicline. Three NRT formulations (gum, lozenge, and transdermal patch) are nonprescription, but the nicotine inhaler, nicotine nasal spray, bupropion, and varenicline require a prescription.

Nicotine Replacement Therapy

NRT is the most commonly used pharmacotherapy for smoking cessation.[30] NRT products are often used to help non-cigarette tobacco users to quit, but these products are only FDA labeled to help cigarette smokers quit. Similar to the nicotine present in tobacco, NRT stimulates the release of dopamine in the central nervous system.[10] The rationale underlying the use of NRT for smoking cessation is twofold. First, NRT provides smokers with a nontobacco source of nicotine to reduce the physiologic symptoms of nicotine withdrawal that typically occur after abstinence from tobacco. Second, by attenuating the symptoms of withdrawal, NRT assists quitters by allowing them to focus on the behavioral and psychological aspects of smoking cessation. A key advantage of NRT is that patients, as well as those in the smoker's environment, are not exposed to the carcinogens and other toxic constituents present in tobacco and tobacco smoke. Furthermore, compared with cigarettes, NRT formulations provide lower, slower, and less-variable plasma nicotine concentrations,[15] thereby eliminating the almost immediate reinforcing effects of nicotine obtained through smoking.

Nicotine is well absorbed (Figure 47–3) from many sites, including the lungs, skin, and nasal and buccal (oral) mucosa. Nicotine absorption is pH dependent, and lower systemic concentrations are achieved under acidic conditions. Nicotine is also well absorbed from the gastrointestinal tract (small intestine)

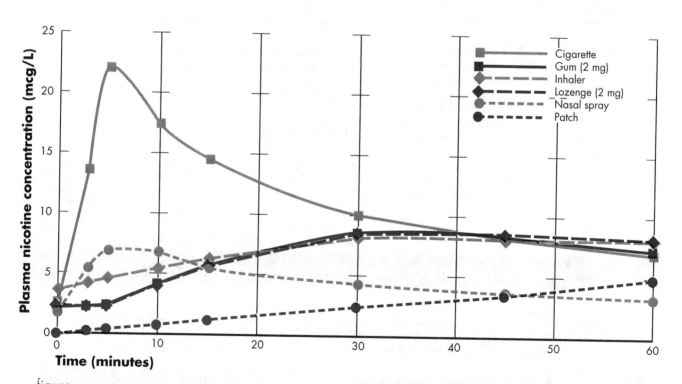

figure 47–3 Plasma nicotine concentrations for various nicotine delivery systems. (*Source:* Reproduced with permission from Rx for Change: Clinician-Assisted Tobacco Cessation program. The Regents of the University of California. Copyright © 1999–2015.)

but undergoes extensive first-pass hepatic metabolism, resulting in negligible systemic levels of nicotine.[15]

The main difference between the various NRT formulations is the site and rate of nicotine absorption (Figure 47–3). Compared with cigarettes, all of the NRT formulations deliver nicotine less rapidly and achieve lower serum nicotine levels, thus lowering the likelihood of developing physical dependence. Peak serum concentrations are achieved most rapidly with the nasal spray (11–18 minutes); followed by the gum, lozenge, and inhaler (30–60 minutes); and then by the transdermal patch (3–12 hours). In contrast, significantly higher peak nicotine levels are attained within 10 minutes of smoking a cigarette.[15]

Patients should be instructed not to smoke cigarettes or use other forms of tobacco (e.g., snuff, chewing tobacco, cigars, and pipes) while using NRT. Use of tobacco in combination with NRT may result in serum nicotine concentrations that are higher than those achieved from tobacco products alone, increasing the likelihood of nicotine-related adverse effects, including nausea, vomiting, hypersalivation, perspiring, abdominal pain, dizziness, weakness, and palpitations.

Nicotine Polacrilex Gum

Nicotine polacrilex gum is a resin complex of nicotine and polacrilin in a sugar-free (<3 calories/piece) chewing gum base. The product is available as 2 mg and 4 mg strengths, in original (tobacco-like, peppery), cinnamon, fruit, mint (various), and orange flavors (Table 47–5). All gum formulations contain buffering agents (sodium carbonate and sodium bicarbonate) to increase salivary pH, thereby enhancing absorption of nicotine across the buccal mucosa. When the 2 mg and 4 mg gums are used properly, approximately 1.6 mg and 2.2 mg of nicotine is absorbed from each dose, respectively. Peak serum concentrations of nicotine are achieved approximately 30 minutes after chewing a single piece of gum and then slowly decline over 2–3 hours.[15]

The recommended dosage of nicotine gum is based on the "time to first cigarette" (TTFC) of the day. Having a strong desire or need to smoke soon after waking is viewed as a key indicator of nicotine dependence. Therefore, patients who smoke their first cigarette of the day within 30 minutes of waking are likely to be more highly dependent on nicotine and require higher dosages than those who delay smoking for more than 30 minutes after waking. Specifically, if the TTFC is 30 minutes or less, therapy should be initiated with the 4 mg gum. If the TTFC is more than 30 minutes, therapy should be initiated with the 2 mg gum. Table 47–5 provides the manufacturer's recommended dosing

schedule. During the initial 6 weeks of therapy, patients should use one piece of gum every 1–2 hours while awake. In general, this amounts to at least 9 pieces of gum daily. Table 47–6 provides specific instructions for proper use of the nicotine gum. The "chew and park" method described in the table allows for the slow, consistent release of nicotine from the polacrilin resin. Patients can use additional pieces of gum (up to the maximum of 24 pieces per day) if cravings occur between the scheduled doses. In general, individuals who smoke heavily will need more pieces to alleviate their cravings.

An important point to note is that patients often do not use enough of the gum to derive its full benefit or they use it incorrectly (e.g., incorrect chewing technique or concurrent consumption of beverages or foods that alter the pH of the mouth). Commonly, patients chew too few pieces per day or shorten the duration of treatment. For this reason, recommending a fixed schedule of administration, tapering over 1–3 months, is preferable to having the patient use the gum as needed to control cravings.[29]

The most common side effects associated with the use of the nicotine gum include unpleasant taste, mouth irritation, jaw muscle soreness or fatigue, hypersalivation, hiccups, and dyspepsia. Many of these side effects can be minimized or prevented by using proper chewing technique.[29] The nicotine polacrilin resin is more viscous than ordinary chewing gum and more likely to adhere to fillings, bridges, dentures, crowns, and braces. Patients should be warned that chewing the gum too rapidly may result in excessive release of nicotine, leading to lightheadedness, nausea, vomiting, irritation of the throat and mouth, hiccups, and indigestion.

Patients with active temporomandibular joint (TMJ) disease should not use the nicotine gum because the highly viscous consistency of the formulation and the need for frequent chewing may exacerbate this condition. In addition, the manufacturer recommends that patients with stomach ulcers or diabetes contact their health care provider before use of the product because these conditions are more serious and might require further monitoring.

Nicotine Polacrilex Lozenge

The nicotine polacrilex lozenge is a resin complex of nicotine and polacrilin in a sugar-free mint- or cherry-flavored lozenge (Table 47–5). The lozenges are available in 2 mg and 4 mg strengths with two different physical sizes (regular and mini) and should be used similarly to other medicinal lozenges or troches (i.e., suck and rotate it within the mouth until it dissolves).

table 47–5	Dosages for Nonprescription Nicotine Polacrilex Gum and Lozenge	
	Gum	**Lozenge**
Product strength	Nicorette: 2 mg, 4 mg; original, cinnamon, fruit, mint (various) Generic: 2 mg, 4 mg; original, fruit, mint, orange	Nicorette (standard): 2 mg, 4 mg; cherry, mint Nicorette (mini): 2 mg, 4 mg; mint Generic (standard): 2 mg, 4 mg; mint
Dose	First cigarette ≤30 minutes after waking: 4 mg First cigarette >30 minutes after waking: 2 mg Weeks 1–6: 1 piece every 1–2 hours Weeks 7–9: 1 piece every 2–4 hours Weeks 10–12: 1 piece every 4–8 hours	First cigarette ≤30 minutes after waking: 4 mg First cigarette >30 minutes after waking: 2 mg Weeks 1–6: 1 lozenge every 1–2 hours Weeks 7–9: 1 lozenge every 2–4 hours Weeks 10–12: 1 lozenge every 4–8 hours

table
47–6 Usage Guidelines for Nicotine Polacrilex Gum

- Do not smoke cigarettes or use other forms of tobacco (e.g., snuff, chewing tobacco, cigars, and pipes) while on nicotine gum therapy. (*Note:* In 2013, the FDA recommended labeling changes that will remove this warning.[47])
- Note that nicotine gum is a nicotine delivery system, not a chewing gum.
- Proper administration technique is necessary when using this product. Nicotine from the gum is released using the "chew and park" method:
  - Chew each piece of gum *slowly* several times.
  - Stop chewing at the first sign of a peppery, minty, fruity, or citrus taste, or after experiencing a slight tingling sensation in the mouth. This usually occurs after about 15 chews, but the onset varies.
  - Park the gum between the cheek and gum to allow absorption of nicotine across the lining of the mouth.
  - When the taste or tingling dissipates (generally after 1–2 minutes), slowly resume chewing.
  - When the taste or tingle returns, stop chewing and park the gum in a different place in the mouth. This will decrease the incidence of mouth irritation.
  - The chew-and-park steps should be repeated until most of the nicotine is gone, which is when the taste or tingle does not return after continued chewing. On average, each piece of gum lasts 30 minutes.
- To minimize withdrawal symptoms, use the nicotine gum on a scheduled basis rather than as needed.
- Follow the dosage regimen carefully; reduce the dosage at the recommended intervals; if needed for longer than 12 weeks of treatment to keep from smoking, talk to your health care provider.
- Do not chew more than 24 pieces per day.
- Acidic beverages such as coffee, juices, wine, or soft drinks may transiently reduce the salivary pH, resulting in decreased absorption of nicotine across the buccal mucosa. Do not eat or drink anything (except water) 15 minutes before or while using the nicotine gum.
- Note that chewing the gum too quickly will result in an unpleasant taste caused by too much nicotine in the saliva and, if the nicotine is swallowed, may cause effects similar to those produced by excessive smoking (e.g., nausea, throat irritation, light-headedness, and hiccups).
- Have nicotine gum readily available at all times. Keep the nicotine gum in the same place you previously kept your cigarettes (e.g., shirt pocket, purse, or desk).
- Keep this product, including used pieces, out of the reach of children and pets.

Because the mini-lozenge is smaller, it is more easily concealed and dissolves more quickly. The pharmacokinetics of the nicotine lozenge and gum formulations are comparable, but a nicotine lozenge delivers approximately 25% more nicotine than an equivalent dose of nicotine gum because of complete dissolution of the dosage form.[33] The lozenge form contains buffering agents (sodium carbonate and potassium bicarbonate) to increase salivary pH, enhancing the buccal absorption of nicotine.

As with nicotine gum, dosing for the lozenge is based on the TTFC. If the TTFC is 30 minutes or less, therapy should be initiated with the 4 mg lozenge. If the TTFC is more than 30 minutes, therapy should be initiated with the 2 mg lozenge.

During the initial 6 weeks of therapy, patients should use 1 lozenge every 1–2 hours while awake. In general, this amounts to at least 9 lozenges daily. Table 47–7 provides further instructions for proper use of the nicotine lozenge. Patients can use additional lozenges (up to 5 lozenges in 6 hours or a maximum of 20 lozenges per day) if cravings occur between the scheduled doses. The manufacturer recommends that patients with stomach ulcers or diabetes contact their health care provider before using the lozenges because these conditions, which are more serious, may require further monitoring.

Side effects associated with the nicotine lozenge include mouth irritation, nausea, hiccups, cough, heartburn, headache, flatulence, and insomnia. Patients who use more than 1 lozenge at a time, continuously use 1 lozenge after another, or chew or swallow the lozenge are more likely to experience heartburn or indigestion.

Nicotine Transdermal Systems (Nicotine Patch)

Nicotine transdermal systems deliver continuous, low levels of nicotine through the skin over 24 hours. The patch consists of a waterproof surface layer, a nicotine reservoir, an adhesive layer, and a disposable protective liner. Currently patients can choose from two marketed products (Table 47–8).

table
47–7 Usage Guidelines for Nicotine Polacrilex Lozenge

- Do not smoke cigarettes or use other forms of tobacco (e.g., snuff, chewing tobacco, cigars, and pipes) while using the nicotine lozenge. (*Note:* In 2013, the FDA recommended labeling changes that will remove this warning.[47])
- Proper administration technique is necessary when using the nicotine lozenge:
  - Place the lozenge in the mouth and allow it to dissolve slowly (20–30 minutes for standard lozenge; 10 minutes for mini-lozenge). As the nicotine is released from the lozenge, you may experience a warm, tingling sensation.
  - To reduce the risk of side effects (e.g., nausea, hiccups, and heartburn), do not chew or swallow the lozenge.
  - Occasionally rotate the lozenge to different areas of the mouth to decrease mouth irritation.
- To minimize withdrawal symptoms, use the nicotine lozenge on a scheduled basis rather than as needed.
- Follow the dosage regimen carefully; reduce the dosage at the recommended intervals; if needed for longer than 12 weeks of treatment to keep from smoking, talk to your health care provider.
- Do not use more than 5 lozenges in 6 hours or more than 20 lozenges per day.
- Acidic beverages such as coffee, juices, wine, or soft drinks may transiently reduce the salivary pH, resulting in decreased absorption of nicotine across the buccal mucosa. Do not eat or drink anything (except water) 15 minutes before or while using the nicotine lozenge.
- Patients who use more than 1 lozenge at a time, continuously use 1 lozenge after another, or chew or swallow the lozenge are more likely to experience heartburn or indigestion.
- Have nicotine lozenges readily available at all times. Keep the nicotine lozenges in the same place you previously kept your cigarettes (e.g., shirt pocket, purse, or desk).
- Keep this product out of the reach of children and pets.

<table>
<tr><td colspan="2">table
47–8   **Dosages for Nonprescription Nicotine Transdermal Systems (Patch)**</td></tr>
</table>

	NicoDerm CQ and Generic Patch
Product strength	7, 14, 21 mg (24 hour)
Dose	**>10 cigarettes/day** 21 mg/day × 6 weeks (NicoDerm CQ; × 4 weeks for generic); 14 mg/day × 2 weeks; 7 mg/day × 2 weeks **≤10 cigarettes/day** 14 mg/day × 6 weeks; 7 mg/day × 2 weeks

The dosing schedules for the nicotine patches vary slightly (Table 47–8). Before recommending a specific product and a dosing schedule, the caregiver should know how many cigarettes the patient smokes per day. In general, heavier smokers will require higher-strength formulations for a longer duration of therapy. Patients experiencing side effects from the patches, such as dizziness, perspiration, nausea, vomiting, diarrhea, or headache, should consider a lower-strength patch. Additional instructions for proper use of the nicotine patch are listed in Table 47–9.

The most common side effects associated with the nicotine patch are local skin reactions (erythema, burning, and pruritus) at the application site, which are generally caused by skin occlusion or sensitivity to the patch adhesives. If this side effect is bothersome, the patient can apply nonprescription hydrocortisone cream to the site or try another manufacturer's product that uses a different adhesive. Other, less common side effects include vivid or abnormal dreams, insomnia, and headache. Sleep disturbances might be caused by nocturnal nicotine absorption. If this side effect becomes troublesome, patients should be instructed to remove the patch at bedtime and apply a new patch as soon as possible after waking the following morning because they may experience increased urges to smoke with the lack of nicotine coverage throughout the night.[29]

Prescription Medications for Smoking Cessation

Detailed information about prescription products for tobacco cessation is outside the scope of this publication. The following information is a summary of key information; for more detailed discussion the reader is encouraged to utilize another reference.

Nicotine Inhaler

The nicotine inhaler consists of a plastic mouthpiece and a nicotine-containing cartridge that delivers 4 mg of nicotine as an inhaled vapor, 2 mg of which is absorbed across the oropharyngeal mucosa. The inhaler reduces nicotine withdrawal symptoms and may give some degree of comfort by providing

<table>
<tr><td colspan="2">table
47–9   **Usage Guidelines for Nicotine Transdermal Systems (Nicotine Patch)**</td></tr>
</table>

- Do not smoke cigarettes or use other forms of tobacco (e.g., snuff, chewing tobacco, cigars, and pipes) while using the nicotine patch. (*Note:* In 2013, the FDA recommended labeling changes that will remove this warning.[47])
- Apply the patch to a clean, dry, hairless area of the skin on the upper body or the upper outer part of the arm at approximately the same time each day.
- The patch should be applied to a different area of skin each day. To minimize the potential for local skin reactions, the same area should not be used again for at least 1 week.
- During application, apply firm pressure to the patch with the palm of the hand for 10 seconds. Be sure that the patch adheres well to the skin, especially around the edges; this is necessary for a good seal.
- Wash your hands after applying or removing the patch.
- The patch should not be left on the skin for more than 24 hours because prolonged use may lead to skin irritation.
- Any adhesive remaining on the skin after patch removal can be removed with rubbing alcohol.
- Water will not reduce the effectiveness of the nicotine patch if it is applied correctly. You may bathe, swim, shower, or exercise while wearing the patch.
- Do not cut patches in half or into smaller pieces to adjust or reduce the nicotine dosage. Nicotine in the patch may evaporate from the cut edges and the patch may be less effective.
- Local skin reactions (e.g., itching, burning, and redness) are common with the nicotine patch. These reactions are generally caused by adhesives; they can be minimized by rotating patch application sites and, if they occur, treated with nonprescription hydrocortisone cream.
- Remove the nicotine patch before having a magnetic resonance imaging (MRI) procedure. Burns from nicotine patches worn during MRIs have been reported and are likely caused by the metallic component in the backing of some patches.
- Individuals experiencing troublesome dreams or other sleep disruptions should remove the patch before bedtime.
- Discard the removed nicotine patch by folding it onto itself, completely covering the adhesive area.
- Keep new and used patches out of the reach of children and pets.

a hand-to-mouth ritual that emulates smoking. However, reinforcing the hand-to-mouth ritual can make quitting more difficult. The inhaler has not been evaluated for use in patients with bronchospastic diseases, such as asthma, so it should be used with caution in these patients because of the risk of exacerbation.[34] Side effects of the inhaler include mild mouth and throat irritation, cough, and rhinitis.

Nicotine Nasal Spray

The nicotine nasal spray is an aqueous solution of nicotine for administration to the nasal mucosa. Each actuation delivers a 0.5 mg bolus of nicotine that is absorbed across the nasal mucosa. Because of its rapid onset of action (relative to other NRT formulations), the spray is a potential option for patients who prefer a medication to manage withdrawal symptoms rapidly; however, in 15%–20% of patients, use of the nasal spray can result in dependence. Some patients with asthma have reported bronchospasm after using the nasal spray, so use of this medication in patients with bronchospastic disease should be avoided.[34] Initially, most patients will experience nose and throat irritation (peppery sensation), watery eyes, sneezing, or coughing when using this product. This product is to be administered without sniffing (i.e., not administered like standard allergy nasal sprays). After the first week, most patients have minimal difficulty with the product, and tolerance generally develops with regular use.

Sustained-Release Bupropion

Sustained-release bupropion was the first non-nicotine medication approved for smoking cessation. This agent is a prescription antidepressant medication that is believed to promote smoking cessation by blocking the reuptake of dopamine and norepinephrine in the brain, thereby decreasing the cravings for cigarettes and symptoms of nicotine withdrawal.[29]

Therapy is started with a dose of 150 mg orally every morning for 3 days, followed by 150 mg twice daily for 7–12 weeks. Because steady-state blood levels are reached after approximately 7 days of therapy, patients set their quit date for 1–2 weeks after starting therapy. Insomnia and dry mouth are the most common side effects reported with bupropion. Because seizures have been reported in approximately 0.1% of patients, bupropion is contraindicated in patients who (1) have a seizure disorder, (2) have a current or prior diagnosis of anorexia or bulimia nervosa, (3) are undergoing abrupt discontinuation of alcohol or sedatives (including benzodiazepines), (4) are currently using or have used a monoamine oxidase inhibitor within the past 14 days, or (5) are currently being treated with any other medications that contain bupropion. Other factors that might increase the odds of seizure and are classified as warnings for this medication include history of head trauma or prior seizure, central nervous system tumor, severe hepatic cirrhosis, and concomitant use of medications that lower the seizure threshold. In July 2009, FDA mandated that the prescribing information for all bupropion-containing products include a black-box warning that highlights the risk of serious neuropsychiatric symptoms, including changes in behavior, hostility, agitation, depressed mood, suicidal thoughts and behavior, and attempted suicide.[35] These additional warnings were based on postmarketing adverse event surveillance reports received by FDA.

Varenicline

Varenicline (Chantix) is a partial agonist and is highly selective for the alpha$_4$beta$_2$ nicotinic acetylcholine receptor. The efficacy of varenicline in smoking cessation is believed to be the result of sustained, low-level agonist activity at the receptor site that is combined with competitive inhibition of nicotine binding. The partial agonist activity induces modest receptor stimulation, leading to increased dopamine levels that attenuate the symptoms of nicotine withdrawal. In addition, by competitively blocking the binding of nicotine to nicotinic acetylcholine receptors in the central nervous system, varenicline inhibits the surges of dopamine release that occur immediately after inhalation of tobacco smoke. The latter mechanism may be effective in preventing relapse by reducing the pleasure associated with smoking.[36]

Similar to sustained-release bupropion, treatment with varenicline should be started 1 week before the patient stops smoking. This regimen allows for gradual escalation of the dose to minimize treatment-related nausea and insomnia. Therapy is generally started at 0.5 mg daily on days 1–3; 0.5 mg twice daily on days 4–7; and 1 mg twice daily for weeks 2–12. Nausea, insomnia, abnormal dreams, and headache are the most commonly reported side effects. In July 2009, FDA mandated that the prescribing information for varenicline contain a black-box warning that highlights the risk of serious neuropsychiatric symptoms, including changes in behavior, hostility, agitation, depressed mood, and suicidal events including ideation, behavior changes, and attempted suicide.[37] These additional warnings were based on continued postmarketing adverse event surveillance reports received by FDA. Although these reports are rare in comparison with the total number of patients exposed to varenicline, providers and patients should monitor for changes in mood and behavior during treatment with varenicline.[37]

A small increased risk of cardiac events has been reported in some patients with existing cardiovascular disease.[38] In December 2012, FDA shared results of a meta-analysis conducted by the manufacturer of varenicline, reporting that a higher occurrence of major adverse cardiovascular events was observed in patients using varenicline compared with placebo (although the increased risk was not statistically significant).[38] The warnings and precautions labeling was updated to include the results of the meta-analysis and included instructions to patients to notify their health care providers of new or worsening cardiovascular symptoms and to seek immediate medical attention if they experience signs and symptoms of myocardial infarction or stroke.[37]

Pharmacotherapeutic Comparison

Few trials have directly compared the various agents for smoking cessation. In general, compared with placebo, regimens with the first-line agents approximately double the long-term quit rates (Table 47–10).[29]

Product Selection Guidelines

Because all first-line, FDA-approved cessation medications enhance quit rates, the choice of therapy is based largely on contraindications or precautions, patient preference, tolerability of the available dosage forms, use during prior quit attempts (i.e., what worked well and what did not, regardless of whether medication was being used correctly or not), and cost. Regardless of the regimen selected, the cost of treatment will be insignificant compared with the costs of continued smoking and the costs of managing the resultant complications.

A number of smokeless tobacco products are now on the market, including snuff, snus, and dissolvable tobacco. Currently no guidelines exist for the treatment of tobacco cessation for individuals using these products. A randomized, clinical trial comparing varenicline to placebo showed positive results; however, more studies are needed.[39]

Special Populations

NRT should be used with caution in patients with serious underlying cardiovascular disease, including those who have had a recent myocardial infarction (i.e., within the preceding 2 weeks), those with serious arrhythmias, and those with serious or worsening angina pectoris.[29] Nicotine may increase the

table 47–10 Methods for Smoking Cessation: Estimates of Treatment Efficacy for First-Line Agents Compared with Placebo at 6 Months after Quitting

Pharmacotherapy	Estimated Odds Ratio[a] (95% CI)	Estimated Abstinence Rate[b] (95% CI)
Placebo	1.0	13.8
Monotherapy (first-line agents)		
Sustained-release bupropion	2.0 (1.8–2.2)	24.2 (22.2–26.4)
Nicotine gum (6–14 weeks)	1.5 (1.2–1.7)	19.0 (16.5–21.9)
Nicotine inhaler	2.1 (1.5–2.9)	24.8 (19.1–31.6)
Nicotine lozenge (2 mg)	2.0 (1.4–2.8)	24.2[c]
Nicotine patch (6–14 weeks)	1.9 (1.7–2.2)	23.4 (21.3–25.8)
Nicotine nasal spray	2.3 (1.7–3.0)	26.7 (21.5–32.7)
Varenicline (2 mg/day)	3.1 (2.5–3.8)	33.2 (28.9–37.8)
Combination Therapy (first-line agents)		
Nicotine patch (>14 weeks) + as-needed NRT (gum, nasal spray, or lozenge[d])	3.6 (2.5–5.2)	36.5 (28.6–45.3)
Nicotine patch + bupropion SR	2.5 (1.9–3.4)	28.9 (23.5–35.1)
Nicotine patch + nicotine inhaler	2.2 (1.3–3.6)	25.8 (17.4–36.5)

Key: C, = Confidence interval; NRT = nicotine replacement therapy; SR = sustained release.

[a] Estimated relative to placebo.

[b] Abstinence percentages for specified treatment.

[c] One qualifying randomized trial; 95% CI not reported in the 2008 clinical practice guideline.

[d] A recent trial, not included in the clinical practice guideline, supports the combination of the nicotine patch and nicotine lozenge.[45]

Source: Reproduced with permission from Rx for Change: Clinician-Assisted Tobacco Cessation program. The Regents of the University of California. Copyright © 1999–2015.

myocardial workload by increasing the heart rate and blood pressure and may constrict coronary arteries, leading to cardiac ischemia.[40] Although most experts believe the risks of NRT in patients with cardiovascular disease are small relative to the risks of continued smoking,[41–43] patients with serious underlying cardiovascular disease are advised to use NRT only while under the supervision of a health care provider.

Prescription forms of nicotine are classified by FDA as Pregnancy Category D, meaning there is evidence of risk to the human fetus.[44] Although NRT may pose a risk to the developing fetus, some experts have argued that NRT use during pregnancy is safer than continued smoking.[43,44] However, because data showing effectiveness of NRT in pregnancy are inconclusive and because nicotine has the potential to cause fetal harm, the 2008 clinical practice guideline states that pregnant women should be encouraged to quit without the use of medication. Instead, providers are advised to offer interventions of person-to-person behavioral counseling for their pregnant patients who smoke.[29]

The efficacy of NRT, sustained-release bupropion, and varenicline has not been established in pediatric or adolescent smokers, and no NRT product is currently indicated for use in these populations.[29] Accordingly, counseling is the recommended treatment method for smokers younger than 18 years.

People older than 65 years can benefit greatly from quitting smoking. Pharmacologic therapy and counseling are recommended. If mobility is an issue, referral to a quit line may be useful.[13,29]

The manufacturers of nicotine gum, lozenge, and patch products recommend that patients taking a prescription medicine for asthma or depression speak with their physician or pharmacist before using nonprescription NRT. Fluvoxamine and theophylline (both now used infrequently) and inhaled corticosteroids have known clinically significant interactions with tobacco smoke (Table 47–2).

For light smokers (those who smoke fewer than 10 cigarettes per day and those who do not smoke every day), counseling is the recommended treatment method for this population.[29] However, the nicotine patch is approved for use in light smokers, and the nicotine lozenge was shown to be effective in individuals smoking 15 or fewer cigarettes daily.[45] Use of smokeless tobacco (e.g., snuff, moist snuff, chewing tobacco, and dissolvable tobacco); cigars; and pipes can produce nicotine addiction and lead to serious health consequences. Behavioral counseling is the recommended treatment method for these tobacco users.[29]

Patient Factors

When recommending a nonprescription agent for smoking cessation, health care providers should determine the patient's smoking patterns, lifestyle habits, and coexisting medical conditions. In general, higher levels of smoking will require higher dosages of NRT and longer durations of treatment.

Some patients might need to use their smoking cessation medication longer than the usual recommended treatment duration. Although the general goal is complete, long-term abstinence from all nicotine-containing products, some smokers may benefit from long-term medication use.[29] If continued use helps prevent relapse, this approach is considered preferable to the patient returning to smoking.[29]

Patients who smoke continuously throughout the day might have better success with a nicotine patch because it provides a sustained, steady release of nicotine. Conversely, patients who smoke intermittently throughout the day or who smoke intensely for short periods of time, followed by long periods of abstinence, might prefer a relatively short-acting formulation, such as a nicotine gum or lozenge, to more closely mimic their tobacco use patterns. For some quitters, frequent gum chewing may not be feasible or socially acceptable. The nicotine patch, which can be concealed under clothing, might be a reasonable choice for these individuals. Others may find nicotine lozenges, which can be used more discreetly, to be an acceptable alternative. Patients with underlying dermatologic conditions (e.g., psoriasis, eczema, or atopic dermatitis) or allergy to adhesive tape are more likely to experience skin irritation and should not use the nicotine patch. The nicotine lozenge or patch is more appropriate than the nicotine gum for patients with TMJ disease or dentures. Finally, patients with serious cardiovascular disease, women who are pregnant or nursing, light smokers, and adolescents should be referred for further evaluation by their primary provider before starting treatment with NRT.

Patient Preferences

Understanding the patient's perceptions and expectations about pharmacotherapy is particularly important, including the ability to adhere to the regimen, previous experience with smoking cessation medications, and concern about weight gain. Because NRT formulations require frequent dosing or nontraditional routes of administration, patient education about proper use of these products is essential. Patients who have difficulty taking multiple doses of medications throughout the day or those who want a simplified regimen might achieve greater success with the nicotine patch. In contrast, the gum or lozenge may be preferable for patients who want to titrate nicotine levels to manage withdrawal symptoms. Some patients may find they need an oral substitute for tobacco; the oral gratification given by the nicotine gum, lozenge, or inhaler might be beneficial in these patients. Other patients may prefer the idea of using a combination of medications, such as the nicotine patch plus gum or lozenge, on an as-needed basis as discussed later in this section.

All smokers making a repeat quit attempt should be queried about their prior use of pharmacotherapy and their perceptions of the treatment options. For patients reporting a favorable past experience with a given product, repeated treatment with the same agent may be appropriate, with consideration given to increasing the dose, frequency of dosing, or duration of therapy. For patients who report a negative experience with a particular medication (e.g., poor adherence, side effects, palatability issues, or cost), a different regimen should be considered. For example, if a patient had short-term success with the patch but discontinued therapy because of intolerable nightmares, he or she may attempt to quit again by using the patch but may remove it at bedtime. A patient who is unable to tolerate nicotine gum because of jaw muscle ache could be advised to switch to the nicotine lozenge or patch. For patients who express concern about postcessation weight gain, the 4 mg nicotine gum or lozenge or the sustained-release bupropion might be particularly

helpful, given that these products were shown to delay weight gain after quitting.[29] Among patients for whom the out-of-pocket expense might be a barrier to pharmacologic treatment, use of the generic formulations is preferable.

Combination therapy should be considered a first-line treatment and might be particularly appropriate in patients who have experienced numerous failed attempts using monotherapy. Combination therapy generally involves the use of a long-acting medication (nicotine patch or sustained-release bupropion) in combination with a short-acting nicotine formulation (nicotine gum, lozenge, inhaler, or nasal spray). The long-acting nicotine formulation, which delivers relatively constant concentrations of drug, is used to prevent the onset of severe withdrawal symptoms, whereas the short-acting nicotine formulation, which delivers nicotine more rapidly, is used as needed to control withdrawal symptoms that may occur during potential relapse situations (e.g., after meals, during episodes of stress, or around other smokers). Research suggests that combination therapy may be somewhat more efficacious than monotherapy.[29,46] Disadvantages of combination therapy are the possibility of more side effects (e.g., nicotine toxicity), difficulty with adherence, and increased cost. In 2013, FDA recommended nonprescription NRT labeling changes that will remove the warning against the concomitant use of nicotine-containing products (including other forms of NRT).[47] For other combination regimens, patients should be referred to their primary care provider to determine the most appropriate option.

Complementary Therapies

Although a variety of herbal and homeopathic products are available to aid cessation, data are lacking to support their safety and efficacy. Many herbal preparations for cessation contain lobeline (*Lobelia inflata*), an herbal alkaloid with partial nicotinic agonist properties. A meta-analysis[48] and a multicenter trial[49] found no evidence to support the role of lobeline as an aid for smoking cessation. Similarly, controlled trials did not find hypnosis or acupuncture to be an effective treatment for smoking cessation.[29,50]

Electronic Cigarettes

More recently, electronic cigarettes (e-cigarettes) have become available in the United States. These devices are being marketed as a substitute for cigarettes in situations that do not allow smoking. Currently, data are insufficient to support their safety or efficacy in reducing or stopping smoking.[51]

Assessment of Tobacco Cessation: A Case-Based Approach

To help patients succeed at tobacco cessation, the provider must assist them in evaluating how they smoke, identify medications and quitting methods they have or have not tried in the past, and determine appropriate cessation therapies. Analysis of the patient's smoking patterns and the triggers for smoking help the provider work with the patient to develop an appropriate treatment plan.

Cases 47–1 and 47–2 illustrate the assessment of patients who want to quit smoking.

case
47–1

Relevant Evaluation Criteria	Scenario/Model Outcome

Information Gathering

1. Gather essential information about the patient's symptoms, including:

   a. description of symptom(s) (i.e., nature, onset, duration, severity, associated symptoms)

   Patient would like information about the various OTC medications for tobacco cessation. He is noticing that he gets more "winded" when he walks, and he is concerned about the effects of smoking on his health. He has smoked one pack per day (or 20 cigarettes) for 21 years. He smokes 2 cigarettes with his morning coffee and smokes in social situations such as when having a few drinks with coworkers. He has not received cessation counseling from a provider. He has tried the nicotine patch and gum in the past and wants to try Chantix (varenicline).

   b. description of any factors that seem to precipitate, exacerbate, and/or relieve the patient's symptom(s)

   He is in a rush because he has to get back to work. He smokes mostly on work breaks and at home in the morning and in the evenings after dinner.

   c. description of the patient's efforts to relieve the symptoms

   He has tried to quit smoking about 5 times to date, 3 times using NRT.

   d. patient's identity

   Kevin Stills

   e. age, sex, height, and weight

   61 years old, male, 5 ft 8 in., 170 lb

   f. patient's occupation

   Accountant

   g. patient's dietary habits

   Reasonably healthy diet; walks 30 minutes daily during his lunch break.

   h. patient's sleep habits

   Sleeps 7 hours/night during the workweek; does not have trouble sleeping.

   i. concurrent medical conditions, prescription and non-prescription medications, and dietary supplements

   Hypertension (controlled on lisinopril 10 mg daily).

   j. allergies

   NKA

   k. history of other adverse reactions to medications

   None

   l. other (describe)

   Married, no kids. His wife is supportive of his attempt to quit. Some close friends and coworkers also smoke.

Assessment and Triage

2. Differentiate patient's signs/symptoms and correctly identify the patient's primary problem(s).

   Patient is a middle-aged male who would like to quit smoking to improve his breathing and overall health.

3. Identify exclusions for self-treatment (Figure 47–2).

   None

4. Formulate a comprehensive list of therapeutic alternatives for the primary problem to determine if triage to a medical provider is required, and share this information with the patient or caregiver.

   Options include:

   (1) Recommend pharmacotherapy and counseling. Pharmacotherapy options include:

   - Nicotine patch.
   - Nicotine gum.
   - Nicotine lozenge.
   - Combination therapy with the nicotine patch plus a short-acting NRT.
   - Referral to PCP for prescription pharmacotherapy (nicotine inhaler, nicotine nasal spray, bupropion SR, varenicline).

   (2) Refer Mr. Stills to telephone counseling (1-800-Quit-Now) because he is in a hurry.

   (3) Recommend that he set a quit date in 1–2 weeks.

   (4) Take no action.

Plan

5. Select an optimal therapeutic alternative to address the patient's problem, taking into account patient preferences.

   Mr. Stills expressed interest in using varenicline. Refer him to his PCP for a prescription.

   For behavioral counseling, refer him to the quit line. (See Tables 47–3 and 47–4.)

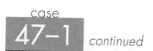

case
47–1 continued

Relevant Evaluation Criteria	Scenario/Model Outcome
6. Describe the recommended therapeutic approach to the patient or caregiver.	"Medication is recommended. Although you have no contraindications or precautions for self-care use, varenicline is available only by prescription."
7. Explain to the patient or caregiver the rationale for selecting the recommended therapeutic approach from the considered therapeutic alternatives.	"Chantix, or varenicline, is considered a first-line treatment for smoking cessation. Because you would like to use this medication and it is available by prescription only, you will need to contact your primary care provider to obtain a prescription. I can also call your provider for you now if you would like. Receiving counseling, in addition to taking Chantix as directed, will increase your chances of success with quitting."

Patient Education

8. When recommending self-care with nonprescription medications and/or nondrug therapy, convey accurate information to the patient or caregiver.	Criterion does not apply in this case.
Solicit follow-up questions from the patient or caregiver.	"What should I do if I am tempted to smoke when I am around my friends?"
Answer the patient's or caregiver's questions.	"The quit line counselor will be able to talk to you about problem-solving and coping skills for your smoking triggers. It is important that your friends and wife support you when you quit. To minimize relapse, reduce or avoid use of alcohol during the first 2 weeks of your quit attempt. The counselor will arrange follow-up contacts after your quit date."

Evaluation of Patient Outcome

9. Assess patient outcome.	Mr. Stills plans to contact his PCP and will return to the pharmacy to fill his prescription. He also set a quit date in 2 weeks with plans to follow up with the quit line.

Key: NKA = No known allergies; NRT = nicotine replacement therapy; OTC = over-the-counter; PCP = primary care provider; SR = sustained release.

case
47–2

Relevant Evaluation Criteria	Scenario/Model Outcome

Information Gathering

1. Gather essential information about the patient's symptoms, including:	
a. description of symptom(s) (i.e., nature, onset, duration, severity, associated symptoms)	Patient quit smoking 7 days ago and is using the generic 21 mg nicotine patch. She complains of trouble sleeping and is experiencing disturbing dreams since starting to use the patch. She had been smoking approximately 1.5 packs per day (~30 cigarettes daily) for 10 years before quitting.
b. description of any factors that seem to precipitate, exacerbate, and/or relieve the patient's symptom(s)	Before quitting, patient used to have a cigarette before even getting out of bed, because she had such intense cravings.
c. description of the patient's efforts to relieve the symptoms	Patient has been using the 21 mg nicotine patch for 7 days. She has not previously tried pharmacotherapy for quitting. She purchased the patch after speaking to a pharmacist. She has not received any formal counseling from a provider. She feels a bit agitated and irritable from time to time during the day; she is very tempted to smoke in the morning when she wakes up. Overall, she likes the patch and is not experiencing any significant skin reactions.
d. patient's identity	Kristen Brady
e. age, sex, height, and weight	28 years old, female, 5 ft 6 in., 140 lb

case
47–2   *continued*

Relevant Evaluation Criteria	Scenario/Model Outcome
f. patient's occupation	Web designer
g. patient's dietary habits	Tries to eat healthy; drinks approximately 8 cups of caffeinated coffee per day.
h. patient's sleep habits	Sleeps 7–8 hours a night. Since using the patch, she has experienced trouble sleeping and disturbing dreams.
i. concurrent medical conditions, prescription and non-prescription medications, and dietary supplements	Not pregnant or breastfeeding; temporomandibular joint (TMJ) disease; acetaminophen 325 mg every 6 hours as needed for pain, but uses rarely.
j. allergies	NKA
k. history of other adverse reactions to medications	None
l. other (describe)	Patient is single. Her boyfriend and roommate are supportive of her desire to quit.

Assessment and Triage

2. Differentiate patient's signs/symptoms and correctly identify the patient's primary problem(s).

Patient quit smoking 1 week ago and is experiencing intolerable side effects from the nicotine patch (i.e., sleep disturbances), daily withdrawal symptoms (i.e., agitation and irritability), and morning cravings.

3. Identify exclusions for self-treatment (Figure 47–2).

None

4. Formulate a comprehensive list of therapeutic alternatives for the primary problem to determine if triage to a medical provider is required, and share this information with the patient or caregiver.

Options include:

(1) Recommend continued pharmacotherapy and counseling. Pharmacotherapy options include:

■ Removal of nicotine patch at night and addition of a lozenge as needed (particularly in the morning upon waking).

■ Alternative NRT, such as lozenge alone.

■ Referral to PCP for prescription pharmacotherapy (nicotine inhaler, nicotine nasal spray, bupropion SR, varenicline).

(2) Take no action.

Plan

5. Select an optimal therapeutic alternative to address the patient's problem, taking into account patient preferences.

Because Ms. Brady has expressed that she thinks the patch is working well to manage her withdrawal symptoms, continue the nicotine patch, but advise her to take the patch off before bedtime. This should help reduce the sleep disturbances and disturbing dreams. She can use combination therapy with a nicotine lozenge, as needed. The nicotine gum would not be a good choice because she has TMJ disease. A 2 mg lozenge dose to be used on an as-needed basis is reasonable.

6. Describe the recommended therapeutic approach to the patient or caregiver.

"It's great that the patch is working for you so far. You have no contraindications or precautions for use of the nicotine patch and as-needed 2 mg lozenge. I have some ideas that should help you with your sleep problems and some other information for you, including how to manage morning cravings."

7. Explain to the patient or caregiver the rationale for selecting the recommended therapeutic approach from the considered therapeutic alternatives.

"You do not have any medical conditions for which nicotine replacement medications should be used with caution (e.g., recent heart attack, serious arrhythmias, or angina). The nicotine patch provides a low, constant level of nicotine to help reduce nicotine withdrawal symptoms. By taking it off at night, you should no longer experience sleep disturbances. The nicotine lozenge should be used only when you experience situations in which you are craving a cigarette, such as when you wake up. Receiving counseling, in addition to taking your medications as directed, will increase your chances of quitting."

case

47–2 *continued*

Relevant Evaluation Criteria	Scenario/Model Outcome

Patient Education

8. When recommending self-care with nonprescription medications and/or nondrug therapy, convey accurate information to the patient or caregiver:

a. appropriate dose and frequency of administration

"Use the 2 mg nicotine lozenge if you experience situations in which you are craving a cigarette, such as when you wake up." (See Tables 47–5 and 47–8.)

b. maximum number of days the therapy should be employed

See Table 47–8.

c. product administration procedures

See Tables 47–7 and 47–9.

d. expected time to onset of relief

"With the lozenge, nicotine levels will peak 30–60 minutes after you start using it. You are already using the nicotine patch, which provides a steady amount of nicotine throughout the day. The blood nicotine levels from the patch and lozenge are lower than those from smoking but should be sufficient to help control your nicotine withdrawal. Most patients find that nicotine withdrawal symptoms peak in the first few days after the last cigarette; withdrawal symptoms then gradually diminish over the next 2–4 weeks."

e. degree of relief that can be reasonably expected

"Over time, you may find you need to use the lozenge less often. Be sure to stick with the recommended daily dosing schedule for the patch and the duration of use needed for the best chance of success. This will help you to be more comfortable while you are quitting."

f. most common side effects

"The most common side effects of the nicotine patch include skin reactions (redness, burning, itching) at the application site and headaches. The sleep disturbances (vivid dreams, insomnia) that you are currently experiencing from the patch should resolve when you remove it before bedtime. The most common side effects of the nicotine lozenge are nausea, hiccups, and heartburn."

g. side effects that warrant medical intervention should they occur

"If you find that reducing your caffeine intake and using the nicotine lozenge do not help relieve your morning cravings and irritability during the day, contact your PCP. If you experience symptoms of nicotine excess (e.g., nausea, vomiting, dizziness, weakness, or rapid heartbeat), also contact your PCP."

h. patient options in the event that condition worsens or persists

"Contact your PCP for the following reasons:

▪ If you experience withdrawal symptoms or severe cigarette cravings, you may need a higher dosage of nicotine.

▪ If you have side effects related to nicotine excess." (see outcome in 8.g.)

i. product storage requirements

"Store the patches and lozenges at room temperature. Keep unused patches in the closed, protective pouch. Keep all new and used patches and lozenges out of the reach of children and pets."

j. specific nondrug measures

"Reduce caffeine use by half to minimize agitation and trouble sleeping. In addition to the counseling I can provide, other counseling programs are available, including the telephone quit line (1-800-QUIT NOW), group classes, and Internet-based programs. We can discuss which options you feel might be useful to you."

Solicit follow-up questions from the patient or caregiver.

"How often can I use the lozenge?"

Answer the patient's or caregiver's questions.

"You should use the lozenge when you feel a strong craving to smoke, such as when you wake up in the morning. The patch will provide a consistent low level of nicotine to help reduce withdrawal symptoms. You should use the nicotine lozenge only when you feel a need, or urge, to smoke. Even though the box says you can use up to 20 lozenges a day, you should not need this many when you use them with the patch. Also remember to switch to the lower 14 mg strength patch after 6 weeks, use this for 2 weeks, then use the 7 mg patch for 2 weeks."

Key: NKA = No known allergies; NRT = nicotine replacement therapy; PCP = primary care provider; SR = sustained release; TMJ = temporomandibular joint.

Patient Counseling for Tobacco Cessation

Smoking is the leading cause of preventable morbidity and mortality in the United States. Substantial benefits of quitting can be realized at any age. Although approximately 70% of adult smokers would like to quit,[52] few are able to do so on their own. Research has shown that tobacco cessation rates can be substantially improved with treatment that includes counseling and pharmacotherapy.[29] (See Nonpharmacologic Therapy for a detailed discussion of counseling.) Health care providers are in an ideal position to identify tobacco users and to either provide assistance throughout the cessation attempt or refer the patient to a tobacco cessation resource. The box Patient Education for Tobacco Cessation describes specific information to provide to patients.

Evaluation of Patient Outcomes for Tobacco Cessation

Follow-up contact is an essential component of treatment for tobacco use and dependence.[29] At each follow-up contact, the provider should do the following:

- Assess a patient's tobacco use status and, if appropriate, evaluate and monitor pharmacotherapy use.
- Congratulate abstinent patients and encourage them to remain tobacco free.

- In cases of relapse, review the specific circumstances; reassess the commitment to abstinence; encourage the patient to learn from his or her mistakes; and identify strategies to prevent future lapses.
- Determine whether the patient is experiencing nicotine withdrawal symptoms or adverse effects from the pharmacotherapy.
- Offer ongoing support. If providing that level of support is not possible, refer the patient to a specialist for more intensive treatment.

Key Points for Tobacco Cessation

- ➤ Apply the 5 A's approach in providing tobacco cessation counseling: ask, advise, assess, assist, and arrange.
- ➤ For a patient who is not ready to quit, provide brief counseling by addressing the 5 R's: relevance, risks, rewards, roadblocks, and repetition.
- ➤ For a patient who is ready to quit, offer counseling and pharmacotherapy. If time is limited, ask about tobacco use, advise the patient to quit, and refer the patient to the toll-free quit line (1-800-Quit-Now).
- ➤ Numerous effective medications are available for tobacco dependence; encourage their use by all patients attempting to quit smoking—except when medically contraindicated or with specific populations for which there is insufficient

---

patient education for
Tobacco Cessation

Tobacco dependence is a chronic disease optimally treated with a combination of counseling and medications. The primary goal of tobacco cessation treatment is to attain complete, long-term abstinence from all nicotine-containing products. For most people, carefully following product instructions and the self-care measures listed here will help ensure optimal treatment outcomes.

Nondrug Methods

- Receiving counseling from a health care provider will increase the success of tobacco cessation. A provider can help develop a tailored tobacco cessation treatment plan.
- Telephone quit lines (e.g., 1-800-Quit-Now) are also available to provide comprehensive counseling services at no cost.

Nonprescription Medications
Nicotine Replacement Therapy (NRT)

- NRT helps relieve and prevent symptoms of nicotine withdrawal by partially replacing the high levels of nicotine that your body is used to obtaining from cigarettes. Use of NRT helps you to focus on changing your smoking routines and to practice new coping skills while decreasing your withdrawal symptoms.
- NRT does not contain any of the harmful tars and other toxins present in tobacco smoke.
- Symptoms of nicotine withdrawal are common and should subside over 2–4 weeks.
- Recommended daily dosages for NRT are shown in Tables 47–5 and 47–8.
- See Table 47–6 for usage guidelines for nicotine gum, Table 47–7 for the nicotine lozenge, and Table 47–9 for the nicotine patch.
- Carefully follow the dosage regimen of the selected product. Failure to do so will increase the chance of having withdrawal symptoms. Discontinuing therapy early might lead to relapse.
- Discontinue the use of any form of NRT if you relapse back to smoking.

- Symptoms of nicotine excess include nausea, vomiting, dizziness, diarrhea, weakness, and rapid heartbeat.
- Do not eat or drink (except water) 15 minutes before or while using the nicotine gum or lozenge.
- Store NRT products at room temperature and protect from light.
- Keep new and used products out of the reach of children and pets.
- For all forms of NRT, consult your primary care provider before use if you have had a recent (in the past 2 weeks) heart attack, experience frequent pain caused by severe angina, have an irregular heartbeat, are pregnant or breast-feeding, are younger than 18 years, or smoke fewer than 10 cigarettes a day.
- You may consider use of the nicotine gum with the patch (gum used only as needed). For other possible medication combinations, speak to your primary care provider first.

When to Seek Medical Attention

- For all forms of NRT, stop use and seek medical attention if irregular heartbeat or palpitations occur, or if you have symptoms of nicotine overdose, such as nausea, vomiting, dizziness, diarrhea, or weakness.
- For nicotine gum: Stop use if mouth, teeth, or jaw problems develop.
- For nicotine lozenge: Stop use if mouth problems, persistent indigestion, or severe sore throat develops.
- For nicotine patch: Stop use if the skin swells, a rash develops, or skin redness caused by the patch does not subside with use of nonprescription hydrocortisone cream or does not go away after 4 days.

evidence of effectiveness (i.e., pregnant women, smokeless tobacco users, light smokers, and adolescents). If a patient has exclusions for self-treatment with NRT, refer the patient to a primary care provider for further assessment.

➤ Advise patients that it is never too late for them to quit, but quitting earlier in life is clearly advantageous. Quitting smoking at any age has immediate as well as long-term benefits by reducing the risk for smoking-related diseases and improving health in general.

REFERENCES

1. U.S. Department of Health and Human Services. *The Health Consequences of Smoking: Cancer. A Report of the Surgeon General*. Rockville, MD: Public Health Service, Office on Smoking and Health; 1982. DHHS Publication No. (PHS) 82-50179.

2. U.S. Department of Health and Human Services. *Adult Cigarette Smoking in the United States: Current Estimate*. Atlanta, GA: U.S. Department of Health and Human Services, Centers for Disease Control and Prevention, National Center for Chronic Disease Prevention and Health Promotion, Office on Smoking and Health; 2012.

3. Centers for Disease Control and Prevention. Smoking-attributable mortality, years of potential life lost, and productivity losses—United States, 2000–2004. *MMWR Morb Mortal Wkly Rep*. 2008;57(45):1226–8.

4. Centers for Disease Control and Prevention. Current cigarette smoking among adults—United States, 2012. *MMWR Morb Mortal Wkly Rep*. 2014;63(02):29–34.

5. Centers for Disease Control and Prevention. Tobacco control state highlights 2012. *Selected indicators for states and ranks*. Accessed at http://www.cdc.gov/tobacco/data_statistics/state_data/state_highlights/2012/pdfs/indicators.pdf, April 7, 2013.

6. Centers for Disease Control and Prevention. Vital signs: current cigarette smoking among adults aged ≥ 18 years with mental illness—United States, 2009–2011. *MMWR Morb Mortal Wkly Rep*. 2013;62(05):81–7.

7. U.S. Department of Health and Human Services. *Healthy People 2020*. Washington, DC: U.S. Department of Health and Human Services; 2010. Accessed at http://www.healthpeople.gov/2020/default.aspx, April 7, 2013.

8. World Health Organization. *Report on the Global Tobacco Epidemic, 2008*. Geneva, Switzerland: World Health Organization; 2008.

9. U.S. Department of Health and Human Services. *The Health Consequences of Smoking: Nicotine Addiction: A Report of the Surgeon General*. Washington, DC: U.S. Government Printing Office; 1988.

10. Benowitz NL. Nicotine addiction. *N Engl J Med*. 2010;362(24):2295–303.

11. U.S. Department of Health and Human Services. *How Tobacco Smoke Causes Disease: The Biology and Behavioral Basis for Smoking-Attributable Disease: A Report of the Surgeon General*. Atlanta, GA: U.S. Department of Health and Human Services, Centers for Disease Control and Prevention, National Center for Chronic Disease Prevention and Health Promotion, Office on Smoking and Health; 2010.

12. Campaign for Tobacco-Free Kids. *Spending vs Tobacco Company Marketing*. Accessed at http://www.tobaccofreekids.org/content/what_we_do/state_local_issues/settlement/FY2013/10.%20State%20Tobacco%20Prevention%20Spending%20vs.%20Tob.%20Co.%20Marketing%2011-27-12.pdf, April 7, 2013.

13. Doll R, Peto R, Boreham J, et al. Mortality in relation to smoking: 50 years' observations on male British doctors. *BMJ*. 2004;328(7455):1519.

14. National Cancer Institute. *Risks Associated with Smoking Cigarettes with Low Machine-Measured Yields of Tar and Nicotine. Smoking and Tobacco Control Monograph No. 13*. Bethesda, MD: U.S. Department of Health and Human Services, National Institutes of Health, National Cancer Institute; 2001. NIH Publication No. 02-5074.

15. Benowitz NL, Hukkanen J, Jacob P 3rd. Nicotine chemistry, metabolism, kinetics and biomarkers. *Handb Exp Pharmacol*. 2009;192:29–60.

16. Benowitz NL. Clinical pharmacology of nicotine: implications for understanding, preventing, and treating tobacco addiction. *Clin Pharmacol Ther*. 2008;83(4):531–41.

17. American Psychiatric Association. *Diagnostic and Statistical Manual of Mental Disorders*. 5th ed. Washington, DC: American Psychiatric Association; 2013.

18. Hughes JR. Effects of abstinence from tobacco: valid symptoms and time course. *Nicotine Tob Res*. 2007;9(3):315–27.

19. U.S. Department of Health and Human Services. *Secondhand Smoke (SHS) Facts*. Atlanta, GA: U.S. Department of Health and Human Services, Centers for Disease Control and Prevention, Coordinating Center for Health Promotion, National Center for Chronic Disease Prevention and Health Promotion, Office on Smoking and Health; 2013.

20. U.S. Department of Health and Human Services. *The Health Consequences of Involuntary Exposure to Tobacco Smoke: A Report of the Surgeon General*. Bethesda, MD: U.S. Department of Health and Human Services, Centers for Disease Control and Prevention, Coordinating Center for Health Promotion, National Center for Chronic Disease Prevention and Health Promotion, Office on Smoking and Health; 2006.

21. Zevin S, Benowitz NL. Drug interactions with tobacco smoking. *Clin Pharmacokinet*. 1999;36(6):425–38.

22. Kroon LA. Drug interactions with smoking. *Am J Health Syst Pharm*. 2007;64(18):1917–21.

23. World Health Organization. *Medical Eligibility Criteria for Contraceptive Use*. 4th ed. Geneva, Switzerland: World Health Organization; 2009:1–121. Accessed at http://www.who.int/reproductivehealth/publications/family_planning/9789241563888/en/, July 1, 2011.

24. Pomp ER, Rosendaal FR, Doggen CJ. Smoking increases the risk of venous thrombosis and acts synergistically with oral contraceptive use. *Am J Hematol*. 2008;83(2):97–102.

25. Tanis BC. Oral contraceptives and the risk of myocardial infarction. *Eur Heart J*. 2003;24(5):377–80.

26. American College of Obstetricians and Gynecologists. ACOG practice bulletin no. 73: use of hormonal contraception in women with coexisting medical conditions. *Obstet Gynecol*. 2006;107(6):1453–72.

27. University of California San Francisco. Rx for Change: Clinician-Assisted Tobacco Cessation. San Francisco, CA: University of California San Francisco; 2004–2014. Accessed at http://rxforchange.ucsf.edu, July 1, 2014.

28. U.S. Department of Health and Human Services. *The Health Benefits of Smoking Cessation. A Report of the Surgeon General*. Rockville, MD: U.S. Department of Health and Human Services, Public Health Service, Office on Smoking and Health; 1990. DHHS Publication No. (CDC) 90-8416.

29. Fiore MC, Jaén CR, Baker TB, et al. *Treating Tobacco Use and Dependence: 2008 Update. Clinical Practice Guideline*. Rockville, MD: U.S. Department of Health and Human Services, Public Health Service; 2008.

30. Shiffman S, Brockwell SE, Pillitteri JL, et al. Use of smoking-cessation treatments in the United States. *Am J Prev Med*. 2008;34(2):102–11.

31. Stead LF, Bergson G, Lancaster T. Physician advice for smoking cessation. *Cochrane Database Syst Rev*. 2008;2:CD000165. doi:10.1002/14651858. CD000165.pub3. Accessed at http://www.thecochranelibrary.com/view/0/index.html.

32. Centers for Disease Control and Prevention. Updated recommendations for prevention of invasive pneumococcal disease among adults using the 23-valent pneumococcal polysaccharide vaccine (PPSV23). *MMWR Morb Mortal Wkly Rep*. 2010;59(34):1102–6.

33. Shiffman S, Dresler CM, Hajek P, et al. Efficacy of a nicotine lozenge for smoking cessation. *Arch Intern Med*. 2002;162(11):1267–76.

34. Stead LF, Perera R, Bullen C, et al. Nicotine replacement therapy for smoking cessation. *Cochrane Database Syst Rev*. 2012;11:CD000146. doi:10.1002/14651858.CD000146.pub4. Accessed at http://www.thecochranelibrary.com/view/0/index.html.

35. GlaxoSmithKline Inc. Zyban [package insert]. Research Triangle Park, NC: GlaxoSmithKline Inc.; September 2010.

36. Foulds J. The neurobiological basis for partial agonist treatment of nicotine dependence: varenicline. *Int J Clin Pract*. 2006;60(5):571–6.

37. Pfizer, Inc. Chantix [package insert]. New York, NY: Pfizer, Inc.; December 2012.

38. U.S. Food and Drug Administration. FDA Drug Safety Communication: Chantix (varenicline) may increase the risk of certain cardiovascular adverse events in patients with cardiovascular disease. July 22, 2011. Accessed at http://www.fda.gov/Drugs/DrugSafety/ucm259161.htm#data, July 23, 2011.

39. Fagerstrom K, Gilljam H, Metcalfe M, et al. Stopping smokeless tobacco use with varenicline: randomized double-blind placebo-controlled trial. *BMJ.* 2010;341:c6549.

40. U.S. Food and Drug Administration. FDA Drug Safety Communication: safety review update of Chantix (varenicline) and risk of cardiovascular adverse events. December 12, 2012. Accessed at http://www.fda.gov/Drugs/DrugSafety/ucm330367.htm, December 14, 2012.

41. Benowitz NL. Cigarette smoking and cardiovascular disease: pathophysiology and implications for treatment. *Prog Cardiovasc Dis.* 2003;46(1):91–111.

42. Joseph AM, Fu SS. Safety issues in pharmacotherapy for smoking in patients with cardiovascular disease. *Prog Cardiovasc Dis.* 2003;45(6):429–41.

43. Henningfield JE, Shiffman S, Ferguson SG, et al. Tobacco dependence and withdrawal: science base, challenges and opportunities for pharmacotherapy. *Pharmacol Ther.* 2009;123(1):1–16.

44. Benowitz N, Dempsey D. Pharmacotherapy for smoking cessation during pregnancy. *Nicotine Tob Res.* 2004;6(suppl 2):S189–202.

45. Shiffman S. Nicotine lozenge efficacy in light smokers. *Drug Alcohol Depend.* 2005;77(3):311–4.

46. Cahill K, Stevens S, Perera R, et al. Pharmacological interventions for smoking cessation: an overview and network meta-analysis. *Cochrane Database Syst Rev.* 2013;5:CD009329. doi:10.1002/14651858. CD009329.

pub2. Accessed at http://www.thecochranelibrary.com/view/0/index.html.

47. U.S. Food and Drug Administration. Nicotine-containing products. *Guidance, Compliance & Regulatory Information.* April 2, 3013. Accessed at http://www.fda.gov/Drugs/GuidanceComplianceRegulatoryInformation/ucm345928.htm?source=govdelivery, April 14, 2013.

48. Stead LF, Hughes JR. Lobeline for smoking cessation. *Cochrane Database Syst Rev.* 2000;2:CD000124. doi:10.1002/14651858.CD000124. Accessed at http://www.thecochranelibrary.com/view/0/index.html.

49. Glover ED, Rath JM, Sharma E, et al. A multicenter phase 3 trial of lobeline sulfate for smoking cessation. *Am J Health Behav.* 2010;34(1):101–9.

50. White AR, Rampes H, Campbell JL. Acupuncture and related interventions for smoking cessation. *Cochrane Database Syst Rev.* 2006;1:CD000009. doi:10.1002/14651858.CD000009. Accessed at http://www.thecochranelibrary.com/view/0/index.html.

51. Cobb NK, Abrams DB. E-cigarette or drug-delivery device? Regulating novel nicotine products. *N Engl J Med.* 2011;365(3):193–5.

52. Centers for Disease Control and Prevention. Cigarette smoking among adults—United States, 2000. *MMWR Morb Mortal Wkly Rep.* 2002; 51(29):642–5.

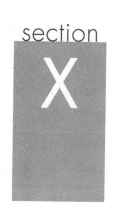
HOME MEDICAL EQUIPMENT

HOME TESTING AND MONITORING DEVICES

Geneva Clark Briggs and Holly Duhon

In 1977, Warner-Lambert introduced the first home pregnancy test kit—an event that had a dramatic effect on the home diagnostics market. Annual sales of home pregnancy tests, excluding Walmart sales, totaled $227 million in 2010.[1] The market continues to grow, with an expanded array of products that are also more user friendly. Forces driving the growth in home diagnostics include (1) increased public interest in health and preventive medicine; (2) reduced health care costs because patients can avoid unnecessary visits to health care providers and can seek earlier treatment of a medical condition; (3) reduced access and availability of health care resources; (4) increased number of available tests; and (5) important advances in technology that have led to simplified, accurate tests that can be easily performed at home.

Home testing and monitoring kits are designed to detect the presence or absence of a medical or physiologic condition and to monitor disease therapy. The Food and Drug Administration (FDA) requires home tests to perform as well as the professional-use equivalent. However, these products must be used properly to achieve accurate results.

This chapter discusses home test kits that aid in detecting the following conditions: pregnancy, female fertility, male fertility, colorectal cancer (fecal occult blood tests), high cholesterol levels, urinary tract infections (UTIs), human immunodeficiency virus (HIV), hepatitis C, and drug abuse. This chapter also covers proper selection and use of blood pressure monitors. In addition, a table of miscellaneous tests is included at the end of the chapter. For other products used in self-monitoring of disorders, see Chapter 8, for vaginal fungal infections, and Chapter 45, for asthma and diabetes mellitus.

Selection Criteria

With the variety of diagnostic and monitoring products available, deciding which test to recommend to a given patient can be challenging. The major product variables to consider include test complexity, ease of reading results, presence of a control, and cost. Table 48–1 addresses these variables as well as the major patient assessment variables, which fall within three general areas:

1. Appropriateness of testing.
2. Ability to accurately conduct the test and interpret the results.
3. Potential interference with test results.

Pregnancy Detection Tests

In 2010, the birth rate in the United States was 13.0 live births per 1000 population. The female fertility rate in women ages 15–44 years was 64.1 births per 1000 women that year.[2] Women are now able to detect pregnancy earlier, including before the day of the missed period because of the heightened sensitivity of at-home pregnancy tests. Early detection of pregnancy is desirable for many reasons, including allowing the woman to make decisions regarding prenatal care and lifestyle changes to avoid potential harm to the fetus.

Physiology of the Female Reproductive Cycle

The female reproductive cycle is approximately 28 days and is hormonally controlled. At the beginning of the cycle (day 1 through approximately day 12), low levels of circulating estrogen and progesterone cause the hypothalamus to secrete gonadotropin-releasing hormone (GnRH). GnRH stimulates release of follicle-stimulating hormone (FSH) and low levels of luteinizing hormone (LH) from the anterior pituitary gland. This combination of hormones promotes development of several follicles within an ovary during each cycle. One follicle continues to mature while the others regress. At midcycle (approximately day 14 or 15), circulating and urinary LH levels significantly increase and cause final maturation of the follicle. Ovulation (rupturing of the follicle and release of the ovum) occurs approximately 20–48 hours after the LH surge. Cells in the ruptured follicle form the corpus luteum, which begins to secrete progesterone and estrogen. For approximately 7–8 days after ovulation, the corpus luteum continues to develop and secrete estrogen and progesterone, inhibiting further secretion of FSH and LH.

Once ovulation occurs, the ovum remains viable for fertilization for only 12–24 hours. Sperm may live up to 72 hours; therefore, optimal days for fertilization to occur include the 2 days before ovulation, the day of ovulation, and the day after ovulation. For the greatest chance of achieving pregnancy, intercourse should take place within 24 hours after the LH surge.

table

48–1   Selection and Use of Home Tests and Devices

- Not all available tests are FDA approved for home use. Check the status of a particular test at www.accessdata.fda.gov/scripts/cdrh/cfdocs/cfIVD/Search.cfm.

- Always check the expiration date before purchasing a product to ensure that reagents are not outdated. For example, a test that has an expiration date of 07/16 expires at the end of July 2016.

- Follow the manufacturer's instructions for storing the tests to ensure that reagents remain stable.

- When selecting a test, consider simplicity of use. Single-step tests are usually desirable because each step is a potential source of error.

- When considering cost, determine the cost per test unit and whether kits with multiple tests are needed. Generic or store-brand kits may cost significantly less.

- When possible, select a test that includes a control to ensure that the test is functioning correctly.

- Read all instructions carefully and completely before attempting to perform a test.

- Note the time of day that the test is to be conducted, the length of time required, and any necessary supplies or equipment; then schedule the best time and place to conduct the test.

- Follow instructions exactly as described and in the order described. If you have questions about the testing procedure or interpretation of the results, consult a health care provider, or call the test manufacturer's toll-free number, if provided, for customer assistance.

- Use an accurate timing device that measures seconds to ensure that you wait the specified length of time between steps. In addition, waiting longer than the specified time to read test results could affect test reliability.

- If the selected test requires observation of a color change, read the test in good lighting. If you have color-defective vision or other visual impairment, ask someone without vision problems to observe the color change and/or read the test results.

- If you have physical limitations that could interfere with performing the test, ask someone to help you perform the test.

- If the test requires a fingerstick and you have a medical condition or take medications that may cause excessive bleeding, consult your health care provider before performing the test.

- Food, medications, and certain diseases or conditions can sometimes interfere with test results.

Key: FDA = Food and Drug Administration.

If fertilization occurs, trophoblastic cells produce human chorionic gonadotropic (hCG) hormone. This hormone causes the corpus luteum to continue to produce progesterone and estrogen, forestalling the onset of menses while the placenta develops and becomes functional. As early as day 7 after conception, the placenta produces hCG, some of which is excreted in the urine. The concentration of hCG continues to increase during early pregnancy, reaching maximum levels 6 weeks after conception. The levels of hCG decline over the following 4–6 weeks and then stabilize for the remainder of the pregnancy.

If fertilization does not occur during a cycle, the corpus luteum degenerates, circulating levels of progesterone and estrogen diminish, and menstruation occurs (days 1–5). Resulting low levels of progesterone and estrogen cause release of GnRH from the hypothalamus, and the hormonal cycle begins again.

Usage Considerations

The hormone produced by the trophoblast of the fertilized ovum, hCG, is detectable in the urine within 1–2 weeks after fertilization. It is composed of multiple forms of hCG, including intact hCG, hyperglycosolated hCG (hCG-H), and free alpha and beta subunits. The primary form detected in early pregnancy is hCG-H.[3] However, most pregnancy tests have a decreased sensitivity for hCG-H and beta subunits, so further improvements are needed to detect pregnancies earlier.[4]

Numerous pregnancy tests with different reaction times and hCG sensitivity are available for home use. Table 48–2 lists some available products that have been tested for accuracy.[5–8] Overall, First Response Early Result may be the best test for detecting

table

48–2   Selected Nonprescription Pregnancy Tests

Trade Name	hCG Sensitivity	Product Features
First Response Early Result	<6.3 mIU/mL	Test stick; best combination of sensitivity and reliability; can test up to 4 days before missed period; First Response Rapid Result produces a result in 1 minute
Clearblue +/– Results	25 mIU/mL	Test stick; can test up to 4 days before missed period; Clearblue digital display test also available
Store brands	100 mIU/mL	Test sticks; some CVS samples failed to work[6]
E.P.T.	100 mIU/mL	Test sticks; some samples failed to work[6]; E.P.T. has digital display test also available
Accu-Clear	>100 mIU/mL	Test sticks or cassettes; 1% of samples failed to work[6]
Fact Plus	>100 mIU/mL	Test sticks or cassettes; can use test sticks to test up to 4 days before missed period

Key: hCG = Human chorionic gonadotropic hormone.
Source: References 5–8.

pregnancy before the fourth week of gestation, when hCG levels are low. After that point, most of the tests are equivalent.

Mechanism of Action

Home pregnancy tests detect hCG in the urine by using monoclonal or polyclonal antibodies in an enzyme immunoassay. The antibodies are bound to a solid surface such as a stick, bead, or filter. If urinary hCG is present, it will form a complex with the antibodies. Another antibody is added, one that is linked to an enzyme and will react with a chromogen to produce a distinctive color. The hCG is sandwiched between the antibody linked to the enzyme and the antibodies bound to the solid surface. Washing or filtering within the testing device removes unbound substances; a chromogen then reacts with the enzyme, causing a color change.

Accuracy Rate

A pregnancy cannot be detected before implantation. Because of natural variability in the timing of ovulation, implantation does not necessarily occur before the expected onset of the next menses. One study found that the highest possible screening sensitivity for an hCG-based pregnancy test conducted on the first day of a missed period is 90% because 10% of women may not have an implanted embryo at that point. Although most pregnancy tests are advertised as 99% accurate, studies estimate that the highest possible screening sensitivity of a home pregnancy test by 1 week after the first day of the missed period is 97%.[9] A test sensitivity for hCG of 12.4 mIU/mL is needed to detect 95% of pregnancies on the expected day of a missed period.[10] The actual accuracy rate of these tests is less because users do not carefully follow the directions; formatting changes and improved instructions could help to improve the patient's ability to use home pregnancy tests and accurately interpret results.[11]

Interferences

A false-positive result may occur if the woman has had a miscarriage or given birth within the previous 8 weeks because hCG may still be present in the body. Medications such as Pergonal (menotropins for injection) and Profasi (chorionic gonadotropin for injection) can produce false-positive results. Unreliable results may occur in patients with ovarian cysts or an ectopic pregnancy. Oral contraceptive use does not affect test results.

Because hCG levels are very low in early pregnancy and may be below the sensitivity of a particular test, false-negative results may occur with home pregnancy tests if they are performed on or before the first day of a missed period. Erroneous results may also result from not allowing refrigerated urine to warm to room temperature before testing, using waxed cups to collect urine, or collecting urine in household containers that contain soap residue.

Usage Guidelines

See the box Patient Education for Pregnancy Tests.

Product Selection Guidelines

Product labeling for most tests states that women may use the test as early as the first day of a missed menstrual period. Some tests that can detect hCG levels at 25 mIU/mL or less can be used 3 days before the missed period. The earlier a pregnancy test is used, the greater the likelihood of a false-negative result. Most pregnancy tests are one-step procedures. Some tests have clear test sticks that allow the woman to see the reaction occurring; this serves as a check that the stick absorbed sufficient urine. Other tests include two devices, which can be helpful if the first test is negative. The newest tests are digital and display the results as "pregnant" or "not pregnant," or "yes" or "no," instead of showing colored lines, which eliminates the need to interpret the results. Test results are generally obtained in 3 minutes.

A study of seven nonprescription pregnancy tests found that First Response Early Result was the most sensitive and most reliable test. It detected hCG at concentrations as low as 6.5 mIU/mL. In addition, this product was expected to detect more than 95% of pregnancies on the first day of a missed period.[6]

Assessment of Pregnancy Test Use

Whether a pregnancy test is appropriate for the patient should be determined first by asking questions about her menstrual cycle and the number of days since intercourse. If product use is appropriate, the patient should be asked about previous use of pregnancy tests and any difficulties the patient had with the tests. Questions about medical disorders and medication use should also be asked to determine whether inaccurate test results are possible or whether special measures may be required to protect the unborn child. Case 48–1 illustrates assessment of a patient who wishes to use a pregnancy test.

Patient Counseling for Pregnancy Tests

During counseling on the use of pregnancy tests, the health care provider should emphasize the importance of following package instructions carefully, especially the instruction for when to begin testing. Pregnancy tests are very sensitive; therefore, the patient should be advised of medical and environmental factors that can cause inaccurate test results. The box Patient Education for Pregnancy Tests lists specific information to provide patients.

Evaluation of Patient Outcomes with Pregnancy Tests

If the pregnancy test result is positive, the woman should assume she is pregnant and contact her health care provider as soon as possible. In addition, if the patient is taking a medication with teratogenic potential (e.g., Accutane or methotrexate) or any medications for chronic conditions, she should be advised to discuss with her health care provider any possible effects the drugs may have on a fetus. If the test result is negative, the woman should review the procedure and make sure she performed the test correctly. She should test again in 1 week if menstrual flow has not begun. If the results of the second test are negative and menses still has not begun, the woman should seek the advice of a health care provider.

case

48-1

Relevant Evaluation Criteria	Scenario/Model Outcome

Information Gathering

1. Gather essential information about the patient's symptoms and medical history, including:

   a. description of symptom(s) (i.e., nature, onset, duration, severity, associated symptoms)

   Patient thinks that she may be pregnant. She has not had a period in 6 weeks according to her calculations, and she has been feeling a little nauseated. She is not due for her annual OB/Gyn checkup for another couple of months.

   b. medical history, including family history

   Menstrual cycle: 29 days; regular cycle in the past. She has regular intercourse with her boyfriend of 1 year.

   c. patient's identity

   Lauren Mason

   d. age, sex, height, and weight

   21 years old, female, 5 ft 5 in., 155 lb

   e. patient's occupation

   College student

   f. concurrent medical conditions, prescription and non-prescription medications, and dietary supplements

   No current medical conditions; multivitamin daily

   g. prior use of diagnostic/monitoring test

   Never used any home diagnostic tests

   h. Potential problems with performing/interpreting test

   Lauren does not know how to use a pregnancy test.

Assessment and Triage

2. Determine if self-testing is appropriate.

   Self-testing is appropriate.

3. Identify exclusions for self-treatment.

   None

4. Formulate a comprehensive list of therapeutic alternatives for the primary problem to determine if triage to a medical provider is required, and share this information with the patient or caregiver.

   Options include:

   (1) Recommend a digital pregnancy test today. Educate the patient to follow all manufacturer's instructions when performing the self-test.

   (2) Advise the patient to make an appointment with her health care provider to verify test results if the test comes back positive.

   (3) Take no action.

Plan

5. Select an optimal therapeutic alternative to address the patient's problem, taking into account patient preferences.

   Because of financial limitations, the patient could try one of the generic store brand tests.

Patient Education

6. Describe the testing procedure to the patient:

   a. specific instructions

   "When you do perform the test, follow the instructions carefully."

   b. how to avoid incorrect results

   See the box Patient Education for Pregnancy Tests.

   Solicit follow-up questions from the patient or caregiver.

   "If the test comes back positive, does this mean I am pregnant?"

   Answer the patient's or caregiver's questions.

   "Most likely. Your medication and medical histories indicate that you would not have a false-positive test result. The test determines whether you have increased hCG levels in your urine. In addition, symptoms of pregnancy are occurring. If the test comes back positive, you should see a health care provider immediately for follow-up."

Evaluation of Patient Outcome

7. Assess patient outcome.

   "You can call if you have any questions while doing the test or are concerned about the results."

Key: hCG = Human chorionic gonadotropic hormone.

Avoidance of Incorrect Results

■ The most accurate results will be obtained by waiting at least 1 week after the date of the expected period. Performing the test too early may produce false-negative results.

■ Be sure to use the urine collection device provided in the kit. Wax particles in waxed cups can clog the test matrix, causing false results. Soap residue in household containers can also interfere with test results.

■ Try to test the urine sample immediately after collection.

■ If the sample must be tested later, store it in the refrigerator but allow the sample to warm to room temperature for 20–30 minutes before testing. Chilled urine may produce false-negative results. Be careful not to redisperse or shake up any sediment present in the sample.

Usage Guidelines

■ Unless package instructions specify otherwise, use the first morning urine because the levels of hCG, if present, will be concentrated at that time.

■ If testing occurs at other times of the day, restrict fluid intake for 4–6 hours before urine collection.

■ Check the expiration date of the packaging. Remove test stick or cassette from packaging just before use. For test sticks, remove cap, if present, from absorbent tip.

■ Apply urine to testing device using whichever of the following methods is specified in package instructions: (1) hold test stick in the urine stream for designated time, (2) urinate into testing well of test cassette, or (3) collect urine in a collection cup and dip the strip in the urine.

■ After the urine is applied, lay the testing device on a flat surface. Wait the recommended time (1–5 minutes) before reading the results. Waiting the maximum allowed time may improve the sensitivity of the test.

■ After reading the results, discard the testing device. If the test result is negative, test again in 1 week if menstruation has not started.

When to Seek Medical Attention

■ If the second test is negative and menstruation has not begun, consult a health care provider.

Source: References 3, 7, and 8.

Female Fertility Tests

Women use basal thermometers and ovulation prediction test kits and devices to time sexual intercourse to coincide with optimal fertility. These tests and devices are also useful for women who want to be more aware of their time of ovulation. However, they are not a reliable means of birth control.

It may take several months of attempting pregnancy for a fertile woman to be successful. Infertility, however, is defined as the medical inability to conceive after 1 year of unsuccessful attempts. Infertility is estimated to occur in 6% of married women ages 15–44 years.[12]

Available nonprescription products for ovulation prediction (Table 48–3) include ovulation detection devices, basal thermometers, and urine tests.[13–18] Each detection method has a different mechanism of action and method of use. Women should pick their own preferred method.

Saliva microscopy and home saliva monitors are also available. These two products are not discussed here because the results obtained are not reliable or the data on accuracy are conflicting.[13]

Basal Thermometry

For many years, women have measured basal body temperature (BBT) to predict the time of ovulation. Resting BBT is usually between 96.0°F (35.5°C) and 97.5°F (36.4°C) during the first part of the female reproductive cycle. Approximately 24–48 hours after ovulation, it rises to a level closer to normal (i.e., 98.6°F [37°C]).[16]

Usage Considerations
Mechanism of Action

When using basal thermometry, women take their temperature (orally, rectally, or vaginally) with a basal thermometer each morning before arising. These temperature measurements are then plotted graphically. A rise in temperature signals that ovulation has occurred. When the increase occurs, women who want to become pregnant should have intercourse as soon as possible to maximize their chances of conception.

Accuracy Rate

The only equipment necessary for monitoring BBT is a basal thermometer, which has smaller gradations than a regular thermometer (i.e., 0.1 degree versus 0.2). Although basal thermometry is a relatively simple method of ovulation prediction, interpreting temperature data can be confusing. The temperature increase that follows ovulation is small (0.4°F–1.0°F [0.2°C–0.6°C]). Women who have trouble reading a thermometer may miss the rise altogether; in this case, a digital model should be used.

Interferences

Several factors, such as emotions, movements, and infections, can influence the basal temperature. Eating, drinking, talking, and smoking should be postponed until after each measurement is obtained.

Usage Guidelines

See the box Patient Education for Ovulation Prediction Tests and Devices.

table 48–3	Selected Nonprescription Ovulation Prediction Tests and Devices	
Trade Name	**Reaction Time**	**Product Features**
Clearblue EasyDigital Ovulation Test	3 minutes	7-day kit or 1-month kit. Urine test sticks; clear and easy to read with no lines to interpret; digital smiley face technology, highly sensitive and easy to read with 97% of study volunteers correctly reading result and considered most preferred test[14]
Clearblue Easy Fertility Monitor	5 minutes	Reusable monitor. Urine test sticks; typically predicts 2-day window of peak or high fertility; stores daily fertility information; easy to read; tests for LH and E3G, an estrogen metabolite
Clearblue Advanced Digital Ovulation Test	5 minutes	1 or 2 month supply available, Urine test sticks + holder, tests for LH and E3G, an estrogen metabolite; typically identifies 4 fertile days
Answer 1-Step Ovulation	5 minutes	7-day kit. Urine test sticks; predicts ovulation within 24–36 hours
Accu-Clear Early Ovulation Predictor Test	3 minutes	5-day kit. Urine test sticks; predicts ovulation within 24–48 hours
First Response 1-Step Ovulation Predictor Test	5 minutes	7-day kit or 1-month supply kit. Urine test sticks; predicts ovulation within 24–36 hours; digital ovulation test also available
Nexcare Basal Thermometer	1 minute	Digital thermometer. Auto memory for last reading; continuous beep to indicate it is working; signals when done; large lighted display
OV-Watch	Measures chloride ions every 30 minutes up to 12 readings	Lightweight watch that is worn during sleep; detects up to 4 days prior to ovulation; easy to use and read

Key: LH = Luteinizing hormone; E3G = estrone-3-glucuronide.
Source: References 13–19.

Product Selection Guidelines

Digital thermometers that track multiple temperature readings for the user are available, although they are more expensive than digital thermometers that lack this feature.

Urinary Hormone Tests

Ovulation prediction tests that use urine samples to estimate the time of ovulation are marketed to women who are having difficulty conceiving and need to pinpoint ovulation.

Usage Considerations
Mechanism of Action

Urine-based ovulation prediction tests use antibodies specific to luteinizing hormone to detect the surge in LH. An enzyme-linked immunosorbent assay (ELISA) elicits a color change that indicates the amount of LH in the urine.[19] The LH surge is revealed by a difference in color or color intensity from that noted on the previous day of testing. The intensity of color on the test stick is directly proportional to the amount of LH in the urine sample. The standard digital test has a similar mechanism of action; when LH is detected in urine, the test stick shows a blue surge line that is read by the digital device. The digital device will display a smiley face, which means that LH has been detected and a woman's chances for conceiving are increased over the next 48 hours. This device also sets an individualized threshold for measuring the user's LH readings and compares them from baseline. The digital device helps to decrease human error. Generally, early morning collection of urine is recommended because the LH surge usually begins early in the day, and the urine concentration is relatively consistent at this time. Some products do not specify a time of day but require only that a consistent time of day be used.

Testing should begin 2–4 days before the estimated day of ovulation. The kit contains directions to determine when to begin testing; the starting date is based on the average length of the past three menstrual cycles. If the cycle varies by more than 3–4 days each month, the woman should use the shortest menstrual cycle to determine the starting date.

The Clearblue Advanced Digital Ovulation Test and Clearblue Fertility Monitor both increase the specificity of ovulation prediction by measuring two hormones, LH and estrone-3-glucuronide (E3G), a component of estrogen. E3G levels rise and fall in a pattern similar to that of LH. The new advanced digital product uses a test holder with disposable test sticks that are designed to detect a user's fertile window. The test holder contains special software that tracks changes in a woman's hormones from baseline in order to display peak and high fertility trends. The Clearblue Fertility Monitor is a small, palm-size device with a light-emitting diode screen that allows the woman to use urine test sticks that she then inserts into the monitor for results. The patient must establish a baseline using data about fluctuations in her hormone levels to accurately predict ovulation. For the first month, the test monitor will instruct the woman to test daily for 10–20 consecutive days, starting on approximately the sixth day after the beginning of menstruation. Using these data, the monitor calculates the time window during which the woman is most likely to conceive. After establishing her baseline, the woman tests for 10–20 days each month, depending on her cycle length. Each day's results are displayed as low, high, or peak fertility. A low result indicates a small chance of conception; a high result indicates an increased chance of conception. This reading is typically displayed for 1–5 days, leading up to the peak fertility period for each cycle. A peak fertility reading indicates the highest chance of conception and is usually observed 2 days before ovulation.[7]

Interferences

Medications used to promote ovulation (e.g., menotropins) artificially elevate LH and may cause false-positive results in ovulation prediction tests that measure only LH. The true LH surge can be detected in patients receiving clomiphene as long as testing does not begin until the second day after the drug therapy ends. Medical conditions associated with high levels of LH, such as menopause and polycystic ovarian syndrome (PCOS), may cause false-positive results for ovulation. Pregnancy can also cause a false-positive result for ovulation. If the patient has recently discontinued using oral contraceptives, the start of ovulation may be delayed for one to two cycles. Therefore, it would not be appropriate to use a home ovulation prediction test until fertilization has been attempted unsuccessfully for 1–2 months after discontinuation of the oral contraceptives.

PCOS, medications that affect the cycle (e.g., oral contraceptives, certain fertility treatments, and estrogen-containing medications), impaired liver or kidney function (which alters levels of E3G), breast-feeding, tetracycline (not oxytetracycline or minocycline), and perimenopause may produce false-positive results with the Clearblue Fertility Monitor. Women who have recently been pregnant, stopped breast-feeding, or stopped using hormonal contraception should consider waiting until they have at least two consecutive natural menstrual cycles (lasting 21–42 days) before using the Clearblue Fertility Monitor.[7]

Usage Guidelines

See the box Patient Education for Ovulation Prediction Tests and Devices.

Product Selection Guidelines

The available ovulation prediction tests vary in the length of time needed to complete the test, method of applying urine to the test stick, number of individual tests provided, and method for reading results. Patients with longer cycles may benefit from purchasing kits that contain more testing sticks.

The Clearblue Fertility Monitor and Clearblue Advanced Digital Ovulation Test have some possible advantages over the traditional ovulation prediction kits, which detect only LH. The traditional kits identify the 24- to 48-hour window around ovulation. Both Clearblue products identify a larger window of several days and do not require that patients interpret color changes. In addition, they measure both LH and E3G, increasing the specificity of ovulation prediction. However, no studies have proved that these advantages increase a woman's chance of accurately identifying ovulation and, ultimately, conceiving. The initial cost of the Clearblue Fertility Monitor is higher than that of the traditional ovulation prediction kits, which detect only LH, but it is reusable for an indefinite period, with only the additional expense of more test sticks.

In an evaluation of 4 ovulation prediction kits, one study found that the Clearblue Digital Ovulation Test was the most preferred by study participants and easiest to read.[14]

Wristwatch Ovulation Prediction Device

OV-Watch, which is worn on the wrist, uses a specialized biosensor to detect and measure the fluctuation of chloride ions to predict ovulation.

Usage Considerations
Mechanism of Action

During a woman's cycle, numerous electrolytes in perspiration fluctuate. One of the electrolytes, chloride, peaks at various times throughout the monthly cycle.[18] Approximately 5 days before ovulation, a chloride ion surge occurs. The OV-Watch has a biosensor that detects the chloride ion surge transdermally. The woman should begin wearing the watch at least 6 hours during sleep, starting on the first, second, or third day of the menstrual cycle. Chloride ion data are recorded every 30 minutes.

Accuracy Rate

The OV-Watch underwent clinical testing to be cleared as an acceptable device by the FDA. Research concluded that the watch was equivalent to the other products that measured LH. However, compared with the other products, the watch detected fertility up to 4 days prior to ovulation. Finally, the data suggest that approximately two-thirds of patients who used the watch were more likely to become pregnant within 6 months.[18]

Interferences

Factors such as excessive moisture, hormonal contraceptives, menopause, liver and kidney disease, breast-feeding, and PCOS can affect the accuracy of the watch.

Usage Guidelines

See the box Patient Education for Ovulation Prediction Tests and Devices.

Product Selection Guidelines

The OV-Watch uses advanced technology to help predict a woman's fertile window. In addition, the more fertile days that a woman can identify, the greater are her chances of becoming pregnant.

Assessment of Female Fertility Test Use

The patient should be asked privately about her reasons for using an ovulation prediction test. If the reason is difficulty in conceiving, the patient should be asked whether she has consulted a health care specialist about a possible fertility problem and whether she has previously used ovulation prediction tests or devices. Questions about other possible pathology and medication use are appropriate to determine possible interferences with test results or temperature measurements.

Patient Counseling for Female Fertility Tests

To use ELISA-based ovulation prediction products effectively, a woman must know approximately when ovulation occurs or be willing to track three menstrual cycles to determine when it occurs. The health care provider should explain hormonal fluctuations during the cycle and how they relate to the use of ovulation prediction tests and devices. The provider should also explain the reason for the number of tests or measurements that must be performed with each type of product. Finally, counseling should emphasize consistent use of the products for at least 3 months to achieve accurate results should. The box Patient Education for Ovulation Prediction Tests and Devices lists specific information to provide patients.

Evaluation of Patient Outcomes with Female Fertility Tests

Ovulation prediction products should not be used for more than 3 months. If conception does not occur within this period, the woman should see a health care provider.

---

patient education for
Ovulation Prediction Tests and Devices

Basal Thermometers
Avoidance of Incorrect Results

- Do not move while taking temperature measurements.
- Emotions can affect temperature measurements.
- If fever is present, discontinue the measurements until resolved. Resume measurements on the first day of the menstrual cycle that occurs after the fever is gone.
- Do not eat, drink, talk, or smoke within 30 minutes before taking temperature measurements.

Usage Guidelines

- Read and follow the instructions thoroughly before using the thermometer.
- Choose one method of taking temperatures (orally, vaginally, or rectally), and use that method consistently.
- Take temperature readings at approximately the same time each morning. Take temperature just before rising each morning after at least 5 hours of sleep. If using a regular basal thermometer, plot the temperatures on a graph. A rise in temperature indicates that ovulation has occurred.

Ovulation Prediction Tests
Avoidance of Incorrect Results

- Fertility medications, PCOS, menopause, and pregnancy can cause false-positive results for ovulation.
- With the Clearblue Easy Fertility Monitor, estrogen-containing medications, impaired liver or kidney function, breast-feeding, tetracycline (but not oxytetracycline or minocycline), and perimenopause can cause false-positive results.
- Recent pregnancy or discontinuation of oral contraceptives or breast-feeding will delay ovulation for one or two cycles. Start testing after two natural menstrual cycles have occurred.

Usage Guidelines (Except Clearblue Easy Fertility Monitor)

- Start using the test 2–3 days before ovulation is expected.
- Follow the manufacturer's specific directions regarding the timing of urine collection. If the first morning urine is not tested, restrict fluid intake for at least 4 hours before testing, and avoid urinating until ready to test the urine so that the urine will not be diluted.
- Test the urine sample immediately after collection.
- If immediate testing is not feasible, refrigerate urine for the length of time specified in the product's directions. Allow refrigerated sample to stand at room temperature for 20–30 minutes before beginning the test.

- Do not shake up any sediment that may be present in the sample.
- If using a kit designed to be passed through the urine stream, either hold a test stick in the urine stream for the specified time, or collect urine in a collection cup and dip the stick in the urine.
- If using a kit not designed to be passed through the urine stream, collect urine in a collection cup, and then place the urine in the testing well using the dropper provided.
- After the urine is placed on the testing device, read the results in 3 to 5 minutes, depending on the manufacturer's instructions.
- Watch for the test's first significant increase in color intensity or, if using a digital test, the display of the "smiley face." Either result indicates that the surge of LH has occurred and that ovulation will occur within 1 or 2 days.
- Once the LH surge is detected, discontinue testing. Remaining tests can be used later, if necessary.
- If the LH surge is not detected, carefully review the testing instructions to ensure that they were performed properly.
- If the testing procedure was accurate, ovulation may not have occurred or testing may have occurred too late in the cycle. Consider testing for a longer period and earlier in the next cycle to increase the chances of detecting the LH surge.

Usage Guidelines for Clearblue Easy Fertility Monitor Test

- For the first month, begin testing on the sixth day after menstruation starts; the monitor will indicate how many total days you should test.
- For subsequent months, test the number of days indicated by the monitor.
- Remove test stick from packaging just before use.
- Hold the test stick in the urine stream; insert stick in monitor.
- Discard test stick after use.

OV-Watch Fertility Predictor Device
Avoidance of Incorrect Results

- Fertility medications, hormonal contraceptives, menopause, impaired liver and kidney function, breast-feeding, and PCOS may interfere with results.
- Do not expose the watch to water or excessive moisture. Wait 1 hour after exercising or showering before wearing the watch.

Usage Guidelines

- Before using the watch, read thoroughly the manufacturer's instructions for attaching the sensor and programming the device.
- Use the watch on the first, second, or third day of the menstrual period.

Key: LH = Luteinizing hormone; PCOS = polycystic ovarian syndrome.
Source: References 15–19.

Male Fertility Tests

Sperm concentration is one of the many factors used to determine male fertility. Because many additional factors play a role in male infertility, a positive test for sperm count is not a guarantee of fertility. Sperm production is influenced by physical, emotional, and psychological factors. Factors such as concentration of hormones, stress, high fever, exercise, travel, surgery, medication, and changes in diet may result in a decreased sperm concentration.

Usage Considerations

The male fertility test measures sperm concentration as either above or below the cutoff of 20 million sperm cells per milliliter, which is the World Health Organization criterion for determining low sperm count.[20] Two test results of fewer than 20 million sperm cells per milliliter obtained at least 3 days apart, but not more than 7 days apart, may indicate male infertility.[21]

Mechanism of Action

The test works by detecting the concentration of a sperm–specific protein (antigen SP-10) in the semen, which is then used to determine the sperm count.[21] The semen is mixed with a buffer to help release the specific protein from the sperm. The mixture then binds to a colloidal gold compound in the test well and flows through the test. If the sample contains more than 20 million cells per milliliter, a reddish line appears, indicating a positive result. The test kit contains all the necessary supplies for the test: a testing device, testing solution, transfer device, and sperm collection cup.

Accuracy Rate

Testing performed by the manufacturer found the overall accuracy of the test to be 98%.[22]

Interferences

There are no known interferences.

Usage Guidelines

See the box Patient Education for Male Fertility Tests.

Product Selection Guidelines

SpermCheck is the only male fertility test currently on the market. Because this test requires the user to determine visually whether a line is present, patients with visual difficulties should seek assistance in interpreting the test results.

Assessment of Male Fertility Test Use

The patient should be asked privately whether he has consulted a health care provider about a possible fertility problem, and whether he has previously used male fertility tests. Questions about possible pathology, medication use, stress, and physical activity are appropriate to determine possible interference with test results.

Patient Counseling for Male Fertility Tests

Because physical, psychological, and emotional factors can affect sperm concentration, the patient should be advised that a positive test does not account for sperm motility, morphology, and other factors that contribute to male fertility. The box Patient Education for Male Fertility Tests lists specific information to provide patients.

Evaluation of Patient Outcomes with Male Fertility Tests

If a negative result is obtained, the patient should contact his health care provider or a fertility specialist. If a negative result is obtained but the patient is trying to increase his sperm count, he can test his fertility every 3 months.

patient education for
Male Fertility Tests

Avoidance of Incorrect Results
- Collect a semen sample between 2 and 7 days after the last ejaculation.
- Test within 3 hours of sample collection.

Usage Guidelines
- The semen sample is collected by masturbation, with semen directed into the liquefaction cup.
- Because freshly ejaculated semen is gel-like, the sample must be allowed to sit for 20 minutes, during which it will thin to a liquid consistency for testing.
- Gently stir the cup with the semen transfer device at least 10 times.
- Insert the semen-transfer device into the sample cup and withdraw semen to the black line, while trying to avoid any air bubbles.
- Gently add the semen to the upright SpermCheck solution bottle. Gently mix the solution by turning the bottle upside down at least

5–10 times. Let the solution bottle stand for 2 minutes before completing the next step.
- Add 6 drops of the solution to the sample well on the SpermCheck Device that is labeled "S."
- Read results exactly 7 minutes after adding the solution.
- To read the test, make sure there is a reddish line beside the "C" (Control) position on the device. If a control line is not present, the test did not work accurately. If a reddish line appears next to the "T" (Test) position on the device, the result is positive (sperm ≥20 million/mL). If no line is present at the test position, the sample is negative (sperm ≤20 million/mL). Do not compare the faintness or darkness of the lines between the control and test positions. The presence of a line is a positive test result.

When to Seek Medical Attention
- If a negative test is obtained, see a health care provider for evaluation and further testing.

Source: Reference 22.

Fecal Occult Blood Tests

Colorectal cancer is the second leading cause of cancer death in the United States. In 2013, the American Cancer Society estimated that 149,880 cases of colorectal cancer would be diagnosed and approximately 51,700 people would die from the disease that year.[23] This disorder may be hard to detect. One early and common symptom of colorectal cancer is rectal bleeding. Checking for hidden (occult) blood in the stool is an easy way to screen for a potential colon problem. Fecal occult blood tests (FOBTs) can be used as an adjunct to more-invasive tests to detect colorectal cancer and other causes of gastrointestinal (GI) bleeding.

Colorectal cancer occurs most commonly in patients with a family history of colorectal cancer, intestinal polyps, or ulcerative colitis. The incidence of colorectal cancer has been associated with advancing age and consumption of high amounts of red and processed meat.[24]

Usage Considerations

Several nonprescription FOBTs are available. They fall into three categories: toilet tests, manual stool application devices, and collection kits that are sent to a laboratory. They are all noninvasive and easy to use in the privacy of the home.

Accuracy Rate

The sensitivity of FOBT for colorectal cancer detection varies from 13%–50%.[25]

Mechanism of Action

The in-home tests detect blood in feces with a colorimetric assay for hemoglobin. The heme portion of hemoglobin acts as an oxidizing agent; it catalyzes oxidation of the test reagent, tetramethylbenzidine, which produces a blue-green color. The appearance of this color indicates a positive test.[26-28]

Blood may be present on the surface or contained within the stool matrix. In general, matrix blood originates in the upper GI tract, whereas surface blood comes from the lower tract. FOBT kits are more likely to detect blood from lower GI abnormalities. The toilet tests use a reagent that is sandwiched between two layers of biodegradable paper. These tests are placed in the toilet bowl after a bowel movement. This type of kit is based on the premise that a significant amount of fecal blood from stool will remain on the surface of the toilet bowl water after a bowel movement. With the stool application device tests, a wooden stick is used to apply stool to two pads or wells. For these tests, the patient should attempt to obtain samples of both surface and inner stool.

Interferences

Blood in the stool can signify a number of conditions in addition to cancer of the colon and rectum, including ulcers, Crohn's disease, colitis, anal fissures, diverticulitis, and hemorrhoids. Any of these conditions can give a positive result for a FOBT.

Women who are menstruating should delay testing until menses has ceased. Menstrual blood that is present in the toilet bowl water or contaminates the stool sample can produce a positive result.

Aspirin, nonsteroidal anti-inflammatory drugs (NSAIDs), and steroids may cause sufficient gastric bleeding to produce positive results. These medications should be avoided for at least 2–3 days before testing and during the test period. One study, however, found that usual doses of aspirin and NSAIDs did not increase the risk of a false-positive FOBT.[29] The study's authors concluded that little concern exists for a false-positive FOBT in patients who cannot safely discontinue aspirin or NSAIDS before specimen collection. Rectally administered medications should also be avoided. However, patients should always consult a health care provider before discontinuing any prescribed medications.

Vitamin C ingestion in excess of 250 mg/day may interfere with the peroxidase action of hemoglobin, causing false-negative results in the ColonTest-Sensitive product.[27] The FOBTs are not specific for human blood and may produce false-positive results if red meat is consumed. A meta-analysis of dietary restriction studies found no difference in response rates between restricting and not restricting meat consumption before testing.[30] Toilet bowl cleaners may also produce false-positive results. The box Patient Education for Fecal Occult Blood Tests lists measures for avoiding inaccurate test results.

Usage Guidelines

See the box Patient Education for Fecal Occult Blood Tests.

Product Selection Guidelines

Patients who want to avoid restricting their diet or stopping vitamin C may prefer the toilet test products, which do not require a diet or medication change. All tests are similar in cost. All products, except ColonTest-Sensitive, have a card on which the patient records results; the patient then gives the card to the health care provider for evaluation.

Assessment of Fecal Occult Blood Test Use

Because of better sensitivity, the American College of Gastroenterology recommends that colonoscopy rather than FOBT be used to screen for colon cancer.[31] For most patients, colonoscopy screening should start at age 50 and be conducted every 5 years; in African Americans, screening should begin at age 45.[31] The American Cancer Society recommends FOBT yearly, colonoscopy every 10 years, or other screening tests such as a virtual colonoscopy every 5 years as options for people ages 50 and over who are at average risk of colon cancer.[32] For those at increased risk, FOBT is not recommended. Patients seeking FOBT information should be assessed for risk factors for colon cancer. Those with risk factors should be encouraged to have a screening test other than FOBT. Determining the potential for false test results is an important consideration. False-negative tests could delay necessary treatment, whereas false-positive tests could cause unwarranted anxiety and expensive follow-up testing.

Avoidance of Incorrect Results

- Do not perform test during times of known bleeding, such as hemorrhoidal or menstrual bleeding.
- Increase dietary fiber intake for several days before testing. Roughage increases the accuracy of the test by stimulating bleeding from lesions that might not otherwise bleed.
- Because bleeding from cancerous lesions may be intermittent, perform the test on three consecutive bowel movements to increase the chance of detecting a possible lesion.
- Complete all three stool tests, even if the first two produce negative results.
- Do not take nonprescription medications such as aspirin and NSAIDs for 2–3 days before testing and during testing.
- Some prescription medications can cause bleeding and may need to be stopped before testing. Consult a health care provider about which medications to stop before performing the test.
- Chemicals in the toilet can interfere with the test. Following the instructions carefully can prevent this problem.

Usage Guidelines

- Do not eat red meat 2–3 days before testing and during the test period because undigested meat may produce a false-positive result.
- Do not take more than 250 mg/day of vitamin C for 2–3 days before and during the test period.

Toilet Test Products (EZ-Detect and Early Detect Colorectal)

- Remove toilet tank cleansers or deodorizers, and flush toilet twice before testing.
- Before testing, use one test pad to perform a water quality check. If any trace of blue appears in the cross-shaped area when the

pad is placed in the toilet water, use another toilet to complete the testing. Perform this water quality check on the second toilet as well.
- Immediately after a bowel movement, place a pad in the toilet bowl, printed side up. After 2 minutes, check for the appearance of a blue cross on the test pad (positive result).
- If color changes differ from the blue cross, discard the pad and repeat the test after the next bowel movement.
- Repeat the test on the next two bowel movements.
- If results are negative for all three tests, use remaining pad to perform a quality check of the test pads using the positive control chemical package that is provided. Flush the toilet and empty the contents of the package into the bowl as it refills. Float the remaining test pad in the water, printed side up. After 2 minutes, check for a blue cross, which indicates the test pads are working properly. If the blue cross does not appear, call the product manufacturer's assistance line provided with the product.

Stool Application Product (ColonTest-Sensitive)

- Open the test device lid. Apply a stool sample to wells A and B. Try to get both surface and inner stool with each sample.
- Close the device lid and press on the space labeled "press last" to break the test ampule.
- Turn the test device over and hold in a vertical position for 15 seconds.
- The test is positive if wells are partially or completely blue. The test is negative if wells are beige or brown.
- Repeat the test on the next two bowel movements.

When to Seek Medical Attention

- Notify a health care provider if any of the three tests is positive.

Source: References 26–28.

Patient Counseling for Fecal Occult Blood Tests

When counseling a patient on the use of FOBTs, the health care provider should emphasize the importance of following package instructions carefully. The box Patient Education for Fecal Occult Blood Tests lists specific information to provide patients.

Evaluation of Patient Outcomes with Fecal Occult Blood Tests

A patient evaluating the results of an FOBT must remember that the test is a screening method and is not specific to a particular disease. A positive test result may indicate any medical condition that causes a loss of blood through the GI system. The primary value of FOBT is to alert patients and health care providers that a thorough workup may be needed. The kits are not intended to replace other diagnostic procedures. Patients should be advised to contact their health care provider if a positive test result is obtained.

Cholesterol Tests

Elevated levels of low-density lipoprotein cholesterol (LDL-C) and triglycerides and low levels of high-density lipoprotein cholesterol (HDL-C) are major contributors to the development of atherosclerotic heart disease, which can result in heart attack and stroke.[33] Fourteen percent of American adults have high cholesterol.[34] The National Cholesterol Education Program recommends that all adults have a lipid profile measured at least every 5 years, starting at age 20.[33] A home cholesterol test is one means of achieving this critical step to minimize the risk for cardiovascular disease. However, this test should not replace a complete lipid panel conducted by a health care provider.

Because elevated cholesterol is a chronic condition that requires lifestyle modification and, frequently, medication for treatment, adhering to a treatment plan can be difficult for patients. Home cholesterol tests can help monitor the efficacy of and adherence to diet, exercise, and medication plans.

Usage Considerations

Some nonprescription cholesterol tests (Table 48–4) measure only total cholesterol, whereas others also measure LDL-C, HDL-C, and triglycerides.[35-40] Individuals with diabetes might want to consider a device such as the CardioChek, which measures glucose levels in addition to cholesterol and triglyceride levels. The CholesTrack and First Check kits allow patients to measure their total blood cholesterol levels at home. Check Up America offers a self-collected, laboratory-performed test for a complete lipid profile.

Mechanism of Action

With the total cholesterol test cassettes, cholesterol present in a blood sample is converted into hydrogen peroxide through a chemical reaction involving cholesterol esterase and cholesterol oxidase.[35,36] The peroxide then reacts with horseradish peroxidase and a dye to produce the color that rises along the cholesterol test's measurement scale. The test cassette has two separate indicator spots that change color to show that the test is functioning properly. One of the indicator spots also indicates completion of the test, signaling that it is time to read the scale.

CardioChek, Accutrend Plus, and Q. Steps Cholesterol Biometer all use a reflectance photometer that reads the color intensity of the chemical test reaction.[37-39] Similar to a glucose meter, the results of the test are displayed on a screen. Check Up America's lipid profile is performed by a Clinical Laboratory Improvement Act (CLIA)–certified laboratory.[40]

Accuracy Rate

The accuracy rate of home cholesterol tests is debated. Except for Check Up America, which is mailed to a laboratory, all products are FDA approved for home use, are CLIA-waived devices, and are rated substantially equivalent to a laboratory-based cholesterol test. A published study of the CholesTrak device found that untrained patients obtained results that correlated well with a laboratory-based cholesterol reference method.[41] Several years ago, *Consumer Reports* tested the CholesTrak, First Check, and CardioChek kits. The first two, which are essentially the same device, gave results that varied no more than 15% from laboratory values. The CardioChek yielded results that were "often wide of the mark."[42] The report provided no more specifics. The professional version of the CardioChek (CardioChek PA) has been tested against another point-of-care device (Cholestech LDX) and laboratory measurements and did not meet the National Cholesterol Education Program (NCEP) accuracy goal.[43]

Interferences

Good fingerstick technique is necessary to avoid erroneous results with cholesterol tests. Two or three hanging drops of blood are needed, but excessive squeezing and milking of the finger will negatively affect the quality of the blood sample. If sufficient blood cannot be obtained from the first fingerstick, the patient should use a different finger. A low cholesterol value may result if the blood sample is too small or if it takes longer than 5 minutes to collect the necessary amount of blood.

The patient should avoid doses of 500 mg or more of vitamin C before the test to avoid obtaining an artificially low result. Vitamin C slows the development of the color reaction by slowing the rate of peroxide production by oxidases.

Usage Guidelines

See the box Patient Education for Cholesterol Tests.

Product Selection Guidelines

Although significantly more expensive than individual total cholesterol test cassette kits, the cholesterol meters are reusable with the purchase of additional testing materials and will store test results. Some of the meters have the ability to test for HDL-C and triglycerides, whereas the other home tests measure only total cholesterol. Check Up America provides a lipid profile done in a certified laboratory, but results are not immediately available.

Assessment of Cholesterol Test Use: A Case-Based Approach

Whether the patient has been diagnosed with or has some reason to be concerned about hypercholesterolemia should be determined before a cholesterol test is recommended. Any factors that could affect the test results should also be determined.

Case 48–2 is an example of assessment of a patient who wishes to use a cholesterol test.

table 48–4	Selected Nonprescription Cholesterol Tests
Trade Name	**Product Features**
CholesTrak AccuMeter Home Cholesterol Test/First Check Home Cholesterol Test	Measures total cholesterol; not reusable; includes test cassette, lancet, and chart for interpreting test results from a drop of blood; chart is specific for test cassette and should not be reused
CardioChek	Measures total cholesterol, HDL-C, and triglycerides; can also measure glucose and ketones; stores results; reusable; separate test strip and corresponding color-coded memory chip required for each type of test
Accutrend Plus and Cholesterol Biometer	Measures total cholesterol; can also measure glucose; stores results; reusable; separate test strip required for each type of test; low and high control solutions (Accutrend Plus only)
Check Up America Cholesterol Panel	Lipid profile (total cholesterol, triglycerides, HDL-C, LDL-C) results are obtained after mailing sample to laboratory; not reusable; contains lancet and sample collection cassette

Key: HDL-C = High-density lipoprotein cholesterol; LDL-C = low-density lipoprotein cholesterol.
Source: References 35–40.

case
48–2

Relevant Evaluation Criteria	Scenario/Model Outcome

Information Gathering

1. Gather essential information about the patient's symptoms and medical history, including:

   a. description of symptom(s) (i.e., nature, onset, duration, severity, associated symptoms)

   b. medical history, including family history

   c. patient's identity

   d. age, sex, height, and weight

   e. patient's dietary habits

   f. concurrent medical conditions, prescription and non-prescription medications, and dietary supplements

   g. prior use of diagnostic/monitoring test

   h. potential problems with performing/interpreting test

Patient recently started a new medication and is interested in knowing whether her cholesterol level has gone down.

She has heart disease, high cholesterol, diabetes, and hypertension. Her health care provider checks her cholesterol level annually.

Sue Esposito

68 years old, female, 5 ft 4 in., 180 lb

Patient says that she tries to stick with low-fat, low-cholesterol diet.

Simvastatin 20 mg, ezetimibe 10 mg, metformin 850 mg, losartan 50 mg, clopidogrel 75 mg daily (adherence verified by refill records)

Sue checks her blood pressure at home but does not check her glucose.

She does have some visual impairment and lives alone.

Assessment and Triage

2. Determine if self-testing is appropriate.

3. Identify exclusions for self-treatment.

4. Formulate a comprehensive list of therapeutic alternatives for the primary problem to determine if triage to a medical provider is required, and share this information with the patient or caregiver.

Self-testing is not appropriate.

Visual impairment, no help at home to read test, and use of clopidogrel

Options include:

(1) Refer patient for cholesterol testing.

(2) Take no action.

Plan

5. Select an optimal therapeutic alternative to address the patient's problem, taking into account patient preferences.

The patient understands why self-testing is not appropriate. She has an appointment with her health care provider in 4 months but will see whether it can be rescheduled to an earlier date.

Evaluation of Patient Outcome

6. Assess patient outcome.

Contact the patient in a day or two to ensure that she made an appointment and sought medical care for repeat testing.

Patient Counseling for Cholesterol Tests

Counseling about cholesterol tests should emphasize the importance of properly collecting blood samples. Patients should also be advised to seek assistance with the fingerstick, if needed. As further assurance of accurate test results, patients should be advised of factors that can cause inaccurate test results. The box Patient Education for Cholesterol Tests lists specific information to provide patients.

Evaluation of Patient Outcomes with Cholesterol Tests

Any patient who obtains a total cholesterol result of 200 mg/dL or greater, an HDL–C of 40 mg/dL or less, or triglycerides of 150 mg/dL or greater should see a health care provider for a full lipid profile and appropriate medical workup. Patients

should not adjust their cholesterol-lowering medications based on a home test without consulting their health care provider.

Urinary Tract Infection Tests

Urinary tract infections (UTIs) are the cause of 4 million visits to health care providers every year.[44] Women have a shorter urethra compared with men and are therefore more likely to contract UTIs because of retrograde migration of bacteria from the skin. Conditions that increase risk of UTIs include pregnancy, diabetes, urinary stones, urinary obstructions such as those caused by an enlarged prostate, presence of urinary catheters, and a history of UTIs.[45]

Avoidance of Incorrect Results

- If two or three hanging drops of blood cannot be obtained, or if it takes longer than 5 minutes to collect this amount of blood, do not perform the test.
- Do not excessively squeeze or milk the finger.
- If taking vitamin C in doses of 500 mg or more, do not take the dose within 4 hours of testing.
- The lancet is a biohazard; dispose of it in a puncture-resistant container.

Usage Guidelines

- Before starting the test, wash your hands thoroughly with soap and warm water, and then dry them.
- To stabilize the cholesterol level, sit and relax for 5 minutes before performing the test.
- CardioChek Test: Insert the memory chip corresponding to the desired test into the meter and turn on the meter.
- Lance the outside of one fingertip, and wipe away the first sign of blood with the gauze pad. Then apply blood to the testing device as quickly as possible. Test cassettes (CholesTrak/First Check): Fill the well of the test cassette. Cholesterol meters: Apply enough blood to cover the testing area of a strip. Check Up America Test:

Place enough blood to fill the well on the test device and to turn the indicator window red.

- Test cassettes: Wait at least 2 minutes, but no more than 4 minutes, before pulling the clear plastic tab on the right side of the cassette. Pull the tab until it clicks into place and a red line appears. Use a timepiece with a second hand for accurate timing. Wait another 10–12 minutes. When the "END" indicator turns green, measure the height of the purple column against the scale printed on the cassette. Use the result chart included in the kit to interpret the reading.
- Cholesterol Meter: A test strip may need to be inserted before applying blood for the meter to read the bar code. The test strip can be removed to apply the blood sample. The meter displays the test results in approximately 1–3 minutes.
- Check Up America Test: Allow blood to dry on the test cassette. Seal the device in the provided mailing pouch along with the completed paperwork. Mail to the laboratory. Results will be available online in approximately 1 week.
- Dispose of the lancet in a puncture-resistant container.

When to Seek Medical Attention

- If the total cholesterol reading is 200 mg/dL or greater, HDL-C is 40 mg/dL or less, or triglycerides are 150 mg/dL or greater, see a health care provider for evaluation and further testing.

Key: HDL-C = High-density lipoprotein cholesterol.
Source: References 35–40.

The gram-negative bacterium *Escherichia coli* is responsible for 80% of UTIs.[44] Other gram-positive and gram-negative bacteria account for the other 20% of causative organisms. Symptoms of a UTI include pain on urination, the sensation of an urgent need to urinate, frequent urination, blood in the urine, and lower abdominal pain or discomfort.

Two primary uses for UTI tests are (1) early detection of an infection in patients with a history of recurrent UTIs or risk factors associated with UTIs and (2) confirmation that an infection has been cured by antibiotic therapy.

Usage Considerations

Two types of UTI tests are available. The mechanism of action is the primary difference between the two.

Mechanism of Action

One type of UTI test (UTI Home Test) detects nitrites in the urine on the basis of the principle that gram-negative bacteria reduce nitrate in the urine to nitrite.[46] In the test strip, arsanilic acid reacts with urinary nitrite to form a diazonium compound, which in turn reacts with another chemical on the strip to produce a pink color. A positive test requires a bacterial concentration of 10^5 per milliliter of urine. This test also detects protein in the urine, another clinical sign of a UTI.

The other type of test (AZO Test Strips, store brands) detects both nitrite and leukocyte esterase (LE), an enzyme unique to leukocytes (white blood cells).[47] White blood cells may be found in the urine when a UTI is present.

Accuracy Rate

In general, nitrite-only tests have low sensitivity (45%–60%) and high specificity (85%–98%).[48] Higher levels of accuracy are achieved in elderly, pregnant, and urology patients. Combining nitrite and LE or urinary protein in one test not only increases overall sensitivity and specificity but also decreases the risk of false-negative results.

Interferences

A strict vegetarian diet that provides insufficient urinary nitrates can cause false-negative nitrite results with a UTI test. Tetracycline may also produce a false-negative reading for nitrites, along with doses of vitamin C in excess of 250 mg because ascorbic acid blocks the nitrite test reaction. The patient should allow 10 hours between the last dose of vitamin C and the test procedure. Doses of vitamin C in excess of 500 mg within 24 hours of testing may result in a false-negative result for the LE test by blocking the development of the color reaction.[47] Dyes or medications such as phenazopyridine, commonly used by patients with UTIs, may cause a false-positive result by changing the sensor pad to pink.

Usage Guidelines

See the box Patient Education for Urinary Tract Infection Tests.

Product Selection Guidelines

The UTI Home Test is a test stick similar to those used in pregnancy tests. Although the AZO test strips have a small handle attached, the longer test sticks may be easier to hold in the urine stream.

Assessment of Urinary Tract Infection Tests

The patient's reason for using a UTI test should be determined before a test is recommended. If the patient is testing for a suspected UTI, the patient's symptoms and risk factors for UTIs should be evaluated. If symptoms of a UTI are present, the patient should be referred to his or her health care provider immediately for evaluation and treatment. If the patient is testing to find out whether a treated UTI has been cured, the patient's adherence to the therapy should be assessed. The patient's diet and medication use are important factors to evaluate for possible interference with test results.

Patient Counseling for Urinary Tract Infection Tests

If the sensor pad is to be immersed in a cup of urine, counseling on the use of UTI tests should emphasize the importance of collecting a clean sample of midstream urine. A patient with visual difficulties should be advised to seek assistance in interpreting test results. As further assurance of accurate test results, patients should be advised of medical and dietary factors that can cause inaccurate test results. The box Patient Education for Urinary Tract Infection Tests lists specific information to provide patients.

Evaluation of Patient Outcomes with Urinary Tract Infection Tests

Because UTI tests will detect only about 90% of infections, the patient should contact a health care provider if a negative result is obtained but UTI symptoms persist. If a positive result is obtained, the patient should contact a health care provider immediately for evaluation and treatment.

Human Immunodeficiency Virus Tests

More than 50,000 new cases of human immunodeficiency virus (HIV) infection occur each year in the United States, and an estimated 18% of individuals with HIV are undiagnosed.[49] Home HIV tests allow a person to test for HIV in privacy.

Acquired immunodeficiency syndrome (AIDS) is an incurable disease caused by the HIV virus. The disease destroys the body's immune system. HIV infection can be contracted by contact with infected body fluids such as blood or semen. People at risk for contracting the virus include those who (1) share needles or syringes for the purpose of injecting drugs, including steroids; (2) have sexual intercourse with a person infected with HIV, with someone who injects drugs, or with multiple partners; (3) had a blood transfusion anytime between 1978 and May 1985; and (4) were born to a mother infected with HIV.

Usage Considerations

Home test kits that require saliva or blood samples for HIV detection are currently available. Home Access HIV Test and Home Access Express HIV Test Systems require a blood sample. A saliva-based kit (OraQuick) was approved for home use in 2012.

Mechanism of Action

The HIV tests detect antibodies to the virus. Because 3 weeks to 6 months may be required for an exposed individual to develop sufficient antibodies for detection, the time of possible exposure to the virus must be considered in determining when to perform the test.

---

patient education for

Urinary Tract Infection Tests

Avoidance of Incorrect Results

- Persons on a strict vegetarian diet or tetracycline may not obtain accurate results.
- Certain dyes or medications, such as phenazopyridine, may cause a false-positive result by changing the sensor pad to pink.
- If using the UTI Home Test, do not take 250 mg or more of vitamin C within 10 hours of testing.
- If using AZO Test Strips, do not take 500 mg or more of vitamin C within 24 hours of testing.
- Women should not use AZO Test Strips during menses because menstrual blood will cause a false-positive result.

Usage Guidelines

- Clean the genital area thoroughly before collecting a urine sample.
- Test the first urine of the morning or, for later testing, use urine held in the bladder for at least 4 hours.

- To improve sensitivity, test on 3 consecutive days if the test on the previous day was negative.
- Depending on the test purchased, pass the test strip or stick through the urine stream.
- Do not touch the sensor pad with your fingers because skin oils can interfere with the test reaction. If urine is collected in a cup, immerse the sensor pad in the cup for 1 second.
- Make sure urine completely covers the pad.
- Wait the indicated time (30–60 seconds), then compare the color on the sensor pad with the color chart provided.
- Wait no longer than 3 minutes to read the test strip, and ignore any color changes that occur after that time.

When to Seek Medical Attention

- Contact a health care provider immediately for evaluation and treatment of any positive test.
- If the test is negative but symptoms persist, see a health care provider immediately for evaluation and treatment.

Source: References 46 and 47.

The saliva test uses technology similar to that used in home pregnancy tests to detect antibodies to both HIV-1 and HIV-2.[50] After collection, the home HIV test blood samples are mailed to a certified laboratory for processing. Positive samples are rescreened twice. Repeated positive samples are confirmed with an immunofluorescent assay.[51]

Interferences

Providing an inadequate blood sample (i.e., incompletely filling the circle on the blood sample card) or inadequately swabbing the gums to provide an adequate saliva sample may cause inaccurate results.

Usage Guidelines

See the box Patient Education for HIV Tests.

Product Selection Guidelines

Many people will prefer to use the saliva test because it gives faster results and does not require a fingerstick. Its price is similar to that of the first Home Access test. For the blood tests, the two available HIV tests differ in price and turnaround time to obtain results. The first test, Home Access, takes approximately 7 business days to obtain the results. The second, Home Access Express, takes approximately 3 business days. The Home Access sample is

sent to the testing laboratory by regular mail, whereas the Home Access Express sample is shipped through Federal Express. Consequently, the Home Access Express version costs more.

Assessment of HIV Test Use

The elapsed time since possible exposure to the HIV virus should be determined before an HIV test is recommended. The patient may not know all the risk factors for HIV infection; therefore, whether the patient has engaged in any activities that increase risk for contracting HIV should be tactfully determined. The patient should be asked about medical disorders that might rule out the use of a fingerstick-based test, such as an anticoagulation or bleeding disorder, or physical limitations that might interfere with performing the test.

Patient Counseling for HIV Tests

Counseling on the use of HIV blood tests should emphasize the importance of applying enough blood on the specimen card to ensure an accurate reading. Patients should also be advised of the fragility of blood samples and not to delay mailing the specimen card. Counseling for the saliva test should emphasize the importance of adequately swabbing the gums with the test stick. The box Patient Education for HIV Tests lists specific information to provide patients.

---

patient education for
HIV Tests

Precautions—Blood Tests
- Do not share the test lancet with other individuals. Do not allow the blood being tested to contact other individuals.
- The lancet is a biohazard; dispose of it in a puncture-resistant container.

Avoidance of Incorrect Results—Saliva Test
- Do not open any of the packets until you are ready to begin the test.
- Do not eat, drink, or use oral care products (such as mouthwash, toothpaste, or whitening strips) for 30 minutes before starting the test.
- Remove dental products such as dentures or retainers that cover gums.
- To prevent a false-positive result, swab each gum only once.

Usage Guidelines—Blood Tests
- Call the product manufacturer's toll-free number to register and receive pretest counseling. The manufacturer's customer representative will ask for the confidential code included in the kit.
- Using alcohol, clean the fingertip chosen for puncture. Allow alcohol to dry.
- Prick the cleaned fingertip using the lancet provided, and place a few drops of blood on the blood specimen card. Fill the circle on the card completely to ensure a readable test. Examine the back of the card to ensure that the blood soaked through. If it did not, place more blood on the front of the card. If a second fingerstick is needed, use the second lancet provided in the kit.
- Allow the card to air dry for 30 minutes; place the sample in the specimen return pouch, and seal the pouch in the prepaid and

addressed shipping package. Be sure that the processing laboratory receives the specimen within 10 days of sampling.
- To obtain the results, call the manufacturer's toll-free number 3–7 business days after mailing the specimen, depending on which test kit was used.
- Note that counseling is available 24 hours a day, for both negative and positive results, and counseling is included in the cost of the testing unit.

Usage Guidelines—Saliva Tests
- A timer or watch is needed.
- Remove the test tube from packaging, pop it open, and insert it into the holder. Hold the test tube upright to avoid spilling the liquid that is inside.
- Remove the test stick from packaging. Do not touch the test pad.
- Swipe the test pad along upper and lower gums. Swipe each gum only once.
- Insert the test stick into the test tube with the test window facing forward. Start timing.
- Read the test result in the test window at 20 minutes. After 40 minutes, the results may be invalid.
- The test kit provides guidelines for reading results and what the results mean. One line at C is negative. A line at C and T is positive.
- Note that counseling on performing the test is available 24 hours a day from the company.

When to Seek Medical Attention
- If the test is positive, see a health care provider immediately for evaluation and treatment. Avoid activities that can result in transfer of blood or other body fluids to other individuals.

Source: References 50 and 51.

Evaluation of Patient Outcomes with HIV Tests

A patient with a positive result should see a health care provider to be retested for confirmation of HIV infection. Infected patients should be counseled on precautions to avoid infecting others. Patients with negative results should confirm that sufficient time has passed since the potential exposure.

Hepatitis C Tests

Hepatitis C (HCV) is one of six identified hepatitis viruses. With an estimated 3.2 million chronically infected individuals, HCV infection is the most common blood-borne infection in the United States.[52]

The following are risk factors for hepatitis C[53]:

- Use of injectable drugs
- Receipt of clotting factor concentrate produced before 1987
- Long-term hemodialysis
- Transfusion or organ transplant before 1992
- Sexual intercourse with multiple partners
- Birth by a mother infected with hepatitis C
- Occupational exposure to blood

Hepatitis C induces liver damage by causing hepatic cell necrosis and inflammation, which over time may progress to fibrosis, cirrhosis, and hepatocellular carcinoma. Of people infected with hepatitis C, 75%–85% are likely to progress to the chronic disease state.[52] Clinically, hepatitis C may go undetected for many years; liver disease may be advanced by the time symptoms arise.

Usage Considerations

Home Access Hepatitis C Check is a single-use test kit containing two lancets, a blood sample card, a gauze pad, an adhesive bandage, and a postage-paid envelope. After collection, the blood sample is mailed to a certified laboratory for processing. Each kit also includes a unique personal identification number, which the purchaser uses to register the kit and access test results.

Mechanism of Action

The kit tests for presence of antibodies to the hepatitis C virus, not the virus itself. The Hepatitis C Check uses an ELISA to test for antibodies and then confirms the results with a recombinant immunoblot assay.[53] Because 6 months may be required to develop sufficient antibodies for detection, the time since possible exposure to the virus must be considered in determining when to perform the test.

Interferences

Providing an inadequate blood sample (i.e., incompletely filling the circle on the blood sample card) may cause inaccurate results.

Usage Guidelines

See the box Patient Education for Hepatitis C Tests.

Product Selection Guidelines

Hepatitis C Check is the only test kit currently available for hepatitis C detection.

Assessment of Hepatitis C Test Use

A patient who recently has been infected may receive a false-negative result because antibodies to the virus have not had sufficient time to form. Clinical studies on file with the manufacturer report no false-positive results.[53] The patient may not know all the risk factors for hepatitis C; therefore, whether the patient has engaged in any activities that can cause the disease should be tactfully determined. The patient should be asked about medical disorders that might rule out use of a fingerstick-based test or physical limitations that could interfere with performing the test.

Patient Counseling for Hepatitis C Tests

Patients should be advised of the fragility of blood samples and not to delay mailing the specimen card. The box Patient Education for Hepatitis C Tests lists specific information to provide patients.

---

patient education for
Hepatitis C Tests

Precautions
- Do not share the test lancet with other individuals.
- Do not allow the blood being tested to contact other individuals.
- The lancet is considered a biohazard; dispose of it in a puncture-resistant container.

Usage Guidelines
- Register the PIN (personal identification number) with the manufacturer by calling the provided toll-free telephone number and following the automated directions.
- Remain seated during the testing process to prevent falling if dizziness occurs.
- Before starting the test, wash your hands thoroughly with soap and warm water, and then dry them.
- Date the blood sample card.

- Lance the side of one of your middle fingers.
- Apply a sufficient number of blood drops until both the front and back of the circular area on the testing card are saturated.
- Allow the sample to dry at least 30 minutes before sealing it in the pouch and mailing.
- Within 4–10 business days after mailing the sample, call the toll-free number provided, using the PIN to access the test results. Test results are available for up to 1 year.
- Note that counseling is included in the cost of the testing unit and is available 24 hours a day, for both negative and positive results.

When to Seek Medical Attention
- If the test is positive, see a health care provider immediately for evaluation and treatment. Avoid activities that can result in transfer of blood or other body fluids to other individuals.

Source: Reference 53.

Evaluation of Patient Outcomes with Hepatitis C Tests

Patients who test positive should be referred to a health care provider, given that treatment options are available only by prescription. Infected patients should be counseled on precautions to avoid infection of others. These patients should also be advised to avoid alcohol and other drugs that may advance the progression of liver disease. They should also be tested for and vaccinated against other forms of hepatitis, such as the hepatitis A and B viruses.

Drug Abuse Tests

An estimated 8.7% of Americans abuse drugs, whether legal or illegal.[34] The symptoms of drug use are varied but may include withdrawal from normal activities, fatigue, red eyes, drowsiness, slurred speech, and chronic cough. The National Institute of Drug Abuse (www.nida.nih.gov) is a good resource for specific symptoms for the various drugs of abuse. Drug abuse tests may allow parents and caregivers to detect drug use early enough to affect the course of addiction.

Usage Considerations

Numerous products for detecting use of drugs are available in retail stores and pharmacies, by telephone, and through the Internet. A number of the tests currently available are not FDA approved for home use. FDA is currently following a policy that the agency proposed and that allows the marketing of non-FDA-approved home test kits if the specimen is mailed to a certified laboratory. Table 48–5 lists some example tests and the substances that each test identifies.

Home drug tests are marketed primarily to parents as an aid for determining drug use in their children. These tests are a means of obtaining results anonymously when drug use is suspected. Home drug testing, however, is not a substitute for open communication between parents and children regarding drug use.

Users of these tests may have questions about how soon drugs can be detected after consumption and how long they can be detected after being used. Clearance rates for common drugs of abuse are given in Table 48–6.[54] These are only guidelines, however, and the times can vary significantly from these estimates based on how long the person has been taking the drug, the amount they use, or the person's metabolism.

Samples of urine or hair are collected at home. The hair tests and some of the urine tests are mailed to a clinical laboratory, with results obtained by telephone or over the Internet. For some of the urine tests, the user conducts a preliminary screening test in the home and then mails positive samples to a laboratory for confirmation. Other urine tests are performed only at home. Saliva tests are available, but they are currently marketed only to drug testing programs and employers.

Some of the test kits include telephone counseling to (1) help parents recognize the signs of drug use, (2) assist in creating a family drug policy, and (3) emphasize that parents should use the test to develop trust and open communication within their families, rather than to intimidate with the threat of random testing. Some telephone counseling programs provide referrals to rehabilitation and counseling services in the family's community.

Mechanism of Action

For the home urine tests, an immunochromatographic assay similar to the home pregnancy and ovulation tests is used for

table **48–5**	**Selected Nonprescription Home Drug Abuse Tests**			
Product (Web site)	**Time to Result**	**Body Site**	**Testing Location**	**Substances Detected**
At Home Drug Test (www. phamatech.com)	10 minutes for initial screen; 5–7 days for laboratory confirmation	Urine	Home; send away for confirmation	Depends on kit purchased; one kit tests for amphetamines, marijuana, cocaine, and opiates; other kits test for a single substance
Dr. Brown's Home Drug Testing System (www. drbrowns.com)	5–7 days	Urine	Send away	Marijuana, cocaine, amphetamines, phencyclidine, codeine, morphine, heroin
PDT-90 Personal Drug Testing Service (www. psychemedics.com)	5–7 days	Hair	Send away	Marijuana, cocaine, opiates, amphetamines, phencyclidine
HairConfirm Regular, Express, and Prescription (www.hairconfirm.com)	5–7 days	Hair	Send away	Marijuana, cocaine, opiates, amphetamines, phencyclidine; in addition to these drugs, Hairconfirm Prescription tests for oxycodone, hydrocodone, hydromorphone; express includes overnight shipping

Source: References 55–58.

table 48-6 Example Estimated Times for Positive Drug Test

Drug	How soon after taking drug will there be a positive drug test?	How long after taking drug will there continue to be a positive drug test?
Amphetamine, methamphetamine	4–6 hours	2–3 days
Barbiturates	2–4 hours	1–3 weeks
Benzodiazepine	2–7 hours	1–4 days
Cocaine	2–6 hours	2–3 days
Ecstacy	2–7 hours	2–4 days
Marijuana	1–3 hours	1–7 days
Methadone	3–8 hours	1–3 days
Opiates	2–6 hours	1–3 days
Oxycodone	1–3 hours	1–2 days
PCP	4–6 hours	7–14 days
Tricyclic antidepressants	8–12 hours	2–7 days

Source: Reference 54.

initial screening of a sample. Available testing devices include (1) a test cassette to which urine is applied and (2) a test device that is placed in the urine sample. In each test, a positive result for a particular drug is the absence of a line next to the drug name in the testing area. For a negative test, a line appears by the drug name and in the control area.

The laboratories use an enzyme-multiplied immuno-assay technique to detect drugs in the urine samples. Gas chromatography–mass spectrometry is then used to identify the specific drug. Positive home urine samples sent to clinical laboratories for confirmation are checked for evidence of adulteration.[55-57] Substances such as water or household chemicals can be added to urine samples in an attempt to mask drug use.

Home urine tests detect drug use that occurred from several hours before testing to within 2–3 days of testing. The amount of drug found in the urine is affected by the time since consumption, the amount taken, and the amount of water consumed before sampling. Test results are reported as only positive or negative for a drug. Quantity or route of ingestion is not determined.

Hair testing detects trace amounts of ingested drugs that become trapped in the core of the hair shaft as it grows at an average rate of ½ inch per month. Drug use over a 90-day period can be determined from a hair sample of 1½ inches.[58] The presence of drugs is determined by radioimmunoassay techniques, and then gas chromatography–mass spectrometry analysis identifies the specific substance. Hair tests report positive or negative results for a drug. Positive results are reported as a number indicating low, medium, or high levels of use for

all drugs except marijuana, which is reported only as positive or negative.

Usage Guidelines

See the box Patient Education for Drug Abuse Tests.

Interferences

Ingestion of decongestants, dextromethorphan, antidiarrheals, or cough medicines containing codeine may cause false-positive results for home drug abuse tests. These items contain substances structurally related to certain drugs of abuse. Consumption of large quantities of poppy seeds or poppy seed paste may or may not cause a false-positive result for opiates, depending on the test's sensitivity. Sensitivity standards for opiates have been raised to reduce the possibility of false-positive results.

Product Selection Guidelines

The criteria for selecting one drug abuse test over another include the drugs that are suspected of being used, the type of suspected use (i.e., casual versus chronic), the length of time since last use, and the possibility that the suspected drug user tampered with the sample. The list of drugs that may be identified varies with each kit. These tests can test for a single drug or up to 12 drugs. Information on FDA approval of a particular drug abuse test for home use is available on the FDA Web site (www. fda.gov/MedicalDevices/ProductsandMedicalProcedures/ InVitroDiagnostics/HomeUseTests).

In general, urine tests are better for detecting low-level, casual drug use. Hair testing detects longer-term use. It takes at least 5–7 days for hair to grow far enough from the scalp for testing purposes.

Urine samples are subject to tampering by adding chemicals, diluting with water, or substituting someone else's urine sample. Some of the test kits include a temperature strip on the urine collection cup to ensure the sample is at body temperature. Hair samples, if taken directly from the person being tested, are not subject to tampering. Parents should weigh the possibility of tampering when deciding which type of test to choose.

Assessment of Drug Abuse Test Use

The length of time of suspected drug use and the types of drugs that are suspected will determine which type of drug abuse test to recommend. Whether the suspected user is likely to tamper with urine samples should also be determined. Finally, whether the suspected user takes legal prescription or nonprescription medications that may interfere with the test should be determined.

Patient Counseling for Drug Abuse Tests

When parents or caregivers ask for assistance in selecting a drug abuse test, health care providers should offer clinical advice and information about family counseling agencies. Counseling should emphasize the limitations of the tests for confirming drug use and, in the case of urine tests, for identifying anything more

patient education for
Drug Abuse Tests

Avoidance of Incorrect Results

- Drug tests on urine samples report only a positive or negative outcome. Neither the quantity of drug taken nor the method in which it was taken is determined.
- Drug tests on hair samples can report a low, medium, or high level of drug use, but the use could have occurred as long as 90 days before testing.
- Cough medications that contain codeine or dextromethorphan, decongestants, antidiarrheals, narcotic analgesics, and possibly poppy seeds may cause false-positive test results.

Usage Guidelines for Urine Drug Abuse Tests

- Collect urine using the collection device included with the test. Do not take urine from the toilet.
- Check the temperature of the urine sample immediately after collection using the temperature strip, if included. If the sample is not between 90°F (32°C) and 100°F (38°C), adulteration may have occurred.
- Immerse the test card in the urine sample for 10 seconds or until visible migration across the test panels has occurred. Place the device on a flat surface or leave it immersed in the sample. Do not allow urine to exceed the "max line."

- Read the results when the "results ready" indicator changes to a pinkish red. Do not read the results 15 minutes or more after this indicator changes color or after the "results expired" indicator changes color.
- If no line appears in the control region, the test is invalid and should be repeated with a new card.

Usage Guidelines for Hair Drug Abuse Tests

- Collect a hair sample, ½-inch wide and one strand deep, from the crown of the head, as close to the scalp as possible.
- Align the cut ends of the hair sample and place the sample in the collection package as directed. Do not collect hair from a hairbrush, comb, or clothing; there is no guarantee that the hair is actually from the person to be tested.
- Results are available approximately 5 days after receipt by the laboratory. To access results, call the manufacturer's toll-free number and provide the code number accompanying the kit.

When to Seek Medical Attention

- If the test is positive, seek the services of a drug rehabilitation organization.

Source: References 55–58.

than the type of drug that is being abused. The box Patient Education for Drug Abuse Tests lists specific information to provide patients.

Evaluation of Patient Outcomes with Drug Abuse Tests

If a positive result is obtained with a drug abuse test, parents or caregivers need to consider potential problems with the test itself before concluding that drug use is confirmed. In addition, they must not assume that a negative result is accurate. Parents should also consider the testing window when evaluating results.

are multiple, but a significant factor is lack of patient motivation to take steps to control blood pressure, especially if the patient is asymptomatic, which leads to nonadherence with treatment strategies.

The consequences of untreated hypertension are well documented. Long-standing elevations in blood pressure can lead to damage to the heart, kidneys, lungs, eyes, and blood vessels, and to an increase in morbidity and mortality.

Treatment of high blood pressure often involves significant lifestyle changes (diet and exercise) and the institution of drug therapies. These measures inevitably produce side effects, so the patient who was without symptoms of disease may become symptomatic. Patient education and empowerment play a large role in improving patient adherence with antihypertensive efforts. Adherence, in turn, helps reduce morbidity and

Blood Pressure Monitors

Hypertension, defined as either a systolic blood pressure greater than 140 mm Hg or a diastolic blood pressure greater than 90 mm Hg, is often an asymptomatic disease.[59] Table 48–7 lists the classification of blood pressures from the seventh report of the Joint National Committee on Prevention, Detection, Evaluation and Treatment of High Blood Pressure (JNC 7).

Thirty-two percent of Americans 20 years of age and older have hypertension.[34] Thirty percent of people with hypertension are unaware of their condition; almost 40% are not receiving treatment; and 66% have not achieved national goals for blood pressure control.[59] The reasons for the lack of adequate control

table 48–7   Classification of Blood Pressure

Category	Systolic BP (mm Hg)		Diastolic BP (mm Hg)
Normal	<120	AND	<80
Prehypertension	120–139	OR	80–89
Hypertension, stage 1	140–159	OR	90–99
Hypertension, stage 2	≥160	OR	≥100

Key: BP = Blood pressure.
Source: Reference 59.

mortality, maintains or improves the patient's quality of life, and improves the patient's use of health care resources.

Teaching patients to take their own blood pressure at home is an excellent means of achieving those goals because home blood pressure monitoring gives patients a sense of control over their health and allows them to measure their progress toward a target blood pressure. Three general advantages of measuring blood pressure at home are the ability to (1) distinguish sustained hypertension from "white-coat hypertension" (measurements affected by being in the health care provider's office), (2) assess response to antihypertensive medication, and (3) improve patient adherence to treatment.

Usage Considerations

Of the three categories of blood pressure monitors (mercury column, aneroid, and digital), the most popular choices for home use are aneroid and digital monitors. Monitors that measure pressure at the wrist and fingers have become popular, but the systolic and diastolic pressures vary substantially in different parts of the arterial tree. Finger monitors have so far been found to be inaccurate and are not recommended.[59,60] Wrist monitors are typically smaller than the arm devices and can be used in obese people because the wrist diameter is little affected by obesity.[60]

Mechanism of Action

Blood pressure readings include two types of pressures: systolic, which indicates pressure at the time of contraction of the heart cavities, and diastolic, which indicates pressure at the time of dilation of the heart cavities. Blood pressure is measured indirectly by two methods: auscultatory (measurement of sound) and oscillometric (measurement of vibration). Mercury column and aneroid meters involve auscultation with the use of a stethoscope to detect Korotkoff's sounds, which are produced by the motion of the arterial wall in response to changes in arterial pressure. Oscillometric sensors, which are often used with digital meters, measure blood pressure by detecting blood surges underneath the cuff as it is deflated. The detection device, which is usually indicated on the cuff with a tab or other marking, is placed directly over the brachial artery. The brachial artery can be found by palpating 1–2 inches above and just to the inside of the antecubital space. As cuff pressure increases during the measurement procedure, the brachial artery is compressed and blood flow is obstructed. As cuff pressure is gradually released, blood flow is reestablished and Korotkoff's sounds can be heard in different phases. Phase I, which corresponds to systolic pressure, can be identified when at least two consecutive "beats" are heard as cuff pressure is decreased. The nature of the sounds changes over the next three phases. Diastolic pressure is identified at the point the sounds disappear (Phase V).

Interferences

Stress, tobacco smoking, and ingestion of caffeine-containing beverages can increase blood pressure. Some medications such as pseudoephedrine may also increase blood pressure.

Usage Guidelines

The actual measurement of blood pressure is a relatively simple procedure; however, many people consistently do it incorrectly. Blood pressure is naturally variable. Therefore, proper technique is essential to reduce measurement variability and improve the quality of results. The normal range for blood pressure was established in patients seated in the resting state; any variation from this setting can produce inaccurate results.

Using the appropriate size cuff is essential to accurately measure a patient's blood pressure (Table 48–8). If the cuff is too small, blood pressure readings can be overestimated significantly by as much as 20–30 mm Hg. Several monitors are supplied with a large cuff; many others allow a large cuff to be purchased separately. For patients with arms too large for the largest size cuff, a wrist monitor may be a useful alternative. To obtain accurate readings with wrist cuffs, the patient must hold the wrist at heart level during the reading. Because these devices are also highly sensitive to changes in the wrist level, it is best to support the arm on a table with a pillow that will raise the wrist to the appropriate level. For the person who is doing the actual monitoring, following the steps outlined in the box Patient Education for Self-Monitoring of Blood Pressure will help improve the accuracy of blood pressure readings, regardless of whether they are taken in the health care provider's office, the pharmacy, or the home.

Product Selection Guidelines

Of the three types of blood pressure–measuring devices, no single one is best for every patient. The choice of device is individualized according to characteristics such as the patient's ability and willingness to learn, physical disabilities, patient preference, and the cost of the device. Mercury column devices are expensive and, as discussed in the next section, have other disadvantages for home use. In general, aneroid devices are the least expensive. Depending on its features, a digital device can cost as much as a mercury column device. A discussion of the pros and cons of all three types of devices follows.

table
48–8 Arm Circumferences to Determine Appropriate Blood Pressure Cuff Size

Arm Circumference (adult)[a]	Cuff Size
22–26 cm	Small adult cuff
27–34 cm	Regular adult cuff
35–44 cm	Large adult cuff
≥45 cm	Thigh cuff[b]

[a] Determine arm circumference by measuring around the midpoint of the upper arm. Remeasure the patient's arm periodically, especially if he or she has recently gained or lost significant weight.

[b] Consider a wrist monitor for patients whose arm circumference is >45 cm.

Source: Reference 60.

Mercury Column Devices

The mercury column blood pressure monitor is still the reference standard in blood pressure measurement. This monitor typically comes with a cuff and an inflation bulb. The tubing from the cuff is attached to a column of mercury encased in a calibrated vertical glass tube.

Although mercury monitors are the most accurate and reliable of the devices, their routine use for home measurement is discouraged because they are cumbersome and pose the risk of mercury toxicity should the glass tubing break. They also require good eyesight and hearing for effective use. If the mercury does not rest at zero when the cuff is lying flat and completely deflated, the device needs recalibration.

Aneroid Devices

Next to mercury column monitors, aneroid devices are the most accurate and reliable. They are light, portable, and very affordable, and they pose no risk from mercury toxicity. They include several features that make patient instruction much easier. First, many devices now come with a stethoscope attached to the cuff, which frees the patient from having to hold the bell of the stethoscope in place. Second, a D-ring on the cuff allows a single user to place the cuff on the arm easily. Third, a few manufacturers offer a gauge attached to the inflation bulb, making it easier to manipulate the equipment because there are fewer pieces to control. These monitors are considered the option of choice for home use, but they do require careful patient instruction and follow-up. Good eyesight and hearing are necessary for accurate readings with standard models. For patients with reduced visual capacity, however, devices with large-type print on the face of the gauge are available.

At the bottom of the face of each aneroid device is a small box. When the cuff is completely deflated and lying on the table, the needle of the gauge should rest in the box. If the needle is outside the box, the gauge needs recalibration. Many manufacturers sell recalibration tools to allow health care providers to adjust the devices.

Digital Devices

With advancing technology, digital devices have become more accurate, reliable, and easy to use; as a result, they have skyrocketed in popularity. These devices include semiautomatic (manually inflating), fully automatic (autoinflating), wrist, and finger blood pressure monitors. Features such as printouts, pulse monitor, digital clock, automated inflation and deflation, memory, large display, and D-ring for the cuff differentiate many of the devices. These features significantly affect the price.

A major drawback to digital monitors is the user's inability to determine whether the device is out of calibration. As a result, many providers recommend the aneroid devices over the easier-to-use digital products. The JNC 7 report notes that home measurement devices should be checked regularly for accuracy[59]; therefore, patients should be advised to have their monitors checked at least yearly by a health care provider.

If recommending a digital device, the provider should check the manufacturer's specifications to ensure that the monitor meets at least the accuracy standards set by the American National Standards Institute (ANSI). The ANSI standards for digital sphygmomanometers state that blood pressure readings between 20 and 250 mm Hg must not differ by more than 3 mm Hg or 2%, whichever is greater.[61]

Assessment of Blood Pressure Self-Monitoring

Assessment should include determination of (1) why a patient wants to use a blood pressure monitor, (2) whether the patient has physical impairments that can interfere with proper use of the monitor, and (3) the patient's ability to comprehend and follow instructions.

Patient Counseling for Blood Pressure Self-Monitoring

The health care provider should emphasize the importance of tracking blood pressure values to monitor control of hypertension. Regular self-monitoring of blood pressure will illustrate positive effects of proper diet, exercise, and medication use in controlling the disorder. This reinforcement can improve patient adherence with prescribed therapies. The patient should be shown the proper technique for blood pressure monitoring and be encouraged to return for a follow-up evaluation of his or her technique. Because of white coat hypertension, patients who measure blood pressure at home usually obtain lower results than those taken at the provider's office. In the home setting, a blood pressure greater than 135/85 mm Hg should be considered elevated.[60] The box Patient Education for Self-Monitoring of Blood Pressure lists specific information to provide patients.

Evaluation of Patient Outcomes for Self-Monitoring of Blood Pressure

Patients measuring blood pressure for diagnostic and monitoring purposes should be instructed on how to track values and how to discuss the values with a health care provider. Patients monitoring their blood pressure should be cautioned not to adjust their medications unless instructed otherwise. Patients should be instructed to immediately contact their health care provider if they obtain elevated values (Table 48–7) and have any symptoms of high blood pressure, such as headache or blurred vision. Patient counseling and follow-up can improve outcomes in hypertensive patients by (1) motivating them to perform home monitoring of blood pressure, (2) guiding them in product selection, (3) training them to use devices appropriately, and (4) facilitating communication between the patient, the patient's family, and the patient's health care provider regarding any antihypertensive therapy.

Miscellaneous Home Tests

As the market for home test products and shopping over the Internet have exploded, new tests are becoming available with increasing frequency. Selected miscellaneous home tests are described in Table 48–9. Instructions for use are generally available from the manufacturer's Web site or a site that sells the product. Following the general guidelines given in this chapter will also help patients obtain accurate results.

patient education for
Self-Monitoring of Blood Pressure

Precautions and Avoidance of Incorrect Results

- Keep a log of blood pressure readings and any circumstances that might have affected the reading (e.g., feeling nervous or being late for work).
- If home readings are being performed for diagnostic purposes, take readings at different times throughout the day and under different circumstances.
- If readings are being done to determine adequacy of antihypertensive therapy, take the reading at the same time of day, preferably in the early morning soon after arising from bed.
- Allow plenty of time to relax before taking a blood pressure reading. Feelings of stress or pressure can elevate the blood pressure.
- Do not use tobacco products or drink caffeine-containing beverages for at least 30 minutes before taking a measurement. These activities can increase blood pressure.
- Wait 10–15 minutes after a bath and 30 minutes after eating to take a measurement. These activities can lower blood pressure.
- Some medications may increase blood pressure. Be alert for possible changes in readings when starting or stopping medications.

Usage Guidelines

- Make sure the room is at a comfortable temperature.
- Sit in a comfortable chair, with your back supported and your feet facing straight ahead and placed flat on the floor.
- If using an arm cuff, place the arm to be measured on a table, making sure your upper arm is at heart level. Remove restrictive clothing from the arm.
- If using a wrist cuff, place pillows under the arm to be measured to bring the wrist up to heart level.

- Place the cuff on the arm to be measured. The cuff should be snug but not tight enough to restrict blood flow. Use the guidelines in Table 48–8 for selecting cuff size.
- Rest for at least 5 minutes in this position.
- Measure the blood pressure as directed by the product instructions. If using a stethoscope, listen for the Korotkoff's sounds as defined:
  - Phase 1: Sound begins as a soft tapping. Record the systolic pressure when two taps are heard in sequence.
  - Phase 2: Tapping sound becomes louder and is accompanied by a swishing sound or murmur.
  - Phase 3: Tapping sounds persist, but the swishing or murmur sound stops.
  - Phase 4: There is muffling or softening of tapping sounds.
  - Phase 5: Sound stops. Record the diastolic pressure when the sound stops.
- Using the same arm, take two to three measurements separated by at least 2 minutes.
- Record the results, arm used, time and date of measurement, and name and time of last dose of any medications, including antihypertensive medications.
- Do not adjust blood pressure medications on the basis of home measurements unless specifically instructed to do so by a health care provider.

When to Seek Medical Attention

- See a health care provider immediately for evaluation and treatment if readings are above limits set by your health care provider or above the limits stated in national guidelines and if you are having symptoms such as headache or blurred vision.

Source: References 59 and 60.

table
48–9 Selected Miscellaneous Nonprescription Home Tests

Test	Purpose	Important Points	Additional Information
Alcohol screening tests (breath and saliva)	Prevent inappropriate alcohol consumption	Put nothing in mouth for 15 minutes before or during the test. Follow timing directions carefully and use a timing device.	Semiquantitative BAC; saliva test strips can be used to detect alcohol in drinks.
Visiderm (visiderm.com)	Monitors moles for changes over time	Use a transparent overlay to trace outline of individual moles; record color and other details. Do subsequent examinations of each mole on same overlay.	Test includes transparent overlays, pen, color chart, instructions, and storage box.
Breast Self-Examination Aid	Makes breast self-examination easier and more comfortable	Examine breasts monthly. Self-examination does not take place of mammogram and professional examination.	Two-layer polyurethane breast shield or glove contains a small amount of silicone lubricant to reduce friction. Some kits come with instructional video (Aware, Sensa Touch).
Vagisil Screening Kit (www.vagisilkit.com)	Detects pH of vaginal secretions	pH 4.5 + symptoms suggest yeast. pH ≥ 5 + symptoms suggest bacterial vaginosis or trichomoniasis.	Those with first-time yeast infection and those with pH ≥ 5 should see HCP for diagnosis. See Chapter 8 for additional information.

table

48–9 Selected Miscellaneous Nonprescription Home Tests *(continued)*

Test	Purpose	Important Points	Additional Information
TobacAlert/NicAlert (www.tobacalert.com, nymox.com)	Detects tobacco use or exposure	Test detects cotine, a metabolite of nicotine; test detects use or exposure in previous 48–72 hours. Dip strip in urine (TobaAlert) or saliva (NicAlert) sample and read results in specified time.	Use of nicotine patch or gum can affect results.
My Allergy Test (www.immunetech.com)	Detects allergy to 10 most common allergens: dust mites, cat, mold (*Alternaria*), ragweed, mountain cedar (juniper), Timothy grass, Bermuda grass, egg white, milk, wheat	If negative result but positive symptoms, see PCP.	Test measures IgE antibodies but tests for only 10 allergens. Results are available by e-mail in 10 days or by regular mail.
IDENTIGENE DNA Paternity Test Collection Kit	Checks paternity of a child	Collect cheek cell samples from each participant: alleged father, child, and biological mother. Swabs are mailed to laboratory.	Cost includes additional ~$120 laboratory fee plus price of kit ($30). Kit is not available in all states. Results are available 3–5 days after sample is received by laboratory. Results are not valid for legal purposes (requires verified collection procedure and additional costs).
EarCheck Middle Ear Monitor (www.earcheck.com)	Detects middle ear fluid (otitis media with effusion)	Device emits sound waves into the ear canal. Some of the sound reflects off the eardrum and travels back to the built-in microphone. The sound is then analyzed to determine whether middle ear fluid is present.	Device is not validated in patients >19 years and cannot be used in those <6 months of age, or in those with ear tubes, known perforation or rupture of the eardrum, or visible drainage of pus or blood in the outer ear canal. If a negative result + symptoms or a positive result is obtained, see HCP.
Menopause Test	Detects FSH in urine	Positive test = FSH level >25 IU/L, which may indicate a woman is menopausal. FSH levels change during the menstrual cycle so the test should be done twice 1–2 weeks apart to confirm results.	Not a definitive diagnostic test for menopause. The diagnosis would need to be confirmed by the woman's health care provider.

Key: BAC = Blood alcohol concentration; FDA = Food and Drug Administration; Ig = immunoglobulin; IOP = intraocular pressure; HCP = health care provider; FSH = follicle-stimulating hormone.

Key Points for Home Testing and Monitoring Devices

➤ To advise patients properly on selecting and using home testing or monitoring products, health care providers must be familiar with the procedures for each available product.

➤ Manufacturers continually introduce new products and modify current ones to provide more user-friendly versions. To keep up-to-date, providers should request product information from manufacturers by calling their toll-free numbers, visiting their Web sites, or contacting their sales representatives.

➤ FDA's Web site should also be checked frequently for problem reports, updates, and news on home tests.

➤ Patients who are using home tests or devices should be encouraged to follow instructions carefully and to contact either their health care provider or the manufacturer's toll-free number for assistance, if needed.

➤ Health care providers should stress that the patient is self-testing, not self-diagnosing. Positive test results should be reported immediately for definitive diagnosis and management. Negative test results should be questioned when the patient is experiencing symptoms of a suspected condition.

➤ If there is any question about the results, the patient should seek the advice of a health care provider.

REFERENCES

1. *The New York Times.* Maker of pregnancy test finds opportunity in personal stories. Accessed at http://www.nytimes.com/2010/05/03/business/media/03adco.html, September 15, 2014.

2. Martin J, Hamilton B, Ventura S, et al. *Births: Final Data for 2010. National Vital Statistics Reports; vol 61 no 1.* Hyattsville, MD: National Center for Health Statistics; 2012.

3. First Response Resource Center. Accessed at http://www.firstresponse.com, April 10, 2013.

4. Cole LA. The utility of six over-the-counter (home) pregnancy tests. *Clin Lab Med.* 2011;49(8):1317–22.

5. Butler SA, Khanlian SA, Cole LA. Detection of early pregnancy forms of human chorionic gonadotropin by home pregnancy test devices. *Clin Chem.* 2001;47(12):2131–6.

6. Cole L, Sutton-Riley J, Khanlian S, et al. Sensitivity of over-the-counter pregnancy tests: comparison of utility and marketing messages. *J Am Pharm Assoc.* 2005;45(5):608–15.

7. Clearblue [product information]. Geneva, Switzerland: Swiss Precision Diagnostics GmbH; 2013.

8. Fact Plus [product information]. Geneva, Switzerland: Swiss Precision Diagnostics GmbH; 2008–12.

9. Wilcox AJ, Baird DD, Dunson D, et al. Natural limits of pregnancy testing in relation to the expected menstrual period. *JAMA.* 2001;286(14):1759–61.

10. Cole L, Khanlian S, Sutton J, et al. Accuracy of home pregnancy tests at the time of a missed menses. *Am J Obstet Gynecol.* 2004;190(1):100–5.

11. Wallace L, Zite N, Homewood V. Making sense of home pregnancy test instructions. *J Womens Health.* 2009;18(3):323–68.

12. Martinez G, Daniels K, Chandra A. Fertility of men and women aged 15–44 years in the United States: National Survey of Family Growth, 2006–2010. *National Health Statistics Reports.* 2012;51. Hyattsville, MD: National Center for Health Statistics.

13. Scolaro KL, Lloyd KB, Helms KL. Devices for home evaluation of women's health concerns. *Am J Health Syst Pharm.* 2008;65(4):299–314.

14. Johnson S, Ellis J, Godbert S, et al. Comparison of a digital ovulation test with three popular line ovulation tests to investigate user accuracy and certainty. *Expert Opin Med Diagn.* 2011;5(6):467–73.

15. Accu-Clear [product information]. Geneva, Switzerland: Swiss Precision Diagnostics GmbH; 2008–12.

16. Nexcare Basal Digital Thermometer [product information]. Franklin Lakes, NJ: 2007.

17. Lennard J, Lind J, Honeywell M. Advanced technology for fertility prediction. *US Pharm.* 2006;12:49–54.

18. OV Watch [product information]. Watersound, FL: Health Watch Systems, Inc; 2011.

19. Eichner S, Timpe E. Urinary-based ovulation and pregnancy: point-of-care testing. *Ann Pharmacother.* 2004;38(2):325–31.

20. Cooper T, Noonan E, Eckardstein S, et al. WHO reference values for human semen characteristics. *Human Reproductive Update* 2010;16(3):231–45.

21. Coppola MA, Klotz KL, Kim KA, et al. SpermCheck Fertility, an immuno-diagnostic home test that detects normozoospermia and severe oligozoospermia. *Hum Reprod.* 2010;25(4):853–61.

22. SpermCheck [product information]. Bellingham, WA: Fairhaven Health; 2012–13.

23. American Cancer Society. *Cancer Facts and Figures 2013.* Accessed at http://www.cancer.org, March 29, 2013.

24. Ferguson LR. Meat and cancer. *Meat Sci.* 2010;84(2):308–13.

25. Health Quality Ontario. Fecal occult blood test for colorectal screening. *Ont Health Technol Assess Ser.* 2009;9(10):1–40.

26. EZ-Detect [product information]. Newport Beach, CA: Biomerica; 2000–1.

27. ColonTest-Sensitive [product information]. Las Vegas, NV: Diagnostica.

28. Early Detect Colorectal [product information]. Irvine, CA: Early Detect; 2007.

29. Kahi CJ, Imperiale TF. Do aspirin and nonsteroidal anti-inflammatory drugs cause false-positive fecal occult blood test results? A prospective study in a cohort of veterans. *Am J Med.* 2004;117(11):837–41.

30. Pignone M, Campbell MK, Carr C, et al. Meta-analysis of dietary restriction during fecal occult blood testing. *Eff Clin Pract.* 2001;4(4):150–6.

31. Rex DK, Johnson DA, Anderson JC, et al. American College of Gastroenterology guidelines for colorectal cancer screening 2008. *Am J Gastroenterol.* 2009;104(3):739–50.

32. American Cancer Society. Recommendations for Colorectal Cancer Early Detection. Accessed at http://www.cancer.org/cancer/colonandrectumcancer/moreinformation/colonandrectumcancerearlydetection/colorectal-cancer-early-detection-acs-recommendations, March 19, 2013.

33. National Institutes of Health. Executive summary. In: *Third Report of the National Cholesterol Education Program (NCEP) Expert Panel on Detection, Evaluation, and Treatment of High Blood Cholesterol in Adults (Adult Treatment Panel III).* Bethesda, MD: National Institutes of Health; May 2001. NIH Publication No. 01-3670.

34. National Center for Health Statistics. *Health, United States, 2011.* Hyattsville, MD: National Center for Health Statistics; 2011.

35. CholesTrak [product information]. Vista, CA: Accutech; 2008.

36. First Check Home Cholesterol Test [product information]. Waltham, MA: Inverness Medical; 2008.

37. CardioChek [product information]. Indianapolis, IN: Polymer Technology Systems; 2010.

38. Accutrend Plus [product information]. Indianapolis, IN: Roche Diagnostics; 2012.

39. Q. Steps Cholesterol Biometer [product information]. Fremont, CA: Biomedix Inc.; 2004.

40. Check Up America Cholesterol Panel [product information]. Hoffman Estates, IL: Home Access Health.

41. McNamara JR, Warnick GR, Leary ET, et al. Multicenter evaluation of a patient-administered test for blood cholesterol measurement. *Prev Med.* 1996;25(5):583–92.

42. Do home cholesterol tests work? *Consum Rep.* August 2003:9.

43. Shephard MD, Mazzachi BC, Shephard AK. Comparative performance of two point-of-care analysers for lipid testing. *Clin Lab.* 2007;53(9–12):561–6.

44. Centers for Disease Control and Prevention. *Urinary Tract Infections.* Accessed at http://www.cdc.gov, March 19, 2013.

45. Gupta K, Trautner BW. Urinary tract infections, pyelonephritis, and prostatitis. In: Longo DL, Fauci AS, Kasper DL, et al., eds. *Harrison's Principles of Internal Medicine.* 18th ed. New York, NY: McGraw-Hill; 2012.

46. UTI Home Test [product information]. Jackson, WI: Consumers Products, Inc.; 2010.

47. AZO Test Strips [product information]. Cromwell, CT: I-Health, Inc.; 2013.

48. Devillé WLMJ, Yzermans JC, van Duijn NP. The urine dipstick test useful to rule out infections. A meta-analysis of the accuracy [serial online]. *BMC Urol.* 2004;4:4.

49. Centers for Disease Control and Prevention. *HIV in the United States: At a Glance.* Accessed at http://www.cdc.gov, March 19, 2013.

50. OraQuick In Home HIV Test. [product information]. Bethlehem, PA: OraSure Technologies, Inc.; 2012.

51. Home Access Express HIV Test System [product information]. Hoffman Estates, IL: Home Access Health.

52. Centers for Disease Control and Prevention. *Hepatitis C Information for Health Professionals.* Accessed at http://www.cdc.gov/hepatitis/HCV/index.htm, March 19, 2013.

53. Home Access Hepatitis C Check [product information]. Hoffman Estates, IL: Home Access Health.

54. U.S. Food and Drug Administration. Drugs of Abuse Home Use Test. Accessed at http://www.fda.gov/MedicalDevices/ProductsandMedicalProcedures/InVitroDiagnostics/HomeUseTests/ucm125722.htm, October 30, 2013.

55. At Home Drug Test [product information]. San Diego, CA: Pharmatech; 2010.

56. Dr. Brown's Home Drug Testing System [product information]. Elan. Accessed at http://www.drbrowns.com, March 19, 2013.

57. PDT-90 Personal Drug Testing Service [product information]. Cambridge, MA: Psychemedics; 2010.

58. HairConfirm [product information]. San Diego, CA: Confirm Biosciences.

59. U.S. Department of Health and Human Services, National Institutes of Health, National Heart, Lung, and Blood Institute, National High Blood Pressure Education Program. *The Seventh Report of the Joint National Committee on the Detection, Evaluation, and Treatment of High Blood Pressure (JNC 7).* Bethesda, MD: U.S. Department of Health and Human Services; 2004. NIH Publication No. 04-5230. Accessed at http://www.nhlbi.nih.gov/files/docs/resources/heart/jnc7full.pdf, September 15, 2014.

60. American Heart Association. AHA scientific statement. Recommendations for blood pressure measurement in humans and experimental animals, part 1: blood pressure measurement in humans: a statement for professionals from the Subcommittee of Professional and Public Education of the American Heart Association Council on High Blood Pressure Research. *Circulation.* 2005;111:697–716.

61. Association for the Advancement of Medical Instrumentation. Manual, Electronic, or Automated Sphygmomanometers. Arlington, VA: American National Standards Institute; 2002:1–66.

ADULT URINARY INCONTINENCE AND SUPPLIES

Christine K. O'Neil

Urinary incontinence (UI) is defined as the complaint of any involuntary leakage of urine.[1] Although often mistakenly thought of as a problem of aging, UI affects people of all ages, socioeconomic backgrounds, and ethnicities. UI is twice as common in women, but men also suffer from the symptoms.[2] An estimated 17 million people in the United States are affected by UI,[3,4] whereas 42.2 million may suffer from overactive bladder (OAB).[5]

UI is an underdiagnosed and underreported condition with major psychosocial and economic effects on society. Feelings of embarrassment, denial, and misinformation prevent many people from seeking help, which may lead to anxiety, depression, and, possibly, social isolation. Severe UI usually results in a loss of self-esteem and the ability to maintain an independent lifestyle. In addition, it is generally recognized as a strong predictor of nursing home admission of older people.[3]

Direct costs associated with UI include the expenses for diagnosis, specific treatment, routine care, rehabilitation, and hospital and nursing home admissions. The direct costs of treating UI in men and women of all ages were estimated at $19.5 billion in 2000.[4]

Several studies have determined the prevalence of UI in nursing homes and the community.[6,7] The reported prevalence rates are approximately 50% for people in nursing homes and range between 2% and 55% for adults living in the community, depending on the type of UI, population characteristics, and methodological approach.[8] Among adults 30–60 years of age, the prevalence of UI is 12%–42% for women and 3%–5% for men. For older people (>60 years of age), prevalence rates for women have been reported as 17%–55% and rates for men as 11%–34%.

Despite the high prevalence of UI, less than half of community-dwelling adults with UI consult with their health care provider.[9] Many accept the symptoms as a natural part of aging and use self-care strategies with little or no health professional guidance. Although they are reluctant to talk about UI, Americans spend $1.1 billion annually on disposable incontinence products (e.g., pads, shields, guards, undergarments, and briefs).[10]

Pathophysiology of Urinary Incontinence

Urination is a complex process, involving a coordinated effort by the bladder, urethra, and muscular components of the lower urinary tract, brain, and spinal cord.[11,12] Urine produced by the kidneys is propelled through the ureters to the bladder. The detrusor muscle, the smooth muscle layer of the bladder, gives tone to the bladder, relaxing as the bladder fills with urine and contracting during urination. The bladder neck, which joins the bladder and the urethra, is surrounded by smooth muscle, referred to as the internal sphincter, which either constricts to hold urine in the bladder or relaxes, permitting urine to flow through the urethra. Voluntary control of urination, or micturition, is maintained by contraction of the external sphincter, a striated muscle located at mid-urethral length. When relaxed, the urethra, which is surrounded by both smooth and striated muscle, allows urine to leave the body.

The bladder and the internal sphincter are innervated by the autonomic nervous system, and the external sphincter is innervated by the somatic or voluntary nervous system. Parasympathetic and sympathetic nerves innervate the smooth muscle of the bladder and urethra. Both alpha-adrenergic and beta-adrenergic receptors are present in the urinary structures. The alpha receptors are located in the base of the bladder and the proximal urethra, and the beta receptors are found primarily in the body of the bladder detrusor. Stimulation of the alpha receptors causes contraction of the smooth muscles in the bladder neck and urethra, thus closing the bladder outlet. Stimulation of the beta receptors results in smooth muscle relaxation and allows the bladder to fill. Thus, sympathetic stimulation causes the bladder to retain urine. Parasympathetic cholinergic receptors are located throughout the bladder. Stimulation of these receptors causes the detrusor to contract, emptying the bladder. The sacral center, lying between vertebrae S2 and S4, acts as the relay center for information to and from the bladder, pelvic floor, and brain.

The capacity of the bladder is approximately 400–500 mL. When the bladder fills, stretch receptors in the detrusor wall transmit signals to the brain through the spinal cord, initiating the urge to urinate when the bladder is approximately half full. Under normal circumstances, adults can delay voiding for 30–60 minutes as a result of the short sacral reflex, which diminishes the urge to urinate by increasing contraction of the external sphincter and relaxing the detrusor muscle of the bladder. Bladder emptying is initiated voluntarily, causing relaxation of the external sphincter and contraction of the detrusor. Normal urination results in complete emptying of the bladder, with little or no residual urine (≤50 mL). Any disruption in the integration of musculoskeletal and neurologic function can lead to loss of control of normal bladder function and UI.[13]

Clinical Presentation of Urinary Incontinence

UI is a symptom that can be caused by external factors and by anatomic, physiologic, and pathologic factors that affect the urinary tract.[2,14–16] In many cases, multiple and interacting factors contribute to UI. The risk of UI is strongly associated with aging. Additional risk factors for UI, some at least partially reversible, have been identified (Table 49–1).[2,14–16] Identification of the cause(s) of UI is essential for the assessment and successful management of UI.

Age-related changes in the bladder and urinary tract may contribute to an older person's vulnerability to UI. With age, the kidney's ability to concentrate urine diminishes, resulting in larger urine volumes. In addition, age-related hypotrophic changes in bladder tissue lead to frequent urination and nocturia, whereas decreased muscle tone of the bladder, as well as the bladder sphincters and pelvic muscles, contributes to the potential for reduced urine control. This loss of control, combined with diminished mobility and reaction time, predisposes older people to UI.[17]

In women, the loss of estrogen causes a decrease in bladder outlet and urethral resistance, as well as a decline in pelvic musculature—all of which increase the likelihood of UI. In addition, estrogen loss results in atrophic changes in the vaginal and urethral mucosa, disrupting the vaginal flora and leading to atrophic vaginitis and chronic urethritis. These conditions, in turn, may cause urinary frequency and urgency, dysuria, urinary tract infections, and UI. The woman's short urethra exerts less resistance to intravesicular pressure compared with the longer male urethra. Consequently, obesity, chronic cough, and jarring exercise, which all increase intra-abdominal pressure, result in an extra load on the bladder. As such, these factors can overwhelm the relatively low resistance offered by the short female urethra. Childbirth, gynecologic procedures, and muscle atrophy from aging also weaken the woman's pelvic floor muscles, thereby decreasing support for the bladder. Without adequate support, positioning of the bladder becomes distorted (known as cystocele or anterior wall prolapse) and can result in urethral kinking, with subsequent poor bladder emptying. These conditions may result in chronic obstruction of the bladder, again leading to UI from urine volume overload.

Men often develop prostatic enlargement beginning in their middle to late 40s, which results in urethral obstruction, leading to decreased urinary flow rates, increased residual volumes, detrusor instability, and possibly overflow incontinence. Paradoxically, prostatectomy to relieve bothersome symptoms related to benign prostatic hyperplasia (BPH) can result in stress incontinence caused by incidental injury to the internal sphincter.

UI can be described broadly as transient or chronic. Transient UI is usually of sudden onset and secondary to acute illness (e.g., urinary tract infections) or to any disease that causes acute confusion (e.g., respiratory disease, myocardial infarction, or septicemia) or immobility, preventing the person from reaching a toilet independently or in time. Many other conditions and medications can cause or contribute to transient UI (Table 49–2).[2,18]

---

table 49–1 Risk Factors for Urinary Incontinence

Medical Disorders or Procedures

BPH/TURP/prostatectomy

Childhood nocturnal enuresis

Diabetes

Fecal impaction

Immobility/chronic degenerative disease

Impaired cognition: acute or chronic

Metabolic disorders (hyperglycemia, hypercalcemia)

Neurologic disorders (spinal cord injury, neuropathy)

Obesity (moderate-morbid)

Pregnancy/vaginal delivery/episiotomy

Stroke

Physiologic Factors

Estrogen depletion

High fluid intake (leading to polyuria and bladder capacity overload)

Low fluid intake (leading to concentrated urine and bladder irritation that worsens symptoms)

Pelvic floor muscle weakness

Lifestyle Factors

High-impact physical activities

Smoking

Other Factors

Caucasian race

Environmental barriers

Medications (Table 49–2)

Key: BPH = Benign prostatic hyperplasia; TURP = transurethral resection of the prostate.
Source: Adapted from references 2 and 14–16.

---

table 49–2 Reversible Conditions That Cause or Contribute to Urinary Incontinence

Conditions Affecting the Lower Urinary Tract

Urinary tract infections, atrophic vaginitis/urethritis, fecal impaction, pelvic floor prolapse, hyperglycemia, hypercalcemia

Drug Side Effects

Polyuria, frequency, urgency: caffeine, diuretics, alcohol, acetylcholinesterase inhibitors

Urinary retention: anticholinergics, antidepressants, hypnotics/sedatives, antipsychotics, narcotics, muscle relaxants, antihypertensives (calcium channel blockers), beta-adrenergic agonists, alpha-adrenergic agonists

Urethral relaxation: alpha-adrenergic blockers

Urethral pressure imbalance (stress incontinence): cough from ACE inhibitors

Increased Urine Production

Metabolic disorders (e.g., hyperglycemia, hypercalcemia), excessive fluid intake, volume overload, venous insufficiency with edema leading to nocturia

Inability or Unwillingness to Reach a Toilet

Dementia, delirium, illness/injury that interferes with mobility, psychological conditions

Key: ACE = Angiotensin-converting enzyme.
Source: References 2 and 18.

Managing these conditions may resolve UI in some patients but only reduce the severity of symptoms in others. Chronic UI is often related to neurologic or other chronic conditions, such as intrinsic sphincter deficiency, BPH, or cystocele.[19] UI can be classified as OAB, stress incontinence, mixed incontinence (OAB plus stress incontinence), overflow incontinence, or functional incontinence, depending on the underlying etiologies.

Recognition of signs and symptoms of UI is an essential first step in providing treatment advice. Patients often delay discussion or do not seek medical evaluation of UI with their health care provider. Therefore, it is important for health care providers to inquire about potential UI symptoms when such conditions are suspected on the basis of clinical evidence or patient inquiries. Open-ended questions such as "What problems are you having, if any, with your bladder?" and "How often do you experience urine leakage?" can be used to begin this dialogue. An awareness of signs such as the odor of urine or appearance of wetness is also necessary to identify potential patients suffering from UI. Table 49–3 lists observed and reported symptoms commonly associated with particular types of UI. Encouraging the use of a 24-hour voiding diary, paper or electronic, is a helpful tool in diagnosing and managing UI.[20,21] Voiding dairies permit the patient to document fluid intake, amount of urine voided, episodes of urine leakage, urge to urinate, and activity at the time of leakage or sense of urgency.

Overactive bladder occurs in both men and women, and its incidence increases with age. OAB is characterized by sudden and profound urinary urgency (strong desire to void), frequency (urinating more than eight times daily), nocturia (two or more awakenings at night to pass urine), or UI; the condition is often, but not always, accompanied by urge incontinence (involuntary urine leakage with urgency).[2,12,13,17] OAB is usually, but not always, attributable to uninhibited contractions of the detrusor muscle, referred to as detrusor instability. Other terms describing detrusor instability are detrusor hyperreflexia, detrusor hyperactivity with impaired bladder contractility, and bladder instability.

Neurogenic causes of detrusor instability include dementia, stroke, parkinsonism, suprasacral spinal cord injury, multiple sclerosis, and medullary lesions. Detrusor instability of neurologic origin is referred to as hyperreflexia. Non-neurogenic causes of detrusor instability include bladder irritation caused by infection or interstitial cystitis (bladder pain syndrome), obstruction (e.g., BPH or cystocele), bladder stones, and tumors. Excessive beverage intake and some therapeutic agents (e.g., diuretics and alcohol) can exacerbate symptoms of urge incontinence as a result of increased filling of the bladder. Bethanechol can also

lead to urge incontinence through cholinergically mediated contraction of bladder smooth muscle.

Stress incontinence is the most frequently encountered type of UI in women, except in the very old (>75 years), in whom OAB is most common. Symptoms of stress incontinence may occur in some men after transurethral resection of the prostate and radical prostatectomy.[13] Stress incontinence is characterized by involuntary leakage of urine with sudden increases in abdominal pressure associated with sneezing, laughing, coughing, exercising, and lifting. Symptoms are exacerbated with pregnancy and obesity, which also increase intra-abdominal pressure. This involuntary leakage is believed to be caused by hypermobility of the bladder neck or weakness of the urethral sphincter and pelvic floor muscles. Hypermobility refers to displacement of the bladder neck and urethra during physical exertion; it occurs when the supporting pelvic muscles have been weakened as a result of vaginal childbirth and aging. The weakening of the urethral sphincter can be secondary to vaginal or urologic surgery, trauma, aging, or inadequate estrogen, or it may be neurologic in etiology.[22] Drug-related causes of stress incontinence include alpha-adrenergic antagonists such as prazosin, terazosin, doxazosin, tamsulosin, and alfuzosin, which cause urethral relaxation (Table 49–2).

Overflow incontinence, an involuntary urine loss associated with overdistention of the bladder, is observed in 7%–11% of incontinent older patients.[2] Symptoms include dribbling, reduced force and caliber of urinary stream, urgency, and a sensation of incomplete voiding. The two main causes are outlet obstruction and/or an underactive bladder (detrusor) muscle. Outlet obstruction can be caused by BPH, urogenital tumors, pelvic organ prolapse, or previous anti-incontinence surgery. Dysfunctional bladder contractility can result from diabetic or alcoholic neuropathy, lower spinal cord injury, radical pelvic surgery, or medications with anticholinergic properties, such as antihistamines, antipsychotics, narcotics, tricyclic antidepressants, muscle relaxants, and medications used to treat urge incontinence. These medications can cause overflow incontinence by blocking cholinergically mediated bladder contractions, thereby inhibiting normal bladder function.

Mixed incontinence, most common in women, consists of the combination of OAB and stress incontinence.[2] Although the term *mixed UI* is generally applied to women, men with outlet obstruction resulting from BPH may exhibit mixed symptoms of OAB and overflow incontinence. Men may also exhibit mixed symptoms as a result of stress UI attributable to radical prostatectomy or transurethral resection of the prostate combined with OAB.

table 49–3	**Common Signs and Symptoms of Urinary Incontinence, by Type**				
Type of UI	**Urgency**	**Frequency**	**Volume of Loss**	**Nocturia**	**Other**
Urge	Frequent	>8 times per day	Large amount of urine loss: >100 mL and may empty completely	>1 time per night	Inability to reach toilet following urge to void
Stress	Occasional	Urine leakage during physical activity, lifting, coughing, sneezing; if severe, urine loss on ambulating	Small-moderate urine loss, depending on level of activity	Rare	Ability to reach toilet in time to complete void
Overflow	Hesitancy	Straining to void	Decreased or incomplete urine stream; dribbling	Frequent	Sensation of bladder or abdominal fullness, and incomplete bladder emptying

Functional incontinence is described as urine loss caused by factors such as physical or cognitive impairment, which interfere with a person's ability to reach toilet facilities in time or to perform toileting tasks.[2,12] Causes of this type of UI are many and include stroke, diminished mobility, impaired cognitive function or perception, environmental barriers, use of sedative and hypotensive agents, poorly controlled severe pain, and psychological unwillingness to release urine in the proper place. Because many functionally impaired people may have other types of UI, functional incontinence should be a diagnosis of exclusion.

The consequences of UI are considerable. Many people are embarrassed by such a condition and refrain from discussing their urinary problems with their primary care providers. Some people with UI believe it is a normal consequence of aging, rather than a symptom of underlying disease or anatomic change. Social isolation occurs because the incontinent patient avoids social interaction to prevent the embarrassment and rejection that often accompany UI. In turn, social isolation leads to depression. Intimate contact and sexual activity with the patient's partner can also decrease. Attempts to limit episodes of involuntary urine loss by restricting fluid intake can cause dehydration and hypotension, whereas skin irritation and ulceration caused by long exposure to urine results in "diaper rash" and possibly pressure ulcers.[2]

The caregivers of incontinent older patients are under stress because of the tedious and time-consuming care needed to deal with the problems of UI at home. Often, the loss of urine control leads to a drastic reduction in quality of life, and in some cases, placement in a nursing home.[2,23] Falls and fractures can result from UI and also with urgency symptoms in the absence of incontinence.

Treatment of Adult Urinary Incontinence

Treatment Goals

The goals of treatment of UI are to cure incontinence or to reduce the severity of symptoms, avoid complications, and improve the patient's quality of life. When incontinence aids are used as part of self-management in UI treatment, additional goals are to control or treat skin breakdown (diaper rash), control the odor of leaked urine, and contain urine in the undergarment.

General Treatment Approach

Treatment is individualized for the type of UI. The four major categories of intervention are behavioral modification, use of devices, pharmacologic treatment, and surgical treatment. Nonsurgical treatments for UI in women have been systematically reviewed in a recent publication.[24] Figure 49–1 outlines the self-management of adult UI.

Nonpharmacologic Therapy

Behavioral techniques decrease the frequency of UI in most patients, have no reported side effects, and do not limit future therapies.[2] To be most successful, these techniques generally require patient and caregiver involvement and continued practice. Three types of behavioral techniques, listed in order of increasing need for patient involvement, are toileting assistance, bladder training, and pelvic floor muscle training. Behavioral techniques are now the accepted first-line therapy in treating all forms of UI except

overflow incontinence.[12] A behavioral modification program involving pelvic floor muscle training and behavioral techniques was found to prevent the development of UI in continent older women.[25] Providers should educate patients about the role of behavioral therapy in the prevention and management of UI.

Toileting assistance includes routine or scheduled voiding performed at fixed, regular intervals (every 2–4 hours); habit training, which is voiding scheduled to match patterns in those who have natural voiding patterns; and prompted voiding. In prompted voiding, patients are trained to void only if the need is voiced on direct questioning. They are checked for wetness and praised for maintaining continence and trying to void.

Bladder training consists of education, scheduled voiding with systematic delay, and positive reinforcement. Patients are taught to delay voiding when the urge occurs and to use tactics to increase urine volume and the interval between voids. Bladder training is recommended for urge or mixed incontinence, but it is often difficult to achieve in cognitively impaired or frail older people.

Pelvic floor muscle training aims to improve urethral closure pressure by activating the striated muscles of the urethra and the underlying pelvic floor muscles. Two components of training have been established. Early improvement (reduction of urine leakage within 1 week of beginning pelvic floor muscle exercises) may be achieved by some women who learn "the knack maneuver," or volitional precontraction. The *knack* describes learning to contract pelvic floor muscles in anticipation of and during increases in intra-abdominal pressure (e.g., coughing). This maneuver alone has demonstrated the capacity to reduce stress incontinence.[26] In addition, pelvic floor muscle training, also known as Kegel exercises or pelvic floor exercises, is designed to strengthen the voluntary periurethral and perivaginal muscles, giving the patient more control of micturition and reducing UI.[2] Kegel exercises, which have been used successfully for stress and OAB, are performed by squeezing the pelvic muscles as if to stop the flow of urine. The contractions should be held for about 10 seconds and then released for 10 seconds; 3–4 sets of 10 contractions per day are generally recommended.[2,27] It is important to advise patients that the response to pelvic muscle exercises is delayed. The exercises may be augmented by the use of vaginal weights or biofeedback techniques. Biofeedback can facilitate learning pelvic muscle exercises. Direct electrical stimulation of the pelvic floor muscles with vaginal or anal probes or surface electrodes has been used with limited success in stress, urge, and mixed UI. Radiofrequency energy treatment (Lyrette, formerly Renessa) is available in a physician's office and is a nonsurgical approach to stress UI. The treatment, which uses low temperature to cause natural collagen to become firmer, produces improvements in 3 of 4 women and nearly 60% can eliminate the use of pads.[28]

Another option available only through a primary care provider's office is the NeoControl Pelvic Floor Therapy System.[29] This is a pulsating magnetic chair that uses directed magnetic fields to induce pelvic muscle contractions. Patients generally require treatments twice a week for about 20–30 minutes for a total of 8 weeks or more. This option is approved by the Food and Drug Administration (FDA) for the treatment of stress, OAB, and mixed UI.

Application of mechanical pressure to support the urethra is evident in the age-old advice to women with stress incontinence to cross their legs before coughing or sneezing to prevent urine leakage.[30] Similarly, various devices have been used for UI, including elevating devices to support the bladder neck (pessary, tampon, or prosthesis); urethral occlusive devices (urethral plug or insert, caps, expandable urethral devices, or urethral shields);

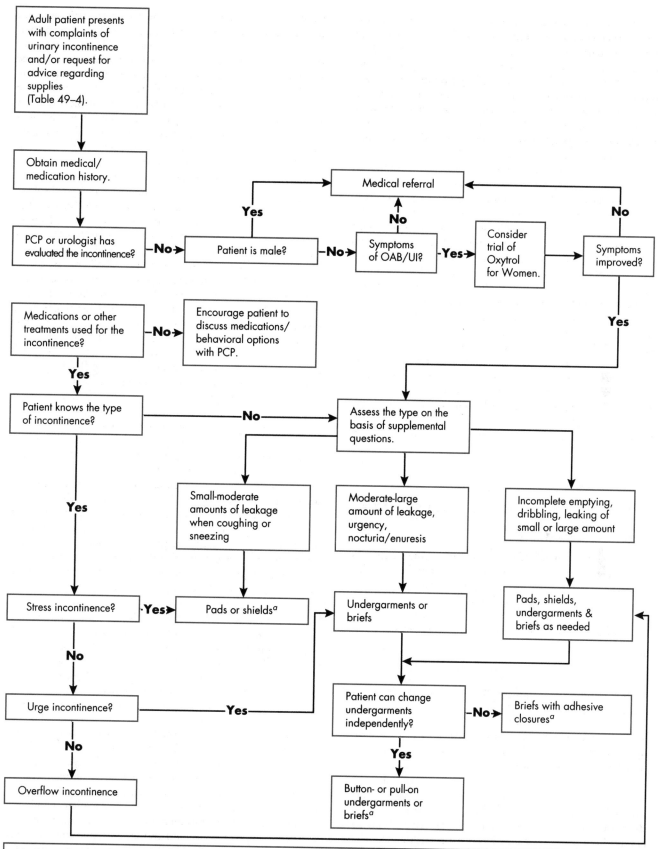

ᵃ Follow up on recommended products (see Evaluation of Patient Outcomes for Urinary Incontinence and Supplies).

figure

49–1   Self-care of adult urinary incontinence. Key: OAB = Overactive bladder; PCP = primary care provider; UI = urinary incontinence.

external collection systems (condom catheters or female urinals); penile compression devices; and catheterization (intermittent, indwelling, or suprapubic).[2] FemSoft, a small single-use product available by prescription for stress urinary incontinence, is the only urethral insert available in the United States. A recent review of mechanical devices found inconsistent results, insufficient evidence to compare one device with another, and no evidence to compare mechanical devices with other forms of treatment.[18]

Surgery is uncommon in the treatment of OAB; however, both stress and overflow incontinence can be treated successfully by surgery. Surgery is an option when other nonpharmacologic and pharmacologic therapies have failed or the patient wants definitive treatment. The aims of continence surgery are to elevate the bladder neck, support the urethra, and increase urethral resistance.[2,31] Some surgical options include urethral bulking agents (collagen), sling operation, tension-free vaginal tape, artificial sphincter insertion, needle bladder-neck suspension, retropubic suspension, urinary diversion, and bladder denervation. It should be noted that surgical treatment for stress incontinence can instigate or exacerbate symptoms of urgency.

Pharmacologic Therapy

The type of UI influences the choice of treatments. For that reason, an overview of the pharmacologic measures for specific types of UI is presented here. Most medications used to treat these disorders are prescription products; however, a nonprescription form of oxybutynin, Oxytrol for Women, was approved in 2013. Inappropriate use of systemic nonprescription products and incorrect use of absorbent undergarments and pads before a proper evaluation may result in unnecessary expense, inappropriate treatment, and possibly unnecessary changes in the patient's lifestyle and psychological well-being.

Overactive bladder or urge incontinence may be treated with anticholinergic medications, which facilitate urine storage by decreasing uninhibited detrusor contractions. Oxytrol for Women provides a nonprescription option for women ages 18 years and older with urinary symptoms consistent with OAB. The patch is applied every 4 days to a clean, dry and smooth area of the skin on the abdomen, hips, or buttocks. Application sites need to be rotated with each patch. Common side effects include skin irritation at the patch application site, constipation, and dry mouth. If symptoms do not improve, women should seek a medical referral.[32] Prescription anticholinergic medications such as darifenacin, oxybutynin chloride, solifenacin, tolterodine, fesoterodine, or trospium are frequently used for OAB and urge UI. Mirabegron, a beta-3 adrenergic agonist approved for the treatment of OAB and urge UI, is an alternative to anticholinergic medications. For patients who do not respond or who cannot take anticholinergic medication, onabolutinumtoxinA offers significant relief from symptoms of OAB and urge UI.[33] Other prescription medications that have less evidence of clinical efficacy and raise concerns about risks of side effects include propantheline, imipramine, hyoscyamine, and nifedipine. Flavoxate, FDA approved for urinary tract symptoms, is not effective according to the results of four placebo-controlled trials.[31] Diphenhydramine (see Chapter 11) and dicyclomine are used occasionally. Providers should counsel patients about the potential side effects that occur more frequently with diphenhydramine than with the prescription products. Sedation, dry mouth (a problem for denture users and patients with gastroesophageal reflux disease, dysphagia, or stroke), dizziness, constipation, and confusion can be significant problems in older patients. Contraindications to the use of diphenhydramine (and

other anticholinergic medications) include many conditions (e.g., narrow-angle glaucoma, peptic ulcer, urinary tract obstruction, gastroesophageal reflux disease, and uncontrolled hyperthyroidism) that occur more often in older patients than in other patients.

Stress incontinence is often treated with agents that increase outflow resistance through alpha-receptor stimulation that enhances contraction of the bladder-neck muscles.[2] A commonly recommended nonprescription drug is pseudoephedrine (see Chapter 11).[2,22] The dose of pseudoephedrine is 15–30 mg 3 times daily, starting with the lowest dose, especially in older people. Use of nonprescription medications for UI is an off-label indication and must be approved by a primary care provider. Caution should be used, however, when initiating such therapy in patients with hypertension and/or cardiac arrhythmias. The provider should advise patients to monitor their blood pressure and pulse, and to report any new occurrences of heart palpitations or fainting. Common adverse effects of pseudoephedrine include insomnia, headache, tachycardia, elevated blood pressure, dizziness, nervousness, agitation, and tremor.

In women, only topical estrogen should be advised because placebo-controlled studies have shown that oral estrogen therapy is not effective and that systemic therapy is associated with potentially serious adverse effects including venous thromboembolism, heart attack, stroke, and breast cancer. Topical vaginal estrogen therapy is most useful in stress UI with underlying vaginitis and urethritis due to estrogen deficiency; several randomized controlled trials of vaginal estrogen have shown a decrease in urgency and incontinence.[34,35] Therapy with estrogen vaginal cream is usually initiated with daily application and tapered to several times weekly applications; benefits are usually seen in 4–6 weeks. Other vaginal estrogen options include the vaginal ring and vaginal tablets. Estrogen can be used in combination with alpha-adrenergic agonists; however, the combination is only slightly more effective and can be associated with more adverse effects and increased therapy cost. The antidepressant imipramine, which also acts as an adrenergic agonist, has been suggested when alpha-adrenergic agonists and estrogens have failed. Duloxetine, a selective serotonin and norepinephrine reuptake inhibitor currently approved for the treatment of depression, post-herpetic neuropathy, and diabetic neuropathy, is moderately effective in managing stress UI.[36] If medical treatment fails, surgical correction may be possible.

The treatment of overflow incontinence is directed by the underlying cause. In BPH, alpha-adrenergic antagonists (terazosin, doxazosin, tamsulosin, alfuzosin, silodosin, or prazosin) or 5-alpha-reductase inhibitors (finasteride or dutasteride) can be used to reduce the degree of outlet obstruction. Alpha-adrenergic antagonists have a much faster onset of effect (several days) compared with 5-alpha-reductase inhibitors. Because of a relatively high rate of orthostatic hypotension, prazosin is not recommended for therapy of UI. Prescription agents such as bethanechol chloride may be initiated if the bladder has insufficient contractile strength, such as after general anesthesia. Its efficacy is not well established in long-standing hypotonic bladder, however, and it is associated with potentially serious adverse effects. In neurogenic bladder, bethanechol appears to be most effective when starting therapy as soon as possible after the occurrence of incontinence following the neurologic event. Surgery for BPH is often necessary. Catheterization, usually intermittent, is combined with frequent attempts to void as a last resort when medical and surgical corrections have failed.

Treatment of functional and iatrogenic incontinence requires evaluating the patient's entire medical status, medication history, and environment. UI resulting from medications can be resolved by initiating alternative treatments. Underlying dysfunctions such as pain related to rheumatoid arthritis and decreased mobility can be remedied by medical and environmental changes that make using the toilet possible or easier within the limitations of the patient's functional status. Often an assessment by physical or occupational therapists can be useful in enhancing physical function.

Use of Urinary Incontinence Supplies

Absorbent undergarments and pads are used to protect clothing, bedding, and furniture while allowing the patient to have independence and mobility. Although absorbent products are beneficial, they should be used only after a thorough and complete physical examination. Prematurely initiating the use of absorbent protective products relieves the discomfort and obscures the cause of UI. Because correction of the cause may be possible, the premature acceptance of UI may have significant financial, social, and psychological consequences.

Product Selection Guidelines

The type of absorbent product selected depends on several factors[2]:

- Type and severity of UI
- Functional status
- Gender
- Availability of caregivers
- Patient preference
- Cost
- Convenience

The health care provider needs to discuss these factors with patients and their caregivers when helping them select absorbent garments and pads, which are available as reusable or disposable products (Table 49–4). This discussion is particularly important for low-income patients, who often do not have the economic flexibility to purchase absorbent products; they may be forced to resort to toilet paper or tissue products, an ineffective substitute. Many people attempt to extend the life of disposable products by layering flushable tissue over the pad. The tissue is also easier to dispose of in public places. However, its reduced wicking capacity can expose the skin to more moisture and thus the potential for breakdown. Some patients may be inclined to use low-cost menstrual pads that may be effective in some cases; however, these products contain materials that are specific to absorbing blood, not urine. Given the wide variety of available products, a resource guide published by the National Association for Continence (NAFC) may be invaluable in helping patients with selection of a product.[37] In 2012, the NAFC recommended the following eight national quality performance standards for disposable adult absorbent products[38]:

1. Rewet rate: a measure of a product's ability to withstand incontinent episodes between changes
2. Rate of acquisition: a measure of the speed at which urine is drawn away from the skin
3. Retention capacity: a measure of a product's capacity to hold fluid
4. Sizing options: sizes ranging from youth and small adult to extra large and XX-large adult

table
49–4   Selected Adult Incontinence Product Features[a]

Trade Name	Absorbency	Size	Characteristics
Undergarments			
Assurance Slip-On Protective Undergarment[b]	For moderate-heavy leakage	One size	One-piece design; no buttons or tapes
Attends Undergarments Super Absorbency	For moderate leakage		Reusable elastic belts
Depend Undergarments Easy Fit Elastic Leg/Adjustable Straps Regular & Extra Absorbency	For moderate leakage	One size; fits hip sizes up to 65 inches	Soft, cloth-like outer cover; reusable hook and loop strap tabs
Depend Undergarments Elastic Leg/Button Straps Regular & Extra Absorbency	For moderate leakage	One size; fits hip sizes up to 65 inches	Soft, cloth-like outer cover; reusable button strap tabs
Depend Undergarments Elastic Leg Extra Absorbency	For moderate leakage	One size	Soft, cloth-like outer cover; reusable button strap tabs
Depend Underwear Extra & Super Plus Absorbency	For heavy leakage	S/M, L	Feels and wears like underwear
Depend Refastenable Underwear Extra & Super Plus Absorbency	For heavy leakage	S/M, L/XL	Feels and wears like underwear; four refastenable tabs
Prevail Underwear	For heavy leakage	S, M, L	For men and women; look and feel like underwear; pull-on
Briefs			
Attends Briefs	For heavy leakage	Y, S, M, L	Refastenable tapes
Attends Briefs with Waistband	For heavy leakage	M, L	Waistband
Depend Fitted Briefs Regular & Overnight Absorbency	For heavy leakage; overnight absorbency absorbs 30% more urine than regular absorbency	M, L	Six refastenable tapes plus elastic leg and waist; wetness indicator
TENA Briefs	For heavy leakage	Y, S, M, L	Refastenable tabs

table 49–4 Selected Adult Incontinence Product Features[a]

Trade Name	Absorbency	Size	Characteristics
Pads			
Attends Pads	For light leakage; medium-, extra-, super absorbency	8.5, 10.5, 12.5 14.5, 18 inches long	
Poise Pantiliners	Very light absorbency	6.5 inches long	
Poise Extra Coverage Pantiliners	Very light absorbency	7.5 inches long	
Poise Thin Pads Light Absorbency	For light leakage	8.5 inches long	Elasticized sides
Poise Pads Regular Absorbency	For light leakage	8.5 inches long	Elasticized sides
Poise Pads Extra Absorbency	For light leakage	9.5 inches long	Elasticized sides; one end wider
Poise Pads Extra Plus Absorbency	For light-moderate leakage	11 inches long	Elasticized sides; one end wider
Poise Pads with Side Shields Ultra Absorbency	For light-moderate leakage	11 inches long	
Poise Pads with Side Shields Ultra Plus Absorbency	For moderate leakage	13 inches long	Pad-like comfort with guard-like absorbency; one end wider
Serenity/TENA Dry Active Liners	For light leakage	Regular and long	
Serenity/TENA Active Ultra Thin Pads	For light-moderate leakage	Regular and long	
Serenity/TENA Stylish Ultra Thin Pads with Wings	For light leakage	One size	Form fitting, sleek, and super absorbent
Serenity/TENA Anywhere Ultra Thin Pads	For heavy leakage	Long	
Serenity/TENA Anywhere Ultra Thin Pads	For moderate leakage	Regular	
Serenity/TENA Pads Moderate	For moderate leakage	Regular and long	
Serenity/TENA Pads Heavy	For heavy leakage	Regular and long	
Serenity/TENA Ultimate Pads	For heavy leakage	One size	
Serenity/TENA Overnight Pads	For heavy leakage; overnight	One size	Longest pad
Serenity/TENA Insta-DRY HEAVY Pads	For heavy leakage	One size	Fast-absorbing pad
Guards			
Attends Guards Super Absorbency	For light-moderate leakage	One size	Curved fit
Conveen Drip Collector	For dribbling or light leakage; adheres to underwear; designed for men	3- and 4-ounce capacity	
Depend Guards for Men	For light-moderate leakage	One size	Anatomic design with elasticized pouch and cup-like fit
Serenity/TENA Guards Super Absorbency	For moderate-heavy leakage	One size	
Serenity Guards Super Plus Absorbency	For heavy leakage	One size	

Key: Y = Youth; S = small; M = medium; L = large.
[a] Products change often; for current product availability, refer to Web sites (i.e., www.depend.com, www.poise.com, www.serenity.com).
[b] Manufacturer markets other products similar to the Depend line but offers a lower price point.

5. Safety: no components, including additives, that are listed in any federal regulatory agency as being considered "unsafe"
6. Presence of a closure system: mechanism that allows the product to be opened and refastened
7. Breathable zones: an acceptable minimum air flow in side "wings" of the product sufficient to release trapped body heat and gaseous body perspiration in the pelvic region
8. Performance of elastics: provision of evidence of fit and the functionality of containment of body waste, without sacrificing comfort

The disposable product market has been a multimillion-dollar industry since the 1990s. These products work in the same manner as children's disposable diapers. They are designed to absorb urine; provide a moisture barrier to protect clothes, bedding, and furniture; and minimize skin contact with urine. For maximum absorbency, products containing an absorptive gel of superabsorbent polymers may be preferable. Urine is jelled in the matrix of the absorbent layer, minimizing its contact with skin. Reusable incontinence undergarments may offer a more affordable option.[39] These resemble underpants with a waterproof crotch and are designed to hold a reusable panty liner. The newest option is reusable incontinence undergarments that resemble standard underwear but have the absorbency of disposable briefs. These undergarments have a unique crotch design made of several layers of wicking fabric that quickly pulls moisture away from the skin. They are available for men and women in a variety of leakage control levels. Reusable incontinence underwear is constructed of waterproof outer fabrics ranging from lace to nylon floral prints, making them an attractive and affordable option for patients with an active lifestyle. A comparative evaluation of the performance and cost-effectiveness of four key absorbent product designs demonstrated significant and substantial differences between products and considerable individual variability in preference. Cost-effective management with absorbent products may best be achieved by allowing users to choose combinations of designs for different circumstances.[40]

The capacity of each disposable product corresponds to the needs of the patient:

- Guards/shields: 2–12 ounces (60–360 mL), light-heavy capacity
- Undergarments: 12–18 ounces (360–540 mL), moderate-heavy capacity
- Briefs: 28–36 ounces (840–1100 mL), moderate-heavy capacity

Patients with small amounts of leakage (e.g., dribbling), as occurs in stress or overflow incontinence and after urologic surgical procedures, may require only a pad or shield.[41,42] A recent systematic review of absorbent products suggested that disposable insert pads are best for leak-through prevention; they are also the most acceptable and preferred design for women with light UI.[43] In a similar study, guards were a preferred product for light UI in men.[44] If larger amounts of urine are lost with UI, as often occurs with detrusor instability, products with a larger capacity would be more appropriate. Many products designed for overnight (heavy) use tend to have the largest capacities.[37] Booster or doubler pads or inserts are also available to prevent leaks and increase the absorbency of current absorbent products.

Another important issue is the functional capacity of the patient. If the patient needs assistance with absorbent garments, the caregiver may find that briefs or diapers with "roll-on" bed application and adhesive closures are useful. Securing the product may be an important issue. Close-fitting underwear is recommended. Some garments or shields have adhesive strips or belts to hold them in place. The use of belts may require assistance from a caregiver. Of course, comfort and leg security from urine leakage are important. Many product lines offer elastic legs or contoured shapes. Caregivers and patients should consider products designed for the differences between male and female anatomy when selecting large-capacity products.[41,42]

Protective underpads are often used in conjunction with briefs and undergarments for extended duration activities, such as sleeping and sitting. Both bed and chair pads are available, and the provider should inquire about the need for additional protection. The underpad should have a known capacity, a waterproof duration of several hours, and an ability to remain intact when wet. Bed pads are available in sizes from 16 by 24 inches to 30 by 36 inches. For chairs, a 16- by 18-inch pad should be used.[42]

Complications from Absorbent Products

Because the use of absorbent products increases the risk of skin irritation and maceration, these products should be checked every 2 hours. With continual urine loss, it is recommended that the absorbent material be changed every 2–4 hours. The use of skin protectants (barrier creams and ointments), as in diaper

rash, is appropriate. If a rash occurs, the same treatment as that described for infants is indicated (see Chapter 35).

Urine odor is an embarrassing problem. Nonprescription products containing chlorophyll (e.g., Derifil, Pals, or Nullo) or vitamin C can be recommended to help decrease urine odor. However, frequent checks and changes are preferable to efforts to mask the odor.

The healing of skin wounds may be delayed in the patient with skin wetted by urine. Any skin breakdown needs to be reported to the primary care provider. This serious complication should not be treated with nonprescription products without medical supervision.

UI products that are not available from the pharmacy or specialty supply store may be obtained by contacting the National Association for Continence, PO Box 1019, Charleston, SC 29402-1019; 1-843-377-0900, 1-800-BLADDER; fax: 1-843-377-0905; or www.nafc.org.

Complementary Therapies

Nutritional deficiencies of protein, calcium, vitamin C, zinc, magnesium, and vitamin B_{12} have been proposed as possibly contributing to the development of UI.[45] Of these, the relationship between vitamin B_{12} deficiency and UI has been established.[46] A B_{12} deficiency may lead to diminished neurosensory input regarding bladder fullness or to inappropriate neurologic stimulation of the bladder, causing detrusor instability. Many factors, such as spicy and acidic foods (e.g., caffeine, alcohol, and tobacco), dyes (e.g., Food Drug and Cosmetic Yellow Dye No. 5), food preservatives, and sugar substitutes (i.e., aspartame), may cause urinary frequency and urgency with the potential for UI.

Several herbal treatments have been suggested for UI, including phytoestrogens (e.g., soybean and flaxseed), saw palmetto and pygeum (African plum), St. John's wort, and bearberry (uva-ursi) teas. Good clinical evidence from recent rigorous studies showed that saw palmetto is not effective in improving lower urinary tract symptoms related to benign prostatic hyperplasia.[47,48] In addition, there is no evidence from controlled studies that other herbal products significantly improve lower urinary tract symptoms of benign prostatic hyperplasia.[49] Patients should be advised to consult with their primary care provider before using any of these products for UI. An in-depth discussion of saw palmetto and pygeum is presented in Chapter 51.

Assessment of Adult Urinary Incontinence and Supplies: A Case-Based Approach

Because of the public's general lack of sufficient medical knowledge about the different types of UI, some patients (or their caregivers) may attempt self-diagnosis and treatment without consulting their primary care provider. Self-diagnosis obviously could lead to inappropriate assessment and treatment. Therefore, it is imperative that providers inquire about a proper medical evaluation before recommending nonprescription products, including absorbent products. A primary care provider must recommend use of nonprescription medications for off-label indications.

Armed with the patient's history and proper diagnosis, the provider can answer questions appropriately and help in the selection and proper use of devices and medications for treating this disorder.

Cases 49–1 and 49–2 illustrate the assessment of adult patients with UI.

case
49–1

Relevant Evaluation Criteria	Scenario/Model Outcome

Information Gathering

1. Gather essential information about the patient's symptoms and medical history, including:

a. description of symptom(s) (i.e., nature, onset, duration, severity, associated symptoms)

Patient complains of episodes of a "weak bladder," and "I have the urge to go more than 8 times in a day, and sometimes I don't make it to the bathroom in time." The first incident occurred 3 months ago. As a result, she has restricted her fluids and limited her activities. She has not seen her primary care provider.

b. description of any factors that seem to precipitate, exacerbate, and/or relieve the patient's symptom(s)

The "leakage" occurs unexpectedly at no particular time.

c. description of the patient's efforts to relieve the symptoms

"I have been using feminine products. I usually can get to the bathroom in time. When leakage does happen, the urine soaks the pads."

d. patient's identity

Mary Ross

e. age, sex, height, and weight

48 years old, female, 5 ft 4 in., 150 lb

f. patient's occupation

Accountant

g. patient's dietary habits

Balanced diet, 1–2 cups of coffee/tea per day; social alcohol use

h. patient's sleep habits

No nighttime awakenings

i. concurrent medical conditions, prescription and nonprescription medications, and dietary supplements

Occasional use of acetaminophen for morning stiffness

j. allergies

NKA

k. history of other adverse reactions to medications

None

l. other (describe) _____

Lives with husband and children.

Assessment and Triage

2. Differentiate patient's signs/symptoms and correctly identify the patient's primary problem(s).

Characteristics of Ms. Ross urine leakage are consistent with overactive bladder with urge incontinence.

3. Identify exclusions for self-treatment.

None. However, Ms. Ross should be encouraged to seek a diagnosis for her UI before relying on incontinence products.

4. Formulate a comprehensive list of therapeutic alternatives for the primary problem to determine if triage to a medical provider is required, and share this information with the patient or caregiver.

Options include:

(1) Recommend a trial of Oxytrol for Women. If symptoms do not improve, seek medical referral.

(2) Refer Ms. Ross to her primary care provider or gynecologist for evaluation of urge incontinence.

(3) Recommend a pad or shield for light urine leakage. Reusable incontinence underwear may also be an option for her active lifestyle.

(4) Suggest avoidance of frequent use of caffeine.

(5) Take no action.

Plan

5. Select an optimal therapeutic alternative to address the patient's problem, taking into account patient preferences.

See Figure 49–1. Ms. Ross should be offered a trial of Oxytrol for Women. She should be advised to consider using pads, shields, or reusable incontinence underwear, as needed, for light urine leakage. These products would offer more protection than feminine pads. She should be counseled on the benefits of caffeine reduction.

6. Describe the recommended therapeutic approach to the patient or caregiver.

"Oxytrol for Women is recommended for the self-care of symptoms of overactive bladder, specifically the sudden and urgent need to urinate. If symptoms persist, a medical referral will be necessary."

7. Explain to the patient or caregiver the rationale for selecting the recommended therapeutic approach from the considered therapeutic alternatives.

"Oxytrol for Women has been shown to be a safe and effective treatment for overactive bladder. Medical evaluation may be necessary for persistent symptoms to determine the type of incontinence and the need for a prescription medication or device."

case
49–1 *continued*

Relevant Evaluation Criteria	Scenario/Model Outcome

Patient Education

8. When recommending self-care with nonprescription medications and/or nondrug therapy, convey accurate information to the patient or caregiver:

"Oxytrol for Women is recommended for the self-care of symptoms of overactive bladder, specifically the sudden and urgent need to urinate."

 a. appropriate dose and frequency of administration

"Apply 1 Oxytrol for Women to the skin every 4 days. It is a thin clear patch."

See the box Patient Education for Adult Urinary Incontinence and Supplies.

 b. maximum number of days the therapy should be employed

"Apply the patch no more than 2 days per week. Select 2 days of the week (e.g., Sunday and Wednesday) and maintain a consistent schedule."

See the box Patient Education for Adult Urinary Incontinence and Supplies.

 c. product administration procedures

"Remove the patch every 4 days and apply a new patch to a different area. The patch may be applied to the abdomen, hip, or buttock. Contact with water when you are bathing, swimming, showering, or exercising will not change the way Oxytrol works."

See the box Patient Education for Adult Urinary Incontinence and Supplies.

 d. expected time to onset of relief

"Symptoms may improve within 3–4 weeks but could be seen as early as 2 weeks. Results are generally seen by 12 weeks."

 e. degree of relief that can be reasonably expected

"Usage may reduce symptoms by as much as 75%."

See the box Patient Education for Adult Urinary Incontinence and Supplies.

 f. most common side effects

"The Oxytrol for Women patch may cause skin irritation where the patch was applied, dry mouth, and constipation. Incontinence pads may cause skin irritation, rash, maceration, and breakdown."

 g. side effects that warrant medical intervention should they occur

"If skin irritation is severe, discontinue product use. You should check for skin irritation every 2 hours." See the box Patient Education for Adult Urinary Incontinence and Supplies.

 h. patient options in the event that condition worsens or persists

"If symptoms persist, see your primary care provider or urologist for further follow-up. If urine loss is continual, change absorbent undergarments every 2–4 hours."

 i. product storage requirements

NA

 j. specific nondrug measures

See the box Patient Education for Adult Urinary Incontinence and Supplies for behavioral measures to reduce and improve incontinence symptoms.

Solicit follow-up questions from patient or caregiver.

(1) "What if the symptoms don't improve?"

(2) "What if the incontinence product does not provide enough protection?"

Answer patient's or caregiver's questions.

(1) "If symptoms do not improve, see your primary care provider. Do not increase the dose or frequency of the patch."

(2) "You may select a product with higher absorbency according to the amount of urine leakage (Table 49–4)."

Evaluation of Patient Outcome

9. Assess patient outcome.

"If symptoms do not improve within 2 weeks of using Oxytrol, consult your primary care provider for further evaluation and treatment."

Key: N/A = Not applicable; NKA = no known allergies.

case
49–2

Relevant Evaluation Criteria	Scenario/Model Outcome

Information Gathering

1. Gather essential information about the patient's symptoms and medical history, including:

   a. description of symptom(s) (i.e., nature, onset, duration, severity, associated symptoms)

   Patient wants to use an herbal product for "dribbling and inability to empty my bladder." The medication prescribed for this problem 2 weeks ago does not "seem to be working." He heard about a product for urinary health during a recent radio broadcast.

   b. description of any factors that seem to precipitate, exacerbate, and/or relieve the patient's symptom(s)

   The dribbling occurs throughout the day. He often wakes up 2–3 times per night to urinate. These symptoms often make his work deliveries late.

   c. description of the patient's efforts to relieve the symptoms

   Frequent trips to the bathroom

   d. patient's identity

   Joe Sample

   e. age, sex, height, and weight

   55 years old, male, 5 ft 8 in., 220 lb

   f. patient's occupation

   Floral delivery driver

   g. patient's dietary habits

   2–3 cups of caffeine-containing beverages per day

   h. patient's sleep habits

   Frequent nighttime awakenings to urinate

   i. concurrent medical conditions, prescription and non-prescription medications, and dietary supplements

   Benign prostatic hyperplasia: Proscar 5 mg daily; hypertension: currently takes lisinopril 10 mg daily

   j. allergies

   NKA

   k. history of other adverse reactions to medications

   None

   l. other (describe) _____

   Married

Assessment and Triage

2. Differentiate patient's signs/symptoms and correctly identify the patient's primary problem(s).

   Joe's urine leakage is consistent with symptoms of BPH. He is currently on Proscar (finasteride) and has not had symptom relief because of the short duration of the therapy. However, considering his work situation and the impact of BPH, he should see his PCP or urologist for reevaluation of the therapy and prior to starting any dietary supplement or any other nonprescription treatment.

3. Identify exclusions for self-treatment.

   Mr. Sample has been evaluated by a PCP or urologist and is currently receiving therapy for BPH.

4. Formulate a comprehensive list of therapeutic alternatives for the primary problem to determine if triage to a medical provider is required, and share this information with the patient or caregiver.

   Options include:

   (1) Refer Joe for further evaluation for BPH therapy.

   (2) Counsel Joe about options for prescription drug treatment. Because of his symptoms and job requirements, advise him to ask his PCP about alpha-adrenergic antagonists for faster relief of his symptoms.

   (3) Counsel on the benefits of avoiding frequent use of caffeine.

   (4) Recommend a guard for persistent urine leakage.

   (5) Take no action.

Plan

5. Select an optimal therapeutic alternative to address the patient's problem, taking into account patient preferences.

   Joe should consult a PCP or other health care provider for further evaluation prior to using any nonprescription medication, prescription medication, or incontinence product.

6. Describe the recommended therapeutic approach to the patient or caregiver.

   "Once current therapy has been evaluated and other causes eliminated, alternative prescription drug therapy may be suggested for reducing the symptoms of BPH. An absorbent guard may be appropriate for persistent symptoms."

7. Explain to the patient or caregiver the rationale for selecting the recommended therapeutic approach from the considered therapeutic alternatives.

   "Medical evaluation is necessary to assess the effectiveness of your current regimen and determine the need for another drug therapy option."

case
49–2 *continued*

Relevant Evaluation Criteria	Scenario/Model Outcome
Patient Education	
8. When recommending self-care with nonprescription medications and/or nondrug therapy, convey accurate information to the patient or caregiver:	
a. appropriate dose and frequency of administration	See the box Patient Education for Adult Urinary Incontinence and Supplies.
b. maximum number of days the therapy should be employed	See the box Patient Education for Adult Urinary Incontinence and Supplies.
c. product administration procedures	See the box Patient Education for Adult Urinary Incontinence and Supplies.
d. expected time to onset of relief	NA
e. degree of relief that can be reasonably expected	See the box Patient Education for Adult Urinary Incontinence and Supplies.
f. most common side effects	"You may experience skin irritation, rash, maceration, and breakdown."
g. side effects that warrant medical intervention should they occur	"You should check for skin irritation every 2 hours."
h. patient options in the event that condition worsens or persists	See the box Patient Education for Adult Urinary Incontinence and Supplies. "If urine loss is continual, change absorbent undergarments every 2–4 hours. See your primary care provider or urologist for further follow-up."
i. product storage requirements	NA
j. specific nondrug measures	See the box Patient Education for Adult Urinary Incontinence and Supplies.
Solicit follow-up questions from patient or caregiver.	"What if the incontinence product does not provide enough protection?"
Answer patient's or caregiver's questions.	"You may select another product with higher absorbency according to the amount of urine leakage (Table 49–4)."
Evaluation of Patient Outcome	
9. Assess patient outcome.	Contact the patient in a day or two to ensure that he made an appointment and sought medical care

Key: BPH = Benign prostatic hyperplasia; NA = not applicable; NKA = no known allergies; PCP = primary care provider.

Patient Counseling for Adult Urinary Incontinence and Supplies

The primary care provider's role in self-treatment of UI includes educating patients about UI; recommending medical evaluation, as appropriate, on the basis of an initial evaluation of signs and symptoms; assisting patients and caregivers in selecting products to reduce the risk of urine leaking to outer garments; and avoiding aggravating factors. Patients should be provided with information to help them understand UI. The box Patient Education for Adult Urinary Incontinence and Supplies lists specific information to provide patients regarding the use of incontinence supplies. An excellent resource for patient education is the Simon Foundation for Continence, PO Box 815, Wilmette, IL 60091; 1-800-23Simon; or www.simonfoundation.org.

Evaluation of Patient Outcomes for Adult Urinary Incontinence and Supplies

At follow-up, the provider should find out whether the pharmacologic therapy is effective and the recommended incontinence product is comfortable and easy to use, and whether leakage from the undergarment or odor is a problem. If leakage is occurring, the absorbency and/or type of product should be reassessed. Patients who have problems with odor may need to use deodorizers. The patient or caregiver should also be asked whether the skin, especially in the perivaginal and perianal areas, is being checked for breakdown. Redness or skin fissures call for the use of skin protectants. Questioning about occurrence of urinary tract or vaginal infections is also appropriate. Such infections may indicate a need to change undergarments more often or to use another type of incontinence product. These measures will prevent prolonged skin contact with urine. In addition, the provider should monitor the effectiveness of other prescription medications and behavioral therapies for UI. The patient should be asked about side effects associated with the specific medication he or she may be prescribed.

Providers should also evaluate whether the use of incontinence products and other treatments has allowed the patient to resume his or her normal lifestyle and social interactions. If these objectives are not being met after an adequate duration of any pharmacotherapy, the medication dose and type should be reviewed. Alternative absorbent products should also be considered. The patient should be encouraged to seek further advice from his or her primary care provider on treatment options.

Key Points for Adult Urinary Incontinence and Supplies

➤ UI is a common treatable condition that is often cured or improved with therapy.

patient education for

Adult Urinary Incontinence and Supplies

The objectives of self-treatment are to (1) reduce or eliminate symptoms of urinary incontinence (UI), (2) control or treat skin irritation caused by contact with urine, (3) control the odor of urine leaked from the bladder, (4) control leakage of urine to outer garments, and (5) prevent other complications such as falls and social isolation. For most patients, carefully following product instructions and the self-care measures listed here will help to ensure optimal therapeutic outcomes.

- Consult a primary care provider or urologist for a thorough examination before resorting to permanent use of absorbent undergarments or shields. Many cases of UI are reversible with treatment.
- These products are designed to absorb urine; to provide a moisture barrier to protect clothes, bedding, and furniture; and to minimize skin contact with urine.
- Base selection of absorbent products on the amount of leaked urine:
  - Guards/shields: 2–12 ounces (60–360 mL), light-heavy capacity
  - Undergarments: 12–18 ounces (360–540 mL), moderate-heavy capacity
  - Briefs: 28–36 ounces (840–1000 mL), moderate-heavy capacity
- Choose briefs or diapers with roll-on bed application and adhesive closures (for patients who are unable to change themselves).
- If additional protection is needed during sleeping and sitting, select absorbent bed or chair pads to use with absorbent undergarments.
- Check skin for irritation or maceration every 2 hours, even when absorbent garments are used.
- If urine loss is continual, change absorbent undergarments every 2–4 hours, and consult your primary care provider or urologist if UI symptoms worsen.
- If desired, use skin protectants labeled for diaper rash to protect the skin.

- If desired, use products containing chlorophyll, such as Derifil, Pals, and Nullo, to help decrease odor. However, continue frequent skin checks and frequent changes of absorbent undergarments.
- If pressure ulcers (open sores) occur in an immobile patient, the caregiver should not attempt to treat the ulcers with nonprescription products and should instead consult a primary care provider.
- Identify and eliminate foods, liquids, or other substances that can irritate the bladder (e.g., coffee, tea, soda, alcohol, chocolate, acidic juices, tomato-based sauces, spicy food, artificial sweeteners, and nicotine).
- Avoid excessive intake of liquid. Drink enough to produce about a cup of urine every 3–4 waking hours on average. Do not drink large amounts of liquid after 5 pm.
- Avoid products that irritate the urethra and bladder. Use cotton underwear, avoid scented powders or bath products, and use white toilet paper.
- Follow instructions for behavioral therapy and medications for incontinence if prescribed by your primary care provider or urologist.

➤ Because the cause of UI may be multifactorial, the patient should receive a comprehensive medical evaluation before a therapy plan is developed.

➤ A variety of treatment options are available, including drug therapy, behavioral therapies, devices, incontinence aids, and surgery.

➤ Incontinence aids are designed to absorb urine; to provide a moisture barrier to protect clothes, bedding, and furniture; and to minimize skin contact with urine.

➤ The selection of absorbent products is based on the amount of urine leakage.

➤ Providers can play an important role in educating patients about UI; performing assessment and triage and referring for medical evaluation, if needed; counseling on the selection and appropriate use of prescription and nonprescription incontinence products and the avoidance of aggravating factors; and monitoring patient response.

REFERENCES

1. Sand PK, Dmochowski R. Analysis of the standardisation of terminology of lower urinary tract dysfunction: report from the standardisation subcommittee of the international continence society. *Neurourol Urodynam.* 2002;21:167–78.
2. Fantl AJ, Newman DK, Lolling L, et al. *Urinary Incontinence in Adults: Acute and Chronic Management, Clinical Practice Guideline.* Rockville, MD: U.S. Department of Health and Human Services, Public Health Service, Agency for Health Care Policy and Research; 1996. Publication No. 96–0682.
3. Gaugler JE, Duval S, Anderson KA, et al. Predicting nursing home admission in the US: a meta-analysis. *BMC Geriatr.* 2007;7:13.
4. Hu T-W, Wagner TH, Bentkover JD, et al. Costs of urinary incontinence and overactive bladder in the United States: a comparative study. *Urology.* 2004;63(3):461–5.
5. Onukwugha E, Zuckerman IH, McNally D, et al. The total economic burden of overactive bladder in the United States: a disease-specific approach. *Am J Manag Care.* 2009;15 (4 suppl):S90–7.
6. Brandeis GH, Baumann MM, Hossain M, et al. The prevalence of potentially remediable urinary incontinence in frail older people: a study using the Minimum Data Set. *J Am Geriatr Soc.* 1997;45(2):179–84.
7. Roberts RO, Jacobsen SJ, Rhodes T, et al. Urinary incontinence in a community-based cohort: prevalence and health care-seeking. *J Am Geriatr Soc.* 1998;46(4):467–72.
8. Thom D. Variation in estimates of urinary incontinence prevalence in the community: effects of differences in definition, population characteristics, and study type. *J Am Geriatr Soc.* 1998;46(4):473–80.
9. Burgio KL, Ives DG, Locher JL, et al. Treatment seeking for urinary incontinence in adults. *J Am Geriatr Soc.* 1994;42(2):208–12.
10. Lee SY, Phanumas D, Fields SD. Urinary incontinence: a primary care guide to managing acute and chronic symptoms in older adults. *Geriatrics.* 2000;55(11):65–72.
11. de Groat WC, Yoshimura N. Pharmacology of the lower urinary tract. *Annu Rev Pharmacol Toxicol.* 2001;41:691–721.
12. Busby-Whitehead J, Johnson TM. Urinary incontinence. *Clin Geriatr Med.* 1998;14(2):285–96.
13. Couture JA, Valiquette L. Urinary incontinence. *Ann Pharmacother.* 2000; 34(5):646–55.
14. Holroyd-Leduc JM, Strauss SE. Management of urinary incontinence in women. *JAMA.* 2004;291(8):986–95.
15. Grodstein F, Fretts R, Lifford K, et al. Association of age, race, and obstetric history with urinary symptoms among women in the Nurses' Health Study. *Am J Obstet Gynecol.* 2003;189(2):428–34.
16. Sampselle CM, Harlow SD, Skurnick J, et al. Urinary incontinence predictors and life impact in ethnically diverse perimenopausal women. *Obstet Gynecol.* 2002;100(6):1230–8.
17. Staskin DR. Overactive bladder in the elderly: a guide to pharmacological management. *Drugs Aging.* 2005;22(12):1013–28.
18. Shaikh S, Ong EK, Glavind K, et al. Mechanical devices for urinary incontinence in women. *Cochrane Database Syst Rev.* 2006;3:CD001756.

doi:10.1002/14651858.CD001576.Accessed at http://www.thecochrane library.com/view/0/index.html.

19. DeLancey JO, Miller JM, Kearney R, et al. Vaginal birth and de novo stress incontinence: relative contributions of urethral dysfunction and mobility. *Obstet Gynecol.* 2007;110(2 pt 1):354–62.

20. American Urogynecological Society Intake and Voiding Diary. Accessed at http://www.oabcentral.org/resources/AUGS_Voiding_Diary.pdf. April 30, 2013.

21. iP voidingdiary. Accessed at http://www.ip-voiding-diary.com, April 30, 2013.

22. Culligan PJ, Heit M. Urinary incontinence in women: evaluation and management. *Am Fam Physician.* 2000;62(11):2433–44.

23. Jackson S. The patient with an overactive bladder: symptoms and quality of life issues. *Urology.* 1997;50(suppl 6A):18–22.

24. Shamilyan TA, Kane, RL, Wyman J, et al. Systematic review: randomized, controlled trials of nonsurgical treatments for urinary incontinence in women. *Ann Intern Med.* 2008;148(6):459–73.

25. Diokno AC, Samselle CM, Herzog AR, et al. Prevention of urinary incontinence by behavioral modification program: a randomized, controlled trial among older women in the community. *J Urol.* 2004;171(3):1165–71.

26. Miller J, Sampselle C, Ashton-Miller J, et al. Clarification and confirmation of the knack maneuver: the effect of volitional pelvic floor muscle contraction to preempt urine expected stress incontinence. *Int Urogynecol J.* 2008;19(6):773–82.

27. Culligan PJ, Neit M. Information from your family doctor: exercising your pelvic muscles. *Am Fam Physician.* 2000;62:2447.

28. Elser D, Mitchell G, Miklos J, et al. Nonsurgical transurethral radio-frequency collagen denaturation: results at three years after treatment *Advances in Urology.* 2011;Vol. 2011:Article ID 872057.

29. NeoControl® Pelvic Floor Therapy System. Accessed at http://www.neocontrol.de/neocontrol.php, April 30, 2013.

30. Norton PA, Baker JE. Postural changes reduce leakage in women with stress urinary incontinence. *Obstet Gynecol.* 1994;84(5):770–4.

31. Smith PP, McCrery RJ, Appell RA. Current trends in the evaluation and management of female urinary incontinence. *CMAJ.* 2006;175(10):1233–40.

32. Oxytrol® For Women. Accessed at http://www.oxytrolforwomen.com, April 30, 2013.

33. Nitti V, Dmochowski R, Herschorn S, et al. OnabotulinumtoxinA for the treatment of patients with overactive bladder and urinary incontinence: results of a phase 3, randomized, placebo controlled trial. EMBARK Study Group. *J Urology.* 2013;189(6):2186–93.

34. Moehrer B, Hextall A, Jackson S. Oestrogens for urinary incontinence in women. *Cochrane Database Syst Rev.* 2003;2:CD001405. doi:10.1002/ 14651858.CD001405.Accessed at http://www.thecochranelibrary.com/view/0/index.html.

35. The North American Menopause Society. The role of local vaginal estrogen for treatment of vaginal atrophy: 2007 position statement of the North American Menopause Society. *Menopause.* 2007;14(3 pt 1):357–69.

36. McCormick PL, Keating GM. Duloxetine: in stress urinary incontinence. *Drugs.* 2004;64(22):2567–73.

37. National Association for Continence. Resource Guide®: Products and Services for Incontinence. Accessed at http://www.nafc.org/online-store/consumer-publications-and-products/nafc-educational-booklets/resource-guide-products-and-services-for-incontinence, May 15, 2011.

38. Muller N, McInnis E. The development of national quality performance standards for disposable absorbent products for adult incontinence. *Ostomy Wound Manage.* 2013;59(9):40–55.

39. Gallo M, Staskin DR. Patient satisfaction with a reusable undergarment for urinary incontinence. *J Wound Ostomy Continence Nurs.* 1997;24(4): 226–36.

40. Fader M, Cottenden A, Getliffe K, et al. Absorbent products for urinary/faecal incontinence: a comparative evaluation of key product designs. *Health Technol Assess.* 2008;12(29):1–208.

41. Newman DK. Bladder dysfunction in women. Products and devices play important role. *Adv Nurse Pract.* 2006;14(5):55–6, 58, 60–2.

42. Brink CA. Absorbent pads, garments, and management strategies. *J Am Geriatr Soc.* 1990;38(3):368–73.

43. Fader M, Cottenden AM, Getliffe K. Absorbent products for light urinary incontinence in women. *Cochrane Database Syst Rev.* 2007;2:CD001406. doi:10.1002/14651858.CD001406.Accessed at http://www.thecochrane library.com/view/0/index.html.

44. Fader M, Macaulay M, Pettersson L, et al. A multi-centre evaluation of absorbent products for men with light urinary incontinence. *Neurourol Urodyn.* 2006;25(7):689–95.

45. Bottomley JM. Complementary nutrition in treating urinary incontinence. *Top Geriatr Rehab.* 2000;16:61–77.

46. Rana S, D'Amico F, Merenstein JH. Relationship of vitamin B_{12} deficiency with incontinence in older people. *J Am Geriatr Soc.* 1998;46(7):931–2.

47. Barry MJ, et al. Effect of increasing doses of saw palmetto extract on lower urinary tract symptoms: a randomized trial. *JAMA.* 2011;306(12):1344–51.

48. Tacklind J, et al. Serenoa repens for benign prostatic hyperplasia. *Cochrane Database Syst Rev.* 2009;(2):CD001423. doi:10.1002/14651858. CD001423.pub2.Accessed at http://www.thecochranelibrary.com/view/0/index.html.

49. Kane CJ, et al. What do I tell patients about saw palmetto for benign prostatic hyperplasia? *Urol Clin N Am.* 2011;38(3):261–77.

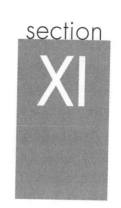
COMPLEMENTARY THERAPIES

INTRODUCTION TO DIETARY SUPPLEMENTS

Candy Tsourounis and Cathi Dennehy

The Food and Drug Administration (FDA) defines *dietary supplements* (DS) as vitamins, minerals, herbs or other botanicals, and amino acids; dietary substances used to supplement the diet by increasing dietary intake or concentrates, metabolites, constituents, and extracts; or any combination of these stated ingredients.[1] Many terms have been used to describe DS, including *nutraceuticals, natural products, supplements, herbs, botanicals,* and *phytochemicals.* Dietary supplements are most often grouped into the natural products category of Complementary and Alternative Medicine (CAM), according to the National Institutes of Health (NIH).[2] For the purposes of this chapter, herbs, vitamins, and similar products will be referred to as DS. This designation is also used by FDA as it relates to the intended use, namely for oral use only and for supplementing the diet. Indeed, DS are used by consumers not only to supplement the diet but also to maintain health and wellness. Some consumers also use DS to treat symptoms of medical conditions, despite FDA legislation that prohibits DS manufacturers from marketing products for this purpose unless the DS have undergone extensive review and been preapproved by FDA for a specified health claim.

Use of Dietary Supplements
Prevalence and Indications for Use

The 2007 National Health Interview Survey (NHIS) surveyed more than 30,000 U.S. citizens; survey results showed that about 18% of adults older than 18 years and 4% of children had used at least one non-vitamin, non-mineral natural product in the previous 12 months.[3] Importantly, this type of product was the most common form of CAM being used when vitamin and mineral products, the top-selling DS class, were excluded. A 2013 consumer survey of approximately 2000 adults conducted by the Council for Responsible Nutrition estimates that DS use in adults is closer to 68%, with 77% of supplement users taking a multivitamin product. The 2007 NHIS survey reported that use of a multivitamin/mineral product in children is 31%.[4,5] The inclusion of vitamin and mineral products accounts for these higher use estimates.

The 2007–2010 National Health and Nutrition Examination Survey (NHANES) examined motivations for adults to use DS.[6] The primary reasons cited were to improve overall health (45%), maintain health (33%), and promote bone health (25%). Among adults ages 60 years and older, DS were used for site-specific conditions involving the bones, heart, and joints, whereas younger adults, ages 20–39, used DS for energy and immunity. Gender differences also existed: women were frequent users of calcium for bone health, whereas men used DS for heart health and lowering of cholesterol levels.

The 2007 NHIS cited primary indications for CAM use in children, in order of prevalence, as pain, head or chest cold, anxiety or stress, musculoskeletal disorders, and attention-deficit/hyperactivity disorder.[3] When DS were considered as a separate CAM modality, indications of use were less specific and involved diverse health conditions.[5]

Top-Selling Dietary Supplements

In 2011, Americans spent an average of $30 billion on DS.[7] Vitamins accounted for 34% of this market, closely followed by specialty products (e.g., products formulated for a specific organ or body function) at 19%, herbs and botanicals at 17%, sports and nutrition products at 12%, meal replacement products at 10%, and minerals at 8%.[7] Although DS sales may be rising, the use of particular DS may be on the decline. Among all DS, multivitamins are the top-selling supplements, primarily because they are used across all life stages. Vitamin D is a market leader, with an increase in sales from $42 million in 2002 to $605 million in 2011.[8] Studies correlating low vitamin D levels and poor health outcomes specific to immunity bone and joint health, and heart health are likely to impact sales. Reports of top DS sales differ according to the purchase location.[7] Sales data, however, may differ from actual consumer use data reported in the 2007 NHIS and the 2007–2010 NHANES study. The most commonly used non-vitamin, non-mineral DS among adults in the 30 days prior to completion of the NHIS survey were fish oil, omega-3 fatty acids or docosahexaenoic acid (37%), glucosamine (20%), echinacea (20%), flaxseed (16%), and ginseng (14%).[3] The NHANES study included vitamins and minerals and cited multivitamin/mineral products as the most frequently used DS, followed by calcium and omega-3 or fish oil supplements.[6]

Attitudes and Predictors of Use

Many studies have measured predictors of CAM use and, more specifically, use of natural products such as DS.[3,6] For most American adults, common predictors for DS use include being a female, ages 50–69 years; having a college education or higher; living in the Western United States (i.e., West North Central, Mountain, and Pacific states); and having a current self-rated health status of very good to excellent.[3,6] Having a higher socio-economic status, defined as not poor or near poor, and having private health insurance are also predictors of high DS use; individuals who were poor, lacked health insurance, or had public health insurance reported low use of DS.[3] Users of DS are also more likely to have a higher number of physician visits and a greater number of health conditions.[3]

Among children, use of non-vitamin, non-mineral natural products was twice as likely to be reported if the parent also used a CAM modality (9% vs. 4%).[3] When vitamins and minerals were included, predictors of use in children included being from a family with a higher level of parental education, being from a family with private health insurance, living in the western United States, and being of White or Asian ethnicity.[5] DS use was more common in children who have a higher disease burden and ill health than in healthier children.[5]

Older adults, ages 61–69 years, are frequent DS users, according to the NHIS survey. They are more likely to have chronic conditions and to use concomitant prescription medications. Individuals who cited general wellness as their rationale for use were 16 times more likely to consume DS. Other factors that appear to be highly predictive of DS use include having an attitude that the DS will work and having a history of receiving health care from CAM providers.[9] The findings suggest that the most important predictor of use is preservation of health, regardless of an individual's assessment of his or her own health status, medical history, or use of concomitant medications.[9]

Television was the most commonly reported source of DS information (73%), followed by magazines and radio (both 30%), newspapers (13%), friends (8%), and store displays (5%).[9] Consistent across several surveys, users of DS tend not to report this use to their health care providers; this nondisclosure is estimated to be as high as 72%.[3] This tendency is especially concerning among older adults in whom concomitant use of prescription drugs and DS is estimated to be between 49% and 74%, raising the risk of potential interactions.[10] These data confirm the importance of obtaining a complete medication history, at all patient encounters, that includes use of DS and prescription and nonprescription drugs. The nondisclosure rate is reported to increase if the provider seems disinterested, appears judgmental of CAM use, or appears to lack sufficient knowledgeable about these therapies. Consumers may also feel that CAM therapies are not relevant to medical care and that the coordination of care is a personal choice.

Legislation and Regulatory Issues

FDA regulates both finished (ready to be sold) DS products and individual dietary ingredients that are used to make a DS product. Importantly, FDA regulates DS under a different set of regulations than those covering conventional foods and medications.

Dietary Supplement Health and Education Act

In 1994, the Dietary Supplement Health and Education Act (DSHEA) was approved by Congress and signed into law.[1] This act allowed FDA to regulate DS under the purview of the Center for Food Safety and Applied Nutrition (CFSAN). As a result, DS were excluded from the strict purity and potency standards that are applied to prescription and nonprescription drugs by the Center for Drug Evaluation Research. DS had to meet only the

standards that applied to food preparation. Any additional standards regarding purity and potency were the sole responsibility of the manufacturer. The lack of strict good manufacturing practice (GMP) standards created problems with DS content, purity, potency, consistency, and actual identity, as well as contamination, herb misidentification, and sub- and supratherapeutic effects. The lack of strict standards and limited oversight of the manufacturing process created a buyer beware market, placing the consumer at risk and often alienating conventional health care providers to the use of CAM therapies, and also led to the misconception that DS are not regulated by FDA.

Another major difference between DS and prescription and nonprescription drugs is the level of evidence required to demonstrate safety and efficacy. For prescription and non-prescription drugs, clinical trials are required to demonstrate evidence of a drug's safety and efficacy prior to its marketing. Although DS manufacturers are prohibited from marketing unsafe or ineffective products, clinical trials are not generally required to prove the safety and efficacy of DS products prior to their marketing; however, some exceptions exist (e.g., new DS ingredients or DS with health and nutrient content claims). The DS manufacturer is responsible for the product's safety and efficacy; however, FDA assumes a post-marketing surveillance role and must prove that a DS is not safe in order to restrict its use or remove it from the market.

New DS Ingredients

DS ingredients that were sold in the United States prior to October 15, 1994, are not required to be reviewed for safety by FDA before being marketed; they are assumed to be safe based on a history of use in humans. For any new DS ingredient (i.e., an ingredient that was not on the market prior to October 15, 1994), a manufacturer must notify FDA 75 days in advance of its intent to market the product and also provide FDA with evidence that the DS is safe in humans when used as directed.[1] Unfortunately, a comprehensive list of DS ingredients that were sold prior to this date is not available. As a result, the decision whether a product contains a new ingredient is left up to the manufacturer. Since DSHEA was approved by the U.S. Congress, nearly 55,000 DS have come on the market, yet FDA has received only 700 premarket notifications during this period.[11] This stark disparity between newly marketed DS and premarket notifications led to the creation of a guidance document for industry regarding new dietary ingredients. In 2011, FDA issued comprehensive guidance that outlines specific recommendations that must be submitted in new dietary ingredient notifications. The guidance document outlines the specific materials that should be submitted to FDA and makes recommendations for the types of safety evidence that should be submitted for new DS ingredients taken short term, long term, or intermittently. Submission of available information on genotoxicity, teratogenicity, mutagenicity, and toxicology for a dietary ingredient is also recommended.[11]

Good Manufacturing Practice

Enactment of DSHEA required establishment of GMP standards for the DS industry. In 2007, FDA issued a final rule on proposed changes to GMP standards for DS.[12] Among the changes, DS must be manufactured in a quality manner without adulterants or impurities, and they must be labeled accurately.

These changes have helped to better regulate manufacturing practices, especially with regard to setting limits on the presence of bacteria, pesticides, and heavy metals. DS manufacturers are required to meet GMP standards as outlined in DSHEA. Most achieve this requirement through their manufacturing and production processes. Some manufacturers take extra steps to have their DS products tested by external quality assurance programs so their product can carry a seal of approval verifying compliance with GMP standards. These programs are discussed in the section Quality Assurance Programs.

Labeling

FDA has primary responsibility for regulating claims found on packaging, package labeling, inserts, and other promotional materials that are distributed at the point of sale. The Federal Trade Commission (FTC) has primary responsibility for advertising claims made through print and broadcast advertisements, infomercials, catalogs, and other direct marketing materials.[13] FTC requires DS claims of safety and efficacy to be supported by "competent and reliable scientific evidence." This evidence is defined as "tests, analyses, research, studies or other evidence based on the expertise of professionals in the relevant area that have been conducted and evaluated in an objective manner by qualified individuals, using procedures generally accepted to yield accurate and reliable results." Complaints against DS advertising may be filed with FTC online.

All DS marketed in the United States must meet supplement labeling requirements.[1] The labels must list (1) the name of the product as well as the word *supplement;* (2) the net quantity of contents; (3) the manufacturer's, packer's, or distributor's name and place of business; and (4) directions for use. In addition, each label must also contain a supplement facts panel that describes the serving size, the list of dietary ingredients, amount per serving size, and the percent daily value, if one is established. (See Figure 50–1 for the Council for Responsible Nutrition's sample label. The label is also available at www.crnusa.org/pdfs/CRN_How_to_read_a_ds_label.pdf.) Plant-based DS should indicate the plant's scientific name, or Latin binomial (i.e., genus and species) and the specific plant part used. Manufacturers may market a combination of DS ingredients as a proprietary blend. Although the individual ingredients in the proprietary blend are listed, the actual quantity of each ingredient is not disclosed. Under DSHEA, the total weight of the blend and the components of the blend, in order of predominance by weight, are required. Fillers, artificial colors, sweeteners, flavors, or binders should also be listed in descending order of predominance. Consistent with the trend in formulating proprietary blends, many multivitamin products are being combined with DS.

When a DS does not follow labeling requirements, the product is considered misbranded.[1] DS manufacturers are not allowed to make claims that their product will diagnose, cure, mitigate, treat, or prevent disease.[1] These claims would require the product to adhere to the regulations related to a drug, and the product would be subject to all the regulatory processes necessary to demonstrate safety and efficacy. Other examples of misbranding include DS that do not conform to labeling requirements; fail to contain the name or place of business of the manufacturer, packer, or distributor; or fail to include accurate statements regarding the quantity of the contents.

The claims for all DS products fall under one of three types: (1) health claim, (2) nutrient content claim, or (3) structure–function claim.[14] Health claims and nutrient content claims require FDA approval, whereas structure–function claims do not. A manufacturer must notify FDA of the exact wording of any structure–function claim within 30 days after the product is marketed. Product labels that contain these claims must also carry a disclaimer: "This statement has not been evaluated by the FDA. This product is not intended to diagnose, treat, cure or prevent disease."

Health claims describe the relationship between a food, food component, or DS ingredient and the resulting reduction in risk of a disease or health-related condition. Claiming that a diet low in saturated fat and cholesterol that includes 25 grams of soy protein daily may reduce the risk of heart disease is an example of an approved health claim. Nutrient content claims describe the relative amount of a nutrient or dietary substance in a product. For example, "very low sodium" means the product is required to have 35 mg or less of sodium per reference amount. Finally, a structure–function claim describes how a product may maintain the normal healthy structure or function of the body without discussing a specific disease state. A supplement manufacturer may claim that the product "supports healthy cholesterol levels" but is prohibited from indicating that the supplement may "reduce high cholesterol levels."

Dietary Supplement and Nonprescription Drug Consumer Protection Act

One of the most important changes to the supplement industry involves the Dietary Supplement and Nonprescription Drug Consumer Protection Act (Public Law 109-462), which was signed into law on December 22, 2006.[15] This law requires manufacturers, packers, or distributors of DS to submit to FDA reports of serious adverse events that are based on specific information received from the public. Serious adverse events are defined as death, a life-threatening situation, a hospitalization, a persistent or significant disability or incapacity, a congenital anomaly or birth defect, or an adverse event that, based on reasonable medical judgment, requires medical or surgical intervention to prevent such serious outcomes. Increased reporting of adverse events may better characterize the frequency and type of serious adverse events associated with DS. FDA actively evaluates trends in serious adverse events so that appropriate corrective action may be taken. Consumers and health care providers are also encouraged to report DS-related adverse events through FDA's MedWatch adverse event reporting program (www.fda.gov/medwatch).[16]

Production Issues
Plant Species and Parts

A health care provider should explain that herbal products typically carry two names, the common name and the Latin binomial. An example would be a product such as St. John's wort (common name), which is also known as *Hypericum perforatum* (Latin genus and species name). Some product labels may list only the Latin name, which can be confusing to a consumer who is unfamiliar with this terminology. When consumers enter a pharmacy and search for an echinacea product, they may encounter single-ingredient products that contain *Echinacea pallida, Echinacea purpurea,* or *Echinacea angustifolia;* products that contain a mixture of two or all of these species; and products that

How do you read a supplement label?

Serving size is the manufacturer's suggested serving expressed in the appropriate unit (tablet, capsule, softgel, packet, teaspoonful).

Amount Per Serving heads the listing of nutrients contained in the supplement, followed by the quantity present in each serving.

International Unit (IU) is a standard unit of measure for fat soluble vitamins (A, D and E).

Milligram (mg) and microgram (mcg) are units of measurement for water soluble vitamins (C and B complex) and minerals. A milligram is equal to .001 grams. A microgram is equal to .001 milligrams.

The list of all ingredients includes nutrients and other ingredients used to formulate the supplement, in decreasing order by weight.

All supplements should be stored in a cool, dry place in their original containers, out of the reach of children and should be used before the expiration date to assure full potency.

Supplement Facts

Serving Size 1 tablet

Suggested Use: Adults, take one tablet per day with meal

Amount Per Serving	% Daily Value
Vitamin A 5000 I.U.	
50% as Beta Carotene	100%
Vitamin C 250 mg	417%
Vitamin D 400 I.U.	100%
Vitamin E 200 I.U.	667%
Vitamin K 80 mcg	100%
Thiamin 5 mg	333%
Riboflavin 5 mg	294%
Niacin 20 mg	100%
Vitamin B_6 5 mg	250%
Folic acid 400 mcg	100%
Vitamin B_{12} 6 mcg	100%
Biotin 150 mcg	50%
Pantothenic Acid 10 mg	100%
Calcium 200 mg	20%
Iron 18 mg	100%
Phosphorus 200 mg	20%
Iodine 150 mcg	100%
Selenium 35 mcg	50%
Magnesium 200 mg	50%
Zinc 15 mg	100%
Copper 2 mg	100%
Boron 150 mcg	*

* Daily Value not established

Ingredients: vitamin A acetate, beta carotene, vitamin D, dl-alpha tocopherol acetate, ascorbic acid, thiamin mononitrate, riboflavin, niacinamide, pyridoxine hydrochloride, vitamin B12, biotin, d-calcium pantothenate, potassium chloride, dicalcium phosphate, potassium iodine, ferrous fumarate, magnesium oxide, copper sulfate, zinc oxide, manganese sulfate, sodium selenate, chromium chloride, sodium molybdate, microcrystalline cellulose, calcium carbonate, sodium carboxymethyl cellulose

Storage: Keep tightly closed in dry place; do not expose to excessive heat

KEEP OUT OF REACH OF CHILDREN

Expiration date: JUN 2016

Company V, Cityville, New York 01010

Percent Daily Value (DV) tells what percentage of the recommended daily intake for each nutrient for adults and children ages 4 and up is provided by the supplement.

An asterisk under the "Percent Daily Value" heading indicates that a Daily Value is not established for that nutrient.

The manufacturer's or distributor's name and place of business or phone number are required to appear on the label.

figure
50–1

Statutory labeling format for certain dietary supplements. (*Source:* Food and Drug Administration. Anatomy of the New Requirements for Dietary Supplement Labels. Accessed at http://www.preventivehealthtoday.com/fda/ fdac/fdac_9811_fdsuppla.pdf, May 18, 2011.)

contain echinacea as one of many listed supplement ingredients. In the case of echinacea, single-ingredient products involving the above-ground parts of *E. purpurea,* formulated as an alcohol extract of the fresh pressed juice, have been the most widely studied. According to one meta-analysis, the above-ground parts of *E. purpurea* demonstrate some evidence of efficacy, albeit weak, in reducing cold symptoms in adults when administered at the first sign of symptoms.[17] The other two species of echinacea and combinations involving these species, with or without *E. purpurea,* have not demonstrated consistent benefits in clinical trials for treating colds.[17]

Common Product Formulations

The content of any DS is based on the raw starting material and how the material is subsequently processed or formulated. Plant-based DS (e.g., echinacea and ginseng) have greater variability in product composition than single-ingredient non-botanical DS (e.g., creatine or melatonin). This variability is due to the chemical composition of botanical DS, which is influenced by the plant's growing conditions, the plant species, the specific plant part used, and the time of harvest.

Knowing which plant species is preferred or which part of the plant to use can be based on historical precedent when clinical trial data are lacking. In developing countries, plant-based medicine is common, and information regarding preferred plant species, preferred plant part, and proper use is handed down from generation to generation, setting a historical precedent for use. An estimated 25% of modern drugs are plant derived, and 50% are derived from natural products (e.g., plants, animals, microbes, and their derivatives).[18] In developing countries, such as those in Africa, the use of plants as drugs is as high as 80%.[18] Use of herbs based on historical precedent is also common in the practice of midwifery. Few clinical trials exist on the use of DS in pregnant women, lactating women, and children. The decision to use DS based on historical precedent is something providers must discuss with their patients.

Method of Preparation

The method in which a DS is manufactured will ultimately affect its final chemical composition and potential efficacy. Some formulations may be well studied, whereas others may not have been studied at all. The most common herbal formulations that a consumer will encounter are made either directly from the fresh plant (e.g., expressed juice, tincture, or tea) or from the dried plant (e.g., fluid extract/tincture, evaporated extract [capsules, tablets], or tea).[19] Tinctures are most commonly prepared by combining chopped herbs with alcohol. This type of formulation should be avoided in persons taking sedating medications or medications that carry disulfiram reaction warnings. Tinctures should also be used cautiously in special populations such as infants, children, and the elderly. Most of the common non–plant-based DS, such as vitamins, minerals, glucosamine, creatine, coenzyme Q10, melatonin, and S-adenosyl-methionine, are manufactured as tablets or capsules; these DS represent compounds that are structurally similar to or identical to compounds naturally found in the human body.

Freshly pressed juice formulations are prepared by pressing the herb and collecting the liquid that is removed.[19] This type of preparation often takes a large amount of the herb to create a substantial portion of juice. In the case of *E. purpurea,* the best-studied formulation is an alcohol extract of the expressed freshly pressed juice.[17] A potential advantage of the alcohol extract is that the presence of alcohol increases the product's shelf life.

Tea formulations can be prepared from the root, leaf, bark, and/or fruit of a plant. Most often they are prepared as an *infusion* by pouring boiling water over the fresh or dried leaf portions of one or more plant species and then letting the herb steep for a small amount of time.[19] This process releases the water-soluble constituents into the tea. The potency is determined by the steeping time and the amount of herb used. The term *decoction* may be used when the plant parts are placed in cold water, brought to a boil, and then simmered for a period of time.[19] Common single-herb tea formulations include chamomile, ginger, peppermint, green tea, and black tea. Multi-ingredient blends that are customized to a specific person's ailment are commonly used in traditional Chinese medicine and may also be administered as teas.

Extracts are intended to concentrate the effects of an herb and can be prepared by soaking fresh or dried plant parts in alcohol, water, alcohol/water mixtures, or oil.[19] The extraction liquid is then reserved and the plant material discarded. Tinctures are fluid extracts in which alcohol is typically used as the extraction medium.[19] Chemicals that seep into the extraction liquid are specific to the solution used. If the extracted liquid is evaporated and dried, it can be formulated into pills or capsules.[19] Extracts and tinctures may list the extraction ratio on the package label. For example, a 5:1 ratio would indicate that 5 parts of herb were used to prepare 1 part of the extract. *Ginkgo biloba* is prepared as a dried extract in tablet form. Ginkgo is typically standardized to a 50:1 extract ratio, meaning that 50 parts of the ginkgo leaf were used to prepare 1 part of the extract.[19] Garlic is available in multiple formulations, the most popular being a dried powdered extract in tablet or capsule form and an aged garlic extract. The chemical composition of the powdered extract will differ from that of the aged extract because of the differences in method of preparation. This variance in composition, in turn, may influence the efficacy of each product.

Standardization

The process of standardization is reserved primarily for plant-based DS because herbs contain many active and inactive constituents. For specific DS, standardization involves identifying specific chemicals or "markers" that may possess therapeutic activity, isolating them, and then formulating them into a final and consistent product. Standardization can occur only if the chemical markers that contribute to the pharmacologic effect have been identified. For example, a *Ginkgo biloba* product may be standardized to contain 6% terpene lactones and 24% flavonoid glycosides, whereas a chastetree berry product may not list any standardized markers at all. The identified active chemical markers may change over time as new research is performed. For example, the active antidepressant marker for St. John's wort was initially thought to be hypericin but is now considered to be hyperforin. Bottles of St. John's wort may list one or both of these standardizations on the package label. Interestingly, no legal or regulatory definition is accepted as it relates to standardization of DS. Claiming that a product is standardized does not necessarily mean a uniform manufacturing process was used. DS verification programs, however, may be helpful in determining compliance with package labeling and actual product composition.

Common Quality Control Issue: Adulteration

According to DSHEA, adulteration of a DS occurs when (1) the DS presents a significant or unreasonable risk of illness or injury when used in accordance with the suggested labeling, (2) the DS is a new entity and lacks adequate evidence to ensure its safety of use, (3) the DS has been declared an imminent hazard by the Secretary of the Department of Health and Human Services, or (4) the DS contains a dietary ingredient that is present in sufficient quantity to render the product poisonous or deleterious to human health, as described for adulterated foods in the Food, Drug, and Cosmetic Act.[1] Adulteration of DS has occurred both intentionally and unintentionally. Examples of unintentional adulterants include heavy metals introduced at the time of cultivation or during the manufacturing process.[20] Heavy metals from environmental pollution can leach from contaminated soil into a plant as the plant grows.[21] In an analysis of 230 Ayurvedic medicines purchased over the Internet, 21% of the Indian-manufactured medicines and 22% of the U.S.-manufactured medicines contained lead, mercury, or arsenic.[20] Heavy metals may also be added to traditional medicine products with the intent of promoting good health. In traditional *rasa shastra* Ayurvedic medicine, addition of heavy metals is standard practice.[21] In this instance, the presence of heavy metals would not be considered adulteration because they were added intentionally and with the intent of promoting good health. However, this practice could still lead to heavy metal contamination of the product user if the content exceeds recommended levels for heavy metal exposure set by state or national health standards.[21]

Intentional adulteration can occur when a manufacturer substitutes a different DS for an ingredient that is in short supply or is too expensive (e.g., economic adulteration). It can also occur when a prescription drug is added to the product to enhance its efficacy. A survey of FDA Class I drug recalls performed between 2004 and 2012 found that 50% of all drug recalls involved DS products.[22] A Class I drug recall involves products containing a drug compound that is likely to result in serious health consequences or death.[22] These recalls most commonly involved products manufactured in the United States and marketed for sexual enhancement, body building, and weight loss. In addition, traditional Chinese medicines have frequently been found to contain heavy metals and undeclared drugs.[23] Violations of GMP standards have been documented for nearly half of the DS manufacturing firms inspected by FDA.[22] The agency is addressing this issue by issuing targeted marketing about adulterated supplements to both consumers and health care providers and by creating multinational enforcement groups who target suppliers of commonly adulterated supplements.[22]

Quality Assurance Programs

Several organizations have developed quality assurance programs to assess analytical reference standards and to certify DS composition. These programs indicate whether the DS product contents match the label contents; unfortunately DS safety or efficacy cannot be ensured. These programs also do not address product quality between different batches or lots because only a single batch is tested at any one time. Most quality assurance programs offer a "voluntary verification program" to manufacturers who pay to have their products tested. Products that pass are then allowed to carry a verification seal on the product label.

United States Pharmacopoeia Dietary Supplement Verification Program

In 2002, the U.S. Pharmacopoeia (USP) initiated a voluntary Dietary Supplement Verification Program.[24] The purpose of the program is to provide consumers with a method for identifying DS that have passed rigorous standards for purity, accuracy of ingredient labeling, and GMP. Products earning USP certification carry a distinctive seal of approval on the product label. These products are certified to contain the listed ingredients in the indicated amounts, to be bioavailable and free of contaminants, and to have been manufactured under appropriate conditions. As of 2013, a total of 13 DS manufacturers are regular program participants. The USP will periodically conduct audits of certified products to ensure continuing adherence to quality standards. Approved products can be found at the USP Web site (www.usp.org/USPVerified/dietarySupplements).

ConsumerLab.com

ConsumerLab.com, LLC (CL) is an independent company that tests products related to health, wellness, and nutrition, such as DS.[25] Products are tested on the basis of identity, purity, and consistency with the labeled ingredients. The test results are posted at www.consumerlab.com/aboutcl.asp, with new results available every 4–6 weeks. Manufacturers are allowed to license the CL seal of approval for a product that passes the review. To continue to carry the approval seal, a product must pass random sample testing every 12 months. The site provides free access to some names of a few products in each category that have passed testing, whereas names of products that fail testing are available only to subscribers. A yearly subscription currently costs $30. The company is not affiliated with manufacturers of any DS, health, or nutrition products.

National Sanitation Foundation International

National Sanitation Foundation (NSF) was established over 66 years ago to standardize sanitation and food safety requirements. Today, NSF International (www.nsf.org) is an independent, nonprofit organization that provides certifications of DS and food and water quality.[26] This organization verifies that the DS product contains the labeled ingredients and that contaminants and unlisted ingredients are not present. Any DS product that meets certification standards is allowed to carry the NSF certification seal of approval on the label. NSF is unique in that it works with professional sports teams to do testing on athletic enhancement supplements.

Hazards from Dietary Supplements
False Advertising/Quackery

Manufacturers who make DS health claims sometimes ignore the regulations established by FDA and FTC and market products using false or misleading claims. FTC requires all advertising to be truthful, not misleading, and based on sound scientific evidence. The weight-loss DS market is one example in which false or misleading health claims are commonly identified.[27] Historically, this type of practice might be considered "quackery," which implies that the person promoting use of the product knows it to be ineffective and is still promoting its use. In the case of some DS, manufacturers may believe, with or without strong clinical support, that their products are effective for a wide variety of ailments. Consumers and providers should be wary of information found on online sites that market DS products. Compared with non-retail online sites, some retail sites have been shown to be unreliable and may list disease claims, may fail to cite the standard disclaimer, and may lack referenced information.[28] Consumers should be wary of products that contain any of the characteristics listed in Table 50–1.[27,29] In addition, consumers should consult a reliable drug information resource, as well as their health care provider, to confirm whether the health claims have a scientific basis. Consumers and providers can go to the NIH Office of Dietary Supplements site and sign up to receive FDA and FTC press releases for products that have been identified as containing adulterants (e.g., prescription drugs) or for manufacturers that have been issued warnings or recalls for product quality.[27] This online site also has tips on how to evaluate health information on the Internet.[27] FDA has also created supplement categories that should be viewed with scrutiny because of a history of prior violations or problems.[29] These supplement categories are listed in Table 50–2. A consumer or provider who wishes to file a complaint related to false advertising should contact FTC.[13]

Hazards Introduced by the Consumer

Exceeding the recommended dietary allowance for a vitamin or mineral supplement or taking more of a supplement than

table

50–1 Characteristics of Supplements Making Fraudulent or Misleading Claims

- List specific disease states or allude to the product's use for a disease usually treated with prescription drug therapy.
- State that supplement's efficacy is similar to, or supplement can be used as an alternative to, a prescription or nonprescription drug.
- List a wide variety of unrelated clinical conditions for use.
- State only benefits and no harmful effects.
- Neglect to provide expiration date, lot number, and contact information for the manufacturer on the package label.
- Use pseudo-medical terminology such as *detoxify, purify,* or *improves body chemistry.*
- Use terms such as *miraculous discovery, revolutionary therapy,* or *breakthrough treatment,* which suggest that the product has superior efficacy to standard care.
- Suggest that the product is more expensive because it works so well.
- Use personal testimonials in place of sound scientific evidence to support product claims.
- Promise quick relief of a health condition.
- Promote natural content as being superior to conventional medicine.
- Provide a money back guarantee or satisfaction guarantee but marketers of fraudulent products often relocate their business location.
- Make accusations that pharmaceutical drug manufacturers and health care providers are working together to defraud consumers and steer consumers away from healthier DS options.

table

50–2 Categories of Supplements That FDA Considers "Clearly Problematic"

- Treatments for life-threatening diseases (e.g., HIV or cancer) or serious medical conditions (e.g., diabetes, Alzheimer's disease)
- Weight-loss products
- Chelation products
- Treatments for behavioral disorders (e.g., attention-deficit/ hyperactivity disorder) or autism
- Treatments for mental retardation or Down syndrome
- Colloidal minerals and silver products
- Supplements for addiction (e.g., smoking, drinking)
- Supplements for body builders
- Supplements for sexual enhancement (e.g., impotence)

Key: FDA = Food and Drug Administration; HIV = human immunodeficiency virus.

is directed on the label can occur intentionally or accidentally. Accidental over-supplementation is more likely to occur when a consumer is taking more than one multi-ingredient product containing similar ingredients. Regardless of how it occurs, over-supplementation should be discouraged because an adverse event may result. Overuse of some DS has serious consequences. For example, overuse of colloidal silver has led to irreversible blue-gray skin discoloration.[30] Overuse of calcium or vitamin D supplements over short periods may cause hypercalcemia. In addition, concern exists that excessive calcium supplementation over long periods of time may contribute to coronary artery calcification.[31] As mentioned previously, adverse events should be reported by consumers and health care professionals to MedWatch.[16] For most DS, individual case reports and postmarketing surveillance provide the best means of identifying adverse events and drug interactions. Consumers should be advised to monitor for acute adverse events for up to 2 weeks after initiating a new DS and to continue the monitoring while using the product.

Product Hazards: Adverse Effects and Drug Interactions

The fact that herbal DS are derived from a natural source does not guarantee safety. Some plants such as poison oak or ivy were never meant to be ingested. Adverse effects are often linked to the pharmacology of the supplement, as was noted when products containing ephedra were removed from the market because of their association with stroke and myocardial infarction.[32] Other DS may be harmful because they contain chemicals that are toxic when ingested. Pyrrolizidine alkaloids present in comfrey, borage, and life root have been associated with case reports of hepatotoxicity.[33] If an adverse event is suspected, product testing is essential to rule out possible plant misidentification; adulteration with prescription or nonprescription drugs; or contamination with heavy metals, microbial contaminants, and pesticides that can occur during production.[34]

Interactions between DS and conventional medications may have a pharmacodynamic or pharmacokinetic basis. Pharmacodynamic interactions can occur when a supplement's pharmacology is similar to or opposite that of a drug the consumer is taking. For example, both St. John's wort and L-tryptophan have been linked to case reports of serotonin syndrome in persons taking these products with prescription psychotropic drugs.[35,36] Additive effects have occurred, or could theoretically occur, in persons combining central nervous system depressants with DS that have sedative properties (e.g., melatonin or valerian) or in persons combining drugs that have antiplatelet or anticoagulant activity with DS that have antiplatelet properties (e.g., fish oil, flaxseed oil, garlic, ginseng, ginkgo, and ginger).[37] Case reports of a DS opposing the effect of a drug or adversely influencing an existing disease state have been reported infrequently in the literature. Theoretical concerns are cited as a reason to avoid DS that enhance immune system activity (e.g., echinacea) in persons who have autoimmune disorders or require immunosuppressants.[38] Finally, DS may have pharmacokinetic interactions. St. John's wort induces multiple cytochrome P450 isoenzymes, as well as the p-glycoprotein drug transporter system.[37] This herb has been reported to induce metabolism of drugs, including oral contraceptives, indinavir, and cyclosporine, thereby lowering drug levels and overall drug efficacy.

Communication Issues
Counseling on Dietary Supplements

The primary consideration in counseling consumers on DS is to recognize the importance of respecting the person's beliefs and values so that a trusting, nonjudgmental relationship can develop. The person must feel comfortable telling the provider about any use of DS. Providers should ask about all therapies being used, including DS, because consumers may not routinely disclose this information. Providers must also be able to provide recommendations regarding DS, when information is available. The risk of adverse effects versus the potential for positive effects must be considered and clearly explained. As an example, if a consumer wishes to take a DS that has *demonstrated both positive and negative outcomes in clinical trials but lacks* documented side effects or drug interactions, a provider may support DS use with the caveat that it may or may not be of benefit. The consumer should be advised to monitor for perceived benefit and side effects. If no benefits are observed within the time frame expected for the DS's onset of action, the DS should be discontinued. Providers should be less inclined to support use of a DS whose efficacy is not supported by EBM and should discourage the use of unsafe products and practices. Importantly, providers do not control access to DS, and consumers may choose to use any available DS. In many instances, providers may be in the position of educating a consumer about DS even though they believe that the product should not be used. In these situations, counseling on expectations and adverse events is essential. For example, educating consumers on the early signs of a serious adverse effect will enable them to recognize a problem and discontinue the DS to minimize harm. Consumers should always be advised to seek medical care for serious conditions.

Consumers should read labels carefully and ask questions. Providers should be aware of the potential for confusion related to DS labels and claims, and counsel consumers in a way that lessens confusion. *Thymus* is an example of a term that might be dangerous if misunderstood. *Thymus vulgaris* is the Latin name for garden thyme. On a supplement label, "*Thymus* extract" may refer to an extract of the herbs thyme, Spanish thyme, or wild thyme, products with relatively few adverse events when used in small doses. However, "thymus extract" may refer to a preparation made from animal thymus gland that is marketed to enhance immune function, a product with considerable quality and safety concerns.

In addition to these broad counseling issues, the following points should be emphasized. First, providers should emphasize that most self-care with DS should be for a limited period. If a problem persists, the consumer should seek medical care. Second, consumers should inform their provider before taking DS for a condition that is also being treated with a prescription drug. Third, consumers should be informed that FDA does not require DS manufacturers to submit data demonstrating efficacy or safety before the product is marketed, unless the product contains a new dietary ingredient (i.e., an ingredient that was not on the market prior to October 15, 1994). Quality and consistency of DS products remain a concern but may improve with the new GMP standards. The following points should be used in counseling consumers who wish to use a DS:

- Purchase products that have either a seal of quality on the label, acquired through a program such as United States Pharmacopeia's Dietary Supplement Verification Program or NSF International's certification program, or that meet their content claim as assessed by ConsumerLab.com.
- Purchase from large, reputable companies. These companies have the resources to meet strict manufacturing standards, have a reputation to uphold, and are more likely to follow quality assurance procedures. Companies that also manufacture prescription or nonprescription drugs (e.g., Bristol-Meyers-Squibb, American Home Products, and drugstore chain store brands) are more likely to have GMP standards in place and to follow these procedures when producing DS.
- Once a quality DS has been selected, continue to use the same brand and formulation. Although this approach does not guarantee a lack of potential quality issues, given that variability between batches can occur, it does increase the likelihood of a consistent product and dose. Providers working with consumers who have not had positive results with use of a DS might consider a trial of a different brand that is appropriate for the specific symptom before determining that the supplement is ineffective for that consumer.
- Know the DS products that you are using and tell your health care provider about them.
- Report any adverse effects related to DS use to your health care provider.

Additional recommendations for counseling can be found in Table 50–3. Cases 50–1 and 50–2 provide examples of how to counsel consumers who wish to treat ailments with DS.

Considerations for Special Population Groups

This section provides a brief overview of issues regarding the use of DS by different consumers. The lack of data on safety and efficacy in these groups, as well as the current regulatory issues, underscores the need for comprehensive assessment of the consumer's health status and knowledgeable counseling.

Older Adults

Although many older adults are healthy and living independently, some may have a significant burden of disease. The latter may have age- and disease-related physiologic declines such as impaired kidney function. Older individuals may be chronically taking multiple prescription and nonprescription drugs, making

table
50-3 General Recommendations for Consumers

Appropriate Use
- Read all labels carefully; never take more than the recommended amount.
- Never share DS with others.
- Do not select a product that lacks dosing recommendations on the label.
- Avoid products that do not carry a lot number or expiration date.
- Discard products 1 year from date of purchase if no other expiration date is present.
- Select products that list the manufacturer's name, address, and telephone number.
- Store products in a dry environment out of direct sunlight and away from young children and pets.

Special Groups
- Always seek the advice of a pediatrician before using a DS in children.
- Avoid DS if you are pregnant or breast-feeding or are trying to become pregnant.
- Speak to your primary care provider if you are trying to treat a life-threatening condition, such as cancer or HIV.

Adverse Effects
- The term *natural* does not mean safe; be diligent and report any unusual experiences to your health care provider.

- If you are allergic to plants, weeds, and/or pollen, ask your provider before using a DS.

Interactions
- If you are taking a prescription medicine, do not take a DS for the same condition.
- When possible, avoid taking multi-ingredient preparations; select single-ingredient products that list the strength per dose.
- Do not take these products with alcohol.
- Check with your primary care provider if you are taking "blood thinning" drugs; some DS may interact with these drugs.
- Always inform your primary care provider of the products you are taking; keep a list if necessary or bring them with you to your appointment.

Expectations
- Never use these products in place of proper rest and nutrition; eat a balanced diet.
- Do not expect a cure or unrealistic results; these agents are not cure-alls.
- If it sounds too good to be true, it probably is; use discretion when evaluating claims.
- Keep a diary to track the effectiveness and side effects of DS.

Key: DS = Dietary supplements; HIV = human immunodeficiency virus.

case
50-1

Patient Complaint/History

Mr. Jones is 72 years old and would like to select a glucosamine product for his knee pain. He has knee osteoarthritis that was diagnosed 10 years ago. His knee pain comes and goes; his stiffness and pain usually last a few weeks and then subside. He has been taking acetaminophen 500 mg for his pain every 6 hours when he has flare ups. His doctor told him that he has degraded cartilage and that he should start taking glucosamine to help strengthen his cartilage. He is taking aspirin 81 mg once daily for heart protection and he has no known drug allergies. He is not taking other medicines and is in excellent health. He walks 3 miles every day except when his arthritis flares up. Mr. Jones noticed many glucosamine products on the shelf and is wondering how to select a quality product.

Clinical Considerations

Mr. Jones appears to be a great candidate for glucosamine because his health care provider has confirmed that Mr. Jones has damaged cartilage in his knee, an area where glucosamine may work. Since Mr. Jones is taking only low-dose aspirin, drug interactions with glucosamine are not likely.

Mr. Jones should select a glucosamine supplement that has been approved by one of the three DS quality assurance programs: United States Pharmacopoeia Dietary Supplement Verification Program, ConsumerLab.com, or National Sanitation Foundation International. Some glucosamine products may carry a seal of approval on the label, but others may not. When a seal of approval is not present, a good way to verify the quality of the product is to visit the Web site of each quality assurance program to verify whether the product is approved.

Mr. Jones should also evaluate the supplement facts panel to help him select a product that follows appropriate labeling recommendations. The product he selects should list the name of the DS, its active ingredients, and the strength of each ingredient provided in each pill. The manufacturer's name and address and the recommended daily dose should also be listed. In some cases, the packer's or the distributor's information may be listed instead. He should review and consider all the DS ingredients listed on the label, paying special attention to ingredients that are not necessary, including added salt (e.g., sodium chloride). If the DS makes any statements regarding the structure or function of the body, in this case "strengthening cartilage", the DS product must also carry the following structure–function claim disclaimer: "This statement has not been evaluated by the Food and Drug Administration. This product is not intended to diagnose, treat, cure or prevent any disease."

Mr. Jones should follow the dosing recommendations on the label and keep a diary of how he is feeling while taking the supplement. He should document his pain, mobility, and stiffness over time. He should also document any side effects and when they began and disappeared. Keeping a glucosamine diary is important because the supplement may take months to work. He should continue to take acetaminophen as his doctor recommended during his acute flare ups because glucosamine is not an analgesic. Before undergoing any surgical procedures, Mr. Jones should be instructed to let his provider know that he is taking glucosamine. Finally, Mr. Jones should be instructed to purchase his supplements from reputable companies. These companies have the resources to meet strict manufacturing standards, have a reputation to uphold, and are more likely to follow strict quality assurance procedures. Companies that also manufacture prescription and nonprescription drugs are more likely to have good manufacturing practices in place and to follow these procedures when producing DS.

case
50–2

Patient Complaint/History

Ms. McDonald is 22 years old. She approaches the pharmacy counter with two empty DS bottles that she has questions about. She says she is looking for something to boost her mood and hands you an empty bottle of a product that a friend gave her. The products are called "CDF body, life and mood" and "CDF body, life and energy." You are familiar with Ms. McDonald because she regularly receives her prescription birth control pills and prescription antidepressant medicine (paroxetine) from your pharmacy. Today she looks more tired and disheveled than usual. For the past month, she had been taking two supplements that a friend gave her and was feeling better, but she ran out of pills a week ago. Her friend purchased the supplements when she traveled home to Canada. Ms. McDonald wanted to know if she could buy them in the United States. She would like your help in selecting supplements that are the same or similar to the ones that her friend gave her.

You ask her if anything has happened in her life recently that has made things more difficult for her. She shares that her pet cat died 3 months ago and that graduate school is stressful and she is not performing as well as she would like. She also shares that her mood has been more up and down over the last 6 months and that she has not shared this information with her health care provider because she did not have the time to make an appointment. You ask if she has been eating the same as usual, and she responds that she has lost some weight because she has been eating less over the past 2 months. She sees this as a positive thing, however, because her boyfriend has complimented her on her slimmer figure.

You evaluate the label on the CDF mood supplement and find that it is a proprietary blend with hypericum perforatum listed as the first ingredient. The energy supplement is also a proprietary blend with Panax ginseng listed as the first ingredient.

Clinical Considerations

The ingredient listed first in a proprietary blend is present in the greatest quantity. In general, the actual amount of each ingredient in a proprietary blend is not listed, but the total weight of the blend is listed. In addition, the contents are listed in the order of the most prevalent to the least prevalent ingredient. Evaluating the first three ingredients in a blend is a good place to start. If the ingredients listed are unfamiliar, one of the drug information resources listed in this chapter can be used to evaluate the ingredients. *Hypericum perforatum* is the Latin binomial name (genus and species) for St John's wort. Compared with placebo, this DS has been shown to be efficacious in relieving symptoms of mild-moderate depression in some clinical trials. The herb's pharmacology increases the levels of brain neurotransmitters such as norepinephrine, dopamine, and serotonin. If taken with paroxetine, which also increases serotonin levels, the herb may cause an additive effect. Too much serotonin can lead to serotonin syndrome. St John's wort is also known to enhance the metabolism of several prescription drugs, including oral contraceptives, leading to reduced efficacy. Panax ginseng does not interact with any of her prescription medicines, but, when compared with placebo, it has not shown any consistent benefit in improving energy in clinical trials.

Ms. McDonald has been feeling better after taking the two products, but she has some symptoms that warrant referral. Although she experienced the loss of a pet about 3 months ago and is currently experiencing stress from her graduate studies, her alterations in mood have been occurring for about 6 months. This could be symptomatic of a worsening of her depression. She also presents with a reduced dietary intake accompanied by weight loss and is tired and disheveled in her appearance, which can by symptomatic of depression. Ms. McDonald should be informed that the mood supplement contains St John's wort as its primary ingredient and that although you sell supplements containing this herb, she should not take this herb in combination with her prescription medications because it can have an additive effect with paroxetine and reduce the efficacy of her birth control pills. She should be informed that taking an energy supplement containing *Panax ginseng* will cause no harm, but this herb has not been shown to have any consistent benefit in improving energy. You should let Ms. McDonald know that you are most concerned that her mood fluctuations and reduced dietary intake may be a sign that her prescription antidepressant needs to be adjusted. You should also advise her not to substitute DS for prescription drug therapy for chronic health conditions without first consulting her provider.

---

a thorough medical history essential. The potential for drug–food and drug–DS interactions, age-related functional declines, and concomitant diseases should be considered in counseling older adults about DS. Products that are likely to be used in older adults include fish oil or omega-3 fatty acids, glucosamine, gingko, garlic, saw palmetto in men, and flaxseed and soy supplements in women.

Children

Use of DS by children presents unique challenges. The central nervous system of a child may be sensitive to many drugs and chemicals. Little research is available regarding the safe and effective use of DS in children, making evidence-based recommendations difficult. In addition, from a practical perspective, an appropriate pediatric dosage of a DS product cannot be determined if the content of the product is in question. Finally, DS should have childproof safety closures because accidental ingestions may occur in young children. The 2007 NHIS found the

most commonly used products in children were echinacea, fish oil, flaxseed, pre- or probiotics, and goldenseal.[3]

Pregnancy and Lactation

Use of DS by a woman who is planning to become pregnant or is already pregnant presents several dilemmas. Throughout the world, herbal DS have been used to maintain health during pregnancy, prevent miscarriages, and induce labor. In the United States, concern has focused on minimizing fetal exposures to prescription and nonprescription drugs, as well as DS. Although many natural products have been used in pregnancy, little published data exist on their safety with regard to the developing embryo and fetus. As part of standard preconception care, a woman should be asked about her use of DS, especially if her nutritional status might be affected at the time of conception (e.g., folic acid intake) or her ability to become pregnant might be affected (e.g., DS effecting ovulation). The most important issue concerning DS use during pregnancy and lactation is the uncertainty about the exact content in any given product batch or brand. Currently, providers should advise women to limit their use of DS to products that have reasonable proof of safety and efficacy for use during pregnancy and lactation. Products that are likely to be used in pregnant women include fish oil, ginger, and tea formulations of raspberry leaf, peppermint, and chamomile.

Kidney Disease

Many Americans have chronic kidney disease (CKD) caused by diseases such as diabetes mellitus. CKD presents many challenges to the safe use of many prescription and nonprescription drugs. Most commonly, the individual may be unable to eliminate the drug appropriately, potentially resulting in supratherapeutic concentrations. This effect is also true for hepatically metabolized drugs with active, renally eliminated metabolites. When a patient with CKD requires dialysis, the absorption, distribution, and hepatic metabolism of drugs may also be altered. In addition, many herbs possess antiplatelet properties that might increase the risk of bleeding in CKD.[37]

Liver Disease

The effects of liver disease on DS pharmacokinetics have not been adequately studied. Many DS products contain combination ingredients; studying and evaluating the effects of liver disease on the pharmacokinetics of combination DS presents unique challenges. For this reason, DS should be avoided or used cautiously in patients with compromised liver function. Some DS products can affect the ability of the liver to metabolize other medications, which can lead to drug interactions. DS products containing known hepatotoxic ingredients should be avoided. No DS have been found to be clinically effective in reversing liver disease or in preventing liver damage.

Surgery

A detailed preoperative history that includes questions related to DS use should be obtained from all patients undergoing surgery. Supplements that are known to affect sedation or platelet function or that may possibly affect the metabolism of anesthetic agents should be discontinued 2 weeks prior to the procedure. Other DS that the patient is taking should be reviewed by the provider to avoid potential harm.

Reliable Information Resources

The following resources may be used for general information, ongoing research, regulatory updates and alerts, and information on DS composition. Among these, AltMedDex, Natural Standard, Natural Medicine's Comprehensive Database, and ConsumerLab require a paid subscription.

AltMedDex, Micromedex

AltMedDex provides drug information on all types of DS, including herbs, vitamins, minerals, Chinese medicine, and acupuncture. This resource provides information about DS dosing, pharmacokinetics, interactions, and clinical use, along with primary literature citations. The content undergoes extensive review and is updated quarterly. The database is searchable only by DS ingredient(s) and not by trade name.[39]

CARDS, Office of Dietary Supplements

The Computer Access to Research on Dietary Supplements (CARDS) database contains federally funded research specific to DS. Information found in CARDS is provided from many government agencies that sponsor DS research, including but not limited to the Office of Dietary Supplements. The database is searchable by DS ingredient, health outcome, study type, or names of research investigators. A record of completed and published research studies on DS is maintained within the database.[40]

Cochrane Database of Systematic Reviews

This Cochrane database is accessible through Medline and offers evidence-based analyses of DS. These reports provide detailed information on trials that were included and excluded from the analysis and on the methodology used.[41] One advantage of this database is that statements that support or refute the use of a specific DS are clearly expressed. A disadvantage is that many providers may have difficulty understanding the style and arrangement of the information that supports the analyses.

ConsumerLab.com

This site provides access to a Natural Products Encyclopedia. The information in this encyclopedia is evidence based and well referenced. It is a useful resource for both consumers and health care providers.[25]

Dietary Supplement Ingredient Database

The Dietary Supplement Ingredient Database (DSID) was created by a group of federal agencies and research organizations to estimate the levels of ingredients found in DS products. The database provides information on analyzed levels of nutrients found in adult multivitamins and minerals used in the United States. The database is intended for use in research applications that are appropriate for conducting population-based studies on nutrient intake as opposed to assessing individual products. The data are grouped by nutrient levels rather than by product name.[42]

Dietary Supplements Labels Database

The Dietary Supplements Labels Database (DSLD) was created by the National Library of Medicine and includes information from the labels of more than 4000 DS products. The database is intended to help consumers and health care professionals identify ingredients found in brand-name DS. Information in this database is based on the ingredients declared by the DS manufacturer and includes both active and inactive ingredients. DS ingredients are linked to MedlinePlus and PubMed to allow users to investigate the dietary ingredients and evaluate the primary literature pertaining to them. For each DS product listed, the database provides the DS manufacturer's name and contact information. The DSLD also provides links to fact sheets published by FDA, the Office of Dietary Supplements, National Center for Complementary and Alternative Medicine (NCCAM), and the National Cancer Institute.[43]

MedlinePlus

MedlinePlus, published by NIH, is designed for consumers and contains information regarding diseases, conditions, and wellness. In addition, drug and DS information is provided in consumer-friendly language. The DS content is based on the Natural Medicines Comprehensive Database and includes both plant-based and other DS. Directories, a medical encyclopedia, and a medical dictionary are available in several languages.[44]

Natural Medicines Comprehensive Database/Natural Standard[38,45]

The Natural Medicines Comprehensive Database is produced by Therapeutics Faculty, Inc., which also publishes *The Pharmacist's Letter* and *The Prescriber's Letter*. In 2013, Natural Medicines Comprehensive Database merged with Natural Standard. The latter is another electronic DS database that represents an international research collaboration of providers from many disciplines, including those trained in Western- and Asian-based forms of care. Combining the two databases into one platform allows a comprehensive listing of single-ingredient and combination DS products and their associated adverse effects, drug–supplement interactions, and more. Recommendations are graded to reflect the type and quality of the clinical evidence on which they are based. In addition to reviews of DS, the database also includes monographs on other CAM modalities and a dictionary of terms. Each monograph has an accompanying consumer handout.

National Center for Complementary and Alternative Medicine

NCCAM is part of NIH and is one of the federal government's leading agencies in promoting evidence-based research on CAM therapies. This online site provides information on clinical trials, opportunities for research and funding, training opportunities for CAM providers, and health information on CAM modalities. DS monographs are in the health information section and provide concise evidence-based summaries.[46]

Office of Dietary Supplements, National Institutes of Health

The NIH Office of Dietary Supplements is a comprehensive site for general information on DS. The online site contains information regarding health and nutrition and decision-making approaches for DS treatment options and nutrient recommendations. Importantly, the site provides evidence-based fact sheets on many DS, including vitamins and botanicals. In addition, the site provides resources for researchers of DS and information on DS training and career development opportunities.[47] In 2013, the My Dietary Supplements (MyDS) free mobile application for consumers was launched; it provides an easy way to track vitamin, mineral, and herbal use and to access science-based information on DS.[47]

PubMed Subset for Dietary Supplements

The NIH Office of Dietary Supplements instituted a joint project with the National Library of Medicine to create the PubMed subset for DS. This subset succeeds the International Bibliographic Information on Dietary Supplements database, which was a collaboration between the Office of Dietary Supplements and the U.S. Department of Agriculture National Agricultural Library. The subset was created to help improve access to DS-related literature and incorporates journals indexed in Medline that contain DS-related content.[48]

Key Points for Dietary Supplements

➤ DS use is common among consumers, making it essential for all providers to be knowledgeable about the most frequently used products. This education should include information about evidenced-based resources and where to report adverse effects, drug interactions, or suspected fraudulent health claims.

➤ Regulation under DSHEA has created a marketplace in which product safety, efficacy, and quality can be uncertain.

➤ Health care providers are in a unique position to counsel consumers on DS and should take an open, nonjudgmental, evidence-based approach.

➤ Obtaining a DS history should be part of the overall drug history.

➤ Counseling recommendations should include consideration of overall scientific support, specific patient groups, potential for adverse effects, and potential for interactions with other medications or medical illnesses.

REFERENCES

1. U.S. Food and Drug Administration. Dietary Supplement Health and Education Act of 1994. Pub L No. 103-417. 103rd Congress. Accessed at http://www.fda.gov/RegulatoryInformation/Legislation/FederalFoodDrugandCosmeticActFDCAct/SignificantAmendmentstotheFDCAct/ucm148003.htm, May 6, 2013.

2. CAM BASICS. What is Complementary and Alternative Medicine? Last update May 2012. Accessed at http://nccam.nih.gov/health/whatiscam, May 6, 2013.

3. Barnes PM, Bloom B, Nahin RL. Complementary and alternative medicine use among adults and children: United States, 2007. Hyattsville, MD: National Center for Health Statistics; 2008. National Health Statistics Reports; No 12.

4. Council for Responsible Nutrition (CRN). The 2013 CRN Consumer Survey on Dietary Supplements, 2013. Accessed at http://www.crnusa.org/consumersurvey/CRN2013CCsurvey-infographic-pages.pdf/, August 5, 2014.

5. Dwyer J, Nahin RL, Rogers GT, et al. Prevalence and predictors of children's dietary supplement use: the 2007 National Health Interview Survey. *Am J Clin Nutr.* 2013;97(6):1331–7. doi: 10.3945/ajcn.112.052373. Epub 2013 Apr 10.

6. Bailey RL, Gahche JJ, Miller PE, et al. Why US adults use dietary supplements. *JAMA Intern Med.* 2013;173(5):355–61.

7. Considering a Post-DSHEA World. *Nutrit Business J.* 2012;17:1–9.

8. Greider K. Has vitamin D been oversold? AARP Bulletin, July 2012. Accessed at http://www.aarp.org/health/drugs-supplements/info-07-2012/how-much-vitamin-d-is-enough.html, May 16, 2013.

9. Marinac JS, Buchinger CL, Godfrey LA, et al. Herbal products and dietary supplements: a survey of use, attitudes and knowledge among older adults. *J Am Osteopath Assoc.* 2007;107:13–23.

10. Nahin RL, Pecha M, Welmerink DB, et al. Concomitant use of prescription drugs and dietary supplements in ambulatory elderly people. *J Am Geriatr Soc.* 2009;57(7):1197–205.

11. U.S. Food and Drug Administration. Draft guidance for industry: dietary supplements: new dietary ingredient notifications and related issues. July 2011. Accessed at http://www.fda.gov/Food/GuidanceRegulation/GuidanceDocumentsRegulatoryInformation/DietarySupplements/ucm257563.htm#iii-scope, May 7, 2013.

12. U.S. Food and Drug Administration. Current good manufacturing practice in manufacturing, packaging, labeling, or holding operations for dietary supplements. Final rule. *Federal Register.* 2007;72:34752–958. Accessed at http://www.fda.gov/regulatoryinformation/legislation/federalfooddrug andcosmeticactfdcact/significantamendmentstothefdcact/ucm148003. htm, June 2, 2011.

13. Federal Trade Commission. Dietary supplements: an advertising guide for industry. Accessed at http://business.ftc.gov/documents/bus09-dietary-supplements-advertising-guide-industry, May 6, 2013.

14. U.S. Food and Drug Administration. Claims that can be made for conventional foods and dietary supplements. September 2003. Accessed at http://www.fda.gov/Food/IngredientsPackagingLabeling/Labeling Nutrition/ucm111447.htm, May 6, 2013.

15. U.S. Food and Drug Administration. Dietary Supplement and Non-Prescription Drug Consumer Protection Act. Pub L No. 109-462. 109th Congress. December 22, 2006. Accessed at http://www.fda.gov/down loads/AboutFDA/CentersOffices/CDER/ucm102797.pdf, May 6, 2013.

16. U.S. Food and Drug Administration. MedWatch: The FDA Safety Information and Adverse Event Reporting Program. Accessed at http://www.fda.gov/medwatch, May 6, 2013.

17. Linde K, Barrett B, Wolkart K, et al. Echinacea for preventing and treating the common cold. *Cochrane Database Syst Rev.* 2014;2:CD000530. doi: 10.1002/14651858.CD000530.pub3. Accessed at http://www.the cochranelibrary.com/view/0/index.html.

18. Gurib-Fakim A. Medicinal plants: traditions of yesterday and drugs of tomorrow. *Mol Aspects Med.* 2006;27(1):1–93.

19. Schulz V, Hansel R, Blumenthal M, eds. *Rational Phytotherapy: A Reference Guide for Physicians and Pharmacists.* 2nd ed. Berlin Heidelberg, Germany: Springer-Verlag; 2004.

20. Saper RB, Phillips RS, Sehgal A, et al. Lead, mercury, and arsenic in U.S. and Indian manufactured Ayurvedic medicines sold via the Internet. *JAMA.* 2008;300(8):915–23.

21. Genius SJ, Schwalfenberg G, Siy AK, et al. Toxic element contamination of natural health Products. *PLoS One.* 2012;7(11):e49676. doi: 10.1371/journal.pone.0049676. Epub 2012 Nov 21.

22. Harel Z, Harel S, Wald R, et al. The frequency and characteristics of dietary supplement recalls in the United States. *JAMA Intern Med.* 2013; 173(10):926–8.

23. Miller GM, Stripp R. A study of western pharmaceuticals contained within samples of Chinese herbal/patent medicines collected from New York City's Chinatown. *Legal Med.* 2007;9:258–64.

24. U.S. Pharmacopeial Convention. USP verification services. Accessed at http://www.usp.org/usp-verification-services, July 25, 2014.

25. Consumer.Lab.com. 2008. Accessed at http://www.consumerlab.com/aboutcl.asp, May 6, 2013.

26. NSF International. Dietary, nutritional and sports supplements verification. Accessed at http://www.nsf.org/consumer-resources/what-is-nsf-certification/dietary-sports-supplements-certification, July 25, 2014.

27. National Institutes of Health Office of Dietary Supplements. Consumer protection. Accessed at http://ods.od.nih.gov/HealthInformation/consumerprotection.sec.aspx, May 31, 2013.

28. Morris CA, Avorn J. Internet marketing of herbal products. *JAMA.* 2003;290(11):1505–9.

29. U.S. Food and Drug Administration: Health Fraud Consumer Updates. Accessed at http://www.fda.gov/ForConsumers/ProtectYourself/Health Fraud/ucm267375.htm#3-tab, May 2, 2013.

30. Chung IS, Lee MY, Jung HR. Three systemic argyria cases after ingestion of colloidal silver solution. *Int J Dermatol.* 2010;49(10):1175–7.

31. Wang L, Manson JE, Sesso HD. Calcium intake and risk of cardiovascular disease: a review of prospective studies and randomized clinical trials. *Am J Cardiovasc Drugs.* 2012;12(12):105–16.

32. Siegner AW Jr. The Food and Drug Administration's actions on ephedra and androstenedione: understanding their potential impacts on the protections of the Dietary Supplement Health and Education Act. *Food Drug Law J.* 2004;59:617–28.

33. Chitturi S, Farrell G. Hepatotoxic slimming aids and other herbal hepatotoxins. *J Gastroenterol Hepatol.* 2008;23(3):366–73.

34. Van Breemen RB, Fong HHS, Farnsworth NR. Ensuring the safety of botanical dietary supplements. *Am J Clin Nutr.* 2008;87(suppl):509S–13S.

35. Schulz V. Safety of St. John's wort extract compared to synthetic antidepressants. *Phytomed.* 2006;13(3):199–204.

36. Fernstrom JD. Effects and side effects associated with the non-nutritional use of tryptophan by humans. *J Nutr.* 2012 Dec;142(12):2236S–2244S.

37. Haller CA. Clinical approach to adverse events and interactions related to herbal and dietary supplements. *Clin Toxicol.* 2006;44(5):605–10.

38. Natural Standard. Foods, Herbs & Supplements [database]. Accessed at http://naturalstandard.com/databases/herbssupplements/all/a/, May 6, 2013.

39. AltMedDex®. Thomson Healthcare. Accessed at http://www.micro medexsolutions.com, July 12, 2013.

40. Office of Dietary Supplements. Computer Access to Research on Dietary Supplements (CARDS) database. Accessed at http://ods.od.nih.gov/Research/CARDS_Database.aspx, May 6, 2013.

41. The Cochrane Database of Systematic Reviews [electronic resource]. Chichester, West Sussex, UK: Wiley; 2010.

42. Office of Dietary Supplements. Dietary Supplement Ingredient Database. Accessed at http://www.dietarysupplementdatabase.usda.nih.gov, May 6, 2013.

43. Office of Dietary Supplements. Dietary Supplements Label Database. Accessed at http://dsld.nlm.nih.gov/dsld, May 6, 2013.

44. National Library of Medicine. Medline Plus. Accessed at http://medline plus.gov, May 6, 2013.

45. Jellin JM, Gregory PJ, Batz F, et al., eds. *Natural Medicines Comprehensive Database.* Stockton, CA: Therapeutic Research Faculty; 2008. Online version accessed at http://www.naturaldatabase.com, July 15, 2013.

46. National Center for Complementary and Alternative Medicine. Accessed at http://nccam.nih.gov, May 6, 2013.

47. Office of Dietary Supplements. Accessed at http://ods.od.nih.gov, May 6, 2013.

48. Office of Dietary Supplements. A new PubMed® subset on dietary supplements. Accessed at http://ods.od.nih.gov/health_information/ibids. aspx, May 6, 2013.

NATURAL PRODUCTS

Cydney E. McQueen and Katherine Kelly Orr

This chapter uses the organ system approach outlined in Table 51–1. The products discussed were chosen because they have evidence to support their use, are widely promoted either with or without evidence supporting use, or present known or theoretical safety concerns. Some information has been adapted from an earlier version of this chapter.[1]

Cardiovascular System

Coenzyme Q10

Coenzyme Q10 (CoQ10, or ubiquinone) is converted to ubiquinol in the body and is found in every cell, primarily in mitochondria.

Therapeutic Uses

Consumers use CoQ10 for cardiovascular conditions and as a general antioxidant. It has been investigated for use in Parkinson's disease, breast cancer, migraine prevention, and reduction of chemotherapy-associated adverse effects.[2]

Physiologic Activity

CoQ10 concentrations are greatest in heart, liver, pancreas, and kidney mitochondria.[2] As the rate-limiting cofactor in mitochondrial adenosine triphosphate (ATP) formation, CoQ10 is involved in many energy production functions and regeneration of other antioxidants such as vitamin E. Statins decrease CoQ10 biosynthesis and lower its serum concentrations, but not always in muscle tissue.[3,4] The extent of the lowering of CoQ10 concentrations differs among statins.[5] CoQ10 stabilizes membranes and may have vasodilatory and inotropic effects.[6]

Dosage and Product Considerations

For heart failure, cardiomyopathy, or hypertension, the CoQ10 dosage has been 100 mg 1–3 times daily, preferably with meals to aid absorption. The dosage is 30–50 mg once daily for patients taking statins. Products meeting United States Pharmacopeia (USP) standards are available.

Safety Considerations

Gastrointestinal (GI) effects from CoQ10 use may be minimized by splitting large (>100 mg) doses. Mild increases in liver enzymes have been reported. The use of CoQ10 should be avoided during pregnancy and lactation because safety information is lacking.

Vitamin K–like procoagulant effects have been theorized because of CoQ10's structural similarity to synthetic vitamin K. Case reports of interactions with warfarin exist, although a placebo-controlled crossover study of CoQ10 noted no differences in international normalized ratio (INR) values in patients taking stable dosages of warfarin.[7] Patients taking warfarin should discuss CoQ10 with their health care providers; if used, the INR should be monitored more frequently until CoQ10's effects are determined.

CoQ10 may possibly decrease effectiveness of radiation therapy.[8,9] Information on interactions changes rapidly, so cancer patients should discuss CoQ10 use with their oncologists.

Table 51–2 provides more information on supplement–medication interactions discussed in the chapter.

Summary of Clinical Evidence

Evidence for CoQ10 in heart failure is contradictory. Studies have shown improvements in markers of cardiovascular health, such as endothelial function and C-reactive protein levels; further, early clinical trials were promising.[10,11] Recent studies have demonstrated contradictory results in overall symptoms, ejection fraction, or oxygen consumption when CoQ10 was added to standard therapy.[12,13] Patients on a heart transplant waiting list experienced significant improvements in multiple symptoms, especially in the 6-minute walk test and in the New York Heart Association functional class, but echocardiography measurements did not change.[12] Although its true efficacy is unknown, CoQ10 has few adverse effects and so might be an option as adjunctive therapy, if carefully monitored.

Preliminary trials have investigated CoQ10 for cardiomyopathy and ischemic heart disease. Risk reduction in adults was minimal, although a 6-month trial in pediatric and adolescent patients with idiopathic cardiomyopathy found improved diastolic function.[14] A 1-year trial examining 120 mg/day CoQ10 in 144 patients who experienced a myocardial infarction (MI) reported a significantly lower rate of cardiac events (24.6% for CoQ10 vs. 45% for B vitamins).[15]

table
51–1 **Discussed Supplements Grouped by Organ Systems**

System	Supplement
Cardiovascular system	Coenzyme Q10
	Garlic
	Fish oil
	Red yeast rice
	Resveratrol
Central nervous system	Butterbur
	Feverfew
	Huperzine
	Ginkgo
	Kava
	Melatonin
	St. John's wort
	Valerian
	5-Hydroxytryptophan
Digestive system	Ginger
	Milk thistle
	Peppermint
Endocrine system	Alpha-lipoic acid
	American ginseng
	Cinnamon
	DHEA
Immune modulators	Colostrum
	Echinacea
	Probiotics
	Elderberry
Physical and mental performance enhancers	Eleuthero
	Ginseng
	Green tea
Kidney, urinary tract, and prostate	African plum
	Cranberry
	Saw palmetto
Musculoskeletal system	Glucosamine sulfate
	Chondroitin sulfate
	MSM
	SAMe
	Devil's claw
Skin and mucous membranes	Melissa (lemon balm)
	Tea tree oil
Women's health	Black cohosh
	Chaste tree berry
	Evening primrose oil
	Fenugreek
	Phytoestrogens

Key: DHEA = Dehydroepiandrosterone; MSM = methylsulfonylmethane; SAMe = S-adenosyl-L-methionine.

Although statins can reduce endogenous CoQ10 concentrations, the clinical significance is not well understood. CoQ10, with or without statin discontinuation, may reverse some statin-associated adverse effects.[16] A study in older athletes taking statins noted improved muscle performance, whereas another study found no difference in development of myalgia.[17,18] Genetic differences may be responsible for the diverse findings with CoQ10.[19]

CoQ10 has a slight blood pressure–lowering effect in patients with hypertension. Evidence is variable but sufficient to support a trial as adjunctive therapy in patients needing small additional decreases in blood pressure.[20,21]

Garlic

Garlic supplements are derived from dried or fresh bulbs of *Allium sativum,* the same plant used as a food or spice.

Therapeutic Uses

Garlic is used to treat hyperlipidemia, hypertension, and type 2 diabetes mellitus, and for improvement of immune function and prevention of various cancers.[22]

Physiologic Activity

Garlic bulbs contain an odorless sulfur-containing amino acid derivative alliin (S-allyl-l-cysteine sulfoxide). When crushed, the enzyme allinase is released, converting alliin to the pungent allicin, the main component of garlic's volatile oil. For supplements, allicin is used as a quality marker but may not be the primary active compound; other organosulfur-containing or phenolic substances may exert pharmacologic effects. The production of alliin actually occurs after ingestion and is lessened by interference of stomach acid with allinase. In animal and in vitro models, garlic possesses hypotensive, hypolipidemic, antiplatelet, antioxidant, and anti-infective properties.[23] Garlic's prevention of lipid oxidation may be as important to cardiovascular health as its hypolipidemic activity.[24]

Dosage and Product Considerations

Research on garlic has been conducted primarily with tablets or capsules of powdered, dehydrated garlic standardized to an allicin content of 1%–1.6%, providing 3–5 mg of allicin per day. These dosages should be recommended.

Garlic supplements vary in their chemical composition, which may contribute to the contradictory study results. An enteric coating will help prevent destruction of alliin by gastric acid and may also help to decrease breath odor. The odorless (aged) products are less likely to contain appropriate amounts of allicin but may contain other compounds that have some activity.[22]

Safety Considerations

Although well tolerated, garlic may cause nausea, vomiting, and heartburn, especially at higher dosages. Bad breath and body odor may also occur. Allergic reactions have been reported.

Garlic should be stopped 10–14 days prior to surgery to reduce the risk of bleeding.[25] Patients taking warfarin or antiplatelet agents should use garlic supplements with caution because of potential bleeding risk; however, dietary amounts do not affect platelet function.[26,27]

Garlic's effect on cytochrome (CYP) P450 isoenzymes is unclear. Garlic decreased concentrations of saquinavir by about 50%. The mechanism may involve P-glycoprotein induction and therefore decreased absorption, rather than increased clearance, because two studies did not find interactions with docetaxel and other CYP3A4 and CYP2D6 substrates.[28,29]

table
51–2 **Selected Herb–Drug Interactions**

Herb	Known Interactions/Results[a]	Theoretical Interactions/Results[b]
African plum (pygeum)		Potential risk for increased adverse effects when combined with finasteride
Alpha-lipoic acid	Increased bioavailability of valproate	SMBG recommended in patients taking antihyperglycemic drugs Potential chelating activity with minerals and antacids Possible interference with conversion of thyroxine to triiodothyronine Possible reduction of effectiveness of some chemotherapy agents
Black cohosh		Possible additive estrogenic activity with ET or OCP May increase toxicity of doxorubicin and docetaxel May decrease effectiveness of cisplatin Possible potentiation of antihypertensive agents Avoid with other hepatotoxic drugs
Butterbur	Substrate of CYP3A4; avoid with known inducers	Possible interaction with anticholinergics or antimigraine medications
Chastetree berry		Minimal evidence for possible interference with hormonal contraceptives Possible interaction with antipsychotics, dopamine agonists, and metoclopramide because of dopaminergic activity
Chondroitin		Possible increased risk of bleeding if taken with antiplatelet agents or warfarin
Coenzyme Q10		Possible vitamin K–like procoagulant effects if taken with warfarin; monitor INR initially
Cranberry		Possible increased INR and risk of bleeding in people taking warfarin Possible CYP2C9 inhibition May alter excretion of weakly alkaline drugs or neutralize effects of antacids
Devil's claw		Possible increased risk of bleeding in patients taking warfarin
DHEA	Triazolam: increased blood levels	Interference with hormonal or antihormonal therapies such as aromatase inhibitors May increase risk of blood clots with OCPs Possible increased levels of CYP3A4 substrates
Echinacea		Possible interaction with immunomodulating therapies CYP3A4 substrates with low oral bioavailability: verapamil, cyclosporine, tacrolimus. Effects on CYP1A2, CYP2C9, or CYP3A4 are likely to be clinically insignificant
Eleuthero ("Siberian ginseng")	Digoxin: possible false elevation in plasma levels (assay dependent) Caffeine: increased CNS stimulation Hexobarbital: inhibited metabolism	SMBG recommended in patients taking antihyperglycemic drugs Possible inhibition of CYP1A2, CYP2C9, CYP3A4, and CYP2D6 (although CYP3A4 and CYP2D6 not affected at normal doses) Variable activity on blood pressure; avoid if taking antihypertensives
Evening primrose oil		Possible additive effects if taken with other antiplatelet agents or herbs Seizure possible if taken with phenothiazines Potential additive effects to antihypertensives
Fenugreek		Possible additive effects if taken with other antiplatelet agents or herbs
Feverfew		Possible additive effects if taken with other antiplatelet agents or herbs Avoid with antihyperglycemic drugs because of additive effects
Garlic	Warfarin: increased INR in case reports Saquinavir: 50% decrease in levels OCPs: decreased effectiveness	Contradictory evidence regarding induction of drugs metabolized through CYP3A4 and CYP2D6

table
51–2   Selected Herb–Drug Interactions *(continued)*

Herb	Known Interactions/Results[a]	Theoretical Interactions/Results[b]
Ginger	Antiplatelet agents: possible additive effect at high dosages (>4 g/day)	Avoid with antihyperglycemic drugs because of additive effects
Ginkgo	Antiplatelet agents: possible additive effect (contradictory evidence) Trazodone: case report of coma in patient taking low-dose trazodone Omeprazole: decreased levels	Ingestion associated with seizures; avoid in patients with a history of seizures or on drugs that may lower seizure threshold Potential additive effects with antihypertensive drugs, although paradoxical hypertension has been reported with HCTZ
Ginseng (*Panax ginseng*)	Glucose-lowering drugs: possible lowered BG levels in type 2 DM; SMBG levels required Phenelzine: possible headache, tremor, and mania in case report	Unpredictable effect on concurrent anticoagulant and antiplatelet agents Possible interference with antipsychotics and immunosuppressants Inhibition of CYP2D6 (not clinically significant)
Ginseng, American (*Panax quinquefolius*)	Warfarin: reduced anticoagulant effect	
Glucosamine	Warfarin: increased bleeding risk in individuals with variant CYP2C9 alleles	SMBG recommended for first few days of use in patients taking antihyperglycemic drugs
Green tea	Decongestants: additive stimulant effects	Possible antagonism of warfarin's effect Possible antagonism of concurrent sedatives related to caffeine content
Fish oil		Possible additive effects if taken with anticoagulant and antiplatelet agents that; occur primarily at dosages > 4 grams daily
5-HTP	SSRIs, tramadol, DM: increased risk of serotonergic adverse effects Carbidopa: decreased peripheral metabolism	
Huperzine A		Possible decreased effectiveness if taken with anticholinergic drugs Possible additive cholinergic effects if taken with acetylcholinesterase inhibitors or cholinergic agents (e.g., bethanechol) Additive effects with drugs causing bradycardia
Kava	Levodopa: reduced efficacy of levodopa Inhibits CYP2E1 Concern over hepatotoxicity contraindicates use with other drugs and supplements that damage liver	Possible increased sedative effect with alcohol and other CNS depressants Possible additive effects with other antiplatelet agents or herbs Preliminary evidence suggests kava may inhibit CYP2C9, CYP2C19, CYP2D6, and CYP3A4 (significance unknown)
Lemon balm (Melissa)		Use of oral lemon balm and sedating supplements and drugs contraindicated
Melatonin	Nifedipine: reduced delivery via the GITS Fluvoxamine, MAOIs, and tricyclic antidepressants: increase melatonin BZDPs and sodium valproate: decrease nighttime levels	Caffeine or OCP use has various effects on melatonin levels Verapamil may decrease melatonin Possible interaction with immunosuppressant drugs related to immunostimulating properties
Milk thistle		Effect on CYP3A4 and CYP2C9 unclear
Peppermint	Decreased absorption of iron salts Premature dissolution of enteric-coated peppermint oil capsules by drugs that increase gastric pH	Decreased activity of CYP3A4 observed during in vitro and in vivo studies; clinical significance is unknown
Phytoestrogens (red clover, others)		Possible increased risk of bleeding in patients taking warfarin with red clover–based products
Probiotics	Separate doses from antibiotics or antifungals by 2 or more hours	
Red yeast rice	Additive activity when used with statins	
SAMe		Possible increased risk of serotonin syndrome if taken with antidepressants and 5-HT₁ agonists Significance on glucocorticoid increases unknown
Saw palmetto		Potential interaction with hormonal or antihormonal therapies Possible additive effects when used with antiplatelet or anticoagulant agents

table

51-2 Selected Herb–Drug Interactions *(continued)*

Herb	Known Interactions/Results[a]	Theoretical Interactions/Results[b]
St. John's wort	CYP3A4 substrates: decreased drug levels and effects (e.g., alprazolam, amitriptyline, atorvastatin, finasteride, imatinib, irinotecan, methadone, nifedipine, simvastatin, tacrolimus, verapamil, warfarin, zolpidem) Antidepressants: increased risk of serotonin syndromes with nefazodone, sertraline, and paroxetine Cyclosporine: decreased blood levels of immunosuppressant, including case reports of transplant graft rejection OCPs and HT: decreased activity Protease inhibitors and nonnucleoside reverse transcriptase inhibitors: decreased serum levels	Possible increased risk of serotonin syndrome if taken with 5-HT$_1$ agonists, DM, meperidine, pentazocine, and tramadol; interaction possibly similar to conventional antidepressants and MAOIs, with increased potential for hypertension, hyperthermia, agitation, and coma Possible decreased levels and effect of amiodarone Monitoring for fexofenadine toxicity recommended if taken concomitantly Morphine: increased narcotic-induced sleep time in animal studies Use with other photosensitizing agents contraindicated
Valerian		Possible increased sedative effect if taken with alcohol or other CNS depressants (BZDPs) May inhibit CYP3A4 (not usually clinically significant)

Key: BG = Blood glucose; BZDP = benzodiazepine; CNS = central nervous system; CYP = cytochrome P450; DM = dextromethorphan; ET = estrogen therapy; GITS = gastrointestinal therapeutic system; HCTZ = hydrochlorothiazide; HT = hormone therapy; 5-HT$_1$ = 5-hydroxytryptamine$_1$; 5-HTP = 5-hydroxytryptophan; INR = international normalized ratio; MAOI = monoamine oxidase inhibitor; OCP = oral contraceptive pill; SAMe = S-adenosyl-L-methionine; SMBG = self-monitoring of blood glucose; SSRI = selective serotonin reuptake inhibitor.

[a] Based on human studies and/or validated case reports.

[b] Extrapolated from animal or in vitro studies.

Summary of Clinical Evidence

Garlic supplements slightly reduce total and low-density lipoprotein (LDL-C) concentrations.[30] Reported reductions range from 4% to 12.4% in total cholesterol (TC), 1% to 16.3% in LDL-C, and 18.6% to 22% in triglycerides (TG).[31,32]

A meta-analysis concluded that, compared with placebo, garlic has greater effects for hypertension; the effects are larger in individuals with higher blood pressures.[33] Mean decreases were 6–12 mm Hg for systolic pressure and 5–9 mm Hg for diastolic pressure, so garlic's usefulness would generally be for mild hypertension. Aged garlic products may be preferred for this use.[34]

Fish Oil

Fish oil is a source of omega-3 fatty acids, primarily docosahexaenoic acid (DHA) and eicosapentaenoic acid (EPA).

Therapeutic Uses

Fish oil is used to lower TG levels, improve cardiac health, and relieve inflammatory conditions, such as rheumatoid arthritis. Average American diets tend to be low in omega-3 fatty acids and high in omega-6 fatty acids; consumers who do not eat fish can take fish oil supplements to aid in normalizing the omega-3:omega-6 intake ratio.

Physiologic Activity

Intake of exogenous EPA and DHA in fish oil influences production and concentrations of inflammatory response cytokines.

Competitive inhibition of arachidonic acid decreases production of thromboxane A_2 and leukotriene B_4, whereas effects at another part of the production cascade increase thromboxane A_3 and prostaglandin E_3. Overall, the fish oil's actions can be summarized as increasing noninflammatory and decreasing proinflammatory cytokines.

Omega-3 fatty acids may decrease intestinal cholesterol absorption and inhibit enzymes involved in synthesis, excretion, and degradation of very low-density lipoproteins (VLDL), thereby decreasing other lipoproteins, including LDL-C.[35] The mechanism of hypotriglyceridemic action through peroxisome proliferator–activated receptors may also be responsible for improvements in glucose concentrations and insulin resistance.[36]

Dosage and Product Considerations

The usual recommendation for fish oil is 1–2 grams daily; for hyperlipidemia, dosages of 2–4 grams per day in divided doses are used. Available fish oil products have varying amounts of EPA and DHA; most studies have used products with an EPA:DHA ratio of 1.2:1 or 1.5:1. EPA and DHA amounts may not equal the stated dose per capsule because of additional product components, such as small quantities of vitamin E and excipients; however, high-quality products will be close to the total. For example, a "1 gram fish oil" product labeled to contain "480 mg EPA and 370 mg of DHA" per capsule would be within the acceptable ratios, whereas a "1 gram fish oil" product with "250 mg EPA and 180 mg of DHA" per capsule would not contain adequate active components. A prescription omega-3 fatty acid product would be more appropriate for severe hypertriglyceridemia because of ensured quality and insurance coverage. For example, a 1 gram Lovaza capsule contains 465 mg of EPA and 375 mg of DHA, with a dosage of 4 capsules per day, given in 1–2 doses.

Anecdotally, some patients have had success with freezing the capsules to minimize the fish burp. Data on mercury and other toxins in fish have increased concerns about quality of fish oil supplements. Because mercury is insoluble in oil, it collects primarily in flesh, whereas most fish oil is extracted from the skin. Supplements tested have had no or barely detectable concentrations of mercury.[37] Dioxin and pesticides can accumulate in the oil, so the use of a high-quality product meeting USP standards may limit toxin exposure.[38]

Safety Considerations

Fish oil products are generally safe; the most common adverse effects are belching, fishy halitosis, and GI distress.[39] Patients taking anticoagulants and antiplatelet agents should use no more than 3 g/day and should be monitored closely.

A recent analysis suggested a possible association between high blood levels of polyunsaturated fatty acids and worsened survival or development of prostate cancer.[40] This finding contrasts with other epidemiological data demonstrating a lower risk of prostate cancer with higher dietary intake of omega-3 fatty acids.[41] Until more data are available, patients with, or known to be at high risk for, prostate cancer should avoid taking more than 1 g/day; dietary intake is preferred over supplements.

Summary of Clinical Evidence

The primary effect of fish oil on lipids and lipoproteins is on TG concentrations. Although some studies have noted 40% reductions in TG concentrations, according to meta-analyses, a decrease of 14%–29% with greater lowering of VLDL is a more reasonable expectation.[42,43] In general, high-density lipoprotein cholesterol (HDL-C) concentrations do not change or they increase slightly (<10%).[44] Effects on LDL-C are variable, with most studies noting slight decreases.

One gram per day of omega-3 fatty acids, generally as fish oil, reduced the risk of adverse cardiac outcomes (mortality, nonfatal MI, and nonfatal stroke) by 20% in the 1999 GISSI-Prevenzione trial.[45] Similar benefits were shown for primary and secondary prevention in a meta-analysis.[46] A recent study found no difference in cardiovascular mortality and/or morbidity.[47] One potential reason for the differences in outcomes is the increasing use of statins. One large study examined omega-3 fatty acids for secondary prevention in statin users and nonusers and found no differences in outcomes among statin users.[48] Earlier trials of patients with metabolic syndrome noted improvement in cardiovascular and inflammatory markers, whereas recent studies have not demonstrated decreased mortality and/or morbidity.[49]

A large trial is currently evaluating benefits of marine omega-3 fatty acid supplements in the primary prevention of cardiovascular disease and cancer.[50] On the basis of data from the earlier trials before statin use was common, the American Heart Association recommends the intake of 1 g/day of omega-3 fatty acids. The recommendation emphasizes the dietary intake of fatty fish at least twice weekly.[51]

Red Yeast Rice

Monascus purpureus, a yeast that grows on fermented rice, is used in traditional Chinese medicine and gives Peking duck its red hue.

Therapeutic Uses

Red yeast rice is used to lower lipid concentrations.

Physiologic Activity

Red yeast rice contains multiple components; monacolin K, a naturally occurring lovastatin analogue, is the most important. The amount of monacolin K component is usually small, with most products containing less than 5 mg/day. As a result, this component cannot be solely responsible for the lipid-lowering effects reported in clinical trials. Other mechanisms such as increased bile acid excretion may also be involved.[52]

Dosage and Product Considerations

For hyperlipidemia, the dosage is 1.2–2.4 g/day in 2 doses. In the United States, certain red yeast rice products were declared illegal in 2000 because they contained an "unauthorized drug."[53] As a result, although red yeast rice products are available, many manufacturers no longer ensure that their products contain a standardized amount of monacolin K, making choice of a high-quality product difficult.[53]

Safety Considerations

Adverse effects associated with red yeast rice include allergic reactions, headache, bloating, flatulence, and heartburn. Increased liver function tests and rhabdomyolysis have been reported, so patients taking red yeast rice should have regular liver function monitoring.[53] Patients ingesting more than two alcoholic drinks should not use red yeast rice because of a potentially increased risk of hepatotoxicity. Red yeast rice is considered Pregnancy Category X.[54]

The *Monascus purpureus* yeast can also generate citrinin, a nephrotoxin, during fermentation.[55] Only brands of red yeast rice that have been tested to be free of citrinin should be used; patients with kidney disease should not use red yeast rice.

At least three studies have found that red yeast rice can be safely used in patients unable to take statins.[56–58] Initial increased monitoring for muscle pain is appropriate if used in a patient with prior statin-induced myalgia.

Summary of Clinical Evidence

Multiple studies have demonstrated that red yeast rice lowers lipid concentrations.[59] A systemic review reported reductions in TC of 10%–44%, in LDL-C of 7%–25%, and in TGs of 13%–44%.[60] In general, increases in the HDL-C concentration have not been significant.

Resveratrol

Resveratrol is a polyphenol present in grapes and wines, bilberries and blueberries, and pistachios. Interest in resveratrol began with research into the cardioprotective effects hypothesized for red wine. Higher dietary intake of resveratrol has been associated with lower levels of lipids, blood pressure, glucose, and heart rate.[61]

Therapeutic Uses

Resveratrol is generally used for cardiovascular health and cancer prevention.

Physiologic Activity

Resveratrol is well absorbed but has low bioavailability because of the extensive first-pass effect. Metabolites may be responsible for some effects, and beta-glucoronidase may repeatedly transform metabolites back to *trans*-resveratrol.[62]

Resveratrol is an antioxidant, decreases LDL-C oxidation, and has anti-inflammatory effects.[63] The greatest effects are improved endothelial function; clinically significant flow-mediated dilation of blood vessels occurs through nitric oxide and prostacyclin mechanisms.[64,65] In addition, insulin sensitivity is improved, possibly from increased phosphorylation of protein kinase, part of the signaling mechanism for insulin.[64]

Dosage and Product Considerations

The optimal dosage of resveratrol is unknown because studies have used varying preparations or extracts. The most recent clinical trial reporting beneficial effects used 10 mg daily, whereas pharmacokinetic studies have used up to 600 mg daily.[63,66]

Safety Considerations

Headache has been reported with the use of resveratrol.[66]

Summary of Clinical Evidence

In cardiovascular disease patients on standard drug therapy, a 3-month trial of 10 mg resveratrol resulted in only slight improvement in left ventricular systolic function, but significant improvement in left diastolic function and flow-mediated dilation was seen. Collagen-induced platelet aggregation significantly decreased from 42.61% to 32.89% and LDL-C concentrations from 122 mg/dL to 104 mg/dL.[63]

A 1-year primary prevention trial in patients with cardiac risk factors used 8 mg of resveratrol daily and examined inflammatory markers known to be associated with cardiovascular risk.[67] Significant decreases were reported for tumor necrosis factor-α (−19.8%), high-sensitivity C-reactive protein (−26%), and plasminogen activator inhibitor type 1 (−16.8%); however, interleukin-10 increased by 19.8%.[67] Large-scale studies evaluating clinical outcomes associated with these markers have not been conducted.

Central Nervous System

Butterbur

Petasites hybridus (L.) Gaertner, Meyer & Scherb, also known as butterbur, is native to marshy areas in northern Asia, Europe, and parts of North America. It is a member of the Asteraceae/Compositae family.

Therapeutic Uses

Butterbur is used to prevent migraines and treat allergic rhinitis and asthma.

Physiologic Activity

Petasin and isopetasin are isolated from butterbur's rhizomes, roots, and leaves. Extracts also contain volatile oils, tannins, flavonoids, and pyrrolizidine alkaloids (PAs). Petasin may reduce spasms in smooth muscle and vascular walls and also inhibit leukotriene synthesis. Isopetasin decreases prostaglandin synthesis, thereby reducing inflammation. Both compounds have an affinity for cerebral blood vessels.[68]

Dosage and Product Considerations

For migraine prevention, studies have used standardized extracts of butterbur containing a minimum of petasin 7.5 mg and isopetasin 7.5 mg per 50 mg tablet or capsule. Dosages of standardized butterbur ranging from 50 to 75 mg twice daily are used for 4–6 months, then tapered until migraine incidence increases; however, maximum study duration has been only 12–16 weeks.[68] Standardized petasin (Ze 339) 8–16 mg has been administered 3–4 times daily for allergic rhinitis.[69,70]

Safety Considerations

Butterbur is generally well tolerated; minor GI complaints are most commonly reported, followed by skin changes and dizziness.[68] PAs and their N-oxides are highly toxic compounds in butterbur extracts that can cause serious hepatotoxicity and carcinogenesis. German manufacturing requirements restrict the content of PAs in butterbur preparations to 1 mcg/day (limited intake to 6 weeks only) or 0.1 mcg/day (no limitations of intake).[71] Patients with an allergy to ragweed and related plants in the Asteraceae/Compositae family should avoid butterbur. Its use should also be avoided during pregnancy and lactation because of the potential for hepatotoxicity.

Summary of Clinical Evidence

The American Academy of Neurology and the American Headache Society consider butterbur effective for the prevention of migraine, with the highest evidence level of A.[72] Studies including children and adolescents have shown similar results.[73,74] In patients with symptoms related to seasonal allergic rhinitis, studies suggest short-term use for less than 14 days may be as effective as cetirizine and fexofenadine.[69,70] Results of one study indicated that butterbur had similar effects as fexofenadine in patients with perennial allergic rhinitis.[75]

Feverfew

Feverfew (*Tanacetum parthenium* [L.] Schultz-Bip.) is a member of the Asteraceae/Compositae family. The plant is native to the Balkans and now is found throughout the world.

Therapeutic Uses

Feverfew is used to prevent migraines and treat dysmenorrhea, arthritis, and psoriasis.

Physiologic Activity

The activity of feverfew for migraine prevention may involve many mechanisms. Parthenolide, a sesquiterpene lactone, is the most abundant and biologically active component and likely contributes anti-inflammatory benefits. Other active components include flavonoids, volatile oils, and additional sesquiterpene lactones. Feverfew may have effects on prostaglandin synthesis, platelet aggregation, serotonin release, histamine release, and vascular smooth muscle contraction.[76]

Dosage and Product Considerations

Studies have used feverfew leaf 50–100 mg daily in divided doses or 6.25 mg CO_2-standardized extract (MIG-99) of 0.2%–0.35% of parthenolide 2–3 times daily.[77,78] Standardization of a product to its parthenolide content does not appear to be necessary. Feverfew must be taken continuously to be effective for migraine prophylaxis and is not effective for treatment of acute migraine attacks.

Safety Considerations

GI adverse effects may result from ingestion of feverfew. Oral ulcers can occur from chewing fresh leaves. Post-feverfew syndrome has been reported after abrupt withdrawal from chronic use, resulting in anxiety, headaches, insomnia, and muscle stiffness. Patients who are allergic to plants in the Asteraceae/Compositae family should avoid use of feverfew, as should women who are pregnant or breast-feeding.[76] Possible antiplatelet effects have been identified; therefore, patients taking oral anticoagulants and antiplatelet agents or herbs should use feverfew with caution.[25,76]

Summary of Clinical Evidence

A Cochrane review of feverfew in preventing migraine headache found insufficient evidence from randomized, double-blind trials to suggest an effect.[77] Newer studies that included MIG-99 have been conducted since this publication. From their evaluation of more recent trials, the American Academy of Neurology and the American Headache Society consider MIG-99 probably effective for prevention of migraine, with an evidence level of B.

Huperzine

Huperzine A is derived from the Chinese club moss (*Huperzia serrata* [Thumb.] Trev.) and is a member of the Lycopodiaceae family. In China, it is approved as a treatment for Alzheimer's disease and vascular dementia.

Therapeutic Uses

Huperzine A has been used to treat Alzheimer's disease and dementia and to enhance cognitive function.

Physiologic Activity

Huperzine A is a sesquiterpene compound; the levorotatory isomer is the most pharmacologically active. This compound is a potent peripherally and centrally acting reversible acetylcholinesterase inhibitor and may have neuroprotective properties.[79]

Dosage and Product Considerations

The dosages for Alzheimer's disease range from 200–400 mcg of huperzine A daily.

Safety Considerations

Adverse effects include sweating, blurred vision, nausea, vomiting, diarrhea, dizziness, bradycardia, and loss of appetite. Theoretically, huperzine A should be avoided in patients with bradycardia, peptic ulcer disease, and increased gastric acid secretion. Concurrent use of anticholinergic drugs such as benztropine may decrease the effectiveness of huperzine A. Additive cholinergic effects may occur if huperzine A is taken with other acetylcholinesterase inhibitors (e.g., donepezil), or cholinergic agents (e.g., bethanechol). In addition, huperzine A can have additive effects in the presence of other drugs that cause bradycardia, including beta-blockers. Huperzine should be avoided during pregnancy and lactation because of the lack of safety information.

Summary of Clinical Evidence

Systematic Cochrane reviews have been conducted to evaluate the use of huperzine A in mild cognitive impairment, vascular dementia, and Alzheimer's disease. No trials met inclusion criteria for mild cognitive impairment and only one trial of patients with vascular dementia was included; the results were not significant.[80,81] The six clinical trials reviewed concluded that huperzine A has some benefit on cognitive function, global clinical status, behavioral disturbance, and functional performance in patients with Alzheimer's disease. However, only one study was of good quality and sufficient size. Huperzine A should not be used in Alzheimer's disease until additional evidence is available.[82]

Ginkgo

Ginkgo biloba L. is a tree and the only living member of the family Ginkgoaceae.

Therapeutic Uses

Ginkgo has been used for Alzheimer's disease, vascular dementia, intermittent claudication, tinnitus, acute mountain sickness, and age-related macular degeneration.

Physiologic Activity

The standardized *Ginkgo biloba* L. (EGb 761) concentrated (50:1) leaf extract contains ginkgolides (A, B, C, and M) and bilobalide. These constituents may be responsible for neuroprotective properties reported with the leaf extract. Ginkgolide B is a potent platelet-activating factor antagonist. The extract also contains bioflavonoids and flavone glycosides, such as quercetin, 3-methyl quercetin, and kaempferol. The flavonoid fractions may possess antioxidant and free radical scavenger effects.[83,84]

Dosage and Product Considerations

Recommended dosages for dementias and intermittent claudication range between 120 and 240 mg daily of ginkgo leaf extract in 2–3 divided doses. EGb 761 is available as 40, 60, or 120 mg capsules or tablets containing 24% ginkgo flavone glycosides and

6% terpenoids.[83,84] The standardized extract EGb 761 is used in many clinical trials. Many ginkgo supplements may contain subtherapeutic amounts of ginkgolides and bilobalide.

Safety Considerations

Mild GI adverse effects, headache, dizziness, and allergic skin reactions have been reported with ginkgo.[85] Recent concerns have been raised from animal studies that showed an increased rate of cancer in the nose and throat.[86] Single case reports have linked the use of gingko with other medications to priapism with risperidone, coma with trazadone, treatment failure of efavirenz, and fatal seizure with valproic acid and phenytoin.[87] Ginkgo has generally been associated with a reduction in blood pressure, although a paradoxical loss of antihypertensive efficacy has also been documented between ginkgo and a thiazide diuretic (Table 51–1).[83] Ginkgo may also increase concentrations of nifedipine.[85] Gingko should be avoided during pregnancy and lactation because of the lack of safety information.

Several case reports have documented a potential link to hemorrhage in patients taking anticoagulants or antiplatelet agents who used unstandardized gingko product.[87,88] In contrast, a meta-analysis of 18 randomized controlled trials comparing EGb 761 against placebo groups found no significant changes in hemostasis outcomes.[89] Patients taking warfarin, antiplatelet agents, and herbs should use ginkgo with caution because of the potential risk for bleeding.[88] The use of ginkgo should also be stopped at least 7–10 days before any surgical procedure.[25]

Summary of Clinical Evidence

A Cochrane review evaluated 36 studies comparing the efficacy and safety of gingko in patients with dementia or cognitive decline. Nine recent studies were of adequate size, totaling over 2000 patients, with duration of at least 6 months and good methodology. Higher-quality trials lacked consistent results that demonstrated benefit on cognition, activities of daily living, mood, depression, and care burden. The subgroup of 925 patients with Alzheimer's disease also showed conflicting results.[90]

Recently, a large randomized placebo-controlled trial, GuidAGE, assessed the prevention of Alzheimer's disease in patients older than 70 years. At 5 years, no significant differences were noted between patients taking 120 mg EGb 761 twice daily or placebo.[91]

The Ginkgo Evaluation of Memory (GEM) study evaluated 120 mg of ginkgo extract twice daily versus placebo in more than 3000 community-dwelling adults ages 72–96 years. At baseline, participants either had no cognitive impairment or only mild disease, and the study had a mean follow-up of about 6 years. The two groups were similar in the rates of change measured by the Modified Mini-Mental State Examination, the cognitive subscale of the Alzheimer Disease Assessment Scale, and the neuropsychological domains of memory, attention, visual–spatial construction, language, and executive functions.[92] Older adults with normal cognition are unlikely to benefit from the use of gingko.

Kava

Kava is derived from the rhizome and roots of *Piper methysticum* G. Forster. A member of the black pepper family (Piperaceae), kava is widely used by Pacific Islanders as a social and ceremonial tranquilizing beverage.

Therapeutic Uses

Kava is used to treat mild anxiety and sleep disturbances.

Physiologic Activity

The pharmacologically active constituents of kava are kavalactones and kavapyrones. The mechanism of action affects sodium and calcium channels, inhibiting central monoamine oxidase (MAO)-B, and modulating gamma-aminobutyric acid (GABA) receptors. Kava may also inhibit reuptake of noradrenaline and dopamine.[93]

Dosage and Product Considerations

The usual daily dosage of kava is equivalent to 60–120 mg of kavapyrones in divided doses or 70–280 mg kavalactones at bedtime. Kava extract is generally standardized to 30% kavalactones. WS 1490 is a standardized kava extract used in many studies at 300 mg per day.[94] Kava-containing products have limited availability because of concerns about the risk of hepatotoxicity as discussed in the next section.

Safety Considerations

Dizziness and drowsiness are most commonly reported with high doses of kava. The use of kava is discouraged during operation of machinery or motor vehicles. Acute overdoses may result in impaired mental status and ataxia.[95] Mouth ulceration and numbness occurs if the raw plant is chewed. Kava dermopathy syndrome, a dry, scaly rash primarily on the palms, soles, forearms, shins, and back, can appear in patients chronically using high-dose kava teas, tablets, or the native plant; the rash is reversible upon discontinuation of use. Hematological findings such as thrombocytopenia, leukopenia, increased red blood cells, and reduced serum albumin have been observed. Kava should be avoided during pregnancy and lactation because of lack of safety information.[94]

In 2002, the Center for Food Safety and Nutrition issued a warning advising consumers and professionals of the risk of severe liver injury associated with kava-containing supplements. Germany, Switzerland, Canada, Australia, and France have restricted the sale of kava products in response to case reports of liver failure associated with use.[96] Several factors are in question as to the origin of liver injury, including aqueous versus acetone or ethanol extracts, continuous high doses, inappropriate raw products, and potential contaminants. No updates to the consumer advisory have been made.[97]

Concomitant use of kava with alcohol and other central nervous system (CNS) depressants (e.g., benzodiazepines, anticonvulsants, opioids, and valerian) could increase the risk of sedation. Kava should not be taken with other hepatotoxic medications, natural products, or alcohol. Kava may interfere with dopamine transmission, resulting in an interaction with levodopa or worsening of symptoms of parkinsonism.[87]

Summary of Clinical Evidence

Small studies have shown kava extracts to be superior to placebo for short-term treatment of anxiety. A 3-week, placebo-controlled, double-blind crossover study of 60 adults with generalized anxiety accompanied by depression used an aqueous extract of

250 mg/day of kavalactones. Results demonstrated a significant impact on scores for the Hamilton Anxiety (HAM-A) Scale and for the Beck Anxiety Inventory and Montgomery-Asberg Depression Rating Scale.[98] A meta-analysis of kava extract WS 1490 reported efficacy (OR 3.3, 95% CI, 2.09–5.22) compared with the placebo change in HAM-A; however, overall HAM-A scores were not significant. Women and younger patients showed the most improvement.[99]

Melatonin

Therapeutic Uses

Melatonin, a hormone produced by the pineal gland, is synthesized from tryptophan via a serotonin pathway. Melatonin has Food and Drug Administration (FDA) orphan drug status for sleep disorders in blind patients. Dietary supplement melatonin is primarily used for insomnia and prevention of jet lag.

Physiologic Activity

Melatonin regulates sleep and circadian rhythms. Its release is induced by darkness and suppressed by light; exogenous administration increases concentrations to stimulate sleep regulation mechanisms. When taken near bedtime, melatonin does not generally cause drowsiness; instead, it makes attempts to sleep more successful. A potent antioxidant, melatonin has regulatory effects on sexual development and ovulation and may have effects on bone regulation.[100–102]

Dosage and Product Considerations

For insomnia, 0.3–5 mg can be taken 30 minutes prior to bedtime. For jet lag, the dosage is 2–5 mg the evening (between 5:00 and 10:00 pm) of arrival day at the destination and at bedtime for the following 2–5 days. The dosage for occasional insomnia remains unclear; even 0.3 mg will produce supraphysiologic concentrations and, although higher doses may not be more effective, dosages of 3 mg or 5 mg are most commonly used.[103]

Most melatonin is produced synthetically. Products extracted from bovine pineal glands are available; these products may carry added risk of bacterial contamination and bovine spongiform encephalitis (mad cow disease), so they should be avoided.

Safety Considerations

Rare adverse effects include nausea and vomiting, headache, tachycardia, irritability, dysthymia and worsening of depressive symptoms, and a morning hangover effect.[100] Long-term use is recommended only under direct supervision of a health care provider.

Melatonin use in children and adolescents is controversial because of potential hormonal effects. Use in children should be discussed first with a health care provider. The use of melatonin should be avoided during pregnancy and lactation.

Several drug interactions are known. Fluvoxamine, MAO inhibitors, and tricyclic antidepressants may increase endogenous melatonin concentrations, whereas benzodiazepines and sodium valproate decrease nighttime concentrations. Oral contraceptives and caffeine have variable effects on melatonin concentrations in women, depending on the reproductive cycle phase.[104] Verapamil may decrease concentrations by increasing melatonin excretion.

Nifedipine's effects are reduced, but whether melatonin affects nifedipine or the gastrointestinal therapeutic system (GITS) delivery method is unclear.[105]

Melatonin may increase effectiveness of some types of chemotherapy or radiotherapy for cancer and help reduce toxicities of doxorubicin and cisplatin.[106,107] Patients should always discuss any melatonin use with their oncologist.

Summary of Clinical Evidence

Evidence of the effectiveness of melatonin for sleep disturbances in healthy people is inconclusive.[100,108] One meta-analysis concluded melatonin had small but clinically significant benefits, whereas another concluded benefit was only for delayed sleep phase syndrome.[103,109] Individuals with developmental or neurologic disorders have had more consistent responses to melatonin, with improved sleep and daytime behaviors.[110] Prolonged-release melatonin in elderly patients has improved sleep quality and daytime alertness or psychomotor performance.[111] Melatonin may benefit depressed patients with sleep disorders.[112,113]

Melatonin can decrease jet lag when crossing five or more time zones; benefit is greater for eastward travel than westward and the amount and timing of exposure to daylight after arrival can decrease the benefit.[114,115] Melatonin may not be as effective as zolpidem for sleep improvement or daytime tiredness.[116]

Despite some positive trial results, evidence does not strongly support melatonin for insomnia caused by shift work, although other delayed sleep phase disorders may benefit.[108]

St. John's Wort

Hypericum perforatum L. is a perennial with more than 400 species that grow wild throughout Europe, Asia, North America, and South America. The yellow flowers and the leaves contain the highest levels of medicinally useful compounds. St. John's wort (SJW) is classified in the Clusiaceae family but may also be listed under the Hypericaceae family.

Therapeutic Uses

SJW is used to treat depression, pain, anxiety, obsessive-compulsive disorder, menopause symptoms, and premenstrual syndrome.

Physiologic Activity

Although hypericin was previously considered to have antidepressant activity, evidence now indicates that hyperforin and related compounds are mainly responsible. Other potential biologically active constituents include flavonoids and its derivatives, as well as procyanides, tannins, volatile oils, amino acids, phenylpropanes, and xanthones. SJW appears to modulate serotonin, dopamine, and norepinephrine. Additional data suggest SJW may also activate GABA and glutamate receptors and potentially inhibit MAO.[117,118]

Dosage and Product Considerations

The dosage of SJW for adults with mild-moderate depression is 900–1800 mg/day of standardized extract of 0.3% hypericin or 2%–5% hyperforin. It should be taken in three divided doses with meals. LI 160, ZE 117, WS 5570, STW3, and STW3-VI are extracts commonly used in clinical studies. The content of hypericin and hyperforin varies in commercial preparations, and products may not be interchangeable.[119] As with prescription antidepressants, the therapeutic effects of SJW are not evident for several weeks. Depression should never be self-diagnosed or self-treated. Patients should seek appropriate medical care for this serious condition before using SJW.

Safety Considerations

An analysis of randomized trials found rates of adverse effects in patients taking SJW that were similar to those for placebo. In addition, rates for SJW were much lower compared with older antidepressants and slightly lower compared with selective serotonin reuptake inhibitors (SSRIs).[120] The most frequently reported adverse effects include paresthesias, headache, nausea, dry mouth, agitation, and skin reactions. SJW should be avoided in patients with bipolar disorder and schizophrenia. Photosensitivity reactions have been reported although evidence is contradictory.[121] Until the potential photosensitivity with SJW is established, patients should limit their exposure to sun and apply sunscreen. As with SSRIs, SJW may cause sexual dysfunction. Abrupt discontinuation after chronic use may result in withdrawal symptoms similar to those of conventional antidepressants. SJW should be avoided during pregnancy and lactation.

Interactions with SJW are well documented and clinically significant (Table 51–2). SJW is a potent inducer of CYP3A4, resulting in significantly lower concentrations of drugs metabolized through this pathway. The extent of CYP3A4 induction may correlate to hyperforin dose and varies among products.[122] SJW may also induce P-glycoprotein transport proteins, resulting in lower serum concentrations of drugs such as digoxin.[122] Additional evidence suggests possible induction of CYP2C19 and CYP2E1.[122] If taken with other serotonergic agents, SJW may also increase the risk of developing serotonin syndrome.[122]

Summary of Clinical Evidence

SJW may be as effective as many antidepressants with fewer adverse effects for mild-moderate depression. A Cochrane review evaluating *Hypericum* extracts for major depression included 18 placebo-controlled trials and 17 studies with an active control. SJW had a significant benefit compared with placebo and similar efficacy to standard antidepressants for mild-moderate depression. The rates for adverse effects and trial discontinuation were also significantly lower with SJW than with older antidepressants, indicating *Hypericum* extract may be more tolerable. In addition, the results vary depending on the country of origin, with German-speaking countries showing more positive outcomes. Conclusions cannot be made regarding severe depression.[123] Similar results have been noted with WS 5572, LI 160, WS 5570, and ZE 117 *Hypericum* extracts when compared with placebo and antidepressants. Evidence supports efficacy for mild-moderate depression, with efficacy comparable to that of fluoxetine, sertraline, and citalopram, but with better tolerability.[124] Preliminary evidence demonstrates potential benefit for treatment of vasomotor symptoms in perimenopausal or postmenopausal women using SJW.[125] (See Women's Health section). However, because of its drug interactions, SJW is not an appropriate choice for many patients.

Valerian

Native to Europe and Asia, valerian grows in most parts of the world. More than 200 plant species belong to the genus *Valeriana*. The most common plant used for medicinal purposes is *Valeriana officinalis* L. from the Valerianaceae family.

Therapeutic Uses

Valerian is used for alleviating insomnia and anxiety.

Physiologic Activity

The CNS activity of valerian may be the result of valepotriates and sesquiterpene constituents of the volatile oils. Other active components include alkaloids, furanofuran ligans, and free amino acids, including GABA. Valeric acid and other components likely interact with GABA receptors in the brain, with valeproates and valeric acid producing sedation.[126] Valerian may also have barbiturate-like CNS depressant effects.

Dosage and Product Considerations

Most clinical trials for insomnia use valerian root extract in a dosage of 400–900 mg, administered 30–120 minutes before bedtime. Teas can be prepared from dried roots, although they often have an unpleasant taste and smell. Combination products with hops or lemon balm are commonly marketed.

Safety Considerations

Valerian is generally well tolerated with headache, excitability, and paradoxical insomnia occurring infrequently. Benzodiazepine-like withdrawal symptoms have been reported after discontinuation of valerian. Residual daytime sedation has been associated with higher dosages. *Valeriana officinalis* preparations are safe despite the known in vitro cytotoxic activity of valepotriates, which are generally not found in products. Chronic administration has been linked to hepatotoxicity, although reports include multi-ingredient products and the role of valerian is unclear. Valerian can potentiate the effects of other CNS depressants and should not be taken concomitantly. Pregnant women should avoid the use of valerian because of potential induction of uterine contractions.

Summary of Clinical Evidence

A meta-analysis of 18 randomized, placebo-controlled trials evaluated the effect of valerian on insomnia. Eight trials were of high quality. Subjective improvements were reported for insomnia, although the overall effectiveness of valerian could not be assessed.[127] A study of older adults found *V. officinalis* to be inferior to temazepam or diphenhydramine.[128]

5-Hydroxytryptophan

Therapeutic Uses

5-Hydroxytryptophan (5-HTP) is used for depression, anxiety, and insomnia.

Physiologic Activity

5-HTP is an intermediary step in the synthesis of serotonin from tryptophan. 5-HTP crosses the blood–brain barrier and can increase levels of several other neurotransmitters, such as dopamine and norepinephrine.[129]

Dosage and Product Considerations

Patients should be counseled that depression, severe anxiety, and panic disorders are not self-treatable conditions; symptoms should be discussed with health care providers. If 5-HTP is used, close monitoring is necessary, and dosages should not exceed 150–300 mg/day.

Safety Considerations

5-HTP is marketed as a safer alternative to tryptophan, which was banned in 1989 after more than 1500 cases of eosinophilia myalgia syndrome (EMS), including 38 deaths, were reported. Cases were originally linked to contamination of tryptophan with peak X (4,5-tryptophan-dione).[130] However, doubt exists about the role of peak X because EMS has also occurred with use of uncontaminated tryptophan and 5-HTP products.[131,132] Until more evidence is available, patients should avoid 5-HTP.

Adverse effects include nausea, vomiting, diarrhea, anorexia, belching, flatulence, and serotonergic effects.[132] 5-HTP should not be used during pregnancy or lactation. In addition, the product should not be used with serotonergic agents or MAOIs because of increased risk of serotonin syndrome or mania.[133] Carbidopa may increase 5-HTP adverse effects by decreasing its peripheral metabolism.[134] Use of 5-HTP may increase urinary 5-hydroxyindole acetic acid levels, resulting in misdiagnosis of carcinoid malignancy.[135]

Summary of Clinical Evidence

Evidence of 5-HTP's efficacy for depression, anxiety, and insomnia is preliminary. Depression studies have been small, and few trials have been conducted in the past decade.[129]

Digestive System

Ginger

Ginger (*Zingiber officinale* Roscoe) is a perennial from the Zingiberaceae family whose rhizomes and roots are used medicinally.

Therapeutic Uses

The primary use of ginger has been to relieve nausea and vomiting associated with pregnancy, motion sickness, chemotherapy, and surgery. Ginger has also been used for indigestion, colic, and arthritis.

Physiologic Activity

Ginger rhizomes possess a volatile oil that contains sesquiterpene hydrocarbons, including zingiberene and alpha-curcumene

with lesser amounts of farnesene, beta-sesquiphellandrene, and beta-bisabolene. Ginger also contains an oleoresin with non-volatile pungent components, including gingerol, shogaols, and zingerone. Galanolactone, a diterpenoid isolated from ginger, and 6-shogaol have anti-5-hydroxytriptamine activity in the GI tract, which possibly contributes to ginger's antiemetic activity. Ginger does not affect GI motility or increase gastric emptying. The 6-shogaol and 6-gingerol components inhibit cyclooxygenase and lipoxygenase pathways, resulting in anti-inflammatory actions and potential inhibition of platelet thromboxane.[136]

Dosage and Product Considerations

Dried ginger 250 mg 4 times daily has been used for nausea and vomiting in pregnancy. For motion sickness, a typical dosage is 2 capsules (500 mg) of dried powdered ginger root taken 30 minutes before travel, followed by 1–2 additional 500 mg capsules as needed every 4 hours. Daily dosages greater than 4 grams should be avoided.

Safety Considerations

Mild heartburn and belching have been reported with ginger.[85] Ginger may increase the risk of hypoglycemia and alter platelet function at dosages greater than 1 g/day. Although findings are mixed, ginger should be used with caution by individuals also taking anticoagulants and antiplatelet agents or natural products.[25,85]

Studies have found no significant adverse effects on pregnancy outcomes between ginger and placebo or pyridoxine.[137,138] A large population-based cohort study, with 1020 of 68,522 women in Norway reporting use of ginger during pregnancy, found no increase in malformations, fetal death, premature birth, low birth weight, or Apgar scores below 7. About 45% ingested ginger during the first trimester, although timing of exposure and dosing is lacking. A small, but significant, increase in vaginal bleeding was noted after week 17 (7.8% vs. 5.8%; p = 0.007) compared with controls.[139] The American College of Obstetricians and Gynecologists includes ginger as an option with beneficial effects (level evidence B) in treating nausea and vomiting in pregnancy.[140]

Summary of Clinical Evidence

Mixed results have been found for ginger's efficacy in the management of postoperative and chemotherapy-induced nausea and vomiting. A meta-analysis evaluated a fixed dose of ginger in the management of postoperative nausea and vomiting.[141] Pooled data from five placebo-controlled trials were included, providing evidence that at least 1 gram of ginger was effective in the management of nausea and vomiting. However, the study with the strongest design did not find a difference between ginger and placebo. A systematic review of five randomized, controlled trials encompassing over 800 subjects compared ginger with metoclopramide or placebo for treatment of chemotherapy-induced nausea and vomiting. Ginger did not control the severity or incidence of acute nausea.[142] However, ginger may be useful as an adjunct in patients receiving highly emetogenic chemotherapy. Both populations, one with children and young adults and the other with only adults, demonstrated a significant delay and reduction in severity of symptoms when ginger powder or oil capsules were used in addition to ondansetron and dexamethasone.[143,144]

A systematic review of pregnancy-induced nausea and vomiting evaluated six randomized controlled clinical trials and one observational study. Five studies were of high quality. In early pregnancy, ginger's efficacy was better than that of placebo and similar to that of pyridoxine.[137] A Cochrane review concluded that ginger may have a role in early pregnancy for nausea and vomiting.[145] The effectiveness of ginger for hyperemesis gravidarum is limited, so ginger should not be recommended for this condition.

Milk Thistle

Milk thistle (*Silybum marianum* [L.] Gaertn.) is a member of the Asteraceae/Compositae family.

Therapeutic Uses

Milk thistle has been used to treat liver disease, including hepatitis and cirrhosis. In Europe, it is used to treat poisoning by the mushroom *Amanita phalloides* (death cap). Milk thistle has been used as a liver protective agent for exposure to alcohol, acetaminophen, and carbon tetrachloride.

Physiologic Activity

Milk thistle's seeds and, to a lesser extent, the leaves and stems contain several compounds, collectively referred to as silymarin. The compounds include silybin, isosilybin, dehydrosilybin, silydianin, and silychristin. These biologically active compounds may have antioxidant, antifibrotic, and anti-inflammatory activity, in addition to other beneficial effects such as regulation of cell permeability and inhibition of mitochondrial injury. Stimulation of nucleolar polymerase A, resulting in increased ribosomal protein synthesis, stimulates liver regeneration and the formation of new hepatocytes. The antioxidant properties of silymarin may be the primary beneficial effect.

Dosage and Product Considerations

The average dosage is silymarin 150 mg 3 times per day for cirrhosis and silybin (silibinin) 240 mg twice daily for hepatitis. Milk thistle preparations contain varying amounts of a concentrated seed extract, standardized to flavonolignans 70%–80% calculated as silymarin; approximately 70% is silybin. Multiple products of silymarin and silybin have been used in clinical studies, but they may not be available in the United States, even with identical standardization. Liver disease resulting from alcohol, acetaminophen, and other drugs or chemicals is potentially fatal, and patients should be cautioned against self-treatment with milk thistle.

Safety Considerations

Neither pregnant women nor patients with an allergy to ragweed and other members of the Asteraceae/Compositae family should use milk thistle. The product may stimulate lactation, although evidence is limited.[146] A potential inhibitory effect of milk thistle on several CYP isoenzymes and p-glycoprotein has been identified in vitro.[87]

Summary of Clinical Evidence

Evidence to support the use of milk thistle in liver disease is limited. A Cochrane review of 18 randomized controlled studies investigated the effect of milk thistle on liver disease caused by alcohol or hepatitis B or C viral infection. Reductions in mortality or complications of liver disease or changes in liver histology were not found. Liver-related mortality was significantly reduced with inclusion of all trials but not in the five high-quality trials.[147] In a well-designed, randomized, placebo-controlled trial of patients with chronic hepatitis C virus who did not respond to interferon therapy, patients took 420 mg or 700 mg of silymarin daily for 6 months; the results did not demonstrate reduction in serum alanine aminotransferase levels, hepatitis C virus RNA levels, or changes in quality of life.[148]

Peppermint

Peppermint (*Mentha piperita* L.) is a member of the mint family Lamiaceae. It has been cultivated for its fragrant volatile oil, which is extracted primarily from its leaves.

Therapeutic Uses

Both peppermint leaf and oil have been used for many purposes, including treatment of irritable bowel syndrome, nonulcerative dyspepsia, colonic spasm, and tension headache.

Physiologic Activity

The activity of peppermint may be a result of its 0.5%–4% essential oil. The oil or leaf preparations should be standardized to contain not less than 44% menthol. Menthol stereoisomers are also present, including 3% *d*-neomenthol and menthone, menthofuran, eucalyptol, and limonene. The mechanism of action of peppermint involves direct relaxation of GI smooth muscle.

Dosage and Product Considerations

The usual dosage of peppermint oil enteric-coated capsules for irritable bowel syndrome is 0.2–0.4 mL (187–374 mg) 3 times a day 15–30 minutes before meals. Enteric-coated preparations reduce risk of heartburn. Clinical trials have studied 8–16 mL of peppermint oil solution as an antispasmodic.[149]

Safety Considerations

Heartburn may be attributed to relaxation of the lower esophageal sphincter. Patients who have severe preexisting gastroesophageal conditions should avoid use of peppermint oil. Peppermint leaf tea or topical products should be used with caution in infants and small children because of possible laryngeal and bronchial spasms from volatilized menthol. The oil may also irritate mucous membranes. Data suggest that peppermint tea and peppermint oil may decrease activity of CYP3A4.[87] The ingestion of peppermint may decrease absorption of iron.[26] Antacids or other medications that increase stomach pH may affect dissolution of enteric-coated capsules.

Summary of Clinical Evidence

Studies evaluating peppermint oil have been positive. Pooled data from one meta-analysis included four trials, three with a Jadad score greater than 4, with about 400 patients demonstrating that peppermint was more effective than placebo. The number needed to treat to prevent persistent symptoms of irritable bowel syndrome in 1 patient was 2.5.[150] A Cochrane review revealed similar results, although the authors used a different method of identifying high-quality trials, finding a significant improvement in global assessment (RR 2.25; 95% CI, 1.70–2.98; 225 patients) and symptom scores (RR 1.94; 95% CI, 1.09–3.46; 269 patients).[151]

Peppermint's efficacy in reducing colonic spasms during procedures has been investigated with positive results. Studies in patients receiving barium enemas have demonstrated that the incidence of spasms is significantly decreased, compared with placebo, and is similar to that of scopolamine butylbromide.[152,153] Compared with intramuscular hyoscyamine, peppermint has also been shown to significantly increase the opening ratio of the pyloric ring during upper endoscopy with fewer adverse effects.[154] A small study administering delayed-release, enteric-coated capsules prior to colonoscopy decreased colonic spasm and pain in patients, while also decreasing procedure time.[155]

Endocrine System

Alpha-Lipoic Acid

Therapeutic Uses

Alpha-lipoic acid (ALA), or thioctic acid, is an endogenous antioxidant promoted for diabetic patients. Intravenous and oral dosage forms have been studied for diabetic peripheral neuropathy.

Physiologic Activity

ALA is a cofactor for glucose metabolism enzymes. Diabetic animals with decreased glucose uptake in muscle tissue have reduced ALA concentrations; theoretically, supplementation would increase enzyme activity and therefore glucose uptake. Animal studies have noted improvements in blood flow and distal conduction of nerves, whereas human studies show improvement in glucose metabolism measurements such as insulin sensitivity.[156]

Dosage and Product Considerations

With oral bioavailability of 30%, 600 mg 3 times daily is comparable to the 600 mg intravenous dosage used in most European trials for diabetic neuropathy.[157] Because food decreases absorption, ALA should be taken on an empty stomach; because of its chelating activity, it should be separated 2–3 hours from antacids or other mineral-containing supplements.[158]

Safety Considerations

Adverse effects include headache, nausea, and rash. Diabetic patients who wish to add ALA to their current regimen should discuss its use with their health care providers because additive hypoglycemic effects may occur. Frequent monitoring of glucose concentrations is necessary, especially during initial weeks of therapy.

ALA can inhibit conversion of thyroxine to triiodothyronine and may displace thyroxine from serum-binding protein. Patients with thyroid conditions should avoid the use of ALA.

Summary of Clinical Evidence

Evidence for oral ALA for diabetic neuropathy is contradictory. Controlled trials have noted improvement in total symptom scores, neuropathy impairment scores, and symptoms of pain and paresthesia in the short term, whereas a 2-year study found improvements in nerve conduction but not neuropathic symptoms.[159–161] The most recent large (n = 460) and rigorous study of 4 years suggests that ALA may be more useful in prevention of progression of neuropathy than in acute treatment.[162]

Reductions in glucose and hemoglobin A1C have not been significant, although studies have noted improvement in insulin sensitivity and glucose disposal rates.[156] Two recent trials documented clinically significant lowering of fasting blood glucose (from 185.4 mg/dL to 156.3 mg/dL) and hemoglobin A1C (−0.6%) when ALA was added to standard antidiabetic medications in poorly controlled patients.[163,164] The 1200 mg daily dosage provided the greatest reduction in the parameters, and body weight was also decreased by 2.1 kg after 8 weeks in one study.[163]

American Ginseng

Therapeutic Uses

American ginseng, *Panax quinquefolius,* is closely related to Asian ginseng, *P. ginseng. P. quinquefolius* is most frequently used to reduce postprandial glucose and to reduce severity of cold and upper respiratory infection symptoms. In traditional Chinese medicine, both ginseng species are considered adaptogens to aid the body in returning to normal function and adapting to stress.

Physiologic Activity

The ginsenosides present in all *Panax* species, triterpene saponins, exert their effects on blood pressure and immune cell function, whereas nonsaponin components are more responsible for hypoglycemic effects.[165,166] The latter compounds are more plentiful in American ginseng.

Dosage and Product Considerations

Trials demonstrating reductions in postprandial glucose concentrations have used 1–9 grams of variously standardized American ginseng products 40–120 minutes before meals.[167–169] The dose should be limited to 1–3 grams taken 40 minutes before meals for safety.

Safety Considerations

American ginseng is better tolerated than other ginseng species, with mild GI effects reported. Ginsenosides often occur in pairs with opposing pharmacologic actions, so adverse effects include both increased and decreased blood pressure and blood glucose concentrations.[165] The opposing actions may explain why two studies found no effects on blood pressure.[170-172] Use in patients with schizophrenia is contraindicated because of reports of worsening symptoms, although one study has shown memory improvement in patients with schizophrenia.[173]

American ginseng may decrease the effectiveness of warfarin. This action may be caused by batch and product variability. As a result, concomitant use should be avoided.

Summary of Clinical Evidence

Clinically significant reductions in postprandial hyperglycemia have been noted in trials, although most were short term and used glycemic loads of 25 grams, smaller than a typical meal.[167,169,174] Overall, long-term effects and value for glucose management are unknown, so American ginseng cannot be recommended for diabetes.

Cinnamon

Therapeutic Uses

Cinnamon, specifically *Cinnamomum cassia* (also called *C. aromaticum*), the type most commonly found in grocery store spice aisles, is used to help lower blood glucose. True cinnamon, *C. verum* (also called *C. zeylanicum*), contains many of the same compounds and has had similar results on blood glucose in rodent studies.[175] However, a human trial of true cinnamon found no effect on glucose or insulin levels, so only *C. cassia* can be recommended as a supplement.[176]

Physiologic Activity

The flavonoids most responsible for hypoglycemic effects are procyanidin type-A polymers of epicatechin and catechin. Prevalent in water extracts, these flavonoids act to increase insulin sensitivity through increased insulin receptor autophosphorylation and cellular glucose uptake.[177] Consequently, tyrosine phosphatase, which inactivates insulin receptors, is inhibited, and anti-inflammatory actions result through changes in multiple cytokines involved in the inflammatory process.[177]

Dosage and Product Considerations

The dosage of aqueous extract, the form that may be most effective, is 0.5–1 gram daily. The dosage of ground cinnamon is 2–6 grams given in divided doses, either in capsules or in food. A half-teaspoonful is about 1 gram.[178]

Safety Considerations

Patients should not confuse cinnamon supplements with cinnamon oil because hypersensitivity reactions to cinnamon oil and pediatric poisoning from its ingestion have occurred.[178] Other than an allergic rash, no adverse events have been reported in supplement trials lasting up to 4 months. Potentiation of hypoglycemic reactions in patients on hypoglycemic medications is possible, so additional glucose monitoring is recommended. Cinnamon supplements may contain varying concentrations of coumarin, a potential hepatotoxin and carcinogen that occurs naturally in cinnamon bark.[179]

Summary of Clinical Evidence

Clinical trials and meta-analyses have had contradictory results. In general, negative trials used 1–1.5 g/day, whereas positive trials used 3–6 grams or equivalent aqueous extract.[180-182] A well-designed trial of 2 g/day of ground cinnamon added to standard antidiabetic medications reduced mean hemoglobin A1C from 8.22% to 7.86% after 12 weeks, a significantly greater reduction than with placebo.[183] Small decreases in blood pressure were also reported. A recent 3-month trial of cinnamon aqueous extract (120 and 360 mg/day) added to sulfonylurea therapy found both dosages significantly reduced hemoglobin A1C (8.9% to 8.23% and 8%, respectively) compared with placebo.[184] Fasting plasma glucose was also reduced, from 162 mg/dL to 144 mg/dL in the 120 mg group and from 202 mg/dL to 173 mg/dL in the 360 mg group. Cinnamon could be considered for adjunctive therapy in some patients with type 2 diabetes.

Dehydroepiandrosterone

Therapeutic Uses

Dehydroepiandrosterone (DHEA) is a steroid hormone secreted by the adrenal cortex that declines with advancing age. The dietary supplement form of DHEA is marketed to treat sexual dysfunction or improve sexual performance, to combat physical and mental symptoms of aging, and to enhance athletic performance or increase muscle mass.

Physiologic Activity

In general, the exogenous use of DHEA in women increases testosterone concentrations more than those of estrogen, whereas in men the reverse is true.[185] The extent to which androgen and estrogen transformation occurs depends partly on a patient's baseline hormone concentrations.

Dosage and Product Considerations

For most uses, the dosage is 25–100 mg once daily. Because of greater risk of adverse effects with dosages over 25 mg, patients should use larger dosages only on the recommendation of a health care provider.[186]

Most DHEA is synthetic, but some animal-based products exist; these should be avoided because of contamination risks. Wild yam products are falsely promoted as DHEA or hormone precursors because wild yam contains diosgenin, once used by pharmaceutical manufacturers to produce estrogens and androgens. However, the necessary chemical reactions do not occur in vivo. To further complicate patient education, some wild yam plants do contain very small amounts of naturally occurring DHEA.

Safety Considerations

Adverse effects are related to sex hormones. Women may experience hirsutism, voice deepening (generally irreversible), increased acne, and menstrual changes. Men have reported gynecomastia and testicular changes. If hormone-associated effects appear, DHEA should be discontinued. Other adverse effects include increased levels of liver function enzymes and possibly HDL-C cholesterol, headache, nasal congestion, and insomnia. At least four reports of mania requiring hospitalization exist, so DHEA is contraindicated in bipolar disorder and probably should be avoided in any mood disorder.[186] DHEA should be avoided by patients who have a history of hormone-sensitive cancer, who are taking hormonal or hormone-blocking medications, or who are pregnant or lactating. One study noted increased levels of 5-alpha-androstane-3-alpha-17-beta-diol glucuronide with DHEA supplementation in healthy young men. This substance may function as a prostate growth factor, so long-term use may have negative effects on prostate health.[187]

Summary of Clinical Evidence

Studies of DHEA have evaluated its effects on blood glucose, lipids, and adipose tissue. Results are contradictory, with one small study in men and women over 60 years noting no improvement in glucose metabolism or body fat and small decreases in both TG and HDL-C concentrations.[188] Another study noted slight decreases in visceral fat and significant improvements in oral glucose tolerance; this trial also found a reduction in HDL-C concentrations in women (not men), but the decrease reversed by the end of the second treatment year.[189]

Oral DHEA does not improve sexual arousal or function in healthy premenopausal women.[190] In postmenopausal women, one small study of 10 mg/day DHEA for 1 year found improved McCoy Female Sexuality Questionnaire total scores and increased intercourse frequency equivalent to those of the hormone therapy group.[191] The evidence of the effectiveness of DHEA for erectile dysfunction is also preliminary. In two trials, improvement was noted for erectile dysfunction related to hypertension or unknown causes but not for diabetes-related or neurologically-induced dysfunction. Men with documented declines in DHEA levels did not have benefits for sexuality, lipids, or body composition.[192,193]

Even high dosages of DHEA do not increase strength, lean body mass, or athletic performance in young healthy men, although strength and body composition may be improved in older men and women when supplementation is combined with exercise.[194-196] Some study patients have noted improved skin health, such as increased epidermal thickness and sebum production; topical use may also beneficially affect aging skin.[193,197] Three trials have noted increases in vertebral bone mineral density, although the benefit is limited to women.[198,199]

Immune Modulators

Colostrum

Therapeutic Uses

Colostrum is the thin, white fluid secreted by mammary glands immediately after birth and prior to milk production. It provides passive immunity against many pathogens until the newborn is able to produce sufficient antibodies. In addition to treatment of different types of diarrhea, colostrum is marketed for general well-being, improved athletic performance, and immune system stimulation.

Physiologic Activity

Colostrum is rich in antibodies, immunoglobulins A and E, and growth factors, which may be the components that provide immune-modulating benefits. Hyperimmune bovine colostrum, which is collected from cows inoculated with pathogens to induce production of specific antibodies and immunoglobulins, has FDA-approved orphan drug status for conditions such as acquired immunodeficiency syndrome (AIDS)-related diarrhea. Dietary supplement bovine colostrum products are generally not collected from inoculated cows. The results of research with hyperimmune colostrum cannot be extrapolated to other types; this section discusses only dietary supplement colostrum products.

Human studies have found that bovine colostrum and colostrum extracts can increase serum concentrations of insulin-like growth factor and immune variables such as interleukins, interferons, and immune globulins, as well as inhibit the absorption of lipopolysaccharide endotoxins from the intestine.[200,201] A preliminary study suggested that bovine colostrum may have beneficial effects on blood glucose and lipid levels in diabetic patients.[202]

Dosage and Product Considerations

Trials have used a wide range of dosages and formulations; dosages of colostrum powder of 20–60 grams once daily are common.

A cow never exposed to a pathogen will not produce antibodies to that pathogen, so immune function benefit is general. Patients should be wary of colostrum marketing claims regarding specific diseases or pathogens.

Products carry a small risk of contamination from diseased cattle. Risk of bovine spongiform encephalitis is almost nil because colostrum is collected from live cattle and should not come in contact with nerve tissue.

Safety Considerations

Adverse effects include increased liver function enzymes in patients with AIDS and GI upset. Individuals with milk allergies and pregnant or lactating women should avoid the use of colostrum.

Summary of Clinical Evidence

Research on bovine colostrum's effects on strength and endurance do not support improvement in athletic performance. Dietary supplement bovine colostrum is promoted to counteract decreases in immune function seen with intense physical exercise. Trials examining the exercise-related decreases and changes in intestinal permeability have noted both no effects and increases in interleukins, interferons, and immune globulins, as well as both increases and decreases in intestinal permeability.[203,204] An Italian trial found bovine colostrum combined with influenza vaccination was 3 times more effective at reducing flu sick days compared with vaccination alone.[205] Another study examined patient logbooks from earlier studies that compared concentrated bovine colostrum versus whey protein (as placebo).[206] Upper respiratory symptoms reported in bovine colostrum and whey protein users were 32% and 48%, respectively.

Echinacea

Echinacea species used in clinical trials include *E. purpurea, E. angustifolia,* and *E. pallida.* Roots, leaves, and flowers are all used medicinally; depending on the species, the above-ground parts may have greater activity.

Therapeutic Uses

Echinacea is used to prevent and treat colds and other respiratory infections.

Physiologic Activity

Echinacea has many different components targeting the nonspecific cellular immune system, including alkylamides, caffeic acid derivatives (e.g., chicoric acid), flavonoids, glycoproteins, and polysaccharides. Multiple mechanisms of action may be involved, including increased cytokine secretion, lymphocyte activity, and phagocytosis. Direct inactivation of viruses, bacteria, and fungi has been observed.[207] Anti-inflammatory activities and decreases in mucin production may be more directly responsible for decreased symptoms of upper respiratory infections.[207]

Dosage and Product Considerations

Products labeled as echinacea may contain chemically different plants or plant parts, making product comparisons difficult. The optimal standardization and dosage for echinacea are unknown. Standardized concentrates, such as Echinaforce, generally perform better in trials. Echinacea is available in single- and multiple-ingredient formulations, such as teas, extracts, juices, throat sprays, capsules, and tablets; each formulation has its own dosing regimen. Many products available in the United States are less concentrated or are labeled for use at dosages much lower than those used in clinical trials. All formulations must be taken at the first sign of illness.

Safety Considerations

Adverse effects include mild GI discomfort, tingling sensation of the tongue, and headache. Allergic reactions may occur. Patients with a history of asthma or atopy should avoid echinacea; a severe allergy to the Asteraceae/Compositae family, which includes ragweed and chrysanthemums, is a contraindication. Use of echinacea should be avoided in patients with severe systemic illnesses, such as human immuno deficiency virus (HIV) infection or AIDS, multiple sclerosis, tuberculosis, and autoimmune disorders, and in patients taking immunosuppressants; this concern, however, is based on case reports and theory.[208] Echinacea exhibits some effects on P-glycoprotein transport and several intestinal and hepatic CYP450 systems; except for drugs with a narrow therapeutic range, these effects are not likely to be significant.[209] A systematic review of use of echinacea during pregnancy found no differences in rates of major malformations during pregnancy.[210]

Summary of Clinical Evidence

A Cochrane review analyzed 16 clinical trials that evaluated echinacea for treatment and prevention of the common cold.[211] For treatment, nine studies reported a significant effect on severity and duration compared with placebo, whereas six showed no benefit. *E. purpurea* demonstrated the best results when administered at the first sign of symptoms. A meta-analysis of 14 randomized placebo-controlled studies found a significant reduction in duration of 1.4 days, and the risk of cold development was reduced by 58%.[212] A trial using a low overall dosage and use of echinacea within 36 hours of the onset of cold symptoms demonstrated a shorter duration of symptoms of less than half a day, which is unlikely to be clinically significant.[213]

For prevention of colds, three comparisons showed no benefit over placebo.[211] An additional 8-week study of echinacea prophylaxis found no benefit over placebo for reducing cold frequency.[214] Overall, results have been inconsistent and a review has proposed a more consistent approach to outcomes measurement for future studies.[215]

A pilot study in adults with respiratory disease compared the rates of influenza- and parainfluenza-like symptoms and respiratory complications in groups prophylactically given influenza vaccine, a hydroalcoholic root extract of *E. angustifolia* roots, or both. Rate decreases were found in the echinacea-only and echinacea+vaccine groups compared with the vaccine-alone group.[216] Parainfluenza-like symptoms occurred in five patients in the vaccine-only group and in only one patient in each of the echinacea-only and echinacea+vaccine groups.

Echinacea throat sprays are commonly sold. A randomized, controlled, double-dummy study compared an echinacea/sage extract spray to a standard lidocaine/chlorhexidine spray. Response rates and symptom decreases were similar between groups, with 50% of patients reaching symptom-free status a half day sooner in the echinacea group than in the lidocaine group; this result was not statistically significant.[217]

Elderberry

Therapeutic Uses

Juice or extracts of the *Sambucus nigra* berry are used for prevention or treatment of influenza and other upper respiratory illnesses.

Physiologic Activity

Elderberries contain many vitamins (e.g., C, B_2, B_6, folic acid, beta-carotene) and multiple flavonoids and anthocyanins.[218] Activities include inhibition of replication of viruses, increased production of anti-inflammatory and inflammatory cytokines, strong antioxidant capacity, and inhibition of hemagglutination of the influenza virus, which prevents entry into cells.[219] Liquid extracts have inhibited growth of several gram-positive and gram-negative bacteria.[220] A rigorous in vitro and animal study determined that in vitro activity against influenza A virus was relatively weak, but viral antibodies significantly increased.[221]

Dosage and Product Considerations

Elderberry is available in multiple dosage forms. Clinical trials have been performed with at least three products: a spray-dried elderberry juice (400 mg 3 times daily, 10% anthocyans), a syrup standardized to flavonoid content (Sambucol), and an encapsulated extract (125 mg anthocyanin).[222-224] The optimal standardization and dosage form have not been determined.

Safety Considerations

Use of appropriate products is important because insufficiently cooked or unripe berries, stems, or leaves contain cyanogenic glycosides metabolized in the GI tract to cyanide; reports exist of not only nausea and vomiting but also dizziness, weakness, and stupor with home-prepared juices and extracts.[218] Commercially available elderberry extracts are well tolerated.

Summary of Clinical Evidence

The first study of elderberry extract (Sambucol) used 30 mL (15 mL for children) daily for 3 days in patients reporting flu symptoms during an outbreak of influenza B. The duration of fever was 4 days versus 6 days in the treatment and placebo groups, respectively. After 3 days "complete cure" was noted in 46.7% of elderberry-treated patients and 16.7% of placebo-treated patients.[223] The second study (n = 60) of elderberry extract (Sambucol) during an influenza A epidemic used a visual analogue scale to assess symptom improvement and found that elderberry-treated patients reached scores closer to "pronounced improvement" (10 on the 0–10 scale) within 3–4 days, whereas placebo-treated patients reached similar scores after 7–8 days.[225] Rescue medications of a nasal spray and analgesic were used by 21 and 26 patients, respectively, in the placebo group and by 5 and 7 patients, respectively, in the elderberry group. The use of elderberry extracts is an option for patients with flu or upper respiratory symptoms.

Probiotics

Therapeutic Uses

The term *probiotics* refers to several types of beneficial bacteria, including *Lactobacillus* spp. and *Bifidobacterium* spp., and one yeast, *Saccharomyces boulardii.* In addition to antibiotic-associated diarrhea and other GI disorders (see Chapter 23), probiotics are also used for atopic dermatitis and allergies and are being investigated for prevention and treatment of upper respiratory infections.

Physiologic Activity

The mechanisms by which probiotics reduce allergic symptoms such as rhinitis or dermatitis are not well understood. Probiotics decrease intestinal permeability, which may help to decrease exposure to allergens. The normalization of gut flora decreases inflammatory responses, but probiotics may have immunomodulating activity. Macrophage and lymphocyte activity are both affected, as are various cytokines, such as increased interferon-alpha and immunoglobulin and decreased tumor necrosis factor. (See Chapter 23, Table 23–8 for an in-depth discussion of other potential physiologic effects with probiotics.)

Dosage and Product Considerations

Many probiotic preparations with one or multiple species and wide dosing ranges are available. Health care providers and consumers should be cautious in selecting products because many species and strains of probiotic bacteria exist; results from studies using one product may not be applicable to different species or strains. (See Chapter 23, Table 23–9.)

For atopy and dermatitis, *Lactobacillus rhamnosus* GG is the most researched and recommended, although *L. acidophilus* and *Bifidobacterium lactis* have also shown benefit.[226,227] *Lactobacillus* and *Bifidobacterium* species are dosed at 1–10 billion colony-forming units per day, given in divided doses. *Saccharomyces boulardii* is dosed at 250–500 mg taken 2–4 times daily. Trials have investigated multiple species, but *Bifidobacterium*-dominant products are generally preferred in infants because they better match the normal flora in this population.

Product quality has been a concern because some studies found products containing few or no live cultures; refrigerated products have been recommended as perhaps less likely to have suffered from degrading temperatures.[228] Recent research suggests that dead probiotics may also offer benefit by triggering gut anti-inflammatory responses.[229,230]

Safety Considerations

GI adverse effects including mild bloating and flatulence subside over time, and titration of doses may minimize these adverse effects. Diarrhea has been reported in children. Although probiotics are being studied in HIV-positive and AIDS patients, immunocompromised patients should avoid their use because of rare reports of systemic infection.[231] No harmful effects have been observed in women in late-stage pregnancy or in breast-feeding infants during long-term use.[232] Doses of antimicrobial agents should be administered several hours apart from probiotics.

Summary of Clinical Evidence

Early trials demonstrated a reduction in the development of eczematous dermatitis, asthma, and atopic sensitization in infants after mothers were treated with probiotics during pregnancy and/or breast-feeding. Several recent trials have not supported any benefit of this practice.[226,233–235] Studies in children with atopic dermatitis have had contradictory results, ranging from no benefit to substantially significant improvement in symptoms and SCORAD (SCOring Atopic Dermatitis) values.[227,236] Adults with atopic dermatitis have also benefitted from probiotic treatments; a recent trial demonstrated significant reductions in SCORAD indices with use of *L. salivarius.*[237]

The most recent meta-analysis of probiotics for reduction of respiratory tract infections in children and adults concluded that the results were greater than placebo.[238] Studies used different single and combination therapies, but *Lactobacillus* species were used most often. A combination of *L. rhamnosus* and *B. adolescentis* in a yogurt product demonstrated changes in cytokines but no significant benefits on symptoms or quality of life scores.[239] Children with asthma and allergic rhinitis had improved pulmonary function and decreased rhinitis symptom scores when treated with *L. gasseri* for 2 months.[240] The low cost and safety of probiotics support their use as a treatment option, alone or in conjunction with standard therapies.

Physical and Mental Performance Enhancers

Eleuthero

Eleutherococcus senticosus from the Araliaceae family is often referred to as *Acanthopanax senticosus* or Siberian ginseng. The plant is not a genus of *Panax,* as are Asian and American ginseng species. *Eleutherococcus* is found in eastern Siberia, northeastern China, Korea, and Hokkaido Island in Japan.

Therapeutic Uses

Eleuthero's traditional use is as an adaptogen for improvement of athletic performance, chronic stress, upper respiratory conditions, and immune deficiency. Other uses include treatment of herpes simplex type 2 infections, blood pressure (hypotension and hypertension), prevention of atherosclerosis, and diabetes mellitus.

Physiologic Activity

The active compounds of eleuthero, derived primarily from the root and leaf, are referred to as eleutherosides (subtypes A to M). Flavonoids, hydroxycinnamates, and other constituents such as sesamin, B-sitosterol, hedarasaponin B, and isofraxidin may also have biological activity. Animal studies and in vitro analysis suggest these compounds have antiplatelet, immunostimulant, and antioxidant properties.[241]

Dosage and Product Considerations

Commercial products are often standardized to eleutheroside B and/or E content at a dosage of 300–400 mg/day. A 33% ethanolic extract 10 mL taken 3 times a day has also been used. After 2 months of daily use, patients should discontinue the product for a minimum of 2 weeks.[241]

Safety Considerations

Both drowsiness and stimulant effects have been reported with eleuthero. Because of its variable effects on blood pressure, eleuthero should be avoided in patients with hypertension. Theoretically, patients with diabetes mellitus should be monitored for hypoglycemia. Eleuthero does not affect activity of CYP2D6 and CYP3A4 at normal dosages.[241] Safety data are lacking for use during pregnancy and lactation. In patients taking digoxin, eleuthero may interfere with digoxin assays because of structural likeness of some of its glycosides.[87]

Summary of Clinical Evidence

Well-designed, randomized clinical trials documenting the safety and efficacy of eleuthero are lacking. In a small 6-month study, *Eleutherococcus* extract taken once daily demonstrated a beneficial effect on frequency, severity, and duration of herpes simplex type 2 infections.[242] A small trial in elderly patients found improvement in social function measures related to quality of life after 4 weeks of use, but not at 8 weeks.[243]

Ginseng (*Panax ginseng*)

The root and rhizome of Asian ginseng (*Panax ginseng* C.A. Meyer) is from the family Araliaceae and is exported primarily from Korea, China, and Japan.

Therapeutic Uses

Asian ginseng has been used to improve mental and physical stress, anemia, diabetes mellitus, immune response, insomnia, and impotence, and for cancer prevention.

Physiologic Activity

The constituents likely responsible for ginseng's adaptogen activity are triterpenoid saponins, including ginsenosides. At least 30 ginsenosides, also referred to as panaxosides, have been identified. Additional constituents include carbohydrates, B vitamins, and flavonoids.[244]

Dosage and Product Considerations

Ginseng extracts are standardized to 4% ginsenosides administered at 200 mg/day in divided doses. Crude powdered root has been used in dosages of 2–3 g/day. Decoctions and tea preparations are also commonly used.[244]

Safety Considerations

Adverse effects include insomnia, headache, blood pressure changes, anorexia, rash, mastalgia, and menstrual abnormalities. Large dosages can result in gastric upset and CNS stimulation. Ginseng should be used with caution in patients with cardiovascular disease, diabetes mellitus, or acute illness. Ginseng's effect on anticoagulant and antiplatelet therapy is not predictable. The use of ginseng with phenelzine or other MAOIs, corticosteroids, or large amounts of stimulants, including caffeine-containing beverages, should be avoided.[85,244] Concurrent use with imatinib has resulted in hepatotoxicity.[87] Ginseng abuse syndrome has been described in long-term ginseng users. Although reports have been discredited, prolonged use of ginseng is not recommended.[244] Ginseng should not be used during pregnancy or lactation because of a lack of data and concern about its potential estrogenic effects.[245]

Summary of Clinical Evidence

Small short-term studies that evaluated Asian ginseng's effect on fasting and postprandial glucose concentrations in patients with type 2 diabetes mellitus yielded mixed results. A systematic review of randomized controlled trials, four of which met inclusion criteria, found a lack of overall effect on fasting blood glucose, hemoglobin A1C, or 2-hour postprandial glucose.[246]

For erectile dysfunction, a systematic review of seven randomized controlled trials found significant benefit with Asian ginseng, although the review noted the limitations of a small sample size and trial quality.[247] A small, randomized, placebo-controlled trial found benefit in improving sexual arousal in menopausal women.[248]

Five trials were included in a Cochrane review of the role of *P. ginseng* for cognition; the majority of subjects were healthy. Because of various dosing regimens, outcomes, and study length, data could not be pooled. Although ginseng benefited some end points related to cognitive function, quality of life, and behavior, available evidence does not support its use.[249]

Green Tea

Native to southeastern Asia, the tea shrub *Camellia sinensis* (L.) Kuntze belongs to the family Theaceae. Tea leaves are heated immediately after harvesting and then mechanically rolled and crushed before drying to produce green tea. From the same plant as green tea, black tea is produced by allowing the leaves to wilt before they are rolled and left in a humid environment for several hours. This process promotes fermentation and a gradual change in color to reddish-brown. Oolong, another commonly available tea, is a partially fermented tea.

Therapeutic Uses

Green tea is considered a performance enhancer because of the stimulant effect from caffeine. Green tea has also been used to prevent cardiovascular disease, cancer, and liver disorders. A topical prescription product, Polyphenon E, made from green tea extract is approved for the treatment of condylomata acuminata.[250]

Physiologic Activity

In addition to caffeine, green tea contains polyphenolic compounds including flavonols (also known as catechins), flavonoids, and phenolic acids. The most prevalent flavonols include epicatechin, epicatechin-3-gallate, epigallocatechin, and epigallocatechin-3-gallate. These components are thought to have antioxidant and antitumor effects.[251] Catechins and caffeine may each contribute to weight loss.[252]

Dosage and Product Considerations

Dosages of green tea in epidemiologic studies vary between 1 and 10 cups daily. The preferred dosage is 3–5 cups per day, or up to 1200 mL/day, including a minimum of 250 mg/day of catechins.[253] Green tea extract supplements standardized to polyphenol content retain effects similar to those of green tea while reducing exposure to caffeine.[251]

Safety Considerations

Ingestion of large quantities of green tea can cause adverse GI symptoms as well as CNS and cardiac stimulation attributed to the caffeine content. One 8-ounce cup of green tea contains 24–40 mg of caffeine. In comparison, an 8-ounce cup of black tea has 14–61 mg of caffeine, and an 8-ounce cup of coffee can range from 95 to 200 mg on average.[254] Green tea should be avoided if other stimulating drugs are ingested. Green tea products have been associated with liver toxicity.[255] Serum folate levels have also been reduced by green tea.[87] Green tea should be used cautiously during pregnancy and lactation because of caffeine consumption and potential folic acid concerns. Green tea in large dosages may antagonize the effects of warfarin because of small amounts of vitamin K.[85]

Summary of Clinical Evidence

Epidemiologic data suggest that daily consumption of green tea may protect against cardiovascular and metabolic diseases.[256] A randomized placebo-controlled trial demonstrated that standardized green tea capsules lowered blood pressure, serum lipids, and serum amyloid alpha in healthy adults at the end of 3 weeks.[257] Another randomized controlled trial of theaflavin-enriched green tea extract demonstrated mild reductions in LDL-C concentrations in patients on diets low in saturated fats.[258] Green and black teas are currently being reviewed for primary prevention of cardiovascular disease by the Cochrane Heart Group.[259] In obese patients, a Cochrane review found green tea products had no significant effects for weight loss and weight maintenance.[252]

Consumption of green tea to reduce the incidence of breast, prostate, lung, bladder, ovarian, digestive, and oral cancers has been studied. A Cochrane review of 51 studies that included 1.6 million subjects was unable to identify a substantive link to green tea consumption and cancer prevention. Most studies were epidemiologic and performed in Asia where green tea consumption is high. The only randomized controlled trial, coupled with higher quality observational studies, found a reduction in prostate cancer risk with consumption of larger quantities. Although data were limited, evidence for prevention of lung, pancreatic, and colorectal cancer was moderate to strong.[253]

Kidney, Urinary Tract, and Prostate

African Plum

African plum is derived from the bark of *Prunus africana* (Hook f.) Kalkman (syn. *Pygeum africanum* Hook f.), a member of the Rosaceae family.

Therapeutic Uses

Pygeum (African plum tree) bark has been used to treat benign prostatic hyperplasia (BPH).

Physiologic Activity

Pygeum bark contains phytosterols; pentacyclic triterpenes, including ursolic and oleanic acids; and ferulic acid esters, including docosanol and tetracosanol. Phytosterols may compete with androgen precursors and inhibit prostaglandin synthesis in the prostate. Triterpenes may have anti-inflammatory properties. Ferulic acid esters reduce concentrations of prolactin and prostate cholesterol, a precursor to testosterone synthesis.[260]

Dosage and Product Considerations

Products are standardized to contain 14% triterpenes and 0.5% *n*-docosanol; the average dosage is 50–100 mg twice daily.[261] Demand for pygeum extract has caused the African plum tree to become a threatened species, with current international trade being monitored under the Convention on International Trade in Endangered Species of Wild Fauna and Flora.[260]

Safety Considerations

Adverse effects include diarrhea, constipation, and gastric pain. Men presenting with prostate symptoms should contact their health care provider before starting pygeum to rule out prostate cancer. It is unclear if pygeum affects prostate-specific antigen concentrations. Adverse effects are increased if pygeum is combined with finasteride.

Summary of Clinical Evidence

Pygeum has improved urinary flow, void volumes, residual volumes, nocturia, daytime frequency, and subjective symptom assessments of BPH. Larger studies that include standardized dosages, active comparisons, and adequate durations are needed to fully assess its efficacy.[262]

Cranberry

Cranberry (*Vaccinium macrocarpon* Ait.) is an evergreen bush native to North America and belongs to the family Ericaceae.

Therapeutic Uses

Cranberry has been used to prevent and treat urinary tract infections (UTIs).

Physiologic Activity

Cranberry contains proanthocyanidins. Epicatechin is the primary proanthocyanidin found in cranberry extracts. Evidence suggests that cranberry blocks bacteria, *Escherichia coli*, in particular, from adhering to bladder, kidneys, and urethra. Fructose found in cranberry juice may also alter bacterial adhesion.[263]

Dosage and Product Considerations

Many studies have used unsweetened cranberry juices. Cranberry juice cocktail is about 30% pure cranberry juice and contains sugar; it is unknown if this product will demonstrate the same effects. Efficacy appears to be based on the proanthocyanidins content, although controlling for this variable in studies is inconsistent. For prevention of UTI, the dosage of cranberry juice is 300–900 mL/day. Encapsulated cranberry formulations at a dosage of about 400 mg twice daily may be preferred to avoid the sugar content of juices.

Safety Considerations

Evidence suggests that regular use of cranberry concentrate tablets might increase risk of kidney stones.[264] Patients may experience diarrhea with large daily doses. Theoretically, cranberry juice may alter excretion of weakly alkaline drugs or neutralize effects of antacids. Case reports have suggested cranberry may cause bleeding in patients taking warfarin; however, pharmacokinetic and pharmacodynamic evidence is lacking.[87,265]

Summary of Clinical Evidence

A Cochrane review of 24 studies, with 13 included in a meta-analysis, concluded preventive use of cranberry products does not significantly reduce the overall risk of UTIs or in subgroups of women or children with recurrent UTIs, older adults, pregnant women, cancer patients, and catheterized patients. A high dropout rate suggests long-term use of cranberry, specifically juice, is not well tolerated.[266] It is unknown if tablet or capsule products included in studies contain enough proanthocyanidins to be effective.[266] Cranberry should not be used to treat UTIs, and patients should be referred to their health care provider.[267]

Saw Palmetto

Saw palmetto (*Serenoa repens* [Michx.] G. Nichols), a dwarf palm tree from the Arecaceae family, is native to the southeast coastal region of the United States.

Therapeutic Uses

Saw palmetto has been used to treat BPH.

Physiologic Activity

The lipophilic extracts from the ripened fruit contain saturated and unsaturated fatty acids and plant sterols. Although the active compounds have not been identified, they are likely present in the lipophilic extract. Saw palmetto does not appear to reduce prostate-specific antigen concentrations. Saw palmetto inhibits 5-alpha-reductase and cytosolic androgen receptor binding; it also has local antiestrogenic and anti-inflammatory effects on the prostate.[268]

Dosage and Product Considerations

The usual dosage is 160 mg twice daily or 320 mg once daily. Saw palmetto products should contain 80%–95% standardized fatty acids.

Safety Considerations

In comparative studies, saw palmetto was better tolerated than finasteride and tamsulosin. GI complaints are most commonly reported. Two reports of pancreatitis have been documented.[269] Significant bleeding has also been reported with saw palmetto; its use in individuals taking other products that might prolong bleeding should be avoided.[85] Patients taking androgenic drugs should also avoid its use. Men with prostate symptoms should contact their provider before starting saw palmetto to rule out prostate cancer. Saw palmetto is occasionally used in multi-ingredient products intended for women. Because of the inhibition of 5-alpha-reductase, it should be considered Pregnancy Category X and also should not be used in lactation.

Summary of Clinical Evidence

Evidence does not support use of saw palmetto for symptoms related to BPH. In a Cochrane review that included 32 randomized controlled trials ranging from 4 to 72 weeks with over 5000 male subjects, saw palmetto was not effective for treating urinary symptoms, increasing peak urine flow, or reducing prostate size. In the updated review, two new high-quality trials of scores of 582 men, based on the American Urological Association Symptom Score Index, demonstrated no difference in lower urinary tract symptoms for those taking saw palmetto compared with placebo. One 72-week study with double or triple the usual dose of 320 mg/day found differences in lower urinary tract symptoms, including nocturnal symptoms, remained insignificant. Three high-quality trials assessing peak urine flow in 667 men also found no change compared with placebo. A 12-month trial of 225 men reported no change in prostate size.[270]

Musculoskeletal System

Chondroitin Sulfate

Therapeutic Uses

Chondroitin sulfate is a glycosaminoglycan found in cartilage. As a dietary supplement, chondroitin sulfate is usually combined with other supplements in osteoarthritis and joint health products.

Physiologic Activity

Chondroitin sulfate's primary activity may be inhibition of leukocyte elastase, an enzyme involved in cartilage degradation. Chondroitin also serves as building material for cartilage production, inhibits resorption by osteoclasts, and may stimulate chondrocytes to produce cartilage.[271,272] The supplement also reduces inflammation via inhibition of the translocation of nuclear factor kappa, which is involved in activating B cells, and serves as a sulfur donor, an essential component for creation of the sulfur bonds used in cartilage synthesis.[271,272]

Dosage and Product Considerations

For osteoarthritis, the common dosage is 1200 mg daily in 1 or divided doses. Combination products with glucosamine may offer increased benefits, but chondroitin has both less evidence of efficacy and greater cost. Patients should begin therapy with glucosamine sulfate. If, after 4–5 months, a benefit is seen but symptoms are still bothersome, chondroitin may be added. Chondroitin should be taken with food if nausea or GI upset occurs.

Chondroitin is often produced from bovine trachea, so a slight microbial contamination risk may exist. Because trachea contains little neural tissue, risk of bovine spongiform encephalitis (mad cow disease) is minimal.

Safety Considerations

Adverse effects include mild GI upset and nausea. Allergic reactions, edema, diarrhea, constipation, nausea, heartburn, and hair loss have also been reported.[273] Use during pregnancy or lactation should be avoided because safety information is inadequate. Although no interactions have been reported in humans, patients taking anticoagulants or antiplatelet agents should be monitored carefully because chondroitin and heparin have some structural similarity.

Summary of Clinical Evidence

Information on the efficacy of chondroitin is limited because few trials have examined monotherapy. A meta-analysis examining three trials with a duration of 2 years concluded that chondroitin alone resulted in a decrease in the rates of knee cartilage degradation.[274] A recent well-designed study using 800 mg/day also noted statistically significant reduction in loss of cartilage volume compared with placebo, although pain and other symptoms were similar to those of the placebo group.[275] Pain, morning stiffness, and the Functional Index for Hand Osteoarthritis scores were all significantly improved over placebo in a 6-month trial using 800 mg/day.[276] Another study examined patients with both knee osteoarthritis and plantar psoriasis; chondroitin demonstrated significant improvement over placebo in pain visual analogue scale, Lequesne index scores, and both patient and physician efficacy ratings after 3 months.[277] Some evidence suggests chondroitin has beneficial effects that persist after discontinuation, and a meta-analysis concluded that long-term use slows radiographic progression of joint space narrowing in osteoarthritis of the knee.[278,279]

Devil's Claw

Therapeutic Uses

Harpagophytum procumbens is an African desert plant. Both dried ground root and standardized extracts are used for arthritis and back and joint pain.

Physiologic Activity

Devil's claw has anti-inflammatory, anticonvulsant, analgesic, and hypoglycemic activity.[280] Harpagoside, an iridoid glycoside, is likely the primary active component although beta-sitosterol may contribute. Effects in arthritis may be linked to inhibition of matrix metalloproteinases, which degrade cartilage. Anti-inflammatory effects on pain and osteoarthritis include inhibition of mRNA expression of tumor necrosis factor alpha, interleukin-6, and cyclooxygenase-2, as well as release of prostaglandin E_2.[281]

Dosage and Product Considerations

Extracts are often standardized to harpagoside content. The dosage is 100 mg/day of harpagoside in an aqueous extract given in divided doses. Evidence has suggested greater efficacy with aqueous extracts over ethanolic extracts.[280]

Safety Considerations

Adverse effects include diarrhea, headache, anorexia, and rash. GI disturbances are related to the stimulation of gastric acid.[282] Devil's claw is not recommended for patients with diabetes or cardiac disease because of blood pressure and glucose reductions identified in animal studies. Its use during pregnancy is not recommended because of the potential to induce uterine contractions.[280] Although only one report for anticoagulants and antiplatelet agents exists, devil's claw should not be used with these agents.

Summary of Clinical Evidence

Several trials have examined the use of devil's claw in osteoarthritis and demonstrated pain relief greater than placebo or equivalent to a prescription analgesic on standard assessment instruments, such as the Western Ontario and McMaster University Osteoarthritis Index (WOMAC) scale.[283] Meta-analyses and systemic reviews support the use of aqueous extracts of devil's claw for osteoarthritis.[280,283]

Devil's claw has been compared with placebo, anti-inflammatory agents, and controls such as massage and acupuncture for treatment of lower back pain. All but one study found greater benefit for devil's claw in pain relief and increased mobility.[280,283] Evidence supports its use for chronic back pain not associated with disk or nerve root conditions.

Glucosamine

Therapeutic Uses

Glucosamine is marketed primarily for osteoarthritis.

Physiologic Activity

Glucosamine is an endogenous mucopolysaccharide. Similar to chondroitin, it increases components available for cartilage synthesis. Glucosamine stimulates chondrocytes to produce cartilage and synoviocytes to produce synovial fluid and hyaluronic acid, inhibits matrix metalloproteinase, and modulates activities of inflammatory cytokines.[284] Glucosamine sulfate and glucosamine hydrochloride have different efficacy profiles, which may be explained by differences in inhibition of gene expression: compared with glucosamine hydrochloride, glucosamine sulfate and combination glucosamine sulfate+chondroitin sulfate stimulate greater increases in the receptor activator of nuclear factor kappa–B ligand to reduce bone resorption by osteoclasts.[285] Glucosamine sulfate may also be a sulfur donor for sulfur bonds used in cartilage production.[286]

Dosage and Product Considerations

For osteoarthritis, the appropriate dosage is 1500 mg daily of glucosamine sulfate, given in 1 or divided doses. Glucosamine will not provide pain relief as quickly as NSAIDs or acetaminophen can, so concurrent analgesic therapy should be continued as needed. Glucosamine sulfate combined with NSAID therapy has been shown to be more effective than glucosamine sulfate alone in reducing pain symptoms over 3 months.[287] Effects may not be experienced for 6–8 weeks, with full benefits not evident for 4–6 months. If benefits are not observed after 6 months of use, therapy should be discontinued.

Optimal product choice may be difficult, as many supplements use the less expensive glucosamine hydrochloride, which is possibly less effective than the sulfate salt form. Many trials demonstrating the efficacy and safety have used crystalline glucosamine sulfate products from Rotta Laboratories.

Safety Considerations

Nausea, stomach upset, constipation, and diarrhea are the most common adverse effects for glucosamine. These symptoms are usually alleviated by taking glucosamine in divided doses with meals. Drowsiness, headache, and skin reactions have been infrequently reported.

Glucosamine is manufactured from shellfish chitin or produced synthetically. Some products claim to be allergen free because processing removes allergenic material. Two studies tested this claim using shellfish-derived products and found no reactions in individuals with documented shellfish allergies.[288] Because a manufacturer's source materials may not remain consistent, patients with severe shellfish allergies should avoid glucosamine.

Because of glucosamine's glucose-based chemical structure, older reference texts still contain cautions regarding hyperglycemia. Multiple studies have found no reason for caution beyond having diabetic patients monitor glucose levels more closely for a few days.[289]

Anecdotal cases of cholesterol elevations have been reported, although evidence from long-term clinical trials and a short-term safety trial do not support this concern.[285] Pregnant or lactating women should avoid glucosamine because safety data are lacking. Drug interactions with glucosamine have not been documented.

Summary of Clinical Evidence

Studies of glucosamine for osteoarthritis can be divided into three general groups: glucosamine sulfate monotherapy, glucosamine hydrochloride monotherapy, and glucosamine of either salt combined with chondroitin sulfate. Conclusions regarding the efficacy of glucosamine have varied, depending on the specific group.

The 2-year Glucosamine/chondroitin Arthritis Intervention Trial (GAIT) funded by the National Institutes of Health is cited both as support that "glucosamine works" and as support that it does not.[290] Five groups in the GAIT compared glucosamine hydrochloride, chondroitin sulfate, glucosamine hydrochloride + chondroitin sulfate, celecoxib, and placebo. The primary outcome measure was a 20% reduction in the WOMAC scale. None of the treatment groups' results were statistically

significantly different from those of the placebo group, although patients in the celecoxib and glucosamine hydrochloride groups did achieve slightly better odds of reaching the outcome measure, 1.21 and 1.16, respectively, than did patients in the chondroitin and combination groups. Of the small number of studies evaluating glucosamine hydrochloride alone for knee osteoarthritis, only one demonstrated partial benefit; overall, changes in pain or function scores were not significant.[291] At this time, the overall evidence does not support the use of glucosamine hydrochloride monotherapy.

Trial results for glucosamine hydrochloride + chondroitin sulfate are contradictory, but overall have shown more benefit than glucosamine hydrochloride monotherapy. One example is a study of low doses of 1200 mg glucosamine hydrochloride and 60 mg chondroitin sulfate per day compared with placebo.[292] Outcome measures included Japanese Orthopaedic Association criteria scores and visual analog scales for knee pain. At 16 weeks, the treatment group had significantly improved scores ($p < 0.5$) for both "walking ability and painfulness" and "stairs – ascending/descending ability and painfulness." Both treatment and placebo groups improved from baseline on the visual analog scale scores of pain, but the treatment group had significantly greater improvement at week 16.

Most glucosamine trials in knee osteoarthritis that demonstrated significant efficacy used glucosamine sulfate alone or with chondroitin sulfate. Multiple early glucosamine sulfate trials found positive results for clinically significant reduction of pain and improvement of movement.[293] Many were criticized for small sample size or association with a glucosamine sulfate manufacturer, although later reviews have supported findings.

Outcome measurements differed as well. Early trials often used the Lequesne Index for symptoms, whereas later trials with negative results or smaller effect sizes used the WOMAC scale. This scale was used in the largest (n = 318) trial that compared glucosamine sulfate with placebo and acetaminophen. Glucosamine sulfate was significantly more effective for symptom reduction compared with placebo on both the Lequesne and WOMAC indices, whereas acetaminophen was not.[294] Additional research is needed to identify the effect size expected from this therapy. Although benefit will likely be smaller than early research indicated, evidence is sufficient to support recommendations for glucosamine sulfate use, either alone or in combination with chondroitin sulfate. Currently, osteoarthritis treatment guidelines from the Osteoarthritis Research Society International and the European League Against Rheumatism include glucosamine as initial options, whereas the American College of Rheumatology considers such recommendations to be premature, and the British National Institute for Health and Care Excellence (NICE) guidelines no longer include glucosamine.[285] The evidence at this time ranks the efficacy for knee osteoarthritis as follows: glucosamine sulfate (monotherapy or in combination with chondroitin sulfate) is greater than glucosamine hydrochloride + chondroitin sulfate, which is much greater than glucosamine hydrochloride monotherapy.

Glucosamine is also used for other types of osteoarthritis and joint issues. A recent well-designed trial of glucosamine sulfate versus placebo in patients with lumbar osteoarthritis and chronic low back pain found no difference in pain or disability scores after 6 months of treatment or a 1 year follow-up.[295] Older studies of glucosamine sulfate or glucosamine hydrochloride + chondroitin sulfate noted some benefit for temporomandibular joint pain or joint noise, but the most recent study, well-designed except for a short duration, demonstrated no benefit of 1500 mg/day of glucosamine sulfate over placebo after 12 weeks of treatment.[296]

Methylsulfonylmethane

Therapeutic Uses

Methylsulfonylmethane (MSM) is a naturally occurring compound in foods and a major metabolite of dimethylsulfoxide (DMSO), an industrial solvent. Arthritic workers began using DMSO topically, and MSM was developed in an attempt to avoid DMSO's toxicity and adverse effects.[297] MSM is included in arthritis supplements despite little clinical evidence for efficacy.

Physiologic Activity

Intestinal bacteria break down MSM to release sulfur, which is then incorporated into amino acids such as cysteine. Sulfur is essential for cartilage bonding, and animal studies have found lower sulfur levels in arthritic cartilage. One study of MSM noted decreased joint disease in a rheumatoid arthritis mice model.[298] Studies in mice tissue have demonstrated anti-inflammatory effects such as reduced production of interleukin-6 and tumor necrosis factor-α, decreased cyclooxygenase-2 expression, and inhibition of nuclear factor kappa B.[299]

Dosage and Product Considerations

The dosages of MSM used in clinical trials have varied from 1500 to 3000 mg/day in 1 or divided doses.[300] A patient choosing to use MSM should not exceed 3000 mg daily. MSM can be destroyed by water or excessive heat during the manufacturing process or storage, so purchasing from a reliable manufacturer and proper storage are essential. Smaller doses of MSM are present in combination products for osteoarthritis than in single-entity products.

Safety Considerations

Adverse effects of MSM use include headache, pruritus, nausea, and diarrhea. Use during pregnancy and lactation should be avoided because of lack of safety information. No drug interactions are known.

Summary of Clinical Evidence

For osteoarthritis, one 12-week trial (n = 118) compared MSM with glucosamine sulfate, placebo, and the combination of MSM and glucosamine sulfate. Pain and functioning improved in all groups but the placebo group. Improvement was greater in the combination group than with MSM or glucosamine sulfate alone.[300] Evidence is insufficient to recommend MSM at this time.

S-Adenosyl-L-Methionine

Therapeutic Uses

S-Adenosyl-L-methionine (SAMe) is an endogenous substance formed from L-methionine and ATP. SAMe is used for osteoarthritis and depression.

Physiologic Activity

SAMe is produced primarily in the liver. Liver disease and low vitamin B_{12} or folate levels may decrease concentrations.[301] For osteoarthritis, SAMe stimulates chondrocytes to produce proteoglycans, may block cartilage degradation enzymes, and has anti-inflammatory effects such as decreased tumor necrosis factor-α.[301,302]

SAMe donates methyl groups to neurotransmitters and catecholamines, and it increases brain neurotransmitter levels, including those of norepinephrine, dopamine, and serotonin, which may contribute to its antidepressant effects.

Dosage and Product Considerations

Most osteoarthritis trials used dosages of 400–800 mg/day in divided doses, whereas dosages for depression are 1200–1600 mg/day.[303]

Safety Considerations

Adverse effects include nausea, diarrhea, and heartburn. Less frequently, dry mouth, headache, dizziness, nervousness, insomnia, cognitive impairment, and a switch to mania in patients with bipolar disorder have been reported.[304] SAMe is also associated with hypomania or severe mania in subjects with no personal or family history of mania or bipolar disorder.[305] A report of mixed mania with suicidal ideation occurred within 2 weeks.[306] The CNS effects may be dose related because mania/hypomania has not been reported in lower-dosage osteoarthritis trials. Until more information is available, SAMe should not be recommended. Patients who use SAMe for osteoarthritis should take the lowest dosage that provides relief and no more than 800 mg/day.

SAMe should not be used with SSRIs or 5-hydroxytryptamine$_1$ (5-HT$_1$) agonists because of a potentially increased risk of serotonin syndrome. The use of SAMe during pregnancy or lactation should also be avoided because of inadequate safety data.

Summary of Clinical Evidence

Early osteoarthritis studies with SAMe that demonstrated positive results were of short duration and poor design, and they used injectable dosage forms or combinations of intravenous and oral therapies.[307] When SAMe was compared with NSAIDs or a cyclooxygenase-2 inhibitor, equivalent results in restoration of functionality and decreased pain were seen, although with a slower onset.[308] A meta-analysis concluded that SAMe's clinical effects may be small.[307] A more rigorously designed trial compared SAMe (1200 mg/day) with nabumetone.[309] Pain on a 40 mm visual analogue scale was significantly decreased to a similar extent in both the SAMe (−13 mm) and nabumetone (−15.7 mm) groups at 8 weeks. The WOMAC index also decreased similarly in the SAMe and nabumetone groups (−6.9 mm and −9.3 mm, respectively; p = 0.459). Changes occurred more slowly in the SAMe group; the WOMAC index change was only −3 mm at 4 weeks compared with −6.4 mm for nabumetone.

Clinical trials for depression have had methodologic problems, including small sample sizes. Two meta-analyses examining results with both intravenous and oral SAMe concluded that SAMe does have efficacy for depression that is possibly comparable to that of tricyclic antidepressants.[303] When SAMe was added in an open-label fashion to SSRIs or venlafaxine in patients who had not responded to antidepressant therapy alone, significant changes in outcome measures resulted.[310] The Hamilton-D-17 score decreased from 17.7 to 10 (p = 0.0001) and the Montgomery Asberg Depression Rating Scale from 23.2 to 13.9 (p = 0.0002).

Skin and Mucous Membrane

Lemon Balm

Lemon balm is derived from the plant *Melissa officinalis* L. of the family Lamiaceae (mint).

Therapeutic Uses

Lemon balm is commonly used as a topical cream for cold sores (herpes labialis) and orally for relaxation, agitation related to dementia, insomnia, or GI complaints.

Physiologic Activity

Lemon balm's effects may be a result of volatile oils extracted from the plant's leaves that are believed to have sedative, antioxidant, and antiviral effects.[311]

Dosage and Product Considerations

For cold sores, studies have used a cream or ointment containing 1% of a 70:1 lyophilized aqueous extract applied 2–5 times daily at first sign of symptoms and until all lesions heal. The treatment does not alter the ability to transmit the infection to others.

Safety Considerations

Hypersensitivity reactions and skin irritation have been associated with topical application. Theoretically, concomitant use of sedative herbs and drugs should not be combined with oral lemon balm. This natural product has been associated with thyroid inhibition and should be used cautiously in individuals with hypothyroid disease. The use of oral lemon balm should be avoided during pregnancy and lactation because of a lack of safety data.[311]

Summary of Clinical Evidence

The application of lemon balm cream has produced significant benefits by reducing the intensity of discomfort and the size and blistering of oral herpes lesions in clinical trials. Chronic use may delay the time to the next herpes flare-up.[312] Combination with valerian has shown efficacy in patients with anxiety and in children with sleep disorders.[313,314]

Tea Tree Oil

Tea tree oil is derived from leaves of the tree *Melaleuca alternifolia* (Maiden & Betche) Cheel from the family Myrtaceae. The tea tree is not related to the plant used to make black and green teas.

Therapeutic Uses

Tea tree oil has been used as a topical anti-infective agent.

Physiologic Activity

Tea tree oil has also demonstrated anti-inflammatory properties in decreasing tumor necrosis factor, interleukin-1, interleukin-8, interleukin-10, and prostaglandin E2.[315]

Dosage and Product Concerns

The oil is applied topically once or twice daily in concentrations of 0.4%–100%, depending on the condition and area of treatment. For acne, a 5% concentration is applied daily. For athlete's foot, tea tree oil cream 25%–50% is applied twice daily for 4 weeks. For fungal toenail infections, tea tree oil 100% has been used twice daily for 6 months.

Safety Considerations

Skin irritation may occur in sensitive patients, especially at higher concentrations. Although the oil can be used safely on oral mucosa, it should not be swallowed; ingesting small amounts may cause confusion, ataxia, and systemic contact dermatitis that resolves slowly.[315] Prepubertal gynecomastia occurred in three boys using topical tea tree and lavender oils and resolved upon discontinuation.[316]

Summary of Clinical Evidence

Randomized controlled trials using tea tree oil 5% body wash have demonstrated success in preventing colonization of *Staphylococcus aureus* and clearing methicillin-resistant *S. aureus* in hospitalized patients compared with standard regimens.[317,318] Nasal colonization was also evaluated with 10% tea tree cream, finding that 2% mupirocin was more effective.[318]

Tea tree oil may be effective for athlete's foot and other fungal infections of the skin, hair (dandruff), and nails.[319-321] For onychomycosis, tea tree oil was compared with clotrimazole 1% solution and after 6 months had similar culture and clinical resolutions. Tea tree oil has also been studied in fluconazole-resistant oral *Candida* infections occurring in patients with AIDS, with 60% of patients demonstrating full or partial resolution in an open-label trial.[322] In the treatment of mild-moderate acne, daily application of a tea tree oil gel 5% for 45 days significantly reduced the total acne lesion count and acne severity index compared with placebo.[323] Tea tree oil is an option for individuals who are not tolerating current therapies for the treatment of athlete's foot, onychomycosis, or acne.

Women's Health

Black Cohosh

Black cohosh is made from the dried rhizome and roots of *Cimicifuga racemosa* (L.) Nutt., formerly *Actaea racemosa*. It is a member of the Ranunculaceae (buttercup) family.

Therapeutic Uses

Black cohosh has been used to treat the symptoms of premenstrual syndrome, dysmenorrhea, menopause, and rheumatoid arthritis.

Physiologic Activity

The primary active components of black cohosh rhizomes are triterpene glycosides, including acetein, cimicifugoside, and 27-deoxyacetin. Isoflavones such as formononetin are often present, but they may be absent from commercial products. Other constituents include isoferulic and salicylic acids, tannins, resin, starch, and sugars.[324] Black cohosh extract may also act as a partial serotonin agonist.[325] Whether black cohosh has estrogenic activity is controversial; it probably does not exhibit estrogenic activity and has no effect on vaginal epithelium, endometrium, or hormone concentrations.[326]

Dosage and Product Considerations

Black cohosh, as a standardized extract, is usually taken as 40 mg daily in 1–2 doses. A common proprietary preparation is Remifemin. The extract is standardized to 1 mg of triterpene glycosides, calculated as 27-deoxyacetin, per 20 mg extract tablet.[327]

Safety Considerations

Adverse effects are mild and include GI complaints, headache, rash, and weight gain. Hepatitis, seizures, and cardiovascular disease have been reported in patients taking multiple herbal products including black cohosh, although causal relationship has not been established.[328] Due to case reports of acute hepatitis with black cohosh, the Dietary Supplement Information Expert Committee recommended a cautionary statement regarding potential hepatotoxicity be placed on product labels.[329] Further evaluations have suggested lack of product quality may have contributed, with the wrong plant being used.[330] The use of black cohosh for longer than 6 months is not recommended because of the lack of long-term safety studies. Data on drug interactions with black cohosh are limited, with the exception of possible additive effects with tamoxifen.[328] Data on concurrent use with estrogens or progestins are not available.[85] The use of black cohosh should be avoided during pregnancy and lactation because of its potential hormonal effects.

Summary of Clinical Evidence

Several clinical trials have evaluated black cohosh alone and combination products for menopausal symptoms, with mixed results. The largest and most recent systematic review of single-entity black cohosh included 16 randomized controlled trials with 2027 perimenopausal or postmenopausal women.[331] Efficacy was determined against placebo, hormone therapy, red clover, and fluoxetine. Analysis found the median dose of 40 mg per day of black cohosh for a mean of 23 weeks. For hot flushes and menopausal scores, no significant difference was noted between black cohosh and placebo; however, hormone therapy significantly reduced these variables compared with black cohosh (95% CI, 0.13–0.51).[331]

Multi-ingredient product comparisons with placebo, hormonal therapy, and fluoxetine lack standardized dosing and have poor methodologic quality or small differences compared with placebo, making it difficult to establish efficacy. Benefits from other constituents in multi-ingredient black cohosh products and SJW may be responsible for improvement in symptoms.[325] Combination

with SJW has demonstrated an impact on climacteric symptoms.[332] Positive results were reported in a meta-analysis, with substantial heterogeneity between studies; six of nine randomized placebo-controlled trials demonstrated a significant improvement of 26% in symptoms related to menopause.[333]

The safety and efficacy of black cohosh in women who have had breast cancer remains controversial. A systematic review in women with a history of breast cancer found inconclusive evidence to support safety and efficacy, although the product did not exert estrogenic effects.[334] The long-term effects on cardiovascular disease, osteoporosis, and breast cancer are unknown.

Chastetree Berry

Chastetree (*Vitex agnus-castus* L.), commonly referred to as vitex, is a member of the Verbenaceae family. The dried ripe fruits, or berries, and the leaves are the medicinally useful parts of the plant.

Therapeutic Uses

Chastetree berry has been used to treat symptoms of premenstrual syndrome, dysmenorrhea, mastalgia, and menopausal symptoms.

Physiologic Activity

The fruits contain essential oils, diterpines, iridoid glycosides, and flavonoids. Effects on menstrual regulation are likely due to the dopaminergic compounds diterpines, which are responsible for suppressing prolactin release by binding to the dopamine-2 receptor. Chastetree berry may have weak estrogenic activity.[335]

Dosage and Product Considerations

Clinical trials have used 20–40 mg of the extract daily. The standardization of chastetree berry has not been well established. It is available alone or in combination products.

Safety Considerations

GI complaints occur occasionally with use of chastetree berry. Other symptoms include dry mouth, headache, rashes, itching, acne, menstrual disorders, and agitation. The use of chastetree berry should be avoided during pregnancy because of potential effects on the uterus. Chastetree berry potentially may interact with dopaminergic antagonists and oral contraceptives, but these interactions have not been documented.[336]

Summary of Clinical Evidence

Clinical evidence for chastetree berry, in combination with other herbals, for menopausal symptoms is mixed. A randomized, double-blind, placebo-controlled parallel trial studied combination SJW (*Hypericum perforatum*) and chastetree berry administered twice daily over 16 weeks in 100 late perimenopausal and postmenopausal women. Symptoms did not differ between the groups regarding the primary end point of hot flushes.[337] A small subgroup analysis of 14 late perimenopausal women found significant improvement in premenstrual syndrome–like symptom scores.[338] Phyto-Female Complex, standardized extracts of black cohosh, dong quai, milk thistle, red clover, American ginseng, and chastetree berry, has been studied in 50 premenopausal and postmenopausal women in a randomized, placebo-controlled trial. Improvements in hot flushes, night sweats, and sleeping quality were reported, with no changes on vaginal ultrasonography, estradiol, follicle-stimulating hormone, liver enzymes, or thyroid-stimulating hormone.[339]

Chaste tree extract may be effective in other reproductive disorders such as premenstrual syndrome, premenstrual dysphoric disorder, and latent hyperprolactinemia. Methodologic quality is a barrier, with limited study sizes and variable treatment measures.[340] A systematic review suggested benefit in cyclic mastalgia, often related to latent hyperprolacteinemia, for at least three cycles.[341]

Evening Primrose Oil

Evening primrose (*Oenothera biennis* L.) is a member of the primrose family Onagraceae and is used for its high content of essential fatty acids. The seed oils of black currant (*Ribes nigrum* L.) and borage (*Borago officinalis* L.) are also used for similar purposes.

Therapeutic Uses

Evening primrose oil has been used for mastalgia, premenstrual syndrome, menopause, preeclampsia, diabetic neuropathy, chronic fatigue syndrome, and atopic dermatitis.

Physiologic Activity

The oil from evening primrose seeds consists of omega-6 essential fatty acids, primarily 65%–75% linoleic acid and 7%–10% gamma-linolenic acid. These components are thought to be responsible for anti-inflammatory activity.[342,343] The seed oil contains smaller amounts of palmitic, oleic, and stearic acids, as well as the steroids campesterol and beta-sitosterol.[343]

Dosage and Product Considerations

In clinical trials, daily dosages of evening primrose oil 2–4 grams have been used as a liquid or capsule. A standardized product, Efamol, a 1 gram capsule is comprised of 0.62 gram linoleic acid, 0.05 gram gamma-linolenic acid, and 0.062 gram oleic acid.[342]

Safety Considerations

Adverse effects include headache, nausea, diarrhea, and occasional abdominal pain. Evening primrose oil products may possess antiplatelet effects and should be used with caution in patients taking anticoagulants and antiplatelet agents or herbs. Seizures have been reported in people taking evening primrose oil; individuals taking anticonvulsants or medications to lower their seizure threshold should avoid its use.[85,87] Use of evening primrose oil for cervical ripening during labor may be associated with adverse pregnancy outcomes, including prolonged rupture of membranes and vacuum extraction.[343]

Summary of Clinical Evidence

Data on evening primrose oil for mastalgia and atopic dermatitis have been contradictory. A randomized pilot placebo-controlled study found improvement in cyclical mastalgia with 3 grams of evening primrose oil, taken alone or in combination with vitamin E 1200 IU over 6 months.[344] A large double-blind, randomized, placebo-controlled trial comparing Efamast with or without antioxidant vitamins found no significant changes

in reported pain in patients with moderate-severe mastalgia. A large placebo effect was noted, with 40% of subjects reporting improvement without therapy.[345]

A Cochrane review of oral evening primrose oil and borage oil concluded neither was effective for the treatment of atopic eczema. Studies analyzed found no improvement in global eczema symptoms or visual analogue scales.[346] Another meta-analysis of 26 randomized, placebo-controlled trials studying Efamol for use in atopic dermatitis demonstrated promising outcomes regarding itch/pruritus, crusting, edema, and erythema in 4–8 weeks of treatment. Comparisons have not been made to current therapies, and evening primrose oil may not be as effective as high-potency topical steroids.[347]

Fenugreek

Fenugreek (*Trigonalla foenum-graecum*) has a long history of use as a spice and a medicine in India, China, and Northern Africa. Both leaves and seeds may have medicinal properties.[348]

Therapeutic Uses

Fenugreek has been used for diabetes, hyperlipidemia, and stimulation of breast milk production.[348]

Physiologic Activity

An active constituent of fenugreek, 4-hydroxyisoleucine, may contribute to the hypoglycemic effects by stimulating glucose-induced insulin release and reducing insulin resistance. Saponins converted to saponogenins in the GI tract may decrease cholesterol levels through activation of biliary cholesterol secretion. Fenugreek seeds are high in fiber, possibly delaying glucose absorption or binding cholesterol.[348] Lactation effects may be the result of increased sweat production impacting the milk duct or by phytoestrogens and diosgenin found in fenugreek.[146]

Dosage and Product Considerations

Dosages have varied, with fenugreek seed powder capsules 2.5 grams twice daily or seed powder 25 grams daily in 2 divided doses used in studies. Defatted seeds have also been used at 100 grams daily in 2 equally divided doses. Fenugreek can also be administered in a tea.[349] For increasing milk supply, 2–3 capsules (580–610 mg per capsule) can be administered 3–4 times per day.[146]

Safety Considerations

Fenugreek is generally safe when used in meal preparation. When fenugreek is consumed, urine, sweat, and breast milk have been noted to smell like maple syrup, which is caused by sotolone excretion. This effect also occurs in breast-feeding infants, which has led to mistaken cases of maple syrup urine disease. Patients with an allergy to chickpeas should avoid fenugreek because of possible cross-reactivity; inhalation of the powder has resulted in bronchospasm. Fenugreek should be avoided during pregnancy because of potential oxytocic and uterine stimulant effects. Hypoglycemia or hypokalemia may result from use. The high-fiber content can bind with drugs and decrease absorption.[348] Fenugreek may increase risk of bleeding in patients taking warfarin.[87]

Summary of Clinical Evidence

Although fenugreek is promoted to stimulate production of breast milk, evidence is limited.[146] A small trial of immediate post-partum mothers and nursing newborns compared a treatment group receiving a tea containing fenugreek with placebo and control groups. Infants in the fenugreek group had significantly less weight loss and regained birth weight earlier, and mothers had higher breast milk volume at 3 days compared with placebo and control groups.[350] Other components present in the tea may have contributed to findings as well.

Phytoestrogens

Phytoestrogens are found in many different plants; supplements have been derived primarily from soy (*Glycine max* [L.] Merrill) and red clover (*Trifolium pratense* L.).

Therapeutic Uses

Phytoestrogens have been used mainly for symptoms associated with menopause and related bone health. Phytoestrogens may also have a role in preventing prostate cancer.

Physiologic Activity

Soy-based phytoestrogens may include isoflavones such as genistein, daidzein, and glycitein. Red clover–based products may include biochanin, genistein, daidzein, and formononetin. These compounds have effects including estrogenic, antiestrogenic, antioxidant, and anticancer activity.

Dosage and Product Considerations

A recommended dosage of phytoestrogen has not been established. Phytoestrogen products contain varying amounts and types of isoflavones. Products derived from soy and red clover sources may have different effects. The benefits from soy are primarily from dietary sources, not from supplements. Soy supplements meeting USP standards are available.

Safety Considerations

Phytoestrogen products derived from soy or red clover are well tolerated. GI complaints and allergic reactions may occur. The long-term safety of phytoestrogens is not established, especially with respect to the risk of estrogen-dependent cancers and thromboembolic disease. The safety of phytoestrogen supplements in women with hormone-sensitive cancers is unknown, and their use should be avoided.[85] Red clover may increase the risk of bleeding, especially if anticoagulants are taken concomitantly, although clear evidence of this interaction is lacking.[87]

Summary of Clinical Evidence

Purported benefits of phytoestrogens, especially soy-based products, are derived from population-based observational studies of dietary patterns. It is simplistic to think that the lifetime risk of any given disease is related solely to the presence or absence of one dietary component such as isoflavones. The phytoestrogen content in foods, especially of the biologically active isoflavones, varies significantly even in soy foods, let alone supplements.

The most common use of phytoestrogens is for managing vasomotor symptoms. Several meta-analyses and systematic reviews of randomized controlled trials have been conducted to evaluate the effectiveness of phytoestrogens, without finding strong evidence to support their usage. Variations in study design, including dosage and phytoestrogen content, makes it difficult to establish clear benefit. Overall safety is promising because endometrial, uterine, and breast cancer risk does not appear to be increased. Dietary soy intake may even be associated with a decrease in endometrial or uterine cancers; however, it should be used with caution until conclusive data support this finding.[351]

The effect of soy isoflavones on the risk of osteoporosis has yielded mixed findings. A double-blind, placebo-controlled study randomized 389 postmenopausal women with osteopenia to receive placebo or genistein 54 mg/day. Significant changes were observed in the anteroposterior lumbar spine, the femoral neck, and urinary markers, with no documented changes in endometrial thickness.[352] A follow-up study at 3 years continued to show benefit for bone loss, with no significant changes in breast health.[353] Soy isoflavones 120 mg/day did not demonstrate a benefit on lumbar spine, total proximal femur, and total body bone mineral density in 432 postmenopausal women without osteoporosis in a double-blind, placebo-controlled trial. Improvement was found only at the femoral neck.[354] Another trial of fixed combination genistein and diadzein compared with placebo found no difference in bone mineral density of the lumbar spine or femur after 2 years of use in Taiwanese postmenopausal women.[355]

The ingestion of at least 25 grams of soy protein daily as part of a diet low in saturated fat and cholesterol may reduce the risk of coronary heart disease. The effect of phytoestrogen dietary supplements on the risk of myocardial infarction is unclear.[356]

Epidemiologic research has indicated consumption of soy products has a role in decreasing breast cancer risk; however, concerns exist that estrogenic activity will increase recurrence. The potential effect likely will depend on the specific isoflavone, timing of exposure, genetic factors, and whether estrogen receptors are positive or negative for cancer. Dietary consumption of soy similar to that in Asian populations does not appear to increase cancer recurrence, nor does it interact with tamoxifen or anastrozole.[357] Epidemiologic data analyzed in a meta-analysis suggest that soy food consumption may play a role in reducing prostate cancer risk.[358]

Assessment of Natural Product Use: A Case-Based Approach

The health care provider should determine the patient's reasons for purchasing a natural product. The appropriateness of supplements must be determined and is essential for a child, a pregnant woman, or an older adult. If a medical condition is being treated and use of a supplement is appropriate, the patient should be encouraged to involve the health care provider in the use of the supplement. Information about possible allergies to plant materials, current drug therapy, and comorbid conditions will identify possible contraindications. For patients who ask about weight loss supplements, the provider can use the information in the box A Word about Weight-Loss Products to counsel them on the safest products to use.

If self-treatment with a natural product is appropriate, the provider should review the length of therapy and recommended dosages with the patient. The efficacy of different dosage forms should also be explained. Cases 51–1 and 51–2 provide examples of assessment of patients who are considering use of a natural product.

a word about
Weight-Loss Products

Hoodia

Hoodia gordonii, a succulent plant found in the Kalahari Desert, is used by the Khoi-San to decrease appetite on long journeys.[359] Animal studies of the P57 glycoside suggest hoodia may affect the hypothalamus to increase satiety and may also affect oral and GI bitter receptors to affect food intake.[359] Drug development of P57 was discontinued because of lack of efficacy and safety concerns over hepatic effects. One human trial with rigorous design, despite a short duration of 15 days, found no significant difference from placebo on caloric intake or weight change but found definite differences in adverse effects.[360] South Africa protects endangered *Hoodia* species with special permits required to grow or harvest plants, so production is very low. One study found 11 of 13 hoodia supplements to contain no hoodia glycosides.[359] Hoodia should be avoided given the lack of efficacy and the potential for adverse effects.

Chitosan

Chitosan is claimed to aid weight loss by blocking intestinal fat absorption. A Cochrane review concluded benefits were slight and likely of no clinical significance.[361] A recent well-designed study combined low-molecular-weight chitosan with a mild exercise program (1 hour twice weekly) and noted clinically relevant weight loss and lipid changes compared with the placebo and exercise groups.[362] Whether the available chitosan supplements are helpful is unanswered, but, fortunately, adverse effects are limited to slight GI effects and cross-reactivity with shellfish allergy. Patients using chitosan should take a multivitamin to prevent deficiencies of fat-soluble vitamins and take any medications at least 2 hours apart from a dose of chitosan.

Stimulants and "Fat Burners"

After FDA banned ephedrine alkaloids from weight-loss supplements, some manufacturers claimed their supplements were "ephedra free" and simply substituted other sources of the ephedrine alkaloids, such as heartleaf and country mallow. Guarana, yerba maté, cola nut, or other caffeine sources are common in these supplements, as is bitter orange (*Citrus aurantium*), a source of synephrine. Bitter orange has been associated with cardiovascular events and ischemic colitis in case reports, although research has found no cardiovascular effects.[363–365] Even though stimulants may provide a slight weight loss, safety issues outweigh the small benefits.

Raspberry Ketone

4-4(hydroxyphenyl)butan-2-one is similar to synephrine in structure. Mechanistic effects such as increased adiponectin secretion in fat cells seem promising, but two animal studies had contradictory results for weight loss.[366] Raspberry ketone cannot be recommended because human studies and information on adverse effects are lacking.

Hydroxycitric Acid

Hydroxycitric acid from the *Garcinia cambogia* plant has been shown in animals to influence satiety through hepatic glucoreceptors, to increase serotonin to affect appetite, and to aid in regulation of leptin and insulin.[367] Short-term human trials have had contradictory results and even positive studies have noted only small benefits compared with placebo.[367] Adverse effects reported in trials have been mild and uncommon. The Hydroxycut brand of weight loss products was reformulated after case reports of hepatotoxicity, although hydroxycitric acid has not been determined to be the actual cause.[367] Until more is known about this possible adverse effect, hydroxycitric acid cannot be recommended; patients should be steered toward other options or closely monitored if they choose to use this supplement.

case
51-1

Relevant Evaluation Criteria	Scenario/Model Outcome
Information Gathering	

1. Gather essential information about the patient's symptoms and medical history, including:

   a. description of symptom(s) (i.e., nature, onset, duration, severity, associated symptoms)

   The patient approaches the pharmacy counter in the electric scooter that she uses occasionally instead of her cane. She says, "My left knee has been extra bad this week." The patient exhibits multiple misshapen joints; you can see that her left knee is more swollen than the right and is also slightly reddened.

   b. description of any factors that seem to precipitate, exacerbate, and/or relieve the patient's symptom(s)

   The patient has severe rheumatoid arthritis affecting all joints. She is under the care of a rheumatologist and follows a daily exercise regimen to preserve mobility and also does water exercise at the local community center several times per week. Her disease state waxes and wanes over time; colder weather and changes in barometric pressure always cause her increased pain and stiffness.

   c. description of the patient's efforts to relieve the symptoms

   "My regular medicines aren't helping—I feel so bad and I really want to try something else." She holds up a couple of combination glucosamine products and adds, "I have two friends who tell me all the time that these work for their arthritis. Which one would be better for me? I know you told me before that I couldn't take glucosamine, but this one says it's OK for people who are allergic to shellfish."

   d. patient's identity

   Gwendolyn Gisingham

case
51–1 | continued

Relevant Evaluation Criteria	Scenario/Model Outcome
e. age, sex, height, and weight	54 years old, female, 5 ft 6 in., 138 lb
f. patient's occupation	Schoolteacher, retired for 3 years because of disability
g. patient's dietary habits	Eats a very healthy diet that is high in vegetables, fruits, whole grains, and small portions of low-fat meats.
h. patient's sleep habits	Occasional insomnia when pain is severe.
i. concurrent medical conditions, prescription and nonprescription medications, and dietary supplements	Hypothyroidism: levothyroxine; rheumatoid arthritis: methotrexate; mild hypertension: hydroxychloroquine, lisinopril; perennial allergic rhinitis: fexofenadine and fluticasone nasal spray daily; daily multivitamin/mineral, calcium + vitamin D (500 mg/200 IU) twice daily, and 1 gram of enteric-coated fish oil daily. She carries an epinephrine auto injector for allergic reactions and has a prescription for generic Percocet for severe rheumatoid arthritis exacerbations, although she uses it only rarely because of concerns of addiction.
j. allergies	She has many environmental allergies and is highly allergic to bee stings, with severe reactions to strawberries and shellfish as well.
k. history of other adverse reactions to medications	None

Assessment and Triage

2. Differentiate patient's signs/symptoms and correctly identify the patient's primary problem(s).	Hypothyroidism, controlled; hypertension, controlled; perennial allergic rhinitis, treated; exacerbation of rheumatoid arthritis; lack of knowledge regarding dietary supplements
3. Identify exclusions for self-treatment.	(1) The patient's symptoms may need additional evaluation and diagnosis. (2) The patient has contraindications to therapies in which she is interested.
4. Formulate a comprehensive list of therapeutic alternatives for the primary problem to determine if triage to a health care provider is required, and share this information with the patient or caregiver.	Options include: (1) Continue current prescription and exercise therapy, and refer patient to rheumatologist for further evaluation. (2) Continue current prescription and exercise therapy, and refer patient to rheumatologist for further evaluation. Suggest increasing fish oil dose as an alternative to the products she is interested in. (3) Continue current exercise therapy, and refer patient to rheumatologist for further evaluation. Encourage patient to utilize pain medication as prescribed during episodes of increased pain. (4) Take no action.

Plan

5. Select an optimal therapeutic alternative to address the patient's problem, taking into account patient preferences.	The patient should make an appointment with the rheumatologist right away; use the generic Percocet to help manage the pain; continue the exercise as long as it is helping to decrease the stiffness and/or pain. If movement is making the left knee worse, it may be better to try rest instead of medicating until she can see her primary care provider.
6. Describe the recommended therapeutic approach to the patient or caregiver.	"A visit to the rheumatologist is needed to determine if you are simply having a worsening of the rheumatoid arthritis or if a different problem, such as infection, is developing and needs to be treated." "Patients who use pain medication as prescribed for occasional or short-term use are extremely unlikely to become addicted. Pain can elevate blood pressure, so it's important for your hypertension to keep pain under control."

case
51-1 *continued*

Relevant Evaluation Criteria	Scenario/Model Outcome
7. Explain to the patient or caregiver the rationale for selecting the recommended therapeutic approach from the considered therapeutic alternatives.	"Your rheumatoid arthritis may simply be getting worse, but because your increased pain and swelling are localized to one knee, it could mean that something else is going on. Your current rheumatoid arthritis medicines might stay the same or be changed."
	"The arthritis products that your neighbors are recommending are for use in osteoarthritis. They have not been shown to have any benefit for rheumatoid arthritis, which has a different cause. They also take a very long time to take effect, and you are having pain now. Even though some glucosamine products do seem to be safe for use by patients with shellfish allergy, their use is recommended only when the reaction is fairly mild, such as a mild rash. Your reaction is severe and could be life threatening. Manufacturers can change the source of their products at any time. One batch might be safe to take, but the next one might contain shellfish allergen and trigger a reaction."

Patient Education

8. When recommending self-care with nonprescription medications and/or nondrug therapy, convey accurate information to the patient or caregiver.	Criterion does not apply in this case.
Solicit follow-up questions from the patient or caregiver.	"Aren't there any supplements I can take to help my rheumatoid arthritis?"
Answer the patient's or caregiver's questions.	"Yes, if you are still interested in a supplement after seeing the doctor and it turns out that your rheumatoid arthritis is worse, we could talk about increasing the dose of your fish oil. High doses of fish oil have been shown to have some benefit on rheumatoid arthritis symptoms."

Evaluation of Patient Outcome

9. Assess patient outcome.	"Call me after you have seen the doctor, and we can talk more about the possibility of using fish oil for your arthritis."

case
51-2

Relevant Evaluation Criteria	Scenario/Model Outcome

Information Gathering

1. Gather essential information about the patient's symptoms and medical history, including:	
a. description of symptom(s) (i.e., nature, onset, duration, severity, associated symptoms)	Patient is inquiring about using a "natural" treatment for prevention of migraines. She is holding individual bottles of feverfew and butterbur. She reports developing migraines 2–3 times per month. She currently has no symptoms.
b. description of any factors that seem to precipitate, exacerbate, and/or relieve the patient's symptom(s)	Her migraines usually present unilaterally with fatigue, nausea, and sensitivity to light. They occur mainly when the patient is fatigued or stressed or prior to her menstrual period.
c. description of the patient's efforts to relieve the symptoms	The patient has taken divalproex, propranolol, and topiramate for prevention, but she discontinued their use because of adverse events. She would like something "more natural."
d. patient's identity	Emme Toce
e. age, sex, height, and weight	36 years old, female, 5 ft 5 in., 150 lb
f. patient's occupation	Nurse coordinator for medical practice
g. patient's dietary habits	Healthy diet; tries to avoid migraine triggers, such as caffeine and alcohol.

case
51–2   continued

Relevant Evaluation Criteria	Scenario/Model Outcome
h. patient's sleep habits	Approximately 6 hours of sleep per night
i. concurrent medical conditions, prescription and non-prescription medications, and dietary supplements	Acute migraine: sumatriptan 50 mg as needed, ibuprofen 400 mg every 4–6 hours as needed for migraine pain; vitamin B_2 daily for migraine prevention (she read it may help).
j. allergies	NKDA
k. history of other adverse reactions to medications	Topiramate: parasthesias, memory loss; divalproex: weight gain, hair loss; propranolol: weight gain, fatigue

Assessment and Triage

2. Differentiate patient's signs/symptoms and correctly identify the patient's primary problem(s).

Recurrent migraines, approximately 2–3 per month. Symptoms are not severe or intractable.

3. Identify exclusions for self-treatment.

No exclusions for self-treatment at this time. She is under medical care for migraines.

4. Formulate a comprehensive list of therapeutic alternatives for the primary problem to determine if triage to a medical provider is required, and share this information with the patient or caregiver.

Options include:

(1) Refer Emme to a neurologist to select another medication for prevention of migraines.

(2) Educate Emme on nonpharmacologic methods to prevent migraines.

(3) Assist in selecting a natural product for prevention of migraines.

(4) Take no action.

Plan

5. Select an optimal therapeutic alternative to address the patient's problem, taking into account patient preferences.

The patient prefers to use feverfew or butterbur to prevent migraines. Confirm that patient does not have an allergy to ragweed (Asteraceae/Compositae family).

6. Describe the recommended therapeutic approach to the patient or caregiver.

"A trial basis of butterbur could be considered in consultation with the health care provider who treats your migraines."

7. Explain to the patient or caregiver the rationale for selecting the recommended therapeutic approach from the considered therapeutic alternatives.

"Evidence based on two well-designed trials suggests that butterbur is effective in preventing migraines. Data to support the effectiveness of feverfew are not as strong. Natural product options for prevention of this condition are limited. Long-term data on safety and efficacy are available for prescription medications."

Patient Education

8. When recommending self-care with nonprescription medications and/or nondrug therapy, convey accurate information to the patient or caregiver:

a. appropriate dose and frequency of administration

"Take 50–75 mg twice per day (petasin 7.5 mg and isopetasin 7.5 mg per 50 mg tablet or capsule)."

b. maximum number of days the therapy should be employed

"Long-term data do not exist for efficacy and safety. Studies support use for 12–16 weeks, although some monographs support use for 4–6 months, then taper off."

c. product administration procedures

"For prevention of migraine headaches, select a high-quality product that does not contain pyrrolizidine alkaloids (PAs)."

d. expected time to onset of relief

"This product is for prevention of migraines."

e. degree of relief that can be reasonably expected

"Recurrence of migraines will be reduced."

f. most common adverse effects

"Minor GI upset, possible dermatologic changes, or dizziness are the most common adverse effects."

g. adverse effects that warrant medical intervention should they occur

"The product is generally well tolerated. See your provider if you suspect liver damage (yellowing of skin, abdominal pain) from the presence of PA."

h. patient options in the event that condition worsens or persists

"If recurrent migraines continue, seek your provider's guidance on prescription options to prevent them."

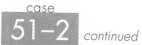

case *continued*

Relevant Evaluation Criteria	Scenario/Model Outcome
i. product storage requirements	"Keep product in an appropriate storage area away from excessive heat and moisture and out of reach of children and pets."
j. specific nondrug measures	"Nonpharmacologic measures to help prevent migraines include avoiding triggers, maintaining regular sleep and eating patterns, and managing stress. Relax in a quiet, dark room when onset occurs. A cool pack or ice pack placed on the forehead or temples may be useful."
Solicit follow-up questions from the patient or caregiver.	"Can I use butterbur to treat a migraine?"
Answer the patient's or caregiver's questions.	"No. Evidence does not support use for an acute migraine. Continue to use medications currently listed for acute migraine."

Evaluation of Patient Outcome

9. Assess patient outcome.	"Please discuss using this product with your doctor prior to its use. Call me after a few weeks to tell me how you are tolerating butterbur and whether you are having fewer migraines."

Key: GI = Gastrointestinal; NKA = no known drug allergies.

REFERENCES

1. Hume AL, Strong KM. Botanical medicines. In: Berardi RR, DeSimone EM, Newton GD, et al, eds. *Handbook of Nonprescription Drugs*. 15th ed. Washington, DC: American Pharmaceutical Association; 2006.

2. Bonakdar RA, Guarneri E. Coenzyme Q10. *Am Fam Phys*. 2005;72: 1065–70.

3. Rundek T, Naini A, Sacco R, et al. Atorvastatin decreases the coenzyme Q10 level in the blood of patients at risk for cardiovascular disease and stroke. *Arch Neurol*. 2004;61:889–92.

4. Laaksonen R, Jokelainen K, Sahi T, et al. Decreases in serum ubiquinone concentrations do not result in reduced levels in muscle tissue during short-term simvastatin treatment in humans. *Clin Pharmacol Ther*. 1995;57:62–6.

5. Toyama K, Sugiyama S, Oka H, et al. Rosuvastatin combined with regular exercise preserves coenzyme Q10 levels associated with a significant increase in high-density lipoprotein cholesterol in patients with coronary artery disease. *Atherosclerosis*. 2011;217:158–64.

6. Turunen M, Olsson J, Dallner G. Metabolism and function of coenzyme Q. *Biochim Biophys Acta*. 2004;1660:171–90.

7. Engelsen J. Effect of coenzyme Q10 and *Ginkgo biloba* on warfarin dosage in stable, long-term warfarin treated outpatients. A randomized, double-blind, placebo-crossover trial. *Thromb Haemost*. 2002;87:1075–6.

8. Lund EL, Quistorff B, Span-Thomsen M, et al. Effect of radiation therapy on small-cell lung cancer is reduced by ubiquinone intake. *Folia Microbiol*. 1998;43:505–6.

9. Mukhopadhyay P, Horvath B, Zsengeller Z, et al. Mitochondrial-targeted antioxidants represent a promising approach for prevention of cisplatin-induced nephropathy. *Free Rad Biol Med*. 2012;52:497–506.

10. Gao L, Mao Q, Cao J, et al. Effects of coenzyme Q10 on vascular endothelial function in humans: a meta-analysis of randomized controlled trials. *Atherosclerosis*. 2012;221:311–6.

11. Okello E, Jiang X, Mohamed S, et al. Combined statin/coenzyme Q10 as adjunctive treatment of chronic heart failure. *Med Hypoth*. 2009; 73:306–8.

12. Khatta M, Alexander B, Krichten C, et al. The effect of coenzyme Q10 in patients with congestive heart failure. *Ann Intern Med*. 2000; 132:636–40.

13. Belardinelli R, Mucaj A, Lacalaprice F, et al. Coenzyme Q10 and exercise training in chronic heart failure. *Eur Heart J*. 2006;27:2675–81.

14. Kocharian A, Shabanian R, Rafiei-Khorgami M, et al. Coenzyme Q10 improves diastolic function in children with idiopathic cardiomyopathy. *Cardiol Young*. 2009;19:501–6.

15. Singh RB, Neki NS, Kartikey K, et al. Effect of coenzyme Q10 on risk of atherosclerosis in patients with recent myocardial infarction. *Mol Cell Biochem*. 2003;246:75–82.

16. Langsjoen PH, Langsjoen JO, Langsjoen AM, et al. Treatment of statin adverse effects with supplemental coenzyme Q10 and statin drug discontinuation. *Biofactors*. 2005;25:147–52.

17. Deichmann RE, Lavie CJ, Dornelles AC. Impact of coenzyme Q-10 on parameters of cardiorespiratory fitness and muscle performance in older athletes taking statins. *Physician Sportsmed*. 2012;40:88–95.

18. Bookstaver DA, Burkhalter NA, Hatzigeorgiou C. Effect of coenzyme Q10 supplementation on statin-induced myalgias. *Am J Cardiol*. 2012;110:526–9.

19. Ruaño G, Windemuth A, Wu, AHB, et al. Mechanisms of stain-induced myalgia assessed by physiogenomic associations. *Atherosclerosis*. 2011;218:451–6.

20. Young JM, Florkowski CM, Molyneux SL, et al. A randomized, double-blind, placebo-controlled crossover study of coenzyme Q10 therapy in hypertensive patients with the metabolic syndrome. *Am J Hypertens*. 2012; 25:261–70.

21. Ho MJ, Bellusci A, Wright JM. Blood pressure lowering efficacy of coenzyme Q10 for primary hypertension. *Cochrane Database Syst Rev*. 2009;4:CD007435. doi: 10.1002/14651858.CD007435.pub2. Accessed at http://www.thecochranelibrary.com/view/0/index.html.

22. Stabler SN, Tejani AM, Huynh F, Fowkes C. Garlic for the prevention of cardiovascular morbidity and mortality in hypertensive patients. *Cochrane Database Syst Rev*. 2012;8:CD007653. doi: 10.1002/14651858. CD007653.pub2. Accessed at http://www.thecochranelibrary.com/view/0/index.html.

23. Lawson LD, Gardener CD. Composition, stability and bioavailability of garlic products being used in a clinical trial. *J Agric Food Chem*. 2005; 53(16):6254–61.

24. Dhawan V, Jain S. Garlic supplementation prevents oxidative DNA damage in essential hypertension. *Mol Cell Biochem*. 2005;275:85–94.

25. Ciocon JO, Ciocon DG, Galindo DJ. Dietary supplements in primary care. Botanicals can affect surgical outcomes and follow-up. *Geriatrics*. 2004;59:20–4.

26. Boullata J. Natural health product interactions with medication. *Nutr Clin Pract*. 2005;20:33–51.

27. Scharbert G, Kalb ML, Duris M, et al. Garlic at dietary doses does not impair platelet function. *Anesth Analg*. 2007;105:1214–8.

28. Markowitz JS, Devane CL, Chavin KD, et al. Effects of garlic (*Allium sativum* L.) supplementation on cytochrome P450 2D6 and 3A4 activity in healthy volunteers. *Clin Pharmacol Ther*. 2003;74:170–7.

29. Cox MC, Low J, Lee J, et al. Influence of garlic (*Allium sativum*) on the pharmacokinetics of docetaxel. *Clin Cancer Res.* 2006;12:4636–40.

30. Alder R, Lookinland S, Berry JA, et al. A systemic review of the effectiveness of garlic as an anti-hyperlipidemic agent. *J Am Acad Nurse Pract.* 2003;15:120–9.

31. Reinhart KM, Talati R, White CM, et al. The impact of garlic on lipid parameters: a systematic review and meta-analysis. *Nutr Res Rev.* 2009; 22:39–48.

32. Sobenin IA, Pryanishnikov VV, Kunnova LM, et al. The effect of timed-released garlic powder tablets on multifunctional cardiovascular risk in patients with coronary artery disease. *Lipids Health Dis.* 2010;9:119.

33. Ried K, Frank OR, Stocks NP, et al. Effect of garlic on blood pressure: a systematic review and meta-analysis. *BMC Cardiovasc Disorders.* 2008;8:13.

34. Ried K, Frank OR, Stocks NP. Aged garlic extract lowers blood pressure in patients with treated but uncontrolled hypertension: a randomized controlled trial. *Maturitas.* 2010;67:144–50.

35. Adkins Y, Kelley DS. Mechanisms underlying the cardioprotective effects of omega-3 polyunsaturated fatty acids. *J Nutr Biochem.* 2010; 21:781–92.

36. Siriwardhana N, Kalupahana NS, Moustaid-Moussa N. Health benefits of n-3 polyunsaturated fatty acids: eicosapentaenoic acid and docosahexaenoic acid. *Adv Food Nutr Res.* 2012;65:211–22.

37. Smutna M, Kruzikova K, Marsalek P, et al. Fish oil and cod liver as safe and healthy food supplements. *Neuroendocrinol Let.* 2009;30(suppl 1):156–62.

38. Melanson SF, Lewandrowski EL, Flood JG, et al. Measurement of organochlorines in commercial over-the-counter fish oil preparations: implications for dietary and therapeutic recommendations for omega-3 fatty acids and a review of the literature. *Arch Pathol Lab Med.* 2005;129:74–7.

39. de Leiris J, de Lorgeril M, Boucher F. Fish oil and heart health. *J Cardiovasc Pharmacol.* 2009;54:378–84.

40. Brasky TM, Darke AK, Song, X, et al. Plasma phospholipid fatty acids and prostate cancer risk in the SELECT Trial. *J Natl Canc Inst.* 2013;105:1132–41.

41. Heinze VM, Actis AB. Dietary conjugated linoleic acid and long-chain n-3 fatty acids in mammary and prostate cancer protection: a review. *Int J Food Sci Nutr.* 2012;63:66–78.

42. Hartweg J, Farmer AJ, Perera R, et al. Meta-analysis of the effects of n-3 polyunsaturated fatty acids on lipoproteins and other emerging lipid cardiovascular risk markers in patients with type 2 diabetes. *Diabetologia.* 2007;50:1593–602.

43. Eslick GD, Howe PRC, Smith C, et al. Benefits of fish oil supplementation in hyperlipidemia: a systematic review and meta-analysis. *Int J Cardiol.* 2009;136:4–16.

44. Lewis A, Lookinland S, Beckstrand RL, et al. Treatment of hypertriglyceridemia with omega-3 fatty acids: a systematic review. *J Am Acad Nurse Pract.* 2004;16:384–95.

45. GISSI-Prevenzione Investigators. Dietary supplementation with n-3 polyunsaturated fatty acids and vitamin E after myocardial infarction: results of the GISSI-Prevenzione trial. *Lancet.* 1999;354:447–55.

46. Wang C, Harris WS, Chung M, et al. n-3 Fatty acids from fish or fish oil supplements, but not alpha-linolenic acid, benefit cardiovascular disease outcomes in primary- and secondary-prevention studies: a systematic review. *Am J Clin Nutr.* 2006;84:5–17.

47. The Risk and Prevention Study Collaborative Group. n-3 fatty acids in patients with multiple cardiovascular risk factors. *N Engl J Med.* 2012; 368:1800–8.

48. Eussen SRBM, Geleijnse JM, Giltay EJ, et al. Effects of *n*-3 fatty acids on major cardiovascular events in stain users and non-users with a history of myocardial infarction. *Eur Heart J.* 2012;33:1582–88.

49. Ebrahimi M, Ghayour-Mobarhan M, Rezaiean S, et al. Omega-3 fatty acid supplements improve the cardiovascular risk profile of subjects with metabolic syndrome, including markers of inflammation and auto-immunity. *Acta Cardiol.* 2009;64:321–7.

50. Manson JE, Bassuk SS, Lee IM, et al. The VITamin D and OmegA-3 trial (VITAL): rationale and design of a large randomized controlled trial of vitamin D and marine omega-3 fatty acid supplements for the primary prevention of cancer and cardiovascular disease. *Contemp Clin Trials.* 2012;33:159–71.

51. American Heart Association. Fish 101. Accessed at http://www.heart.org/HEARTORG/GettingHealthy/NutritionCenter/Fish-101_UCM_305986_Article.jsp, September 28, 2013.

52. Ma K-Y, Zhang Z-S, Zhao S-X, et al. Red yeast rice increases excretion of bile acids in hamsters. *Biomed Environment Sci.* 2009;22:269–77.

53. Gordon RY, Cooperman T, Obermeyer W, Becker DJ. Marked variability of monacolin levels in commercial red yeast rice products. *Arch Int Med.* 2010;170:1722–7.

54. Kazmin A, Garcia-Bournissen F, Koren G. Risks of statin use during pregnancy: a systematic review. *J Obstet Gynaecol Can.* 2007;29:906–8.

55. Patakova P. Monascus secondary metabolites: production and biological activity. *J Indust Microbiol Biotech.* 2013;40:169–81.

56. Venero CV, Venero JV, Wortham DC, et al. Lipid-lowering efficacy of red yeast rice in a population intolerant to statins. *Am J Cardiol.* 2010;105:664–6.

57. Halbert SC, French B, Gordon RY, et al. Tolerability of red yeast rice (2,400 mg twice daily) versus pravastatin (20 mg twice daily) in patients with previous statin intolerance. *Am J Cardiol.* 2010;105:198–204.

58. Becker DJ, Gordon RY, Halbert SC, et al. Red yeast rice for dyslipidemia in statin-intolerant patients. *Ann Intern Med.* 2009;150:830–9.

59. Liu J, Zhang J, Shi Y, et al. Chinese red yeast rice (*Monascus purpureus*) for primary hyperlipidemia: a meta-analysis of randomized controlled trials. *Chin Med.* 2006;1:4.

60. Huang J Frohlich J, Ignaszewski AP. The impact of dietary changes and dietary supplements on lipid profile. *Can J Cardiol.* 2011;27:488–505.

61. Zamora-Ros R, Urpi-Sarda M, Lamuela-Raventós RM, et al. High urinary levels of resveratrol metabolites are associated with a reduction in the prevalence of cardiovascular risk factors in high-risk patients. *Pharmacol Res.* 2012;65:315–20.

62. Nunes T, Almeida L, Rocha J-F, et al. Pharmacokinetics of *trans*-resveratrol following repeated administration in healthy elderly and young subjects. *J Clin Pharmacol.* 2009;49:1477–82.

63. Magyar K, Halmosi R, Palfi A, et al. Cardioprotection by resveratrol: a human clinical trial in patients with stable coronary artery disease. *Clin Hemorheol Microcirc.* 2012;50:179–87.

64. Brasnyó P, Molnár GA, Mohás M, et al. Resveratrol improves insulin sensitivity, reduces oxidative stress and activates the Akt pathway in type 2 diabetic patients. *Brit J Nutr.* 2011;106:383–9.

65. Lekakis J, Rallidis LS, Andreadou I, et al. Polyphenolic compounds from red grapes acutely improve endothelial function in patients with coronary heart disease. *Eur J Cardiovasc Prevent Rehab.* 2005; 12:596–600.

66. Almeida L, Vaz-da-Silva M, Falcão A, et al. Pharmacokinetic and safety profile of trans-resveratrol in a rising multiple-dose study in healthy volunteers. *Mol Nutr Food Res.* 2009;53(suppl 1):S7–15.

67. Tomé-Carneiro J, Gonzálvez M, Larrosa M, et al. One-year consumption of a grape nutraceutical containing resveratrol improves the inflammatory and fibrinolytic status of patients in primary prevention of cardiovascular disease. *Am J Cardiol.* 2012;110:356–63.

68. Sutherland A, Sweet BV. Butterbur: an alternative therapy for migraine prevention. *Am J Health Syst Pharm.* 2010;67:705–11.

69. Schapowal A. Randomised controlled trial of butterbur and cetirizine for treating seasonal allergic rhinitis. *BMJ.* 2002;321:1–4.

70. Schapowal A. Treating intermittent allergic rhinitis: a prospective, randomized, placebo and antihistamine-controlled study of butterbur extract Ze 339. *Phytother Res.* 2005;19:530–7.

71. Avula B, Wang YH, Wang M, Smillie TJ, Khan IA. Simultaneous determination of sesquiterpenes and pyrrolizidine alkaloids from the rhizomes of Petasites hybridus (L.) G.M. et Sch. and dietary supplements using UPLC-UV and HPLCTOF-MS methods. *J Pharm Biomed Anal.* 2012;70:53–63.

72. Holland S, Silberstein SD, Freitag F, et al. Evidence-based guideline update: NSAIDs and other complementary treatments for episodic migraine prevention in adults: report of the Quality Standards Subcommittee of the American Academy of Neurology and the American Headache Society. *Neurology.* 2012;78:1346–53.

73. Pothmann R, Danesch U. Migraine prevention in children and adolescents: results of an open study with a special butterbur root extract. *Headache.* 2005;45:196–203.

74. Oelkers-Ax R, Leins A, Parzer P, et al. Butterbur root extract and music therapy in the prevention of childhood migraine: an explorative study. *Eur J Pain*. 2008;12:301–13.

75. Lee D, Gray R, Robb F, et al. A placebo-controlled evaluation of butterbur and fexofenadine on objective and subjective outcomes in perennial allergic rhinitis. *Clin Exp Allergy*. 2004;34:646–9.

76. Pareek A, Suthar M, Rathore GS, et al. Feverfew (Tanacetum parthenium L.): A systematic review. *Pharmacogn Rev*. 2011;5:103–10.

77. Pittler M, Ernst E. Feverfew for preventing migraine. *Cochrane Database Syst Rev*. 2004;1:CD002286. doi: 10.1002/14651858.CD002286. Accessed at http://www.thecochranelibrary.com/view/0/index.html.

78. Diener HC, Pfaffenrath V, Schnitker J, et al. Efficacy and safety of 6.25 mg t.i.d. feverfew CO2-extract (MIG-99) in migraine prevention: a randomized, double-blind, multicentre, placebo-controlled study. *Cephalalgia*. 2005;25:1031–41.

79. Ha GT, Wong RK, Zhang Y. Huperzine a as potential treatment of Alzheimer's disease: an assessment on chemistry, pharmacology, and clinical studies. *Chem Biodivers*. 2011;8:1189–204.

80. Yue J, Dong BR, Lin X, et. al. Huperzine A for mild cognitive impairment. *Cochrane Database Syst Rev*. 2012;12:CD008827. doi: 10.1002/14651858. CD008827.pub2. Accessed at http://www.thecochranelibrary.com/view/0/index.html.

81. Hao Z, Liu M, Liu Z, et. al. Huperzine A for vascular dementia. *Cochrane Database Syst Rev*. 2009;2:CD007365. doi:10.1002/14651858.CD007365. pub2. Accessed at http://www.thecochranelibrary.com/view/0/index.html.

82. Li J, Wu HM, Zhou RL, et al. Huperzine A for Alzheimer's disease. *Cochrane Database Syst Rev*. 2008;2:CD005592. doi: 10.1002/14651858. CD005592.pub2.Accessed at http://www.thecochranelibrary.com/view/0/index.html.

83. Sierina VS, Wollschlaeger B, Blumenthal M. Ginkgo biloba. *Am Fam Physician*. 2003;68:923–6.

84. Chan PC, Xia Q, Fu PP. Ginkgo biloba leave extract: biological, medicinal, and toxicological effects. *J Environ Sci Health C Environ Carcinog Ecotoxicol Rev*. 2007;25(3):211–44.

85. Ulbricht C, Chao W, Costa D, et al. Clinical evidence of herb-drug interactions: a systematic review by the natural standard research collaboration. *Curr Drug Metab*. 2008;9:1063–120.

86. National Toxicology Program. Toxicology and carcinogenesis studies of Ginkgo biloba extract (CAS No. 90045-36-6) in F344/N rats and B6C3F1/N mice (Gavage studies). *Natl Toxicol Program Tech Rep Ser*. 2013;578:1–183.

87. Izzo AA. Interactions between herbs and conventional drugs: overview of the clinical data. *Med Princ Pract*. 2012;21:404–28.

88. Stanger MJ, Thompson LA, Young AJ, et al. Anticoagulant activity of select dietary supplements. *Nutr Rev*. 2012;70:107–17.

89. Kellermann AJ, Kloft C. Is there a risk of bleeding associated with standardized Ginkgo biloba extract therapy? A systematic review and meta-analysis. *Pharmacotherapy*. 2011;31:490–502.

90. Birks J, Grimley Evans J. Ginkgo biloba for cognitive impairment and dementia. *Cochrane Database Syst Rev*. 2009;1:CD003120. doi: 10.1002/14651858.CD003120.pub3. Accessed at http://www.thecochranelibrary.com/view/0/index.html.

91. Vellas B, Coley N, Ousset PJ, et al. Long-term use of standardised Ginkgo biloba extract for the prevention of Alzheimer's disease (GuidAge): a randomised placebo-controlled trial. *Lancet Neurol*. 2012;11:851–9.

92. Snitz BE, O'Meara ES, Carlson MC, et al.; for Ginkgo Evaluation of Memory (GEM) Study Investigators. *Ginkgo biloba* for preventing cognitive decline in older adults: a randomized trial. *JAMA*. 2009;302:2663–70.

93. Sarris J, LaPorte E, Schweitzer I. Kava: a comprehensive review of efficacy, safety, and psychopharmacology. *Aust N Z J Psychiatry*. 2011;45:27–35.

94. Ulbricht C, Basch E, Boon H, et al. Safety review of kava (*Piper methysticum*) by the Natural Standard Research Collaboration. *Expert Opin Drug Saf*. 2005;4:779–94.

95. Perez J, Holmes JF. Altered mental status and ataxia secondary to acute kava ingestion. *J Emerg Med*. 2005;28:49–51.

96. Centers for Disease Control and Prevention. Hepatic toxicity possibly associated with kava-containing products—United States, Germany, and Switzerland, 1999–2002. *MMWR Morb Mortal Wkly Rep*. 2002;51:1065–7.

97. Teschke R, Lebot V. Proposal for a kava quality standardization code. *Food Chem Toxicol*. 2011;49:2503–16.

98. Sarris J, Kavanagh DJ, Byrne G, et al. The kava anxiety depression spectrum study (KADSS): a randomized, placebo-controlled crossover trial using an aqueous extract of *Piper methysticum*. *Psychopharmacology*. 2009;205:399–407.

99. Witte S, Loew D, Gaus W. Meta-analysis of the efficacy of the acetonic kava-kava extract WS1490 in patients with non-psychotic anxiety disorders. *Phytother Res*. 2005;19:183–8.

100. Dennehy CE, Tsourounis C. Dietary supplements & herbal medicines. In: Katzung BG, Masters SB, Trevor AJ, eds. *Basic and Clinical Pharmacology*. 12th ed. New York, NY: Lange/McGraw Hill; 2012:1125–37.

101. Luboshitzky R, Lavie P. Melatonin and sex hormone interrelationships—a review. *J Ped Endocrinol*. 1999;12:355–62.

102. Kotlarczyk MP, Lassila HC, O'Neil CK, et al. Melatonin osteoporosis prevention study (MOPS): a randomized, double-blind, placebo-controlled study examining the effects of melatonin on bone health and quality of life in perimenopausal women. *J Pineal Res*. 2012;52:414–26.

103. Brzezinski A, Vangel MG, Wurtman RJ, et al. Effect of exogenous melatonin on sleep: a meta-analysis. *Sleep Med*. 2005;9:41–50.

104. Wright KP Jr, Myers BL, Plenzler SC, et al. Acute effects of bright light and caffeine on nighttime melatonin and temperature levels in women taking and not taking oral contraceptives. *Brain Res*. 2000;873:310–7.

105. Lusardi P, Piazza E, Fogari R. Cardiovascular effects of melatonin in hypertensive patients well controlled by nifedipine: a 24-hour study. *Br J Pharmacol*. 2000;49:423–7.

106. Wang Y, Jin B, Ai F, et al. The efficacy and safety of melatonin in concurrent chemotherapy or radiotherapy for solid tumors: a meta-analysis of randomized controlled trials. *Canc Chemother Pharmacol*. 2012;69:1213–20.

107. Sanchez-Barcelo EJ, Mediavilla MD, Alonso-Gonzalez C, Reiter RJ. Melatonin uses in oncology: breast cancer prevention and reduction of the side effects of chemotherapy and radiation. *Expert Opin Investig Drugs*. 2012;21:819–31.

108. van Geijlswijk IM, Korzilius HPL, Smits MG. The use of exogenous melatonin in delayed sleep phase disorder: a meta-analysis. *Sleep*. 2010;33:1605–14.

109. Buscemi N, Vandermeer B, Hooton N, et al. Effects of exogenous melatonin on sleep: a meta-analysis. *Sleep Med Res*. 2005;9:41–50.

110. Braam W, Didden R, Maas AP, et al. Melatonin decreases daytime challenging behavior in persons with intellectual disability and chronic insomnia. *J Intellect Disab Res*. 2010;54:52–9.

111. Luthringer R, Muzet M, Zisapel N, et al. The effect of prolonged-release melatonin on sleep measures and psychomotor performance in elderly patients with insomnia. *Intl Clin Psychopharmacol*. 2009;24:239–49.

112. Serfaty MA, Osborne D, Buszewicz MJ, et al. A randomized double-blind placebo controlled trial of treatment as usual plus exogenous slow-release melatonin (6 mg) or placebo for sleep disturbance and depressed mood. *Intl Clin Psychopharmacol*. 2010;25:132–42.

113. Rahman SA, Kayumov L, Shapiro CM. Antidepressant action of melatonin in the treatment of delayed sleep phase syndrome. *Sleep Med*. 2010;11:131–6.

114. Pandi-Perumal SR, Trakht I, Spence DW, et al. The roles of melatonin and light in the pathophysiology and treatment of circadian rhythm sleep disorders. *Nature Clin Pract*. 2008;4:436–47.

115. Herxheimer A, Petrie K. Melatonin for the prevention and treatment of jet lag. *Cochrane Database Syst Rev*. 2002;2:CD001520. doi: 10.1002/14651858.CD001520.pub2. Accessed at http://www.thecochranelibrary.com/view/0/index.html.

116. Suhner A, Schlagenhauf P, Höfer I, et al. Effectiveness and tolerability of melatonin and zolpidem for the alleviation of jet lag. *Aviation Space Environ Med*. 2001;72:638–46.

117. Butterweck V, Schmidt M. St. John's wort: role of active compounds for its mechanism of action and efficacy. *Wien Med Wochenschr*. 2007;157:356–61.

118. Linde K. St. John's wort—an overview. *Forsch Komplementmed*. 2009;16:146–55.

119. Wurglics M, Westerhoff K, Kaunzinger A, et al. Batch-to-batch reproducibility of St. John's wort preparations. *Pharmacopsychiatry*. 2001;34:S152–6.

120. Knuppel L, Linde K. Adverse effects of St. John's wort: a systematic review. *J Clin Psychiatry.* 2004;65:1470–9.

121. Schulz HU, Schürer M, Bässler D, et al. Investigation of the effect on photosensitivity following multiple oral dosing of two different hypericum extracts in healthy men. *Arzneimittelforschung.* 2006;56:212–21.

122. Borrelli F, Izzo A. Herb-drug interactions with St. John's wort (Hypericum perforatum): an update on clinical observations. *AAPS J.* 2009;11:710–27.

123. Linde K, Berner M, Kriston L. St. John's wort for major depression. *Cochrane Database Syst Rev.* 2008;4:CD000448. doi:10.1002/14651858. CD000448.pub3. Accessed at http://www.thecochranelibrary.com/view/0/index.html.

124. Kasper S, Caraci F, Forti B, et al. Efficacy and tolerability of Hypericum extract for the treatment of mild to moderate depression. *Eur Neuropsychopharmacol.* 2010;11:747–65.

125. Abdali K, Khajehei M, Tabatabaee HR. Effect of St John's wort on severity, frequency, and duration of hot flashes in premenopausal, peri-menopausal and postmenopausal women: a randomized, double-blind, placebo-controlled study. *Menopause.* 2010;17:326–31.

126. Hadley S, Petry JJ. Valerian. *Am Fam Physician.* 2003;67:1755–8.

127. Fernández-San-Martín MI, Masa-Font R, Palacios-Soler L, et al. Effectiveness of valerian on insomnia: a meta-analysis of randomized placebo-controlled trials. *Sleep Med.* 2010;11:505–11.

128. Glass J, Sproule B, Herrmann N, et al. Acute pharmacological effects of temazepam, diphenhydramine, and valerian in healthy elderly subjects. *J Clin Psychopharmacol.* 2003;23:260–8.

129. Iovieno N, Dalton ED, Fava M, Mischoulon D. Second-tier natural antidepressants: review and critique. *J Affect Disorders.* 2011;130:343–57.

130. Michelson D, Page SW, Casey R, et al. An eosinophilia-myalgia syndrome related disorder associated with exposure to L-5-hydroxytryptophan. *J Rheumatol.* 1994;21:2261–5.

131. Das YT, Bagchi M, Bagchi D, et al. Safety of 5-hydroxy-L-tryptophan. *Toxicol Lett.* 2004;150:111–22.

132. Shaw K, Turner J, Del Mar C. Tryptophan and 5-hydroxytryptophan for depression. *Cochrane Database Syst Rev.* 2002;1:CD003198.pub2. Accessed at http://www.thecochranelibrary.com/view/0/index.html.

133. Pardo JV. Mania following addition of hydroxtryptophan to monoamine oxidase inhibitor. *Gen Hosp Psychiatry.* 2012;34:102.e.13–102.e.14.

134. Gijsman HJ, van Gerven JM, de Kam ML, et al. Placebo-controlled comparison of three dose-regimens of 5-hydroxytryptophan challenge test in healthy volunteers. *J Clin Psychopharmacol.* 2002;22:183–9.

135. Preshaw RM, Hoag G. The dietary supplement 5-hydroxytryptophan and urinary 5-hydroxyindole acetic acid. *CMAJ.* 2008;178:993.

136. Chrubasik S, Pittler MH, Roufogalis BD. *Zingiberis rhizoma:* a comprehensive review on the ginger effect and efficacy profiles. *Phytomed.* 2005;12:684–701.

137. Borelli F, Capasso R, Aviello G, et al. Effectiveness and safety of ginger in the treatment of pregnancy-induced nausea and vomiting. *Obstet Gynecol.* 2005;105:849–56.

138. Ding M, Leach M, Bradley H. The effectiveness and safety of ginger for pregnancy-induced nausea and vomiting: A systematic review. *Women Birth.* 2013;26:e26–30.

139. Heitmann K, Nordeng H, Holst L. Safety of ginger use in pregnancy: results from a large population-based cohort study. *Eur J Clin Pharmacol.* 2013;69:269–77.

140. American College of Obstetricians and Gynecologists. Nausea and vomiting of pregnancy. *Obstet Gynecol.* 2004;103:803–15

141. Chaiyakunapruk N, Kitikannakorn N, Nathisuwan S, et al. The efficacy of ginger for the prevention of postoperative nausea and vomiting: a meta-analysis. *Am J Obstet Gynecol.* 2006;194:95–9.

142. Lee J, Oh H. Ginger as an antiemetic modality for chemotherapy-induced nausea and vomiting: a systematic review and meta-analysis. *Oncol Nurs Forum.* 2013;40:163–70.

143. Pillai AK, Sharma KK, Gupta YK, et al. Anti-emetic effect of ginger powder versus placebo as an add-on therapy in children and young adults receiving high emetogenic chemotherapy. *Pediatr Blood Cancer.* 2010;56:234–8.

144. Ryan JL, Heckler CE, Roscoe JA, et al. Ginger (Zingiber officinale) reduces acute chemotherapy-induced nausea: a URCC CCOP study of 576 patients. *Support Care Cancer.* 2012;20:1479–89.

145. Matthews A, Dowswell T, Haas DM, et al. Interventions for nausea and vomiting in early pregnancy. *Cochrane Database Syst Rev.* 2010;9:CD007575.

doi: 10.1002/14651858.CD007575.pub2. Accessed at http://www.thecochranelibrary.com/view/0/index.html.

146. Forinash AB, Yancey AM, Barnes KN, et al. The use of galactogogues in the breastfeeding mother. *Ann Pharmacother.* 2012;46:1392–404.

147. Rambaldi A, Jacobs BP, Gluud C. Milk thistle for alcoholic and/or hepatitis B or C virus liver diseases. *Cochrane Database Syst Rev.* 2007;4:CD003620. doi:10.1002/14651858.CD003620.Accessed at http://www.thecochranelibrary.com/view/0/index.html.

148. Fried MW, Navarro VJ, Afdhal N, et al. Effect of silymarin (milk thistle) on liver disease in patients with chronic hepatitis C unsuccessfully treated with interferon therapy: a randomized controlled trial. *JAMA.* 2012;308:274–82.

149. Keifer D, Ulbricht C, Abrams TR, et al. Peppermint (Mentha piperita): an evidence-based systematic review by the Natural Standard Research Collaboration. *J Herb Pharmacother.* 2007;7:91–143.

150. Ford AC, Talley NJ, Spiegel BM, et al. Effect of fibre, antispasmodics, and peppermint oil in the treatment of irritable bowel syndrome: systematic review and meta-analysis. *BMJ.* 2008;337:a2313.

151. Ruepert L, Quartero AO, de Wit NJ, et al. Bulking agents, antispasmodics and antidepressants for the treatment of irritable bowel syndrome. *Cochrane Database Syst Rev.* 2011;(8):CD003460. doi:10.1002/14651858. CD003460.pub3. Accessed at http://www.thecochranelibrary.com/view/0/index.html.

152. Mizuno S, Kato K, Ono Y, et al. Oral peppermint oil is a useful antispasmodic for double-contrast barium meal examination. *J Gastroenterol Hepatol.* 2006;21:1297–301.

153. Asao T, Kuwano H, Ide M, et al. Spasmolytic effect of peppermint oil in barium during double-contrast barium enema compared with Buscopan. *Clin Radiol.* 2003;58:301–5.

154. Hiki N, Kurosaka H, Tatsutomi Y, et al. Peppermint oil reduces gastric spasm during upper endoscopy: a randomized, double-blind, double-dummy controlled trial. *Gastrointest Endosc.* 2003;57:475–82.

155. Shavakhi A, Ardestani SK, Taki M, et al. Premedication with peppermint oil capsules in colonoscopy: a double blind placebo-controlled randomized trial study. *Acta Gastroenterol Belg.* 2012;75(3):349–53.

156. Kamenova P. Improvement of insulin sensitivity in patients with type 2 diabetes mellitus after oral administration of alpha-lipoic acid. *Int J Endocrinol Metab.* 2007;5:251–8.

157. Tiechert J, Kern J, Tritschler HJ, et al. Investigations on the pharmacokinetics of alpha-lipoic acid in healthy volunteers. *Int J Clin Pharmacol Ther.* 1998;36:625–8.

158. Gleiter CH, Schug BS, Hermann R, et al. Influence of food intake on the bioavailability of thioctic acid enantiomers. *Eur J Clin Pharmacol.* 1996;50:513–4.

159. Reljanovic M, Reichel G, Rett K, et al. Treatment of diabetic polyneuropathy with the antioxidant thioctic acid (α-lipoic acid): a two year multicenter randomized double-blind placebo-controlled trial (ALADIN II). *Free Radic Res.* 1999;31:171–9.

160. Zeigler D, Ametov A, Barinov A, et al. Oral treatment with alpha-lipoic acid improves symptomatic diabetic polyneuropathy. *Diab Care.* 2006;29:2365–70.

161. Hahm JR, Kim, BJ, Kim KW. Clinical experience with thioctacid (thioctic acid) in the treatment of distal symmetric polyneuropathy in Korean diabetic patients. *J Diabetes Complications.* 2004;18:79–85.

162. Ziegler D, Low PA, Litchy WJ, et al. Efficacy and safety of antioxidant treatment with alpha-lipoic acid over 4 years in diabetic polyneuropathy. *Diab Care.* 2011;34:2054–60.

163. Ansar H, Mazloom Z, Kazemi F, Hajazi N. Effect of alpha-lipoic acid on blood glucose, insulin resistance, and glutathione peroxidase of type 2 diabetic patients. *Saudi Med J.* 2011;32:584–8.

164. Porasuphatana S, Suddee S, Nartnampong A, et al. Glycemic and oxidative status of patients with type 2 diabetes mellitus following oral administration of alpha-lipoic acid: a randomized double-blinded placebo-controlled study. *Asia Pac J Clin Nutr.* 2012;21:12–21.

165. Lü J-M, Yao Q, Chen C. Ginseng compounds: an update on their molecular mechanisms and medical applications. *Curr Vasc Pharmacol.* 2009;7:293–302.

166. Sievenpiper JL, Arnason JT, Leiter LA, et al. Decreasing, null and increasing effects of eight popular types of ginseng on acute postprandial

glycemic indices in healthy humans: the role of ginsenosides. *J Am Coll Nutr.* 2004;23:248–58.

167. Vuksan V, Sievenpiper JL, Koo VY, et al. American ginseng (*Panax quinquefolius* L) reduces postprandial glycemia in nondiabetic subjects and subjects with type 2 diabetes mellitus. *Arch Intern Med.* 2000;160:1009–13.

168. Vuksan V, Stavro MP, Sievenpiper JL, et al. American ginseng improves glycemia in individuals with normal glucose tolerance: effect of dose and time escalation. *J Am Coll Nutr.* 2000;19:738–44.

169. Vuksan V, Sievenpiper JL, Wong J, et al. American ginseng (*Panax quinquefolius* L.) attenuates postprandial glycemia in a time-dependent but not dose-dependent manner in healthy individuals. *Am J Clin Nutr.* 2001;73:753–8.

170. Stavro PM, Woo M, Leiter LA, et al. Long-term intake of North American ginseng has no effect on 24-hour blood pressure and renal function. *Hypertension.* 2006;47:791–6.

171. Stavro PM, Woo M, Heim TF, et al. North American ginseng exerts a neutral effect on blood pressure in individuals with hypertension. *Hypertension.* 2005;46:406–11.

172. Yuan C-S, Wei G, Dey L, et al. American ginseng reduces warfarin's effect in healthy patients. *Ann Intern Med.* 2004;141:23–7.

173. Chen EYH, Hui CLM. HT001, a proprietary North American ginseng extract, improves working memory in schizophrenia: a double-blind, placebo-controlled study. *Phytother Res.* 2012;26:1166–72.

174. Dascalu A, Sievenpiper JL, Jenkins AL, et al. Five batches of Ontario-grown American ginseng root produce comparable reductions of postprandial glycemia in healthy individuals. *Can J Physiol Pharmacol.* 2007;85:856–64.

175. Lu Z, Jia Q, Wang R, et al. Hypoglycemic activities of A- and B-type procyanidin oligomer-rich-extracts from different cinnamon barks. *Phytomed.* 2011;18:298–302.

176. Wickenberg J, Lindstedt S, Berntorp K, et al. Ceylon cinnamon does not affect postprandial plasma glucose or insulin in subjects with impaired glucose tolerance. *Brit J Nutr.* 2012;107:1845–9.

177. Rafehi H, Ververis K, Karagiannis TC. Controversies surrounding the clinical potential of cinnamon for the management of diabetes. *Diab Obes Metab.* 2012;14:493–9.

178. Chase CK, McQueen CE. The use of cinnamon in diabetes. *Am J Health Syst Pharm.* 2007;64:1033–5.

179. Abraham K, Wohrlin F, Lindtner O, Heinemeyer G, Lampen A. Toxicology and risk assessment of coumarin: focus on human data. *Molecular Nutr Food Res.* 2010;54(2):228–39.

180. Leach MJ, Kumar S. Cinnamon for diabetes mellitus. *Cochrane Database Systemic Rev.* 2012;9:CD007170. doi: 10.1002/14651858.CD007170.pub2. Accessed at http://www.thecochranelibrary.com/view/0/index.html.

181. Akilen R, Tsiami A, Devendra D, Robinson N. Cinnamon in glycaemic control: systemic review and meta analysis. *Clin Nutr.* 2012;31:609–15.

182. Davis PA, Yokoyama W. Cinnamon intake lowers fasting blood glucose: meta-analysis. *J Med Food.* 2011;14:884–9.

183. Akilen R, Tsiami A, Devendra D, Robinson N. Glycated haemoglobin and blood pressure-lowering effect of cinnamon in multi-ethnic type 2 diabetic patients in the UK: a randomized, placebo-controlled, double-blind clinical trial. *Diabetic Med.* 2010;27:1159–67.

184. Lu T, Sheng H, Wu J, et al. Cinnamon extract improves fasting blood glucose and glycosylated hemoglobin level in Chinese patients with type 2 diabetes. *Nutr Res.* 2012;32:408–12.

185. Arlt W, Callies F, van Vlijmen JC, et al. Dehydroepiandrosterone replacement in women with adrenal insufficiency. *N Engl J Med.* 1999;341:1013–20.

186. Dean CE. Prasterone (DHEA) and mania. *Ann Pharmacother.* 2000;34:1419–22.

187. Acacio BD, Stanczyk FZ, Mullin P, et al. Pharmacokinetics of dehydroepiandrosterone and its metabolites after long-term daily oral administration to healthy young men. *Fertil Steril.* 2004;81:595–604.

188. Jankowski CM, Gozansky WS, Van Pelt RE, et al. Oral dehydrodoepiandrosterone replacement in older adults: effects on central adiposity, glucose metabolism and blood lipids. *Clin Endocrinol.* 2011;75:456–63.

189. Weiss EP, Villareal DT, Fontana L, et al. Dehydroepiandrosterone (DHEA) replacement decreased insulin resistance and lowers inflammatory cytokines in aging humans. *Aging.* 2011;3:533–42.

190. Panjari M, Davis SR. DHEA for postmenopausal women: a review of the evidence. *Maturitas.* 2010;66:172–9.

191. Genazzani AR, Stomati M, Valentino V, et al. Effect of 1-year, low-dose DHEA therapy on climacteric symptoms and female sexuality. *Climacteric.* 2011;14:661–8.

192. Arlt W, Callies F, Koehler I, et al. Dehydroepiandrosterone supplementation in healthy men with an age-related decline of dehydroepiandrosterone secretion. *J Clin Endocrinol Metab.* 2001;86:4686–92.

193. Reiter WJ, Pycha A, Schatzl G, et al. Dehydroepiandrosterone in the treatment of erectile dysfunction: a prospective, double-blind, randomized, placebo-controlled study. *Urology.* 1999;53:590–4.

194. Kenny AM, Boxer RX, Kleppinger A, et al. Dehydroepiandrosterone combined with exercise improves muscle strength and physical function in frail older women. *J Am Geriatr Soc.* 2010;58:1707–14.

195. von Mühlen D, Laughlin GA, Kritz-Silverstein D, et al. Effect of dehydroepiandrosterone supplementation on bone mineral density, bone markers, and body composition in older adults: the DAWN trial. *Osteoporosis Int.* 2009;19:699–707.

196. Villareal DT, Holloszy JO. DHEA enhances effects of weight training on muscle mass and strength in elderly women and men. *Am J Physiol Endocrinol Metab.* 2006;291:E1003–8.

197. El-Alfy M, Deloche C, Azzi L, et al. Skin responses to topical dehydroepiandrosterone: implications in antiageing treatment? *Brit J Derm.* 2010;163:968–76.

198. Jankowski CM, Gozansky WS, Schwartz RS, et al. Effects of dehydroepiandrosterone replacement therapy on bone mineral density in older adults: a randomized, controlled trial. *J Clin Endocrinol Metab.* 2006;91:2986–93.

199. Weiss EP, Shah K, Fontana L, et al. Dehydroepiandrosterone replacement therapy in older adults: 1- and 2-year effects on bone. *Am J Clin Nutr.* 2009;89:1459–67.

200. Jensen GS, Patel D, Benson KF. A novel extract from bovine colostrum whey supports innate immune functions. II. Rapid changes in cellular immune function in humans. *Prevent Med.* 2012;54:5124–9.

201. Struff WG, Sprotte G. Bovine colostrum as a biologic in clinical medicine: a review—Part II: clinical studies. *Int J Clin Pharmacol Therap.* 2008;46:211–25.

202. Kim JH, Jung WS, Choi N-J, et al. Health-promoting effects of bovine colostrum in type 2 diabetic patients an reduce blood glucose, cholesterol, triglyceride and ketones. *J Nutr Biochem.* 2009;20:298–303.

203. Carol A, Witkamp RF, Wichers HJ, Mensink M. Bovine colostrum supplementation's lack of effect on immune variable during short-term intense exercise in well-trained athletes. *Int J Sport Nutr Exer Metab.* 2011;21:135–45.

204. Marchbank T, Davison G, Oakes JR, et al. The nutriceutical bovine colostrum truncates the increase in gut permeability caused by heavy exercise in athletes. *Am J Physiol Liver Physiol.* 2011;300:G477–84.

205. Cesarone MR, Belcaro G, Di Renzo A, et al. Prevention of influenza episodes with colostrum compared with vaccination in healthy and high-risk cardiovascular subjects: the epidemiologic study in San Valentino. *Clin Appl Thromb Hemost.* 2007;13:130–6.

206. Brinkworth GD, Buckley JD. Concentrated bovine colostrum protein supplementation reduces the incidence of self-reported symptoms of upper respiratory tract infection in adult males. *Eur J Nutr.* 2003;42:228–32.

207. Hudson JB. Applications of the phytomedicine *Echinacea purpurea* (purple coneflower) in infectious diseases. *J Biomed Biotech.* 2012;2012:769896. doi: 10.1155/2012/769896. Epub 2011 Oct 26.

208. Lee A, Werth V. Activation of autoimmunity following use of immunostimulatory herbal supplements. *Arch Dermatol.* 2004;140:723–7.

209. Hermann R, von Richter O. Clinical evidence of herbal drugs as perpetrators of pharmacokinetic drug interactions. *Planta Med.* 2012;78:1458–77.

210. Perri D, Dugoua JJ, Mills E, et al. Safety and efficacy of echinacea (*Echinacea angustafolia, E. purpurea* and *E. pallida*) during pregnancy and lactation. *Can J Clin Pharmacol.* 2006;13:e262–7.

211. Linde K, Barrett B, Wölkart K, et al. Echinacea for preventing and treating the common cold. *Cochrane Database Syst Rev.* 2006;1:CD000530. doi: 10.1002/14651858.CD000530.pub2. Accessed at http://www.thecochranelibrary.com/view/0/index.html.

212. Shah SA, Sander S, White CM, et al. Evaluation of echinacea for the prevention and treatment of the common cold: a meta-analysis. *Lancet Infect Dis.* 2007;7:473–80.

213. Barrett B, Brown R, Rakel D, et al. Echinacea for treating the common cold: a randomized trial. *Ann Intern Med.* 2010;153:769–77.

214. O'Neil J, Hughes S, Lourie A, et al. Effects of echinacea on the frequency of upper respiratory tract symptoms: a randomized, double-blind, placebo-controlled trial. *Ann Allergy Asthma Immunol.* 2008;100:384–8.

215. Woelkart K, Linde K, Bauer R. Echinacea for preventing and treating the common cold. *Planta Med.* 2008;74:633–7.

216. Di Pierro F, Rapacioli G, Ferrara T, Togni S. Use of a standardized extract from *Echinacea angustifolia* (Polinacea®) for the prevention of respiratory tract infections. *Altern Med Rev.* 2012;17:36–41.

217. Schapowal A, Burger D, Klein P, Suter A. Echinacea/sage or chlorhexidine/lidocaine for treating acute sore throats: a randomized double-blind trial. *Eur J Med Res.* 2009;14:406–12.

218. Vlachojannis JE, Cameron M, Chrubasik S. A systematic review on the *Sambuci fructus* effect and efficacy profiles. *Phytother Res.* 2010;24:1–8.

219. American Botanical Council. The ABC clinical guide to elder berry. Accessed at http://abc.herbalgram.org/site/DocServer/Elderberry-scr.pdf?docID=165, September 27 28, 2013.

220. Krawitz C, Abu Mraheil M, Stein M, et al. Inhibitory activity of a standardized elderberry liquid extract against clinically-relevant human respiratory bacterial pathogens and influenza A and B viruses. *BMC Complement Altern Med.* 2011;11:16.

221. Kinoshita E, Hayashi K, Katayama H, et al. Anti-influenza virus effects of elderberry juice and its fractions. *Biosci Biotechnol Biochem.* 2012;76:1633–8.

222. Murkovic M, Abuja PM, Bermann AR, et al. Effects of elderberry juice on fasting and postprandial serum lipids and low-density lipoprotein oxidation in healthy volunteers: a randomized, double-blind, placebo-controlled study. *Eur J Clin Nutr.* 2004;58:244–9.

223. Zakay-Rones Z, Varsano N, Zlotnik M, et al. Inhibition of several strains of influenza virus in vitro and reduction of symptoms by an elderberry extract (*Sambucus nigra* L.) during an outbreak of influenza B Panama. *J Altern Complement Med.* 1995;1:361–9.

224. Curtis PJ, Kroom PA, Hollands WJ, et al. Cardiovascular disease risk biomarkers and liver and kidney function are not altered in postmenopausal women after ingesting and elderberry extract rich in anthocyanins for 12 weeks. *J Nutr.* 2009;139:2266–71.

225. Zakay-Rones Z, Thom E, Wollan T, et al. Randomized study of the efficacy and safety of oral elderberry extract in the treatment of influenza A and B virus infections. *J Int Med Res.* 2004;32:132–40.

226. Betsi GI, Papadavid E, Falagas ME. Probiotics for the treatment or prevention of atopic dermatitis. *Am J Clin Dermatol.* 2008;9:93–103.

227. Gerasimov SV, Vasjuta VV, Myhovych OO, Bondarchuk LI. Probiotic supplement reduces atopic dermatitis in preschool children. *Am J Clin Dermatol.* 2010;11:351–61.

228. Temmerman R, Scheirlinck I, Huys G, et al. Culture-independent analysis of probiotic products by denaturing gradient gel electrophoresis. *Appl Environ Microbiol.* 2003;69:220–6.

229. Adams CA. The probiotic paradox: live and dead cells are biological response modifiers. *Nutr Res Rev.* 2010;23:37–46.

230. Moroi M, Uchi S, Nakamura K, et al. Beneficial effect of a diet containing heat-killed *Lactobacillus paracasei* K71 on adult type atopic dermatitis. *J Dermatol.* 2011;38:131–9.

231. Liong M-T. Safety of probiotics: translocation and infection. *Nutr Rev.* 2008;66:192–202.

232. Rautava S, Kainonen E, Salminen S, Isolauri E. Maternal probiotic supplementation during pregnancy and breastfeeding reduces the risk of eczema in the infant. *J Allergy Clin Immunol.* 2012;130:1355–60.

233. van der Aa LB, Heymans HAS, van Aalderen WMC, et al. Probiotics and prebiotics in atopic dermatitis: review of the theoretical background and clinical evidence. *Pediatr Allergy Immunol.* 2010;21:e355–67.

234. Boyle RJ Ismail IH, Kivuori S, et al. *Lactobacillus* GG treatment during pregnancy for the prevention of eczema: a randomized controlled trial. *Exp Allergy Immunol.* 2011;66:509–16.

235. Dotterud CK, Storrø O, Johnsen R, Øien T. Probiotics in pregnant women to prevent allergic disease: a randomized, double-blind trial. *Brit J Dermatol.* 2010;163:616–23.

236. Gore C, Custovic A, Tannock GW, et al. Treatment and secondary prevention effects of the probiotics *Lactobacillus paracasei* or *Bifidobacterium* on early infant eczema: randomized controlled trial with follow-up until age 3 years. *Clin Exp Allergy.* 2011;42:112–22.

237. Drago L, Iemoli E, Rodighiero V, et al. Effects of *Lactobacillus salivarius* LS01 (DSM 22775) treatment on adult atopic dermatitis: a randomized placebo-controlled study. *Int J Immunopathol Pharmacol.* 2011;24:1037–48.

238. Hao Q, Lu Z, Dong BR, et al. Probiotics for preventing acute upper respiratory tract infections. *Cochrane Database Systemic Rev.* 2011;9: CD006895.pub2. doi: 10.1002/14651858.CD006895. Accessed at http://www.thecochranelibrary.com/view/0/index.html.

239. Koyama T, Kirjavainen PV, Fisher C, et al. Development and pilot evaluation of a novel probiotic mixture for the management of seasonal allergic rhinitis. *Can J Microbiol.* 201;56:730–8.

240. Chen Y-S, Jan R-L, Lin Y-L, et al. Randomized placebo-controlled trial of *Lactobacillus* on asthmatic children with allergic rhinitis. *Ped Pulmonol.* 210;45:1111–20.

241. Anonymous. Eleutherococcus senticosus. Monograph. *Altern Med Rev.* 2006;11:151–5.

242. Williams M. Immunoprotection against herpes simplex type II infection by eleutherococcus root extract. *Int J Altern Complement Med.* 2001;13:9–12.

243. Cicero AF, Derosa G, Brillante R, et al. Effects of Siberian ginseng (*Eleutherococcus senticosus* maxim.) on elderly quality of life: a randomized clinical trial. *Arch Gerontol Geriatr Suppl.* 2004;9:69–73.

244. Anonymous. *Panax ginseng.* Monograph. *Altern Med Rev.* 2009;14:172–6.

245. Seely D, Dugoua JJ, Perri D, et al. Safety and efficacy of *Panax ginseng* during pregnancy and lactation. *Can J Clin Pharmacol.* 2008;15:e87–94.

246. Kim S, Shin BC, Lee MS, et al. Red ginseng for type 2 diabetes mellitus: a systematic review of randomized controlled trials. *Chin J Integr Med.* 2011;17:937–44.

247. Jang DJ, Lee MS, Shin BC, et al. Red ginseng for treating erectile dysfunction: a systematic review. *Br J Clin Pharmacol.* 2008;66:444–50.

248. Oh KJ, Chae MJ, Lee HS, et al. Effects of Korean red ginseng on sexual arousal in menopausal women: placebo-controlled, double-blind crossover clinical study. *J Sex Med.* 2010;7(4 pt 1):1469–77.

249. Geng J, Dong J, Ni H, et al. Ginseng for cognition. *Cochrane Database Syst Rev.* 2010;(12):CD007769. doi: 10.1002/14651858.CD007769.pub2. Accessed at http://www.thecochranelibrary.com/view/0/index.html.

250. Tzellos TG, Sardeli C, Lallas A, et al. Efficacy, safety and tolerability of green tea catechins in the treatment of external anogenital warts: a systematic review and meta-analysis. *J Eur Acad Dermatol Venereol.* 2011;25:345–53.

251. Henning S, Niu Y, Lee N, et al. Bioavailability and antioxidant activity of tea flavanols after consumption of green tea, black tea, or green tea extract supplement. *Am J Clin Nutr.* 2004;80:1558–64.

252. Jurgens TM, Whelan AM, Killian L, et al. Green tea for weight loss and weight maintenance in overweight or obese adults. *Cochrane Database Syst Rev.* 2012;12:CD008650. doi: 10.1002/14651858.CD008650.pub2. Accessed at http://www.thecochranelibrary.com/view/0/index.html.

253. Boehm K, Borrelli F, Ernst E, et al. Green tea (*Camellia sinensis*) for the prevention of cancer. *Cochrane Database Syst Rev.* 2009;3:CD005004. doi: 10.1002/14651858.CD005004.pub2. Accessed at http://www.thecochranelibrary.com/view/0/index.html.

254. The Mayo Clinic. Caffeine content for coffee, tea, soda and more. Accessed at http://www.mayoclinic.com/health/caffeine/AN01211, September 28, 2013.

255. Sarma DN, Barrett ML, Chavez ML, et al. Safety of green tea extracts: a systematic review by the US Pharmacopeia. *Drug Saf.* 2008;31:469–84.

256. Wolfram S. Effects of green tea and EGCG on cardiovascular and metabolic health. *J Am Coll Nutr.* 2007;26:373S–88S.

257. Nantz MP, Rowe CA, Bukowski JF, et al. Standardized capsule of *Camellia sinensis* lowers cardiovascular risk factors in a randomized, double-blind, placebo-controlled study. *Nutrition.* 2009;25:147–54.

258. Maron D, Lu G, Cai N, et al. Cholesterol lowering effect of a theaflavin-enriched green tea extract: a randomized controlled trial. *Arch Intern Med.* 2003;163:1448–53.

259. Hartley L, Flowers N, Clarke A. et al. Green and black tea for the primary prevention of cardiovascular disease. *Cochrane Database Syst Rev.* 2012;6:CD009934. doi: 10.1002/14651858.CD009934.pub2. Accessed at http://www.thecochranelibrary.com/view/0/index.html.

260. Strong KM. African plum and benign prostatic hypertrophy. *J Herb. Pharmacother.* 2004;4:41–6.

261. Anonymous. *Pygeum africanum* (*Prunus africana*) (African plum tree). *Altern Med Rev.* 2002;7:71–4.

262. Wilt T, Ishani A, MacDonald R, et al. *Pygeum africanum* for benign prostatic hyperplasia. *Cochrane Database Syst Rev.* 2002;1:CD001044. doi: 10.1002/14651858.CD001044. Accessed at http://www.thecochranelibrary.com/view/0/index.html.

263. Howell AB. Bioactive compounds in cranberries and their role in prevention of urinary tract infections. *Mol Nutr Food Res.* 2007;51:732–7.

264. Terris MK, Issa MM, Tacker JR. Dietary supplementation with cranberry concentrate tablets may increase the risk of nephrolithiasis. *Urology.* 2001;57:26–9.

265. Haber SL, Cauthon KA, Raney EC. Cranberry and warfarin interaction: a case report and review of the literature. *Consult Pharm.* 2012;27:58–65.

266. Jepson R, Williams G, Craig J. Cranberries for preventing urinary tract infections. *Cochrane Database Syst Rev.* 2012;10:CD001321. doi:10.1002/14651858.CD001321. Accessed at http://www.thecochranelibrary.com/view/0/index.html.

267. Jepson RG, Mihaljevic L, Craig J. Cranberries for treating urinary tract infections. *Cochrane Database Syst Rev.* 2010;2:CD001322. doi: 10.1002/14651858.CD001322. Accessed at http://www.thecochranelibrary.com/view/0/index.html.

268. Fong YK, Milani S, Djavan B. Role of phytotherapy in men with lower urinary tract symptoms. *Curr Opin Urol.* 2005;15:45–8.

269. Wargo KA, Allman E, Ibrahim F. A possible case of saw palmetto-induced pancreatitis. *South Med J.* 2010;103:683–5.

270. Tacklind J, Macdonald R, Rutks I, et al. Serenoa repens for benign prostatic hyperplasia. *Cochrane Database Syst Rev.* 2012;12:CD001423. doi: 10.1002/14651858.CD001423.pub3. Accessed at http://www.thecochranelibrary.com/view/0/index.html.

271. Volpi N. Anti-inflammatory activity of chondroitin sulphate: new functions from an old natural molecule. *Inflammopharmacol.* 2011;19:299–306.

272. Martel-Pelletier J, Tat SK, Pelletier J-P. Effects of chondroitin sulfate in the pathophysiology of the osteoarthritic joint: a narrative review. *Osteoarthr Cart.* 2010;18:S7–11.

273. Mazieres B, Combe B, Phan Van A, et al. Chondroitin sulfate in osteoarthritis of the knee: a prospective, double-blind, placebo-controlled multicenter clinical study. *J Rheumatol.* 2001;28:173–81.

274. Hochberg MC. Structure-modifying effects of chondroitin sulfate in knee osteoaerthritis: an updated meta-analysis of randomized placebo-controlled trials of 2-year duration. *Osteoarthr Cart.* 2010;18:S28–31.

275. Wildi LM, Raynauld J-P, Martel-Pelletier J, et al. Chondroitin sulphate reduces both cartilage volume and bone marrow lesions in knee osteoarthritis patients starting as early as 6 months after initiation of therapy: a randomized, double-blind, placebo-controlled pilot study using MRI. *Ann Rheum Dis.* 2011;70:982–9.

276. Gabay C, Medinger-Sadowski C, Gascon D, et al. Symptomatic effects of chondroitin 4 and chondroitin 6 sulfate on hand osteoarthritis. *Arth Rheumatism.* 2011;63:3383–91.

277. Möller I, Pérez M, Monfort J, et al. Effectiveness of chondroitin sulphate in patients with concomitant knee osteoarthritis and psoriasis: a randomized, double-blind, placebo-controlled study. *Osteoarthr Cart.* 2010;18:S32–40.

278. Uebelhart D, Malaise M, Marcolongo R, et al. Intermittent treatment of knee osteoarthritis with oral chondroitin sulfate: a one-year, randomized, double-blind, multicenter study versus placebo. *Osteoarthr Cart.* 2004;12:269–76.

279. Lee YH, Woo J-H, Choi SJ, et al. Effect of glucosamine or chondroitin sulfate on the osteoarthritis progression: a meta-analysis. *Rheumatol Int.* 2010;30:357–63.

280. Mncwangi N, Chen W, Vermaak I, et al. Devil's claw—a review of the ethnobotany, phytochemistry and biological activity of *Harpagophytum procumbens. J Ethnopharmacol.* 2012;143:755–71.

281. Fiebich BL, Muñoz E, Rose T, et al. Molecular targets of the anti-inflammatory *Harpagophytum procumbens* (devil's claw): inhibition of TNFα and COX-2 gene expression by preventing activation of AP-1. *Phytother Res.* 2012;26:806–11.

282. Vlachojannis J, Roufogalis BD, Chrubasik S. Systemic review on the safety of *Harpagophytum* preparations for osteoarthritic and low back pain. *Phytother Res.* 2008;22:149–52.

283. Sanders M, Grundmann O. The use of glucosamine, devil's claw (*Harpagophytum procumbens*), and acupuncture as complementary and alternative treatments for osteoarthritis. *Altern Med Rev.* 2011;16:228–38.

284. Nagaoka I, Igarashi M, Sakamoto K. Biological activities of glucosamine and its related substances. *Adv Food Nutr Res.* 2012;65:337–52.

285. Henrotin Y, Mobasheri A, Marty M. Is there any scientific evidence for the use of glucosamine in the management of human osteoarthritis? *Arthritis Res Ther.* 2012;14:201.

286. Hoffer LJ, Kaplan LN, Hamadeh MJ, et al. Sulfate could mediate the therapeutic effect of glucosamine sulfate. *Metab Clin Exp.* 2001;50:767–70.

287. Selvan F, Rajiah K, Nainar M S-M, Mathew EM. A clinical study on glucosamine sulfate versus combination of glucosamine sulfate and NSAIDs in mild to moderate knee osteoarthritis. *Sci World J.* 2012;2012:902676. doi: 10.1100/2012/902676. Epub 2012 Apr 1.

288. Villacis J, Rice TR, Bucci LR, et al. Do shrimp-allergic individuals tolerate shrimp-derived glucosamine? *Clin Exper Allergy.* 2006;36:1457–61.

289. Simon RR, Marks V, Leeds AR, Anderson JW. A comprehensive review of oral glucosamine use and effects on glucose metabolism in normal and diabetic individuals. *Diabetes Metab Res Rev.* 2011;27:14–27.

290. Sawitzke AD, Shi H, Finco MF, et al. Clinical efficacy and safety of glucosamine, chondroitin sulfate, their combination, celecoxib or placebo taken to treat osteoarthritis of the knee: 2-year results from GAIT. *Ann Rheum Dis.* 2010;69:1459–64.

291. Wandel S, Jüni P, Tendal B, et al. Effects of glucosamine, chondroitin, or placebo in patients with osteoarthritis of hip or knee: network meta-analysis. *BMJ.* 2010;34:c4675.

292. Kanzaki N, Saito K, Maeda A, et al. Effect of a dietary supplement containing glucosamine hydrochloride, chondroitin sulfate and quercetin glycosides on symptomatic knee osteoarthritis: a randomized, double-blind, placebo-controlled study. *J Sci Food Agric.* 2012;92:862–9.

293. Reginster J-Y, Neuprez A, Lecart M-P, et al. Role of glucosamine in the treatment for osteoarthritis. *Rheumatol Int.* 2012;32:2959–67.

294. Herrero-Beaumont G, Ivorra JAR, Trabado MC, et al. Glucosamine sulfate in the treatment of knee osteoarthritis symptoms. *Arthritis Rheum.* 2007;56:555–67.

295. Wilkens P, Scheel IB, Grundnes O, et al. Effect of glucosamine on pain-related disability in patients with chronic low back pain and degenerative lumbar osteoarthritis. *JAMA.* 2010;304:45–52.

296. Cahlin BJ, Dahlström L. No effect of glucosamine sulfate on osteoarthritis in the temporomandibular joints—a randomized, controlled, short-term study. *Oral Surg Oral Med Oral Pathol Oral Radiol Endod.* 2011;112:760–6.

297. Ely A, Lockwood B. What is the evidence for the safety and efficacy of dimethylsulfoxide and methylsulfonylmethane in pain relief? *Pharmaceutical J.* 2002;269:685–7.

298. Moore RD, Morton JI. Diminished inflammatory joint disease in MRL/1pr mice ingesting dimethylsulfoxide (DMSO) or methylsulfonylmethane (MSM). *Fed Proc.* 1985;44:530, 692.

299. Kim YH, Kim DH, Lim H, et al. The anti-inflammatory effects of methylsulfonylmethane on lipopolysaccharide-induced responses in murine macrophages. *Biol Pharm Bull.* 2009;32:651–6.

300. Brien S, Prescott P, Bashir N, et al. Systematic review of the nutritional supplements dimethylsulfoxide (DMSO) and methylsulfonylmethane (MSM) in the treatment of osteoarthritis. *Osteoarth Cart.* 2008;16:1277–88.

301. Hosea Blewett HJ. Exploring the mechanisms behind S-adenosylmethionine (SAMe) in the treatment of osteoarthritis. *Crit Rev Food Sci Nutr.* 2008;48:458–63.

302. Lopez HL. Nutritional interventions to prevent and treat osteoarthritis. Part II: focus on micronutrients and supportive nutraceuticals. *PM R.* 2012;4:S155–68.

303. Williams A, Girard C, Jui D, et al. S-Adenosylmethionine (SAMe) as treatment for depression: a systematic review. *Med Clin Exp.* 2005;28:132–9.

304. Brown RP, Gerbarg P, Bottiglieri T. S-Adenosylmethionine (SAMe) for depression. *Psychiatric Ann.* 2002;1:29–44.

305. Kagan BL, Sultzer DL, Rosenlicht N, et al. Oral *S*-adenosylmethionine in depression: a randomized, double-blind, placebo-controlled trial. *Am J Psychiatry.* 1990;147:591–5.

306. Gorén JL, Stoll AL, Damico KE, et al. Bioavailability and lack of toxicity of S-adenosyl-l-methionine (SAMe) in humans. *Pharmacotherapy.* 2004;24:1501–7.

307. Rutjes AWS, Nüesch E, Reichenbach S, et al. S-Adenosyl-l-methionine for osteoarthritis of the knee or hip. *Cochrane Database Syst Rev.*

2009;4:CD007321.pub2. doi: 10.1002/14651858.CD007321. Accessed at http://www.thecochranelibrary.com/view/0/index.html.

308. Najm WI, Reinsch S, Hoehler F, et al. S-Adenosyl methionine (SAMe) versus celecoxib for the treatment of osteoarthritis symptoms: a double-blind cross-over trial. *BMC Musculoskelet Disord.* 2004;5:6. Accessed at http://www.biomedcentral.com/1471-2474/5/6, September 28, 2013.

309. Kim J, Lee EY, Koh E-M, et al. Comparative clinical trial of S-adenosyl-l-methionine versus nabumetone for the treatment of knee osteoarthritis: an 8-week, multicenter, randomized, double-blind, double-dummy, phase IV study in Korean patients. *Clin Therapeut.* 2009;31:2860–72.

310. Alpert JE, Papakostas G, Mischoulon D, et al. S-Adenosyl-l-methionine (SAMe) as an adjunct for resistant major depressive disorder: an open trial following partial or nonresponse to selective serotonin reuptake inhibitors or venlafaxine. *J Clin Psychopharmacol.* 2004;24:661–4.

311. Ulbricht C, Brendler T, Gruenwald J, et al. Lemon balm (Melissa officinalis L.): an evidence-based systematic review by the Natural Standard Research Collaboration. *J Herb Pharmacother.* 2005;5:71–114.

312. Gaby AR. Natural remedies for Herpes simplex. *Altern Med Rev.* 2006;11:93–101.

313. Kennedy DO, Little W, Haskell CF, et al. Anxiolytic effects of a combination of Melissa officinalis and Valeriana officinalis during laboratory induced stress. *Phytother Res.* 2006;20:96–102.

314. Müller SF, Klement S. A combination of valerian and lemon balm is effective in the treatment of restlessness and dyssomnia in children. *Phytomedicine.* 2006;13:383–7.

315. Pazyar N, Yaghoobi R, Bagherani N, et al. A review of applications of tea tree oil in dermatology. *Int J Dermatol.* 2012;52:784–90.

316. Henley DV, Lipson N, Korach KS, et al. Prepubertal gynecomastia linked to lavender and tea tree oils. *N Engl J Med.* 2007;356:479–85.

317. Thompson G, Blackwood B, McMullan R, et al. A randomized controlled trial of tea tree oil (5%) body wash versus standard body wash to prevent colonization with methicillin-resistant *Staphylococcus aureus* (MRSA) in critically ill adults: research protocol. *BMC Infect Dis.* 2008;8:161.

318. Dryden MS, Dailly S, Crouch M. A randomized, controlled trial of tea tree topical preparations versus a standard topical regimen for the clearance of MRSA colonization. *J Hosp Infect.* 2004;56:283–6.

319. Satchell AC, Saurajen A, Bell C, et al. Treatment of interdigital tinea pedis with 25% and 50% tea tree oil solution: a randomized, placebo-controlled, blinded study. *Australas J Dermatol.* 2002;43:175–8.

320. Buck DS, Nidorf DM, Addino JG. Comparison of two topical preparations for the treatment of onychomycosis: *Melaleuca alternifolia* (tea tree) oil and clotrimazole. *J Fam Pract.* 1994;38:601–5.

321. Satchell AC, Saurajen A, Bell C, et al. Treatment of dandruff with 5% tea tree oil shampoo. *J Am Acad Dermatol.* 2002;47:852–5.

322. Vazquez JA, Zawawi AA. Efficacy of alcohol-based and alcohol-free melaleuca oral solution for the treatment of fluconazole-refractory oropharyngeal candidiasis in patients with AIDS. *HIV Clin Trials.* 2002;3:379–85.

323. Enshaieh S, Jooya A, Siadat AH, et al. The efficacy of 5% topical tea tree oil gel in mild to moderate acne vulgaris: a randomized, double-blind placebo-controlled study. *Indian J Dermatol Venereol Leprol.* 2007;73:22–5.

324. Li JX, Yu ZY. Cimicifugae rhizoma: from origins, bioactive constituents to clinical outcomes. *Curr Med Chem.* 2006;13:2927–51.

325. Palacio C, Masri G, Mooradian AD. Black cohosh for the management of menopausal symptoms: a systematic review of clinical trials. *Drugs Aging.* 2009;26:23–36.

326. Roberts H. Safety of herbal medicinal products in women with breast cancer. *Maturitas.* 2010;66:363–9.

327. Kligler B. Black cohosh. *Am Fam Physician.* 2003;68:114–6.

328. Borrelli F, Ernst E. Black cohosh (Cimicifuga racemosa): a systematic review of adverse events. *Am J Obstet Gynecol.* 2008;199:455–66.

329. Mahady GB, Low Dog T, Barrett ML, et al. United States Pharmacopeia review of the black cohosh case reports of hepatotoxicity. *Menopause.* 2008;15(4 pt 1):628–38.

330. Teschke R, Schwarzenboeck A, Schmidt-Taenzer W, et al. Herb induced liver injury presumably caused by black cohosh: a survey of initially purported cases and herbal quality specifications. *Ann Hepatol.* 2011; 10:249–59.

331. Leach MJ, Moore V. Black cohosh (Cimicifuga spp.) for menopausal symptoms. *Cochrane Database Syst Rev.* 2012;9:CD007244.pub2. doi:

10.1002/14651858.CD007244. Accessed at http://www.thecochrane library.com/view/0/index.html.

332. Laakmann E, Grajecki D, Doege K, et al. Efficacy of Cimicifuga racemosa, Hypericum perforatum and Agnus castus in the treatment of climacteric complaints: a systematic review. *Gynecol Endocrinol.* 2012;28:703–9.

333. Shams T, Setia MS, Hemmings R, et al. Efficacy of black cohosh-containing preparations on menopausal symptoms: a meta-analysis. *Altern Ther Health Med.* 2010;16:36–44.

334. Walji R, Boon H, Guns E, et al. Black cohosh (*Cimicifuga racemosa* [L.] Nutt.): safety and efficacy for cancer patients. *Support Care Cancer.* 2007;15:913–21.

335. van Die MD, Burger HG, Teede HJ, et al. Vitex agnus-castus (Chaste-Tree/Berry) in the treatment of menopause-related complaints. *J Altern Complement Med.* 2009;15:853–62.

336. Daniele C, Thompson Coon J, Pittler MH, et al. *Vitex agnus castus:* a systematic review of adverse events. *Drug Saf.* 2005;28:319–32.

337. van Die MD, Burger HG, Bone KM, et al. *Hypericum perforatum* with *Vitex agnus-castus* in menopausal symptoms: a randomized, controlled trial. *Menopause.* 2009;16:156–63.

338. van Die MD, Bone KM, Burger HG, et al. Effects of a combination of *Hypericum perforatum* and *Vitex agnus-castus* on PMS-like symptoms in late-perimenopausal women: findings from a subpopulation analysis. *J Altern Complement Med.* 2009;15:1045–8.

339. Rotem C, Kaplan B. Phyto-Female Complex for the relief of hot flushes, night sweats and quality of sleep: randomized, controlled, double-blind pilot study. *Gynecol Endocrinol.* 2007;23:117–22.

340. van Die MD, Burger HG, Teede HJ, et al. Vitex agnus-castus extracts for female reproductive disorders: A systematic review of clinical trials. *Planta Med.* 2012;79:562–75.

341. Carmichael AR. Can *Vitex agnus castus* be used for the treatment of mastalgia? What is the current evidence? *Evid Based Complement Alternat Med.* 2008;5:247–50.

342. Bayles B, Usatine R. Evening primrose oil. *Am Fam Physician.* 2009; 80(12):1405–8.

343. Stonemetz D. A review of the clinical efficacy of evening primrose. *Holist Nurs Pract.* 2008;22:171–4.

344. Pruthi S, Wahner-Roedler DL, Torkelson CJ, et al. Vitamin E and evening primrose oil for management of cyclical mastalgia: a randomized pilot study. *Altern Med Rev.* 2010;15:59–67.

345. Goyal A, Mansel RE. Efamast Study Group. A randomized multicenter study of gamolenic acid (Efamast) with and without antioxidant vitamins and minerals in the management of mastalgia. *Breast J.* 2005;11:41–7.

346. Boehm K, Pittler MH, Wilson N, et al. Oral evening primrose oil and borage oil for atopic eczema. *Cochrane Database Syst Rev.* 2009;4: CD004416. doi: 10.1002/14651858.CD004416. Accessed at http://www.thecochranelibrary.com/view/0/index.html.

347. Morse NL, Clough PM. A meta-analysis of randomized, placebo-controlled clinical trials of Efamol evening primrose oil in atopic eczema. Where do we go from here in light of more recent discoveries? *Curr Pharm Biotechnol.* 2006;7:503–24.

348. Ulbricht C, Basch E, Burke D, et al. Fenugreek (*Trigonella foenum-graecum* L. Leguminosae): an evidence-based systematic review by the natural standard research collaboration. *J Herb Pharmacother.* 2007;7:143–77.

349. Basch E, Ulbricht C, Kuo G, et al. Therapeutic applications of fenugreek. *Altern Med Rev.* 2003;8:20–7.

350. Turkyılmaz C, Onal E, Hirfanoglu IM, et al. The effect of galactagogue herbal tea on breast milk production and short-term catch-up of birth weight in the first week of life. *J Altern Complement Med.* 2011;17:139–42.

351. Eden JA. Phytoestrogens for menopausal symptoms: A review. *Mauritas.* 2012;72:157–9.

352. Marini H, Minutoli L, Polito F, et al. Effects of the phytoestrogen genistein on bone metabolism in osteopenic postmenopausal women: a randomized trial. *Ann Intern Med.* 2007;146:839–47.

353. Marini H, Bitto A, Altavilla D, et al. Breast safety and efficacy of genistein aglycone for postmenopausal bone loss: a follow-up study. *J Clin Endocrinol Metab.* 2008;93:4787–96.

354. Alekel DL, Van Loan MD, Koehler KJ, et al. The soy isoflavones for reducing bone loss (SIRBL) study: a 3-y randomized controlled trial in postmenopausal women. *Am J Clin Nutr.* 2010;91:218–30.

355. Tai TY, Tsai KS, Tu ST, et al. The effect of soy isoflavone on bone mineral density in postmenopausal Taiwanese women with bone loss: a 2-year randomized double-blind placebo-controlled study. *Osteoporos Int.* 2012;23:1571–80.

356. Sacks FM, Lichtenstein A, Van Horn L, et al. Soy protein, isoflavones, and cardiovascular health: an American Heart Association Science Advisory for professionals from the Nutrition Committee. *Circulation.* 2006;113:1034–44.

357. Magee PJ, Rowland I. Soy products in the management of breast cancer. *Curr Opin Clin Nutr Metab Care.* 2012;15:586–91.

358. Yan L, Spitznagel EL. Soy consumption and prostate cancer risk in men: a revisit of a meta-analysis. *Am J Clin Nutr.* 2009;89:1155–63.

359. Vermaak I, Hamman J, Viljoen A. *Hoodia gordonii:* an up-to-date review of a commercially important anti-obesity plant. *Planta Med.* 2011;77:1149–60.

360. Blom WAM, Abrahamse SL, Bradford R, et al. *Am J Clin Nutr.* 2011; 94:1171–81.

361. Jull AB, Ni Mhurchu C, Dunshea-Mooij C, et al. Chitosan for overweight or obesity. *Cochrane Database Syst Rev.* 2008;3:CD003892. doi: 10.1002/14651858.CD003892.pub3.

362. Cornelli U, Belcaro G, Cesarone MR, et al. Use of polyglucosamine and physical activity to reduce body weight and dyslipidemia in moderately overweight subjects. *Minerva Cardioangiol.* 2008;56(suppl 1): 71–8.

363. Gange CA, Madias C, Felix-Getzik EM, et al. Variant angina associated with bitter orange in a dietary supplement. *Mayo Clin Proc.* 2006; 81:54518.

364. Sultan S, Spector J, Mitchell RM. Ischemic colitis associated with use of a bitter orange-containing dietary weight-loss supplement. *Mayo Clin Proc.* 2006;81:1630–1.

365. Stohs SJ, Preuss HG, Shara M. The safety of *Citrus aurantium* (bitter orange) and its primary protoalkaloid *p*-synephrine. *Phytother Res.* 2011;25:1421–8.

366. Scott GN. Is raspberry ketone effective for weight loss? *Medscape.* December 11, 2012. Accessed at: www.medscape.com/viewarticle/775741, September 28, 2013.

367. Márquez F, Babio N, Bulló M, Salas-Salvadó J. Evaluation of the safety and efficacy of hydroxycitric acid or *Garcinia cambogia* extracts in humans. *Crit Rev Food Sci Nutr.* 2012;52:585–94.

COMMON COMPLEMENTARY AND ALTERNATIVE MEDICINE HEALTH SYSTEMS

Catherine Ulbricht

The term *complementary and alternative medicine* (CAM) refers to a broad group of healing philosophies, diagnostic approaches, and therapeutic products that do not conform to the conventional Western health system.[1] *Alternative therapies* have been defined as those used in place of conventional practices, whereas *complementary* or *integrative medicine* is used in combination with mainstream approaches.[2,3] Other terms used to describe CAM include *folkloric, holistic, irregular, nonconventional, non-Western, traditional, unorthodox,* and *unproven* medicine. Some common CAM therapies and health systems include homeopathy, naturopathy, traditional Chinese medicine (TCM), acupuncture, chiropractic care, Ayurveda, and massage. This chapter presents an overview of common complementary and alternative modalities other than dietary supplements, which are discussed in Chapters 51.

Overview of Common CAM Health Systems

Major Categories

In the United States, the National Center for Complementary and Alternative Medicine (NCCAM) classifies CAM therapies into three broad categories, which are neither formally defined nor exclusive:

1. *Natural Products.* This category includes herbal medicines or botanicals, minerals, vitamins, and other natural products such as probiotics.
2. *Mind–Body Medicine.* According to NCCAM, the CAM modalities in this category are diverse and feature procedures or techniques that are taught or conducted by a trained practitioner or teacher. Examples of mind–body medicine include acupuncture, guided imagery, hypnotherapy, *qi gong, tai chi,* yoga, massage therapy, movement therapies, and spinal manipulation.
3. *Other CAM Practices.*
   a. *Traditional healers* use "methods based on indigenous theories, beliefs, and experiences handed down from generation to generation," according to the National Institutes of Health (NIH).[4] Native American healers (e.g., medicine men) and shamans are examples.
   b. *Energy therapies* use various energy fields to promote health. Veritable energies such as light and magnetism are measurable forces that may be used to treat patients. In contrast, putative energy fields, also known as biofields, are not measurable but are instead based on theories that humans contain vital energies or life forces, which include *qi* in traditional Chinese medicine and *prana* in Ayurveda. Practices such as healing touch, *qi gong,* and reiki are purported to manipulate these forces.
   c. *Whole medical systems* are "complete systems of theory and practice that have evolved over time in different cultures apart from conventional or Western medicine."[4] Ancient whole medical systems include Ayurveda and TCM, whereas homeopathy and naturopathy are examples of modern whole medical systems.

Healing systems encompass complete sets of theories and practices. A system centers on a philosophy or lifestyle, such as the power of nature or the presence of energy in the body. Some CAM therapies have become widely integrated into conventional medicine. Many prescription drugs originally came from natural products; examples include digoxin from the foxglove plant, paclitaxel from the bark of the yew tree, yohimbine from yohimbe bark, oseltamivir from Chinese star anise, and artemether from sweet wormwood.[5,6]

Potential Risks and Benefits

CAM is often considered a form of preventive medicine and is widely used to maintain health and reduce disease risk.[2] The attraction of CAM includes the potential to treat diseases for which conventional therapies have been ineffective. CAM may also provide an increased sense of patient empowerment and participation, and there is a widespread belief that CAM represents safe and natural therapeutic approaches. Cancer patients have cited the media as influencing their decisions to try CAM therapies.[7] In addition, some patients use CAM techniques such as meditation and prayer to cope with chronic or untreatable illnesses.[3]

Although some CAM therapies are supported by basic science and clinical evidence, many CAM therapies have not been subjected to rigorous clinical testing.[5] Because they often contain pharmacologically active constituents, natural products may potentially cause adverse effects or have clinically significant interactions with drugs, foods, or other dietary supplements.[5,8] Therefore, CAM should not be used concurrently with drugs, or in place of proven conventional therapies, without medical supervision.

Research Issues

Many CAM approaches have not been fully evaluated. In 1992, the U.S. Congress established the Office of Alternative Medicine within NIH and provided a budget of $2 million to rigorously evaluate CAM practices. In 1998, after the creation of NCCAM, Congress elevated the status of the Office of Alternative Medicine to a NIH center with a budget of $50 million for fiscal year 1999. In 2012, the Federal appropriations for NCCAM reached $128 million. The mission of NCCAM is to "define, through rigorous scientific investigation, the usefulness and safety of complementary and alternative medicine interventions and their roles in improving health and health care."[9]

In addition, the National Cancer Institute (NCI) established the Office of Cancer Complementary and Alternative Medicine (OCCAM) in October 1998 to coordinate and enhance the activities of NCI and to increase the amount of high-quality cancer research and information on the use of CAM. According to OCCAM, in fiscal year 2010, NCI supported approximately $114,460,116 in CAM-related research. This represents more than 406 projects in the form of grants, cooperative agreements, supplements, or contracts. Other NIH institutes also contribute funds to CAM research, with estimates of almost $500 million for all institutes and centers combined.[1]

Evidence on the safety and efficacy of CAM may be difficult to obtain. This challenge may be partly related to the fact that many CAM studies are reported in foreign languages and in journals that are not peer reviewed. To conduct evidence-based assessments on CAM, authors of systematic reviews and meta-analyses often broaden literature searches to include languages other than English. Several databases may be searched in addition to PubMed or MEDLINE. Researchers may also use guides and validated scales, such as the Jadad scale, which has been used to rate the quality of many available studies concerning CAM therapies.[10]

Another issue in evaluating CAM research is the lack of standardization. Many individual therapies involve a variety of techniques or dosages, making comparisons difficult. Some types of CAM such as Ayurveda do not require providers to be licensed or formally trained, which may contribute to the variable research results.

Experimental design is the most problematic issue in CAM research. The metaphysical aspects of some CAM therapies, such as the harmony between the body and the universe in Ayurveda, are difficult to test with scientific methods.[11] Critical elements of clinical research such as placebo control and double blinding are difficult in many CAM studies. For example, the participatory nature of meditation therapy prevents blinding of the subject to the active treatment.[12] Double blinding is a central problem with modalities such as acupuncture because this therapy cannot be easily delivered by a provider blinded to the intervention. The Jadad score is sometimes modified for application to acupuncture studies because of the difficulty in blinding the acupuncturist.[13] In such cases, modified Jadad scoring may include awarding one point if the trial is single blinded or if outcomes are assessed by a blinded investigator rather than the acupuncturist.

With respect to the challenge of a placebo control for CAM therapies such as acupuncture, researchers have developed sham treatments to approximate subject blinding. For acupuncture, sham treatment typically involves placement of needles at non-active sites or at a specific distance, usually about 1 inch, from the active sites in the study, whereas depth and stimulation remain the same. Other sham acupuncture techniques involve treatment at actual acupuncture points but without needle penetration. Critics of this approach argue that even pressure at acupuncture points may elicit effects. Although some studies have demonstrated that sham procedures achieved blinding of subjects, methods used to create sham acupuncture vary widely. Sham acupuncture often is not regarded as a true placebo because the patient is subjected to physical stimulation, and studies have shown this technique to also elicit effects.[14]

Working with CAM Providers

Ideally, conventional and CAM providers should work collaboratively for the benefit of the patient. Pharmacists and other health care providers should have an objective attitude toward CAM providers, especially given that some techniques are now provided in conventional medical centers. An example of an integrative approach is a clinic that includes both conventional and CAM providers. To meet patient demand, conventional providers may refer patients to CAM therapies, such as therapeutic massage or acupuncture.[15]

Individuals who use CAM may also lack a clear understanding about the therapies. A survey among users of homeopathy in England showed that nearly 10% of users were confused about what constitutes a homeopathic product.[16] Patients should feel comfortable discussing potential CAM therapies with their conventional health care providers, and an increasing number of conventional providers now integrate certain evidence-based CAM techniques into their own practices.

Homeopathy

Homeopathy is a distinct system of medicine with its own pharmacopoeia and principles of practice. The term *homeopathy* comes from the two Greek words *homoios* (similar) and *pathos* (suffering or disease). Dr. Samuel Hahnemann developed homeopathy in the early 1800s and also coined the term *allopathy* as a synonym for conventional medicine. Homeopathy is based on the principle of "like cures like" or the "law of similars." This principle maintains that if a substance produces the symptoms of an illness in large doses, that same substance can cure it in very small doses. The more dilute a homeopathic medicine is, the greater is its potency. The efficacy of homeopathic medicines is believed to depend not only on the dilution factor but also on vigorous shaking, or succussion, which is performed with each dilution.

The homeopathic principle of like cures like is often compared with vaccination, which involves administration of antigenic material to induce immunity to infectious agents. However, this comparison is not entirely accurate. Vaccines typically contain measurable levels of attenuated or killed pathogens (or their purified antigens) and are used for prophylaxis. In contrast, homeopathic preparations are often so dilute that they contain statistically negligible amounts of the purported active ingredients. In addition, homeopathic remedies are generally used to treat an existing illness rather than for prophylaxis. One exception is Oscillococcinum, a homeopathic preparation derived from wild duck heart and liver, which is used to both prevent and treat influenza, although evidence of its efficacy is lacking.[17]

Although homeopathic medicines are generally intended to be ingested, they are not classified as dietary supplements. The

Food and Drug Administration (FDA) regulates homeopathic medicines under Sections 201(g) and 201(j) of the Federal Food, Drug, and Cosmetic Act as drugs recognized in the official *United States Pharmacopoeia* (USP), *Homoeopathic Pharmacopoeia of the United States* (HPUS), or *National Formulary* (NF). For homeopathic drugs, the premarket approval process is distinct from the approval process for conventional drugs.[18] Homeopathic drugs are approved with the publication of a monograph by the Homeopathic Pharmacopoeia Convention of the United States (HPCUS) in the HPUS. For a homeopathic drug to be included in the HPUS, it must be manufactured according to approved methods of preparation and determined by HPCUS to be safe and effective. The safety and efficacy of a homeopathic drug is determined by procedures called provings (or research procedures in the HPUS), which determine dosages necessary to induce symptoms in healthy individuals. Evidence from homeopathic provings is subject to verification by conventional clinical research methods; however, according to FDA, "compliance with requirements of the HPUS, USP, or NF does not establish that it has been shown by appropriate means to be safe, effective, and not misbranded for its intended use."[18]

As with conventional drugs, homeopathic remedies may be sold over the counter if they are intended to treat self-limiting conditions such as headaches and colds. Most homeopathic remedies are available without a prescription, whereas about 5% require prescriptions from medical care providers.[18] Homeopathic medicines are commonly found in integrative pharmacies that stock dietary supplements and alternative remedies along with standard drugs. Chain pharmacies and health food markets may also carry homeopathic medicines, including pediatric and veterinary formulations.

Sales of homeopathic drugs are estimated to be about 0.26% of the U.S. drug market, and their sales increase at a rate of about 8% per year, with estimated sales of $450 million in 2003.[18] According to the 2007 National Health Interview Survey, nearly 4 million adults and 1 million children used homeopathy in the previous year.[19] Despite the widespread use of homeopathic products, particularly in children, surveys have demonstrated that confusion exists about what constitutes a homeopathic product, which suggests that providers need to dispense better patient education.[16]

Technique

Medicines used in homeopathy are derived from many substances, including botanical, mineral, pharmaceutical, and zoological sources. These substances are serially diluted and succussed (or triturated) to increase the strength or potency of the medication. This process is called attenuation or potentization. After each attenuation step, the preparation is given a higher number, so a substance that was attenuated 4 times would be designated as 4X, 4C, or LM4 depending on the dilution factor.[18] The decimal (1:10 dilutions) and centesimal (1:100 dilutions) scales of attenuation are used to make X and C potencies, respectively (Figure 52–1). The letter M means 1000C, not the use of 1:1000 dilutions in the attenuation process. A 1:50,000 dilution is represented by the potency LM, which is derived by combining Roman numerals L and M for 50 and 1000, respectively (although the actual Roman numeral LM means 1000 minus 50, or 950). The method for preparing LM potencies is illustrated in Figure 52–2. Although many homeopathic medicines are derived from highly toxic materials such as aconite and arnica, the final preparations are often so dilute that they are well below toxic dosages.

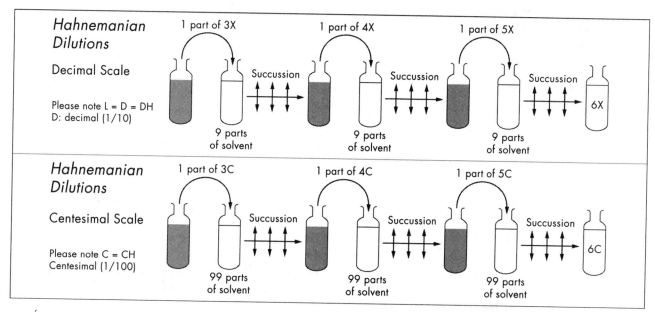

figure

52–1 Method for making homeopathic X and C potencies. Decimal scale, designated by an *X* or *D*, involves dilutions of 1:10 for each attenuation (dilution with succussion) step taken to make the desired X potency. Centesimal scale, designated by *C*, involves dilutions of 1:100 for each attenuation step taken to make the desired C potency. (*Source:* Reprinted with permission from *Introduction to Homeopathic Medicines for Pharmacists.* New Town Square, PA: Boiron Institute; 2001:9.)

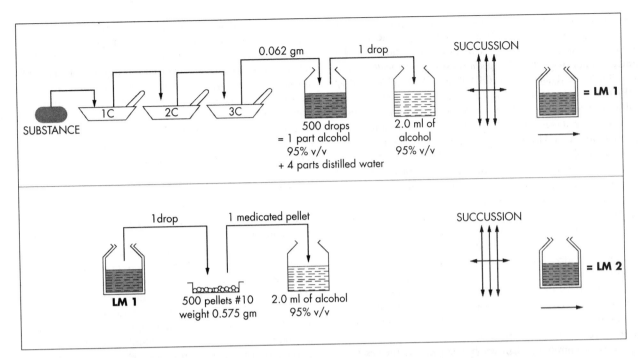

figure

52-2   Method for making homeopathic LM potencies. The 50-Millesimal scale, designated by LM or Q, involves a complex attenuation process using incremental dilutions of 1:50,000 with succussion. (*Source:* Reprinted with permission from *The Homeopathic Pharmacopoeia of the United States*. Southeastern, PA: The Homeopathic Pharmacopoeia Convention of the United States Revision Service; December 2004:40.)

Training

More than 30 schools in North America offer training in homeopathy, and the Accreditation Commission for Homeopathic Education in North America (ACHENA, formerly Council on Homeopathy Education [CHE]) continually develops professional standards for homeopathic education. The Council for Homeopathic Certification offers a Certificate in Classical Homeopathy (CCH) and provides listings of certified homeopathic practitioners on their Web sites for use by other health care providers to identify qualified homeopaths.

Certification with CCH is not recognized by any state as a license to practice homeopathy. Arizona, Connecticut, and Nevada require that homeopaths also be licensed allopathic or osteopathic physicians. Health freedom acts in some states, such as Senate Bill 577 of the State of California, protect the rights of professionals without medical licenses to practice homeopathy and other modalities that the state deems harmless. Most other states lack specific regulatory language for homeopathy; therefore, homeopathy falls under the statutes regulating the practice of medicine.

Theory/Evidence

Because homeopathic preparations contain little-to-no active ingredient, critics argue that any demonstrated efficacy is simply a placebo effect.[20] Proponents of homeopathy state that trials have demonstrated effectiveness in infants or animals, and that these subjects are unlikely to have preconceived expectations that may influence their perceptions. Overall, the effectiveness of homeopathy has not been demonstrated consistently in randomized controlled trials.[21,22] A 2010 analysis of six reviews in the Cochrane Database of Systematic Reviews concluded that the evidence suggests the effects of homeopathic therapies are similar to those of placebo.[22] Citing the contradictory results of clinical trials and the overall lack of evidence determined by systematic reviews and meta-analyses, NCCAM has stated that homeopathy has not been definitively proven to treat any clinical condition. Similarly, both the American Medical Association and the American Academy of Pediatrics have neither accepted nor rejected homeopathy in the treatment of any medical condition.[23]

Safety

For most homeopathic medicines, the risk of toxicity is low because of the extremely dilute nature of the homeopathic remedies.[18] Studies have suggested that adverse effects are less frequent in patients receiving homeopathic treatments than in those receiving conventional care.[18,24] The popular cold remedy Zicam has been labeled homeopathic, but some formulations contain significant levels of zinc. The nasal spray formulation containing zinc gluconate is known to cause irreversible damage to human nasal tissue.[25] According to FDA, more than 100 reports of loss of sense of smell have been associated with the use of this product, and this dosage form has since been withdrawn from the U.S. market.

Naturopathy

The term *naturopathy* was coined in the late 1890s by German priest Sebastian Kneipp, who practiced herbal medicine and water therapies. Dr. Benedict Lust, who studied under Kneipp, purportedly purchased the rights to naturopathic medicine from another of Kneipp's students. In 1902, Dr. Lust opened the American Institute of Naturopathy in New York City. Because he was instrumental in promoting this field of medicine, Dr. Lust is generally credited as the founder of naturopathy.

Traditional naturopathy is a philosophy of life and an approach to living that encourages lifestyles and therapies as close to nature as possible. A system of naturopathic therapy employs natural forces such as light, heat, air, water, and massage. Naturopathy focuses primarily on building health rather than on treating disease.

The practice of naturopathic medicine emerges from six underlying principles of healing that distinguish the profession from other medical approaches. These principles are based on the observation of the nature of health and disease and are continually reexamined in light of scientific analysis. The first principle is that the body has the inherent ability to maintain and restore health. Second, the naturopathic physician aims to identify and treat the cause rather than the symptoms of a disease. The third principle states that methods designed to treat only the symptoms may be harmful and should be avoided or minimized. Fourth, the physician treats the whole person, taking into account the physical, spiritual, mental, and social aspects of the individual. The fifth principle is that the naturopath educates and encourages patients to take responsibility for their own health. Finally, the naturopath assesses risk factors and hereditary susceptibility to disease and makes appropriate interventions to avoid further harm or risk to patients.

Technique

In most cases of disease or wellness, nutritional counseling and support are major components of naturopathic treatments. Naturopathic physicians use dietetics, fasting, and nutritional supplementation in practice. Botanical medicine and homeopathy may be used in naturopathy.

Naturopathic medicine has its own methods of therapeutic manipulation of the muscles, bones, and spine. Physicians use ultrasound, diathermy (electrically induced heat), exercise, massage, water, heat, cold, air, and gentle electrical pulses. Naturopathic physicians also provide natural childbirth care. They offer prenatal and postnatal care using modern diagnostic techniques. In some states, naturopaths may perform minor outpatient surgeries, such as repair of superficial wounds or removal of foreign bodies or cysts.

Because naturopaths believe that mental attitudes and emotional states may influence or cause physical illnesses, they may incorporate counseling, nutritional balancing, stress management, hypnotherapy, biofeedback, and other therapies to help patients heal on the psychological level.

Naturopaths may prescribe substances that are deemed appropriate by the Naturopathic Formulary Advisory Peer Committee. Listed substances depend on state law and vary among states. Some state-specific regulations, such as the Naturopathic Physician Practice Act Rule of Utah[26] and those set forth by the Office of Professional Regulation in Vermont,[27] allow naturopaths to prescribe only medicines listed in the *Naturopathic Physician Formulary*.

Training

In North America, seven schools offer training for the Doctor of Naturopathic Medicine (ND) degree. These include Bastyr University (Seattle, Washington), Boucher Institute of Naturopathic Medicine (Vancouver, British Columbia), the Canadian College of Naturopathic Medicine (Toronto, Ontario), National College of Natural Medicine (Portland, Oregon), National University of Health Sciences (Chicago, Illinois), Southwest College of Naturopathic Medicine (Phoenix, Arizona), and University of Bridgeport College of Naturopathic Medicine (Bridgeport, Connecticut).

Similar to allopathic medical schools, admission into a naturopathic training program requires 4 years of undergraduate study that includes premedical coursework. The ND degree consists of 4 years of postgraduate training, which includes about 4500 hours of academic and clinical training. Academic training includes courses such as anatomy, biochemistry, microbiology, and pathology. Clinical training encompasses various alternative modalities, including herbal therapy and homeopathy, in addition to mainstream clinical training such as that in cardiology and nutrition. Naturopathic physicians are educated in modern methods of diagnostic testing and imaging, including X-ray, ultrasound, and other imaging techniques. Some naturopaths may participate in residency programs, including integrative programs that train NDs in conventional medical settings.

In addition to a standard medical curriculum, a naturopath must study holistic therapies with a strong emphasis on preventing disease and optimizing wellness. The ND is required to complete training in clinical nutrition, acupuncture, homeopathic medicine, botanical medicine, psychology, and counseling. Before they can practice, naturopathic physicians must pass board examinations set by the North American Board of Naturopathic Examiners, and most states require NDs to complete continuing education hours to renew their licenses.

The licensing of naturopathic physicians varies among states. According to the Association of Accredited Naturopathic Medical Colleges (AANMC; aanmc.org/careers/licensure/) and the Council on Naturopathic Medical Education (CNMD; www. cnme.org/faq.html), NDs are licensed to practice in Alaska, Arizona (where they are known as Natural Medical Doctors, or NMDs), California, Connecticut, Hawaii, Idaho, Kansas, Maine, Minnesota, Montana, New Hampshire, North Dakota, Oregon, Utah, Vermont, and Washington as well as in Alberta, British Columbia, Manitoba, Ontario, and Saskatchewan. In addition, naturopaths are licensed in the District of Columbia, Puerto Rico, and the Virgin Islands. According to the AANMC, legislation for state/province licensing is pending for Colorado, Illinois, Iowa, Massachusetts, New York, North Carolina, Nova Scotia, Wisconsin, and Pennsylvania. Naturopathy is prohibited in the states of South Carolina and Tennessee. In all other states, laws currently do not regulate the practice of naturopathy.

Because of the popularity of naturopathy, more physicians trained in conventional medicine or other CAM fields are incorporating naturopathic treatments into their practices. Health care providers who hold degrees in osteopathy, chiropractic, acupuncture, dentistry, and veterinary medicine may seek additional training in naturopathy; they sometimes use terms such as *holistic, natural,* or *integrative* to promote their practices.

Theory/Evidence

The individual methods used in naturopathic medicine vary in their effectiveness. For instance, a proper diet may help prevent heart disease; this measure is recommended in both conventional and naturopathic medicine. Other forms of naturopathic treatment may not be more effective than conventional medicine. For example, acupuncture may help to reduce pain in some instances, but it is not widely recommended for use in place of standard analgesics for extreme pain or in surgery.[28] On the other hand, compared with psychotherapy, some naturopathic treatments may be more effective than conventional therapies for certain conditions, as shown with a combination naturopathic treatment for anxiety (nutrition counseling, relaxation techniques, and vitamin/herbal supplementation).[29]

Safety

The safety of naturopathic remedies depends on the treatment and the condition. Naturopathic methods are generally considered safer alternatives to some conventional drugs or treatments. However, herbal remedies are not free from adverse effects, and interactions may occur with drugs, supplements, or foods.[1,5,30] The safety of other naturopathic modalities, such as fasting or other dietary restrictions, depends on the individual. As with all CAM therapies, naturopathic treatments should not be used in place of proven therapies for serious medical conditions. Case 52–1 illustrates assessing the appropriateness of naturopathic treatments in a patient trying to cope with stress and anxiety.

Traditional Chinese Medicine

Chinese medicine is a broad term encompassing many different modalities and traditions of healing, including herbal medicine and acupuncture.[6,31] These therapies share a common root in Chinese philosophy, including Taoism, Confucianism, and Buddhism, and may date back more than 5000 years.

In the 1940s and 1950s, the Chinese government undertook an effort to coalesce diverse forms of Chinese medicine into a unified system to be officially defined as traditional Chinese medicine (TCM). The intent was to integrate traditional providers into an organized health system and to provide care for a large population by using familiar and inexpensive methods.

Although TCM is considered to be complementary or alternative medicine in most of the Western world, in China the term for TCM literally means "central medicine." TCM and Western medicine are commonly used side by side in modern China. As a result, compared with Western countries, China is relatively advanced in using integrative medicine. TCM features prominently in the treatment of major illnesses, including cancer and heart disease. According to the World Health Organization, TCM is fully integrated into the Chinese health system and is practiced in 95% of Chinese hospitals.[32]

Technique

TCM emphasizes herbal medicine. Herbs are usually given as pills, extracts, capsules, tinctures, or powders, which may be used directly or combined with food or other treatments. More than 2000 different types of herbs are used in Chinese medicine, with 400 frequently used and 50 considered "fundamental" herbs.[33,34] Some Chinese herbs have received attention in Western medicine for treating serious disorders. For example, the *Monascus purpureus* fungus, found in red yeast rice, is a natural source of lovastatin. Bevirimat, derived from the Chinese herb *Syzygium claviflorum,* is in a new class of drugs called maturation inhibitors and is being investigated in ongoing clinical trials in HIV.[35]

TCM incorporates not only herbs but also minerals, metals, and animal products into therapeutic preparations. The use of animal products has become more infrequent in recent years, in part because of restrictions on certain species, particularly endangered species.

Acupuncture is also considered a form of TCM, although it is regarded as more of a supportive treatment to herbal therapy. Many varieties of acupuncture exist both in Chinese and Western medicine. Classic acupuncture, also known as five-element acupuncture, uses a different needling technique and relies on acupuncture without the use of herbs. Needles used in Japanese acupuncture are smaller than those of other forms of acupuncture. Medical acupuncture refers to acupuncture practiced by a conventional physician. Auricular acupuncture treats the entire body through acupuncture points in the ears only, and electro-acupuncture uses electrical currents attached to acupuncture

---

case 52–1

Common CAM Health Systems

Patient Complaint/History

PF is a 43-year-old man who has been experiencing significant amounts of stress and anxiety related to the recent diagnosis of illness in a family member. He comes to your pharmacy and seeks your advice. He likes his primary care provider but thinks the provider is too busy to listen to his concerns and is likely just to prescribe more prescription drugs. The patient states that he does not want to become like his father who takes more than 15 different drugs every day for various chronic illnesses. PF currently takes glipizide for type 2 diabetes (A1C of 6.5%) and low-dose aspirin for prevention of heart disease. He also takes fish oil because his neighbor told him it is good for health. He is interested in any therapies that might ease his anxiety.

Recommendation

Many CAM approaches are available to ease PF's anxiety and stress. He may consider seeing a naturopath to discuss a holistic approach to his anxiety and health. Compared with psychotherapy, some naturopathic treatments may be more effective than conventional therapies for certain conditions, as has been shown with a combination naturopathic treatment for anxiety (nutrition counseling, relaxation techniques, and vitamin/herbal supplementation). Naturopathic methods are generally considered safer alternatives to some conventional drugs or treatments. However, herbal remedies are not free from adverse effects, and interactions may occur with drugs, supplements, or foods. As with all CAM therapies, naturopathic treatments should not be used in place of proven therapies for serious medical conditions. PF should be encouraged to tell his health care provider about his use of CAM.

Key: A1C = Glycosylated hemoglobin; CAM = complementary and alternative medicine.

case

52-2

Common CAM Health Systems

Patient Complaint/History

RA is a 49-year-old man with a history of lower back pain. He has been treated with various modalities, including nonsteroidal anti-inflammatory drugs and chiropractic treatment. He tells you that he previously took Vioxx (rofecoxib), but since it was taken off the market, he has not tried any other drug. He also adds that he does not like the "cracking" sound when he goes to his chiropractor. RA has a history of type 2 diabetes and takes metformin 1000 mg twice daily; he also has depression, for which he takes St. John's wort. He tells you that his regular (allopathic) primary care provider is also trained in several CAM techniques.

Recommendation

Scientific evidence supports the use of acupuncture for several indications, including various types of pain. Adverse events rarely occur with acupuncture, even with cupping and moxibustion procedures. In normal office practice, acupuncture is commonly used in combination with herbs or supplements. As with many therapies, acupuncture may require multiple treatments and long-term follow-up for symptom improvement and health maintenance. Reassure RA that acupuncture is worth exploring, and provide him with reliable sources of information from which he can acquire more information on which to make an informed decision. After researching the available information, he should discuss his suitability for acupuncture with his allopathic physician.

Key: CAM = Complementary and alternative medicine.

needles. As with many forms of TCM, acupuncture may require multiple treatments and long-term follow-up for symptom improvement and health maintenance. Case 52–2 illustrates assessing the appropriateness of acupuncture for a patient with lower back pain.

Cupping and moxibustion are commonly used to complement acupuncture, but these techniques may also be used independently in TCM. They share the principle of using heat to stimulate circulation to break up congestion or stagnation of blood and *chi* (*qi*), which is the life force central to health and well-being in TCM. Cupping has some relation to the massage technique *tuina,* which uses rapid skin pinching at points on the back to break up congestion and stimulate circulation. Cupping may also be used over acupuncture points or elsewhere. Popular in the United States, moxibustion involves the burning of dried moxa (mugwort), either on or near the skin, and sometimes in conjunction with cupping or acupuncture on specific points.[36]

TCM providers may use other modalities such as meditation and martial arts. *Tai chi chuan* (or *tai chi*) is a meditative form of martial arts that incorporates the theories of *yin* and *yang* from both Taoism and Confucianism. *Tai chi* is practiced to improve balance, coordination, and relaxation, and overall well-being. TCM may also incorporate *feng shui,* which is the art of arranging furniture and objects to increase health and prosperity.

Training

The Accreditation Commission of Acupuncture and Oriental Medicine (ACAOM) accredits professional acupuncture programs and is recognized by the U.S. Department of Education. According to the ACAOM, acupuncture and Oriental medicine is a 3- or 4-year master's degree program, offered by over 60 accredited or candidate colleges in the United States (www.naturalhealers.com/natural-health-careers/article/acupuncture-licensure). The National Certification Commission for Acupuncture and Oriental Medicine (NCCAOM) offers four independent certification programs, including Acupuncture, Chinese Herbology, Oriental Medicine, and Asian Bodywork

Therapy (www.nccaom.org; select Certification Brochure). Acupuncturists who pass national examinations administered by NCCAOM are entitled to identify themselves as board certified in their discipline and as diplomates of the NCCAOM.

Licenses to practice acupuncture are granted by individual states. Although requirements vary, many states require acupuncturists to pass the NCCAOM examinations and obtain continuing education.

Theory/Evidence

Taoism, Confucianism, and Buddhism provided the basis for the development of Chinese medical theory. According to these philosophies, nature and the laws that govern the ongoing, harmonious flow of life energy through the natural world also govern the body and health. The person is viewed as an ecosystem that is embedded in the larger ecosystem of nature and is therefore subject to the same laws. The life force called *chi* (or *qi*) circulates through the body and enlivens it. Health is a function of a balanced, harmonious flow of chi, and illness results when there is a blockage or an imbalance in the flow of chi. *Yin* and *yang* are opposite and complementary qualities of life energy (*qi*). *Yin* is regarded as the feminine principle and *yang* the masculine principle. The human being has a system of pathways called meridians, which may also be referred to as channels, through which *chi* flows. Meridians correspond with specific organs or organ systems (organ networks). Health is an ongoing process of maintaining balance and harmony of the circulation of *chi* through all the organs and systems of the body. The body has five organ networks, each corresponding with a particular element.

Despite the growing popularity of TCM in the West, its effectiveness remains debatable. Scientific evidence supports the use of acupuncture for several indications including osteoarthritis and various types of pain and nausea.[5] The American Cancer Society states "clinical studies have found acupuncture may help treat nausea caused by chemotherapy drugs and surgical anesthesia." Moxibustion, which is traditionally used to turn breech babies, has been used with some success, although systematic reviews and meta-analyses have yielded insufficient evidence to support its efficacy.[36] In general, few well-designed trials of TCM herbal formulas have been conducted,[31] and the need for improving the methodological quality of TCM research has been identified.[37–39]

Safety

Adverse events with acupuncture are rare, including acupuncture with cupping and moxibustion.[35] Needles must be sterile and disposable needles are often used to reduce the risk of disease transmission. Acupuncture should be avoided or used cautiously in individuals with heart disease, seizures, infections, bleeding disorders, or neurologic disorders, or among individuals using antithrombotic drugs because of theoretical or reported adverse effects.[5] Acupuncture should be avoided on areas that have received radiation therapy and for conditions of unknown medical origin. Caution is advised during pregnancy. Frail older adults or otherwise medically complex patients should use acupuncture with caution. Electroacupuncture should be avoided in patients with an arrhythmia or seizure disorder and in patients with pacemakers.

Cupping commonly leaves a temporary bruising of the skin. Moxibustion may also leave a temporary discoloration on the skin, which may be washed off or will disappear on its own. Historically, some traditional providers of moxibustion have intentionally employed more aggressive use of the technique to an extent that might leave minor scarring, but this aggressive form of practice is not regularly used in the West.

Chinese herbs have been associated with adverse effects. According to a 2004 FDA ruling, more than 1500 cases of serious toxicity, including death related to the use of ephedra or ma huang (*Ephedra sinica*) have been reported. Some Chinese herbal products have contained toxins or heavy metals. In addition, prescription drugs such as corticosteroids have been included in the preparations but not listed as ingredients.[40] Patients should purchase Chinese herbs from trustworthy sources and should be aware that Chinese herbs can interact with other herbs, foods, and drugs.

Chiropractic Care

Chiropractic focuses on the relationship between spinal structure and body function mediated by the nervous system. It originated in 1895 with D. D. Palmer, a popular hands-on healer practicing in Davenport, Iowa. The formulation of *chiropractic* combined the Greek *cheir* (hand) and *praxis* (practice). Palmer's original philosophy described the approach as connecting "man the spiritual" to "man the physical" by eliminating interference to the flow of "Innate Intelligence" through each individual. This innate intelligence, an almost metaphysical phenomenon, flows through the nervous system. The clearer the nervous system is, the more the innate intelligence can express itself and fully enliven the person's body and organs.[41]

Important distinctions exist between the profession of chiropractic, chiropractic care, and spinal manipulation. A chiropractor delivers chiropractic care that is a full range of treatment delivered in one or more therapeutic encounters. Treatment includes procedures and techniques of assessment and a tailored mix of therapeutic interventions to improve a patient's health status. The term *spinal manipulation* or *spinal adjustment* does not operationally define the profession or chiropractic care, although it is a well-known procedure. Chiropractic care also includes other procedures, such as exercise, dietary advice, ergonomic and lifestyle advice, supplements, all forms of physical therapy and rehabilitation intervention, and referral to other providers as necessary.

Techniques

Patients usually lie face down on a Cox table, which is similar to a massage table with an open space in which to place the face. Depending on the technique used, chiropractic visits may last 15 minutes to 1 hour or more. Chiropractors may see clients up to 3 times a week initially and then less frequently over time.

Patients can be diagnosed by different procedures including X-ray, computed tomography, magnetic resonance imaging, electrical current, and ultrasound therapy. Thermography may also be used, followed by treatment with ice packs and heat packs.

More than 100 chiropractic and spinal manipulative adjusting techniques may be employed. Spinal manipulative therapy uses many techniques to apply force to an area of the spine joint. Massage or mobilization of soft tissue is used in techniques such as myofascial trigger point therapy, cross-friction massage, active release therapy, muscle stripping, Rolfing, or other forms of structural integration. Mechanical traction or the use of external resistance on the spine may also be used. The cracking sound has typically been associated with cavitation in the spinal zygapophyseal (the neural arch between the joint processes) joints. The cracking or popping of a joint has not been proven to be essential to a clinically effective manipulation.

Training

Chiropractic is one of the largest and best-established professions of CAM in the United States. According to the U.S. Department of Labor, the estimated employment of chiropractors in 2012 was 27,740 practitioners.[42] The Council on Chiropractic Education accredits programs and institutions offering the Doctor of Chiropractic degree, which currently includes 15 schools in the United States and 2 in Canada (www.cce-usa.org/DCP_Representatives.html). According to the Federation of Chiropractic Licensing Boards, all 50 states have formal statutes that recognize and regulate the practice of chiropractic (http://directory.fclb.org/Statistics.aspx).

According to the American Chiropractic Association, a typical applicant to a chiropractic college has completed 4 years of undergraduate coursework. The curriculum of a chiropractic college includes didactic coursework and clinical training totaling a minimum of 4200 hours. Clinical training with actual patients typically lasts a minimum of 1 year. Specialty training is available through residency programs, which may require an additional 2–3 years of clinical training. Before they are allowed to practice, doctors of chiropractic must pass national board examinations and become licensed. Chiropractors generally do not prescribe drugs, but those who are also licensed naturopaths or other health care professionals may prescribe remedies according to the respective guidelines in the state in which they practice (www.acatoday.org/patients/index.cfm; select FAQs).

Theory/Evidence

Designing clinical trials to evaluate the efficacy of chiropractic is difficult, primarily because of the issues in developing an appropriate control. Other major issues include a potentially strong placebo effect and the high rate of spontaneous recovery. In addition, patients often seek chiropractic treatment for conditions with poorly understood pathologies, such as fibromyalgia; available evidence is insufficient to support the use of chiropractic for this condition.[43] For low back pain, sufficient evidence from both blinded and nonblinded trials supports the use of spinal manipulation, although the benefits are modest and of uncertain clinical significance.[44] Chiropractic has been used to treat many conditions including asthma, colic, ear infection, headache, whiplash, and hypertension, although evidence is insufficient to support efficacy for these conditions.[20]

Safety

The safety of chiropractic is controversial. Some systematic reviews show that spinal manipulation is associated with mild-moderate adverse effects. The most common serious adverse effects with spinal manipulation are vertebral artery dissection and stroke (VADS).[45] A 2010 review revealed 26 deaths associated with chiropractic spinal manipulation, and many more fatalities may be unpublished.[46] However, despite the increasing popularity of chiropractic and its association with potentially fatal adverse events such as VADS, myelopathy, vertebral disc extrusion, and epidural hematoma, few studies have properly evaluated the safety of chiropractic.[47] Whether the adverse effects are directly related to spinal manipulation or to sampling bias of patients is unclear. Case-control studies suggested a causal role,[46] although patients predisposed to VADS may be more likely to seek chiropractic treatment, suggesting a potential sampling bias.[48] A 2009 systematic review showed that adverse events occurred with a frequency of 33%–60.9%, but serious adverse events were rare (as few as 1.46 serious adverse events and 2.68 deaths for every 10 million manipulations).[47] Although this study did not support a strong causal relationship between chiropractic manipulation and the adverse events, the authors stated further high-quality studies are needed to assess its safety.

Patients with osteoporosis or any type of acute arthritis should either avoid chiropractic adjustment or use it cautiously because of the risk of fracture. Caution is also warranted in patients with bleeding disorders, migraines, and tumors or metastases to the spine. Patients with symptoms of vertebrobasilar vascular insufficiency, aneurysms, arteritis, or unstable spondylolisthesis should avoid chiropractic care. Patients receiving anticoagulant therapy should also be advised to avoid chiropractic care.[5]

A final consideration with this health system is that chiropractors have traditionally discouraged the use of routine vaccinations.[49] Although this attitude may be less likely now, Western health care providers, including pharmacists, should be aware of this aspect of chiropractic care.

Ayurveda

Ayurveda originated in India more than 5000 years ago and is probably the world's oldest system of natural medicine.[50] When translated, *Ayurveda* means science of life, which stems from the spiritual teachings known as the Vedas. Ayurveda may be the original basis for Chinese medicine and is an integrated system of specific theories and techniques that employ diet, herbs, exercise, meditation, yoga, and massage or bodywork. The goal of Ayurveda is to achieve optimal health on physical, psychological, and spiritual levels.

In India, Ayurveda involves the eight principal branches of medicine: pediatrics, gynecology, obstetrics, ophthalmology, geriatrics, otolaryngology, general medicine, and surgery. In Western countries, the practice of Ayurveda is less focused on its spiritual roots than on its use as a form of CAM. Ayurveda relies on the individual's willingness to participate in lifestyle and behavior changes.

Technique

Ayurveda teaches that vital energy (*prana*) is the basis of all life and healing.[50] As *prana* circulates throughout the human body, it is governed by the five elements of earth, air, fire, water, and ether. The five elements combine with one another into pairs called *doshas* that include *vata* (ether and air), *pitta* (fire and water), and *kapha* (earth and water). Health is a state of balance and harmony among the five elements, and illness occurs when there is an imbalance or lack of harmony among them.

The regulation of diet as a form of therapy is a central idea in Ayurveda. An individual's temperament and mental and spiritual development can be influenced by the quality and quantity of food consumed. An important principle in Ayurveda is that "there is nothing in the world that is not a medicine or food." Foods and herbs are described in terms of their energetic qualities rather than chemical properties. Sweet foods (called *madhura*) provide nourishment and coolness and also aid in increasing body weight. Sour foods (called *amla*) provide warmth and aid in weight gain. Salty foods (*lavana*) provide warmth, stimulate the senses, and aid weight gain. In contrast, bitter foods (*katu*) provide coolness and help weight loss. Pungent foods (*tikta*) also aid in weight loss but provide warmth and stimulation. Numerous herbs and spices including turmeric and cumin are used in Ayurveda.[50]

Ayurveda holds that each 24-hour cycle is divided into 4-hour segments governed by the *doshas*. These time periods are believed to correspond with nature. Ayurvedic providers guide patients to plan their activities to be in harmony with these natural principles of timing.[50]

A provider usually interviews the patient about his or her medical history. The provider then palpates the patient's wrist to determine subtle qualities of the pulse. Providers may also evaluate the appearance of the tongue, face, lips, nails, or eyes. Laboratory tests of blood, urine, and stools may be used to help with diagnosis. The initial consultation is usually the longest and lasts from 45 to 90 minutes or longer. Follow-up consultations may be spaced by several weeks or months to monitor the individual's progress. Follow-up will usually be brief office visits involving a diagnostic review and an adjustment of the regimen.[50]

Training

In India, more than 150 undergraduate and 30 postgraduate institutions for Ayurvedic medicine exist, and according to the NCCAM, the standard length of training is at least 5 years. Despite the abundance of institutions, the standard of Ayurvedic education in India is poorly structured and largely unregulated, which has resulted in a global negative perception of the practice.[51]

According to NCCAM, no national standard for Ayurvedic training or certification exists in the United States. Ayurveda is practiced in Western medicine by health care providers who are licensed in a variety of disciplines.[50] Allopathic and osteopathic physicians, naturopaths, acupuncturists, nurses, massage therapists, and chiropractors may all practice Ayurveda. Health counselors, educators, or consultants may also incorporate Ayurveda into their practices without specific licensing. In Western countries, two major approaches to training and practice exist. The first is offered by diverse teachers and providers, many of whom are either from India or were trained there. The second consists of devotees of Maharishi Mahesh Yogi, the Indian spiritual teacher who introduced Transcendental Meditation (TM) to the West. In 1980, this group coined the term *Maharishi Ayur-Ved,* a practice that incorporates TM as part of an Ayurvedic approach.

Theory/Evidence

Some of the more metaphysical aspects of Ayurveda, such as harmony between the body and the universe, are difficult to assess with modern scientific methods.[11] Several herbal formulations have been studied in Western-style clinical trials; currently, evidence is inadequate to recommend Ayurveda for any indication.

Safety

Many different Ayurvedic herbs exist, and they are frequently taken in combination with other herbs and/or minerals. Safety and toxicity will vary depending on the herb and its preparation. In general, Ayurvedic herbal medicines should be used cautiously because their potencies may not be tested or standardized. Therapeutic levels of sildenafil have been detected in Ayurvedic herbal preparations used for aphrodisiac purposes.[52] Patients should purchase Ayurvedic herbs from trustworthy sources and should be aware that Ayurvedic herbs can interact with other herbs, foods, and drugs. For example, ginger, which is commonly used in Ayurveda, may increase the risk of bleeding when used with anticoagulants or antiplatelet drugs.[8]

Heavy metal contamination continues to be a concern in Ayurvedic medicines. In addition to herbs, Ayurvedic formulas known as *rasa shastra* may also contain metals such as arsenic, mercury, or zinc. Providers claim that these medicines are safe when properly prepared and administered. However, from 1978 to 2009, at least 80 cases of heavy metal poisoning worldwide have been linked to Ayurvedic medicine.[53] According to the U.S. Centers for Disease Control and Prevention, 12 cases of lead poisoning in five states were associated with Ayurvedic medicines from 2000 to 2003. Even herbal Ayurvedic formulas may contain heavy metals; a recent study found that approximately 20% of purported herb-only formulas contained detectable metals compared with 40% of *rasa shastra* medicines.[54] Consequently, patients are advised to use Ayurvedic herbs cautiously. Products that have USP seals of quality approval have been tested and should not contain unacceptable levels of harmful metals. Product testing information is also available from sites such as ConsumerLab (see Chapter 50).

Massage

Soft tissue manipulation has been practiced for thousands of years in diverse cultures. Chinese use of massage dates to 1600 BC, and Hippocrates referred to the importance of physicians being experienced with "rubbing" as early as 400 BC.[5]

Massage spread throughout Europe during the Renaissance and was introduced in the United States in the 1850s. By the early 1930s, massage became a less prominent part of Western medicine. Interest in therapeutic massage resurged in the 1970s, particularly among athletes to promote well-being, relaxation, analgesia, stress relief, healing of musculoskeletal injuries, sleep enhancement, and quality of life. Massage is one of the most common forms of CAM therapy used in the United States.[19]

A common goal of massage therapy is to help the body heal itself. Touch is fundamental to massage therapy and is used by therapists to locate painful or tense areas, to determine how much pressure to apply, and to establish a therapeutic relationship with clients. The term *toxic touch* refers to techniques with detrimental effects.

Technique

Different therapeutic techniques can be classified as massage therapy. Most involve the application of fixed or moving pressure or manipulation of the clients' muscles and connective tissues. Providers may use their hands or other areas such as forearms, elbows, or feet. Lubricants may be used to aid the smoothness of massage strokes. Examples of massage therapy include Swedish massage, sports massage, deep tissue massage, and trigger point massage.

Training

Training requirements for massage therapy vary in the United States, but they generally involve 500–1000 hours for certification by the National Certification Board for Therapeutic Massage and Bodywork. Over 1000 massage training programs exist, and some have received accreditation by the Commission on Massage Therapy Accreditation, which is recognized by the U.S. Department of Education as a specialized accrediting agency. Upon fulfilling the necessary requirements, massage therapists receive the designation of Nationally Certified in Therapeutic Massage and Bodywork. A national examination is available from the National Certification Board for Therapeutic Massage and Bodywork. Most states require massage therapists to be certified before practicing.

Theory/Evidence

Research on massage therapy is limited, and published studies frequently use a variety of techniques and trial designs. The effectiveness of massage has not been established for any health condition, although it remains popular for improving relaxation, mood, and overall well-being, particularly in palliative care.[55]

Safety

Few adverse effects have been reported with massage.[5] Fractures, discomfort, bruising, swelling of massaged tissues, and liver hematoma have been reported. Vigorous massage should be avoided in patients with bleeding disorders, peripheral vascular disease, or thrombocytopenia, or in those receiving antithrombotic therapy. According to preliminary data, blood pressure may increase in healthy patients following vigorous massage (e.g., trigger point therapy, which focuses on painful muscle knots); however, in patients with hypertension, massage may lower blood pressure. Areas that should not be massaged include those with osteoporotic and other fractures, open/healing skin wounds, skin infections,

table

52–1 Common Health Issues with Evidence of Benefit from CAM

Condition	CAM Treatment
Osteoarthritis	Acupuncture
Chronic pain, fibromyalgia, postoperative pain	Acupuncture
Nausea	Acupressure
Low back pain	Chiropractic
Quality of life in cancer patients	Massage
Anxiety and stress	Therapeutic touch

Key: CAM = Complementary and alternative medicine.

recent surgery, or blood clots. Massage and other touch-based therapies should be used cautiously in patients with a history of physical abuse. Women who are pregnant should consult their obstetrician before beginning massage therapy. Allergies or skin irritation can occur with the oils used in massages, such as olive and mineral oil.

Massage has not been evaluated as a method to diagnose medical conditions. Massage should not be used as a substitute for more proven therapies for medical conditions.

Conclusion

Patients increasingly seek care from CAM providers and health systems. Although some historical and scientific evidence supports the effectiveness of some approaches, general statements are difficult to make on the safety and efficacy of CAM. Important components of clinical trials, such as placebo controls and blinding, are difficult to achieve and, as a result, evidence is limited. Because the use of CAM continues to increase, both patients and providers should be informed about the potential risks and benefits of CAM techniques. (See Table 52–1 for common evidence-based uses of CAM health systems.)

More patients are using the Internet for health information before consulting health care providers. As information has become increasingly available, patients have increased their responsibility for their health decisions and should be encouraged to tell their health care providers whether they are also using any CAM approaches to their health. Similarly, all Western health care providers, including pharmacists, must be knowledgeable about CAM health systems and the evidence that supports or refutes their use.

Key Points for CAM Health Systems

➤ The term *complementary and alternative medicine* (CAM) is generally regarded as a broad group of healing philosophies, diagnostic approaches, and therapeutic interventions that do not conform to the conventional Western health system. The most common CAM therapies and health systems include homeopathy, naturopathy, traditional Chinese medicine (TCM)/acupuncture, chiropractic care, Ayurveda, and massage.

➤ Homeopathy is based on the principle of "like cures like," which states that if a substance produces the symptoms of an illness in large doses, that same substance can cure it in very minute dosages. The effectiveness of homeopathy currently cannot be determined for any clinical condition, although the risk of toxicity is low.

➤ Naturopathy employs natural forces such as light, heat, air, water, and massage; this therapy focuses on building health rather than on treating disease. Naturopathy is based on six principles: (1) the healing power of nature, (2) identifying and treating the cause, (3) doing no harm, (4) treating the whole person, (5) the physician as teacher, and (6) preventing disease. The licensing of naturopathic doctors varies depending on state laws.

➤ TCM includes herbal medicine as well as various techniques such as acupuncture, moxibustion, and cupping. TCM is dependent on the life force (*qi*), which circulates through the body through meridians (channels) connecting all major organs. *Qi* consists of *yin* and *yang*, which are opposite and complementary qualities. Illness results when these forces are unbalanced. An acupuncturist inserts sterilized needles into channels of energy to try to restore balance to the patient's *qi*.

➤ Chiropractic focuses on the relationship between spinal structure and body function mediated by the nervous system. The most common adverse event is mild localized discomfort, although adverse events including death have been reported.

➤ Ayurveda is an integrated system employing diet, herbs, exercise, meditation, yoga, and massage or bodywork. Ayurveda teaches that vital energy (*prana*) is the basis of all life and healing. As *prana* circulates throughout the body, it is governed by the five elements of earth, air, fire, water, and ether. The five elements combine with one another into pairs called *doshas*, which include *vata* (ether and air), *pitta* (fire and water), and *kapha* (earth and water). Ayurvedic herbs may interact with other drugs, herbs, and foods.

➤ Touch is fundamental to massage therapy and is used by therapists to locate painful or tense areas, to determine how much pressure to apply, and to establish a therapeutic relationship with clients.

REFERENCES

1. Ulbricht CE, Cohen L, Lee R. Complementary, alternative, and integrative therapies in cancer care. In: Devita VT, ed. *Devita, Hellman, and Rosenberg's Cancer: Principles & Practice of Oncology.* 8th ed. Philadelphia, PA: Wolters Kluwer/Lippincott Williams & Wilkins; 2008.
2. Vickers A, Zollman C. ABC of complementary medicine. Massage therapies. *BMJ.* 1999;319(7219):1254–7.
3. Cassileth BR. 'Complementary' or 'alternative'? It makes a difference in cancer care. *Complement Ther Med.* 1999;7:35–7.
4. U.S. Department of Health and Human Services, National Institutes of Health. CAM basics. What is complementary and alternative medicine? May 2012. Accessed at http://nccam.nih.gov/sites/nccam.nih.gov/files/D347_05-25-2012.pdf, July 28, 2014.
5. Natural Standard: The Authority on Integrative Medicine. 2013. Accessed at http://www.naturalstandard.com, August 19, 2013.
6. Ulbricht C, Seamon E. *Natural Standard Herbal Pharmacotherapy: An Evidence-Based Approach.* St. Louis, MO: Mosby/Elsevier; 2009.
7. Mercurio R, Eliott JA. Trick or treat? Australian newspaper portrayal of complementary and alternative medicine for the treatment of cancer. *Support Care Cancer.* 2011;19(1):67–80.
8. Ulbricht C, Chao W, Costa D, et al. Clinical evidence of herb-drug interactions: a systematic review by the natural standard research collaboration. *Curr Drug Metab.* 2008;9(10):1063–120.

9. National Center for Complementary and Alternative Medicine (NCCAM). NCCAM facts-at-a-glance and mission. Accessed at http://nccam.nih.gov/about/ataglance, July 28, 2014.

10. Jadad AR, Moore RA, Carroll D, et al. Assessing the quality of reports of randomized clinical trials: is blinding necessary? *Control Clin Trials.* 1996;17(1):1–12.

11. Valiathan MS, Thatte U. Ayurveda: the time to experiment. *Int J Ayurveda Res.* 2010;1(1):3.

12. Mehling WE, DiBlasi Z, Hecht F. Bias control in trials of bodywork: a review of methodological issues. *J Altern Complement Med.* 2005; 11(2):333–42.

13. Schnyer RN, Allen JJ. Bridging the gap in complementary and alternative medicine research: manualization as a means of promoting standardization and flexibility of treatment in clinical trials of acupuncture. *J Altern Complement Med.* 2002;8(5):623–34.

14. Birch S. A review and analysis of placebo treatments, placebo effects, and placebo controls in trials of medical procedures when sham is not inert. *J Altern Complement Med.* 2006;12(3):303–10.

15. Wong LY, Toh MP, Kong KH. Barriers to patient referral for complementary and alternative medicines and its implications on interventions. *Complement Ther Med.* 2010;18(3–4):135–42.

16. Thompson EA, Bishop JL, Northstone K. The use of homeopathic products in childhood: data generated over 8.5 years from the Avon Longitudinal Study of Parents and Children (ALSPAC). *J Altern Complement Med.* 2010;16(1):69–79.

17. Ulbricht C, Chao W, Clark A, et al. Oscillococcinum (Anas barbariae hepatis et cordis extractum 200CK HPUS). *Altern Comp Ther.* 2011;17:41–9.

18. Borneman JP, Field RI. Regulation of homeopathic drug products. *Am J Health Syst Pharm.* 2006;63(1):86–91.

19. Barnes PM, Bloom B, Nahin RL. Complementary and alternative medicine use among adults and children: United States, 2007. *Natl Health Stat Rep.* 2008;12:1–23.

20. Ernst E, Gilbey A. Chiropractic claims in the English-speaking world. *N Z Med J.* 2010;123(1312):36–44.

21. Merrell WC, Shalts E. Homeopathy. *Med Clin North Am.* 2002;86(1): 47–62.

22. Ernst E. Homeopathy: what does the "best" evidence tell us? *Med J Aust.* 2010;192(8):458–60.

23. Stehlin I. Homeopathy: real medicine or empty promises? *FDA Consum.* 1996;30:15–9.

24. Marian F, Joost K, Saini KD, et al. Patient satisfaction and side effects in primary care: an observational study comparing homeopathy and conventional medicine. *BMC Complement Altern Med.* 2008;8:52.

25. Lim JH, Davis GE, Wang Z, et al. Zicam-induced damage to mouse and human nasal tissue. *PLoS One.* 2009;4(10):e7647.

26. Utah Department of Administrative Services, Division of Administrative Rules. Naturopathic Physician Practice Act Rule. Accessed at http://www.rules.utah.gov/publicat/code/r156/r156-71.htm, July 28, 2014.

27. Vermont Secretary of State. Administrative Rules for Naturopathic Physicians. Accessed at https://www.sec.state.vt.us/media/166567/NAT_Rules.pdf, July 28, 2014.

28. Wang SM, Kain ZN, White P. Acupuncture analgesia, I: the scientific basis. *Anesth Analg.* 2008;106(2):602–10.

29. Cooley K, Szczurko O, Perri D, et al. Naturopathic care for anxiety: a randomized controlled trial ISRCTN78958974. *PLoS One.* 2009;4(8):e6628.

30. Skalli S, Zaid A, Soulaymani R. Drug interactions with herbal medicines. *Ther Drug Monit.* 2007;29(6):679–86.

31. Shea JL. Applying evidence-based medicine to traditional Chinese medicine: debate and strategy. *J Altern Complement Med.* 2006;12(3):255–63.

32. Xutian S, Zhang J, Louise W. New exploration and understanding of traditional Chinese medicine. *Am J Chin Med.* 2009;37(3):411–26.

33. Wong M. La Medecine Chinoise par les Plantes. Paris: Tchou; 1976.

34. Hucker CO. *China's Imperial Past: an Introduction to Chinese History and Culture.* Stanford, CA: Stanford University Press; 1997.

35. Yu D, Morris-Natschke SL, Lee KH. New developments in natural products-based anti-AIDS research. *Med Res Rev.* 2007;27(1):108–32.

36. Coyle ME, Smith CA, Peat B. Cephalic version by moxibustion for breech presentation. *Cochrane Database Syst Rev.* 2005;2:CD003928. doi: 10.1002/14651858.CD3928. Accessed at http://www.thecochranelibrary.com/view/0/index.html.

37. Xue CC, Zhang AL, Greenwood KM, et al. Traditional Chinese medicine: an update on clinical evidence. *J Altern Complement Med.* 2010; 16(3):301–12.

38. Wen BL, Jia CS, Liu WH, et al. [Thinking about academic development of acupuncture and moxibustion in recent ten years]. *Zhongguo Zhen Jiu.* 2009;29(12):949–54.

39. Xiao X, Xiao P, Wang Y. [Some key issues about scientific research on traditional Chinese medicine]. *Zhongguo Zhong Yao Za Zhi.* 2009;34(2):119–23.

40. Keane FM, Munn SE, du Vivier AW, et al. Analysis of Chinese herbal creams prescribed for dermatological conditions. BMJ. 1999 Feb 27; 318(7183):563–4.

41. Holisticonline. Chiropractic, History. Accessed at holisticonline.com/chiropractic/chiro_history.htm, July 28, 2014

42. U.S. Department of Labor, Bureau of Labor Statistics. May 2012 National Occupational Employment and Wage Estimates: United States. Accessed at http://www.bls.gov/oes/2012/may/oes_nat.htm#29-0000, July 28, 2014.

43. Ernst E. Chiropractic treatment for fibromyalgia: a systematic review. *Clin Rheumatol.* 2009;28(10):1175–8.

44. Walker BF, French SD, Grant W, et al. Combined chiropractic interventions for low-back pain. *Cochrane Database Syst Rev.* 2010;4:CD005427. doi: 10.1002/14651858.CD005427.pub2. Accessed at http://www.thecochranelibrary.com/view/0/index.html.

45. Paciaroni M, Bogousslavsky J. Cerebrovascular complications of neck manipulation. *Eur Neurol.* 2009;61(2):112–8.

46. Ernst E. Deaths after chiropractic: a review of published cases. *Int J Clin Pract.* 2010;64(8):1162–5.

47. Gouveia LO, Castanho P, Ferreira JJ. Safety of chiropractic interventions: a systematic review. *Spine.* 2009;34:E405–13.

48. Murphy DR. Current understanding of the relationship between cervical manipulation and stroke: what does it mean for the chiropractic profession? *Chiropr Osteopat.* 2010;18:22.

49. Busse JW, Wilson K, Campbell JB. Attitudes towards vaccination among chiropractic and naturopathic students. *Vaccine.* 2008;26(49):6237–43.

50. Sharma H, Chandola HM, Singh G, et al. Utilization of Ayurveda in health care: an approach for prevention, health promotion, and treatment of disease, part 1: Ayurveda, the science of life. *J Altern Complement Med.* 2007;13(9):1011–9.

51. Patwardhan K, Gehlot S, Singh G, et al. Global challenges of graduate level Ayurvedic education: a survey. *Int J Ayurveda Res.* 2010;1(1):49–54.

52. Savaliya AA, Shah RP, Prasad B, et al. Screening of Indian aphrodisiac ayurvedic/herbal healthcare products for adulteration with sildenafil, tadalafil and/or vardenafil using LC/PDA and extracted ion LC-MS/TOF. *J Pharm Biomed Anal.* 2010;52(3):406–9.

53. Kales SN, Saper RB. Ayurvedic lead poisoning: an under-recognized, international problem. *Indian J Med Sci.* 2009;63(9):379–81.

54. Saper RB, Phillips RS, Sehgal A, et al. Lead, mercury, and arsenic in US- and Indian-manufactured Ayurvedic medicines sold via the Internet. *JAMA.* 2008;300(8):915–23.

55. Gray RA. The use of massage therapy in palliative care. *Complement Ther Nurs Midwifery.* 2000;6(2):77–82.

FDA PREGNANCY RISK CATEGORIES FOR SELECTED NONPRESCRIPTION MEDICATIONS AND NUTRITIONAL SUPPLEMENTS

Drug therapy during pregnancy may sometimes be necessary. However, because most drugs cross the placenta to some extent, a mother who takes a drug might expose her fetus to it. Medications should be used during pregnancy only under the supervision of a physician and only when the potential benefits outweigh the potential risks.

The table on the following pages contains Food and Drug Administration (FDA) categories for evaluating the safety of drugs during pregnancy for many of the nonprescription medications discussed in this book. The listed categories pertain to the particular strengths or formulations in which the nonprescription medications are available. Prescription strengths or formulations of a medication may have different pregnancy risk categories. Categories that bear a subscript M (e.g., C_M) were assigned by the manufacturer. The majority of the remaining categories were assigned by drug information sources based on available clinical information. *Drugs in Pregnancy and Lactation: A Reference Guide to Fetal and Neonatal Risk* is the primary information source. The pregnancy risk categories are defined as follows:

A Adequate studies in pregnant women have not demonstrated a risk to the fetus in the first trimester of pregnancy, and there is no evidence of risk in later trimesters.

B Animal studies have not demonstrated a risk to the fetus, but there are no adequate studies in pregnant women ... or ... Animal studies have shown an adverse effect, but adequate studies in pregnant women have not demonstrated a risk to the fetus during the first trimester of pregnancy, and there is no evidence of risk in later trimesters.

C Animal studies have shown an adverse effect on the fetus, but there are no adequate studies in humans; the benefits from the use of the drug in pregnant women may be acceptable despite its potential risks ... or ... There are no animal reproduction studies and no adequate studies in humans.

D There is evidence of human fetal risk, but the potential benefits from the use of the drug in pregnant women may be acceptable despite its potential risks.

X Studies in animals or humans demonstrate fetal abnormalities, or adverse reaction reports indicate evidence of fetal risk. The risk of use in a pregnant woman clearly outweighs any possible benefit. Use of drugs with this rating is contraindicated in women who are or may become pregnant.

Medication	Pregnancy Risk Category Rating
Acesulfame potassium	No rating[b]
Acetaminophen	B
Alcloxa	No rating[b]
Alpha galactosidase	No rating[b]
Alpha hydroxy acid	No rating[b]
Aluminum acetate	No rating[b]
Aluminum chloride	C[a]
Aluminum hydroxide	C[a]
Aluminum sulfate	No rating[b]
Aminobenzoic acid (PABA)	C[a]
Ammonium chloride	B
Ammonium lactate	B[M]
Antazoline	No rating[b]

(Continued)

Medication	Pregnancy Risk Category Rating
Ascorbic acid	See Vitamin C
Aspartame	B (C in women with phenylketonuria)
Aspirin	No rating[b] (D if full doses taken in 3rd trimester)
Avobenzone	No rating[b]
Bacitracin	C
Bentonite	No rating[b]
Benzocaine	C_M
Benzoyl peroxide	C
Benzyl alcohol	B_M
Beta-carotene	C
Biotin	B[a] (30 mcg/day recommended during pregnancy)
Bisacodyl	B
Bismuth	C
Brompheniramine	C_M
Butamben picrate	No rating[b]
Butenafine	C_M
Butoconazole	C_M
Caffeine	B
Calamine	No rating[b]
Calcium carbonate	C[a]
Calcium citrate	C[a]
Calcium gluconate	C_M
Calcium polycarbophil	No rating[b]
Camphor	C
Capsaicin	B_M
Carbamide peroxide	No rating[b]
Casanthranol	C
Cascara sagrada	C
Castor oil	C (avoid; oxytocic effects)
Cetirizine	B_M
Charcoal, activated	No rating[b]
Chlophedianol	No rating[b]
Chlorhexidine gluconate	B
Chlorpheniramine	B
Choline	C[a]
Chromium	No rating[b]
Cimetidine	B_M
Cinoxate	No rating[b]
Clemastine	B_M
Clotrimazole	B
Coal tar	C[a]
Codeine	C (D if used for prolonged periods or in high doses at term)
Colloidal oatmeal	No rating[b]
Copper	No rating[b]
Cromolyn	B_M
Cyanocobalamin	See Vitamin B_{12}
Cyclizine	B

Medication	Pregnancy Risk Category Rating
Dexbrompheniramine	C
Dexchlorpheniramine	B_M
Dexpanthenol	C_M
Dextromethorphan	C
Dibucaine	No rating[b]
Dimenhydrinate	B_M
Dimethisoquin hydrochloride	No rating[b]
Dioxybenzone	No rating[b]
Diphenhydramine	B_M
Docosanol	B[a]
Docusate calcium	C
Docusate potassium	C
Docusate sodium	C
Doxylamine	A
Dyclonine	C_M
Ecamsule (terephthalyidene dicamphor sulfonic acid)	No rating[b]
Ensulizole (phenyl benzimidazole sulfonic acid)	No rating[b]
Ephedrine	C
Epinephrine	C
Esomeprazole	C
Ethanol	D (X if used in large amounts or for prolonged periods)
Ethyl alcohol	See Ethanol
Famotidine	B_M
Fexofenadine	C_M
Fluoride	C[a] (doses up to 2 mg fluoride/day)
Folic acid	A (C if doses exceed RDA)
Fructose	No rating[b] (natural sources in diet)
Glycolic acid	No rating[b]
Glycerin	C_M
Homosalate	No rating[b]
Hydrocortisone	C (D if used in the 1st trimester)
Hydrogen peroxide	C[a]
Hydroquinone	C_M
Ibuprofen	B (D if used in 3rd trimester or near delivery)
Insulin	B (nonprescription insulins only)
Iodine	See Potassium iodide
Ipecac syrup	C[a]
Iron (fumarate, gluconate, and sulfate salts)	A (C if doses exceed RDA)[a]
Isopropyl alcohol in anhydrous glycerin	No rating[b]
Kaolin	C
Ketoconazole	C_M
Ketotifen	C_M
Lactic acid	C[a]
Lanolin	B[a]
Lansoprazole	B_M
Levmetamfetamine (L-desoxyephedrine)	No rating[b]

(Continued)

Medication	Pregnancy Risk Category Rating
Lidocaine	B_M
Loperamide	C_M
Loratadine	B_M
Magnesium citrate	C^b
Magnesium hydroxide	C^b
Magnesium salicylate	No rating[b]
Manganese	A (RDA during pregnancy is 2 mg/day; no rating if doses exceed RDA[b])
Meclizine	B_M
Menthol	No rating[b]
Meradimate (menthyl anthranilate)	No rating[b]
Methylcellulose	No rating[b]
Miconazole	C
Mineral oil	C
Minoxidil	C_M
Molybdenum	No rating[b]
Naphazoline	C_M
Naproxen sodium	C (D if used in 3rd trimester or near delivery)
Neomycin	C
Neotame	No rating[b]
Niacin	See Vitamin B_3
Niacinamide (nicotinamide)	A (C if doses exceed RDA)
Nicotine transdermal system	D_M
Nicotine polacrilex gum	C_M
Nizatidine	B_M
Nonoxynol-9	B^a
Octoxynol-9	No rating[b]
Octocrylene	C^a
Octinoxate (octyl methoxycinnamate)	C^a
Octisalate (octyl salicylate)	No rating[b]
Omeprazole	C_M
Orlistat	X
Oxybenzone	No rating[b]
Oxymetazoline	C
Padimate O	No rating[b]
Pamabrom	No rating[b]
Pantothenic acid	A (C if doses exceed RDA)
Permethrin	B_M
Petrolatum	C^a (poor dermal absorption)
Pheniramine	C
Phenol	No rating[b]
Phenylephrine hydrochloride	C
Phospholipids	No rating[b]
Phosphorus	No rating[b] (an essential nutrient)
Polyethylene glycol	C_M
Polymyxin B	B
Potassium iodide	D
Povidone–iodine	D

Medication	Pregnancy Risk Category Rating
Pramoxine	C_M
Propylene glycol	C^a
Propylhexedrine	No rating[b]
Pseudoephedrine	C
Psyllium	No rating[b]
Pyrantel pamoate	C
Pyrethrins	C
Pyridoxine	See Vitamin B_6
Pyrilamine	C
Pyrithione zinc	B^a
Ranitidine	B_M
Resorcinol	B^a
Riboflavin	See Vitamin B_2
Saccharin	C
Salicylic acid	No rating[b] (D if full doses used in 3rd trimester)
Selenium	No rating[b] (an essential element)
Selenium sulfide	C_M
Senna	C
Sennosides	See Senna
Simethicone	C
Sodium bicarbonate	C_M
Sodium chloride	C_M
Sodium citrate	No rating[b]
Sodium fluoride	C^a (doses up to 2 mg fluoride/day)
Sodium phosphate	No rating[b]
Sodium salicylate	C^a
Sorbitol	C_M
Sucralose	B^a
Sulfur	No rating[b]
Sulisobenzone	No rating[b]
Terbinafine	B_M
Tetracaine	C
Thiamine	See Vitamin B_1
Tioconazole	C_M
Titanium dioxide	C^a (does not cross placenta)
Tolnaftate	No rating[b]
Triethanolamine	No rating[b]
Tripelennamine	B
Trolamine salicylate	No rating[b]
Undecylenic acid	No rating[b]
Urea	C
Vitamin A	A (X if doses exceed RDA)
Vitamin B_1 (thiamine)	A (C if doses exceed RDA)
Vitamin B_2 (riboflavin)	A (C if doses exceed RDA)
Vitamin B_3 (niacin)	A (C if doses exceed RDA; C_M for doses used to treat hyperlipidemia)
Vitamin B^6 (pyridoxine)	A

(Continued)

Medication	Pregnancy Risk Category Rating
Vitamin B$_{12}$ (cyanocobalamin)	A (C if doses exceed RDA)
Vitamin C (ascorbic acid)	A (C if doses exceed RDA)
Vitamin D (calcitriol)	C$_M$ (D if used in doses above the RDA)
Vitamin D$_2$ (ergocalciferol)	A (D if doses exceed RDA)
Vitamin D$_3$ (cholecalciferol)	C (D if used in doses above the RDA)
Vitamin E (tocopherols)	A (C if doses exceed RDA)
Vitamins, multiple	A (risk factor varies for amounts exceeding RDAs)
Witch hazel	No rating[b]
Xylometazoline	C[a]
Xylitol	No rating[b] (natural sources in diet)
Zinc acetate	No rating[b] (RDA 15 mg/day)
Zinc oxide	C[a] (poor dermal absorption)

[a] Source references did not provide pregnancy risk category. Category is instead based on available clinical information.

[b] Source references did not provide pregnancy risk category. Insufficient clinical information is available to support a rating.

Sources:

Briggs GG, Freeman RK, Yaffe SJ. *Drugs in Pregnancy and Lactation: A Reference Guide to Fetal and Neonatal Risk.* 8th ed. Philadelphia, PA: Lippincott Williams & Wilkins; 2008.

Wickersham RM, Scott JA, Novak KK, managing eds. *Drug Facts and Comparisons.* St. Louis, MO: Wolters Kluwer Health, Inc.; 2011.

Lexi-Drugs Online™ [subscription database]. Hudson, OH: Lexi-Comp, Inc.; 2011. Accessed at http://online.lexi.com.

Micromedex® Healthcare Series [subscription database]. Greenwood Village, CO: Thomson Reuters (Healthcare) Inc. Updated periodically. Accessed at http://www.thomsonhc.com.

SAFETY ISSUES WITH THE USE OF SELECTED NATURAL PRODUCTS IN PREGNANCY

Natural Product	Pregnancy Risk Category Rating	Risk Summary
Black cohosh	None	A case report of a woman given a mixture of black cohosh and blue cohosh during labor reported the birth of an infant with severe neurologic impairments. Blue cohosh is unrelated to black cohosh. Black cohosh was associated with estrogenic changes in vaginal cells at 12 weeks in one study and no changes in another. Studies are also mixed for in vitro assays of estrogen activity.
Butterbur	Not recommended	Metabolites of butterbur have been shown to inhibit endocrine function. Butterbur should also be avoided in pregnancy because of its potential hepatotoxicity.
Chastetree berry	Not recommended	Chastetree berry is reported to be a uterine stimulant, so its use in pregnancy should be avoided. Mastodynon (a product containing chastetree berry) was administered to rats at 80 times the human dose, without any noted adverse effects. Teratogenic studies using Mastodynon also found no anomalies in the fetuses. Chastetree berry products may reduce prolactin levels, which has been demonstrated in both animal and human trials.
Chondroitin	C (no human data; probably compatible)	Injection of pregnant mice during gestation produced an increase in cleft palate and tail abnormalities in offspring. In another study, no adverse effects were seen in offspring after administration of chondroitin.
Colostrum	No human data	No studies that document use in humans or animals are available.
Devil's claw	Not recommended	Devil's claw has oxytocic effects in animals; therefore, its use in pregnancy is not recommended.
DHEA	None	DHEA-S (in the sulfated form) has been reported to facilitate midtrimester abortion. It has also been used for the induction of labor at term. No teratogenic effects were observed among the offspring of pregnant rabbits treated with DHEA at doses as high as 125 mg/kd/day. Studies in mice and rats, however, have shown androgenic effects such as masculinization of the external genitalia of female pups. DHEA also inhibits pregnancy development in mice when administered early in the pregnancy.
Echinacea	C (limited human data)	No animal reproductive study has been conducted to examine the effects of echinacea or its components. A prospective cohort study documented the use of echinacea by 206 pregnant women. Of these, 112 women documented use during the first trimester. After matching of data between the study and control arms, no statistically significant differences were observed in live births, spontaneous abortions, induced abortions, gestational age, birth weight, fetal distress, or major malformations. This led the authors to conclude that echinacea posed no major risk of an anomaly.
Eleuthero	None	Secondary resources have not reported teratogenic effects with eleuthero use in mink, sheep, or rats. This effect was determined to be without regard to dose or trimester of pregnancy.
Evening primrose oil	C (probably compatible)	In 2003, a review of pregnancy outcomes in patients taking herbal medications concluded that evening primrose oil (EPO) was safe for use in the induction of labor. A randomized, double-blind, placebo-controlled trial compared the effect of evening primrose oil versus placebo on the Bishop score and cervical length. No adverse affects of EPO were observed in fetuses. The effects of EPO in other stages of pregnancy have not been evaluated. Its use during pregnancy has not been recommended.

(Continued)

Natural Product	Pregnancy Risk Category Rating	Risk Summary
Fenugreek	No human data	In a study of rats fed fenugreek seeds as 30% of their diets, a reduction in litter size and weight was noted. Male rabbits were also noted to have reduced testes, damaged seminiferous tubules and interstitial tissue, and reduced androgen and sperm production.
Feverfew	Not recommended	A preliminary study found no adverse effects in rats receiving high doses of feverfew. The study, however, was limited by a small sample size. Feverfew has also been rumored to be an abortifacient. Use in pregnancy is not currently recommended.
Ginger	C (compatible, but recent data have suggested concern)	In a reproductive study in rats, consumption of ginger tea was associated with early embryonic loss at a rate double that of the control. Surviving fetuses were heavier and had more advanced skeletal growth. Another study administered ginger extract at a dose of 1000 mg/kg/day during organogenesis in rats; no differences in adverse effects or teratogenicity were noted. The use of ginger for hyperemesis gravidarum was studied in 27 women who reported relief of symptoms. No adverse effects were noted in the women, and no congenital abnormalities were noted in the 25 infants. One woman elected abortion for an unspecified reason, and another had a miscarriage in the 12th week of gestation.
Ginkgo	C (data suggest low risk)	Reproductive studies in animals have revealed no teratogenicity or mutagenicity. Doses as high as 1600 mg/kg were administered to pregnant rats without observing toxic effects. No mutagenic effects were observed in animal or human sperm exposed to *Ginkgo biloba*. Data are limited, however, and no trials have yet been conducted in humans.
Ginseng (tea)	B (animal data suggest low risk)	A reproductive study examined the effect of *Panax ginseng* on two generations of rats and noted no differences in behavior and in histopathologic examination at autopsies. Another study examined the use of *P. ginseng* as a fetal protectant for the compound hexavalent chromium in rats. Rats receiving *P. ginseng* for protection had better outcomes, such as fewer implantation losses, stillbirths, and skeletal anomalies. Three small reports have described estrogen-like effects such as vaginal bleeding in postmenopausal women taking ginseng. A retrospective study of 88 pregnant women taking ginseng and 88 matched controls found no differences in birthweight, preterm delivery, and stillbirths. No congenital malformations were observed.
Glucosamine	C (probably compatible, although information is limited)	In 1956, a study found no teratogenicity when glucosamine was administered to mice and rabbits. In a brief abstract in 2005, the exposure of pregnant women to glucosamine was documented. The study included 55 women; data are available for 34 subjects. Of the remainder, some pregnancies were still ongoing (20), and no data were provided for 1. For all subjects, a total of 33 live births and 3 spontaneous abortions were reported. The timing of exposures was not noted, and a correlation was not determined. Glucosamine is suspected to inhibit protein, RNA, and DNA synthesis. The percentage of free drug at the maternal/fetal interface is limited, and very little would have the potential to cross into the placenta.
Green tea	None	In two abstracts, tea drinking was associated with neural tube defects, but details on exposure or extent of association have not surfaced. Epigallocatechin gallate is a component of green tea that has some anticancer activity. In rats, this product did not affect embryo development or fertility, despite the subjects receiving very high doses. The caffeine content of green tea should also be considered.
5-HTP	No human data	No studies that document use in humans or animals are available.
Huperzine	No human data	No studies that document use in humans or animals are available.
Juniper tea	X (berries)	Juniper berries are abortifacient; juniper oil stimulates uterine contractions.
Lactobacillus	None	In a study of 127 women, use of *Lactobacillus* in the third trimester was not associated with adverse effects in fetuses, including congenital anomalies. However, insufficient data are available at this time to rule out fetal risk.
Lemon balm	Not recommended	Lemon balm is contraindicated in pregnancy because it causes menstrual flow. In one study, lemon balm was used as an antimutagen for amino acid pyrolysate and was found to have 100% effect in the Ames test.
Melatonin	C (no human data; animal data suggest moderate risk)	No study in pregnant women that documented the use of melatonin was found. However, there is a trial that documents its use as a human contraceptive. Use was associated with decreased levels of blood luteinizing hormone (LH), estradiol, and progesterone. A study in six rats evaluated their female offspring after the ingestion of melatonin at about 2–10 times the usual human dose. The offspring had lower LH levels and late vaginal opening. Another study in rats during gestation used 143–1400 times the usual human dose and found no increased maternal or fetal risk. The data are limited and somewhat contradictory; the use of melatonin is not recommended and should be avoided.

Natural Product	Pregnancy Risk Category Rating	Risk Summary
Milk thistle	Not recommended	A published abstract reported the use of milk thistle by 15 pregnant women, but outcome data on the infants were not reported. In a reproductive teratology study, pregnant rats and rabbits were administered milk thistle at high doses (1000 mg/kg), and no congenital anomalies were noted in the offspring. However, data are inadequate to evaluate the safety of use in pregnancy.
MSM	No human data	MSM was administered to pregnant rats at varying doses during organogenesis. Neither biologically significant alterations in the fetus or maternal weight nor any anomalies were observed.
Red rice yeast	X[a]	No studies that document use of red rice yeast (RRY) in humans or animals are available. The RRY products may contain monacolin K, a naturally occurring lovastatin-like analogue. The use of RRY products should be avoided in pregnancy.
SAMe	Limited data	One study reported the use of SAMe in pregnant women, but the details on use and data on teratogenicity were not available. Adverse effects were not expected because of SAMe's similarity to methionine. SAMe is the naturally occurring methylated form of methionine, an essential amino acid.
Saw palmetto	X[a]	Effects of saw palmetto have not been studied in pregnant women or other species, but the antiandrogenic activity for which it is used is of concern in the development of male fetuses.
St. John's wort	C (limited human data)	There are no data that document the animal or placental transfer of hypericin or other constituents of St. John's wort (SJW). In a randomized, placebo-controlled, reproductive study in mice, the pups exposed to SJW had lower birth weights and lower performance on the negative geotaxis task, which is a measure of behavioral development. The data were driven by a significant effect in male pups. No other differences were noted, and by day 5 all pups were similar in weight and performance. A case report described the use of SJW in a pregnant 38-year-old during her first trimester. Other than late onset thrombocytopenia, the pregnancy was unremarkable. The physical examination and laboratory results of the fetus were normal. Neonatal jaundice developed on day 5 but responded to brief phototherapy. Behavioral assessments were normal. The case study did not report on the presence or absence of physical anomalies. The use of SJW is widespread and dates back many years, with no reports of teratogenicity or other reproductive toxicity.
Valerian	B (limited human data)	Reproductive studies in animals using valerian have shown no negative effects on ovulation, fertility, and embryonic development. Five female mice were bred after exposure to didrovaltrate, a metabolite of valerian. Each had a normal pregnancy and normal offspring. In humans, two cases of attempted suicide in pregnant women taking valerian are documented, with the women going on to give birth. Of the two infants, one was of normal weight and cognition, whereas the other had impaired cognition and low birth weight after being delivered at 36 weeks gestation. The mother of the second infant attempted suicide during her next pregnancy, with similar results. Two other cases in pregnant women record the use of valerian at weeks 3 and 4 gestation. The infants were born with no abnormalities. Another concern with valerian is its potential to induce uterine contractions. Because of the uncertainty about this risk and the actual content of the products, the use of valerian should be avoided during pregnancy.

Key: DHEA, dehydroepiandrosterone; 5-HTP, 5-hydroxytryptophan; MSM, methyl-sulfonyl-methane; SAMe, *S*-adenosyl-l-methionine.

[a] Rating is based on prescription drugs that contain very similar ingredients: red rice yeast (lovastatin) and saw palmetto (finasteride).

Source:

Briggs GG, Freeman RK, Yaffe SJ. *Drugs in Pregnancy and Lactation: A Reference Guide to Fetal and Neonatal Risk.* 8th ed. Philadelphia, PA: Lippincott Williams & Wilkins; 2008.

Micromedex® Healthcare Series, REPRORISK® System [subscription database]. Greenwood Village, CO: Thomson Reuters (Healthcare) Inc. Updated periodically. Accessed at http://www.thomsonhc.com.

Micromedex® Healthcare Series, AltMedDex® System [subscription database]. Greenwood Village, CO: Thomson Reuters (Healthcare) Inc. Updated periodically. Accessed at http://www.thomsonhc.com.

Blumenthal M, Goldberg A, Brinckmann J, eds. *Herbal Medicine, Expanded Commission E Monographs.* 1st ed. Newton, MA: Integrated Medicine Communications, 2000.

Newall C, Anderson L, Phillipson J. *Herbal Medicines: A Guide for Health-Care Professionals.* London, England; The Pharmaceutical Press; 1996.

Index

Page numbers followed by *t* and *f* indicate tables and figures, respectively. The abbreviation *CP* followed by a number indicates a photograph identified by that number in the color photograph plates, which are inserted near the middle of the book.

A

AAP. *See* American Academy of Pediatrics
5 A's approach to smoking cessation, 873–875
abbreviated NDA (ANDA), 50
A-B-C-D system, 702
abdominal bloating
    intestinal gas, 227, 229–230
    premenstrual, 143
abrasions, 725
    corneal, 548
abrasive dentifrices, 574
Abreva, 601
absorbent products
    for anorectal disorders, 291
    for ostomy pouches, 348
    for urinary incontinence, 927*t*–928*t*, 927–929
A1C, 818
acacia honey, 125*t*
Acanthopanax senticosus. See Siberian ginseng
access to health care, 8–10
ACCP (American College of Chest Physicians), 202
Accreditation Commission for Homeopathic Education in North America (ACHENA), 998
Accreditation Commission of Acupuncture and Oriental Medicine (ACAOM), 1001
acculturation, 36
ACD. *See* allergic contact dermatitis
acesulfame potassium, 494*t*, 815
acetaminophen
    adult dosages, 68*t*
    for breastfeeding patients, 74, 136
    for burns, 735
    for colds, 178
    dosage forms, 67, 68*t*
    drug interactions, 69, 69*t*
    for dysmenorrhea, 134, 136, 136*t*
    for fever, 88–90
    for headache, 67–69
    for musculoskeletal pain, 101–102
    for pediatric patients, 25, 67*t*–68*t*, 74
    pharmacotherapeutic comparison, 74, 90

for pregnant patients, 74
selected products, 68*t*, 73*t*
in sleep aids, 856, 857*t*
toxicity, 67–69, 329
for wounds, 735
acetic acid (vinegar)
    for dermatitis, 646
    vaginal douching with, 128
    for water-clogged ears, 560–561
acetylcholine, 380, 382
ACHENA (Accreditation Commission for Homeopathic Education in North America), 998
Achilles tendonitis, 786*f*, 787*t*
aching feet. *See* tired, aching feet
acid neutralizing capacity (ANC), 217
acne, 685–697
    assessment of, 688*t*, 693–696
    clinical presentation of, 688, CP–22, CP–23
    epidemiology of, 685
    exacerbating factors, 687, 687*t*
    information resources, 696, 696*t*
    key points for, 697
    outcome evaluation, 697
    pathophysiology of, 685–688, 686*f*
    patient counseling for, 690, 693, 696
    treatment of, 688–693
        complementary therapy, 692–693
        goals and general approach, 688, 693*f*
        nonpharmacologic, 688–689
        pharmacologic, 689–692, 691*t*, 692*t*
ACOG (American College of Obstetrics and Gynecologists), 320
acquired immunodeficiency syndrome (AIDS). *See* HIV
Actaea racemosa. See black cohosh
activated charcoal
    adverse effects, 333
    contraindications, 332*t*, 333
    dosage guidelines, 233*t*, 333, 333*t*
    for intestinal gas, 231–232, 234*t*
    pharmacotherapeutic considerations, 333–334
    for poisoning, 332–334
    selected products, 234*t*
acupressure wristbands, 319*t*, 320, 321

acupuncture, 1000–1002
    for dysmenorrhea, 136
    for headache, 75
    for insomnia, 858
    for musculoskeletal pain, 101
AD. *See* atopic dermatitis
AD (Alzheimer's disease), 960–961
ADA (American Dental Association), 571–572
ADA (American Diabetes Association), 811, 816, 818
ADA (American Dietetic Association), 243, 427, 429, 432, 434
adenosine triphosphate (ATP), 428, 437
adenoviruses, 171
adequate intakes (AIs), 367, 368*t*–370*t*
    of dietary fiber, 406
    for pediatric patients, 368*t*–370*t*, 450*t*, 450–451
adherence. *See* patient adherence
adhesives
    for heat therapy, 101
    for ostomy pouches, 348, 348*t*
    for wart removal, 766
    wound dressings, 732*t*, 735
adhesive removers, for ostomy pouches, 348, 348*t*
adipose tissue, 490
adjunctive therapy
    dietary supplements as, 366
    nonprescription products as, 5
adolescents
    acne in (*See* acne)
    contraception for, 166
    diabetes in, 822
    exercise recommendations, 495*t*
    menstrual disorders in, 132, 144
    pregnancy in, 151, 166
    sexually transmitted infections in, 151, 166
    sleep aids for, 857–858
    tobacco cessation by, 884
adsorbents
    for anorectal disorders, 291
    for poisoning, 332–334
adulteration, of dietary supplements, 499
adult urinary incontinence. *See* urinary incontinence
adverse event reporting, 56–57

adverse reactions. *See also* drug interactions; *specific drug*
    to dietary supplements, 945–946
    in geriatric patients, 27–28
    in pediatric patients, 26
    in pregnant patients, 29
advertising
    of dietary supplements, 944–945, 945*t*
    regulation of, 55–56
aerosols, antiseptic, 736*t*, 738, 738*t*
Affordable Care Act (2010), 6, 57
African Americans
    cultural characteristics of, 41–42, 42*t*
    mistrust of health care system, 36–40
African geranium, 180*t*
African plum (pygeum), 972–973
    drug interactions, 955*t*
    for urinary incontinence, 929
AGA (androgenetic alopecia), 797, 799*t*. *See also* hair loss
Agency for Healthcare Research and Quality (AHRQ), 44
age spots (solar lentigines), 713
aging population, 6–7. *See also* geriatric patients
aging process. *See also* photoaging
    pharmacokinetics and, 27–28
AHA (American Heart Association), 71, 487, 840, 958
AHAs. *See* alpha-hydroxy acids
AHRQ (Agency for Healthcare Research and Quality), 44
AIDS. *See* HIV
airborne drugs, contact lenses and, 546
air vent systems, for ostomy pouches, 348*t*
AIs. *See* adequate intakes
ALA (alpha-lipoic acid), 955*t*, 966
albendazole, 303
alcloxa, 290*t*
alcohol-based sanitizers, 174
alcohol consumption
    caffeine and, 863
    by diabetic patients, 815
    drug interactions, 11, 12*t*, 67, 69*t*, 71, 75
    home testing for, 917*t*
    for insomnia, 857
alcohol poisoning, 88
ALE (artichoke leaf extract), 220